HANDBOOK OF CLINICAL AUDIOLOGY

SIXTH EDITION

HANDBOOK OF CLINICAL AUDIOLOGY

SIXTH EDITION

EDITOR-IN-CHIEF

JACK KATZ
Director
Auditory Processing Service
Prairie Village, Kansas
and Research Professor
University of Kansas Medical Center
Kansas City, Kansas and Professor Emeritus
University at Buffalo State University of New York
Buffalo, New York

EDITOR

LARRY MEDWETSKY, Ph.D.
Vice President of Clinical Services
Rochester Hearing and Speech Center
Rochester, New York

ROBERT BURKARD, Ph.D.
Professor and Chair
Department of Rehabilitation Science
University at Buffalo
Buffalo, New York

LINDA J. HOOD, Ph.D.
Department of Hearing and Speech Sciences
Vanderbilt Bill Wilkerson Center
Vanderbilt University
Nashville, Tennessee

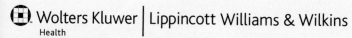

Wolters Kluwer | Lippincott Williams & Wilkins
Health

Philadelphia · Baltimore · New York · London
Buenos Aires · Hong Kong · Sydney · Tokyo

Acquisitions Editor: Peter Sabatini
Editorial Manager: Eric Branger
Managing Editor: Kevin C. Dietz/Jennifer Glazer
Marketing Manager: Allison Noplock
Compositor: Aptara, Inc.
Printer: RR Donnelley-Willard

Library of Congress Cataloging-in-Publication Data

Handbook of clinical audiology / editor-in-chief, Jack Katz ; editors, Robert Burkard, Linda Hood, Larry Medwetsky. – 6th ed.
   p. ; cm.
 Includes bibliographical references and index.
 ISBN-13: 978-0-7817-8106-0
 ISBN-10: 0-7817-8106-X
1. Audiology–Handbooks, manuals, etc.   2. Hearing disorders–Diagnosis–Handbooks, manuals, etc.   I. Katz, Jack.   II. Title: Clinical audiology.
 [DNLM: 1. Hearing Disorders. WV 270 H2363 2009]
 RF291.H36 2009
 617.8–dc22

                                                              2008019853

*This book is dedicated to four exemplary
audiologists who have contributed for many
years to the field of audiology and to the
Handbook of Clinical Audiology.
Moe Bergman
Frederick Martin
Mark Ross
Laura Ann Wilber*

FOREWORD

From our pre-technology beginnings to today's complex and sophisticated field of audiology; a brief historical account.

In preparation for this assignment, I first scanned my decades in this field, beginning with the experiences I participated in and the technology I used in the early and mid-20th century. Prior to World War II, we did not yet have a name for the field, which was often referred to simply as "aural rehabilitation". As that name implied; it centered mainly on the learning of lip (speech) reading, with additional attention on improving the interpretation of auditory signals (auditory training). In short, in the absence of effective amplification the burden of rehabilitation for auditory problems was shifted onto the hearing impaired individual, who was expected to work hard to develop new communication skills. We teachers of lip reading were always discouraged by our apparent lack of success at this task in teaching deaf children, even when the teacher was the brilliant therapist, Louis Di Carlo. Lou's classes were electric, but it would be hard to document the improved communication abilities of his "students" in their everyday lives.

The *raison d'etre* of the field, and its non-medical practitioners of that time, was clearly to augment the defective auditory channel for verbal communication by enhancing the visual information available on the face of the talker.

In diagnostics we had not yet emerged from the tuning fork period. They had been used routinely for medical diagnosis since the late 19th century to differentiate middle ear from inner ear pathology. In time, we pre-audiologists proudly employed the new "pure tone audiometer", either for screening or for follow-up threshold audiometry. (I lugged a 68-pound "portable" version, the WE 2A audiometer, from school to school to test children's hearing, air conduction only.) Some time later we began to use the bone conduction unit of the audiometer, as the controlled version of tuning forks. The time of quantification and calibration for hearing tests had arrived, but the main purpose remained for diag-

nostic site-of-lesion, rather than the assessment of auditory function.

These modest beginnings, in what I think of as the pre-technology period of our field, carried over into the military "aural rehabilitation" clinics (referred to in one soldier patient's letters home as "rural rehabiliation" (sic)), but the remarkable infusion in those clinics of personnel who had been university-trained and active in speech communication research brought about an almost instant metamorphosis. The revised view of diagnosis and the "selection" of hearing aids spurred the appearance of new equipment, with an emphasis on calibration, measurability and repeatability. The die was cast. Importantly we included intensive auditory training with speech recordings and also generated sound stimuli for identification and tolerance training. We integrated much advice and explanation in these training sessions. I recall that Grant Fairbanks attempted to quantify the program efficacy for the Oklahoma clinic and I believe that Bill Hardy did the same for the navy program. Regardless, it was readily apparent that in contrast to our pre-war experiences a high percentage of our soldier patients left our hospitals using their new hearing aids and, by all accounts, for years afterwards.

After the war the new instrumentation-based concepts were quickly introduced in college-level courses at leading universities, under the recently-coined term "Audiology", and our field took off! Increasingly complex technology began to reveal detailed information about physiological dysfunction, while rehabilitative efforts centered on the rapidly improving and, at the same time, shrinking hearing aid.

The "new" audiology expanded – nay, exploded – quickly, and very soon it was the inspiration for numerous publications, the most comprehensive of which was the Handbook of Clinical Audiology. Suddenly there was enough material for authoritative presentations in dozens of chapters, as the written expression of a lively and exciting newcomer among the university disciplines and professions. The training for such a flourishing science-based profession was on the post-baccalaureate level, and soon warranted a doctoral level degree for many audiologists. Today, the Doctor of Audiology (Au.D.) degree is accepted as the education and training level for entry into clinical practice in this field.

As with all vibrant professions their focus and responsibilities are dynamic. New areas of interest emerge, requiring new knowledge to replace or augment previous areas. This revised edition of the "bible" for audiologists indicates that our specialty continues to evolve, including, logically, the rest of the hearing and balance organ in the vestibular system, and updating our information about the rehabilitation of adults.

The breadth and sophistication of "Clinical Audiology" in this 21st century, which is only one working lifetime away from our humble beginnings that I found so stimulating early in our history, is encapsulated more than ever in this new edition of the Handbook of Clinical Audiology.

Moe Bergman, Ed.D.

PREFACE

Over the past 35 years, the *Handbook of Clinical Audiology* (HOCA) has maintained an important role in the education of graduate students in audiology, both in North America and throughout the world. It also serves as a useful reference for audiologists, otologists and speech-language pathologists who wish to have a comprehensive and practical guide to the current practices in audiology.

Each edition of the HOCA has been an update of the previous one, but we have also striven to make the newer edition better than the one that came before. For this edition, there were three highly skilled and knowledgeable editors plus one senior editor. We have worked together to select highly qualified contributors on topics that are both core and current for students and professionals in audiology. Online appendices have been added to this edition to enable the reader to go beyond the basic scope of this book.

THE FOREWORDS

The previous edition of the Handbook contained the first foreword for HOCA. It was written by Delbert Ault, Au.D., founder of the National Association of Future Doctors of Audiology (NAFDA). Forming this vibrant organization was an important contribution of Dr. Ault's to the field of audiology, and we also appreciate his continued support for the HOCA.

By contrast, the foreword for the Sixth Edition is written by a distinguished gentleman with many years of audiology behind him. Moe Bergman, Ed.D., was in the very first group of audiologists who began this discipline more than 60 years ago. Starting prior to World War II and for decades following, Dr. Bergman was a clinician, administrator, professor, researcher, and writer, and after he retired from Hunter College in New York City, he went to Israel to establish audiology as a profession there. For many years, Dr. Bergman has continued to be active as an advisor and an officer in international professional organizations. His clarity about the events and developments so many years ago (see Bergman, 2002, reference in Chapter 1) makes him a treasured link to our roots. Dr. Bergman's foreword is a must read.

SECTIONS, CHAPTERS, AND CONTRIBUTORS

The strength of HOCA has always been the knowledge and expertise of the contributors in the many aspects of audiology. They have both research and clinical credentials in the topics they write about. Audiologists looking down the list of contributors will recognize familiar and highly respected colleagues. They have contributed much to the field in the past and now contribute again by providing important and readable materials for both colleagues and students. We have made every effort to provide up-to-date, accurate, and clinically applicable information.

Each of the three main editors of this book has a distinguished record of teaching, research, writing, and clinical work. Each one took responsibility for roughly one-third of the chapters. Linda Hood, our most recent editor, was responsible for most of the basic clinical topics, which are applicable to just about all individuals who are seen by audiologists, and some chapters dealing with special populations. Robert Burkard, as in the previous edition of HOCA, was responsible for all of the physiologic chapters. Larry Medwetsky, who contributed to the two previous editions of this book, dealt with all of the management chapters as well as some special populations. Jack Katz filled in here and there and saw to the overall manuscript issues.

The book is divided into four sections. There are seven chapters dealing with Introduction, Basic Tests, and Principles. Laura Wilber is singled out in this section because she has contributed the Calibration chapters in each of the previous five editions, and in this edition, she coauthored the chapter with Robert Burkard. Other top-notch audiologists wrote on Puretone Air Conduction, Bone

Conduction, and Speech Audiometry, as well as Masking and Case History.

The second section is made up of 15 chapters dealing with Physiologic Principles and Measures. We are glad to welcome back Chuck Berlin who contributed to the First Edition of HOCA. He and Linda Hood wrote a new chapter for this book dealing with the Physiologic Bases of Audiologic Interpretation and Management. This second section of the book, which has many previous and new contributors, is arguably the one that contains the most changes in content since the Fifth Edition. Doug Keefe and Pat Feeney discuss the principles of immittance, but also introduce peripheral anatomy and physiology, as well as a new contribution to HOCA, the topic of wideband acoustic reflectance.

The third section is devoted to a wide variety of Special Populations. It contains 11 chapters beginning with Assessment of Hearing Loss in Children and Educational Audiology/Hearing Screening and ending with Hearing Loss in the Elderly and Tinnitus/Hyperacousis. It is a pleasure to welcome back Fred Martin who, along with Dr. Wilber, has contributed to each of the six editions of the HOCA. A new and important chapter for the Handbook is one on Tinnitus/Hyperacousis that was written by Richard Tyler and his colleagues.

The final section, Management of Hearing Disorders, is made up of 10 chapters. Five of the chapters deal with hearing aids and cochlear implants, three focus on management and counseling, and the remaining two are on Room Acoustics and Assistive Technologies as well as Building a Successful Audiologic Practice. We welcome back Gus Mueller who contributed chapters to several previous editions of the HOCA.

Sadly, during the writing of their chapters two wonderful people and highly respected colleagues died. They are Carl Crandell and Moneca Price. Their deaths are a great loss to audiology and to this handbook (see dedications at the end of Chapters 34 and 36).

■ TERMINOLOGY

The following is an explanation of some of the spelling conventions used in the HOCA and why we chose them.

■ COMPOUND WORDS

In clinical audiology, as well as in English generally, compound words (two words written as one) are common. Compound words are simplifications of words that are frequently used together. For example, *brain* and *stem* are combined in the term *auditory brainstem response*. Two separate words, when frequently used to express a certain meaning, in time, may be connected by a hyphen and eventually joined together into a single word (base ball, base-ball, baseball).

Puretone

Audiologists have used the term *pure tone* to convey a specific meaning since our inception. It is one of the terms we use most frequently, and thus, this encouraged us to combine it into a compound word, *puretone*. It also provides a simplification and a consistency that we do not have at the present time. For example, when the words *pure tone* appear before a noun, as they often do, we are to hyphenate them (e.g., *pure-tone threshold*), but not at other times. Some audiologists follow these conventions consistently, other inconsistently and still others not at all which produces unnecessary variability in reports and even publications. We think it is time to make *puretone* into a compound word in order to simplify the writer's task and to increase consistency from audiologist to audiologist.

A quick check of a previous edition of the HOCA shows dozens of compound words that we often use that have been simplified (e.g., bandwidth, earphone, hardwire, headroom, noisemakers, nonorganic, overmasking, waveform). It is both logical and practical and perhaps overdue to use *puretone* as a single word because we use the term *puretone* so frequently.

Sensory-Neural

On the one hand, there is good reason to use *puretone* as a compound word, but on the other hand, it would be beneficial for the term *sensorineural* to be hyphenated as *sensory-neural* because the term represents two separate and often contrasting entities for audiologists and thus can and does lead to misinterpretation. When some students and even faculty members were asked about the meaning of *sensorineural*, they assumed that it was just cochlear (the sensory part only). This confusion cannot be easily avoided when the word is spoken but can be more clearly separated when written as *sensory-neural* and conceptualized as two separate regions with different characteristics and influences that are treated very differently. In fact, for a draft of a previous edition of the HOCA, one author wrote "... sensorineural hearing loss produces recruitment." Only the *sensory* cases have recruitment and not those with *neural* lesions.

This is not a purely academic concern. Often when referral sources see that the person has a *sensorineural* loss, they are inclined to be relieved that it is not *retrocochlear*. We need a term that will both designate a nonconductive problem and do a better job in clarifying that there are two distinct alternatives. Although the hyphenated version *sensory-neural* will not completely eliminate the ambiguity, it will surely be clearer than using *sensorineural*. For this reason, we recommend that we return to the earlier spelling, *sensory-neural*, for greater precision.

EPILOG

We are pleased that the *Handbook of Clinical Audiology* (HOCA) is used widely by audiologists around the world. Interestingly when the HOCA first came out, we were living in the Turkish Republic. There the word *hoca* (pronounced, /h o○↗ ≜/) means a religious leader or a revered teacher. While HOCA is certainly not a religious leader, we do hope it will be a revered teacher for the many students and colleagues that read this book.

 ACKNOWLEDGMENTS

We would like to thank the editors of Lippincott Williams & Wilkins, Andrea Klinger, Jennifer Glazer, Kevin Dietz and especially Eric Branger, not only for their editing of this book but also for advising us and keeping us to our deadlines. In addition, Tom Zalewski was kind enough to review material when an outside reader was needed, and Irma Katz maintained the files and kept track of 43 chapters and more than 70 authors and coauthors.

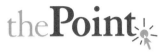

There are supplemental materials for Chapter 23 on thePoint companion website at http://thepoint.lww.com/Katz6e.

CONTRIBUTORS

PAUL J. ABBAS, Ph.D.
Professor and Chair
Department of Communication Sciences and Disorders
University of Iowa
Iowa City, Iowa

DANIEL A. ABRAMS, Ph.D.
Postdoctoral Fellow
Department of Psychiatry and Behavioral Sciences
Stanford Medical School
Palo Alto, California

JAMES BAER, Au.D.
Assistant Professor and Director of Audiology
Department of Speech and Hearing Science
Lamar University
Beaumont, Texas

ADITYA BARDIA, M.D.
Research Assistant
Department of Otolaryngology
University of Iowa
Iowa City, Iowa

KAMRAN BARIN, Ph.D.
Assistant Professor
Department of Otolaryngology-Head and Neck Surgery and
Department of Speech and Hearing Science
Director, Balance and Disorders Clinic
The Ohio State University
Columbus, Ohio

DOUGLAS L. BECK, Au.D.
Director of Professional Relations
Oticon, Inc.
Somerset, New Jersey

RUTH A. BENTLER, Ph.D.
Professor
Department of Communication Sciences and Disorders
University of Iowa
Iowa City, Iowa

CHARLES I. BERLIN, Ph.D.
Director Emeritus, Kresge Hearing Research Lab
LSU Health Sciences Center
Kenneth and Frances Barnes Bellington Professor of Hearing
Science, Emeritus
Research Professor
Departments of Communication Science and Disorders
Otolaryngology Head and Neck Surgery
University of South Florida
Tampa, Florida

ARLENE STREDLER BROWN, M.A.
Adjunct Faculty
University of Colorado
Boulder, Colorado

CAROLYN J. BROWN, Ph.D.
Professor
Department of Communication Sciences and Disorders
University of Iowa
Iowa City, Iowa

ROBERT BURKARD, Ph.D.
Professor and Chair
Department of Rehabilitation Science
University at Buffalo
Buffalo, New York

ANTHONY T. CACACE, Ph.D.
Professor
Department of Communicative Sciences and Disorders
Wayne State University
Detroit, Michigan

MARSHALL CHASIN, Au.D.
Director of Auditory Research
Musician's Clinics of Canada
Toronto, Ontario, Canada

CLAUDIA BARROS COELHO, M.D., Ph.D.
Research Scientist
Department of Otolaryngology
University of Iowa
Iowa City, Iowa

WILLIAM COLE, BASc, PEng
President
Etymonic Design Inc.
Dorchester, Ontario, Canada

BARBARA CONE, Ph.D.
Professor
Department of Speech, Language and Hearing Sciences
University of Arizona
Tucson, Arizona

CARL CRANDELL, Ph.D.*
Department of Communication Sciences and Disorders
University of Florida
Gainesville, Florida
*Deceased

DAVID CUNNINGHAM, Ph.D.
Professor
Division of Audiology
Department of Surgery
University of Louisville School of Medicine
Louisville, Kentucky

ALLAN O. DIEFENDORF, Ph.D.
Associate Professor and Director
Indiana University School of Medicine
Carmel, Indiana

ANDREW DIMITRINJEVIC, Ph.D.
Adjunct Professor of Neurology
University of California, Irvine
Irvine, California

MANUEL DON, Ph.D.
Head, Electrophysiology Department, Scientist III
House Ear Institute
Los Angeles, California

JOHN D. DURRANT, Ph.D.
Professor and Vice Chair
Department of Communication Science and Disorders
Professor, Department of Otolaryngology and Rehabilitation
    Science and Technology
University of Pittsburgh
Pittsburgh, Pennsylvania

KRIS ENGLISH, Ph.D.
Associate Professor
University of Akron/NOAC
Akron, Ohio

SUSAN ERLER, Ph.D.
Coordinator, Doctor of Audiology Program
Northwestern University
Evanston, Illinois

M. PATRICK FEENEY, Ph.D.
Associate Professor and Chief of Audiology
Department of Otolaryngology, Head and Neck Surgery
Virginia Merrill Bloedel Hearing Research Center
University of Washington
Seattle, Washington

JAMES FEUERSTEIN, Ph.D.
Professor of Audiology and Chair
Department of Communication Sciences & Disorders
Nazareth College of Rochester
Rochester, New York

TRACY FITZGERALD, Ph.D.
Assistant Professor
Department of Hearing and Speech Sciences
University of Maryland-College Park
College Park, Maryland

DEAN GARSTECKI, Ph.D.
Professor
Audiology and Hearing Science and
Otolaryngology-Head and Neck Surgery
Northwestern University
Evanston, Illinois

STANLEY A. GELFAND, Ph.D.
Professor
Linguistics & Communication Disorders
Queens College of CUNY
Doctoral Program in Speech and Hearing Sciences
Graduate School of CUNY
Flushing, New York

GEORGE HASKELL, Ph.D.
Audiologist
Department of Otolaryngology
University of Iowa
Iowa City, Iowa

THERESA HNATH-CHISOLM, Ph.D.
Professor and Chair
Department of Communication Sciences & Disorders
University of South Florida
Tampa, Florida

LINDA HOOD, Ph.D.
Professor
Vanderbilt Bill Wilkerson Center
Department of Hearing and Speech Sciences
Vanderbilt University
Nashville, Tennessee

BRENDA HOOVER, M.A.
Research Audiologist
Boys Town National Research Hospital
Omaha, Nebraska

MARTYN L. HYDE, Ph.D.
Professor
Department of Otolaryngology
University of Toronto
Director, Research and Development
Hearing, Balance and Speech Department
Mt. Sinai Hospital
Toronto, Ontario, Canada

ANDREW JOHN, Ph.D.
Department of Communication Sciences and Disorders
University of Oklahoma Health Sciences Center
Oklahoma City, Oklahoma

CHERYL DECONDE JOHNSON, Ed.D. CEO
The ADVantage – Audiology, Deaf-Education Vantage
  Consulting
Greeley, Colorado

JACK KATZ, Ph.D.
Professor Emeritus, University at Buffalo
Director, Auditory Processing Service
Prairie Village, Kansas
Research Professor
University of Kansas Medical Center
Kansas City, Kansas

DOUGLAS H. KEEFE, Ph.D.
Staff Scientist, IV
Boys Town National Research Hospital
Omaha, Nebraska

NINA KRAUS, Ph.D.
Hugh Knowles Professor
Communication Sciences; Neurobiology and Physiology,
  Otolaryngology
Northwestern University
Evanston, Illinois

BRIAN KREISMAN, Ph.D.
Department of Audiology, Speech-Language Pathology and
  Deaf Studies
Towson University
Towson, Maryland

NICOLE KREISMAN, Ph.D.
Department of Audiology, Speech-Language Pathology and
  Deaf Studies
Towson University
Towson, Maryland

BETTY KWONG, M.S.
Research Associate
Electrophysiology Department
House Ear Institute
Los Angeles, California

FREDERICK N. MARTIN, Ph.D.
Lillie Hage Jamail Centennial Professor Emeritus
Department of Communication Sciences & Disorders
Jesse H. Jones Communication Center
The University of Texas at Austin
Austin, Texas

WILLIAM MARTIN, Ph.D.
Professor of Otolaryngology/Head & Neck Surgery
Professor of Public Health and Preventive Medicine
Oregon Hearing Research Center
Oregon Health and Science University
Portland, Oregon

RACHEL MCARDLE, Ph.D.
Chief, Audiology and Speech Pathology Service
Bay Pines VA Healthcare System
Bay Pines, FL

DENNIS J. MCFARLAND, Ph.D.
Research Scientist
Laboratory of Nervous System Disorders
Wadsworth Center
New York State Health Department
Albany, New York

KATHLEEN SZALDA MCNERNEY, Ph.D.
Research Assistant Professor
Department of Rehabilitation Science
University at Buffalo
Buffalo, New York

LARRY MEDWETSKY, Ph.D.
VP, Clinical Services
Rochester Hearing and Speech Center
Rochester, New York

H. GUSTAV MUELLER, Ph.D.
Professor
Department of Hearing and Speech Science
Vanderbilt University
Nashville, Tennessee

PEGGY NELSON, Ph.D.
Associate Professor
Department of Speech-Language-Hearing Sciences
University of Minnesota
Minneapolis, Minnesota

WILLIAM NOBLE, Ph.D.
Professor of Psychology
University of New England
Armidale, Australia

BETH PRIEVE, Ph.D.
Associate Professor
Department of Communication Sciences and Disorders
Syracuse University
Syracuse, New York

MONECA PRICE, M.ClSc., Reg. CASLPO*
Senior Audiologist
The Canadian Hearing Society
Ottawa, Ontario, Canada
*Deceased

LAURA RIDDLE, Ph.D.
Assistant Professor
Department of Communication Sciences and Disorders
Nazareth College of Rochester
Rochester, New York

ROBERT SCHLAUCH, Ph.D.
Associate Professor
Department of Speech-Language-Hearing Sciences
University of Minnesota
Minneapolis, Minnesota

JANET E. SHANKS, Ph.D.
Manager, Audiology Clinic
VA Long Beach Healthcare System
Long Beach, California

NEIL T. SHEPARD, Ph.D.
Director, Dizziness & Balances Disorders Program, Mayo Clinic
Professor of Audiology, Mayo College of Medicine
Rochester, Minnesota

YONGBING SHI, M.D., Ph.D.
Assistant Professor
Department of Otolaryngology/Head & Neck Surgery
Oregon Health & Science University
Portland, Oregon

JACK A. SHOHET, M.D.
Associate Clinical Professor
Department of Otolaryngology-Head and Neck Surgery
University of California-Irvine
Shohet Ear Associates Medical Group, Inc.
Newport Beach, California

YVONNE S. SININGER, Ph.D.
Professor, Division of Head & Neck Surgery
University of California Los Angeles
David Geffen School of Medicine
Los Angeles, California

JOSEPH SMALDINO, Ph.D.
Professor and Chair
Department of Communication Sciences and Disorders
Illinois State University
Normal, Illinois

DAVID STAPELLS, Ph.D.
Professor
School of Audiology & Speech Sciences
University of British Columbia
Vancouver, British Columbia, Canada

PATRICIA G. STELMACHOWITZ, Ph.D.
Director of Audiological and Vestibular Services
Boys Town National Research Hospital
Omaha, Nebraska

ANNE MARIE THARPE, Ph.D.
Professor
Vanderbilt Bill Wilkerson Center
Department of Hearing and Speech Sciences
Vanderbilt University
Nashville, Tennessee

KIM L. TILLERY, Ph.D.
Associate Professor and Chair
Department of Speech Pathology and Audiology
State University of New York at Fredonia
Fredonia, New York

RICHARD S. TYLER, Ph.D.
Professor and Director of Audiology
Department of Otolaryngology
Roy J & Lucille A Carver College of Medicine
University of Iowa
Iowa City, Iowa

L. MAUREEN VALENTE, Ph.D.
Director of Audiology Studies
Assistant Professor of Otolaryngology
Program in Audiology and Communicative Sciences
Washington University School of Medicine
St. Louis, Missouri

MICHAEL VALENTE, Ph.D.
Professor of Clinical Otolaryngology
Department of Otolaryngology and Head-Neck Surgery
Director of Adult Audiology
Program in Audiology and Communicative Sciences
Washington University School of Medicine
St. Louis, Missouri

BARBARA A. VENTO, Ph.D.
Assistant Professor
Department of Communication Science & Disorders
University of Pittsburgh
Pittsburgh, Pennsylvania

BARBARA E. WEINSTEIN, Ph.D.
Professor and Executive Office
Health Sciences Doctoral Programs-Audiology,
    Nursing Sciences, Physical Therapy, Public Health
Graduate Center, CUNY
New York, New York

LAURA ANN WILBER, Ph.D.
Professor Emeritus
Communication Sciences and Disorders
Northwestern University
Evanston, Illinois

WILLIAM YACULLO, Ph.D.
Professor and Chair
Department of Communication Disorders
Governors State University
University Park, Illinois

TERESA A. ZWOLAN, Ph.D.
Clinical Associate Professor
Director, University of Michigan Cochlear Implant
    Program
Department of Otolaryngology
University of Michigan Health System
Ann Arbor, Michigan

CONTENTS

SECTION I

INTRODUCTION AND BASIC TESTS AND PROCEDURES

Clinical Audiology

Jack Katz

▧ INTRODUCTION

Very few students will read the introductory chapter of an audiology textbook voluntarily. They are often eager to learn about tests, devices, remediation procedures, and even basic science aspects of the field but may view the introduction as mere chaff. One student complained after reading the assigned chapter, "But it's just philosophy!" as though philosophy was not part of the practice of audiology. Whether or not the student was correct that the introduction was simply philosophy, it does provide some context for the book and hopefully will serve as an introduction to the field of audiology for the student.

▧ WHAT IS AUDIOLOGY?

Audiology means the study of hearing. Just as several professions led to the development of audiology, two languages led to the name *audiology*. The prefix is Latin, and the suffix is Greek. Audiology is broader than its name implies because it includes not only hearing, but also the vestibular system and how heard information is managed by the central nervous system.

It is important to remember that clinical audiology is a helping profession. In addition to assessing hearing and hearing disorders, audiologists are charged with helping people to cope with and improve their auditory and vestibular limitations. Because of our knowledge, experience, and compassion, patients who consult with us are able to leave better than when they came in.

▧ WHERE WE CAME FROM

During World War II, servicemen and women who suffered hearing losses were referred to what we now call "audiologists" for evaluation and rehabilitation. Fortunately for the patients and the profession that grew out of that work, it was an interdisciplinary team of professionals that coalesced to form audiology. The professionals were primarily in the fields of speech correction, education of the deaf, psychology, and medicine. Each profession, to our benefit, left its unique mark on our field, and where we have gone from there continues to evolve.

The focus of audiology during and immediately after that war was to provide very basic hearing tests and then to help remediate the adverse effects of the hearing losses. What is so remarkable is the enormous success with which those early audiologists accomplished their goals. Although the hearing aids were archaic by today's standards, the servicemen and women were trained and educated so that years after the conflict, by and large, they were still effective speech readers and hearing aid users and were well adjusted to their hearing difficulties (Ross, 2007).

Pretty soon, it became obvious that our discipline lacked important diagnostic tests that not only could accurately describe the extent of loss and puretone configuration, but also could assess the person's clarity for hearing and determine whether the individual was performing in an authentic manner (i.e., likely had an organic hearing loss and not a nonorganic problem). Within 20 years, audiologists had developed a wide variety of behavioral diagnostic procedures as well as a number of physiologic tests that could provide site-of-lesion information as well as an "objective assessment of hearing." During this period of rapid development, the emphasis was on evaluation to the exclusion of remediation of the consequences of hearing loss. However, a few voices spoke out that we should not neglect nonmedical management—a most important function of audiology (Ross, 1997). In time, there was a gradual broadening of interest to include rehabilitative aspects of the field. The greatest impetus to the rehabilitative component was the reversal of American Speech-Language-Hearing Association (ASHA) policy that prohibited audiologists from dispensing hearing aids. Once freed from this restriction, audiologists began returning to their roots to improve the lives of those who were hard of hearing. This included not only providing hearing aids and assistive devices but also counseling of patients and their families. More recently, audiologists have become involved in vestibular as well as auditory therapies.

Major milestones in audiology along the way are archived in the previous editions of the *Handbook of Clinical Audiology* (also see Robinette, 1994). They include the introduction of site-of-lesion measures to distinguish cochlear from eighth-nerve lesions and central auditory function tests. This led to work with auditory processing disorders and the widespread use of physiologic measures (e.g., tympanometry and acoustic reflexes), followed by the introduction of auditory brainstem response (ABR), vestibular testing, and more recently, otoacoustic emissions (OAE). Intraoperative monitoring has been a more recent advance in the diagnostic-monitoring end of the field. Cochlear implants have produced miraculous results for patients with prelingual as well as postlingual deafness. This development has added importantly to the work of audiologists in the evaluation prior to surgery and afterwards in mapping and monitoring the implants, and in training. This long list of audiologic activities also includes school and industrial hearing screenings, infant hearing screening programs, and many other developments and applications.

The minimum age for testing hearing has gotten younger and younger. I remember 50 years ago being told not to test deaf or hard-of-hearing children until they were 10 years old! At that age, it was said, they are "not so wild and you can get a decent audiogram." We know now that early identification is critical and that, by 10 years of age, the children would have lost so much time that it would be difficult, if not impossible, to reclaim it later on. Fortunately, we now have the capability of newborn hearing screenings and programs to immediately intervene to bring about greatly improved speech, language, and learning potential. The best outcomes with cochlear implantation of the prelingually deaf child are at or before 18 months of age (Hammes, 2002).

THE PRACTICE OF AUDIOLOGY

Audiology is a science-art. It has a scientific base starting with the physics of sound and anatomy as well as electrophysiology of the auditory system and auditory perception. It also includes clinical understanding, which deals with the bases and knowledge of both testing and remedial procedures. However, although that information is necessary, it is not sufficient without the art of audiology. This requires the ability to work well with people and to utilize professional procedures skillfully. Thus, knowledge alone is insufficient

to make an able audiologist. We must also develop and hone our interpersonal and technical skills to be fully capable of this work.

Audiology encompasses a broad range of endeavors. Of course, we administer test procedures and evaluate the results. Audiologists also dispense hearing aids and assistive devices and provide counseling and therapy for a variety of problems. Audiologists are educators as well, in teaching patients and their families, our professional colleagues, and the public about topics in our field. Years ago, I was influenced by a sign on my physical therapist's door, "If I *treat* you today I will help you today. If I *teach* you today I will help you forever." While *forever* is more than audiologists can ethically promise, teaching patients and their families will help them to understand the problem and aid them in finding additional solutions on their own.

PREDICTIONS AND THE FUTURE OF AUDIOLOGY

Previous Predictions

This writer has always felt more confident about describing the past than predicting the future. My assumption was that, over the years, my batting average was probably below .500, but to my surprise, after reviewing those predictions, they were better than I had assumed. The following shows where we were 35 and 20 years ago as well as some predictions for the future.

The prediction in the First Edition stated, "It is obvious that the 70's will demonstrate a broader approach to the auditory system including many areas of the cerebrum and cerebellum which are not now within the province of the audiologist" (Katz, 1972, p 9). This prediction was partly correct, as we added approaches such as acoustic reflexes and regions of the brain such as the corpus callosum that were outside of our purview when the prediction was made. However, the cerebellar aspect of my prediction remains unfulfilled even 35 years later (but I am not giving up).

Another prediction was, "... brain stem will be as common a term as VIII nerve is to us today" (Katz, 1972, p 9). This was true for the most part with the advent of brainstem behavioral tests, ABR, and more recently, brainstem implants. "Another trend will be to pick up problems at the earliest possible time. This will call for refinements of the present tests and the development of new ones. What we have learned with cooperative adult patients will be applied downward to younger and younger children and [upward to] older and older adults" (p 9). These were pretty good predictions. While the use of amplification for younger and younger children was correct, of course, we could not possibly have imagined the newborn hearing screenings that we have today and almost immediate intervention. In addition, we have seen the continually increasing emphasis on the use of amplification and training for the elderly and even those who are very elderly.

It seemed, back then, that we would need more stringent criteria for what was considered normal hearing for children than those used for adults. This was a correct prediction, although I am surprised that not everyone seems to be aware of the more stringent threshold norms for children. In that same vein, it seemed that audiologists were likely to provide, "amplification and training for adults and children [who are] considered too mild for it by today's standards" (Katz, 1972, p 9). This prediction certainly came true, and the tendency to fit hearing aids for milder and milder losses continues. "Audiology, no doubt, will spread through school systems" (p 9). Audiology did indeed spread in the schools and currently represents an important aspect of our field. Educational audiologists have important advantages because they are not generally constrained by third-party reimbursements and they are more conveniently located to their clients.

Finally, "The line between the functions of hearing becomes finer as the line between 'auditory perception' and 'language' begins to erode" (Katz, 1972, p 9). The delineation (e.g., outer and inner hair cells) and interdependence among hearing functions and anatomic regions (e.g., processing centers of the brain) have certainly become clearer. Indeed the very thin line between auditory processing and language has created theoretical questions and practical challenges in scope of practice for audiologists and speech-language pathologists that were not present in 1972 (Duchan and Katz, 1983).

Given enough time, almost any prediction can come true. Some of this writer's predictions in the Third Edition in 1985 are yet to happen. Some of these predictions involved computer audiometers (this came true) using digitized speech lists (this is also available), smart hearing aids designed for the individual's hearing and perceptual dysfunctions (to date, this prediction is partially correct), and noise reduction circuits (yes, this has happened). Those were pretty good predictions, but we will have to wait a bit longer for the hearing aids to be carefully tailored to the individual's processing characteristics. Considering the progress in speech recognition capabilities and the sophistication in hearing aid technology, it seems that this prediction, though delayed, will be coming to fruition in the not too distant future.

One Last Prediction from the Past

In the First Edition, I wrote that there was beginning to be a turnaround in audiology in the direction of auditory rehabilitation. Although it has taken a long time, the trend has continued slowly. We started as a rehabilitation field and then made a right turn to concentrate almost exclusively on diagnostics. Now because of hearing aids, cochlear implants, counseling, vertigo, tinnitus, and auditory processing, we are establishing a better balance in our profession between evaluation and management. It is a natural progression.

Many audiologists see patients for evaluation and refer them elsewhere for therapy. Could we be doing an equally, or more, effective job ourselves in aspects of counseling and in other therapeutic activities? Many audiologists do already. Not only does this make good clinical sense, but instead of explaining to another professional what is wrong and what needs to be done, we could actually do it ourselves (with appropriate training of course). It also makes economic and patient satisfaction sense because rehabilitation is not a one time visit. Thus, for the audiologist, this represents repeat business and a more satisfied customer, whether it is orienting a patient after a hearing aid fitting or providing vestibular therapy.

From personal experience, working with patients over time and seeing their progress is extremely gratifying. There is every reason to believe that the trend for greater involvement in rehabilitative services will continue for the betterment of our patients and our profession.

What the Future Holds

From the very beginning of audiology to today, the field has grown in number, scope, knowledge, and expertise. During this period of time, there were apparent obstacles that caused some to wonder if they meant the demise of audiology. Each problem came and went, and audiology continued its forward momentum. There was a period of hostility from some in the medical profession. Then, computed tomography (CT) scans and magnetic resonance imaging (MRI) threatened us. Also, not being able to dispense hearing aids was a great concern, and when we were finally were able to do so, there were concerns about that too. A decade ago, there was fear about changing to an Au.D. degree and the training of audiology technicians. None of these issues materialized into death blows to audiology and generally resulted in furthering our profession. However, we should never rest on our laurels, but rather redouble our efforts to make our profession an ever more important contributor to the health and welfare of our communities.

It is likely that the future will hold some surprises for us, but if the past teaches us anything, we can expect to broaden our caseload up and down the age range, for more and less severe as well as different problems, specifying more of the auditory anatomy and physiology, and using techniques with greater effectiveness. There will be increased use of physiologic tests, but I believe that behavioral procedures will remain the mainstay of our field for the foreseeable future. Hearing aids have had evolutions and revolutions and will, no doubt, continue to provide better and better performance. Hearing assistive devices (HAT) will be used more than they currently are and thereby broadening our scope to more and more children and adults. Surely audiologists will continue to provide aural rehabilitation and, hopefully, with more emphasis on teaching/training (Katz, 2006). I believe the advent of the Au.D. has made our profession in the United States more viable than it was before and better able to find new paths for our efforts in the future.

Audiology training and practices vary throughout the world. Some countries are ahead of us in some aspects and not as advanced in others. Because the world is shrinking, it seems that we will surely share our ideas more freely with time.

To the students who read this chapter, thank you. My hope is that you will enjoy the practice of audiology as much as the many contributors of this book have enjoyed it.

REFERENCES

Duchan J, Katz J. (1983) Language and auditory processing: top-down plus bottom-up. In: Lasky E, Katz J, eds. *Central Auditory Processing Disorders: Problems of Speech, Language and Learning*. Baltimore: University Park Press.

Hammes DM, Novack MA, Rotz LA, Willis M, Edmonson DM, Thomas JF. (2002). Early identification and cochlear implantation: critical factors for spoken language development. *Ann Otol Rhinol Laryngol Suppl*. 189, 74–78.

Katz J. (1972) Clinical audiology. In: Katz J, ed. *Handbook of Clinical Audiology*. Baltimore: Williams & Wilkins.

Katz J. (2006) Relationship enhancement and educational audiology. *Educ Audiol Rev*. 23, 15–17.

Robinette MS. (1994) Integrating audiometric results. In: Katz J, ed. *Handbook of Clinical Audiology*. 4th ed. Baltimore: Williams & Wilkins; pp 181–186.

Ross M. (1997) A retrospective look at the future of aural rehabilitation. *J Acad Rehabil Audiol*. 30, 11–28.

Ross M. (2007) The state of the science of aural rehabilitation. *Hearing Loss*. 28, 32–35.

Calibration: Puretone, Speech, and Noise Signals

Laura Ann Wilber and Robert Burkard

WHY CALIBRATE?

In some ways, calibration can be compared to exercising. We know it is good for us, but some of us would prefer not to participate. However, unlike exercising, if one does not calibrate, it hurts others (our clients) more than it does us. For years, many clinicians felt that calibration was something that researchers did but that such procedures were not necessary in the clinic. Today, that basic attitude has changed dramatically. The Occupational Safety and Health (OSHA) regulations (1983) require that audiometric equipment be regularly checked. Some state regulations for hearing aid dispensers and/or for audiologists also require that equipment calibration (and records of calibration) be maintained. Furthermore, many state health departments concerned with school screening also insist on having calibration checked on a routine basis. Thus, we *must* calibrate if we are to meet the current regulations, and we *should* calibrate to make sure our results are within specified tolerances.

Most clinicians recognize that the initial audiometric calibration provided by the manufacturer is insufficient to guarantee that the audiometer will function correctly over time. Although today's digitally-based audiometers are less likely to arrive out of calibration and less likely to develop problems later than the older vacuum tube machines, even brand new audiometers that have just arrived from the factory, as well as audiometers that were in perfect calibration when they were new, can show variations in sound level, frequency, distortion, etc. Often the problems are related to the transducers (earphones, bone vibrators, loudspeakers), but occasionally, the electronic components lead to the audio-

meter failing to remain in calibration. If you have ever worked with a computer, you realize that even digitally-based instrumentation does not always provide error-free performance. Regardless of whether the audiometer is new or has been in use for some time, it is the responsibility of the user (i.e., the audiologist) to either check its calibration personally or to arrange for regular calibration of the equipment by an outside service. Checking calibration is necessary to be sure that an audiometer produces a pure tone at the specified level and frequency, that the signal is present only in the transducer to which it is directed, and that the signal is free from excessive distortion or unwanted noise interference. The audiologist who has demonstrated that the clinic equipment is "in calibration" can then feel confident in reporting the obtained results. Calibration checks can determine if an audiometer meets appropriate standards and also whether the instrument has changed over time.

The purpose of this chapter is to show the audiologist or student who does not have an extensive electronic background how to check audiometers to determine if they meet current national (or international) standards. A chapter on the topic of calibration is a necessary ingredient in a book on audiology. Because we generally cannot control the error of measurement produced by the client, we must put our efforts into controlling the two other major sources of error to ensure the best possible results: (1) personal calibration—educating the audiologist; and (2) electronic calibration—checking the audiometer. The other chapters in this book are devoted to educating (or calibrating) the audiologist. This chapter is devoted to calibrating the audiometer.

Throughout this chapter, we will refer to various standards. For the most part, we rely on standards that have been approved by the American National Standards Institute (ANSI), but we will also reference standards promulgated by the International Electrotechnical Committee (IEC) and the International Organization for Standardization (ISO). Since these standards do not have the status of law, it is important to understand how, and perhaps why, they are developed. Simply stated, standards are developed so that manufacturers of equipment (from all countries) and users of the equipment are all on the same page. According to its Website (http://ansi.org/about_ansi/overview/overview.aspx?menuid=1), ANSI is "a private, nonprofit organization (501(c) 3) that administers and coordinates the U.S. voluntary standardization and conformity assessment system." Its "mission is to enhance both the global competitiveness of U.S. business and the U.S. quality of life by promoting and facilitating voluntary consensus standards and conformity assessment systems, and safeguarding their integrity" (ANSI, 2004a). Some values (for example, the "0" hearing level) have both international and national approval. The procedures for developing standards are fairly rigid but may be explained in a rather simple manner. For purposes of this chapter, we will only discuss the ANSI procedure. The international procedures are similar but require the additional step of approval by the various countries that belong to IEC and ISO. In most cases, ANSI standards and ISO and IEC standards are very similar because this similarity (in current jargon, this is called harmonization) enhances commercial interchange between nations. If, for example, the ANSI audiometer standard was radically different from the IEC standard, manufacturers would have to build instruments solely for the American market and solely for the European, or World, market. In a relatively small-volume industry (such as audiometric instrumentation), this would be impractical at best.

To start the procedure of developing a new standard, if an individual or company believes that a standard should exist for a piece of equipment or a test procedure, the request is forwarded to the chair of the standards section that deals with the area. For example, when bone conduction was first used in audiometers, there were no standards for threshold values, and more importantly, there were no standards for the equipment on which to measure the bone vibrators. Once an artificial mastoid was developed, it was suggested that such a standard should exist. At this point, the chair of the appropriate standards committee (in this case, S3 Bioacoustics) and the standards secretariat (this is held by the Acoustical Society of America (ASA) for the four ANSI Accredited Standards Committees dealing with acoustics: S1 Acoustics, S2 Shock and Vibration, S3 Bioacoustics, and S12 Noise) prepare a ballot. This ballot is sent to the voting membership of the S3 committee to see if it is agreed that such a standard should be written. A first discussion is often held at the annual meeting of S3 (held during the spring meeting of the ASA). If it appears that the idea is a good one, then the members vote to approve the work. At this point, the person who suggested the standard (or the chair of S3 or the secretariat) will recommend that the work be given to an existing working group or that a new working group be formed to develop the standard. The chair of S3 (in consultation with the secretariat and usually the person who suggested the standard) will ask a particular person to chair the working group that will develop the standard. That person is contacted, and if they agree, they will ask others (or others may be suggested by the chair of S3, the secretariat, or other knowledgeable people) to participate in the working group. The working group must have broad representation of all interested parties. For example, it would be desirable for a working group on hearing aids to include not only manufacturers of hearing aids, but also audiologists. It must be emphasized that all of this is voluntary. There is **no** compensation for the chair of S3 or for the chair or the members of the working group. The group will meet face-to-face or will correspond (via phone, fax, mail, or e-mail) until a draft is written. After the working group has agreed on the draft, it will be forwarded to S3 for vote by the members of S3. Each Accredited Standards Committee has a group of individual experts who are also asked to review the proposed standard. Various companies and national organizations that might have a stake (direct and material interest) in such standards are voting members of S3 and the other committees; there is a rather substantial annual fee for membership. If there are negative comments (and votes) by the members, then the chair of the working group (often with the assistance of the chair of the Accredited Standards Committee) will try to revise the proposed standard to obtain agreement by all voting members. At one time, it was necessary to obtain unanimous agreement; however, today, "consensus" is reached when the vast majority of those voting approve, and every effort has been made to address the concerns of those who voted against the standard. Although the individual experts do not vote, they may comment, and their comments are considered in the revision of the draft standard. At this stage, the standard is sent out for comment by the general public. Once the public comment period is over and any comments have been considered, the standard is forwarded to ANSI by the secretariat for a final decision. Normally, ANSI will approve the document for publication and dissemination.

It should be pointed out that those who have a stake, interest, or knowledge will be encouraged to participate in the writing of the standard. The first author of this chapter learned the procedure firsthand when, after sitting in on a working group meeting and asking questions and challenging some of the assertions made by members, she was asked to become a member of the working group on the spot. It is not in the best interests of any standards developer to allow only limited participation in the working groups. However, it is also not in the best interests of the group to include large numbers of people with limited knowledge about the proposed standard or those who have very strong opinions and/or closed minds. This can bog down discussion and prolong the completion of the standard. All standards are reviewed periodically. If they are reaffirmed (and not changed), then the standard will read, for example, ANSI S3.39-1987 (R2002). This means the standard was approved in 1987 and was reaffirmed in 2002. If the standard is revised, then the date changes (e.g., ANSI S3.6-2004, which was previously ANSI S3.6-1997). An announcement is made when the standard is going to be voted on so that interested parties can obtain a copy and comment to the person or persons who will be voting. For example, audiologists might contact the American Speech-Language-Hearing Association (ASHA), which is a voting member. This is the basic procedure for development and approval of standards. For more information on the standards process, the reader is referred to Melnick (1973) and Wilber (2004).

Finally, if you are going to check the calibration of audiometric instrumentation, you must purchase the current editions of the relevant standards. Although those who work on developing the standards volunteer their time, the standards process is not free. There are costs to the secretariat for being members of ANSI and for coordinating the creation, modification, and dissemination of standards. There are three primary sources of funding for the production of standards in acoustics: financial support from ASA, fees paid by the voting members of an Accredited Standards Committee, and income from the sales of standards. Through your purchase of standards, you are supporting the efforts of those professionals who donate their time and effort to develop and maintain ANSI standards. Current contact information for the secretariat of ANSI S1, S2, S3, and S12 is:

Acoustical Society of America
ASA Secretariat
35 Pinelawn Road, Suite 114E
Melville, NY 11747-3177
Phone: (631) 390-0215
Fax: (631) 390-0217
E-mail: asastds@aip.org

PARAMETERS OF CALIBRATION

Much "how to calibrate" information is available in the manuals that accompany the audiometric equipment and the pieces of equipment used in checking or calibrating equipment. Although many of us seem to live by the slogan "When all else fails, read the manual," the first step in learning how to check calibration should always be to read the appropriate manual(s). Additional resources include electronic parts stores that often have basic manuals on test equipment, ASHA, and ASA. A number of books have also discussed procedures for acoustic measurements and equipment that might be used in such measurements (Decker and Carrel, 2004; Beranek, 1988; Silverman, 1999). The United States Government Printing Office is also a good source of information on basic test procedures. The specific parameters that

must be checked in an audiometer are outlined in standards provided by the ANSI and the IEC. See Table 2.1 for a listing of applicable standards. ANSI also lists and sells IEC and ISO standards. Generally, the ANSI, ISO, and IEC standards are in close agreement. When differences do exist, it is wise to use the ANSI standard when in the United States. The ISO and IEC standards are normally used by the rest of the world. It is beyond the scope of this chapter to discuss each area of calibration in detail. Therefore, it behooves the reader to purchase copies of the latest standards to verify the exact parameters to be checked and their permissible variability. To better understand the procedures for checking calibration, one must first understand the parameters that need to be checked as well as the basic equipment with which this is done. For puretone and speech audiometers, the three parameters are: (1) frequency, (2) sound pressure level (SPL), and (3) time (both phase and signal duration). These parameters apply whether one is using a portable audiometer, a standard diagnostic audiometer, or a computer-based audiometric system.

American standards for some instruments do not yet exist (for example, equipment used for auditory brainstem response [ABR] or otoacoustic emissions), but several basic parameters should be measured nevertheless, so that one can determine whether the equipment has changed over time. When such standards are developed (and currently both of the above are being developed by working groups), one can then ascertain if past tests are likely to have been valid. Although not discussed here, appropriately programmed computers interfaced with appropriate electroacoustic instrumentation may be used to check audiometric equipment. Some organizations, such as ASHA and OSHA, specify time intervals at which calibration checks should be made. It is the first author's opinion that, with current solid state electronic circuitry (as opposed to vacuum tubes), frequency and time parameters should be checked when the audiometer is first acquired and at yearly intervals thereafter. Older equipment should be checked at least biannually. It is the opinion of the first author that the output levels of all transducers (for both current and older audiometers) should be checked at trimonthly intervals or sooner if there is reason to suspect the audiometer output has changed. It is the opinion of the second author that the output of the transducers should be verified at least annually, unless there is reason to suspect that the output has changed. His opinion differs from the first author's for two reasons. First, it is his belief that most clinics only perform an electroacoustic analysis of transducer output annually (i.e., during the full annual calibration). Second, there is no compelling data to suggest that there are substantial changes in transducer output when the daily biologic calibration does not suggest an output change. Research facilities generally check calibration more often than specified earlier during the running of an experiment. In addition to regularly scheduled checks, audiometers should be tested *whenever* the clinician notices anything unusual in their performance.

TABLE 2.1   ANSI, IEC, and ISO standards for audiometers and audiometric testing

Number	Title
ANSI S3.1-1999 (R2003)	Maximum Permissible Ambient Noise for Audiometric Test Rooms
ANSI S3.2-1989 (R1999)	Method for Measuring the Intelligibility of Speech Over Communication Systems
ANSI S3.6-2004	Specification for Audiometers
ANSI S3.7-1995 (R2003)	Coupler Calibration of Earphones, Method for
ANSI S3.13-1987 (R2007)	American National Standard Mechanical Coupler for Measurement of Bone Vibrators
ANSI S3.20-1995 (R2003)	Bioacoustical Terminology
ANSI S3.21-2004	Method for Manual Pure-Tone Threshold Audiometry
ANSI S3.25-1989 (R2003)	American National Standard for an Occluded Ear Simulator
ANSI S3.36-1985 (R2006)	Specification for a Manikin for Simulated In Situ Airborne Acoustic Measurements
ANSI S3.39-1987 (R2007)*	Specifications for Instruments to Measure Aural Acoustic Impedance and Admittance (Aural Acoustic Immittance)
ANSI S1.4-1983 (R2006)	Specifications for Sound Level Meters
IEC 60645-1 2001	Audiological Equipment: Part 1—Pure-Tone Audiometers
IEC 60645-2 1993	Audiometers: Part 2—Equipment for Speech Audiometry
IEC 60645-3 1994	Audiometers: Part 3—Auditory Test Signals of Short Duration for Audiometric and Neuro-Otological Purposes
IEC 60645-4 1994	Audiometers: Part 4—Equipment for Extended High-Frequency Audiometry
IEC 60645-5 2004	Audiometric Equipment: Part 5—Instruments for the Measurement of Aural Acoustic Impedance/Admittance
IEC 60318 1998	Electroacoustics: Simulators of Human Head and Ear. Part 1—Ear Simulator for the Calibration of Supra-Aural Earphones
IEC 60318 2007	Electroacoustics: Simulators of Human Head and Ear. Part 6—Mechanical coupler for the measurement on bone vibrators
IEC 60711 1981	Occluded-Ear Simulator for the Measurement of Earphones Coupled to the Ear by Ear Inserts
ISO 6189, 1983	Acoustics: Pure Tone Air-Conduction Threshold Audiometry for Hearing Conservation Purposes
ISO 8253-1, 1989	Acoustics: Audiometric Test Methods. Part 1: Basic Pure-Tone and Bone Conduction Threshold Audiometry
ISO 389, 1964	Acoustics: Standard Reference Zero for the Calibration of Pure-Tone Audiometers
ISO 389-1, 1998	Acoustics: Reference Zero for the Calibration of Audiometric Equipment. Part 1: Reference Equivalent Threshold Sound Pressure Levels for Pure Tones and Supra-Aural Earphones
ISO 389-2, 1994	Acoustics: Reference Zero for the Calibration of Audiometric Equipment. Part 2: Reference Equivalent Threshold Sound Pressure Levels for Pure Tones and Insert Earphones
ISO 389-3, 1994	Acoustics: Reference Zero for the Calibration of Audiometric Equipment. Part 3: Reference Equivalent Threshold Force Levels for Pure Tones and Bone Vibrators
ISO 389-4, 1994	Acoustics: Reference Zero for the Calibration of Audiometric Equipment. Part 3: Reference Equivalent Levels for Narrow-Band Masking Noise
ISO 389-5, 1998	Acoustics: Reference Zero for the Calibration of Audiometric Equipment. Part 5: Reference Equivalent Threshold Sound Pressure Levels for Pure Tones in the Frequency Range 8 kHz to 16 kHz
ISO 389-6, 2007	Acoustics: Standard Reference Zero for the Calibration of Pure-Tone Audiometers
ISO 389-7, 2005	Acoustics: Reference Zero for the Calibration of Audiometric Equipment: Part 7: Reference Threshold of Hearing under Free-Field and Diffuse-Field Listening Conditions
ISO 389-8, 2004	Acoustics: Reference Zero for the Calibration of Audiometric Equipment. Part 8: Reference Equivalent Threshold Sound Pressure Levels for Pure Tones and Circumaural Earphones

ANSI, American National Standards Institute; ASHA, American Speech-Language-Hearing Association; IEC, International Electrotechnical Commission; ISO, International Standards Organization.
* Currently being revised.

Sometimes test results themselves reveal the need for an immediate calibration check (for example, when the same air-bone gap is obtained for two successive patients). It is always better to check the audiometer first rather than assume the problem lies with the client or clinician. A quick biologic check (described later) can always be performed. If this confirms the probability of an equipment problem, then a more elaborate electronic check should be carried out.

If the audiologist discovers that the frequency or time components of the audiometer are out of calibration, then the manufacturer or a local representative should be contacted for immediate repair and proper calibration of the instrument. Only a qualified electronics technician should attempt to take the machine apart to rectify the problem. However, if there is a stable deviation in output level at a given frequency, calibration corrections can be made either by adjusting the trim pots (potentiometers) on the audiometer, by using the audiometer's self-calibrating mechanism, or by posting a note on the front of the audiometer indicating the corrections. If paper corrections must be used, then the adjustment in decibels (plus or minus) that should be made at the various frequencies should be shown for each transducer. Note that if the SPL output is too high (e.g., by 5 dB), then you must increase their audiometric threshold (e.g., by 5 dB hearing level [HL]). Most modern audiometers provide some sort of internal calibration system for earphones, and many also provide this for bone conduction or sound field. If one plans to use bone vibrators for both mastoid and frontal bone testing or two sets of earphones with the same audiometer (for example supra-aural earphones and insert receivers), it is probably advisable to use "paper corrections," rather than trying to adjust trim pots between each transducer's use. Unstable SPL variations or lack of attenuator linearity may require further investigation by a qualified technician. Furthermore, if the trim pots need frequent adjustment, it is probably wise to check with a qualified technician.

INSTRUMENTATION

As mentioned earlier, the calibration of an audiometer requires the use of various pieces of electroacoustic and electronic instrumentation. Most, if not all, graduate audiology programs will have the instrumentation needed to at least evaluate whether the audiometer meets the reference equivalent threshold sound pressure level (RETSPL), frequency, linearity, and distortion standards specified in ANSI S3.6 Specification for audiometers. In this section, we will review the use of several basic instruments, including the sound level meter, a multimeter, a frequency counter, an oscilloscope, and a digital spectrum analyzer. More details on acoustics and instrumentation can be found in numerous texts (e.g., Curtis and Schultz, 1986; Speaks, 1996; Rosen and Howell, 1991; Richards, 1976; Decker and Carrell, 2004; Harris, 1998).

Multimeter

The term multimeter indicates that this device can be used to make multiple measurements. In most cases, a multimeter will allow you to make measurements of voltage, current, and resistance. Each of these measurements is made differently, and we will limit our discussion herein to making voltage measurements. To measure voltage, we must make the measurement in parallel (across) the device of interest. For example, if we are interested in attenuator linearity, we want to place the leads of the multimeter across the earphone leads. We can replace the earphone with an equivalent impedance (in most cases, a 10-, 50-, or 300-ohm resistor for ER-3A, TDH-39, TDH-49, or TDH-50 earphones). Simply unplugging the earphones and plugging in the multimeter may produce inaccurate results, because this approach likely changes the load impedance of the audiometer output. It is important to purchase a true root mean square (RMS) multimeter for accurate voltage readings. A true RMS multimeter actually calculates and displays RMS voltage. It is important to set the meter to AC, or alternating current (vs. DC, or direct current), voltage. The meter is most accurate when set to the lowest voltage range possible. In most cases, the voltage range is set in powers of 10, where the listed voltage is the highest voltage possible for that voltage range. When this highest voltage is exceeded, an overload is indicated (see multimeter manual for the overload indicator for your multimeter). You adjust the multimeter range until you have the most sensitive range (lowest maximum voltage) where the output is NOT overloaded.

Frequency Counter

This might be a stand-alone device, or it might be an option on your multimeter. In the case of a stand-alone device, a frequency counter will often have a trigger adjust (the voltage level and direction: positive-going or negative-going) that determines when an event is triggered. It is important that each "event" or "cycle" is counted and counted only once. This is because the frequency counter combines an event counter with an accurate clock. The ratio of events (i.e., cycles) divided by the time elapsed gives you the frequency (in Hz). Thus, if 100 events are measured in 100 ms (one-tenth of a second), then the cycles per second (or Hz) = 100 cycles/0.1 s = 1,000 cycles/s (Hz). If the counter does not trigger (no events counted), you need to reduce the trigger level or turn up the signal (e.g., increase the dB HL on the audiometer dial). If the frequency counter reads a number substantially larger than expected, then it is possible that the trigger level is set so low (or the signal presented is set so high) that multiple triggers per cycle are occurring. In this case, turning the signal level down or increasing the trigger level of the frequency counter should correct this problem. If the frequency counter is an option in a multimeter, there is often no trigger function, and the signal level must be changed in order to correctly trigger the counter function.

Sound Level Meter

The sound level meter (SLM) is actually multiple instrumentation components provided in a single instrument. It is possible that you can combine separate instruments into a usable device when an SLM is not available. At a minimum, for checking the calibration of the RETSPL (i.e., 0 dB HL values on the audiometer), you need an acoustic calibrator, an appropriate coupler (2 cc and/or 6 cc), a microphone, and the SLM. SLMs used for checking the calibration of audiometers should be Type 1, as should microphones used for such calibrations. The most commonly used Type 1 microphone is a condenser microphone. Condenser microphones come in four standard sizes (referring to their diameter): 1/8″, 1/4″, 1/2″, and 1″. In general, the smaller the microphone is, the higher its upper frequency cutoff and the less its sensitivity. Sensitivity is a measure of its efficiency transferring sound pressure into voltage and is commonly reported as mV/Pa. Condenser microphones are either prepolarized or require application of an external polarization voltage. Many nonprepolarized condenser microphones require a DC polarization voltage of 200 volts. Microphones also come as pressure microphones (to be used in a coupler), free-field microphones (to be used in sound field recordings such as when measuring the ambient noise in the sound booth), or random-incidence microphones (for measures in, for example, reverberant environments). More information about microphones and SLMs can be found in Johnson et al. (1998) and Yeager and Marsh (1998). It is important that your SLM and microphone be compatible, or equipment damage and/or incorrect SPL measures may result. In addition to providing the correct polarization voltage, the SLM contains amplifiers (whose gain is changed when you change the SPL range), time-weighting circuits (for fast, slow, and possibly impulse and peak time weightings), various filter settings (e.g., dBA, dBC, and octave and/or third-octave band filters) as well as a display function (this could be a VU meter, an LED indicator, and/or a digital readout). The gain of an amplifier in the SLM must be adjusted to account for the sensitivity of each microphone. For example, a 1″ microphone might have a sensitivity of 50 mV/Pa, while a 1/4″ microphone might have a sensitivity of 1 mV/Pa. If the SLM were adjusted appropriately for the 1/4″ microphone, then when 1 Pa of pressure was presented to the microphone diaphragm, the SLM would read 94 dB SPL [20log(1 Pa/0.0002 Pa) = 94 dB SPL]. If we replaced the 1/4″ microphone with the 1″ microphone but did not change the SLM amplifier gain, the 1″ microphone would read 128 dB SPL [94 dB SPL + 20log(50 mV/1 mV)]. How, then, do we calibrate the SLM? In most instances, we use a device that presents a known SPL to the diaphragm of the microphone. Two types of calibration devices are commercially available for this purpose: pistonphones and acoustic calibrators. The former produces sound by a mechanical piston, while the latter uses an electrical oscillator and a transducer to produce the tone. Each calibrator produces a specified SPL at a specified frequency, and this calibrator should be periodically sent back to the manufacturer to assure it remains within specified tolerances of frequency and SPL. These calibrators can accommodate a variety of microphone sizes by inserting nesting adapters. Turn on the SLM, place the calibrator snugly over the microphone, and turn on the calibrator. Making sure that the frequency response of the SLM is wideband (flat, or dBC if flat weighting is not available), adjust the gain of the SLM (by trimming a calibration potentiometer using a screwdriver or via software-based procedures) until the specified output of the calibrator (e.g., 114 dB SPL) is displayed on the SLM.

Once the SLM is calibrated, you must remove the acoustic calibrator (or pistonphone) and place an appropriate coupler over the microphone: a 2-cc coupler for insert earphones (e.g., Etymotic ER3A earphones) or a 6-cc coupler for supra-aural earphones (such as TDH-39, TDH-49, or TDH-50 earphones). ANSI S3.6-2004 has RETSPL values for both insert and supra-aural earphone for several 6-cc and 2-cc couplers.

Oscilloscope

The oscilloscope, in its most common display mode, presents voltage as a function of time. Oscilloscopes come in analog and digital types. In the analog oscilloscope, the output of an electron gun transiently phosphoresces (lights up) the screen of a cathode ray tube. Freezing the display on the oscilloscope screen involves repeated triggering of the oscilloscope on a fixed phase of the stimulus. Specialized analog oscilloscopes that can freeze a display for prolonged periods of time are called storage oscilloscopes. A digital oscilloscope is similar to an analog oscilloscope, except that instead of electron guns and a cathode ray tube, the signal is recorded by an analog-to-digital converter and displayed on a flat panel display. Digital oscilloscopes often have features that are not typically available on analog oscilloscopes (e.g., storage of waveforms, cursor functions, and summary statistics such as peak-to-peak and RMS voltage calculations). Simple amplitude and voltage measurements are easily performed on a signal using an oscilloscope. Manipulations of the time base (in time per division) and amplitude (in volts per division), as well as the appropriate adjustment of the trigger, allow the "freezing" of the signal on the oscilloscope. To measure, for example, peak-to-peak voltage, one counts the number of vertical divisions (usually a division is a centimeter) extending from the positive to the negative extremes and multiplies this number of divisions by the voltage per division to obtain the peak-to-peak voltage. For example, if the peak-to-peak amplitude of a sine wave is four divisions and each division is equal to 5 volts, then the peak-to-peak voltage is 20 volts (four divisions × 5 volts/division). To measure the period of the sine wave, you count the number of divisions for one cycle (e.g., from one positive peak to the next positive peak) and multiply by the specified time per division. For example, if the number of divisions per cycle is two divisions and the time base specifies 1 ms/division, then the period of this sine wave is 2 ms (two divisions × 1 ms/division). To convert to frequency (in Hz), you convert the milliseconds to seconds (2 ms = 0.002 s) and then take the inverse (1/0.002 s) to arrive at the frequency (500 Hz). It should be noted that measurements made on an analog oscilloscope are assumed to have an error of 5% or more.

Spectrum Analyzer

Numerous devices can be used to provide a frequency domain representation of a signal (including the octave or third-octave band filters available on many SLMs). In this section, we will limit our discussion to instruments referred to as digital spectrum analyzers. These instruments may be stand-alone hardware devices or might be part of a computer-based hardware/software application. These devices convert an analog input signal to digital format by use of an analog-to-digital converter. For a more detailed discussion of the limitations of analog-to-digital conversion, see Chapter 11 in this volume. For our present purposes, it is important that the reader understand that if the sampling rate used during analog to digital conversion is too slow, it can cause the generation of "false frequencies" in a process called aliasing. Many spectrum analyzers preclude aliasing by judicious use of a low-pass filter (called an antialiasing filter). It should also be noted that not all possible signal amplitudes can be encoded following analog-to-digital conversion, but signal level is rounded off ("quantized"), and that the magnitude of possible quantization error is related to the voltage range and the resolution (related to the number of bits) of the analog-to-digital converter. The time-domain signal is digitized over a limited time period, called the time window or the time epoch. Once the signal is digitized into a time epoch, it is converted into the frequency domain by Fourier transformation. (See Rosen and Howell [1991] for a more complete explanation of aliasing, antialiasing, quantizing, and digitization). Many readers have heard of the Fast Fourier Transform (FFT), which is one of many algorithms that have been developed to convert a time-domain (voltage over time) signal into a frequency-domain (amplitude across frequency) signal. Another term for the frequency domain representation is the spectrum. In addition to the possibility of quantization errors and aliasing, you must be aware that signal processing prior to Fourier transformation can have an influence on the results. Due to some underlying assumptions about the periodic nature of the discretely sampled signal, the spectrum of the signal is distorted unless an integer number of cycles of all frequencies is contained in the time epoch over which the signal is digitized. To prevent such distortion (often called leakage) that occurs when a noninteger number of cycles is contained in the time epoch, the digitized time epoch can be shaped. This shaping multiplies the signal by values at or near zero near the beginning and end of the time window and weights them at or near 1 near the middle of the signal. One popular windowing function is the Hanning window. A given windowing function trades amplitude uncertainty for frequency resolution. Once the data are converted to the frequency domain, the amplitude of a given Fourier coefficient (e.g., frequency) can be determined using a cursoring function. It should be noted that Fourier transformation produces multiple discrete harmonically related (i.e., integer multiples) spectral components. The lowest frequency (fundamental frequency) and, hence, the frequency interval between components are related to the recorded time-domain signal. If the time-domain signal is, for example, 500 ms (0.5 s), then the lowest frequency is 1/0.5 s, or 2 Hz. The longer the time window is, the better the spectral resolution.

⊠ BASIC EQUIPMENT

The basic calibration equipment for checking output levels of an audiometer should include: (1) a voltmeter or multimeter; (2) condenser microphones (both pressure and free-field types); (3) acoustic calibrator; (4) a 6-cc coupler (National Bureau of Standards [NBS] 9-A or IEC 60318); (5) a 2-cc coupler (ANSI HA-1 or HA-2 or IEC 60711); (6) a 500-g weight; (7) a mechanical coupler for bone vibrator measurements (artificial mastoid); and (8) an SLM (or equivalent piece of equipment) that allows one to read the output from an attached microphone input (ANSI, 1995; IEC, 1998; IEC, 1981; ANSI, 1987a; ANSI, 1983). When purchasing any of the above components, it is wise to check with others who use similar types of equipment to find the best specific brands available locally.

Other equipment such as a digital oscilloscope, frequency counter, and/or a spectrum analyzer will also prove to be invaluable in checking the acoustic parameters of audiometers. In many instances, this equipment can be shared by more than one facility. Certainly their expense is such that a single-person facility is unlikely to want to bear the cost of this less frequently used electronic equipment. A rule of thumb is that, if one has only one audiometer, a service contract is most sensible. If one has two to five pieces of audiometric test equipment, an SLM (with appropriate couplers, microphone(s), and acoustic calibrator) and a multimeter should be purchased and used. With more than five pieces of audiometric equipment, a more elaborate array of electronic equipment is probably desirable. If the accuracy of the audiometer is questioned, it necessitates shutting down the equipment or retesting patients at a later date. This translates into time and financial loss, not to mention more serious consequences in surgical or medicolegal cases. In a busy practice, such a loss would surely be equivalent to the cost of one or more pieces of electronic test equipment that would prevent this problem.

CHECKING THE CALIBRATION OF PURETONE AUDIOMETERS

Basic Signal

As soon as one obtains a new audiometer, the manual should be read and calibration instructions, if any, followed. Be as thorough as possible. These instructions describe the most effective way to check the performance of the audiometer. Perhaps the most common mistake made by the audiologist is to assume that the audiometer is so simple that it is not necessary to read the instructions. While that may be true for the operation of the machine, it is not necessarily true for its initial setup.

Biologic Check

After the audiometer has been installed, plugged in, turned on, and allowed to warm up, the operator should listen to the signal at different dial settings through each transducer (earphone, loudspeaker, and bone vibrator). Although few audiologists are equipped with "golden ears," with a little practice, one can hear basic faults in the equipment. A vague complaint to the audiometer technician or distributor that it "sounds funny" is as futile as telling an auto-repair person the same thing. However, a specific description of the sound and circumstances under which it occurs can help determine the source of the trouble. If the technician is given a detailed description of the problem, then the fault may be found immediately, without wasting their time and your money.

A great deal of information on the source of the problem may also be obtained by inspecting the audiometer. Following are some areas of potential malfunction that the audiologist should check periodically (normally on a daily basis).

1. Check the power, attenuator, earphone, and vibrator cords for signs of wearing or cracking. One way to determine if the transducer cord is defective is to listen to the tone through the transducer at a comfortable level while twisting and jiggling the cords. A defective cord will usually produce static or will cause the tone to be intermittent. Sometimes tightening the earphone screws or resoldering the phone plug connections is all that is necessary. If this does not alleviate the problem, it is wise to replace the cord.

2. If the audiometer has dials, check for loose dials or for dials that are out of alignment. If such faults exist, the dial readings will be inaccurate. Defective dials should be repaired immediately (sometimes this simply requires tightening the set screws that hold the dial to the audiometer), and the audiometer should be recalibrated to determine outputs at the "new" dial settings. Check to see that incremental changes are correctly reflected in the readout.

3. The audiologist should listen for audible mechanical clicks through the earphone when the dials or switches

are manipulated. The ANSI S3.6-2004 standard (section 5.4.4.1) suggests that two normal-hearing listeners should listen at a distance of 1 meter from the audiometer with the earphones in place but disconnected and with a proper resistive load (coinciding with the impedance of the earphone at 1,000 Hz) across the circuit while manipulating the presenter/interrupter switch, etc., to make sure that there are no audible signals that would clue the subject to the presence of the test signal. A mechanical click can often be detected more easily by listening than through the use of electronic equipment.

4. To determine if electronic transients are audible, it is wise to listen to the output both at a moderate hearing level (e.g., 60 dB) and below the threshold of hearing. Electronic transients will show up on an oscilloscope as an irregularity when the problem switch or dial is manipulated. The danger of an audible transient, whether mechanical or electronic, is that the patient may respond to the transient rather than the stimulus tone. Sometimes an antistatic or contact-cleaner spray can alleviate the problem of electronic transients.

5. The audiologist should listen for hum or static at high dial hearing levels, both when a stimulus signal is present and when it is absent. One should not hear static or hum at levels below 60 dB HL on the dial.

6. "Cross-talk" may occur between earphones; that is, the signal that is sent to one earphone may be heard in the contralateral earphone. Such a problem could greatly affect the measurements obtained on that audiometer, especially for cases with unilateral hearing loss. Cross-talk may be detected by disconnecting a phone jack and sending a signal to that phone. As before, when removing the earphone, a proper resistive load must be put in its place. The signal at a supra-threshold dial setting (e.g., 70 dB HL) should not be heard in the opposite earphone when a signal is presented in the normal manner. Cross-talk may be caused by faulty external wiring between the examiner's booth and that of the test subject or within the audiometer itself. Cross-talk must be corrected before any testing is carried out.

7. The clinician should listen to the signal while the attenuation dial is changed from maximum to minimum levels. For instance, a tone may be present at 20 dB HL on the dial, whereas no tone is present at 15 dB HL on the dial. In some cases, the tone stays at the same hearing level from 20 dB HL to –10 dB HL on the dial. These problems are easily detected by listening to the audiometer.

8. Finally, the threshold of the clinician (or a person with known hearing thresholds) should be checked with the earphones and bone vibrators to make sure that the output is approximately correct. If the levels are not within 10 dB of the previous threshold values, the output levels should be checked electronically.

Audiometer Serial #								
Date:								
Time:								
Checked By:								
Earphone Cords								
Power Cord								
Attenuator Cord								
Hum								
Dials								
Frequency								
Attenuation								
Intensity Right Phone								
Intensity Left Phone								
Tone Interrupter								
Tone Pulse Rate								
Cross-Talk								
Acoustic Radiation								
Bone Vibrator(s)								
Loudspeakers								
Other Comments								

FIGURE 2.1 Form for biologic check of audiometer.

Aside from these gross problems, which can be detected by looking or listening (see Fig. 2.1 for an example of a form that may be used to aid the clinician in carrying out the listening check), the precise accuracy of the output levels must be evaluated when the audiometer is first purchased and at regular intervals thereafter. Frequency, output level, linearity of attenuation, and percentage of distortion should all be checked electronically, in addition to the biologic check. Section 5.4 of ANSI S3.6-2004 describes various checks for unwanted sound from the transducer or audiometer.

Frequency Check

The frequency output from the audiometer should be checked by using an electronic frequency counter. This instrument will tell the exact frequency of the output signal. Fortunately, the cost of adequate frequency counters has been reduced significantly since the first edition of this book. Indeed, quite accurate frequency counters are often included in a digital multimeter. Thus, it is not really necessary to rely on other less precise procedures. The output from the audiometer may be sent directly to the instrument because the frequency is determined by an oscillator in the audiometer rather than the transducer. By using an electronic frequency counter, one can easily determine if the output from the audiometer corresponds to the nominal frequency. The standard for audiometers allows a tolerance of $\pm$ 1% of the indicated frequency value for Type 1 and 2 audiometers; $\pm$ 2% for Type 3 and 4 audiometers, and $\pm$ 3% for Type 5 audiometers. For example, if the audiometer dial reads 500 Hz, then the actual output must be between 495 and 505 Hz for a standard diagnostic (Type 1) audiometer.

Frequency should be checked on initial receipt of the audiometer and at yearly intervals thereafter. Nevertheless, it is appropriate to listen to the audiometer each day to judge whether the frequencies are maintaining reasonably good accuracy. Figure 2.2 presents a worksheet that can be used to record the frequency for a fixed-frequency audiometer.

Distortion Check

Linearity measurements may also help detect distortion in a transducer or in the audiometer itself. Distortion may appear as a lack of linear attenuation, especially at high output

YEARLY AUDIOMETER CALIBRATION CHECK for TYPE I AUDIOMETER

PART I

Audiometer: _____   Place: _____

Date: _____   Checked By: _____

TRANSDUCER   *EARPHONES*   *BONE*

Channel		I	II		I	I	II	II		I	II
				Allowed Percent					Allowed Percent		
Ear	Allowed Variation in Hz.			Total Harm. Distort.	Level	RT	LF	RT	LF	Total Harm. Distort.	Level		I	II
FREQUENCY:														
125	1.25			2.5%	75									
250	2.5			2.5%	90					5.5%	20			
500	5.0			2.5%	110					5.5%	50			
750	7.5			2.5%	110					5.5%	50			
1000	10.0			2.5%	110					5.5%	60			
1500	15.0			2.5%	110					5.5%	60			
2000	20.0			2.5%	110					5.5%	60			
3000	30.0			2.5%	110					5.5%	60			
4000	40.0			2.5%	110					5.5%	60			
6000	60.0			2.5%	90									
8000	80.0			2.5%	90									

Figure 2.2A Yearly calibration worksheet for puretone frequency, total harmonic distortion, and rise-fall time.

Rise/Fall - Allowable (20 - 200 msec.) Channel I _____/_____   Channel II _____/_____
(See p. 16, ANSI S3.6 - 1996 for details)

levels (90 dB HL and above). Harmonic distortion must be checked through the transducer itself. Excessive harmonic distortion is rarely caused by the audiometer but often arises in the various transducers. The maximum permissible total harmonic distortion in the current standard (ANSI S3.6-2004) is 2.5% for earphones and 5.5% for bone vibrators. The standard also shows the maximum permissible distortion for the second, third, fourth, and higher harmonics, as well as the subharmonics, across audiometric frequency. Total harmonic distortion can be recorded on the worksheet provided as Figure 2.2A.

Rise-Fall Time

The rise-fall time of the tone is a basic parameter of the audiometer, which may be checked by taking the output directly from the audiometer and routing it into a digital or storage oscilloscope. When gating the signal on, rise time is the length of time it takes for the signal to increase from −20 to −1 dB (10% to 90%) of its final steady-state value. The

fall time is the converse, or the length of time between −1 and −20 dB (90% to 10%) relative to its steady-state value. This is usually checked at a hearing level of 60 dB HL or less. ANSI S3.6-2004 specifies a rise time as well as a fall time of not less than 20 ms and not more than 200 ms. A detailed description of the rise and fall characteristics is given in section 7.5.3 of ANSI S3.6-2004 (ANSI, 2004b). A place to record the rise-fall time is provided at the bottom of Figure 2.2A.

Linearity Check

Attenuator linearity (the hearing level dial) may be checked electrically, directly from the audiometer, or acoustically through its transducer (earphone or bone vibrator). If measurements are to be made electrically, the earphone should remain in the circuit, and the voltage should be measured in parallel to the earphone, or a dummy load that approximates the earphone impedance should replace the transducer. To check linearity, the audiometer should be turned to its maximum output and then attenuated in 5-dB steps until the

Yearly Audiometer Calibration Check
Yearly - Part III

Audiometer: _____   Place: _____

Serial No.: _____   Date: _____   Checked By: _____

Attenuation Check 1K Rt. Phone   *Comments: Steps may not differ by more than 1 dB.*

Level	Ch. I	Ch. II
110		
105		
100		
95		
90		
85		
80		
75		
70		
65		
60		
55		
50		
45		
40		
35		
30		
25		
20		
15		
10		
5		
0		

Listening Check:
Mechanical Click: Yes: _____ No: _____ (Where) _____
Attenuation Complete: Ch. I: Yes: _____ No: _____
Attenuation Complete: Ch. II: Yes: _____ No: _____
Earphone Cords: OK: ____ Worn: _____ Crackle: _____ Need Replacing: _____
Bone Vibrator Cords: OK: ____ Worn: _____ Crackle: _____ Need Replacing: _____
Power Cord: OK: ____ Worn: _____ Crackle: _____ Need Replacing: _____

Figure 2.2B   Attenuator Linearity

output can no longer be read. Each attenuator on the audiometer should be checked separately. In order to meet the ANSI S3.6-2004 standard, the attenuator should be linear within 0.3 of the interval step or by 1 dB, whichever is smaller. That is, if you change the level in 5-dB steps, the audiometer must attenuate between 4 and 6 dB per step. If the attenuation step is 2 dB, then the reading should be between 1.4 and 2.6 dB per step (0.3 × 2 dB = 0.6 dB, which is less than 1 dB).

Attenuator linearity should be checked annually. If a "fixed loss pad" (i.e., a device that automatically changes the signal level by a set amount, e.g., 20 dB) is present in the audiometer, its attenuation must also be checked. If the audiometer attenuates in 1- or 2-dB steps, then these smaller attenuation steps should be checked if they are used clinically. Unfortunately, not all calibration equipment is accurate enough to allow one to check intervals of less than 1 dB (with an acceptable range of 0.7 to 1.3 dB) with confidence.

Therefore, more accurate (and therefore more expensive) equipment might be required if finer accuracy is necessary. Figure 2.2B is a worksheet that can be used when evaluating attenuator linearity.

EARPHONE LEVEL CALIBRATION

Real Ear Methods

There are two basic approaches for the calibration of earphones. One is the "real ear" method, and the other is the "artificial ear" or coupler method. With the original real ear method, one simply tested the hearing of a group of normal-hearing persons, averaged the results, and checked to see that the average hearing of this group was at zero on the dial for each frequency. Although this is theoretically feasible with a large population sample, it is not a recommended procedure. ANSI S3.6-2004, Appendix D, describes probe tube, loudness balance, and threshold procedures that may be used for this purpose. Clearly, these procedures are possible but quite unwieldy, especially if they are to be followed weekly or monthly. It should be noted that this procedure is essentially the procedure used for determination of normal hearing level (nHL) for auditory evoked potentials when using click or tone burst procedures. Furthermore, for audiometers, this approach is technically incorrect because the ISO 389-1, 1998 reference (which is also used in ANSI S3.6-2004) is not tied to normal hearing per se, but simply refers to an arbitrarily accepted SPL (i.e., the RETSPL or force level). If the audiologist wishes to use a new earphone (that is not listed in the ANSI standard or its appendix), a real ear procedure might be the only way to check calibration, but if generally accepted earphones are used, it is much easier and more efficient to use an artificial ear/coupler method.

Artificial Ear (Coupler) Methods

The most commonly used procedure today is that of the "artificial ear," which consists of a condenser microphone and a 6-cc coupler (for supra-aural earphones) or 2-cc coupler (for insert earphones). The 6-cc coupler was originally chosen because it was thought that the enclosed volume was approximately the same as the volume under a supra-aural earphone for a human ear (Corliss and Burkhard, 1953). However, since volume displacement is only one component of acoustic impedance, it cannot be assumed that the coupler actually represents a human ear. Burkhard and Corliss (1954) pointed out that the impedance characteristics of a 6-cc coupler probably simulate the impedance of the human ear over only a small part of the frequency range. Because the 6-cc coupler does not replicate the impedance of the human ear, it cannot be considered a true artificial ear. Subsequent work by Zwislocki (1970, 1971), Killion (1978), Cox (1986), and Hawkins et al. (1990) has quantified the differences between real ear and coupler values. In an attempt to solve this problem, the IEC 318 coupler was developed. However, there is still some disagreement as to the accuracy of this ear simulator (formerly called an artificial ear) because its impedance characteristics are also not exactly those of a real human ear. However, it is clearly more accurate than the present NBS 9-A coupler.

In addition to the problem of acoustic impedance characteristics, the NBS 9-A coupler is known to have a natural resonance at 6,000 Hz (Rudmose, 1964). This interferes with the measurement of the output of an audiometer earphone around that frequency. Other coupler problems are its size, its shape, and the hard walls that permit the possibility of standing waves at frequencies above 6,000 Hz. Despite these difficulties, the 6-cc coupler remains the accepted device (by ANSI S3.6-2004) for measuring the acoustic output from the audiometer through a supra-aural earphone. A coupler

developed by Zwislocki (1970, 1971, 1980) appears to very closely approximate the acoustic impedance of the human ear. It is used in KEMAR (a manikin that has a pinna and an ear canal, as well as a coupler and microphone) (Burkhard and Sachs, 1975, Burkhard, 1978). This manikin is described in ANSI S3.25-1989 (ANSI, 1989), but RETSPLs are not given for supra-aural or insert receivers using the Zwislocki coupler or the manikin.

When checking the audiometer earphone output, the supra-aural earphone is placed on the coupler and a 500-g weight is placed on top of it. If using an SLM (rather than a microphone preamplifier), the output is read in dB SPL, where $SPL = 20\log P/P_{ref}$ (where P is the observed sound pressure, and $P_{ref} = 20\ \mu Pa$). After the earphone is placed on the coupler, a low-frequency tone (125 or 250 Hz) is introduced, and the earphone is reseated on the coupler until the highest SPL value is read. This helps assure optimal earphone placement on the coupler. The output from the earphone is then compared to the expected values at each frequency. The standard SPL values that are used are given in (1) ISO 389-1 (1998), often referred to as ISO-1964 because of its initial publication date, and (2) ANSI S3.6-2004. These values evolved through a "round robin" in which several earphones were measured on various couplers at a group of laboratories throughout the world (Weissler, 1968).

The current ANSI standard includes RETSPLs for the TDH type earphones, as well as insert earphones. It also provides values for both the IEC and NBS couplers for supra-aural earphones and values for insert phones using an occluded ear simulator or HA-1 or HA-2 coupler. Figure 2.3 shows an audiometer earphone calibration worksheet, which contains the expected values at each frequency with TDH-39 or TDH-49 (or TDH-50) earphones in Telephonics type 51 cushions on an NBS 9-A coupler and insert receivers using an HA-1–type coupler. ANSI S3.6-2004 allows a tolerance from the listed values of ± 3 dB from 125 to 5,000 Hz and ± 5 dB at 6,000 Hz and higher.

The supra-aural output measurements referred to above are only valid when a supra-aural–type earphone cushion (which touches the pinna) such as the Telephonics 51 is used and not when a circumaural cushion (which encircles the pinna) is used. The lack of an approved reference threshold for circumaural earphone cushions has been pointed out by Benson et al. (1967) and by Zwislocki et al. (1988). Although it is possible to place the earphone receiver on a coupler, this does not ensure that the SPL at the eardrum will be the same when the earphone is placed in a circumaural cushion. Procedures for and the outcomes of such measurements have been described by Shaw and Thiessen (1962), Stein and Zerlin (1963), and Tillman and Gish (1964). Vilchur (1970) has also described a circumaural earphone and a procedure for calibration. ANSI S3.6-2004 provides information in Annex C for the calibration of circumaural earphones. This includes the dimensions of the earphone, the type of coupler (IEC 318 with adapter), and expected RETSPLs.

AUDIOMETER EARPHONE CALIBRATION SHEET

Audiometer: _____ S # _____ Earphone: _____ Channel: _____ Room: _____

Calibrated By: _____ Date: _____ Equipment: _____

FREQUENCY	125	250	500	750	1000	1500	2000	3000	4000	6000	8000
1. SPL*											
2. Audiometer Dial Setting											
3. Nominal Ref. SPL (Line 1 - Line 2)											
4. Equipment & Mike Correction											
5. Corrected Ref. SPL (Line 3 - Line 4)											
6a. TDH - 49/50 Earphones**	47.5	26.5	13.5	8.5	7.5	7.5	11.0	9.5	10.5	13.5	13.0
TDH - 39	45.0	25.5	11.5	8.0	7.0	6.5	9.0	10.0	9.5	15.5	13.0
6b. ER 3-A Earphones***	26.5	14.5	6.0	2.0	0.0	0.0	2.5	2.5	0.0	-2.5	-3.5
7. Calibration Error (Line 5 - Line 6)											
8. Corrections @											

* SPL = Sound Pressure Level in dB re 20 μ PA
** TDH-49/50 values from **ANSI S3.6-1996,** p. 18 (see standard for coupler, and cushions)
*** ER 3-A values from **ANSI S3.6-1996,** p.20 using HA-1 type coupler (see standard for different coupler values)
@ Correction - Rounded to the nearest 5 dB; – = audiometer weak, make threshold better
+ = audiometer strong, make threshold poorer

Figure 2.3 Earphone calibration worksheet.

When the output of the audiometer through the earphone has been established, it is compared to the appropriate standard to determine whether it is in calibration or not. If possible, the audiometer trim pots (or by software adjustments in newer digital audiometers) should be used to bring the audiometer into calibration. However, when this is not possible or when different earphones will be used with the same audiometer, and when corrections are less than 15 dB, a calibration correction card may be placed on the audiometer showing the discrepancy from the established norm. It should be noted that, if the output of the audiometer is, for example, 10 dB too low, then the dB HL correction sheet must be decreased by 10 dB. Such corrections must then be taken into consideration when an audiogram is plotted. If an audiometer is off by more than 15 dB at any frequency or by 10 dB at three or more frequencies, it is advisable to have the audiometer put into calibration by the audiometer manufacturer or their representative. If the audiometer is new, it should meet ANSI S3.6-2004 tolerances. With current digital audiometers, deviations in desired output are usually due to the transducer rather than the audiometer, so sometimes it is better to simply replace the offending transducer(s).

From time to time, people have suggested calibrating and presenting audiograms in SPL instead of HL. This would be feasible for air conduction. However, because air and bone conduction values differ in rather complex ways (e.g., bone conduction is in force level and air conduction is in SPL; force levels are referenced to 1 μN rather than 20 μPa; RETSPLs and reference equivalent threshold force levels [RETFL] vary quite differently across frequency), we would have to get used to assessing air-bone gaps in a completely different way. In addition, the re-education of audiologists and physicians would probably be quite difficult. Thus, we appear to be stuck with HL for the foreseeable future.

Others have suggested using each person as his/her own control by placing a probe tube near the tympanic membrane and measuring the air-conduction output at threshold. The difficulty here is the fact that each individual canal has its own unique resonance pattern and each eardrum has its own unique impedance, which could lead to incorrectly interpreted results. In addition, it is very difficult to obtain accurate SPL estimates using the probe tube procedure for sounds as faint as 10 dB SPL, as would be the case when thresholds are within the normal range at some frequencies. Finally, there are standing waves in the ear canal with high-frequency, steady-state stimuli, resulting in differences in SPL at the tympanic membrane as compared to the SPL at the location of the probe microphone in the ear canal, which cannot be controlled.

BONE VIBRATOR CALIBRATION

Real Ear Procedures

Checking the calibration of a bone vibrator presents a different problem than that of an earphone. While earphones can be checked easily using a microphone as a pickup, bone vibrators cannot. The original technique for checking bone vibrator calibration was a real ear procedure (American Medical Association, 1951), which was somewhat different than that used for earphones. The method assumes that air- and bone-conduction thresholds are equivalent. If six to 10 normal-hearing subjects are tested for both air and bone conduction with an audiometer whose air-conduction system is in proper calibration, bone-conduction corrections for the audiometer can be determined by using the difference obtained between air- and bone-conduction thresholds. This procedure makes a few assumptions that are not always met. For example, it presupposes that true thresholds can be obtained for all the normal-hearing subjects using the given audiometer. Because (1) many audiometers do not go below 0 dB HL and (2) the ambient noise in test booths often does not allow assessment below 0 dB HL, it is not always possible to determine the true threshold. To avoid these problems, Roach and Carhart (1956) suggested using individuals with pure sensorineural losses for subjects in the real ear procedure. Such an approach eliminates the problems of ambient noise and lack of audiometric sensitivity, thus increasing the probability that one will obtain "true" thresholds. A problem arises when trying to find a group of subjects with "pure sensorineural" losses who have no conductive component and who have thresholds that do not extend beyond the bone-conduction limits of the audiometer. However, the more basic problem with real ear bone vibrator calibration is the supposition that air- and bone-conduction thresholds are equivalent in the absence of conductive pathology. While this is certainly true, on average, for a large group of people, it cannot be expected to be true for any individual or for small groups (Studebaker, 1967; Wilber and Goodhill, l967).

Artificial Mastoid Procedure

The preferred procedure for calibrating bone vibrators involves the use of a mechanical coupler, often referred to as an artificial mastoid. Artificial mastoids were proposed as early as 1939 by Hawley (1939). However, it was not until Weiss (1960) developed his artificial mastoid that they became commercially available. Just as replication of the acoustic impedance of the human ear is difficult with a coupler, replication of the mechanical impedance of the head is difficult with an artificial mastoid. Because no commercially available artificial mastoid met the mechanical impedance requirements of the ANSI (S3.13-1972) or IEC (IEC 60373-1971) standards, both the ANSI and IEC standards were revised to conform more closely to an artificial mastoid that *is* available (ANSI S3.13-1987; IEC 60373-1990). ANSI S3.6-2004 gives threshold values (RETFLs) that are appropriate for a bone vibrator such as the B-71 or B-72 or one meeting the physical requirements described in 9.4.3 of ANSI S3.6-2004. The ISO standard (ISO 389-3 1994) gives one set of values that are to be used for all bone vibrators having the circular tip described in the ANSI and IEC documents (ISO, 1994b). These values are also used in the ANSI standard. It is important to recognize that both the ANSI and the ISO values are based on unoccluded ears using contralateral masking. Thus, the values presuppose that masking will be used in the contralateral ear when obtaining threshold. Figure 2.4 shows a sample calibration worksheet for bone vibrators, incorporating the ANSI S3.6 values. In both earphone and bone vibrator calibration, it is important to check distortion as well as overall level through the transducer. Distortion may be measured directly with (1) a distortion meter (connected to the output from the artificial mastoid) or (2) a frequency analyzer. An oscilloscope provides a visual picture of the time-domain wave, but it is not possible to determine the exact percentage of distortion this way. As mentioned earlier, allowable distortion values for bone vibrators are more lenient than for earphones. This is because bone vibrators have more distortion than earphones. In addition to the earlier mentioned physical measurement procedures, the importance of just listening to the audiometer cannot be overly stressed. The normal ear (with audiologist attached) should be able to perceive gross attenuation and distortion problems. The electronic procedures, however, serve to precisely describe the problems that the human ear only approximates.

SPEECH AUDIOMETERS

Because running speech fluctuates in SPL (as well as frequency content) over time, the preferred method is to introduce a pure tone (1,000 Hz) into the microphone, tape, or compact disc (CD) input of the speech audiometer. For purposes of calibration, when an electronic signal is introduced in older audiometers, the input impedance of the audiometer must be matched by the output impedance of the oscillator. In most newer audiometers, these audiometer inputs are buffered with high-impedance operational amplifiers (op-amps), and such impedance matching is unnecessary. The input level should be adjusted so that the monitoring meter on the face of the audiometer reflects the appropriate level, usually 0 dB. The output from the

CALIBRATION WORKSHEET FOR BONE VIBRATORS

Audiometer: _____ Channel:_____ Vibrator: _____

Place: _____

Date: _____ Calibrated By: _____

Equipment Used: _____ + B& K Mastoid _____

FREQUENCY:	250	500	750	1000	1500	2000	3000	4000
1. dB re 1 μN								
2. N.U. B&K Correction								
3. Line 1 ± Line 2								
4. Audiometer Dial	40	60	60	60	60	60	60	60
5. Line 3 − Line 4								
6. B-71 (Mastoid)*	47.0	38	28.5	22.5	16.5	11.0	10.0	15.5
7. Line 5 − Line 6								
8. Corrections @								
9. FBC-MBC Difference	12.0	14.0	13.0	8.5	11.0	11.5	12.0	8.0
10. Frontal Correction								

*based on ANSI S3.6-1996 (Specification for Audiometers)

@ Correction - Rounded to the nearest 5 dB; − = audiometer weak, make threshold better
+ = audiometer strong, make threshold poorer

Figure 2.4 Bone vibrator calibration worksheet.

transducer is then measured. If an oscillator is not available, you can use the 1,000-Hz tone, which precedes the test words on most commercially available speech material recordings for checking the tape and CD circuits. A tone from another audiometer might be used to check the microphone circuit. Details concerning the calibration of the speech circuit of an audiometer are given in Section 6.2 of ANSI S3.6-2004.

ANSI S3.6-2004 states that the output for the 1,000-Hz tone at 0 dB HL should be 12.5 dB above the RETSPL for the earphone at 1,000 Hz. Bone vibrators should be calibrated separately. All subsequent speech testing must be carried out with the monitoring meter peaking at the same point as during the calibration check. If, for example, one

prefers −3 dB on the meter rather than 0 dB, then calibration of the 1,000-Hz tone must be peaked at −3 dB, or an appropriate correction must be made in reporting measurements.

The required flatness of the frequency response of the speech audiometer circuit is defined as ± 3 dB for the frequencies of 250 to 4,000 Hz and from 0 to −10 dB between 125 and 250 Hz and ± 5 dB between 4,000 and 6,000 Hz. ANSI S3.6-2004 gives specific requirements for checking the microphone circuit as well as the other speech input circuits. If the puretone and speech audiometers are separate machines, then the speech audiometer must also be checked for cross-talk, internal noise, and attenuator linearity as described earlier.

MONITORING METER

Monitoring meters are indicators of signal level and are found on the face of most audiometers. The monitoring meter is calibrated relative to the input signal that it monitors and should not be interpreted as yielding any absolute values such as 0 dB SPL. On a speech audiometer, the meter is used to monitor the speech signal or to aid the audiologist in adjusting the input calibration tone that precedes the recorded speech materials. The exact specifications for the meters may be found in Section 6.2.10 of ANSI S3.6-2004. In general, it is important that the meter be stable, that there is minimal undershoot or overshoot of the needle indicator relative to the actual signal, and that any amplitude change is accurately represented on the meter. The audiologist may check the meter and its entire accompanying input system as described below.

A puretone should be fed from an oscillator through an electronic switch to the input of the audiometer. The tone should be monitored by a voltmeter or an oscilloscope. By activating the electronic switch to produce a rapidly interrupted signal, one can watch the meter to ascertain whether there is any overshoot or undershoot relative to the signal in its steady-state. One must also check the response time of the needle on the VU meter. A computer-generated or tape-recorded tone may be used to ensure that the needle reaches its 99% state deflection in 350 ms ± 10 ms. In addition, the overshoot should be no more than 1.5%. One can insert a linear attenuator in the line between the oscillator and the audiometer input, one may reduce the output from the oscillator and the audiometer input, or one may reduce the output from the oscillator by a known amount (as monitored by a voltmeter or oscilloscope). The change in input should be accurately reflected by a corresponding change on the monitoring meter.

SOUND FIELD TESTING

ANSI S3.6-2004 describes the primary characteristics of sound field testing in Section 9.5. This includes the test room, frequency response, method for describing the level of the speech signal, and the location of the speakers. Table 9 of the standard also gives specific RETSPL values for band-limited stimuli (frequency-modulated tones or narrow bands of noise) for binaural and monaural listening. An ASHA working group prepared a tutorial for sound field testing that discusses some of the problems of setting up the test procedure (ASHA, 1991). Characteristics of the frequency-modulated signals are given in Section 6.1.3 of ANSI S3.6-2004. In addition, the characteristics of narrowband noise levels are presented in Table 5 of the standard. The level for speech in sound field should be comparable to the corrected free-field response for earphones.

When calibrating stimuli presented in the sound field, it is important to place some sort of marker (such as a ring suspended from the ceiling) at the place where the subject's head will be. A free-field microphone should be placed so that the diaphragm is facing toward the direction of the plane-propagated wave (called frontal incidence). If a pressure microphone is used, the microphone diaphragm should be placed facing at a right angle to the direction of the place propagated wave (called grazing incidence). In either case, the microphone should be placed at the place where the subject's head will be during testing. There should be nothing between the speaker and the calibration equipment.

The amplifier hum or internal noise of the loudspeaker system should be checked. This may be done by adjusting the attenuator dial to some high setting (between 80 and 90 dB HL) and then measuring the output from the loudspeaker when no signal is present. That is, everything is in normal position for testing except that there is no signal (warble tone or noise, etc.) presented to the speaker. The equipment noise should be at least 50 dB below the dial setting (i.e., if the dial reads 80 dB HL, then the equipment noise should be <30 dB SPL).

Figure 2.5 shows a worksheet that may be used to check the output from the loudspeakers.

CALIBRATION OF ANCILLARY EQUIPMENT

Masking Generator

ANSI S3.6-2004 defines white noise, weighted random noise for masking of speech, and narrowband noise. Instead of HL, masking noise is discussed in terms of effective masking (dB EM), meaning that, for example, a 20-dB EM noise is that noise level that perceptually masks a 20-dB HL signal. The bandwidths for narrow bands are specified by frequency with RETSPL corrections for third-octave and half-octave measurements. Cutoff values are given in the standard (Table 5). When checking the bandwidth of the narrowband noise, it is necessary to have a frequency analyzer or spectrum analyzer (or a computer program that allows one to produce a Fourier analysis of the noise) to determine if the noise bandwidths from the audiometer conform to specifications. The same transducer that will be used when delivering the masking sound should be used to make final calibration measurements. However, because the characteristics of various transducers are quite different from one another, it is sensible to first do an electronic check directly from the audiometer to verify that any variation from the bandwidth is due to the transducer rather than the electrical output of the audiometer.

The masking sound should be checked periodically through the transducers used to present it. The examiner should be careful to use a signal that is high enough in level to avoid interference by ambient room noise (generally about 80 dB HL). In the case of narrowband noise,

CALIBRATION WORKSHEET FOR SOUND FIELD AUDIOMETRY - 45° AZIMUTH

Audiometer: _____ Channel: _____ SN#: _____ Earphone: _____ Room #: _____

Calibrated By: _____ Date: _____ Equipment: _____

FREQUENCY:	125	250	500	750	1000	1500	2000	3000	4000	6000	8000
1. SPL											
2. Audiometer Dial	50	60	70	80	70	70	70	70	70	70	70
3. Line 1 - Line 2											
4. Equip. & Mike Correct.											
5. Corrected Ref. SPL (Line 3 - Line 4)											
6. FM Tone (or NB noise) @ 45° Azimuth	23.5	12.0	3.0	0.5	0.0	-1.0	-1.5	-9.0	-8.5	-3.0	8.0
7. Calibration Error Line 5 - Line 6											
8. Correction*											

SPL = Sound Pressure Level in dB re 20μPa coupler in sound field at 45° Azimuth using Frequency Modulated (FM) tones or narrow bands of noise
*Correction - Rounded to nearest 5 dB [- = audiometer weak, make threshold better; + = audiometer strong, make threshold poorer]
based on ANSI S3.6 - 1996 (Specifications for Audiometers)

Figure 2.5 Sound-field measurement calibration worksheet.

the SPL values measured should be within ± 3 dB of the RETSPLs for the geometric center frequency and corrected appropriately for masker bandwidth. A worksheet for recording the upper and lower cutoff frequencies of one-third octave bandwidth noise is given in Figure 2.6. If white noise (noise that has equal level across frequency) is the only masking signal on the audiometer, one need only check the output through the earphone with a linear setting (no filter) on the SLM. The overall output and attenuation characteristics should be checked in the same basic manner as described for puretones using an artificial ear.

The audiologist should be aware that, when making noise measurements, the characteristics of the measuring equipment are critical. Since noise is not a "clean" (i.e., uniform and unvarying) signal, it is highly susceptible to errors of overshoot and undershoot on a meter and to damping on a graphic level recorder. A spectrum analyzer that is capable of frequency-domain averaging and with storage capabilities is optimal for checking calibration of noise. Unfortunately, most clinics do not have such sophisticated equipment.

COMPACT DISC AND TAPE PLAYERS

CD or tape players that are used in a clinic for reproducing speech signals, filtered environmental sounds, or other test stimuli should be checked electroacoustically at least once every 12 months. However, if the CD or tape player is in regular use, weekly maintenance should be carried out (such as cleaning and demagnetizing the heads for tape players). The instruction manuals normally outline the procedures to be used with the particular tape or CD player. If not, any good audio-equipment dealer can explain the procedure. In addition, the frequency response and time characteristics of the tape player should be checked.

At present, there are no standards for tape players used with audiometers per se. However, the frequency response and time characteristics of the tape player may be checked by using a standard commercial tape recording of puretones of various frequencies. If you do not have access to such a tape, it is possible to make one by introducing puretones from an audio oscillator into the machine, recording them, and playing them back. This enables the operator to check both the record and playback sections of the tape recorder. Unfortunately, if both the record and playback are equally reduced (or increased) in frequency, the output will appear at the nominal frequency. The output from the oscillator should be monitored with a voltmeter to make certain that a constant voltage signal is used. Distortion of the puretone from the tape player should also be checked. If none of this is possible, the speed of the tape player can be checked grossly by marking a tape and then, after timing a segment as it goes across the tape head, measuring to see how many inches passed over the heads per second. Also, if the machine is badly out of calibration, it will be audible as a pitch

MASKING CALIBRATION

Audiometer: _____Channel___ Room: _____ Date: _____

Calibrated by: _____ Equipment Used: _____

| FREQUENCY: | LOWER Cut-Off Freq. | | | UPPER Cut-off Freq. | | | RIGHT | | LEFT | |
	Min.	Max.	Actual	Min.	Max.	Actual	Expect. Level	Actual Level	Expect. Level	Actual Level
125	105	111		140	149		47.5		47.5	
250	210	223		281	297		26.5		26.5	
500	420	445		561	595		13.5		13.5	
750	631	668		842	892		8.5		8.5	
1000	841	891		1120	1190		7.5		7.5	
1500	1260	1340		1680	1780		7.5		7.5	
2000	1680	1780		2240	2380		11.0		11.0	
3000	2520	2670		3370	3570		9.5		9.5	
4000	3360	3560		4490	4760		10.5		10.5	
6000	5050	5350		6730	7140		13.5		13.5	
8000	6730	7130		8980	9510		13.0		13.0	

Figure 2.6 Masker calibration worksheet.

change in the recorded speech (higher if too fast, lower if too slow).

It must be remembered that the CD or tape player used to reproduce speech materials is an integral part of the audiometer system. Thus, it should not be ignored when checking calibration.

AUTOMATIC AUDIOMETERS

A calibration check of automatic (or Bekesy) audiometers begins with frequency, level, cross-talk, and other aspects described for manual puretone audiometers. In addition, the attenuation rate and interruption rate for pulsed signals should be checked. ANSI S3.6-2004 requires that a rate of change of 2.5 dB/s be provided for Type 1, 2, and 3 audiometers. Permissible rates for all types of audiometers are given in the ANSI S3.6-2004 standard. As in manual audiometers, the permissible variance in level per step is 1 dB or 0.3 of the indicated step size, whichever is smaller. The attenuation rate may be measured quite easily with a stopwatch. After starting the motor, a pen marking on the chart is started at the same instant as a stopwatch is started. One reads the chart to determine how far the signal was attenuated (or increased) during the measured time interval. By dividing the duration (in seconds) into the dB change in level, one can find the dB per second attenuation rate. The audiometer should be checked for signals both increasing and decreasing in level.

To check the pulsed stimulus duration, one may go from the "scope sync" output on the back of the audiometer (if such exists) to an electronic counter, or if that is not available, one can record across the terminals of the timing mechanism inside the audiometer. It is difficult to check the pulse speed on a graphic level recorder because of pen damping, but it is possible to check it on a digital or storage oscilloscope. It is not difficult to estimate whether there is roughly a 50% duty cycle (on half the time and off half the time), but it is quite difficult to judge whether the signal is on for 200 ms versus 210 ms. The characteristics of the pulsed tone are described in Section 7.5.4 of ANSI S3.6-2004.

If both pulsed and continuous signals are used, it is important to check the relative level of the pulsed and continuous signals. If they are not equal, this should be corrected. The relative levels can be compared by observing the envelope of the waveform on an oscilloscope or by recording the output with a graphic level recorder if there is no damping problem. The attenuation rate and pulse rate should be checked annually unless there is a reason to suspect a problem earlier.

AUDITORY EVOKED POTENTIAL INSTRUMENTS

As of this writing, there are no ANSI standards for auditory evoked potential (AEP) instrumentation. However, an ANSI working group is trying to develop such a standard. In the absence of an accepted "HL" for acoustic transients such as clicks or tone bursts, most investigators recommend the determination of an nHL for one's own unit. There is an IEC standard for auditory test signals of short duration for audiometric and neuro-otologic purposes (IEC-60645-3; IEC, 1994a). Until such time as ANSI adopts the IEC standard or develops its own standard, one should check the equipment to make sure that it does not change over time, as well as to obtain data to allow comparison of results obtained on equipment at other centers.

The basic parameters of the acoustic signals are the same as for conventional audiometry. One must check output level, frequency, and time. When calibrating acoustic transients from an AEP instrument, the instrumentation used to calibrate an audiometer may be inappropriate. It is especially important to check the output from the AEP unit acoustically as well as electrically. It is easy to display the electrical output from the AEP unit on an oscilloscope, but to analyze that display, one needs to repeat it very rapidly or, preferably, use a digital or storage oscilloscope. Determination of the acoustic level of these acoustic transients requires an SLM that can record true peak SPL (pSPL) or a microphone system or SLM that allows routing the output to an oscilloscope to determine pSPL or peak equivalent SPL (peSPL). See Chapter 11 for details concerning calibration of transient signals.

In addition to the overall level, it is important to determine the frequency characteristics of the signal (i.e., its spectrum) as it is played through the transducer. One can never assume that an electronic representation of the frequency characteristics of this brief signal has more than a passing resemblance to the signal after it has been passed through a transducer. This is because each system has its own transfer function (i.e., filtering characteristics), and the acoustic spectra of the stimuli will be affected by both the earphone and the coupler used to couple the earphone to the SLM microphone. The spectrum of the signal can be measured by routing the acoustic signal through a coupler, condenser microphone, and microphone conditioner/preamplifier or SLM. Finally, the output of the microphone conditioner/amplifier or SLM is routed to a spectrum analyzer with storage capabilities or to an analog-to-digital converter to a computer that is programmed to do a Fourier analysis of the signal. In each case, a display of the spectrum of each signal type can be obtained. For completeness, also obtain the spectrum directly from the AEP unit (bypassing the transducer), so that if a change occurs, one can determine whether the AEP unit or the transducer has changed. Spectral analysis of acoustic transients is discussed in more detail in Chapter 11.

The third dimension, time, can be checked directly from the AEP unit by feeding the signal into a digital oscilloscope or through an analog-to-digital converter into the computer. One should determine the duration of the individual signal (i.e., click, tone burst) and the interval between stimuli. Next, determine the accuracy of the signal analysis system of the AEP unit itself by introducing a fixed signal with a specified temporal/amplitude pattern. Eventually, we will probably be able to simulate a "typical" ABR response pattern with known time-voltage relationships in order to see whether the unit correctly assesses (in time) where each simulated peak occurs. Unfortunately no standard ANSI or IEC AEP waves exist yet, but clinicians can construct them for their own equipment to thus serve as a standard lab (or clinic) reference.

Eventually, other parameters of the AEP stimulus and the response measurement will, no doubt, be specified and a standard developed. Until that time, the provided suggestions should at least allow one to determine the consistency of the AEP equipment and perhaps facilitate exchange of data among clinicians and researchers. Certainly one should not be so overwhelmed by the complexity of the equipment that one fails to make any attempt to check it.

OTOACOUSTIC EMISSION DEVICES

As reported earlier with AEP units, there are currently no ANSI standards for otoacoustic emission (OAE) devices. However, there is a working group that is developing such a standard. Until such time as a standard does exist, the clinician should carefully measure the output of the signal in terms of its amplitude and spectral characteristics. If one is using a click, some of the procedures described in the IEC standard might be applicable. If one is using distortion product otoacoustic emissions (DPOAEs), one should at least check to see that the primary signals are those indicated by the machine. One may use an electronic frequency counter or spectrum analyzer to make sure that each primary tone signal is near the nominal frequency. In as much as the DPOAE response is an intermodulation distortion product (typically the cubic difference tone), it is critical to measure the amplitude of the distortion at this frequency in a hardwalled cavity in order to know when measured distortion in fact represents distortion in the instrumentation itself. The reader is referred to Chapter 21 for more details concerning OAEs.

ACOUSTIC IMMITTANCE DEVICES

The standard for acoustic immittance (impedance/admittance) devices is ANSI S3.39-1987 (ANSI, 1987b). Note that there is also an IEC standard, IEC 60645-5, for measurement of aural acoustic impedance/admittance (IEC, 2004). ANSI S3.39-1987 describes four types of units for measuring acoustic immittance (listed simply as Types 1, 2, 3, and 4). The specific minimum mandatory requirements are given for Types 1, 2, and 3. There are no minimum requirements for the Type 4 device. Types 1, 2, and 3 must have at least a 226-Hz probe signal, a pneumatic system (manual or automatic), a way of measuring static acoustic immittance, tympanometry, and the acoustic reflex. Thus, to check the acoustic immittance device, one may begin by using a frequency counter to determine the frequency of the probe signal(s). The frequency should be accurate within 3% of the nominal value. The total harmonic distortion shall not exceed 5% of the fundamental frequency level when measured in an HA-1–type coupler (this is commonly called a 2-cc coupler). The probe signal shall not exceed 90 dB SPL as measured in that coupler. This is to try and minimize the possibility that the probe signal will elicit an acoustic reflex. The range of acoustic admittance and acoustic impedance values that should be measurable varies by instrument type. The accuracy of the acoustic immittance measurements should be within 5% of the indicated value or $\pm 10^{-9}$ cm^3/Pa (0.1 acoustic mmhos), whichever is greater. The accuracy of the acoustic immittance measurement can be determined by connecting the probe to the test cavities and checking the accuracy of the output at specified temperatures and ambient barometric pressures. A procedure for checking the temporal characteristics of the acoustic immittance instrument is described by Popelka and Dubno (1978) and by Lilly (1984).

Air pressure may be measured by connecting the probe to a manometer or "U" tube and then determining the water displacement as the immittance device air pressure dial is rotated. If the SI unit of decapascals (daPa) is used, then an appropriate measuring device must also be used. The air pressure should not differ from that stated on the device (i.e., 200 daPa) by more than ± 10 daPa or $\pm 15\%$ of the reading, whichever is greater. The standard states that the air pressure should be measured in cavities with volumes of 0.5 to 2 cm^3.

Finally, one should check the reflex-activating system. In checking the activation of a contralateral or ipsilateral reflex, normally an insert receiver will be used that may be measured on a standard HA-1 coupler. The frequency of the activator can be measured electrically directly from the acoustic immittance device. In this case, one uses a frequency counter as described earlier for checking the frequency of puretones in audiometers. Frequency should be $\pm 3\%$ of the stated value, and harmonic distortion should be less than 3% at specified frequencies for earphones and 5% or less for the probe tube transducer or insert receiver. Noise bands should also be checked if they are to be used as activating stimuli. Broadband noises should be uniform within ± 5 dB for the range between 250 and 6,000 Hz for supra-aural earphones. This can be checked by sending the output through the transducer connected to a coupler, a microphone, and a graphic level recorder or spectrum analyzer. The SPL of tonal activators should be within ± 3 dB of the stated value for frequencies from 250 to 4,000 Hz and within ± 5 dB for frequencies of 6,000 to 8,000 Hz and for noise. The rise and fall times should be the same as those described for audiometers and may be measured in the same way. One should have daily listening checks as well as periodic tests of one or two persons with known acoustic immittance to check tympanograms and acoustic reflex thresholds to catch any gross problems.

In summary, acoustic immittance devices should be checked as carefully as one's puretone audiometer. Failure to do so can lead to variability in measurement, which may invalidate the immittance measurement. The reader is referred to Chapters 8, 9, and 10 for more details concerning acoustic immittance measures.

TEST ROOM STANDARDS

It is insufficient to limit the periodic calibration checks to the audiometric equipment. The environment in which the test is to be carried out must also be evaluated. ANSI S3.1-1999 (ANSI, 1999) provides criteria for permissible ambient noise during audiometric testing. ISO 6189-1983 (ISO, 1984) also specifies appropriate ambient noise levels. The ambient level in the test room is checked by using an SLM that is sensitive enough to allow testing to levels as low as 8 dB SPL. Many modern SLMs can measure to levels of 5 dB SPL or less. However, if the SLM is not that sensitive, an additive procedure of combining dB allows one to check how much sound is added in the ambient noise condition. For example, if the noise floor of the SLM is 7 dB SPL and we read 10 dB SPL in the sound booth, we can estimate that the actual level in the sound room is 7 dB SPL because when two uncorrelated (independent) sounds are presented together, their total output is 3 dB more than each individual sound. In this example, the noise floor of the SLM is 7 dB SPL, the room noise is 7 dB SPL, and they sum to 10 dB SPL. One should place the SLM (preferably using a free-field microphone) in the place where the subject is to be seated. The doors of the test room should be closed when making the measurements. If one plans to use monitored live voice testing, the ambient levels in the examiner's room should also be checked. However, there are no standards concerning acceptable noise levels in the examiner's room. ANSI S3.1-1999 provides acceptable ambient noise values for threshold estimation at 0 dB HL, for one- and third-octave bandwidths, for use with supra-aural and insert earphones, and for free-field (or bone conduction) testing. These values vary with the range of audiometric frequencies investigated (due to downward spread of masking). If the level prescribed by ANSI S3.1-1999 is exceeded, then the minimum dB HL value that can be recorded is increased from 0 dB HL. This is (more or less) a linear function, so if the accepted ambient noise level in a given band is exceeded by 5 dB, then the minimum dB HL value that you can measure is increased to 5 dB HL.

CONCLUSIONS

This chapter has emphasized that the first responsibility of the audiologist is to listen to the output of the equipment.

There are many problems that can be detected by a trained human ear. However, the listener is simply not good enough to check the auditory equipment with the precision that is needed to ensure that it is working properly. Thus, it has been stressed that, to determine the precise characteristics of the equipment, routine electronic checks must be carried out. Even when there are no current standards (as is the case for AEPs and OAEs), one should at least check the stability of one's equipment. Because the test results that one obtains are no more accurate than the equipment on which they are performed, both clinical and calibration equipment must be chosen and maintained with care. The ultimate responsibility for the accuracy of the test results lies with the audiologist. Therefore, the audiologist must make sure that the equipment is working properly by carrying out routine calibration checks. And perhaps, like daily exercise, one might even learn to enjoy this procedure.

REFERENCES

American Medical Association. (1951) Specifications of the Council of Physical Medicine and Rehabilitation of the American Medical Association. *J Am Med Assoc.* 146, 255–257.

American National Standards Institute. (2004) About ANSI overview. Accessed December 26, 2004. Available at: http://ansi.org/about_ansi/overview/overview.aspx?menuid=1.

American National Standards Institute. (1999) Maximum Permissible Ambient Noise for Audiometric Test Rooms. ANSI S3.1-1999 (R2003). New York: American National Standards Institute, Inc.

American National Standards Institute. (1987a) Mechanical Coupler for Measurement of Bone Vibrators. ANSI S3.13-1987. New York: American National Standards Institute, Inc.

American National Standards Institute. (1987b) Specifications for Instruments to Measure Aural Acoustic Impedance and Admittance (Aural Acoustic Immittance). ANSI S3.39-1987 (R2002). New York: American National Standards Institute, Inc.

American National Standards Institute. (1995) Method for Coupler Calibration of Earphones. ANSI S3.7-1995 (R2003). New York: American National Standards Institute, Inc.

American National Standards Institute. (1989) Occluded Ear Simulator. ANSI S3.25-1989 (R2003). New York: American National Standards Institute, Inc.

American National Standards Institute. (2004) Specifications for Audiometers. ANSI S3.6-2004. New York: American National Standards Institute, Inc.

American National Standards Institute. (1983) Specifications for Sound Level Meters. ANSI S1.4-1983 (R1997). New York: American National Standards Institute, Inc.

American Speech-Language-Hearing Association. (1991) *Sound Field Measurement Tutorial.* Rockville, MD: American Speech-Language-Hearing Association.

Benson R, Charan K, Day J, Harris J, Niemoller J, Rudmose W, Shaw E, Weissler P. (1967) Limitations on the use of circumaural earphones. *J Acoust Soc Am.* 41, 713–714.

Beranek LL. (1988) *Acoustical Measurements.* New York: American Institute of Physics.

Burkhard MD. (1978) *Manikin Measurements–Conference Proceedings.* Elk Grove Village, IL: Industrial Research Products.

Burkhard MD, Corliss ELR. (1954) The response of earphones in ears and couplers. *J Acoust Soc Am.* 26, 679–685.

Burkhard MD, Sachs RM. (1975) Anthropometric manikin for acoustic research. *J Acoustic Soc Am.* 58, 214–222.

Corliss ELR, Burkhard MD. (1953) A probe tube method for the transfer of threshold standard between audiometer earphones. *J Acoust Soc Am.* 25, 990–993.

Cox R. (1986) NBS-9A coupler-to-eardrum transformation: TDH-39 and TDH-49 earphones. *J Acoust Soc Am.* 79, 120–123.

Curtis J, Schultz M. (1986) *Basic Laboratory Instrumentation for Speech and Hearing.* Toronto: Little, Brown and Co.

Decker TN, Carrell TD. (2004) *Instrumentation: An Introduction for Students in the Speech and Hearing Sciences.* Mahwah, NJ: Lawrence Erlbaum Associates.

Harris C. (1998) *Handbook of Acoustical Measurements and Noise Control.* 3rd ed. Woodbury, NY: Acoustical Society of America.

Hawkins DB, Cooper WA, Thompson DJ. (1990) Comparisons among SPLs in real ears, 2 cm³ and 6 cm³ couplers. *J Am Acad Audiol.* 1, 154–161.

Hawley MS. (1939) An artificial mastoid for audiophone measurements. *Bell Lab Rec.* 18, 73–75.

International Electrotechnical Commission. (2001) Audiologic Equipment: Part 1—Pure-Tone Audiometers. IEC 60645-1 2001. Geneva: International Electrotechnical Commission.

International Electrotechnical Commission. (1993) Audiometers: Part 2—Equipment for Speech Audiometry. IEC 60645-2 1993. Geneva: International Electrotechnical Commission.

International Electrotechnical Commission. (1994a) Audiometers: Part 3—Auditory Test Signals of Short Duration for Audiometric and Neuro-Otologic Purposes. IEC 60645-3 1994. Geneva: International Electrotechnical Commission.

International Electrotechnical Commission. (1994b) Audiometers: Part 4—Equipment for Extended High-Frequency Audiometry. IEC-60645-4 1994. Geneva: International Electrotechnical Commission.

International Electrotechnical Commission. (2004) Electroacoustics: Audiometric Equipment: Part 5—Instruments for the Measurement of Aural Acoustic Impedance/Admittance. IEC 60645-5 2004. Geneva: International Electrotechnical Commission.

International Electrotechnical Commission. (1998) Electroacoustics: Part 1—Ear Simulator for the Calibration of Supra-Aural Earphones. IEC 60318 1998. Geneva: International Electrotechnical Commission.

International Electrotechnical Commission. (1990) Mechanical Coupler for Measurements of Bone Vibrators. IEC 60373 1990. Geneva: International Electrotechnical Commission.

International Electrotechnical Commission. (1981) Occluded Ear-Simulator for the Measurement of Earphones Coupled to the Ear by Ear Inserts. IEC 60711 1981. Geneva: International Electrotechnical Commission.

International Standards Organization. (1984) Acoustics: Pure Tone Air-Conduction Threshold Audiometry for Hearing Conservation Purposes. ISO/DIS 6189.2-1983. Geneva: International Standards Organization.

International Standards Organization. (1998) Acoustics: Reference Zero for the Calibration of Audiometric Equipment. Part 1: Reference Equivalent Threshold Sound Pressure Levels for Pure Tones and Supra-Aural Earphones. ISO 389-1 1998. Geneva: International Standards Organization.

International Standards Organization. (1994a) Acoustics: Reference Zero for the Calibration of Audiometric Equipment. Part 2: Reference Equivalent Threshold Sound Pressure Levels for Pure Tones and Insert Earphones. ISO 389-2 1994. Geneva: International Standards Organization.

International Standards Organization. (1994b) Acoustics: Reference Zero for the Calibration of Audiometric Equipment. Part 3: Reference Equivalent Threshold Force Levels for Pure Tones and Bone Vibrators. ISO 389-3 1994. Geneva: International Standards Organization.

International Standards Organization. (1994c) Acoustics: Reference Zero for the Calibration of Audiometric Equipment. Part 4: Reference Equivalent Levels for Narrow-Band Masking Noise. ISO 389-4 1994. Geneva: International Standards Organization.

International Standards Organization. (1998) Acoustics: Reference Zero for the Calibration of Audiometric Equipment. Part 5: Reference Equivalent Threshold Sound Pressure Levels for Pure Tones in the Frequency Range 8 kHz to 16 kHz. ISO 389-5 1998. Geneva: International Standards Organization.

International Standards Organization. (1981) Acoustics: Reference Zero for the Calibration of Audiometric Equipment. Part 7: Reference Threshold of Hearing Under Free-Field and Diffuse-Field Listening Conditions. ISO 389-7 1981. Geneva: International Standards Organization.

Johnson D, Marsh A, Harris C. (1998) Acoustic measurement instruments. In: Harris C, ed. *Handbook of Acoustical Measurements and Noise Control*. 3rd ed. Woodbury, NY: Acoustical Society of America; pp 5.1–5.21

Killion MD. (1978) Revised estimate of minimum audible pressure: where is the "missing 6 dB?" *J Acoust Soc Am*. 63, 1501.

Lilly DJ. (1984) Evaluation of the response time of acoustic-immittance instruments. In: Silman S, ed. *The Acoustic Reflex*. New York: Academic Press.

Melnick W. (1973) What is the American National Standards Institute? *ASHA*. 10, 418–421.

Occupational Safety and Health Administration. (1983) Occupational Noise Exposure, Hearing Conservation Amendment. Rule and Proposed Regulation. Federal Register, United States Government Printing Office, Washington, DC. Popelka GR, Dubno JR. (1978) Comments on the acoustic-reflex response for bone-conducted signals. *Acta Otolaryngol (Stockh)*. 86, 64–70.

Richards A. (1976) *Basic Instrumentation in Psychoacoustics*. Baltimore: University Park Press.

Roach R, Carhart R. (1956) A clinical method for calibrating the bone-conduction audiometer. *Arch Otolaryngol*. 63, 270–278.

Rosen S, Howell P. (1991) *Signals and Systems for Speech and Hearing*. London: Academic Press.

Rudmose W. (1964) Concerning the problem of calibrating TDH-39 earphones at 6kHz with a 9 A coupler. *J Acoust Soc Am*. 36, 1049.

Shaw EAG, Thiessen GJ. (1962) Acoustics of circumaural earphones. *J Acoust Soc Am*. 34, 1233–1246.

Silverman FH. (1999) *Fundamentals of Electronics for Speech-Language Pathologists and Audiologists*. New York: Allyn and Bacon.

Speaks C. (1996) *Introduction to Sound. Acoustics for the Hearing and Speech Sciences*. 2nd ed. San Diego: Singular Publishing.

Stein L, Zerlin S. (1963) Effect of circumaural earphones and earphone cushions on auditory threshold. *J Acoust Soc Am*. 35, 1744–1745.

Studebaker G. (1967) Intertest variability and the air-bone gap. *J Speech Hear Disord*. 32, 82–86.

Tillman TW, Gish KD. (1964) Comments on the effect of circumaural earphones on auditory threshold. *J Acoust Soc Am*. 36, 969–970.

Villchur E. (1970) Audiometer-earphone mounting to improve inter-subject and cushion-fit reliability. *J Acoust Soc Am*. 48, 1387–1396.

Weiss E. (1960) An air-damped artificial mastoid. *J Acoust Soc Am*. 32, 1582–1588.

Weissler P. (1968) International standard reference zero for audiometers. *J Acoust Soc Am*. 44, 264–275.

Wilber LA. (2004) *What Are Standards and Why do I care? Seminars in Hearing – Current Topics in Audiology: A Tribute to Tom Tillman*. Stuttgart, Germany: Thieme; pp 81–92.

Wilber LA, Goodhill V. (1967) Real ear versus "artificial mastoid" methods of calibration of bone-conduction vibrators. *J Speech Hear Res*. 10, 405–416.

Yeager D, Marsh A. (1998) Sound levels and their measurement. In: Harris C, ed. *Handbook of Acoustical Measurements and Noise Control*. 3rd ed. Woodbury, NY: Acoustical Society of America; pp 11.1–11.18.

Zwislocki JJ. (1970) An acoustic coupler for earphone calibration. Rep. LSC-S-7, Lab Sensory Commun. Syracuse, NY: Syracuse University.

Zwislocki JJ. (1971) An ear-like coupler for earphone calibration. Rep. LSC-S-9, Lab Sensory Commun. Syracuse, NY: Syracuse University.

Zwislocki JJ. (1980) An ear simulator for acoustic measurements. Rationale, principles, and limitations. In: Studebaker G, Hochberg I, eds. *Acoustical Factors Affecting Hearing Aid Performance.* Baltimore: University Park Press.

Zwislocki J, Kruger B, Miller JD, Niemoeller AF, Shaw EA, Studebaker G. (1988) Earphones in audiometry. *J Acoust Soc Am.* 83, 1688–1689.

Puretone Evaluation

Robert S. Schlauch and Peggy Nelson

INTRODUCTION

When most persons outside the profession of audiology think about hearing assessment, puretone audiometry is probably what comes to mind. After all, most people who attended primary school in the United States and in other industrialized nations have experienced puretone testing firsthand as a method to screen for hearing loss. Also, when audiology is depicted in films, such as Woody Allen's award-winning movie *Hannah and Her Sisters* or the more recent film *Wind Talkers*, puretone threshold testing is shown. These casual experiences with audiology may give lay people the false impression that audiology is a narrow profession and that puretone threshold assessment is always simple and straightforward.

The 43 chapters of this book are evidence that audiology is much more than puretone threshold testing, but most audiologists would likely agree that puretone thresholds represent a key component of the assessment battery. Proper administration and interpretation of puretone threshold tests require considerable knowledge. The goal of this chapter is to introduce readers to the complexity of puretone threshold testing as well as to provide clinicians with a reference for clinical applications.

WHAT ARE PURETONES, AND HOW ARE THEY SPECIFIED?

Puretone thresholds represent the lowest level that a person responds to a tonal stimulus some fixed percentage of time. Puretones are the simplest of sounds but unlikely to occur in nature. Puretones are described by their frequency, amplitude, phase, and duration. The most important of these characteristics for puretone audiometry are frequency and amplitude (or level).

Puretone frequency is perceived as pitch, the characteristic of sound that determines its position on a musical scale (Moore, 2003). Young persons with normal hearing are able to perceive frequencies between 20 Hz and 20,000 Hz. Human hearing is much more sensitive (better) in the range of frequencies between 500 Hz and 8,000 Hz than it is at either extreme of the audible range of frequencies. Conventional puretone audiometry typically assesses thresholds for frequencies between 250 (or 125) Hz and 8,000 Hz. The frequency range for conventional audiometry is very similar to the range of frequencies (100 Hz to 6,000 Hz) that is important for speech understanding (French and Steinberg, 1947).

Puretone amplitude or level is usually quantified in decibels. Decibels, abbreviated as dB, represent the logarithm of a ratio of two values; the term is meaningless without a reference. Two commonly used decibel scales are sound pressure level (SPL) and hearing level (HL). The reference level for dB SPL is 20 μPa, a pressure value. This reference value for SPL was selected to correspond to the faintest pressure that is audible in the frequency region where hearing is most sensitive. The frequency is not specified in the reference level for dB SPL; all sounds expressed in units of dB SPL share the same reference of 20 μPa. The SPL scale is frequently used in audiology to compare the level of speech or other sounds at different frequencies to a person's thresholds for those same frequencies. Such comparisons are critical for prescribing and evaluating hearing aids. HL, a second decibel scale, is used to plot an audiogram, the accepted clinical representation of puretone thresholds as a function of frequency. The reference for dB HL is the median threshold for a particular frequency for young adults with no history of ear problems. Unlike dB SPL, the zero reference level for dB HL varies with frequency because humans have more sensitive hearing at

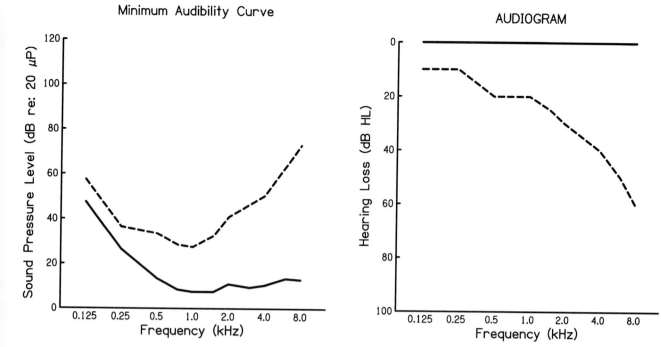

FIGURE 3.1 Thresholds in dB sound pressure level (SPL; left panel) and dB hearing level (HL; right panel) as a function of frequency. The solid line represents average normal hearing; the dashed line represents a person's threshold who has a high-frequency hearing loss.

some frequencies than others. Because the reference is normal human hearing, thresholds that deviate from 0 dB HL at each frequency show how much one's hearing deviates from this normal value.

Figure 3.1 illustrates thresholds displayed in dB SPL and dB HL. The left panel shows hearing thresholds plotted in dB SPL as a function of frequency. Thresholds plotted in this way constitute a minimum audibility curve. The right panel shows a conventional audiogram plotted in dB HL. Note that on the dB SPL scale, larger decibel values are plotted higher on the graph. By contrast, larger values in dB HL are plotted lower on the audiogram. To illustrate the relationship between dB SPL and dB HL, the reference values for 0 dB HL (average normal hearing) for a specific earphone are plotted in dB SPL as a solid line. Illustrated with a dashed line on these same two figures are the thresholds for a person with a high-frequency hearing loss. Note in the figure on the left that the separation between the solid line and the dashed line represent values for dB HL on the audiogram.

WHY PURETONE THRESHOLDS?

The reader might be wondering why audiologists test hearing using puretones at specific frequencies when the most meaningful stimulus is speech. Two important reasons are that puretone thresholds provide information about the type of hearing loss as well as quantify frequency-specific

threshold elevations that result from damage to the auditory system.

Puretone thresholds provide quantification of amount of loss due to problems with the outer and middle ear (the conductive system) separately from the cochlea and the auditory nerve (the sensory-neural system). This division helps in diagnosis and guides audiologists and physicians with important details for the design and implementation of treatment strategies.

Damage to the auditory system often results in a loss of sensitivity that is frequency specific. For instance, changes in the stiffness and mass properties of the middle ear affect the relative amount of loss in the low and high frequencies (Johanson, 1948). For air-conduction thresholds, an increase in stiffness results in a greater low-frequency loss, whereas an increase in mass results in a greater loss in the high frequencies. Thresholds for puretones (or other narrowband sounds) also provide us with diagnostic information about the integrity of different channels in the sensory-neural pathway. The auditory system is organized tonotopically (i.e., a frequency-to-place mapping) from the cochlea to the cortex (Pickles, 1988). The tonotopic organization of the cochlea is a result of the frequency tuning of the basilar membrane. A gradual change in the stiffness properties of a healthy basilar membrane results in a continuous representation of frequency, with high frequencies represented at the basal end and low frequencies at the apical end (Pickles, 1988). Damage to sensory cells of the cochlea at a specific place along the basilar membrane can result in a loss of hearing that corresponds to the frequencies coded by that place. For this reason, puretone threshold tests provide details that would otherwise remain unknown if a broadband stimulus such as speech were used.

In addition to providing audiologists with critical diagnostic information about the amount and type of loss, puretone thresholds find applications for estimating the degree of handicap, as a baseline measure for hearing conservation programs, for monitoring changes in hearing following treatment or progression of a disease process, for screening for hearing loss, for determining candidacy for a hearing aid or a cochlear implant, and for selecting the frequency-gain characteristics of a hearing aid. Puretone thresholds also provide a reference level for presentation of supra-threshold speech testing and for the meaningful interpretation of other audiologic tests, such as evoked otoacoustic emissions and acoustic reflex thresholds.

TUNING FORK TESTS

Tuning forks provide a simple means to assess hearing. A struck tuning fork produces a sustained puretone that decays in level over time. Unlike an audiometer, tuning forks cannot present a calibrated signal level to a listener's ear. Despite this shortcoming, tuning fork tests provide qualitative information that can help determine whether a hearing loss is conductive or sensory-neural. Tuning fork tests are promoted by some as an important supplement to puretone audiometry. In a recently published book, otologists are advised to include tuning fork tests as an integral part of the physical examination for conductive hearing loss (Yoshikawa et al., 2005).

The two best known tuning fork tests are the Weber and Rinne. Judgments about the type of hearing loss are made by comparing the pattern of results on both tests. Air conduction (AC) is tested by holding the fork at the opening of the ear canal, and bone conduction (BC) is tested by placing the fork on the mastoid process (the bony area behind the pinna) or on the forehead or incisors (British Society of Audiology, 1987). For the Weber test, a client judges whether sound is perceived in one or both ears when the fork is placed on the forehead. For the Rinne test, the client judges whether sound is louder when presented by AC or by BC. From this, the tester can determine the type of loss. Ideally, conductive hearing losses produce a pattern of responses that is uniquely different from the one for sensory-neural hearing losses.

Some recommend tuning fork tests to check the validity of audiograms (Gabbard and Uhler, 2005) or to confirm the audiogram prior to conducting surgery on an ear (Sheehy et al., 1971). However, it is important to recognize that tuning fork tests administered to persons with known conductive losses have shown that these procedures are often ineffective (Snyder, 1989; Browning, 1987). Although only about 5% of persons with normal hearing or sensory-neural losses are falsely identified as having conductive losses with the Rinne test, this test misses many persons with significant conductive losses (Browning, 1987). In a group of children with otitis media, the Rinne tuning fork test failed to identify 50% of children with 20-dB to 35-dB air-bone gaps, the measure used to quantify middle ear problems. Other studies with adult clients revealed that the problem with the Rinne test is not due to the young age of the participants in the otitis media study. In adults with otosclerosis, the Rinne test identified correctly only 50% of persons with 20-dB air-bone gaps and 75% of persons with 30-dB air-bone gaps. The air-bone gap had to reach 40 dB before 90% of the conductive losses were identified correctly. The Weber test fares equally poorly. Studies report that a majority of children with conductive losses give inappropriate responses on the Weber test. From these studies, one must conclude that tuning fork tests are not a replacement or even a supplement to audiometry. Audiometry is capable of identifying nearly 100% of air-bone gaps as small as 15 dB.

PURETONE AUDIOMETRY

Audiometers are used to make quantitative measures of puretone AC and BC thresholds. AC thresholds assess the entire auditory pathway and are usually measured using earphones. When sound is delivered by an earphone, the hearing sensitivity can be assessed in each ear separately. BC thresholds are measured by placing a vibrator on the skull, and ears are assessed separately, usually by applying masking noise to the nontest ear. The goal of BC testing is to bypass the outer and middle ears and to stimulate the cochlea directly. A comparison of thresholds measured by AC and BC provides separate estimates of the status of the conductive and sensory-neural systems. If thresholds are elevated equally for sounds presented by AC and BC, then the outer and middle ear are not contributing to a hearing loss. By contrast, if thresholds are poorer by AC than by BC, then the source of at least some of the loss is the outer or middle ear. Figure 3.2 illustrates the AC and BC pathways and how hearing thresholds are affected by damage to these structures.

Equipment

AUDIOMETERS

Puretones are generated within an audiometer. Audiometers have the ability to select tonal frequency and intensity level. They also have the ability to route tones to the left or right earphone. All audiometers also have an interrupter switch that presents the stimulus to the examinee. The American National Standards Institute (ANSI) Specification for Audiometers (ANSI, 2004) describes four types of audiometers, with Type 1 having the most features and Type 4 having the fewest features. A Type 1 audiometer is a full-featured diagnostic audiometer. A Type 1 audiometer has earphones, bone vibrator, loud speakers, masking noise, and other features. A Type 4 audiometer is simply a screening device with

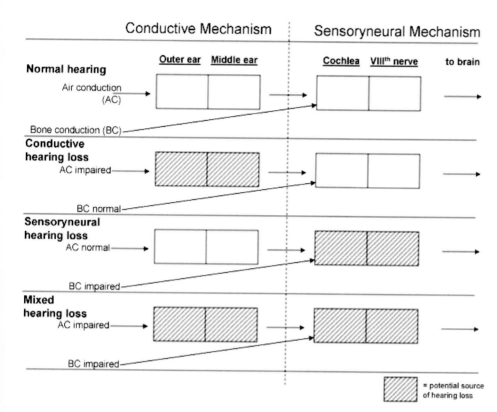

FIGURE 3.2 Conductive and sensorineural pathways. (Adapted from Martin [1994]).

earphones but none of the other special features. The Type 1 audiometer also is able to test a wider range of frequencies and levels than a Type 4 audiometer. The ANSI standard also describes the minimum requirements for audiometers that are able to test puretones in the high frequencies beyond the normal audiometric range.

Type 1 (full-featured, diagnostic audiometer) has the ability to assess puretone AC thresholds for frequencies ranging from 125 to 8,000 Hz and BC thresholds for frequencies ranging from 250 to 6,000 Hz. If an audiometer has extended high-frequency capability, frequencies between 8,000 Hz and 16,000 Hz will be present, but only for AC thresholds. Maximum output levels for AC testing are as high as 120 dB HL for frequencies where hearing thresholds are most sensitive. By contrast, distortion produced by bone oscillators at high intensities limit maximum output levels for BC thresholds to values nearly 50 dB lower than those for AC thresholds for the same frequency.

TRANSDUCERS

Earphones

Earphones are generally used to test puretone AC thresholds. A pair of supra-aural earphones is illustrated in Figure 3.3. For decades, supra-aural earphones, ones in which the cushion rests on the pinna, were the only choice for clinical audiology. The popularity of supra-aural phones was mainly due to their ease of calibration and the lack of other types of commercially available earphones. In the past few

years, insert earphones and circumaural earphones have become available and provide some useful applications for puretone assessment.

Insert earphones are coupled to the ear by placing a probe tip, typically a foam plug, into the ear canal. The commercially available model that has a standardized calibration method for audiology is the Etymotic model ER-3A, which is illustrated in Figure 3.4. These earphones have gained popularity in the past few years because they offer distinct advantages over supra-aural earphones. One major advantage is that insert earphones yield higher levels of interaural

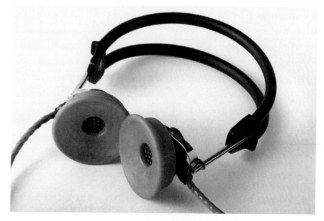

FIGURE 3.3 Telephonics model TDH-39, an example of supra-aural earphones.

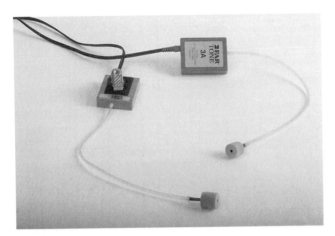

FIGURE 3.4 Etymotic model ER3A insert earphones.

attenuation than supra-aural earphones (Killion and Villchur, 1989). Interaural attenuation represents the decibel reduction of a sound as it crosses the head from the test ear to the nontest ear. The average increase in interaural attenuation is roughly 20 dB. This reduces the need for masking the nontest ear and decreases the number of masking dilemmas, situations for which thresholds cannot be assessed because the presentation level of the masking noise is possibly too high. Another important advantage of insert earphones over supra-aural earphones is lower test-retest variability for thresholds obtained at 6.0 kHz and 8.0 kHz; variability for other frequencies is comparable.[1] Given that thresholds for 6.0 kHz and 8.0 kHz are important for documenting changes in hearing due to noise exposure and for identifying acoustic tumors, lower variability should increase the diagnostic precision. A third advantage that insert earphones offer is elimination of collapsed ear canals (Killion and Villchur, 1989). In about 4% of clients, supra-aural earphones cause the ear canal to narrow or be closed off entirely when the cushion presses against the pinna (Lynne, 1969). This results in false hearing thresholds, usually in the high frequencies (Figure 3.5) (Ventry et al., 1961; Chandler, 1964). Because insert earphones keep the ear canal open, collapsed canals are eliminated. A fourth advantage of insert earphones is that they can be easily used with infants and toddlers who cannot or will not tolerate supra-aural earphones. Although insert earphones offer a hygienic advantage over supra-aural earphones because the foam tips that are placed into a client's ear canal are disposable, the replacement cost of those tips

---

[1] The data from which these conclusions are made regarding test-retest variability at 6,000 and 8,000 Hz are from separate studies—one assessed insert earphones, and the other assessed supra-aural earphones. Schumuziger et al.'s (2004) study of insert earphones had a large sample size and found no difference in test-retest variability for frequencies between 250 and 8,000 Hz. All studies of TDH-style supra-aural earphones, and there are several, show greater variability at 6,000 and 8,000 Hz than for lower frequencies. Although the sample size is large (138 participants) in Schumuziger et al.'s study of insert earphones, which gives one assurance that the result is valid, ideally both earphone types should be compared in a single study to draw more definitive conclusions.

is prohibitive for many applications. In addition to higher costs, insert earphones also yield errant thresholds in persons with eardrum perforations, including pressure-equalization tubes (Voss et al., 2000). (See Figure 3-14 for additional information about perforations.) Insert earphones also have maximum output levels that are lower than those produced by supra-aural earphones for some frequencies. Because of these differences, many diagnostic clinics keep both earphone types on hand and switch between them depending on the application.

Circumaural earphones, a third type, have cushions that encircle the pinna. ANSI S3.6 (2004) describes reference equivalent threshold SPL values (SPL values corresponding to 0 dB HL) for Sennheiser model HDA200 and Koss model HV/1A earphones. These earphones are the only ones in the current standard that have reference values covering the extended high frequencies (8.0 to 20 kHz).

Current standards for earphone calibration specify the level based on measures obtained with the earphone attached to an acoustic coupler or artificial ear. These couplers are designed to approximate the ear canal volume of an average person. Given that some clients have very small (e.g., infants) or very large ear canals (e.g., some postsurgical clients and persons with perforated eardrums), coupler measures may produce erroneous results, regardless of the earphone type (Voss et al., 2000; Voss and Herman, 2005). For these cases, measuring the SPL at the eardrum to specify the level presented to an individual patient would improve the accuracy of hearing thresholds. The probe-tube microphones necessary for these types of measures already exist, and hopefully, this technology will be incorporated into some future models of diagnostic audiometers.

Speakers

AC thresholds can be measured using speakers as the transducer. Thresholds so obtained are known as sound field thresholds. Sound field thresholds are unable to provide ear-specific sensitivity estimates. In cases of unilateral hearing losses, the listener's better ear determines threshold. This limitation and others dealing with control over stimulus level greatly limit clinical applications involving sound field thresholds. Applications for sound field thresholds are screening infant hearing or demonstrating to the parents their child's hearing ability. Sound field thresholds also may be desirable for a person wearing a hearing aid.

In sound field threshold measures, the orientation of the listener to the speaker has a large effect on stimulus level presented at the eardrum. A person's head and torso as well as the external ear (e.g., pinna, ear canal, concha, etc.) affect sound levels (Shaw, 1974). Differences in SPL at the eardrum are substantial for speaker locations at different distances and different angles relative to the listener. For this reason, sound field calibration takes into consideration these factors. A mark is usually made on the ceiling (or floor) of the room to indicate the location of the listener during testing. Even at the desired location, stimulus level at the eardrum

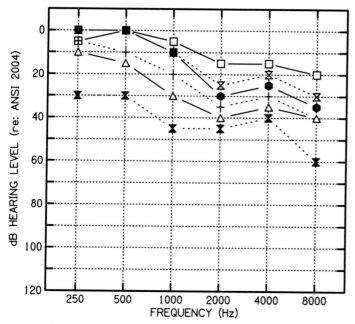

Occlusion	Symbol
80.5%	□
91.6%	✖
94.4%	●
98.3%	+
99.3%	△
100%	✕

FIGURE 3.5 Air conduction (AC) thresholds (in dB hearing level [HL]) for different percentages of ear canal occlusion. One hundred percent indicates that the ear canal is completely occluded. Deviations from 0 dB HL represent the loss due to occlusion. (Adapted from Chandler [1964]).

for some frequencies can vary as much as 20 dB or more by simply having the listener move his or her head (Shaw, 1974). Calibration assumes the listener will always be facing the same direction relative to the sound source (ANSI S3.6, 2004). Furniture and other persons in the sound field also affect the stimulus level at a listener's eardrum (Morgan et al., 1979). All of these factors add to the challenge of obtaining accurate sound field thresholds.

Another important consideration in sound field threshold measures is the stimulus type. Thresholds corresponding to different frequencies are desired for plotting an audiogram, but puretones can exhibit large differences in level at different positions in a testing suite as a result of standing waves. Standing waves occur when direct sound from the speaker interacts with reflections, resulting in regions of cancellation and summation. Differences in stimulus level due to standing waves are minimized by using narrowband noise or frequency-modulated (FM) tones as the stimulus (Morgan et al., 1979). FM tones, also known as warbled tones, are tones that vary in frequency over a range that is within a few percent of the nominal frequency. This variation occurs several times per second. Under earphones, thresholds obtained with these narrowband stimuli are nearly identical to thresholds obtained with puretones; with some exceptions.[2] FM tones and narrowband noise are the preferred stimuli for sound field threshold measures.

Bone Vibrators

A bone vibrator is a transducer that is designed to apply force to the skull when placed in contact with the head. Puretone

BC thresholds are measured with a bone vibrator like the one illustrated in Figure 3.6. A separation of 15 dB or more between masked AC and BC thresholds, with BC thresholds being better than AC thresholds, is often evidence of a conductive hearing loss. Other possible explanations for air-bone gaps and bone-air gaps, such as equipment miscalibration and test-retest variability.

Bone vibrators are typically placed behind the pinna on the mastoid process or on the forehead for threshold measurements. Although forehead placement produces slightly lower intrasubject and intersubject threshold differences (Dirks, 1994), placement on the mastoid process is preferred by 92% of audiologists (Martin et al., 1998). Mastoid placement is preferred mainly because it produces between 8- and 14-dB lower (better) thresholds than forehead placement for the same power applied to the vibrator, depending on the

---

[2] A steeply sloping hearing loss or large variations in threshold due to threshold microstructure (Long and Tubis, 1988) may produce different results with puretones and FM tones because the listener's threshold changes substantially with frequency.

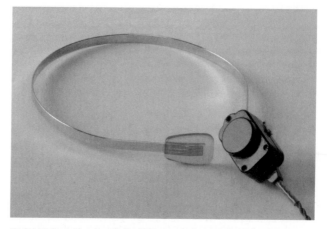

FIGURE 3.6 A clinical bone conduction vibrator (Radioear Model B-72).

frequency (ANSI S3.43, 1992). The median difference is 12 dB. Given that the maximum output limits for bone vibrators with mastoid placement are as much as 50 dB lower than that for AC thresholds, forehead placement would yield an even a larger difference. The inability to measure BC thresholds for higher levels means that a comparison of AC and BC thresholds is ambiguous in some cases. That is, when BC thresholds indicate no response at the limits of the equipment (e.g., 70 dB HL) and AC thresholds are poorer than the levels where no response was obtained (e.g., 100 dB HL), the audiologist cannot establish from these thresholds whether the loss is purely sensory-neural or whether it has a conductive component.

Test Environment

Hearing tests ideally are performed in specially constructed sound-treated chambers with very low background noise. A sound-treated room is not a soundproof room. High-level external sounds can penetrate the walls of a sound-treated room and may interfere with test results. Because test tones near threshold can be easily masked by extraneous, external noise, test chambers have strict guidelines for maximum permissible ambient noise levels. Low background noise levels are particularly important for BC testing, when the ears remain uncovered. When testing is done in a room that meets the ANSI guidelines, the audiogram reflects that by citing ANSI S3.1 (1999), the standard governing permissible ambient noise levels. Table 3.1 shows the minimum levels of ambient noise measured in octave bands encompassing the test frequency that enable valid hearing threshold measurements at 0 dB HL.

At times, audiologists must estimate hearing thresholds in rooms that do not meet the guidelines for minimal ambient noise. Some patients in hospital rooms or nursing homes must be tested at bedside. In those cases, test results should be clearly marked so that others know the conditions under which the test was done. When possible, these bedside tests

TABLE 3.1	Maximum Permissable Ambient Noise Levels for Puretone Threshold Testing	
Octave band center frequency (Hz)	Max dB SPL with ears covered	Max dB SPL with ears uncovered
125	39	35
250	25	21
500	21	16
1,000	26	13
2,000	34	14
4,000	37	11
8,000	37	14

Adapted from ANSI (1999). Octave band levels cannot exceed the tabled values to measure valid thresholds at 0 dB HL or lower.

should be performed using insert earphones, which provide a greater amount of attenuation in low frequencies where ambient noise is typically more of a problem. In these environments, BC testing, particularly in the low frequencies, may not be valid.

Measuring Puretone Thresholds

Psychophysics is the field of study that relates the physical world with perception (Gescheider, 1997). Puretone thresholds are an example of a psychophysical measure relating the physical characteristics of a tone to a behavioral threshold.

A psychophysical procedure describes the specific method used to obtain behavioral thresholds. The most common one used in puretone audiometry is a modified method of limits. In the method of limits, the tester has control over the stimulus. A threshold search begins with the presentation of a tone at a particular frequency and intensity that is often specified by the procedure. After each presentation of the tone (or a short sequence of pulsed tones), the tester judges whether or not the listener heard it based upon the listener's response or lack of response. Each response determines the subsequent decibel level presentation. If a tone on a given presentation is not heard, then the task is made easier by raising its level. If a tone is heard, the task is made harder by lowering the level. The rules of the psychophysical procedure govern the amount of the level change following each response as well as knowing when to stop the threshold search and for determining threshold. The procedure, which is described in detail in subsequent sections, may be modified based on the clinical population (e.g., the age of the listener).

COOPERATIVE LISTENERS AGE 5 YEARS TO ADULT (EARPHONES)

Guidelines for Manual Puretone Audiometry is a publication that describes a uniform method for measuring thresholds (American Speech-Language-Hearing Association [ASHA], 2005). The goal of the guideline is to standardize procedures across clinics that should minimize intertest differences. The committee that drafted this consensus document understood that its recommendations represent general guidelines and that clinical populations may require variations of the procedure.

Instructions

Puretone audiometry begins with instructing the individual being tested. The instructions are a critical part of the puretone test because thresholds measured using this clinical procedure are biased by the willingness of a person to respond. Some listeners wait for a tone to be distinct before they respond, which leads to higher thresholds than for someone who responds whenever they hear any sound that could be the tone. This bias is controlled in the instructions by informing listeners to respond any time they hear the tone no matter how faint it may be. A study by Marshall and Jesteadt (1986) shows that response bias controlled for in this manner plays only a small role (a few dB at most) in puretone thresholds obtained using the ASHA guideline. Marshall and Jesteadt (1986) also reported that the response bias of elderly listeners was not different than that of a group of younger persons. Before the study by Marshall and Jesteadt (1986), it was believed that elderly persons might adopt an extremely conservative response criterion, resulting in artificially elevated thresholds.

According to the ASHA guideline (ASHA, 2005), the instructions should also include the response task (e.g., raise your hand or finger or press a button), the need to respond when the tone begins and to stop responding when it ends, and that the two ears are tested separately. Although not in the ASHA guideline, instructions asking the examinee to indicate which ear the sound is heard in may be useful. This is especially important in cases of unilateral or asymmetrical hearing losses where cross-hearing is possible.

The examiner should present the instructions prior to placement of earphones. Earphones attenuate external sounds, which increases speech understanding problems in persons with hearing loss. Listeners should also be queried after the instructions are presented to determine if they understood what was said. Sample instructions are given below:

You are going to hear a series of tones that sound like whistles, first in one ear and then the other. I would like you to respond to the tones by raising your finger when one comes on and lowering it as soon as it goes off. Some of the tones will be very faint, so listen carefully and respond each time you hear one. Do you have any questions?

Earphone Placement

The earphones should be placed by the examiner. For convenience, earphones are color coded; red and blue correspond to the right and left ears, respectively. Prior to placement of earphones, clients are asked to remove jewelry such as earrings and glasses if they will interfere with the placement of the earphone. This is particularly relevant for supra-aural earphones.

For circumaural and supra-aural earphones, the diaphragm of the earphone should be centered over the ear canal. The examiner should view each ear while the phone is being placed (Flottorp, 1995). Immediately after placement, the headband is tightened enough to make the earphone perpendicular to the floor when the examinee is sitting upright.

The first step in placement of insert earphones is to attach a spring-loaded clip that holds the transducer in place to the examinee's clothing. The clip can be attached to clothing near the shoulder (or behind a child's neck) to keep the plug from being pulled out of the ear. The audiologist depresses the foam plug and inserts it into the ear canal so that its outer edge lines up with the tragus.

Placement of the Bone-Conduction Vibrator

Although some recommend forehead placement (Dirks, 1994), typically audiologists place the BC oscillator on the most prominent part of the mastoid process. While holding the oscillator against the mastoid process with one hand, the headband is fit over the head to hold the oscillator in place using the other hand. The oscillator surface should be set directly against the skin, not touching the pinna, and with no hair or as little hair as possible between the oscillator and the skin. Some audiologists play a continuous low-frequency tone while moving the oscillator slightly side to side, asking the listener to report the location at which the tone is the strongest.

Audiometric Procedure for Threshold Measurement

The ASHA Guideline (2005) recommends starting a threshold search from either well below threshold or using a suprathreshold tone that familiarizes the participant with the stimulus. Most clinicians prefer the familiarization method. For the familiarization approach, testing usually begins at 1000 Hz at 30 dB HL unless prior knowledge of the examinee's hearing suggests otherwise (ASHA, 2005). At 1,000 Hz, an examinee is more likely to have residual hearing than at a higher frequency, and test-retest reliability is excellent. Testing begins with an examinee's self-reported better ear. If the examinee believes both ears are identical, testing begins by convention with the right ear. The better ear is tested first to provide a reference to know whether masking needs to be delivered to obtain a valid estimate of threshold for the poorer ear.

Tonal duration is an important factor in a puretone test. On most audiometers, the option exists to select either pulsed or manual presentation. A 1- to 2-second duration tone is recommended for manual presentation (ASHA, 2005). The duration is determined by the amount of time the interrupter switch is held down. Pulsed tones are achieved by selecting this option on the audiometer's front panel. If pulsed tones are selected, then the audiometer alternately presents the tone followed by a short silent interval (typically 225 ms on followed by 225 ms off) for as long as the interrupter switch is depressed. The minimum duration for a single pulse of the tone is critical. Numerous psychoacoustic studies have shown that tonal durations between roughly 200 ms and 1 second or more yield nearly identical thresholds (Plomp and Bouman, 1959; Watson and Gengel, 1969). By contrast, the same studies show that durations less than 200 ms result in poorer thresholds. For this reason, audiometers are designed to have a nominal pulse duration of 225 ms (ANSI, 2004). Pulsed and manually presented tones presented from audiometers that maintain tonal durations between 200 ms and 2 seconds yield nearly identical thresholds, as the psychoacoustic studies suggest. However, pulsed tones are preferred for two reasons. Most patients prefer pulsed tones (Burk and Wiley, 2004), and pulsed tones also reduce the number of presentations required to find threshold in persons with cochlear hearing loss who have tinnitus (Mineau and Schlauch, 1997). Apparently, pulsed tones help patients to distinguish the puretone signal from the continuous or slowly fluctuating noises generated from within their auditory system (tinnitus), thereby reducing false-positive responses. False-positive responses can lengthen test time

(Mineau and Schlauch, 1997), which is costly to an audiology practice.

Thresholds are obtained using a modified Hughson-Westlake up-down procedure, which is a specific implementation of a method-of-limits procedure (Carhart and Jerger, 1959; Hughson and Westlake, 1944). The examiner begins the threshold-finding procedure by presenting a tone at 30 dB HL (ASHA, 2005). If the listener responds, the level of the tone is decreased in 10-dB steps until the listener no longer responds. If the listener does not respond to this initial 30-dB tone, the examiner raises the tone in 20-dB steps until a response is obtained. After every response to a tone, the level of the tone is decreased in 10-dB steps until there is no response. For subsequent presentations when there is no response, the examiner raises the level of the tone in 5-dB steps until a response is obtained. Following this "down-10/up-5" rule, the tester continues until the threshold is bracketed a few times, and a threshold estimate is obtained. ASHA (2005) recommends that threshold should correspond to the level at which responses were obtained for two ascending runs, which is what most clinicians based their thresholds on even when the ASHA (1978) Guideline recommended that thresholds be based on three ascending runs. Research based on computer simulations of clinical procedures (Marshall and Hanna, 1989) supports the clinician's position and that of the new ASHA (2005) Guideline. The computer simulations of thresholds based on three ascending showed only a minimal reduction of the variability when compared to thresholds based on two ascending runs. Listeners who produce inconsistent responses are an exception, and for these listeners, additional measurements can be made to confirm the threshold estimate.

After a threshold is measured at 1,000 Hz, the next frequencies that are examined depend on the goal, but the higher frequencies are typically tested prior to the lower frequencies. For diagnostic audiometry, thresholds are measured at octave intervals between 250 and 8000 Hz, along with 3000 Hz and 6000 Hz. Intra-octave thresholds between 500 Hz and 2000 Hz should be measured when thresholds differ by 20 dB or more between two adjacent octaves. ASHA also recommends that 1,000 Hz be tested twice as a reliability check. Consult the ASHA guidelines for specifics about the recommended protocol and Chapter 6 for details about the use of masking noise to eliminate the participation of the nontest ear. Masking noise is needed whenever the threshold difference between ears is equal to or exceeds the lowest possible values for interaural attenuation. For BC testing, masking is needed to verify results anytime an air-bone gap in the test ear of greater than 10 dB is observed. For AC testing, masking is needed when the difference between the AC threshold in the test ear and the BC threshold of the nontest ear is greater than or equal to 40 dB for supra-aural earphones, and considerably more for insert earphones, especially in the low frequencies (Killion and Villchur, 1989). Specific recommendations for insert earphones cannot be made until a study with a larger sample size is completed.

TESTING CHILDREN YOUNGER THAN AGE 5 YEARS AND PERSONS WITH SPECIAL NEEDS

For most children younger than age 5 years, audiologists have special procedures that they employ to measure puretone thresholds. Some of these same procedures are also appropriate for persons older than 5 who have cognitive deficits. Chapter 23 on pediatric hearing assessment describes these procedures and their interpretation.

Audiometric Interpretation

Puretone thresholds are sometimes displayed in tabular format, but they are usually plotted on an audiogram. ASHA (1990), in a publication entitled *Guidelines for Audiometric Symbols*, suggests a standardized form for the audiogram. Although other formats for plotting audiograms are acceptable, it is helpful to use a standardized format for ease of interpretation across clinics. The audiogram recommended in the ASHA guidelines (1990) is shown in Figure 3.7 along with recommended symbols in Figure 3.8. This audiogram only covers the conventional frequencies. Thresholds for extended high frequencies are usually plotted in units of dB SPL because frequency-specific reference equivalent threshold SPLs corresponding to 0 dB HL were just recently published for two commercially available earphones (ANSI, 2004). Additionally, average extended high-frequency thresholds vary over a wide range with the age of the listener, making SPL a better reference than dB HL for comparing thresholds to norms for listeners of different ages.

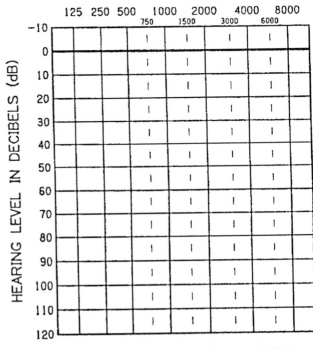

FIGURE 3.7 Recommended audiogram (ASHA, 1990).

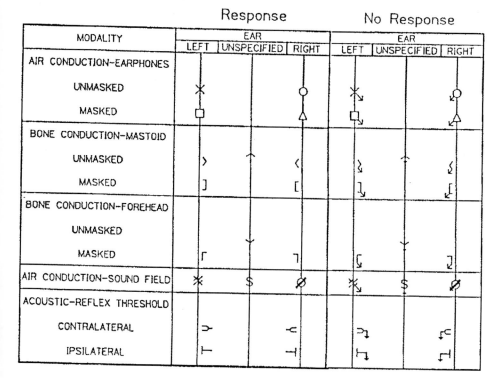

FIGURE 3.8 Audiometric symbols recommended by ASHA (1990).

Audiograms are often classified by categories based on the degree of hearing loss. A number of authors have published schema for the classification of hearing loss based on the average AC thresholds for three frequencies. The frequencies used for this purpose are usually 500, 1,000, and 2,000 Hz, often referred to as the three frequency puretone average. Table 3.2 shows the categories for the degree of loss based on this puretone average for three different authors (Goodman [1965], Northern and Downs [2002], and Jerger and Jerger [1980]). The first category is normal hearing. Note that none of the three authors agree on the upper limit for normal, which ranges from 15 to 25 dB HL. Northern and Downs (2002) suggest using 15 dB HL as the upper limit for normal hearing for children between 2 and 18 years of age and a higher limit for adults. Regardless of the value used

as an upper limit for normal hearing, bear in mind that an ear-related medical problem can still exist even though all thresholds fall within the defined normal range. For example, the presence of a significant air-bone gap might indicate the presence middle ear pathology even though all AC thresholds fall within normal limits.

The original intent of classification schema for severity of loss based on a three-frequency puretone average was to express, in a general way, the degree of handicap associated with the magnitude of the loss. These categories are only somewhat successful at achieving this goal because (1) handicap is dependent on many factors related to an individual's needs and abilities, (2) only some of the speech frequencies are assessed using this three-frequency average (speech frequencies range from 125 to 6,000 Hz), and

TABLE 3.2 Classification of degree of hearing loss calculated from the average of thresholds for 500, 1,000, and 2,000 Hz[a]

Degree of Loss	Northern and Downs (2002)	Goodman (1965)	Jerger and Jerger (1980)
None	<16	<26	<21
Slight	16–25		
Mild	26–30	26–40	21–40
Moderate	30–50	41–55	41–60
Moderately severe		56–70	
Severe	51–70	71–90	61–80
Profound	>70	>90	>80

[a] Although all three references cited differ in the value accepted as a profound loss, a loss of 90 dB HL or more is widely accepted as representing a qualitative as well as a quantitative boundary between hearing and deafness.

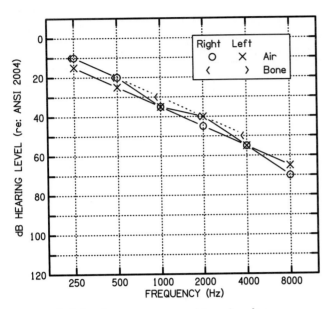

FIGURE 3.9   A sensory-neural hearing loss.

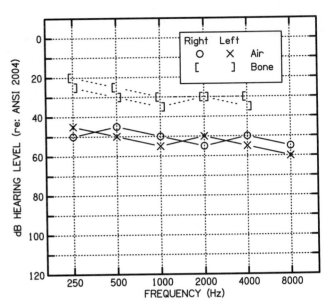

FIGURE 3.11   A mixed hearing loss.

(3) identical amounts of hearing loss sometimes result in large differences in the ability to understand speech and, as a consequence, the degree of disability associated with the loss. Despite these limitations, many audiologists use these categories routinely to summarize the amount of loss in different frequency regions of an audiogram when describing results to other professionals or to a client during counseling.

Another method of classifying audiograms is by the type of hearing loss. The type of hearing loss is determined by comparing the amount of hearing loss for air and BC thresholds at the same frequency. A sensory-neural hearing loss has an equal amount of loss for AC and BC thresholds (Fig. 3.9).

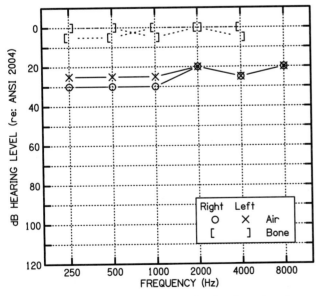

FIGURE 3.10   A bilateral conductive hearing loss. The plotted values represent the average loss reported by Fria et al. (1985) in a group of children with otitis media.

By contrast, a conductive loss has better BC thresholds than AC thresholds (Fig. 3.10). The amount of a conductive loss is described by the decibel difference between air and BC thresholds. This difference is known as the air-bone gap, a value that has a maximum of about 65 dB[3] (Rosowski and Relkin, 2001). Due to test-retest differences, an air-bone gap needs to exceed 10 dB before it is considered significant. A mixed hearing loss shows a conductive component and a sensory-neural component. In other words, a mixed loss has an air-bone gap, and the thresholds for BC fall outside the range of normal hearing (Fig. 3-11).

Still another way that audiograms are classified is by the hearing loss configuration. The configuration takes into account the shape of the hearing loss. A description of the configuration of the loss helps in summarizing the loss to patients and to other professionals and often provides insight into the etiology or cause of the loss. Some typical shapes and the criteria used to describe them are shown in Table 3.3.

An audiogram is summarized verbally by the degree, type, and configuration of the hearing loss for both ears. If a person has normal thresholds in one ear and a hearing loss in the other ear, this is known as a unilateral hearing loss. A loss in both ears is described as a bilateral hearing loss. Bilateral losses are described as symmetric (nearly equal thresholds in both ears) or asymmetric.

Some Limitations of Puretone Testing

TEST-RETEST RELIABILITY

Puretone thresholds are not entirely precise. Consider a cooperative adult whose AC thresholds are measured twice at

---

[3] Physiologic models suggest that the maximum air-bone gap occurs when there is an intact tympanic membrane and a disarticulated ossicular chain (Rosowski and Relkin, 2001).

TABLE 3.3	Criteria for classifying audiometric configurations
Term	**Description**
Flat	<5-dB rise or fall per octave
Gradually falling	5- to 12-dB increase per octave
Sharply falling	15- to 20-dB increase per octave
Precipitously falling	Flat or gradually sloping, then threshold increasing at 25 dB or more per octave
Rising	>5-dB decrease in threshold per octave
Peaked or saucer	20-dB or greater loss at the extreme frequencies, but not at the mid frequencies
Trough	20-dB or greater loss in the mid frequencies (1,000–2,000 Hz), but not at the extreme frequencies (500 or 4,000 Hz)
Notched	20-dB or greater loss at one frequency with complete or near-complete recovery at adjacent octave frequencies

Modified from Carhart (1945) and Lloyd and Kaplan (1978).

octave intervals between 250 and 8,000 Hz. For these two measures, assume too that the earphones are removed and replaced between tests. For this situation, the probability of obtaining identical thresholds at each frequency is small. This is due to test-retest variability. Test-retest variability is also responsible for BC thresholds not always lining up with AC thresholds in persons with pure sensory-neural losses. As reported by Studebaker (1967), test-retest variability causes false air-bone gaps and false bone-air gaps (BC thresholds poorer than AC thresholds). The source of this variability is a combination of variations in the person's decision process, physiologic or bodily noise, a shift in the response criterion, and differences in transducer placement. It is assumed that the equipment is calibrated correctly for successive tests.

The inherent variability of puretone thresholds poses a problem for audiologists who are faced with making clinical decisions based on these responses. Audiologists frequently need to assess whether hearing has changed significantly since the last test, whether hearing is significantly better in one ear than the other, and whether an air-bone gap is significant.

A good place to begin with understanding test-retest variability is to consider the standard deviation (SD) of test-retest differences at a single frequency. Following Studebaker (1967), let's assume that test-retest differences are normally distributed with an SD of 5 dB. Assume, too, that the mean test-retest difference (or mean air-bone gap in sensory-neural losses) is 0 dB. From these assumptions, Studebaker

calculated the percentage of expected thresholds falling into discrete intervals corresponding to the 5-dB steps used to measure thresholds. Accordingly, nearly 87% of thresholds on retest are within ± 5 dB of the first one (or air and bone will agree within 5 dB 87% of the time). By contrast, 10-dB differences occur roughly 12% of the time, and still larger differences should be rare. These calculations for the proportion of thresholds differing on retest by a given amount are based on measurements for a single frequency. When complete audiograms are assessed, the likelihood of obtaining a large threshold difference on retest increases. For example, 15-dB or greater differences on retest are expected only 1.24% of the time when the threshold for a single frequency is assessed. When thresholds for six frequencies are assessed in each ear (octave intervals between 0.25 and 8.0 kHz), 14% of the persons tested would be expected to have at least one threshold differing by 15 dB or more (Schlauch and Carney, 2007). Thus, differences of 15 dB or more in these applications would be much more commonplace than those predicted by the SD of intertest differences for a single frequency.

Several methods have been proposed to assess the significance of threshold differences for complete audiograms (Schlauch and Carney, 2007). These methods usually require that thresholds for more than one frequency contribute to the decision process, although some accept a large change for a single frequency, such as 20 dB or more, as a significant difference. One of these methods defines a significant threshold shift by a minimal change in a puretone average. For instance, the Occupational Safety and Health Administration (1983) defines a notable threshold shift (in their terminology, a Standard Threshold Shift) as a 10-dB or greater change in the puretone average based on thresholds for 2.0, 3.0, and 4.0 kHz in either ear. These frequencies were selected because they are ones susceptible to damage by occupational noise. A second commonly used approach requires threshold differences to occur at adjacent frequencies. One rule that is applicable to many situations defines a significant threshold shift as one for which two adjacent thresholds differ by 10 dB or more on retest. This criterion has been applied widely in audiometric studies (e.g., Mori et al., 1985) and is sometimes combined with other criteria to arrive at a decision (ASHA, 1994). A third approach recommends repeating threshold measurements during a single session to improve audiometric reliability (e.g., National Institute for Occupational Safety and Health, 1998). This method is paired with a rule or rules defining the criterion for a significant threshold shift. The notable difference between this method and the others described earlier is that the criterion defining a threshold shift must be repeatable to be accepted as significant.

The examples in this section on the variability of puretone thresholds have assumed a fixed SD of test-retest differences of ± 5 dB for all audiometric frequencies. Although 5 dB is a reasonable average value for many situations, studies show that the SD varies with the time between tests and even with audiometric frequency. For insert earphones and short intertest intervals of a few weeks or less, SDs are roughly 3 dB for audiometric frequencies between 500 and 8,000 Hz (Schmuziger et al., 2004). For supra-aural earphones, short intertest intervals result in SDs of about 3 dB up to 4 kHz and 5 dB or more for 6 kHz and 8 kHz (Jervall and Arlinger, 1986). Intertest intervals of 3 months produce SDs of 4 to 5 dB up to 4.0 kHz and nearly 8 dB for 6.0 kHz. An intertest interval of 3 years produces SDs of 5 to 6 dB and 9 dB for frequencies up to 4.0 kHz and 6.0 kHz, respectively (Burns and Hinchcliff, 1957; Burns et al., 1964). For large time intervals between tests, it is possible that the larger SDs reflect, in part, changes in the hearing sensitivity of the persons being tested and not simply the routine factors contributing to test-retest variability.

VIBROTACTILE THRESHOLDS

In persons with significant hearing losses, sound vibrations produced by earphones and bone vibrators may be perceived through the sense of touch. Such thresholds are known as vibrotactile thresholds.

Figure 3.12 illustrates the range of levels found to yield vibrotactile thresholds for a supra-aural earphone and a bone vibrator. A threshold occurring within the range of possible vibrotactile thresholds is ambiguous; it could be a hearing threshold or a vibrotactile threshold. Because relatively low vibrotactile thresholds are observed for BC at 250 and 500 Hz, a false air-bone gap is likely to occur in persons with significant sensory-neural losses at these frequencies. Boothroyd and Calkwell (1970) recommend asking the client if they

"feel" the stimulus or "hear" the stimulus as a means to differentiate between these two outcomes. Persons with experience with auditory sensations can usually make this distinction.

The values for vibrotactile thresholds illustrated in Figure 3.12 are based on only nine listeners. A more detailed study needs to be conducted to specify these ranges more precisely for the transducers in current use.

BONE-CONDUCTION THRESHOLDS: NOT A PURE ESTIMATE OF SENSORY-NEURAL RESERVE

The goal of BC testing is to obtain an estimate of sensory-neural reserve, but BC thresholds sometimes are influenced by the properties of the external and middle ears. The BC vibrator sets the skull into vibration, which stimulates the cochlea, but this does not happen in isolation. When the skull is vibrated, the middle ear ossicles are also set into motion, and this inertial response of the ossicular chain contributes to BC thresholds. Changes in the external and middle ear can modify the contribution of the inertial response, which may result in significant changes in BC thresholds (Dirks, 1994).

A classic example of a middle ear problem that influences BC thresholds is otosclerosis. Otosclerosis frequently causes the footplate of the stapes to become ankylosed or fixed in the oval window. This disease process and some other types of conductive losses (e.g., glue ear) (Kumar et al., 2003) reduce the normal inertial response of the ossicles to BC hearing. The result is poorer thresholds that form a depressed region of BC hearing known as Carhart's notch (Carhart, 1950). This notch, which typically shows poorer BC thresholds between 500 and 4,000 Hz with a maximum usually at 2,000 Hz of 15 dB, disappears following successful middle ear surgery. The finding that BC thresholds improve following middle ear surgery is strong evidence that these poorer BC thresholds observed in stapes immobilization are due to a middle ear phenomenon rather than a change in the integrity of the cochlea.

A frequently observed example of middle ear problems affecting BC thresholds occurs in persons with otitis media with effusion. In this group, falsely enhanced BC thresholds in the low frequencies (1,000 Hz and below) are seen often. The magnitude of the enhancement can be as much as 25 dB (Snyder, 1989). Upon resolution of the middle ear problem, these previously enhanced BC thresholds become poorer and return to their premorbid values.

Similarly, enhancement in BC thresholds occurs for low frequencies with occlusion of the external ear canal by a supra-aural ear phone. This low-frequency BC enhancement, known as the occlusion effect, must be considered when occluding the nontest ear to present masking noise during BC testing. However, when the masking noise is presented using an insert earphone with the foam plug inserted deeply into the ear canal, the amount of the low-frequency enhancement is smaller than it is when supra-aural earphones are used to deliver the masking noise (Dean and Martin, 2000).

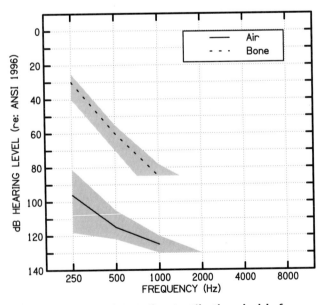

FIGURE 3.12 Mean vibrotactile thresholds for bone conduction (dashed line) and air conduction (solid line). The range of responses is indicated by the shaded region. (Adapted from Boothroyd and Cawlkwell, 1970.)

Special Populations

TINNITUS

Many people who come for hearing testing experience tinnitus, the sensation of hearing internal sounds when no sound is present (see Chapter 33). These listeners, and others who may be confused by the instructions, may tend to give a large number of false-positive responses when no test tone has been presented. False-positive responses can produce an inaccurate (too sensitive) threshold estimation. Some listeners simply require additional instruction and encouragement to wait until they are more certain they have heard a test tone. In some cases, the audiologist can present a clearly audible tone at the test frequency to remind the listener of the test tone. For more intractable cases, the examiner can present a series of pulsed tones and ask the listener to count the number of tones. It is important with listeners who are giving false-positive responses to avoid a fixed presentation rhythm and to provide irregular intervals of "no trial" silence to confirm that their responses are, in fact, responses to test tones.

In rare cases, patients have tinnitus resulting from blood flowing nearby auditory structures. Blood flowing through a vein or artery sometimes produces masking noise or "bruit" that can elevate thresholds for low-frequency tones (Champlin et al., 1990). On the audiogram, this form of tinnitus may produce an apparent sensory-neural loss. The loss occurs because the tinnitus masks AC and BC thresholds. Bruit is documented by audiologists by measuring sound levels in the ear canal. This problem is treatable when the problem is caused by a vein. In a case study reported by Champlin et al. (1990), the patient received some reduction in tinnitus loudness before surgery by applying pressure to her neck. Surgical ligation of the vein responsible for the tinnitus was shown to be an effective treatment. Surgery reduced tinnitus loudness, SPLs of the bruit measured in the ear canal were lower, and the audiogram showed significantly improved thresholds.

PSEUDOHYPACUSIS

Pseudohypacusis, also known as functional hearing loss and nonorganic hearing loss, is the name applied to intratest and intertest inconsistencies that cannot be explained by medical examinations or a known physiologic condition (Ventry and Chaiklin, 1965). Most persons who present with this condition are feigning a hearing loss for monetary or psychological gain, but a very small percentage of persons have subconscious motivations related to psychological problems (see Chapter 31).

Persons presenting with pseudohypacusis are often identified from inconsistencies in their responses to the puretones. In addition to general poor reliability during threshold searches, there is a tendency for the threshold to become poorer as more presentations are made (Green, 1978). Methods of identifying the pseudohypacusis by comparing puretone thresholds with other measures and the use of special tests are covered in Chapter 31.

AUDITORY NEUROPATHY

Auditory neuropathy (or auditory dys-synchrony) is presumed to be a relatively rare condition that may occur in up to 10% of cases of childhood hearing loss (Scott, 2003). Information about this disorder may be found in Chapter 22. Many of these children appear to be severely hard of hearing because of very poor speech recognition; however, puretone thresholds do not follow any specific pattern. Puretone hearing thresholds for these children range from minimal to profound losses. Individuals with auditory neuropathy classically show very inconsistent audiometric responses during a test and between tests.

AGING

Presbycusis is a term that describes the loss of hearing that gradually occurs in most individuals as they grow older. Studies suggest (Schuknecht, 1974; Schuknecht and Gacek, 1993) that several different types of damage can occur to the auditory system because of aging. Hearing loss due to aging typically causes a gently sloping, high-frequency sensory-neural hearing loss that tends to be slightly greater in men than in women. Figure 3.13 shows the average amount of threshold elevation expected based on aging in men who have had limited exposure to intense sounds. Even among this select group of participants, large individual differences are often observed.

ACOUSTIC TUMORS

An acoustic tumor (acoustic neuroma/neurinoma or vestibular schwannoma) is a rare disorder. Once identified, these tumors are usually removed surgically because they

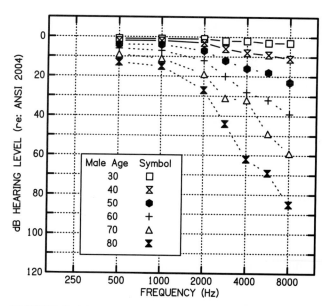

FIGURE 3.13 Average audiograms for adult males for different decades of life. Data from National Institute on Deafness and Other Communication Disorders (2005).

can compress the brainstem and threaten life. Early diagnosis and removal lessens the risk of complications during surgery and increases the opportunity to preserve hearing if that approach is pursued.

Magnetic resonance imaging (MRI) is the definitive test for acoustic tumors. Unfortunately, it is expensive and only becomes cost effective when a screening test is used to assess which patients should receive an MRI. Puretone audiometry should be considered as part of that screening procedure. When the auditory nerve is compressed by the tumor, it often, but not always (Magdziarz et al., 2000), results in a unilateral or asymmetrical hearing loss. Because the fibers on the outside of the auditory nerve code high frequencies, the hearing loss is associated with the high frequencies (Schlauch et al., 1995). Studies have shown that a screening test that compares the average threshold difference between ears for 1.0, 2.0, 4.0, and 8.0 kHz is most effective (Mangham, 1991; Schlauch et al., 1995). Threshold differences between ears for this puretone average that exceed 15 dB or 20 dB maximize identification of persons with these tumors while minimizing false-positive diagnoses of persons with cochlear losses. The pass-fail criterion (e.g., requiring a 20-dB difference between ears) may differ depending on the money available for follow-up tests. A pass-fail criterion requiring 15-dB or greater differences between ears identifies more tumors than one requiring 20-dB or larger differences, but the smaller difference also yields more false-positive responses. False-positive responses (in this case, persons with cochlear losses identified incorrectly as having tumors) place a burden on the health care system because follow-up tests such as MRI or auditory evoked potentials are expensive.

The effectiveness of a screening test based on the threshold asymmetries between ears is dependent on the clinical population. This test was found to be ineffective in a Veterans hospital where many patients are males who have presbycusis and noise-induced hearing loss (Schlauch et al., 1995). By contrast, preliminary data from young women with normal hearing in their better ear suggest that true-positive rates and false-positive rates for this test are comparable to those for auditory brainstem response (Schlauch et al., 1995). It should also be noted that a small percentage of persons (<3%) with acoustic tumors have no hearing loss or hearing threshold asymmetry (Magdziarz et al., 2000).

MÉNIÈRE'S DISEASE

Ménière's disease is diagnosed based on the symptoms of sensory-neural hearing loss, vertigo, tinnitus, and aural fullness (Committee on Hearing and Equilibrium, 1995) as well as the exclusion of other known diseases. Adding to the diagnostic challenge, the four symptoms do not occur all at once, and some of them may occur only during the intermittent attacks that characterize this disease. It takes, on average, 1 year after the first symptom occurs before all of the symptoms are experienced by a person stricken with this disease. Ménière's disease rarely occurs before age 20 and is most

likely to begin between the fourth and sixth decades (Pfaltz and Matefi, 1981).

Ménière's disease usually begins as a unilateral sensory-neural hearing loss, but the frequency of bilateral involvement increases with disease duration (Stahle and Klockhoff, 1986). Although audiometric configuration is not too helpful in diagnosing Ménière's disease, a peaked audiogram is most common (roughly 60% of involved ears), and a rising audiogram is also seen quite frequently, especially in the earliest stages of the disease. However, the peaked audiogram is also seen in 13% of ears with acoustic tumors (Ries et al., 1998).

NOISE-INDUCED HEARING LOSS AND ACOUSTIC TRAUMA

Exposure to intense sound levels can cause permanent or temporary hearing loss due to hair cell damage. When a narrowband sound is presented at a level high enough to result in damage, a loss occurs at a frequency roughly one-half octave above the frequency of exposure (Henderson and Hamernik, 1995). Most people who are exposed to damaging noise levels in their work or recreational endeavors are exposed to broadband sounds, but their losses, especially during early stages of noise-induced hearing loss, are characterized by a "notch" (a drop in hearing) on the audiogram. The greatest hearing loss typically occurs in the region of 3,000 to 6,000 Hz. The susceptibility of these frequencies is a result of sound amplification by the external ear (Gerhardt et al., 1987). The amplification is mainly a result of the ear canal resonance, which increases the level of sound by 20 dB or more. Temporary hearing loss is referred to as temporary threshold shift (TTS), and permanent changes are referred to as permanent threshold shifts (PTS).

Changes in hearing threshold can be slowly progressive, as listeners are exposed to high sound levels over months and years (Ward et al., 2000), or they can be rapidly changing, such as noise trauma after a sudden explosion or impulsive sound (Kerr and Byrne, 1975; Orchik et al., 1987; Taylor and Williams, 1966). Shooting a rifle results in a greater loss in the ear closest to the muzzle of the gun. In right-handed persons, the left ear is exposed directly to the muzzle, and the right ear is protected from the direct blast by the head.

OTOTOXICITY

Regular monitoring of puretone thresholds is particularly important for patients who take drugs known to be ototoxic. (For example, certain powerful antibiotics and cancer-fighting drugs are known to cause cochlear and vestibular damage in many patients.) Monitoring hearing sensitivity during treatment could allow a physician to consider alternative treatments that might preserve hearing. Ototoxic drugs typically cause reduction in high-frequency hearing prior to having any adverse effect on hearing for the speech range. For this reason, extended high-frequency hearing testing is recommended for ototoxic monitoring test protocols. Several studies have demonstrated the effectiveness of early identification of ototoxic hearing loss by monitoring thresholds for frequencies higher than 8,000 Hz (e.g., Dreschler et al., 1985; Fausti et al., 1992).

OTITIS MEDIA

Young children are susceptible to temporary, recurring middle ear inflammations (otitis media) that are often accompanied by fluid in the middle ear (effusion). Otitis media, often referred to as a middle ear "infection," may be viral or bacterial but is most often serous (noninfected fluid). Otitis media is the most common medical diagnosis for children, accounting for 6 million office visits in 1990 for children between the ages of 5 and 15 years (Stoll and Fink, 1996). Adults, too, may have otitis media with effusion, although the prevalence decreases significantly with age (Fria et al., 1985). During the active infection, often lasting a month or more, a patient's hearing loss may fluctuate, usually varying between 0 and 40 dB. The average degree of hearing loss is approximately 25 dB. Figure 3.10, which was used earlier in this chapter to illustrate an audiogram for a conductive loss, shows an audiogram derived from the average thresholds from a group of children diagnosed with otitis media.

TYMPANIC MEMBRANE PERFORATIONS

Tympanic membrane perforations are caused by trauma, disease, or surgery. The diameter and location of perforation and the involvement of other middle ear structures determine the amount of conductive hearing loss, if any. For instance, a myringotomy and the placement of pressure-equalization tubes represent a physician-induced perforation that results in a minimal air-bone gap in successful surgeries.

The measurement of AC thresholds in the presence of tympanic membrane perforations requires special consideration. Figure 3.14 shows an audiogram obtained in a single

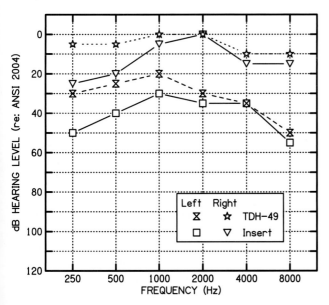

FIGURE 3.14 Audiograms obtained with two types of earphones from the same child who had bilateral perforations.

session from a school-age child who has a tympanic membrane perforation in the left ear and a pressure-equalization tube in the right ear. Thresholds were measured twice in each ear, once with supra-aural earphones and again with insert earphones. Note that the low-frequency thresholds obtained from insert earphones were as much as 15 to 25 dB poorer than the ones obtained with supra-aural earphones. This outcome is typical and is predicted because insert earphones are more susceptible to calibration problems in the presence of perforations than are supra-aural earphones (Voss et al., 2000). The thresholds obtained using the supra-aural earphones are more accurate in this instance and in any situations in which the effective volume of the ear canal is significantly larger than is typical.

Relation between Puretone Thresholds and Speech Measures

Puretone thresholds are often compared with speech audiometric test results. The two most common comparisons are with speech thresholds and supra-threshold word recognition scores.

Speech thresholds obtained using spondaic words (or spondees) agree well with puretone thresholds for low frequencies. Spondees are easily recognized; listeners only need to recognize the vowels to identify these words correctly. Because of the importance of the vowels at low intensities, spondee thresholds are found to agree closely with the average of puretone thresholds for 500 and 1,000 Hz (Carhart and Porter, 1971). In the event of a rising audiogram, better agreement between the spondee and puretone thresholds is the average for 1,000 and 2,000 Hz. Spondee thresholds and a two-frequency puretone average, as noted earlier, nearly always agree within ± 10 dB in cooperative examinees. This agreement makes the threshold for spondaic words an excellent check on the validity and reliability of the audiogram. This comparison is important for most children. It is also a valuable tool for assessing the reliability of puretone thresholds in adults who demonstrate inconsistent puretone responses or who may present with pseudohypacusis (Schlauch et al., 1996).

Supra-threshold word recognition scores provide a more valid evaluation of speech understanding than thresholds for a limited set of spondaic words (Wilson and Margolis, 1983), but word recognition scores are correlated with puretone audiometric thresholds in persons with cochlear losses (Rankovic, 1997; Pavlovic et al., 1986). Word recognition performance assesses a listener's ability to repeat back a list of monosyllabic words. Persons with mild cochlear hearing loss are expected to have high word recognition scores, and those with severe to profound losses are likely to have fairly low scores. This may not be the case for some persons with retrocochlear losses, who may demonstrate word recognition scores that are poorer than expected for their puretone average. Dubno et al. (1995) and Yellin et al. (1989) have published tables relating word recognition scores and the average of puretone thresholds for 500, 1,000, and 2,000 Hz for groups of persons with cochlear losses. Persons with scores that are abnormally low for a given puretone average are suspected of having a retrocochlear loss.

Automated Audiometry

Clinical researchers automated the measurement of routine hearing thresholds to increase clinical efficiency (Rudmose, 1963; Hughes, 1972). Devices were developed for this purpose, and several machines were manufactured and sold commercially. Some of these automated audiometers had the ability to vary intensity and frequency during a hearing test.

The Bekesy audiometer is an automated audiometer that was a common piece of equipment in major clinical and research settings in the 1960s. In its routine application, AC thresholds were assessed for interrupted tones and sustained tones for frequencies ranging from 100 Hz to 10 kHz. Frequency was swept through its range over time, typically at a rate of one octave per minute. The examinee controlled the level of the sound by depressing a handheld switch for as long as he or she heard a tone and released it when none was heard. The resulting brackets around threshold were recorded on an audiogram. Patterns of responses for sustained tones and interrupted tones were found to distinguish between different etiologies of hearing loss (see Chapter 31 on pseudohypacusis), but in recent years, Bekesy audiometry has fallen into disuse.

Within the past few years, a new generation of automated audiometers has been developed (Margolis, 2005). The new automated audiometers are capable of measuring masked AC and BC thresholds, as well as word recognition scores, with only a single placement of the earphones and BC oscillator. Computer-based rules control the presentation of stimuli, examinee responses, and the plotting of thresholds. The goal is to automate threshold collection for routine cases, which will free audiologists to perform more complex measures or to work with difficult-to-test populations. Extensive clinical trials will determine the success of these devices.

Calibration

Clinical data require accurate stimulus specification, or the results are meaningless. When most persons think of calibration of audiometers, the obvious examples include the accuracy of puretone frequency and level. However, puretone calibration involves much more, including an assessment of attenuator linearity, harmonic distortion, rise and fall times, and more. Consult ANSI S3.6 (2004) and Chapter 2 on calibration in this book to learn more about this topic.

Puretone Thresholds and the Audiologic Test Battery

Puretone thresholds are measured on nearly everyone entering a diagnostic audiology clinic, but the test sequence and the extent of the measurements often differ across clinics. Most of these differences in protocol are implemented to save testing time, which contributes to the cost of running a clinic. ASHA's guide to manual puretone threshold audiometry (2005) makes no recommendation concerning the puretone test sequence. In 2000, the Joint Audiology Committee on Practice Algorithms and Standards recommended an algorithm that listed puretone AC testing (with appropriate masking applied) followed by puretone BC testing with appropriate masking. They acknowledged that the assessment process may vary "based on patient need and the assessment setting." Furthermore, they stated that "decision-making…occurs(s) throughout this process."

Based on informal surveys of clinicians in a variety of settings, it seems that there is considerable variability in test protocols among clinics. In many clinics, BC thresholds are not usually obtained from persons with normal AC thresholds (near 0 dB HL) unless the case history or risk of middle ear problems suggests otherwise. BC threshold testing is also omitted in some clinics for returning patients with pure sensory-neural losses if their AC thresholds match those of the prior visit. A common alternative test sequence is to begin with puretone AC thresholds followed by suprathreshold word recognition testing. After word recognition testing, BC thresholds are measured. Although it would be useful to have puretone BC thresholds prior to AC thresholds to know how much masking noise can be presented safely, this advantage is outweighed by the inconvenience of having to enter the booth multiple times to reposition the BC vibrator and earphones. Valid, masked AC thresholds can be obtained successfully from most clients prior to obtaining BC thresholds.

A few clinics begin with immittance testing, which usually includes a tympanogram and acoustic reflex thresholds. If the case history does not indicate a middle ear problem and these tests of middle ear function are normal, then BC thresholds may not be performed, and the loss, if present, is assumed to be a sensory-neural loss. A possible risk of this strategy is that, in rare instances, persons with middle ear problems have normal immittance measures. In this situation, a conductive loss would be missed. This approach also adds the expense of immittance testing for each client. Studies should be done using an evidence-based practice model to determine whether administration of the immittance battery to each client is justified. Another time-saving strategy might be to measure BC thresholds at two frequencies, a low and a high frequency, and if an air-bone gap is not observed, BC thresholds are not measured for other frequencies. A low frequency, such as 500 Hz, would assess stiffness-related middle ear pathologies. A high frequency, such as 4,000 Hz, would identify mass-related middle ear pathologies and collapsed canals. Since this method requires placement of the BC vibrator, the amount of time actually saved would be limited.

Despite the observed variability, it seems that it is possible for audiologists to obtain important diagnostic information about the degree, type, and configuration of hearing losses using a variety of valid, evidence-based puretone audiometric methods. Although at first glance the puretone test procedure may appear elementary, it is clear that well-informed test procedures using appropriate and calibrated test equipment provides a necessary part of the complete audiologic test battery and forms the basis for clinical decision making.

REFERENCES

American National Standards Institute. (1999) Maximum Permissible Ambient Noise for Audiometric Test Rooms. ANSI S3.1-1999. New York: American National Standards Institute, Inc.

American National Standards Institute. (2004) Specifications for Audiometers. ANSI S3.6-2004. New York: American National Standards Institute, Inc.

American National Standards Institute. (1992) Standard Reference Zero for Calibration of Pure Tone Bone Conduction Audiometers. ANSI S3.43-1992. New York: American National Standards Institute, Inc.

American Speech-Language-Hearing Association. (1978) Guidelines for manual pure-tone audiometry. *ASHA.* 20, 297–301.

American Speech-Language Hearing Association. (1990) Guidelines for audiometric symbols. *ASHA.* 32, 25–30.

American Speech-Language-Hearing Association. (1994) Guidelines for the audiologic management of individuals receiving cochleotoxic drug therapy. *ASHA.* 36, 11–19.

American Speech-Language-Hearing Association. (2005) Guidelines for manual pure-tone threshold audiometry. Available from www.asha.org/policy/html/GL2005-00014.html.

Boothroyd A, Cawkwell S. (1970) Vibrotactile thresholds in pure tone audiometry. *Acta Otolaryngol.* 69, 381–387.

British Society of Audiology. (1987) Recommended procedure for the Rinne and Weber tuning-fork tests. *Br J Audiol.* 21, 229.

Browning GG. (1987) Is there still a role for tuning-fork tests? *Br J Audiol.* 21, 161–163.

Burk MH, Wiley TL. (2004) Continuous versus pulsed tones in audiometry. *Br J Audiol.* 13, 54–61.

Burns W, Hinchcliff R. (1957) Comparison of the audiometric threshold as measured by individual pure tone and by Bekesy audiometry. *J Acoust Soc Am.* 29, 1274–1277.

Burns W, Hinchcliff R, and Littler TS. (1964) An exploratory study of hearing and noise exposure in textile workers. *Ann Occup Hyg.* 7, 323–333.

Carhart R. (1945) An improved method of classifying audiograms. *Laryngoscope.* 5, 1–15.

Carhart R. (1950) Clinical application of bone conduction. *Arch Otolaryngol.* 51, 789–807.

Carhart R, Jerger J. (1959) Preferred method for clinical determination of pure-tone thresholds. *J Speech Hear Disord.* 24, 330–345.

Carhart R, Porter LS. (1971) Audiometric configuration and prediction of threshold for spondees. *J Speech Hear Res.* 14, 486–495.

Champlin CA, Muller SP, Mitchell SA. (1990) Acoustic measurements of objective tinnitus. *J Speech Hear Res.* 33, 816–821.

Chandler JR. (1964) Partial occlusion of the external auditory meatus: it's effect upon air and bone conduction hearing acuity. *Laryngoscope.* 74, 22–54.

Committee on Hearing and Equilibrium. (1995) Committee on Hearing and Equilibrium guidelines for the diagnosis and evaluation of Ménière's disease. *Otolaryngol Head Neck Surg.* 113, 181–185.

Dean MS, Martin FN. (2000) Insert earphone depth and the occlusion effect. *Am J Audiol.* 9, 131–134.

Dirks D. (1994) Bone-conduction thresholds testing. In: Katz J, ed. *Handbook of Clinical Audiology.* 4th ed. Baltimore: William & Wilkins; pp 132–146.

Dix MR, Hallpike CS, Hood JD. (1948) Observations upon the loudness recruitment phenomenon, with special reference to the differential diagnosis of internal ear and VIII nerve. *Proc R Soc Med.* 41, 516–526.

Dreschler WA, van der Hulst RJAM, Tange RA, Urbanus NAM. (1985) The role of high-frequency audiometry in early identification of ototoxicity. *Audiology.* 24, 387–395.

Dubno JR, Lee F, Klein A, Matthews L, Lam CF. (1995) Confidence limits for maximum word-recognition scores. *J Speech Hear Res.* 38, 490–502.

Fausti SA, Henry JA, Schaffer HI, Olson DJ, Frey RH, McDonald WJ. (1992) High frequency audiometric monitoring for early detection of ototoxicity. *J Infect Dis.* 165, 1026–1032.

Flottorp G. (1995) Improving audiometric thresholds by changing the headphone position at the ear. *Audiology.* 34, 221–231.

French NR, Steinberg JC. (1947) Factors governing the intelligibility of speech sounds. *J Acoust Soc Am.* 19, 90–119.

Fria TJ, Cantekin EI, Eichler JA. (1985) Hearing acuity of children with otitis media with effusion. *Arch Otolaryngol.* 111, 10–16.

Gabbard SA, Uhler K. (2005) The hearing evaluation. In: Jafek BW, Murrow BW, eds. *ENT Secrets.* 3rd ed. Philadelphia: Elsevier Mosby.

Gerhardt KJ, Rodriguez GP, Hepler EL, Moul ML. (1987) Ear canal volume and variability in patterns of temporary threshold shifts. *Ear and Hearing.* 8, 316–321.

Gescheider GA. (1997) *Psychophysics: The Fundamentals.* Mahwah, NJ: Lawrence Ehrlbaum Associates.

Goodman A. (1965) Reference zero levels for pure tone audiometer. *Am Speech Hear Assoc.* 7, 262–263.

Green DS. (1978) Pure tone air conduction testing. In: Katz J, ed. *Handbook of Clinical Audiology.* 2nd ed. Baltimore: Williams and Wilkins.

Henderson D, Hamernik RP. (1995) *Occupational Medicine: State of the Art Reviews, Biologic Bases of Noise-induced Hearing Loss.* Philadelphia: Hanley & Belfus, Inc.

Hughes RL. (1972) Bekesy audiometry. In: Katz J, ed. *Handbook of Clinical Audiology.* Baltimore: Williams and Wilkins.

Hughson W, Westlake H. (1944) Manual for program outline for rehabilitation of aural casualties both military and civilian. *Trans Am Acad Ophthalmol Otolaryngol Suppl.* 48, 1–15.

Jerger J, Jerger S. (1980) Measurement of hearing in adults. In: Paperella MM, Shumrick DA, eds. *Otolaryngology.* 2nd ed. Philadelphia: W.B. Saunders.

Jerger J, Shedd J, Harford E. (1959) On the detection of extremely small changes in sound intensity. *Arch Otolaryngol.* 69, 200–211.

Jervall L, Arlinger S. (1986) A comparison of 2-dB and 5-dB step size in pure-tone audiometry. *Scand Audiol.* 15, 51–56.

Johanson H. (1948) Relation of audiograms to the impedance formula. *Acta Otolaryngol Suppl.* 74, 65.

Joint Audiology Committee on Practice Algorithms and Standards. (2000) Clinical Practice Guidelines and Statements. *Audiology Today,* Special Issue.

Kerr AG, Byrne JET. (1975) Concussive effects of bomb blast on the ear. *J Laryngol Otol.* 89, 131–143.

Killion MC, Villchur E. (1989) Comments on "Earphones in audiometry." *J Acoust Soc Am.* 85, 1775–1778.

Kumar M, Maheshwar S, Mahendran A, Oluwasamni A, Clayton MI. (2003) Could the presence of a Carhart notch predict the presence of glue at myringotomy? *Clin Otolaryngol.* 28, 183–186.

Lloyd LL, Kaplan H. (1978) *Audiometric Interpretation: A Manual for Basic Audiometry.* Baltimore: University Park Press.

Long GR, Tubis A. (1988) Investigations into the nature of the association between threshold microstructure and otoacoustic emissions. *Hear Res.* 36, 125–136.

Lynne GE. (1969) Effects of collapsed auditory canals during audiometry. *Maico Audiological Library Series.* 7, 25–28.

Magdziarz DD, Wiet RJ, Dinces EA, Adamiec LC. (2000) Normal audiologic presentations in patients with acoustic neuroma: an evaluation using strict audiologic parameters. *Otolaryngol Head Neck Surg.* 122, 157–162.

Mangham CA. (1991) Hearing threshold differences between ears and risk for acoustic tumor. *Otolaryngol Head Neck Surg.* 105, 814–817.

Margolis RM. (2005) Automated audiometry: progress or pariah? Available: http://www.audiologyonline.com/articles/arc_disp.asp?id=1328.

Marshall L, Hanna TE. (1989) Evaluation of stopping rules for audiological ascending test procedures using computer simulations. *J Speech Hear Res.* 32, 265–273.

Marshall L, Jesteadt W. (1986) Comparison of pure-tone audibility thresholds obtained with audiological and two-interval forced-choice procedures. *J Speech Hear Res.* 29, 82–91.

Martin FN. (1994) *Introduction to Audiology.* 5th ed. Boston: Allyn and Bacon.

Martin FN, Champlin CA, Chambers JA. (1998) Seventh survey of audiometric practices in the United States. *J Am Acad Audiol.* 9, 95–104.

Mineau SM, Schlauch RS. (1997) Threshold measurement for patients with tinnitus: pulsed or continuous tones. *Am J Audiol.* 6, 52–56.

Moore BCJ. (2003) *An Introduction to the Psychology of Hearing.* 5th ed. London: Academic Press.

Morgan DE, Dirks DD, Bower DR. (1979) Suggested threshold sound pressure levels for frequency-modulated (warble) tones in the sound field. *J Speech Hear Disord.* 44, 37–54.

Mori N, Asai A, Suizu Y, Ohta K, Matsunaga T. (1985) Comparison between electrocochleography and glycerol test in diagnosis of Ménière's disease. *Scand Audiol.* 14, 209–213.

National Institute for Occupational Safety and Health. (1998) Criteria for a recommended standard: occupational noise exposure: revised criteria. Cincinnati: National Institute for Occupational Safety and Health, US Department of Health and Human Services Report 98-126.

National Institute on Deafness and Other Communication Disorders. (2005) Presbycusis. Available at: http://www.nidcd.nih.gov/health/hearing/presbycusis.asp.

Northern JL, Downs MP. (2002) *Hearing in Children.* 5th ed. New York: Lippincott Williams & Wilkins.

Occupational Safety and Health Administration. (1983) Occupational noise exposure: hearing conservation amendment. Occupational Safety and Health Administration, 29 CFR 1910.95; 48 *Federal Register,* 9738–9785.

Orchik DJ, Schmaier DR, Shea JJ Jr, Emmett JR, Moretz WH Jr, Shea JJ. (1987) Sensorineural hearing loss in cordless telephone injury. *Otolaryngol Head Neck Surg.* 96, 30–33.

Pavlovic CV, Studebaker GA, Sherbecoe RL. (1986) An articulation index based procedure for predicting the speech recognition performance of hearing-impaired subjects. *J Acoust Soc Am.* 80, 50–57.

Pfaltz CR, Matefi L. (1981) Ménière's disease – or syndrome? A critical review of diagnose criteria. In: Vosteen KH, Schuknecht H, Pfaltz CR, et al., eds. *Ménière's Disease.* New York: Thieme.

Pickles JO. (1988) *An Introduction to the Physiology of Hearing.* 2nd ed. New York: Academic Press.

Plomp R, Bouman MA. (1959) Relation between hearing thresholds and duration for tone pulses. *J Acoust Soc Am.* 31, 749–758.

Rankovic CM. (1997) Prediction of speech reception for listeners with sensorineural hearing loss. In: Jesteadt W, ed. *Modeling Sensorineural Hearing Loss.* Mahwah, NJ: Erlbaum; pp 421–431.

Ries DT, Rickert M, Schlauch RS. (1998) The peaked audiometric configuration in Ménière's disease: disease related? *J Speech Lang Hear Res.* 42, 829–843.

Rosowski JJ, Relkin EM. (2001) Introduction to analysis of middle-ear function. In: Jahn AF, Santos-Sacchi J, eds. *Physiology of the Ear.* 2nd ed. San Diego: Singular.

Rudmose W. (1963) Automatic audiometry. In: Jerger J, ed. *Modern Developments in Audiometry.* New York: Academic Press.

Schlauch RS, Arnce KD, Olson LM, Sanchez S, Doyle TN. (1996) Identification of pseudohypacusis using speech recognition thresholds. *Ear Hear.* 17, 229–236.

Schlauch RS, Carney E. (2007) A multinomial model for identifying significant pure-tone threshold shifts. *J Speech Hear Res.* 150, 1391–1403.

Schlauch RS, Levine S, Li Y, Haines S. (1995) Evaluating hearing threshold differences between ears as a screen for acoustic neuroma. *J Speech Hear Res.* 38, 1168–1175.

Schlauch RS, Wier CC. (1987) A method for relating loudness-matching and intensity-discrimination. *J Speech Hear Res.* 30, 13–20.

Schmuziger N, Probst R, Smurzynski J. (2004) Test-retest reliability of pure-tone thresholds from 0.5 to 16 kHz using Sennheiser HDA 200 and Etymotic Research ER-2 earphones. *Ear Hear.* 25, 127–132.

Schuknecht HF. (1974) *Pathology of the Ear.* Cambridge, MA: Harvard University Press.

Schuknecht HF, Gacek MR. (1993) Cochlear pathology in presbycusis. *Ann Otol Rhinol Laryngol.* 102, 1–16.

Scott TM. (2003) Auditory neuropathy in children. Available at: http://www.asha.org/NR/rdonlyres/C00C842E-CBD4-4F6E-BFA8-338951132D1F/0/D9AuditoryNeuropathy.pdf.

Shaw EAG. (1974) The external ear. In: Kleidel WD, Neff WD, eds. *Handbook of Sensory Physiology*. Berlin: Springer; pp 455–490.

Sheehy JL, Gardner G Jr, Hambley WH. (1971) Tuning fork tests in modern otology. *Arch Otolaryngol*. 94, 132.

Snyder JM. (1989) Audiometric correlations in otology. In: Cummings CW, Fredrickson JM, Harker LS, et al., eds. *Otolaryngology Head and Neck Surgery: Update*. St Louis: Mosby.

Stahle J, Klockhoff I. (1986) Diagnostic procedures, differential diagnosis, and general conclusions. In: Pfaltz CR, ed. *Controversial Aspects of Ménière's Disease*. New York: Goerg Thieme.

Stoll L, Fink D. (1996) *Changing Our Schools*. Buckingham, United Kingdom: Open University Press.

Studebaker G. (1967) Intertest variability and the air-bone gap. *J Speech Hear Disord*. 32, 82–86.

Taylor GD, Williams E. (1966) Acoustic trauma in the sports hunter. *Laryngoscope*. 76, 863–879.

Ventry IM, Chaiklin JB. (1965) Multidisciplinary study of functional hearing loss. *J Aud Res*. 5, 179–272.

Ventry IM, Chaiklin JB, Boyle WF. (1961) Collapse of the ear canal during audiometry. *Arch Otolaryngol*. 73, 727.

Voss SE, Herman BS. (2005) How does the sound pressure generated by circumaural, supraaural and insert earphones differ for adult and infant ears. *Ear Hear*. 26, 636–650.

Voss SE, Rosowski JJ, Merchant SN, Thornton AR, Shera CA, Peake WT. (2000) Middle ear pathology can affect the ear-canal sound pressure generated by audiologic earphones. *Ear Hear*. 21, 265–274.

Ward WD, Royster JD, Royster LH. (2000) Auditory and nonauditory effects of noise. In: *The Noise Manual*. 5th ed. Fairfax, VA: AIHA Press; pp 123–147).

Watson CS, Gengel RW. (1969) Signal duration and signal frequency in relation to auditory sensitivity. *J Acoust Soc Am*. 46, 989–997.

Wilson RH, Margolis RH. (1983) Measurements of auditory thresholds for speech stimuli. In: Konkle DF, Rintelmann WF, eds. *Principles of Speech Audiometry*. Baltimore: University Park Press.

Yellin MW, Jerger J, Fifer RC. (1989) Norms for disproportionate loss in speech intelligibility. *Ear Hear*. 10, 231–233.

Yoshikawa N, Murrow BW, Cass SP. (2005) Conductive hearing loss. In: Jafek BW, Murrow BW, eds. *ENT Secrets*. 3rd ed. Philadelphia: Elsevier Mosby.

Assessing Bone Conduction Thresholds in Clinical Practice

B.A. Vento and J.D. Durrant

▧ INTRODUCTION

Measuring bone-conduction (BC) thresholds is a well-established part of the traditional "basic battery" used in audiology. It is well known that vibrations from the stem of a tuning fork or from an audiometric device, called the bone vibrator, when pressed against the skull results in the perception of a sound. It would appear that these vibrations are able to bypass the outer and middle ear and stimulate the cochlear fluids. Indeed, BC threshold measurement is essential to evaluate the sensitivity of the sensory-neural system and allows us to differentiate outer and middle ear from cochlear pathology. However, as straightforward as BC testing may seem, there are complex underlying mechanisms and technical difficulties that influence the clinical assessment of BC thresholds. The purpose of this chapter is to present various aspects of BC theory and insights into clinical application of BC theory to aid audiologists in optimal interpretations of their test findings.

▧ THEORY OF BONE CONDUCTION—UNDERLYING MECHANISMS

The membranous labyrinth of the cochlea and semicircular canals is housed within the temporal bone of the skull; therefore, application of a vibrating source on any bone of the skull will result in vibration of the temporal bone. Logically, this should lead to effective stimulation of the hearing organ. However, stimulation of the organ of Corti is only accomplished by sufficient displacement of the basilar membrane, which is produced by pressure differential between the scala vestibuli and scala tympani. In air-conduction (AC) hearing, this happens when displacement of the stapes footplate causes volume displacement of the incompressible perilymph, which is relieved by bulging of the flexible round window membrane. It is not obvious that mere vibration of the temporal bone should lead to effective stimulation of the hearing organ. How, then, can BC hearing be explained?

Traveling Waves Run "North"

Before considering specific mechanisms of BC, it is useful to recall an experiment of Wever and Lawrence (1952) completed over a half century ago. These pioneers in physiologic acoustics considered, in an animal model, the simple question of whether it matters at which end of the cochlea the stapes is situated. Creating an artificial window in the bony wall of the scala vestibuli toward the apex, they found fundamentally the same cochlear microphonics (electrical response of the hair cells) whether vibrating the natural stapes at the base or the artificial stapes at the more apical site. These results confirmed that vibratory energy delivered to the cochlear fluids, at any point along the cochlear structure, will result in the creation of mechanical waves that progress uniquely from base to apex along the basilar membrane. This is quite good news since the problem of finding a particular path into the cochlea for efficient acoustic stimulation seems not to be particularly critical. It is the pressure differential across the cochlear partition (i.e., scala media, its boundary membranes, and its contents) that is essential to the initiation of traveling waves, ultimately causing vibration of the hair cells.

What then is the "path" by which BC leads to creation of the pressure differential across the cochlear partition? Actually, the more appropriate question is, "What are the *paths* of BC stimulation?" Traditionally, hearing scientists suggest three modes of BC stimulation: (1) the compression/distortion or osseous mechanism; (2) the inertial mechanism; and (3) the external canal or osseotympanic mechanism. The earliest theories of BC hearing were provided by Herzog and Krainz (1926) and Barany (1938) and carefully detailed by Tonndorf (1968). More recently, others (Freeman et al., 2000; Sohmer et al., 2000; Sohmer and Freeman, 2004) have proposed yet a fourth, nonosseous mechanism of BC involving the fluid pathways derived from the contents of the skull.

Compression Mode

The *compression* mechanism of BC, coined the "distortion" mechanism by Tonndorf, was first described by Herzog and Krainz (1926). Specifically, they proposed that vibration of the bones of the skull resulted in the stimulation of the basilar membrane due to the compression of the cochlear shell. This theory was later modified by Tonndorf (Tonndorf, 1968; Tonndorf and Tabor, 1962) based on experiments in animals and cochlear models. The theory of Herzog and Krainz depended on a flexible round window because (again) the cochlear fluids cannot be compressed; the round window is commonly illustrated as in Figure 4.1 The round window is more elastic than the oval window, providing at least one way to develop a pressure difference between the perilymphatic scalae. However, as shown in Figure 4.1, an even greater pressure differential and, therefore, a greater deflection of the cochlear partition are produced by the additional involvement of the volume of fluid in the semicircular canals. Tonndorf and Tabor (1962) carried out an experiment in cats in which they occluded both the oval and round windows. The results showed that, when these windows were occluded,

BC was only slightly impaired. This provided early support for the notion of a "third cochlear window" that would allow for basilar membrane displacement. In an additional experiment, using a cochlear model, Tonndorf (1968) concluded that simple symmetrical compression of the cochlear shell is a less accurate description of this mechanism than some form of "distortion" of the cochlea, which does not necessarily imply symmetry of compression of the cochlear shell. In fact, nonuniform distortion would allow for development of a pressure differential across the cochlear partition, causing excitation even with both cochlear windows occluded. Whatever the exact mix of these several "compression paths," the contribution of the compression mode of vibration to BC hearing is clear and appears to provide a robust mechanism by which to stimulate the organ of Corti directly via skull vibration.

Inertial Mode

The second mode is *inertial* BC, first described by Barany (1938). The basis of this mode of stimulation is the fact that the ossicles are suspended by ligaments in the middle ear space and form a folded lever made up of the manubrium of the malleus and the long crus of the incus. In general, the ossicular chain is built to vibrate independently from the skull. Inertial BC derives from the mass of the ossicles and occurs most efficiently in the low frequencies where the skull will vibrate side-to-side as a whole, thereby setting up relative motion between the ossicular chain and the skull, resulting in vibration of the stapes footplate in the oval window. This is the normal course of events in AC stimulation of the cochlear partition; consequently, the inertial mode leads to excitation of traveling waves in the conventional manner. Because the ossicular chain does not constitute merely a dangling mass (like a simple pendulum), it follows that the exact contribution of inertial BC to the total BC response is determined further by the impedance characteristics of the ossicular chain, including effects of the rest of the middle-ear system (e.g., air within the middle ear space) and the external canal to which it is connected via the tympanic membrane (Tonndorf, 1966; Tonndorf, 1968). In short, the latter factors are exactly the same as those influencing the efficiency of AC, so BC audiometry is not exclusively a test of the inner ear.

Ear Canal Contribution to Bone-Conduction Sensitivity

Perhaps no effect more emphatically demonstrates the point of potential noncochlear influences on BC hearing than the third mode of BC—the *osseotympanic* mode—based on observations in humans and results of animal experiments on the *occlusion effect* (Tonndorf, 1964). The occlusion effect is the improvement of hearing sensitivity or increased loudness lateralized to the side of a blocked ear canal upon application of a bone vibrator to the skull (see Chapter 6). The lateralization effect is independent of the site of application

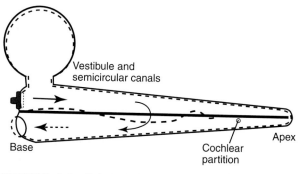

Vestibule and semicircular canals

Base

Cochlear partition

Apex

FIGURE 4.1 Schematic representation of the combined effects of the compression/distortion mechanism of bone conduction and volume displacement in the vestibular portion of the labyrinth, resulting in greater displacement of the cochlear partition than compression of the cochlear wall alone.

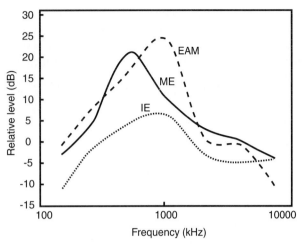

FIGURE 4.2 Frequency response of relative contributions to bone conduction from the external auditory meatus (EAM), middle ear (ME), and inner ear (IE). Based on data from the cat (Tonndorf et al. [1966]). While different response characteristics and magnitude of effects are expected in the human, the point is an appreciation of the complexity of bone conduction mechanistically, including the frequency dependence of their contributions.

of the bone vibrator. The results of Tonndorf showed that vibration of the skull results in radiation of sound energy (from the vibrating skull) into the external meatus, namely from vibration of the walls of the canal. Findings of more recent experiments by Stenfelt et al. (2003) suggest that only the vibration of the cartilaginous ear canal, not the bony portion, is a significant energy source for this mechanism. Once the cartilaginous canal is vibrating, the sound waves created in the canal excite hearing via the normal AC route. Unoccluded (open ear canal situation), the energy derived from this mode of BC stimulation is effectively high-pass filtered, wherein low-frequency energy "leaks" out from the ear canal. Clinically, we take advantage of this effect in hearing aid fittings when we use vented earmolds (see Chapter 38).

The results of subsequent animal experiments by Tonndorf (Tonndorf, 1968) are displayed in Figure 4.2 and show the relative contributions of these several modes of BC stimulation and their (relative) frequency-response characteristics. Specifically, the ear canal response is dominant in the low frequencies, the inertial response dominates the low to the mid-frequency range, and the compression mode is largely dominant at high frequencies.

Nonosseous Mode of Bone Conduction—Effect of Vibrating Fluid Contents of the Skull

More recently, Freeman et al. (2000) reported findings from an experiment in animals demonstrating auditory brainstem responses (ABRs) recorded in response to a bone vibrator

applied to the surface of the cerebrum via a craniotomy. In fact, thresholds of detection of the ABR obtained with the bone vibrator placed on the brain itself were quite similar in appearance, latency, and sensitivity as those obtained via placement on the skull (Freeman et al., 2000). Sohmer et al. (2000) completed a similar experiment in humans comparing BC ABRs in neonates to those of older children undergoing neurosurgery. Thresholds of BC ABRs compared favorably between the infants, in whom the vibrator was placed over the fontanelle, and those of the pediatric neurosurgical patients, in whom the bone vibrator was placed on the brain's surface. It was concluded that placement of the bone vibrator on the skull not only results in the activation of the classical BC pathways described earlier, but also a fluid pathway is stimulated. Specifically, the vibrating bone oscillator initiates audio-frequency pressure waves in the cerebral spinal fluid (CSF), which stimulates (effectively) the cochlear fluids, resulting in basilar membrane activation (Freeman et al., 2000; Sohmer et al., 2000; Sohmer and Freeman, 2004). Presumably, this is another manifestation of the compression mode.

Consideration of these results also points to the reality that the total mechanical load to the bone vibrator is not correctly viewed as though it were coupled to the skull alone. The living skull has elaborate soft tissue and fluid contents and is covered by a multilayered tissue—skin. The skull and all of its contents thus must be vibrated sufficiently to effectively stimulate the hearing organ. An overly simplified perception of BC risks errors that can confound the clinician's interpretation of findings in some clinical cases (for example, those times when seemingly anomalous air-bone gaps are encountered in diagnostic testing). However, with the various BC mechanisms in mind, such admittedly unusual cases prove not to be anomalous, per se, and can be explained reasonably well, as discussed later in this chapter. However, various technical issues and concepts relevant to BC testing should be considered first.

▨ TESTING CONSIDERATIONS

Bone Vibrator Placement—Forehead Versus Mastoid

The most commonly used bone vibrator (Radioear B-71) is shown in Figure 4.3A, mounted on a standard head band. Unlike the earphone, the construction of the bone vibrator allows it to be placed nearly anywhere on the skull. There are two primary sites for placement of the bone vibrator that have been used clinically and/or are recommended (via texts and standards such as American National Standards Institute [ANSI] S3.6-1996)—the mastoid and the forehead. Mastoid placement is used most frequently, being the closest site to the cochlea and an easy to maintain position on the patient/client. Mastoid placement yields lower thresholds than those obtained with forehead placement. This was confirmed by Durrant and Hyre (1993b) using real-head accelerometer

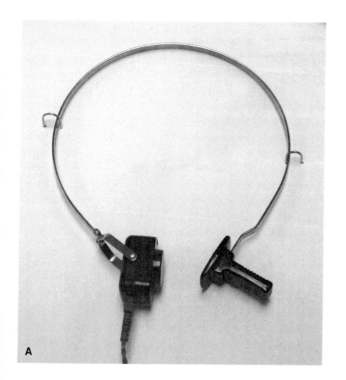

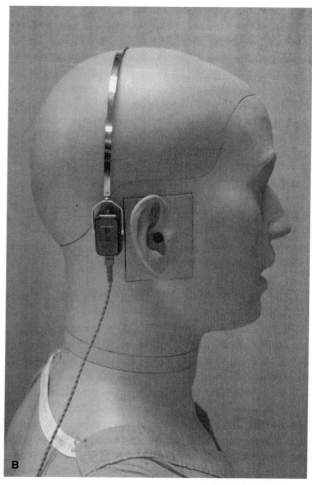

FIGURE 4.3 **A, Radioear B-71 bone conduction vibrator with head band. (Note: two small clips were used to open the headband slightly for this photograph, reflecting its spring-like quality.) B, Demonstration of correct placement of the bone vibrator using the KEMAR manikin; precise placement is adjusted for best compromise of location of the mastoid tip, surface flatness, and headband stability.**

measurements; forehead stimulation was seen to be approximately 10 dB less efficient overall. Yet, some scholars have suggested that the forehead might actually be the placement of choice. The reasons offered supporting forehead placement include less variability of thresholds (at least at some frequencies), less contribution of the middle ear mechanism to BC thresholds, and less impact of individual variables, such as subcutaneous fat and hair that can confound findings using mastoid placement (Dirks, 1964; Dirks & Malmquist, 1969; Goodhill et al., 1970; Studebaker, 1962). These rationales warrant detailed consideration; it will be seen that such claims of superiority of forehead placement are largely unsubstantiated.

LESS INTERSUBJECT VARIABILITY?

Anatomic variables appear to be simplified at the forehead compared with the mastoid process. Most notably, the forehead is essentially flat when compared with the mastoid prominence, which is inherently knobby. Consequently, consistent mechanical interface between skull and vibrator

seems more likely at the forehead than at the mastoid. However, modifications in bone vibrators have been made over the years, resulting in improved contact of the vibrator with the mastoid. This has reduced the variances in BC thresholds at both sites (Dirks, 1964; Studebaker, 1962). Still, as noted earlier, there are differences in BC thresholds between these two sites, and this must be taken into account in clinical applications.

IMPROVED TEST-RETEST RELIABILITY IN BONE-CONDUCTION THRESHOLDS?

Initially, lack of standards in bone vibrator construction could have contributed to greater test-retest variability in BC thresholds with mastoid placement. Specifically, early BC vibrators lacked standardization of their frequency response, as well as other mechanical characteristics. In addition, the contact area for the bone vibrator with the skull was very small, which further contributed to threshold variability (Hart and Naunton, 1961). However, with both the improved shape and the size of the contact area of the vibrator (see next page),

TABLE 4.1   Mean Differences between forehead and mastoid, providing bone-conduction threshold correction factors at various frequencies[a]

	Frequency in Hz					
	250	500	1,000	2,000	3,000	4,000
	Forehead-mastoid corrections in dB					
ANSI S3.43-1992	12.0	14.0	8.5	11.5	12.0	8.0
Frank (1982)	14.3	14.7	8.7	12.0	12.4	13.5

ANSI, American National Standards Institute.
[a] The correction should be subtracted from the forehead thresholds to approximate mastoid thresholds.

the test-retest reliability factor for mastoid placement was less significant than originally believed (Studebaker, 1962; Dirks, 1964).

Is there less hearing loss in cases of conductive pathology?

The issue of variability between placement sites relates to the inertial theory of BC, described earlier. It has been suggested that the direction of skull vibration—side-to-side versus front-to-back—could account for the differences in thresholds in relation to placement site (Dirks & Malmquist, 1969). Specifically, stimulation at the forehead, presumably favoring front-to-back vibration might be assumed to result in less middle ear contribution to the reported BC threshold (Dirks & Malmquist, 1969; Goodhill et al., 1970; Studebaker, 1962). Of some concern were reports of BC thresholds being 5 dB worse with mastoid placement in cases with middle ear pathology. However, results of a recent study in cadavers by Stenfelt et al. (2002) challenge this theory. Their investigation showed that, regardless of the direction of stimulation (that is, presumed replacement), the effective vibration at the cochlear input was the same.

The primary disadvantages of forehead placement is the reduced dynamic range and need for a different set of calibration values (Studebaker, 1962). Table 4.1 shows the recommended correction values for forehead placement as recommended by ANSI S3.43-1992, derived from results of an investigation by Frank (1982). The clinical impact of the reduced dynamic range is especially troublesome. For example, the forehead-to-mastoid difference is worth 15 dB at 500 Hz (see Table 4.1). Given that BC thresholds already are limited to 70 dB hearing level (HL) or less with decreasing frequency (notably below 1 kHz), an additional reduction of output would limit the useful range of bone vibrator output (e.g., 55 dB).

Based on the above discussion, it appears that the better choice for BC vibrator placement is the mastoid. This is consistent with current clinical practice. However, forehead placement does lend itself to another variation of BC testing—the Sensorineural Acuity Level (SAL) test. Although this test never gained popularity for clinical use, the SAL is still useful both from a theoretical perspective and possibly for special applications (e.g., in testing the ABR; see Ysunza and Cone-Wesson, 1987).

Sensorineural Acuity Level Procedure

The SAL test (Jerger and Tillman, 1960) is based on the work of Rainville (1959). It was anticipated that this approach would avoid ambiguities encountered in some cases. Jerger and Tillman (1960) reported a variation of the BC test to make it more appropriate and usable in clinic practice. The SAL test requires a constant and relatively high level of masking noise to be presented through a BC vibrator that is placed on the forehead. Then, AC thresholds are obtained for each ear with the constant BC masking level. These masked AC thresholds are then compared to unmasked AC thresholds to determine the BC thresholds.

Although the SAL technique eliminates the need for contralateral masking, it is equally vulnerable to the occlusion effect as more basic, conventional BC audiometry. The variability of the occlusion effect among individuals also has not permitted the development of a correction factor. Due to the perceived cumbersome nature of the procedure, the SAL test has never become a part of standard clinical practice (Jerger and Jerger, 1965; Tillman, 1963). Still, the SAL procedure has been advocated for use in determining conductive hearing loss in children using ABR testing (Ysunza and Cone-Wesson, 1987). Yet, this too has not found favor in standard clinical practice.

Vibrator Application Force and Surface Area

In general, the greater the application forces of the BC vibrator to the skull, the lower (more sensitive) the BC threshold. The best thresholds have been reported with forces between 750 and 1,000 grams. However, this amount of force is impractical and difficult to maintain in clinical practice, as well as very uncomfortable for the patient. Therefore, the recommended force for clinical practice is a minimum of 400 grams (Dirks, 1964) or 5.4 ± 0.5 N (ANSI S3.6-1996).

As suggested earlier, the surface area of the BC vibrator has a significant impact on BC threshold sensitivity. In experiments conducted by Khanna et al. (1976) and Queller and Khanna (1982), the contact area of the BC vibrator was varied systematically. The results showed an improvement in threshold sensitivity in the mid-frequency range by as much as 35 dB with increasing contact area. The use of a relatively large and standard contact area, as expected, reduced the variability seen in clinical BC testing.

Figure 4.3B shows correct mastoid placement for routine, clinical BC testing. The ideal placement area is on the skin behind and not touching the pinna and avoiding hair. It is a good idea to ask the patient to remove glasses, hair decorations, etc., that may interfere with either the vibrator or the headband. The headband crosses to the other side of the patient's head. Years of clinical experience have demonstrated that placing the end of the headband anterior to the patient's opposite ear will adequately secure the bone vibrator in place. With children or in cases of extremely small heads, placing a folded washcloth on top of the individual's head, under the band, can improve stability. Cases of extremely large heads tend to be more of a challenge. The audiologist must place the vibrator as close as possible to the mastoid where the headband can securely anchor the vibrator. Given that placement will influence BC thresholds (as in forehead vs. mastoid placement), unusual placements of the vibrator should be avoided or clearly noted on the audiogram if unavoidable.

The Occlusion Effect

It should be clear at this juncture that the occlusion effect is a pervasive factor in BC testing and theory and so deserves dedicated consideration. To review, when the ear canal is occluded and the skull is vibrated, the usual path for low-frequency release of the energy of the vibrating cartilaginous ear canal is eliminated. Clinically, this results in better BC thresholds than expected, particularly in lower frequencies through 1,000 Hz. The occlusion effect is readily demonstrated on oneself by simply pushing the tragus to cover the opening of the external meatus of one ear and humming, whereupon the humming sound lateralizes to the occluded ear. Occluding both ears greatly amplifies the sound of chewing, especially when "noisy" foods or chewing activities (i.e., chewing gum) are involved.

In clinical testing, when masking for BC, the occlusion effect is created inadvertently when placing an earphone over or inserted into the nontest ear. Thus, this effect must be taken into consideration in clinical masking paradigms, as discussed in greater depth in Chapter 6 .The occlusion effect varies with type of earphone and can be somewhat reduced by deep insertion when using insert earphones; namely, the amount of decrease in the occlusion effect is related to the depth of insertion of the ear plug. From earlier discussion in this chapter, the insert phone clearly must block the ear canal to the end of the cartilaginous canal to truly eliminate the occlusion effect (Dean and Martin, 2000). This is also true of earplug-type ear defenders and hearing aids (see Chapters 30 and 38), although such insertion depth may not be well tolerated by the examinee in these applications.

Tuning Fork Tests

While originally developed for the tuning of musical instruments, in 1825 the Weber brothers, Ernest and Wilhelm, reported that a tuning fork placed on the center of the skull (the vertex) was heard in the better ear for normal-hearing or sensory-neural loss cases and in the poorer hearing ear in cases of conductive hearing loss. Heinrich Rinne reported in 1855 that a tuning fork was heard longer by AC than BC in normal-hearing or sensory-neural loss cases. Later in 1885, Schwabach noted that, in those instances when BC was perceived longer than AC, the individual usually had a conductive hearing loss (Girgis and Shambaugh, 1988). The final commonly used tuning fork test, the Bing test, uses the occlusion effect to predict type of hearing loss (Stankiewicz and Mowry, 1979). Until the development of the clinical audiometer, tuning forks were the practitioner's only method of evaluating the auditory system. Even today, most otolaryngologists will use tuning forks to try to discriminate between conductive and sensory-neural pathology. In the hands of experienced examiners, tuning forks can provide useful information on auditory function but cannot replace pure-tone AC and BC audiometry for completeness and precision as well as for determining the type of hearing impairment (Stankiewicz and Mowry, 1979). Still, information about the tuning fork tests, which are discussed in the following sections, provides useful concepts for audiologists.

THE WEBER TEST

The Weber tuning fork test is conducted using a low-frequency (256-Hz) tuning fork. After striking the tines, the handle of the fork is placed on the patient's forehead near the hairline. The patient is asked to indicate which ear is "hearing" the tone. If the tone lateralizes, it will lateralize to the better hearing ear or the ear with a conductive hearing loss. If the tone is perceived at midline, it is indicative of normal hearing or equal sensation in both ears.

THE RINNE TEST

The Rinne test is also conducted using a 256-Hz tuning fork. After striking the tines, the fork is alternately held to the patient's mastoid and then lateral to (but not touching) the external ear, while asking the patient to indicate when he or she hears the tone. If the patient hears the tone longer by AC, then the Rinne test is said to be "positive." A positive result is found for normal or sensory-neural hearing loss. A Rinne test is "negative" if the patient hears the tone longer when the handle is placed on the mastoid. A "negative" Rinne test is an indication for conductive hearing loss.

THE BING TEST

Again, using a low-frequency tuning fork, the fork is struck, and the stem is held against the mastoid. The examiner (or the patient) then covers the external auditory canal, and the patient is asked whether the tone is louder. The Bing test is "positive" if the patient says the tone is louder when the ear is occluded. A "positive" Bing test is expected for normal or

TABLE 4.2   Tuning fork interpretation guidelines

Tuning fork test	Results and interpretation		
Weber	Heard at midline—Normal Lateralize to "better" ear—Sensory-neural Lateralize to ear with conductive loss		
Rinne	Positive	Heard longer by air conduction	Normal or sensory-neural
	Negative	Heard longer by bone conduction	Conductive
Bing	Positive	Heard louder when ear is occluded	Normal or sensory-neural
	Negative	Louder or unchanged when occluded	Conductive

sensory-neural hearing loss. A Bing test is "negative" if the patient reports that there is no change in loudness or that the sound is louder when the ear canal is not occluded.

Accuracy of Tuning Fork Tests

By virtue of the procedures just summarized, accuracy of tuning fork tests is greatly dependent on the individual patient's ability to make the required judgments and the examiner's expertise with the test protocols. In addition, the need for masking when attempting these tests has been suggested, yet there is no strong evidence that masking improves the accuracy of these tests. In a randomized controlled trial, Miltenberg (1994) evaluated the validity of the Weber, Bing, and masked and unmasked Rinne tests. He reported that the Rinne test showed a sensitivity of 84% independent of type of hearing loss and that masking did not improve test performance. The Bing and Weber tests were not found to be clinically useful diagnostic tools (Miltenburg, 1994).

Certainly, clinical audiologists must be conversant with the methods and interpretation of tuning fork tests because many otolaryngologists continue to rely on them to "confirm" the type of hearing loss. Audiologists should be able to explain, based on their knowledge of BC theory and hearing loss, what may appear to be discrepancies between tuning fork tests and behavioral test results. See Table 4.2 for an overview of tuning forks tests and interpretation.

⬛ EQUIPMENT AND CALIBRATION CONSIDERATIONS

Principle of the Tuning Fork

For the normal-hearing listener or individual with purely sensory-neural hearing loss, bone vibration does not account significantly for the hearing of airborne sounds due to the relatively high impedance of the skull (compared to the low impedance of air), which largely scatters or reflects sound waves. This ancient device—the tuning fork—is well suited to stimulate the auditory system both by AC and BC and has served piano tuners, as well as physicians, for centuries. The workings of the tuning fork can also be instructive for the audiologist. This device is essentially a bar that is bent and attached to a handle at its middle, giving the appearance of a fork (Fig. 4.4). The bend and added mass at the middle,

however, have important physical consequences. The fork forms a standing wave (Fig. 4.4). Because the ends of the bar (prongs of the fork) are relatively freely displaced, they make for highly efficient sound generators as they support standing-wave components of relatively large peak displacements or antinodes. In contrast, the more massive middle part supports only a foreshortened standing-wave component and a much lower displacement antinode. The handle is not efficient for sound-wave generation. This is good because

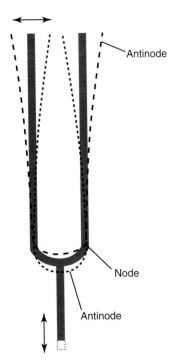

FIGURE 4.4 Bases of the ability of the tuning fork to stimulate the ear nearly equally effectively by air or bone conduction in humans. Essentially, when struck, a folded bar's natural (or first) mode of vibration is due to the formation of a standing wave with displacement antinodes occurring at each end, where large displacements are relatively easily achieved, and an antinode in the middle, where its much more dense and rigid structure limits displacement. The former represents a relatively low impedance source that is well-suited for delivering vibratory energy to air, whereas the latter is more appropriate for imparting vibratory energy to solids, like wood and bone.

it gives the tuning fork a much higher impedance at its middle, allowing it to be held with little damping of the vibration. It is fortunate that the impedance of the handle matches well the impedance of skull bones because this makes the tuning fork nearly as efficient at stimulating the cochlea by air as it is by BC.

The Bone Conduction Vibrator

The BC vibrator is fundamentally the same transducer as the conventional supra-aural earphone standardized for audiometric testing. However, instead of the transducer element (an electromagnetic device) driving a diaphragm to move air molecules, it is anchored and encased in a small plastic box or shell attached to a headband (see Fig. 4.3A), so as to provide a vibrating surface pressed against the skull. The distinctive characteristic of the modern bone vibrator is a protruding circular disk on one side of the shell, forming the contact surface of the device. The round contact surface represents a modification of the device originally standardized for BC testing, wherein the contact surface was the entire side of the shell, which had in turn a slight curved surface. The curvature was presumed to conform well to the less than perfectly flat mastoid. However, in the current design, the emphasis is on uniformity of contact across subjects, hence the disk-shaped "tip" of the current design. Indeed, both international and national standards recommend such a contact area and that the area should be no larger than 1.75 cm (ANSI S3.13; International Electrotechnical Commission [IEC] 29/592/CD). The Radioear B-71 is the vibrator that is used most often for BC testing and conforms to this standard.

Calibration of the Bone Conduction Vibrator

Calibration of the bone vibrator is maintained via electroacoustic checks using a so-called artificial mastoid, a mechanical coupler for the measurement of the device's output, in accordance with ANSI and IEC standards (ANSI S3.13; IEC 29/592/CD). The 6- and 2-cc couplers, used for earphone calibration, are only rough models of the real ear, whereas the artificial mastoid reflects an effort to model the impedance load offered to the bone vibrator by the real mastoid. The respective calibration curves for bone vibrators (tested on the artificial mastoid) and audiometric earphones (tested on the 6- or 2-cc coupler) thus cannot be compared directly; however, it is possible to make a direct comparison between transducers via behavioral measures (Fig. 4.5). The findings of Durrant and Hyre (1993b) show that, with effective stimulation of the cochlea using a B-71 bone vibrator versus an ER-3A earphone, the artificial mastoid underestimates effective BC output in the high frequencies and exaggerates the effective output in the low frequencies. Durrant and Hyre's results are as predicted by Gorga and Thornton (1989), who noted that the common audiometric limits of BC output are more severe for lower than higher fre-

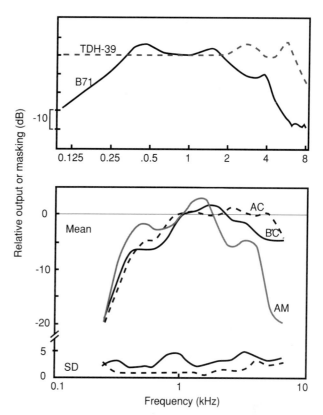

FIGURE 4.5 Upper panel, frequency-response comparison between a bone vibrator (B-71) and a headphone (TDH-39) as commonly used and calibrated for hearing testing (i.e. via a 6-cc coupler and artificial mastoid, respectively). Lower panel, effective frequency response for air- (AC) versus bone-conduction (BC) transducers deduced from masking efficiency of an AC- versus BC-delivered noise on an AC test stimulus (delivered by a tubal-insert earphone), compared in turn to the response measured on the artificial mastoid (AM) at the same frequencies. The frequency responses estimated thus appear much more similar between BC and AC than expected from the AM versus 6-cc coupler responses, and the BC curve is poorly represented by the AM results. Lower plots correspond to BC and AC means (above) and provide standard-deviations (SD) of BC and AC masking, respectively, indicating greater inherent variance of the estimated frequency response of BC, than AC, stimulation of the hearing organ. (Based on data of Durrant and Hyre, 1993b.)

quencies (as typically noted on the dB-HL dial of the clinical audiometer).

Clinical Issues

The Basics

There are several factors that might interfere with a proper comparison between BC and AC thresholds in actual clinical practice for individual cases. First, there is an acoustic delay in all transducers. This concept is most apparent in going from supra-aural earphones to tubal insert earphones or from earphones to loudspeakers—the farther from the eardrum the source is, the greater the delay between initiation of the stimulus and its arrival at the eardrum, and the more latent the recorded response. Acoustic delays are not unique to tubal insert earphones or loudspeakers but also are measurable for supra-aural devices, although involving much shorter delays (a few tenths of a millisecond vs. approximately 1 ms or longer). Although less clear cut, there is also a delay for BC stimulation, presumably due to complexities of vibration of the skull (Durrant and Hyre, 1993b). In addition to similarities between overall effective spectra of AC and BC stimulation between a TDH-39 and B-71, Durrant and Hyre (1993a) found a serendipitous similarity of stimulation delays for the TDH-39 supra-aural and ipsilateral BC vibrator placement on the mastoid, given equal sensation levels of stimulation. Still, results with BC were found to be substantially more variable (Fig. 4.5, lower panel, lower plots). The acceptance of agreement within some range (e.g., ± 5 dB) as effectively equivalent AC and BC thresholds is thus a "necessary evil" of clinical practice. Indeed, "reverse" air-bone gaps are not uncommon and should not go unreported on the audiogram. Such variances between BC and AC thresholds and/or seemingly counterintuitive effects (like BC poorer than AC thresholds) presumably reflect inevitable differences in effective coupling of the two transducers and other nuances of each mode of stimulation. In other words, substantial individual differences in relative input impedances for AC versus BC transducers are likely the rule. Perhaps of most pragmatic influence here is the simple fact that calibration standards represent averages, thus obscuring individual differences in air versus bone thresholds. These then emerge in the individual audiogram to challenge the clinician's interpretational skills and/or ingenuity in seeking corroborating measure(s) via other test modalities and, thereafter, to raise the dilemma of accepting versus rejecting the validity of the BC thresholds observed.

Variance in the air-bone gap is a third factor, as seen in Figure 4.5 (lower panel, lower plots), and indeed is not trivial. The variance of effective BC stimulation across frequency is twice that of AC and much less flat across frequency in some cases. Variance or noise in measurements is troubling enough, but "variance of variance" or nonstationarity, as depicted here, is considered to be one of the nightmares of statistical analysis (i.e., in addition to problems such as bimodal distributions, skewing, and the like). In fact, from this perspective, not only is the occasional air-bone gap likely to be observed in cases truly free of conductive pathology (as suggested earlier), but the reverse air-bone gap is expected with equal probability. Still, the clinician must carefully scrutinize observations of BC/AC differences, especially the reverse air-bone gap, with healthy skepticism. Such findings equally may indicate invalid measurements via one or the other mode (i.e., a technical problem) or suggest nonorganic involvement (i.e., a behavioral problem).

Finally, the patient's age is a factor in comparing BC and AC findings, as the head's size and bone density change with age, and this may influence BC coupling effectiveness. This is an area that begs more extensive research. A problem in defining developmental changes, in particular, is that the major changes in skull dimensions occur early on, namely when subjects are less reliably testable by conventional audiometry. Still, clear indications of the complexity of the matter are seen in results of studies of the ABR in young infants (vs. adults). Indeed, BC in ABR testing, as a popular tool for evoked response audiometry, warrants special attention.

BONE-CONDUCTION AUDITORY BRAINSTEM RESPONSE TESTING

The potential testing confound mentioned earlier—transducer delay as related to BC vibrator placement, potentially resulting in AC/BC differences—is of particular concern when measuring BC-ABR. The ABR may be affected in terms of overall magnitude, wave morphology, and/or latency, even to relatively small changes in stimulus level and/or spectrum. Equivalent ABRs cannot be expected between modes of stimulation unless, in fact, SL is identical between modes. This is not readily achievable in most practical cases of interest (e.g., testing young children) where sensation levels are not readily assessable and adequate BC vibrator placement may be difficult to attain. In ABR testing, age-dependent latency differences in AC-click- versus BC-click–elicited responses are especially evident over early development (e.g., see Yang et al., 1987). Unfortunately, BC thresholds and air-bone gaps are not well established in very young infants, and AC/BC agreement is likely to be confounded by such maturational changes, not only in BC-evoked responses but also in maturation changes in middle ear power reflectance over the first year or two of life (Keefe et al., 1993). These points are not meant to discourage use of BC in ABR testing but rather to caution the need for the interested clinician to be well informed of the nuances involved. Although methods involved are beyond the scope here, BC testing can help to rule out conductive impairment in ABR testing, just as in conventional BC audiometry, although precise quantification of the air-bone gap is even more elusive.

■ CLINICAL MANIFESTATIONS OF BONE CONDUCTION THEORY

The audiologist is responsible for the functional assessment of the auditory system; the more quantitatively precise the results and the more specific the interpretation of the findings, the more likely that a definitive diagnosis is forthcoming. The traditional classification of hearing loss—conductive, sensory-neural, or mixed—is the major goal of the basic test battery, and this decision readily transcends professional lines of interest. The otologist thus looks to the audiogram to provide information on the integrity of the sensory-neural system when deciding on surgical intervention. In such a case, it is generally assumed that, in a purely conductive hearing loss, BC thresholds should be within normal limits and the difference between AC and BC thresholds should accurately represent the magnitude of the conductive impairment. Acoustic immittance measurements also provide the means to detect middle ear dysfunction and certainly are a highly quantitative (and objective) method, but tympanometric results do not provide a quantitative assessment of conductive loss. Although clinical BC findings may seem imprecise at times, an understanding of the mechanisms of BC, especially the role of the external and middle ear in BC testing, can provide a logical basis for interpreting the results.

Perhaps the earliest report of questionable BC results regarding the air-bone gap was the description of "Carhart's notch," which was frequently found in cases of otosclerosis (Carhart, 1950). Carhart's notch is an apparent sensory-neural loss implied by reduction in BC sensitivity observed around 2,000 Hz, given that a completely conductive hearing loss is expected (unless there has been invasion of the otic capsule—cochlear otosclerosis). Figure 4.6 provides an example of pre- and postoperative stapedectomy audiograms from a patient presenting with a Carhart's notch preoperatively. Postoperatively (Fig. 4.6, bottom panel), the threshold at 2,000 Hz is seen to improve to within normal limits for both bone- and air-conducted stimuli. Because the treatment is not reasonably expected to improve cochlear function (indeed, the surgeon must work very skillfully to avoid acoustic trauma–like damage to the hearing organ), such results strongly suggest that the original estimate of the sensory-neural reserve was biased. Indeed, this effect can be attributed to restriction of the inertial BC response due to the fixation of the stapes in the oval window. The frequency most impacted by stapes fixation turns out to be the resonant frequency of the ossicular chain, 2,000 Hz (Tonndorf, 1966).

Other pathologies are now known to create anomalous BC findings, and although otosclerosis is an adult disease, similar problems can occur in pediatric populations. One such clinical population is patients afflicted by large vestibular aqueduct (LVA) syndrome (Govaerts et al., 1999; Madden et al., 2003; Nakashima et al., 2000). The LVA syndrome is a congenital disorder in which the vestibular aqueduct is larger than 1.5 mm (Emmett, 1985; Valvassori and Clemis, 1978). Although the hearing loss often associated with this disorder is fundamentally sensory-neural (by site of lesion), there are consistent reports of cases that present mixed hearing losses, namely suggesting a low-frequency conductive component. In fact, a low-frequency conductive component may occur in 17% to 38% of patients (Govaerts et al., 1999; Madden

et al., 2003). Three explanations have been offered for this effect of LVA. The first is that there is abnormal endolymphatic pressure, which adversely affects cochlear mechanics (Govaerts et al., 1999; Nakashima et al., 2000; Valvassori, 1983). This explanation is supported by results of an experiment completed by Govaerts et al. (1999). They completed three middle ear explorations in subjects presenting with conductive hearing loss and normal tympanometric findings. In these cases, they discovered unrestricted movement of the ossicular chain and an absent round window effect. They concluded that the low-frequency conductive loss in LVA patients was most likely due to endocochlear mechanical problems related to pressure imbalance in the inner ear, presumably adversely affecting the compression-distortion mechanism (Fig. 4.1).

The second explanation is that the stapes is fixated in the oval window. Shirazi et al. (1994) reported a single case where they found the stapes fixated in the oval window with LVA.

The third and final explanation, suggesting incomplete development of the stapes, was proposed by Nakashima et al. (2000). They argued that if stapes mobility was restricted, one would expect a higher resonant frequency, as measured by multifrequency tympanometry (Shahnaz and Polka, 1997). However, the patients of Nakashima et al., in fact, showed lower than expected resonant frequencies. Therefore, given that LVA has been associated with Mondini-type cochlear malformations and misshapen ossicles, this could be a cause of air-bone gaps in LVA. This is further supported by multifrequency tympanometric findings that show a reduced resonant frequency in cases of ossicular discontinuity (Shanks, 1984). However, there is no conclusive evidence for any of the three theories of air-bone gap in LVA. Figure 4.7 is a clinical example of a young male with documented bilateral LVA. This case is a good example of the potential for asymmetry and variability in hearing loss associated with LVA.

Low-frequency air-bone gaps with normal middle ear structures have also been reported in cases of superior semicircular canal dehiscence syndrome (SSCD). Patients presenting with SSCD often have balance problems that can be triggered by middle ear pressure change or even loud sound. Clinically, sound-evoked vestibular myogenic potentials are observed at lower thresholds (see Chapters 19 and 20). Confirmation of SSCD is by computerized tomography (CT) scan (Mikulec et al., 2004; Minor, 2000). These clinical findings have been theorized to be the result of a virtual "third window" to the inner ear that allows the air-conducted signal to be shunted away from the cochlea, resulting in increased AC thresholds as illustrated in Figure 4.8 (Rosowski et al., 2004; Sohmer et al., 2004). Specifically, for AC, the thinning of the superior semicircular canal allows for the energy to be shunted from the cochlea. Clinically, this presents as a low-frequency AC loss. BC thresholds are less affected by the SSCD due to exaggeration of the compression mechanism of BC. This point is underscored by the observation of

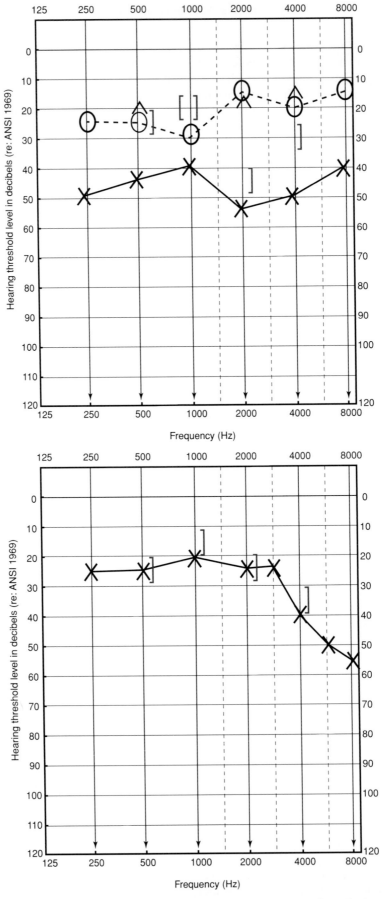

FIGURE 4.6 Upper panel, re-operative audiogram for patient with otosclerosis. Lower panel, post-operative audiogram. Note improvement in bone conduction threshold at 2000 Hz.

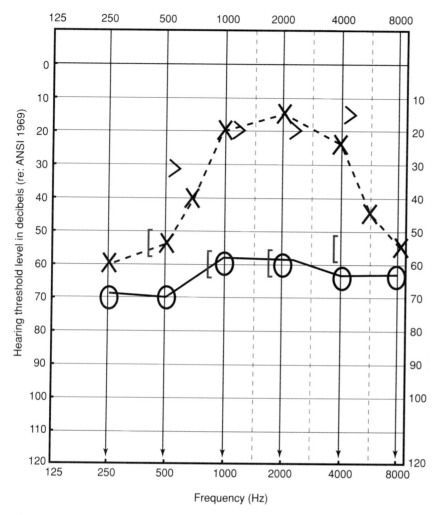

FIGURE 4.7   Example of low frequency air-bone gaps in case of bilateral large vestibular aqueduct (LVA). This case shows the variability of configuration of hearing loss in LVA and the presence of air-bone gaps at 500 Hz for both ears.

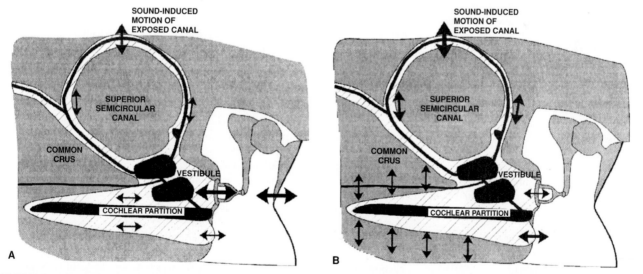

FIGURE 4.8   Schematic representation of semicircular canal dehissence (SSCD) from Mikulec et al. (2004). Panel A shows vibratory energy delivered via air conduction being shunted away from the cochlea, namely to the superior semicircular canal. The outcome from this defect is elevated air conduction thresholds. Panel B shows bone conduction stimulation of the cochlear shell resulting in greater-than-expected cochlear fluid motion and, consequently, an air-bone gap in the absence of middle-ear pathology. (Reprinted with permission from Lippincott Williams & Wilkins.)

negative BC thresholds in the lower frequencies. This theory was offered as a fourth possible explanation for the air-bone gaps experienced in cases of LVA (Mikulec et al., 2004; Rosowski et al., 2004).

These cases of apparent incongruities point out the importance of anomalies on both sides of the air-bone gap. Middle ear pathology can potentially bias AC or BC threshold estimates. For example, Kruger and Tonndorf (1978) found AC thresholds to be overestimated (i.e., appear poorer than they are) in animals given large tympanic membrane perforations. They proposed that, in some cases, it is likely that the earphone may no longer be in calibration, in effect, due to the unusually increased acoustic volume loading the transducer. Consequently, incongruous findings may well challenge the clinician for a rational explanation and interpretation, but they do not evade understanding and/or a sense of congruity once all of the diagnostic facts are in, as in the case of LVA.

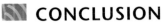 ## CONCLUSION

Several take-home messages can be derived from consideration of the theory and clinical findings from BC testing. First, there are three or perhaps four mechanisms of BC that contribute to the clinical assessment of the air-bone gap and/or sensory-neural reserve. Second, common explanations for variability and inconsistencies in BC thresholds or presumed difference in air and bone stimulation are not entirely as they may seem (namely, the variability of bone vibrator placement or differences between respective transducers). BC threshold testing is inherently more variable than AC threshold testing. Finally, understanding the mechanisms of BC allows the audiologist to better understand the apparent incongruities in findings from the basic battery that occur across the diverse clinical populations likely to be examined by the clinical audiologist.

REFERENCES

American National Standards Institute. (1992) Standard Reference Zero for Calibration of Pure Tone Bone Conduction Audiometers. ANSI S3.43-1992. New York: American National Standards Institute, Inc.

Barany E. (1938) A contribution to the physiology of bone conduction. *Acta Otolaryngol.* 26.

Carhart R. (1950) Clinical application of bone conduction. *Arch Otolaryngol.* 51, 798–807.

Dean MS, Martin F. (2000) Insert earphone depth and the occlusion effect. *Am J Audiol.* 9, 1–4.

Dirks D. (1964) Factors related to bone conduction reliability. *Arch Otolaryngol.* 79, 551–558.

Dirks D, Malmquist C. (1969) Comparison of frontal and mastoid bone-conduction threshold in various conductive lesions. *J Speech Hear Res.* 12, 725–746.

Durrant J, Hyre R. (1993a) Observations on temporal aspects of bone-conduction clicks: real head measurements. *J Am Acad Audiol.* 4, 213–219.

Durrant J, Hyre R. (1993b). Relative effective frequency response of bone versus air conduction stimulation examined via masking. *Audiology.* 32, 175–184.

Emmett J. (1985) The large vestibular aqueduct syndrome. *Am J Otol.* 6, 387–415.

Frank T. (1982) Forehead versus mastoid threshold differences with a circular tipped vibrator. *Ear Hear.* 3, 91–92.

Freeman S, Sichel J, Sohmer H. (2000) Bone conduction experiments in animals—evidence for a non-osseous mechanism. *Hear Res.* 146, 72–80.

Girgis T, Shambaugh G. (1988) Tuning for tests: forgotten art. *Am J Audiol.* 9, 64–69.

Goodhill V, Dirks D, Malmquist C. (1970) Bone-conduction thresholds. Relationships of frontal and mastoid measurement in conductive hypacusis. *Arch Otolaryngol.* 91, 250–256.

Gorga M, Thornton A. (1989) The choice of stimuli for ABR measurements. *Ear Hear.* 10, 217–230.

Govaerts P, Casselman J, Daemers K, De Ceulaer G, Somers TH, Offeciers F. (1999) Audiological findings in large vestibular aqueduct syndrome. *Int J Pediatr Otorhinolaryngol.* 51, 157–164.

Hart C, Naunton R. (1961) Frontal bone conduction tests in clinical audiometry. *Laryngoscope.* 71, 24–29.

Herzog H, Krainz W. (1926) Das knochenleitungsproblem. *Z Hals Usw Heilk.* 15, 300–306.

Jerger J, Jerger S. (1965) Critical evaluation of SAL audiometry. *J Speech Hear Res.* 8, 103–127.

Jerger J, Tillman T. (1960) A new method for the clinical determination of sensorineural acuity level (SAL). *Arch Otolaryngol.* 71, 948–953.

Keefe DH, Bulen J, Arehart K, Burns E. (1993) Ear-canal impedance and reflection coefficient in human infants and adults. *J Acoust Soc Am.* 94, 2617–2638.

Khanna S, Tonndorf J, Queller J. (1976) Mechanical parameters of hearing by bone conduction. *J Acoust Soc Am.* 60, 139–154.

Kruger B, Tonndorf J. (1978) Tympanic membrane perforations in cats: configurations of losses with and without ear canal extensions. *J Acoust Soc Am.* 63, 436–441.

Madden C, Halsted M, Benton C, Greinwald J, Choo D. (2003) Enlarged vestibular aqueduct syndrome in the pediatric population. *Otol Neurotol.* 24, 625–632.

Mikulec A, McKenna M, Ramsey M, Rosowski J, Herrmann B, Rauch S, et al. (2004) Superior semicircular canal dehiscence presenting as conductive hearing loss without vertigo. *Otol Neurotol.* 25, 121–129.

Miltenburg D. (1994) The validity of tuning fork tests in diagnosing hearing loss. *J Otolaryngol.* 23, 254–259.

Minor L. (2000) Superior canal dehiscence syndrome. *Am J Otol.* 21, 9–19.

Nakashima T, Ueda H, Furuhashi A, Sato E, Asahi K, Naganawa S, et al. (2000) Air-bone gap and resonant frequency in large vestibular aqueduct syndrome. *Am J Otol.* 21, 671–674.

Queller J, Khanna S. (1982) Changes in bone conduction thresholds with vibrator contact area. *J Acoust Soc Am.* 71, 1519–1526.

Rainville M. (1959) New method of masking for the determination of bone conduction curves. *Trans Beltone Inst Res.* 11.

Rosowski J, Songer J, Nakajima H, Brinsko K, Merchant S. (2004) Clinical, experimental, and theoretical investigations of the effect of superior semicircular canal dehiscence on hearing mechanisms. *Otol Neurotol.* 25, 323–332.

Shahnaz N, Polka L. (1997) Standard and multifrequency tympanometry in normal and otosclerotic ears. *Ear Hear.* 18, 326–341.

Shanks, J. (1984) Tympanometry. *Ear Hear.* 5, 268–281.

Shirazi A, Fenton J, Fagan P. (1994) Large vestibular aqueduct syndrome and stapes fixation. *J Laryngol Otol.* 108, 989–990.

Sohmer H, Freeman S. (2004) Further evidence for a fluid pathway during bone conduction auditory stimulation. *Hear Res.* 193, 105–110.

Sohmer H, Freeman S, Geal-Dor M, Adelman C, Savion I. (2000) Bone conduction experiments in humans—a fluid pathway from bone to ear. *Hear Res.* 146, 81–88.

Sohmer H, Freeman S, Perez R. (2004) Semicircular canal fenestration—improvement of bone- but not air-conducted auditory thresholds. *Hear Res.* 187, 105–110.

Stankiewicz J, Mowry H. (1979) Clinical accuracy of tuning fork tests. *Laryngoscope.* 89, 1956–1963.

Stenfelt S, Hato N, Goode RL. (2002) Factors contributing to bone conduction: the middle ear. *J Acoust Soc Am.* 111, 947–959.

Stenfelt S, Wild T, Hato N, Goode RL. (2003) Factors contributing to bone conduction: the outer ear. *J Acoust Soc Am.* 113, 902–913.

Studebaker G. (1962) Placement of vibrator in bone-conduction testing. *J Speech Hear Res.* 5, 321–331.

Tillman T. (1963) Clinical applicability of the SAL test. *Arch Otolaryngol.* 78, 20–32.

Tonndorf J. (1964) Animal experiments in bone conduction: clinical conclusions. *Ann Otol Rhinol Laryngol.* 73, 658–678.

Tonndorf J. (1966) Bone conduction. Studies in experimental animals. *Acta Otolaryngol.* 213 (suppl), 132.

Tonndorf J. (1968) A new concept of bone conduction. *Arch Otolaryngol.* 87, 595–600.

Tonndorf J, Tabor J. (1962) Closure of the cochlear windows: its effect upon air- and bone-conduction. *Ann Otol Rhinol Laryngol.* 71, 5–29.

Valvassori G. (1983) The large vestibular aqueduct and associated anomalies of the inner ear. *Otolaryngol Clin North Am.* 16, 95–101.

Valvassori G, Clemis J. (1978) The large vestibular aqueduct syndrome. *Laryngoscope.* 88, 723–728.

Wever E, Lawrence M. (1952) Sound conduction in the cochlea. *Trans Am Otol Soc.* 40, 168–179.

Yang EY, Rupert AL, Moushegian G. (1987) A developmental study of bone conduction auditory brainstem response in infants. *Ear Hear.* 8, 244–251.

Ysunza A, Cone-Wesson B. (1987) Bone conduction masking for brainstem auditory-evoked potentials (BAEP) in pediatric audiological evaluations. Validation of the test. *Int J Pediatr Otorhinolaryngol.* 12, 291–302.

Speech Audiometry

Rachel McArdle and Theresa Hnath-Chisolm

▨ INTRODUCTION

Auditory assessment using speech stimuli has a long history in the evaluation of hearing. As early as 1804, there were scientific attempts to study hearing sensitivity for speech by assessing which classes of speech sounds an individual could hear: (1) vowels; (2) voiced consonants; or (3) voiceless consonants. In 1821, Itard, who is well-known for his contributions to deaf education, differentiated individuals who were hard of hearing from those who were deaf by whether a person could understand some or none of a spoken message (Feldmann, 1970). This early focus on hearing for speech continued through the 19th century, and by the mid-1920s, the first speech audiometer, the Western Electric 4A, which incorporated a phonograph with recorded digit speech stimuli, was employed in large-scale hearing screenings (Feldmann, 1970).

Hearing and understanding speech have unique importance in our lives. For children, the ability to hear and understand speech is fundamental to the development of oral language. For adults, difficulty in detecting and understanding speech limits the ability to participate in the communication interactions that are the foundation of numerous activities of daily living. Measures of sensitivity and understanding form the basis of speech audiometry. This chapter is focused on providing information that can lead to the implementation of evidence-based best practices in speech audiometry.

▨ WHAT IS SPEECH AUDIOMETRY?

Speech audiometry refers to procedures that use speech stimuli to assess auditory function (Konkle and Rintelmann, 1983). Since the classic work of Carhart (1951), speech

audiometry has involved the assessment of sensitivity for speech as well as assessment of clarity when speech is heard. These concepts were described by Plomp (1978), in his framework of hearing loss, as an audibility component (i.e., loss of sensitivity) and a distortion component (i.e., loss of clarity). The audibility component is quantified through assessment of speech thresholds. The distortion component is a reduction in the ability to understand speech, especially in a background of noise, regardless of the presentation level. Quantifying the distortion component typically involves percent correct recognition at supra-threshold levels for the speech recognition score (SRS). More recently, the signal-to-noise ratio (S/N) at which 50% correct recognition is achieved has been recommended instead of the traditional SRS (Nilsson et al., 1994; Killion et al., 2004; Wilson, 2003). Prior to discussing measurement of speech thresholds and speech recognition in quiet and noise, general considerations in speech audiometry related to terminology, stimulus calibration, presentation methods, response modes, and presentation levels are discussed.

▨ SPEECH AUDIOMETRY TERMINOLOGY

There are two types of threshold measures using speech stimuli: speech detection threshold (SDT) and speech recognition threshold (SRT). SDT, as defined by the American Speech-Language-Hearing Association (ASHA) (1988), is an estimate of the level at which an individual perceives speech to be present 50% of the time and should be reported in decibels hearing level (dB HL). SDTs are commonly used to establish the level for awareness of speech stimuli by infants, young children, or adults who cannot respond verbally or whose speech recognition ability is so poor that they are unable to recognize spondaic (i.e., compound) words to obtain an SRT. SDT is sometimes called a speech awareness threshold (SAT), although SDT is the term preferred by ASHA (1988).

The SRT is an estimate of the level at which an individual can repeat back spondaic words (e.g., hotdog, baseball) 50% of the time; it is most commonly reported in dB HL or decibels sound pressure level (dB SPL). The most common supra-threshold measure in quiet is the SRS or word recognition score and is generally measured in percent correct at a level (dB HL) relative to either the SRT or an average of puretone thresholds. Word recognition has been referred to as speech discrimination; however, discrimination infers that an individual is judging between two or more specific stimuli, which is not the task in most supra-threshold speech recognition measures.

GENERAL CONSIDERATIONS FOR SPEECH AUDIOMETRY

A number of factors can affect the accuracy of threshold and supra-threshold speech measures. Instrumentation used to administer a test is one of the major factors that can affect the precision of these measurements (Schiavetti and Metz, 2002). Historically, audiometers that employed speech stimuli were called speech audiometers. These audiometers presented either recorded speech or live voice through a microphone. The speech stimuli were then passed through an amplifier, where the level could be adjusted, and were routed to either loudspeakers or to earphones. Currently most clinical audiometers come standard for testing speech stimuli, and the term speech audiometer is no longer used.

Audiometers have to meet calibration standards set forth by the American National Standards Institute (ANSI) (1996). In addition, recorded materials used as stimuli for speech audiometry must meet the ANSI standards (ANSI, 1996, Annex B). In order to reduce error of measurement and increase consistency from clinic to clinic, speech measures should employ accepted calibration procedures, methods and modes of presentation, test instructions, and response modes.

Calibration

STIMULI

Speech recordings must have a calibration tone of 1,000 Hz that is set at the same level as the speech materials (ANSI, 1996). Typically the calibration tone reflects the peak level of the spondaic words and the average level of the carrier phrase used with monosyllabic stimuli. The purpose of the calibration tone is to permit the tester to view the stimulus level via the monitoring meter (or volume unit [VU] meter) of the audiometer and to adjust the level to 0 dB on the meter. It should be noted that brief acoustic events, such as monosyllabic words whose speech energy is sustained for less than 350 ms, may not register properly on the meter even if the calibration tone has been properly set on the monitoring meter (Wilson and Strouse, 1999).

TRANSDUCERS

The standard reference SPL for words and short sentences should be 12.5 dB above the reference equivalent threshold sound pressure level (RETSPL) at 1,000 Hz for a given transducer. For each stimulus and transducer, RETSPL is the SPL value representing 0 dB HL. TDH-type earphones have an RETSPL at 1,000 Hz of 7.5 dB; therefore, when the 1,000-Hz calibration tone for recorded stimuli is set to 0 on the monitoring meter and the attenuator is set to 0 dB HL, the SPL of the speech signal is 20 dB SPL. The RETSPL for insert phones is either 5.5 dB or 0 dB depending on the coupler producing a standard reference for speech stimuli through insert phones of 18 or 12.5 dB (ANSI, 1996).

Loudspeakers are the transducers used in a sound field. One or more are set up in the sound-treated room at certain angles or, in this case, azimuths. The azimuth describes the angle of the sound source relative to the head of the listener. As shown in Figure 5.1, when the sound source is at 0° azimuth, the signal is directly in front of the listener. When the sound source is at 90°, 180°, and 270° azimuth, the signal is adjacent to the right ear, directly behind the listener, and adjacent to the left ear, respectively. The RETSPL for 1,000 Hz when listening binaurally in sound field is 2.0 dB, making the standard reference SPL 14.5 dB. For monaural presentations of speech stimuli in sound field, the RETSPL values for 1,000 Hz are 4.0, 0.0, and –1.5 dB for 0°, 45°, and 90° azimuth, respectively. The corresponding standard reference SPL values for 0°, 45°, and 90° azimuth are 16.5, 12.5, and 11 dB (ANSI, 1996).

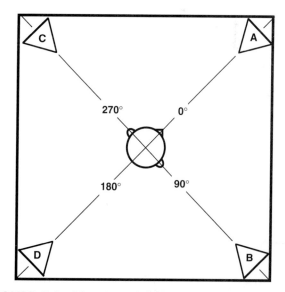

FIGURE 5.1 Diagram of the common loudspeaker azimuth locations (*triangles A-D*) used for sound field testing with reference to the listener.

Method of Presentation

Historically, VU meters were used for the tester to "monitor" the energy of his or her voice while presenting speech stimuli via the speech audiometer. The development of analog audiotape followed by compact disc technology was instrumental in facilitating standardization of word lists used in speech audiometry (Wilson et al., 1990). ASHA guidelines (1988) for speech thresholds indicate that the use of recorded stimuli is preferred. The majority of audiologists, however, who responded to a survey of audiometric practices (Martin et al., 1998) still report using monitored live speech to determine thresholds for speech. Of the 218 audiologists who completed the survey, 94% reported using monitored live voice test methods.

We feel that it is even more important to use recorded speech for SRSs. Digitized speech recordings improve both the intrasubject and intersubject precision of threshold and supra-threshold measures by providing a consistent level for all test items and consistent speech patterns between patients. The reliability of a given set of speech stimuli can vary across speakers and across test time for a single speaker. Hood and Poole (1980) found that a speaker had a significant impact on the difficulty of particular monosyllabic word lists. Similarly, Penrod (1979) reported that speech recognition performance differences among speakers were not attributed to a single speaker, but rather the variability was related to talker-listener interactions. Other studies have found variability in recognition performance as a function of speaker-list interactions (Hirsh et al., 1954; Asher, 1958) such that the acoustic waveforms of two speakers can cause differences in recognition performance even when the word lists are the same. The reported contribution of the speaker to the recognition performance of each listener reinforces previous reports by Kruel et al. (1969), who stated that word lists should be thought of as a group of utterances and not as a written list of words because speaker differences may affect a person's performance on a particular list.

Presentation Level

PSYCHOMETRIC FUNCTION

Understanding the influence of presentation level on performance is best described by psychometric functions (also known as performance-intensity functions). In simple terms, a function is when you measure a change in a dependent variable (y-axis; e.g., percent correct) based on changes of an independent variable (x-axis; e.g., dB level). A psychometric function provides a means for interpreting some parameter of a physical variable (x) on performance of a psychological variable (y). In speech audiometry, the physical variable (x-axis) is generally the level of the speech signal, expressed in dB SPL, dB HL, or dB S/N. Performance is usually measured in percent correct along the y-axis. Figure 5.2 is a graphic display of a generic psychometric function. Level is graphed along the x-axis in dB HL, whereas percent correct perfor-

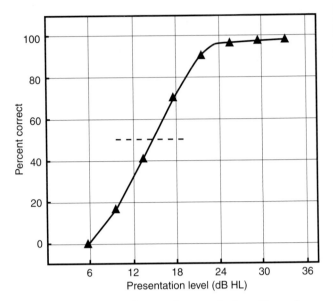

FIGURE 5.2 Sample psychometric function of word recognition performance measured in percent correct (ordinate) for a listener with normal hearing as a function of presentation level (abscissa). The dashed line indicates the 50% point or the speech recognition threshold.

mance is graphed along the y-axis. As can be seen, the percent correct is low when the level is low, and as the level is increased, the percent correct increases. The dashed line in Figure 5.2 highlights the 50% point on the function and indicates that an SRT was obtained at 15 dB HL. Also illustrated in Figure 5.2 is that the maximum point of performance (100%) was reached at approximately 26 dB HL. As the level is increased above 26 dB HL, no change in performance is observed. The highest percent correct score obtained by an individual is often referred to as PB$_{max}$, because historically SRSs were obtained using phonetically balanced (PB) word lists. Further discussion of PB word lists can be found later in this chapter under the section titled "Speech Recognition in Quiet."

Since listeners with normal hearing, on average, achieve maximal performance at 30 to 40 dB sensation level (SL) re:SRT, clinicians will often test their patients at one of these levels, assuming this will result in maximal performance for the listener. Assessing only a single level may provide limited diagnostic or rehabilitative information. Conversely, assessing performance at multiple levels for individuals with sensory-neural hearing loss provides greater diagnostic information as demonstrated by the example functions drawn in Figure 5.3. In the top panel of Figure 5.3, curve #2 shows a function that reaches maximum performance (88%) at 80 dB HL and plateaus through 100 dB HL. In the bottom panel of Figure 5.3, curve #4 shows a function that reaches maximum performance (85%) at approximately 60 dB HL, and then performance decreases as level is increased, which is depicted by a rollover in the shape of the function.

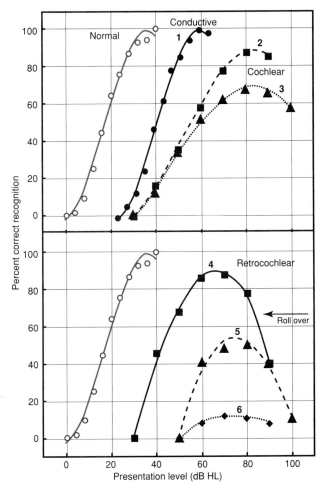

FIGURE 5.3 Psychometric functions of word recognition performance illustrating various types of hearing loss can be seen in both panels as a function of percent correct (ordinate) and presentation level (abscissa). The top panel illustrates a sample psychometric function for a listener with normal hearing (*open circles*), conductive hearing loss (curve #1), and cochlear hearing loss (curves #2 and #3). The bottom panel shows possible psychometric functions for retrocochlear hearing loss (curves #4, #5, and #6). (Adapted from Department of Veterans Affairs, 1997.)

Also of importance when describing performance in terms of the psychometric function is the slope of the function. The slope of the function is typically calculated from the dynamic portion of the function that ranges between 20% and 80%. Scores below 20% are often affected by floor effects because the task difficulty is too great to show subtle changes in performance, whereas scores above 80% are often affected by ceiling effects because the task difficulty is too easy to be sensitive to performance changes. For an individual with a steep slope, the measurements should be made in small (dB) steps to obtain valid results, whereas a shallow function allows for larger step sizes to obtain valid results.

When selecting test material, it is best to choose stimuli that produce a steep function, which suggests the materials are homogenous with respect to the task (Wilson and Margolis, 1983).

Response Mode

The response mode for speech audiometry is generally verbal. However, for SDT, the response mode can be similar to that of puretone thresholds, where the person can push a button or raise their hand when they hear the speech stimuli. A written response is generally avoided because of the increased test time and reliance on the patient's ability to write and spell. For testing children or nonverbal individuals, see Chapters 23 and 29.

Redundancy and Uncertainty

English is a highly redundant language, such that far more information or linguistic cues are found in the structure of the language than necessary to convey a specific meaning. Redundancy is easily explained through the relative frequencies of verbal elements. For example, English can be transcribed using approximately 40 phonemes; however, nine of these 40 phonemes make up more than half of our vocal behavior. Similarly, 12 syllables of the more than 1,370 syllables that can be found in the English language make up 25% of our verbal behavior. Redundant languages are more verbose and less efficient but also are more dependable under adverse conditions (Miller, 1951).

A fair amount of redundancy is required for a reliable language. The absence of redundancy within a language leads to uncertainty. Redundancy and uncertainty are inversely proportional, such that as redundancy is increased, uncertainty is decreased. Miller (1951) emphasized the importance of maximizing redundancy and minimizing uncertainty to improve the ability to understand speech, especially in difficult listening situations.

Bocca and Calearo (1963) further defined redundancy as it relates to language as intrinsic and extrinsic redundancies. According to Bocca and Calearo, intrinsic redundancy refers to the physiologic redundancy provoked by a message at the level of the auditory centers in the brain. Incoming auditory information stimulates the cochlea, where numerous synaptic events between the afferent and efferent pathways electrically transmit the message. Intrinsic redundancies are influenced for an individual by their experience with the language. Extrinsic redundancies can range from probabilistic phonotactics to semantic, syntactic, and pragmatic rules of a language that help to convey the message.

Boothroyd and Nittrouer (1988) examined the effect of extrinsic redundancy on speech recognition and derived mathematical constants related to the constraints imposed at the phonemic level (j factor) and contextual constraints imposed at the sentence level (k factor). As stated earlier, successive words in English are not unrelated. j and k factors represent numerically the interdependencies among successive items in a message, whether they are successive phonemes (probabilistic phonotactics) or successive words (linguistic context).

Intrinsic and extrinsic redundancies decrease uncertainty and increase recognition performance, as does word frequency. Many studies have documented that word frequency is highly correlated with recognition performance, such that the more frequent a word is used in the English language, the easier it is to recognize (Luce, 1986; Marslen-Wilson, 1987). Similarly, word familiarity has an effect on recognition performance, such that words that are highly familiar are easier to recognize, especially in adverse listening situations (Gernsbacher, 1984).

SPEECH RECOGNITION THRESHOLD

Stimuli

Spondaic words are generally used for obtaining SDTs and SRTs and are recommended by ASHA (1988). Spondaic (adjective) words or spondees (noun) are two-syllable words with equal stress on both syllables. Lists of spondaic words for assessing hearing loss for speech were first developed at the Harvard Psychoacoustic Laboratories by Hudgins et al. (1947). Criteria for selection of words included a high level of word familiarity, phonetic dissimilarity, and homogeneity with respect to audibility. Of the original 42 spondees identified by Hudgins et al. (1947), 36 of the most familiar were used in the development of the Central Institute for the Deaf (CID) W-1 and W-2 tests (Hirsh et al., 1952). Currently, ASHA (1988) recommends the use of 15 of the original 36 spondees used in the CID W-1 and W-2 tests for obtaining SRTs. These 15 words, shown in Table 5.1, are the most homogenous with respect to audibility (Young et al., 1982), as is the list of 20 easily pictured spondees for use with children (Frank, 1980).

Recommended SRT Testing Protocol

The SRT measurement involves four steps: (1) instructions; (2) familiarization; (3) initial and test phase for the descending technique; and (4) calculation of threshold. Wilson et al. (1973) originally described these steps, which were subsequently set forth by ASHA (1988) as a guideline for determining an SRT.

STEP 1: INSTRUCTIONS

Patients need to be instructed regarding what stimuli will be used (i.e., spondaic words from the list) and how to respond during the testing procedure (i.e., written or verbal response). Also, it is important to make patients aware that the level of the stimulus will become quite soft and to encourage them to guess throughout the testing procedure.

TABLE 5.1	Spondaic words recommended by ASHA (1988)
15 Most Homogenous Re: Audibility (Young et al., 1982)	**20 Most Easy to Picture (Frank, 1980)**
Toothbrush	Toothbrush
Inkwell	Hotdog
Playground	Baseball
Sidewalk	Airplane
Railroad	Cupcake
Woodwork	Popcorn
Baseball	Bathtub
Workshop	Fire truck
Doormat	Football
Grandson	Mailman
Eardrum	Snowman
Northwest	Ice cream
Mousetrap	Sailboat
Drawbridge	Flashlight
Padlock	Bluebird
	Toothpaste
	Reindeer
	Shoelace
	Seesaw

STEP 2: FAMILIARIZATION

Each patient should be familiarized with the word list to be used during the testing procedure by listening to the list of test words at a level that is easily audible and repeating back each word as a demonstration of word recognition. If a patient is unable to repeat back a particular spondaic word from the test list, then that word should be removed from the test list. Another method of familiarization is to give the patient a written list of the test words to read.

Previous research has shown differences in SRT values obtained with and without familiarization (Conn et al., 1975; Tillman and Jerger, 1959). Specifically, Tillman and Jerger (1959) found poorer SRTs of almost 5 dB HL when individuals were not familiarized with the test list. The ASHA guideline strongly suggests that familiarization not be eliminated from the test protocol.

STEP 3: DETERMINATION OF THRESHOLD

(a) Initial starting level—Present one spondaic word at a level 30 to 40 dB HL above the anticipated SRT. If a correct response is received, drop the level in 10-dB steps until an incorrect response occurs. Once an incorrect response is received, present a second spondaic word at the same level. If the second word is repeated correctly, drop down by 10-dB steps until two words are missed at the same level. Once you reach the level where two spondees are missed, increase the level by 10 dB. This is the starting level.

(b) Threshold estimation—Thresholds have been estimated using 2-dB or 5-dB steps since most audiometers are equipped with those step sizes. Previous studies have shown that threshold differences as a function of step size are too small to be clinically significant (Chaiklin and Ventry, 1964; Wilson et al., 1973).

(2-dB step size)—Present two spondaic words at the starting level. Drop the level by 2 dB, and present two spondaic words. An individual should get the first five out of six words correct or else the starting level needs to be increased by 4 to 10 dB. If at least five of the first six words are correct, continue dropping the level by 2 dB until the individual misses five of six presentations.

(5-dB step size)—Present five spondaic words at the starting level. An individual should get the first five spondaic words correct at the starting level. Drop the level by 5 dB, and present five spondaic words. Continue dropping the level by 5 dB until the individual misses all five spondaic words at the same level.

STEP 4: CALCULATION OF THRESHOLD

Calculation of an SRT is based on the Spearman-Kärber equation (Finney, 1952). An SRT is calculated by subtracting the number of words repeated correctly from the starting level and adding a correction factor of 1 dB when using the 2-dB step size and a correction factor of 2 dB when using the 5-dB step size. For a 5-dB step example, with a starting level of 40 dB, the patient got all five words; at 35 dB, three of the words were correct; and at 30 dB, none were correct. Eight of the 15 words were correct. Therefore, the SRT calculation would be $40 - 8 = 32$, $+ 2$ for the correction, equals 34 dB HL.

Clinical Functions of SRT

The most recent surveys of audiometric practices in the United States reported that 99.5% (Martin et al., 1998) and 83% (ASHA, 2000) use SRT as part of their basic audiologic assessment. The reasons stated for using SRT were: (1) cross validation for puretone thresholds; (2) measurement of communication disability; and (3) reference for supra-threshold measures. Unfortunately, most of the historical purposes lack scientific evidence to support routine clinical use of an SRT (see Wilson and Margolis, 1983). In addition, only 58% of audiologists complete the familiarization step of the test protocol, and 60% do not follow the recommended ASHA protocol (ASHA, 1988) but, instead, determine an SRT using a modified Hughson-Westlake procedure with a two out of three criterion (Martin et al., 1998). These observations are of concern because the SRT is a valid and reliable procedure when standardized recorded materials are used with a specified testing procedure. The SRT is also particularly useful when assessing response reliability in an individual who appears to be malingering (see Chapter 31).

SPEECH RECOGNITION IN QUIET

The purpose of speech recognition testing in quiet is to assess how well a person can understand speech in a quiet environment when the level of the speech is loud enough to obtain a maximum SRS (PB_{max}). The level necessary for a person with hearing loss to perform maximally is highly variable from person to person and is dependent on the materials used to obtain the SRS (Carhart, 1965; Jerger and Hayes, 1977). We feel that it is unfortunate that, in most audiology clinics, speech recognition testing is assessed only at one presentation level (Wiley et al., 1995). The majority of audiologists select a single presentation level 30 to 40 dB SL re:SRT, meaning that the materials are presented 30 to 40 dB above the SRT (Martin et al., 1998; Wiley et al., 1995). Kamm et al. (1983) found that speech recognition testing at 40 dB SL re:SRT did not approximate maximal performance for 40% of their 25 subjects with hearing loss. Evidence suggests that evaluating speech recognition abilities at more than one level captures a portion of the psychometric function and allows a better estimation of performance at PB_{max}. A procedure suggested by Wilson (2005) suggests the use of at least two levels with 25 words presented at each level. For persons with normal hearing or mild hearing loss as evidenced by a puretone average (PTA) of ≤ 35 dB HL for 500, 1,000, and 2,000 Hz, the first level should be 50 dB HL followed by the second level of 70 dB HL. For persons with greater hearing loss, the first level should be 10 dB greater than their PTA of 500, 1,000, and 2,000 Hz, and the second level should be 20 dB greater than the first level. If you are unable to raise the second level 20 dB greater than the first level because of loudness discomfort issues, raise the second level as high as possible over the first level.

Several types of materials are used to assess speech recognition ability in quiet such as sentences, nonsense syllables, and the most commonly used stimuli, monosyllabic words. Previous research has shown that nonsense syllables are the most difficult of the three aforementioned materials for individuals to recognize, whereas sentences are the easiest (e.g., Miller, 1951). Recognition performance of monosyllabic words falls on the performance continuum somewhere between nonsense syllables and sentences. Although monosyllables are the most commonly used stimuli in clinical settings for measuring speech recognition performance in quiet, it is important to note that empirical data (e.g., Bilger, 1984; Boothroyd and Nittrouer, 1988) support that speech recognition performance is a single construct and performance at one level of linguistic complexity (e.g., sentences) can be predicted by performance at another level (e.g., monosyllabic words).

The systematic relationship between recognition performances at various levels of linguistic complexity by adults with acquired hearing losses was demonstrated by Olsen et al. (1997). Performance for phonemes, words in isolation, and words in sentences was measured for 875 listeners with sensory-neural hearing loss. They found that the scores for words in isolation and in sentences were predictable from the phoneme recognition scores, with mean prediction errors of only 6% and 12%, respectively. Thus, for example, a person scoring 60% correct on a phoneme recognition task would be predicted to score 22% ($\pm$ 6%) for the recognition of words in isolation and 42% ($\pm$ 12%) for the recognition of words in sentences.

Monosyllabic Words

Historically, word lists, such as the Northwestern University Auditory Test Number 6 (NU No. 6; Tillman and Carhart, 1966), the CID Auditory Test W-22 (CID W-22; Hirsh et al., 1952), and the Phonetically-Balanced 50 (PB-50; Egan, 1948) have been used to assess word recognition performance in a quiet background during audiologic evaluations.

The initial work of Egan (1944) outlined six principal criteria that the Psychoacoustics Lab at Harvard used to develop the PB-50 word lists. The six criteria were: (1) monosyllabic structure, (2) equal average difficulty of lists, (3) equal range of difficulty of lists, (4) equal phonetic composition of lists, (5) representative sample of American English, and (6) familiar words. According to Hood and Poole (1980), it was assumed by Egan that meeting criteria 1, 4, 5, and 6 would ensure criteria 2 and 3. Further work to revise the PB-50 word lists by Hirsh et al. (1952) and Tillman et al. (1963) utilized the six criteria to create the W-22 word lists and the NU No. 6 word lists, respectively.

PB-50

The initial use of monosyllabic words for speech recognition testing is attributed to Egan (1948) who worked in the Psychoacoustic Laboratories (PAL) at Harvard University. His original pool of 1,000 words was divided into 20 lists of 50 words, which collectively are known as the PAL PB-50 word lists. Each list was considered to be phonetically balanced such that the 50 words that composed a list were a proportionally correct representation of the phonetic elements in English discourse.

CID W-22

Hirsh et al. (1952) had five judges rate the familiarity of the 1,000 monosyllabic words selected by Egan for the PB-50 word lists, and 120 of the PB-50s were selected along with 80 other words to compose the new word lists. These 200 very common words were selected and phonetically balanced into four 50-word lists known as the CID W-22 word lists. The CID W-22 word lists were recorded onto magnetic tape as spoken by Ira Hirsh who monitored his voice on a VU meter stating the carrier phrase "You will say" and letting each target word naturally fall at the end of the phrase. The CID W-22 word lists are some of the most popular word lists used by audiologists for measuring supra-threshold word recognition ability in quiet.

NU No. 6

Lehiste and Peterson (1959) devised lists of CNCs [consonant–syllable nucleus (vowel)–consonant] that were phonemically balanced versus phonetically balanced. That is, lists that were developed to be phonetically balanced did not take into account the position of the sound in a word and how the acoustic realization of the sound would be affected by coarticulatory factors. Lehiste and Peterson argued that phonemic balancing could be accomplished by allowing for the frequency of occurrence of each initial consonant, vowel nucleus, and final consonant to be similar across CNC word lists. The Lehiste and Peterson lists were condensed into four lists of 50 words known today as the NU No. 6.

Historically, 50 words were included in each test list in order to facilitate phonetic balancing and to allow for a simple conversion from number correct to percent correct following testing. Studies have examined the benefits of abbreviating the number of words used per list from 50 to 25 with mixed results in terms of test-retest reliability (Elpern, 1961; Beattie et al., 1978). The most important work regarding this issue of half versus full lists was the examination of speech recognition data as a binomial variable by Thornton and Raffin (1978). As discussed in the earlier section on psychometric functions, performance ability between 20% and 80% is the most variable, while performance ability is least variable at either extreme of the function (Egan, 1948). The results of Thornton and Raffin (1978) support these early views on performance using the binomial distribution to mathematically model word recognition performance. It indicates that the accuracy between scores for the same listener depends on the number of words used per list and the listener's level of performance. In addition, Thornton and Raffin created a table of the lower and upper limits of the 95% critical differences for percentage scores as a function of test items. Table 5.2 shows the critical differences a retest score would need to exceed to be considered statistically different for the original test score. As seen in Table 5.2, as the number of items increases, the range decreases, suggesting that as the set size increases, the variability in the scores decreases, allowing for the detection of more subtle differences in performance. One way to increase set size without increasing test time is to move from whole-word scoring to phoneme scoring (Boothroyd, 1968). In a 25-word list of monosyllables, you have 25 items to score using whole-word scoring, whereas you would have 50 to 75 possible items to score using phoneme scoring.

Sentence Tests

Sentence level tests were developed at Bell Laboratories (Fletcher and Steinberg, 1929) and were used during World War II to evaluate military communication equipment (Hudgins et al., 1947). Until the development of the CID Everyday Sentences (Silverman and Hirsh, 1955), no sentence test had received clinical acceptance. The CID sentences consist of 10 lists of 10 sentences each with 50 key words in each list. Interrogative, imperative, and declarative sentences are

TABLE 5.2	Critical difference ranges (95%) for select percent correct scores as a function of number of test items		
% Correct	10 Words	25 Words	50 Words
0	0–20	0–8	0–4
10	0–50		2–24
20	0–60	4–44	8–36
30	10–70		14–48
40	10–80	16–64	22–58
50	10–90		32–68
60	20–90	36–84	42–78
70	30–90		52–86
80	40–100	56–96	64–92
90	50–100		76–98
100	80–100	92–100	96–100

From Thornton and Raffin, 1978.

included. Responses can be spoken or written and are scored as the percentage of key words correctly recognized.

The basis for the use of sentences in the clinical assessment of speech recognition abilities is that sentences provide a more "realistic" listening condition for everyday communication than does the use of isolated words or nonsense syllables (Silverman and Hirsh, 1955; Bess, 1983). Although sentences may have greater face validity than other stimuli, they also provide semantic, syntactic, and lexical clues, (i.e., extrinsic redundancies). Thus it is difficult to distinguish individuals who do well on a speech recognition task because they have good speech recognition skills or because they make good use of top-down (linguistic, cognitive) processing skills. Another complication of the use of sentence materials is that, as length exceeds seven to nine syllables, memory constraints, particularly in the elderly, may impact performance (Miller, 1956). Despite these potential limitations, several clinically useful sentence tests have been developed. Since the ability to use context is preserved even in older adults with hearing loss, for most patient populations, sentence tests are typically too easy (ceiling effect) and, therefore, fail to distinguish among levels of difficulty. However, they are well suited as adaptive noise procedures (see "Speech Recognition in Noise" section) instead of suprathreshold quiet procedures. An exception to this trend is the use of sentence tests in quiet for individuals with severe-to-profound hearing losses.

For the profoundly impaired patient population, the City University of New York (CUNY) Sentences (Boothroyd et al., 1988), which consist of 72 sets of topic-related sentences, were designed to assess the use of cochlear implants and tactile aids as supplements to speech reading. Each sentence in a set is about one of 12 topics: food, family, work, clothes, animals, homes, sports/hobbies, weather, health, seasons/holidays, money, or music. Each set contains four statements, four questions, and four commands and one

sentence of each length from three to 12 words, for a total of 102 words per set. Performance is scored as the number of words correct. Original recordings were on laservideo disc and were presented via the Computer Assisted Speech Perception Software (CASPER; Boothroyd, 1987) program. The CUNY Sentences are being converted to DVD format with upgrades to the CASPER software as part of current work at the Rehabilitation Engineering Research Center (RERC) on Hearing Enhancement at Gallaudet University (http://www.hearingresearch.org/).

Nonsense Syllable Tests/Phoneme Recognition Tests

The effects of lexical context and word familiarity on test performance can be minimized by the use of nonsense syllable and/or closed-set phoneme recognition tests. Nonsense syllables were one of the first materials used to assess speech recognition ability during the development of telephone circuits at Bell Telephone Laboratories (Campbell, 1910; Fletcher, 1922; Fletcher and Steinberg, 1929). However, clinical use of nonsense syllables for those with hearing loss did not occur until the 1970s when two carefully developed tests became available—The CUNY Nonsense Syllable Test (CUNY-NST; Levitt and Resnick, 1978) and the Nonsense Syllable Test (NST; Edgerton and Danhauer, 1979). The CUNY-NST is a closed-set test consisting of seven subtests, each of which has seven to nine consonant-vowel (CV) or vowel-consonant (VC) syllables. The CUNY-NST assesses perception of the consonants most likely to be confused by individuals with hearing loss using three vowel contexts. The Edgerton-Danhauer NST is an open-set test consisting of 25 nonsense bisyllabic CVCV items, allowing for assessment of the perception of 50 consonant and 50 vowel stimuli. More recently, Boothroyd et al. (1988) described the Three Interval Forced Choice Test of speech pattern contrast perception (THRIFT), a nonsense syllable test that can be used with children 7 years of age or older (Hnath-Chisolm et al., 1998). The THRIFT measures the perception of nine speech pattern contrasts presented in varying phonetic context. Contrasts include: intonation; vowel height and place; and, initial and final consonant voicing, continuance, and place. In addition to minimizing the effects of lexical context and word familiarity on performance, the use of nonsense syllables allows for detailed examination of phonetic errors. Despite these advantages, nonsense syllables lack face validity with regard to being representative of every day speech communication.

Minimization of lexical context and word familiarity effects, while allowing for the analysis of errors and confusions, can also be accomplished through the use of closed-set tests using real word stimuli. Classic tests of phoneme recognition include the Modified Rhyme Test (MRT; House et al., 1955; Kruel et al., 1968) and its variations (i.e., Rhyming Minimal Contrasts Test; Griffiths, 1967; and Distinctive Features Discrimination Test; McPherson and Pang-Ching, 1979) and the California Consonant Test (CCT; Owens and Schubert,

1977). The MRT consists of 50 test items each with six response alternatives. Twenty-five of the items differ by the initial consonant (i.e., bent, went, sent, tent, dent, and rent), and the other 25 items differ by the final consonant (i.e., peas, peak, peal, peace, peach, and peat). The CCT also consists of 100 items but uses a four-choice, rather than a six-choice, response format in assessing perception of 36 initial consonant items and 64 final consonant items. The perception of medial vowels as well as initial and final consonants was added in the University of Oklahoma Closed Response Speech Test by Pederson and Studebaker (1972).

A closed-set format is also used in the Speech Pattern Contrast test (SPAC; Boothroyd, 1984), which was designed to assess the ability to perceive both supra-segmental (i.e., stress and intonation) as well as segmental phonologically (i.e., vowel height and place, initial and final consonant voicing, continuance, and place) relevant distinctions. Test length of SPAC is minimized by combining two segmental contrasts in one subset (e.g., final consonant voicing and continuance) with four items (e.g., seat-seed-cease-sees). Although the SPAC as well as other speech feature tests and nonsense syllable tests are not routinely used in clinical audiology, the information provided about the details of an individual's speech perception ability can be quite useful when assessing the need for and the benefits of hearing aids and cochlear implants for both children and adults.

SPEECH RECOGNITION IN NOISE

One of the most common complaints expressed by individuals with hearing loss is the inability to understand a speaker when listening in an environment of background noise. In 1970, Carhart and Tillman suggested that an audiologic evaluation should include some measure of the ability of an individual to understand speech when in a background of speech noise. Prior to the revival of the directional microphone in the late 1990s, however, the information gained from a speech-in-noise task for most rehabilitative audiologists was not pertinent to the selection of amplification due to the fact that most hearing aids were mainly selected based on gain, slope, and output curves. Thus in the technology-driven field of audiology, speech-in-noise testing failed to gain a place in the traditional audiologic evaluation. The revolution of digital hearing aids and their multitude of features, such as directional microphones, noise reduction strategies, and digital signal processing strategies, have created an important reason for utilizing speech-in-noise tasks on a routine basis when evaluating an individual with hearing loss.

For the past 40 years, researchers have observed that listeners with hearing loss show a greater disadvantage when listening in a competing speech background compared with listeners with normal hearing, such that the signal-to-noise ratio (S/N) needed for the listener with hearing loss is 10 to 15 dB greater than that needed by listeners with normal hearing (e.g., Groen, 1969; Olsen and Carhart, 1967; Carhart

and Tillman, 1970). Plomp (1978) reported that for every 1-dB increase in signal over the competing noise, a listener with hearing loss would receive, on average, an improvement of 3% in terms of ability to recognize the signal. Thus, a 10-dB improvement in S/N should add 30% in terms of intelligibility as measured by open-set, speech recognition tests for listeners with hearing loss.

The addition of background noise to a speech recognition task has been shown to improve the sensitivity and validity of the measurement (Findlay, 1976; Beattie, 1989; Willott, 1991; Sperry et al., 1997; Wiley and Page, 1997). In terms of improving sensitivity, the addition of multiple S/Ns increases the difficulty of the task and allows for separation between individuals with normal hearing and those with hearing loss (Beattie, 1989; McArdle et al., 2005b). Typically, individuals with sensory-neural hearing loss require the signal to be 10 to 12 dB higher than the noise to obtain 50% performance on the psychometric function, whereas individuals with normal hearing on average obtain 50% performance at an S/N of 2 to 6 dB. McArdle et al. (2005a; 2005b) found mean performance on the Words-in-Noise (WIN) test (Wilson, 2003) to be 12.5-dB S/N and 6.0-dB S/N for 383 listeners with hearing loss and 24 listeners with normal hearing, respectively. Similarly, under similar experimental conditions, Dirks et al. (1982) and Beattie (1989) who used CID W-22 word lists in noise found 50% points of 12-dB S/N and 11.3-dB S/N, respectively, for listeners with hearing loss.

Several studies have examined the possibility of predicting the ability of an individual to understand speech in noise using puretone audiograms and SRSs in quiet without success (Cherry, 1953; Groen, 1969; Carhart and Tillman, 1970; Plomp, 1978; Plomp and Mimpen, 1979; Dirks et al., 1982; Beattie, 1989; Killion and Niquette, 2000; Wilson, 2003). The data in Figure 5.4 were compiled from two studies (McArdle et al., 2005a; 2005b). In the figure, performance on a word recognition in quiet task at 80 dB HL is graphed on the ordinate as a function of 50% points on the WIN test along the abscissa. The same words spoken by the same speaker were used for both the recognition task in quiet and in noise. The shaded area of the figure represents the range of performance by 24 listeners with normal hearing on the WIN.

Two main observations can be seen in the data in Figure 5.4: (1) only five out of 387 listeners with hearing loss performed in the normal range on both the recognition task in quiet and in noise; and (2) 45.5% of the 387 listeners with hearing loss had word recognition scores in quiet at 80 dB HL that were ≥90% correct. Thus it is of interest to note that, although 73% of the listeners with hearing loss had word recognition scores in quiet ≥80%, the overwhelming majority of these listeners displayed abnormal performance on a word recognition task in noise. In addition, it is clear that word recognition ability in noise is not easily predicted by word recognition in quiet for listeners with hearing loss other than to say that listeners with poor recognition ability in quiet also perform poorly on word recognition tasks in noise. Because we are unable to predict the ability of an individual to understand speech in a noisy background,

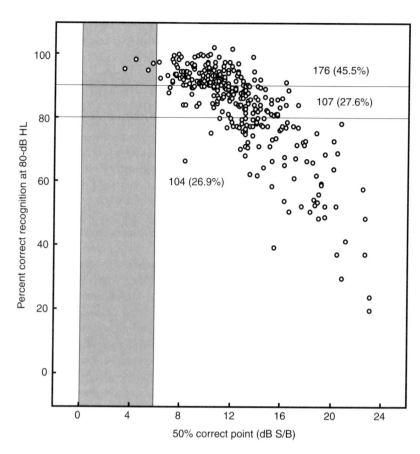

FIGURE 5.4 A plot of word recognition performance in quiet in percent correct (y-axis) versus the 50% point of recognition performance in multi-talker babble on the Words-in-Noise (WIN) test (x-asis). The shaded area of the figure defines the range of performances (10th to 90th percentiles) obtained by listeners with normal hearing on the WIN test. The numbers represent the number of listeners who had word recognition scores in quiet ≥90%, ≥80%, and ≥70% correct on the words in quiet. The data are combined from McArdle et al. (2005a; 2005b). (Reprinted with permission from the *Journal of Rehabilitative Research and Development*.)

audiologists should use the tests available for quantifying the S/N needed by the listener to understand speech in noise. Several materials, described in the following section, have been developed to measure speech-in-noise performance.

Materials

Initially, efforts in speech-in-noise testing were focused on sentence-level materials in order to make the task more of a real-world experience; however, normal everyday sentences were too easy, and further manipulation of the sentences was needed to obtain the 50% correct point of performance for a listener on a speech-in-noise task. Speaks and Jerger (1965) developed the Synthetic Sentence Identification (SSI) test to minimize the effect of contextual cues that often made it easy to understand sentence-level materials even in a background of noise. The stimuli are called synthetic sentences because they are not actual sentences, but rather, they contain normal English phonemes and syntax but no semantic context. An example of a sentence is *"Small boat with a picture has become."* The task of the listener is to select which one of 10 sentences displayed on a response form is perceived when presented against a competing story describing the life of Davy Crockett. The competing story can be presented either contralaterally or ipsilaterally.

Another interesting sentence-level test, the Speech Perception in Noise (SPIN) test (Kalikow et al., 1977), varies the amount of semantic context that leads to the last word of each

sentence, which is a monosyllabic target word. The SPIN test has eight forms of 50 sentences each that are presented at a fixed S/N of 8 dB. The target word in 25 of the sentences has low predictability (LP) given the limited clues from the preceding context, and the other 25 have high predictability (HP) from the preceding sentence context. Recognition performance is scored as the percentage of LP and HP words correctly perceived. By providing both LP and HP scores, the SPIN test not only allows for the assessment of the acoustic-phonetic components of speech but also examines the ability of an individual to utilize linguistic context.

In the 1980s, two additional tests designed to assess recognition of everyday speech based on correct word recognition performance in sentence length stimuli were developed. The Connected Speech Test (CST; Cox et al., 1987), which was developed as a criterion measure in studies of hearing aid benefit, consists of 48 passages of conversationally produced connected speech. Each passage is about a familiar topic and contains 10 sentences. Sentence length varies from seven to 10 words, and there is a total of 25 key words in each passage. Sentences are presented at an individually determined signal-to-noise ratios, and performance is scored as the number of key words correct.

The most recent application of sentence length stimuli is in tests that are scored in terms of the decibel-to-noise ratio required to achieve 50% correct performance. The two most common tests are the Hearing in Noise Test (HINT; Nilsson et al., 1994) and the Quick Speech in Noise Test (QuickSIN;

Killion et al., 2004). The two tests vary in the type of sentences and type of noise used. The HINT uses the Bamford-Kowal-Bench (BKB) Standard Sentence Lists (Bench et al., 1979) that were compiled from the utterances of hearing-impaired children and contain straightforward vocabulary and syntax. Sentences are presented in sets of 10 sentences, and the listener must repeat the entire sentence correctly to receive credit. The noise used is speech-spectrum noise that is held constant while the signal is varied to find the 50% correct point. The QuickSIN uses the Harvard Institute of Electrical and Electronics Engineers (IEEE; 1969) sentences, which are a collection of low-context, meaningful sentences, whose phonetic balance is similar to that of English. In the QuickSIN, there are six sentences per list, and each sentence contains five key words. All sentences are presented in multi-talker babble with the five key words in each sentence scored as correct or incorrect. Recently, the BKB-SIN test (Etymotic Research, 2005) was developed for use with children (ages 5 and up), cochlear implant patients, and adults for whom the QuickSIN test is too difficult.

More recently, monosyllabic and digit materials in multitalker babble have been developed at the Auditory Research Lab of the James H. Quillen Veterans Affairs Medical Center (Wilson, 2003; Wilson and Weakley, 2004; Wilson and Strouse, 2002). The word and digit materials have been shown to be sensitive to the different recognition abilities of normal-hearing and hearing-impaired adults in multitalker babble (Wilson et al., 2003; Wilson and Weakley, 2004).

McArdle et al. (2005b) examined the effect of material type (i.e., digits, words, and sentences) on S/N loss for young listeners with normal hearing and older listeners with hearing impairment. The three speech-in-noise tests that were examined included: (1) QuickSIN (Etymotic Research, 2001); (2) Words-in-Noise Test (WIN) (Wilson and Strouse, 2002; Wilson, 2003); and (3) digit triplets-in-multitalker babble (Wilson and Weakley, 2004). As expected, the younger listeners performed better than the older listeners on all three tasks. For the older listeners with hearing loss, the S/N required for 50% recognition of each material type presented was –4 dB S/N, 12.4 dB S/N, and 11.7 dB S/N for digits, words, and sentences, respectively. Figure 5.5 shows a bivariate plot of the 50% points for the older listeners with hearing loss on both the QuickSIN (abscissa) and the WIN (ordinate). The diagonal line in Figure 5.5 represents equal performance on both QuickSIN and the WIN. As can be seen, mean performance, as indicated by the bold filled circle, is close to the diagonal line, suggesting that either the use of monosyllabic words or IEEE sentences in this population provided a similar measure of performance in noise. More importantly, the performance difference at the 50% point between normal-hearing listeners and hearing-impaired listeners was 7.6 dB for both words and sentences, suggesting that words and sentences in a descending speech-in-noise task were equally sensitive to the effects of hearing loss. For a more in-depth discussion of the use of words or sentences in speech-in-noise testing see Wilson and McArdle (2005).

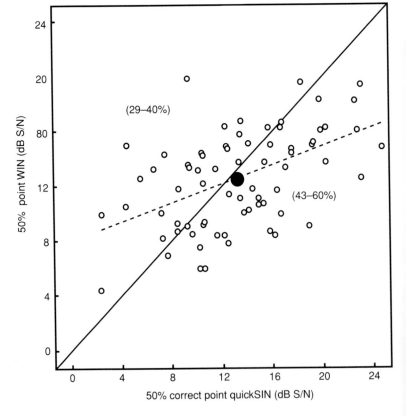

FIGURE 5.5 Bivariate plot of the 50% points (in dB S/N) on the Words-in-Noise (WIN) test (ordinate) and on the Quick Speech in Noise (QuickSIN) test (abscissa). The diagonal line represents equal performance, with the larger filled symbol indicating the mean datum point. The dashed line is the linear regression fit to the data. The numbers in parentheses are the number of performances above and below the line of equal performances. (Reprinted with permission from the *Journal of Rehabilitative Research and Development*.)

A new body of literature has evolved in the area of speech-in-noise testing focused on informational masking, which is defined as nonenergetic masking that increases threshold as a result of uncertainty. Although the term informational masking is more recent, the construct was described by Carhart et al. (1969) and termed perceptual masking. Energetic masking is described in the literature as peripheral masking, such that a stimulus interferes with the perception of a second stimulus making the first stimulus a "masker." Nonenergetic masking, or informational masking, occurs when the target stimulus is similar to the masking stimulus, creating uncertainty for the listener as to whether he or she is hearing the target or the masker. Informational masking can occur at different processing levels (e.g., phonetic, semantic) and is greater for a speech masker than noise, especially when the talker is the same gender or, even worse, the same talker for both the target and the masker (Brungart, 2001). Informational masking has a greater effect when the masker is a single speaker versus a background of multiple talkers since once you add more than a couple speakers the background "information" in the masker becomes hard to distinguish. Most commercially available speech-in-noise tests involve multitalker babble, which decreases the effects of informational masking but future studies in this area are warranted.

CONSIDERATIONS FOR SPEECH AUDIOMETRY IN CHILDREN AND OTHER SPECIAL POPULATIONS

Speech stimuli are used for the behavioral assessment of the auditory function of a child from birth onward. With very young infants, speech stimuli might be used to elicit a startle response, and as the infant develops, SDTs and SRTs can be obtained using a variety of behavioral techniques, such as visual response audiometry or play audiometry. The technique used will be dependent on the motor capabilities of the child. In addition to considering the motor capacity of the child for responding (e.g., head turn, picture pointing), the phonologic, receptive, and expressive language skills of the child need to be considered during speech recognition testing. For example, by the time a child can function at about a 5-year-old level, conventional SRTs can be obtained as long as the spondee words used are within the receptive vocabulary of the child (ASHA, 1988). Similarly, several supra-threshold pediatric speech recognition tests, such as the Word Intelligibility Picture Identification (WIPI) test (Ross and Lerman, 1970) and the Northwestern University Children's Perception of Speech (NU-CHIPS) test (Elliot and Katz, 1980), are comprised of words expected to be within the receptive vocabulary of a child.

A variety of speech recognition tests are available for use with children. For example, both the WIPI and NU-CHIPS

use monosyllabic words presented in a closed-set format. Other test paradigms allow for the assessment of the perception of speech feature contrasts (e.g., Imitative Test of Speech Pattern Contrast Perception [IMSPAC]; Kosky and Boothroyd, 2003; Visually Reinforced Audiometry Speech Pattern Contrast Perception [VRASPAC]; Eisenberg et al., 2004), syllabic pattern and stress (e.g., Early Speech Perception [ESP] test; Moog and Geers, 1990), lexically easy versus lexically hard words (e.g., the Lexical Neighborhood Test [LNT]; Kirk et al., 1995), and words in sentences presented in quiet (e.g., BKB sentences; Bamford and Wilson, 1979) and in noise (e.g., BKB-SIN test; Etymotic Research, 2005), a task which requires word and sentence recognition in both quiet and noise (e.g., Pediatric Speech Intelligibility [PSI] test; Jerger and Jerger, 1984).

In addition to children, special consideration also needs to be given to the assessment of speech perception abilities in profoundly hearing-impaired adults, nonverbal patients, and multilingual patients (Wilson and Strouse, 1999). Profoundly hearing impaired adults typically obtain scores of zero on standard speech recognition tests. As a result, batteries such as the Minimal Auditory Capabilities (MAC) battery have been developed (Owens et al., 1985). Tasks included in the MAC battery involve discrimination of syllabic number, noise versus voice, and statements versus questions; recognition of spondaic words and consonants and vowels in real words in closed-set tasks; and more standard open-set recognition of words in isolation and sentences.

Nonverbal patients are often encountered in medical settings where patients may have medical conditions such as laryngectomies or cerebral vascular accidents. For these patients, written responses or picture pointing tasks may be appropriate. Increases in the ethnic diversity of the US population can result in the audiologist assessing a patient who speaks little to no English. Limited knowledge of English could impact on speech perception performance in the same way that the developing linguistic abilities of a child are important to consider in assessment. Although recorded materials are available in languages such as Spanish (e.g., Wesilender and Hodgson, 1989), unless the audiologist speaks Spanish, errors could be made in determining correct from incorrect responses. Wilson and Strouse (1999) suggest the use of a multimedia approach similar to that used by McCullough et al. (1994) with nonverbal patients. Stimulus words are presented in the patient's native language, and the person responds by selecting the perceived word from a closed set of alternatives shown on a touch-screen monitor. Scoring could be done automatically through a software program.

CLINICAL FUNCTIONS OF SPEECH RECOGNITION MEASURES

One of the historical purposes for the use of speech recognition testing in the clinical test battery was as a diagnostic tool for determining the location of peripheral auditory pathology. Figure 5.3 illustrates typical psychometric functions obtained in quiet for the recognition of monosyllabic words by listeners with normal auditory function as well as those with conductive, sensory (cochlear), and neural (retrocochlear) hearing losses. For normal-hearing listeners, regardless of word recognition materials used, when the presentation level is about 30 dB higher than the dB level needed for 50% performance (i.e., SRT), a score of 90% or better can be expected. For individuals with hearing loss, when listening at a moderate level, scores may range anywhere from 100% correct to 0% correct. Due to this wide dispersion of speech recognition performance across individuals with various types of hearing loss, speech recognition testing provides only limited diagnostic information if testing is done at only one intensity level (see, for discussion, Bess, 1983; Penrod, 1994). When testing is completed at several intensity levels, however, certain patterns of performance can be expected with certain hearing losses (Wilson and Strouse, 1999).

Individuals with conductive hearing loss tend to exhibit little difficulty on speech recognition tests, with performance typically at 90% or better when testing is conducted at moderate SLs (curve #1 of Fig. 5.3). A patient with a sensory-neural hearing loss will generally have poorer SRSs than would a person with the same degree of hearing loss due to conductive pathology. Although a very wide range of scores is found across patients with cochlear as well as retrocochlear hearing losses, SRSs tend to be poorest among those with retrocochlear pathology. While some individuals with cochlear losses will demonstrate a slight decrease in recognition performance when intensity levels are increased beyond the initial level needed for obtaining maximum performance (curve #3 of Fig. 5.3), marked decreases in performance with increasing intensity after maximum performance is achieved are typically characteristic of a neural loss (curves #4 and #5 of Fig. 5.3). The phenomenon of reduced SRSs with increasing intensity that occurs with retrocochlear pathology is referred to as the "rollover" effect (Dirks et al., 1977; Jerger and Jerger, 1971). In addition to rollover, retrocochlear pathology would be suspected in the presence of a significant discrepancy in SRSs between two ears or lower than expected performance at all presentation levels (curve #6 of Fig. 5.3).

Assessment of the central auditory system also uses measures of speech recognition performance. Tasks can be presented either monaurally or binaurally. Monaural tasks use distorted, degraded, or low-redundancy speech stimuli to reduce extrinsic redundancies. Methods of degradation include filtering (e.g., Bocca et al., 1954; Bocca et al., 1955), time compression (e.g. Beasley et al., 1972; Wilson et al., 1994), and reverberation (e.g., Moncur and Dirks, 1967; Nabelek and Robinson, 1982). Binaural tests were designed to assess the ability of the central auditory nervous system to integrate or resynthesize the different parts of a signal that are presented to each of the two ears. For example, in the Bin-

aural Fusion test (Matzker, 1959), a low-pass filtered version of a word is presented to one ear, while a high-pass filtered version of the same word is presented to the opposite ear. A normal-functioning central auditory nervous system is able to integrate the information from each ear and respond with the correct target word. On the other hand, binaural dichotic tasks involve the presentation of different speech signals simultaneously to both ears. The patient must repeat either or both of the signals depending on the test used. Common clinical dichotic tests include Dichotic Digits (Kimura, 1961), the Staggered Spondaic Word test (Katz, 1962), and the Dichotic Sentence Identification test (Fifer et al., 1983). The interpretation of performance on tests designed to assess auditory processing abilities is beyond the scope of the present chapter and is discussed in detail in Chapters 25 and 27.

In addition to diagnostic applications, speech recognition testing has an important role in estimating the adequacy and effectiveness of communication and in the planning and evaluation of (re)habilitative efforts, including the selection and fitting of hearing aids and cochlear implants. For example, many audiologists label speech recognition performance for monosyllabic words presented in quiet performance as "excellent," "good," "fair," or "poor" in an attempt to link performance to the adequacy of communication in everyday settings. However, research designed to demonstrate systematic relationships between recognition performance in quiet and actual everyday communication has been largely unsuccessful (e.g., Davis, 1948; High et al., 1964; Giolas et al., 1979). A better estimate of the impact of a hearing loss on daily communication might be obtained with the use of speech-in-noise tests such as the WIN, QuickSIN, or HINT. As Wilson and McArdle (2005) discuss, speech-in-noise testing allows for the assessment of the most common complaint of patients—the inability to understand speech in background noise; and thus, test results provide important information for use in counseling. Furthermore, test results can provide insight into the use of appropriate amplification and/or cochlear implant speech processing strategies.

In addition to testing in noise, Brandy (2002) points out that audiologists can gain insight into the (re)habilitative needs of patients through recording incorrect word responses, with subsequent examination of speech feature error patterns (e.g., fricatives, stops, glides, etc.). Other rehabilitative applications of speech audiometry include the use of materials that allow for the assessment of use of linguistic context (e.g., Erber, 1992; Flynn and Dowell, 1999) and auditory-visual performance (e.g., Boothroyd, 1987) and for the determination of most comfortable and uncomfortable listening levels (Punch et al., 2004). Information obtained with a variety of materials presented in a variety of paradigms can be useful in determining optimal device settings, starting points for therapeutic intervention, and directions for patient counseling.

▓ REFERENCES

American Speech-Language-Hearing Association. (1988) Guidelines for determining threshold level for speech. *ASHA*. 30, 85–89.

American Speech-Language-Hearing Association. (2000) Audiology survey. Rockville, MD: American Speech-Language-Hearing Association.

American National Standards Institute. (1996) Specifications for Audiometers. S3.6-1996. New York: American National Standards Institute.

Asher WJ. (1958) Intelligibility tests: a review of their standardization, some experiments, and a new test. *Speech Monogr*. 25, 14–28.

Bamford J, Wilson I. (1979) Methodological considerations and practical aspects of the BKB sentence lists. In: Bench J, Bamford JM, eds. *Speech-Hearing Tests and the Spoken Language of Hearing Impaired Children*. London: Academic Press.

Beasley DS, Forman B, Rintelmann WF. (1972) Perception of time-compressed CNC monosyllables by normal listeners. *J Aud Res*. 12, 71–75.

Beattie RC. (1989) Word recognition functions for the CID W-22 Test in multitalker noise for normally hearing and hearing-impaired subjects. *J Speech Hear Disord*. 54, 20–32.

Beattie RC, Svihovec DA, Edgerton BJ. (1978) Comparison of speech detection and spondee thresholds and half- versus full-list intelligibility scores with MLV and taped presentation of NU-6. *J Am Aud Soc*. 3, 267–272.

Bench J, Kowal A, Bamford J. (1979) The BKB (Bamford Kowal-Bench) sentence lists for partially-hearing children. *Br J Audiol*. 13, 108–112.

Bess FH. (1983) Clinical assessment of speech recognition. In: Konkle DF, Rintelmann WF, eds. *Principles of Speech Audiometry*. Baltimore: University Park Press; pp 127–201.

Bilger RC. (1984) Speech recognition test development. In: Elkins E, ed. *Speech Recognition by the Hearing Impaired. ASHA Reports*. 14, 2–7.

Bocca E, Calearo C. (1963) Central hearing processes. In: Jerger J, ed. *Modern Developments in Audiology*. New York: Academic Press; pp 337–368.

Bocca E, Calearo C, Cassinari V. (1954) A new method for testing hearing in temporal bone tumors. *Acta Otolaryngol*. 44, 219–221.

Bocca E, Calaero C, Cassinari V, Migilavacca F. (1955) Testing "cortical" hearing in temporal lobe tumors. *Acta Otolaryngol*. 45, 289–304.

Boothroyd A. (1984) Auditory perception of speech contrasts by subjects with sensorineural hearing loss. *J Speech Hear Res*. 27, 134–144.

Boothroyd A. (1987) CASPER: Computer Assisted Speech Perception Evaluation and Training. Proceedings of the 10th Annual Conference on Rehabilitation Technology. Washington, DC, Association for the Advancement of Rehabilitation Technology.

Boothroyd A. (1968) Developments in speech audiometry. *Sound*. 3–10.

Boothroyd A, Hnath-Chisolm T, Hanin L, Kishon-Rabin L. (1988) Voice fundamental frequency as an aid to the speechreading of sentences. *Ear Hear*. 9, 335–341.

Boothroyd A, Nittrouer S. (1988) Mathematical treatment of context effects in phoneme and word recognition. *J Acoust Soc Am*. 84, 101–114.

Brandy WT. (2002) Speech audiometry. In: Katz J, ed. *Handbook of Clinical Audiology*. 4th ed. Baltimore: Lippincott Williams & Wilkins; pp 96–110.

Brungart DS. (2001) Informational and energetic masking effects in the perception of two simultaneous talkers. *J Acoust Soc Am*. 109, 1101–1109.

Campbell GA. (1910) Telephonic intelligibility. *Philosophical Magazine*. 19, 152–159.

Carhart R. (1951) Basic principles of speech audiometry. *Acta Otolaryngol*. 40, 62–71.

Carhart R. (1965) Problems in the measurement of speech discrimination. *Arch Otolaryngol*. 82, 253–260.

Carhart R, Tillman TW. (1970) Interaction of competing speech signals with hearing losses. *Arch Otolaryngol*. 91, 273–279.

Carhart R, Tillman TW, Greetis ES. (1969) Perceptual masking in multiple sound backgrounds. *J Acoust Soc Am*. 45, 694–703.

Chaiklin JB, Ventry, IM. (1964) Spondee threshold measurement: a comparison of 2- and 5-dB methods. *J Speech Hear Disord*. 29, 47–59.

Cherry EC. (1953) Some experiments on the recognition of speech with one and with two ears. *J Acoust Soc Am*. 25, 975–979.

Conn MJ, Dancer J, Ventry IM. (1975) A spondee list for determining speech reception threshold without prior familiarization. *J Speech Hear Disord*. 40, 388–396.

Cox RM, Alexander GC, Gilmore C. (1987) Development of the connected speech test (CST). *Ear Hear*. 8, 119S–126S.

Davis H. (1948) The articulation area and the social adequacy index for hearing. *Laryngoscope*. 58, 761–778.

Department of Veterans Affairs. (1997) *The Audiology Primer for Students and Health Care Professionals*. Mountain Home, TN: Veterans Affairs Medical Center.

Dirks D, Kamm D, Bower D, Betsworth A. (1977) Use of performance intensity function in diagnosis. *J Speech Hear Disord*. 27, 311–322.

Dirks DD, Morgan DE, Dubno JR. (1982) A procedure for quantifying the effects of noise on speech recognition. *J Speech Hear Disord*. 47, 114–123.

Edgerton BJ, Danhauer JL. (1979) *Clinical implications of speech discrimination testing using nonsense stimuli*. Baltimore: University Park Press.

Egan JP. (1944) *Articulation testing methods*, II. OSRD report no. 3802. Cambridge, MA: Psychoacoustic Laboratory, Harvard University.

Egan JP. (1948) Articulation testing methods. *Laryngoscope*. 58, 955–991.

Eisenberg LS, Martinez AS, Boothroyd A. (2004) Perception of phonetic contrasts in infants. In: Miyamoto RT, ed. *Cochlear Implants: International Congress Series 1273*. Amsterdam: Elsevier; pp 364–367.

Elliot L, Katz D. (1980) *Northwestern University Children's Perception Speech (NU-CHIPS)*. St. Louis: Auditec.

Elpern BS. (1961) The relative stability of half-list and full-list discrimination tests. *Laryngoscope*. 71, 30–36.

Erber NP. (1992) Effects of a question-answer format on visual perception of sentences. *J Acad Rehab Aud*. 25, 113–122.

Etymotic Research. (2005) BKB-SINTM (Compact Disc). Elk Grove Village, IL: Etymotic Research.

Etymotic Research. (2001) QuickSINTM (Compact Disc). Elk Grove Village, IL: Etymotic Research.

Feldmann H. (1970) A history of audiology: a comprehensive report and bibliography from the earliest beginnings to the present. Translations for the Beltone Institute for Hearing Research, 22, 1–111. [Translated by J. Tonndorf from Die geschichtliche entwicklung der horprufungsmethoden, kuze darstellung and bibliographie von der anfongen bis zur gegenwart. In: Leicher L, Mittermaiser R, Theissing G, eds. *Zwanglose Abhandlungen aus dem Gebiet der Hals-Nasen-Ohren-Heilkunde.* Stuttgart, Germany: Georg Thieme Verlag; 1960.]

Fifer RC, Jerger JF, Berlin CI, Tobey EA, Campbell JC. (1983) Development of a dichotic sentence identification test for hearing-impaired adults. *Ear Hear.* 4, 300–305.

Findlay RC. (1976) Auditory dysfunction accompanying noise-induced hearing loss. *J Speech Hear Disord.* 41, 374–380.

Finney DJ. (1952) *Statistical Method in Biological Assay.* London: C. Griffen.

Fletcher H. (1922) The nature of speech and its interpretation. *J Franklin Inst.* 193, 729–747.

Fletcher H, Steinberg J. (1929) Articulation testing methods. *Bell System Technical Journal.* 8, 806–854.

Flynn MC, Dowell RC. (1999) Speech perception in a communicative context: an investigation using question/answer pairs. *J Speech Lang Hear Res.* 42, 540–552.

Frank T. (1980) Clinically significance of the relative intelligibility of pictorially represented spondee words. *Ear Hear.* 1, 46–49.

Gernsbacher MA. (1984) Resolving 20 years of inconsistent interactions between lexical familiarity and orthography, concreteness, and polysemy. *J Exp Psychol Gen.* 113, 256–281.

Giolas TG, Owens E, Lamb SH, Schubert ED. (1979) Hearing performance inventory. *J Speech Hear Disord.* 44, 169–195.

Griffiths JD. (1967) Rhyming minimal contrasts: a simplified diagnostic articulation test. *J Acoust Soc Am.* 42, 236–241.

Groen JJ. (1969) Social hearing handicap: its measurement by speech audiometry in noise. *Int Audiol.* 8, 182–183.

High WS, Fairbanks G, Glorig A. (1964) Scale for self-assessment of hearing handicap. *J Speech Hear Disord.* 29, 215–230.

Hirsh IJ, Davis H, Silverman SR, Reynolds EG, Eldert E, Benson RW. (1952) Development of materials for speech audiometry. *J Speech Hear Disord.* 17, 321–337.

Hirsh IJ, Palva T, Goodman A. (1954) Difference limen and recruitment. *AMA Arch Otolaryngol.* 60, 525–540.

Hnath-Chisolm T, Laipply E, Boothroyd A. (1998) Age-related changes on speech perception capacity. *J Speech Hear Res.* 41, 94–106.

Hood JD, Poole JP. (1980) Influence of the speaker and other factors affecting speech intelligibility. *Audiology.* 19, 434–455.

House AS, Williams CE, Hecker MHL, Kryter KD. (1955) Articulation-testing methods: consonantal differentiation with a closed-response set. *J Acoust Soc Am.* 37, 158–166.

Hudgins CV, Hawkins JE Jr., Karlin JE, Stevens SS. (1947) The development of recorded auditory tests for measuring hearing loss for speech. *Laryngoscope.* 57, 57–89.

Institute of Electrical and Electronics Engineers. (1969) IEEE recommended practice for speech quality measurements. *IEEE Trans Audio Electroacoustics.* 17, 227–246.

Jerger J, Hayes D. (1977) Diagnostic speech audiometry. *Arch Otolaryngol.* 103, 216–222.

Jerger J, Jerger S. (1971) Diagnostic significance of PB word functions. *Arch Otolaryngol.* 93, 573–580.

Jerger S, Jerger J. (1984) *Pediatric Speech Intelligibility Test.* St. Louis: Auditec.

Kalikow DN, Stevens KN, Elliot LL. (1977) Development of a test of speech intelligibility in noise using sentence materials with controlled word predictability. *J Acoust Soc Am.* 61, 1337–1351.

Kamm CA, Morgan DE, Dirks DD. (1983) Accuracy of adaptive procedure estimates of PB-max level. *J Speech Hear Disord.* 48, 202–209.

Katz J. (1962) The use of staggered spondaic words for assessing the integrity of the central auditory nervous system. *J Aud Res.* 2, 327–337.

Killion MC, Niquette PA. (2000) What can the pure-tone audiogram tell us about a patient's SNR loss? *Hear J.* 53, 46–53.

Killion MC, Niquette PA, Gudmundsen GI, Revit LJ, Banerjee S (2004). Development of a quick speech-in-noise test for measuring signal-to-noise ratio loss in normal-hearing and hearing-impaired listeners. *J Acoust Soc Am.* 116, 2395–2405.

Kimura D. (1961) Some effects of temporal lobe damage on auditory perception. *Can J Psychol.* 15, 157–1165.

Kirk KI, Pisoni DB, Osberger MJ. (1995) Lexical effects of unspoken word recognition by pediatric cochlear implant users. *Ear Hear.* 16, 470–481.

Konkle DF, Rintelmann WF. (1983) Introduction to speech audiometry. In: Konkle DF, Rindtelman WF, eds. *Principles of Speech Audiometry.* Baltimore: University Park Press; pp 1–10.

Kosky C, Boothroyd A. (2003) Validation of an on-line implementation of the Imitative Test of Speech Pattern Contrast Perception (IMSPAC). *J Am Acad Audiol.* 14, 72–83.

Kruel EJ, Bell DW, Nixon JC. (1969) Factors affecting speech discrimination test difficulty. *J Speech Hear Res.* 12, 281–287.

Kruel EJ, Nixon JC, Kryter KD, Bell DW, Lang JS, Schubert ED. (1968) A proposed clinical test of speech discrimination. *J Speech Hear Res.* 11, 536–552.

Lehiste I, Peterson G. (1959) Linguistic considerations in the study of speech intelligibility. *J Acoust Soc Am.* 31, 280–286.

Levitt H, Resnick S. (1978) Speech reception by the hearing impaired. *Scand Audiol.* 6 (suppl), 107–130.

Luce PA. (1986) Neighborhood of words in the mental lexicon. In: *Research on Speech Perception (Tech Rep No. 6).* Bloomington, IN: University of Indiana, Department of Psychology, Speech Research Laboratory.

Marslen-Wilson WD. (1987) Functional parallelism in spoken word-recognition. In: Frauenfelder UH, Tyler LK, eds. *Spoken Word Recognition.* Cambridge, MA: MIT Press; pp 71–102.

Martin FN, Champlin CA, Chambers JA. (1998) Seventh survey of audiometric practices in the United States. *J Am Acad Audiol.* 9, 95–104.

Matzker J. (1959) Two new methods for the assessment of central auditory functions in cases of brain disease. *Ann Otol Rhinol Laryngol.* 68, 1185–1197.

McArdle R, Chisolm TH, Abrams HB, Wilson RH, Doyle PJ. (2005a) The WHO-DAS II: measuring outcomes of hearing aid intervention for adults. *Trends Amplif.* 9, 127–143.

McArdle R, Wilson RH, Burks CA. (2005b) Speech recognition in multitalker babble using digits, words, and sentences. *J Am Acad Audiol.* 16, 726–739.

McCullough JA, Wilson RH, Birck JD, Anderson LG. (1994) A multimedia approach for estimating speech recognition in multilingual clients. *Am J Audiol.* 3, 19–22.

McPherson DF, Pang-Ching GK. (1979) Development of a distinctive feature discrimination test. *J Aud Res.* 19, 235–246.

Miller GA. (1951) *Language and Communication.* New York: McGraw-Hill.

Miller GA. (1956) The magical number seven, plus or minus two: some limits on our capacity for processing information. *Psychol Rev.* 63, 81–97.

Moncur JP, Dirks DD. (1967) Binaural and monaural speech intelligibility in reverberation. *J Speech Hear Res.* 10, 186–195.

Moog JS, Geers AE. (1990) *Early Speech Perception Test for Profoundly Deaf Children.* St. Louis: Central Institute for the Deaf.

Nabelek A, Robinson P. (1982) Monaural and binaural speech perception in reverberation for listeners of various ages. *J Acoust Soc Am.* 71, 1242–1248.

Nilsson M, Soli S, Sullivan J. (1994) Development of the Hearing in Noise Test for the measurement of speech reception thresholds in quiet and in noise. *J Acoust Soc Am.* 95, 1085–1099.

Olsen WO, Carhart R. (1967) Development of test procedures for evaluation of binaural hearing aids. In: *Bulletin of Prosthetics Research: Prosthetic and Sensory Aids Service.* Washington, DC: Department of Medicine and Surgery, Veterans Administration; pp 22–49.

Olsen WO, Van Tassell DJ, Speaks CE. (1997) Phoneme and word recognition for words in isolation and in sentences. *Ear Hear.* 18, 175–188.

Owens E, Kessler DT, Raggio MW, Schubert ED. (1985) Analysis and revision of the minimum auditory capabilities (MAC) battery. *Ear Hear.* 6, 280–290.

Owens E, Schubert ED. (1977) Development of the California Consonant Test. *J Speech Hear Res.* 20, 463–474.

Pederson OT, Studebaker GA. (1972) A new minimal-contrast closed-response-set speech test. *J Aud Res.* 12, 187–195.

Penrod JP. (1994) Speech threshold and word recognition/discrimination testing. In: Katz J, ed. *Handbook of Clinical Audiology.* 4th ed. Baltimore: Williams & Wilkins; pp 147–164.

Penrod JP. (1979) Talker effects on word-discrimination scores of adults with sensorineural hearing impairment. *J Speech Hear Disord.* 44, 340–349.

Plomp R. (1978) Auditory handicap of hearing impairment and the limited benefit of hearing aids. *J Acoust Soc Am.* 63, 533–549.

Plomp R, Mimpen AM. (1979) Speech-reception threshold for sentences as a function of age and noise level. *J Acoust Soc Am.* 66, 1333–1342.

Punch J, Joseph A, Rakerd B. (2004) Most comfortable and uncomfortable loudness levels: six decades of research. *Am J Audiol.* 13, 144–157.

Ross M, Lerman J. (1970) A picture identification task for hearing-impaired children. *J Speech Hear Res.* 13, 44–53.

Schiavetti N, Metz DE. (2002) *Evaluating Research in Communicative Disorders.* 4th ed. Boston: Allyn & Bacon; 2002.

Silverman SR, Hirsh IJ. (1955) Problems related to the use of speech in clinical audiometry. *Ann Otol Rhinol Laryngol.* 64, 1234–1244.

Speaks C, Jerger J. (1965) Performance-intensity characteristics of synthetic sentences. *J Speech Hear Res.* 9, 305–312.

Sperry JL, Wiley TL, Chial MR. (1997) Word recognition performance in various background competitors. *J Am Acad Audiol.* 8, 71–80.

Thornton AR, Raffin MJM. (1978) Speech-discrimination scores modeled as a binomial variable. *J Speech Hear Res.* 21, 507–518.

Tillman TW, Carhart R. (1966) An expanded test for speech discrimination utilizing CNC monosyllabic words. Northwestern University Auditory Test No. 6. Brooks Air Force Base, TX: US Air Force School of Aerospace Medicine.

Tillman TW, Carhart R, Wilber L. (1963) A test for speech discrimination composed of CNC monosyllabic words. Northwestern University Auditory Test No. 4. Technical Documentary Report No. SAM-TDR-62-135. Brooks Air Force Base, TX: US Air Force School of Aerospace Medicine.

Tillman TW, Jerger JF. (1959) Some factors affecting the spondee threshold in normal-hearing subjects. *J Speech Hear Res.* 2, 141–146.

Wesilender P, Hodgson WR. (1989) Evaluation of four Spanish word recognition ability lists. *Ear Hear.* 10, 387–392.

Wiley TL, Page AL. (1997) Summary: current and future perspectives on speech perception tests. In: Medel LL, Danhauer JL, eds. *Audiologic Evaluation and Management and Speech Perception Assessment.* San Diego: Singular Publishing Group; pp 201–210

Wiley TL, Stoppenbach DT, Feldhake LI, Moss KA, Thordardottir ET. (1995) Audiologic practices: what is popular versus what is supported by evidence. *Am J Audiol.* 4, 26–34.

Willott JF. (1991) *Aging and the Auditory System.* San Diego: Singular Publishing Group.

Wilson RH. (2003) Development of a speech in multitalker babble paradigm to assess word-recognition performance. *J Am Acad Audiol.* 14, 453–470.

Wilson RH. (2005) Personal communication.

Wilson RH, Abrams HB, Pillion AL. (2003) A word-recognition task in multitalker babble using a descending presentation mode from 24 dB to 0 dB in signal to babble. *J Rehab Res Dev.* 40, 321–328.

Wilson RH, Margolis RH. (1983) Measurements of auditory thresholds for speech stimuli. In: Konkle DF, Rintelmann WF, eds. *Principles of Speech Audiometry.* Baltimore: University Park Press; pp 79–126.

Wilson RH, McArdle R. (2005) Speech signals used to evaluate the functional status of the auditory system. *J Rehabil Res Dev.* 42 (suppl 2), 79–94.

Wilson RH, Morgan DE, Dirks DD. (1973) A proposed SRT procedure and its statistical precedent. *J Speech Hear Disord.* 38, 184–191.

Wilson RH, Preece JP, Salamon DL, Sperry JL, Bornstein SP. (1994) Effects of time compression and time compression plus reverberation on the intelligibility of Northwestern University Auditory Test No. 6. *J Am Acad Audiol.* 5, 269–277.

Wilson RH, Preece JP, Thornton AR. (1990) Clinical use of the compact disc in speech audiometry. *ASHA.* 32, 3247–3251.

Wilson RH, Strouse A. (1999) Auditory measures with speech signals. In: *Contemporary Perspectives in Hearing Assessment.* Needham Heights, MA: Allyn & Bacon.

Wilson RH, Strouse A. (2002) Northwestern University Audiology Test #6 in multitalker bubble: a preliminary report. *J Rehabil Res Dev.* 39, 105–113.

Wilson RH, Weakley DG. (2004) The use of digit triplets to evaluate word-recognition abilities in multitalker babble. *Semin Hear.* 25, 93–111.

Young L, Dudley B, Gunter MB. (1982) Thresholds and psychometric functions of the individual spondaic words. *J Speech Hear Res.* 25, 586–593.

Clinical Masking

William S. Yacullo

A major objective of the basic audiologic evaluation is assessment of auditory function of each ear. There are situations during both air-conduction and bone-conduction testing when this may not occur. Although a puretone or speech stimulus is being presented through a transducer to the test ear, the nontest ear can contribute partially or totally to the observed response. Whenever it is suspected that the nontest ear is responsive during evaluation of the test ear, a masking stimulus must be applied to the nontest ear in order to eliminate its participation.

THE NEED FOR MASKING

Air-Conduction Testing

Cross hearing occurs when a stimulus presented to the test ear "crosses over" and is perceived in the nontest ear. There are two parallel pathways by which sound presented through an earphone (i.e., an air-conduction transducer) can reach the nontest ear. Specifically, there are both bone-conduction and air-conduction pathways between an air-conduction signal presented at the test ear and the sound reaching the nontest ear cochlea (Studebaker, 1979). First, the earphone can vibrate with sufficient force to cause deformations of the bones of the skull. An earphone essentially can function as a bone vibrator at higher sound pressures. Because both cochleas are housed within the same skull, the outcome is stimulation of the nontest ear cochlea through bone conduction. Second, sound from the test earphone can travel around the head to the nontest ear, enter the opposite ear canal, and finally reach the nontest ear cochlea through an air-conduction pathway. Because the opposite ear typically is covered during air-conduction testing, sound attenuation provided by the earphone will greatly minimize or eliminate the contribution of the air-conduction pathway to the process of cross hearing.

Consequently, cross hearing during air-conduction testing is considered primarily a bone-conduction mechanism.

Cross hearing is the result of limited interaural attenuation (IA). IA refers to the "reduction of energy between ears." Generally, it represents the amount of separation or the degree of isolation between ears during testing. Specifically, it is the decibel difference between the hearing level (HL) of the signal at the test ear and the HL reaching the nontest ear:

$$IA = dB\ HL_{Test\ Ear} - dB\ HL_{Nontest\ Ear}$$

Consider the following hypothetical examples presented in Figure 6.1. You are measuring puretone air-conduction threshold using traditional supra-aural earphones. A puretone signal of 90 dB HL is presented to the test ear. Because of limited IA, a portion of the test signal can reach the nontest ear cochlea. If IA is 40 dB, then 50 dB HL theoretically is reaching the nontest ear.

$$IA = dB\ HL_{Test\ Ear} - dB\ HL_{Nontest\ Ear}$$
$$= 90\ dB\ HL - 50\ dB\ HL$$
$$= 40dB$$

If IA is 80 dB, then only 10 dB HL is reaching the nontest ear. It should be apparent that a greater portion of the test signal can reach the nontest ear when IA is small. Depending on the hearing sensitivity in the nontest ear, cross hearing can occur.

IA during earphone testing is dependent on three factors: transducer type, frequency spectrum of the test signal, and individual subject. There are three major types of earphones currently used during audiologic testing: supra-aural, circumaural, and insert (American National Standards Institute [ANSI], 2004b). Supra-aural earphones use a cushion that makes contact solely with the pinna. Circumaural earphones use a cushion that encircles or surrounds the pinna, making contact with the skin covering the cranial

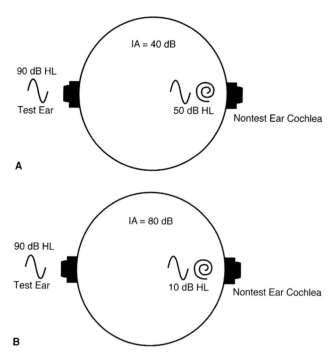

A

B

FIGURE 6.1 Interaural attenuation (IA) is calculated as the difference between the hearing level (HL) of the signal at the test ear and the HL reaching the nontest ear cochlea. A puretone signal of 90 dB HL is being presented to the test ear through traditional supra-aural earphones. Example A: If interaural attenuation is 40 dB, then 50 dB HL is reaching the nontest ear cochlea. Example B: If interaural attenuation is 80 dB, then 10 dB HL is reaching the nontest ear cochlea. (From Yacullo WS. [1996] *Clinical Masking Procedures.* Boston, MA: Allyn & Bacon; p 3. Copyright © 1996 by Pearson Education. Adapted by permission of the publisher.)

skull. Insert earphones are coupled to the ear by insertion into the ear canal.

Generally, IA increases as the contact area of the transducer with the skull decreases (Zwislocki, 1953). More specifically, IA is greater for supra-aural than circumaural earphones. Furthermore, IA is greatest for insert earphones (Killion et al., 1985; Sklare and Denenberg, 1987), partly because of their smaller contact area with the skull. (The reader is referred to Killion and Villchur [1989] and Zwislocki et al. [1988] for a review of advantages and disadvantages of earphones in audiometry.) Because supra-aural and insert earphones are most typically used during audiologic testing, they will be the focus of this discussion.

There are different approaches to measuring IA for air-conducted sound (e.g., "masking" method, "compensation" method, method of 'best beats'; the reader is referred to Zwislocki [1953] for discussion). The most direct approach, however, involves measurement of transcranial thresholds (Berrett, 1973). Specifically, IA is measured by obtaining unmasked air-conduction (AC) thresholds in subjects with

unilateral, profound sensory-neural hearing loss and then calculating the threshold difference between the normal and impaired ears:

$$IA = Unmasked\ AC_{Impaired\ Ear} - Unmasked\ AC_{Normal\ Ear}$$

For example, if unmasked air-conduction thresholds are obtained at 60 dB HL in the impaired ear and 0 dB HL in the normal ear, then IA is calculated as 60 dB:

$$IA = 60\,dB\,HL - 0\,dB\,HL$$
$$= 60\,dB$$

There is the assumption that air- and bone-conduction thresholds are equal (i.e., no air-bone gaps) in the ear with normal hearing.

Figure 6.2 illustrates the expected *unmasked* puretone air-conduction thresholds in an individual with normal hearing in the left ear and a profound sensory-neural hearing loss in the right ear. Unmasked bone-conduction thresholds, regardless of bone vibrator placement, are expected at HLs consistent with normal hearing in the left ear. If appropriate contralateral masking is not used during air-conduction testing, then a shadow curve will result in the right ear. Because cross hearing is primarily a bone-conduction mechanism, unmasked air-conduction thresholds in the right ear will "shadow" the bone-conduction thresholds in the left (i.e., better) ear by the amount of IA. For example, if IA for air-conducted sound is equal to 60 dB at all frequencies, then unmasked air-conduction thresholds in the right ear theoretically will be measured 60 dB above the bone-conduction thresholds in the better ear. The shadow curve does not represent true hearing thresholds in the right ear. Rather, it reflects cross-hearing responses from the better (i.e., left) ear.

When using supra-aural earphones, IA for puretone air-conducted signals varies considerably, particularly across subjects, ranging from about 40 dB to 85 dB (Berrett, 1973; Chaiklin, 1967; Coles and Priede, 1970; Killion et al., 1985; Sklare and Denenberg, 1987; Smith and Markides, 1981; Snyder, 1973). Your assumption about IA will influence a decision about the need for contralateral masking. The use of a smaller IA value assumes that there is smaller separation between ears. Consequently, contralateral masking will be required more often. When making a decision about the need for contralateral masking during clinical practice, a single value defining the lower limit of IA is recommended (Studebaker, 1967a).

Based on currently available data, a conservative estimate of IA for supra-aural earphones is 40 dB at all frequencies.

Although this very conservative estimate will take into account the IA characteristics of all individuals, it will result in the unnecessary use of masking in some instances.

Commonly used insert earphones are the Etymotic Research ER-3A (Killion, 1984) and the E-A-RTONE 3A (E-A-R Auditory Systems, 1997). The ER-3A and the E-A-RTONE 3A insert earphones are considered functionally

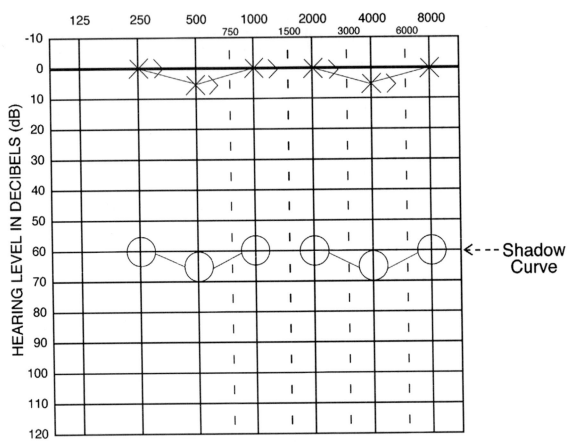

FIGURE 6.2 Expected unmasked puretone air- and bone-conduction thresholds in an individual with normal hearing in the left ear and a profound sensory-neural hearing loss in the right ear. Without the use of appropriate contralateral masking, a shadow curve will result in the right ear. Unmasked air-conduction thresholds in the right ear will shadow the bone-conduction thresholds in the better (i.e., left) ear by the amount of interaural attenuation. (From Yacullo WS. [1996] *Clinical Masking Procedures*. Boston, MA: Allyn & Bacon; p 7. Copyright © 1996 by Pearson Education. Adapted by permission of the publisher.)

equivalent because they are built to identical specifications (Frank and Vavrek, 1992). Each earphone consists of a shoulder-mounted transducer, a plastic sound tube of specified length, a nipple adaptor, and a disposable foam eartip. A major advantage of the 3A insert earphone is increased IA for air-conducted sound, particularly in the lower frequencies (Hosford-Dunn et al., 1986; Killion et al., 1985; Sklare and Denenberg, 1987; Van Campen et al., 1990). This is clearly illustrated in the results of a study by Killion et al. (1985) (Fig. 6.3).

Increased IA with 3A insert earphones is the result of two factors: (1) reduced contact area of the transducer with the skull; and (2) reduction of the occlusion effect. Zwislocki (1953) evaluated IA for three types of earphones: circumaural, supra-aural, and insert. Results suggested that IA for air-conducted sound increased as the contact area of the earphone with the skull decreased. When an acoustic signal is delivered through an earphone, the resultant sound pressure acts over a surface area of the skull determined by the earphone cushion. The surface area associated with a small eartip will result in a smaller applied force to the skull, resulting in reduced bone-conduction transmission.

Chaiklin (1967) also has suggested that IA may be increased in the low frequencies with a deep insert because of a reduction of the occlusion effect. ANSI (2004b) defines the occlusion effect as an increase in loudness for bone-conducted sound at frequencies below 2,000 Hz when the outer ear is covered or occluded. There is evidence that the occlusion effect influences the measured IA for air-conducted sound (e.g., Berrett, 1973; Chaiklin, 1967; Feldman, 1963; Killion et al., 1985; Littler et al., 1952; Van Campen et al., 1990; Zwislocki, 1953). In fact, there is an inverse relationship between magnitude of the occlusion effect and the measured IA in the lower frequencies. Specifically, an earphone that reduces the occlusion effect will exhibit increased IA for air-conducted sound. If the opposite ear is occluded and exhibits a normal occlusion effect, then IA will be increased in magnitude by the size of the occlusion effect (Berrett, 1973). Recall that cross hearing occurs primarily through the mechanism of bone conduction. When the nontest ear is covered or occluded by an air-conduction transducer, the presence of an occlusion effect will enhance hearing sensitivity for bone-conducted sound in that ear. Consequently, the separation between ears is reduced, and the measured IA

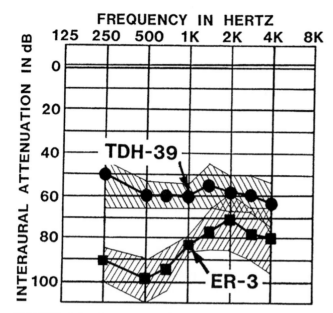

FIGURE 6.3 Average and range of interaural attenuation values obtained on six subjects using two earphones: TDH-39 encased in MX-41/AR supra-aural cushion (•) and ER-3A insert earphone with deeply inserted foam eartip (■). (From Killion MC, Wilber LA, Gudmundsen Gl. [1985] Insert earphones for more interaural attenuation. *Hearing Instruments.* 36, 34. Copyright © 1985. *Hearing Instruments* is a copyrighted publication of Advanstar Communications Inc. All rights reserved. Reprinted by permission of the publisher.)

is increased. The increased IA for air-conducted sound observed in the lower frequencies when using 3A insert earphones (with deeply inserted foam eartips) is primarily related to the significant reduction or elimination of the occlusion effect. The occlusion effect is presented in greater detail later in this chapter in the section on clinical masking procedures during bone-conduction audiometry.

If increased IA is a primary goal when selecting an insert earphone, then the 3A is the transducer of choice. Evidence suggests that the 3A insert earphone provides significantly greater IA, particularly in the lower frequencies, than the "button" transducer (Blackwell et al., 1991; Hosford-Dunn et al., 1986). Blackwell et al. (1991) compared the IA obtained with a standard supra-aural earphone (TDH-50P) and a button transducer fitted with a standard immittance probe cuff. Although greater IA was observed with the button transducer, the difference between the insert and supra-aural earphone did not exceed 10 dB at any frequency.

There are only limited data available regarding IA of 3A insert earphones using deeply or intermediately inserted foam eartips. IA values vary across subjects and frequency, ranging from about 75 dB to 110 dB at frequencies of ≤1,000 Hz and about 50 dB to 95 dB at frequencies >1,000 Hz

(Killion et al., 1985; Sklare and Denenberg, 1987; Van Campen et al., 1990). Based on Studebaker's (1967a) recommendation, we again will use the smallest IA values reported when making a decision about the need for contralateral masking. In order to take advantage of the significantly increased IA proved by the 3A insert in the lower frequencies, a single value of IA will not be employed across the frequency range.

Based on currently available data, conservative estimates of IA for 3A insert earphones with deeply inserted foam eartips are 75 dB at ≤1,000 Hz and 50 dB at frequencies >1,000 Hz.

The IA values recommended clinically for 3A earphones assume that deeply inserted foam eartips are used. Maximum IA is achieved in the low frequencies when a deep eartip insertion is used (Killion et al., 1985). The recommended deep insertion depth is achieved when the outer edge of the eartip is 2 to 3 mm inside the entrance of the ear canal. Conversely, a shallow insertion is obtained when the outer edge of the eartip protrudes from the entrance of the ear canal (E-A-R Auditory Systems, 1997). An intermediate insertion is achieved when the outer edge of the eartip is flush with the opening of the ear canal (Van Campen et al., 1990). There are limited data suggesting that IA is similar for either intermediate or deep insertion of the foam eartip. However, a shallow insertion appears to significantly reduce IA (Killion et al., 1985; Sklare and Denenberg, 1987; Van Campen et al., 1990). Remember that a major factor contributing to superior IA of the 3A insert earphone is a significantly reduced occlusion effect. There is evidence that the occlusion effect is negligible when using either deeply or intermediately inserted insert earphones. In fact, the advantage of a greatly reduced occlusion effect is lost when a shallow insertion is used (Berger and Kerivan, 1983). In order to achieve maximum IA with 3A insert earphones, deeply inserted eartips are strongly recommended.

Recently, E-A-R Auditory Systems (2000a; 2000b) introduced a next-generation insert earphone, the E-A-RTONE 5A. The lengthy plastic sound tube that conducted sound from the body level transducer of the 3A has been eliminated in the 5A model; rather, the foam eartip is coupled directly to an ear level transducer. Very limited data obtained with only two subjects (unpublished research by Killion, 2000, as cited in E-A-R Auditory Systems, 2000b) suggest that the average IA for puretone stimuli ranging from 250 to 4,000 Hz is equivalent (within approximately 5 dB) to the average values reported for the 3A insert earphone (Killion et al., 1985).

IA for speech typically is measured by obtaining speech recognition thresholds (SRT) in individuals with unilateral, profound sensory-neural hearing loss. Specifically, the difference in threshold between the normal ear and impaired ear without contralateral masking is calculated:

$$IA = Unmasked\ SRT_{Impaired\ Ear} - SRT_{Normal\ Ear}$$

Recall that SRT represents the lowest HL at which speech is recognized 50% of the time (ANSI, 2004b; American

Speech-Language-Hearing Association [ASHA], 1988). IA for spondaic words presented through supra-aural earphones varies across subjects and ranges from 48 dB to 76 dB (Martin and Blythe, 1977; Sklare and Denenberg, 1987; Snyder, 1973). Again, a single value defining the lower limit of IA is recommended when making a decision about the need for contralateral masking (Studebaker, 1967a). A conservative estimate of IA for spondees, therefore, is 45 dB when using supra-aural earphones (Konkle and Berry, 1983). The majority of audiologists measure SRT using a 5-dB step size (Martin et al., 1998). Therefore, the IA value of 48 dB is typically rounded down to 45 dB.

There is considerable evidence that speech can be detected at a lower HL than that required to reach SRT. Speech detection threshold (SDT) is defined as the lowest HL at which speech can be detected or "discerned" 50% of the time (ASHA, 1988). The SRT typically requires an average of about 8 to 9 dB greater HL than that required for the detection threshold (Beattie et al., 1978; Chaiklin, 1959; Thurlow et al., 1948). Given this relationship between the two speech thresholds, Yacullo (1996) has suggested that a more conservative value of IA may be appropriate when considering the need for contralateral masking during measurement of SDT.

Consider the following hypothetical example. You are measuring speech thresholds in a patient with normal hearing in the right ear and a profound, sensory-neural hearing loss in the left ear. If the patient exhibits the minimum reported IA value for speech of 48 dB, then an SRT of 0 dB HL would be measured in the right ear and an *unmasked* SRT of 48 dB HL would be measured in the left ear. If an unmasked SDT is subsequently measured in the left ear, it is predicted that the threshold would occur at an HL about 8 to 9 dB lower than the unmasked SRT. An unmasked SDT would be expected to occur at about 39 to 40 dB HL. Comparison of the unmasked SDT in the impaired ear with the SRT in the normal ear theoretically would result in measured IA of approximately 39 to 40 dB. When an unmasked SDT is measured and the response is compared to the SRT in the nontest ear, a more conservative estimate of IA for speech may be appropriate.

It should be noted that the actual IA for speech does not change during measurement of speech detection and recognition thresholds. Rather, a different response task when measuring *different* speech thresholds in each ear (i.e., SDT in one ear and SRT in the other) can affect the measured IA for speech. Comparison of SRTs between ears or SDTs between ears generally should result in the same measured IA. Smith and Markides (1981) measured IA for speech in 11 subjects with unilateral, profound hearing loss. IA was calculated as the difference between the SDT in the better ear and the unmasked SDT in the poorer ear. The range of IA values was 50 to 65 dB. It is interesting to note that the lowest IA value reported for speech using a detection task in each ear was 50 dB, a value comparable to the lowest minimum reported IA value (i.e., 48 dB) for spondaic words (e.g., Martin and Blythe, 1977; Snyder, 1973).

There is also some evidence that it may be appropriate to use a more conservative estimate of IA when making a decision about the need for contralateral masking during assessment of supra-threshold speech recognition. Although IA for the speech signal remains constant during measurement of threshold or supra-threshold measures of speech recognition (i.e., the decibel difference between the level of the speech signal at the test ear and the level at the nontest ear cochlea), differences in the performance criterion for each measure must be taken into account when selecting an appropriate IA value for clinical use. SRT is defined relative to a 50% response criterion. However, supra-threshold speech recognition performance can range from 0% to 100%.

Konkle and Berry (1983) provide an excellent rationale for the use of a more conservative estimate of IA when measuring supra-threshold speech recognition. They suggest that the fundamental difference in percent correct criterion requires the specification of nontest ear cochlear sensitivity in a different way than that used for threshold measurement. If supra-threshold speech recognition materials are presented at an HL equal to the SRT, then a small percentage of the test items can be recognized. It should be noted that the percentage of test words that can be recognized at an HL equal to SRT is dependent on the type of speech stimuli, as well as on the talker and/or recorded version of a speech recognition test. Regardless of the type of speech stimulus (e.g., meaningful monosyllabic words, nonsense syllables, or sentences) and the specific version (i.e., talker/recording) of a speech recognition test, 0% performance may not be established until an HL of about −10 dB relative to the SRT. Konkle and Berry (1983) recommend that the value of IA used for measurement of supra-threshold speech recognition should be estimated as 35 dB. That is, the IA value of 45 dB (rounded down from 48 dB) based on SRT measurement is adjusted by subtracting 10 dB. This adjustment in the estimate of IA reflects differences in percent correct criterion used for speech threshold and supra-threshold measurements.

The majority of audiologists use an IA value of 40 dB for all air-conduction measurements, both puretone and speech, when making a decision about the need for contralateral masking (Martin et al., 1998). The use of a single IA value of 40 dB for both threshold and supra-threshold speech audiometric measurements can be supported. Given the smallest reported IA value of 48 dB for spondaic words, a value of 40 dB is somewhat too conservative during measurement of SRT. However, it should prove adequate during measurement of SDT and supra-threshold speech recognition when a more conservative estimate of IA (by around 10 dB) may be appropriate.

Unfortunately, there are only very limited data available about IA for speech when using insert earphones. Sklare and Denenberg (1987) reported IA for speech (i.e., SRT using spondaic words) in seven adults with unilateral, profound sensory-neural hearing loss using ER-3A insert earphones.

IA ranged from 68 to 84 dB. It should be noted that the smallest reported value of IA for spondaic words (i.e., 68 dB) is 20 dB greater when using 3A insert earphones with deeply inserted foam eartips (Sklare and Denenberg, 1987) than when using supra-aural earphones (i.e., 48 dB) (Martin and Blythe, 1977; Snyder, 1973). Therefore, a value of 60 dB represents a very conservative estimate of IA for speech when using 3A insert earphones. This value is derived by adding a correction factor of 20 dB to the conservative IA value used with supra-aural earphones (i.e., 40 dB) for all threshold and supra-threshold measures of speech.

Based on currently available data, conservative estimates of IA for all threshold and supra-threshold measures of speech are 40 dB for supra-aural earphones and 60 dB for 3A insert earphones with deeply inserted foam eartips.

Bone-Conduction Testing

There are two possible locations for placement of a bone vibrator (typically, the Radioear B-71) during puretone threshold audiometry: the mastoid process of the temporal bone and the frontal bone (i.e., the forehead). Although there is some evidence that a forehead placement produces more reliable and valid thresholds than a mastoid placement (see Dirks [1994] for further discussion), the majority (92%) of audiologists in the United States continue to place a bone-conduction transducer on the mastoid process (Martin et al., 1998).

IA is greatly reduced during bone-conduction audiometry. IA for bone-conducted sound when using a bone vibrator placed at the forehead is essentially 0 dB at all frequencies; IA when using a mastoid placement is approximately 0 dB at 250 Hz and increases to about 15 dB at 4,000 Hz (Studebaker, 1967a). Regardless of the placement of a bone vibrator (i.e., mastoid vs. forehead), it is generally agreed that IA for bone-conducted sound at all frequencies is negligible and should be considered 0 dB (e.g., Dirks, 1994; Hood, 1960; Sanders and Rintelmann, 1964; Studebaker, 1967a). When a bone vibrator, regardless of its location, sets the bones of the skull into vibration, both cochleas potentially can be stimulated. Consequently, an unmasked bone-conduction threshold can reflect a response from either cochlea or perhaps both. Although a bone vibrator may be placed at the side of the test ear, it cannot be assumed that the observed response is in fact from that ear.

Consider the following example. You have placed a bone vibrator at the right mastoid process. A puretone signal of 50 dB HL is presented. If IA is considered to be 0 dB, then it should be assumed that a signal of 50 dB HL potentially is reaching both cochleas. It should be apparent that there essentially is no separation between the two cochleas during unmasked bone-conduction audiometry.

Based on currently available data, a conservative estimate of IA for bone-conducted sound is 0 dB at all frequencies.

WHEN TO MASK

Contralateral masking is required whenever there is the possibility that the test signal can be perceived in the nontest ear. IA is one of the major factors that will be considered when evaluating the need for masking. The basic principles underlying the decision-making processes of when to mask during puretone and speech audiometry will now be addressed.

Puretone Audiometry: Air Conduction

When making a decision about the need for masking during puretone air-conduction testing, three factors need to be considered: (1) IA, (2) unmasked air-conduction threshold in the test ear (i.e., HL at the test ear), and (3) bone-conduction hearing sensitivity (i.e., threshold) in the nontest ear. Recall that when cross hearing occurs, the nontest ear is stimulated primarily through the bone-conduction mechanism. When a decision is made about the need for contralateral masking, the unmasked air-conduction threshold in the test ($AC_{Test\ Ear}$) is compared to the bone-conduction threshold in the nontest ear ($BC_{Nontest\ Ear}$). If the difference between ears equals or exceeds IA, then air-conduction threshold in the test ear must be remeasured using contralateral masking. The rule for when to mask during puretone air-conduction testing can be stated as follows:

Contralateral masking is required during puretone air-conduction audiometry when the unmasked air-conduction threshold in the test ear equals or exceeds the apparent bone-conduction threshold (i.e., the unmasked bone-conduction threshold) in the nontest ear by a conservative estimate of IA:

$$AC_{Test\ Ear} - BC_{Nontest\ Ear} \geq IA$$

This rule is consistent with the guidelines for manual puretone threshold audiometry recommended by ASHA (2005).

Note that the term "apparent" bone-conduction threshold is considered when making a decision about the need for masking. Remember that an unmasked bone-conduction threshold does not convey ear-specific information. It is assumed that the bone-conduction response can originate from either or both ears. Therefore, the unmasked bone-conduction response is considered the apparent or possible threshold for either ear.

Consider the unmasked puretone audiogram[1] presented in Figure 6.4. Because IA for bone-conducted sound is considered 0 dB, unmasked bone-conduction thresholds traditionally are obtained at only one mastoid process. During air-conduction threshold testing, the potential for cross hearing is greatest when there is a substantial difference in hearing sensitivity between the two ears and when a stimulus is presented at higher HLs to the poorer ear.

---

[1] The puretone audiogram and audiometric symbols used throughout this chapter are those recommended in ASHA's (1990) most recent guidelines for audiometric symbols (see Chapter 3).

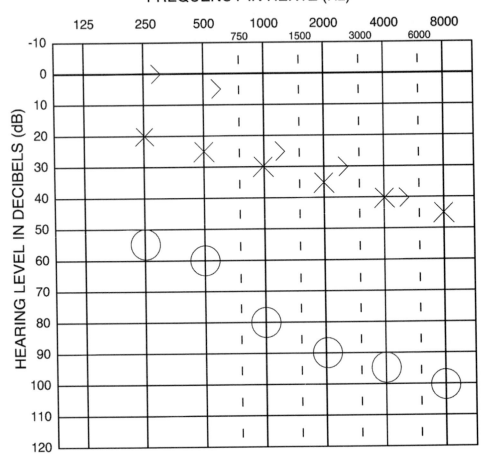

FIGURE 6.4 Audiogram illustrating the need for contralateral masking during puretone air-conduction audiometry. See text for discussion.

Consequently, there is greater potential for cross hearing when measuring puretone thresholds in the right ear.

First consider the need for contralateral masking assuming that air-conduction thresholds were measured using supra-aural earphones. A conservative estimate of IA is 40 dB. We will use the following equation when making a decision about the need for contralateral masking:

$$AC_{Test\ Ear} - BC_{Nontest\ Ear} \geq IA$$

Because it is not possible to measure bone-conduction threshold at 8,000 Hz, it is necessary to predict an unmasked threshold given the findings at other test frequencies. In this particular example, unmasked bone-conduction threshold at 8,000 Hz will probably have a similar relationship with the air-conduction thresholds in the better (i.e., left) ear. Because there is no evidence of air-bone gaps at the adjacent high frequencies, we will assume that a similar relationship exists at 8,000 Hz. Therefore, our estimate of unmasked bone-conduction threshold is 45 dB HL.

It will be necessary to remeasure puretone thresholds at all test frequencies in the right ear using contralateral masking because the difference between ears equals or exceeds our estimate of IA.

Right ear (Test ear)		Masking needed?
250 Hz	55 − 0 ≥ 40?	Yes
500 Hz	60 − 5 ≥ 40?	Yes
1,000 Hz	80 − 25 ≥ 40?	Yes
2,000 Hz	90 − 30 ≥ 40?	Yes
4,000 Hz	95 − 40 ≥ 40?	Yes
8,000 Hz	100 − 45 ≥ 40?	Yes

However, contralateral masking is not required when testing the left ear. The difference between ears does not equal or exceed the estimate of IA.

Left ear (Test ear)		Masking needed?
250 Hz	25 − 0 ≥ 40?	No
500 Hz	25 − 5 ≥ 40?	No
1,000 Hz	30 − 25 ≥ 40?	No
2,000 Hz	35 − 30 ≥ 40?	No
4,000 Hz	40 − 40 ≥ 40?	No
8,000 Hz	45 − 45 ≥ 40?	No

Many audiologists will obtain air-conduction thresholds prior to measurement of bone-conduction thresholds. A preliminary decision about the need for contralateral masking can be made by comparing the air-conduction thresholds of the two ears.

Contralateral masking is required during puretone air-conduction audiometry when the unmasked air-conduction threshold in the test ear ($AC_{Test Ear}$) equals or exceeds the air-conduction threshold in the non-test ear ($AC_{Nontest Ear}$) by a conservative estimate of IA:

$$AC_{Test Ear} - AC_{Nontest Ear} \geq IA$$

It is important to remember, however, that cross hearing for air-conducted sound occurs primarily through the mechanism of bone conduction. Consequently, it will be necessary to re-evaluate the need for contralateral masking during air-conduction testing following the measurement of unmasked bone-conduction thresholds.

Consider again the audiogram presented in Figure 6.4. Let us assume that we have not yet measured unmasked bone-conduction thresholds. We can make a preliminary decision about the need for contralateral masking by considering the difference between air-conduction thresholds in the two ears. Based on the air-conduction responses only, it appears that contralateral masking is needed only when testing the right ear at octave frequencies from 1,000 through 8,000 Hz. Yet, once unmasked bone-conduction thresholds are measured, it becomes apparent that contralateral masking also will be required when testing the right ear at 250 Hz and 500 Hz.

It is conventional to obtain air-conduction thresholds prior to bone-conduction thresholds. However, an alternative (and recommended) approach involves obtaining unmasked bone-conduction thresholds prior to obtaining unmasked air-conduction thresholds. Decisions about the need for masking during air-conduction testing then can be made using the important bone-conduction responses.

3A insert earphones are often substituted for the supra-aural configuration during audiometric testing. We will now take a second look at the audiogram in Figure 6.4 and assume that air-conduction thresholds were obtained with 3A insert earphones. Recall that conservative estimates of IA for 3A insert earphones with deeply inserted foam eartips are 75 dB at ≤1,000 Hz and 50 dB at frequencies >1,000 Hz. Previously, we determined that contralateral masking was not required when testing the better (i.e., left) ear using supra-aural earphones. Given the greater IA offered by 3A insert earphones, it is easy to understand that contralateral masking again should not be required when testing the left ear. However, a different picture results when considering the need for contralateral masking when testing the right ear.

Right ear (Test ear)		Masking needed?
250 Hz	55 − 0 ≥ 75?	No
500 Hz	60 − 5 ≥ 75?	No
1,000 Hz	80 − 25 ≥ 75?	No
2,000 Hz	90 − 30 ≥ 50?	Yes
4,000 Hz	95 − 40 ≥ 50?	Yes
8,000 Hz	100 − 45 ≥ 50?	Yes

Because of the greater IA provided by 3A insert earphones in the lower frequencies, the need for contralateral masking is eliminated at 250, 500, and 1,000 Hz. It should be apparent that the process of evaluating the need for contralateral masking when using either supra-aural or insert earphones is the same. The only difference is the substitution of different values of IA in our equations.

Puretone Audiometry: Bone Conduction

Remember that a conservative estimate of IA for bone-conducted sound is 0 dB. Theoretically, masked bone-conduction measurements are always required if ear-specific information is needed. However, given the goal of bone-conduction audiometry, contralateral masking is not always required. Generally, bone-conduction thresholds are primarily useful for determining gross site of lesion (i.e., conductive, sensory-neural, or mixed). The presence of air-bone gaps suggests a conductive component to a hearing loss.

The major factor to consider when making a decision about the need for contralateral masking during bone-conduction audiometry is whether the unmasked bone-conduction threshold (Unmasked BC) suggests the presence of a significant conductive component in the test ear.

The use of contralateral masking is indicated whenever the results of unmasked bone-conduction audiometry suggest the presence of an air-bone gap in the test ear (Air-Bone Gap $_{Test Ear}$) of 15 dB or greater:

$$\text{Air-Bone Gap}_{Test Ear} \geq 15\,dB$$

where

$$\text{Air-Bone Gap} = AC\,Test\,Ear - Unmasked\,BC$$

ASHA (2005) recommends that contralateral masking should be used whenever a potential air-bone gap of 10 dB or greater exists. When taking into account the variability inherent in bone-conduction measurements (Studebaker, 1967b), however, a criterion of 10 dB may be too stringent. There is a certain degree of variability between air- and bone-conduction thresholds, even in individuals without conductive hearing loss. If we assume that there is a normal distribution of the relationship between air- and bone-conduction thresholds in individuals without significant air-bone gaps, then an air-bone difference of ± 10 dB is not unexpected.

If unmasked bone-conduction thresholds suggest air-bone gaps of 10 dB or less, then contralateral masking is not required. Although unmasked bone-conduction thresholds do not provide ear-specific information, we have accomplished our goal for bone-conduction testing. If unmasked bone-conduction thresholds suggest no evidence of significant air-bone gaps, then we have ruled out the presence of a significant conductive component. Consequently, our assumption is that the hearing loss is sensory-neural in nature.

Figure 6.5 provides three examples of the need for contralateral masking during bone-conduction audiometry. Unmasked air- and bone-conduction thresholds are provided in each case.

Example A: Contralateral masking is not required during bone-conduction testing in either ear. When we compare the unmasked bone-conduction thresholds to the air-conduction thresholds in each ear, there are no potential air-bone gaps of 15 dB or greater. For example, consider the thresholds at 2,000 Hz. Comparison of the unmasked bone-conduction thresholds to the air-conduction thresholds suggests a potential air-bone gap of 5 dB in the right ear and 0 dB in the left ear. Because the unmasked bone-conduction thresholds do not suggest the presence of significant air-bone gaps in either ear, our conclusion is that the hearing loss is sensory-neural bilaterally. Obtaining masked bone-conduction thresholds, although they would provide ear-specific information, would not provide additional diagnostic information.

Example B: Comparison of unmasked bone-conduction thresholds to the air-conduction thresholds in the left ear does not suggest the presence of significant air-bone gaps. Consequently, masked bone-conduction thresholds are not required in the left ear. Our conclusion is that the hearing loss is sensory-neural.

However, masked bone-conduction thresholds will be required in the right ear. Comparison of unmasked bone-conduction thresholds to the air-conduction thresholds in the right ear suggests potential air-bone gaps ranging from 25 to 35 dB. The unmasked bone-conduction thresholds may reflect hearing in the better (i.e., left) ear. Bone-conduction thresholds in the right ear may be as good as the unmasked responses. They also may be as poor as the air-conduction thresholds in that ear. Because we do not have ear-specific information for bone-conduction thresholds, the loss in the right ear can be either mixed or sensory-neural. In order to make a definitive statement about type of hearing loss, it will be necessary to obtain masked bone-conduction thresholds in the right ear.

Example C: There is evidence that contralateral masking will be required when measuring bone-conduction thresholds in both ears. Comparison of unmasked bone-conduction thresholds to the air-conduction thresholds suggests potential air-bone gaps ranging from 30 to 35 dB in each ear. As in the previous example, bone-conduction thresholds in each ear may be as good as the unmasked responses. They also may be as poor as the air-conduction thresholds in that

ear. In order to make a definitive statement about type of hearing loss, it will be necessary to obtain masked bone-conduction thresholds in both ears.

Speech Audiometry

Because speech audiometry is an air-conduction procedure, the rules for when to mask will be similar to those used during puretone air-conduction audiometry. There are three factors to consider when making a decision about the need for contralateral masking during speech audiometry: (1) IA, (2) presentation level of the speech signal (in dB HL) in the test ear, and (3) bone-conduction hearing sensitivity (i.e., threshold) in the nontest ear.

Contralateral masking is indicated during speech audiometry whenever the presentation level of the speech signal (in dB HL) in the test ear (Presentation Level $_{\text{Test Ear}}$) equals or exceeds the best puretone bone-conduction threshold in the nontest ear (Best BC$_{\text{Nontest Ear}}$) by a conservative estimate of IA:

$$\text{Presentation Level}_{\text{Test Ear}} - \text{Best BC}_{\text{Nontest Ear}} \geq \text{IA}$$

Because speech is a broadband signal, it is necessary to consider bone-conduction hearing sensitivity at more than a single puretone frequency. Konkle and Berry (1983) and Sanders (1991) recommend the use of the bone-conduction puretone average of 500, 1,000, and 2,000 Hz or some other average that is predictive of the SRT. ASHA (1988) recommends that the puretone bone-conduction thresholds at 500, 1,000, 2,000, and 4,000 Hz should be considered. Martin and Blythe (1977) suggest that 250 Hz can be eliminated from any formula for determining the need for contralateral masking when measuring the SRT. Yet, the nontest ear bone-conduction threshold at 250 may be an important consideration when measuring the SDT. Olsen and Matkin (1991) state that the SDT may be most closely related to the best threshold in the 250 to 4,000 Hz range when audiometric configuration steeply rises or slopes. Therefore, following the recommendation of Coles and Priede (1975), the most conservative approach involves considering the best bone-conduction threshold in the 250- to 4,000-Hz frequency range.

The examples presented in Figures 6.6 and 6.7 illustrate the need for contralateral masking during threshold and supra-threshold speech audiometry, respectively. First consider the audiogram presented in Figure 6.6. Audiometry was performed using supra-aural earphones. Puretone testing (using appropriate contralateral masking during both air- and bone-conduction audiometry) reveals a severe-to-profound, sensory-neural hearing loss of gradually sloping configuration in the right ear. There is a very mild, sensory-neural hearing loss of relatively flat configuration in the left ear. Given the difference between ears observed during puretone audiometry, it is anticipated that contralateral masking may be needed during assessment of SRT in the poorer ear.

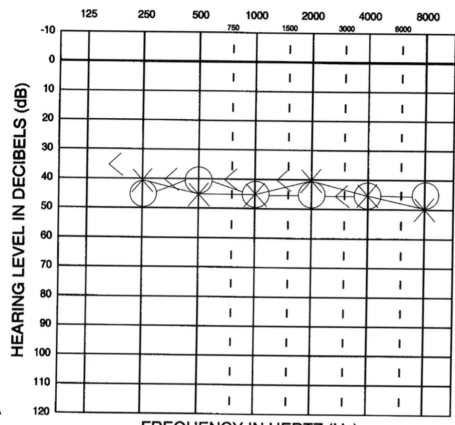

A

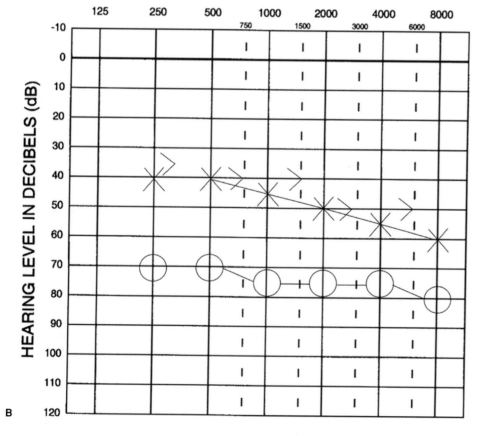

B

FIGURE 6.5 Audiogram illustrating the need for contralateral masking during bone-conduction audiometry. Example A: Masked bone-conduction thresholds are not required in either ear. Example B: Masked bone-conduction thresholds are required only in the right ear. Example C: Masked bone-conduction thresholds are potentially required in both ears. See text for further discussion.

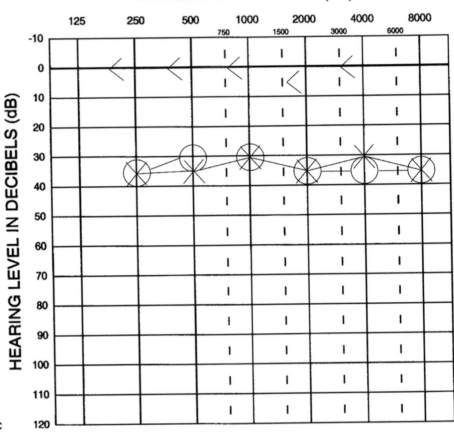

FIGURE 6.5   (Continued)   C

There are different approaches that can be used when determining the need for contralateral masking during measurement of SRT. The most efficient and recommended approach involves predicting the speech threshold using the puretone threshold data in the poorer ear and, on that basis, determining the need for contralateral masking. For example, SRT is measured at 20 dB HL in the left ear, a finding consistent with the puretone results. Given the relatively low HL at which the SRT was established in the better (i.e., left) ear, it is expected that contralateral masking will not be required when measuring the SRT. Specifically, the SRT of 20 dB HL in the left ear does not equal or exceed the best bone-conduction threshold of 55 dB HL in the nontest ear by a conservative estimate of IA (40 dB):

$$\text{Presentation Level}_{\text{Test Ear}} - \text{Best BC}_{\text{Nontest Ear}} \geq \text{IA}$$

$$20\,\text{dB HL} - 55\,\text{dB HL} \geq 40\,\text{dB?}\ \underline{\text{No}}$$

However, if we predict that an SRT will be measured at about 80 dB HL in the right ear (based on the puretone average), then contralateral masking will be required because the estimated speech threshold of 80 dB HL equals or exceeds the best bone-conduction threshold of 15 dB HL in the nontest ear by 40 dB, our estimate of IA for speech:

$$\text{Presentation Level}_{\text{Test Ear}} - \text{Best BC}_{\text{Nontest Ear}} \geq \text{IA}$$

$$80\,\text{dB HL} - 15\,\text{dB HL} \geq 40\,\text{dB?}\ \underline{\text{Yes}}$$

Stated differently, the difference between the predicted presentation level in the test ear and the best bone-conduction threshold in the nontest ear equals or exceeds our estimate of IA. It is important to note, however, that a decision about the need for contralateral masking during measurement of speech threshold must always take into account not only the presentation level at the measured SRT, but also all suprathreshold levels used during threshold measurement. This will be discussed further in the section addressing selection of masking levels during speech audiometry.

During our earlier discussion of the need for contralateral masking during puretone air-conduction audiometry, it was indicated that a correct decision about the need for contralateral masking sometimes can be made by simply comparing the air-conduction thresholds of the two ears. Similarly, a decision about the need for contralateral masking during measurement of speech thresholds can often be made by comparing speech thresholds in the two ears.

Contralateral masking is required during measurement of speech threshold when the speech threshold in the test ear (ST $_{\text{Test Ear}}$) equals or exceeds the speech threshold in the nontest ear (ST $_{\text{Nontest Ear}}$) by a conservative estimate of IA:

$$\text{ST}_{\text{Test Ear}} - \text{ST}_{\text{Nontest Ear}} \geq \text{IA}$$

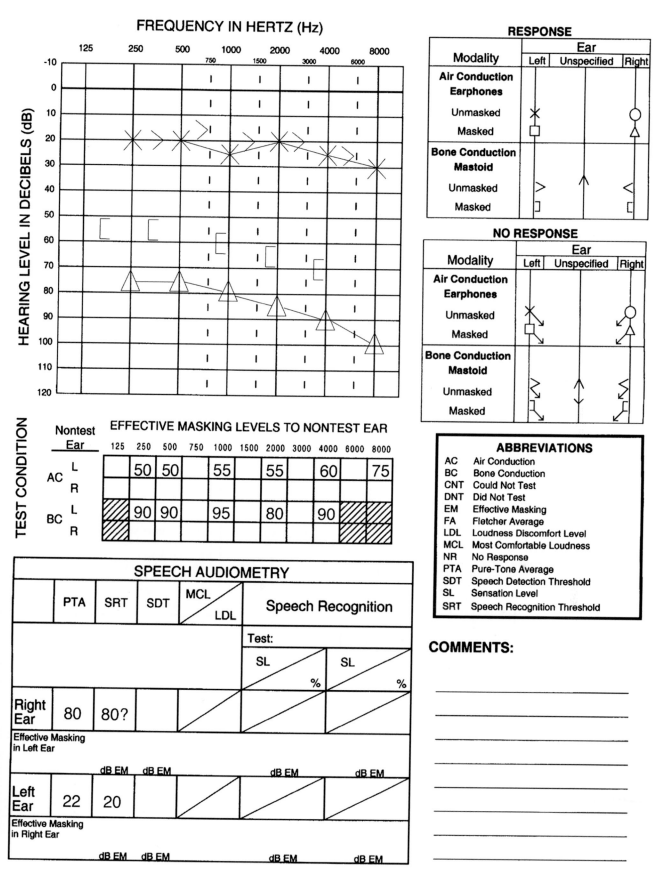

FIGURE 6.6 Audiogram illustrating the need for contralateral masking during measurement of speech recognition threshold (SRT). See text for further discussion.

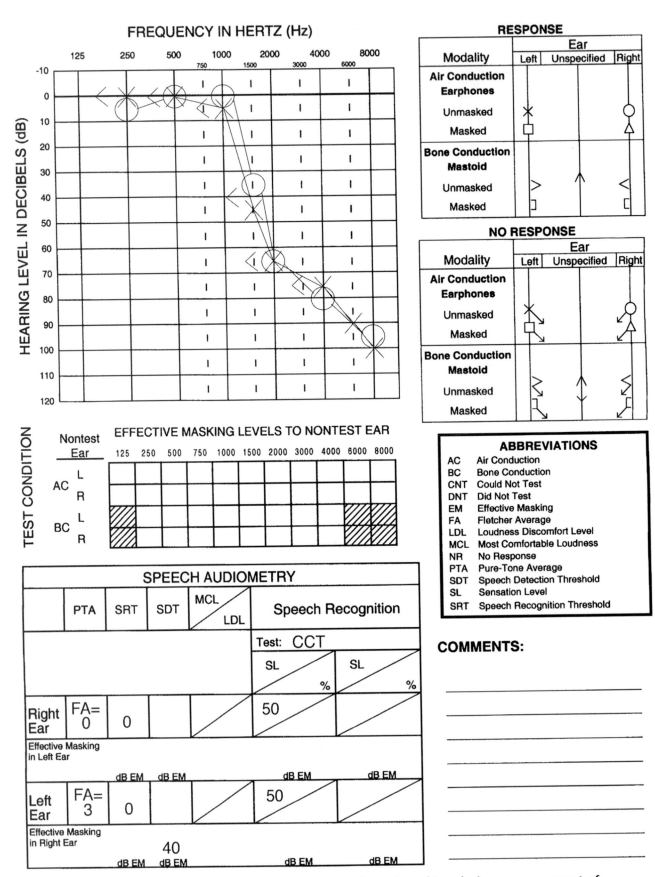

FIGURE 6.7 Audiogram illustrating the need for contralateral masking during measurement of supra-threshold speech recognition. See text for further discussion.

Consider again the audiogram presented in Figure 6.6. Recall that we predicted that SRT would be measured at about 80 dB HL in the right ear. In this particular example, comparison of the two speech thresholds (i.e., the measured SRT of 20 dB HL in the left ear and the predicted SRT of 80 dB HL in the right ear) would lead us to a correct decision about the need for contralateral masking when measuring SRT in the poorer ear without the need to consider bone-conduction hearing sensitivity in the nontest ear. The difference between the predicted SRT in the right ear (80 dB HL) and the measured SRT in the left ear (20 dB HL) equals or exceeds 40 dB, our estimate of IA for speech:

$$ST_{Test\ Ear} - ST_{Nontest\ Ear} \geq IA$$

$$80\ dB\ HL - 20\ dB\ HL \geq 40\ dB?\ \underline{Yes}$$

An alternative approach that can be used when making a decision about the need for contralateral masking during assessment of SRT involves measuring unmasked speech thresholds in both ears. Consider again the example presented in Figure 6.6. Assume that unmasked SRTs were measured at 65 dB HL and 20 dB HL in the right and left ears, respectively. Again there is an indication that contralateral masking will be required when measuring the SRT in the right ear: The presentation level of 65 dB HL (i.e., the unmasked SRT) in the test ear equals or exceeds the best bone-conduction threshold of 15 dB HL in the nontest ear by 40 dB, our estimate of IA for speech:

$$Presentation\ Level_{Test\ Ear} - Best\ BC_{Nontest\ Ear} \geq IA$$

$$65\ dB\ HL - 15\ dB\ HL \geq 40\ dB?\ \underline{Yes}$$

Similarly, the difference between the unmasked SRT in the right ear (65 dB HL) and the measured SRT in the left ear (20 dB HL) equals or exceeds our estimate of IA (40 dB). Although this approach can sometimes provide the audiologist with a more accurate estimate of the patient's IA for speech (which may be useful when selecting appropriate masking levels), it often just increases the number of steps needed to establish the true SRT in the test ear.

The audiogram presented in Figure 6.7 illustrates the need for contralateral masking during assessment of supra-threshold speech recognition. Puretone testing reveals normal hearing through 1,000 Hz, steeply sloping to a severe-to-profound sensory-neural hearing loss in the high frequencies bilaterally. SRTs were measured at 0 dB HL in both ears, a finding consistent with the puretone findings. Contralateral masking was not required during puretone and speech threshold audiometry. Supra-threshold speech recognition will be assessed using the California Consonant Test (CCT). This is a closed-set word recognition test that is sensitive to the speech recognition difficulties of individuals with high-frequency hearing loss (Owens and Schubert, 1977). If we use the recommended sensation level (SL) of 50 dB (Schwartz and Surr, 1979), then presentation level for both ears will be 60 dB HL (i.e., 50 dB relative to the SRT of 10 dB HL).

Let us now consider the need for contralateral masking during assessment of supra-threshold speech recognition. We will consider the need for masking using two types of air-conduction transducers: supra-aural and 3A insert earphones. The advantage of insert earphones will become apparent.

Let us assume that supra-aural earphones are being used during speech audiometry. Contralateral masking will be required when assessing supra-threshold speech recognition in both ears because the difference between the presentation level of 50 dB HL in the test ear and the best puretone bone-conduction threshold of 0 dB HL in the nontest ear equals or exceeds 40 dB, our conservative estimate of IA for speech:

$$Presentation\ Level_{Test\ Ear} - Best\ BC_{Nontest\ Ear} \geq IA$$

Right Ear $\quad$ 50 dB HL − 0 dB HL $\geq$ 40 dB? $\underline{Yes}$

Left Ear $\quad$ 50 dB HL − 0 dB HL $\geq$ 40 dB? $\underline{Yes}$

A different outcome results if we substitute 3A insert earphones for the supra-aural arrangement. Because of the greater separation between ears offered by 3A insert earphones, contralateral masking will not be required when assessing supra-threshold speech recognition in either ear. Specifically, the difference between the presentation level of 50 dB HL in the test ear and the best puretone bone-conduction threshold of 0 dB HL in the nontest ear does not equal or exceed 60 dB, our conservative estimate of IA for speech:

$$Presentation\ Level_{Test\ Ear} - Best\ BC_{Nontest\ Ear} \geq IA$$

Right Ear 50 dB HL − 0 dB HL $\geq$ 60 dB? $\underline{No}$

Left Ear 50 dB HL − 0 dB HL $\geq$ 60 dB? $\underline{No}$

The example presented in Figure 6.7 illustrates two important concepts related to assessment of supra-threshold speech recognition. First, it should not be assumed that contralateral masking is never required when assessing individuals with symmetrical sensory-neural hearing loss. Second, the need for contralateral masking often can be eliminated by using an air-conduction transducer that provides greater IA (i.e., 3A insert earphone).

▨ MASKING CONCEPTS

Before proceeding to a discussion of clinical masking procedures, a brief review of basic masking concepts, including masking noise selection and calibration, will be presented. Generally, masking relates to how sensitivity for one sound is affected by the presence of another sound. The American National Standards Institute (ANSI, 2004b) defines masking as follows:

> The process by which the threshold of hearing for one sound is raised by the presence of another (masking) sound. The amount by which the threshold of hearing for one sound is raised by the presence of another (masking) sound, expressed in decibels (pp 6–7).

Consider the following example. Absolute threshold for a 1,000-Hz puretone stimulus is initially determined to be 40 dB HL. Another sound, white noise, is now presented simultaneously to the same ear. Absolute threshold for the 1,000-Hz signal is redetermined in the presence of the white noise and increases to 60 dB HL. Sensitivity to the puretone signal has been affected by the presence of the white noise. This increase in threshold of one sound in the presence of another is defined as masking. Because the puretone threshold was raised by 20 dB (i.e., a threshold shift of 20 dB), the white noise has produced 20 dB of masking.

There are two basic masking paradigms: ipsilateral and contralateral. In an ipsilateral masking paradigm, the test signal and the masker are presented to the same ear. In a contralateral masking paradigm, the test signal and masker are presented to opposite ears. Masking is used clinically whenever it is suspected that the *nontest* ear is participating in the evaluation of the test ear. Consequently, masking is always applied to the nontest or contralateral ear. Masking reduces sensitivity of the nontest ear to the test signal. The purpose of contralateral masking, therefore, is to raise the threshold of the nontest ear sufficiently so that its contribution to a response from the test ear is eliminated.

Masking Noise Selection

Standard diagnostic audiometers provide three types of masking stimuli: narrowband noise, speech spectrum noise, and white noise. Our clinical goal is to select a masker that is efficient (Hood, 1960). An efficient masker is one that produces a given effective level of masking with the least overall sound pressure level.

In order to better understand this concept of masker efficiency, let us review the classic masking experiment conducted by Fletcher (1940). White noise is a broadband stimulus that contains equal energy across a broad range of frequencies. Because of its broadband spectrum, it has the ability to mask puretone stimuli across a broad range of frequencies (Hawkins and Stevens, 1950). Fletcher addressed which frequency components of broadband noise contribute to the masking of a tone.

Fletcher (1940) conducted what is known as a centered masking experiment. Initially, a very narrow band of noise was centered around a puretone signal. The bandwidth of the noise was progressively widened, and the masking effect on the puretone signal was determined. Fletcher observed that the masked puretone threshold increased as the bandwidth of the masking noise was increased. However, once the noise band reached and then exceeded a "critical bandwidth," additional masking of the puretone signal did not occur.

This concept of the critical band as first described by Fletcher (1940) consists of two components:

1. When masking a puretone with broadband noise, the only components of the noise that have a masking effect on the tone are those frequencies included within a narrow band centered around the frequency of the tone.

2. When a puretone is just audible in the presence of the noise, the total noise power present in the narrow band of frequencies is equal to the power of the tone.

The first component of the critical band concept has clinical implications when selecting an appropriate masker during puretone audiometry. The second component has relevance when calibrating the effective masking (EM) level of the masking stimulus.

White noise is adequate as a masker for puretone stimuli. However, it contains noise components that do not contribute to the effectiveness of the masker. The additional noise components outside the tone's critical band simply add to the overall level (and loudness) of the masking stimulus. Therefore, the most efficient masker for puretone stimuli is a narrow band of noise with a bandwidth slightly greater than the critical band surrounding the tone. It provides the greatest masking effect with the least overall intensity. Sanders and Rintelmann (1964) confirmed that narrowband noise was a far more efficient masker for puretone stimuli than white noise. For a given sound pressure level (50, 70, and 90 dB SPL), narrowband noise centered at the frequency of the puretone signal (ranging from 250 to 4,000 Hz) consistently produced a greater masking effect (about 10 to 20 dB) than white noise.

The masking noise typically used during puretone audiometry, therefore, is narrowband noise centered geometrically around the audiometric test frequency. ANSI (2004b) specifies the band limits (i.e., the upper and lower cut-off frequencies) of narrowband masking noise. In order to minimize the perception of tonality that is often associated with very narrow bands of noise, the bands specified by ANSI are somewhat wider than the critical bands for effective masking. The goal is to avoid confusion of the masker with the signal.

Speech spectrum noise (i.e., weighted random noise for the masking of speech) is typically used as a masker during speech audiometry. Speech is a broadband stimulus that requires a broadband masker. Although white noise is an adequate masker, it is not the most efficient. Speech spectrum noise is white noise that has been filtered to simulate the long-term average spectrum of speech. The average spectrum of speech contains the greatest energy in the low frequencies with spectrum level decreasing as a function of increasing frequency (Dunn and White, 1940). Speech spectrum noise has a more limited bandwidth than white noise. It is a more efficient masker than white noise, producing a masking advantage of 8 dB (Konkle and Berry, 1983). ANSI (2004b) specifies that the spectrum of weighted random noise for the masking of speech should have a sound pressure spectrum level that is constant from 100 to 1,000 Hz, decreasing at a rate of 12 dB per octave from 1,000 to 6,000 Hz.

Calibration of Effective Masking Level

When a masking noise is presented to the nontest ear, we are interested in how much masking is produced. Consequently, masking noise is calibrated in EM level (dB EM).

ANSI (2004b) defines EM level for puretones as "the sound pressure level of a band of noise, whose geometric center frequency coincides with that of a specific puretone that masks the puretone to 50% probability of detection" (p 7). (Reference EM levels, calculated by adding an appropriate correction value to the reference equivalent threshold sound pressure level [RETSPL] at each frequency, are provided in the current ANSI specification for audiometers.) It is also indicated that, in individuals with normal hearing, "the amount of effective masking is equal to the number of decibels that a given band of noise shifts a puretone threshold. . . .when the band of noise and the puretone are presented simultaneously to the same ear" (ANSI, 2004b, p 7).

Stated differently, effective masking (in dB EM) refers to:

1. The HL (dB HL) to which puretone threshold is shifted by a given level of noise; and
2. The puretone threshold shift (in dB) relative to 0 dB HL provided by a given level of noise.

Although contralateral masking is used clinically during hearing assessment, the following examples of ipsilateral masking will facilitate an understanding of the concept of EM level.

Example 1: A puretone air-conduction threshold is measured at 0 dB HL in the right ear. A narrow-band noise geometrically centered at the test frequency is presented to the same ear at 50 dB EM. This EM level of 50 dB will shift puretone threshold to 50 dB HL.

Example 2: A puretone air-conduction threshold is measured at 30 dB HL in the right ear. A narrowband noise geometrically centered at the test frequency is presented to the same ear at 50 dB EM. This EM level of 50 dB will shift puretone threshold to 50 dB HL.

These examples illustrate two important points. First, a given level of EM will shift all unmasked puretone thresholds to the same dB HL. Of course, if unmasked puretone threshold is greater than a particular level of EM, then no threshold shift will occur. For example, a masker of 50 dB EM will not have a masking effect if the unmasked puretone threshold is 70 dB HL. Second, EM refers to the amount of threshold shift only relative to 0 dB HL.

Speech spectrum noise is also calibrated in EM level. Just as HL for speech (dB HL) is specified relative to the SRT, EM level is also referenced to the SRT. Specifically, EM for speech refers to the dB HL to which the SRT is shifted by a given level of noise. ANSI (2004b) defines EM level for speech as the "sound pressure level of a specified masking noise that masks a speech signal to 50% probability of recognition" (p 7). (If the speech spectrum noise has spectral density characteristics as specified by ANSI and if the sound pressure level of the masker is equal to the RETSPL for speech, then the masker is calibrated in dB EM.) ANSI (2004b) also states that, in individuals with normal hearing, "the amount of effective masking is equal to the number of decibels that a masking noise shifts a SRT. . . .when the masking noise and speech signal are presented simultaneously to the same ear" (p 7).

Consider the following example. SRT is measured at 0 dB HL. Speech spectrum noise is then presented to the same ear at 50 dB EM. This EM level of 50 dB will shift the SRT to 50 dB HL.

Calibration of masking noise in EM level greatly simplifies clinical masking procedures. When masking noise is calibrated in dB EM, then the decibel value indicated on the masking level control will indicate the masking effect produced in the nontest ear. This clearly facilitates the selection of appropriate masking levels during clinical testing.

▨ CLINICAL MASKING PROCEDURES

All approaches to clinical masking address two basic questions. First, what is the minimum level of noise that is needed in the nontest ear to eliminate its response to the test signal? Stated differently, this is the *minimum masking level* that is needed to avoid *undermasking* (i.e., even with contralateral masking, the test signal continues to be perceived in the nontest ear). Second, what is the maximum level of noise that can be used in the nontest ear that will not change the true threshold or response in the test ear? Stated differently, this is the *maximum masking level* that can be used without overmasking (i.e., with contralateral masking, the true threshold or response in the test ear has been changed). Because of limited IA for air-conducted sound, the masking stimulus presented to the nontest ear can also cross over to the test ear and produce masking of the test signal (i.e., overmasking). Stated simply, the purpose of clinical masking is to make the test signal inaudible in the nontest ear without affecting the true response to the signal in the test ear. Therefore, the major goal of any clinical masking procedure is the avoidance of both undermasking and overmasking.

Studebaker (1979) has identified two major approaches to clinical masking: psychoacoustic and acoustic. Psychoacoustic procedures are "those based upon observed shifts in the measured threshold as a function of suprathreshold masker effective levels in the nontest ear" (Studebaker, 1979, p 82). These approaches also are identified as threshold shift or shadowing procedures. Acoustic procedures are "those based upon calculating the approximate acoustic levels of the test and masker signals in the two ears under any given set of conditions and on this basis deriving the required masking level" (Studebaker, 1979, p 82). These procedures also are referred to as calculation or formula methods. Psychoacoustic approaches are considered appropriate for threshold measurements, whereas acoustic methods typically are most efficient for supra-threshold measurements.

Puretone Audiometry

Formulas and equations have been presented for the calculation of minimum and maximum masking levels during puretone audiometry (Lidén et al., 1959; Martin, 1967, 1974; Studebaker, 1962; 1964). A brief discussion of these formulas will facilitate an understanding of the manner in which appropriate levels of masking are selected during puretone threshold testing.

MINIMUM MASKING LEVEL

Lidén et al. (1959) and Studebaker (1964) offered formulas for calculating minimum masking level during puretone air-conduction audiometry that include consideration of IA, HL of the test signal, and air-bone gaps in the nontest ear. Although this "formula" approach to calculating minimum masking level is necessary during administration of supra-threshold auditory tests (this approach will be discussed later in the section addressing masking in speech audiometry), it proves somewhat disadvantageous during threshold audiometry. First, it can be time consuming. Second, the clinician may not have all required information to accurately calculate minimum masking level at that point in time. (The reader is referred to Yacullo [1996] for further discussion of the derivation of these equations and formulas.)

The simplified method described by Martin (1967; 1974) is recommended for clinical use. Martin has suggested that formulas are unnecessary during threshold audiometry and has simplified the calculation of minimum masking level. Specifically, the "initial" masking level (in dB EM) during air-conduction threshold testing is simply equal to air-conduction threshold (in dB HL) of the nontest ear (i.e., AC$_{\text{Nontest Ear}}$). It should be noted that the initial masking level is calculated in the same manner regardless of the air-conduction transducer being used (i.e., supra-aural earphone or 3A insert earphone).

The audiometric data presented in Figure 6.8 will be used to facilitate an understanding of the calculation of masking levels during puretone threshold audiometry. Audiometry was performed using supra-aural earphones. Unmasked air- and bone-conduction thresholds at 500 Hz are provided; masked air- and bone-conduction thresholds are also included for later discussion. Unmasked puretone air-conduction testing suggests that contralateral masking will be required only when measuring air-conduction threshold in the left ear. Specifically, the unmasked air-conduction threshold of 65 dB HL in the left ear equals or exceeds the threshold (both air and bone conduction) in the nontest ear by a conservative estimate of IA (i.e., 40 dB). According to Martin (1967; 1974), the initial masking level (in dB EM) is equal to 5 dB EM (i.e., AC$_{\text{Nontest Ear}}$).

Martin (1967; 1974) explains the derivation of this simplified equation in the following way. A signal detected at

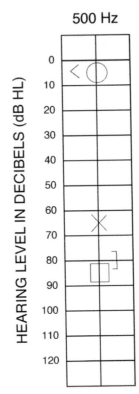

FIGURE 6.8 An example illustrating the calculation of initial and maximum masking levels during puretone threshold audiometry. See text for further discussion.

threshold is assumed to have an SL of 0 dB, regardless of whether it is perceived in the test or nontest ear. Therefore, a cross-hearing response during puretone threshold testing theoretically represents a *threshold* response in the nontest ear. Given this assumption, the initial masking level required is one that will just mask a signal of 0 dB SL (i.e., threshold) in the nontest ear. Because of the manner in which masking stimuli are calibrated clinically (i.e., EM level, dB EM), a masker presented at a level (in dB EM) equal to the air-conduction threshold (in dB HL) in the nontest ear should just mask the threshold response in the nontest ear. Given the example presented in Figure 6.8, a masker level of 5 dB EM (which is equal to the air-conduction threshold in the right ear) should be sufficient to just mask a threshold response to the test signal in the right ear. Martin also indicates that the simplified approach will lead to the selection of the same masker level as when using the more complex formulas for calculating minimum masking level.

Martin (1974) recommends that approximately 10 dB should be added to the initial masking level to account for intersubject variability. Remember that dB EM refers to the HL (dB HL) to which threshold is shifted by a given level of noise. Calibration of EM is based on the averaged responses of a group of normal-hearing subjects. Therefore, a given EM level will not prove equally effective for all subjects. If masked thresholds are normally distributed around the average effective level and if the standard deviation of the distribution is about 5 dB, then Studebaker (1979) recommends that a safety factor of not less than 10 dB should be added to the calculated minimum masking level. Given this recommendation, Martin's simplified equation for initial masking level (in dB EM) during air-conduction threshold audiometry can be stated as follows:

Initial Masking Level $= AC_{Nontest\ Ear} + 10\ dB$

Considering again the example presented in Figure 6.8, initial masking level is now calculated as 15 dB EM:

$$Initial\ Masking\ Level = AC_{Nontest\ Ear} + 10\ dB$$
$$= 5\ dB\ HL + 10\ dB$$
$$= 15\ dB\ EM$$

It is important to differentiate the terms *minimum masking level* and *initial masking level* during air-conduction threshold audiometry. Earlier in this discussion, a general definition of minimum masking level was provided. Minimum masking level was defined as the minimum level of noise needed in the nontest ear to eliminate its response to the test signal. Related to puretone threshold audiometry, a more specific definition of minimum masking level can be offered: Minimum masking level is the minimum level of noise needed to eliminate the contribution of the nontest ear *in order to establish the true or correct threshold in the test ear*. Initial masking level is simply the first level of noise introduced to the nontest ear. This initial level of masking often is not sufficient to establish the threshold in the test ear; higher levels of masking often are required. This concept will be addressed again in our discussion of the recommended clinical masking procedure during puretone threshold audiometry.

Lidén et al. (1959) and Studebaker (1964) also have offered formulas for minimum masking level during bone-conduction testing that are derived from the same theoretical constructs used during air-conduction testing (see Yacullo [1996] for further discussion). Again, the formula approach during bone-conduction threshold audiometry is not clinically practical. The use of Martin's simplified approach is recommended. Specifically, initial masking level during bone-conduction audiometry is equal to the air-conduction threshold of the nontest ear. However, we will need to add the occlusion effect (OE) to the initial masking level in order to compensate for covering (i.e., occluding) the nontest ear with an earphone (Martin, 1967; 1974; Studebaker, 1964). Martin's simplified equation for initial masking level (in dB EM) during bone-conduction threshold testing can be stated as follows:

Initial Masking Level $= AC_{Nontest\ Ear} + OE + 10\ dB$

Bone-conduction thresholds are always obtained with the test ear unoccluded or uncovered. However, when an earphone covers or occludes the nontest ear during masked bone-conduction audiometry, an occlusion effect can be created in the nontest ear. The nontest ear consequently can

become more sensitive to bone-conducted sound for test frequencies below 2,000 Hz, particularly when using supra-aural earphones (Berger and Kerivan, 1983; Berrett, 1973; Dean and Martin, 2000; Dirks and Swindeman, 1967; Elpern and Naunton, 1963; Goldstein and Hayes, 1965; Hodgson and Tillman, 1966). During the application of contralateral masking, there is increased probability that the nontest ear will respond when obtaining a masked bone-conduction threshold in the test ear. Studebaker (1979) points out that the occlusion effect does not actually affect hearing sensitivity of the occluded ear, but rather increases the sound pressure level of the signal reaching the cochlea. The reader is referred to Tonndorf (1968; 1972) for further discussion of the contribution of the external auditory meatus to bone-conduction thresholds.

There is evidence suggesting that the occlusion effect is decreased significantly when using deeply inserted insert earphones (Berger and Kerivan, 1983; Chaiklin, 1967; Dean and Martin, 2000). Berger and Kerivan (1983) and Dean and Martin (2000) studied the magnitude of the occlusion effect in normal-hearing subjects using E-A-R foam eartips and supra-aural earphones as occluding devices. Their overall results are remarkably similar. First, the average occlusion effects in the low frequencies are greatly reduced when occluding the ear using an E-A-R foam eartip with deep insertion. Second, the advantage of a greatly reduced occlusion effect for the E-A-R foam eartip is lost when a partial or shallow insertion is used. Third, partial or shallow insertion of an E-A-R foam eartip yields average occlusion effects that are similar to those measured with supra-aural earphones. Different theories have been offered to explain the reduced occlusion effect for an occluding device that is deeply inserted into the ear canal. The reader is referred to Berger and Kerivan (1983), Tonndorf (1972), and Yacullo (1996) for further discussion.

The clinician can use either individually determined (Martin et al., 1974; Dean and Martin, 2000) or fixed occlusion effect values (i.e., based on average data reported in the literature) when calculating initial masking level. Based on the largest average occlusion effects reported in the literature (Berger and Kerivan, 1983; Berrett, 1973; Dean and Martin, 2000; Dirks and Swindeman, 1967; Elpern and Naunton, 1963; Goldstein and Hayes, 1965; Hodgson and Tillman, 1966), the following values are recommended for clinical use.

When using supra-aural earphones, the following fixed occlusion effect values are recommended: 30 dB at 250 Hz, 20 dB at 500 Hz, and 10 dB at 1,000 Hz. When using 3A insert earphones with deeply inserted foam eartips, the following values are recommended: 10 dB at 250 and 500 Hz and 0 dB at frequencies of 1,000 Hz or higher.

It should be noted that the occlusion effect is decreased or absent in ears with conductive hearing impairment (Martin et al., 1974; Studebaker, 1979). If the nontest ear exhibits a potential air-bone gap of 20 dB or more, then the occlusion effect should not be added to the initial masking level at that frequency.

Consider again the example presented in Figure 6.8. Assume that we have subsequently measured a masked air-conduction threshold of 85 dB HL in the left ear. A masked bone-conduction threshold will also be required in the left ear. Comparison of the unmasked bone-conduction threshold of 5 dB HL with the masked air-conduction threshold of 85 dB HL in the left ear suggests a potentially significant air-bone gap (i.e., ≥15 dB). Initial masking level is calculated in the same manner regardless of the air-conduction transducer used for the delivery of the masking stimulus. The only difference in calculation relates to applying a different correction factor for the occlusion effect when testing in the lower frequencies. Using the recommended fixed occlusion effect values for supra-aural earphones, initial masking level during bone-conduction testing at 500 Hz is calculated as follows:

$$\text{Initial Masking Level} = AC_{\text{Nontest Ear}} + OE + 10 \text{ dB}$$
$$= 5 \text{ dB HL} + 20 \text{ dB} + 10 \text{ dB}$$
$$= 35 \text{ dB EM}$$

In this particular example, it is appropriate to account for the occlusion effect because there is no evidence of a significant air-bone gap in the nontest (i.e., right) ear. The use of a supra-aural earphone for delivery of masking in the lower frequencies, however, will result in greater initial masking levels than when using a 3A insert because of a larger occlusion effect correction factor.

MAXIMUM MASKING LEVEL

Maximum masking level refers to the maximum level of noise that can be used in the nontest ear that will not shift or change the true threshold in the test ear. Two factors influence maximum masking level during puretone audiometry: (1) the bone-conduction threshold of the test ear ($BC_{\text{Test Ear}}$), and (2) IA of the air-conducted masking stimulus (Lidén et al., 1959). Maximum masking level (M_{Max}), based on the original concept described Lidén et al., can be summarized using the following equation:

$$M_{\text{Max}} = BC_{\text{Test Ear}} + IA - 5 \text{ dB}$$

If $BC_{\text{Test Ear}}$ + IA is just sufficient to produce overmasking, then clinically, we want to use a masking level that is somewhat less than the calculated value. Consequently, 5 dB is subtracted from the level that theoretically produces overmasking. Because we are concerned about an undesired masking effect in the test ear, bone-conduction sensitivity in that ear must be considered. As a result, overmasking is more of a potential problem when bone-conduction sensitivity is very good in the test ear. Overmasking, on the other hand, is generally not an issue when bone-conduction hearing sensitivity is poor. The poorer the bone-conduction hearing sensitivity is in the test ear, the greater the levels of masking that can be used without overmasking.

The following two points are important to remember. First, the equation for maximum masking level is the same for both air- and bone-conduction audiometry. Masking noise is always delivered through an air-conduction transducer (e.g., insert or supra-aural earphone) regardless of the transducer used for measuring puretone threshold (i.e., air- or bone-conduction transducer). Second, maximum masking level generally is higher when using 3A insert earphones because of increased IA, particularly in the lower frequencies.

Consider again the example presented in Figure 6.8. We will now calculate the maximum masking level that can be used during both masked air- and bone-conduction audiometry:

$$M_{\text{Max}} = BC_{\text{Test Ear}} + IA - 5 \text{ dB}$$
$$= 80 \text{ dB HL} + 60 \text{ dB} - 5 \text{ dB}$$
$$= 135 \text{ dB EM}$$

Rather than using the very conservative IA estimate of 40 dB when using supra-aural earphones, in this case, we will use the more accurate estimate of 60 dB. If bone-conduction threshold in the right (i.e., nontest) ear is assumed to be 5 dB HL (i.e., the unmasked bone-conduction threshold) and unmasked air-conduction threshold in the left ear is 65 dB HL, then there is evidence that IA is at least 60 dB. If 140 dB EM is just sufficient to produce overmasking (i.e., $BC_{\text{Test Ear}}$ + IA), then 135 EM is the maximum level of noise that can be used in the nontest ear that will not shift or change the true threshold in the test ear. It should be noted that 135 dB EM is a level that significantly exceeds the output limits for standard audiometers.

Generally, it is neither time efficient nor necessary to calculate maximum masking level during puretone threshold audiometry, particularly when using psychoacoustic or threshold shift masking procedures (which will be described shortly). In addition, the estimated maximum masking level is typically very conservative and not an accurate indication of the true maximum. In the above example, we calculated a relatively accurate estimate by using a more accurate value of IA (rather than the conservative value) and the actual bone-conduction threshold in the test ear (i.e., 80 dB HL). However, the true bone-conduction threshold (obtained with appropriate contralateral masking) in the test ear typically is not known when maximum masking level is estimated during both air- and bone-conduction threshold audiometry. Because only an unmasked bone-conduction threshold is available at the time that masking levels are determined, we are required to use the unmasked threshold as the estimate of bone-conduction hearing sensitivity in the test ear. Let us calculate again M_{Max} using the unmasked bone-conduction response as the estimate of bone-conduction threshold:

$$M_{\text{Max}} = 5 \text{ dB HL} + 60 \text{ dB} - 5 \text{ dB}$$
$$= 60 \text{ dB EM}$$

Clearly in this case, our calculation based on the unmasked bone-conduction threshold (i.e., 60 dB EM) is an underestimate of the actual maximum level (i.e., 135 dB EM).

Whenever an unmasked bone-conduction threshold is used during determination of maximum masking, the resultant value is typically smaller than the masking level that will actually result in overmasking. Although the actual calculation of maximum masking level during puretone threshold audiometry is often of limited use, consideration of the maximum level of noise that can be used in the nontest ear can alert the audiologist to the possibility of overmasking, particularly in cases of conductive hearing loss when bone-conduction hearing sensitivity is very good.

RECOMMENDED CLINICAL PROCEDURE

The most popular method for measuring masked puretone thresholds was first described by Hood in 1957 (Hood, 1960). The Hood method, also referred to as the plateau, threshold shift, or shadowing procedure, is a psychoacoustic technique that relies on observations about the relationship between masker level in the nontest ear and measured threshold in the test ear. Hood originally described a masking procedure that was applicable for measurement of masked bone-conduction thresholds. However, it proves equally effective for measurement of air-conduction thresholds as well.

The example presented in Figure 6.9 will help facilitate an understanding of the underlying concept of the threshold shift procedure. Unmasked puretone air-conduction thresholds, obtained using supra-aural earphones, were measured at 10 dB HL in the right ear and 60 dB HL in the left ear (Fig. 6.9A). Contralateral masking will be required when testing the left ear because there is a difference between the test and nontest ears that equals or exceeds a conservative estimate of IA (i.e., 40 dB). An initial masking level of 20 dB EM (i.e., $AC_{Nontest\ Ear} + 10$ dB) is now presented to the right ear, and puretone threshold is re-established. Recall that the purpose of contralateral masking is to raise the threshold of the nontest ear sufficiently to eliminate its contribution when measuring a response in the test ear. Assuming that overmasking is not occurring, then contralateral masking should have an effect only on the responsiveness of the nontest ear.

There are two possible outcomes when puretone threshold is re-established in the presence of contralateral masking: (1) no measured puretone threshold shift (e.g., puretone threshold remains constant at 60 dB HL; Fig. 6.9B), or (2) a measured puretone threshold shift (e.g., puretone threshold shifts from 60 to 70 dB HL; Fig. 6.9C). If contralateral masking in the nontest ear does not produce a masking effect, then it is concluded that the unmasked puretone threshold represents a response from the test ear. Conversely, if contralateral masking in the nontest ear does produce a masking effect, then it is concluded that the unmasked puretone threshold represents a response from the nontest ear. The underlying concept of the Hood procedure is that the introduction of masking to the nontest ear will produce a masking effect (i.e., a threshold shift) only if the nontest ear is contributing

to the observed response. Decisions about which ear is contributing to the measured threshold are based on whether a threshold shift occurs when masking is introduced to the nontest ear.

Hood (1960) outlined two essential steps of the plateau masking procedure: (1) demonstration of the shadowing effect, and (2) identification of the changeover point. The hypothetical example presented in Figure 6.10 illustrates basic concepts of the plateau masking procedure. Puretone testing using supra-aural earphones reveals unmasked air-conduction thresholds of 0 dB HL in the right ear and 40 dB HL in the left ear (Fig. 6.10A). Unmasked bone-conduction threshold is 0 dB HL. Because there is a 40-dB difference between ears, contralateral masking will be required when measuring air-conduction threshold in the left ear. (Masked air- and bone-conduction thresholds in the left ear are included for later discussion.)

The masking function presented in Figure 6.10B shows the relationship between measured puretone threshold (in dB HL) in the test ear and EM level (in dB EM) in the nontest ear. Masking noise is introduced at an initial masking level of 10 dB EM (i.e., $AC_{Nontest\ Ear} + 10$ dB), and puretone threshold is re-established. Threshold shifts to 50 dB HL. When the masker level is raised sequentially to 20 dB EM and 30 dB EM, puretone threshold continues to shift by 10 dB. A shadowing effect has occurred because the masked puretone threshold "shadows" the threshold of the nontest or masked ear with each increment in EM level. Because a threshold shift occurs when masking level is raised, it is concluded that the masking noise and the tone are restricted to the nontest ear.

When the masker is raised from 30 dB EM to 100 dB EM, puretone threshold no longer shifts and remains stable at 70 dB HL. A plateau has been reached. Because there is no additional masking effect (i.e., a threshold shift) when masker level is increased, it is concluded that the nontest ear is no longer contributing to the observed response. Puretone threshold of the test ear (i.e., 70 dB HL) has been reached. Hood (1960) refers to the initial point on the masking function where puretone threshold remains stable with increasing masking level as the "changeover point." In this example, the changeover point of 30 dB EM also corresponds to minimum masking level, the minimum amount of noise required to establish the true threshold in the test ear. Masker levels that result in no threshold shift (i.e., the plateau) represent adequate masking (i.e., 30 dB EM through 100 dB EM). Masker levels less than 30 dB EM represent undermasking. That is, there is insufficient masking to establish the true puretone threshold in the test ear.

When the masker level exceeds 100 dB EM (i.e., 110 dB EM and 120 dB EM), however, a puretone threshold shift with each increment in masking level is again observed. Overmasking is now occurring. The masking noise has reached the test ear through cross hearing, and a masking effect (i.e., a threshold shift) is observed in the test ear. Assuming that a masked bone conduction is measured subsequently in the left ear at 65 dB HL, then an estimate of maximum masking

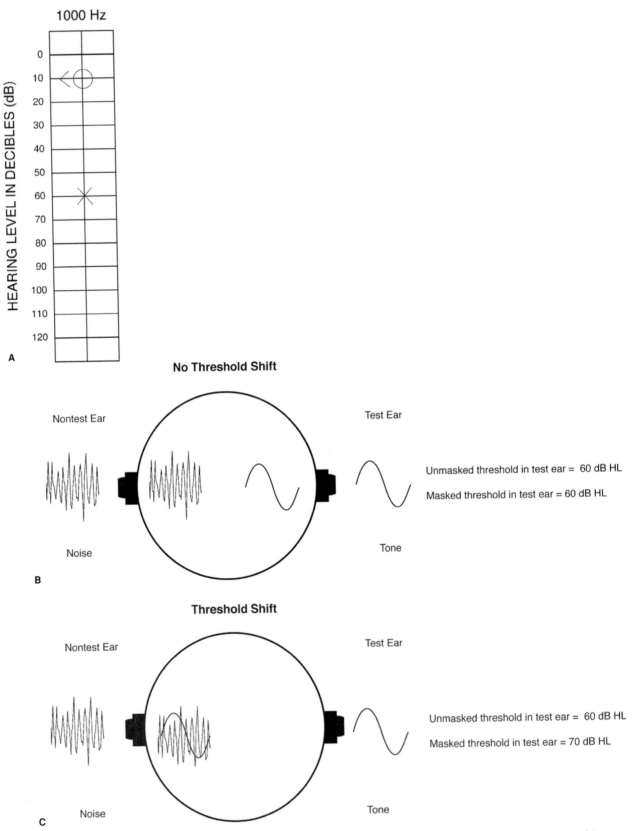

FIGURE 6.9 Example illustrating the underlying concept of the plateau or threshold shift masking procedure. See text for further discussion. (From Yacullo WS. [1996] *Clinical Masking Procedures*. Boston, MA: Allyn & Bacon; p 69. Copyright © 1996 by Pearson Education. Adapted by permission of the publisher.)

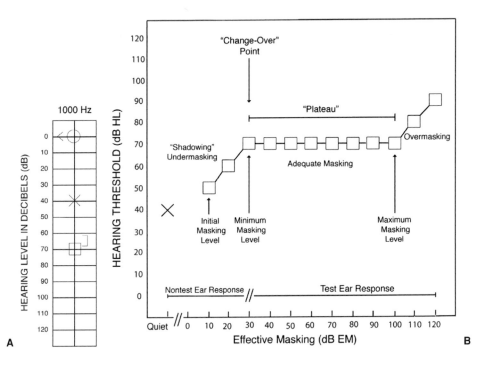

FIGURE 6.10
Hypothetical example illustrating the concepts of undermasking, adequate masking, and overmasking using the threshold shift or plateau masking procedure. See text for explanation. (From Yacullo WS. [1996] *Clinical Masking Procedures.* **Boston, MA: Allyn & Bacon; p 72. Copyright © 1996 by Pearson Education. Adapted by permission of the publisher.)**

level is 100 dB EM ($BC_{Test\,Ear}$ + IA − 5 dB: 65 dB HL + 40 dB − 5 dB). While the plateau and overmasking portions of the masking function represent responses from the test ear, the undermasking or shadowing portion represents responses from the nontest ear. It should be apparent from the masking function in Figure 6.10 that the width of the masking plateau is defined by the minimum and maximum masking levels.

The clinical goal of the plateau procedure is to establish the HL at which puretone threshold remains unchanged with increments in masking level. Two important variables that relate to the plateau procedure are (1) the magnitude of the masker increment, and (2) the number of masker increments needed to establish a masking plateau. Although Hood (1960) originally recommended that masker level be changed in increments of 10 dB, others have suggested that the level should be a 5-dB step size (Martin, 1980; Silman and Silverman, 1991). Martin (1980) suggests that accuracy is increased somewhat by using a masker increment of 5 dB. It is somewhat arbitrary whether a 5-dB or 10-dB step size is used for increasing masker level. Either step size is acceptable. However, the smaller step size of 5 dB is strongly recommended whenever the masking plateau is narrow and there is increased risk of overmasking (i.e., cases of bilateral conductive hearing loss).

Hood (1960) did not specify the number of masker increments needed to establish a masking plateau. Clinically, it is neither time efficient nor necessary to measure the entire masking plateau. It is generally agreed that a masking "plateau" has been established when masker level can be increased over a range of at least 15 to 20 dB without shifting puretone threshold (Kaplan et al., 1993; Martin, 1980; Sanders, 1991; Silman and Silverman, 1991).

The recommended clinical procedure (Yacullo, 1996; 2004), based on the major components of Hood's shadowing technique, is summarized as follows:

1. Masking noise is introduced to the nontest ear at the initial masking level. Puretone threshold then is reestablished.

2. Level of the tone or noise is increased subsequently by 5 dB. If there is a response to the tone in the presence of the noise, the level of the noise is increased by 5 dB. If there is no response to the tone in the presence of the noise, the level of the tone is increased in 5-dB steps until a response is obtained.

3. A plateau has been reached when the level of the noise can be increased over a range of 15 to 20 dB without shifting the threshold of the tone. This corresponds to a response to the tone at the same HL when the masker is increased in three to four consecutive levels.

4. Masked puretone threshold corresponds to the HL of the tone at which a masking plateau has been established.

If a 10-dB step size is used for increasing masking level, then the plateau corresponds to a range of 20 dB (i.e., a response to the tone at the same HL when the masker is increased in two consecutive levels).

The recommended procedure for establishing a masking plateau does not require that puretone threshold be formally established each time that the masking level is increased. This approach would significantly increase the time required to establish a masking plateau. Rather, the tone is presented once at the same HL as the previous response. If no response occurs, the tone is increased in 5-dB steps until audibility is achieved. However, the HL of the tone may be increased inappropriately because of a decision-making process based on a single response. This may lead to imprecision when measuring the masked threshold. Therefore, it is recommended that masked puretone threshold be re-established using a standardized threshold procedure (ANSI, 2004a; ASHA, 2005) in the presence of the final level of masking noise that resulted in a plateau. This sometimes leads to a 5-dB improvement in the masked puretone threshold. However, the decision to re-establish masked puretone threshold at the end of the plateau procedure will be influenced by time considerations.

Remember that the goal of the plateau procedure is to establish the HL at which puretone threshold remains unchanged with increments in masking level. Given this goal, there are three major outcomes that can result when measuring puretone threshold. These outcomes are illustrated in the three examples presented in Figure 6.11. In each example, the unmasked puretone thresholds are the same. Unmasked puretone air-conduction thresholds, obtained using 3A insert earphones, were measured at 15 dB HL in the right ear and 75 dB HL in the left ear. Contralateral masking will be required when measuring air-conduction threshold in the left ear; an initial masking level of 25 dB EM is presented to the right ear, and puretone threshold is re-established.

In the first outcome, the unmasked puretone threshold of 75 dB HL remains unaffected with increasing masking level. The level of the noise was increased over a range of 20 dB without shifting the threshold of the tone. In this example, the initial masking level occurs at the masking plateau. Contralateral masking has confirmed that the unmasked puretone threshold represents a response from the test ear.

In the second outcome, the initial masking level produces a puretone threshold shift. A masking plateau is reached, however, when masking level is increased from 35 dB EM to 55 dB EM (i.e., a masking range of 20 dB). Because masked puretone threshold remains stable at 95 dB HL with increasing masking level, puretone threshold is recorded as 95 dB HL. Contralateral masking has confirmed that the unmasked puretone threshold represents a cross-hearing response from the nontest ear.

In the third outcome, the initial masking level again produces a puretone threshold shift. However, puretone threshold continues to shift to the output limits of the audiometer with increasing masking level. A plateau is not obtained. Therefore, it is concluded that there is no measurable hearing in the left ear. This conclusion is correct assuming that overmasking has not occurred.

Turner (2004a; 2004b) has described a masking method that can replace the plateau procedure in some masking situations. A disadvantage of the plateau method is that it can be time consuming. The "optimized" masking method described by Turner reportedly can reduce the number of required masking levels. However, there are some masking situations where the optimized approach is not recommended. The reader is referred to the two articles by Turner (2004a; 2004b) for further discussion.

THE MASKING DILEMMA

There are clinical situations where minimum masking levels can result in overmasking. Studebaker (1979) states that a "masking dilemma" results when the width of the masking plateau is very narrow or nonexistent. Remember that the width of the masking plateau is defined by minimum and maximum masking levels. Generally, a masking dilemma results whenever there is a significant hearing loss in the nontest ear and a conductive hearing loss in the test ear. The presence of significant hearing loss in the nontest ear requires higher initial masking levels; the presence of a conductive hearing loss in the test ear (i.e., normal bone-conduction hearing sensitivity) decreases the maximum masking level. The consequence of a reduced or nonexistent masking plateau is the inability to establish correct masked thresholds in the test ear.

The classic example of a masking dilemma is demonstrated with a bilateral, mild-to-moderate conductive hearing loss. The possibility for overmasking exists when measuring masked air- and bone-conduction thresholds in both ears. Naunton (1960) states that, in some cases of bilateral conductive hearing loss, it is not possible to mask the nontest ear without simultaneously producing a masking effect in the test ear.

One solution to the masking dilemma is the use of insert earphones (Coles and Priede, 1970; Hosford-Dunn et al., 1986; Studebaker, 1962; 1964). Recall that the use of 3A insert earphones significantly increases IA for air-conducted sound, particularly in the lower frequencies (Killion et al., 1985; Sklare and Denenberg, 1987). There are two advantages of using insert earphones in cases of bilateral conductive hearing loss. First, the need for masking during measurement of air-conduction thresholds is often eliminated because of greater IA for air-conducted sound. Second, the use of insert earphones reduces the probability of overmasking in cases where contralateral masking is required. The use of an air-conduction transducer with increased IA increases the range between the minimum and maximum masking levels, thereby increasing the width of the masking plateau and the range of permissible masking levels (Studebaker, 1962).

CENTRAL MASKING

The introduction of contralateral masking can produce a small threshold shift in the test ear even when masking level is insufficient to produce overmasking. Wegel and Lane (1924) referred to this phenomenon as central masking. It has been hypothesized that threshold shifts in the presence of low levels of masking are mediated through central nervous system processes (Lidén et al., 1959). Central masking has been reported to influence thresholds measured during both puretone and speech audiometry (Dirks and Malmquist, 1964; Lidén et al., 1959; Martin, 1966; Martin et al., 1965; Martin and DiGiovanni, 1979; Studebaker, 1962). Although the threshold shift produced by central masking is generally considered to be approximately 5 dB (Konkle and Berry, 1983;

Outcome 1

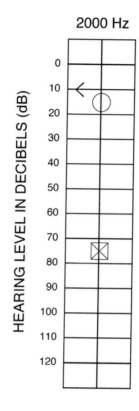

2000 Hz

dB EM	dB HL
--	75
25	75
30	75
35	75
40	75
45	75

Threshold = 75 dB HL

Outcome 2

2000 Hz

dB EM	dB HL
--	75
25	85
30	90
35	95
40	95
45	95
50	95
55	95

Threshold = 95 dB HL

FIGURE 6.11 Examples illustrating the use of the plateau method for measuring masked puretone air-conduction thresholds. The unmasked air- and bone-conduction thresholds are the same in each example. Three different outcomes can result when using the threshold shift procedure. See text for discussion. (From Yacullo WS. [1996] *Clinical Masking Procedures*. Boston, MA: Allyn & Bacon; pp 75–77. Copyright © 1996 by Pearson Education. Adapted by permission of the publisher.)

Outcome 3

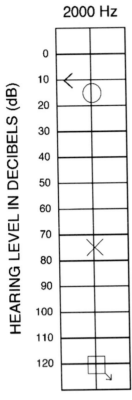

dB EM	dB HL
--	75
25	85
30	90
35	95
40	100
45	105
50	110
55	115
60	120
65	NR

No response at 120 dB HL

FIGURE 6.11   (Continued)

Martin, 1966), variable results have been reported across subjects and studies. There is also some indication that central masking effects increase with increasing masking level (Dirks and Malmquist, 1964; Martin et al., 1965; Studebaker, 1962).

There currently is no agreed upon procedure that accounts for central masking effects during threshold audiometry. However, it generally is not recommended that the effect of central masking be subtracted from masked thresholds. First, it is difficult to determine an appropriate correction factor given the variability of the central masking effect across subjects. Second, the typical central masking effect size of about 5 dB is considered to be within good test-retest reliability during threshold measurements. It is important to remember that the use of contralateral masking can somewhat influence the measured masked thresholds and should be taken into account when interpreting audiometric test results. For example, a difference of 5 dB between unmasked and masked thresholds is generally not considered significant. This difference may simply reflect (1) central masking effects and/or (2) normal variability related to test-retest reliability.

MASKED AUDIOGRAM INTERPRETATION

Unmasked and masked puretone thresholds are typically recorded on the same audiogram. Therefore, audiogram interpretation will involve consideration of both masked and unmasked responses. ASHA (1990) has published guidelines for audiometric symbols and procedures for graphic representation of frequency-specific audiometric findings. These guidelines have been followed throughout this chapter.

Figure 6.12 presents an audiogram in which contralateral masking was required when obtaining both air- and bone-conduction thresholds in the left ear. Air-conduction audiometry was performed using supra-aural earphones. Puretone testing reveals a mild conductive hearing loss of flat configuration in the right ear. Masked air- and bone-conduction responses indicate a severe-to-profound, sensory-neural hearing loss of gradually sloping configuration in the right ear.

It should be noted that the unmasked air-conduction thresholds in the left ear are not considered when interpreting hearing status. Because a significant threshold shift (i.e., >5 dB) occurred when contralateral masking was introduced to the nontest ear, the unmasked air-conduction responses in the left ear actually represent cross-hearing responses from the better (i.e., right) ear. In this case, the unmasked air-conduction thresholds should not be connected with lines. In cases where contralateral masking is required, it is acceptable to record only the masked thresholds (ASHA, 1990).

Although the results of unmasked bone-conduction audiometry suggested that masked bone-conduction thresholds were required in both ears because of potential air-bone gaps, contralateral masking was required only

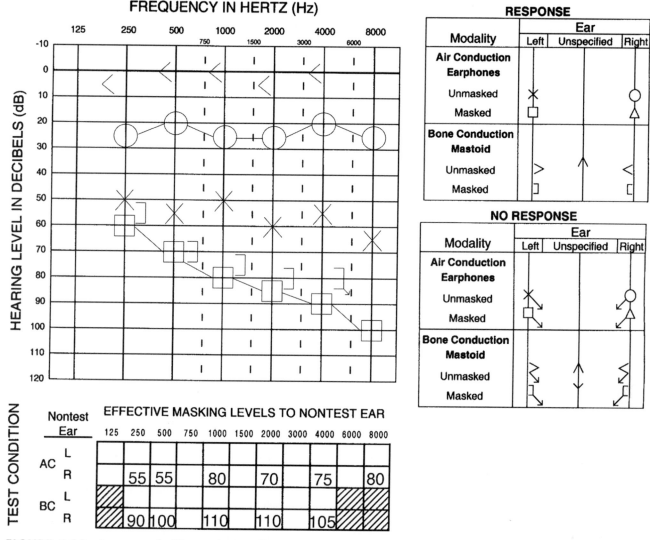

FIGURE 6.12 An example illustrating audiogram interpretation using unmasked and masked puretone thresholds.

when testing the left ear. Whenever there is an asymmetrical hearing loss, it is traditional to first measure masked bone-conduction thresholds in the poorer ear. There is the assumption that the unmasked bone-conduction thresholds may more likely reflect hearing in the better ear. When masked bone-conduction thresholds were subsequently measured in the left ear, results suggested a sensory-neural hearing loss. Consequently, we can correctly assume that the unmasked responses are originating from the better (i.e., right) ear. Depending on the outcome when measuring masked bone-conduction thresholds in the poorer ear, it is not always necessary to also measure masked thresholds in the opposite ear. As the above example illustrates, ear-specific information can be inferred from unmasked bone-conduction responses in some cases.

It is traditional to record masking levels when obtaining masked air- and bone-conduction thresholds. Assuming that the clinician has used the recommended thresh-

old shift (i.e., plateau) procedure, then a range of masking levels will be used when establishing threshold. ASHA (1990) recommends that the final level of masking used to obtain masked threshold should be recorded for the nontest ear. A table for recording EM levels to the nontest ear typically is provided on an audiogram form. Consider again the audiogram presented in Figure 6.12. For example, a masked puretone air-conduction threshold was measured at 85 dB HL at 2,000 Hz in the left ear; this threshold was obtained with a final masking level of 70 dB EM in the right ear.

Speech Audiometry

The speech audiometry test battery traditionally is comprised of two major components: (1) measures of hearing sensitivity for speech (i.e., speech threshold), and (2) measures of supra-threshold speech recognition. Although the psychoacoustic or threshold shift procedure proves efficient when measuring SDT, the acoustic masking procedure is the method of choice when assessing threshold and supra-threshold speech recognition.

PSYCHOACOUSTIC MASKING PROCEDURES

Recall that the psychoacoustic or threshold shift masking procedures rely on observation of shifts in the measured threshold in the test ear as a function of masking levels in the nontest ear. The plateau procedure can be applied easily during measurement of speech thresholds (Konkle and Berry, 1983; Studebaker, 1979). A major advantage of the plateau procedure is that information about bone-conduction hearing sensitivity in each ear is not required when selecting appropriate masking levels. Although the plateau procedure can be applied during measurement of both masked recognition and detection thresholds, it proves most efficient during measurement of SDT because of the nature of the response task (i.e., detection rather than recognition).

ASHA's most recent guidelines for determining threshold level for speech were published in 1988. Recommended procedures for measuring both detection and recognition thresholds are described. Given that determination of SDT involves a detection task that is similar to the one used in puretone threshold audiometry, ASHA recommends using a test procedure that follows published guidelines for measuring puretone threshold (e.g., ANSI, 2004a; ASHA, 2005). Therefore, the plateau masking procedure recommended earlier for use during puretone threshold audiometry can be used equally effectively when measuring masked SDT.

Consider the example presented in Figure 6.13. Audiometry was performed using 3A insert earphones. Puretone testing reveals normal hearing in the right ear. There is a profound sensory-neural hearing loss of fragmentary configuration in the left ear. (Contralateral masking was required during measurement of air- and bone-conduction thresholds in the left ear.) An SRT of 5 dB HL was measured in the right ear, a finding that supports the puretone results. When spondaic words were presented at supra-threshold levels in the left ear, the patient was not able to correctly recognize any words. Consequently, a decision was made to measure an SDT.

An unmasked SDT is measured at 75 dB HL in the left ear. Because the difference between the unmasked SDT in the test ear (i.e., 75 dB HL) and the SRT in the nontest ear (i.e., 5 dB HL) clearly exceeds our conservative estimate of IA for speech (i.e., 60 dB) when using 3A insert earphones, contralateral masking will be required.

Using the recommended plateau masking procedure, speech spectrum noise is introduced to the nontest ear at an initial masking level, that is, an EM level (in dB EM) equal to the speech threshold of the nontest ear ($SRT_{Nontest Ear}$) plus a 10-dB safety factor:

$$\text{Initial Masking Level} = SRT_{Nontest Ear} + 10 \text{ dB}$$

In this example, initial masking level is equal to 15 dB EM. SDT is then re-established in the nontest ear in the presence of the initial masking level. Depending on the patient's response to the speech in the presence of the noise, the level of the speech or noise is increased by 5 dB until a masking plateau has been reached. Remember that it is acceptable to use a 10-dB masker increment when establishing a masking plateau. In this particular case, the risk of overmasking is essentially nonexistent because of the poor bone-conduction hearing sensitivity in the test ear (and the use of an air-conduction transducer with increased IA for presenting the masking noise). Therefore, the use of a 10-dB masker increment can be easily justified. Masked SDT is subsequently measured at 90 dB HL (using 40 dB EM).

Although the plateau masking procedure can be used during assessment of masked SRT, it can prove very time consuming. Recall that only a single detection response to speech is required when measuring masked SDT before making a decision about increasing the level of the speech or masker. The use of the plateau procedure for measuring masked SRT, however, requires that threshold be re-established (i.e., 50% correct recognition of spondaic words) at each masking level until a plateau is reached. The acoustic method proves to be the method of choice when measuring masked SRT because of its greater time efficiency (Konkle and Berry, 1983; Studebaker, 1979) and will be discussed in the following section.

ACOUSTIC MASKING PROCEDURES

Recall that acoustic masking procedures are based on calculating the estimated acoustic levels of the test and masking stimuli in the two ears during a test condition and, on this basis, selecting an appropriate masking level. A major disadvantage of the acoustic or formula approach is that the application requires knowledge about air-bone gaps in both test and nontest ears (Konkle and Berry, 1983; Studebaker, 1979). Knowledge about air-bone gaps in the nontest ear is required to calculate minimum masking level. Information about bone-conduction hearing sensitivity in the test ear is required to calculate maximum masking level. Assuming that complete puretone threshold data are available prior to performing speech audiometry, however, formula approaches for calculating required masking levels prove very effective during measurement of both threshold and supra-threshold speech recognition.

The underlying concepts of minimum and maximum masking levels for speech are similar to those offered earlier for puretone stimuli. Minimum masking level for speech (M_{Min}), originally described by Lidén et al. (1959), can be defined using the following equation:

$$M_{Min} = \textbf{Presentation Level}_{TestEar} - \textbf{IA}$$
$$+ \textbf{Largest Air-Bone Gap}_{Nontest Ear}$$

Presentation Level$_{Test Ear}$ represents the HL (dB HL) of the speech signal at the test ear, IA is equal to IA for speech,

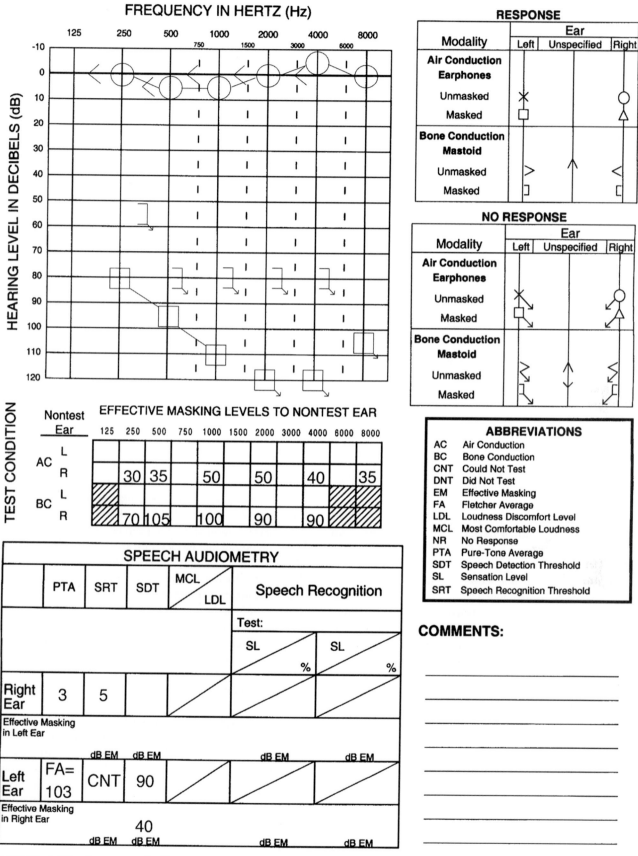

FIGURE 6.13 An example illustrating the use of the threshold shift masking procedure for determining speech detection threshold.

and Largest Air-Bone Gap$_{Nontest Ear}$ represents the largest air-bone gap in the nontest ear in the 250- to 4,000-Hz frequency range. Presentation Level$_{Test Ear}$ – IA, an estimate of the HL of the speech signal reaching the test ear, represents the minimum masking level required. The presence of air-bone gaps in the nontest (i.e., masked) ear, however, will reduce the effectiveness of the masker. Consequently, minimum masking level must be increased by the size of the air-bone gap.

Lidén et al. (1959) recommended that the *average* air-bone gap in the nontest ear, calculated using frequencies of 500, 1,000, and 2,000 Hz, be accounted for when determining the minimum masking level. Coles and Priede (1975) suggested a more conservative approach and recommended that the largest air-bone gap at any frequency in the range from 250 to 4,000 Hz be considered. Remember that speech is a broadband signal. Therefore, bone-conduction hearing sensitivity across a range of frequencies in the nontest ear must be considered. There is the assumption that the largest air-bone gap will have the greatest effect on masking level. Following the conservative recommendation of Coles and Priede (1975), it is recommended that the largest air-bone gap across the frequency range in the nontest ear be accounted for when determining minimum masking level.

Maximum masking level (M$_{Max}$) for speech, originally described by Lidén et al. (1959), can be defined using the following equation:

$$M_{Max} = Best\ BC_{Test\ Ear} + IA - 5\ dB$$

Best BC$_{Test Ear}$ represents the best bone-conduction threshold in the test ear in the frequency range from 250 to 4,000 Hz, and IA is equal to IA for speech. If Best BC$_{Test Ear}$ + IA represents a level that will just produce overmasking in the test ear, then a slightly lower masking level should be used clinically. Consequently, a value of 5 dB is subtracted from the calculated level.

Lidén et al. (1959) originally recommended that the *average* puretone bone-conduction threshold in the test ear, again calculated using frequencies of 500, 1,000, and 2,000 Hz, should be accounted for when estimating maximum masking level. However, a more conservative approach includes consideration of the *best* bone-conduction threshold in the test ear (Martin, 1997) over a wider range of frequencies (i.e., 250 to 4,000 Hz). There is the assumption that the best bone-conduction threshold in the test ear is the most susceptible to the effects of overmasking.

The optimal masking level during speech audiometry is one that occurs above the minimum and below the maximum masking levels (Konkle and Berry, 1983; Lidén et al., 1959; Studebaker, 1979). Minimum and maximum masking levels represent respectively the lower and upper limits of the masking plateau. Studebaker (1979) states that a major goal of the acoustic or formula approach is to apply rules that will place the masking level at approximately the middle of the range of correct values (i.e., the middle of the masking plateau). This concept was originally discussed by Luscher and König in 1955 (cited by Studebaker, 1979).

Studebaker (1962) first described an equation for calculating midmasking level during puretone bone-conduction audiometry. The basic concepts underlying the midplateau procedure, however, can be easily applied during speech audiometry. Yacullo (1999) states that a simple approach to calculating the midmasking level (M$_{Mid}$) involves determining the arithmetic mean of the minimum and maximum masking levels:

$$M_{Mid} = (M_{Min} + M_{Max})/2$$

For example, if M$_{Min}$ is equal to 40 dB EM and M$_{Max}$ is equal to 80 dB EM, then M$_{Mid}$, the masking level that falls at midplateau, is 60 dB EM. When a masking level falls at the middle of the acceptable masking range (i.e., midmasking level), then the risk of undermasking and overmasking is minimized (Studebaker, 1962). It should be noted that midplateau actually represents a range of values surrounding the midmasking level. Consequently, there is some flexibility in using a somewhat higher or lower masking level.

Yacullo (1999) states that there are two major advantages of the midplateau masking procedure. First, IA is eliminated as a source of error when determining an appropriate masking level. Masking levels are often determined using very conservative estimates of IA. However, IA has equal yet opposite effects on minimum and maximum masking levels. Although the value of IA used for determining minimum and maximum masking levels will influence the width of the masking plateau, the midmasking level remains the same.

Second, midmasking level can be determined for both threshold and supra-threshold speech measures by using the same formula approach (Konkle and Berry, 1983). The midplateau procedure avoids a potential problem during measurement of supra-threshold speech recognition that is related to calibration of EM level and percent correct response criterion. Recall that EM level for speech is specified relative to the SRT (i.e., 50% correct recognition of spondaic words) (ANSI, 2004b). Supra-threshold speech recognition performance, however, can range from 0% to 100%. Konkle and Berry (1983) indicate that a major advantage of the midplateau procedure is that the middle of the masking plateau (i.e., the optimal masking level) is not influenced by different listener response criteria used during assessment of threshold and supra-threshold speech recognition. The reader is referred to Konkle and Berry (1983) and Studebaker (1979) for more detailed discussion.

Studebaker (1979) has described a somewhat different acoustic masking procedure for use during speech audiometry that is consistent with the goal of selecting a masking level that occurs at midplateau. Specifically, the recommended masking level is equal to the presentation level of the speech signal in dB HL at the test ear, adjusted appropriately for air-bone gaps in the test and nontest ears. In cases where there are no air-bone gaps in either ear, the selected masking level is simply equal to the HL of the speech signal. In order to avoid the use of very high levels of contralateral masking that can sometimes result, Studebaker indicates that it is permissible to reduce the masking level by 20 to 25 dB below the presentation level of the speech signal. The reader is referred to Studebaker (1979) for a more comprehensive discussion.

According to the results of a survey of audiometric practices in the United States, many audiologists "base their masking level for word-recognition testing on the stimulus level presented to the test ear and subtract a set amount, such as 20 dB" (Martin et al., 1998, p 100). Although selection of a masking level that is equal to the presentation level at the test ear minus 20 dB may appear somewhat arbitrary, it actually can be supported by sound theoretical constructs.

Yacullo (1996; 1999) has described a simplified approach, based on the underlying concepts of both the midplateau and Studebaker acoustic procedures, that can be used when selecting contralateral masking levels during speech audiometry. Although this approach was originally described for use during assessment of supra-threshold speech recognition (Yacullo, 1996), it also proves equally effective during measurement of SRT (Yacullo, 1999). Stated simply, EM level is equal to the presentation level of the speech signal in dB HL at the test ear minus 20 dB:

$$dB\ EM = \text{Presentation Level}_{\text{Test Ear}} - 20\ dB$$

Given two prerequisite conditions (which will be discussed shortly), the selected masking level will fall approximately at midplateau. Unfortunately, inappropriate use of this simplified approach can result in undermasking or overmasking.

Jerger and associates (Jerger and Jerger, 1971; Jerger et al., 1966) appear to be the first to report the use of a masking procedure that involved presenting contralateral masking noise at a level 20 dB less than the presentation level of the speech signal at the test ear. Specifically, it was reported that "whenever the speech level to the test ear was sufficiently intense that the signal might conceivably cross over and be heard on the nontest ear, the latter was masked by white noise at a level 20 dB less than the speech presentation level on the test ear" (Jerger and Jerger, 1971, p 574). It should be noted, however, that Jerger and associates used white noise as a contralateral masker rather than the typically used speech spectrum noise. In addition, the white noise was not calibrated in EM level for speech.

More recently, Hannley (1986) and Gelfand (2001) have also briefly discussed the simplified approach to masking. Gelfand indicates, however, that using an EM level equal to the HL of the speech signal at the test ear minus 20 dB generally proves most effective in cases of sensory-neural hearing loss. In fact, the desired outcome may not occur when there are significant air-bone gaps in the nontest ear (e.g., conductive hearing loss).

Yacullo (1999) states that the simplified masking procedure when used appropriately can significantly reduce the calculations required for the determination of optimal (i.e., midmasking) masking level. Specifically, the method proves effective given the following two conditions: (1) there are no significant air-bone gaps (i.e., ≥ 15 dB) in either ear, and (2) speech is presented at a moderate SL (i.e., 30 to 40 dB SL) relative to the measured or estimated SRT. If these two prerequisites are met, then the selected masking level should occur approximately at midplateau.

Acoustic masking procedures are recommended when assessing threshold and supra-threshold speech recognition. The following two examples help illustrate the use of the midplateau masking procedure, as well as the simplified approach when applicable, for measurement of supra-threshold speech recognition and SRT.

The example presented in Figure 6.14 illustrates the use of the midplateau masking procedure during assessment of supra-threshold speech recognition. Puretone testing reveals a mild, sensory-neural hearing loss of flat configuration in the right ear. There is a moderate-to-severe, sensory-neural hearing loss of gradually sloping configuration in the left ear. SRTs were measured at 35 dB HL in the right ear and 55 dB HL in the left ear, findings that support the puretone results. Supra-threshold speech recognition will be assessed at 40 dB SL using Central Institute for the Deaf (CID) W-22 monosyllabic word lists.

Let us first consider the situation where supra-aural earphones are being used during audiometry. Contralateral masking will be required only when measuring supra-threshold speech recognition in the left ear. Specifically, the presentation level of 95 dB HL (i.e., SRT of 55 dB HL + 40 dB SL) exceeds the best bone-conduction threshold of 30 dB HL in the nontest ear by a conservative estimate of IA for speech (i.e., 40 dB).

$$\text{Presentation Level}_{\text{Test Ear}} - \text{Best BC}_{\text{Nontest Ear}} \geq IA$$

$$95\ dB\ HL - 30\ dB\ HL \geq 40\ dB$$

$$65\ dB\ HL \geq 40\ dB$$

We will use the midplateau masking procedure to select an appropriate contralateral masking level. Remember that the midplateau masking procedure involves a three-step process: calculation of (1) minimum masking level (M_{Min}), (2) maximum masking level (M_{Max}), and (3) midmasking level (M_{Mid}).

$$M_{Min} = \text{Presentation Level}_{\text{Test Ear}} - IA$$
$$+ \text{Largest Air-Bone Gap}_{\text{Nontest Ear}}$$
$$= 95\ dB\ HL - 40\ dB + 5\ dB$$
$$= 60\ dB\ EM$$

$$M_{Max} = \text{Best BC}_{\text{TestEar}} + IA - 5\ dB$$
$$= 45\ dB\ HL + 40\ dB - 5\ dB$$
$$= 80\ dB\ EM$$

$$M_{Mid} = (M_{Min} + M_{Max})/2$$
$$= (60 + 80)/2$$
$$= 70\ dB\ EM$$

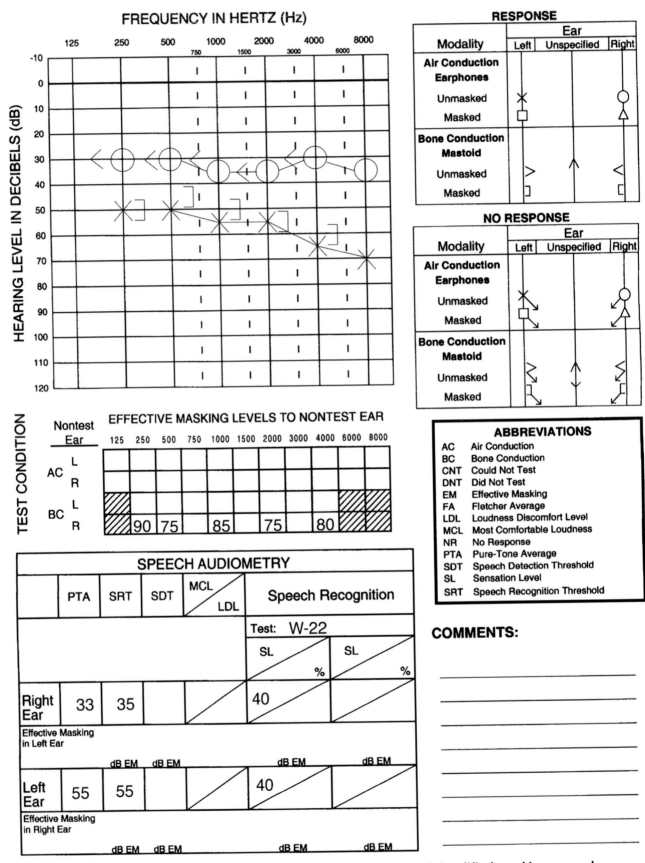

FIGURE 6.14 An example illustrating the use of the midplateau and simplified masking procedures during assessment of supra-threshold speech recognition.

An EM level of 70 dB EM is appropriate for three reasons. First, it occurs at midplateau. Second, it occurs at least 10 dB above the calculated minimum. Remember that a safety factor of at least 10 dB or greater should be added to the calculated minimum value in order to account for intersubject variability with respect to masker effectiveness (Martin, 1974; Studebaker, 1979). Finally, it does not exceed the calculated maximum masking level.

It should be noted that the width of the masking plateau is typically underestimated when a conservative estimate of IA is used for determining the minimum and maximum masking levels. If IA is actually greater than the conservative estimate of 40 dB, then the width of the masking plateau will increase. For example, if this patient actually exhibits IA for speech of 55 dB (rather than the conservative estimate of 40 dB), then the minimum level will be decreased and the maximum level will be increased by the same amount (i.e., 15 dB). Although the width of the masking plateau increases, the midmasking level remains the same. As stated earlier, a major advantage of the midplateau method is that IA is eliminated as a source of error when selecting an appropriate masking level.

We will now take another look at the example presented in Figure 6.14 and substitute 3A insert earphones for the supra-aural arrangement. Contralateral masking will also be required when assessing supra-threshold speech recognition in the left ear. The presentation level of 95 dB HL (i.e., SRT of 55 dB HL + 40 dB SL) exceeds the best bone-conduction threshold of 30 dB HL in the nontest ear by a conservative estimate of IA for speech (i.e., 60 dB). We again will use the midplateau masking procedure to select an appropriate level of contralateral masking. The calculations are the same for both supra-aural and 3A insert earphones with the exception that an IA value of 60 dB will be substituted in our equations for minimum and maximum masking levels. Masking levels for use with insert earphones are summarized below.

$$M_{Min} = 40 \text{ dB EM}$$

$$M_{Max} = 100 \text{ dB EM}$$

$$M_{Mid} = 70 \text{ dB EM}$$

It should be apparent that an increase in IA has equal yet opposite effects on minimum and maximum masking levels. Because IA is increased by 20 dB when using insert earphones, the width of the masking plateau is increased by 40 dB. The midmasking level, however, remains the same.

We will now take one last look at the example presented in Figure 6.14 and consider the use of the simplified masking approach. Because the two prerequisite conditions are met, the simplified approach should result in the selection of an optimal masking level (i.e., midmasking level). Recall that EM level is simply calculated as the presentation level of the speech signal in dB HL at the test ear minus 20 dB. The same equation will be applicable when using any earphone (i.e., 3A and supra-aural).

$$\text{dB EM} = \text{Presentation Level}_{Test Ear} - 20 \text{ dB}$$
$$= 95 \text{ dB HL} - 20 \text{ dB}$$
$$= 75 \text{ dB}$$

It should be noted that the masking level of 75 dB HL calculated using the simplified approach is in good agreement (i.e., ±5 dB) with the value (i.e., 70 dB EM) determined using the midplateau procedure.

Yacullo (1999) indicates that there are two major advantages to using the simplified masking approach with 3A insert earphones, which are the result of a wider masking plateau. First, there is greater flexibility in deviating somewhat from the calculated midmasking level while still remaining within an acceptable range of midplateau. It should be noted that the midplateau actually represents a small range of values surrounding the midmasking level. This range of acceptable values essentially increases when using 3A insert earphones. The use of the simplified masking approach can sometimes result in the selection of high masking levels, even though overmasking is not occurring. Consequently, the audiologist can certainly justify subtracting a value of greater than 20 dB (e.g., 25 or 30 dB) from the presentation level at the test ear when using insert earphones. In the example presented in Figure 6.14, an EM level equal to the presentation level in the test ear minus 25 or 30 dB (e.g., 65 or 70 dB EM) would still result in an acceptable masking level that falls within the vicinity of midplateau, yet clearly exceeds the minimum level by a sizeable amount.

Second, there is greater flexibility in deviating slightly from the recommended prerequisite conditions (i.e., no air-bone gaps in either ear, use of moderate SLs) while still remaining within an acceptable range of midplateau and without significantly increasing the potential for overmasking. Consequently, there is greater margin for error when selecting an appropriate level of masking.

The example presented in Figure 6.15 illustrates the application of the midplateau and simplified masking procedures during measurement of SRT. Audiometry was performed using 3A insert earphones. Puretone testing reveals normal hearing in the right ear. There is a severe sensory-neural hearing loss of flat configuration in the left ear. Based on the puretone findings, it is predicted that SRTs will be measured at approximately 0 dB HL in the right ear and 70 dB HL in the left ear. Prior to measurement of speech thresholds, we can accurately predict whether contralateral masking will be required. Contralateral masking will be required only when measuring SRT in the left ear because the estimated speech threshold of 70 dB HL exceeds the best bone-conduction threshold of 0 dB HL in the nontest ear by a conservative estimate of IA for speech (i.e., 60 dB). An unmasked SRT is subsequently measured in the left ear at 0 dB HL, a finding consistent with the puretone results.

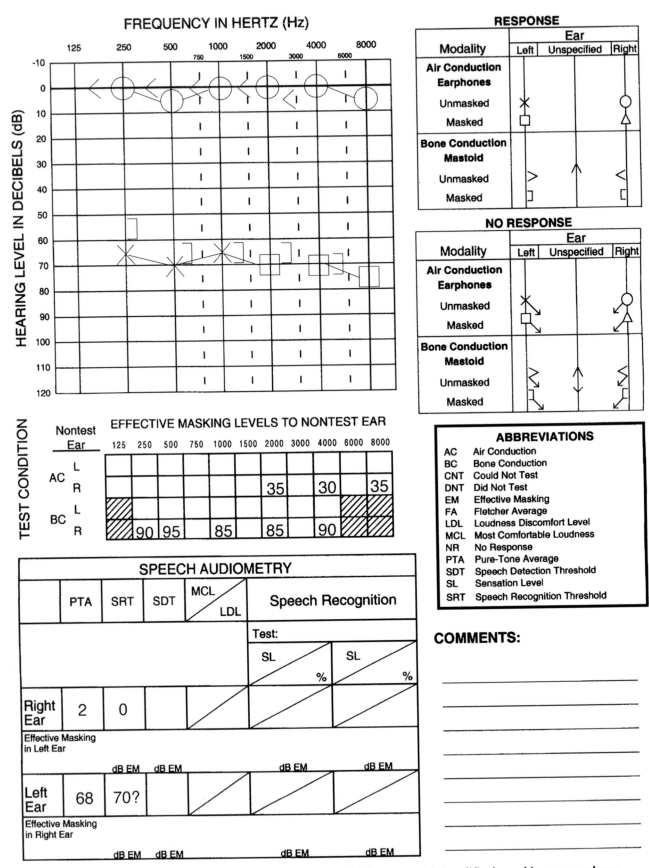

FIGURE 6.15 An example illustrating the use of the midplateau and simplified masking procedures during assessment of speech recognition threshold.

It has already been demonstrated that the simplified masking procedure proves very effective during assessment of supra-threshold speech recognition. However, it also can be applied effectively during measurement of SRT. When selecting an appropriate contralateral masking level when measuring SRT, it is important to consider not only the HL at which the speech threshold is finally established, but also the highest presentation levels used throughout the threshold procedure. Regardless of the SRT procedure used, spondaic words are presented typically at both supra-threshold and threshold levels.

For example, ASHA (1988) recommends a descending threshold technique for measuring SRT that is based on the earlier work of others (Hirsh et al., 1952; Hudgins et al., 1947; Tillman and Olsen, 1973; Wilson et al., 1973). The initial phase involves familiarizing the patient with the spondaic words at a comfortable, supra-threshold HL. (Familiarization with test words is strongly recommended regardless of the SRT procedure.) The preliminary phase involves setting the HL to 30 to 40 dB above the estimated or predicted SRT prior to descending in 10-dB decrements until two words are missed. In fact, an HL of 30 to 40 dB above the predicted SRT typically results in a comfortable listening level for most patients during the familiarization phase. The test phase involves initially presenting test words at HLs approximately 10 dB higher than the calculated SRT. The calculation of threshold, based on a statistical precedent, takes into account the patient's responses at higher HLs.

Consider again the example presented in Figure 6.15. If the ASHA-recommended procedure is used to measure SRT, then the highest HLs employed (during the familiarization and preliminary phases) will be about 30 to 40 dB above the estimated SRT. In this example, we will use a moderate SL of 30 dB above the estimated SRT (i.e., 70 dB HL + 30 dB SL = 100 dB HL) during the familiarization and preliminary phases.

The use of the simplified approach to selecting an appropriate level of contralateral masking should prove effective in this case because both prerequisite conditions have been met. First, there are no significant air-bone gaps in either ear. Second, speech is presented at a moderate SL (i.e., 30 dB) when the highest HLs are used during the test procedure (i.e., familiarization and preliminary phases). Assuming that 100 dB HL is the highest presentation level used during our test procedure, then EM level in the nontest ear is calculated as follows.

$$\text{dB EM} = \text{Presentation Level}_{\text{Test Ear}} - 20 \text{ dB}$$

$$= 100 \text{ dB HL} - 20 \text{ dB}$$

$$= 80 \text{ dB}$$

We can verify the appropriateness of the selected masking level by using the midplateau method.

$$M_{\text{Min}} = \text{Presentation Level}_{\text{Test Ear}} - \text{IA}$$

$$+ \text{Largest Air-Bone Gap}_{\text{Nontest Ear}}$$

$$= 100 \text{ dB HL} - 60 \text{ dB} + 0 \text{ dB}$$

$$= 40 \text{ dB EM}$$

$$M_{\text{Max}} = \text{Best BC}_{\text{TestEar}} + \text{IA} - 5 \text{ dB}$$

$$= 55 \text{ dB HL} + 60 \text{ dB} - 5 \text{ dB}$$

$$= 110 \text{ dB EM}$$

$$M_{\text{Mid}} = (M_{\text{Min}} + M_{\text{Max}})/2$$

$$= (40 + 110)/2$$

$$= 75 \text{ dB EM}$$

The masking level of 80 dB EM selected using the simplified approach is in good agreement (i.e., ± 5 dB) with the value determined using the midplateau approach (i.e., 75 dB EM). Although spondees will be presented at lower HLs when measuring the SRT, it is not necessary to decrease the original level of masking. First, the selected masking level is appropriate for the highest HLs used during all phases of threshold determination. Second, the selected masking level does not exceed the maximum masking level (i.e., overmasking will not occur).

It can be argued that the simplified approach (as well as the midplateau method) can result in the use of unnecessarily high masking levels during measurement of SRT. As was discussed earlier, the midplateau represents a range of masking levels. The audiologist can justify subtracting a value of greater than 20 dB (e.g., 25 or 30 dB) from the presentation level at the test ear, particularly when using insert earphones. In this example, a masking level of 70 or 75 dB EM (rather than the original level of 80 dB EM) still falls within an acceptable range of midplateau, while still occurring significantly higher than the minimum.

Yacullo (1999) states that the simplified masking approach during speech audiometry has wide applicability. First, it can be used with a large and diverse patient population, including those with normal hearing and sensory-neural hearing loss. Second, it can be used equally effectively when using either supra-aural and insert earphones. Third, the procedure can be used in clinical situations where moderate SLs are used. For example, the majority of audiologists in the United States continue to administer supra-threshold word recognition tests at a specified SL referenced to the SRT (Martin et al., 1994; Martin et al., 1998; Martin and Morris, 1989), typically 30 or 40 dB (Martin et al., 1994; Martin and Morris, 1989). Finally, it can be applied effectively during both threshold and supra-threshold measures of speech recognition.

Direct calculation of midmasking level is strongly recommended in cases where there is potential risk of overmasking. Yacullo (1999) states that any factor that increases minimum masking level or decreases maximum masking level will reduce the width of the masking plateau and increase the probability of overmasking. For example, the presence of significant air-bone gaps in the in the nontest ear and/or the use of higher SLs (i.e., ≥ 50 dB) will increase minimum masking level. The presence of significant air-bone gaps in the test ear will decrease maximum masking level. In cases where the masking plateau is either very narrow or nonexistent (e.g., unilateral or bilateral conductive hearing loss), knowledge about minimum and maximum masking levels will allow the clinician to make well-informed decisions about appropriate contralateral masking levels.

REFERENCES

American National Standards Institute. (2004a) Methods for Manual Pure-Tone Threshold Audiometry. ANSI S3.21-2004. New York: American National Standards Institute.

American National Standards Institute. (2004b) Specification for Audiometers. ANSI S3.6-2004. New York: American National Standards Institute.

American Speech-Language-Hearing Association. (2005) Guidelines for manual pure-tone threshold audiometry. Available at: http://www.asha.org/docs/pdf/GL2005-00014.pdf.

American Speech-Language-Hearing Association. (1988) Guidelines for determining threshold level for speech. *ASHA*. 30, 85–89.

American Speech-Language-Hearing Association. (1990) Guidelines for audiometric symbols. *ASHA*. Suppl 2, 25–30.

Beattie RC, Svihovec DV, Edgerton BJ. (1978) Comparison of speech detection and spondee thresholds for half- versus full-list intelligibility scores with MLV and taped presentations of NU-6. *J Am Audiol Soc*. 3, 267–272.

Berger EH, Kerivan JE. (1983) Influence of physiological noise and the occlusion effect on the measurement of real-ear attenuation at threshold. *J Acoust Soc Am*. 74, 81–94.

Berrett MV. (1973) Some relations between interaural attenuation and the occlusion effect. Unpublished doctoral dissertation. Iowa City: University of Iowa.

Blackwell KL, Oyler RF, Seyfried DN. (1991) A clinical comparison of Grason Stadler inserts earphones and TDH-50P standard earphones. *Ear Hear*. 12, 361–362.

Chaiklin JB. (1959) The relation among three selected auditory speech thresholds. *J Speech Hear Res*. 2, 237–243.

Chaiklin JB. (1967) Interaural attenuation and cross-hearing in air-conduction audiometry. *J Aud Res*. 7, 413–424.

Coles RRA, Priede VM. (1970) On the misdiagnosis resulting from incorrect use of masking. *J Laryngol Otol*. 84, 41–63.

Coles RRA, Priede VM. (1975) Masking of the non-test ear in speech audiometry. *J Laryngol Otol*. 89, 217–226.

Dean MS, Martin FN. (2000) Insert earphone depth and the occlusion effect. *Am J Audiol*. 9, 131–134.

Dirks DD. (1994) Bone-conduction threshold testing. In: Katz J, ed. *Handbook of Clinical Audiology*. 4th ed. Baltimore: Williams & Wilkins; pp 132–146.

Dirks DD, Malmquist C. (1964) Changes in bone-conduction thresholds produced by masking in the non-test ear. *J Speech Hear Res*. 7, 271–278.

Dirks DD, Swindeman JG. (1967) The variability of occluded and unoccluded bone-conduction thresholds. *J Speech Hear Res*., 10, 232–249.

Dunn HK, White SD. (1940) Statistical measurements on conversational speech. *J Acoust Soc Am*. 11, 278–288.

E-A-R Auditory Systems. (1997) Instructions for the use of E-A-RTONE 3A insert earphones. Revised ed. Indianapolis: E-A-R Auditory Systems.

E-A-R Auditory Systems. (2000a) Instructions for the use of E-A-RTONE 5A insert earphones. Indianapolis: E-A-R Auditory Systems.

E-A-R Auditory Systems. (2000b) Introducing the new E-A-RTONE® 5A insert earphone [Brochure]. Indianapolis: E-A-R Auditory Systems.

Elpern BS, Naunton RF. (1963) The stability of the occlusion effect. *Arch Otolaryngol*. 77, 376–382.

Feldman AS. (1963) Maximum air-conduction hearing loss. *J Speech Hear Disord*. 6, 157–163.

Fletcher H. (1940) Auditory patterns. *Rev Modern Phys*. 12, 47–65.

Frank T, Vavrek MJ. (1992) Reference threshold levels for an ER-3A insert earphone. *J Am Acad Audiol*. 3, 51–58.

Gelfand SA. (2001) *Essentials of Audiology*. 2nd ed. New York: Thieme Medical Publisher, Inc.

Goldstein DP, Hayes CS. (1965) The occlusion effect in bone-conduction hearing. *J Speech Hear Res*. 8, 137–148.

Hannley M. (1986) *Basic Principles of Auditory Assessment*. Needham Heights, MA: Allyn & Bacon.

Hawkins JE, Stevens SS. (1950) Masking of pure tones and of speech by white noise. *J Acoust Soc Am*. 22, 6–13.

Hirsh IJ, Davis H, Silverman SR, Reynolds EG, Eldert E, Benson RW. (1952) Development of materials for speech audiometry. *J Speech Hear Disord*. 17, 321–337.

Hodgson W, Tillman T. (1966) Reliability of bone conduction occlusion effects in normals. *J Aud Res*. 6, 141–151.

Hood JD. (1960) The principles and practice of bone-conduction audiometry. *Laryngoscope*. 70, 1211–1228.

Hosford-Dunn H, Kuklinski AL, Raggio M, Haggerty HS. (1986) Solving audiometric masking dilemmas with an insert masker. *Arch Otolaryngol Head Neck Surg*. 112, 92–95.

Hudgins CV, Hawkins JE Jr., Karlin JE, Stevens SS. (1947) The development of recorded auditory tests for measuring hearing loss for speech. *Laryngoscope*. 57, 57–89.

Jerger J, Jerger S. (1971) Diagnostic significance of PB word functions. *Arch Otolaryngol*. 93, 573–580.

Jerger J, Jerger S, Ainsworth J, Caram P. (1966) Recovery of auditory function after surgical removal of cerebellar tumor. *J Speech Hear Disord*. 31, 377–382.

Kaplan H, Gladstone VS, Lloyd LL. (1993) *Audiometric Interpretation*. 2nd ed. Needham Heights, MA: Allyn & Bacon.

Killion MC. (1984) New insert earphones for audiometry. *Hear Instr*. 35, 28, 46.

Killion MC, Villchur E. (1989) Comments on "Earphones in audiometry" [Zwislocki et al., J. Acoust. Soc. Am. 83, 1688–1689)]. *J Acoust Soc Am*. 85, 1775–1778.

Killion MC, Wilber LA, Gudmundsen GI. (1985) Insert earphones for more interaural attenuation. *Hear Instr*. 36, 34, 36.

Konkle DF, Berry GA. (1983) Masking in speech audiometry. In: Konkle DF, Rintelmann WF, eds. *Principles of Speech Audiometry*. Baltimore: University Park Press; pp 285–319.

Lidén G, Nilsson G, Anderson H. (1959) Masking in clinical audiometry. *Acta Otolaryngol.* 50, 125–136.

Littler TS, Knight JJ, Strange PH. (1952) Hearing by bone conduction and the use of bone-conduction hearing aids. *Proc R Soc Med.* 45, 783–790.

Martin FN. (1966) Speech audiometry and clinical masking. *J Aud Res.* 6, 199–203.

Martin FN. (1967) A simplified method for clinical masking. *J Aud Res.* 7, 59–62.

Martin FN. (1974) Minimum effective masking levels in threshold audiometry. *J Speech Hear Disord.* 39, 280–285.

Martin FN. (1980) The masking plateau revisited. *Ear Hear.* 1, 112–116.

Martin FN. (1997) *Introduction to Audiology.* 6th ed. Needham Heights, MA: Allyn & Bacon.

Martin FN, Armstrong TW, Champlin CA. (1994) A survey of audiological practices in the United States in 1992. *Am J Audiol.* 3, 20–26.

Martin FN, Bailey HAT, Pappas JJ. (1965) The effect of central masking on threshold for speech. *J Aud Res.* 5, 293–296.

Martin FN, Blythe ME. (1977) On the cross hearing of spondaic words. *J Aud Res.* 17, 221–224.

Martin FN, Butler EC, Burns P. (1974) Audiometric Bing test for determination of minimum masking levels for bone conduction tests. *J Speech Hear Disord.* 39, 148–152.

Martin FN, Champlin CA, Chambers JA. (1998) Seventh survey of audiometric practices in the United States. *J Am Acad Audiol.* 9, 95–104.

Martin FN, DiGiovanni D. (1979) Central masking effects on spondee threshold as a function of masker sensation level and masker sound pressure level. *J Am Aud Soc.* 4, 141–146.

Martin FN, Morris LJ. (1989) Current audiologic practices in the United States. *Hear J.* 42, 25–44.

Naunton RF. (1960) A masking dilemma in bilateral conduction deafness. *Arch Otolaryngol.* 72, 753–757.

Olsen WO, Matkin ND. (1991) Speech audiometry. In: Rintelmann WF, ed. *Hearing Assessment.* Needham Heights, MA: Allyn & Bacon; pp 39–140.

Owens E, Schubert ED. (1977) Development of the California consonant test. *J Speech Hear Res.* 20, 463–474.

Sanders JW. (1991) Clinical masking. In: Rintelmann WF, ed. *Hearing Assessment.* Needham Heights, MA: Allyn & Bacon; pp 141–178.

Sanders JW, Rintelmann WF. (1964) Masking in audiometry. *Arch Otolaryngol.* 80, 541–556.

Schwartz DM, Surr R. (1979) Three experiments on the California consonant test. *J Speech Hear Disord.* 64, 61–72.

Silman S, Silverman CA. (1991) *Auditory Diagnosis: Principles and Applications.* San Diego: Academic Press.

Sklare DA, Denenberg LJ. (1987) Interaural attenuation for Tubephone insert earphones. *Ear Hear.* 8, 298–300.

Smith BL, Markides A. (1981) Interaural attenuation for pure tones and speech. *Br J Audiol.* 15, 49–54.

Snyder JM. (1973) Interaural attenuation characteristics in audiometry. *Laryngoscope.* 73, 1847–1855.

Studebaker GA. (1962) On masking in bone-conduction testing. *J Speech Hear Res.* 5, 215–227.

Studebaker GA. (1964) Clinical masking of air- and bone-conducted stimuli. *J Speech Hear Disord.* 29, 23–35.

Studebaker GA. (1967a) Clinical masking of the non-test ear. *J Speech Hear Disord.* 32, 360–371.

Studebaker GA. (1967b) Intertest variability and the air-bone gap. *J Speech Hear Disord.* 32, 82–86.

Studebaker GA. (1979) Clinical masking. In: Rintelmann WF, ed. *Hearing Assessment.* Baltimore: University Park Press; pp 51–100.

Thurlow WR, Silverman SR, Davis H, Walsh TE. (1948) A statistical study of auditory tests in relation to the fenestration operation. *Laryngoscope.* 58, 43–66.

Tillman TW, Olsen WO. (1973) Speech audiometry. In: Jerger J, ed. *Modern Developments in Audiology.* 2nd ed. New York: Academic Press; pp 37–74.

Tonndorf J. (1968) A new concept of bone conduction. *Arch Otolaryngol.* 87, 49–54.

Tonndorf J. (1972) Bone conduction. In: Tobias JV, ed. *Foundations of Modern Auditory Theory.* Volume II. New York: Academic Press; pp 197–237.

Turner RG. (2004a) Masking redux I: an optimized masking method. *J Am Acad Audiol.* 15, 17–28.

Turner RG. (2004b) Masking redux II: a recommended masking protocol. *J Am Acad Audiol.* 15, 29–46.

Van Campen LE, Sammeth CA, Peek BF. (1990) Interaural attenuation using Etymotic ER-3A insert earphones in auditory brain stem response testing. *Ear Hear.* 11, 66–69.

Wegel RL, Lane GI. (1924) The auditory masking of one pure tone by another and its probable relation to the dynamics of the inner ear. *Physics Rev.* 23, 266–285.

Wilson R, Morgan D, Dirks D. (1973) A proposed SRT procedure and its statistical precedent. *J Speech Hear Disord.* 38, 184–191.

Yacullo WS. (1996) *Clinical Masking Procedures.* Boston, MA: Allyn & Bacon.

Yacullo WS. (1999) Clinical masking in speech audiometry: a simplified approach. *Am J Audiol.* 8, 106–116.

Yacullo WS. (2004) Clinical masking. In: Kent RD, ed. *The MIT Encyclopedia of Communication Disorders.* Cambridge, MA: MIT Press; pp 500–504.

Zwislocki J. (1953) Acoustic attenuation between the ears. *J Acoust Soc Am.* 25, 752–759.

Zwislocki J, Kruger B, Miller JD, Niemoeller AR, Shaw EA, Studebaker G. (1988) Earphones in audiometry. *J Acoust Soc Am.* 83, 1688–1689.

7 Case History

Douglas L. Beck

INTRODUCTION

The case history is relevant and focused information concerning an individual that facilitates an appropriate diagnosis and treatment plan. Obtaining and using the case history requires skill, patience, and knowledge.

It has often been said that there are two key ingredients to a correct differential diagnosis: (1) an excellent case history, and (2) a thorough physical exam. Given those two pieces of information, the differential diagnosis often "emerges" to the trained professional as the only clear conclusion.

Audiologists are charged with the responsibility of diagnosing and nonmedically treating hearing loss (American Academy of Audiology [AAA], 2004; American Speech-Language-Hearing Association [ASHA], 2004). Therefore, we must look critically and judiciously at all information related to hearing loss to render an appropriate diagnosis. Case history gathering is an important skill that facilitates the correct differential diagnosis.

In general, if you are not looking for something, you probably will not find it. A likely corollary is also true: If you are looking for zebras in a cow pasture, you probably will not find them. To find the correct solution to a given problem, we must pose the right question, formulate reasonable options and alternatives, and ultimately, choose the most probable alternative.

When gathering and assembling case histories, health care professionals must narrow the focus and filter the information available to gather what is most important quickly and efficiently. The case history should be reasonable, result driven, and provide an evidence-based outcome.

In health care, the method of choice for obtaining the case history is the "medical model." The medical model efficiently directs the professional to the "chief complaint" and helps organize information into a rational hierarchy with the most important or likely concerns at the top.

Researchers have designed decision trees and analysis weightings and other complex models that are powerful and accurate and, theoretically, will assist in finding the correct diagnosis. However, when the audiologist is working one-on-one in the examination room with the patient, assembling the case history is essentially a person-to-person event.

CASE HISTORY TOOLS

There are three primary tools used to create a case history: interviews, questionnaires, and the Subjective, Objective, Assessment, and Plan (SOAP) format. These three tools are typically used in tandem but can certainly be used as preferred by the professional.

As a licensed health care professional, the audiologist has a legal obligation to the patient regarding his or her health and well-being. The audiologist must be aware of the warning signs of dangerous and treatable medical and surgical conditions and should refer appropriate patients based on "red flags." Red flags include sudden hearing loss, ear pain, draining or bleeding ears, unilateral symptoms of hearing loss or tinnitus, conductive hearing loss, dizziness, and other referral criteria. Assembling the case history provides an opportunity to identify any red flags while considering a multitude of diagnostic and treatment alternatives.

Interview Techniques

Of course, there is no "one correct way" to interview patients. Flexibility is the key, as professionals, patients, work settings, and the particulars of each situation vary. Nonetheless, it is always a good idea to proceed in an orderly and professional manner. Interviews should be patient centered, friendly, and private, in accordance with applicable laws, rules, and regulations (see Health Insurance Portability and Accountability Act [HIPPA], 2006).

While gathering the case history, ascertaining an "index of suspicion" regarding the chief complaint is an important part of the interview. If the index of suspicion for the item highest on our list is low, we generally need to look for more probable alternatives. If the index of suspicion is high, we ask further questions to confirm or refute our suspicions.

For example, a patient presenting with a fluctuating low-frequency sensory-neural hearing loss and tinnitus in the same ear, with aural fullness and occasional vertigo, has a low index of suspicion for otosclerosis but has a reasonably high index of suspicion for Ménière's disease. The high index of suspicion for Ménière's disease would lead us to ask probing questions to see whether the presenting symptomatology is in agreement with a Ménière's disease profile or would lead us in another direction, such as an acoustic neuroma.

The competent professional understands the probabilities of certain things occurring and the related signs and symptoms of each. Although Ménière's disease is a relatively rare disorder, occurring in less than 1% of the general population, it is a common diagnosis for patients with the symptoms described earlier. Knowing the symptoms of Ménière's disease, the professional asks appropriate questions to increase or decrease the index of suspicion, ultimately leading to the primary diagnosis.

Three scenarios follow to illustrate the interview technique.

SCENARIO ONE

Review any/all assembled paperwork (chart, lab notes, test results, history, etc.) before meeting the patient for the initial consultation. Shake hands and greet the patient, their spouse, significant other, family, and so on, and always introduce yourself. This is an amazingly simple protocol, but it is often overlooked, and when it is overlooked, it sets a bad tone for the rest of the encounter. I usually say, "Good morning. My name is Dr. Beck, I'm an audiologist. Please come in Mr. Smith."

After exchanging greetings and after sitting down in the office, inquire as to why the patient scheduled today's visit.

"Thanks for coming in today Mr. Smith. What brings you to the office?"

Mr. Smith: *"I would like a comprehensive audiometric evaluation to confirm my bilateral sensory-neural noise-induced hearing loss that my otolaryngologist diagnosed last week. I am very interested in acquiring two digital hearing aids, and by the way, I am wealthy and do not have insurance. I pay cash, and money is no object. I want to hear everything as best I can."*

Because this patient has already been seen and diagnosed by the ear, nose, and throat (ENT) specialist, the index of

suspicion for some other disease process or a medical/surgical issue is extremely low.

SCENARIO TWO

Mr. Smith: *"Well doc, you know how it is. My wife always complains I have the TV up too loud and it drives her outta the room. I like to be able to hear the darn thing so I keep it a little loud. The same thing happens with the car radio when we're driving to the store. When she sets the volume, I just hear noise and can't tell anything about what they're saying. When I was a boy, I could hear a pin drop from 40 paces."*

"I understand. How long have you been playing the TV and radio louder than your wife enjoys it?"

"Let's see, I started working at the steel fabrication factory 14 years ago, and my son was born 8 years ago ... so yeah, it's been at least 8 or 10 years. When I let her set the volume, I can hear the voices, but I really can't understand what they're saying. That drives me nuts. I told her and I'm telling you too, I ain't gonna wear no hearing aids."

Given the information presented in this scenario, one can make several, reasonable, assumptions. We could assume that Mr. Smith has a noise-induced sensory-neural hearing loss, likely impacting 4,000 Hz, and because he cannot hear the consonant sounds (high frequencies), he cannot clearly understand the words spoken to him. We might also assume that Mr. Smith is not going to wear hearing aids and that there is little we can do to assist. However, there are other options and protocols to employ:

"Mr. Smith, have you had a hearing test before?"

"Not since the Army, back some 20 years ago."

"Do both ears seem about the same, or is one ear better than the other?"

"The left ear is terrible—can't hear thunder with that one."

"I see. Do you have any ear pain?"

"None at all. My ears feel fine."

"Okay then. May I take a look?"

"Sure, help yourself."

At this point, the audiologist has a rather low index of suspicion for a tumor, such as an acoustic neuroma, because they occur in some 0.00001% of the population, but a higher index of suspicion for more likely possibilities, including a unilateral sudden sensory-neural loss that went undiagnosed (or maybe Mr. Smith works with his left ear toward a loud machine while wearing hearing protection only in the right ear, or perhaps he experienced head trauma on the left or an explosion near his left side during boot camp; there are lots of possibilities). The examination of the pinna, concha, ear canal, and tympanic membranes is normal in appearance. The audiologist says, "Okay, your ears look fine," and the interview continues to determine which diagnosis has the highest index of suspicion.

"Mr. Smith, let me make sure I understand... the right ear is the better ear and the left ear has been bad for a long time. Have you ever had the left ear checked?"

"Yes. I had the doctor look at it a year or two ago when it went bad. He put me on antibiotics and that was the end of it. It didn't get better though, so I left it alone."

"Okay. What about drainage, anything coming out of your ears?"

"No sir."

"Any dizziness or spinning sensations?"

"Not any more. Well, maybe a little. When my left ear was going bad, I had some dizziness, but the doctor looked in it and put me on antibiotics, and the dizziness got better after a while."

"So both the dizziness started and the left ear went bad all about a year or two ago?"

"That's right."

"Okay, very good. Are you on any medications?"

"Just a cholesterol pill and a baby aspirin, that's about it."

"Okay, and one last thing I'd like to ask you before we do the hearing test—do you have any ringing or buzzing noises in your ears?"

"Yeah, the darn left ear can't hear anything, but it sure makes a racket. Kinda like a "shhhhh" noise going on in there. Keeps me up at night sometimes."

The audiologist does a comprehensive audiometric evaluation and determines the following audiometric profile.

Right ear: Normal hearing. Tympanogram normal (type A), ipsi reflex within normal limits (WNL). Word recognition score (WRS) = 96%. Speech reception threshold (SRT) = 15 dB.

Left ear: Flat 85 dB sensory-neural (SN) loss. Tympanogram normal (type A), ipsi reflex absent @105 dB stim. WRS = 8%, SRT = SAT (Speech Awareness Level used because speech understanding was severe in this ear) = 80 dB.

The index of suspicion for a left retrocochlear disorder is very high at this point. The case history supports this possibility, and the test results indicate a possible retrocochlear diagnosis for the left ear.

The audiologist refers the patient to an otolaryngologist (preferably an otologist or neurotologist) based on the high index of suspicion for a retrocochlear hearing loss. The otologist meets with and interviews the patient and refers the patient for a magnetic resonance imaging (MRI) study with contrast (gadolinium). A 3-cm vestibular schwannoma (acoustic neuroma) is diagnosed. Mr. Smith is scheduled for surgery 3 weeks later, and the tumor is removed via the translabyrinthine approach.

SCENARIO THREE

Mr. Smith: *"Let's see, I started working at this really noisy factory 14 years ago, and my son was born 8 years ago... so yeah, it's been at least 8 or 10 years. When my wife sets the TV, it sounds like everyone is mumbling; I can hear the voices, but I really can't understand what they're saying. That drives me nuts. I told her and I'm telling you too, I ain't gonna wear no hearing aids."*

Given the information presented above, one can make several assumptions. We could assume Mr. Smith has a noise-induced sensory-neural hearing loss, impacting frequencies around 4,000 Hz, and because of the reduced amplitude and distortion affecting mostly the high-frequency consonant sounds, he cannot clearly hear the words spoken to him. We can also be pretty sure that Mr. Smith is not going to wear hearing aids, so this reduces what we can do to assist. However, there are other options and protocols to explore.

"Mr. Smith, have you had a hearing test before?"

"Not since the Army, back some 20 years ago."

"Do both ears seem about the same, or is one ear better than the other?"

"They're just about the same"

"I see. Any ear pain?"

"None at all. My ears feel fine."

"That's good. May I take a look?"

"Sure doc, knock yourself out."

The pinna, concha, ear canal, and tympanic membranes are normal in appearance. The audiologist says, "Your ears look fine," and the interview continues.

"Okay, what about drainage? Is there anything coming out of your ears?"

"No sir."

"Any dizziness or spinning sensations"

"Nope."

"Very good. Are you on any medications?"

"Just a cholesterol pill and a baby aspirin, that's about it."

"The last thing I'd like to ask you before we do the hearing test is do you have any ringing or buzzing noises in your ears?"

"Yeah... maybe a little when it's really quiet, nothing that really bothers me though."

The audiologist does a comprehensive audiometric evaluation and determines the following audiometric profile:

Right ear: Moderate high-frequency sensory-neural hearing loss. Tympanogram normal (type A), ipsi reflex within normal limits (WNL). WRS = 96%. SRT = 45 dB.

Left ear: Moderate high-frequency sensory-neural hearing loss. Tympanogram normal (type A), ipsi reflex WNL. WRS = 92%. SRT = 45 dB.

"Mr. Smith, I'd like to review the results of today's tests with you. Would you like to have your wife join us while I review the results?"

"Sure, that would be great. She's in the waiting room."

"Hi Mrs. Smith, please join us while I review the results of today's exam. This way, the two of you will have the chance to learn about the results, and I can address your questions."

In this third scenario, the index of suspicion for a noise-induced hearing loss is high, and there are no red flags and no indications of a medical or surgical problem.

In essence, the same patient, in three different scenarios, has three separate sets of circumstances, each of which are typically revealed through an interview-based case history, which is more or less driven by the index of suspicion.

Questionnaires

Another very useful and efficient case history tool is the health questionnaire. A well-designed questionnaire is highly focused, simple, takes just a few minutes to fill out, and quickly directs the professional to the area(s) of greatest concern. Questionnaires regarding hearing health care can be presented to patients verbally, as a pencil and paper presentation, or on a computer.

VERBAL PRESENTATIONS

Remember, if you are giving a patient a verbal presentation of a hearing questionnaire, there is already a reasonable index of suspicion for hearing loss. Therefore, sit about 3 feet away from the patient in a well-lit room, face the patient, be sure there is no background noise or visual distractions, and be sure to have the patients' full attention.

PENCIL AND PAPER PRESENTATIONS

Keep in mind that, because the majority of patients seen by audiologists are over 55 years of age, large font, dark print, and maximal contrast between the printed words and the background page are preferred and appreciated. Black print on a white background will be the easiest to read. Another important consideration is to use and/or design questionnaires that are easily assessed and tabulated, so the professional can scan the page to find the "positive" results, which will need to be considered.

In 2005, the Centers for Medicare and Medicaid Services (CMS) added a new benefit under Medicare Part B that will likely increase the quantity of pencil and paper–based hearing and balance screenings offered to patients. This benefit is "bundled" within the "Welcome to Medicare" exam. The exam has seven screening sections for physicians, nurses, or nurse practitioners to employ when addressing new patients. Importantly, the Medicare rules state that the screening tests must be in the form of questions or questionnaires and that the selected screening tests must be recognized by a national medical professional organization.

The AAA and ASHA have recommended that the following questionnaire be used for this purpose: Hearing Handicap Inventory–Screening Version (HHIE-S; Ventry and Weistein, 1982). In addition, AAA recommends the National Institute for Deafness and Communication Disorders (NIDCD) Screening Test (NIDCD, 2006), the Hearing Health Quick Test (AAA, 2008), and the Dizziness Handicap Inventory–Screening Version (DHI-S; Jacobson and Calder, 1998). ASHA has also recommended: Five Minute Hearing Test (American Academy of Otolaryngology–Head and Neck Surgery, 2002).

There is likely to be greater popularity for screening tests. Therefore, audiologists should be familiar with the above-noted questionnaires and their format, scoring, and importance.

COMPUTER-BASED QUESTIONNAIRES

The Internet has many health-related questionnaires available. The major advantage to online hearing questionnaires is the instant scoring feature, which allows the patient to immediately determine his or her results. The following online questionnaire was designed by this author (D.L.B.) and is available at www.healthyhearing.com; it is free, and it self-scores immediately.

Please answer ALL questions as they pertain to you.

1. Do you often think "my hearing is not as good as it used to be?"
   - ○ Yes, most of the time
   - ○ Yes, sometimes
   - ○ Maybe
   - ○ No, almost never
   - ○ No, this never happens
2. Do women and children seem to "mumble?"
   - ○ Yes, most of the time
   - ○ Yes, sometimes
   - ○ Maybe
   - ○ No, almost never
   - ○ No, this never happens
3. Do you get in arguments or in difficult situations with your spouse (or friends or family) because you thought they said one thing, and they say they said another?
   - ○ Yes, most of the time
   - ○ Yes, sometimes
   - ○ Maybe
   - ○ No, almost never
   - ○ No, this never happens

4. Do you have difficulty understanding some voices and words on the phone?
   - ○ Yes, most of the time
   - ○ Yes, sometimes
   - ○ Maybe
   - ○ No, almost never
   - ○ No, this never happens

5. Do you have difficulty hearing the words from your grandchildren (or other children)?
   - ○ Yes, most of the time
   - ○ Yes, sometimes
   - ○ Maybe
   - ○ No, almost never
   - ○ No, this never happens

6. Do you have ringing in one or both ears?
   - ○ Yes, most of the time
   - ○ Yes, sometimes
   - ○ Maybe
   - ○ No, almost never
   - ○ No, this never happens

7. Do you have a history of industrial, work-related, or recreational noise exposure, like working in a factory, as a firefighter, as a musician, at an airport, firing weapons, target practice, or other noisy sources?
   - ○ Yes, most of the time
   - ○ Yes, sometimes
   - ○ Maybe
   - ○ No, almost never
   - ○ No, this never happens

8. Do you sometimes say "people don't speak clearly any more, they don't pronounce the words as clearly as they used to"?
   - ○ Yes, most of the time
   - ○ Yes, sometimes
   - ○ Maybe
   - ○ No, almost never
   - ○ No, this never happens

9. Do you sometimes feel embarrassed about asking for repeats?
   - ○ Yes, most of the time
   - ○ Yes, sometimes
   - ○ Maybe
   - ○ No, almost never
   - ○ No, this never happens

10. Do you get frustrated easily with unfamiliar and soft voices?
    - ○ Yes, most of the time
    - ○ Yes, sometimes
    - ○ Maybe
    - ○ No, almost never
    - ○ No, this never happens

11. Do you find that you sometimes "fake it" by trying to nod in agreement, even though you weren't sure what was said?
    - ○ Yes, most of the time
    - ○ Yes, sometimes

- ○ Maybe
- ○ No, almost never
- ○ No, this never happens

12. Do you think you can hear "loud enough" but cannot understand the words?
    - ○ Yes, most of the time
    - ○ Yes, sometimes
    - ○ Maybe
    - ○ No, almost never
    - ○ No, this never happens

13. Do you have a hard time hearing normal conversation in noisy backgrounds, such as at a restaurant or a cocktail party?
    - ○ Yes, most of the time
    - ○ Yes, sometimes
    - ○ Maybe
    - ○ No, almost never
    - ○ No, this never happens

14. Do you have a hard time understanding whispers?
    - ○ Yes, most of the time
    - ○ Yes, sometimes
    - ○ Maybe
    - ○ No, almost never
    - ○ No, this never happens

15. Do you listen to the TV louder than most people?
    - ○ Yes, most of the time
    - ○ Yes, sometimes
    - ○ Maybe
    - ○ No, almost never
    - ○ No, this never happens

16. Do you have difficulty hearing the words during religious services or at large meetings?
    - ○ Yes, most of the time
    - ○ Yes, sometimes
    - ○ Maybe
    - ○ No, almost never
    - ○ No, this never happens

17. Do you have difficulty determining where the sounds are coming from?
    - ○ Yes, most of the time
    - ○ Yes, sometimes
    - ○ Maybe
    - ○ No, almost never
    - ○ No, this never happens

18. Do your ears hurt or drain, or does one ear hear better than the other?
    - ○ Yes, most of the time
    - ○ Yes, sometimes
    - ○ Maybe
    - ○ No, almost never
    - ○ No, this never happens

19. Do you have difficulty understanding when there are more than two people talking at the same time?
    - ○ Yes, most of the time
    - ○ Yes, sometimes
    - ○ Maybe

○ No, almost never
○ No, this never happens

20. Do you turn the volume up on the public telephone systems to hear better?

○ Yes, most of the time
○ Yes, sometimes
○ Maybe
○ No, almost never
○ No, this never happens

The Internet is the largest, most significant, least expensive, and most efficient venue for the transfer of information. Exploration of additional Internet-based screening mechanisms is encouraged. It is likely that many patients have taken an online hearing screening prior to visiting a hearing professional, and this trend is expected to increase.

Subjective, Objective, Assessment, and Plan

Another way to gather useful case history information quickly is to use the standard SOAP format. SOAP is an acronym for Subjective, Objective, Assessment, and Plan. The SOAP format is essentially a "medical model" case history–gathering tool. There are many variations on the SOAP format used by clinics, medical schools, and often, military health care facilities.

Critics believe the SOAP format is impersonal and does not recognize the patient as a whole person. In addition, the SOAP format tends to treat the person as if he or she was the disease/disorder/problem, and it calls for the use of jargon and related abbreviations. Although jargon is common in health professions, it can vary from location to location, and it may be nearly impossible for even the most well-educated colleagues to interpret. In the following examples, abbreviations will be used along with their explanations, which will immediately follow in parenthesis.

SUBJECTIVE

The subjective section provides a brief subjective history, often focusing on the chief complaint (CC) as well as other clinical observations. The patients' medical and audiology history would be placed in this section. Other entries in this section would be notes the patient/relative/friends offer regarding pain or discomfort and related miscellaneous symptoms. An example follows:

Pt (patient) is 56-year-old, Caucasian, divorced female. NKA (no known allergies).
Pt has one adult daughter (age 26 years).
Pt has HBP (high blood pressure) that has been under control via meds for 3 years. Pt takes daily multivitamin.
No other known medical issues.
Pt consumes ETOH (alcohol) daily (one glass), stopped smoking 15 years ago.

Previous surgery: C-section 26 years ago. Ingrown toenail (left big toe) operated on 22 years ago.
Today CC – hearing loss AD (right ear) × 1 months with tinnitus, no spinning/vertigo, no complaints AS (left ear).
Pt presents for AE (audiometric evaluation).

OBJECTIVE

In medical charts, the objective section often includes measures of temperature, blood pressure, skin color, swelling, and other "objective" data that can be obtained in the office easily and quickly. This section is where the audiologist would write the "objective" test results. An example follows:

Puretones:
65 dB SN (sensory-neural) HL (hearing loss) AD (right)
AS (left) WNL (within normal limits)
SRT (speech reception threshold):
70 dB AD, 15 dB AS
SAT (speech awareness threshold):
60 dB AD
15 dB AS
WRS (word recognition score):
24% AD at SAT plus 35 dB with masking contra
100% AS
OAEs (otoacoustic emissions):
AD ABS (absent)
AS WNL
Tympanograms:
WNL AU (within normal limits, both ears)

ASSESSMENT

The assessment section is where the physician or audiologist would make a statement about the probable "working" diagnosis, or the final diagnosis, and prognosis. For example:

Pt presents with probable AD SNHL (right sensory-neural hearing loss), possibly from untreated sudden SNHL, possibly retrocochlear?

PLAN

The plan is the "plan" as of this moment, moving forward. The physician may write the recommended prescriptions or may order blood tests, lab work, or radiology tests, as needed. The audiologist might write:

Refer pt. to ENT for AD asymmetric, SNHL to R/O (rule out) retrocochlear origin or other medical/surgical concerns. Assuming medical/surgical is R/O, proceed with hearing aid trial AD.

Although the SOAP format is a quick and efficient way to gather the history and related information, it may ignore more global problems, while attending primarily to the chief complaint.

SUMMARY

Gathering an efficient and thorough case history requires human understanding, patience, and knowledge of hearing, hearing loss, and related disorders. Although there are options regarding the preferred method with which to gather a case history, there is no alternative to accuracy.

Whichever protocol(s) is chosen, the clinician has the responsibility of assembling the information in a meaningful and relevant way to maximally address the needs, concerns, and well-being of the patient.

REFERENCES

American Academy of Audiology. (2004) Audiology: scope of practice. Available at: http://www.audiology.org/publications/documents/practice/.

American Academy of Audiology. (2008) Hearing Health Quick Test. Available at: http://www.audiology.org/aboutaudiology/consumered/guides/quicktest.htm

American Academy of Otolaryngology – Head and Neck Surgery. (2002) Five Minute Hearing Test. Available at: www.entnet.org/healthinfo/hearing/hearing_test.cfm.

American Speech-Language-Hearing Association. (2004) Scope of Practice in Audiology. Available at: http://www.asha.org/NR/rdonlyres/036AC2B1-FB02-4124-8709-80881C1079A6/0/18752_1.pdf.

Health Insurance Portability and Accountability Act. (2006) Office for Civil Rights, HIPAA Medical Privacy. National Standards to Protect the Privacy of Personal Health Information. Available at: http://www.hhs.gov/ocr/hipaa/finalreg.html.

Jacobson GP, Calder JH. (1998) screening version of the Dizziness Handicap Inventory (DHI-S). *Am J Otol.* 19, 804–808.

National Institute for Deafness and Communication Disorders. (2006) National Institute for Deafness and Communication Disorders Screening Test. Available at: http://www.nidcd.nih.gov/health/hearing/10ways.asp.

Ventry IM, Weinstein BE. (1982) The hearing handicap inventory for the elderly: a new tool. *Ear Hear.* 3, *128–134.*

SECTION II

PHYSIOLOGICAL PRINCIPLES AND MEASURES

Principles of Acoustic Immittance and Acoustic Transfer Functions

Douglas H. Keefe and M. Patrick Feeney

◼ INTRODUCTION

This chapter provides an overview of the human anatomy of the outer and middle ear; reviews of vibration, signals, and acoustics; a description of acoustic transfer functions and their relation to acoustic immittance; and an introduction to traditional clinical tests of middle ear function such as tympanometry and acoustic stapedius reflex (ASR) measurement. The latter are described in detail in Chapters 9 and 10. This chapter also discusses the function and potential uses of emerging measurement systems that provide expanded dimensions of middle ear assessment across a wide range of frequencies. For the reader interested in a historical treatment of middle ear measurements, excellent reviews are provided by Shallop (1976) and Van Camp et al. (1986).

◼ BASIC ANATOMY AND PHYSIOLOGY OF THE OUTER AND MIDDLE EARS

The peripheral anatomy of the human ear is illustrated in Figure 8.1. The pinna or auricle and external auditory canal form the outer ear. The tympanic membrane, middle ear ossicles, tympanic muscles, and an air pocket, with access to the mastoid cavity and the Eustachian tube, form the middle ear. The smallest ossicle, the stapes, connects the middle ear with the cochlea via the oval window to the fluid-filled vestibule of the inner ear.

The pinna is a cartilaginous structure covered with squamous epithelium, which has characteristic cavities and folds shown in Figure 8.2. The pinna has vestigial muscles, which are not useful for moving the pinna toward a sound source, as they are used in many mammals, although they may allow the pinnae to wiggle for some individuals. Due to its shape and orientation on the head, the pinna increases the efficiency with which sound is collected by the ear. The cavum concha has a resonance near 5,000 Hz, and the small folds of the helix have even higher resonance frequencies (Shaw, 1974).

The squamous epithelium of the external auditory canal is contiguous with the pinna on its lateral aspect and the tympanic membrane on its medial aspect. Dead cells from the outer layer of epithelium of the external ear canal form debris that migrates out of the external canal. Ceruminous glands in the lateral portion of the canal produce cerumen, which is mostly composed of sebum, a waxy substance that lubricates and protects the canal. The canal functions acoustically to increase the sound pressure level (SPL) at the tympanic membrane in the frequency region near 3,000 Hz (Shaw, 1974).

The cone-shaped tympanic membrane consists of an annular cartilaginous ring that anchors the perimeter of the membrane to the bony canal. The lateral layer of the tri-layer membrane is composed of squamous epithelium, which is supported throughout the pars tensa by a middle fibrous layer consisting of radial and circular fibers. The third mucosal layer is contiguous with the middle ear mucosa. When the normal drum is viewed with an otoscope placed in the ear canal, one arm of the most lateral ossicle, the manubrium of the malleus, can be viewed through the translucent drum. The manubrium terminates near the middle of the conical drum at the umbo. In otoscopic viewing of the normal healthy drum, a cone of light is typically observed to emanate from the umbo due to reflection of the light from the

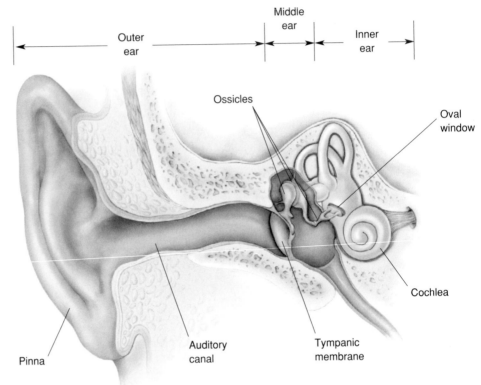

FIGURE 8.1 The outer, middle, and inner ear. (From Bear MF, Connors BW, Parasido MA. [2001] *Neuroscience: Exploring the Brain.* 2nd ed. Philadelphia: Lippincott Williams & Wilkins.)

membrane. The lateral process of the malleus may also be observed at the superior portion of the manubrium just below the pars flaccida of the membrane (Fig. 8.3).

The malleus, incus, and stapes form the ossicular chain (Fig. 8.4). The most lateral bone, the malleus, is attached to the fibrous layer of the tympanic membrane, which permits the transfer of sound-produced membrane movement to the ossicular chain. The head of the malleus lies in the attic of

the middle ear space and is held in place by anterior and posterior ligaments, which form an axis of rotation for the malleus during sound-induced movements of the tympanic membrane. The head of the middle ossicle, the incus, is attached to the head of the malleus at the malleo-incudal joint in the attic space of the middle ear. The long process of the incus is connected to the head of the diminutive stapes at the incudostapedial joint. The ossicles are connected with

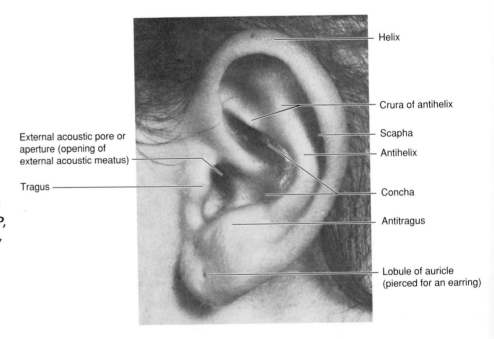

FIGURE 8.2 The parts of the pinna. (From Janfaza P, Nadol JB Jr., Galla R, et al., eds. [2001] *Surgical Anatomy of the Head and Neck.* Philadelphia: Lippincott Williams & Wilkins; p 425, with permission.)

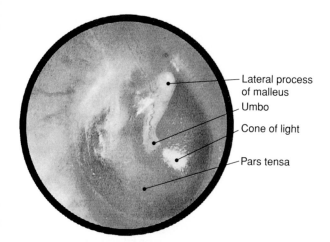

FIGURE 8.3 Otoscopic view of right tympanic membrane. (From Bickley LS, Szilagyi P. [2003] *Bates' Guide to Physical Examination and History Taking.* **8th ed. Philadelphia: Lippincott Williams & Wilkins.)**

flexible joints, which allow some slippage during middle ear pressure changes (Huttenbrink, 1988) and during sound transfer to the inner ear (Goode et al., 1994). Movement of the incus induces a complex, level-dependent rocking motion of the stapes footplate in the oval window, producing vibrations of the fluid of the vestibule of the inner ear. These

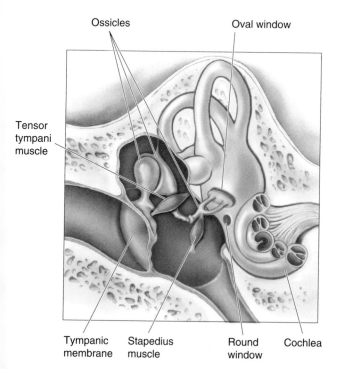

FIGURE 8.4 The ossicles of the middle ear. (From Janfaza P, Nadol JB Jr., Galla R, et al., eds. [2001] *Surgical Anatomy of the Head and Neck.* **Philadelphia: Lippincott Williams & Wilkins; p 443, with permission.)**

vibrations induce a traveling wave on the basilar membrane of the cochlea. A reverse wave generated within the cochlea produces movement of the ossicular chain and tympanic membrane, producing sound pressure in the external auditory canal, which can be measured as low-level otoacoustic emissions (see Chapter 21).

There are two muscles in the middle ear. The tensor tympani has its origin in the Eustachian tube before emerging from the medial wall of the middle ear to insert in the manubrium of the malleus. This muscle is innervated by cranial nerve V, or trigeminal nerve. Contraction of the tensor tympani stiffens the tympanic membrane through its connection with the malleus. This may occur during general body movement or as part of a startle response.

The stapedius muscle is housed in a bony pyramid, which emerges from the posterior wall of the middle ear. The tendon of the stapedius muscle inserts in the neck of the stapes. Bilateral contraction of the stapedius muscle may occur in response to high-level sounds presented to either or both ears and is known as the ASR. This is a three- to four-neuron arc in the low brainstem, involving afferent activity in the VIIIth nerve, cochlear nucleus, and superior olivary complex and efferent activity via the motor nucleus of the VIIth (facial) cranial nerve to the VIIth nerve, resulting in contraction of the stapedius muscle. This acts on the head of the stapes in a direction towards the posterior wall of the middle ear and pulls the footplate at its juncture with the oval window. The annular ligament of the stapes is thereby stiffened (Pang and Peake, 1985). This results in a reduction in energy flow to the cochlea at frequencies below about 1,000 Hz in adults on the order of 10 dB, depending on the activator level (Rabinowitz, 1977). Larger unmasking effects on the response of high-frequency VIIIth cranial nerve fibers (as high as 40 dB) have also been reported (Pang and Guinan, 1997), in which unmasking refers to a reduction in the masking of high-frequency sounds by low-frequency sounds through stapedius muscle contractions.

▧ VIBRATION AND ACOUSTICS

Overview

Acoustics is the science of sound, including its properties related to generation, transmission, and reception. *Sound*, in its physical aspect, is an example of a *wave*, which is a collective disturbance in space and time. Sound waves are generated by the vibration of a *source*. A *vibration* is a back-and-forth motion of an object such as a small mass or diaphragm. The vibration of a sound source at audio rates produces a sound wave in air that travels away from the source. A wave travels in a medium, which for the case of sound waves in air, is the atmosphere. Vibrations and waves are each an example of a *signal*, which is a form of energy that conveys information. Familiar examples of vibrating objects include the diaphragm of a loudspeaker and the vibrating rod of a tuning fork. A loudspeaker is an example of a *transducer*, which is a device that converts one form of energy into another. A *loudspeaker* converts an electrical signal into an acoustic signal or sound wave. Sound waves deliver energy to sound *receivers*. A familiar example of a sound receiver is a *microphone*, which converts an acoustic signal into an electrical signal.

The ear is the human organ of hearing and functions as a transducer that converts sound energy into a neural signal encoding the listener's sound field. Audiologists measure acoustic responses in the ear canal in order to assess the functional status of the ear's ability to receive, or collect, sound energy. One such family of acoustic responses, which is called an *acoustic immittance* response, is of fundamental concern to audiologic testing and is the subject of this chapter.

The subject of acoustic immittance is developed by first reviewing the properties of vibrating systems followed by the properties of acoustic systems. Topics from signal processing are introduced as needed, which enables a description of signal properties either as a function of time or as a function of frequency. Another theme is the use of systems analysis comprised of a single input and a single output. The system can be described by specification of its system transfer function, which is the ratio of the output signal to its input signal. Finally, the acoustic immittance is defined in terms of a set of acoustic transfer functions.

Review of Vibrations and Signals

Vibrating objects are simpler to visualize and think about than acoustic waves. Many vibrations are *oscillatory* in nature, meaning that the pattern of vibration in time is repetitive, or approximately so. There are two aspects to vibration, a description of the motion of the vibrating object (called *kinematics*) and a description of the forces producing that motion (called *dynamics*). Consider as an example of a vibrating system a child in a swing, which is in a free, back-and-forth, or oscillatory motion. We can measure the motion of the child in terms of the *displacement* of the child from the resting position, in which the swing is stationary at its lowest position relative to the ground. A plot of the displacement of the child versus time would be a displacement *waveform*. The displacement would be zero at those times in which the swing passes through the resting position. Alternatively, we can measure the *velocity* of the child. A plot of the velocity versus time would be a velocity waveform. The velocity would be zero at those times at which the swing is at its farthest distance from the resting position. Examples of such displacement and velocity waveforms are shown in the top and middle panels of Figure 8.13 and are further discussed later in this chapter.

The force producing the oscillatory motion of the swing is the *restoring force* of gravity. Whenever the child's swing is displaced away from its resting position, gravity acts in a downward direction to push the swing back toward the resting position. As the swing moves upward, gravity acts in the opposite direction to the swing velocity. The swing velocity slows to zero and reverses direction at the maximum displacement of the swing. As the swing begins to move in the opposite direction, gravity initially acts in the same direction as the swing velocity, and the swing is accelerated (i.e., its velocity increases). Once the swing passes through the resting position, the force of gravity reverses its direction and acts to decelerate, or reduce the velocity of, the swing. Thus, the force of gravity acts to maintain the vibration. Another force acting on the swing is the force of *friction*, which acts in a direction opposite to that of the velocity of the swing. Frictional forces dissipate energy and attenuate the amplitude of motion over time.

There are two types of energies in this oscillating system. The first is the energy of motion or *kinetic energy*, which is proportional to the mass—mainly that of the child—and proportional to the square of the velocity. At the extremes of swing displacement, the kinetic energy is zero because the velocity is instantaneously zero. At the resting point of the swing, the oscillating swing has its maximum kinetic energy because the velocity is highest at this time. The second type of energy is stored energy or *potential energy*, which is a measure of the capacity (or potential) to perform work. At the extremes of swing displacement, the potential energy is at a maximum because the stored energy of the swing has the capacity to accelerate the child's mass. At the resting point of the swing, the potential energy is zero because all of the stored energy has been converted into the kinetic energy of the moving mass. Thus, a simple oscillator, such as the child on the swing, can be envisioned as an oscillation, or alternation, between stored potential energy and released kinetic energy. The total energy of the oscillating system is the sum of kinetic and potential energies and is constant in the absence of friction or of any external forces. In the presence of friction, the total energy of the oscillating system decays over time.

A more abstract example of a simple oscillator is a mass m connected to a spring, in which the mass is free to move on a nearly frictionless plane. Like gravity on the child's swing, the spring exerts a restoring force on the moving mass, which acts to restore the mass to its resting position. This restoring force F_s increases linearly with increasing displacement x away from the resting position and acts in the opposite direction of the displacement. This relation can be expressed mathematically as:

$$F_s = -kx, \qquad [1]$$

in which k is the spring *stiffness*. The negative sign represents the fact that the restoring force acts in the opposite direction of the displacement. The stiffer the spring, the greater is the restoring force exerted by the spring on the mass. There is a frictional force F_f that acts in the opposite direction to the velocity v of the mass and that can be expressed mathematically by

$$F_f = -Rv, \qquad [2]$$

in which R is the frictional *resistance*. This simple oscillator is completely described by the mass m, the spring stiffness k, and the resistance R.

When frictional forces are negligible, the motion of the oscillator repeats after a time interval T called the *period* of oscillation. The period is related to the properties of the oscillator by $T = 2\pi \sqrt{m/k}$. The period of oscillation is increased by increasing mass or decreasing stiffness. The real number called π occurs in the above equation as it does in many relations involving oscillatory motion. The oldest definition of π is that it is the ratio of the circumference of a circle (i.e., the distance around its perimeter) to its diameter, so that 2π is the ratio of its circumference to its radius. The approximate numerical value of π is 3.14.

Imagine the child's older sister on a skateboard moving around a circular track at a fixed speed. This is a form of periodic motion, inasmuch as the motion is repeated each time the circular track is traversed. The angular displacement of the skateboard around the circle can be measured in units corresponding to the circumferential path length of a circle of radius one (in your favorite unit of length). When the skateboarder makes one complete revolution, this corresponds to a length of 2π units around the circumference of this unit circle. We say that her angular displacement is 2π radians. When she makes one-half of a revolution, her angular displacement is π radians. Thus, one revolution is 360 degrees of rotation or 2π radians of angular displacement. This angular displacement is the phase of the signal in the general case of an oscillating system. As the oscillation proceeds

through each repetition, the *phase* of the oscillation rotates through one revolution or 2π radians (or 360 degrees).

The resonance, or natural, frequency f_0 of the oscillation is defined as the inverse of the period, $f_0 = 1/T$. The resonance frequency is the number of repetitions of the vibration per unit time. The resonance frequency is related to the properties of the oscillator by $f_0 = (1/2\pi) \sqrt{k/m}$. The resonance frequency increases as the stiffness (k) increases or mass (m) decreases.

Some elementary signals are of special interest. One elementary signal is the *impulse* (or *click*), which is a signal of zero amplitude at all times except for an extremely short interval of time in which it has a nonzero amplitude. Another elementary signal is the *sinusoid*, which is a signal representing an object vibrating with a single frequency f. An example of sinusoidal signal is shown in the top row of Figure 8.5. The waveform repeats each millisecond (ms), so that its period of oscillation is 1 ms (0.001 s) and its natural frequency is 1 kHz (1,000 Hz). The lower two panels show the effect of damping, or frictional forces, on the motion of the oscillator. The period is changed only slightly, but the amplitude of oscillation decays over time. The oscillation is said to be more highly damped in the lowest panel because its motion decays more rapidly.

Sinusoids of the same frequency and amplitude can differ in their phase. For example, one sinusoidal signal may have a cosine shape, in which the amplitude is a maximum at time $t = 0$ (as in the top panel of Fig. 8.5), and another sinusoidal signal may have a sine shape, in which the

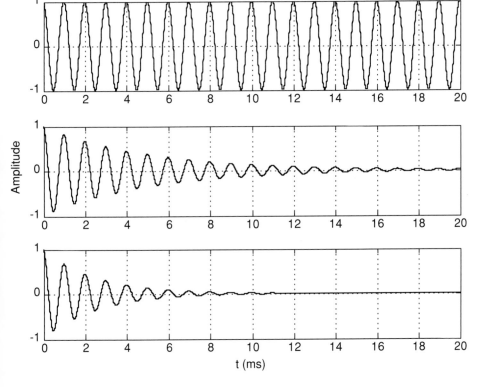

FIGURE 8.5 Top: Displacement waveform of an undamped sinusoidal oscillation with an amplitude of 1 (in arbitrary units) and period of 1 ms (same in all plots). **Middle:** Displacement waveform of a sinusoidal oscillation with damping, which reduces the maximum amplitude over time. **Bottom:** Displacement waveform of a sinusoidal oscillation with more damping than that in middle plot.

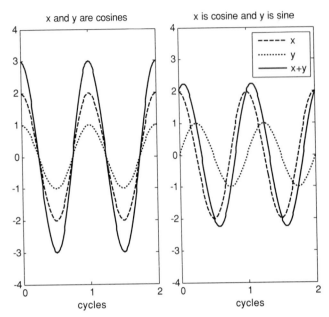

FIGURE 8.6 Addition of a sinusoid *x* in cosine phase to a sinusoid *y* of the same frequency in cosine phase (left panel) and in sine phase (right panel). The resulting sum *x* + *y* is a sinusoid of the same frequency, but its magnitude and phase differ according to the phase of *y* relative to *x*.

amplitude is zero at time $t = 0$ and increasing at later times. When two sinusoids are added together, the relative phase between the sinusoids affects the magnitude of their sum. For example, Figure 8.6 shows, in the left panel, a sinusoid x with an amplitude of 2 and cosine phase (dashed line) that is added to another sinusoid y with an amplitude of 1 and cosine phase (dotted line). Their sum $(x + y)$ at each instant of time is also a sinusoid with cosine phase (solid line), and its amplitude is 3. Suppose that signal y is changed to sine phase, as shown in the right panel of Figure 8.6. In this case, y has its peak amplitude one-quarter (0.25) of a cycle later than does x. This is always the case with sine phase. When the signals are added together at each instant of time to form $x + y$, their sum is a waveform with a sinusoidal shape and a smaller amplitude, which for the previous example has a maximum value of approximately 2.2 instead of 3. The phase of the sum $x + y$ is neither cosine phase nor sine phase because its peak amplitude occurs after 0 cycles and before 0.25 cycles. The magnitude and phase of a sinusoid are independent parameters.

It is apparent in the right panel of Figure 8.6 that y can be described as lagging x by 0.25 cycles because each maximum of y occurs 0.25 cycles earlier than each corresponding maximum of x and similarly for their minima. Irrespective of their relative magnitudes, the sine-phase signal y has a *phase lag* relative to the cosine-phase signal x of 0.25 cycles, which also corresponds to a phase lag of 90 degrees or $\pi/2$ radians.

Consider again the child on a swing. The resonant frequency is the repetition rate of the oscillation when the child is freely swinging in the absence of anyone pushing the swing. The term *resonance* applies to the case that a parent is pushing the swing at a variety of repetition rates, or frequencies. The force exerted by the parent on the child now plays the role of an external sinusoidal force acting on a simple oscillator. If the parent pushes the swing at a frequency f that is much less than the resonance frequency f_0 of the swinging child, the swing will remain at a small amplitude of vibration, and the child will be displeased. If the parent pushes the swing at a frequency f that is much greater than the resonance frequency, the swing will again have a small amplitude of vibration. The sweet spot is to push the swing at a frequency f close to the resonance frequency f_0. The child is now very pleased because the swing will begin to oscillate with a large amplitude of vibration. This increase in the motion of the vibrating oscillator when the external forcing frequency is close to the resonance frequency of the oscillator is the phenomenon of resonance.

Consider now the simple oscillator comprised of a stiffness, mass, and damping. Its resonance frequency f_0 is assumed to be 1,000 Hz. An external sinusoidal force of frequency f acts on the mass. The forcing frequency is varied, while the magnitude of the external force is kept constant. The displacement amplitude (or magnitude) of the mass is measured as a function of forcing frequency and plotted in Figure 8.7 (top panel). Like the child on the swing, the displacement is at maximum when the forcing frequency coincides with the resonance frequency at 1,000 Hz. The thicker curves represent less damping and smaller resistance than do the thinner curves, and the amplitude of motion is larger with less damping. The bottom plot shows the phase of the displacement of the mass relative to the phase of the force as a function of forcing frequency. At low frequencies, the phase is close to 0 degrees, so that the displacement of the mass is in phase with the force. That is, the mass moves toward the right when the force is directed toward the right, and vice versa. At high frequencies, the phase is close to -180 degrees, which means that the displacement of the mass lags behind the force by one-half cycle. This means that the mass moves toward the right when the force is directed toward the left, and vice versa. The phase varies most rapidly at frequencies close to the resonance frequency, and the phase is -90 degrees at resonance.

Because the force was maintained at constant amplitude and phase as a function of frequency, the magnitude and phase response in Figure 8.7 is an example of a transfer function (TF), which, in this case, is the ratio of the displacement of the mass to the force. Each plot is also an example of a *spectrum*, which is a representation of the signal response as a function of frequency. The simple oscillator is an example of a *single-input, single-output system*, in which the input variable is the external force and the output variable is the displacement of the mass. The system transfer function $TF(f)$ at each frequency f is generally defined as the ratio of the output variable to the input variable, in which the input variable is a sinusoid at frequency f. For a linear system

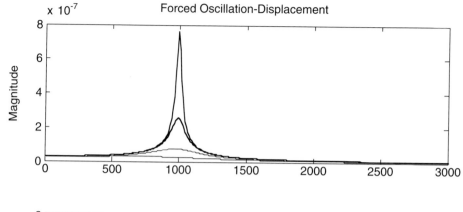

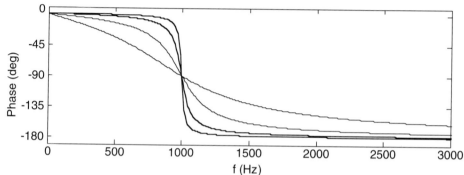

FIGURE 8.7
Displacement transfer function (TF) magnitude (top) and phase (bottom) of a mass in a simple oscillator driver by a sinusoidal external force. In this and subsequent plots, a thicker line represents a simple oscillator with lower damping.

such as the acoustic functioning of the middle ear below the level of the middle ear muscle reflex, the output response to a sinusoidal input is also sinusoidal at the same frequency f.

The motion of the mass may also be described using velocity rather than displacement. An experiment is performed in which the force is varied over frequency, and the resulting velocity TF of mass velocity to force is shown in Figure 8.8. Like the displacement TF, the velocity TF magnitude is peaked at resonance and is more sharply peaked when the resistance is small. The velocity TF phase varies from

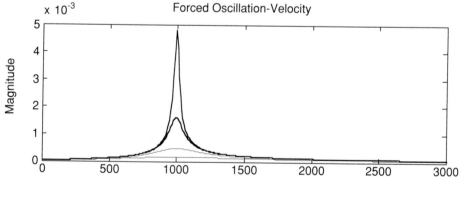

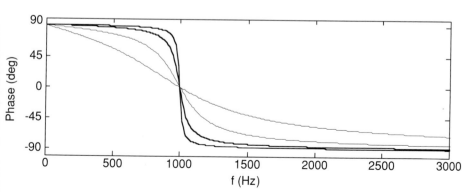

FIGURE 8.8 Velocity transfer function (TF) magnitude (top) and phase (bottom) of a mass in a simple oscillator driver by a sinusoidal external force.

+90 degrees at low frequencies to 0 degrees at resonance to −90 degrees at high frequencies. This means that the simple oscillator is stiffness controlled at low frequencies, resistance controlled at resonance, and mass controlled at high frequencies. In hearing measurements, it is customary to plot responses on a frequency axis in which the octaves are equally spaced, such that a physical *octave* represents a doubling of frequency. Such a frequency axis is logarithmic in frequency. It is also customary to transform an amplitude A into a level L in what is called a decibel (dB) unit through the formula, $L = 20 \log_{10} A$. The resonance responses in the top panels of Figures 8.7 and 8.8 are replotted in the top and bottom panels of Figure 8.9. These level spectra remain sharply peaked at the resonance frequency of the oscillator, but their slopes take a simpler form. The displacement TF has a slope of 0 dB/octave at low frequencies and a slope of −12 dB/octave at high frequencies. A straight dashed line that approximately corresponds to each slope is shown in Figure 8.9. A slope of −12 dB/octave means that the level decreases by 12 dB (i.e., the amplitude decreases by a factor of one-fourth) for each octave increase in frequency. The velocity TF is symmetrical with respect to the resonance frequency; its slope is +6 dB/octave at low frequencies and −6 dB/octave at high frequencies (i.e., the amplitude decreases by a factor of one-half).

The lines corresponding to different damping levels are labeled in Figure 8.9 as having a quality factor Q of 1, 3, 10, and 30 for oscillators of decreasing damping. The Q of a resonator is a convenient, dimensionless measure of the amount of damping. The most commonly used definition is that Q is the ratio of the resonance frequency f_0 to the bandwidth (BW) of the resonance. The BW is measured at frequencies above and below the resonance frequency for which the level is 3 dB lower than the peak level. Thus, $Q = f_0/BW$. This is shown in Figure 8.10 for an oscillator with $Q = 10$; the resonance frequency $f_0 = 1$ kHz, and the bandwidth at the 3-dB frequencies is $BW = 0.1$ kHz. The higher the Q, the more sharply tuned is the resonance. Another common measure of damping is called $Q10$, which is defined as the ratio of f_0 to the bandwidth of the resonance Δf at the 10-dB down frequencies ($Q10 = f_0/\Delta f$). In the example of Figure 8.10, the bandwidth is 300 Hz so that $Q10$ is 3.3.

Review of Acoustics

An advantage of devoting so much attention to vibrations is that many concepts are shared with concepts in acoustics. While acoustics involves wave motion in space and time, we can place a microphone at a particular location in the sound field and measure the response of that local region of space as a function of time. One complication is that oscillations associated with each local region are coupled to one another, such that acoustic waves propagate from one place to another at the speed of sound, called more formally the acoustic phase velocity c. Under typical atmospheric conditions, c is approximately 344 m/s. Associated with each region, or small volume of air, are mass-like and stiffness-like components, which play roles analogous to that of the mass and stiffness in the simple oscillator. The mass-like component is the equilibrium density of air, which is the mass per unit volume of air. The stiffness-like component is the inverse acoustic bulk modulus of air, which assesses the compressibility, or "springiness," of air. Air is compressible, as evidenced by filling a basketball with air and then sitting on

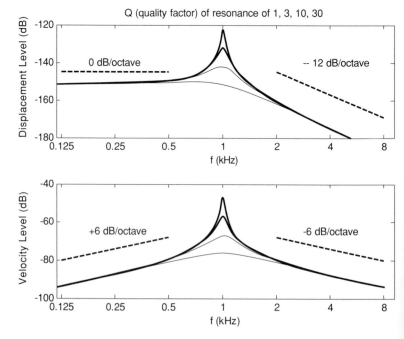

FIGURE 8.9
Displacement transfer function (TF) level spectrum (top) and velocity TF level spectrum (bottom) for a simple forced oscillator. The dashed lines indicate the constant slopes at frequencies distant from the resonance frequency of 1 kHz.

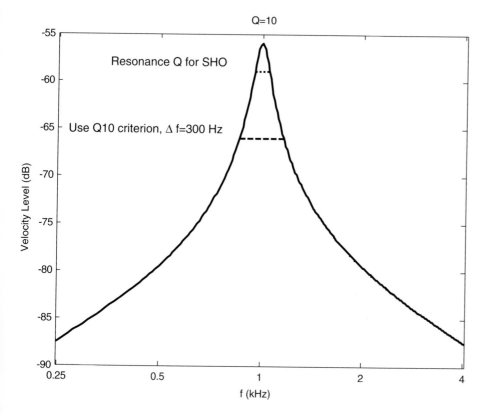

FIGURE 8.10 Resonance bandwidths used to define Q (3 dB down from peak) and *Q10* (10 dB down from peak). Q for SHO denotes the Q for simple harmonic oscillator model described in the text.

it. It takes both the properties of inertia and compressibility for sound waves to exist in air.

Local acoustic motions are produced by local forces acting over the bounding surface of each small volume of air. The *acoustic pressure* is the force per unit area acting on such a surface. In a typical microphone, the local pressure produces a net oscillatory force on the microphone diaphragm, which is displaced and, in turn, produces a fluctuating electrical signal that can be recorded and analyzed.

An acoustic wave is a *longitudinal* wave, which means that the acoustic motion is along the same axis as the direction of energy propagation. The acoustic motion involves an alternating compression and rarefaction (note: compression refers to an increase in air density, and rarefaction refers to a reduction in air density) of the local regions of space aligned in the direction of wave propagation. When the acoustic pressure is slightly larger in a particular local region than the ambient static pressure of the atmosphere, the air is compressed in that region. Half an oscillatory cycle later, the acoustic pressure is slightly smaller in that region than ambient pressure, and the air density is reduced. For a traveling acoustic wave produced by a sinusoidal source of frequency f, the distance between each alternating pair of regions of compression and rarefaction is called the wavelength λ. A fundamental relation of wave motion, which links the oscillating temporal and spatial patterns to the phase velocity, is $c = f\lambda$. For example, a 100-Hz sinusoid has a wavelength of 344 cm, a 1-kHz sinusoid has a wavelength of 34.4 cm, and a 10-kHz sinusoid has a wavelength of 3.44 cm.

A sound that traverses the external pinna and concha of an ear and enters the ear canal is said to be an *incident* sound. The energy in an incident sound is traveling toward the tympanic membrane. The ear canal terminates at the tympanic membrane, where the fluctuating acoustic pressure of the sound wave exerts fluctuating forces on the tympanic membrane, causing it to vibrate. This vibrating motion of the tympanic membrane is the input to the air-conduction pathway of the middle ear.

ACOUSTIC TRANSFER FUNCTIONS

The acoustic pressure at any location in the ear canal and at any time is a sum of a *forward*-traveling wave moving toward the tympanic membrane, which includes the incident sound, and a *reverse*-traveling wave moving away from the tympanic membrane. This pressure sum is the total acoustic pressure; a microphone at this location measures this total pressure. An external sound source creates a forward-traveling wave incident on the tympanic membrane, in particular, a sinusoidal signal at frequency f. At the tympanic membrane, part of this incident wave energy is absorbed by the middle ear, and part is reflected as a reverse-traveling wave that moves away from the tympanic membrane. At a particular ear canal location, the ratio of the reverse-traveling wave amplitude to the forward-traveling wave amplitude is defined as the (ear canal) *pressure reflectance* $r_a(f)$.

The *energy reflectance* $ER(f)$ is defined as the squared magnitude $|r_a(f)|^2$ of the pressure reflectance; it is the ratio of the reflected energy (in the reverse wave) to the incident energy (in the forward wave). Energy reflectance is sometimes called power reflectance. Power dissipation is the rate at which energy is dissipated. The energy reflectance has the important property that its value is independent of location within the ear canal as long as the ear canal walls are rigid and negligible sound energy is dissipated at the walls. These conditions are satisfied in the ear canals of adults and older children. The principle of energy conservation requires that the incident energy is equal to the sum of the energy reflected at the tympanic membrane and the energy absorbed by the middle ear at the tympanic membrane. It follows that the ratio of the energy absorbed by the middle ear to the incident energy is $EA(f) = 1 - ER(f)$, a quantity which is called the *energy absorbance*, which is the ratio of absorbed energy to incident energy. The term energy absorbance signifies that this is energy absorbed by the middle ear of the incident sound. If there were no energy dissipation within the middle ear, then the energy absorbance would equal the proportion of the incident energy transmitted to the cochlea (except for effects of otoacoustic emissions). For this reason, the energy absorbance has sometimes been called energy transmittance, but the term transmittance should be reserved to denote the transmission of energy through the middle ear (forward transmittance from ear canal to cochlea, and reverse transmittance from cochlea to ear canal in the form of an otoacoustic emission).

The energy reflectance assesses the ability of the middle ear to absorb sound energy from a sound stimulus; it is a dimensionless variable with values between 0 and 1. If all the energy is reflected from the tympanic membrane, then the energy reflectance is equal to 1, and no sound energy is absorbed by the middle ear. If no energy is reflected from the tympanic membrane, then the energy reflectance is equal to 0, and all of the sound energy is absorbed by the middle ear.

Even though measurements in sound fields are usually based on pressure measurements using microphones, the sound field can equally be well expressed in terms of the acoustic volume velocity. The *acoustic volume velocity* is the rate at which the acoustic displacement over a surface varies with time (i.e., the volume swept out per unit time). For example, the volume velocity of a conventional cone loudspeaker is essentially the product of the area of the cone and the oscillatory velocity of the cone. Suppose that the total volume velocity and total pressure are measured at a particular location for a sinusoidal sound stimulus of frequency f. The *acoustic admittance* $Y_a(f)$ at that location is defined as the ratio of the total acoustic volume velocity to the total acoustic pressure. Another commonly used acoustic TF is the

acoustic impedance $Z_a(f)$, which is defined as the inverse of acoustic admittance: $[Z_a(f) = 1/Y_a(f)]$.

Each of the acoustic reflectance, acoustic admittance, and acoustic impedance responses is an *acoustic transfer function (ATF)*. The acoustic pressure reflectance is the output reverse-wave pressure component for a system driven at its input by an input forward-wave pressure component. The acoustic admittance is the acoustic volume-velocity response of a system driven by an acoustic pressure input. The acoustic impedance is the acoustic pressure response of a system driven by an acoustic volume velocity input.

Acoustic, Mechanical, and Electrical Circuit Analogies

The literature refers to *analogies* between system descriptions of vibration and acoustics. One such analogy involves the velocity TF of a vibrating system, which was shown for a simple oscillator in Figure 8.8 and the bottom panel of Figure 8.9. This velocity TF is analogous to the acoustic admittance function, inasmuch as each velocity TF is a ratio of some type of velocity to some type of force. The acoustic admittance is a ratio of acoustic volume velocity in response to an external pressure. Because acoustic pressure is the force per unit area, pressure can be considered as an acoustic analog of mechanical force.

There are also analogies between *electrical* systems, more properly called electromagnetic systems, and their counterparts in mechanical and acoustic systems. One such family of analogies regards electrical current (measured in amperes in Standard International [SI] units) as a generalized velocity, which is akin to linear velocity in mechanics and volume velocity in acoustics, and electrical voltage (measured in volts) as a generalized force, which is akin to force in mechanics and pressure in acoustics. The electrical impedance, which is defined as the ratio of voltage to current, is analogous to the acoustic impedance. The use of these analogies is sufficiently common that the unit of electrical impedance is the ohm, whereas the unit of acoustic impedance common in audiology is called the *acoustic ohm*, and, in particular, the acoustic CGS ohm, when the acoustic variables are measured in the centigrade-gram-seconds (CGS) system. Table 8.1 lists these analogies between acoustic, mechanical, and electrical systems.

Signals and Transfer Functions on the Complex Plane

This section introduces the topic of representing signals and TFs using the complex plane, which enables a precise characterization of effects such as a compliance-dominated immittance or a mass-dominated immittance. The level of mathematics is higher in this section than in the remainder of the chapter, although no calculus is required, and the treatment is reasonably self-contained. Some students may wish to review the aural acoustic immittance and ATF responses

TABLE 8.1   Electrical, mechanical, and acoustic analogies

Response	Electrical	Mechanical	Acoustical
Generalized force	Voltage (V)	Force (F)	Pressure (P)
Generalized velocity	Current (I)	Velocity (v)	Volume Velocity (u)
Generalized impedance	Electrical impedance ($Z_e = V/I$)	Mechanical impedance ($Y_m = F/v$)	Acoustical impedance ($Z_a = P/u$)
Generalized admittance	Electrical admittance ($Y_e = I/V$)	Mechanical mobility ($Y_m = v/F$)	Acoustical admittance ($Y_a = u/P$)

defined in Table 8.2 or simply skip over this section. The more advanced reader will find that the introduction of the so-called complex exponential function is a powerful tool in understanding signal analysis and the principles of ATFs.

We learned earlier that sinusoidal signals can have the same magnitude and still differ in phase and that the sine signal can be regarded as a cosine signal that has been delayed by 0.25 cycles or $\pi/2$ radians (or 90 degrees). Any sinusoidal signal can be expressed as a sum of cosine and sine signals at frequency f. We also learned that a sinusoidal signal can be expressed in terms of its magnitude and phase, so there must be a close connection between representing a sinusoidal signal using magnitude and phase or using cosine and sine components.

Working with TFs, we learned that a TF can be expressed in terms of its magnitude and phase response. Selecting the acoustic impedance as a particular case, this impedance was defined for sinusoids as the ratio of acoustic pressure p to volume velocity u by $Z_a = p/u$. From the standpoint of a single-input, single-output system, u is the input, and p is the output. The output p is the product of the ATF and the input u (i.e., $p = Z_a u$). Without any loss of generality (because we are free to use whatever phase reference we like), we adopt the convention that the input variable u is a cosine signal. Depending on the TF phase, the output variable p is a sinusoid with arbitrary cosine and sine components.

These sorts of relationships can be visualized by representing the impedance as a *phasor*, as shown in Figure 8.11, in which the impedance may be acoustic, mechanical, or electrical. The impedance Z is represented by the open circle in the figure labeled by Z, as well as by the ray drawn from the origin with its arrow tip pointing at the open circle. The impedance magnitude $|Z|$ has a value equal to the length of the phasor (i.e., the length of the ray). The impedance phase ϕ_z is the angle of the phasor with respect to the positive horizontal axis, as shown by the arc. This arc is drawn in a counter-clockwise direction. The projection of Z onto the horizontal axis is shown by the vertical dashed line, and the distance from the origin to the point where this dashed line intersects the horizontal axis is R, which is the *resistance* or resistive component of the impedance. This resistance is positive because it lies to the right of the origin. The projection of Z onto the vertical axis is shown by the horizontal dashed line, and the distance from the origin to the point

of intersection is X, which is the *reactance*, or the reactive component of the impedance. This reactance is positive because it lies above the origin. Thus, we can represent the impedance on a plane in polar form as its magnitude and phase ($|Z|$, ϕ_z), or in Cartesian or rectangular form as its resistance and reactance (R, X).

The polar components can be expressed in terms of the rectangular components by

$$|Z| = \sqrt{R^2 + X^2},$$
$$\tan\phi_z = \frac{X}{R}. \qquad [3]$$

These relations come from the fact that there is a right triangle in Figure 8.11, in which the side adjacent to the angle has a length R, the side opposite the angle has a length X, and the hypotenuse has a length $|Z|$. The top equation states that the square of the hypotenuse is the sum of the squares of each of its lengths. The bottom equation defines the tangent of the angle as the ratio of the opposite side to the adjacent side.

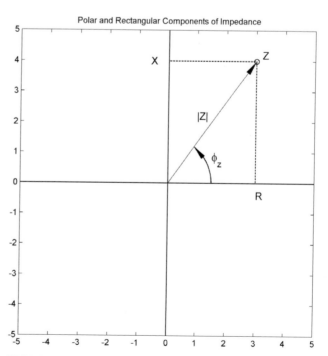

FIGURE 8.11   A phasor representing the impedance Z on the complex plane.

The rectangular components are expressed in terms of the polar components by

$$R = |Z| \cos \phi_z,$$
$$X = |Z| \sin \phi_z. \qquad [4]$$

The top equation is the definition of the cosine of an angle within a right triangle; namely, the cosine of the angle is the ratio of the adjacent side (R) to the hypotenuse ($|Z|$). The bottom equation is the definition of the sine of an angle within a right triangle; namely, the sine of the angle is the ratio of the opposite side (X) to the hypotenuse.

There is a third representation in which the impedance can be written, namely, as $Z = R + jX$, in which j is the unit imaginary number, $j = \sqrt{-1}$. In this case, the plane in Figure 8.11 is called the complex plane, in which the horizontal axis is called the real axis and the vertical axis is called the imaginary axis. In accord with this graphical representation, R is the real part of Z, and X is the imaginary part of Z. This is consistent with the representation $Z = R + jX$, with the convention that the real part includes any part of the right-hand side of the equation independent of j, and the imaginary part includes any part of the right-hand side that is multiplied by j.

The phase of the TF, acoustic impedance in this case, equals the phase of the output sinusoid relative to the phase of the input sinusoid. The fact that the acoustic impedance varies with frequency means that the phasor in Figure 8.11 will also vary in length and orientation (i.e., its phase) with frequency. Another important property is that the resistance is always positive for any system, like the middle ear, that dissipates energy. In terms of Figure 8.11, the case of $R > 0$ is the right side of the plane, so that a phasor representing an impedance always lies on the right half of the complex plane.

The admittance Y is represented as a phasor in Figure 8.12. The admittance magnitude is $|Y|$, and its phase is ϕ_y, for which the subscript y is used to differentiate it from the impedance phase. Note that the admittance Y at the tip of the ray lies below the horizontal axis in this example, so that the phase angle ϕ_y drawn counter-clockwise from the horizontal axis extends more than three-quarters of the way around the circle. Equivalently, the phase angle can be drawn in the clockwise direction from the horizontal axis and labeled as $-\phi_y$. The rectangular components of the admittance are called the conductance G and the susceptance B. The conductance is positive and the susceptance is negative ($B < 0$) because Y lies below the horizontal axis. The polar components of admittance are expressed in terms of its rectangular components by

$$|Y| = \sqrt{G^2 + B^2},$$
$$\tan \phi_y = \frac{B}{G}. \qquad [5]$$

The rectangular components are expressed in terms of the polar components by

$$G = |Y| \cos \phi_y,$$
$$B = |Y| \sin \phi_y. \qquad [6]$$

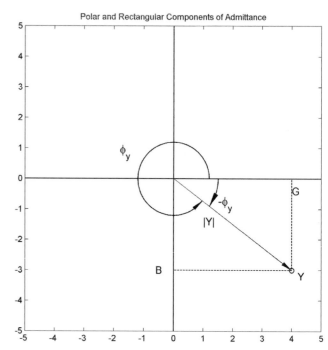

Polar and Rectangular Components of Admittance

FIGURE 8.12 A phasor representing the admittance *Y* on the complex plane.

The admittance can also be written in complex form as $Y = G + jB$, in which G is called the real part of the admittance and B is the imaginary part of the admittance. The conductance is positive ($G > 0$) for any system like the middle ear in which frictional forces are dominant in dissipating energy, so that the admittance phasor lies in the right half of the complex plane in Figure 8.12.

We return to the simple oscillator to understand the relationships between the displacement, velocity, and acceleration of the mass. The simple oscillator is composed of a moving mass acted on by a spring, which acts to restore the mass to its equilibrium resting position, and a resistance, which acts to dissipate the oscillatory energy of the moving mass. An analogy of this simple oscillator is the child on the swing. Figure 8.13 shows the displacement, velocity, and acceleration waveforms of the child on the swing for a case in which resistance is negligible. The resonance frequency in this example is $f_0 = 1$ Hz, which corresponds to a period of 1 s.

The displacement waveform in Figure 8.13 (top panel) shows a sinusoidal oscillation that has zero displacement at time $t = 0$ s; this time origin is identified by the vertical dashed line and labeled as time A. The displacement waveform $d(t)$ has sine phase, because the sine signal is zero at $t = 0$ s and has increasing amplitude at slightly later times, and may be written as

$$d(t) = D \sin 2\pi f_0 t. \qquad [7]$$

This displacement amplitude $D = 10$ cm and corresponds to the maximum absolute value of the waveform. The

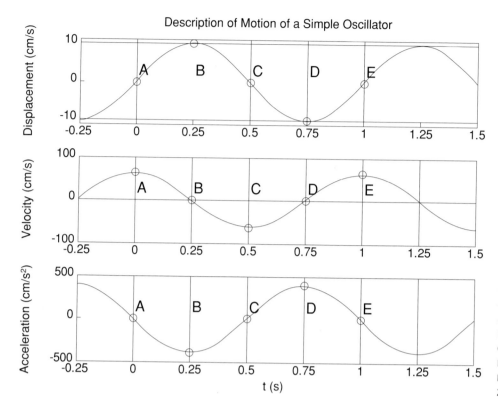

FIGURE 8.13
Sinusoidal oscillation waveforms for a simple oscillator for displacement (top), velocity (middle), and acceleration (bottom). The letters A through E denote times over a single period of oscillation in which the displacement waveform amplitude is zero, a maximum in the positive direction, zero, a maximum in the negative direction, and zero, respectively.

argument of the sine function is $2\pi f_0 t$. As time t progresses through 1 period of oscillation, the sine phase varies by 2π radians or one cycle (or 360 degrees) of oscillation. This is the reason why factors of 2π show up so often in descriptions of vibration and acoustics.

Time B at $t = 0.25$ s is exactly ¼ cycle later than time A. The swing has its maximum displacement of 10 cm at time B. We know that, when a swing is at its maximum displacement, the velocity is instantaneously 0. The velocity waveform in Figure 8.13 (middle panel) has an instantaneous value of 0 cm/s at time B. At slightly later time, the displacement remains in the positive direction, but the swing is moving back towards the center and thus has a velocity in the negative direction. This is shown in Figure 8.13 by the velocity having a negative value at times slightly later than time B.

Just as the velocity is the rate of change of displacement with time, the *acceleration* is defined to be the rate of change of velocity with time. When we speed up while driving a car, the acceleration is positive; when we hit the brakes to slow down, the acceleration is negative. When we travel at constant speed in a particular direction, the velocity is constant, and the acceleration is zero. At time B, the velocity (middle panel of Fig. 8.13) begins at zero and becomes more negative with increasing time. This corresponds to a negative acceleration, as shown in Figure 8.13 (bottom panel) at time B.

Time C at $t = 0.5$ s is ½ cycle later than time A. This is the time at which the displacement is zero, corresponding to the swing moving back through its equilibrium position. The swing is now moving with the maximum speed, and this is shown as the maximum negative amplitude of the

velocity waveform (middle panel of Fig. 8.13) at time C. The speed is the velocity amplitude but does not include the information on the direction of the motion, which is in the negative direction at time C. The acceleration is zero at time C (lower panel of Fig. 8.13) because the speed has reached its maximum value and, thus, its velocity is hardly changing at times close to time C. The displacement, velocity, and acceleration at time C each differs from its respective value at time A (or time E) by a factor of −1 (or else is 0) because the time difference is ½ cycle.

Time D at $t = 0.75$ s is ¾ cycle later than time A. The swing is now at the maximum displacement (upper panel of Fig. 8.13) in the negative direction, its instantaneous velocity is again zero (middle panel of Fig. 8.13), and its acceleration is at a maximum value in the positive direction (lower panel of Fig. 8.13). This positive acceleration means that the swing velocity is about to increase in the positive direction, which is indicated by the positive velocity at times slightly later than time D. Finally, time E at $t = 1$ s is one cycle later than time A. The displacement, velocity, and acceleration (upper, middle, and lower panels of Fig. 8.13) at time E are each identical to the corresponding variable at time A—this is what is meant by a periodic motion.

The acceleration waveform (lower panel of Fig. 8.13) is reversed in direction from the displacement waveform (upper panel of Fig. 8.13) (i.e., it is multiplied by −1). Because the displacement waveform has sine phase, the acceleration waveform $a(t)$ has negative sine phase, i.e.,

$$a(t) = -A_0 \sin 2\pi f_0 t. \qquad [8]$$

The factor of –1 on the right-hand side of the equation expresses the reversal in direction and A_0 is the amplitude of the acceleration. But what about the velocity, which is a maximum at time A? A cosine signal has a maximum (with value 1) at time $t = 0$ and decreases at slightly later times. Thus, the velocity signal (middle panel) in Figure 8.13 has cosine phase and amplitude V_0 and is written as:

$$v(t) = V_0 \cos 2\pi f_0 t. \qquad [9]$$

We know from the example of the child on the swing that the velocity and acceleration amplitudes should be proportional to the displacement amplitude. For example, the larger the displacement amplitude, the larger is the velocity amplitude (i.e., its maximum speed). This is true for any simple oscillator as well.

Instead of a child on a swing, take a piece of string (or imagine taking it) and tie an object of some mass to one end. Start the miniature swing with an initial peak displacement amplitude D_0 and observe its period of oscillation. Next, shorten the length of the swing and use the same initial displacement D_0. You will observe that the period of oscillation is shorter for the shorter swing, so that its resonance frequency f_0 is higher. You should also be able to observe that the object moves with a faster speed when the string is shorter than when it is the original length—it has to traverse a back-and-forth motion in a shorter period than before. Thus, the velocity amplitude or speed V_0 increases with increasing resonance frequency f_0, and it increases with increasing displacement amplitude D_0. The exact relation is that $V_0 = 2\pi f_0 D_0$, which can also be written as $D_0 = \frac{V_0}{2\pi f_0}$. The factor of 2π is always present with f_0, just as it is in the earlier waveform equations; it is convenient to define the *resonance radian frequency* ω_0, which is a lowercase Greek letter omega with subscript 0, by

$$\omega_0 = 2\pi f_0. \qquad [10]$$

The units of ω_0 are radians per second, so that the argument $\omega_0 t$ of the sine and cosine signals has a dimensionless unit of radians (abbreviated *rad*). Because the acceleration is the rate of change of velocity, the larger velocity amplitude with increasing f_0 also produces an increased acceleration amplitude, so that $A_0 = 2\pi f_0 V_0$. It is not customary to start the child's swing with an initial velocity, but this is a simple matter for an object on a string. Simply strike the object with a small hammer or other object, thereby imparting an initial velocity to the object on the string. This is like striking a tuning fork or a piano string with a hammer. In the example in Figure 8.13, $f_0 = 1$ s so that $\omega_0 = 2\pi \approx 6.28$ rad/s. The displacement amplitude $D_0 = 10$ cm, so that $V_0 = 2\pi \times 1 \times 10 \approx 62.8$ cm/s. The acceleration amplitude is $A_0 = 2\pi V_0 = 2\pi f (2\pi f D_0) = (2\pi \times 1)^2 \times 10 \approx 395$ cm^2/s.

The summary in mathematical form of the kinematics of the simple oscillator is

$$\begin{aligned} d(t) &= \frac{1}{\omega_0} V_0 \sin \omega_0 t, \\ v(t) &= V_0 \cos \omega_0 t, \\ a(t) &= -\omega_0 V_0 \sin \omega_0 t. \end{aligned} \qquad [11]$$

These relations will be useful later.

We have described the complex plane already in the representation of impedance (Fig. 8.11) and admittance (Fig. 8.12), in which the real component of each complex quantity is its value along the horizontal axis and the imaginary component of its value along the vertical axis. Because each real component is a real number and each imaginary component is also a real number (tricky terminology!), a complex number is represented on a complex plane by an ordered pair of real numbers specifying the real and imaginary parts. Figure 8.14 shows the *unit circle*, which is a circle of radius 1 on the complex plane. The figure also shows a particular point z on the unit circle, whose real part is x and whose imaginary part is y. The complex number z is thus represented by the *ordered pair* (x, y) as the Cartesian coordinates on the plane. It is also expressed in terms of the unit imaginary number j as $z = x + jy$, which means the same thing as $z = (x, y)$. Because this particular point z is on the unit

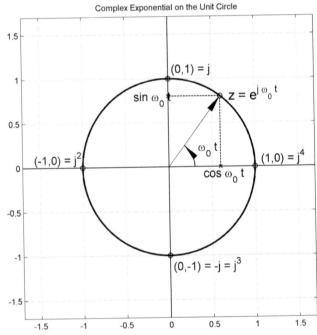

FIGURE 8.14 The complex exponential plotted as a phasor on the complex plane. The complex exponential lies on a circle of radius one, with phase corresponding to a counter-clockwise rotation on the complex plane relative to the positive real (i.e., horizontal) axis. The four other points plotted on the complex plane refer to values of +1, +j, –1 and –j, respectively, as the phase angle varies over one revolution.

circle, its magnitude (denoted $|z|$) is equal to 1, i.e., $|z| = \sqrt{x^2 + y^2} = 1$ (the radius of the unit circle).

The angle ϕ of the phasor with respect to the positive real axis is shown in Figure 8.14, and we define it to have the value $\phi = \omega_0 t$. This enables us to connect the unit circle on the complex plane with the motion of the simple oscillator. For fixed radian resonance frequency, the phase $\omega_0 t$ increases linearly with increasing time t. An increasing phase angle corresponds to a rotation in the counterclockwise direction around the unit circle, and such a rotation corresponds to a sinusoidal waveform. Because the unit circle has a hypotenuse equal to 1, the real component is $x = \cos \phi = \cos \omega_0 t$, and the imaginary component is $y = \sin \phi = \sin \omega_0 t$ (recall that the cosine is the adjacent side over the hypotenuse, and the sine is the opposite side over the hypotenuse).

It is exceedingly useful in describing systems to represent the original complex number z on the unit circle in terms of its phase angle. This is a third way to express z alongside (x, y) and $x + jy$ for the case that z is on the unit circle. We rewrite the expression $z = x + jy$ as

$$e^{j\omega_0 t} = \cos \omega_0 t + j \sin \omega_0 t. \qquad [12]$$

The expression on the left-hand side is defined as the *complex exponential function*. The right-hand side is the point z on the unit circle of the complex plane, such that the real part is the cosine of the angle $\omega_0 t$ and the imaginary part is the sine of the angle (see Fig. 8.14). The magnitude of the complex exponential $\left|e^{j\omega_0 t}\right| = 1$, as it must be for any point on the unit circle. The *real part* of a complex number z is denoted as $Re(z)$, and the *imaginary part* is denoted as $Im(z)$. It follows from Equation 12 that

$$\begin{aligned} Re\left(e^{j\omega_0 t}\right) &= \cos \omega_0 t, \\ Im\left(e^{j\omega_0 t}\right) &= \sin \omega_0 t. \end{aligned} \qquad [13]$$

Most readers have earlier encountered the *real exponential function* and the irrational number e. Many hand calculators have a key representing e, which represents the exponentiation of another number that is the argument of the exponential function. The real exponential function describes the exponential growth and decay of a waveform (as shown for decay in the curves in Fig. 8.5).

Remember that j was defined to be the imaginary number that, when squared, is equal to –1, so that $j = \sqrt{-1}$. It follows that $j^2 = -1$. If we multiple j^2 by itself, then we have the result that $j^4 = j^2 \times j^2 = (-1) \times (-1) = 1$. We can express j^3 as $j^3 = j^2 \times j = (-1) \times j = -j$. These points are labeled on Figure 8.14 and correspond to points on the unit circle. Starting with the real value 1 on the positive real axis [i.e., the ordered pair $z = (1, 0)$], a rotation by 90 degrees or $\pi/2$ radians arrives at the intersection of the unit circle with the positive imaginary axis. This is the unit imaginary number j. A second rotation by $\pi/2$ radians arrives at the intersection of the unit circle with the negative real axis with value –1. From the above relations, this point is also j^2. A third rotation by $\pi/2$ radians arrives at the intersection of the unit circle with the negative imaginary axis with value

$-j$. The above relations show that this point is equal to j^3. A fourth rotation by $\pi/2$ radians arrives at the intersection of the unit circle with the positive real axis with value 1. This point is also equal to j^4. One result is that a rotation on the complex plane by $\pi/2$ radians is equivalent to multiplication of the complex number by j. Another result is that $1/j = -j$, which is proved by multiplying each side by j and using the fact that $-j^2 = 1$.

Using these properties, we form the product of j times $e^{j\omega_0 t}$ as

$$\begin{aligned} j\, e^{j\omega_0 t} &= j\ (\cos \omega_0 t + j \sin \omega_0 t) \\ &= j \cos \omega_0 t + j^2 \sin \omega_0 t \\ &= -\sin \omega_0 t + j \cos \omega_0 t. \end{aligned} \qquad [14]$$

As seen here, algebra with complex numbers is the same as with real numbers, except for these additional rules for handling terms with j or powers of j. Any terms multiplied or divided by powers of j can always be reduced to a sum of real terms or of terms that are multiplied by j. Real terms and imaginary terms are maintained separately as the real and imaginary components of the complex number (e.g., $z = x + jy$). With reference to Figure 8.14, the complex number $j e^{j\omega_0 t}$ corresponds to a rotation by $\pi/2$ radians of $e^{j\omega_0 t}$ because multiplication by j is equivalent to that rotation. The last line of Equation 14 can also be written as

$$\begin{aligned} Re\left(j\, e^{j\omega_0 t}\right) &= -\sin \omega_0 t, \\ Im\left(j\, e^{j\omega_0 t}\right) &= \cos \omega_0 t. \end{aligned} \qquad [15]$$

We form the product of $1/j$ and $e^{j\omega_0 t}$ with the result

$$\begin{aligned} \frac{1}{j}\, e^{j\omega_0 t} &= -j\, e^{j\omega_0 t} \\ &= -j\ (\cos \omega_0 t + j \sin \omega_0 t) \\ &= \sin \omega_0 t - j \cos \omega_0 t. \end{aligned} \qquad [16]$$

This phasor corresponds to a *clockwise* rotation of $e^{j\omega_0 t}$ by $\pi/2$ radians. This equation can also be written as

$$\begin{aligned} Re\left(\frac{1}{j}\, e^{j\omega_0 t}\right) &= \sin \omega_0 t, \\ Im\left(\frac{1}{j}\, e^{j\omega_0 t}\right) &= -\cos \omega_0 t \end{aligned} \qquad [17]$$

The "trick" to using the complex plane to represent motion and forces, as well as all the generalized motions and generalized forces in Table 8.1, is to first embed the physically measured signal in the complex plane, then perform intermediate analyses in the complex plane, and finally take the real part of the final expression as the physically measured variable. We take the velocity cosine waveform in Equation 9 as an example. All that embedding this waveform in the complex plane means is to represent the signal as a new complex signal $\tilde{v}(t)$ whose real part is the original velocity $v(t)$. The superscript tilde is used to denote that the variable is defined on the complex plane. Using the top relation in Equation 13, we can re-write Equation 9 as

$$\tilde{v}(t) = V_0\, e^{j\omega_0 t},$$

$$v(t) = Re\,(\tilde{v}(t)) = V_0\, \cos\omega_0 t. \qquad [18]$$

According to the top relation in Equation 11, the displacement waveform $d(t) = \frac{V_0}{\omega_0}\sin\omega_0 t$ is a sine waveform of positive direction (or polarity), and Equation 17 shows that $\sin\omega_0 t$ can be represented as the real part of $(1/j)e^{j\omega_0 t}$. The complex displacement waveform $\tilde{d}(t)$ is thus written as

$$\tilde{d}(t) = \frac{1}{\omega_0}\, V_0 \times \frac{1}{j}\, e^{j\omega_0 t}$$

$$= \frac{1}{j\omega_0}\, V_0\, e^{j\omega_0 t}$$

$$= \frac{1}{j\omega_0}\, \tilde{v}(t). \qquad [19]$$

The last relation follows the definition of $\tilde{v}(t)$ in Equation 18. This affords a new way to think about pairs of sinusoidal displacement and velocity signals in the complex plane at any radian frequency $\omega = 2\pi f$ defined in terms of a frequency f. The displacement is the velocity divided by $j\omega$, and the velocity is $j\omega$ times the displacement.

According to the bottom relation in Equation 11, the acceleration waveform $a(t) = -\omega_0\, V_0 \sin\omega_0 t$ is a sine waveform of negative polarity, and Equation 15 shows that such a negative sine function can be represented as the real part of $j\, e^{j\omega_0 t}$. The complex displacement waveform $\tilde{a}(t)$ is thus written as

$$\tilde{a}(t) = \omega_0\, V_0 \times je^{j\omega_0 t}$$

$$= j\omega_0\, \left(V_0\, e^{j\omega_0 t}\right)$$

$$= j\omega_0\, \tilde{v}(t). \qquad [20]$$

The velocity is the acceleration divided by $j\omega$, and the acceleration is $j\omega$ times the velocity.

IMPEDANCE AND ADMITTANCE COMPONENTS

The impedance is next described using this complex-variable formulation, with initial emphasis on mechanical systems important in vibrations. The mechanical system is a simple oscillator circuit comprised of a mass m, which is acted on by a resistive force with resistance R, and a restoring force with stiffness k, and is driven by a sinusoidal external force $F(t)$ of the form

$$F(t) = F_0 \cos\omega t. \qquad [21]$$

The driving frequency is f, so the corresponding driving radian frequency is $\omega = 2\pi f$. The simple oscillator described previously was a free oscillator (i.e., an oscillator whose motion was free of external forces). The presence of the external force makes this system a *forced oscillator*. The first step is to embed the external force in the complex plane as the variable $\tilde{F}(t)$ whose real part is the physically measurable force:

$$F(t) = Re\left(\tilde{F}(t)\right). \qquad [22]$$

It follows from Equation 13 that the complex force is equal to the complex exponential with magnitude F_0:

$$\tilde{F}(t) = F_0\, e^{j\omega t}. \qquad [23]$$

With this choice, the real force has the correct cosine phase.

Newton's laws of mechanics state that the sum of forces acting on a mass is equal to the mass times its acceleration. The intuitive concept is that the acceleration of the mass is the change in its motion, and such changes in motion are due to the forces acting on the mass. This equation is written using complex variables as

$$m\tilde{a}(t) = -R\tilde{v}(t) - k\tilde{d}(t) + \tilde{F}(t) \qquad [24]$$

The right-hand side of this equation is the sum of forces acting on the mass and includes the frictional force from Equation 2, the spring force from Equation 1, and the external force. Since the external force is sinusoidal, the resulting motion of the mass will also be sinusoidal after any initial transient has decayed. It is this continuous motion that we wish to calculate. The tilde on each variable indicates that each variable is embedded in the complex plane with radian frequency ω. Forms of Equations 19 and 20 are used at this radian frequency to express the displacement and acceleration in terms of the velocity with the result:

$$j\omega m\, \tilde{v}(t) = -R\tilde{v}(t) - \frac{k}{j\omega}\tilde{v}(t) + \tilde{F}(t). \qquad [25]$$

The terms proportional to $\tilde{v}(t)$ are collected on the left side of the equation with the result:

$$\left[j\omega m + R + \frac{k}{j\omega}\right]\tilde{v}(t) = \tilde{F}(t). \qquad [26]$$

The system TF Y_m is the ratio of the output signal to the input sinusoidal signal, which in this example is the ratio of the velocity to the force (i.e., the mechanical mobility in Table 8.1):

$$Y_m = \frac{\tilde{v}(t)}{\tilde{F}(t)}. \qquad [27]$$

Solving Equations 26 and 27 for Y_m leads to

$$Y_m = \frac{1}{\left[j\omega m + R + \frac{k}{j\omega}\right]}. \qquad [28]$$

This equation is said to be *in the frequency domain* because of its dependence on frequency f via $\omega = 2\pi f$ and its independence of time. This TF depends on the mass, stiffness, and resistance of the simple oscillator.

The mechanical impedance is the inverse of mechanical mobility, namely,

$$Z_m = \frac{1}{Y_m} = j\omega m + R + \frac{k}{j\omega}$$

$$= R + j\left(\omega m - \frac{k}{\omega}\right). \qquad [29]$$

In the top line, the impedance of a mass m is $j\omega m$, the impedance of a resistance is R, and the impedance of a stiffness is $-jk/\omega$ (remember that $1/j = -j$). The bottom line shows that the real part of the impedance is the resistance. The imaginary part of the impedance, which is called the mechanical reactance X_m is

$$X_m = \omega m - k/\omega. \qquad [30]$$

The mechanical compliance C_m is defined as the inverse of the stiffness ($C_m = 1/k$), so that the impedance of a compliant component is $1/j\omega C_m$. Resonance is defined as the frequency $\omega = \omega_0$ at which the reactance is zero, and this zero occurs when the mass and stiffness components (or, equivalently, mass and compliance components) exactly cancel ($\omega m - k/\omega = 0$). This resonance radian frequency and resonance frequency are

$$\omega_0 = \sqrt{\frac{k}{m}} = \frac{1}{\sqrt{mC_m}},$$

$$f_0 = \frac{1}{2\pi}\sqrt{\frac{k}{m}} = \frac{1}{2\pi}\frac{1}{\sqrt{mC_m}}. \qquad [31]$$

In the simple oscillator, the resonance frequency increases when the mass decreases and when the stiffness increases or the compliance decreases. In immittance tympanometry at 226 Hz, we frequently refer to a stiffness-dominated or mass-dominated behavior. A *stiffness-dominated* or *compliance-dominated* behavior occurs when the reactance is negative. This is seen in Equation 30 when the negative term on the right-hand side with the stiffness k is larger than the positive term with mass m. A *mass-dominated* behavior occurs when the reactance is positive. This is seen in Equation 30 when the positive term on the right-hand side with mass m is larger than the stiffness term. The terms ωm and $-k/\omega$ vary as frequency, and therefore, radian frequency ω increases from zero. The mass term is proportional to ω, so it is small when the frequency is low. The stiffness term is proportional to $1/\omega$, so it is large when the frequency is low. The important conclusion is that the simple oscillator is stiffness dominated at low frequencies and mass dominated at high frequencies. When the driving frequency ω is equal, or nearly equal, to the resonance frequency ω_0, the simple oscillator is *resistance dominated*. This occurs at frequencies for which the resistive component R in Equation 29 is larger than the reactive component.

The frequency behavior of the forced oscillator is shown in Figure 8.8 for different levels of resistance and a resonant frequency $f_0 = 1000$ Hz. The phase response of Y_m shown in the figure is stiffness dominated at low frequencies (approximately 90 degrees or $\pi/2$ radians) and mass dominated at high frequencies (approximately -90 degrees or $-\pi/2$ radians). At resonance, $Z_m = R$, so that $Y_m = 1/R$. Smaller values of R produce larger peak values of $|Y_m|$ corresponding to the higher Q peaks in Figure 8.8 (i.e., R and Q are inversely related). A more detailed discussion of the forced oscillator shows that Q is related to its mass, stiffness, and damping parameters by

$$Q = \frac{m\omega_0}{R} = \frac{\sqrt{km}}{R}. \qquad [32]$$

This analysis of mechanical vibrations shows that the elementary impedance and admittance components, or circuit elements, include a mass impedance, stiffness (or compliance) impedance, and a resistance. Similar elementary impedance and admittance components are found in acoustics. The *acoustic compliance C_a* of a small volume V of enclosed air is

$$C_a = \frac{V}{\beta_a},$$

$$\beta_a = \rho c^2, \qquad [33]$$

in which the bulk modulus of air is β_a, the equilibrium (mass) density of air is ρ, and the phase velocity of sound is c. The bulk modulus and density are thermodynamic constants for air. Sound waves may be present in any medium (i.e., any gas or fluid that has a particular bulk modulus and mass density). The top relation of Equation 33 states that the compliance decreases as the bulk modulus of a gas increases.

For example, the bulk modulus of air under standard atmospheric conditions is approximately 1.4×10^5 Pa, whereas the bulk modulus of water is approximately 2.2×10^9 Pa, which is larger than the bulk modulus of air by a factor of 1.6×10^4. This means that the acoustic compliance of water is 16,000 times less than the acoustic compliance of air. This is why water is often assumed to be *incompressible* in hearing science compared to air (e.g., in understanding pathologies such as middle ear fluid or understanding the mechanics of the fluid-filled cochlea). This is simply an approximation because sound waves *are* present in water; for example, underwater sounds are produced and received by marine animals as a means of communication. The bottom relation of Equation 33 is the defining relation for the speed of sound, namely, $c = \sqrt{\beta_a/\rho}$. The density of air at standard room temperature is approximately 1.2 kg/m³, whereas the density of water is approximately 1,000 kg/m³ (i.e., water is almost a thousand times denser than air). The speed of sound in air at atmospheric pressure and a temperature similar to that in the ear canal is 344 m/s, whereas the speed of sound in water is approximately 1,500 m/s. Even though the bulk modulus and density differ by 3 to 4 orders of magnitude in air and water, their sound speeds differ by less than a factor of 5. The audiologic literature often simplifies Equation 33 by defining the acoustic compliance of a volume of air whose dimensions are small compared to the acoustic wavelength as $C_a = V/\rho c^2$.

A probe inserted into a small coupler of volume 2 cm³ acts as an acoustical compliance at a typical probe frequency of 226 Hz. The acoustic impedance Z_a and acoustic admittance $Y_a = 1/Z_a$ of such a compliance is

$$Z_a = \frac{1}{j\omega C_a},$$

$$Y_a = j\omega C_a. \qquad [34]$$

The lower equation states that the susceptance of a small volume is $B_a = Im(Y_a) = 2\pi f V/\rho c^2$. This susceptance evaluated for a 1-cm^3 volume of air at 226 Hz under standard atmospheric conditions (i.e., at sea level) is approximately equal to 0.001 CGS mho (a mho is the inverse of an ohm), or 1 CGS mmho (a millimho, or 1 mho/1,000). The widespread use of 226 Hz in tympanometry is based, in part, on this happy coincidence, which equates a 1-cm^3 volume compliance with a 1-mmho susceptance. This relation is formalized by defining an additional ATF called the *equivalent volume* V_{ea} in terms of the susceptance or the compliance as follows:

$$V_{ea} = \frac{\rho c^2 B_a}{2\pi f} = \rho c^2 C_a. \qquad [35]$$

The equivalent volume varies, in general, with frequency and need not correspond with the acoustic characteristics of a small volume. When measured in an adult ear canal with a mid-canal probe seal, $V_{ea}(f)$ is positive at low frequencies and negative at higher frequencies.

The acoustical analogy to a mass impedance in mechanics is based on the *acoustic inertance* I_a. The root word of inertance is inertia, which is a synonym for mass. The acoustic inertance associated with the moving air of mass density ρ in a narrow cylindrical tube of length L and cross-sectional area S is

$$I_a = \frac{\rho L}{S}. \qquad [36]$$

The acoustic impedance and admittance of an inertance are given by

$$Z_a = j\omega I_a,$$
$$Y_a = \frac{1}{j\omega I_a} \qquad [37]$$

These relations are analogous in their frequency dependence via $j\omega$ to the mass-like impedance and admittance as found in Equations 28 and 29 (after setting resistance and stiffness equal to zero). The acoustic analogy to a resistance is an acoustic resistance $Z_a = R = 1/Y_a$, which in general may vary with frequency but is always independent of j.

The *Helmholtz resonator* is an acoustic resonator, which was devised and used extensively for acoustic measurements by the multidisciplinary scientist Hermann Helmholtz in the 19th century. It is constructed as an enclosed volume of air to which is joined a narrow tube open at its end. The Helmholtz resonator is an acoustic analog to the simple oscillator. The enclosed volume provides the acoustic compliance C_a, the narrow tube provides the inertance I_a, and the acoustic damping associated with wall losses and sound radiation provides the resistance. The resonance frequency of the Helmholtz resonator is

$$f_0 = \frac{1}{2\pi} \frac{1}{\sqrt{I_a C_a}}, \qquad [38]$$

which is analogous to the corresponding expression for a mechanical simple oscillator in Equation 31. A perforation

in the tympanic membrane acts as an acoustic inertance, which, coupled with the volume of air in the middle ear cavities, can act as a Helmholtz resonator.

Table 8.2 shows a summary of quantities used for measurement of ATFs, including acoustic impedance, acoustic admittance, and acoustic reflectance. For all quantities summarized under acoustic impedance and acoustic admittance, the notation is that of American National Standards Institute (ANSI) S3.39 (ANSI, 1987).

It is sometimes necessary to transform acoustic impedance into acoustic admittance, or vice versa. From the preceding discussion, the impedance components are expressed in terms of admittance components by

$$|Z_a| = 1/|Y_a|,$$
$$\phi_z = -\phi_{y,}$$
$$R = \frac{G}{G^2 + B^2},$$
$$X = \frac{-B}{G^2 + B^2}, \qquad [39]$$

Similarly, the admittance components are expressed in terms of impedance components by

$$|Y_a| = 1/|Z_a|,$$
$$\phi_y = -\phi_{z,}$$
$$G = \frac{R}{R^2 + X^2},$$
$$B = \frac{-X}{R^2 + X^2}, \qquad [40]$$

REFLECTANCE COMPONENTS

The concept of the characteristic impedance of a tube of constant cross-sectional area is preliminary to calculating the reflectance. A special acoustic termination is an *anechoic* termination, which literally means an echo-free termination. It is realized by inserting a probe microphone and loudspeaker into the end of a long cylindrical tube, the cross-section area S of which is similar to that of a human ear canal. A typical diameter of an adult ear canal is 0.8 cm, corresponding to an area of 0.5 cm^2. The criterion for an anechoic termination is that it be sufficiently long that the measurement signal at the microphone receives no acoustical echo from the loudspeaker-generated input signal during the measurement interval. In practice, the loudspeaker outputs a brief sound that ends before the first reflection from the end of the tube returns to the microphone. The acoustic impedance of such an anechoic termination is called the *characteristic impedance* Z_c of the cylindrical tube. Neglecting acoustic dissipation at the walls of the tube or ear canal, this characteristic impedance is real (i.e., a resistive component) and defined by

$$Z_c = \frac{\rho c}{S}. \qquad [41]$$

The characteristic impedance of the ear canal is calculated in terms of its cross-section area.

TABLE 8.2   Aural acoustic immittance transfer functions and their components[a]

Acoustic Immittance Transfer Function	Related Transfer Function Components	Description	Symbol
Acoustic Impedance		Pressure response to volume-velocity input	$Z_a = R_a + jX_a = |Z_a|\, e^{j\phi_z}$
	Acoustic resistance	Energy-dissipating part of impedance	$R_a = Re(Z_a) \geq 0,$ $= |Z_a|\cos\phi_z$
	Acoustic reactance	Energy-storage part of impedance	$X_a = Im(Z_a),$ $= |Z_a|\sin\phi_z$
	Acoustic impedance magnitude	Magnitude of acoustic impedance	$|Z_a| = \sqrt{R_a^2 + X_a^2} \geq 0$
	Acoustic impedance phase	Phase of acoustic impedance	$\phi_z,$ with $\tan\phi_z = \dfrac{X_a}{R_a},$ $-\dfrac{\pi}{2} \leq \phi_z \leq \dfrac{\pi}{2}$
	Acoustic inertance	Acoustic mass of air motion	I_a
	Mass acoustic reactance	Mass-like impedance of acoustic inertance	$j\omega\, I_a$
	Acoustic compliance	Acoustic compressibility of volume of air	C_a
	Compliant acoustic reactance	Compliance-like impedance	$-\dfrac{j}{\omega\, C_a}$
	Acoustic stiffness	Inverse of acoustic compliance	$K_a = 1/C_a$
Acoustic Admittance		Volume-velocity response to pressure input	$Y_a = G_a + jB_a = |Y_a|\, e^{j\phi_y}$
	Acoustic conductance	Energy-dissipating part of admittance	$G_a = Re(Y_a) \geq 0,$ $= |Y_a|\cos\phi_y$
	Acoustic susceptance	Energy-storage part of admittance	$B_a = Im(Y_a),$ $= |Y_a|\sin\phi_y$
	Acoustic admittance magnitude	Magnitude of acoustic admittance	$|Y_a| = \sqrt{G_a^2 + B_a^2} \geq 0$
	Acoustic admittance phase	Phase of acoustic admittance	$\phi_y,$ with $\tan\phi_y = \dfrac{B_a}{G_a},$ $-\dfrac{\pi}{2} \leq \phi_y \leq \dfrac{\pi}{2}$
	Mass acoustic susceptibility	Mass-like admittance of acoustic inertance	$-\dfrac{j}{\omega\, I_a}$
	Compliant acoustic susceptibility	Compliance-like admittance	$j\omega\, C_a$
	Acoustic equivalent volume	Equivalent volume is compliance in units of volume	$V_{ea} = \rho c^2\, C_a$
Acoustic Pressure Reflectance		Ratio of reflected to incident pressure	r_a
	Energy reflectance	Ratio of reflected to incident energy	$ER = |r_a|^2,\ 0 \leq ER \leq 1$
	Energy absorbance	Ratio of absorbed to incident energy	$EA = 1 - ER,\ 0 \leq EA \leq 1$

[a] The table uses the radian frequency $\omega = 2\pi f$, which is defined in terms of the frequency f. Other constants used are the equilibrium density of air ρ and the phase velocity of sound c.

Suppose the complex acoustic impedance Z_a is measured in the ear canal at one or more frequencies at the probe tip. Then, the (complex) acoustic pressure reflectance r_a at the probe tip is defined by

$$r_a = \frac{Z_a - Z_c}{Z_a + Z_c}, \qquad [42]$$

and the (real) acoustic energy reflectance $ER = |r_a|^2$ is calculated from the acoustic impedance by

$$ER = \left| \frac{Z_a - Z_c}{Z_a + Z_c} \right|^2. \qquad [43]$$

Acoustic immittance is a term unique to aural measurements that refers collectively to the acoustic impedance, the acoustic admittance, or both quantities (ANSI S3.39-1987). From a systems point of view, the acoustic impedance and the acoustic admittance are both examples of an ATF or, more specifically, of a single-point ATF. The single-point ATF refers to the fact that the two variables comprising an impedance or admittance, which are the acoustic pressure and acoustic volume velocity, are measured at the same location. A two-point ATF is one in which the input variable is measured at one location and the output variable is measured at another location. For example, an important transfer ATF in middle ear mechanics is the forward pressure TF, which is the ratio of the acoustic pressure in the cochlear vestibule to the acoustic pressure just in front of the tympanic membrane in the ear canal in response to a sound source in the ear canal. However, there are also reverse TFs depending on the source and receiver locations (e.g., the reverse middle ear pressure TF is the ratio of the output pressure in the ear canal in response to an input pressure source in the cochlear vestibule and is important in understanding the transmission of an otoacoustic emission from the cochlea back into the ear canal). An acoustic immittance is taken to refer only to a single-point ATF at a measurement location in the ear canal for the case in which the sound source is a stimulus in the ear canal. Given the fact that pressure reflectance and energy reflectance are also single-point ATFs, it is useful to generalize the concept of acoustic immittance in audiology and hearing science to include these reflectance functions.

TYMPANOMETRY

Tympanometry is defined in the ANSI S3.39 (1987) standard as a measure of acoustic immittance in the ear canal as a function of varying air pressure within the ear canal. The *excess pressure* (p_s) in the ear canal is the difference in the static pressure within the ear canal with respect to atmospheric pressure. The excess pressure is produced using a static pump that is connected to a port in a probe assembly that is sealed in the ear canal. The SI unit of pressure is the pascal (Pa), but it is convenient to express the excess pressure in tympanometry using the dekapascal (daPa) unit, such that 1 daPa = 10 Pa. The tympanometric range of excess pressures does not exceed −800 to 600 daPa, and a typical subrange would be −300 to 200 daPa. Standard atmospheric pressure at sea level is 1.01×10^6 daPa, so that an excess pressure of ± 100 daPa is only ± 0.01% of standard atmospheric pressure.

A single-frequency tympanogram is an acoustic admittance response measured as a function of static pressure varied within the ear canal using a single probe frequency; typical frequencies include 226 and 1,000 Hz. A multifrequency tympanogram is an acoustic admittance response measured as a function of static pressure at multiple frequencies. These clinical tympanograms are admittance tympanograms inasmuch as the underlying aural ATF is acoustic admittance.

A generalized definition of tympanometry is proposed to refer to a measurement of an aural single-point ATF as a function of varying air pressure within the ear

canal. This includes the single-point aural ATFs of acoustic impedance, acoustic admittance, acoustic pressure reflectance, and acoustic energy reflectance or absorbance. Such reflectance tympanograms have been measured using wideband stimuli over a frequency range from 0.25 to 8 kHz or higher. There appears to be little distinction with regard to middle ear assessment whether a lower frequency of 250 Hz (0.25 kHz) or 226 Hz is used.

⬛ ANSI S3.39

The ANSI S3.39 (1987) addresses specifications for instruments designed to measure the middle ear. This standard uses a generic term immittance to indicate an acoustic measurement of middle ear function. This encompasses measurements of Z_a and its reciprocal, Y_a. Most clinical systems today measure Y_a or its components, G_a and B_a. ANSI S3.39 (1987) uses SI units, and thus, the units for admittance are $m^3/Pa \cdot s$. This converts to the unit of a mmho, the traditional unit of measure in the CGS system, such that 1 mmho = 1 $cm^5/dynes \cdot s$. Aural acoustic immittance instruments are designed to measure a number of characteristics of the external and middle ear. For the purposes of this discussion, we will refer to Y_a measurements made with a 226-Hz probe tone, which is the only probe frequency specified by the standard, although Z_a could also be used. Admittance instruments must include the capability for the measurement of static Y_a, which refers to the measurement of Y_a at a fixed ear canal pressure, and dynamic Y_a, which refers to the measurement of Y_a during changes in ear canal pressure or during the activation of middle ear muscle reflexes. ANSI S3.39 (1987) provides minimum mandatory characteristics of admittance instruments for obtaining static Y_a, for the generation of tympanograms, and for the ASR activating system. Type 1 instruments have the most features, providing manual and automatic control of air pressure, analog or digital output proportional to air pressure, and measurement plane, as well as compensated static Y_a at the tympanic membrane. Type 2 instruments typically offer either manual or automatic control of pressure, compensated static acoustic admittance, and puretone reflex activating signals. Type 3 instruments do not offer compensated admittance measurements and have either a noise or tonal reflex activating signal. There are no minimum requirements for Type 4 admittance instruments.

Measurement tolerances are also specified in ANSI S3.39 (1987). For example, for instruments measuring static or dynamic Y_a, the accuracy of measurement must be within ± 5% of the indicated value or ± 0.1 acoustic mmho, whichever is greater. The minimum range of Y_a magnitude measurement for Type 1 and Type 2 instruments is 0.0 to 2.0 mmho, whereas Type 3 instruments may have a reduced range of 0.0 to 1.2 mmho.

Although a 226-Hz probe signal must be provided in Type 1, 2, and 3 instruments, additional probe frequencies may also be provided. Several commercial systems provide higher probe frequencies such as 678 Hz and 1,000 Hz. The ANSI S3.39 specifies that at least three calibration cavities of specified volumes are provided with Type 1, 2, and 3 instruments, but the ratio of the length of the cavity to its inside diameter is allowed to range between 1 and 3. Measurements in these cavities are required in order to transform acoustic pressure measurements in the ear into measurements of acoustic immittance. Such variability in cavity design may limit the accuracy of the calibrations at higher probe frequencies. For example, inaccurate estimates of middle ear impedance in the 800-Hz region in a clinical immittance device were concluded to be due to calibration errors related to the design of the calibration cavities (Margolis et al., 1999).

ANSI S3.39 (1987, p 7) states that, "An interaction may exist between the level of the probe tone and the threshold of the acoustic reflex. Ideally, all probe signals should be delivered at levels that will not affect significantly the tonus of the middle-ear muscles." A recent study has shown that the level of the 226-Hz probe used currently in clinical systems (85 to 90 dB SPL) may facilitate the ASR, thus resulting in lower reflex thresholds. Day and Feeney (in press) used an experimental admittance instrument to measure contralateral ASR thresholds in 40 young adult subjects. The system permitted a 226-Hz probe level to be varied from 70 to 85 dB SPL in 5-dB steps. Forty young adults served as subjects. A 226-Hz probe level of 85 dB SPL produced 1,000 Hz contralateral reflex thresholds that averaged 2.3 dB lower than those obtained for a probe level of 70 dB SPL. Individual ASR thresholds were as much as 15 dB lower for the 85-dB

SPL probe than for the 70-dB SPL probe. Similar findings of facilitation on ASR input-output functions for a low-frequency probe tone were reported by Terkildsen et al. (1970). These results suggest that there is an interaction between the level of the 226-Hz probe tone in current clinical use and ASR thresholds.

TYPES OF CLINICAL MEASUREMENTS OF ACOUSTIC IMMITTANCE

Single-Frequency Tympanometry

As indicated earlier, tympanometry is a dynamic measurement of middle ear function, which tracks admittance during changes in ear canal pressure. Most current commercial instruments are single-component tympanometers that provide a measurement of Y_a as a function of ear canal air pressure. Several instruments are also capable of measuring multiple components, G_a and B_a, as a function of pressure to create multicomponent tympanograms. These systems may also provide additional probe frequencies to allow for multicomponent, multifrequency tympanometry (discussed below). More details about tympanometry can be found in Chapter 9.

The basic tympanometric probe consists of a miniature loudspeaker used to generate a probe tone, a microphone to monitor the level of the probe tone, and a pump to change ear canal pressure (Fig. 8.15). A hermetic seal is obtained

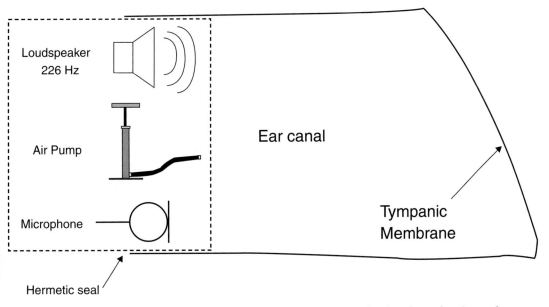

FIGURE 8.15 The basic components of a tympanometer. The loudspeaker introduces a 226-Hz tone to the ear canal while the pump varies the air pressure in the canal above and below atmospheric pressure. The microphone records the level of the tone at various ear canal pressures, and those levels are converted to Ya in mmho. For a constant volume velocity source, Ya varies with the sound pressure by the formula Ya = u/p, where u equals the volume velocity and p equals the sound pressure of the 226-Hz tone.

between the probe and the ear canal, which allows for air pressure changes to be transferred to the tympanic membrane. In the normal ear, pressure changes in the ear canal decrease the admittance of the middle ear, which tends to increase the 226-Hz probe level. An automatic gain control feedback mechanism is used to maintain the level of the probe tone as the pressure is changed. The output of the microphone signal is amplified and compared to the output of the probe amplifier. The change in admittance at the probe tip during the static pressure changes of a tympanometric test is proportional to the change in voltage required to keep the probe tone at a constant level. The magnitude and phase of admittance are calculated based on a comparison with calibration measurements in a hard-walled cavity. Figure 8.16 illustrates a normal adult tympanogram with admittance magnitude $|Y_a|$ at 226 Hz as a function of ear canal pressure.

CHOICE OF PROBE FREQUENCY

Why is a 226-Hz probe frequency specified in the ANSI S3.39 (1987) standard? As discussed earlier, the admittance magnitude of a 1-cm³ volume of air is approximately equal to 1 mmho at 226 Hz at sea level and room temperature. Thus, the admittance magnitude of the enclosed air space in mmho is equivalent to its volume in cm³ but only at 226 Hz. This is a convenient relation in audiology that allows us to express the acoustic admittance magnitude in units of cm³ (equivalent volume). ANSI S3.39 indicates that, to calibrate an admit-

tance instrument with a 226-Hz probe tone, we can use a cylindrical, hard-walled cavity, with an air-tight seal around the probe tip. With this arrangement, a calibration cavity with a volume of 2 cm³ yields an admittance measurement of 2.0 mmho when using a 226-Hz probe tone. This calibration varies with changes in altitude from sea level and must be accounted for (Lilly and Shanks, 1981).

STATIC ACOUSTIC ADMITTANCE

Static Y_a is the measurement of admittance in the ear canal at a specified air pressure. This may be compensated for the admittance of the ear canal volume by subtracting the admittance of the ear canal itself from the overall admittance. This compensated static Y_a is assumed to be equal to the Y_a at the lateral surface of the tympanic membrane. If the admittance of the ear canal is not removed from the measurement, the differences in individual ear canal size create so much variability in the measurement of middle ear function that the uncompensated static admittance is not a useful measurement. The ear canal admittance is measured during a condition of high or low air pressure introduced to the canal using a pneumatic pump to stiffen the tympanic membrane. This is subtracted from the admittance measured at peak pressure, resulting in peak admittance magnitude. The resulting difference is called the peak-compensated static acoustic admittance magnitude (*Peak Y_{tm}*), which is the most common measure of middle ear admittance and used widely as a screening measure of middle ear function (American Speech-Language-Hearing Association [ASHA], 1997).

EQUIVALENT VOLUME

The acoustic compliance C_a is defined in terms of the acoustic susceptance B_a at frequency f by $C_a = B_a/(2\pi f)$. The acoustic equivalent volume V_{ea} is defined in turn by $V_{ea} = C_a/\rho c^2$. It follows that the acoustic equivalent volume of a volume V of air in which acoustic losses are neglected is simply $V_{ea} = V$. Measurements of V_{ea} are useful in the assessment of the integrity of the tympanic membrane and the status of pressure equalization (PE) tubes, which are surgically inserted through the tympanic membrane in patients with chronic otitis media to ventilate the middle ear space. A larger than normal volume measurement suggests either a perforation of the tympanic membrane or a patent PE tube.

TYMPANOGRAM PEAK PRESSURE

The air pressure at which a maximum in the tympanogram occurs is referred to as the tympanogram peak pressure (TPP). This measurement offers an estimate of middle ear pressure, which is often negative in cases of eustachian tube dysfunction. However, TPP has not been found to be useful for the diagnosis of middle ear disorders (Shanks et al., 1988), and it is not recommended as a screening tool for assessing middle ear disorders (ASHA, 1997).

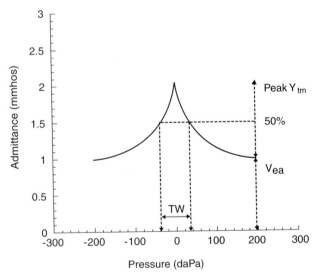

FIGURE 8.16 **Normal admittance tympanogram for an adult (solid line). The vertical dashed lines with arrows on the right of the graph indicate the equivalent volume of the ear canal, V$_{ea}$, and the peak compensated static acoustic admittance, Peak Y$_{tm}$. The horizontal dashed line at 50% of Peak Y$_{tm}$ bisects the tympanogram. The vertical dashed lines drawn to the baseline from these points indicate the tympanometric width (TW) in daPa.**

TYMPANOMETRIC WIDTH

The tympanometric width (TW) is the pressure range over which the tympanogram attains 50% of its peak in admittance. This is measured by obtaining the pressure range between points marked by a line that bisects the 50% point from peak to tail on the tympanogram (Fig. 8.16). This is typically obtained in clinical systems using the positive tail of the tympanogram. Broad TW is associated with middle ear effusion and has proven to be a useful screening measurement (ASHA, 1997; Nozza et al., 1994).

Multifrequency Tympanometry

Several commercial tympanometers offer the use of multiple probe frequencies. The examination of middle ear function using a series of probe frequencies for Y_a, B_a, and G_a tympanograms may provide information about the middle ear resonance frequency. Higher probe frequencies result in notched tympanograms in normal ears. Vanhuyse et al. (1975) developed a model to demonstrate that, in the normal ear, a systematic pattern of notching should occur in multifrequency, multicomponent tympanograms. This model has proven useful in the assessment of middle ear disorders. For example, middle ear resonance for ears with an ossicular disarticulation occurs at a lower frequency than normal, causing notching in tympanograms at a lower than normal frequency, whereas middle ear resonance for ears with otosclerosis occurs at a higher than normal frequency (Lilly, 1984).

Measurement of the Acoustic Stapedius Reflex

Another dynamic measure of middle ear function is the measurement of middle ear muscle reflexes discussed earlier. The ASR requires a functional cochlea, VIIIth cranial nerve, brainstem, and VIIth cranial nerve and a normal middle ear. Absence or elevation of the reflex may point to an abnormality in one or more of these systems. A more detailed description of the acoustic reflex can be found in Chapter 10.

The ASR results in a stiffening of the ossicular chain and thus a decrease in the magnitude of Y_a in the low frequencies. An indirect measurement of the ASR can be made by monitoring Y_a during the presentation of a reflex-activating stimulus. The monitoring (probe) frequency per ANSI S3.39 (1987) is the 226-Hz tone. The activators used clinically are pure tones (i.e., sinusoidal tones) or bands of noise presented to the same ear being monitored (ipsilateral reflex) or to the opposite ear (contralateral reflex). The most common measure is the ASR threshold, which is defined as the lowest level at which an activator evokes an ASR. The patterns of ASR threshold results for the ipsilateral and contralateral tests are compared to yield a powerful diagnostic test of auditory function. Elevated or absent ASR thresholds may indicate a hearing loss of cochlear origin, a retrocochlear or brainstem lesion, a VIIth cranial nerve lesion, or a middle ear conductive problem, depending on the ear of stimulation and presentation mode (ipsilateral vs. contralateral).

Following the establishment of the ASR threshold, a measure of ASR decay may be completed. In this context, the reflex is used to monitor adaptation to the activator stimulus at a level 10 dB above reflex threshold. A reduction in reflex amplitude of 50% or more for mid- and low-frequency activator tones over 5 or 10 seconds is considered a sign of abnormal reflex adaptation and may suggest a retrocochlear lesion.

▨ RESEARCH USING WIDEBAND AMBIENT-PRESSURE ACOUSTIC TRANSFER FUNCTION TESTS

The use of single-frequency tympanometry became widespread clinically following the work of Terkildsen and Thomsen (1959) and Terkildsen and Nielsen (1960), who recorded the impedance at a single low-frequency probe tone (220 Hz) as a function of excess pressure in the ear canal. In addition to limitations of electronics in the era of the 1960s to 1970s, there were two other problems that had to be overcome. One problem was the need to calibrate the tympanometric device so that sound pressure measurements by the microphone could be analyzed as complex admittance or impedance responses. Such calibration is inherently simpler at 220 Hz than at higher frequencies. Another problem was the need to calculate the acoustic immittance at the tympanic membrane, based on a measurement of the acoustic immittance at the probe tip. The admittance at the tympanic membrane is the compensated admittance described earlier. The procedure to compensate for the effect of the internal volume of air between the probe tip and the tympanic membrane is simple at 226 Hz because the volume of air acts as an acoustic compliance at this frequency. This is not the case at higher frequencies (>1.5 kHz in adults) because of the effect of standing waves in the ear canal, which are manifested as maxima and minima in the SPL at particular locations between the probe and the tympanic membrane. While multifrequency tympanometry has extended the range of probe frequencies up to 2 kHz, these two problems have not been addressed in existing clinical devices, and the existing ANSI S3.39 standard is concerned with the parameters and tolerances of aural immittance devices only for the use of a 226-Hz probe tone.

The limitation of such devices is that the bandwidth of human hearing extends far above 226 Hz, and the higher frequencies of normal hearing extend above the maximum frequency of 2 kHz in multifrequency tympanometric devices as well. A single-frequency tympanogram assesses the middle ear response at one probe frequency across a range of excess pressures. Alternatively, a wideband ambient-pressure ATF assesses the middle ear response across a wide range of frequencies, typically 0.25 to approximately 8 kHz, and a single ambient pressure, which corresponds to atmospheric pressure or zero excess pressure in the ear canal. The intent of wideband ATF measurements is to assess middle ear functioning over much of the bandwidth of human hearing. This is similar to the wideband characteristic of behavioral audiograms, otoacoustic emission (OAE) measurements, and auditory brainstem response (ABR) measurements. Acoustic impedance responses have been measured over various bandwidths at ambient pressure and often referenced to the eardrum, by numerous early investigators, in adults (Metz, 1946; Zwislocki, 1957; Moller, 1960; Mehrgardt and Mellert, 1977; Rabinowitz, 1981) and children (Okabe et al., 1988). While some of these reports predate the invention of tympanometry, difficulties in calibration at higher frequencies, a lack of portability of instrumentation, and the relative clinical success of 226-Hz tympanometry in middle ear diagnostics limited clinical utilization of the ambient-pressure ATF tests.

The use of energy reflectance in aural acoustic measurements was introduced by Stinson et al. (1982) and the use of pressure reflectance by Hudde (1983). These reports showed that, unlike acoustic impedance and admittance, the energy reflectance at the tympanic membrane can be measured in adult ears at frequencies above 2 kHz based on mid-canal microphone recordings at ambient pressure and that the energy reflectance is relatively insensitive to anatomic irregularities of the ear canal above 2 kHz. However, their

measurement procedures were not intended for clinical applications. Keefe et al. (1992) described a rapid (inasmuch as responses can be acquired in a few seconds), noninvasive technique to measure wideband acoustic reflectance, impedance, and admittance responses in human ears, which are collectively termed wideband ATF responses. The wideband impedance-measurement calibration technique used by Keefe et al. (1992) was based on a technique used to measure aural impedance in cats (Allen, 1985). Wideband ATF responses were obtained with rapid, noninvasive techniques in normal-hearing adults ears (Keefe et al., 1993; Voss and Allen, 1994, Margolis et al., 1999; Feeney et al., 2003a; Keefe and Simmons, 2003).

Wideband ATF measurements in infants, children, and adults show a developmental gradient in middle ear functioning. Wideband energy reflectance and admittance responses have been measured as means over populations of normal-hearing subjects over the age range from neonates (Keefe et al., 2000), to children of age of 1, 3, 6, 12, 24 months, and adults (Keefe et al., 1993). The adult energy reflectance in Figure 8.17 (thickest solid line) is close to 1 at low frequencies, which means that little energy is transmitted into the middle ear. There is a broad minimum near 2 to 4 kHz, and the energy reflectance increases at frequencies up to 8 kHz. The reflectance decreases above 8 kHz with increasing frequency. Energy reflectance is similar in the 2- to 4-kHz range across age, except that the minimum is approximately 0.2 in older children compared with 0.4 in adults. Energy reflectance at

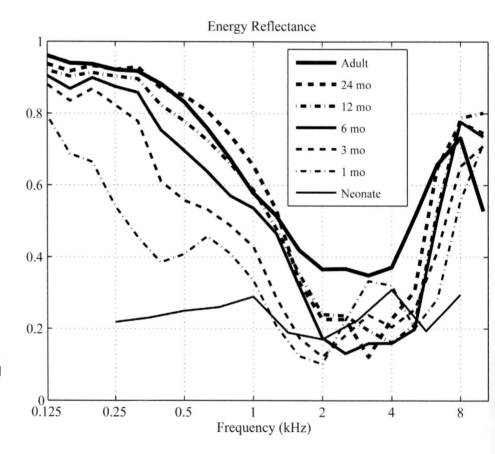

FIGURE 8.17 Energy reflectance measured in adults and in children of ages listed in the symbol legend. (Reprinted from Keefe [2007] with permission of Thieme Publishers.)

low frequencies exceeds 0.8 for older children and adults, but the response for 1-month-old children is approximately 0.55 at 0.25 kHz compared to 0.2 for neonates (thinnest solid line) across a broad frequency range. Reflectance at 0.25 kHz increases with age, which may be due in part to a sound-induced motion of the ear canal walls in younger children. Middle ear transmission may be easier to assess in younger children using frequencies at and above 1 kHz. Functional immaturity may help explain why low-frequency tympanograms are difficult to interpret in young children. Energy reflectance decreased in adults older than 60 years from 0.8 to 2.0 kHz, but increased near 5 kHz (Feeney and Sanford, 2004). This suggests a conductive component to presbycusis.

Wideband ATF tests are capable of identifying ears with otitis media with effusion (OME) (Piskorski et al., 1999; Feeney et al., 2003a). ATF tests were used by Piskorksi et al. (1999) to predict the presence of a conductive hearing loss in a population of 161 ears of children at risk for OME. The criterion for conductive hearing loss was whether the maximum air-bone gap across the octave frequencies between 500 and 4,000 Hz was ≥15 dB. The area under the receiver operating characteristic (ROC) curve is an unbiased measure of the accuracy of a clinical test in classifying a response as normal or impaired, with a perfectly accurate test having an ROC area of 1.0 and a random-choice test having an ROC area of 0.5. The ROC area was larger for the ATF predictor (0.93) than either gradient or static admittance of the 226-Hz tympanometric predictors (0.84). At a fixed sensitivity of 80%, the ATF predictor achieved 93% specificity, whereas the best predictor based on 226-Hz tympanometry achieved 70% specificity. Thus, ambient-pressure ATF was a more effective predictor of conductive hearing loss than 226-Hz tympanometry in a population of children at risk for OME.

The pattern of the wideband ATFs at ambient pressure may be useful in the differential diagnosis of conductive hearing loss. Feeney et al. (2003a) examined wideband reflectance ATFs in a small sample of patients with a variety of middle ear disorders using the system developed by Keefe et al. (1993). Figure 8.18 shows average data from that study for four patients with otitis media and two patients with otosclerosis. Also shown are data from one patient with ossicular discontinuity. The shaded area in the figure represents the 5th to 95th percentile of energy reflectance as a function of frequency for a group of 40 young adults with normal hearing. The pattern of energy reflectance in ears with otitis media tended to be near 1.0 across the frequency range of 250 to 8,000 Hz, except for a narrow high-frequency notch of low energy reflectance. The patients with otosclerosis tended to have a more normal shape to the energy reflectance pattern; however, there was higher energy reflectance than the 90% range at frequencies below 1,000 Hz, with a lower than average notch in energy reflectance near 4,000 Hz. The subject with the ossicular discontinuity had an energy reflectance pattern that was very different from the other disorders, with a deep notch

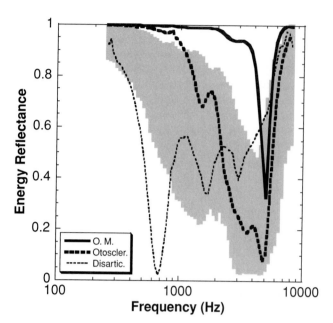

FIGURE 8.18 Energy reflectance results for patients with middle ear disorders. The data were averaged for four patients with otitis media (OM) with effusion and two patients with otosclerosis. There was one patient with an ossicular disarticulation. The shaded area represents the 5th to 95th percentile for 40 young adults with normal hearing. (Based on data from Feeney et al. [2003a].)

in energy reflectance in the low frequencies and with energy reflectance returning to the normal range at higher frequencies. In combination with puretone audiometric data, these patterns of energy reflectance may be helpful in diagnosing various middle ear pathologies. More data are needed from patients with a variety of disorders to be able to assess the utility of this approach.

Norton et al. (2000) described the relative test performance of click-evoked (CE) OAEs, distortion-product (DP) OAEs, and ABRs in newborn hearing screening (NHS) programs. An additional study was performed to evaluate whether a wideband ATF test helped interpret CEOAE, DPOAE, and ABR tests in newborns. It was found that infants with high energy reflectance in the 2- to 8-kHz range tended to have low DPOAE and CEOAE levels. As much as 28% of the variance in OAEs and 15% of variance in ABR latencies was explained by ATF responses, suggesting that ATF responses are more closely coupled to OAE than ABR responses (Keefe et al., 2003b).

An important problem in NHS programs is to identify whether an infant failing the NHS test has failed because of a sensorineural hearing loss or because of middle ear dysfunction. Transient middle ear dysfunction is common in infants tested within 48 hours of birth and in infants residing for extended periods in neonatal intensive care units. An ear that fails the NHS test but is later found to have normal hearing is called a *false positive*. An ATF test of middle ear dysfunction identified false positives with an ROC area of 0.86 (Keefe et al., 2003a). This middle ear dysfunction test was applied for the National Institutes of Health–recommended two-stage hearing screeners—an OAE test followed by an ABR test if the ear fails the OAE test. Both DPOAE/ABR and CEOAE/ABR screening protocols resulted in a 5% false-positive rate. Including the ATF test of middle ear dysfunction reduced the false-positive rate to 1% for each protocol. Thus, an ATF test of middle ear dysfunction accounted for four of five false positives resulting from a two-stage OAE/ABR NHS protocol (Keefe et al., 2003a). A more extended description of the ATF results in the NHS study and their relation to OAE testing is presented elsewhere (Keefe, 2007).

RESEARCH USING ACOUSTIC TRANSFER FUNCTION TYMPANOMETRY TESTS

A wideband ATF tympanometry test was developed and used to measure responses in the ears of adults and young children (Keefe and Levi, 1996). One finding was that some children aged 3 to 6 months old had flat 226-Hz tympanograms but a normal reflectance response. Another study (Margolis et al., 1999) using 20 normal-hearing adults provided results similar to clinical multifrequency tympanometry in terms of tympanometric patterns and resonant frequency estimates up to the 2-kHz limit of the clinical instrument. Admittance tympanograms above 2 kHz did not provide an orderly sequence of patterns such as predicted by the model of Vanhuyse et al. (1975). Energy reflectance tympanograms recorded in 20 subjects did progress through an orderly sequence of patterns as frequency increased from 0.25 to 11.3 kHz. This orderly behavior in energy reflectance tympanograms may provide a useful and simpler framework for detecting middle ear pathology. The following section compares the ability of wideband ATF tympanometry to improve the performance of predicting conductive hearing loss.

Energy Absorbance Predicts Conductive Hearing Loss in Older Children and Adults

Wideband ambient-pressure ATF and ATF tympanogram responses were measured in a group of 60 ears to compare test performance with that of 226-Hz tympanometry in predicting conductive hearing loss (Keefe and Simmons, 2003). There were 18 conductive-impaired ears, including both pure conductive and mixed losses. The age range of all subjects included older children (age ≥10 years) and adults. Each subject had an intact tympanic membrane and no mastoid bowl cavity, the latter of which is an outcome of a surgical procedure (modified radical mastoidectomy) to eradicate chronic mastoid and middle ear disease in which the posterior portion of a patient's ear canal and mastoid air cells are

removed. Energy absorbance (see Table 8.2) was chosen as the ATF response variable because it shows a central peak on the two-dimensional plane of frequency and static pressure, whereas energy reflectance shows a dip. The relevance of this property is described below.

A typical energy-absorbance tympanogram for a normal-hearing ear is shown in Figure 8.19 (upper left panel). Each response was obtained in a 40-s measurement. The normal response shows a peak in absorbance along a ridge of static pressure close to 0 daPa and a maximum of absorbance near 4 kHz. The frequency maximum in energy absorbance corresponds with the minimum in energy reflectance at 4 kHz in the ambient-pressure responses in Figure 8.17 and in the gray baseline band in Figure 8.18. Thus, the energy absorbance tympanogram is "upside down" with respect to an energy reflectance tympanogram. This is because energy absorbance is a measure of how much sound enters the middle ear, whereas energy reflectance is a measure of how much sound does not enter (i.e., is reflected by) the middle ear system. The impaired ear with the approximately

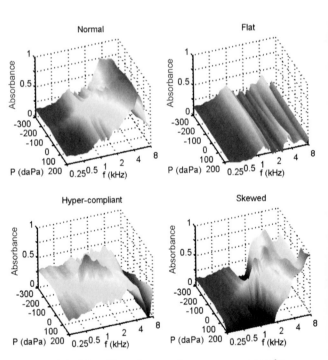

FIGURE 8.19 Absorbance tympanograms in adults for a normal-hearing ear (upper left) and three ears with a conductive hearing loss: an ear with a flat 226-Hz clinical tympanogram (upper right), an ear with a hyper-compliant 226-Hz tympanogram (lower left), and an ear with a skewed response with respect to positive and negative static pressures (lower right). Each tympanogram is plotted as a function of static pressure in the ear canal and frequency, with energy absorbance values coded both by vertical elevation on an axis between 0 and 1 and by grayscale.

flat, low-absorbance tympanogram (Fig. 8.19, upper right panel) also had a flat 226-Hz tympanogram, and the insensitivity in this ear to static pressure variations extended up to 8 kHz in the absorbance tympanogram. An impaired ear had a hyper-compliant 226-Hz tympanogram (Fig. 8.19, lower left panel), and the absorbance shows a local maximum close to 1 kHz followed by reduced absorbance at higher frequencies. The impaired ear with the absorbance that is skewed with respect to variations in static pressure, particularly at and above 4 kHz, had a normal 226-Hz tympanogram along with a conductive hearing loss (Fig. 8.19, lower right panel). While these absorbance tympanograms appear to have useful properties, a pattern-classification approach is needed to simplify their interpretation.

Classification of Multifrequency Tympanograms Using Vanhuyse Patterns

Pattern classification techniques are useful in understanding admittance tympanograms at low frequencies by classifying tympanograms according to the number of extrema in the conductance and susceptance tympanograms (Vanhuyse et al., 1975; Van Camp et al., 1986). Multifrequency tympanograms, measured clinically up to 2 kHz, have been classified in terms of a sequence of Vanhuyse patterns of increasing complexity with increasing frequency. From a study in 56 adult ears with normal hearing, Margolis and Goycoolea (1983) concluded that almost all tympanometric patterns were predicted as a sequence of Vanhuyse patterns, although irregular patterns that did not fit the Vanhuyse model occurred with increasing prevalence at higher frequencies. A description of Vanhuyse tympanogram patterns can be found in Chapter 9.

Classification of Wideband Acoustic Transfer Function Tympanograms Using Moments

The Vanhuyse pattern classification technique has not proven useful with wideband ATF tympanograms, and an alternative pattern classification technique using a moment analysis has been devised (Keefe and Simmons, 2003). This objective method is based on a moment analysis of the tympanogram in the two dimensions of static pressure and frequency. Such a moment analysis may be familiar in terms of moments defined in statistical descriptions of data. For example, in a central probability distribution $p(x)$ that is a function of a single variable x, the moment of order 0 represents the normalization condition that the probabilities sum to 1, the moment of order 1 is the mean of x, and the moment of order 2 is used to define the standard deviation of x. If the probability distribution $p(x, y)$ is a joint function of two variables x and y, then the moment orders are well defined for both x and y.

A tympanometric variable $T(P, f)$ is a two-dimensional distribution over the pair of variables excess pressure P in the ear canal and frequency f. The *pressure moments* over the various moment orders of P and the *frequency moments* over the various moment orders of f are defined just as for the statistical distribution above.

The 0th-order pressure moment, which is called the *pressure-averaged response*, is defined at each frequency as the average value of the response over all static pressures. The 1st-order pressure moment, which is called the *mean pressure*, is defined at each frequency by taking the average of P weighted by $T(P, f)$. This variable is the analog to the TPP in conventional tympanometry. The 2nd-order pressure moment, which is calculated as the variance of the pressure with respect to the mean pressure, is also defined at each frequency. Its square root is defined as the standard deviation (SD) of the pressure and is called the *pressure breadth* (in daPa). This SD is most useful if the underlying distribution has a central-peaked response, akin to that of a normal probability distribution. Thus, the moments are calculated for energy absorbance, which has a central maximum [i.e., $EA = T(P, f)$], rather than for a variable such as energy reflectance, which has a central minimum. The pressure breadth is the analog to the TW of a conventional tympanogram.

The 0th-order frequency moment, which is called the *frequency-averaged response*, is defined at each static pressure as the average value of the response over all frequencies. The other frequency moments are defined at each static pressure and have similar definitions to the corresponding pressure moments. They are called the *mean frequency* (in kHz) and the *frequency breadth* (in kHz).

These six pressure and frequency moments were calculated for each ear in the normal (N = 42) and impaired (N = 18) groups (described earlier). The 10th to 90th percentiles in the normal group were calculated for each of the moments, providing a normal baseline against which to interpret the moments calculated for each impaired ear. With individual line curves in Figure 8.20 representing moments for each impaired ear relative to the normal baseline moment percentiles shown as a gray band, the pressure and frequency moments are plotted in the left and right columns, respectively. The moment plots reduce the complexity of a wideband tympanogram to a much smaller number of simpler functions.

For the normal group, the pressure-averaged absorbance (Fig. 8.20, top left panel, gray band) has a similar frequency dependence to that of the absorbance tympanogram (Fig. 8.19). Like the TPP, the mean pressure (middle left panel) in normal ears is close to 0 daPa. Analogous to TW, but with a different normalization, the median pressure breadth (lower left panel) in the normal group is approximately 130 daPa. The frequency-averaged absorbance (top right panel) is the average absorbance over all frequencies, and the plot versus static pressure shows a pattern like that of a single-peaked tympanogram. The absorbance is higher near 0 daPa in normal ears, corresponding to higher transmission of energy into the middle ear. The normal-group median of the mean

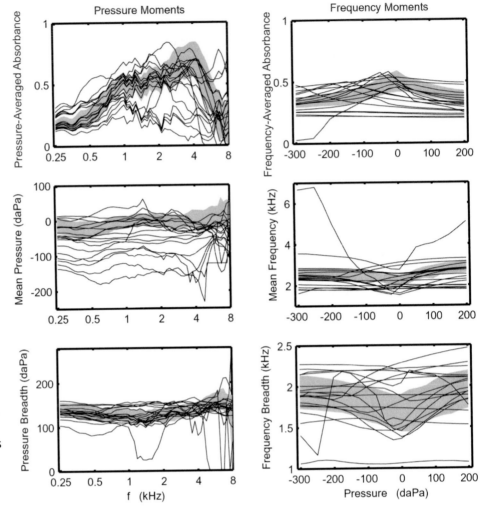

FIGURE 8.20 Based on group measurements of absorbance tympanograms, the pressure moments are plotted versus frequency (left column) and the frequency moments are plotted versus static pressure in the ear canal (right column) for groups of normal-hearing ears and ears with conductive hearing loss. The 10th to 90th percentiles of the normal-hearing group are plotted as a gray background; the moments of each individual conductive-impaired ear are plotted as separate lines.

frequency (middle right panel) varies between 2.3 and 2.6 kHz and represents the spectral centroid of the absorbance at each static pressure. The frequency breadth (lower right panel), which estimates the absorbance bandwidth about its mean frequency, varies between 1.75 and 1.9 kHz.

Clinical Signal Detection of Conductive Hearing Loss

It is apparent in Figure 8.20 that the impaired-ear moments were often outside the 10th to 90th percentiles of the normal responses. This observation led to the creation of an error function to predict conductive hearing loss using both the tympanometric and ambient-pressure energy absorbance responses. For each ear, a difference function was calculated for each pressure moment at each frequency and for each frequency moment at each pressure. This difference function was 0 if the moment was within the normal baseline and, otherwise, was proportional to its distance outside the normal baseline range. The error function was calculated as the average of the difference functions across all the moments.

An "ideal" normal ear would always lie within the normal baseline and would have an error function equal to 0. The impaired ears tended to lie outside the normal baseline in more moments at more frequencies or pressures, and so their error functions tended to be much larger than those of normal ears.

This error function was used in a clinical signal detection theory approach to calculate the ROC area for the ambient-pressure and the pressurized energy absorbance functions. Using a fixed specificity of 0.90, the sensitivity of static admittance, which was calculated from the 226-Hz tympanogram using the pass/fail guidelines of ASHA (1990), was compared to the sensitivities of the ambient-pressure and tympanometric energy absorbance functions.

In predicting the presence of a conductive hearing loss, the ROC area for energy absorbance tympanometry was 0.95, while that for ambient-pressure energy absorbance was 0.90. At a fixed specificity of 0.90, the sensitivity of energy absorbance tympanometry was 0.94, the sensitivity of ambient-pressure energy absorbance was 0.72, and the sensitivity of static admittance was 0.28. Thus, either of the absorbance responses more accurately predicted conductive hearing loss than did static admittance at 226 Hz. Moreover, energy absorbance tympanometry more accurately predicted a conductive hearing loss than did ambient-pressure absorbance. Ambient-pressure ATFs may have sufficient accuracy to use in hearing screening applications for which pressurization of the ear canal is determined to be unwarranted, whereas ATF tympanograms may have additional accuracy that may be appropriate for hearing diagnostic applications.

There may be instances in which a frequency-specific weighting of moments, or an unequal weighting of the contributions of different moments, leads to improved performance. Some middle ear pathologies have a characteristic frequency-specific effect on an ATF. For example, the impedance and the SPL may be helpful in identifying ears with a perforated tympanic membrane (Voss et al., 2001a; 2001b). An unequal-weighting approach has been used in the studies reviewed earlier to predict conductive hearing loss associated with OME (Piskorski et al., 1999) and to predict transient middle ear dysfunction in neonates (Keefe et al., 2003a). Feeney et al. (2003a) described distinct patterns across frequency in ambient-pressure energy reflectance responses measured in ears with middle ear disorders including OME, otosclerosis, ossicular discontinuity, and perforation of the tympanic membrane (see Fig. 8.18).

These examples illustrate the ability to extract useful information from wideband reflectance or absorbance responses that may or may not be reducible to the moments presented in the results of Figure 8.20. The advantage of these pressure and frequency moments is that they provide an objective means of accurately detecting the presence or absence of a conductive hearing loss based on a wideband ATF test.

Research Using Wideband Acoustic Transfer Functions to Measure the Acoustic Stapedius Reflex

Traditional measurement of the ASR involves monitoring the change in middle ear admittance during the presence of a reflex-activating stimulus using a 226-Hz probe tone in the ear canal. However, the ASR evokes a change in middle ear admittance at frequencies as high as 2,000 Hz (Rabinowitz, 1977), and thus, much of the information regarding the presence of an ASR is ignored in the traditional test. Feeney and Keefe (1999) reported on the use of wideband reflectance, admittance, and power absorption to measure the ASR. The probe loudspeaker delivered a wideband signal of 40-ms duration and bandwidth of 0.25 to 10 kHz at an overall level of 65 dB SPL. The average pressure response to eight such signals was used to measure energy reflectance. The data in Figure 8.21 show wideband shifts in energy reflectance induced by the ASR for a young adult subject with normal hearing as a function of a contralateral 2,000-Hz reflex-activating stim-

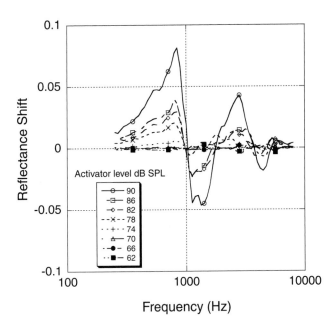

FIGURE 8.21 Wideband shifts in energy reflectance induced by the acoustic stapedius reflex for a young adult subject with normal hearing as a function of the contralateral 2,000-Hz reflex-activating stimulus. The acoustic stapedius reflex threshold was obtained at 74 dB sound pressure level (SPL), which is 12 dB lower than the clinical reflex threshold for this subject.

ulus. The activator level ranged from 4 dB above the ASR threshold (which was 86 dB SPL) obtained with a clinical admittance instrument using a 226-Hz probe tone to 24 dB below the clinical ASR threshold in 4-dB steps.

To obtain an estimate of the ASR threshold from wideband ATF measurements, Feeney and Keefe (2001) developed two statistical tests: a correlation test and a magnitude test. The correlation test examined the cross correlation between reflex-induced shifts in ATFs for higher activator levels compared with lower activator levels across one-twelfth octave data bins for several bandwidths (250 to 1,000 Hz, 250 to 2,000 Hz, 250 to 4,000 Hz, and 250 to 8,000 Hz). Since the wideband shape of the response is similar for lower and higher activator levels (Fig. 8.21), a high positive cross correlation, which exceeded a criterion value, was taken as evidence for the presence of the reflex for responses to both activator levels. The test was conducted for consecutive activator levels in 4-dB steps. The reflex threshold was taken as the lowest activator level for which there was a significant cross correlation with the response to next higher activator level using the 4-dB step size. The second statistical test, the magnitude test, evaluated the magnitude of the shift in the ATF in presence of an activator stimulus compared to the magnitude of shifts due to normal variability. The activator-induced shift in the ATF response had to be larger than some criterion value for a reflex to be judged present. The final estimate of reflex threshold was the lowest activator level for which the correlation test and the magnitude test both agreed that a reflex was present. Further details are described in Feeney and Keefe (2001).

The ASR threshold for the data in Figure 8.21 was obtained by this method at an activator level of 74 dB SPL, which is 12 dB lower than the clinical reflex threshold. This decrease in reflex threshold is similar to that reported by Feeney et al. (2003b) for contralateral ASR thresholds for 1,000- and 2,000-Hz activators in 34 young adults measured with both admittance and energy reflectance wideband ATFs. Thus, one advantage of using wideband ATFs to measure the ASR appears to be an improvement in measurement sensitivity.

This method may be applied to the measurement of the ASR in infants, which varies with probe frequency as a function of development (Weatherby and Bennett, 1980; Bennett and Weatherby, 1982). Because it captures the middle ear response to the ASR across a broad range of frequencies, the wideband ATF method may allow a measurement of the reflex that is independent of changes in the acoustic response of the middle ear across development. This has implications for developing improved clinical normative data for ASR thresholds in infants. Feeney and Sanford (2005) measured contralateral reflex thresholds for a band of noise in a group of 6-week-old infants and adults. The correlation method was used to detect the ASR. The detection of the infant ASR occurred most frequently by examining the correlations across ATF responses from 1,000 to 8,000 Hz, whereas adult ASRs were more likely detected in the frequency band from 250 to 2,000 Hz. More work is needed in this area to examine the development of the ASR threshold in infants.

Wideband ATFs have also been used to measure the ipsilateral ASR by band limiting the ATF measurement to a frequency region different from the activator (Feeney et al., 2004). This resulted in ASR thresholds that were similar to those obtained with a clinical system using a 226-Hz probe tone. The ipsilateral wideband probe stimulus may be more effectively employed by interleaving the probe and activator in time.

▨ LASER DOPPLER VIBROMETRY

Laser Doppler vibrometry (LDV) is a relatively new technique that is also being used to make wideband measurements of middle ear function. LDV is a measurement of the Doppler shift in a laser beam reflected from a moving object, which is used to detect the velocity of the moving object. In the case of middle ear measurements, movement of middle ear structures is obtained in the presence of an acoustic stimulus comprised of a high-level, tonal complex. Recently, measurements have been made at several research centers in normal-hearing subjects and patients with conductive hearing loss. By focusing the laser on or near the umbo, these measurements provide an estimate of sound-induced velocity of the ossicular chain (Goode et al., 1996; Huber et al., 2001, Rosowski et al., 2003; Whittemore et al., 2004). This technique holds promise for studying normal middle ear function and providing diagnostic information about lesions affecting the ossicular chain. LDV measurements in normal-functioning ears appear to contain similar information to acoustic admittance functions estimated at the tympanic membrane (Keefe, 2007). More research is needed to compare these LDV measurements with wideband ATF measurements of middle ear disorders (Feeney et al., 2003a). LDV measurements have particular potential for use in assessing middle ear function during middle ear surgery.

▨ CLINICAL MIDDLE EAR ASSESSMENT: PRESENT AND FUTURE TRENDS

This chapter has laid the groundwork for understanding single-point ATFs of the middle ear. Because of the noninvasive nature of these measurements, they have developed into a standard part of the clinical test battery. However, the most common method of obtaining these measurements, with a 226-Hz probe tone, has been shown to provide reduced test performance compared to newer methods using wideband ATFs. Multifrequency and multicomponent admittance tympanometry provides additional information regarding middle ear resonance frequency, but this approach has often been slow to be accepted clinically perhaps, in part, because of the difficulty in interpreting results and also because of the perceived limited applicability. An example of an application to newborn hearing screening with potential promise is the recent use of 1,000-Hz tympanometry in the middle ear assessment of young infants (Margolis et al., 2003).

Over the last 10 years, there has been significant interest in and development of wideband ATF measures of middle ear function. These techniques, along with LDV tests, offer a new view of middle ear function across the frequency range important for speech perception. The use of wideband reflectance and other ATF responses has shed light on the development of middle ear function (Keefe et al., 1993), which has been difficult to characterize using more traditional measures (Holte et al., 1991). This technology holds promise as a test to rule out middle ear disorders in neonates undergoing newborn hearing screening and for the assessment in infants under 4 months of age (Keefe et al., 2003a). This technology also holds promise for the detection of conductive hearing loss (Keefe and Simmons, 2003) and the diagnosis of middle ear disorders (Feeney et al., 2003a). Finally, the use of wideband ATFs for the measurement of the ASR may result in a more sensitive measurement of the ASR threshold and provide more information on the ASR across a broader frequency range.

REFERENCES

Allen JB. (1985) Measurement of eardrum acoustic impedance. In: Allen JB, Hall J, Hubbard A, Neely S, Tubis A, eds. *Peripheral Auditory Mechanisms.* New York: Springer-Verlag.

American National Standards Institute. (1987) ANSI Specifications for Instruments to Measure Aural Acoustic Impedance and Admittance (Aural Acoustic Immittance). ANSI S3.39-1987. New York: American National Standards Institute.

American Speech-Language-Hearing Association. (1990) Guidelines for screening for hearing impairments and middle-ear disorders. *ASHA.* 32 (suppl 2), 17–24.

American Speech-Language-Hearing Association. (1997) *Guidelines for Audiologic Screening.* Rockville, MD: American Speech-Language-Hearing Association.

Bennett MJ, Weatherby LA. (1982) Newborn acoustic reflexes to noise and pure-tone signals. *J Speech Hear Res.* 25, 383–387.

Day JE, Feeney MP. (in press). The effects of 226-Hz probe level on contralateral acoustic reflex thersholds. *J Speech Lang Hear Res.*

Feeney MP, Grant IL, Marryott LP. (2003a) Wideband energy reflectance measurements in adults with middle-ear disorders. *J Speech Lang Hear Res.* 46, 901–911.

Feeney MP, Keefe DH. (1999) Acoustic reflex detection using wideband acoustic reflectance, admittance and power measurements. *J Speech Lang Hear Res.* 42, 1029–1041.

Feeney MP, Keefe DH. (2001) Estimating the acoustic reflex threshold from wideband measures of reflectance, admittance and power. *Ear Hear.* 22, 316–332.

Feeney MP, Keefe DH, Marryott LP. (2003b) Contralateral acoustic reflex thresholds for tonal activators using wideband reflectance and admittance measurements. *J Speech Lang Hear Res.* 46, 128–136.

Feeney MP, Keefe DH, Sanford CA. (2004) Wideband reflectance measures of the ipsilateral acoustic stapedius reflex threshold. *Ear Hear.* 25, 421–430.

Feeney MP, Sanford CA. (2004) Age effects in the human middle ear: wideband acoustical measures. *J Acoust Soc Am.* 116, 3546–3558.

Feeney MP, Sanford CA. (2005) Detection of the acoustic stapedius reflex in infants using wideband energy reflectance and admittance. *J Am Acad Audiol.* 16, 280–292.

Goode RL, Ball G, Nishihara S, Nakamura K. (1996) Laser Doppler vibrometer (LDV): a new clinical tool for the otologist. *Am J Otol.* 17, 813–822.

Goode RL, Killion M, Nakamura K, Nishihara S. (1994) New knowledge about the function of the human middle ear: development of an improved analog model. *Am J Otol.* 15, 145–154.

Holmquist J, Bergstrom B. (1977) Eustachian tube function and size of the mastoid air cell system in middle ear surgery. *Scand Audiol.* 15, 3–8.

Holte L, Margolis RH, Cavanaugh RM. (1991) Developmental changes in multifrequency tympanograms. *Audiology.* 30, 1–24.

Huber AM, Schwab C, Linder T, Stoeckli SJ, Ferrazzinin M, Dillier N, Fisch U. (2001) Evaluation of eardrum laser Doppler interferometry as a diagnostic tool. *Laryngoscope.* 111, 501–507.

Hudde H. (1983) Measurement of the eardrum impedance of human ears. *J Acoust Soc Am.* 73, 242–247.

Huttenbrink KB. (1988) The mechanics of the middle-ear at static air pressures: the role of the ossicular joints, the function of the middle-ear muscles and the behaviour of stapedial prostheses. *Acta Otolaryngol Suppl.* 451, 1–35.

Keefe DH. (2007) Influence of middle-ear function and pathology on otoacoustic emissions. In: Robinette MS, Glattke TJ, eds. *Otoacoustic Emissions: Clinical Applications.* 3rd ed. New York: Thieme.

Keefe DH, Bulen JC, Arehart KH, Burns EM. (1993) Ear-canal impedance and reflection coefficient in human infants and adults. *J Acoust Soc Am.* 94, 2617–2638.

Keefe DH, Folsom RC, Gorga MP, Vohr BR, Bulen JC, Norton SJ. (2000) Identification of neonatal hearing impairment: ear-canal measurements of acoustic admittance and reflectance in neonates. *Ear Hear.* 21, 443–461.

Keefe DH, Gorga MP, Neely ST, Zhao F, Vohr BR. (2003a) Ear-canal acoustic admittance and reflectance measurements in human neonates. II. Predictions of middle-ear in dysfunction and sensorineural hearing loss. *J Acoust Soc Am.* 113, 407–422.

Keefe DH, Levi E. (1996) Maturation of the middle and external ears: acoustic power-based responses and reflectance tympanometry. *Ear Hear.* 17, 361–373.

Keefe DH, Ling R, Bulen JC. (1992) Method to measure acoustic impedance and reflection coefficient. *J Acoust Soc Am.* 91, 470–485.

Keefe DH, Simmons JL. (2003) Energy transmittance predicts conductive hearing loss in older children and adults. *J Acoust Soc Am.* 114, 3217–3238.

Keefe DH, Zhao F, Neely ST, Gorga MP, Vohr B. (2003b) Ear-canal acoustic admittance and reflectance effects in human neonates. I. Predictions of otoacoustic emission and auditory brainstem responses. *J Acoust Soc Am.* 113, 389–406.

Lilly DJ. (1984) Multiple frequency, multiple component tympanometry: new approaches to an old diagnostic problem. *Ear Hear.* 5, 300–308.

Lilly DJ, Shanks JE. (1981) Acoustic admittance of an enclosed volume of air. In: Popelka CR, ed. *Hearing Assessment with the Acoustic Reflex.* New York: Grune & Stratton; pp 145–160.

Margolis RH, Bass-Ringdahl S, Hanks WD, Holte L, Zapala DA. (2003) Tympanometry in newborn infants—1 kHz norms. *J Am Acad Audiol.* 14, 383–392.

Margolis RH, Goycoolea HG. (1993) Multifrequency tympanometry in normal adults. *Ear Hear.* 14, 408–413.

Margolis RH, Saly GL, Keefe DH. (1999) Wideband reflectance tympanometry in normal adults. *J Acoust Soc Am.* 106, 265–280.

Mehrgardt S, Mellert V. (1977) Transformation characteristics of the external human ear. *J Acoust Soc Am.* 61, 1567–1576.

Metz O. (1946) The acoustic impedance measured in normal and pathological ears. *Acta Otolaryngol.* Suppl 63.

Moller AR. (1960) Improved technique for detailed measurements of the middle ear impedance. *J Acoust Soc Am.* 32, 250–257.

Norton SJ, Gorga MP, Widen JE, Folsom RC, Sininger Y, Cone-Wesson B, Vohr BR, Mascher K, Fletcher KA. (2000) Identification of neonatal hearing impairment: evaluation of transient evoked otoacoustic emission, distortion product otoacoustic emission, and auditory brainstem response test performance. *Ear Hear.* 21, 508–528.

Nozza RJ, Bluestone CD, Kardatzke D, Bachman R. (1994) Identification of middle ear effusion by aural acoustic admittance and otoscopy. *Ear Hear.* 15, 310–323.

Okabe K, Tanaka S, Hamada H, Miura T, Funai H. (1988) Acoustic impedance measurement on normal ears of children. *J Acoust Soc Jpn.* 6, 287–294.

Pang XD, Guinan JJ Jr. (1997) Effects of stapedius-muscle contractions on the masking of auditory-nerve responses. *J Acoust Soc Am.* 102, 3576–3586.

Pang XD, Peake WT. (1985) How do contractions of the stapedius muscle alter the acoustic properties of the ear? In: Allen JB, Hall JL, Hubbard A, Neely ST, Tubis A, eds. *Peripheral Auditory Mechanisms.* New York: Springer-Verlag; pp 36–43.

Piskorski P, Keefe DH, Simmons JL, Gorga MP. (1999) Prediction of conductive hearing loss based on acoustic ear-canal response using a multivariate clinical decision theory. *J Acoust Soc Am.* 105, 1749–1764.

Rabinowitz WM. (1977) Unpublished Doctoral Dissertation. Boston: Massachusetts Institute of Technology.

Rabinowitz WM. (1981) Measurements of the acoustic input immittance of the human ear. *J Acoust Soc Am.* 70, 1025–1035.

Rosowski JJ, Mehta RP, Merchant SN. (2003) Diagnostic utility of laser-Doppler vibrometry in conductive hearing loss with normal tympanic membrane. *Otol Neurotol.* 24, 165–175.

Shallop JK. (1976) The historical development of the study of middle ear function. In: Feldman AS, Wilber LA, eds. *Acoustic Impedance and Admittance: The Measurement of Middle Ear Function.* Baltimore: Williams & Wilkins; pp 8–48.

Shanks JE, Lilly DJ, Margolis RH, Wiley TL, Wilson RH. (1988) Tympanometry. *J Speech Hear Disord.* 53, 354–377.

Shaw EAG. (1974) The external ear. In: Keidel WD, Neff WD, eds. *Handbook of Sensory Physiology.* Volume 5. Berlin: Springer-Verlag; pp 455–490.

Stinson MR, Shaw EAG, Lawton BW. (1982) Estimation of acoustical energy reflectance at the eardrum from measurements of pressure distribution in the human ear canal. *J Acoust Soc Am.* 72, 766–773.

Terkildsen K, Nielsen SS. (1960) An electroacoustic impedance measuring bridge for clinical use. *Arch Otolaryngol.* 72, 339–346.

Terkildsen K, Osterhammel P, Nielsen SS. (1970) Impedance measurements: probe-tone intensity and middle-ear reflexes. *Acta Otolaryngol.* 263, 205–207.

Terkildsen K, Thomsen KA. (1959) The influence of pressure variations on the impedance of the human ear drum. *J Laryngol Otol.* 73, 409–418.

Van Camp KH, Margolis RH, Wilson RH, Creten WL, Shanks JE. (1986) *Principles of Tympanometry.* Rockville, MD: American Speech-Language-Hearing Association.

Vanhuyse VJ, Creten WL, Van Camp KJ. (1975) On the W-notching of tympanograms. *Scand Audiol.* 4, 45–50.

Voss SE, Allen JB. (1994) Measurement of acoustic impedance and reflectance in the human ear canal. *J Acoust Soc Am.* 95, 372–384.

Voss SE, Rosowski JJ, Merchant SN, Peake WT. (2001a) Middle-ear function with tympanic-membrane perforations. I. Measurements and mechanisms. *J Acoust Soc Am.* 110, 1432–1444.

Voss SE, Rosowski JJ, Merchant SN, Peake WT. (2001b) Middle-ear function with tympanic-membrane perforations. II. A simple model. *J Acoust Soc Am.* 110, 1445–1452.

Weatherby LA, Bennett MJ. (1980) The neonatal acoustic reflex. *Scand Audiol.* 9, 103–110.

Whittemore KR, Merchant SN, Poon BB, Rosowski JJ. (2004) A normative study of tympanic membrane motion in humans using a laser Doppler vibrometer (LDV). *Hear Res.* 187, 85–104.

Zwislocki JJ. (1957) Some measurements of the impedance at the eardrum. *J Acoust Soc Am.* 29, 349–356.

Editor's Note

Devices to measure an acoustic reflectance of the ear can be obtained from such companies as Interacoustics and Mimosa Acoustics, Inc.

9

Tympanometry in Clinical Practice

Janet Shanks and Jack Shohet

HISTORY AND DEVELOPMENT OF TYMPANOMETRY

Two "must read" articles on the development of clinical tympanometry are Terkildsen and Thomsen (1959) and Terkildsen and Scott-Nielsen (1960). Their interest in estimating middle-ear pressure and in measuring recruitment with the acoustic reflex had a profound effect on the development of clinical instruments. Each time I read these articles, I am struck first by the incredible amount of information in the articles, and second, by the lack of scientific data to support their conclusions. Most amazing of all, however, is that the principles presented in these two articles have stood up for nearly 50 years, and provide the basis for commercial instruments and tympanometry procedures still in use today.

These articles laid the foundation for the use of hard-walled calibration cavities and the term "equivalent volume of air", compensation of ear-canal volume, and the selection of a single low-frequency probe tone. You should be surprised to read that the probe tone "frequency of 220 cps was chosen partly at random" (Terkildsen and Scott-Nielsen, 1960, p. 341). A low-frequency probe tone was preferred because the current day microphones were nonlinear at high frequencies and the probe tone level could be increased without eliciting an acoustic reflex. In other words, the selection of a 220 Hz probe tone was made without any consideration of its diagnostic value in evaluating middle-ear function. Finally, these articles also set the precedent for measuring only the magnitude of complex acoustic immittance rather than both magnitude and phase angle. Phase angle measurements were abandoned because the middle ear is so stiffness controlled at 220 Hz that phase angle did not vary considerably in either normal or pathological middle ears.

The focus of Terkildsen and Thomsen (1959) was on estimating middle-ear pressure. They adapted an electroacoustic impedance instrument to allow for variation in ear-canal pressure over a range of ±300 mm H_2O and described the first "tympanogram" as a uniform pattern "... with an almost symmetrical rise and fall, attaining a maximum at pressures equaling middle ear pressures" (p. 413). They further noted that, "... the smallest impedance always corresponded exactly to the zone of maximal subjective perception of the test tone" (p. 413). In other words, the probe tone was the most audible and the tympanogram peaked when the pressure was equal on both sides of the eardrum.

In addition, these authors recognized that although the measure of interest was the acoustic immittance in the plane of the eardrum, for obvious reasons, the measurements had to be made in the ear canal. They introduced the clinical procedure used to compensate for the volume of air enclosed between the probe tip and the eardrum. "Under conditions where the ear drum is under considerable tension, the impedance volume measured is dominated by the volume of the ear canal space itself. With decreasing tension of the ear drum the influence of the middle ear space gradually increases, attaining a maximum under conditions where the pressures in both spaces are identical". "... the difference between highest and lowest impedance volumes as obtained by variations of the pressure, is thought to some extent to indicate the vibrating characteristics of the individual ear drum" (p. 414). The difference between the highest and lowest impedances, therefore, was attributed to the middle-ear system, absent the effects of the ear canal. Here, they laid the basis for estimating ear-canal volume and calculating peak compensated static acoustic admittance.

Instead of reporting tympanograms in acoustic ohms, Terkildsen and Thomsen (1959) reported them in terms of an equivalent volume of air with units in milliliters (ml) or cubic centimeters (cc or cm^3). This precedent was followed because at low frequencies such as 220 Hz, the ear functions

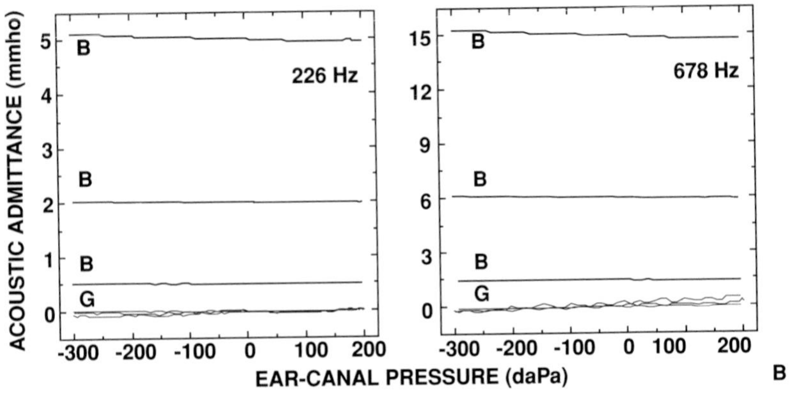

FIGURE 9.1 Uncompensated acoustic susceptance (B) and conductance (G) tympanograms recorded at 226 Hz (A) and 678 Hz (B) in calibration cavities with volumes of 0.5, 2.0, and 5.0 cm³.

like a hard-walled cavity of air. Although the use of equivalent volumes is acceptable at low frequencies, its use is not appropriate at high frequencies where the middle ear is no longer stiffness dominated. Instead of simplifying measurements, the term equivalent volume of air continues to be a source of confusion.

Based largely on these early studies, the electroacoustic immittance systems developed in the early 1960's measured only the magnitude of acoustic impedance for a single, low-frequency probe tone of 220 Hz. The first generation of instruments, like the popular Madsen ZO70, did not incorporate an automatic gain control (AGC) circuit to maintain the sound pressure level of the probe tone at a constant level. As a result, the amplitude of the tympanogram, reported in arbitrary units from 1 to 10, was partially dependent on ear-canal volume. The sound pressure level of the probe tone and the height of the tympanogram were higher in small ear canals than in large ear canals *even when the acoustic immittances of both middle ears were identical* (see Shanks, 1984: Figure 4). Not surprisingly, quantifying the height of tympanograms in arbitrary units was not useful clinically.

To circumvent this problem, the next generation of instruments incorporated AGC circuits to maintain a constant probe tone level in ear canals of all sizes. Measurements no longer were reported in arbitrary units but rather in absolute physical units, the acoustic mmho. In 1970, Grason Stadler introduced a new instrument (Model 1720) with two probe-tone frequencies, 220 and 660 Hz, and two admittance components, acoustic susceptance (B_a) and conductance (G_a). Feldman (1976b) used this instrument to collect 220 and 660 Hz tympanograms from ears with a variety of middle-ear pathologies, and clearly demonstrated the advantage of a high-frequency probe tone in evaluating mass related pathologies of the middle ear. Despite findings such as these, high-frequency tympanometry has never become routine.

The latest generation of computer-based instruments (e.g., Virtual, Model 310; Grason Stadler TympStar, Version 2[1]; Madsen OTOflex 100) continued to offer multiple frequency probe tones (e.g., 226, 678, and/or 1000 Hz) and

multiple admittance components [e.g., acoustic admittance magnitude (Y_a), phase angle (φ), B_a, and G_a]. These instruments are extremely versatile and have the added convenience of being able to store commonly used tympanometry protocols and several records of patient data. By the end of this chapter, you will hopefully recognize several applications for the under utilized high frequency options on these instruments.

CALIBRATION

ANSI S3.39 requires that three calibration cavities (0.5, 2.0, and 5.0 cm³) be provided with each instrument. Measuring the acoustic admittance of these calibration cavities provides a convenient introduction to tympanometry estimates of ear-canal volume, compensated for ear-canal volume versus uncompensated tympanograms, and flat tympanograms. Figure 9.1 shows acoustic susceptance (B) and conductance (G) tympanograms in the three calibration cavities for 226 Hz (Panel A) and 678 Hz (Panel B) probe tones. For the smallest cavity at 226 Hz, the B and G tympanograms are straight lines at 0.5 and 0 acoustic mmho, respectively. Similarly, for the 2.0 and 5.0 cm³ cavities, G at 226 Hz remains at 0 acoustic mmho and B is equal to the volume of the cavities. Because G=0 in these calibration cavities, admittance magnitude (Y) also would be identical to B (see Eq. 8.5) and equal to the volumes of the calibration cavities. At 678 Hz, the results are the same except B is increased by a factor of 3 to 1.5, 6.0, and 15.0 acoustic mmho while G remains at 0 acoustic mmho in all three cavities. You should further notice that the B tympanograms slope slightly upward as pressure decreases. This is expected because the acoustic susceptance (B_a) of an enclosed volume of air increases slightly as the density of air decreases (Beranek, 1954; Lilly and Shanks, 1981).

Hard-walled cavities are used for calibration because they can be constructed as an ideal acoustic element. That is, at sea level, an enclosed cavity of air with certain constraints placed on the radius and length of the cavity can be modeled as pure acoustic compliance (or inversely, stiffness) with negligible mass and resistance up to approximately 1000 Hz (Beranek, 1954; Lilly and Shanks, 1981; Margolis and Smith, 1977; Moller, 1960, 1972; Rabinowitz, 1981; Shanks and Lilly, 1981; Shaw, 1974). The low-frequency probe tone was

---

[1] Grason Stadler, a division of VIASYS Healthcare, Inc. supported this endeavor by providing test equipment for research by the second author.

increased from 220 to 226 Hz in the 1987 standard because under standard atmospheric conditions, the acoustic admittance of a 1 cm^3 cavity is equal to 1 acoustic mmho at 226 Hz (see Lilly and Shanks [1981] for further discussion). This "happy coincidence" discussed in Chapter 8 simplifies calibration.

The dimensions of calibration cavities are more constraining for high-frequency probe tones. The Grason Stadler TympStar, for example, uses all three cavities to calibrate at 226 Hz, uses the 0.5 and the 2.0 cm^3 cavities to calibrate at 678 Hz, and uses only the 0.5 cm^3 cavity to calibrate at 1000 Hz. A fourth, high-resistance cavity is provided for high-frequency calibration. Although this is an unsealed cavity that cannot hold pressure, measurements in this cavity also are instructive. With the probe inserted in this cavity and the starting pressure set to 0 daPa, high conductance (G_a) with minimal susceptance (B_a) is recorded briefly before the procedure is aborted due to an inadequate seal. This is the opposite B_a to G_a relationship recorded in the three sealed cavities.

The exercise depicted in Figure 9.1 should help to clarify the term acoustic immittance of an equivalent volume of air (in ml or cm^3) that is shown on the y-axis of some low-frequency tympanograms. This convention developed because measurements made with early instruments showed that at 220 Hz, the admittance of the middle ear was primarily determined by its stiffness with comparatively low mass and resistance. In other words, the ear practically functioned like a hard-walled cavity, and therefore, the measurements were reported relative to the immittance of an enclosed volume of air. If both panels in Figure 9.1 were replotted in equivalent volumes, the B_a (and Y_a) tympanograms at both 226 and 678 Hz would completely overlap rather than being three times larger at 678 Hz.

As mentioned briefly, the density of air has an effect on the acoustic admittance of a volume of air. Density changes only slightly with changes in ear-canal pressure during tympanometry, but changes significantly with elevation. The tympanograms in Figure 9.1 were recorded at sea level, but these values would not be recorded at higher elevations. For example, at 5000 feet, B_a in the 0.5 cm^3 cavity should read 0.61 acoustic mmho at 226 Hz and 1.83 acoustic mmho at 678 Hz (see Lilly and Shanks, 1981 for correction factors).

Although equipment calibration in most Audiology clinics is contracted, calibration should be checked periodically by recording tympanograms on the calibration cavities. Calibration, particularly at high frequencies, is sensitive to debris in the probe device. The probe should be cleaned regularly according to the procedure specified by the manufacturer and should be visually inspected before recording each tympanogram.

CONSTRAINTS OF TYMPANOMETRY

Prior to analyzing tympanograms, Zwislocki's (1976) simple block diagram of the middle ear depicting sound transmission from the ear canal to the cochlea reminds us of two important constraints. First, acoustic immittance measures the acoustic energy that flows *into* the middle ear, and not what flows *through* the middle ear to the cochlea. Some acoustic energy is lost or absorbed in the decoupled portion of the eardrum and in the ossicular joints, and is not passed on to the cochlea. Tympanometry, therefore, should not be used to make assumptions regarding hearing sensitivity. An ear with atrophic scarring of the eardrum is a prime example of a case where tympanometry can be grossly abnormal with minimal effect on hearing.

Second, when the immittance probe is sealed into the ear canal, measurements are made into a virtual "black box". The measured input admittance cannot be used to determine which specific middle-ear structure/s in the ear contributed to a change in stiffness or a change in mass. The measurements simply reflect the total contribution from all of the individual elements. Just as a sum of 10 can be derived from adding 2+3+5 or from adding 1+9+0, the same input admittance can be derived from different pathologies. In other words, do not expect a 1:1 correspondence between a specific middle-ear abnormality and a specific tympanogram pattern. In reality, the same pathology can produce several different tympanogram patterns, and conversely, the same tympanogram pattern can arise from different middle-ear pathologies. Middle-ear disease changes along a continuum and not in identical discrete steps for every individual. In the case of otitis media, for example, the middle-ear mucosa can become inflamed and negative middle-ear pressure can develop with or without middle-ear fluid, or the middle-ear cavity can contain a small amount of thin serous fluid or can be completely filled with thick fluid. In all cases, the ear might be classified as having otitis media, but the tympanogram pattern will not be identical in all phases of the disease process. Similarly, a tympanogram can be flat when the eardrum is immobilized by fluid or by a fixed malleus. Expectations from tympanometry must be realistic and must be analyzed in conjunction with all available information including case history, otoscopy, and the magnitude and configuration of the hearing loss.

NORMAL 226 HZ ADMITTANCE TYMPANOGRAMS

This section discusses the most commonly used tympanometry procedure that has remained virtually unchanged since 1970. Figure 9.2 demonstrates two methods, one qualitative and one quantitative, for analyzing Y_a tympanograms at 226 Hz.

Qualitative Analysis

The qualitative typing procedure popularized by Jerger is shown in Figure 9.2A (Jerger, 1970; Liden, 1969; Liden et al., 1970, 1974). Notice that no measurement units are shown on the y-axis. Recall that the most commonly used instrument at

FIGURE 9.2 Two methods for analyzing 226 Hz Y_a tympanograms, a qualitative analysis (A) of tympanogram shape in arbitrary units (arb) designated as Type A, B, or C after Jerger (1970) and a quantitative analysis (B) of equivalent ear canal volume (V_{ea} in cm³), peak static acoustic admittance (peak Y_{tm} in mmho), tympanogram peak pressure (TPP in daPa), and tympanogram width (TW in daPa).

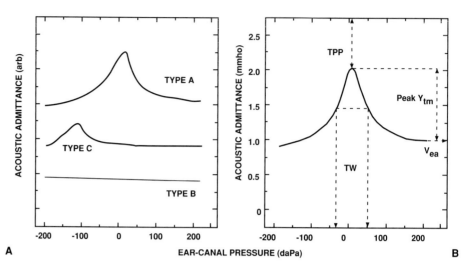

the time, the Madsen ZO70, expressed tympanogram amplitude in arbitrary units (arb); the height of the tympanogram was partly dependent on the volume of the ear canal rather than solely on conditions encountered in the plane of the eardrum. Tympanogram amplitude, therefore, could not be quantified meaningfully, and instead tympanogram shape was categorized into one of three patterns based on simple visual inspection.

A normal tympanogram with a peak near 0 daPa was designated Type A. Subcategories of the Type A were Type A_S for a "shallow" peak (i.e., low admittance) and Type A_D for a "deep" peak (i.e., high admittance) (Jerger et al., 1972). Type A_S tympanograms were associated with otosclerosis and Type A_D tympanograms were associated with ossicular discontinuity or atrophic scarring of the eardrum. The Type C tympanogram was characterized by negative peak pressure, and the Type B tympanogram was flat. Flat tympanograms were recorded from ears with middle-ear effusion (MEE) and eardrum perforation. No amplitude norms were presented to differentiate among Type A, A_S, and A_D tympanograms recorded in arbitrary units, and no pressure norms were presented to differentiate between Type A and C tympanograms. Feldman (1976a) criticized this coding strategy because it implied that everyone was conversant with the typing procedure. To communicate the pertinent information without confusion, he recommended a descriptive analysis of tympanometry peak pressure (e.g., normal, absent, −100 daPa), amplitude (e.g., normal, flaccid, stiff), and shape (e.g., normal, peaked, flat, notched). The typing convention popularized by Jerger, however, is deeply engrained after 35+ years of use and is unlikely to change.

Quantitative Analysis

When AGC circuits were introduced to keep the level of the probe tone in the ear canal constant, tympanograms could be measured in absolute units and quantified. Figure 9.2B shows that tympanogram shape can be precisely described by four numbers.

EAR-CANAL VOLUME

The goal in tympanometry is to measure the acoustic immittance of the middle ear. The probe device, however, cannot be placed at the eardrum but instead must be sealed in the ear canal. The admittance measured at the probe tip (Y_a), then, is the sum of the admittance of the ear-canal volume (Y_{ec}) plus the admittance in the plane of the tympanic membrane (Y_{tm}). If Y_{ec} can be measured independently of the middle ear, then Y_{tm} can be calculated.

Recall from the previous discussion that Terkildsen and Thomsen (1959) proposed that an ear-canal pressure of 200 daPa places the eardrum and middle ear under "considerable tension", and theoretically, all of the energy of the probe tone is reflected at the surface of the eardrum. In other words, Y_{tm} at 200 daPa is 0 acoustic mmho, and the admittance measured at the probe tip is attributed solely to the ear canal, i.e., $Y_a = Y_{ec}$. In Figure 9.2B, Y_a at 200 daPa is 1.0 acoustic mmho for an ear-canal volume (V_{ea}) of 1.0 cm³. As the volume of the ear canal changes, the Y_a tympanogram simply shifts higher or lower on the y-axis without altering the shape of the tympanogram. This is the primary advantage of measuring acoustic-admittance components rather than acoustic-impedance tympanograms. Acoustic-impedance tympanograms not only shift along the y-axis, but also change shape when ear-canal volume changes (Shanks and Lilly, 1981). In other words, the ear canal has a linear effect on admittance tympanograms but a nonlinear effect on impedance tympanograms. The interested reader is referred to Lilly (1972a), Margolis (1981), and Van Camp et al. (1986) for a discussion of series versus parallel acoustic admittances and impedances that accounts for this difference.

Several observations reveal that tympanometry overestimates ear-canal volume by as much as 24% to 39% (Margolis and Smith, 1977; Moller, 1965; Rabinowitz, 1981; Shanks and Lilly, 1981; Vanpeperstraete et al., 1979). Listen to the level of the probe tone as you record a tympanogram from your own ear. Although the probe tone is noticeably softer at both extreme positive and negative pressures, the tone is always audible. If an ear canal pressure of 200 daPa were enough to decrease Y_{tm} to 0 acoustic mmho, the probe tone would not be audible and Y_a at 200 daPa would be the lowest point on the tympanogram. V_{ea} calculated from the negative tail of a 226 Hz tympanogram, however, is up to 0.2 cm^3 lower than the positive tail. The asymmetry has been attributed to eardrum movement, distension of the cartilaginous portion of the ear canal, movement of the probe tip, and residual middle-ear effects (Elner et al., 1971; Margolis and Popelka, 1975; Van Camp et al., 1986; Vanpeperstraete, et al., 1979).

Although 200 daPa does not produce the most accurate estimate of V_{ea}, it is historically the most commonly used pressure. Even more important than selecting the most precise procedure is utilizing a consistent procedure so that estimates of V_{ea} can be compared across clinics and patients. With the advent of computer-based instruments, estimating V_{ea} at 200 daPa has become more practical. The software automatically estimates V_{ea} at the selected starting pressure. Descending pressure changes ($+/-$) are preferred because they result in fewer seal problems in neonates (Holte et al., 1991; Sprague et al., 1985) and produce more consistent tym-

panogram morphology, particularly when high-frequency probe signals are used (Margolis et al., 1985; Wilson et al., 1984). If a descending pressure sweep is desired, then V_{ea} automatically will be estimated at a positive starting pressure.

The most important application of V_{ea} is to differentiate between intact and perforated eardrums or between blocked and functioning tympanostomy tubes (TT). Table 9.1 shows normal mean and 90% ranges for the measures depicted in Figure 9.2B. Unless otherwise indicated, the following recording procedures were used: V_{ea} estimated at 200 daPa from Y226 Hz tympanograms, $+/-$ pressure direction, and a pump speed of 200 daPa/s near the peak. V_{ea} changes both with gender and age. V_{ea} is smaller in females than in males at all ages and averages a difference of 0.2 cm^3 in adulthood (Haapaniemi, 1996; Margolis and Heller, 1987; Roup et al., 1998; Shahnaz and Davies, 2006; Shanks et al., 1992; Wan and Wong, 2002; Wiley et al., 1996). In view of the large range of normal variability, separate norms are not needed for males and females. Different norms, however, are required for children and adults. Table 9.1 shows that V_{ea} increases from an average of 0.6 cm^3 for children less than

TABLE 9.1   226 Hz tympanometry norms from several large scale studies[a]

Study	No. of (years)	Sex	Age (years)	V_{ea} (cm^3) Mean	V_{ea} (cm^3) 90% Range	Y_{tm} (mmho) Mean	Y_{tm} (mmho) 90% Range	TW (daPa) Mean	TW (daPa) 90% Range
Shanks et al., 1992	668	B	0.15–6.7	0.58	0.3–0.9				
Roush et al. 1995	1827	B	.5–2.5			0.45	0.2–0.7	148	102–204
Margolis & Heller 1987	47	M	2.8–5.8	0.8		0.49		105	
	42	F	2.8–5.8	0.7		0.52		95	
	92	B	2.8–5.8	0.75	0.42–0.97	0.5	0.22–0.81	100	59–151
Koebsell & Margolis 1986[b]	88	B	3.7–5.8					133	80–200
Nozza 1992[c], 1994[d,e]	130	B	3–16	0.9	0.6–1.35	0.78	0.40–1.39	104	60–168
Haapaniemi 1996	942	B	6–15	0.8	0.5–1.2	0.5	0.3–1.1		
Hanks & Rose 1993	316	B	6–15	1	0.6–1.5	0.7	0.3–1.5		
Shanks 1985	63	M	Adult	1.59	0.75–2.0				
Margolis & Heller 1987[e]	49	M	19–61	1.14		0.77		79	
	38	F	19–61	0.93		0.65		74	
	87	B	19–61	1.05	0.63–1.46	0.72	0.27–1.38	77	51–114
Wiley et al. 1996	825	M	48–90	1.49	1.0–2.2	0.72	0.2–1.6	73	35–125
	1322	F	48–90	1.28	0.9–1.9	0.62	0.2–1.4	76	40–120
	2147	B	48–90	1.36	0.9–2.0	0.66	0.2–1.5	75	35–125
Holte 1996	136	B	20–90			0.84	0.3–1.8	84	38–141

V_{ea}, ear canal volume; Y_{tm}, admittance in the plane of the tympanic membrane; TW, tympanogram width; B, both male and female; M, male; F, female.
[a] Unless indicated, V_{ea} was estimated at 200 daPa from tympanograms recorded using descending pressure changes at a rate of 200 daPa/s.
[b] minV_{ea}
[c] 300V_{ea}
[d] 400V_{ea}
[e] Handheld probe

7 years (Shanks et al., 1992) to 0.8 cm^3 between 6 and 15 years (Haapaniemi, 1996) to 1.4 cm^3 in adulthood (Wiley et al., 1996).

When the eardrum is perforated, V_{ea} is comprised of the ear canal plus the middle-ear space, antrum, and the mastoid air cell system. Middle-ear volume estimates in patients undergoing stapes mobilization (Zwislocki, 1962) and in cadaver temporal bones (Molvaer et al., 1978) averaged 6.5 to 8.7 cm^3. These large volumes are due predominantly to the mastoid air cell system, which is minimal in newborns and grows rapidly in 2 to 7 year olds (Bentler, 1989; Dolan, 1979; Eby and Nadol, 1986). The normal mastoid is not fully aerated in girls until 10 to 15 years and in boys until 11 to 19 years (Ars, 1989; Diamant, 1965; Dolan, 1979; Eby and Nadol, 1986; O'Donoghue et al., 1986; O'Tuama and Swanson, 1986; Rubensohn, 1965). The relevance of the size of the mastoid air cell system and Eustachian-tube function has been the subject of endless research. Debate continues on whether a small mastoid air cell system is the cause or the result of chronic middle-ear disease. Evidence from animal studies does suggest that chronic middle-ear disease inhibits pneumatization, particularly when it occurs at a very young age (Ikarashi and Nakano, 1988). Andreasson (1977) also showed that longstanding chronic otitis media (COM) with recurrent drainage reduced the volume by shutting off the mastoid air cell system. This is supported by a comparison of volume estimates from ears with perforated eardrums due to COM versus trauma. Lindeman and Holmquist (1982) and Andreasson (1977) reported volumes of 9.7 versus 3.3 cm^3 for perforated eardrums due to trauma versus COM, respectively.

Although several investigators have reported normal ranges for V_{ea}, few have reported V_{ea} in ears with known perforations or patent tympanostomy tubes (TT). Shanks et al. (1992) compared V_{ea} before and after placement of TT in 668 ears of children between 6 weeks and 6.7 years. Average V_{ea} increased from 0.6 cm^3 preoperatively to 2.3 cm^3 6 to 7 weeks after placement of the TT. In addition, post-operative V_{ea} was significantly larger in males than in females and increased as a function of age for both males and females, reflecting continued development of the mastoid air cell system in children under seven years old. The range in post-operative V_{ea} was large and often exceeded the 7 cm^3 recording limits of the equipment. Comparing V_{ea} in the two ears, particularly in cases where V_{ea} falls at the upper end of the normal range, also can be helpful in identifying eardrum perforation. For children under 7 years of age, Shanks et al. (1992) suggested criteria of $V_{ea} > 1.0$ cm^3 or a pre/post difference ≥ 0.4 cm^3. Wilber and Feldman (1976) suggested V_{ea} exceeding 1.5 to 2.0 cm^3 in children or a difference between ears > 0.5 cm^3 is consistent with eardrum perforation. In adult males, $V_{ea} > 2.5$ cm^3 is consistent with a perforated eardrum (Shanks, 1985).

V_{ea} is an under-utilized measure. Although several applications have been suggested, many clinicians do not even obtain tympanograms in ears with eardrum perforation or

TT. Studies that have monitored V_{ea} following placement of TT have found a gradual increase in volume coincident with resolution of fluid and mucosal edema in the middle ear and with growth of the mastoid air cell system in young children (Sederberg-Olsen et al., 1983; Tashima et al., 1986). Other investigators have noted that recurrence of secretory otitis media following extrusion of TT and failed tympanoplasty are more likely to occur in ears with small mastoid air cell systems (Andreasson and Harris, 1979; Diamant, 1965; Holmquist, 1970; Holmquist and Bergstrom, 1977; Jackler and Schindler, 1984; Sederberg-Olsen et al., 1983). An inverse relationship between the size of the mastoid air cell system and risk of otitis media in adults or risk of barotrauma in scuba divers also has been reported (Holmquist, 1970; Sade and Fuchs, 1996; Uzun et al., 2002).

Shanks (1985) cautioned that although $V_{ea} > 2.5$ cm^3 clearly is indicative of a perforated eardrum in adults, a volume < 2.5 cm^3 does not necessarily rule out a perforated eardrum. V_{ea} was measured in 24 adult males scheduled for tympanoplasty to repair a perforated eardrum. Half of the patients had normal middle ears and half had cholesteatoma, granulation tissue, or contracted, sclerotic mastoid air cells. Only 1 of 12 patients with surgically confirmed normal middle ears had a $V_{ea} < 2.5$ cm^3, whereas 6 of the 12 patients in the abnormal group had $V_{ea} < 2.5$ cm^3. A small V_{ea} with a known eardrum perforation indicates the need for more frequent post-surgical follow up.

TYMPANOGRAM PEAK PRESSURE

As the ear-canal pressure is decreased from 200 daPa, more and more of the acoustic energy of the probe tone flows into the middle ear. Energy flow into the middle ear (and the loudness of the probe tone) reaches a maximum when the pressures on both sides of the eardrum are equal. The pressure that coincides with peak admittance, then, provides an estimate of middle-ear pressure. In the normal ear, atmospheric or ambient pressure (0 daPa) is maintained within the middle-ear space by the periodic opening of the Eustachian tube during swallowing. The tympanogram in Figure 9.2B has a normal tympanogram peak pressure (TPP) of 5 daPa and falls well within the normal range of ± 50 daPa. In contrast, when the Eustachian tube does not open properly, negative pressure builds up within the middle-ear space and MEE sometimes develops. In addition to this popular ex vacuo theory proposed by Politzer in the 19th century, several other mechanisms have been identified that contribute to pressure fluctuations in the middle ear. See Sade and Amos (1997) and Margolis and Hunter (1999) for a review of these mechanisms.

TPP can overestimate middle-ear pressure by 30 to 70 daPa, particularly in ears with small middle-ear volumes or highly compliant eardrums (Eliachar and Northern, 1974; Flisberg et al., 1963; Renvall and Holmquist, 1976). Middle-ear pressure also is slightly overestimated due to hysteresis or lag effects related both to the pressure transducer and to the viscoelastic properties of the eardrum and middle ear (Decraemer et al., 1984; Van Camp et al., 1986). Both effects are on the order of 10 to 30 daPa and are in the direction of the pressure change. That is, TPP is shifted more positive for ascending (−/+) pressure changes and more negative for descending (+/−) pressure changes. Some of the new computer-based instruments employ an "x-axis offset" on the order of 25 daPa to correct for instrument hysteresis at fast pump speeds.

Aside from small inaccuracies in equating TPP with middle-ear pressure, extreme deviations in TPP from 0 daPa do reflect true changes in middle-ear pressure. The clinical relevance of negative middle-ear pressure, however, has changed over the years. The 1979 ASHA guideline for acoustic-immittance screening recommended medical referral for TPP in excess of −200 daPa. Many of the children referred for medical treatment, however, had no evidence of middle-ear pathology (Lous, 1982; Roush and Tait, 1985). Middle-ear pressure has been found to fluctuate greatly in children and is no longer considered to be an indication of significant disease (Fiellau-Nikolajsen, 1983; Haughton, 1977; Lildholdt, 1980; Margolis and Heller, 1987; Nozza et al., 1994; Paradise et al., 1976). In the absence of abnormal findings from other tympanometry measures, otoscopy, hearing test, or case history, medical referral on the basis of TPP alone has led to a high over-referral rate and is no longer recommended. Children with high negative pressure, however, are more likely than those with normal TPP to develop MEE and should be monitored closely (Antonio et al., 2002).

Positive TPP greater than 50 daPa is recorded in approximately 1.7% of patients with middle-ear complaints and has been associated with acute otitis media (Ostergard and Carter, 1981). Marked positive TPP also is recorded in ears with pinhole perforations of the eardrum (Fowler and Shanks, 2002; Kessler et al., 1998; Kobayashi and Okitsu, 1986; Kobayashi et al., 1987). To differentiate between the two conditions, tympanograms with positive TPP should be recorded with descending pressure changes and then again with ascending changes. In an ear with a pinhole perforation, TPP from the two pressure sweeps can differ by several hundred daPa in comparison with an expected difference of less than 30 daPa in a normal ear.

PEAK COMPENSATED STATIC ACOUSTIC ADMITTANCE

The next calculation shown in Figure 9.2B is peak compensated static acoustic admittance (peak Y_{tm}). Peak Y_{tm} is the difference in admittance between the peak and 200 daPa. "Compensated" implies that the effects of the ear-canal volume have been removed from the measurement. Most new instruments have the option of recording tympanograms already corrected for ear-canal volume. To do so, the baseline function is turned on, and the tympanogram is zeroed at the selected starting pressure. If the tympanogram in Figure 9.2B had been recorded with the baseline on, the tympanogram would have been shifted down to 0 acoustic mmho at 200

daPa, and the peak Y_{tm} of 1 acoustic mmho could have been read directly from the y-axis.

Mean and 90% ranges for Y_{tm} are shown in Table 9.1. It has become commonplace to report 90% ranges rather than standard deviations or confidence intervals because peak Y_{tm} values are positively skewed (Shahnaz and Polka, 1997; Wilson et al., 1981; Zwislocki and Feldman, 1970). The values can be normalized by performing a logarithmic transformation or by simply reporting the 90% range. Peak Y_{tm} below the 5th percentile indicates an abnormally stiff middle ear. In children under seven years of age, the most common cause is MEE. Examples of low admittance in adults include MEE, otosclerosis, a thickened eardrum, and malleus fixation. High peak Y_{tm} is recorded from ears with eardrum pathology (e.g., atrophic scarring or tympanosclerotic plaques), ossicular replacement prostheses, or ossicular discontinuity. Abnormally high peak Y_{tm} is an indication for medical referral only in the presence of a significant conductive/mixed hearing loss.

The clinical value of peak Y_{tm} has been controversial since tympanometry became routine. The primary criticisms are high normal variability and significant overlap with pathological middle ears. Using consistent recording parameters can help to reduce normal variability. For example, Y_{tm} is greatly affected by the ear-canal pressure used to estimate V_{ea}; peak Y_{tm} is lower when V_{ea} is estimated at 200 daPa than at −400 daPa. Because this is such an important variable, using the ANSI (1987) convention of specifying the ear-canal pressure used to calculate Y_{tm} is recommended, e.g., 200 Y_{tm} versus −400 Y_{tm}. The rate and direction of pressure change, and the number of consecutive pressure sweeps, also affect peak Y_{tm}. In general, Y_{tm} will increase slightly for ascending versus descending pressure sweeps, as the rate of pressure change increases, and as the number of consecutive tympanogram sweeps increases. These procedural variables have a greater effect on high frequency tympanometry and are discussed in more detail later.

TYMPANOGRAM WIDTH

Brooks (1968) was the first to suggest a measure that describes the sharpness of the tympanogram peak. This calculation was popularized when it was observed that tympanograms frequently were broadly rounded in ears with MEE (Brooks, 1969; Fiellau-Nikolajsen, 1983; Haughton, 1977; Paradise et al., 1976). Three measures of the steepness of the tympanogram peak have been suggested over the years (Brooks, 1969; de Jonge, 1986; Paradise et al., 1976). The calculation of tympanogram width (TW) proposed by de Jonge is easy to calculate and is the most widely used. TW demonstrated in Figure 9.2B is the pressure interval (in daPa) encompassing one half peak Y_{tm}. Koebsell and Margolis (1986) confirmed de Jonge's findings. They compared eight different measures of tympanogram slope in 3 to 6 year olds. TW was the preferred measure because it had a narrow normal distribution that was independent of pump speed and a low correlation with peak Y_{tm} that provided complementary rather than redundant information about the middle-ear transmission system. Of the four calculations depicted in Figure 9.2B, TW has been the single most valuable measure in identifying ears with MEE (Fiellau-Nikolajsen, 1983; Haughton, 1977; Nozza et al., 1994).

Effects of Gender, Age, and Race

Some investigators have reported slightly lower peak Y_{tm} and broader TW in females versus males (Jerger et al., 1972; Roup et al., 1998; Wiley et al., 1996; Zwislocki and Feldman, 1970), whereas others have found no gender effect (Holte, 1996; Margolis and Goycoolea, 1993; Margolis and Heller, 1987; Wan and Wong, 2002). Even if present, gender effects are clinically insignificant and do not warrant the added inconvenience of separate norms for males and females.

The effect of race on acoustic admittance measures recently has been investigated. Two studies comparing Caucasian and Chinese adults concluded that a decrease in peak Y_{tm} and an increase in TW in Chinese adults could be attributed to a smaller body size (Shahnaz and Davies, 2006; Wan and Wong, 2002). Different norms, therefore, may be required for Chinese children enrolled in screening programs. Wan and Wong (2002) pointed out that 48% of Chinese children failed tympanometry screening when norms developed on Caucasians were used.

Countless studies also have focused on the effect of age on peak Y_{tm} and TW (Blood and Greenberg, 1977; Holte, 1996; Jerger et al., 1972; Margolis and Heller, 1987; Wiley et al., 1996). Although some small age differences have been reported for adults, any clinically significant differences appear to be masked by the large range of normal variability. Convincing age effects in infants and small children, however, have resulted in separate norms for infants (ASHA, 1997). The ASHA recommendation is based on the data of Roush et al. (1995) who measured broader TW and lower peak Y_{tm} in children less than 1 year of age. They attributed the difference to residual effects of otitis media so prevalent in that age group. DeChicchis et al. (2000) similarly reported a systematic increase in peak Y_{tm} and decrease in TW with increasing age from 6 months to 5 years of age, with the biggest changes occurring during the first 3 years. These authors attributed the differences to anatomic and physiologic changes in the developing ear.

Screening For Middle Ear Effusion

Despite the high prevalence of MEE in children, particularly during the winter months, most cases of MEE are transient and do not necessitate medical intervention (Antonio et al., 2002; Bluestone, 2004; Fiellau-Nikolajsen, 1983; Tos and Poulsen, 1980). For example, Bluestone (2004) reported that 80% of ears with MEE resolved within two months without any medical treatment. A small number of cases, however, do become chronic and require medical management.

Differentiating between these two populations is the challenge facing programs that screen for middle-ear disease and is one reason why the ASHA guideline has undergone three revisions.

The goal of the initial ASHA (1979) screening guideline was to identify children with MEE. Immediate medical referral was recommended for children with flat tympanograms or TPP <-200 daPa with an absent 1000 Hz acoustic reflex (AR). By the time many of these children received medical follow up, the MEE had resolved, and the screening protocol was criticized for unacceptably high over-referral rates (Lous, 1982; Roush and Tait, 1985).

A major goal of the revised ASHA (1990) guideline was to decrease the high over-referral rate by eliminating medical referral for transient, self-resolving, secretory otitis media. Both TPP and the AR were dropped from the revised guideline. As previously discussed, TPP fluctuates widely and is a poor determinant of MEE, and the AR can be absent for reasons other than middle-ear disease (e.g., sensorineural hearing loss, a poor seal, or excessive baseline noise). These two admittance measures were replaced with the following three quantitative measures: $200Y_{tm}$, V_{ea}, and TW. A second major change to the screening protocol was the addition of the following three components: history of otalgia (ear pain) or otorrhea (ear discharge); visual inspection for structural defects; and screening audiometry. Rescreening in 4–6 weeks was recommended when any of the tympanometry measures was abnormal in an attempt to exclude self-resolving cases of MEE. Immediate medical referral without conducting tympanometry was recommended only for previously undetected/untreated structural defects, perforated eardrum, otalgia, or otorrhea.

One problem encountered at the time of the revision was that large scale, quantitative tympanometry studies had been conducted on children with normal middle ears but not with confirmed middle-ear disease. Publication of the ASHA (1990) screening guideline was the catalyst for a series of studies on the sensitivity and specificity of various tympanometry measures in identifying children with confirmed MEE (Nozza et al., 1992, 1994; Roush et al., 1992; Roush et al., 1995; Silman et al., 1992; Silverman and Silman, 1995).

Perhaps the most important finding of the Nozza et al. (1992, 1994) studies that compared tympanometry with myringotomy results was that there are not two but three distinct populations encountered when screening for middle-ear disease: normal middle ears from the general population, ears with MEE, and ears without MEE but with a history of chronic or recurrent otitis media. The pass-fail criteria are different for each population. When the interim norms from the general population were applied to ears with a history of chronic or recurrent MEE, the false-positive rate increased from 5% to 75% (Nozza et al., 1994). In comparison with the general population, children with a history of recurrent otitis media with effusion have lower Y_{tm} and wider TW even when the middle ears were effusion free. TW >275 daPa was the single best (81% sensitivity and 82% specificity)

TABLE 9.2 **ASHA (1997) and AAA (1997) screening criteria for abnormal V_{ea}, Y_{tm}, and TW in children from 4 months to 7 years of age**

	Study	Age	V_{ea} (cm³)	Y_{tm} (mmho)	TW (daPa)
ASHA (1997)	Roush et al., 1995	4–12 mos		<0.2	>235
	Nozza et al., 1992; 1994	1–7 yrs		<0.3	>200
	Shanks et al., 1992	1–7 yrs	>1.0		
AAA (1997)		3–7 yrs		<0.2	>250

ASHA, American Speech-Language-Hearing Association; AAA, Americal Academy of Audiology; V_{ea}, ear canal volume; Y_{tm}, admittance in the plane of the tympanic membrane; TW, tympanogram width.

tympanometry measure to differentiate between ears with and without MEE when a history of chronic or recurrent otitis media was present, followed by peak Y_{tm}, the AR, and TPP.

Silman et al. (1992) tested the ASHA (1990) tympanometry criteria using an experienced otoscopist as the gold standard. The ultimate "gold standard" for studies on MEE is myringotomy and aspiration, although this is not always practical. Otoscopy and surgical findings agree 79% to 86% of the time (Paradise et al., 1976; Nozza et al., 1994). Otoscopy misses few ears with MEE, but has a slightly higher false-positive rate.

Silman et al. (1992) reported that the ASHA (1990) protocol had 81.5% sensitivity and 79% specificity, and that performance improved to 90% sensitivity and 92.5% specificity when TPP and the ipsilateral AR were put back into the screening protocol. There still is no consensus on the value of including TPP and AR in screening programs. Nozza et al. (1992) and Silman et al. (1992) reported good performance of these two measures, whereas other investigators reported excessive false-positive rates (Roush and Tait, 1985). Although the AR performed well, its use in screening is limited because 28% of the normal population either failed the test or could not be tested (Nozza et al., 1992).

An interesting finding of the Silman et al. (1992) study was that when MEE resulted in failed hearing screening, all of the tympanometry measures were effective in identifying MEE. MEE, however, does not always result in significant hearing loss. Estimates of failed hearing screenings with verified MEE have ranged from 35% to 80% (Lyons et al., 2004; Roush and Tait, 1985; Silman et al., 1992). The condition of the middle ear changes along a continuum from a normal ear to a completely fluid-filled ear with significant hearing loss. All tympanometry screening measures were effective in correctly identifying the two extremes, but were less successful in identifying ears falling in the middle. Ears with a history of chronic or recurrent otitis media but without MEE also fall into this challenging middle range and tend to have high false-positive rates for both tympanometry and otoscopy (Nozza et al., 1992, 1994; Roush et al., 1995; Silverman and Silman, 1995). These same ears probably account for the 15-27% incidence of dry taps in ears undergoing myringotomy (Saeed et al., 2004; Watters et al., 1997).

In response to the growing database of sensitivity data, the ASHA guideline for middle-ear screening underwent another revision in 1997. The targeted population is children under seven years of age with chronic or recurrent middle-ear effusion with the potential to cause significant medical and developmental consequences. The primary change is that the tympanometry criteria have been modified to reflect the age and population specific data now available. The new ASHA (1997) and the AAA (1997) criteria are shown in Table 9.2. The AAA criteria are more conservative than the ASHA criteria in minimizing false-positive rates in 3 to 7 year olds. The consensus reflected in all the guidelines is that a test-battery approach is better than any single measure in identifying children requiring medical intervention. As such, the guidelines are changing more from screening to identification guidelines. The guidelines also recognize that the criteria used to identify MEE are highly dependent on the population being tested and recommend that program administrators continually monitor and adjust referral criteria for acceptable pass-fail rates.

REVIEW OF ACOUSTIC IMMITTANCE PRINCIPLES

The remainder of the chapter focuses on multiple-frequency tympanometry (MFT). The principles discussed in Chapter 8 will be reviewed briefly. Additional recommended readings in this area include an excellent chapter by Margolis (1981) and chapters by Lilly (1972a,b) and Van Camp et al. (1986). For students who would like a more basic review of acoustic immittance measurements with an extensive bibliography, a book by Wiley and Fowler (1997) is recommended.

Recall from the preceding chapter that three elements contribute to admittance, spring (also termed compliance or inversely stiffness), mass, and resistance. When an identical sinusoidal force (F) is applied to these three elements, each responds with a unique velocity (V). These unique force velocity relationships are depicted in Figure 9.3 (adapted from Fowler and Shanks, 2002).

An element with pure resistance dissipates or absorbs energy due to friction. The velocity of a purely resistive element is in phase with the applied force. In admittance

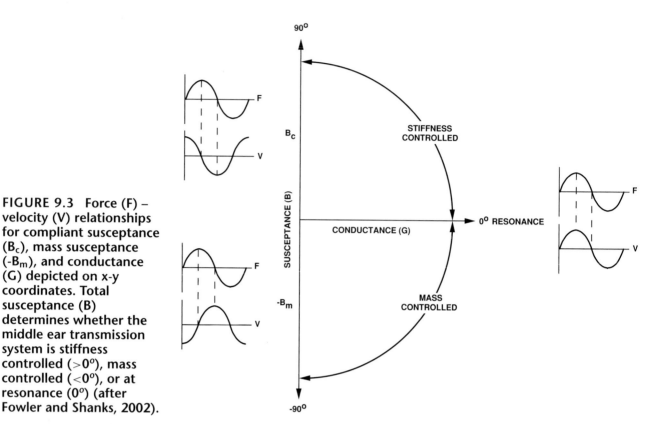

FIGURE 9.3 Force (F) – velocity (V) relationships for compliant susceptance (B_c), mass susceptance ($-B_m$), and conductance (G) depicted on x-y coordinates. Total susceptance (B) determines whether the middle ear transmission system is stiffness controlled ($>0°$), mass controlled ($<0°$), or at resonance ($0°$) (after Fowler and Shanks, 2002).

terminology, the "real" or in phase component of complex acoustic admittance is called acoustic conductance (G_a) and is represented along the x-axis in Figure 9.3. Resistance can never be negative, so only the positive x-axis is shown in the figure.

The other two elements, a spring (or compliant) element and a mass element, both store energy, and their responses are out of phase with the applied force. The velocity of a spring or compliance element *leads* the applied force by $90°$ whereas the velocity of a mass element *lags* force by $90°$. In other words, for the same applied force, the velocities of spring and mass elements are $180°$ out of phase, and are similarly represented at $90°$ and $-90°$ on the y-axis. Compliant or positive susceptance (B_c) is the admittance offered by a compliant element, and mass or negative susceptance ($-B_m$) is the admittance offered by a mass element.

A system like the ear, that contains both compliant and mass susceptance, functions like a system with a single element whose total susceptance (B_a) is equal to the algebraic sum of the two out-of-phase components. All two-component admittance instruments measure total susceptance. If compliant susceptance (B_c) is larger than mass susceptance ($-B_m$), total susceptance is positive. The ear is described as stiffness controlled, and the admittance vector will be in the upper quadrant of Figure 9.3. Conversely, if mass susceptance ($-B_m$) is larger than compliant susceptance (B_c), total susceptance is negative. The ear is described as mass controlled, and the admittance vector will be in the lower quadrant of Figure 9.3. When compliant and mass susceptance are equal, total susceptance is 0 acoustic mmho

and the middle ear is in resonance. The resonant frequency (f_o) of the normal middle ear is between 800 and 1200 Hz. Below f_o, the ear is described as stiffness controlled, and above f_o, the ear is described as mass controlled.

If pathology such as otosclerosis increases the stiffness of the middle-ear transmission system, the ear remains stiffness controlled at higher than normal frequencies and f_o increases. Conversely, if pathology such as ossicular discontinuity increases the mass (or descreases the stiffness) of the middle-ear transmission system, the ear becomes mass controlled at a lower than normal frequency and f_o decreases. These effects frequently are reflected in the audiogram. An increase in stiffness decreases transmission for low frequencies, and the audiogram demonstrates a stiffness tilt. Conversely, an increase in mass decreases transmission for high frequencies, and the audiogram demonstrates a mass tilt.

NORMAL 226 AND 678 HZ TYMPANOGRAMS

Figure 9.4 shows uncompensated acoustic admittance (Y_a), susceptance (B_a), and conductance (G_a) tympanograms at 226 Hz (top) and 678 Hz (bottom) from a normal 40-year-old male. Peak compensated static acoustic admittance is plotted in both polar and rectangular formats to the right of the tympanograms. First, calculate peak $200B_{tm}$ and $200G_{tm}$, i.e., subtract the admittance values at 200 daPa from the respective peak values. At 226 Hz, B_{tm} is 0.57

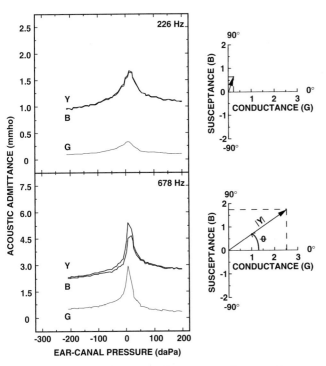

FIGURE 9.4   Normal uncompensated acoustic admittance (Y), susceptance (B), and conductance (G) tympanograms at 226 Hz (top panel) and 678 Hz (bottom panel) with corresponding peak compensated static acoustic admittance plotted in both rectangular (susceptance [B] and conductance [G]) and polar (admittance [|Y|] and phase angle [φ]) formats on the right.

gle of 34°. Measuring only Y_{tm} without phase information is analogous to giving someone directions to your home by saying drive 5 miles. Similarly, specifying only Y_{tm} puts the vector anywhere between the 90° axis (straight up) and the −90° axis (straight down). It is common practice, however, to measure only Y_{tm} when a 226 Hz probe signal is used because the ear is very stiffness dominated, and the admittance vector lies close to the 90° axis. Note in the top panel of Figure 9.4 that the Y_a and B_a tympanograms at 226 Hz basically overlap and G_a contributes minimally to Y_a. This is not the case at 678 Hz, however, where the Y_a tympanogram deviates significantly from the B_a tympanogram near the peak. When high-frequency probe tones are used, both B_a and G_a contribute to complex acoustic admittance and must be specified; phase angle can no longer be assumed to approximate 90°. Although B_{tm} and Y_{tm} are essentially equal at 226 Hz, they are much different at 678 Hz, and in fact, Y_{tm} is closer in magnitude to conductance than to susceptance. Remember that Y_{tm} is a vector quantity and will *always* be larger than either of the contributing rectangular components (B or G). Susceptance is the primary contributor to Y_{tm} at 226 Hz, but conductance is the primary contributor at 678 Hz. If only Y_{tm} were measured at 678 Hz, you would have no idea which component, B_{tm} or G_{tm}, contributed more to its magnitude. Specifying only Y_{tm} at high frequencies presents an incomplete description of the acoustic admittance of the middle ear.

■ MULTIPLE-FREQUENCY TYMPANOMETRY

Normal 226 Hz tympanograms, no matter which admittance component is measured, are always single peaked. As probe frequency increases, however, tympanograms begin to notch in a systematic and predictable manner. The normal multiple-frequency tympanograms in Figure 9.5 were recorded from the same 40-year-old man as shown in Figure 9.4. Notice the change in the shapes of each of the four uncompensated admittance component tympanograms (G_a, B_a, Y_a, φ_a) as probe frequency increases from 226 to 1243 Hz[2]. At low frequencies, the tympanograms all are single peaked; the amplitude at the peak gradually increases with frequency and then develops a notch at the peak. As frequency increases further, the central notch deepens. For the B_a tympanograms, the notch deepens and then develops a secondary notch at the peak. Next, notice the probe frequency at which notching first occurs for each of the admittance components, i.e., B_a at 904 Hz, G_a and Y_a at 1017 Hz, and φ_a at 1130 Hz[3].

(i.e., 1.68 − 1.11) and G_{tm} is 0.21 (i.e., 0.32 − 0.11) acoustic mmho. B_{tm} is plotted on the y-axis and G_{tm} is plotted on the x-axis to the right of the 226 Hz tympanogram. Make the same two calculations on the 678 Hz B_a and G_a tympanograms in the lower panel; $200B_{tm}$ and $200G_{tm}$ are 1.72 (i.e., 4.50 − 2.78) and 2.58 (i.e., 2.96 − 0.38) acoustic mmho, respectively. Perpendicular lines drawn from the x and y axes intersect at a point in the complex admittance plane that describes the peak compensated static acoustic admittance of this 40-year-old male. The intersecting lines form a rectangle when B_a and G_a are plotted in *rectangular* format.

The point where the two perpendicular lines intersect also can be described in *polar* format by drawing a vector from the origin, or x-y intercept, to the same point in the complex plane. The length or magnitude of the admittance vector (Y_{tm} or |Y|) and the phase angle (φ) of Y_{tm} with respect to the x-axis describe acoustic admittance in *polar* format. The vertical bars sometimes are used to indicate that the admittance vector is an absolute value and has no sign. The rectangular components of acoustic admittance can be transformed to polar format using the Pythagorean theorem or Equation 8.5 and converting from radians to degrees. At 226 Hz, Y_{tm} is 0.60 acoustic mmho with a phase angle of 70°, and at 678 Hz, Y_{tm} is 3.10 acoustic mmho with a phase an-

---

[2] An upper range of 1243 rather than 2000 Hz was used because of unstable calibration at higher frequencies.

[3] All the tympanograms in Figure 9.5 are uncompensated for ear-canal volume. Although the shapes of the susceptance and conductance tympanograms are the same compensated and uncompensated, ear-canal volume does not have the same linear effect on admittance and phase angle tympanograms. See Shanks and Lilly (1981) and Shanks et al. (1988) for further discussion.

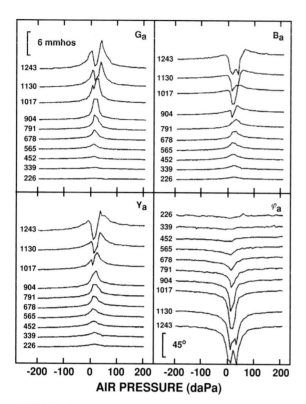

FIGURE 9.5 Uncompensated multiple frequency conductance (G_a), susceptance (B_a), admittance (Y_a), and phase angle (φ_a) tympanograms recorded from a normal, 40-year-old male.

Figure 9.6 demonstrates two ways to plot peak compensated static acoustic admittance for the family of normal tympanograms shown in Figure 9.5. Panel A shows $200B_{tm}$, G_{tm}, and Y_{tm} as a function of frequency.[4] First examine the magnitude relationship between B_{tm} (open squares) and G_{tm} (filled diamonds). B_{tm} is larger than G_{tm} for probe frequencies less than 678 Hz. Stated differently, the peak-to-tail amplitudes of the susceptance tympanograms in Figure 9.5 are larger than the peak-to-tail amplitudes of the conductance tympanograms for probe frequencies of 226 through 565 Hz. The B_{tm} and G_{tm} functions in Figure 9.6A cross when the amplitudes of the B and G tympanograms are equal, i.e., when the admittance vector is at 45° as indicated by the dashed vertical line near 580 Hz. Beginning at 678 Hz, the amplitude of the G_{tm} tympanogram now is greater than the B_{tm} tympanogram, and the conductance function (filled diamonds) now rises above the susceptance function (open squares). As the amplitude of the conductance tympanogram continues to increase, the susceptance tympanogram develops a notch and begins to decrease to 0 acoustic mmho near 850 Hz. Recall that the resonant frequency (f_o) of the middle ear, indicated by the second vertical dashed line, occurs when stiffness susceptance (B_c) and mass susceptance (B_m)

are equal. The ear is stiffness controlled below f_o and mass controlled above f_o. Stated differently, peak B_{tm} is positive below resonance and negative above resonance. In contrast, G_{tm} increases until a notch develops at 1017 Hz and then decreases sharply but can never be negative. Now examine the Y_{tm} function (filled circles) in Figure 9.6A. Recall that both susceptance and conductance contribute to Y_{tm}, so admittance magnitude will always be greater than the larger of the two rectangular components. For low frequencies such as 226 Hz, Y_{tm} is similar in magnitude to B_{tm}, but for frequencies near f_o, Y_{tm} is similar to G_{tm} and reaches a maximum near f_o. As frequency increases above f_o, G_{tm} decreases and Y_{tm} again is similar in magnitude to B_{tm}, but of course will never be negative.

Figure 9.6B shows exactly the same data as shown in Panel A, but plotted in polar format. This format clearly shows that the admittance vector rotates in a very orderly pattern as probe frequency increases from 226 Hz to 1243 Hz. When the admittance vector is above the 0° axis (i.e., between 90° and 0°), B_{tm} is positive, and the middle ear is described as stiffness controlled. At resonance, the admittance vector lies along the x-axis at 0°. Although the probe frequency did not coincide exactly with f_o in this particular ear, the admittance vector crosses the x-axis at about 850 Hz. Above 850 Hz, the admittance vector rotates into the negative susceptance quadrant between 0° and −90°, and the middle ear is described as mass controlled. If only Y_{tm} without phase angle is measured, you cannot tell whether the ear is stiffness controlled or mass controlled, i.e., the admittance vector could be anywhere in the 180° plane.

Plotting only what happens at a single point on the tympanogram ignores valuable information about tympanogram shape. In contrast, plotting the entire tympanogram allows you to analyze both the shape and static admittance. 226 Hz Y_a tympanograms provide information on the stiffness characteristics of the middle ear including volume estimates, and 678 Hz B_a and G_a tympanograms provide more information on the mass characteristics and resonance of the middle ear. At 226 Hz, Y_a tympanograms are almost always single peaked and require calculations to differentiate between normal and pathological middle ears. Analysis of 678 Hz tympanograms is much different, but also much simpler, thanks to a model developed by Vanhuyse and his Belgian colleagues (1975).

The Vanhuyse Model

Notched 678 Hz tympanograms were not completely understood until the paper of Vanhuyse et al. (1975). The Vanhuyse model began with some basic assumptions about the normal shapes and magnitude relationships of acoustic resistance (R_a) and acoustic reactance (X_a) tympanograms recorded by Moller (1965). The R_a tympanogram decreased monotonically from high negative pressures to high positive pressures, and the X_a tympanogram was a parabolic function

---

[4] Although frequency typically is incremented and plotted logarithmically, linear scaling was chosen to enhance plotting resolution.

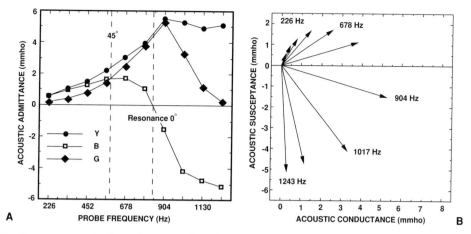

FIGURE 9.6 Peak compensated static acoustic admittance calculated from the normal multiple frequency tympanograms in Figure 9.5. Peak 200B$_{tm}$ (*open squares*), 200G$_{tm}$ (*filled diamonds*), and 200Y$_{tm}$ (*closed circles*) are plotted in rectangular format as a function of probe frequency in Panel **A**; the rectangular admittance values corresponding to phase angles of 45° and 0° are indicated by dashed lines. Rotation of the admittance vector as a function of probe frequency is plotted in polar format in Panel **B**.

symmetric around 0 daPa. The R$_a$ tympanogram was kept constant, and the X$_a$ tympanogram was progressively shifted from stiffness-controlled to mass-controlled conditions. For each of four shifts in the X$_a$ tympanogram, B$_a$ and G$_a$ tympanograms were calculated (Eq. 8.40) and replotted. Although the shapes of the R$_a$ and X$_a$ tympanograms remained constant, the four resultant B$_a$ and G$_a$ tympanograms became increasingly complex with each shift in X$_a$. [See Margolis and Shanks (1985), Shanks (1984), Shanks et al. (1988) and Van Camp et al. (1986) for a more in depth review of the Vanhuyse model].

The left half of Figure 9.7 shows the four tympanogram patterns predicted by the Vanhuyse model. The B$_a$ and G$_a$ tympanograms change shape for each 45° rotation of the admittance vector. When the admittance vector is between 90° and 45°, both the B and G tympanograms are single peaked and are designated 1B1G. When the vector rotates between 45° and 0°, a notch develops in the B tympanogram, but the G tympanogram remains single peaked; this pattern is designated 3B1G. The "3" indicates that there are 3 extrema or direction changes in the peak of the B tympanogram. The vertical lines with the arrows indicate the "peak" of the notched tympanograms and the pressure at which peak compensated static acoustic admittance is calculated. Because acoustic resistance tympanograms are markedly asymmetric, peak pressures for B$_a$ and G$_a$ tympanograms differ slightly (Margolis and Popelka, 1977; Moller, 1965; Van Camp et al., 1978; Van Camp et al., 1986). The horizontal lines with the arrows indicate that the tympanograms have been compensated for ear-canal volume, i.e., baseline corrected. Note that the notch in the 3B tympanogram is still above the baseline, and therefore, peak 200B$_{tm}$ is positive and the middle-ear is stiffness controlled. If the center of the notch had fallen exactly on the baseline, peak 200B$_{tm}$ would equal 0 acoustic mmho and indicate resonance.

As the admittance vector rotates between 0° and −45°, the conductance tympanogram also develops a notch and is designated 3B3G. Look at the susceptance (B) tympanogram and note that the center notch now is below the zero baseline. 200B$_{tm}$ is negative, and the middle ear is mass controlled. When the admittance vector rotates between −45° and −90°, a 5B3G tympanogram is recorded. The notch in the conductance tympanogram deepens and the susceptance tympanogram develops a secondary notch. Note that static acoustic susceptance is calculated using the peak value in the secondary notch as indicated by the vertical arrow. Again, susceptance is negative, and the ear remains mass controlled.

The Vanhuyse model also predicted that a normal admittance magnitude tympanogram (Y$_a$) has only two shapes: a single-peaked tympanogram in a stiffness-controlled middle ear when the vector is >0° and a notched tympanogram in a mass-controlled middle ear when the vector is <0°. In other words, the Y$_a$ tympanogram notches at or above f$_o$.

All four tympanogram patterns in the left half of Figure 9.7 are normal. Tympanograms recorded with descending pressure changes conform best to the Vanhuyse model (Margolis et al., 1985). At 678 Hz, normal B/G tympanograms are distributed as follows: 75% 1B1G, 8% 3B1G, 4% 3B3G, and 13% 5B3G. Notch width for 3B and 5B tympanograms is 36 and 51 daPa, respectively (Creten et al., 1985). In polar format, 83% are 1Y and 89% are 1φ (Creten et al., 1985; Wilson et al., 1984).

Although the Vanhuyse model originally was developed to explain the four normal tympanogram patterns recorded at 678 Hz, the model also is useful in accounting for changes in tympanogram shape as a function of frequency (Margolis et al., 1985). The incidence of notching increases for higher frequency probe tones. For example, at 1000 Hz approximately 80% of normal adult ears have 3B1G tympanograms (Calandruccio et al., 2006).

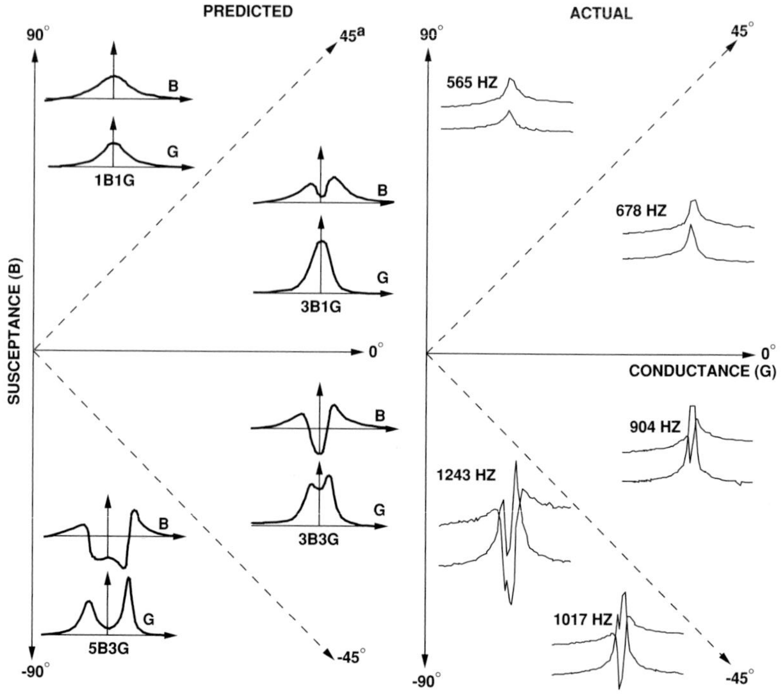

FIGURE 9.7   A comparison of susceptance (B) and conductance (G) tympanograms predicted by the Vanhuyse et al. (1975) model (Predicted) versus actual tympanograms measured from a 40-year-old male with a normal middle-ear transmission system (Actual). The actual tympanograms are from the same person whose data are depicted in Figures 9.4 through 9.6.

In the right half of Figure 9.7, the predicted Vanhuyse patterns are compared with samples of actual MFT previously shown in Figure 9.5. In each tympanogram pair, susceptance (B) is always the top function and conductance (G) is the lower function. Deviations from the predicted model tend to occur at the transitions between patterns, particularly for the 1B1G and 5B3G patterns (Margolis et al., 1985). One very common pattern that is not accounted for by the Vanhuyse model was recorded at 678 Hz. Note that G_{tm} is greater than B_{tm}, although the model predicts that the B_a tympanogram should notch when the admittance vector rotates below 45°. In this example, the phase angle is 34°, but the B_a tympanogram remains single peaked. Similarly, a 3B1G pattern was recorded at 904 Hz when the admittance vector was at an angle of −16°; the model predicts a 3B3G pattern when the middle ear is mass controlled. At 1017 Hz, a 3B3G pattern was recorded even though the phase angle was at −51°; the Vanhuyse model predicts a 5B3G pattern when the admittance phasor is between −45° and −90°. In all cases, the small deviations from the model occurred close to the transition angles of 45°, 0°, and −45°. Despite these small differences, the Vanhuyse model has been invaluable in understanding changes in the shapes of 678 Hz tympanograms across normal subjects and as a function of probe frequency.

This same group of Belgian researchers defined abnormal notching of B_a and G_a tympanograms. Simply determining whether an ear is stiffness controlled, mass controlled, or at resonance is not very diagnostic because the range of normal variability is so large. Examining the characteristic of the notching, however, can be diagnostic. Van de Heyning et al. (1982) quantified the number of extrema and the pressure interval between the outermost extrema to define abnormal notching as follows:

- more than 5 extrema in the susceptance (B) tympanogram,
- more than 3 extrema in the conductance (G) tympanogram,
- notch width >75 daPa for 3B tympanograms,
- notch width >100 daPa for 5B tympanograms, or
- notch width >60 daPa for 3Y tympanograms.

A simple shape analysis also can be used to identify 1B1G tympanograms that are abnormally stiff. Simply compare the relative peak-to-tail amplitudes of the single-peaked B and G tympanograms. Only one of the following three magnitude relationships is possible:

If $B_{tm} > G_{tm}$, then the admittance vector is >45°.
If $B_{tm} < G_{tm}$, then the admittance vector is <45°.
If $B_{tm} = G_{tm}$, then the admittance vector is =45°.

Clinical experience with a 678 Hz probe tone in an adult male population shows that the admittance vector normally is ≤45°. If the vector is closer to the positive y-axis, i.e., between 90° and 45°, then $B_{tm} > G_{tm}$ and the ear is abnormally stiff. Refer again to the 678 Hz susceptance (B) and conductance (G) tympanograms in the lower half of Figure 9.4. In this example, $B_{tm} < G_{tm}$ at 678 Hz, the admittance vector is <45°, and the middle ear is normally stiffness controlled. In contrast to 226 Hz tympanograms, 678 Hz tympanograms can be classified as normal, abnormally stiff, or abnormally mass controlled from a simple visual comparison of the magnitude relationship of B_a and G_a.

The Vanhuyse model lays the foundation for understanding other MFT procedures. Lilly (1984) provides an excellent review of experimental MFT procedures that were the precursors to current clinical techniques. In general, MFT can be categorized as sweep-pressure or sweep-frequency procedures. Traditional tympanometry uses a sweep-pressure technique. In sweep-frequency tympanometry, the probe-tone frequency is swept at discrete ear-canal pressures. Although the shapes of the tympanograms look similar, the estimates of f_0 for the two techniques are different.

Sweep-Pressure Tympanometry

Colletti (1975, 1976, 1977) introduced a sweep-pressure procedure for estimating the resonant frequency of the middle-ear transmission system. He used a custom device to measure uncompensated Z_a tympanograms (i.e., inverted Y_a tympanograms) for probe frequencies of 200 to 2000 Hz. Colletti noted that the shape of the Z_a tympanograms varied systematically from single peaked, to notched, to inverted as frequency increased. The frequency range corresponding to the emergence of the notched tympanogram was the most distinctive and easiest to classify. Recall from the Vanhuyse et al. (1975) model that a notched 3Y pattern emerges near the resonant frequency (f_o) of the middle ear. In normal ears, notched Z_a tympanograms were observed over a 300 Hz frequency interval beginning at an average of 1000 Hz with a normal range of 650 to 1400 Hz. The same three tympanogram patterns were recorded in pathological ears, but the frequency range where the notched pattern first emerged was different from normal ears. In general, the notched pattern emerged at higher than normal frequencies (850 to 1650 Hz) in ears with increased stiffness due to otosclerosis and lower than normal (500 to 850 Hz) in ears with increased mass due to ossicular discontinuity. Although considerable overlap occurred between the normal and otosclerotic ears, little overlap was found between ears with otosclerosis and ossicular discontinuity.

Sweep-Frequency Tympanometry

The MFT option on the Virtual (Model 310) and Grason Stadler (Model 33 and Tympstar) instruments is based on a sweep frequency procedure developed by Funasaka et al. (1984). They used a custom-built instrument to measure the difference in the sound pressure level and phase of a sweep frequency probe tone at 0 daPa versus −200 daPa. They identified four characteristics of the difference curves that were effective in differentiating among middle-ear pathologies. One of the most effective measures was the 0 crossing of the SPL difference curve, which averaged 1500 Hz in normal ears, <720 Hz in ears with ossicular discontinuity, and >1880 Hz in ears with ossicular fixation (Funasaka and Kumakawa, 1988). Their results again reflect an increase in f_o for pathologies that increase stiffness and a decrease in f_o for pathologies that increase mass or conversely, decrease stiffness. 83% of ears with ossicular discontinuity and malleus/incus fixation and 55% of ears with stapedial fixation were correctly identified. Malleus and incus fixations result in very high impedance and typically are easier to detect than the more lateral pathology of stapes fixation. In contrast, at 220 Hz, only 32% of ears with ossicular fixation and 42% with ossicular discontinuity were identified correctly. Overall, 220 Hz tympanometry identified 35% of patients with ossicular discontinuity and fixation, whereas sweep-frequency measures identified 68%.

F_o estimated in the Funasaka studies (1984, 1988) is lower than that reported in the Colletti studies (1975, 1976, 1977) because measurements were made at ambient rather than at peak pressure. The steep slope of tympanograms near the peak results in large differences between Y_{tm} calculated at peak versus 0 daPa. Y_{tm} is about 20% lower at 0 daPa than at peak, so estimates of f_o will be higher at 0 daPa than at peak (Wilson et al., 1984). Although some investigators logically argue that measurements at 0 daPa present the most accurate picture of how an ear functions in the daily environment, measurements at peak are preferred because of better intra- and inter-test agreement (Margolis and Popelka, 1975; Porter and Winston, 1973; Wilson et al., 1984).

Both the Virtual (Model 310) and Grason Stadler (Model 33 and TympStar Version 2) instruments have a test option similar to that described by Funasaka et al. (1984), except the measurements are done at TPP rather than at 0 daPa. To run the multiple-frequency feature on the Grason-Stadler instruments, acoustic admittance first is measured as probe frequency is increased from 250 Hz to 2000 Hz at the selected starting pressure, typically at 200 daPa. Next, a 226 Hz tympanogram is recorded to identify TPP, and then a second frequency sweep is performed at peak. The Grason-Stadler instrument always plots the difference in phase angle between the starting and peak pressures ($\Delta\varphi$) and plots a second difference function of your choice, which logically should be susceptance (ΔB). The difference in acoustic susceptance between peak and 200 daPa is simply a plot of $200B_{tm}$ as a function of frequency (see Fig. 9.6A). F_o is indicated at the 0 crossing of the ΔB function.

The value of the $\Delta\varphi$ function, however, is questionable. Valvik et al. (1994) concluded that $\Delta\varphi$ provides no information of any value. Although *compensated* phase angle is 0° at resonance, $\Delta\varphi$ is derived by simply subtracting two uncompensated phase angles and is not a measure of the phase of the middle-ear transmission system. In contrast, the Virtual instrument plotted true peak compensated phase angle by correcting for ear-canal volume in rectangular format (susceptance and conductance) and then converting back to polar format. In this case, the probe frequency corresponding to a phase angle of 0° provided an estimate of f_o. Although this is a mathematically sound procedure, in practice the procedure was susceptible to artifacts and the test-retest reliability was not very good. Holte (1996) noted errors in estimating f_o with this procedure by as much as 2 octaves.

The mathematics governing complex numbers can be confusing. In contrast to the rectangular components of acoustic admittance (B_a and G_a), the polar components (Y_a and φ_a) cannot be compensated to the plane of the tympanic membrane by simply subtracting the values at 200 daPa from the peak values (Shanks et al., 1993). Stated differently, a Y_a tympanogram baselined at 200 daPa (200Y_a) is not the same as 200Y_{tm} particularly when high-frequency probe tones are used. Simply baselining a Y_a tympanogram at 200 daPa can result in a 200Y_a value that is 0 acoustic mmho or even negative. You know from previous discussions that Y_a is a magnitude value that can never be equal to 0 or negative. Unlike B_a and G_a, the shapes of Y_a and phase-angle tympanograms are different in the plane of the probe tip versus the plane of the tympanic membrane, and must be compensated using vector mathematics (Shanks et al., 1988).

Age and Gender Effects

Wiley et al. (1996; 1999) reported small gender differences with slightly higher f_o in women than in men, except among the 80 to 90 year olds. Other studies reported no age or gender effects on f_o (Ferekidis et al., 1999; Hanks and Mortenson, 1997; Hanks and Rose, 1993; Holte, 1996; Margolis and Goycoolea; 1993; Shahnaz and Davies, 2006). In view of the wide normal range for f_o, small gender and age effects are not clinically significant and do not justify the inconvenience of separate norms.

Procedural Variables

Several procedural variables affect tympanogram amplitude and shape and must be considered when norms are established. In general, procedural variables have a greater effect on the tympanogram peak than on the tails, and have a greater effect at high frequencies than at low frequencies.

RATE AND DIRECTION OF PRESSURE CHANGE

Pump speed has a significant effect on Y_{tm} but little effect on V_{ea} and TW (Creten and Van Camp, 1974; Koebsell and Margolis, 1986; Margolis and Heller, 1987; Shanks and Wilson, 1986). Single-peaked tympanograms increase in amplitude with increasing rates of pressure change. For example, Margolis and Heller (1987) measured a 10–14% increase in Y_{tm} for an increase in pump speed from 200 daPa/s to 400 daPa/s. In addition, the incidence, depth, and complexity of notching increases at high rates of pressure change.

The amplitude and shape of tympanograms also are affected by the direction of pressure change, particularly at high frequencies. Tympanograms recorded in the negative to positive direction ($-/+$) typically result in higher Y_{tm} than the positive to negative ($+/-$) direction and exhibit more complex notching (Alberti and Jerger, 1974; Creten and Van Camp, 1974; Margolis and Smith, 1977; Shanks and Wilson, 1986; Van Camp et al., 1980; Wilson et al., 1984). Wilson et al. (1984) and Shanks and Wilson (1986) reported

that 38% to 46% of 678 Hz tympanograms were notched for ascending pressure changes and only 21% to 25% were notched for descending pressure changes. The descending pressure change is preferred because the notched patterns are more consistent with the Vanhuyse et al. (1975) model. More recently, other studies have shown that ranges of f_o are smaller and test-retest reliability is higher for descending ($+/-$) than for ascending ($-/+$) pressure changes (Margolis and Goycoolea, 1993; Wiley et al., 1999).

COMPENSATION OF EAR-CANAL VOLUME

The pressure used to estimate V_{ea} is the single most important procedural variable to control in establishing norms. Because of tympanogram asymmetry, V_{ea} almost always is larger when estimated from the positive rather than the negative tail of the tympanogram. This in turn results in lower peak Y_{tm} and a lower f_o by 150 to 400 Hz (Hanks and Mortensen, 1997; Holte 1996; Margolis and Goycoolea, 1993; Shahnaz and Polka; 1997; Shanks et al., 1993; Wiley et al., 1999). More importantly, these same studies found that the 90% range for f_o is smaller, with smaller inter- and intra-subject variability for positive versus negative pressure compensation. This provides additional strong support for ear-canal compensation at a positive starting pressure.

NUMBER OF CONSECUTIVE PRESSURE SWEEPS

Y_{tm} also increases with the number of pressure sweeps, especially during the first three to five tympanograms (Osguthorpe and Lam, 1981; Vanpeperstraete et al., 1979; Wilson et al., 1984). An 18% increase in Y_{tm} at 226 Hz from sweep one to sweep ten was attributed to alterations in the viscoelastic properties of the eardrum and middle ear with repeated pressurization (Wilson et al., 1984). This variable is a consideration when sweep-pressure MFT is employed.

SWEEP-PRESSURE VERSUS SWEEP-FREQUENCY TYMPANOMETRY

Margolis and Goycoolea (1993) discussed a myriad of procedural variables that affect the estimate of f_0. They compared eight tympanometry estimates of f_0 in order to identify the measure with the highest test-retest reliability and lowest inter-subject variability. For both sweep-pressure and sweep-frequency tympanometry, f_0 was 78 to 151 Hz higher for Y_a versus B_a tympanograms. In addition, sweep-pressure tympanometry produced lower estimates of f_0 than sweep-frequency tympanometry. Mean f_0 was 990 Hz with a 90% range of 630 to 1400 Hz and 1135 Hz with a 90% range of 800 to 2000 Hz for sweep-pressure and sweep-frequency tympanometry, respectively. Similarly, Hanks and Mortensen (1997) reported a 400 Hz difference in f_0 between sweep-pressure and sweep-frequency tympanometry in young adults. The difference in f_0 could result from multiple consecutive pressure sweeps during sweep-pressure tympanometry (Osguthorpe and Lam, 1981; Vanpeperstraete et al., 1979; Wilson et al., 1984). To maximize the range of possible abnormal values, Margolis and Goycoolea (1993) suggested using sweep-pressure tympanometry to evaluate stiff ears and sweep-frequency tympanometry to evaluate mass-controlled ears. Another consideration in choosing between the two options is time; sweep-frequency tympanometry is faster, and the effects of the direction and rate of pressure change are not issues.

Even when procedural variables are controlled, the normal 90% range of f_o is wide. In general, f_o is shifted higher when stiffness is increased and is shifted lower when mass is increased or conversely, stiffness is decreased. Although the f_o can help to categorize middle-ear pathologies into two broad categories, i.e., stiffness- versus mass-related pathologies, f_o is not very useful in differentiating among pathologies within each broad category. As will be demonstrated with several case studies in the final section of this chapter, tympanogram morphology, particularly TW and notch width, can be more discriminating than f_o.

TESTING NEONATES

Several investigators in the early 1970's noted that conventional 226 Hz tympanometry yielded different patterns in newborns compared with older infants and adults. 226 Hz tympanograms frequently were notched and resembled patterns usually recorded at higher probe-tone frequencies in adults (Bennett, 1975; Keith, 1973, 1975). The atypical, notched tympanograms were hypothesized to reflect hypermobile eardrums (Bennett, 1975; Keith, 1973; 1975), distensible ear-canal walls (Paradise et al., 1976), or developmental changes in the ear (Keith, 1973). In contrast, single-peaked tympanograms were recorded from some infants with otoscopically/surgically confirmed middle-ear effusion (Paradise et al., 1976; Shurin et al., 1976). As a result of these early studies, low-frequency tympanometry was not considered reliable in neonates and infants less than 6 months of age.

Later studies used high-frequency probe tones and the Vanhuyse model to quantify developmental changes in the tympanogram patterns of neonates. At 226 Hz, notched tympanograms (e.g., 3B1G, 3B3G, 5B3G) were recorded in 50% to 83% of neonate ears (Himelfarb et al., 1979; Holte et al., 1991; McKinley et al., 1997; Sprague et al., 1985). Examination of even the 1B1G tympanograms at 226 Hz showed that the magnitude relationship between B_a and G_a was similar to that typically recorded in adult ears at 678 Hz, that is, phase angle was <45° rather than >70° typically found in older children and adults. In contrast, 678 Hz tympanograms in neonates frequently were described as flat or "bizarre" and could not be classified by the Vanhuyse model (Himelfarb et al., 1979; McKinley et al., 1997; Sprague et al., 1985).

These atypical tympanograms converted quite rapidly from notched to 1B1G during the first few weeks of life. All 226 Hz tympanograms were notched in 5 to 11 hour old newborns, decreasing to 70% notched at one week, to 30%

to 46% at two weeks, and to 24% at 1 to 2 months (Bennett, 1975; Calandruccio et al., 2006; Holte et al., 1991). By 2 to 4 months, most 226 Hz tympanograms converted to 1Y or 1B1G and were similar to patterns recorded in adult ears (Himelfarb et al., 1979; Holte et al., 1991; Marchant et al., 1986; Meyer et al., 1997).

The reason for the low-frequency notched tympanograms in neonates is still being debated. One possible difference, in addition to the obvious size difference, is that the ear canal of neonates is entirely cartilaginous at birth and highly distensible under pressure from pneumatic otoscopy or tympanometry. Holte et al. (1991) conducted a study to examine the effect of ear-canal distention on the shapes of multiple-frequency tympanograms. Pneumatic video otoscopy revealed up to a 70% change in ear-canal diameter in 1- to 5-day-old newborns. Although the osseous portion of the ear canal is not fully formed until about 1 year of age, only a minimal change in ear-canal dimension was measured beyond one month of age. Importantly, Holte et al. found no correlation between the distention of the ear canal and the complexity of 226 Hz tympanograms. Ear-canal effects were primarily evidenced in tympanogram asymmetry at the tails but not at the peak.

Although flaccidity of the ear canal did not account for the notching of 226 Hz tympanograms, it did frequently cause ear-canal collapse around the probe tip, particularly for high negative pressures and ascending pressure changes (Holte et al., 1991; Sprague et al., 1985). Collapse occurs most frequently during the first week after birth and is indicated when acoustic admittance abruptly decreases toward 0 acoustic mmho when negative ear-canal pressures are applied during tympanometry. Another effect of the cartilaginous ear canal in newborns is that the ear canal cannot be modeled as a hard-walled cavity or pure acoustic compliance at extreme pressures as it can be in adults. Recall that phase angle at extreme ear-canal pressures should approach 90° in order to accurately estimate the acoustic admittance of the ear canal and compensate measures to the plane of the eardrum. This condition frequently is not met in neonates and makes the calculation of peak Y_{tm} suspect when ear-canal phase angle is less than about 70° (Holte et al., 1991; Sprague et al., 1985). A tympanometry procedure that does not rely on compensated measures, therefore, may be preferable in neonates.

Holte et al. (1991) concluded that the notched 226 Hz tympanograms reflected increased mass and resistance with a concomitant decrease in resonant frequency in newborns. They reported the occurrence of two resonances at 450 and 710 Hz that increased to a single resonance at 900 Hz in older infants. A possible contributor to the decreased f_o in neonates is the presence of fluid/debris in the ear canal and middle ear. At birth, the ear canal contains varying amounts of vernix caseosa, and the middle ear contains residual mesenchyme and amniotic fluid (Eavey, 1993). Renvall et al. (1975) demonstrated in temporal bones that low fluid levels in the middle ear result in broadly notched, mass-controlled tympanograms. Both the vernix and mesenchyme decrease precipitously in the first few days after birth and likely contribute to the shift toward single-peaked tympanograms and increase in f_o in the first few weeks of life (Himelbarb et al., 1979; Holte et al., 1991; Keith, 1975; Meyer et al., 1997). Whether notched 226 Hz tympanograms common in the first few days after birth are due to anatomical/developmental differences or simply to the effects of residual ear-canal and middle-ear fluid is unknown.

The ideal probe-tone frequency and admittance component for use in neonates and infants is likely to be debated for some time. Despite the notching of low-frequency tympanograms in neonates, Holte et al. (1991) recommended a 226 Hz probe tone because tympanogram patterns were the least affected by maturational changes and were most consistent with the Vanhuyse model. Other investigators have argued in favor of high-frequency probe tones after noting that many newborns who failed OAE/ABR screening had flat B_a or Y_a tympanograms at 678, 800, or 1000 Hz (Hirsch et al., 1992; Kei et al., 2003; Marchant et al., 1986; Margolis et al., 2003; McKinley et al., 1997; Rhodes et al., 1999; Sutton et al., 1996). Although sensitivity was higher for high-frequency probe tones in comparison with 226 Hz, flat tympanograms also were recorded from many ears that passed OAE screening (McKinley et al., 1997; Sutton et al., 1996). For example, Sutton et al. (1996) found that half of the ears with flat Y 678 Hz tympanograms passed OAE testing. Their results showed high sensitivity but low specificity for probe-tone frequencies around 678 Hz. Specificity was improved by increasing the probe tone to 1000 Hz (McKinley et al., 1997; Rhodes et al., 1999; Sutton et al., 1996).

As a result of these findings, admittance magnitude (Y_a) measures at 1000 Hz are becoming the measure of choice in testing neonates and young infants (Kei et al., 2003; Margolis et al., 2003; Purdy and Williams, 2000; Sutton et al., 1996). This measure is especially appealing because Y_a tympanograms at 1000 Hz tend to be single peaked or flat, making it easier to differentiate between normal and abnormal ears (Kei et al., 2003; McKinley et al., 1997; Rhodes et al., 1999). Kei et al. (2003) recorded 1Y tympanograms in 92% of newborns and flat tympanograms in 6%. Although all newborns passed TEOAE screening, the newborns with flat tympanograms were associated with less robust TEOAEs. Similarly, Rhodes et al. (1999) reported that 92% of 1000 Hz tympanograms were single peaked and that three ears with flat 1000 Hz tympanograms failed hearing screening.

A quantitative analysis of Y_a at 1000 Hz as suggested by Margolis et al. (2003) is more challenging, largely because it relies on an accurate estimate of ear-canal volume, agreement on what constitutes tympanogram peak, and compensation of a single-component magnitude measurement. Holte et al. (1991) calculated Y_{tm} only when the phase angle at the tail value exceeded 70°, i.e., a B: G magnitude relationship of ≥ 3. This condition frequently is not met in neonates. Although V_{ea} routinely is estimated at 200 daPa, Margolis et al. (2003) recommended a pressure of −400 daPa so that V_{ea} would

be smaller, and therefore Y_{tm} would be larger with a wider range of normal values.

The second consideration is what to designate as "peak" on notched tympanograms. Sutton et al. (2002) recommended the negative notch peak, Margolis et al. (2003) used the positive notch peak, and the Vanhuyse model uses the center notch. In order to minimize variability, a consistent procedure must be adopted.

Third, compensation of admittance magnitude theoretically is not possible without phase information. Recall from the previous discussion that vector quantities like Y_a cannot be subtracted using simple mathematics. Because both components of complex acoustic admittance were not available, Margolis et al. (2003) chose an alternative method of expressing tympanogram amplitude by simply reporting the peak: tail amplitude. Although this may prove to be a valid measure, it is important to recognize that this is not equivalent to $-400Y_{tm}$. To avoid confusion, this calculation should be designated as $-400Y_a$ to indicate that it is an expression of uncompensated Y_a amplitude.

Reaching consensus on a tympanometry protocol for neonates is extremely challenging because "normal" is difficult to define and "abnormal" is nearly impossible to verify. Sensitivity/specificity data are difficult to establish in newborns because there is no "gold standard" for this population. Although otoscopy and surgical findings traditionally are used to validate tympanometry in children and adults, neither is appropriate in newborns. Myringotomies typically are not performed in children under one year of age and otoscopy is unreliable in virtually all newborns either because a view of the eardrum is obscured by vernix or because the eardrum is not "normal" in appearance (Eavey, 1993; Himelfarb et al., 1979; Rhodes et al., 1999; Shurin et al., 1976). Shurin et al. (1976) reported that 5 of 10 newborns identified with MEE otoscopically had dry ears on tympanocentesis.

In the absence of a gold standard, many of the recent studies have used the presence of OAE as an indication of normal middle-ear function. Vernix and residual mesenchyme, however, also are confounding factors in screening newborns with ABR and OAE and have been linked to failed screening (Keefe et al., 2000; McKinley et al., 1997). Pass rates tend to be higher in newborns a few days to two weeks old, after the ear canals and middle ears have had a chance to clear (Margolis et al., 2003; McKinley, et al., 1997; Purdy and Williams, 2000; Sininger, 2003; Sutton et al., 2002).

Considerable work remains before a tympanometry protocol for newborns and infants under four months of age can be established. Special attention should be placed on age *in days* because the ears of neonates change so rapidly. Beyond one month of age, when most of the debris has cleared from the ear and the canal walls show little movement (<10%) under pressurization, peak Y_{tm} may be a more valid measure. It may be necessary to have one protocol for neonates and another for infants over one month. By 3 to 4 months of age, conventional tympanometry may be appropriate (Himelfarb et al., 1979; Holte et al., 1991; Marchant et al., 1986).

CASE STUDIES

The final section of the chapter will reinforce the principles and applications discussed throughout the chapter. Case history, otoscopy, audiometric tuning forks, acoustic reflexes, and the configuration and magnitude of the conductive component are used together in evaluating tympanograms. A test battery approach is advocated because there is not a 1:1 correspondence between a specific tympanometry pattern and middle-ear pathology. Middle-ear pathology changes along a continuum and can involve multiple pathologies. When all available information is used together, however, tympanometry can contribute unique information about the middle-ear transmission system that is not available from any other audiometric test.

Otosclerosis

Otosclerosis is a progressive disease manifesting in early adulthood that results from abnormal otic capsule bone remodeling (Cherukupally et al., 1998; Chole and McKenna, 2001; Shohet and Sutton, 2001). The first stage of the disease is characterized by resorption of bone and replacement with spongy, highly vascularized bone. The disease progresses to bony fixation of the anterior stapes footplate and then diffuse ankylosis of the entire circumference of the footplate. Hearing loss also progresses over several years from a mild low-frequency conductive hearing loss ≤ 30 dB HL to a flat, severe conductive/mixed hearing loss in the late stages of the disease. Although otosclerosis most commonly leads to a conductive hearing loss, a sensorineural component also can result, possibly through enzymatic secretion of the disease into the membranous labyrinth. A positive family history is present in approximately 50% of cases, and 70% to 80% are bilateral. Otosclerosis affects females twice as often as males and is rare in Blacks and Asians. Clinical otosclerosis develops in less than 1% of the population, although 8–11% of temporal bones show histological evidence of the disease at autopsy.

Considerable attention has focused on otosclerosis because of its relatively high prevalence and frustration over an inability to consistently differentiate this population from normal, even in the presence of large air-bone gaps. On a group basis, ears with otosclerosis demonstrate significantly lower Y_{tm} and higher f_0 than normal ears. On an individual basis, however, there is 26% to 56% overlap with the normal population. Muchnik et al. (1989) reported that only 25% of ears with otosclerosis exhibited increased stiffness and 25% actually had higher than normal admittance; results were equally discouraging at 220 and 660 Hz. Several other investigators, however, reported that the two populations are best differentiated when high-frequency probe tones are used (Jacobsen and Mahoney, 1977; Shahnaz and Polka, 2002; Wada et al., 1998; Zhoa et al., 2002). Other studies focused on identifying the optimal acoustic immittance components to measure. Burke and Nilges (1970) reported that peak compensated static acoustic compliance and resistance below

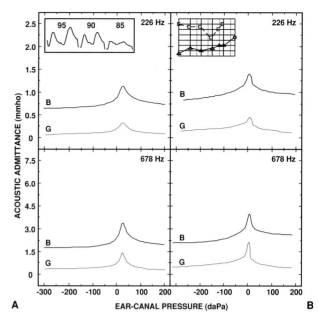

FIGURE 9.8 Susceptance (B) and conductance (G) tympanograms at 226 Hz (top panels) and 678 Hz (bottom panels) recorded from DK with otosclerosis. Panel A shows tympanograms recorded in the early stages of the disease with a biphasic acoustic-reflex response shown in the inset, and Panel B shows tympanograms recorded 18 years later with a pure tone audiogram shown in the inset.

750 Hz differentiated 76% to 89% of the otosclerotic ears from normal. Others reported that φ_{tm} was the single best component to identify otosclerosis (Shahnaz and Polka, 1997; Shanks, 1990; Van Camp and Vogeleer, 1986). In the end, a diagnosis of otosclerosis is based on a finding of normal-appearing tympanograms in conjunction with large air-bone gaps, typically greater in the low-frequency range. In general, tympanometry is less effective in identifying pathologies like otosclerosis that do not directly affect the eardrum.

Figure 9.8 shows tympanograms from DK, a 32-year-old female, who volunteered for a research study on MFT in normal ears. Preliminary screening for study inclusion revealed normal hearing in the left ear and a mild hearing loss in the right ear with air-bone gaps of 15 to 20 dB at 250 and 500 Hz, a classic stiffness tilt on the audiogram. Upon questioning, DK reported that family members across several generations had otosclerosis. 226 Hz and 678 Hz tympanograms were recorded from the right ear at the initial evaluation (Panel A) and again 18 years later (Panel B). The tympanograms in the Panel A are typical of early otosclerosis. At first glance, the tympanograms appear completely normal. At 226 Hz, $200B_{tm}$ (or $200Y_{tm}$) is stiffer than average, but falls well within the normal 90% ranges for adults in Table 9.1. Analysis of the 678 Hz tympanograms, however, shows that the ear is abnormally stiff. A comparison of the peak-to-tail (i.e., compensated) amplitudes of the susceptance (B) and conductance (G) tympanograms reveals that peak $200B_{tm}$ is greater than $200G_{tm}$. In other words, the admittance vector is at $>45°$ and the ear is abnormally stiff. A second finding seen only in early otosclerosis is shown in the inset of Panel A. Although no significant air-bone gaps were measured, biphasic or "on-off" acoustic reflexes were recorded from the right ear (Bennett and Weatherby, 1979). This reflex pattern, characterized by a brief increase in admittance with a return to baseline both at the onset and the offset of the eliciting tone, has been attributed to the elasticity of the stapes (Bel et al., 1975; Ciardo et al., 2005).

The audiogram inset in Figure 9.8B shows that hearing loss in the right progressed considerably in 18 years. The bone conduction thresholds show a classic Carhart notch at 2000 Hz that is attributed to a shift in the resonance of the ossicular chain caused by the disease process (Carhart, 1962). A Carhart notch is not a definitive indication of otosclerosis; as subsequent cases will show, most middle-ear pathology will alter the normal resonance characteristics of the ossicular chain and will result in the smallest air-bone gaps near 2000 Hz.

A comparison of 678 Hz peak $200B_{tm}$ versus $200G_{tm}$ in Panel B shows that conductance is greater than susceptance, and therefore, the admittance vector now is in the normal region at $<45°$. This change in admittance seems counterintuitive; the middle ear is actually less stiff now than it was 18 years ago. Note also that the TW, especially at 678 Hz, is very narrow. Several reports of "peaky" tympanograms in ears with ossicular fixation have been reported in the literature and provide additional evidence for a diagnosis of otosclerosis. An example of narrow tympanogram width can be found in Shanks (1984) and Shanks and Shelton (1991), and also has been noted by Ivey (1975), Dieroff (1978), and Shahnaz and Polka (1997).

In summary, tympanograms in ears with otosclerosis can be normal, abnormally stiff, or have a narrow TW. Any of these patterns in combination with a significant low-frequency conductive hearing loss with normal TPP and otoscopy, and in some cases a positive family history, point to a diagnosis of otosclerosis.

Ossicular Discontinuity

In the absence of a history of otologic surgery or trauma, patients with ossicular discontinuity are difficult to distinguish from those with otosclerosis simply on the basis of case history and otoscopy. Although high resolution CT scanning (Meriot et al., 1997) may aid in the diagnosis, tympanometry with a suggestive history are almost pathognomonic.

Ossicular discontinuity is encountered frequently in the clinical setting, but typically not as an isolated pathology. Discontinuity at the level of the incus most commonly occurs as a sequela of chronic otitis media (COM) and more rarely due to head trauma. Discontinuity associated with COM results from decalcification of the long process of the incus, often leaving only a fibrous band connecting the incus to the stapes (Terkildsen, 1976). Cholesteatoma, eardrum

perforation, and otorrhea also may occur as complications of COM. Surgical intervention in these patients very often is two-staged to remove the disease and repair the eardrum perforation in the first surgery, and to reconstruct the ossicular chain with either a total or partial ossicular replacement prosthesis (TORP or PORP) or bone cements in the second surgery (Babu and Seidman, 2004; Fisch, 1980). Hearing frequently is poorer than pre-surgical levels after the first surgery and then improves following reconstruction of the ossicular chain during the second surgery. Longitudinal fracture of the temporal bone following head trauma also can result in ossicular discontinuity at the incudo-stapedial joint. Head trauma is one of the rare instances when ossicular discontinuity is seen as an isolated pathology.

Figures 9.9A and B show tympanograms recorded from two ears with ossicular discontinuity and intact eardrums. As shown on the inset audiograms, ossicular discontinuity gives rise to a maximum conductive hearing loss. Surprisingly, the cause of the ossicular discontinuity in these two cases was not clear. Figure 9.9A shows tympanograms from RP, a 21-year-old male who suffered head trauma at age 17, but reported that the hearing loss was present prior to the head trauma. Surgical findings revealed complete incudo-stapedial joint separation with degeneration of the long process of the incus. Figure 9.9B shows another case (GS) of ossicular discontinuity with unknown etiology in a 34-year-old male. Surgical intervention again revealed erosion of the long process of the incus, this time with fibrous connections to the head of the stapes.

First, examine the 226 Hz tympanograms in the upper halves of Figures 9.9A and B. The rectangular admittance components, acoustic susceptance (B_a) and conductance (G_a), were recorded in Panel A, whereas admittance magnitude (Y_a) was recorded in Panel B. Y_{tm} calculated using Equation 8.5 is 2.6 acoustic mmho for RP (Panel A) and 2.4 acoustic mmho for GS (Panel B). In this case, conversion of B_{tm} and G_{tm} to Y_{tm} was not necessary to determine whether or not Y_{tm} is abnormal. Recall that B_{tm} and Y_{tm} at 226 Hz are nearly equal because the middle-ear is very stiffness dominated. In addition, Y_{tm} will *always* be greater than either of the two rectangular components; if B_{tm} is abnormally high, Y_{tm} also must be abnormally high. In both cases of ossicular discontinuity, $200Y_{tm}$ is higher than 90% of normal adults, no matter whose norms in Table 9.1 are used. Although 226 Hz TW is wider for GS (Panel B) than for RP (Panel A), both are <200 daPa and fall well within the normal range (see Table 9.2).

Now examine the corresponding 678 Hz tympanograms for these two cases of ossicular discontinuity. Even a cursory glance at these tympanograms reveals that both sets of tympanograms are abnormally mass controlled. First, the 678 Hz susceptance tympanograms are mass controlled because $200B_{tm}$ is negative. Stated differently, B_a in the center notch falls below B_a at 200 daPa. This finding alone does not make these tympanograms abnormal, but the complexity of the notching does. The pattern of the notching is very irregular

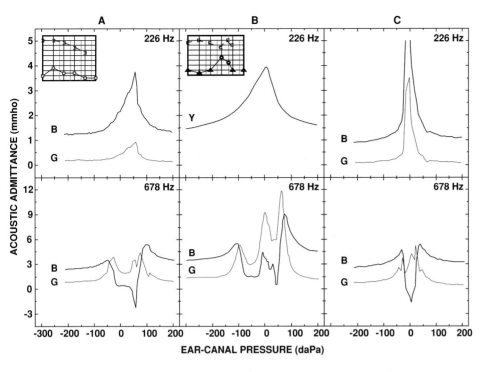

FIGURE 9.9 Susceptance (B) and conductance (G) tympanograms at 226 Hz (top panels) and 678 Hz (bottom panels) recorded from RP and GS with ossicular discontinuity (**A and B**) and from DJC with atrophic scarring of the eardrum (**C**). The audiograms for the two patients with ossicular discontinuity are shown as insets; the audiogram for DJC was normal and is not shown.

with more than five extrema for B_a and more than three extrema for G_a. In addition, the pressure interval between the outmost susceptance extrema exceeds 100 daPa. Both tympanograms are clearly outside the normal range defined by the Vanhuyse model (see Figure 9.7A). In contrast to 226 Hz, the pathology at 678 Hz is so obvious that no calculation is necessary. These abnormally mass-controlled 678 Hz tympanograms in conjunction with 60 to 70 dB air-bone gaps and normal otoscopy indicate ossicular discontinuity.

The presenting findings, however, are not always so clear-cut. As stated previously, many middle ears have multiple pathologies. When multiple pathologies are present, tympanometry will be dominated by the most lateral pathology (Chesnutt et al., 1975). As an example, a case of surgically confirmed ossicular discontinuity with intact eardrum was seen in a 16-year-old girl who suffered a temporal bone fracture with facial paralysis and bleeding into the middle-ear cavity following a motor-vehicle accident. When tympanograms were recorded shortly after the accident, she had a hemotympanum (i.e., blood filled middle-ear cavity) that immobilized the eardrum and completely masked the ossicular discontinuity. Her tympanograms were flat and reflected the immobile eardrum and not the more medial ossicular discontinuity that was confirmed at surgery. Similarly, when a perforated eardrum occurs in conjunction with ossicular discontinuity, tympanograms will reflect only the perforated eardrum and will be flat with a large V_{ea}.

Eardrum Pathology

Figure 9.9C is included in the same figure as ossicular discontinuity to emphasize the importance of otoscopy before analyzing tympanograms. Although eardrum pathology fre-

quently has little or no effect on hearing, it can have a dramatic effect on tympanogram shape. Two of the most common conditions are atrophic scarring secondary to healed eardrum perforation and tympanosclerosis of the eardrum. Several excellent examples of these eardrum pathologies are available in text form and online (Ballachanda, 1995; Hawke and McCombe, 1995; Kavanagh, 2006; Sullivan, 2006).

Small eardrum perforations usually heal spontaneously, typically within 6–8 weeks for ears with traumatic perforation and healthy middle ears, and within 3 to 4 months when associated with otitis media (Hawke and McCombe, 1995). The new membrane, referred to as a neomembrane, a monomeric eardrum, or atrophic scar, however, typically is thinner than the surrounding eardrum because the central, fibrous layer of the eardrum does not regenerate. A monomeric or atrophic eardrum is visible otoscopically, and in some cases, is so thin that it is difficult to differentiate from a perforation unless the eardrum is placed under pressure during pneumatic otoscopy or tympanometry.

In tympanosclerosis, an inflammatory process in the middle ear produces calcified plaques in the middle-ear space and on the medial surface of the eardrum (Forseni et al., 1997). With involved cases affecting the middle-ear space, conductive hearing loss can result that can be challenging to treat surgically. In severe cases, tympanoplasty with or without ossiculoplasty may be required (Bayazit et al., 2004). Frequently, however, tympanosclerotic plaques are a sequela of middle-ear disease in childhood, and are of little medical consequence in adulthood.

Figure 9.9C shows tympanograms from DJC, a 27-year-old male with a history of COM until age 7. During childhood, he was treated with multiple myringotomies without

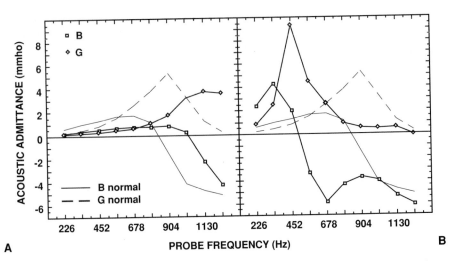

FIGURE 9.10 Peak $200B_{tm}$ (*open squares*) and $200G_{tm}$ (*open diamonds*) as a function of probe-tone frequency from a patient with otosclerosis (**A**) and from a patient with ossicular discontinuity (**B**). For comparison, normal $200B_{tm}$ and $200G_{tm}$ functions are shown in both panels by the solid and dashed lines, respectively.

tympanostomy tubes (TT). Children with a history of TT in childhood, whether or not atrophic scarring is obvious during otoscopy, tend to have higher than average $200Y_{tm}$ in adulthood (de Beer et al., 2005). At age 20, DJC dove into a swimming pool and perforated the left eardrum, which healed spontaneously. Otoscopy revealed atrophic scarring in the posterior-superior quadrant of the left eardrum; no significant conductive component was measured.

Panel C shows mass-controlled tympanograms typical of an ear with eardrum pathology. Y_{tm} at 226 Hz is abnormally high (>4.0 acoustic mmho) and exceeded the upper range of the equipment. At 678 Hz, the tympanograms are mass controlled and irregular as they were in the two cases of ossicular discontinuity. The main difference in tympanogram morphology in cases with ossicular discontinuity versus eardrum pathology is the TW or notch width. 226 Hz TW typically is narrower in ears with eardrum pathology in comparison with ossicular discontinuity. Although all three tympanograms in this figure are abnormally mass controlled at 678 Hz, the pressure interval between the outermost susceptance extrema is abnormal in ossicular discontinuity (>125 daPa) but normal (80 daPa) in the ear with eardrum pathology. Similar tympanogram patterns are recorded from ears that have undergone stapedectomy or stapedotomy for surgical treatment of otosclerosis (Colletti, 1976; Colletti et al., 1993; Liden et al., 1970). Audiometry, case history, and otoscopy are crucial in differentiating eardrum pathology and post-surgical ears from ossicular discontinuity.

Feldman (1974) revealed an important consequence of eardrum pathology: high-admittance eardrum pathology can completely mask a more central low-admittance pathology. In an ear with ossicular fixation and eardrum pathology, for example, the high admittance eardrum will completely dominate tympanometry measures and mask the effect of ossicular fixation. [See Margolis (1981) for a discussion of input impedances in parallel versus series circuits.] The importance of otoscopy in interpreting tympanograms cannot be overstated.

OTOSCLEROSIS VERSUS OSSICULAR DISCONTINUITY

Figures 9.8B and 9.9A showed 226 and 678 Hz tympanograms in patients with otosclerosis and ossicular discontinuity. Figure 9.10 shows an alternative analysis of peak compensated static acoustic admittance at 10 frequencies in these same two ears. Peak $200B_{tm}$ (squares) and $200G_{tm}$ (diamonds) as a function of frequency are displayed for DK with otosclerosis (Panel A) and RP with ossicular discontinuity (Panel B). For comparison, $200B_{tm}$ and $200G_{tm}$ functions from the normal 40 year old depicted in Figures 9.4 to 9.6 are shown in both panels by the solid and dashed lines, respectively. Two points on the functions that are easy to compare are the frequencies corresponding to phase angles of 45° and 0° (resonance). Recall that the admittance vector is at 45° when $200B_{tm}$ and $200G_{tm}$ are equal, i.e., the frequency where the two-component functions cross near 580 Hz. Resonance (f_o) occurs when mass and stiffness susceptance are equal in magnitude and sum to 0 acoustic mmho, i.e., the frequency where the B functions cross the zero axis near 850 Hz. In contrast, the ear with otosclerosis in Panel A remained stiffness controlled over a broader frequency range than normal. This is reflected in higher frequencies for both the 45° point (~700 Hz) and resonance (~1020 Hz). When plotted in this format, the results show that the ear with otosclerosis (Fig. 9.10A) is more clearly separated from the normal ear at high probe frequencies, and that the separation is smallest for the most commonly used probe frequency of 226 Hz.

In contrast to otosclerosis, the ear with ossicular discontinuity (Fig. 9.10B) is mass controlled at a *lower* than normal frequency. The 45° point occurred near 345 Hz and resonance occurred near 500 Hz. There is clear differentiation between otosclerosis with an f_o of 1020 Hz and disarticulation with an f_o of 500 Hz.

Although the ear with the monomeric eardrum in Figure 9.9C is not shown in Figure 9.10, his B_{tm} and G_{tm} functions are indistinguishable from the ear with ossicular discontinuity. This demonstrates a strong advantage of recording tympanograms rather than only one point (peak) from the tympanogram. Even a cursory glance at tympanogram shapes at 678 Hz differentiates all three patients from normal in Figure 9.9, with no calculation needed. When only peak compensated static acoustic admittance is plotted, the shape of the tympanogram and broadness of the notching is lost. Notch width is particularly important and helps to differentiate between an ear with eardrum pathology and one with ossicular discontinuity. As subsequent examples will show, the width and depth of the notch in 678 Hz tympanograms is relied on to differentiate between normal and abnormal mass-controlled ears.

Otitis Externa

Another example of mass-related pathology that can have a marked effect on high-frequency tympanometry, but little effect on hearing, is otitis externa (OE). Ear-canal infections, or OE, often occur in hearing-aid wearers or after water exposure, giving rise to the lay term "swimmer's ear." Common OE presents with significant otalgia, particularly with manipulation of the pinna. Moist, edematous skin with squamous debris or purulent material typically is evident with otoscopy (see examples in Ballachanda, 1995; Hawke and McCombe, 1995; Kavanagh, 2006; Sullivan, 2006). Bacteria are the most common infecting agent, although fungus is often found in chronic cases. Chronic dermatologic conditions of the external auditory canal skin can give rise to itching and occasionally acute infection. A history of trauma, either with a fingertip or Q-tip, preceding the infection often is elicited. Treatment is with appropriate ototopical antibiotics, occasionally with the addition of steroids, as well as water precautions, and pain medications. Diabetic patients with OE require medical referral. These patients may develop a more aggressive form of OE, malignant OE, in which the infection extends beyond the soft tissues of the ear canal and into the surrounding bone. Skull-base osteomyelitis is a sequela and often causes cranial-nerve deficits and even death if not treated expeditiously.

Figure 9.11A shows tympanograms from MR, a 49-year-old male swimmer who reported recurrent otalgia and discharge from his right ear over the past 2 years. Otoscopy revealed otitis externa with greenish discharge in the ear canal and against the eardrum. The audiogram in the inset shows a definite mass tilt. The 226 Hz tympanogram has a $200Y_{tm}$ of 0.35 acoustic mmho with a broad TW. This tympanogram demonstrates a problem encountered in calculating TW from asymmetric tympanograms. In this example, the negative tail never quite reaches the one-half peak value so TW cannot be calculated. The 678 Hz tympanogram shows a shallow, mass-controlled 5B3G pattern with an abnormal notch width in excess of 100 daPa. This pattern is typical of a mass-loaded eardrum and indicates that the discharge is against the eardrum.

Figure 9.11B shows another case of abnormal mass. These tympanograms were recorded from a 76-year-old male (JP) who was seen the day before for earmold impressions.

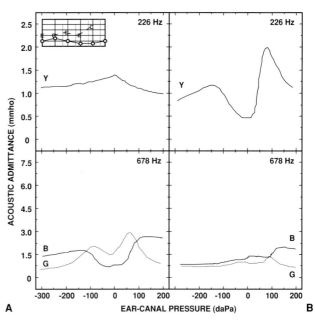

FIGURE 9.11 Susceptance (B), conductance (G), and admittance (Y) tympanograms at 226 Hz (*top panels*) and 678 Hz (bottom panels) recorded from MR with otitis externa and debris against the eardrum (**A**) and from JP with blood filling the ear canal (**B**); the audiogram for MR is shown in the inset but no audiogram was available for JP.

The patient returned to the clinic the next day and reported that on the drive home from his appointment, he noted bleeding from his right ear. Otoscopy showed fresh blood filling much of the ear canal and obscuring a view of the eardrum. Tympanometry was completed to document the status of the eardrum. The 226 Hz acoustic admittance tympanogram shows a V_{ea} of 1.1 cm^3 and verified an intact eardrum. What is so unusual in this case is that the 226 Hz tympanogram was broadly notched and mass controlled; notching typically is recorded only at high-probe frequencies. This patient was immediately referred to ENT. Examination under a microscope revealed bleeding along the inferior, lateral wall of the ear canal; the lesion was cauterized with AgNO.

Otitis Media

Otitis media (OM) associated with immature Eustachian tubes is the most common illness among children receiving medical care. Acute OM presents with otalgia and fever whereas COM presents with a conductive hearing loss and aural fullness. Otoscopy findings can range from bulging, erythematous eardrums with purulence in the middle ear to retracted, opaque eardrums with air-fluid levels or even bubbles in the middle ear. Recurrent or persistent disease is often an indication for myringotomy with TT. Acute OM is more appropriately treated with observation if it is non-suppurative, but is treated with antibiotics if fever and purulent material are noted in the middle ear.

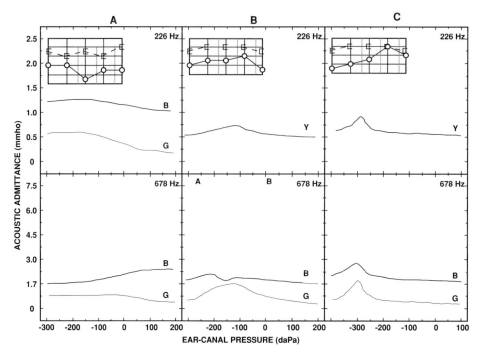

FIGURE 9.12 Susceptance (B), conductance (G), and admittance (Y) tympanograms at 226 Hz (*top panels*) and 678 Hz (*bottom panels*) recorded during three stages of otitis media, SC with a fluid-filled middle ear in Panel **A**; and CC with resolving, low level middle-ear fluid in Panel **B**, improving to resolution of middle-ear fluid with a slightly retracted eardrum in Panel **C**. The corresponding audiograms are shown as insets.

An adult who presents with a chronic serous otitis media should be evaluated for nasopharyngeal pathology. Masses in the nasopharynx can exert extrinsic pressure on the Eustachian tube and cause obstruction. Careful endoscopic examination or imaging can help to rule out significant pathology. Adults having undergone radiation therapy to the head and neck, especially the nasopharynx, parotid, or temporal bone often develop chronic serous otitis media as a result of deleterious effects on the Eustachian tube by the radiation therapy. Treatment often consists of placement of a TT.

Figure 9.12A shows tympanograms recorded from SC, a 6-year-old male with a history of bilateral MEE. Although this tympanogram pattern typically is described as flat with a normal V_{ea} of 1.0 cm³, the B_a and G_a tympanograms have a distinctive sloping pattern. Feldman (1976b) describes this tympanogram pattern, which is indicative of MEE, as "converging 220 Hz and 660 Hz susceptance tympanograms", (p. 126). That is, the 226 Hz tympanograms rise and the 678 Hz tympanograms fall with decreasing pressures. Berry et al. (1975) reported that this distinctive sloping pattern at 660 Hz was indicative of effusion in 100% of the ears. They further concluded that 660 Hz tympanometry was a better indicator of MEE than 220 Hz.

Figure 9.12B and 9.12C show tympanograms recorded from my daughter CC when she was four years old. She had a cold and fever and briefly complained of an earache. All symptoms resolved within a few days. A short time later, her pediatrician saw her for a preschool check up and noted

that she had fluid in her right ear. She not only had flat tympanograms similar to those in Panel A, but she also had 45–55 dB air-bone gaps in the right ear; her left ear was normal. Although her hearing improved slightly and air-bone gaps decreased to 25 dB, her tympanograms remained flat for several months. After four months with no resolution of the fluid, she was scheduled to have TT. A few days prior to the scheduled surgery, the tympanograms shown in Figure 9.13B were recorded. The 226 Hz tympanogram was abnormally stiff (<0.3 acoustic mmho) with an abnormally wide TW (>250 daPa). The 678 Hz tympanograms indicated that finally there was some air in the middle-ear space, although fluid still was present as evidenced by the shallow, broadly notched 678 Hz tympanograms and by the conductive hearing loss greatest in the high-frequency range. Two weeks later, the tympanograms shown in the Figure 9.12C were recorded. Note that the hearing loss improved in the high frequencies, indicating resolution of the mass-loading fluid. Negative pressure of −300 daPa was present, resulting in small low-frequency air-bone gaps, but the amplitude of the tympanogram at 226 Hz was normal and the amplitude relationship between susceptance and conductance at 678 Hz was normal, i.e., $200G_{tm}$ was greater than $200B_{tm}$ and phase angle was <45°. Both the audiogram and tympanograms in Figure 9.12C indicate that the pathology was strictly negative middle-ear pressure with no significant fluid.

Caution, however, must be taken in inferring etiology when interpreting tympanograms. Flat tympanograms with

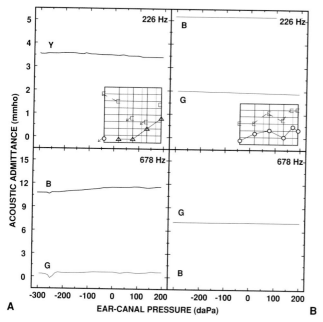

FIGURE 9.13 Susceptance (B), conductance (G), and admittance (Y) tympanograms at 226 Hz (*top panels*) and 678 Hz (*bottom panels*) recorded from AD with a perforated eardrum following ear lavage in an ear with a history of chronic otitis media and multiple TT (Panel **A**), and from BH with a traumatic eardrum perforation from a high-powered squirt gun (Panel **B**).

normal volumes are not always indicative of middle-ear effusion. Other causes of flat tympanograms include a thickened eardrum, malleus fixation, and middle-ear tumors that are discussed in a subsequent section. In other words, if the motion of the eardrum is completely restricted for any reason, the tympanograms will be flat.

Eardrum Perforation

Eardrum perforation can result as a complication of OM, from trauma, or from extruded TT. Historically, there has been little agreement on the relationship between the size and location of an eardrum perforation and the degree and configuration of hearing loss. With the exception of trauma, eardrum perforation rarely occurs as an isolated pathology. When perforation occurs as a sequela of OM, for example, other middle-ear structures such as the ossicles, middle-ear space, and mastoid air cell system also are involved and contribute to the magnitude of the conductive component. Most studies, however, do agree that the larger the perforation, the larger the air-bone gaps (Voss et al., 2001).

At least four different tympanogram patterns have been recorded from ears with eardrum perforation. Figure 9.13A shows tympanograms from AD, a 19-year-old male with a history of COM and multiple TT as a child. He reported to the clinic with a large, 40% posterior-inferior perforation of the right eardrum that occurred following cerumen removal by

lavage. When a flat tympanogram is recorded, the first observation should be the V_{ea} at 200 daPa. Remember from the calibration discussion that the volume of an enclosed cavity can be represented as pure acoustic compliance, and therefore, is most accurately estimated using a low-frequency probe tone such as 226 Hz. Also recall that an ideal hard walled cavity has $G_a = 0$ acoustic mmho, and therefore, V_{ea} will be the same whether estimated from a B_a or Y_a tympanogram. In this example, a V_{ea} of 3.5 cm^3 was estimated from 200Y_a. When the eardrum is perforated, the volume is comprised of the ear canal, the middle-ear space, and the mastoid air cell system. $V_{ea} > 2.5$ cm^3 in an adult male is consistent with eardrum perforation.

Tympanograms in Figure 9.13A are typical of those recorded in ears with a history of COM. V_{ea} estimated at both 226 and 678 Hz are similar to those measured in calibration cavities. V_{ea} estimated from the 678 Hz B_a tympanogram at 200 daPa is 3.7 cm^3 (i.e., 11.1 acoustic mmho divided by 3) and is essentially equal to the corresponding volume estimate of 3.5 cm^3 at 226 Hz. Conductance at 678 Hz is close to 0 acoustic mmho. In other words, this ear functioned like a calibration cavity (refer to Figure 9.1). This finding most likely occurs because the mastoid air cell system is poorly aerated in ears with COM. That is, the mastoid air cell system is functionally shut off from the rest of the middle ear so that the volume of the ear canal plus the middle-ear space closely resembles a hard walled cavity with a uniform cross-sectional area.

In contrast, Figure 9.13B depicts a traumatic eardrum perforation in BH, a 30-year-old male who was hit in the ear with water from a high powered squirt gun. Otologic exam showed a 50% perforation in the posterior-inferior quadrant. The inset audiogram shows a flat 25 dB conductive component. At 226 Hz, the B_a tympanogram was flat and exceeded equipment limits (i.e., >7 acoustic mmho) and G_a was flat at 2 acoustic mmho. This ear did not function like a calibration cavity, particularly at the high-probe frequency. At 678 Hz, B_a in a hard-walled cavity is three times greater than at 226 Hz, and G_a remains at 0 acoustic mmho. The 678 Hz B_a and G_a tympanograms in this ear, however, are the opposite of readings expected in a hard-walled cavity. The B_a tympanogram in this perforated ear was flat and off scale in the *negative* direction, and the G_a tympanogram was flat at 7.0 acoustic mmho.

This "atypical" pattern first was noted in 1982 when recording tympanograms with an Otolaryngology resident on a normal temporal bone following perforation of the eardrum. This pattern can only be seen if the two rectangular components of acoustic admittance are recorded and would not have appeared out of the ordinary if only Y_a had been recorded. Recall that Y_a is always larger than the larger of the two rectangular components (B_a and G_a), so the tympanogram would mirror the G_a tympanogram rather than the B_a tympanogram as typically occurs. The maximum susceptance reading at 226 Hz indicates that the volume being measured is very large. The minimum susceptance reading at 678 Hz indicates that the volume being measured cannot be modeled as pure acoustic compliance. In an ear with a traumatic eardrum perforation, the volume being estimated is comprised of the ear canal, the middle-ear space, and narrow aditus leading to the mastoid air cell system. This combined volume does not begin to approximate a volume with a uniform cross-sectional area. These irregular cavities and narrow aditus introduce mass and resistance, and therefore, make an accurate estimate of volume impossible, particularly when using high-frequency probe tones.

This atypical tympanogram pattern is indicative of a "healthy" middle-ear transmission system and functional mastoid air cell system. Ears with large middle-ear volumes and a large, communicating mastoid air cell system have a better prognosis for successful tympanoplasty and less chance for recurrence of middle-ear disease and post-surgical complications than patients with small volumes (Andreasson, 1977; Holmquist, 1970; Holmquist and Bergstrom, 1977; Lindeman and Holmquist, 1982).

A second "bizarre" tympanogram pattern also was identified while making recordings on temporal bones. The question posed by a resident was, how large does a perforation have to be to result in a flat tympanogram? The resident made a tiny hole in the eardrum, decided it was too large, and then used a needle to rough up the edges of the perforation and draw them closer together. Surprisingly, the tympanogram, which was recorded from 200 daPa to −300 daPa, was not flat, but had a normal peak at an extreme *positive* pressure of 150 daPa. When the direction of the recording was reversed, the peak shifted to an extreme *negative* pressure of −250 daPa. When a high positive pressure is applied to an ear with a small perforation, the pressure stresses the perforation and allows positive pressure to momentarily flow into the middle-ear space. Similarly, an extreme negative starting pressure again stresses the perforation and allows negative pressure to enter the middle ear space. See Figure 12.7 in Fowler and Shanks (2002) for an example of this tympanogram pattern. Be alert to the presence of pinhole perforations. If a significant positive TPP is recorded, it is a simple matter to reverse directions and record a Y 226 Hz tympanogram using ascending pressures to rule out the presence of a pinhole perforation.

Middle Ear Tumors

Flat tympanograms also can be recorded from ears with middle-ear masses or tumors. Two examples are cholesteatoma with or without eardrum perforation and glomus tumor. The shape of the tympanograms is dependent on how much eardrum movement is restricted.

CHOLESTEATOMA

Cholesteatoma is a disorder characterized by squamous (skin) epithelium being trapped in the middle ear or mastoid. It can occur as a sequela of chronic suppurative otitis media by a migration of squamous epithelium from the ear

canal through an eardrum perforation, or from a deep retraction of the pars flaccida or other weakened area of the eardrum as a result of chronic Eustachian tube dysfunction. Cholesteatoma also can arise congenitally by means of an epithelial rest of tissue being trapped behind the eardrum during embryologic development (Shohet and de Jong, 2002). In either event, cholesteatoma has locally invasive properties and can destroy adjacent bone including the ossicles, middle and posterior fossa dura plates, and the bony labyrinth. A bacterial superinfection amplifies the destructive properties of a cholesteatoma and can present as chronic otorrhea refractory to antibiotics; it is usually painless. The treatment is surgical resection with a tympanoplasty or tympanomastoidectomy procedure and has a recurrence rate of between 30% and 50%.

Figure 9.14A shows the fourth tympanogram pattern that can be recorded from an ear with a perforated eardrum. BM is a 62-year-old male referred for pre-operative testing prior to undergoing a tympanomastoidectomy in the left ear. He had a history of eardrum perforation and COM, accompanied by periodic drainage for more than 20 years. His audiogram showed a maximum low-frequency conductive hearing loss with decreasing air-bone gaps with increasing frequency. Surgical findings revealed a cholesteatoma filling the middle-ear space and extending into the attic. The malleus was eroded and the incus was absent. The

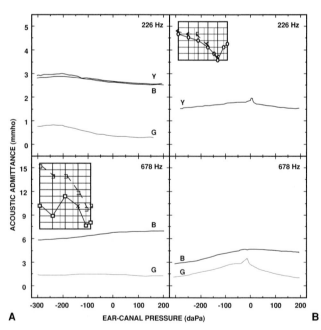

FIGURE 9.14 Susceptance (B), conductance (G), and admittance (Y) tympanograms at 226 Hz (*top panels*) and 678 Hz (*bottom panels*) recorded from BM with a perforated eardrum and cholesteatoma filling the middle-ear space and extending into the attic (Panel A) and from MC with a pulsating glomus tumor visible behind the eardrum (Panel B).

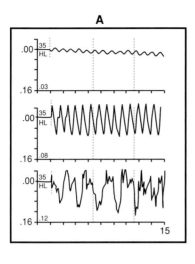
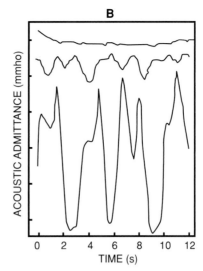

FIGURE 9.15   Changes in acoustic admittance at TPP recorded over 12-15 s in the acoustic reflex mode with the acoustic reflex stimulus at a minimum. The top trace in Panel A shows normal vascular perturbations, the middle trace shows high-magnitude vascular perturbations in MC with the glomus tumor in Figure 9.14B, and the bottom trace shows very large perturbations coincident with breathing in a patient with a patulous Eustachian tube. Panel B shows three tracing from RE with a patulous Eustachian tube. The top trace was recorded while holding his breath, the middle trace while breathing normally, and the bottom trace during forced, closed mouth breathing.

cholesteatoma was removed and ossicular reconstruction was planned for a second surgery. Y_a, B_a and G_a tympanograms at 226 and B_a and G_a tympanograms at 678 Hz are shown in Figure 9.14A. V_{ea} estimated from either the 226 Hz Y_a or B_a tympanogram was 2.5 cm^3 and was at the upper range for normal ear-canal volume in adult males. Although BM had a known eardrum perforation, the cholesteatoma filled the middle-ear space and effectively cut off the middle ear from the ear canal. This is not an uncommon finding with chronic middle-ear disease and serves as a caution when interpreting flat tympanograms. A flat tympanogram with a 226 Hz volume estimate exceeding 1.0 cm^3 in children <7 years of age and exceeding 2.5 cm^3 in adults indicates a perforated eardrum or patent TT, but a flat tympanogram with a normal V_{ea} does not necessarily rule out a perforated eardrum. Tympanometry in conjunction with otoscopy and an otologic exam, however, can be informative and alert the examiner to a space-occupying lesion.

GLOMUS TUMOR

Glomus tumors or paragangliomas are typically benign tumors derived from supporting nerve tissue around the jugular bulb or in the middle ear. Although approximately 95% of glomus tumors are benign and slow growing, they are highly vascular and invasive. Patients often present with pulsatile tinnitus and with conductive or complete hearing loss in approximately 61% of the patients (Manolidis et al., 1999). Otoscopy may reveal a red mass behind the tympanic membrane. Because of their location, these tumors can cause significant morbidity including difficulties swallowing and phonating. Treatment is usually surgical resection, although radiation

therapy may be reserved for patients unable to undergo a prolonged surgical procedure.

MC is a 72-year-old female who complained of aural fullness and a muffled quality to sound in her right ear for the past month. She also had roaring, pulsating tinnitus with vertigo and nausea. Otoscopy revealed a pulsating mass behind the right eardrum. A subsequent MRI showed a 2.4-cm mass in the right temporal bone extending into the right middle ear. Only minimal low-frequency air-bone gaps were measured. The tympanograms displayed in Figure 9.14B were atypical with low normal Y_{tm} at 226 Hz and restricted TW, but the recordings did not reflect the pulsating eardrum noted on otoscopic exam. Others have reported tympanograms in ears with glomus tumors ranging from flat to pulsatile (see Fig. 6.17 in Feldman, 1976b).

In this case, the pulsation was detected when the instrument was put in the AR mode. The AR mode can be used as a very sensitive extension of tympanometry. With the acoustic-reflex stimulus turned off during tone-decay testing, static acoustic admittance at TPP can be measured over time, typically 12 to 15 seconds. Figure 9.15 shows two applications of the AR mode. The top trace in Panel A shows normal vascular perturbations. The rate of oscillation in the top trace is 56 beats per minute and indicates a slight vascular change. The second trace was recorded from MC who complained of pulsatile tinnitus associated with the glomus tumor. When switched to the more sensitive AR mode, the vascular pulsation became very obvious and was greater in magnitude than normally recorded. In contrast to the vascular changes in the top two traces, the bottom trace of Figure 9.15A shows perturbations coincident with breathing in another patient with a patulous Eustachian tube.

Patulous Eustachian Tube

While most Eustachian tube (ET) dysfunction involves a ET that does not open properly, a patulous ET is one that remains open. Movement of the eardrum coincident with breathing can sometimes be detected during otoscopy or noted during tympanometry and AR testing. Patients sometimes complain of aural fullness and autophonia, a sensation of hearing one's own voice louder than normal, although in many cases, the patient is symptom free. Patulous Eustachian tube occurs in approximately 7% of adults and frequently is misdiagnosed as OM because of the similarity in symptoms (Henry and DiBartolomeo, 1993). Precipitating factors include sudden weight loss, inappropriate use of decongestants, and fatigue. Some cases of patulous ET are transient and self-resolving. In persistent cases, treatment is challenging and not always effective. Several methods have been proposed to make the diagnosis, including video endoscopy of the nasopharyngeal opening of the ET and even audiometry of tones presented in the nasal cavity (Kano et al., 2004; Poe et al., 2001; Virtanen and Palva, 1982). The easiest method, however, is a tympanometry procedure that takes advantage of increased instrument sensitivity in the acoustic-reflex mode (Finkelstein et al., 1988; Henry and DiBartolomeo, 1993).

Figure 9.15B shows RE, a 40-year-old male who complained of decreased hearing in both ears and a constant, mild headache for the past 3 to 4 months. Perturbations coincident with respiration were noted when attempting to measure AR thresholds. To verify patulous Eustachian tube, three traces were obtained at peak admittance with the reflex stimulus turned off. The top flat trace was recorded with RE holding his breath. The second trace was obtained during normal breathing, and the third trace was recorded during forced breathing with the mouth closed. Four to six large perturbations should be recorded during the 12- to 15-s time window. Occasionally, movement of the eardrum coincident with respiration can be noted otoscopically. One case encountered with a patulous Eustachian tube had a large atrophic area on the eardrum that moved in and out with normal respiration. That patient had no aural complaints and was not treated.

■ SUMMARY AND CONCLUSIONS

Universal hearing screening has had a positive impact on tympanometry and has focused renewed attention on high frequency measurements. Hopefully, the reader will finally be convinced of the power of high-frequency and MFT tympanometry in evaluating middle-ear disease. In almost every case, pathology that is either absent of subtle at 226 Hz is accentuated at 678 Hz or 1000 Hz. Prepare for the next generation of measurements by utilizing the MFT options already available on commercial instruments and realizing their advantages and applications.

■ REFERENCES

American Academy of Audiology. (1997) Identification of hearing loss & middle-ear dysfunction in preschool & school-age children. *Audiol Today.* 9, 21–23.

American National Standards Institute. (1987) Specifications for instruments to measure aural acoustic impedance and admittance (aural acoustic immittance). ANSI S3.39–1987. New York: American National Standards Institute.

American Speech-Language-Hearing Association. (1979) Guidelines for acoustic immittance screening of middle-ear function. *ASHA.* 21, 283–288.

American Speech-Language-Hearing Association. (1990) Guidelines for screening for hearing impairment and middle-ear disorders. *ASHA.* 32, 17–32.

American Speech-Language-Hearing Association. (1997) Guidelines for audiologic screening. Rockville MD: American Speech-Language-Hearing Association.

Alberti P, Jerger J. (1974) Probe-tone frequency and the diagnostic value of tympanometry. *Arch Otolaryn.* 99, 206–210.

Andreasson L. (1977) Correlation of tubal function and volume of mastoid and middle ear space as related to otitis media. *Acta Otolaryn.* 83, 29–33.

Andreasson L, Harris S. (1979) Middle ear mechanics and Eustachian tube function in tympanoplasty. *Acta Otolaryngol.* 360, 141–147.

Antonio SM, Don D, Doyle WJ, Alper CM. (2002) Daily home tympanometry to study the pathogenesis of otitis media. *Pediatr Infect Dis J.* 21, 882–885.

Ars B. (1989) Organogenesis of the middle ear structures. *J Laryng Otol.* 103, 16–21.

Babu S, Seidman MD. (2004) Ossicular reconstruction using bone cement. *Otol Neurotol.* 25, 98–101.

Ballachanda BB. (1995) The Human Ear Canal: Theoretical Considerations and Clinical Applications Including Cerumen Management. San Diego: Singular Publishing Group.

Bayazit YA, Ozer E, Kara C, Gokpinar S, Kanlikama M, Mumbuc S. (2004) An analysis of the single-stage tympanoplasty with over-underlay grafting in tympanosclerosis. *Otol Neurotol.* 25, 211–214.

Bel J, Causse J, Michaux P. (1975) Paradoxical compliances in otosclerosis. *Audiology.* 14, 118–129.

Bennett M. (1975) Acoustic impedance bridge measurements with the neonate. *Brit J Audiol.* 9, 117–124.

Bennett MJ, Weatherby LA. (1979) Multiple probe frequency acoustic reflex measurements. *Scand Audiol.* 8, 233–239.

Bentler RA. (1989) External ear resonance characteristics in children. *J Speech Hear Res.* 54, 264–268.

Beranek LL. (1954) *Acoustics.* New York: McGraw-Hill.

Berry QC, Andrus WS, Bluestone CD, Cantekin EI. (1975) Tympanometric pattern classification in relation to middle ear effusion. *Ann Otol.* 84, 56–63.

Blood I, Greenberg HJ. (1977) Acoustic admittance of the ear in the geriatric person. *J Am Aud Soc.* 2, 185–187.

Bluestone CD. (2004) Studies in otitis media: Children's Hospital of Pittsburgh-University of Pittsburgh progress report-2004. *Laryngoscope.* 114: 1–26.

Brooks DN. (1968) An objective method of determining fluid in the middle ear. *Int Audiol.* 7, 280–286.

Brooks DN. (1969) The use of the electro-impedance bridge in the assessment of middle ear function. *Int Audiol*. 8, 563–565.

Burke K, Nilges T. (1970) A comparison of three middle ear impedance norms as predictors of otosclerosis. *J Aud Res*. 10, 52–58.

Calandruccio L, Fitzgerald TS, Prieve BA. (2006) Normative multifrequency tympanometry in infants and toddlers. *J Am Acad Audiol*. 17, 470–480.

Carhart R. (1962) Effects of stapes fixation on bone-conduction response. In: Otosclerosis. Boston: Little & Brown, 175–197.

Cherukupally SR, Merchant SN, Rosowski JJ. (1998) Correlations between pathologic changes in the stapes and conductive hearing loss in otosclerosis. *Ann Otol Rhinol Laryngol*. 107, 319–326.

Chesnutt B, Stream RW, Love JT, McLarey DC. (1975) Otoadmittance measures in cases of dual ossicular disorders. *Arch Otolaryn*. 101, 109–113.

Chole RA, McKenna M. (2001) Pathophysiology of otosclerosis. *Otol Neurotol*. 22, 249–257.

Ciardo A, Garavello W, Leva M, Graziano B, Gaini RM (2005) Reversed ipsilateral acoustic reflex: A study on subjects treated with muscle relaxants. *Ear Hear*. 26, 96–103.

Colletti V. (1975) Methodological observations on tympanometry with regard to the probe tone frequency. *Acta Otolaryn*. 80, 54–60.

Colletti V. (1976) Tympanometry from 200 to 2000 Hz probe tone. *Audiology*. 15, 106–119.

Colletti V. (1977) Multifrequency tympanometry. *Audiology*. 16, 278–287.

Colletti V, Fiorino FG, Sittoni V, Policante A. (1993) Mechanics of the middle ear in otosclerosis and stapedoplasty. *Acta Otolarngol*. 113, 637–641.

Creten WL, Van Camp KJ. (1974) Transient and quasi-static tympanometry. *Scand Audiol*. 3, 39–42.

Creten WL, Van de Heyning PH, Van Camp KJ. (1985) Immittance audiometry: Normative data at 220 and 660 Hz. *Scand Audiol*. 14, 115–121.

de Beer B, Snik A, Schilder A, Graamans K, Zielhuis GA. (2005) The effect of otitis media in childhood on the development of middle ear admittance on reaching adulthood. *Arch Otolaryngol Head Neck Surg*. 131, 777–781.

De Chicchis AR, Todd NW, Nozza RJ. (2000) Developmental changes in aural acoustic admittance measurements. *J Am Acad Audiol*. 11, 97–102.

Decraemer WF, Creten WL, Van Camp KJ. (1984) Tympanometric middle ear pressure determination with two component admittance meters. *Scand Audiol*. 13. 165–172.

Dieroff HG. (1978) Differential diagnostic value of tympanometry in adhesive processes and otosclerosis. *Audiol*. 17, 77–86.

de Jonge R. (1986) Normal tympanometric gradient: A comparison of three methods. *Audiol*. 25, 299–308.

Diamant M. (1965) The "pathologic size" of the mastoid air cell system. *Acta Otolaryn*. 60, 1–10.

Dolan K. (1979) Mastoid pneumatization. In: Sade J, ed. Secretory otitis media and its sequelae. New York: Churchill Livingstone, 298–314.

Eavey RD. (1993) Abnormalities of the neonatal ear: Otoscopic observations, histological observations, and a model for contamination of the middle ear by cellular contents of amniotic fluid. *Laryngoscope*. 103, 1–31.

Eby T, Nadol J. (1986) Postnatal growth of the human temporal bone: Implication for cochlear implants in children. *Ann Otol Rhinol Laryngol*. 95, 356–364.

Eliachar I, Northern JL. (1974) Studies in tympanometry: Validation of the present technique for determining intra-tympanic pressures through the intact eardrum. *Laryngoscope*. 84, 247–255.

Elner A, Ingelstedt S, Ivarsson A. (1971) The elastic properties of the tympanic membrane. *Acta Otolaryng*. 72, 397–403.

Feldman AS. (1974) Eardrum abnormality and the measurement of middle-ear function. *Arch Otolaryn*. 99, 211–217.

Feldman AS. (1976a) Tympanometry: Application and interpretation. *Ann Otol Rhinol Laryngol*. 85, 202–208.

Feldman AS. (1976b) Tympanometry–procedures, interpretations and variables. In: Feldman AS, Wilbur LA, eds. Acoustic Impedance and Admittance: The Measurement of Middle Ear Function. Baltimore: Williams & Wilkins, 103–155.

Ferekidis E, Vlachou S, Douniadakis D, Apostolopoulos N, Adamopoulos G. (1999) Multiple-frequency tympanometry in children with acute otitis media. *Otolaryn-Head Neck Surg*. 121, 797–801.

Fiellau-Nikolajsen M. (1983) Tympanometry and secretory otitis media. Observations on diagnosis, epidemiology, treatment, and prevention in prospective cohort studies of three-year-old children. *Acta Otolaryn Suppl*. 394, 1–73.

Finkelstein Y, Talmi Y, Rubel Y, Zohar Y. (1988) An objective method for evaluation of the patulous Eustachian tube by using the middle ear analyzer. *Arch Otolaryn*. 114, 1134–1138.

Fisch U. (1980) Tympanoplasty and Stapedectomy. A manual of techniques. New York: Thieme-Stratton.

Flisberg K, Ingelstedt S, Ortegren U. (1963) On middle ear pressure. *Acta Otolaryng*. 182, 43–56.

Forseni M, Eriksson A, Bagger-Sjoback D, Nilsson J, Hultcrantz M. (1997) Development of tympanosclerosis: Can predicting factors be identified? *Am J Otol*. 18, 298–303.

Fowler CG, Shanks JE. (2002) Tympanometry. In: Katz J, ed. Handbook of Clinical Audiology. Baltimore: Lippincott Williams & Wilkins: 175–204.

Funasaka S, Funai H, Kumakawa K. (1984) Sweep-frequency tympanometry: Its development and diagnostic value. *Audiology*. 23, 366–379.

Funasaka S, Kumakawa K. (1988) Tympanometry using a sweep-frequency probe tone and its clinical evaluation. *Audiology*. 27, 99–108.

Haapaniemi JJ. (1996) Immittance findings in school-aged children. *Ear Hear*. 17, 19–27.

Hanks WD, Mortensen BA. (1997) Multifrequency tympanometry: effects of ear canal volume compensation on middle ear resonance. *J Am Acad Audiol*. 8, 53–58.

Hanks WD, Rose KJ. (1993) Middle ear resonance and acoustic immittance measures in children. *J Speech Hear Res*. 36, 218–222.

Haughton P. (1977) Validity of tympanometry for middle ear effusions. *Arch Otolaryn*. 103, 505–513.

Hawke M, McCombe A. (1995) Diseases of the Ear: A Pocket Atlas. Ontario, Canada: Manticore Communication.

Henry DF, DiBartolomeo JR. (1993) Patulous Eustachian tube identification using tympanometry. *J Am Acad Audiol*. 4, 53–57.

Himelfarb MZ, Popelka GR, Shanon E. (1979) Tympanometry in normal neonates. *J Speech Hear Res*. 22, 179–191.

Hirsch JE, Margolis RH, Rykken JR. (1992) Comparison of acoustic reflex and auditory brain stem response screening of high-risk infants. *Ear Hear*. 13, 181–186.

Holmquist J. (1970) Size of mastoid air cell system in relation to healing after myringoplasty and to Eustachian tube function. *Acta Otolaryn*. 69, 89–93.

Holmquist J, Bergstrom B. (1977) Eustachian tube function and size of the mastoid air cell system in middle ear surgery. *Scand Audiol*. 6, 87–89.

Holte L. (1996) Aging effects in multifrequency tympanometry. *Ear Hear*. 17, 12–18.

Holte L, Margolis RH, Cavanaugh RM. (1991) Developmental changes in multifrequency tympanograms. *Audiol*. 30, 1–24.

Ikarashi H, Nakano Y. (1988) Relation between the onset of chronic middle ear inflammation and the development of the middle ear air cell system. *J Otorhinolaryngol Relat Spec*. 50, 306–312.

Ivey R. (1975) Tympanometric curves and otosclerosis. *J Speech Hear Res*. 18, 554–558.

Jackler RK, Schindler RA. (1984) Role of the mastoid in tympanic membrane reconstruction. *Laryng*. 94, 495–500.

Jacobson JT, Mahoney TM. (1977) Admittance tympanometry in otosclerotic ears. *J Am Aud Soc.* 3, 91–98.

Jerger J. (1970) Clinical experience with impedance audiometry. *Arch Otolaryn.* 92, 311–324.

Jerger J, Jerger SJ, Mauldin L. (1972) Studies in impedance audiometry: I. Normal and sensorineural ears. *Arch Otolaryn.* 96, 513–523.

Kano S, Kawase T, Baba Y, Sato T, Kobayashi T. (2004) Possible new assessment of patulous Eustachian tube function: audiometry for tones presented in the nasal cavity. *Acta Otolaryngol.* 124, 431–435.

Kavanagh K. (2006) Eardrum & Middle Ear Photographs. Online at *http://www.entusa.com/eardrum_and_middle_ear.htm.*

Keefe DH, Folsom RC, Gorga MP, Vohr BR, Bulen JC, Norton SJ. (2000) Identification of neonatal hearing impairment: ear-canal measurements of acoustic admittance and reflectance in neonates. *Ear Hear.* 21, 443–461.

Kei J, Allison-Levick J, Dockray J, Harrys R, Kirkegard C, Wong J, Maurer M, Hegarty J, Young J, Tudehope D. (2003) High-frequency (1000 Hz) tympanometry in normal neonates. *J Am Acad Audiol.* 14, 20–28.

Keith R. (1973) Impedance audiometry with neonates. *Arch Otolaryngol.* 97, 465–467.

Keith R. (1975) Middle ear function in neonates. *Arch Otolaryngol.* 101, 376–379.

Kessler J, MacDonald CB, Cox LC. (1998) Bizarre "sawtooth" tympanogram in a patient with otitis media. *J Am Acad Audiol.* 9, 272–274.

Kobayashi T, Okitsu T. (1986) Tympanograms in ears with small perforations of the tympanic membranes. *Arch Otolaryngol Head Neck Surg.* 112, 642–645.

Kobayashi T, Okitsu T, Takasaka T. (1987) Forward-backward tracing tympanometry. *Acta Otolaryn.* 435:, 100–106.

Koebsell KA, Margolis RH. (1986) Tympanometric gradient measured from normal preschool children. *Audiology.* 25, 149–157.

Liden G. (1969) Tests for stapes fixation. *Arch Otolaryn.* 89, 215–219.

Liden G, Harford E, Hallen O. (1974) Automatic tympanometry in clinical practice. *Audiology.* 13, 126–139.

Liden G, Peterson JL, Bjorkman G. (1970) Tympanometry: A method for analysis of middle ear function. *Acta Otolaryn.* 263, 218–224.

Lildholdt T. (1980) Negative middle ear pressure: Variations by season and sex. *Ann Otol Rhinol Laryngol.* 89, 67–70.

Lilly DJ. (1972a) Acoustic impedance at the tympanic membrane: A review of basic concepts. In: Rose D, Keating L, eds. Proceedings of the Mayo Impedance Symposium. Rochester, MN: Mayo Foundation, 1–34.

Lilly DJ. (1972b) Acoustic impedance at the tympanic membrane: A overview of clinical applications. In: Rose D, Keating L, eds. Proceedings of the Mayo Impedance Symposium. Rochester, MN: Mayo Foundation, 51–74.

Lilly DJ. (1984) Multiple frequency, multiple component tympanometry: New approaches to an old diagnostic problem. *Ear Hear.* 5, 300–308.

Lilly DJ, Shanks JE. (1981) Acoustic immittance of an enclosed volume of air. In: Popelka GR, ed. Hearing Assessment with the Acoustic Reflex. New York: Grune & Stratton, 145–160.

Lindeman P, Holmquist J. (1982) Volume measurement of middle ear and mastoid air cell system with impedance audiometry on patients with eardrum perforations. *Am J Otol.* 4, 46–51.

Lous J. (1982) Three impedance screening programs on a cohort of seven-year-old children. *Scand Audiol Suppl.* 17, 60–64.

Lyons A, Kei J, Driscoll C. (2004) Distortion product otoacoustic emissions in children at school entry: a comparison with pure-tone screening and tympanometry results. *J Am Acad Audiol.* 15, 702–715.

Manolidis S, Shohet JA, Jackson CG, Glasscock ME. (1999) Malignant glomus tumors. *Laryngoscope.* 109, 30–34.

Marchant CD, McMillan PM, Shurin PA, Johnson CE, Turczky VA, Feinstein JC, Panek DM. (1986) Objective diagnosis of otitis media in early infancy by tympanometry and ipsilateral acoustic reflex thresholds. *J Pediat.* 109, 590–595.

Margolis RH. (1981) Fundamentals of acoustic immittance. In: Popelka GR, ed. Hearing Assessment with the Acoustic Reflex. New York: Grune & Stratton, 117–144.

Margolis RH, Bass-Ringdahl S, Hanks WD, Holte L, Zapala DA. (2003) Tympanometry in newborn infants—1 kHz norms. *J Am Acad Audiol.* 14, 383–392.

Margolis RH, Goycoolea HG. (1993) Multifrequency tympanometry in normal ears. *Ear Hear.* 14, 408–413.

Margolis RH, Heller JW. (1987) Screening tympanometry: Criteria for medical referral. *Audiology.* 26, 197–208.

Margolis RH, Hunter LL. (1999) Tympanometry: Basic principles and clinical implications. In: Musiek FE, Rintelmann WF, eds. Contemporary Perspectives in Hearing Assessment. Boston: Allyn & Bacon, 89–130.

Margolis RH, Popelka GR. (1975) Static and dynamic acoustic impedance measurements in infant ears. *J Speech Hear Res.* 18, 435–443.

Margolis RH, Popelka GR. (1977) Interactions among tympanometric variables. *J Sp Hear Res.* 20, 447–462.

Margolis RH, Shanks JE. (1985) Tympanometry. In: Katz J ed. Handbook of Clinical Audiology, 3rd ed. Baltimore: Williams & Wilkins, 438–475.

Margolis RH, Smith P. (1977) Tympanometric asymmetry. *J Speech Hear Res.* 20, 437–446.

Margolis RH, Van Camp KJ, Wilson RH, Creten WL. (1985) Multifrequency tympanometry in normal ears. *Audiology.* 24, 44–53.

McKinley AM, Grose, JH, Roush J. (1997) Multifrequency tympanometry and evoked otoacoustic emissions in neonates during the first 24 hours of life. *J Am Acad Audiol.* 8, 218–223.

Meriot P, Veillon F, Garcia JF, Nonent M, Jezequel J, Bourjat P, Bellet M. (1997) CT appearances of ossicular injuries. *Radiographics.* 17, 1445–54.

Meyer SE, Jardine CA, Deverson W. (1997) Developmental changes in tympanometry: A case study. *Br J Audiol.* 31, 189–195.

Moller AR. (1960) Improved technique for detailed measurements of the middle ear impedance. *J Acoust Soc Am.* 32, 250–257.

Moller AR. (1965) An experimental study of the acoustic impedance of the middle ear and its transmission properties. *Acta Otolaryngol.* 60, 129–149.

Moller AR. (1972) The middle ear. In: Tobias J, ed. Foundations of Modern Auditory Theory. New York: Academic Press, 135–194.

Molvaer O, Vallersnes F, Kringlebotn M. (1978) The size of the middle ear and the mastoid air cell. *Acta Otolaryngol.* 85, 24–32.

Muchnik C, Hildesheimer M, Rubinstein M, Gleitman Y. (1989) Validity of tympanometry in case of confirmed otosclerosis. *J Laryngol Otol.* 103, 36–38.

Nozza RJ, Bluestone CD, Kardatze D, Bachman R. (1992) Towards the validation of aural acoustic immittance measures for diagnosis of middle ear effusion in children. *Ear Hear.* 13, 442–453.

Nozza RJ, Bluestone CD, Kardatze D, Bachman R. (1994) Identification of middle ear effusion by aural acoustic immittance measures for diagnosis of middle ear effusion in children. *Ear Hear.* 15, 310–323.

O'Donoghue G, Jackler R, Jenkins W, Schindler R. (1986) Cochlear implantation in children: The problem of head growth. *Otolaryngol Head Neck Surg.* 94, 78–81.

Osguthorpe JD, Lam C. (1981) Methodologic aspects of tympanometry in cats. *Otolaryngol Head Neck Surg.* 89, 1037–1040.

Ostergard CA, Carter DR. (1981) Positive middle ear pressure shown by tympanometry. *Arch Otolaryngol.* 107, 353–356.

O'Tuama LA, Swanson MS. (1986) Development of paranasal and mastoid sinuses: A computed tomographic pilot study. *J Child Neurol.* 1, 46–49.

Paradise JL, Smith CG, Bluestone CD. (1976) Tympanometric detection of middle ear effusion in infants and young children. *Pediatrics.* 58, 198–210.

Poe DS, Abou-Halawa A, Abdel-Razek O. (2001) Analysis of the dysfunctional eustachian tube by video endoscopy. *Otol Neurotol.* 22, 590–595.

Porter TA, Winston ME. (1973) Methodological aspects of admittance measurements of the middle ear. The Reflex. Concord, MA: Grason-Stadler.

Purdy SC, Williams MJ. (2000) High frequency tympanometry: A valid and reliable immittance test protocol for young infants? *New Zeal Audiol Soc Bull.* 10, 9–24.

Rabinowitz WM. (1981) Measurement of the acoustic input immittance of the human ear. *J Acoust Soc Am.* 70, 1025–1035.

Renvall U, Holmquist J. (1976) Tympanometry revealing middle ear pathology. *Ann Otol Rhinol Laryngol.* 85, 209–215.

Renvall U, Liden G, Bjorkman G. (1975) Experimental tympanometry in human temporal bones. *Scand Audiol.* 4, 135–144.

Rhodes MC, Margolis RH, Hirsch JE, Napp AP. (1999) Hearing screening in the newborn intensive care nursery: A comparison of methods. *Otolaryngol Head Neck Surg.* 120, 799–808.

Roup CM, Wiley TW, Safady SH, Stoppenback DT. (1998) Tympanometric screening norms for adults. *Am J Audiol.* 7, 55–60.

Roush J, Bryant K, Mundy M, Zeisel S, Roberts J. (1995) Developmental changes in static admittance and tympanometric width in infants and toddlers. *J Am Acad Audiol.* 6, 334–338.

Roush J., Drake A, Sexton JE. (1992) Identification of middle ear dysfunction in young children: A comparison of tympanometric screening procedures. *Ear Hear.* 13, 63–69.

Roush J, Tait CA. (1985) Pure tone and acoustic immittance screening of preschool-aged children: An examination of referral criteria. *Ear Hear.* 6, 245–249.

Rubensohn G. (1965) Mastoid pneumatization in children at various ages. *Acta Otolaryngol.* 60, 11–14.

Sade J, Amos AR. (1997) Middle ear and auditory tube: Middle ear clearance, gas exchange, and pressure regulation. *Otolaryngol Head Neck Surg.* 116, 499–524.

Sade J, Fuchs C. (1996) Secretory otitis media in adults: I. The role of mastoid pneumatization as a risk-factor. *Ann Otol Rhinol Laryngol.* 105, 643–647.

Saeed K, Coglianese CL, McCormick DP, Chonmaitree T. (2004) Otoscopic and tympanometric findings in acute otitis media yielding dry tap at tympanocentesis. *Ped Infect Dis J.* 23, 1030–1034.

Sederberg-Olsen J, Sederberg-Olsen A, Jensen A. (1983) The prognostic significance of the air volume in the middle ear for the tendency to recurrence of secretory middle ear condition. *Int J Ped Otorhinolaryngol.* 5, 179–187.

Shahnaz N, Davies D. (2006) Standard and multifrequency tympanometric norms for Caucasian and Chinese young adults. *Ear Hear.* 27, 75–90.

Shahnaz N, Polka L. (1997) Standard and multifrequency tympanometry in normal and otosclerotic ears. *Ear Hear.* 18, 326–341.

Shahnaz N, Polka L. (2002) Distinguishing healthy from otosclerotic ears: effect of probe-tone frequency on static immittance. *J Am Acad Audiol.* 13, 345–355.

Shanks JE (1984). Tympanometry. *Ear Hear.* 5, 268–280.

Shanks JE. (1985) Tympanometric volume estimates in patients with intact and perforated eardrums. Presented at the annual meeting of the American Speech-Language Hearing Association, Washington D.C.

Shanks JE. (1990) Multiple frequency tympanometry: Findings in otosclerosis. Presented at the annual meeting of the American Academy of Audiology, New Orleans.

Shanks JE, Lilly DJ. (1981) An evaluation of tympanometric estimates of ear canal volume. *J Speech Hear Res.* 24, 557–566.

Shanks JE, Lilly DJ, Margolis RH, Wiley TL, Wilson RH. (1988) Tutorial: Tympanometry. *J Speech Hear Dis.* 53, 354–377.

Shanks JE, Shelton C. (1991) Basic principles and clinical applications of tympanometry. *Otolaryngol Clin North Am.* 24: 299–328.

Shanks JE, Stelmachowicz PG, Beauchaine KL, Schulte L. (1992) Equivalent ear canal volumes in children pre- and post-tympanostomy tube insertion. *J Speech Hear Res.* 35, 936–941.

Shanks JE, Wilson RH. (1986) Effects of direction and rate of ear-canal pressure changes on tympanometric measures. *J Speech Hear Res.* 29, 11–19.

Shanks JE, Wilson RH, Cambron NK. (1993) Multiple frequency tympanometry: Effects of ear canal volume compensation on static acoustic admittance and estimates of middle ear resonance. *J Speech Hear Res.* 36, 178–185.

Shaw EAG. (1974) Transformation of sound pressure level from the free field to the eardrum in the horizontal plane. *J Acoust Soc Amer.* 56, 1848–1861.

Shohet JA, de Jong AL. (2002) The management of pediatric cholesteatoma. *Otolaryngol Clin North Am.* 35, 841–51.

Shohet JA, Sutton F. (2001) "Middle Ear, Otosclerosis". *Emedicine Otolaryngology and Facial Plastic Surgery* Online Textbook.

Shurin PA, Pelton SI, Klein JO. (1976) Otitis media in the newborn infant. *Ann Otol Rhinol Laryngol.* 85, 216–222.

Silman S, Silverman CA, Arick DS. (1992) Acoustic-immittance screening for detection of middle-ear effusion in children. *J Am Acad Audiol.* 3, 262–268.

Silverman CA, Silman S. (1995) Acoustic-immittance characteristics of children with middle-ear effusion: Longitudinal investigation. *J Am Acad Audiol.* 6, 339–345.

Sininger YS. (2003) Audiologic assessment of infants. *Curr Opin Otolaryngol Head Neck Surg.* 11, 378–382.

Sprague BH, Wiley TL, Goldstein R. (1985) Tympanometric and acoustic-reflex studies in neonates. *J Speech Hear Res.* 28, 265–272.

Sullivan RF. (2006) Audiology Forum: Video Otoscopy. Online at *www.rcsullivan.com/www/ears.htm.*

Sutton G, Baldwin M, Brooks D, Gravel J, Thornton R. (2002) Tympanometry in neonates and infants under 4 months: A recommended test protocol. The Newborn Hearing Screening Programme, UK; online at *www.nhsp.info.*

Sutton GJ, Gleadle P, Rowe SJ. (1996) Tympanometry and otoacoustic emissions in a cohort of special care neonates. *Br J Audiol.* 30, 9–17.

Tashima K, Tanaka S, Saito H (1986) Volumetric changes of the aerated middle ear and mastoid after insertion of tympanostomy tubes. *Am J Otolaryngol.* 7, 302–305.

Terkildsen K. (1976) Pathologies and their effect on middle ear function. In: Feldman AS & Wilbur LA, eds. Acoustic Impedance and Admittance: The Measurement of Middle Ear Function. Baltimore: Williams & Wilkins, 78–102.

Terkildsen K, Scott Nielsen S. (1960) An electroacoustic impedance measuring bridge for clinical use. Arch Otolaryngol. 72, 339–346.

Terkildsen K, Thompsen KA. (1959) The influence of pressure variations on the impedance of the human ear drum. *J Laryngol Otol.* 73, 409–418.

Tos M, Poulsen G. (1980) Screening tympanometry in infants and two-year-old children. *Ann Otol Rhinol Laryngol Suppl.* 68, 217–222.

Uzun C, Adali MK, Koten, M, Yagiz R, Aydin S, Cakir B, Karasalihoglu A. (2002) Relationship between mastoid pneumatization and middle ear barotraumas in divers. *Laryngoscope.* 112, 287–291.

Valvik B, Johnson M, Laukli E. (1994) Multifrequency tympanometry. *Audiology.* 33, 245–253.

Van Camp KJ, Creten WL, Vanpeperstraete PM, Van de Heyning PH. (1980) Tympanometry-detection of middle ear pathologies. *Acta Otol Rhinol Laryngol.* 34, 574–583.

Van Camp KJ, Margolis RH, Wilson RH, Creten W, Shanks JE. (1986) Principles of tympanometry, (Monograph No. 24) Rockville MD: American Speech-Language-Hearing Association.

Van Camp KJ, Vanhuyse VJ, Creten WL, Vanpeperstraete PM. (1978) Impedance and admittance tympanometry. II. Mathematical approach. *Audiology.* 17, 108–119.

Van Camp KJ, Vogeleer M. (1986) Normative multifrequency tympanometric data on otosclerosis. *Scand Audiol.* 15, 187–190.

Van de Heyning P H, Van Camp K J, Creten WL, Vanpeperstraete PM. (1982) Incudo-stapedial joint pathology: A tympanometric approach. *J Speech Hear Res.* 25, 611–618.

Vanhuyse VJ, Creten WL, Van Camp KJ. (1975) On the W-notching of tympanograms. *Scand Audiol.* 4, 45–50.

Vanpeperstraete PM, Creten WL, Van Camp KJ. (1979) On the asymmetry of susceptance tympanograms. *Scand Audiol.* 8, 173–179.

Virtanen H, Palva T. (1982) The patulous Eustachian tube and chronic middle ear disease. *Acta Otolaryngol.* 93, 49–53.

Voss SE, Rosowski JJ, Merchant SN, Peake WT. (2001) Middle-ear function with tympanic-membrane perforations. I. Measurements and mechanisms. *J Acoust Soc Am.* 110, 1432–1444.

Wada H, Koike T, Kobayashi T. (1998) Clinical applicability of the sweep frequency measuring apparatus for diagnosis of middle ear diseases. *Ear Hear.* 19, 240–249.

Wan IK, Wong LL. (2002) Tympanometric norms for Chinese young adults. Ear Hear. 23, 416–421.

Watters GWR, Jones JE, Freeland AP. (1997) The predictive value of tympanometry in the diagnosis of middle ear effusion. Clin Otolaryngol. 22, 343–345.

Wilber LA, Feldman AS. (1976) The middle ear measurement battery. In: Feldman AS and Wilbur LA, eds. Acoustic Impedance and Admittance: The Measurement of Middle Ear Function. Baltimore: Williams & Wilkins, 345–377.

Wiley TL, Cruickshanks KJ, Nondahl DM, Tweed TS. (1999) Aging and middle ear resonance. *J Am Acad Audiol.* 10, 173–179.

Wiley TL, Cruickshanks KJ, Nondahl DM, Tweed TS, Klein R, Klein BEK. (1996) Tympanometric measures in older adults. *J Am Acad Audiol.* 7, 260–268.

Wiley TL, Fowler CG. (1997) Acoustic Immittance Measures in Clinical Audiology: A Primer. San Diego: Singular Publishing Group.

Wilson RH, Shanks JE, Kaplan SK. (1984) Tympanometric changes at 226 Hz and 678 Hz across 10 trials and for two directions of ear canal pressure change. *J Speech Hear Res.* 27, 257–266.

Wilson RH, Shanks JE, Velde TM. (1981) Aural acoustic-immittance measurements: Inter-aural differences. *J Speech Hear Dis.* 46, 413–421.

Zhao F, Wada H, Koike T, Ohyama K, Kawase T, Stephens D. (2002) Middle ear dynamic characteristics in patients with otosclerosis. *Ear Hear.* 23, 150–158.

Zwislocki J. (1962) Analysis of the middle-ear function. Part I: Input impedance. *J Acoust Soc Am.* 34, 1514–1523.

Zwislocki J. (1976) The acoustic middle ear function. In: Feldman AS and Wilbur LA, eds. Acoustic Impedance and Admittance: The Measurement of Middle Ear Function. Baltimore: Williams & Wilkins, 66–77.

Zwislocki J, Feldman AS. (1970) Acoustic impedance of pathological ears. Monograph No. 15. Rockville, MD: American Speech-Language-Hearing Association.

10 The Acoustic Reflex

Stanley A. Gelfand

INTRODUCTION

The acoustic reflex refers to the reflexive contraction of the intratympanic muscles resulting from sound stimulation. Acoustic reflex tests are used in concert with the tympanometric measures discussed in Chapter 9 to comprise what might be called acoustic immittance assessment, impedance audiometry, or any of several other designations. Acoustic immittance measures are a class of physiologic tests that are part of almost every basic audiologic evaluation and make major contributions to differential diagnosis. This chapter provides the reader with a clinically relevant overview of the many testing methods and applications involving the acoustic reflex, along with the principal clinical findings associated with these tests.

ANATOMY AND PHYSIOLOGY OF THE ACOUSTIC REFLEX

The middle ear contains two muscles, the stapedius and tensor tympani, both of which attach to the ossicular chain. The stapedius muscle is innervated by the seventh cranial (facial) nerve. It is the smallest of the skeletal muscles, measuring only 6 mm long and 5 mm^2 in cross-sectional area. The muscle itself is contained completely inside of a bony canal within the pyramidal eminence, located on the posterior wall of the tympanic cavity. The stapedius tendon exits from the apex of the pyramidal eminence and proceeds in an anterior direction to insert on the posterior surface of the neck of stapes, just above the posterior crus. Contraction of the stapedius muscle thus pulls the stapes in the posterior direction.

The tensor tympani muscle is supplied by the fifth cranial (trigeminal) nerve. This muscle is approximately 25 mm long and 5.85 mm^2 in cross-sectional area. It is located inside of the tensor tympani semicanal within the anterior wall of the tympanic cavity, just above the Eustachian tube from which it is separated by the septum canalis musculotubarii. The tensor tympani tendon exits the middle ear wall, making a turn around the cochleariform process in order to follow a lateral course ending at the top of the manubrium of the malleus. As a result, the malleus is pulled anteriorly and medially when the tensor tympani muscle contracts.

It is tempting to think of the stapedius and tensor tympani muscles as antagonists because they pull the ossicles in essentially opposite directions. However, they actually work synergistically because both muscles exert pulls on the ossicles that are perpendicular to their normal manner of rotation, and their principal effect is to stiffen the middle ear transmission system, thereby increasing its impedance.

The middle ear muscles are activated by vocalizations (talking, yelling) and activities such as chewing and yawning, as well as in response to acoustic activation produced by relatively intense sounds (the acoustic reflex), and by tactile and similar stimulation of the ears and parts of the face (the nonacoustic reflex). The acoustic reflex involves both intratympanic muscles in many animals. However, the human acoustic reflex is a stapedius reflex. It involves just the stapedius muscle unless the stimulating sound is sufficiently intense and unexpected to produce a startle response, in which case, the tensor tympani also contracts as part of the startle reaction (Borg et al., 1984; Møller, 1984; Gelfand, 1984, 1998).

Acoustic Reflex Pathways

The acoustic reflex arc is well described (Borg, 1973; Lyons, 1978) and involves the *bilateral* contraction of the middle ear muscles in response to a high-level sound that is

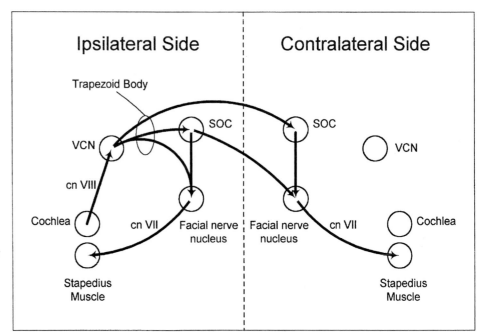

FIGURE 10.1 Schematic diagram of the ipsilateral and contralateral acoustic (stapedius) reflex pathways. cn VIII, auditory nerve; cn VII, motor branch of facial nerve; VCN, ventral cochlear nucleus; SOC, superior olivary complex.

presented to either ear. The ipsilateral (uncrossed) and contralateral (crossed) pathways of the acoustic (stapedius) reflex are shown in Figure 10.1. Notice that there are actually four distinguishable reflex arcs beginning with the stimulation of one cochlea, two that lead to contraction of the ipsilateral stapedius muscle and two that activate the stapedius muscle on the opposite side. The sensory part of the acoustic reflex goes from the stimulated cochlea via the auditory nerve (eighth cranial nerve [CNVIII]) to the *ipsilateral* ventral cochlear nucleus. Second-order neurons from the ventral cochlear nucleus pass through the trapezoid body leading to two ipsilateral and two contralateral reflex pathways.

One ipsilateral pathway goes from the ventral cochlear nucleus to the ipsilateral facial nerve nucleus, from which motor neurons of the facial nerve (CN VII) proceed to the stapedius muscle on the same side as the stimulated cochlea. The second uncrossed pathway goes from the ventral cochlear nucleus to the *ipsilateral* superior olivary complex (more specifically, the medial superior olive). From here, third-order neurons proceed to the *ipsilateral* facial nerve nucleus, from which motor neurons of CN VII activate the *ipsilateral* stapedius muscle.

One of the contralateral acoustic reflex pathways goes from the *ipsilateral* ventral cochlear nucleus to the *ipsilateral* superior olivary complex, from which third-order neurons cross to the *contralateral* facial nerve nucleus. In the second crossed pathway, neurons from the *ipsilateral* ventral cochlear nucleus cross to the *contralateral* superior olivary complex, which sends third-order neurons to the *contralateral* facial nerve nucleus. For both contralateral pathways, the motor leg of the reflex arc goes from the *contralateral* facial nerve nucleus via CN VII to the stapedius muscle in the ear opposite to the simulated cochlea.

Nonacoustic Reflexes

A nonacoustic stapedius reflex is elicited by tactile or electrocutaneous stimulation of most of the areas of skin on the sides of the face and the sides of the head around the pinna, and both the stapedius and tensor tympani muscles are activated when the orbital area is stimulated by an air puff or a quick and sudden lifting of the upper eyelids (Klockhoff and Anderson, 1960; Klockhoff, 1961; Djupesland, 1964, 1967, 1975, 1981; Djupesland et al., 1977).

The nonacoustic reflex arc is less clearly known but appears to involve the following components (Torvik, 1956; Djupesland, 1964, 1967, 1975). The afferent leg of the nonacoustic reflex arc includes CN V (trigeminal), VII (facial), IX (glossopharyngeal), and/or X (vagus), depending on where the skin is stimulated. These nerves project to the nucleus of the solitary fasciculus and to the reflex center in the dorsolateral reticular formation, which in turn communicates with the VIIth CN motor nucleus, activating the stapedius muscle via the facial nerve.

Middle Ear Muscle and Reflex Theories

Even though our interests are with the clinical aspects of the acoustic reflex, it is difficult to avoid wondering about why intratympanic muscles and an acoustic reflex exist in the first place—an issue that is still not resolved. For this reason, we will briefly mention several of the better known theories before proceeding with more practical matters. The interested student will find discussions of these theories elsewhere (Jepsen, 1963; Simmons, 1964; Borg et al., 1984).

The *protection theory* states that acoustic reflex protects the cochlea from damage due to overstimulation by lowering the amount of sound energy reaching the inner ear. The *accommodation theories* hold that the purpose of the middle ear muscles is to modify the conductive mechanism in order to optimize hearing sensitivity in general or to selectively enhance sounds in certain frequency ranges. The *ossicular fixation theories* posit that the stapedius and tensor tympani muscles maintain the proper positioning and rigidity of the ossicular chain. According to Simmons' (1964) *perceptual theory*, the middle ear muscles improve an animal's auditory perception by: (1) smoothing the frequency response of the conductive mechanism by the tonus of the intratympanic muscles; (2) improving attention to the acoustic environment by varying the frequency and intensity characteristics of environmental sounds through modulation of muscle tonus; and (3) attenuating the animal's low-frequency internal sounds without reducing the higher frequency sounds in the environment by activation of the muscles. The latter constitutes an improvement in signal-to-noise ratio and is consistent with Borg's notion that the acoustic reflex improves the dynamic range of the auditory system by attenuating lower frequency sounds.

Borg et al. (1984) proposed a multifunctional *desensitization, interference, injury protection theory* based on a review of existing theories of the nature of middle ear muscle and reflex activity in both human and animal species. The major hypotheses are as follows. Desensitization is prevented because middle ear muscle contractions elicited by eating, talking, yelling, and other vocalizations reduce the noises produced by these activities, which could otherwise reduce sensitivity and/or the alertness to salient aspects of the acoustic environment. Interference is prevented because the attenuation of the low frequencies by intratympanic muscle contractions reduces their masking of the higher frequencies (e.g., reducing the masking produced by the low-frequency components of one's own speech). Finally, potential injury to hearing is avoided by the attenuation of intense sounds.

ACOUSTIC REFLEX ASSESSMENT

Most of the parameters and considerations involved in acoustic reflex testing will be introduced in the context of the tests to which they apply, beginning with the acoustic reflex threshold (ART), which is the most basic, extensively studied, and widely used acoustic reflex measurement. However, several issues will be introduced first, either because they are fundamental to the general process of reflex assessment or because they are too easily overlooked.

Acoustic Reflex Measurement

Acoustic reflex assessment involves the presentation of tonal and/or noise stimuli to elicit a reflex response of the stapedius muscle. The resulting changes in the immittance of the ear are monitored using the same instrumentation as for tympanometry (see Chapters 8 and 9), with the addition of sound sources to present the stimuli. Acoustic reflex testing generally uses a 220- or 226-Hz probe tone unless neonates are being tested, in which case higher frequency probe tones are needed (see section titled "Acoustic Reflexes in Newborns"). Acoustic reflexes have also been measured using wideband energy reflectance methods to measure both contralateral and ipsilateral acoustic reflexes (Feeney and Keefe, 1999, 2001; Feeney et al., 2003; Feeney et al., 2004; see also Chapter 8), although this approach is not yet in general clinical use.

Stimulus levels used for acoustic reflex testing may be expressed in terms of sound pressure level (SPL), hearing level (HL), or sensation level (SL). Two considerations should be kept in mind. First, when dealing with the acoustic reflex, "sensation level" can mean *either* the number of decibels above the patient's hearing threshold *or* the number of decibels above the patient's ART. The SL of an ART refers to the former, conventional meaning. However, when we say that a reflex decay test is administered at 10 dB SL, we mean 10 dB above the ART (sometimes written as 10 dB SL re: ART). Second, the expression of ARTs in dB SL is not recommended because, among other reasons (Gelfand, 1984), it complicates the comparison of a patient's test results to applicable norms (especially 90th percentiles).

Recall that stimulation of one ear leads to reflex contractions in both ears. Thus, we can stimulate either the ear that contains the immittance probe via a receiver built into the probe assembly itself or the opposite ear using an earphone or insert receiver. The ear with the probe assembly is called the probe ear, and the ear receiving the stimulus sound is called the stimulus ear. Ipsilateral (uncrossed) acoustic reflex testing involves stimulating the probe ear, which is also the ear in which the acoustic immittance is being measured. Contralateral or crossed acoustic reflex testing involves presenting the stimulus to one ear and monitoring the acoustic immittance in the opposite (probe) ear.

Because the stimulus ear and the probe ear are the same with ipsilateral testing, there is no question about which ear and reflex pathways are being tested. However, the conventional meaning of a "test ear" is not applicable with contralateral reflexes, which assesses both ears and the crossed reflex pathways between them. For this reason, we will identify reflexes by the stimulus ear and configuration: "right contralateral" indicates that the stimulus is in the right ear and the probe is in the left ear; "left contralateral" means that the stimulus is in the left ear and the probe is in the right ear; "right ipsilateral" means that the stimulus and probe are in the right ear; and "left ipsilateral" means that the stimulus and probe are in the left ear (Fig. 10.2).

Contralateral and Ipsilateral Reflex Testing

The diagnostic power of acoustic reflexes is maximized with the combined use of contralateral and ipsilateral reflexes because diagnostically significant reflex patterns result when

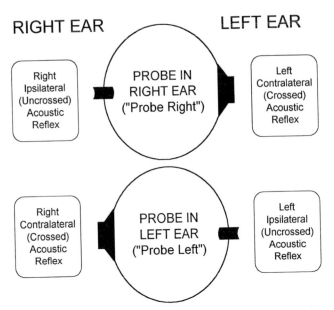

FIGURE 10.2 Nomenclature used to identify acoustic reflexes.

they are combined and also because each type of testing offers its own advantages in terms of sensitivity to particular types of disorders. However, there are applications for which either contralateral or ipsilateral testing is more appropriate to the specific goals of a particular kind of assessment or when practical considerations make it necessary to choose between them. Thus, the clinician should be aware of the relative strengths and limitations of contralateral versus ipsilateral acoustic reflex testing (Green and Margolis, 1984; Silman and Silverman, 1991).

Contralateral testing enjoys at least three major advantages over ipsilateral testing. First, contralateral reflexes are sensitive to disorders involving the crossed reflex pathways, which is not true for ipsilateral reflexes. As a result, some retrocochlear disorders (e.g., intra-axial brainstem lesions) can be missed if ipsilateral testing is used alone. Second, ipsilateral acoustic reflex testing is highly susceptible to artifacts (see below) because the stimulus signal and the probe tone are presented to the same ear, whereas contralateral tests are much less prone to (although certainly not free from) artifacts. Related to the artifact issue is the fact that the maximum stimulus levels that can be used with contralateral tests are much higher than those possible with ipsilateral testing. Third, more extensive normative data are available for contralateral tests.

Ipsilateral reflex testing offers major benefits, as well. In particular, ipsilateral acoustic reflexes are very sensitive to middle ear pathology because they are affected by both the stimulus ear effects and the probe ear effects of conductive disorders. Also, each ear is tested independently of the other one because the stimulus and probe are in the same ear. The latter point means that ipsilateral testing in one ear is not limited (or confounded) by disorders affecting the opposite ear. In addition, ipsilateral testing may be possible in young children or difficult-to-test patients whose behavior precludes the use of the headset (or the two sets of ear inserts) used with contralateral testing.

If contralateral testing is done with a standard supra-aural audiometric earphone on the stimulus ear, then it is prone to the same collapsed ear canal artifacts that affect audiometric tests. As a result, a false conductive hearing loss due to a collapsed ear canal during audiometry can be "confirmed" by an equally artifactual elevated or absent contralateral reflex. Ipsilateral testing avoids this problem because the probe tip prevents ear canal collapse in the test ear. However collapsed ear canals are also avoided with contralateral reflex testing if the stimulus is presented with an insert receiver.

Hermetic Seal and Ear Canal Pressure

Whenever possible, acoustic reflexes should be obtained at the point of tympanometric peak pressure, which usually requires the probe tip to be inserted to provide an air-tight seal of the ear canal. It is often possible to obtain similar ARTs with or without a hermetic seal of the ear canal in normal ears and those with sensorineural hearing losses (Surr and Schuchman, 1976; Kaplan et al., 1980; Ruth et al., 1982b), principally because tympanometric peak pressure is typically close to atmospheric pressure in these cases. However, this is often not the case when there is negative pressure (e.g., in ears with resolving conductive disorders) (Surr and Schuchman, 1976). In these cases, ARTs would be slightly elevated at or close to tympanometric peak pressure but require a hermetic seal. Without a seal, the reflexes would be absent.

Several investigators have studied the effect of ear canal pressures on acoustic reflex measurements (Martin and Coombes, 1974; Rizzo and Greenberg, 1979a; Ruth et al., 1982b). The general finding has been that ARTs are elevated as the pressure in the ear canal deviates from tympanometric peak pressure over a pressure range of about ± 240 daPa. The effect is typically rather small (10 dB or less), but there are cases in which acoustic reflexes are absent at the larger pressure deviations.

The implications of these findings are that, although it is possible to do acoustic reflex tests without a hermetic seal or with ear canal pressures that deviate from tympanometric peak pressure, the results are interpretable only if they are within the normal range. However, we cannot confidently tell whether an elevated or absent reflex is due to pathology, a technical problem when testing without an air-tight seal, or testing at ear canal pressures that deviate from tympanometric peak pressure.

Biphasic Responses

The acoustic reflex response is generally conceptualized as an increase in impedance (or a decrease in admittance) over its entire duration, as depicted by the monophasic response in Figure 10.3b. However, many normal reflex responses are actually biphasic, with a brief drop in impedance at the

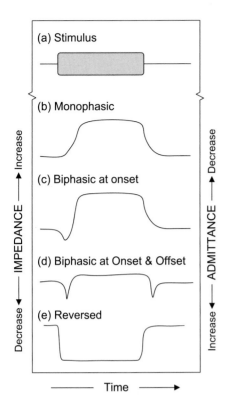

FIGURE 10.3 Idealized representations of the (a) activating stimulus, and reflex response time courses that are (b) monophasic, (c) biphasic at onset only, (d) biphasic at onset and offset, and (e) reversed.

onset of the response, followed by increased impedance for the remainder of its duration (Fig. 10.3c). This impedance decrease at the onset of the reflex response is explained as follows (Møller, 1961; Borg, 1968; Bennett, 1984). The resistance component of the ear's impedance is attributed to the cochlear fluids. A reduction in resistance occurs at the onset of the reflex response as the muscle contraction momentarily changes the coupling between the stapedius footplate and the cochlear fluids.

A different kind of biphasic pattern involves impedance drops at both the onset and offset of the reflex response (Fig. 10.3d). This abnormal pattern of biphasic response is associated with otosclerosis, especially in its earlier stages (Flottorp and Djupesland, 1970; Terkildsen et al., 1973; Jerger and Jerger, 1981). It has also been reported to occur in Cogan's syndrome, congenital stapes fixation, and osteogenesis imperfecta (Djupesland et al., 1974). The abnormal double biphasic response pattern has been attributed to elasticity changes in the stapes and annular ligament, which are associated with the partial fixation of the footplate at the oval window (Bel et al., 1976). In addition, whereas biphasic responses at both onset and offset occur in normal ears when the probe tone frequency is in the 600- to 700-Hz range, the abnormal biphasic response associated with otosclerosis occurs at all probe frequencies. For detailed findings and

theoretical explanations, see Bennett and Weatherby (1979) and Bennett (1984).

Artifact Responses

Recall that an acoustic reflex is inferred from changes in acoustic immittance during stimulus delivery. In other words, we assume that deflections represent immittance changes attributable to the acoustic reflex. However, it is also possible for deflections to be caused by other activity picked up by the instrument, as opposed to what we think we are measuring. These are artifacts. Artifacts are a problem because they can be confused for real reflex responses or alter the appearance of a real reflex response, leading to false or ambiguous test outcomes. Some artifacts are related to, for example, extraneous movements. However, a particularly troublesome class of artifacts is of acoustic origin. Acoustic artifacts occur when the stimulus sound interacts with the probe tone in ways that affect the level of the probe tone, which in turn appear as changes in acoustic immittance on the instrument. Unfortunately, these artifacts are often observed when the stimuli are presented at levels expected to produce real acoustic reflexes. These artifacts can occur when measuring both ipsilateral and contralateral reflexes (Gelfand, 1984; Green and Margolis, 1984). However, they are most likely to occur with ipsilateral testing because the stimulus and probe tone are being presented to the same ear.

Two other commonly known artifacts that can affect acoustic reflex measurement are additive and subtractive (eardrum) artifacts (Kunov, 1977; Lutman, 1980; Lutman and Leis 1980). An *additive artifact* results when the stimulus and probe tones combine in a way that increases the level of the probe tone measured by the immittance device, appearing as a deflection that mimics an increase in impedance, much like what we typically expect from the acoustic reflex. A *subtractive artifact* occurs when the two signals combine in a way that causes a decrease in the level of the probe tone, appearing as a deflection that mimics a decrease in impedance, which can also occur due to the acoustic reflex.

Additive and subtractive artifacts occur almost instantaneously because they are due to physical interactions between the stimulus and probe. In contrast, immittance changes due to real acoustic reflexes are the result of a sequence of physiologic events, so they rarely have latencies shorter than about 40 ms (Bosatra et al., 1984). Also, the earliest reflex latency within the 95% normal ranges reported by Qiu and Stucker (1997) is about 51 ms. Thus, the definitive marker of an additive or subtractive artifact is a latency in the vicinity of about 0 ms. Consequently, a conclusive distinction between an artifact and a real acoustic reflex necessitates comparing the time course of the stimulus and the apparent response on a dual channel storage oscilloscope. The direction of immittance change does not distinguish between a real reflex and an artifact because both alternatives can produce positive or negative deflections on the immittance device.

Why do additive and subtractive artifacts occur? Additive artifacts are easily understood if one knows that immittance devices separate the probe tone from the stimulus and other sounds by measuring the probe tone through a filter. A 226-Hz probe is passed through a narrow filter around 226 Hz, and a 678-Hz probe goes through a narrow filter around 678 Hz. If the stimulus also gets through the filter, then its level will be combined with that of the probe tone, leading to an artificially higher measurement. Hence, additive artifacts are more likely to occur as the stimulus frequency gets closer to the frequency of the probe tone. Additive artifacts can occur in both hard-walled cavities as well as membranous cavities.

Subtractive artifacts occur as the outcome of intermodulation distortion, which can be introduced by nonlinear systems like the membranous cavity formed by the ear canal ending at the eardrum. If we call the frequency of the probe tone $f1$ and the frequency of the stimulus tone $f2$, then intermodulation distortion between the stimulus and probe produces new components (distortion products) at frequencies such as $f1 + f2$ and $f2 - f1$. The energy needed to produce these new components is taken from the original tones, one of which is the probe. In other words, the distortion process lowers the SPL of the probe tone, which appears as a deflection on the immittance device.

Most immittance devices attempt to minimize additive artifacts either by limiting maximum stimulus levels or by indicating the lowest stimulus levels where the artifacts are likely to occur, based on measurements in a hard-walled 2-cc coupler. However, clinicians must be cognizant of two important limitations. First, these limits apply to additive artifacts only; subtractive artifacts can still occur. Second, because SPL increases as the size of a cavity decreases, additive artifacts can occur below these "official maxima" if the patient's ear volume is smaller than 2 cc, which is quite common, especially in small children. To address these limitations, it has been suggested that clinicians determine for their own instrumentation the lowest stimulus levels capable of producing measurable artifacts in various sizes (as small as 0.5 cc) of both hard-walled and membranous cavities (Silman and Silverman, 1991).[1]

An effective and practical method of minimizing artifacts is to employ an immittance device that includes a multiplexing circuit, especially for ipsilateral testing. Multiplexing simply means that the stimulus sound and the probe tone are alternated rapidly, so that they are not both on at the same time. As a result, the likelihood of artifacts due to the interactions between the probe and stimulus is minimized.

Reversed Ipsilateral Acoustic Reflexes

Fria et al. (1975) described a "reversed ipsilateral acoustic reflex" (RIAR), which has recently been studied by Ciardo et al. (2003; 2005). These responses involve an increase (rather than a decrease) in admittance when the reflex stimulus and the probe tone are in the same ear, have latencies much shorter than those of real acoustic reflexes, and are obtained when using stimuli over about 90 dB HL (Ciardo et al., 2003; see Fig. 10.3e).

Ciardo et al. (2003) found that RIARs occurred in normal ears, in ears with monaural deafness or otosclerosis with normal otoscopy and type A tympanograms, and in ears on the side of facial nerve palsy. In contrast, RIARs were not found in cases of otitis media with effusion, eardrum perforation, or radical mastoidectomy. The response was also absent in hard-walled test cavities but was not tested for in a membranous cavity. In a subsequent study, Ciardo et al. (2005) administered a muscle relaxant to block stapedius reflex activity during surgery. The muscle relaxant did not obliterate the RIARs of otosclerotic patients, but it did block the real ipsilateral reflexes of patients with normal middle ear functioning, who then exhibited the reversed pattern. Based on these observations, one is drawn to the conclusion that the RIAR is due to the subtractive (eardrum) artifact rather than representing a clinical entity.

Drug Influences

The acoustic reflex is affected by several classes of drugs. The acoustic reflex may be affected by barbiturates and alcohol, albeit with a considerable degree of intersubject variability. Barbiturates have been reported to produce elevated ARTs (Borg and Møller, 1967; Robinette et al., 1974), with a greater effect contralaterally than ipsilaterally (Borg and Møller, 1967), as well as increases in acoustic reflex latency (Bosatra et al., 1984). Ethyl alcohol results in elevated ARTs. This effect is similar for both contralateral and ipsilateral reflexes (Borg and Møller, 1967) but is larger for broadband noise (BBN) than for puretone stimuli (Cohill and Greenberg, 1977; Bauch and Robinette, 1978). Moreover, Spitzer and Ventry (1980) reported a higher incidence of absent acoustic reflexes among alcoholics compared to matched controls.

Other drugs affect the acoustic reflex, as well. For example, acoustic reflex magnitudes are reduced and ARTs are elevated by curare (Smith et al., 1966; Ruth et al., 1980; Ruth et al., 1982a). In addition, elevated ARTs have also been reported to be produced by the antipsychotic drug chlorpromazine (Simon and Pirsig, 1973). For an informative discussion of drug and related effects see Mangham (1984).

▨ ACOUSTIC REFLEX THRESHOLD

The ART is the lowest level of a sound stimulus that elicits an acoustic reflex response (i.e., a measurable change in acoustic

---

[1] Laboratory suppliers sell microliter syringes that provide for a wide range of hard-wall cavity sizes and are also indispensable for many accurate immittance calibrations, particularly when reflex magnitude is of interest. Calibration cavities for membranous artifact measurements can be fabricated by cutting common hypodermic syringes to a variety of volume sizes and attaching a latex (or similar) membrane to the far end of each cavity. See Lilly (1984), Silman (1984), and Silman and Silverman (1991).

Stimulus Presentation (Event) Markers and Sound Pressure Levels:

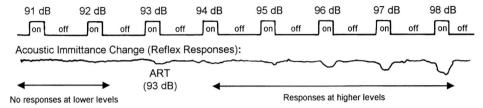

FIGURE 10.4 Acoustic reflex responses (below) produced by various levels of a stimulus sound (above). The acoustic reflex threshold (ART) is the lowest stimulus level producing a time-locked immittance change (93 dB here), and the magnitude of the reflex gets larger as the stimulus level is raised above this level. (From Gelfand SA. [1997] *Essentials of Audiology.* New York: Thieme Medical Publishers, by permission.)

immittance). Stimulus presentations above the ART should also produce reflex responses, which generally become larger as the stimulus level increases. These principles are illustrated in Figure 10.4.

Measurement of Acoustic Reflex Thresholds

In clinical practice, ARTs are usually tested with tonal stimuli at 500, 1,000, and 2,000 Hz, and sometimes using BBN. Testing at 4,000 Hz is not recommended because many normal-hearing young adults experience elevated ARTs at this frequency, probably due to rapid adaptation (Gonay et al., 1974; Gelfand, 1984; Silman and Silverman, 1991).

ARTs do not appear to be affected by the direction in which the stimulus level is changed. Even though Jepsen (1963) found that ARTs were occasionally lower when measured with a descending technique compared to an ascending method, subsequent findings revealed no significant differences between descending and ascending reflex thresholds (Peterson and Liden, 1972; Wilson, 1979).

ARTs are affected by the sensitivity of the instrumentation, the size of the stimulus level increments, and how the responses are monitored (Gelfand, 1984). The instrumentation must be sensitive enough to resolve the lowest ART we expect to encounter. Because of the normal range of ARTs, the immittance device should be sensitive enough to permit the detection of reflex responses elicited by BBN stimuli as low as roughly 60 dB SPL.

Let us consider step size and monitoring method in terms of the two extremes, bearing in mind that choices in these matters fall along a continuum. Laboratory measurements of the ART usually involve (1) changing the stimulus level in 1-dB or 2-dB increments, and (2) hardcopy recordings of the responses, usually with an event marker to indicate when the stimuli were presented (Fig. 10.4). This approach permits a fine-grained determination of the smallest stimulus-related immittance change that can be detected against the background activity or that meets a predetermined minimum size (typically 0.01 to 0.02 mmho). In contrast, clinical ART testing has traditionally involved (1)

changing the stimulus level in 5-dB steps, and (2) visual monitoring of the responses (i.e., watching for deflections in the immittance value shown on the immittance device meter or screen as they are occurring).

The method of choice depends on the accuracy needed for the application at hand, which is clinical assessment, and is affected by the size of the reflex response at and just above the ART (Gelfand, 1984; see also the section in this chapter titled "Acoustic Reflex Magnitude and Growth"). Consequently, 5-dB steps and visual monitoring are quite acceptable when the stimuli are *puretones*. However, ARTs for *BBN* stimuli should be tested with 1-dB or 2-dB steps and recorded (not just visually monitored) because, in this case, the size of the reflex response is very small at and just above the ART (Gelfand and Piper, 1981; Popelka, 1981; Silverman et al., 1983; Gelfand, 1984). It is stressed that contemporary instruments make it easy and practical to use on-screen and hardcopy recordings of reflex responses, as well as different step sizes, in daily clinical practice. See Gelfand (1984) for a detailed discussion of step size and monitoring method considerations.

Reliability

Forquer (1979) reported a high degree of test-retest reliability for multiple acoustic reflex measurements over several days. For example, the widest difference between any two ART means was only 2.4 dB for the normal-hearing group, and there was similar agreement for the group with sensory-neural losses. Silman and Gelfand (1981a) found the mean ART measurements made under clinical conditions by four experienced audiologists to be less than 2 dB apart and not significantly different. Reflex thresholds obtained using laboratory methods (recorded measurements with 1- to 2-dB stimulus steps) are usually less than 2 dB apart from test to retest (Silman and Silverman, 1991).

Normal Acoustic Reflex Thresholds

Numerous studies have established that normal ARTs range from about 85 to 100 dB SPL for puretone stimuli and are

TABLE 10.1   Contralateral and ipsilateral acoustic reflex thresholds (ARTs) in dB HL for puretone and broadband noise (BBN) stimuli in normal-hearing subjects.

	Contralateral ART (in dB HL)		Ipsilateral ART (in dB HL)	
	Mean	Standard deviation	Mean	Standard deviation
500 Hz	84.6	6.3	79.9	5.0
1,000 Hz	85.9	5.2	82.0	5.2
2,000 Hz	84.4	5.7	86.2	5.9
4,000 Hz	89.8	8.9	87.5	3.5
BBN	66.3	8.8	64.6	6.9

Data based on the findings of Wiley et al. (1987).

roughly 20 dB lower for BBN (see Gelfand [1984] for a detailed review). Representative means and standard deviations of normal contralateral and ipsilateral ARTs expressed in dB HL are shown in Table 10.1. There do not appear to be any significant differences between the ARTs of males and females (Jerger et al., 1972; Osterhammel and Osterhammel, 1979; Silverman et al., 1983).

Wilson et al. (1981) found no significant differences between the ears for ARTs in normal individuals, with 80% normal ranges for left-right differences of 6.3 dB at 500 Hz, 6.9 dB at 1,000 Hz, 7.7 dB at 2,000 Hz, and 8.3 dB using BBN stimuli. Inter-ear differences collapsed across frequency (250 to 4,000 Hz) have been reported to be 0 to 5 dB for 22.5%, 0 to 10 dB for 52.2%, and 0 to 15 dB for 70.2% of normal-hearing listeners (Chiveralls et al., 1976; Chiveralls, 1977).

The normal 20-dB noise-tone difference is observed for the two youngest groups in Figure 10.5 as the distance between the tonal ARTs (above) and the BBN ARTs measured with 1-dB steps (filled triangles, below). As expected from the discussion of step size, also notice that the BBN ARTs obtained with 5-dB steps (open triangles) are higher than those obtained with 1-dB steps. As a result, the normal noise-tone difference fails to achieve the expected size of 20 dB when BBN is tested with 5-dB steps. The lower ARTs for BBN are associated with the bandwidth effect of the acoustic reflex, which may be described as follows. Beginning with a

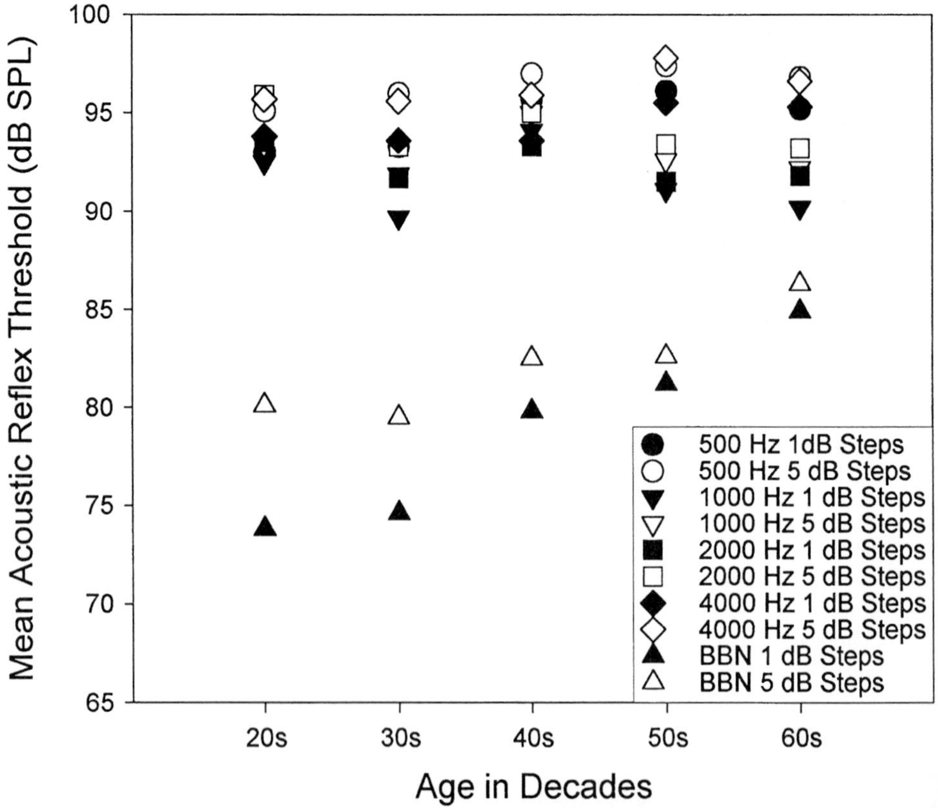

FIGURE 10.5   Mean acoustic reflex thresholds for tonal and broadband noise (BBN) stimuli presented in 1-dB and 5-dB steps at various ages in normal-hearing individuals. SPL, sound pressure level. (Based on data by Silverman et al. [1983].)

puretone, widening the bandwidth of the stimulus does not affect the ART *until* a certain bandwidth is reached, beyond which the ART gets lower as the bandwidth gets wider (Flottorp et al., 1971; Djupesland and Zwislocki, 1973; Popelka et al., 1976). (For further discussion of the bandwidth effect, see Gelfand [1984, 1998].)

Effects of Aging

Tonal ARTs do not change with increasing age in normal-hearing adults, whereas ARTs for BBN do increase with increasing age (Jerger et al., 1972; Handler and Margolis, 1977; Osterhammel and Osterhammel, 1979; Silman, 1979; Thompson et al., 1980; Gelfand and Piper, 1981; Silman and Gelfand, 1981b; Wilson, 1981; Silverman et al., 1983; Gelfand, 1984). These relationships can be seen in Figure 10.5. Notice that ARTs for BBN become noticeably elevated beginning in the age range of 40 to 49 years, with the breakpoint at about 44 years of age, on a statistical basis (Silverman et al., 1983).

Acoustic Reflexes in Newborns

The ability to obtain acoustic reflexes in neonates is heavily dependent on probe frequency. When 220- or 226-Hz probe tones are used, the common findings are a high proportion of absent reflexes and elevated ARTs among those that are present (Keith, 1973; Bennett, 1975; Abahazi and Greenberg, 1977; Himmelfarb et al., 1978; Keith and Bench, 1978; Stream et al., 1978; McMillan et al., 1985; Sprague et al., 1985). On the other hand, the probability of present acoustic reflexes becomes greater and ARTs become lower (better) when higher frequency probe tones are used (Weatherby and Bennett, 1980; Bennett and Weatherby, 1982; McMillan et al., 1985; Sprague et al., 1985). Examples of acoustic reflex data for newborns are shown for 1,000 Hz and BBN activators in Table 10.2 and for 500- to 4,000-Hz tones in Figure 10.6,

which also reveal that the ipsilateral results were superior to the contralateral findings.

Facilitated Reflex Thresholds

There are some conditions under which ARTs have been found to occur at lower levels that those typically encountered. The ART for a stimulus tone can be lowered if it is sensitized or preactivated by a facilitator, which is a second tone presented at a level just below its own reflex threshold (Sesterhenn and Breuninger, 1976; Blood and Greenberg, 1981; Jeck et al., 1983). The basic approach is as follows. A preliminary step is to find the reflex threshold for the facilitator, which is a high-frequency tone (e.g., 4,000 or 6,000 Hz). Then the reflex threshold for the stimulus tone is measured twice: (1) all by itself, and (2) when preactivated by the facilitator. The reflex threshold is lower when the stimulus is presented with the facilitator. For example, Blood and Greenberg (1981) found that a 4,000-Hz facilitator lowered average reflex thresholds for 500- to 2,000-Hz stimuli by about 17 to 22 dB for normal subjects and 5 to 6 dB for subjects with sensory-neural losses. However, the amount of facilitation is not consistent among studies, with means ranging from 12.4 to 29.4 dB at 500 Hz, 10.2 to 25 dB at 1,000 Hz, and 11.8 to 28 dB at 2,000 Hz for the investigations cited here.

Lowered ARTs have also been reported with the use of pulsed stimuli (Tietze, 1969; Sesterhenn and Breuninger, 1976), but other findings have not been consistent with these (Feldman and Katz, 1978; Johnsen and Terkildsen, 1980). More recent studies using click trains found significantly lower ipsilateral reflex thresholds as click rates increased from 50 to 300 per second, even when the total signal energy was constant (Rawool, 1995, 1996b). This effect is similar in normal young children (Rawool, 1996a), but it appears to be affected by aging (Fielding and Rawool, 2002).

In addition, a few studies found that computer averaging resulted in atypically low ARTs, probably by improving the

---

TABLE 10.2   Percentages of occurrence and mean thresholds in dB HL for normal neonates using 1,000-Hz versus broadband noise (BBN) stimuli and 220-Hz versus 660-Hz probe tones

Probe Frequency	Percentage of present reflexes		Mean reflex thresholds (dB HL)	
	220 Hz	660 Hz	220 Hz	660 Hz
Ipsilateral acoustic reflex				
1,000-Hz stimulus	43	81	82.6	81.7
BBN stimulus	51	74	60.9	54.6
Contralateral acoustic reflex				
1,000-Hz stimulus	34	60	92.2	89.1
BBN stimulus	49	83	70.0	70.1

Based on data by Sprague et al. (1985).

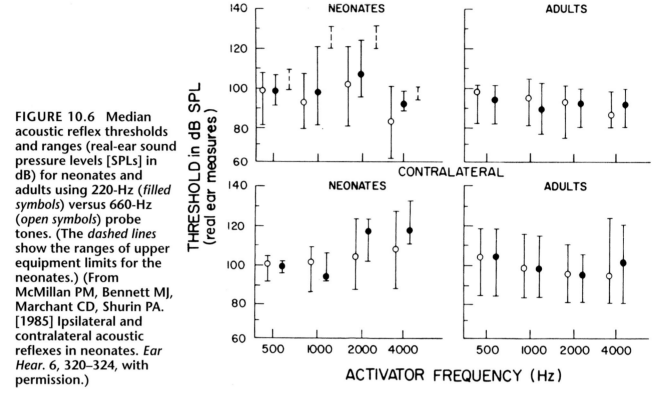

FIGURE 10.6 Median acoustic reflex thresholds and ranges (real-ear sound pressure levels [SPLs] in dB) for neonates and adults using 220-Hz (*filled symbols*) versus 660-Hz (*open symbols*) probe tones. (The *dashed lines* show the ranges of upper equipment limits for the neonates.) (From McMillan PM, Bennett MJ, Marchant CD, Shurin PA. [1985] Ipsilateral and contralateral acoustic reflexes in neonates. *Ear Hear.* 6, 320–324, with permission.)

signal-to-noise ratio of responses (Draf and Leitner, 1972; Zito and Roberto, 1980). However, this has not been the typical finding among most studies using averaged acoustic reflexes (Jerger et al., 1977; Johnsen and Terkildsen, 1980), and it is not clear whether the low-level averaged reflexes were real or artifacts.

ACOUSTIC REFLEXES IN CONDUCTIVE DISORDERS

Conductive impairments are associated with elevated and/or absent acoustic reflexes. An ART is considered to be elevated if it is higher than it would have been if there was no conductive disorder. The acoustic reflex is considered absent when a response cannot be obtained at the highest available stimulus level, which is typically 125 dB HL for contralateral stimulation.

Basic Principles

It is convenient to summarize the effects of conductive loss disorders in terms of two fundamental principles. First, the *probe ear principle* states that acoustic reflexes are usually absent when there is conductive pathology in the probe ear. In this case, the conductive pathology prevents us from being able to monitor changes in acoustic immittance at the probe tip (even though the stapedius muscle may be contracting). This principle is the reason why Jerger et al. (1974a) found

that the probability of being able to register an acoustic reflex was only 50% when the probe ear had an average air-bone gap of just 5 dB. Second, the *stimulus ear principle* states that a conductive disorder in the stimulus ear reduces the stimulus level reaching the cochlea by the amount of the air-bone gap. As a result, the ART is elevated by the amount of the air-bone gap and will be absent if it is elevated beyond the maximum available stimulus level. According to Jerger et al. (1974a), the contralateral ART was absent in 50% of those with air-bone gaps of 27 dB in the stimulus ear.

Unilateral Conductive Disorders

To illustrate the stimulus ear principle, consider two otherwise normal people, both with ARTs of 85 dB HL. One of them develops a 30-dB conductive loss in the stimulus ear, and the other develops a 45-dB conductive loss in the stimulus ear. In the first case, the stimulus level must be raised by 30 dB to overcome the air-bone gap, so that the ART is elevated to 85 + 30 = 115 dB HL. However, the acoustic reflex is absent in the second case because the ART is now elevated to 85 + 45 = 130 dB HL, which exceeds the maximum available stimulus level of 125 dB HL. At first glance, the 30-dB loss example might seem to contradict Jerger et al.'s (1974a) finding that the chances of registering an acoustic reflex fell to 50% when the stimulus ear had an average air-bone gap of 27 dB. But both examples are actually completely consistent because the maximum stimulus level available to Jerger et al. (1974a) was 110 dB HL. On average, combining the 27-dB

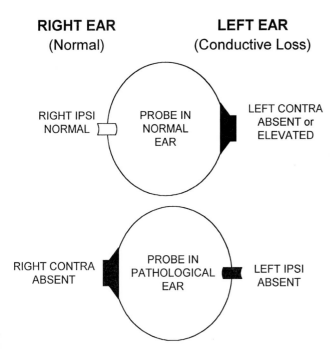

FIGURE 10.7 The typical configuration of contralateral and ipsilateral acoustic reflex outcomes associated with unilateral conductive impairments.

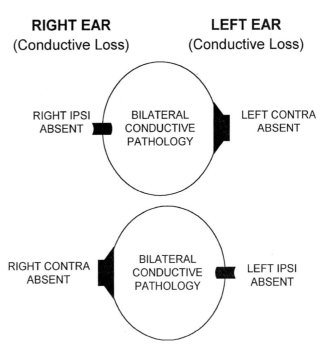

FIGURE 10.8 The typical configuration of contralateral and ipsilateral acoustic reflex outcomes associated with bilateral conductive impairments.

air-bone gap with a typical ART of 85 dB HL elevates the ART to 112 dB HL, which exceeded their maximum level. However, contemporary equipment extends the testing range by 15 dB (up to 125 dB HL), which in turn extends the size of the air-bone gap associated with a 50% chance of absent reflexes to 42 dB (Gelfand, 1984).

As expected from the principles just outlined, conductive disorders are associated with the following clinical configurations, which are conceptualized in Figures 10.7 and 10.8. With a unilateral conductive impairment, contralateral acoustic reflexes are (1) elevated and/or absent when stimulating the pathologic ear (the probe is in the normal ear) due to the stimulus ear principle, and (2) absent when the probe is in the pathologic ear (due to the probe ear principle). However, ipsilateral reflexes will be absent in the pathologic ear because both principles are operative: The effective stimulus delivered to the cochlea is attenuated by the air-bone gap, plus the ability to register an immittance change is precluded by the pathology. This double effect is why ipsilateral acoustic reflexes are so sensitive to conductive disorders. Of course, the ipsilateral reflexes will be normal in the normal ear. Figure 10.9 illustrates these concepts in a representative clinical case.

Bilateral Conductive Disorders

With a bilateral conductive disorder, both contralateral and ipsilateral reflexes are absent in both ears because every test arrangement involves stimulating a pathologic ear combined with trying to monitor a reflex response in a pathologic ear. A typical clinical case is shown in Figure 10.10.

Ossicular Chain Discontinuities

In the typical case, ossicular chain discontinuities are lateral to the insertion of the stapedius muscle on the stapes, so that the effects of its contraction are not transmitted to the tympanic membrane, resulting in absent acoustic reflexes (the probe ear principle). However, *certain* ossicular disruptions produce the opposite, "paradoxical" finding of present contralateral acoustic reflexes with an air-bone gap in the probe ear. This exception occurs if (1) the ossicular interruption is bridged by some type of connection, such as fibrous adhesions, or (2) the disruption affects the stapes at a point that is medial to where the stapedius muscle inserts (Hayes, 1977; Jenkins et al., 1980; Isenberg and Tubergen, 1980; Shapiro et al., 1981). In these cases, the ossicular discontinuity produces an air-bone gap, but the effects of stapedius muscle contractions can still be transmitted to the eardrum. As a result, stimulation of the normal ear is able to elicit a present contralateral acoustic reflex monitored by the probe in the pathologic ear, as illustrated in Figure 10.11. Stimulation of the pathologic ear (probe in the opposite ear) results in either elevated and/or absent acoustic reflexes, depending on the size of the air-bone gap (the stimulus ear principle). Figure 10.12 shows a clinical

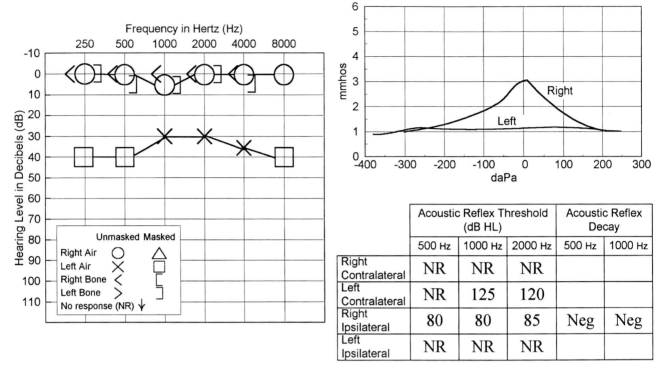

	Acoustic Reflex Threshold (dB HL)			Acoustic Reflex Decay	
	500 Hz	1000 Hz	2000 Hz	500 Hz	1000 Hz
Right Contralateral	NR	NR	NR		
Left Contralateral	NR	125	120		
Right Ipsilateral	80	80	85	Neg	Neg
Left Ipsilateral	NR	NR	NR		

FIGURE 10.9   Acoustic reflex results in a typical clinical case of a unilateral conductive disorder (otitis media in the left ear).

example of these results in a patient with an ossicular discontinuity bridged by fibrous adhesions in the right ear. Notice that the left contralateral reflex is present despite the fact that there is conductive pathology in the right (probe) ear.

Screening for Middle Ear Disorders

Despite its sensitivity to the presence of conductive pathology, there has been considerable controversy over the issue of including ipsilateral acoustic reflex testing to screen

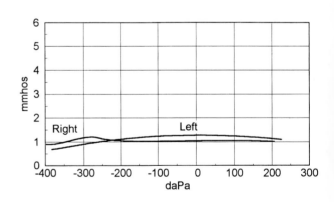

	Acoustic Reflex Threshold (dB HL)			Acoustic Reflex Decay	
	500 Hz	1000 Hz	2000 Hz	500 Hz	1000 Hz
Right Contralateral	NR	NR	NR		
Left Contralateral	NR	NR	NR		
Right Ipsilateral	NR	NR	NR		
Left Ipsilateral	NR	NR	NR		

FIGURE 10.10   Acoustic reflex results in a typical clinical case of a bilateral conductive disorder (bilateral otitis media).

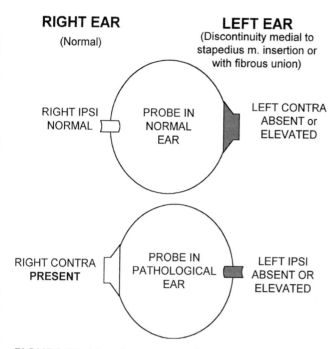

RIGHT EAR
(Normal)

LEFT EAR
(Discontinuity medial to stapedius m. insertion or with fibrous union)

RIGHT IPSI NORMAL

PROBE IN NORMAL EAR

LEFT CONTRA ABSENT or ELEVATED

RIGHT CONTRA **PRESENT**

PROBE IN PATHOLOGICAL EAR

LEFT IPSI ABSENT OR ELEVATED

FIGURE 10.11   The apparently paradoxical configuration of acoustic reflex outcomes associated with an ossicular discontinuity medial to the stapedius muscle insertion or with a fibrous union enabling the effects of the reflex contraction to be conveyed to the eardrum. Notice that the right contralateral reflex is present even though the probe is in the pathologic (left) ear.

for middle ear disorders. An ipsilateral reflex test using a 1,000-Hz stimulus tone presented at 105 dB SPL was included in the American Speech-Language-Hearing Association (ASHA) (1979) screening guidelines, but reflex testing was removed from the ASHA (1990) screening guidelines because it was associated with unacceptably high false-positive rates (Lucker, 1980; Lous, 1983; Roush and Tait, 1985). In this context, a false-positive refers to finding an absent reflex in a normal ear, leading to overreferral. Consequently, the immittance screening criteria suggested by ASHA (1990) include only abnormally low static acoustic admittance and/or abnormally wide tympanometric width.

Silman et al. (1992) compared several screening protocols for middle ear disorders. They found that the sensitivity of the ASHA (1990) immittance protocol was 81.5% for children with middle ear effusion and that its specificity is 79% for children who are free of ear disease. However, sensitivity increased to 90% and specificity increased to 92.5% when tympanometric criteria were supplemented with a 1,000-Hz (activator) ipsilateral reflex test at 110 dB SPL using an instrument with multiplexing (alternated stimulus and probe tones to minimize artifacts). The screening criteria proposed by Silman et al. (1992) are as follows:

A. Tympanometric criteria (50 daPa/s pump speed)
  (1) Tympanometric width >180 daPa, *and/or*
  (2) Static middle ear admittance <0.35 mmho, *and/or*
  (3) Tympanometric peak pressure $\leq$ −100 daPa

PLUS

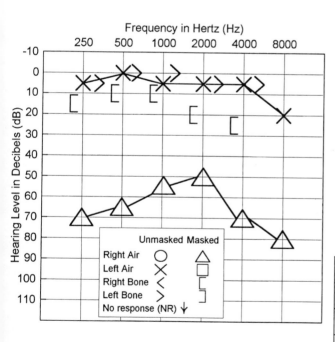

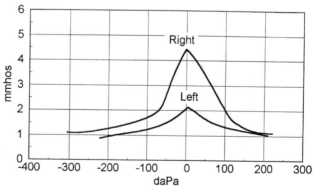

	Acoustic Reflex Threshold (dB HL)			Acoustic Reflex Decay	
	500 Hz	1000 Hz	2000 Hz	500 Hz	1000 Hz
Right Contralateral	NR	NR	125		
Left Contralateral	95	95	95	Neg	Neg
Right Ipsilateral	NR	NR	NR		
Left Ipsilateral	85	85	80		

FIGURE 10.12   Acoustic reflex findings in a case of severe conductive hearing loss in the right ear caused by an ossicular interruption that is bridged by fibrous adhesions (see text).

B. Absent ipsilateral acoustic reflex for 1,000-Hz activator at 110 dB HL (with multiplexing)

Tympanometric criteria (1) and (2) are fundamentally the same as the ASHA (1990) protocol except that the recommended pump speed and cutoff values are those employed by Silman et al. (1992) instead of those in the ASHA (1990) protocol (200 daPa/s pump speed, static admittance <0.2, tympanometric width >150 daPa, for young children).

Convincing findings by Sells et al. (1997) have largely resolved the discrepancies about the viability of ipsilateral reflex testing in the screening protocol for middle ear disorders. They found that the high false-positive rates previously reported for ipsilateral reflex screening tests are most likely attributable to instrumentation factors. Specifically, they found a 31% false-positive rate for ipsilateral reflexes tested using the *screening mode* of a contemporary immittance device compared to the *diagnostic mode* of the same instrument on the same control (i.e., normal) subjects (who all produced normal reflex results in the diagnostic mode). The diagnostic mode uses multiplexing of the probe and stimulus tones and allows decisions based on the smallest detectable immittance change, whereas the screening mode presents the probe and stimulus tones concurrently and uses a relatively large preset immittance change as the decision criterion for whether a reflex is "present" or "absent." These findings, of course, support the use of ipsilateral reflex testing in the middle ear screening protocol.

ACOUSTIC REFLEXES IN SENSORY-NEURAL DISORDERS

Sensory-neural hearing loss of cochlear origin is related to ARTs in a manner that depends on hearing sensitivity

and whether the reflex is elicited using puretones or BBN (Popelka, 1981; Silman and Gelfand, 1981a; Gelfand et al., 1983; Gelfand, 1984; Gelfand and Piper, 1984; Gelfand et al., 1990). The fundamental relationships are illustrated in Figure 10.13, which shows how ARTs depend on hearing thresholds along a continuum of auditory sensitivity from 0 dB HL through 90 dB HL. Notice that puretone ARTs are essentially constant with increasing thresholds up to about 50 dB HL, beyond which the ARTs increase as the hearing thresholds increase. In contrast, ARTs produced by BBN stimuli become higher as hearing thresholds increase up to about 50 dB HL, beyond which the ARTs remain essentially constant. We will concentrate on the implications of puretone ARTs here. Large-sample norms for contralateral ARTs elicited by 500-, 1,000-, and 2,000-Hz stimuli have been developed for individuals with normal hearing and cochlear impairments (Silman and Gelfand, 1981a; Gelfand, 1984; Gelfand et al., 1983; Gelfand and Piper, 1984; Gelfand et al., 1990) and are illustrated inFigure 10.14 in the form of ART medians, 10th percentiles, and 90th percentiles as a function of hearing threshold. Equivalent large-sample norms for ipsilateral ARTs are not available.

IDENTIFYING RETROCOCHLEAR DISORDERS WITH ACOUSTIC REFLEX THRESHOLDS

Retrocochlear pathologies are associated with ARTs that are elevated compared to what they would have been in normal or cochlear-impaired ears, often to the extent that they are absent at the maximum stimulus levels (Anderson et al., 1970; Jerger et al., 1974c; Sanders et al., 1974; Sheehy and Inzer,

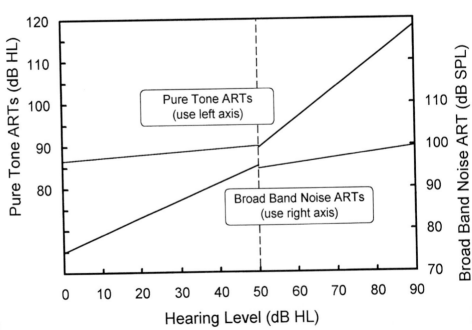

FIGURE 10.13 Idealized representation of how acoustic reflex thresholds (ARTs) depend on hearing sensitivity for puretone and broadband noise (BBN) stimuli, based on data by Popelka (1981) for BBN and Gelfand et al. (1990) for puretones. Use left axis for puretone ARTs and right axis for BBN ARTs. (From Gelfand SA. [1997] *Essentials of Audiology.* **New York: Thieme Medical Publishers, by permission.)**

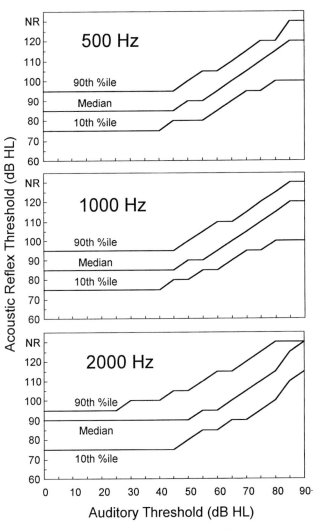

FIGURE 10.14 Medians, 10th, and 90th percentiles for the contralateral acoustic reflex elicited by (A) 500-Hz, (B) 1,000-Hz, and (C) 2,000-Hz stimuli as a function of hearing threshold in a subject with normal hearing and sensory-neural impairments of cochlear origin. NR, no response. (Adapted from Gelfand SA, Schwander T, Silman S. [1990] Acoustic reflex thresholds in normal and cochlear-impaired ears: effects of no-response rates on 90th percentiles in a large sample. *J Speech Hear Dis.* **55, 198–205, with permission of the American Speech-Language-Hearing Association.**

The 90th percentiles of the distributions of ARTs in normal and cochlear-impaired ears, like those shown in Figure 10.14, provide effective cutoff values to determine what constitutes an abnormal elevation of the ART (Silman and Gelfand, 1981a; Gelfand, 1984; Olsen et al., 1983; Sanders, 1984; Gelfand et al., 1990; Silman and Silverman, 1991). Table 10.3 shows two sets of 90th percentile cutoff values that are in common use (Silman and Gelfand, 1981a; Gelfand et al., 1990) that may be used for this purpose. The procedure is to compare each ART to the 90th percentile corresponding to the stimulus frequency and the patient's hearing threshold at that frequency. Reflex thresholds at or below the applicable 90th percentiles are considered to be essentially within the distributions for normal hearing and/or cochlear disorders. Reflex thresholds are considered elevated if they exceed the relevant 90th percentiles because ARTs so high are uncommon among ears with normal hearing and/or cochlear disorders, occurring less than 10% of the time. In that case, the patient is considered at risk for retrocochlear pathology in the stimulus ear, providing that the elevated ART is not attributable to a conductive abnormality.

Prototypical acoustic reflex outcomes associated with cochlear versus retrocochlear disorders are illustrated by the two clinical cases in Figures 10.15 and 10.16. The case of cochlear impairment (Fig. 10.15) has ARTs that are within the 90th percentile cutoff values for the magnitude of hearing loss at each respective frequency and negative reflex decay (see below). In contrast, the case of an eighth-nerve tumor in the left ear (Fig. 10.16) has ARTs that are higher than the applicable 90th percentiles (seen as elevated and/or absent) and positive reflex decay (when testable) when stimulating the left ear (left contralateral and left ipsilateral).

It has been suggested that inter-ear comparisons of acoustic reflex results can assist in the identification of retrocochlear disorders (Chiveralls, 1977; Chiveralls et al., 1976; Mangham et al., 1980; Prasher and Cohen, 1993). Figure 10.17 shows the extent of inter-ear symmetry for tonal ARTs for individuals with normal hearing and cochlear disorders. Consequently, Chiveralls (1977) suggested that retrocochlear involvement should be suspected when inter-ear reflex threshold differences exceed 15 dB at more than one frequency. However, Prasher and Cohen (1993) recommended that the criterion should be an inter-ear difference greater than 10 dB at two adjacent frequencies (500 and 1,000 Hz, 1,000 and 2,000 Hz, and 4,000 Hz). Figure 10.18 shows that the two approaches have similar specificity, but the Prasher and Cohen criteria afford substantially better sensitivity. However, notice that the sensitivity actually achieved appears to depend on whether contralateral and/or ipsilateral reflexes are used and which frequencies are considered. In this context, recall that maximum testable levels are lower for ipsilateral than contralateral reflexes and that 4,000 Hz is not a recommended frequency for most acoustic reflex assessments.

1976; Chiveralls, 1977; Johnson, 1977; Hayes and Jerger, 1980; Mangham et al., 1980; Olsen et al., 1981; Gelfand, 1984; Silman and Silverman, 1991; Prasher and Cohen, 1993; Ferguson et al., 1996). This principle relies on two assumptions. First, a conductive disorder must be ruled out as the reason for the abnormal reflex result. Second, there must be a standard for what constitutes an elevated reflex (including elevation to the extent that the reflex is absent).

TABLE 10.3 Ninetieth percentile cutoff values for contralateral acoustic reflex thresholds at 500, 1,000, and 2,000 Hz as a function of the threshold of hearing at the stimulus frequency in ears with normal hearing and cochlear impairments[a]

Auditory threshold (dB HL)	Acoustic reflex thresholds 90th percentiles (dB HL)					
	Silman & Gelfand (1981a)			Gelfand, Schwander, & Silman (1990)		
	500 Hz	1,000 Hz	2,000 Hz	500 Hz	1,000 Hz	2,000 Hz
0	95	100	95	95	95	95
5	95	100	95	95	95	95
10	95	100	100	95	95	95
15	95	100	100	95	95	95
20	95	100	100	95	95	95
25	95	100	100	95	95	95
30	100	100	105	95	95	100
35	100	100	105	95	95	100
40	100	105	105	95	95	100
45	100	105	105	95	95	105
50	105	105	110	100	100	105
55	105	105	110	105	105	110
60	105	110	115	105	110	115
65	105	110	115	110	110	115
70	115	115	125	115	115	120
75	115	115	125	120	120	125
80	125	125	125	120	125	>125
85	125	125	125	>125	>125	>125
≥ 90	125	125	125	>125	>125	>125

Based on data by Silman and Gelfand (1981a) and Gelfand et al. (1990).
[a] Absent reflexes were excluded from the distributions leading to the 1981 norms and included in the distributions leading to the 1990 norms. The 1990 norms assume that there are measurable hearing thresholds (≤110 dB HL) at all three stimulus frequencies.

ACOUSTIC REFLEX DECAY (ADAPTATION)

Acoustic reflex decay, or adaptation, is the reduction in the magnitude of the acoustic reflex response during the presentation of a sustained stimulus. The typical clinical procedure is to record the acoustic reflex response during the presentation of a puretone stimulus for 10 seconds at a level 10 dB above the ART, as illustrated in Figure 10.19. Clinical testing is limited to 500 and 1,000 Hz because rapid adaptation of the reflex response is quite common at higher frequencies. Reflex decay is determined according to whether the response falls to ≤50% of its initial magnitude during the 10-second stimulus. Acoustic reflex decay is usually tested contralaterally. Ipsilateral reflex decay has received less attention (Alberti et al., 1977; Oviatt and Kileny, 1984). In general, ipsilateral results are similar to those for contralateral testing, although slightly more reflex decay appears to occur ipsilaterally.

Abnormally rapid reflex decay is associated with retrocochlear disorders (e.g., Fig. 10.15 vs. Fig. 10.16), and the combined use of ARTs and reflex decay results in 85% to 95% sensitivity, depending on the sample and criteria used (Anderson et al., 1969, 1970; Jerger et al., 1974c; Olsen et al., 1975, 1981, 1983; Thomsen and Terkildsen, 1975; Sheehy and Inzer, 1976; Silman et al., 1978a; Mangham et al., 1980; Sanders et al., 1981; Bergenius et al., 1983; Sanders, 1984; Wilson et al., 1984; Silman and Silverman, 1991). For example, it has been shown that the combined use of ARTs (with 90th percentile criteria) with reflex decay achieves 85% sensitivity with a false-positive rate of just 11% (Silman and Silverman, 1991). There is some evidence that the sensitivity and specificity of reflex decay may be improved if the stimulus level is raised to 20 dB above ART (Mangham et al., 1980).

There is some controversy about the exact criteria for abnormal reflex decay in terms of whether the decay occurs within the first 5 seconds or any time during the 10-second stimulus presentation and whether decay occurs at just 500 Hz versus 500 and/or 1,000 Hz (Anderson et al., 1969, 1970; J. Jerger et al., 1974c; Jerger, 1975; Olsen et al., 1975; Segal, 1978; Silman and Gelfand, 1982a; Wilson et al., 1984; Silman and Silverman, 1991). It is difficult to resolve this issue for

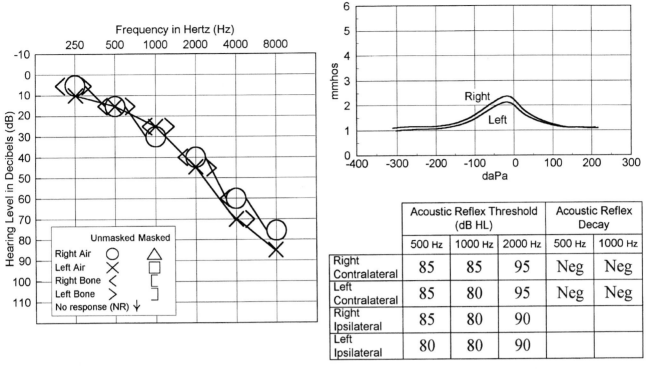

	Acoustic Reflex Threshold (dB HL)			Acoustic Reflex Decay	
	500 Hz	1000 Hz	2000 Hz	500 Hz	1000 Hz
Right Contralateral	85	85	95	Neg	Neg
Left Contralateral	85	80	95	Neg	Neg
Right Ipsilateral	85	80	90		
Left Ipsilateral	80	80	90		

FIGURE 10.15   Acoustic reflex thresholds within the applicable 90th percentiles and negative reflex decay in a typical case of cochlear impairment.

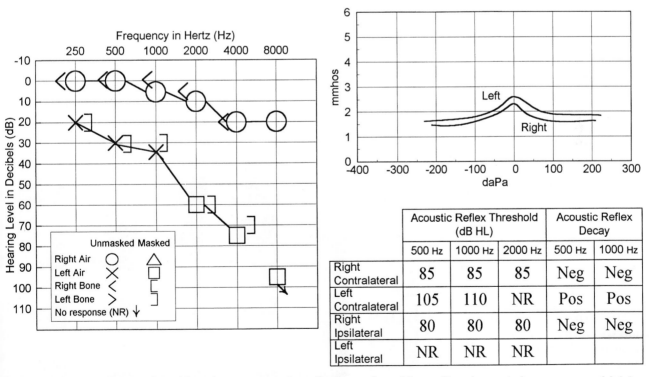

	Acoustic Reflex Threshold (dB HL)			Acoustic Reflex Decay	
	500 Hz	1000 Hz	2000 Hz	500 Hz	1000 Hz
Right Contralateral	85	85	85	Neg	Neg
Left Contralateral	105	110	NR	Pos	Pos
Right Ipsilateral	80	80	80	Neg	Neg
Left Ipsilateral	NR	NR	NR		

FIGURE 10.16   Elevated and/or absent acoustic reflexes and positive reflex decay (where measurable) in a case of retrocochlear pathology (left eighth-nerve tumor).

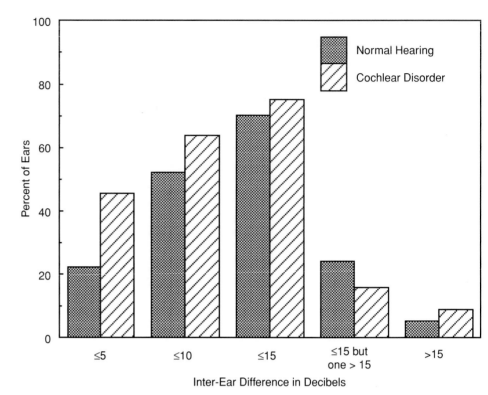

FIGURE 10.17 Percentages of subjects with normal hearing and cochlear disorders having various inter-ear differences in acoustic reflex thresholds for pure tones collapsed across frequency from 250 to 4,000 Hz. (Based on data of Chiveralls et al. [1976] and Chiveralls [1977].)

several reasons. For example, reflex decay testing is limited because absent and elevated reflexes are so common in cases of retrocochlear pathology. Weighted averages across several representative studies (based on Wilson et al. [1984]) suggest that roughly 57% of retrocochlear cases have absent reflexes, in addition to which reflex decay is positive in about 25% using the 5-second method and 29% with the 10-second method. The accumulated evidence suggests that the index of suspicion for retrocochlear pathology is stronger when

reflex decay occurs at 500 Hz than at 1,000 Hz and within the first 5 seconds than during the second 5 seconds of the 10-second test (Olsen et al., 1975, 1981). However, considering both frequencies and the total 10-second interval does improve sensitivity without a major rise in false positives. In addition, reported false-positive rates vary between roughly 8% and 26% in smaller sample studies but are about 3% or less in large-sample studies (Olsen et al., 1975, 1981, 1983; Anderson et al., 1969, 1970; Chiveralls, 1977; Sanders, 1984).

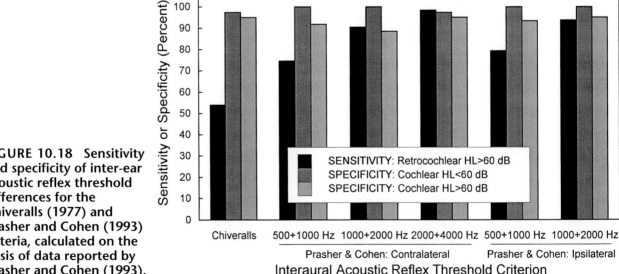

FIGURE 10.18 Sensitivity and specificity of inter-ear acoustic reflex threshold differences for the Chiveralls (1977) and Prasher and Cohen (1993) criteria, calculated on the basis of data reported by Prasher and Cohen (1993).

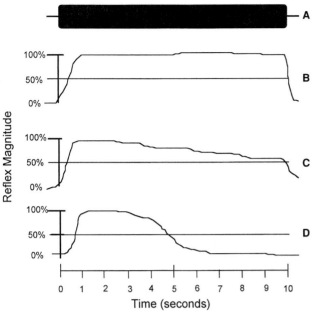

FIGURE 10.19 Measurement of acoustic reflex decay or adaptation. (a) Stimulus tone. (b) Negative reflex decay, with essentially no decay of reflex magnitude over the 10-second period. (c) Negative reflex decay, with reflex magnitude falling by less than 50% over the 10-second period. (d) Positive reflex decay, with reflex magnitude decaying by 50% or more within 10 seconds.

Defining ≥50% reflex decay within 5 seconds as positive and ≤50% decay in 6 to 10 seconds as negative, Ferguson et al. (1996) found that reflex adaptation at 1,000 Hz had 99% specificity (for 110 nontumor cases). All things considered, the most prudent approach is to consider reflex decay

abnormal if it occurs at 500 and/or 1,000 Hz, according to the 10-second criterion.

ACOUSTIC REFLEX MAGNITUDE AND GROWTH

Acoustic reflex magnitude is simply the size of the response (i.e., the amount of immittance change caused by the reflex) (Silman and Gelfand, 1982b; Silman, 1984; Gelfand, 1998). As we saw in Figure 10.4, acoustic reflex magnitude increases as the stimulus level increases above the reflex threshold. This relationship is described as the acoustic reflex growth function and has been described in considerable detail (Møller, 1962; Hung and Dallos, 1964; Peterson and Liden, 1972; Wilson and McBride, 1978; Silman et al., 1978b; Thompson et al., 1980; Silman and Gelfand, 1981b; Sprague et al., 1981; Wilson, 1981; Silman, 1984; Lutolf et al., 2003).

Reflex magnitude and acoustic reflex growth functions are subject to a considerable degree of variability. Moreover, reflex magnitudes are quantified in different ways, from raw values to various kinds of normalized values (e.g., percentage of maximum magnitude). An important but often overlooked source of variability is that reflex magnitude depends on the static acoustic immittance of the ear, which can be controlled by expressing reflex magnitudes in decibels (Silman and Gelfand, 1981b). See Silman (1984) for a discussion of these issues and methods for quantifying reflex magnitudes.

The acoustic reflex growth functions in Figure 10.20 illustrate the fundamental relationships between reflex magnitude (expressed in dB) and stimulus level. The normal acoustic reflex growth function for puretone stimuli shows that reflex magnitude increases linearly with stimulus level. The normal acoustic reflex growth function for BBN stimuli has two segments: Beginning from the reflex threshold, reflex magnitude increases very little with increasing noise

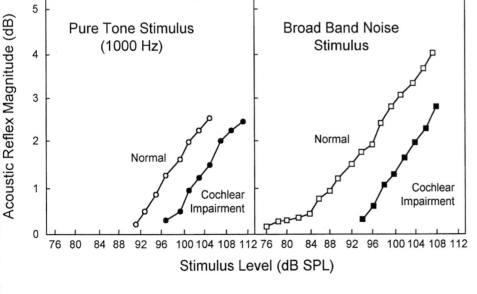

FIGURE 10.20 Acoustic reflex magnitude as a function of stimulus level for puretone and broadband noise (BBN) activating signals. Response magnitude is expressed in dB = 20 log x/y, where x is the magnitude of acoustic impedance during reflex contraction, and y is static acoustic impedance. (Replotted from data reported by Silman et al. [1978b].)

level over a range of roughly 10 dB, above which the BBN growth function rises linearly with further increases in noise level. In other words, the normal BBN growth function has a curvilinear "tail" with little or no reflex growth on its low end, followed by linear growth.

The clinician should be aware of several parameters that might influence the measurement and interpretation of acoustic reflex magnitude and growth. Puretone acoustic reflex growth functions are not affected by stimulus frequency in the 500- to 2,000-Hz range (Møller, 1962; Silman et al., 1978b; Sprague et al., 1981). The acoustic reflex growth function is affected by the aging process, so that the elderly have lower reflex magnitudes and growth functions with shallower slopes than their younger counterparts (Thompson et al., 1980; Silman and Gelfand, 1981b; Wilson, 1981). Ipsilateral stimulation appears to produce steeper growth functions than contralateral stimulation (Møller, 1961, 1962; Jerger et al., 1978). As already mentioned, reflex magnitude depends on the static acoustic immittance of the ear. It is affected by probe-tone frequency and the particular immittance component being measured (Wilson and McBride, 1978; Sprague et al., 1981).

The manner in which reflex magnitude and growth are affected by hearing loss due to cochlear disorders is also shown in Figure 10.20. Notice that the acoustic reflex growth function for ears with cochlear impairment is quite similar to the normal function, except that it is shifted rightward, reflecting their higher reflex thresholds (i.e., it rises linearly with stimulus level). However, in addition to being shifted rightward compared to the normal function, the BBN growth function in ears with cochlear impairments is also missing the curvilinear "tail."

In contrast to cochlear disorders, reflex magnitude and growth are reduced by eighth-nerve and brainstem pathologies affecting the acoustic reflex pathways (Borg, 1977; Bosatra, 1977; Silman et al., 1978a; Mangham et al., 1980; Lew and Jerger, 1991). Significantly reduced acoustic reflex growth functions have also been reported in a case of a cerebellar tumor causing indirect pressure on the reflex pathways, which returned to normal after the tumor was removed (Harrison et al., 1989). Acoustic reflex magnitude is also reduced in the affected ears of patients with unilateral facial paralysis when the facial nerve lesion is proximal to the portion of the facial nerve innervating the stapedius muscle (Ruth et al., 1978).

Figure 10.21 shows reflex responses from both ears of a patient with a unilateral eighth-nerve tumor. The bottom tracing (c) is from the patient's normal ear and shows the normal pattern of increasing reflex magnitude as the stimulus is raised above the reflex threshold. In contrast, the top tracing (a) shows no growth of reflex magnitude at 500 Hz in the pathologic ear. A close look reveals that reflex magnitude actually decreased above 10 dB SL (re: ART). The middle tracing (b) shows that the pathologic ear in this example did have the normal pattern of reflex growth at 1,000 Hz, at least as high as 10 dB SL re: ART, where the maximum testable

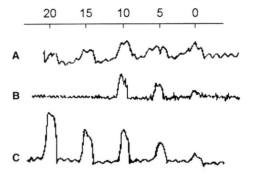

FIGURE 10.21 Acoustic reflex magnitude plotted as a function of increasing stimulus levels (dB re: reflex threshold) for a patient with a unilateral eighth-nerve tumor. Tracings (a) and (b) show reflex magnitudes at 500 Hz and 1,000 Hz in the pathologic ear, and (c) shows results at 500 Hz for the opposite, normal ear. See text. (From Silman S, Gelfand SA, Chun T. [1978a] Some observations in a case of acoustic neuroma. *J Speech Hear Dis.* 43, 459–466, with permission of the American Speech-Language-Hearing Association.)

limits were reached. (The ART here was 115 dB HL, and the maximum testable level was 125 dB HL.)

Mangham et al. (1980) found that reflex magnitudes in patients with eighth-nerve tumors were lower than those of high-risk patients shown not to have tumors. Extensive overlap in the absolute reflex magnitudes of the two groups prevented this measure from distinguishing between them, even though the mean values were smaller for the tumor group. In order to improve the ability to distinguish between tumor and nontumor cases, Mangham et al. (1980) used the ratio of the reflex magnitude in the test ear over the reflex magnitude in the nontest ear to produce a normalized value. This approach is actually a form of inter-ear comparison, in which 1.0 means the two ears have equal reflex magnitudes. All of the normalized values for the tumor cases were less than 0.75; and this approach distinguished between the tumor and nontumor groups without overlap when the stimuli were presented at 10 dB SL re: reflex threshold or higher.

ACOUSTIC REFLEX LATENCY

Acoustic reflex latency refers to how long it takes for the acoustic reflex to occur after the stimulus is presented. This delay is measured from the onset of the stimulus until the beginning of the reflex response. However, instead of being an abrupt change, the immittance change due to the reflex emerges from the prestimulus immittance value and builds up over a certain amount of time, eventually achieving some maximum magnitude. As a result, there are a variety of different ways to define the start of the reflex response for latency measurement and related purposes (Mangham et al.,

1982; Silman and Gelfand, 1982b; Bosatra et al., 1984; Lilly, 1984; Jerger et al., 1986b; Qiu and Stucker, 1997). For example, the beginning of the reflex might be considered the moment when the immittance deviates from the prestimulus baseline or when the immittance change rises to 10% of its eventual maximum value. Latency values will be affected by this definition, as well as by the sensitivity and temporal characteristics of the immittance device being used (Bosatra et al., 1984; Lilly, 1984; Jerger et al., 1986b). Computer averaging improves the ability to visualize the time course of the reflex, so that latency and related measures are facilitated (Silman and Gelfand, 1982b; Stach and Jerger, 1984), but this approach has not been generally adopted clinically.

Acoustic reflex latencies can be as short as about 12 ms if the contractions of the stapedius muscle are being measured directly by electromyography (Zakrisson et al., 1974). However, clinical acoustic reflex latencies are much longer because we are monitoring the immittance changes caused by the mechanical effects of the muscle contraction. Table 10.4 shows normal acoustic reflex latency means and 95% normal ranges for puretone, BBN, and click stimuli presented 10 dB above the ART, which is the level typically used for clinical purposes. These norms were obtained using the Grason-Stadler GSI-33 Middle Ear Analyzer, with latency defined at the point where the reflex response magnitude reaches 10% of its eventual maximum value. Latencies become shorter as the stimulus level increases (Bosatra et al., 1984), and the measured values depend on how latency is defined as well as the electroacoustic characteristics of the instrument itself. Acoustic reflex latencies appear to be similar with age through the fifties but become lengthened with increasing age beginning in the sixties (Bosatra et al., 1984).

Acoustic reflex latencies tend to be within the normal range for ears with cochlear disorders but are substantially longer (often exceeding 200 ms) for ears with retrocochlear pathologies (Strasser, 1975; Clemis and Sarno, 1980; Mangham and Lindeman, 1980; Mangham et al., 1980; Bosatra et al., 1984). However, there is evidence that the interpretation of acoustic reflex latencies can be compromised by complex interactions among a variety of parameters. For example, Jerger and Hayes (1983) found large latency differences between the normal and abnormal ears of four patients with unilateral eighth-nerve tumors for stimuli presented at 10 dB above ART and at equal SPLs but found little if any latency differences when the stimulus levels were adjusted to produce equal reflex magnitudes for both ears. Acoustic reflex latency appears to be normal in patients with cortical lesions and inconsistent among patients with brainstem disorders, so that it does not appear to provide diagnostically useful information when dealing with central auditory pathologies (Bosatra et al., 1984).

ACOUSTIC REFLEXES IN CENTRAL NERVOUS SYSTEM DISORDERS

Extra-Axial Brainstem Disorders

For the most part, the retrocochlear lesions already discussed have focused on eighth-nerve and/or the other cerebellopontine angle tumors that are outside of the brainstem itself, or extra-axial. Figure 10.22 conceptualizes the general configuration of acoustic reflex outcomes associated with eighth-nerve tumors and other extra-axial disorders. This is, of course, the very situation illustrated by the clinical case in Figure 10.16. Notice how the reflex abnormality is found whenever the pathologic ear is stimulated, which is for the left contralateral and left ipsilateral reflexes in these figures.

Intra-Axial Brainstem Disorders

Abnormal acoustic reflex results are also associated with intra-axial brainstem pathologies (i.e., lesions occurring within the brainstem proper) that involve the reflex pathways (Greisen and Rasmussen, 1970; Jerger and Jerger, 1974, 1975, 1977, 1981; Jerger et al., 1975; Stephens and Thornton, 1976; Bosatra et al., 1984; Gelfand, 1984). Because intra-axial

---

TABLE 10.4   Means and 95% normal ranges of acoustic reflex latencies[a] (in milliseconds) of normal-hearing individuals for tonal, broadband noise (BBN), and click stimuli presented at 10 dB above the acoustic reflex threshold

Stimulus:	500 Hz	1,000 Hz	2,000 Hz	4,000 Hz	BBN	Clicks (50/s)
Contralateral						
Mean	102.8	101.9	127.7	147.3	132.3	156.7
95% range	56.0–149.6	51.7–152.1	66.5–188.9	77.9–216.7	59.7–204.9	107.0–206.3
Ipsilateral						
Mean	104.4	102.0	115.2	144.2		
95% range	59.2–149.6	51.4–152.0	70.6–159.8	74.8–213.6		

Data obtained using the Grason-Stadler GSI-33 Middle Ear Analyzer, with latencies defined as the point where the acoustic reflex response magnitude achieves 10% of its eventual maximum value. Based on findings by Qiu and Stucker (1997).
[a] Measured for the admittance (Y) component with a 226-Hz probe tone.

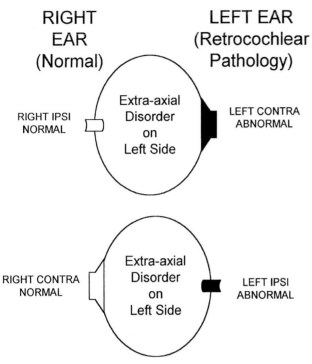

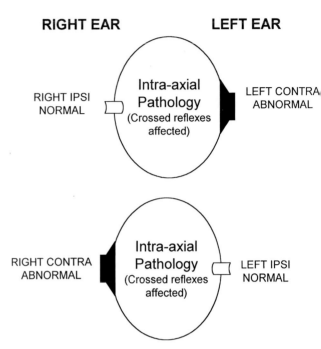

FIGURE 10.22 The typical configuration of contralateral and ipsilateral acoustic reflex outcomes associated with a unilateral retrocochlear disorder, such as an acoustic tumor or extra-axial brainstem lesion. Notice that reflex abnormalities are seen for both the crossed (contralateral) and uncrossed (ipsilateral) conditions in which the pathological side is stimulated.

FIGURE 10.23 The typical configuration of contralateral and ipsilateral acoustic reflex outcomes associated with an intra-axial brainstem lesion. Notice that reflex abnormalities are seen for the crossed (contralateral) conditions, whereas the uncrossed (ipsilateral) conditions may be unaffected.

brainstem lesions often damage one or both of the crossed reflex pathways, they are often associated with abnormal contralateral reflexes without affecting the ipsilateral responses, as illustrated conceptually in Figure 10.23 and clinically in Figure 10.24.

Demyelinating and Neuromuscular Disorders

Abnormalities of reflex thresholds, magnitude, and/or time course have been reported to occur in demyelinating diseases such as multiple sclerosis (Colletti, 1975; Bosatra et al., 1976, 1984; Stephens and Thornton, 1976; Hess, 1979; Mangham, 1984; Wilson et al., 1984; Jerger et al., 1986a; Keith et al., 1987) and neuromuscular disorders like myasthenia gravis (Blom and Zakrisson, 1974; Kramer et al., 1981; Piccolo et al., 1977; Gelfand, 1984; Mangham, 1984; Wilson et al., 1984; Smith and Brezinova, 1991; Tóth et al., 2000).

Cortical Disorders

Disorders superior to the reflex pathways do not appear to affect acoustic reflex results. Although lowered ARTs have been

reported in a few patients with cortical disorders (Downs and Crum, 1980), the preponderance of the evidence and clinical experience indicates that cortical lesions do not affect the acoustic reflex (Jerger and Jerger, 1981; Gelfand and Silman, 1982; Gelfand, 1984, 1997; Silman and Silverman, 1991).

▨ AUDITORY NEUROPATHY OR DYSSYNCHRONY DISORDER

Patients with auditory neuropathy or dyssynchrony disorder usually present with speech recognition performance that is atypically low when viewed in the context of their audiograms. Physiologic tests show abnormal functioning of the auditory nerve and/or lower auditory brainstem along with normal functioning of the outer hair cells, and there is no radiologic evidence of retrocochlear lesions. Normal outer hair cell functioning is demonstrated by normal otoacoustic emissions and/or cochlear microphonics, and the disorder of synchronous neural coding is revealed by abnormal auditory brainstem responses and/or acoustic reflexes (Sininger et al., 1995; Starr et al., 1996; Shivashanker et al., 2003).

The importance of acoustic reflex testing in the identification of auditory neuropathy is highlighted by its inclusion in almost every audiologic evaluation. Moreover, one cannot help but wonder about how many abnormal acoustic reflex findings that turned out to be "false positives" for

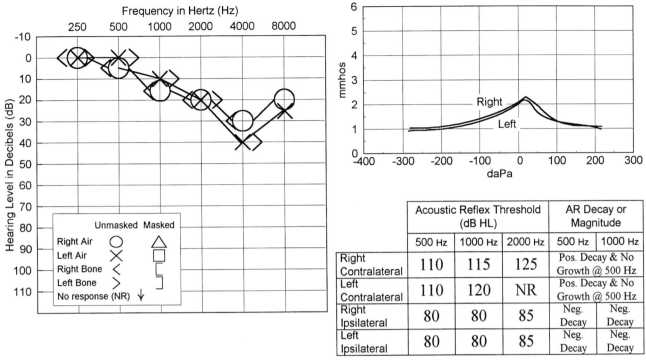

	Acoustic Reflex Threshold (dB HL)			AR Decay or Magnitude	
	500 Hz	1000 Hz	2000 Hz	500 Hz	1000 Hz
Right Contralateral	110	115	125	Pos. Decay & No Growth @ 500 Hz	
Left Contralateral	110	120	NR	Pos. Decay & No Growth @ 500 Hz	
Right Ipsilateral	80	80	85	Neg. Decay	Neg. Decay
Left Ipsilateral	80	80	85	Neg. Decay	Neg. Decay

FIGURE 10.24   Abnormal contralateral and normal ipsilateral acoustic reflex findings in a case with an intra-axial brainstem lesion.

space-occupying retrocochlear lesions were actually hits for neural dyssynchrony disorders.

FACIAL NERVE DISORDERS

Acoustic reflex abnormalities are associated with facial nerve disorders when the probe is located in the affected ear, as illustrated in Figure 10.25 (Alford et al., 1973; Citron and Adour, 1978; Ruth et al., 1978; Wiley and Block, 1984; Silverman et al., 1986; Silman et al., 1988). This is not surprising, because the stapedius muscle is innervated by CN VII.

Because seventh-nerve disorders are usually revealed by other neurologic findings that are readily observable (e.g., facial paralysis), the principal acoustic reflex application in this arena used to be as a tool to monitor the recovery process in cases of Bell's palsy (idiopathic facial nerve palsy). However, it has been shown that seventh-nerve disorders can produce the constellation of ipsilateral and contralateral reflex decay (with the probe on the affected side), even when there are no observable facial abnormalities and when the ARTs are within the applicable 90th percentiles (Silverman et al., 1986; Silman et al., 1988). An illustrative case is shown in Figure 10.26. These findings emphasize the diagnostic potential of acoustic reflex tests with regard to facial nerve disorders and imply that clinicians should consider also testing for ipsilateral reflex decay when reflex decay is observed with contralateral testing.

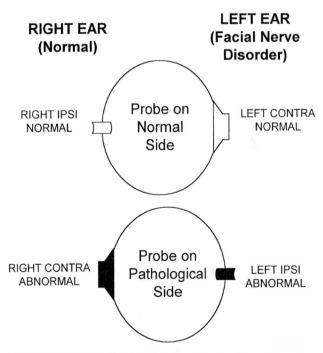

FIGURE 10.25   The typical configuration of contralateral and ipsilateral acoustic reflex outcomes associated with a unilateral facial nerve disorder. Notice that reflex abnormalities are seen for both the crossed (contralateral) and uncrossed (ipsilateral) conditions in which the probe is located on the pathologic side.

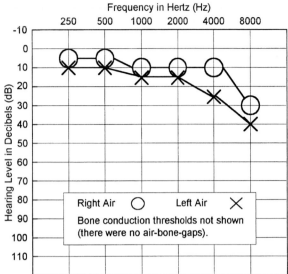

	Right Ear	Left Ear
Tympanometric Peak Pressure	-20 daPa	-70 daPa
Static Admittance	0.60 mmho	0.81 mmho

	Acoustic Reflex Threshold (dB HL)			Acoustic Reflex Decay	
	500 Hz	1000 Hz	2000 Hz	500 Hz	1000 Hz
Right Contralateral	85	85	80	Neg	Neg
Left Contralateral	90	85	75	Pos	Pos
Right Ipsilateral	80	80	80	Pos	Pos
Left Ipsilateral	85	80	85	Neg	Neg

FIGURE 10.26   Acoustic reflex findings in a case with vascular compression of the right facial nerve. This example corresponds to case 1 in Silman et al. (1988). Positive reflex decay occurred for both conditions with the probe on the pathologic right side (right ipsilateral and left contralateral) even though the reflex thresholds were within applicable 90th percentiles and there were no observable signs of facial paralysis. The reliability of the reflex decay results is shown by the double (test and retest) tracings in the upper right-hand frame, which is adapted from Silman S, Silverman CA, Gelfand SA, Lutolf J, Lynn DJ. (1988) Ipsilateral acoustic-reflex adaptation testing for detection of facial-nerve pathology: three case studies. J Speech Hear Dis. 53, 378–382, with permission of the American Speech-Language-Hearing Association.

▧ CLINICAL IMPLICATIONS OF NONACOUSTIC REFLEXES

Recall that the stapedius reflex can be elicited by tactile or electrocutaneous stimulation of the sides of the face and head, and both middle ear muscles are activated as a startle response by stimulating the orbital region. In contrast to the sophisticated measurements we use with acoustic reflexes, nonacoustic reflex tests are limited to determining whether the responses are *present* or *absent.* Moreover, they are lacking in norms and can be prone to artifact when elicited by tactile stimulation. Artifacts are avoided with electrocutaneous stimulation methods, which are described elsewhere (Djupesland et al., 1977; Djupesland and Tvete, 1979; Djupesland, 1981). However, the author has never come across instances of electrocutaneous stimulation of the nonacoustic reflex in actual clinical practice.

Despite these limitations, nonacoustic reflexes may provide useful supplemental diagnostic information when the acoustic reflex is absent, principally because nonacoustic stimulation circumvents the afferent aspects of the acoustic reflex (Klockhoff, 1961; Djupesland, 1964, 1975, 1981; Djupesland et al., 1977; Wiley and Block, 1984; Mulder et al., 1993). The presence versus absence of nonacoustic responses may help the clinician determine whether an abnormality of the afferent (sensory) versus efferent (motor) aspects of the acoustic reflex was responsible for its absence. In these cases, it appears that the most feasible means of nonacoustic stimulation would be to touch the ipsilateral ear canal or pinna (for a stapedius response) and to use an appropriately delivered air puff to the orbit area (for a combined stapedius and tensor tympani response), while being alert to the possibility of movement and other artifacts.

The diagnostic constellations involving nonacoustic stimulation are fundamentally as follows, all of which *assume the acoustic reflex is absent.* A present nonacoustic stapedius reflex suggests that the abnormality is attributable to the afferent side of the acoustic reflex arc. This finding would implicate the eighth nerve on the acoustically stimulated side, but it could also reflect a cochlear or conductive hearing loss large enough to account for the absent acoustic reflex. An absent nonacoustic stapedius reflex is expected when there is a facial nerve, stapedius muscle, or middle ear disorder in the probe ear. Which choice is the most probable involves considering the reflex results in light of the other clinical findings.

Some supplemental information may be generated by nonacoustically stimulating both the tensor tympani and stapedius muscles. Obtaining a response of this kind, when the nonacoustic stapedial reflex is absent, suggests that a seventh-nerve or stapedius muscle disorder is more likely and a middle ear disorder is less likely. Here is why: First, if the *combined* nonacoustic response is present and the *stapedius alone* nonacoustic reflex is absent, then we must credit the combined response to the tensor tympani muscle and trigeminal nerve and conclude that there is a problem with the stapedius muscle and/or facial nerve. Second, had there been middle ear pathology, then we should not be able to monitor an immittance change in the probe ear regardless of which muscle(s) contracted (recall the "probe ear rule"). However, exceptions do occur (see Mulder et al. [1993]).

HEARING LOSS IDENTIFICATION AND PREDICTION

Tonal and Broadband Stimuli

Various techniques using tonal and/or BBN ARTs have been proposed as methods for the prediction of hearing losses in patients who are difficult or impossible to test behaviorally due to age or physical, cognitive, and/or other factors (Popelka, 1981; Silman and Gelfand, 1982a, 1982b; Silman et al., 1984a, 1987). Most of these methods depend on the ways in which puretone and/or BBN ARTs are affected by sensory-neural hearing loss, as illustrated in Figure 10.13.

Several relationships are revealed in this figure. First, tonal ARTs are essentially independent of auditory threshold for hearing losses up to approximately 50 to 60 dB HL, above which the tonal ARTs rise as the magnitude of the hearing loss increases. (Fig. 11.13 shows an arbitrary breakpoint at 50 dB HL.) Second, BBN ARTs increase with increasing sensory-neural hearing loss up to roughly 50 to 60 dB HL but do not continue to rise with further increases in the magnitude of the hearing loss. Third, ARTs are lower for BBN stimuli compared to tonal stimuli, constituting what is called the *noise-tone difference*. Fourth, the noise-tone difference is approximately 20 dB wide in normal-hearing individuals (seen as the distance between the two curves when the auditory threshold is 0 dB HL). Finally, the size of the noise-tone difference depends on the amount of hearing loss in a complex way, because the BBN and tonal ARTs are related to the amount of the hearing loss in different ways. Specifically, the noise-tone difference becomes smaller as the amount of hearing loss increases up to roughly 50 dB (seen as the convergence of the curves in the figure), but it becomes pro-

gressively larger again with further increases in hearing loss (seen as the divergence of the curves).

PREDICTING HEARING LOSS WITH ACOUSTIC REFLEXES

Early ART-based methods for predicting hearing loss attempted to determine the magnitude of hearing loss. The Niemeyer and Sesterhenn (1974) approach provided a hearing loss prediction in decibels. In contrast, the SPAR (Sensitivity Prediction from the Acoustic Reflex) method and its revisions predicted hearing loss categories, such as normal, mild-moderate, severe, and profound (Jerger et al., 1974b, 1978). Computational procedures for these germinal approaches can be found in the original papers and in the review by Silman et al. (1984a). In addition to the prediction methods based on the noise-tone difference, other approaches have used regression analyses as the basis for trying to predict hearing loss from ARTs (Baker and Lilly, 1976; Rizzo and Greenberg, 1979b).

These early approaches were plagued by large false-positive and false-negative rates and large errors in the accuracy with which hearing loss was predicted (Hall and Koval, 1982; Silman et al., 1984a). At least three factors probably accounted for the limitations of these methods (Popelka, 1981; Silman et al., 1984a; Gelfand, 1998). First, the ARTs associated with a given amount of hearing loss are subject to considerable variability, spanning a range of approximately 20 dB or more. Second, tonal and BBN ARTs have a peculiar relationship to the degree of hearing loss, so that the noise-tone difference first converges and then diverges over the course of the hearing threshold continuum. Thus, for example, the size of the noise-tone difference can be the same for a normal ear and one with a severe hearing loss. Third, using regression to predict hearing threshold from the ART involves reversing the actual relationship among the independent and dependent variables.

IDENTIFYING HEARING LOSS WITH ACOUSTIC REFLEXES

Identification

Using the acoustic reflex to *identify* the *existence* of a significant degree of hearing impairment provides a more successful, albeit more conservative, approach compared to trying to *predict* the *amount* of hearing loss. Keith (1977) proposed an elegantly straightforward method capitalizing on the principle that even small amounts of sensory-neural hearing loss elevate the ART for BBN. He found that 87% of normal-hearing subjects had BBN ARTs at 85 dB SPL or below, whereas 97% of hearing-impaired subjects had BBN ARTs higher than 85 dB SPL. Thus, he proposed using a BBN ART of 85 dB SPL as the cutoff value for hearing loss identification with the acoustic reflex. Subsequent findings confirmed that Keith's approach effectively separated those with normal hearing from those with substantial degrees of sensory-neural hearing loss among young adults and in patients with cerebral palsy, although patients with mild or high-frequency hearing losses can have BBN ARTs falling on either side of the 85-dB SPL criterion (Silman et al., 1984a, 1984b; Emmer and Silman, 2003).

Bivariate Approaches

Popelka and Trumph (1976) introduced the widely used bivariate approach to hearing loss identification, which capitalizes on how both BBN and puretone ARTs, as well as the relationship between them, are related to sensory-neural hearing loss. The term bivariate is used because the ART results for an ear are represented by a point plotted on an x-y graph, as illustrated in Figure 10.27. Each point is based on the ARTs obtained at 500, 1,000, and 2,000 Hz and for BBN.

The first phase in the use of the bivariate method is to obtain and plot normative ART data from a sample of subjects with known hearing thresholds. A set of lines is then drawn to separate these points into "normal" and "abnormal" areas, according to some practical, compromise criterion. The plotting procedure itself involves the following basic steps (although variations do exist): All of the ARTs are expressed in dB SPL. The ARTs for 500, 1,000, and 2,000 Hz are then averaged. To arrive at the x-coordinate, the BBN ART is divided by the average of the tonal ARTs, the result of which is multiplied by 100 to produce a convenient numerical value. The y-coordinate is simply the average of the tonal ARTs.

Once the cutoff lines have been established, ARTs obtained from patients can be plotted as points on the same bivariate graph and are interpreted according to where they fall relative to the cutoff lines. In the original bivariate plotting procedure, the cutoff lines were drawn so that ≥90% of the data from young normal ears fell in the area to the left of the lines, which effectively placed the data from young patients with puretone averages of ≥32 dB HL in the region to the right of the lines (Popelka and Trumph, 1976; Popelka, 1981).

Although quite effective for separating normal ears from those with relatively substantial losses, the original approach is less effective when the patient population includes adults with mild losses and/or high-frequency losses, especially for patients above approximately 45 years of age (Silman and Gelfand, 1979; Silman et al., 1984a, 1984b; Silverman et al., 1983). Some of these limitations are alleviated by the modified bivariate method (Silman et al., 1984a, 1984b). In contrast to the original approach, the modified bivariate method involves placing the cutoff lines so that (1) the separation of normal and impaired ears is maximized, and (2) at least 90% of ears with mild and/or sloping losses are placed outside of the normal region. Silman et al. (1984a, 1984b) found correct identification rates for adults between 20 and 44 years of age to be 97% for normal adults but only 69% for the hearing-impaired adults using the original bivariate method, compared with 86% and 96%, respectively, for the modified bivariate approach. Unfortunately, the modified method was also lacking when used with patients ≥45 years old. For this age range, Silman et al. (1984a, 1984b) suggested that a hearing impairment should be suspected when (1) the BBN ART is greater than 95 dB SPL, or (2) the 1,000- or 2,000-Hz ART is 105 dB SPL or higher. These criteria result in correct identification rates of 93% for normal-hearing individuals and 77% for patients with hearing impairments (Wallin et al., 1986).

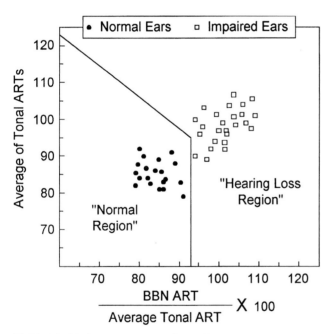

FIGURE 10.27 An example of the bivariate method showing representative acoustic reflex results obtained from ears with normal hearing and various degrees of hearing loss. Each point represents one ear and is considered relative to the line segments that separate the normal and hearing loss regions of the graph.

FUNCTIONAL HEARING LOSS

The possibility of a functional hearing loss may be suspected if a patient's ARTs are atypically low when considered in light of their voluntary auditory thresholds (Alberti, 1970; Feldman, 1963; Lamb and Peterson, 1967; Silman et al., 1984a; Silman, 1988; Gelfand, 1994). The situation is straightforward when the ART is at or below the patient's hearing thresholds, but some reasonable criterion is needed for what constitutes "too low" if the reflex threshold is higher than the hearing threshold. Recall that the recommended criterion for an elevated ART is whether it exceeds the 90th percentile. Based on the same premise, it has been recommended that an ART be considered unusually low if it falls *below* the 10th

TABLE 10.5	Acoustic reflex tenth percentile cutoff values as a function of auditory threshold at 500 Hz, 1,000 Hz, and 2,000 Hz		

Auditory	Acoustic reflex threshold (dB HL)		
Threshold (dB HL)	500 Hz	1,000 Hz	2,000 Hz
<60		(not recommended)	
60	85	85	85
65	90	90	90
70	95	95	90
75	95	95	95
80	100	100	100
85	100	100	110
≥ 90		(10 dB above auditory threshold)	

Based on data by Gelfand et al., 1990.

percentile of the ART distribution for normal and cochlear-impaired individuals, shown in Table 10.5 and by the lower curves in Figure 10.14 (Gelfand and Piper, 1984; Silman et al., 1984a; Silman, 1988; Gelfand et al., 1990; Gelfand, 1994).

The feasibility of using 10th percentiles to identify functional hearing losses was studied by Gelfand (1994). It was found that 10th percentiles are useful in the identification of functional losses, providing the patient's voluntary hearing threshold is *at least* 60 dB HL at the reflex test frequency but not when the voluntary threshold is less than 60 dB HL at that frequency. It is not surprising that 10th percentiles do not contribute to the distinction between organic and

nonorganic impairments when the hearing threshold is ≤55 dB HL because tonal ARTs are essentially unaffected by the magnitude of hearing loss up to about 50 to 60 dB HL, as previously discussed. For this reason, only the 10th percentiles applicable to hearing losses ≥60 dB (at the reflex test frequency) are shown in Table 10.5. The clinical example in Figure 10.28 shows an example from a patient with a bilateral functional hearing loss. Notice that the ARTs are below the 10th percentiles associated with the exaggerated puretone thresholds in the functional audiogram but are consistent with the presumably organic thresholds obtained after the functional overlay was resolved.

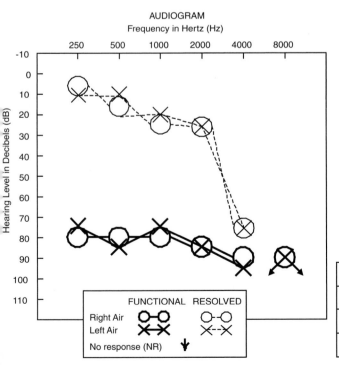

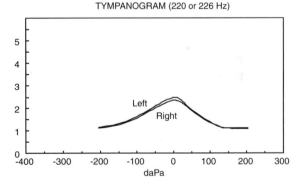

FIGURE 10.28 Acoustic reflex thresholds below the 10th percentiles for the voluntary puretone thresholds in a case of functional hearing loss.

Another ART-based technique that may be used to assess the possibility of the functional impairments is provided by the modified bivariate method for hearing loss identification (Silman et al., 1984a; Silman, 1988). The bivariate method relies on the BBN reflex threshold, which is affected by sensory-neural hearing loss and aging, as already discussed. For this reason, it is effective as a test for functional impairment when the patient is less than 45 years old and does not have an underlying organic hearing loss of any significant degree.

In light of these considerations, Gelfand (1994) proposed several guidelines for interpreting acoustic reflex tests as indicators of possible functional impairment in patients who have a significant degree of hearing loss. First, a functional loss is suggested if the tonal ART is at or below the patient's auditory threshold at the same frequency. Second, results falling inside the "normal region" of the modified bivariate plot imply a functional impairment and underlying hearing sensitivity that is roughly within the normal range. Third, a functional impairment may be suspected if the ART

is below the applicable cutoff values shown in Table 10.5, provided that the voluntary hearing threshold is 60 dB HL or higher at the test frequency. Fourth, a functional impairment cannot be ruled out by negative results (i.e., ARTs at or above the 10th percentiles and/or modified bivariate results inside the "impaired region").

CONCLUDING REMARKS

The intention of this chapter has been to provide both students and practicing audiologists with a clinically relevant overview of acoustic reflex principles and methods. One cannot help but be impressed by the extensive amount of information provided by acoustic reflex measurements, especially when one realizes that this clinical yield is provided by rapid tests that are typically incorporated into routine evaluations. It is hoped that the readers come away with an appreciation for the scope of acoustic reflex applications and become motivated to take full advantage of them.

REFERENCES

Abahazi DA, Greenberg HJ. (1977) Clinical acoustic reflex threshold measurements in infants. *J Speech Hear Dis.* 42, 515–519.

Alberti P. (1970) New tools for old tricks. *Ann Otol Rhinol Laryngol.* 79, 800–807.

Alberti P, Fria J, Cummings F. (1977) The clinical utility of ipsilateral stapedius reflex tests. *J Otolaryngol.* 6, 466–472.

Alford B, Jerger J, Coats A, Peterson C, Weber S. (1973) Neurophysiology of facial nerve testing. *Arch Otolaryngol.* 97, 214.

American Speech-Language-Hearing Association. (1979) Guidelines for acoustic immittance screen of middle-ear function. *ASHA.* 21, 550–558.

American Speech-Language-Hearing Association. (1990) Guidelines for screening for hearing impairment and middle-ear disorders. *ASHA.* 32 (suppl 2), 17–24.

Anderson H, Barr B, Wedenberg E. (1969) Intra-aural reflexes in retrocochlear lesions. In: Hamberger A, Wersäll J, eds. *Disorders of the Skull Base Region (Nobel Symposium 10).* Stockholm: Almqvist Wikell; pp 48–54.

Anderson H, Barr B, Wedenberg E. (1970) Early diagnosis of VIIIth-nerve tumors by acoustic reflex tests. *Acta Otolaryngol.* 262, 232–237.

Baker S, Lilly DJ. (1976) Prediction of hearing level from acoustic reflex data. Presented at the Convention of American Speech-Language-Hearing Association, Houston, TX.

Bauch CD, Robinette MS. (1978) Alcohol and the acoustic reflex: effects of stimulus spectrum, subject variability, and sex. *J Am Aud Soc.* 4, 104–112.

Bel J, Causse P, Michaux P, Cézard R, Canut T, Tapon J. (1976) Mechanical explanation of the on-off effect (diphasic impedance change) in otospongiosis. *Audiology.* 15, 128–140.

Bennett MJ. (1975) Acoustic impedance measurements with the neonate. *Br J Audiol.* 9, 117–124.

Bennett MJ. (1984) Impedance concepts relating to the acoustic reflex. In: Silman S, ed. *The Acoustic Reflex: Basic Principles and Clinical Applications.* Orlando: Academic Press; pp 35–61.

Bennett MJ, Weatherby LA. (1979) Multiple probe frequency acoustic reflex measurements. *Scand Audiol.* 8, 233–239.

Bennett MJ, Weatherby LA. (1982) Newborn acoustic reflexes to noise and puretone signals. *J Speech Hear Res.* 25, 383–387.

Bergenius J, Borg E, Hirsch A. (1983) Stapedius reflex test, brainstem audiometry and optovestibular tests in diagnosis of acoustic neurinomas. *Scand Audiol,* 12, 3–9.

Blom S, Zakrisson JE. (1974) The stapedius reflex in the diagnosis of myasthenia gravis. *J Neurol Sci.* 21, 71–76.

Blood IM, Greenberg HJ. (1981) Low-level acoustic reflex thresholds. *Audiology.* 20, 244–250.

Borg E. (1968) A quantitative study of the effect of the acoustic stapedius reflex on sound transmission through the middle ear of man. *Acta Otolaryngol.* 66, 461–472.

Borg E. (1973) On the neuronal organization of the acoustic middle ear reflex. A physiological and anatomical study. *Brain Res.* 49, 101–123.

Borg E. (1977) The intra-aural muscle reflex in retrocochlear pathology: a model study in the rabbit. *Audiology.* 16, 316–330.

Borg E, Counter SA, Rösler G. (1984) Theories of middle-ear muscle function. In: Silman S, ed. *The Acoustic Reflex: Basic Principles and Clinical Applications.* Orlando: Academic Press; pp 63–99.

Borg E, Møller AR. (1967) Effect of ethyl alcohol and pentobarbital sodium on the acoustic middle ear reflex in man. *Acta Otolaryngol.* 64, 415–426.

Bosatra A. (1977) Pathology of the nervous arc of acoustic reflexes. *Audiology.* 16, 307–315.

Bosatra A, Russolo M, Poli P. (1976) Oscilloscopic analysis of the stapedius muscle reflex in brain stem lesions. *Arch Otolaryngol.* 102, 284–285.

Bosatra A, Russolo M, Silverman CA. (1984) Acoustic-reflex latency: state of the art. In: Silman S, ed. *The Acoustic Reflex: Basic Principles and Clinical Applications.* Orlando: Academic Press; pp 301–328.

Chiveralls K. (1977) A further examination of the use of the stapedius reflex in diagnosis of acoustic neuroma. *Audiology.* 16, 331–337.

Chiveralls K, FitzSimons R, Beck GB, Kernohan H. (1976) The diagnostic significance of the stapedius reflex. *Br J Audiol.* 10, 122–128.

Ciardo A, Garavello W, Leva M, Graziano B, Gaini RM. (2005) Reversed ipsilateral acoustic reflex: a study on subjects treated with muscle relaxants. *Ear Hear.* 26, 96–105.

Ciardo A, Garavello W, Rosetti A, Manghisi PV, Merola S, Gaini RM. (2003) The reversed ipsilateral acoustic reflex: clinical features and kinetic analysis. *Acta Otolaryngol.* 123, 65–70.

Citron D, Adour K. (1978) Acoustic reflex and loudness discomfort in acute facial paralysis. *Arch Otolaryngol.* 104, 303–308.

Clemis JD, Sarno CN. (1980) The acoustic reflex latency test: clinical application. *Laryngoscope.* 90, 601–611.

Cohill EN, Greenberg HJ. (1977) Effects of ethyl alcohol on the acoustic reflex threshold. *J Am Aud Soc.* 2, 121–123.

Colletti V. (1975) Stapedius reflex abnormalities in multiple sclerosis. *Audiology.* 14, 63–71.

Djupesland G. (1964) Middle ear muscle reflexes elicited by acoustic and nonacoustic stimulation. *Acta Otolaryngol.* 188 (suppl), 287–292.

Djupesland G. (1967) Contraction of the tympanic muscles in man. Thesis. Oslo, Norway: Universitetsforlaget.

Djupesland G. (1975) Advanced reflex considerations In: Jerger J, ed. *Handbook of Clinical Impedance Audiometry.* Dobbs Ferry, NY: American Electromedics; 85–126.

Djupesland G. (1981) Diagnostic application of impedance audiometry in testing the middle ear function. Proceedings of the Fourth International Symposium on Acoustic Impedance Measurements, Lisbon, Portugal, pp 217–239.

Djupesland G, Flottorp G, Hansen E, Sjaastad O. (1974) Cogan's syndrome: the audiological picture. *Arch Otolaryngol.* 99, 218–225.

Djupesland G, Flottorp G, Sundby A. (1977) Impedance changes elicited by electrocutaneous stimulation. *Audiology.* 16, 355–364.

Djupesland G, Tvete O. (1979) Impedance changes elicited by tactile and electrocutaneous stimulation. *Scand Audiol.* 8, 243–245.

Djupesland G, Zwislocki JJ. (1973) On the critical band in the acoustic stapedius reflex. *J Acoust Soc Am.* 54, 1157–1159.

Downs DW, Crum MA. (1980) The hyperactive acoustic reflex: four case studies. *Arch Otolaryngol.* 106, 401–404.

Draf W, Leitner H. (1972) Klinischer vergleich von impedanzmessung und anderen recruitment prufmethoden. *Zeitschrift fur Laryagologie, Rhinologie, Otologie Ihre Grenzgebiete.* 51, 700–709.

Emmer MB, Silman S. (2003) The prediction of hearing loss in persons with cerebral palsy using contralateral acoustic reflex threshold for broad-band noise. *Am J Audiol.* 12, 91–95.

Feeney MP, Keefe DH. (1999) Acoustic reflex detection using wideband acoustic reflectance, admittance, and power measurements. *J Speech Lang Hear Res.* 42, 1029–1041.

Feeney MP, Keefe DH. (2001) Estimating the acoustic reflex threshold from wideband measures of reflectance, admittance, and power. *Ear Hear.* 22, 316–332.

Feeney MP, Keefe DH, Marryott LP. (2003) Contralateral acoustic reflex thresholds for tonal activators using wideband energy reflectance and admittance. *J Speech Lang Hear Res.* 46, 128–136.

Feeney MP, Keefe DH, Sanford CA. (2004) Wideband reflectance measures of the ipsilateral acoustic stapedius reflex threshold. *Ear Hear.* 25, 421–430.

Feldman AS. (1963) Impedance measurements at the ear-drum as an aid to diagnosis. *J Speech Hear Res.* 6, 315–327.

Feldman AS, Katz D. (1978) Effects of stimulus duration and stimulus off time on the auditory and acoustic reflex thresholds. *J Speech Hear Res.* 21, 74–78.

Ferguson MA, Smith PA, Lutman ME, Mason SM, Coles RRA, Gibbin KP. (1996) Efficiency of tests used to screen for cerebellopontine angle tumours: a prospective study. *Br J Audiol.* 30, 159–176.

Fielding ED, Rawool VW. (2002) Acoustic reflex thresholds at varying click rates in children. *Int J Pediatr Otorhinolaryngol.* 63, 243–252.

Flottorp G, Djupesland G. (1970) Diphasic impedance change and its applicability in clinical work. *Acta Otolaryngol.* 263, 200–204.

Flottorp G, Djupesland G, Winther F. (1971) The acoustic stapedius reflex in relation to critical bandwidth. *J Acoust Soc Am.* 49, 457–461.

Forquer BD. (1979) The stability of and the relationship between the acoustic reflex and uncomfortable loudness levels. *J Am Aud Soc.* 5, 55–59.

Fria T, LeBlanc J, Dristensen R, Alberti PW. (1975) Ipsilateral acoustic reflex stimulation in normal and sensorineural impaired ears: a preliminary report. *Can J Otolaryngol.* 4, 695–703.

Gelfand SA (1984) The contralateral acoustic reflex. In: Silman S, ed. *The Acoustic Reflex: Basic Principles and Clinical Applications.* Orlando: Academic Press; pp 137–186.

Gelfand SA. (1994) Acoustic reflex threshold tenth percentiles and functional hearing impairment. *J Am Acad Audiol.* 5, 10–16.

Gelfand SA. (1997) *Essentials of Audiology.* New York: Thieme Medical Publishers.

Gelfand SA. (1998) *Hearing: An Introduction to Psychological and Physiological Acoustics.* 3rd ed. New York: Marcel Dekker.

Gelfand SA, Piper N. (1981) Acoustic reflex thresholds in young and elderly subjects with normal hearing. *J Acoust Soc Am.* 69, 295–297.

Gelfand SA, Piper N. (1984) Acoustic reflex thresholds: variability and distribution effects. *Ear Hear.* 5, 228–234.

Gelfand SA, Piper N, Silman S. (1983) Effects of hearing levels at the stimulus and other frequencies upon the expected levels of the acoustic reflex threshold. *J Speech Hear Dis.* 48, 11–17.

Gelfand SA, Schwander T, Silman S. (1990) Acoustic reflex thresholds in normal and cochlear-impaired ears: effects of no-response rates on 90th percentiles in a large sample. *J Speech Hear Dis.* 55, 198–205.

Gelfand SA, Silman S. (1982) Acoustic reflex thresholds in brain damaged patients. *Ear Hear.* 3, 93–95.

Gonay P, Dutillieux D, Matz T. (1974) La dynamique de la contraction du muscle de etrier en fonction de l'age. *Rev Electrodiagnostic-Therapie.* 11, 17–22.

Green KW, Margolis RH. (1984) The ipsilateral acoustic reflex. In: Silman S, ed. *The Acoustic Reflex: Basic Principles and Clinical Applications.* Orlando: Academic Press; pp 275–299.

Greisen O, Rasmussen PE. (1970) Stapedius muscle reflexes and otoneurological examinations in brainstem tumors. *Acta Otolaryngol.* 70, 365–378.

Hall JW, Koval CB. (1982) Accuracy of hearing prediction by the acoustic reflex. *Laryngoscope.* 92, 140–149.

Handler SD, Margolis RH. (1977) Predicting hearing loss from stapedial reflex thresholds in patients with sensorineural impairment. *Ann Otol Rhinol Laryngol.* 84, 425–431.

Harrison T, Silman S, Silverman CA. (1989) Contralateral acoustic-reflex growth function in a patient with cerebellar tumor: a case study. *J Speech Hear Dis.* 54, 505–509.

Hayes D. (1977) Resident's page. *Arch* Otolaryngol. 103, 502–503.

Hayes D, Jerger J. (1980) The effect of degree of hearing loss on diagnostic test strategy. *Arch Otolaryagol.* 106, 266–268.

Hess K. (1979) Stapedius reflex in multiple sclerosis. *J Neurol Neurosurg Psychiatry.* 42, 331–337.

Himmelfarb MZ, Shanon E, Popelka GR, Margolis RH. (1978) Acoustic reflex evaluation in neonates. In: Gerber SE, Mencher GT, eds. *Early Diagnosis of Hearing Loss.* New York: Grune Stratton.

Hung IJ, Dallos P. (1964) Study of the acoustic reflex in human beings. I. Dynamic characteristics. *J Acoust Soc Am.* 52, 1168–1180.

Isenberg SF, Tubergen LB. (1980) An unusual congenital middle ear ossicular anomaly. *Arch Otolaryngol.* 106, 179–181.

Jeck LT, Ruth RA, Schoney ZG. (1983) High-frequency sensitization of the acoustic reflex. *Ear Hear.* 4, 98–101.

Jenkins HA, Morgan DE, Miller RH. (1980) Intact acoustic reflexes in the presence of ossicular disruption. *Laryngoscope.* 90, 267–273.

Jepsen O. (1963) Middle-ear muscle reflexes in man. In: Jerger J, ed. *Modern Developments in Audiology.* New York: Academic Press; 193–239.

Jerger J. (1975) Diagnostic use of impedance measures. In: Jerger J, ed. *Handbook of Clinical Impedance Audiometry.* Dobbs Ferry, NY: Morgan Press; 149–174.

Jerger J, Anthony L, Jerger S, Mauldin L. (1974a) Studies in impedance audiometry. III. Middle ear disorders. *Arch Otolaryngol.* 99, 165–171.

Jerger J, Burney P, Mauldin L, Crump B. (1974b) Predicting hearing loss from the acoustic reflex. *J Speech Hear Dis.* 39, 11–22.

Jerger J, Harford E, Clemis J, Alford B. (1974c) The acoustic reflex in eighth nerve disorders. *Arch Otolaryngol.* 99, 409–413.

Jerger J, Hayes D. (1983) Latency of the acoustic reflex in eighth-nerve tumor. *Arch Otolaryngol.* 109, 1–5.

Jerger J, Hayes D, Anthony L, Mauldin L. (1978) Factors influencing prediction of hearing level from the acoustic reflex. *Maico Mongrs Contemp Audiol.* 1, 1–20.

Jerger J, Jerger S. (1974) Auditory findings in brain stem disorders. *Arch Otolaryngol.* 99, 342–350.

Jerger J, Jerger S, Mauldin L. (1972) Studies in impedance audiometry. I. Normal and sensorineural ears. *Arch Otolaryngol.* 96, 513–523.

Jerger J, Mauldin L, Lewis N. (1977) Temporal summation of the acoustic reflex. *Audiology.* 16, 177–200.

Jerger J, Oliver TA, Chmiel RA, Rivera VM. (1986a) Patterns of auditory abnormality in multiple sclerosis. *Audiology.* 25, 193–209.

Jerger J, Oliver TA, Stach B. (1986b) Problems in the clinical measurement of acoustic reflex latency. *Scand Audiol.* 15, 31–40.

Jerger S, Jerger J. (1975) Extra- and intra-axial brain stem auditory disorders. *Audiology.* 14, 93–117.

Jerger S, Jerger J. (1977) Diagnostic value of crossed vs uncrossed acoustic reflexes: eighth nerve and brain stem disorders. *Arch Otolaryngol.* 103, 445–453.

Jerger S, Jerger J. (1981) *Auditory Disorders.* Boston: Little, Brown Co.

Jerger S, Neely JG, Jerger J. (1975) Recovery of crossed acoustic reflexes in brain stem auditory disorders. *Acta Otolaryngol.* 101, 329–332.

Johnsen NJ, Terkildsen K. (1980) The normal middle ear reflex thresholds for white noise and acoustic clicks in young adults. *Scand Audiol.* 9, 131–135.

Johnson EW. (1977) Auditory test results in 500 cases of acoustic neuroma. *Arch Otolaryngol.* 103, 152–158.

Kaplan H, Babecki S, Thomas C. (1980) The acoustic reflex without a hermetic seal. *Ear Hear.* 1, 83–86.

Keith R. (1973) Impedance audiometry with neonates. *Arch Otolaryngol.* 97, 465–467.

Keith R. (1977) An evaluation of predicting hearing loss from the acoustic reflex. *Arch Otolaryngol.* 103, 419–424.

Keith R, Bench R. (1978) Stapedial reflex in neonates. *Scand Audiol.* 7, 187–191.

Keith RW, Garza-Holquin Y, Smolak L, Pensak ML. (1987) Acoustic reflex dynamics and auditory brain stem responses in multiple sclerosis. *Am J Otol.* 8, 406–413.

Klockhoff I. (1961) Middle ear muscle reflexes in man. A clinical and experimental study with special reference to diagnostic problems in hearing impairment. *Acta Otolaryngol.* Suppl 164.

Klockhoff I, Anderson H. (1960) Reflex activity in the tensor tympani muscle recorded in man. *Acta Otolaryngol.* 51, 184–188.

Kramer LD, Ruth RA, Johns ME, Sanders DB. (1981) A comparison of stapedial reflex fatigue and repetitive stimulation and single-fiber EMG in myasthenia gravis. *Ann Neurol.* 9, 531–536.

Kunov H. (1977) The "eardrum artifact" in ipsilateral reflex measurements. *Scand Audiol.* 6, 163–166.

Lamb LE, Peterson JL. (1967) Middle ear reflex measurements in pseudohypacusis. *J Speech Hear Dis.* 32, 46–51.

Lew H, Jerger J. (1991) Diagnostic applications of suprathreshold acoustic reflex morphology. *Hear Instr.* 42, 21–23.

Lilly DJ. (1984) Evaluation of the response time of acoustic-immittance instruments. In: Silman S, ed. *The Acoustic Reflex: Basic Principles and Clinical Applications.* Orlando: Academic Press; pp 101–135.

Lous J. (1983) Three impedance screening programs on a cohort of seven-year-old children. *Scand Audiol.* Suppl 17, 60–64.

Lucker JR. (1980) Application of pass fail criteria to middle-ear screening results. *ASHA.* 22, 839–840.

Lutman ME. (1980) Real-ear calibration of ipsilateral acoustic reflex stimuli from five types of impedance meters. *Scand Audiol.* 9, 137–145.

Lutman ME, Leis BR. (1980) Ipsilateral acoustic reflex artifacts measured in cadavers. *Scand Audiol.* 9, 33–39.

Lutolf JJ, O'Malley H, Silman S. (2003) The effects of probe-tone frequency on the acoustic-reflex growth function. *J Am Acad Audiol.* 14, 109–118.

Lyons MJ. (1978) The central location of the motor neurons to the stapedius muscle in the cat. *Brain Res.* 143, 437–444.

Mangham CA. (1984) The effect of drugs and systemic disease on the acoustic reflex. In: Silman S, ed. *The Acoustic Reflex: Basic Principles and Clinical Applications.* Orlando: Academic Press; pp 441–468.

Mangham CA, Burnett PA, Lindeman RC. (1982) Standardization of acoustic reflex latency. *Ann Otol Rhinol Laryngol.* 91, 169–174.

Mangham CA, Lindeman RC. (1980) The negative acoustic reflex in retrocochlear disorders. *Laryngoscope.* 90, 1753–1761.

Mangham CA, Lindeman RC, Dawson WR. (1980) Stapedius reflex quantification in acoustic tumor patients. *Laryngoscope.* 90, 242–250.

Martin FN, Coombes S. (1974) Effect of external ear canal pressure on the middle-ear muscle reflex threshold. *J Speech Hear Res.* 17, 526–530.

McMillan PM, Bennett MJ, Marchant CD, Shurin PA. (1985) Ipsilateral and contralateral acoustic reflexes in neonates. *Ear Hear.* 6, 320–324.

Møller AR. (1961) Network model of the middle ear. *J Acoust Soc Am.* 35, 1526–1534.

Møller AR. (1962) The sensitivity of contraction of tympanic muscle in man. *Ann Otol Rhinol Laryngol.* 71, 86–95.

Møller AR. (1984) Neurophysiological basis of the acoustic middle-ear reflex. In: Silman S, ed. *The Acoustic Reflex: Basic Principles and Clinical Applications.* Orlando: Academic Press; pp 1–34.

Mulder J, Vantrappen G, Snik A, Manni J. (1993) The use of the startle reflex measurement in patients with various types of fixation of the ossicular chain. *Scand Audiol.* 22, 257–260.

Niemeyer W, Sesterhenn G. (1974) Calculating the hearing threshold from the stapedius reflex threshold for different sound stimuli. *Audiology.* 13, 421–427.

Olsen WO, Bauch CD, Harner SG. (1983) Application of Silman and Gelfand (1981) 90th percentile levels for acoustic reflex thresholds. *J Speech Hear Dis.* 48, 330–332.

Olsen WO, Noffsinger D, Kurdziel SA. (1975) Acoustic reflex and reflex decay. *Arch Otolaryngol.* 101, 622–625.

Olsen WO, Stach BA, Kurdziel SA. (1981) Acoustic reflex decay in 10 seconds and in 5 seconds for Ménière's disease patients and for VIIIth nerve tumor patients. *Ear Hear.* 2, 180–181.

Osterhammel D, Osterhammel P. (1979) Age and sex variations for the normal stapedial reflex thresholds and tympanometric compliance values. *Scand Audiol.* 8, 153–158.

Oviatt DL, Kileny P. (1984) Normative characteristics of ipsilateral acoustic reflex adaptation. *Ear Hear.* 5, 145–152.

Peterson JL, Liden G. (1972) Some static characteristics of the stapedial muscle reflex. *Audiology.* 11, 97–114.

Piccolo G, Cosi V, Precerutti G. (1977) Stapedius reflex test in diagnosis of myesthenia. *Acta Neurologica.* 32, 150–172.

Popelka GR. (1981) *Hearing Assessment with the Acoustic Reflex.* New York: Grune & Stratton.

Popelka GR, Margolis RH, Wiley TL. (1976) Effect of activating signal bandwidth in acoustic-reflex thresholds. *J Acoust Soc Am.* 59, 153–159.

Popelka GR, Trumph A. (1976) Stapedial reflex thresholds for tonal and noise activating signals in relation to magnitude of hearing loss in multiple-handicapped children. Presented at the Convention of American Speech-Language-Hearing Association, Houston, TX.

Prasher D, Cohen M. (1993) Effectiveness of acoustic reflex threshold criteria in the diagnosis of retrocochlear pathology. *Scand Audiol.* 22, 11–18.

Qiu WW, Stucker FJ. (1997) Characteristics of acoustic reflex latency in normal-hearing subjects. *Scand Audiol.* 27, 43–49.

Rawool VW. (1995) Click-rate induced facilitation of the acoustic reflex using constant number of pulses. *Audiology.* 35, 171–179.

Rawool VW. (1996a) Effect of aging on the click-rate induced facilitation of acoustic reflex thresholds. *J Geron A Bio Sci Med Sci.* 51, B124–B131.

Rawool VW. (1996b) Ipsilateral acoustic reflex thresholds at varying click rates in humans. *Scand Audiol.* 24, 199–205.

Rizzo S Jr, Greenberg HJ. (1979a) Influence of ear canal pressure on acoustic reflex threshold. *J Am Aud Soc.* 5, 21–24.

Rizzo S Jr, Greenberg HJ. (1979b) Predicting hearing loss from the acoustic reflex data. Presented at the Convention of American Speech-Language-Hearing Association, Boston, MA.

Robinette MS, Rhoads DP, Marion ME. (1974) Effects of secobarbital on impedance audiometry. *Arch Otolaryngol.* 104, 31–37.

Roush J, Tait C. (1985) Pure-tone and acoustic immittance screening of preschool aged children: an examination of referral criteria. *Ear Hear.* 6, 245–249.

Ruth RA, Arora NS, Gal TJ. (1982a) Stapedius reflex in curarized subjects—an index of neuromuscular weakness. *J Appl Physiol.* 82, 416–420.

Ruth RA, Johns ME, Gal TJ. (1980) Acoustic reflex response during curare-induced weakness. *Ann Otol Rhinol Laryngol.* 89, 188–193.

Ruth RA, Nilo ER, Mravec JJ. (1978) Consideration of acoustic reflex magnitude (ARM) in cases of idiopathic facial paralysis. *J Otol Rhinol Laryngol.* 86, 215–220.

Ruth RA, Tucci DL, Nilo ER. (1982b) Effects of ear canal pressure on threshold and growth of the acoustic reflex. *Ear Hear.* 3, 39–41.

Sanders JW (1984) Evaluation of the 90th percentile levels for acoustic reflex thresholds. Presented at the Convention of American Speech-Language-Hearing Association. San Francisco, CA.

Sanders JW, Josey AF, Glasscock ME. (1981) Audiologic evaluation in cochlear and eighth nerve disorders. *Arch Otolaryngol.* 100, 283–289.

Sanders JW, Josey AF, Glasscock ME, Jackson C. (1974) The acoustic reflex in cochlear and eighth nerve pathology ears. *Laryngoscope.* 91, 787–793.

Segal A. (1978) Letter to the editor. *J Am Aud Soc.* 3, 227.

Sells JP, Hurley RM, Morehouse CR, Douglas JE. (1997) Validity of the ipsilateral acoustic reflex as a screening parameter. *J Am Acad Audiol.* 8, 132–136.

Sesterhenn G, Brueninger H. (1976) The acoustic reflex at low sensation levels. *Audiology.* 15, 523–533.

Shapiro I, Canalis RF, Firemark R, Bahna M. (1981) Ossicular discontinuity with intact acoustic reflex. *Arch Otolaryngol.* 107, 576–578.

Sheehy JL, Inzer BE. (1976) Acoustic reflex test in neuro-otologic diagnosis: a review of 24 cases of acoustic tumors. *Arch Otolaryngol.* 102, 647–653.

Shivashanker N, Satishchandra P, Shashikala HR, Gore M. (2003) Primary auditory neuropathy—an enigma. *Acta Neurol Scand.* 108, 130–135.

Silman S. (1979) The effects of aging on the stapedius reflex thresholds. *J Acoust Soc Am.* 66, 735–738.

Silman S. (1984) Magnitude and growth of the acoustic-reflex. In: Silman S, ed. *The Acoustic Reflex: Basic Principles and Clinical Applications.* Orlando: Academic Press; pp 225–274.

Silman S. (1988) The applicability of the modified bivariate plotting procedure to subjects with functional hearing loss. *Scand Audiol.* 17, 125–127.

Silman S, Gelfand SA. (1979) Prediction of hearing levels from acoustic reflex thresholds in persons with high-frequency hearing losses. *J Speech Hear Res.* 22, 697–707.

Silman S, Gelfand SA. (1981a) The relationship between magnitude of hearing loss and acoustic reflex threshold levels. *J Speech Hear Dis.* 46, 312–316.

Silman S, Gelfand SA. (1981b) Effect of the sensorineural hearing loss on the stapedius reflex growth function in the elderly. *J Acoust Soc Am.* 69, 1099–1106.

Silman S, Gelfand SA. (1982a) The acoustic reflex in diagnostic audiology–Part 1. *Audiology.* 7, 111–124.

Silman S, Gelfand SA. (1982b) The acoustic reflex in diagnostic audiology–Part 2. *Audiology.* 7, 125–138.

Silman S, Gelfand SA, Chun T. (1978a) Some observations in a case of acoustic neuroma. *J Speech Hear Dis.* 43, 459–466.

Silman S, Gelfand SA, Emmer M. (1987) Acoustic reflex in hearing loss identification and prediction. *Semin Hear.* 8, 379–390.

Silman S, Gelfand SA, Piper N, Silverman CA, VanFrank L. (1984a) Prediction of hearing loss from the acoustic-reflex threshold. In: Silman S, ed. *The Acoustic Reflex: Basic Principles and Clinical Applications.* Orlando: Academic Press; pp 187–223.

Silman S, Popelka GR, Gelfand SA. (1978b) Effect of sensorineural hearing loss on acoustic stapedius reflex growth functions. *J Acoust Soc Am.* 64, 1406–1411.

Silman S, Silverman CA. (1991) *Auditory Diagnosis: Principles and Applications.* San Diego: Academic Press.

Silman S, Silverman CA, Arick DS. (1992) Acoustic-immittance screening for detection of middle-ear effusion. *J Am Acad Audiol.* 3, 262–268.

Silman S, Silverman CA, Gelfand SA, Lutolf J, Lynn DJ. (1988) Ipsilateral acoustic-reflex adaptation testing for detection of facial-nerve pathology: three case studies. *J Speech Hear Dis.* 53, 378–382.

Silman S, Silverman CA, Showers T, Gelfand SA. (1984b) The effect of age on prediction of hearing loss with the bivariate plotting procedure. *J Speech Hear Res.* 27, 12–19.

Silverman CA, Silman S, Gelfand SA, Lutolf J. (1986) The efferent acoustic reflex adaptation pattern. Presented at the Convention of American Speech-Language-Hearing Association, Detroit, MI.

Silverman CA, Silman S, Miller MH. (1983) The acoustic reflex threshold in aging ears. *J Acoust Soc Am.* 73, 248–255.

Simmons BF. (1964) Perceptual theories of middle ear muscle function. *Ann Otol Rhinol Laryngol.* 73, 724–740.

Simon U, Pirsig W. (1973) Influence of chlorpromazine on audiometric tests. *Scand Audiol.* 3, 99–105.

Sininger YS, Hood LJ, Starr A, Berlin CI, Picton TW. (1995) Hearing loss due to auditory neuropathy. *Audiol Today.* 7, 10–13.

Smith MJ, Brezinova V. (1991) Stapedius reflex decay test in diagnosis of myasthenia gravis (MG). *Electromyog Clin Neurophysiol.* 31, 317–319.

Smith RP, Loeb M, Fletcher JL, Thomas DM. (1966) The effects of moderate doses of curare on certain auditory functions. *Acta Otolaryngol.* 62, 101–108.

Spitzer JB, Ventry IM. (1980) Central auditory dysfunction among chronic alcoholics. *Arch Otolaryngol.* 106, 224–229.

Sprague BA, Wiley TA, Block MA. (1981) Dynamics of acoustic reflex growth. *Audiology.* 20, 15–40.

Sprague BH, Wiley TL, Goldstein R. (1985) Tympanometric and acoustic-reflex studies in neonates. *J Speech Hear Res.* 28, 265–272.

Stach BA, Jerger J. (1984) Acoustic reflex averaging. *Ear Hear.* 5, 289–296.

Starr A, Picton TW, Sininger YS, Hood LJ, Berlin CI. (1996) Auditory neuropathy. *Brain.* 119, 741–753.

Stephens SDG, Thornton ARD. (1976) Subjective and electrophysiologic tests in brain-stem lesions. *Arch Otolaryngol.* 102, 608–613.

Strasser DH. (1975) Contralateral and ipsilateral acoustic reflex latency measures in various otologic pathologies. PhD dissertation. Salt Lake City: University of Utah.

Stream RW, Stream KS, Walker JR, Breningstall G. (1978) Emerging characteristics of the acoustic reflex in infants. *Otolaryngology.* 86, 628–636.

Surr RK, Schuchman GI. (1976) Measurement of the acoustic reflex without a pressure seal. *Arch Otolaryngol.* 102, 160–161.

Teitze G. (1969) Einige eigenschaften des akustischen reflexes bei reizung mit tonimpulsen. *Archiv fuer Klinische und Experimentelle Ohrem-, Nasen- und Kehlkopfheilkunde.* 193, 53–69.

Terkildsen K, Osterhammel P, Bretau P. (1973) Acoustic middle ear muscle reflexes in patients with otosclerosis. *Arch Otolaryngol.* 98, 152–155.

Thompson DJ, Sills JA, Recke KS, Bui DM. (1980) Acoustic reflex growth in the aging adult. *J Speech Hear Res.* 23, 405–418.

Thomsen J, Terkildsen K. (1975) Audiological findings in 125 cases of acoustic neuroma. *Arch Otolaryngol.* 80, 353–361.

Torvik A. (1956) Afferent connections to the sensory trigeminal nuclei, the nucleus of the solitary tract and adjacent structures. An experimental study in the rat. *J Comp Neurol.* 106, 51–141.

Tóth L, Lampé I, Diószeghy P, Répássy G. (2000) The diagnostic value of stapedius reflex and stapedius reflex exhaustion in myasthenia gravis. *Electromyog Clin Neurophysiol.* 40, 17–20.

Wallin A, Mendez-Kurtz L, Silman S. (1986) Prediction of hearing loss from acoustic-reflex thresholds in the older adults population. *Ear Hear.* 7, 400–404.

Weatherby LA, Bennett MJ. (1980) The neonatal acoustic reflex. *Scand Audiol.* 9, 103–110.

Wiley TL, Block MG. (1984) Acoustic and nonacoustic reflex patterns in audiologic diagnosis. In: Silman S, ed. *The Acoustic Reflex: Basic Principles and Clinical Applications.* Orlando: Academic Press; pp 287–411.

Wiley TL, Oviatt DL, Block MG. (1987) Acoustic-immittance measures in normal ears. *J Speech Hear Res.* 330, 161–170.

Wilson RH. (1979) Factors influencing the acoustic-immittance characteristics of the acoustic reflex. *J Speech Hear Res.* 22, 480–499.

Wilson RH. (1981) The effects of aging on the magnitude of the acoustic reflex. *J Speech Hear Res.* 24, 406–413.

Wilson RH, McBride LM. (1978) Factors influencing the acoustic-immittance characteristics of the acoustic reflex. *J Acoust Soc Am.* 63, 147–154.

Wilson RH, Shanks JE, Lilly DJ. (1984) Acoustic-reflex adaptation. In: Silman S, ed. *The Acoustic Reflex: Basic Principles and Clinical Applications.* Orlando: Academic Press; pp 329–386.

Wilson RH, Shanks JE, Velde TM. (1981) Aural acoustic-immittance measurements: inter-aural differences. *J Speech Hear Dis.* 46, 413–421.

Zakrisson JE, Borg E, Bloom S. (1974) The acoustic impedance change as a measure of stapedius muscle activity in man: a methodologic study with electromyography. *Acta Otolaryngol.* 78, 357–364.

Zito F, Roberto M. (1980) The acoustic reflex pattern studied by the averaging technique. *Audiology.* 19, 395–403.

11 Introduction to Auditory Evoked Potentials

Robert Burkard and Kathleen McNerney

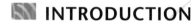 INTRODUCTION

The sixth edition of the *Handbook of Clinical Audiology* includes eight chapters specifically dealing with auditory evoked potentials (AEPs). The chapters range from the very short latency response components from electrocochleography (ECoG) through the long latency responses. These responses vary in terms of generators, time epochs, stimulus and response dependencies, and clinical applications. However, they share a number of commonalities in terms of the common (but not exclusive) use of acoustic transients, as well as the use of differential amplification and time domain signal averaging in order to observe a response that is small when compared to the magnitude of the background electroencephalographic (EEG) activity. This chapter is a revision of the chapter by Burkard and Secor in the fifth edition of Katz's *Handbook of Clinical Audiology* (2002). The present chapter will: (1) present a brief overview of the central auditory nervous system from the eighth nerve through the brainstem, (2) provide a brief overview of the various AEPs and their clinical applications, (3) present an introduction to the instrumentation and principles underlying the acquisition of AEPs, and (4) review the normative aspects of the auditory brainstem response (ABR) as an introduction to the clinical applications of the ABR presented in Chapters 13, 14, and 16.

THE EIGHTH NERVE AND AUDITORY BRAINSTEM

For threshold estimation, it is not very important to know the generators of a particular AEP peak. In contrast, for such clinical applications as site-of-lesion testing (see Chapter 13) or intraoperative monitoring (see Chapter 16), knowledge of the generators of a particular peak can be invaluable. Much of what we know about the physiologic responses from the eighth nerve and auditory brainstem arise from single unit responses in animals. This is for the simple reason that such studies are invasive and hence cannot be used in humans. Early work focusing on the ABR peak generators (Buchwald and Huang, 1975) used lesioning studies in animals (cats) and related the loss of peaks (or changes in amplitude) to the level of the lesion. This led to a mapping of a given ABR peak to a specific generator. This mapping was problematic for two reasons. First, other than for the first peak (generated by the eighth nerve), multiple regions of the auditory nervous system were activated in a temporally overlapping fashion, making a one-to-one mapping of peak to generator impossible. Second, even though in the animal studies it was often possible to identify the dominant contributor to a given peak, the generalization to humans was confounded by the unusually long auditory nerve in humans compared to other mammals (Moller, 1994). Despite these difficulties, our current knowledge of ABR peak generators allows us to make useful clinical decisions for site-of-lesion testing, as well as to interpret changes in the ABR during intraoperative monitoring.

The auditory nerve, one branch of the vestibulocochlear (eighth) cranial nerve, projects from the hair cells to the cochlear nuclei (CN). According to Spoendlin (1972), 90% to 95% of auditory nerve fibers are type I fibers, and 5% to 10% are type II fibers. Type I afferent dendrites innervate inner hair cells (IHCs), while the distal processes of type II afferents innervate outer hair cells (OHCs). Type I fibers are bipolar and heavily myelinated, whereas type II afferents are sparsely myelinated and are pseudomonopolar. The cell bodies of both are contained in the spiral ganglion. Based on number alone, it is clear that IHCs and type I afferents deliver most of the auditory information to the central auditory nervous system. The auditory nerve passes through the internal auditory meatus of the cochlea, and upon entering the posterior fossa, it projects to the lateral aspect of the brainstem, near the pontomedullary junction. These fibers bifurcate and terminate in the CN of the caudal pons. There are three divisions of the CN: the anteroventral cochlear nucleus (AVCN), the posteroventral cochlear nucleus (PVCN), and the dorsal cochlear nucleus (DCN). Each of these nuclei is tonotopically organized (i.e., each has a map specifically relating place in the nucleus to a specific frequency, called the characteristic or best frequency, which responds at the lowest sound level). Indeed, a tonotopic organization is a characteristic of many auditory nuclei. Each of the various subnuclei of the CN has unique anatomic cell types, unique electrophysiologic response patterns, and unique connections. Auditory nerve fibers are uniform in cell type (mostly type I afferents) and present fairly uniform response properties (sustained responses showing adaptation but differing in terms of best frequency and spontaneous discharge rate). However, at the level of the CN, such homogeneity is no longer seen. Multiple cell types are present in the CN, with input from various structures. Similarly, response properties vary greatly, reflecting, among other things, differing membrane properties and combinations of excitatory and inhibitory input. The details of these response properties go well beyond the scope of the present review. (Detailed reviews of the anatomy and physiology of the auditory nervous system can be found in Webster et al. [1992] and Popper and Fay [1992]).

The three subnuclei of the CN have major projections (called acoustic striae) to more rostral regions of the brainstem: (1) The dorsal acoustic stria arises from the DCN and projects to the contralateral inferior colliculus (IC). (2) The ventral acoustic stria projects from the AVCN to the superior olivary complex (SOC). (3) The intermediate acoustic stria projects from the PVCN to the SOC. The SOC is also comprised of multiple subnuclei. The periolivary nuclei are integral to the descending auditory system, which projects to the OHCs or the type I afferents beneath the IHCs via the crossed and uncrossed olivocochlear bundles. This descending system modulates cochlear function, and this can be measured by suppression of otoacoustic emissions (see Chapter 21). In terms of the ascending system, three SOC subnuclei are of importance and include: the medial superior olive (MSO), the lateral superior olive (LSO), and the medial nucleus of the trapezoid body (MNTB). The SOC is where input from both ears first converges. Information from the right and left CN projects to medial and lateral dendritic tufts of the MSO. Single unit responses from the MSO show similar tuning curves from both ears, suggesting convergence of excitatory input from similar best frequency regions from

the right and left CN. The LSO receives direct input from the ipsilateral CN, while the contralateral CN projects first to the contralateral MNTB and then to the LSO. There is evidence that the input from the MNTB is inhibitory. Both MSO and LSO are tonotopically organized. The SOC clearly adds binaural processing to the monaural CN input.

From the SOC, the major output is via the lateral lemniscus (LL). There are two subnuclei of the LL: the dorsal nucleus of the LL (DNLL) and the ventral nucleus of the LL (VNLL). The LL terminate in the IC. The IC are on the dorsal aspect of the midbrain and appear as a pair of protuberances just below the paired superior colliculi. There are several subnuclei of the IC, but the main division is the central nucleus (CNIC). The CNIC is tonotopically organized, with a laminar arrangement. You can visualize the isofrequency (same frequency) laminae like the layers of an onion, with each layer of onion having a narrow range of best frequencies. The other regions of the IC have units with broader tuning curves, making determination of their frequency organization complicated. These other divisions appear to respond to not only auditory input, but also to somatosensory and visual input.

Now that we know something about the auditory nerve and brainstem, we can briefly provide a listing of the primary generators of the various ABR peaks. The human ABR is comprised of a series of up to seven vertex-positive peaks that occur within 10 ms of stimulus onset in adults to moderate-level click stimuli. The first five peaks have received the most attention scientifically and clinically, and these waves are labeled in sequential capital Roman numerals (I, II, III, IV, and V), after the convention of Jewett. Based largely on the studies performed by Moller and Jannetta during intraoperative monitoring, we can assign the following peak generators: Wave I arises from the distal auditory nerve, wave II arises from the proximal eighth nerve, wave III is primarily generated by the CN, wave IV appears to be generated by the SOC, wave V (the peak) appears to emanate from the LL, and the trough following wave V comes predominantly from the IC (Moller, 1994).

AN OVERVIEW OF AUDITORY EVOKED POTENTIALS

If you were to simultaneously measure the responses from all auditory nervous system structures following presentation of an acoustic stimulus, you would record activity in the cochlea, auditory nerve, auditory brainstem, medial geniculate body, and auditory cortex. Multiple brain regions would be activated at the same time. However, it would be true that the more caudal structures in the auditory nervous system would have shorter onset latencies than the more rostral structures. This latency increase for more rostral structures is the result of the finite action potential conduction velocity and the delay as the activity passes through chemical synapses. While we have no noninvasive way of recording

TABLE 11.1	Terminology used for very large and very small values		
Prefix	**Scientific notation**	**Terminology**	**Example**
Giga	10^9	Billion	Gigabyte
Mega	10^6	Million	Megahertz
Kilo	10^3	Thousand	Kilogram
Milli	10^{-3}	One-thousandth	Millimeter
Micro	10^{-6}	One-millionth	Microvolt
Nano	10^{-9}	One-billionth	Nanosecond
Pico	10^{-12}	One-trillionth	Picotesla

Reprinted from Burkard R, Secor C. (2002) Overview of auditory evoked potentials. In: Katz J, ed. *Handbook of Clinical Audiology*. 5th ed. Baltimore: Lippincott Williams & Wilkins; pp 233–248, with the permission of Lippincott Williams & Wilkins.

from these various auditory nuclei directly, it is possible to record a series of responses from the scalp (using noninvasive surface electrodes) that have latencies ranging from one one-thousandth to several tenths of a second. Table 11.1 shows the time and amplitude units that will be used in this chapter. A millisecond (one-thousandth of a second) and a microsecond (one-millionth of a second) will be convenient time units. Microvolts (one-millionth of a volt) will be convenient amplitude units. Reference to Table 11.1 will prove useful for those unfamiliar with metric units. Due to the progressive latency increase of responses from more rostral auditory structures, it is popular to classify AEPs by their response time following the onset of a transient stimulus.

Electrocochleography (ECoG) refers to the responses from the cochlea and auditory nerve, using a recording electrode located in close proximity to the inner ear. Two responses arise from the hair cells: the cochlear microphonic (CM) and the summating potential (SP) (Dallos, 1973; Davis, 1976). Each has a very short latency (1 ms or so), which is basically the delay from stimulus onset to hair cell excitation. The CM has the same waveform as the stimulus, so a 2,000-Hz tone burst will produce a CM with spectral energy primarily at 2,000 Hz. The SP is a direct current (DC) response, which continues for the duration of the eliciting stimulus. The response from the acoustic portion of the eighth cranial nerve is called either the whole-nerve action potential (WNAP) or the compound action potential (CAP). The first two negative peaks of the CAP are labeled N1 and N2. Unlike the CM and SP, which continue for the duration of the stimulus, the WNAP (CAP) occurs at stimulus onset (and sometimes offset). Many AEPs (CAP, ABR, middle latency response [MLR], and slow vertex potential [SVP]) are onset responses. The CAP has a latency roughly 1 ms longer than the CM or SP, which is the result of the synaptic delay from hair cell depolarization to the onset of auditory nerve fiber discharge. Unlike the other AEPs, the ECoG responses are typically NOT measured with scalp electrodes, but rather

from electrodes placed in the ear canal, on or near the tympanic membrane, or on the promontory or round window of the inner ear (see Chapter 12).

The auditory brainstem response (ABR), as its name indicates, is a series of five to seven peaks arising from auditory nerve and brainstem structures (Moller, 1994), occurring within 10 ms of the onset of a moderate-intensity click stimulus in otologically, audiologically, and neurologically intact adults. Most investigators follow the peak-labeling convention of Jewett and Williston (1971) and label the peaks with capital Roman numerals (I through VII). Based on its time window rather than its generators, the ABR is also referred to as the early or short latency AEP. An ABR from a normal adult is shown in Figure 11.1. The ABR is, without question, the most clinically useful AEP at the present time. It can be used for estimating hearing threshold (Chapter 14), differential diagnosis of peripheral and central abnormalities (Chapter 13), and intraoperative monitoring (Chapter 16).

MLRs are usually recorded over a time window of 80 to 100 ms, and peak latencies range from roughly 12 to 65 ms. Generators are thought to include thalamus and auditory cortex (Chapter 17; Moller, 1994; Kraus et al., 1994). Unlike ECoG and ABR, the MLR appears to be affected to some extent by subject variables like attention and arousal. Peak

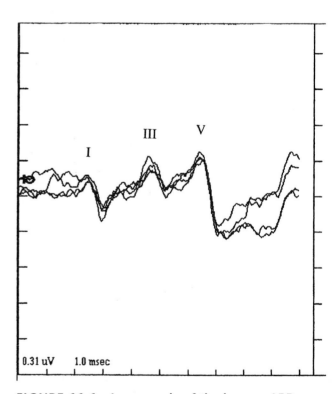

FIGURE 11.1 An example of the human ABR. Waves I, III, and V are labeled. (Reprinted from Burkard R, Secor C. [2002] Overview of auditory evoked potentials. In: Katz J, ed. *Handbook of Clinical Audiology*. 5th ed. Baltimore: Lippincott Williams & Wilkins; pp 233–248, with the permission of Lippincott Williams & Wilkins.)

labeling nomenclature varies somewhat with investigator, but the polarity of the peak is typically indicated by a capital P or N (positive or negative), followed by lowercase early letters of the alphabet (e.g., Pa, Nb, etc.). Due to the recognition of MLR peaks before Pa and Na, the earliest MLR peaks may be labeled Po and No. AEP responses occurring beyond roughly 75 ms are collectively called the slow vertex potential (SVP) or late component responses. These responses are commonly labeled with a capital N or P to indicate peak polarity followed by an Arabic number indicating which SVP peak of that polarity it is (e.g., P1 is the first positive SVP peak). Alternatively, an Arabic number indicating average peak latency may be used as a subscript. For example, N200 would be the negative peak with a mean latency of 200 ms. The various SVP terminology and peak-labeling conventions are reviewed in Hyde (1994b). The SVP is very sensitive to attention and arousal (see Chapter 18). The term event-related potential (ERP) is often used when referring to long latency responses that are strongly dependent on the attention and arousal of the subject (Kraus and McGee, 1994). Innovative paradigms have been developed to study complex constructs such as attention and arousal. One such paradigm is called the oddball paradigm. The oddball paradigm involves the use of two different stimuli, one that occurs frequently and another that occurs infrequently. Responses to the frequent and infrequent stimuli are averaged and displayed separately. There are differences in the responses to the frequent and infrequent stimuli, with these differences depending on whether the subject is attending to the stimuli or not. If attending, there is an additional response called the P3 or P300 response to the infrequent stimulus. This response can be used as an index of a cognitive construct that is related to attention. Both the P3 and the mismatch negativity are discussed in Chapter 18.

A relative newcomer to the family of AEP responses is the auditory steady-state response (ASSR). This response represents a sustained response and can be elicited by trains of clicks, noise bursts, or tone bursts; amplitude-modulated (AM) and/or frequency-modulated stimuli; as well as two-tone stimuli. This response has been extensively investigated in recent years (see Chapter 15).

CLINICAL APPLICATIONS OF AUDITORY EVOKED POTENTIALS

There are a number of clearly defined clinical uses of AEPs. First, and perhaps foremost, AEPs can be used for hearing screening and to estimate hearing thresholds of difficult-to-test populations. The ABR is currently the most popular AEP for hearing screening and threshold estimation in the United States (see Chapter 14). However, it should be noted that, in recent years, there has been a lot of interest in applying the ASSR to the problem of threshold estimation (see Chapter 15). ECoG is more invasive than the ABR (or ASSR), especially if you use a transtympanic electrode, while the middle

and long latency responses have the disadvantage of being at least somewhat dependent on attention and arousal (see Chapters 17 and 18). While there are time and expense advantages in using otoacoustic emissions (OAEs) rather than ABRs for hearing screening, OAEs appear to be less than optimal for threshold estimation, and OAEs in isolation will not allow identification of those patients with auditory neuropathy (see Chapters 13 and 22).

Another clinical application of AEPs is for site-of-lesion testing. The ABR is useful for differentiating conductive, sensory-neural, and retrocochlear disorders (see Chapter 13). While imaging procedures such as magnetic resonance imaging (MRI) might eventually replace the ABR for the identification of central nervous system (CNS) lesions, the current cost of an MRI makes it an expensive alternative to electrophysiologic measures in the early stages of the diagnostic regimen. There are also changes in auditory function that do not produce a lesion recognizable by MRI, although some of these lesions may be revealed by functional MRI. For example, recent studies have revealed a clinical entity termed "auditory neuropathy" (Starr et al., 1996; Hood, 1998). Subjects with auditory neuropathy often have abnormal or missing ABRs, missing acoustic reflexes, normal OAEs but missing contralateral suppression of OAEs, and speech discrimination that is often poorer than predicted by the threshold audiogram. These patients show no evidence of CNS lesions by conventional MRI. The diagnosis is made based on the unusual pattern of audiologic results including OAEs and AEPs, not on diagnostic imaging procedures. Auditory neuropathy will be discussed in more detail in Chapters 13 and 22.

A third clinical application of AEPs is for intraoperative monitoring. Both ECoG and ABR have been used for intraoperative monitoring (see Chapter 16) and are in common use for monitoring during posterior fossa surgery. For intraoperative monitoring, you use the patient's baseline responses as the basis for monitoring changes during surgery. Criterion response degradation is used to warn the surgeon that damage is being done to the auditory system, giving the surgeon the opportunity to modify their procedures.

The above list of clinical uses of AEPs is not exhaustive but does reflect the most common uses of AEPs in clinical audiology today. AEPs are now being used in the mapping of cochlear implants in the pediatric population (see Chapter 12). It is likely that ERPs such as the P3 (also called the P300) and the mismatch negativity (MMN) will find a place in the diagnosis and perhaps in the efficacy of treatment of such complex clinical entities as central auditory processing disorder.

THE TECHNICAL DETAILS

A block diagram of the instrumentation used to obtain an AEP is shown in Figure 11.2. You must present an acoustic stimulus to elicit an AEP. In order to record the AEP, you must

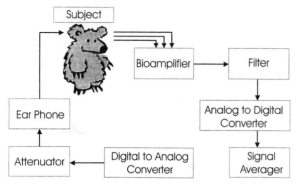

FIGURE 11.2   A block diagram of the instrumentation needed to obtain auditory evoked potentials. (Reprinted from Burkard R, Secor C. [2002] Overview of auditory evoked potentials. In: Katz J, ed. *Handbook of Clinical Audiology*. 5th ed. Baltimore: Lippincott Williams & Wilkins; pp 233–248, with the permission of Lippincott Williams & Wilkins.)

record the electrical response from the human scalp (or, for ECoG, from the ear canal, tympanic membrane, or round window/promontory). Electrodes serve as the interface between the scalp (or ear) and the electronic instrumentation. Because AEPs are small in amplitude, we must use special amplifiers (called bioamplifiers) to make these signals large enough for further signal processing. It is also common to get rid of undesirable electrical activity by the use of filtering. Finally, the scalp-recorded electrical activity must be converted

into a binary format so that it can be utilized by a digital computer. The device that accomplishes this transformation is an analog-to-digital converter (ADC). Once in binary form, the data can be manipulated by a digital computer. This manipulation can include additional filtering (called digital filtering) and the elimination of responses deemed to be too noisy (called artifact rejection) and includes a synchronization of stimulus onset and response recording that herein we will refer to as time-domain signal averaging. In the sections that follow, we will review the stimuli used to elicit AEPs (and the calibration of these stimuli), electrodes, bioamplifiers, filters, artifact rejection, analog-to-digital conversion, and time-domain signal averaging.

Stimuli Typically Used to Elicit Auditory Evoked Potentials

Many AEPs are elicited by presentation of brief acoustic transients. The two most common transients used clinically are clicks and tone bursts. A click is produced by exciting a transducer with a brief-duration (typically 100 μs for human studies) electrical pulse. In a pulse with duration d, there are spectral zeroes (energy at that frequency dips toward zero) at frequencies that are integer multiples of 1/d. Thus, for an electrical pulse with a duration of 100 μs, the first spectral zero occurs at 10,000 Hz, with spectral zeroes occurring at 20,000, 30,000, 40,000 Hz, etc. The time-domain representation of a 100-μs pulse is shown in the upper panel of Figure 11.3. The amplitude spectrum of this pulse is shown in the lower panel of Figure 11.3. The amplitude spectrum

FIGURE 11.3   Time-domain waveform (*upper panel*) and spectrum (*lower panel*) of an electrical pulse with a duration of 100 μs. (Reprinted from Burkard R, Secor C. [2002] Overview of auditory evoked potentials. In: Katz J, ed. *Handbook of Clinical Audiology*. 5th ed. Baltimore: Lippincott Williams & Wilkins; pp 233–248, with the permission of Lippincott Williams & Wilkins.)

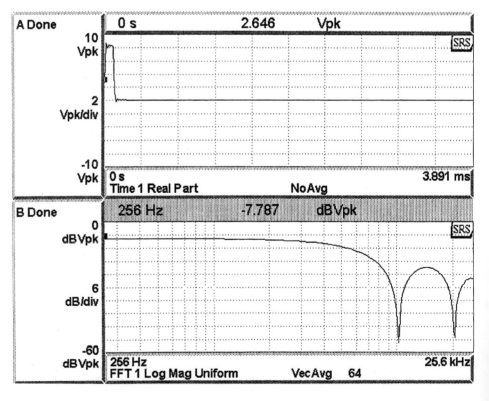

is a frequency-domain representation and is plotted as amplitude over time. In this example, voltage (y-axis) is plotted across frequency in kHz (x-axis). The acoustic representation of this 100-μs pulse, as recorded through a TDH-50 earphone in a 6-cc coupler, is shown in Figure 11.4. The spectrum of the acoustic pulse (the upper panel of Fig. 11.4) has been changed by the acoustic or electroacoustic properties of the earphone, coupler, and microphone (compare to lower panel of Fig. 11.3). The spectrum of this pulse reveals basically a low-pass filter function with a cutoff frequency of approximately 5 kHz. Indeed, if the duration of the electrical pulse is suitably brief, the acoustic spectrum of the click approximates the frequency response of the transducer. The acoustic spectrum of the 100-μs pulse (Fig. 11.4, upper panel) is quite similar to the frequency response of the transducer/recording system as determined by excitation with a broadband noise (Fig. 11.4, lower panel). This demonstrates that the 100-μs pulse, in this example, has a broad enough bandwidth so that the upper cutoff of the acoustic spectrum is limited by the frequency response of the transducer. This, of course, is dependent on the transfer function of the transducer and the spectrum of the stimulus. It is important for the reader to understand that the click has energy over a wide range of frequencies and is a broadband stimulus.

Clicks are often the stimuli of choice for hearing screening (Chapter 14), site-of-lesion testing (Chapter 13), and intraoperative monitoring (Chapter 16). In contrast, if you are interested in obtaining an electrophysiologic estimate of the behavioral audiogram, then a broadband stimulus is not optimal. In this case, a tone burst can be used to elicit AEPs. American National Standards Institute (ANSI) S3.6-2004 (ANSI, 2004), which reviews technical specifications for audiometers (see Chapter 2), states that, for audiometric purposes, a tone must be presented for a duration of not less than 200 ms and have a rise time and fall time ranging between 25 and 100 ms. Figure 11.5 (upper panel) shows a tone burst with a carrier frequency of 2,000 Hz. The time required for the tone burst envelope to increase from zero to its maximal amplitude is termed its rise time. The time that the tone burst envelope remains at this maximal amplitude is called its plateau time. The time required for the tone burst envelope to decrease from its maximal amplitude to zero amplitude is called its fall time. Figure 11.5 (lower panel) shows the amplitude spectrum (i.e., frequency domain representation) of this tone burst. A tone that is infinitely long in duration only has energy at the carrier frequency (i.e., the frequency of the sine wave). For the tone burst, you can see that there is significant energy over a range of frequencies centered at 2,000 Hz. This spread of energy to frequencies above and below the carrier frequency is referred to as spectral splatter. The stimuli used to elicit AEPs differ from those used audiometrically because many of the AEPs that are used clinically are onset responses. Onset responses are elicited by the first few milliseconds of the stimulus onset and hence are affected by the stimulus rise time. Because these responses are sensitive to changes in the envelope of the stimulus, with a long enough plateau time, often offset responses (at response termination) can be observed too. The very fast onset time

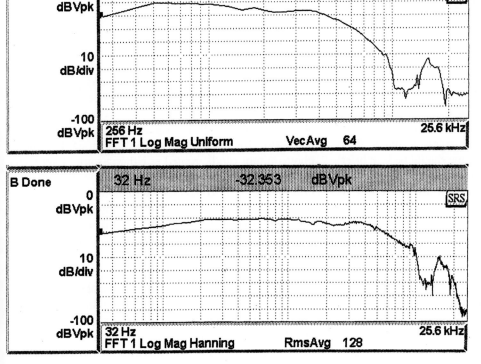

FIGURE 11.4 The acoustic spectra to 100-μs pulses (*upper panel*) and to continuous white noise (*lower panel*) as measured through a TDH-50 earphone in a 6-cc coupler, 1-inch pressure microphone, Larson-Davis 800B and Stanford Research System model SR785 dynamic signal analyzer. (Reprinted from Burkard R, Secor C. [2002] Overview of auditory evoked potentials. In: Katz J, ed. *Handbook of Clinical Audiology*. 5th ed. Baltimore: Lippincott Williams & Wilkins; pp 233–248, with the permission of Lippincott Williams & Wilkins.

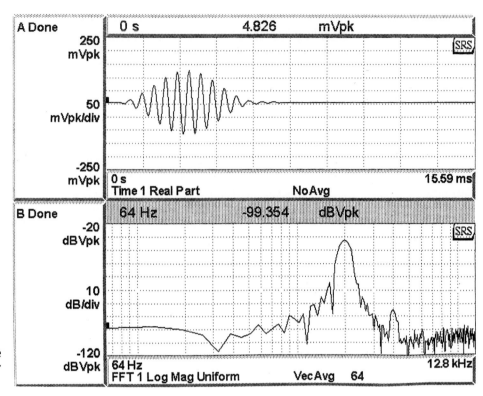

FIGURE 11.5 The time-domain representation of a tone burst is shown in the *upper panel*. The frequency-domain representation of this tone burst is shown in the *lower panel*.

of a click stimulus (as well as its broad spectrum) leads to the generation of large-amplitude CAP and ABR (as well as other AEP) responses. Therefore, when using tone burst stimuli, we use stimuli that are a compromise between an audiometric tone (long duration, long rise/fall times, and a very narrow spectrum) and a click (short duration, very fast rise/fall times, and very broad spectrum). To add even more complexity to this topic, there are many unique gating functions that can be used to shape the onset and offset of the tone burst, including linear, Blackman, and Hanning (cosine^2) functions. There is no compelling evidence showing a clear advantage of one gating function over another for AEP use. Suzuki and Horiuchi (1981) demonstrated that the first few cycles of a tone burst envelope determine ABR peak latency, amplitude, and threshold. Based on these findings, an optimal tone burst envelope, at least for the ABR, is a two-cycle rise/fall time. Plateau time should be kept brief (e.g., zero to two cycles), as longer plateau durations represent shorter off times between stimuli, which will, under at least some circumstances, reduce AEP peak amplitudes.

Calibration of Acoustic Transients

There are no ANSI standards that specify how to measure the sound pressure level (SPL) of an acoustic transient; also, there are no reference equivalent threshold SPLs (the dB SPL values for 0 dB hearing level [HL] used in audiometry) available for brief-duration stimuli. You must calibrate the acoustic signal using specialized instrumentation and procedures. You must

also determine your own in-house normative thresholds for the clicks and/or tone burst stimuli used in your lab/clinic. Alternatively, you can adopt threshold values reported by another clinic or laboratory, but you should at the very least obtain some in-house data on normal-hearing subjects to make sure the normative data from another clinic or laboratory are in the ballpark of your own in-house thresholds. For clinical procedures, it is prudent to use earphones that can be coupled to either a 6-cc or 2-cc coupler. TDH-39s, TDH-49s, and TDH-50s housed in MX 41/AR or Telephonics type 51 cushions can be coupled to a 6-cc (NBS-9a) coupler. Etymotic insert earphones (ER-1, ER-2, ER-3A) can be coupled to a 2-cc coupler. At the base of a 2-cc or 6-cc coupler is a space designed to house a 1-inch condenser pressure microphone. Should you choose to use smaller diameter microphones (1/2″, 1/4″, 1/8″), suitable adapters can be used. The microphone output can be routed to either a sound level meter or to a conditioning amplifier that provides the polarization voltage for the condenser microphone and (in some instruments) provides voltage amplification (gain). The measurement of the SPL of an acoustic transient with a sound level meter is complicated by the time constants used for the SPL measurement. Most sound level meters have at least two exponential-time-weighted averaging modes: fast and slow. Fast exponential-time-weighted averaging has a measurement time constant of 125 ms, while slow exponential-time-weighted averaging has a measurement time constant of 1,000 ms (Yeager and Marsh, 1998). In either case, clicks or tone bursts have durations that are much shorter than the time constant of even the fast exponential-time weighting, and you will underestimate the true SPL of the tone burst using fast (or worse yet, slow) exponential-time-weighted averaging. There are several solutions to this measurement problem. First, if you can turn your tone burst on for several seconds, you can record the level of the tone in the fast or slow exponential-time-weighted averaging mode. If you measure over three time constants (375 ms in fast, 3,000 ms in slow), the recorded value will closely approximate the true SPL of the stimulus. This is one method to obtain what is commonly referred to as the peak equivalent SPL (peSPL) of the tone burst. This approach will not work for a click stimulus because increasing the duration of the electrical pulse dramatically alters the spectrum of the stimulus. A second approach for determining the level of an acoustic transient is to purchase a sound level meter that records the largest instantaneous pressure (the "peak" pressure) and "holds" this value in the display until the meter is reset. This peak-hold measurement may vary with the specific sound level meter because the measurement interval over which this "peak" is evaluated (the time constant) varies with the particular sound level meter. It is desirable to use a meter with a peak SPL time constant of several tens of microseconds or less. A third approach can be used if you have an oscilloscope and a sound level meter that has an analog (AC) output. This type of output allows you to route the analog voltage output of the microphone to the oscilloscope. This technique can be used with any transient, including a click, and this approach is another method to determine the peSPL. Figure 11.6 is adapted from Burkard (1984) and diagrams two procedures for determining click peSPL. In the first procedure, which we will refer to as the baseline-to-peak peSPL procedure, you route the click (in this case) or other transient through the earphone, coupler, microphone, and sound level meter to the oscilloscope. First, you present a click stimulus and measure the baseline-to-peak voltage on the oscilloscope. Next, making sure not to change the SPL range on the sound level meter, you put a tonal stimulus through the earphone and adjust the level of the tone until the baseline-to-peak voltage is identical to that measured for the click. Finally, you read the SPL on the sound level meter. This reading is the baseline-to-peak peSPL of the click. The second method of determining peSPL involves measuring the peak-to-peak voltage of the click on the oscilloscope and adjusting the sine wave until its peak-to-peak voltage is equal to the peak-to-peak voltage of the click. The SPL value displayed on the sound level meter is recorded as the peak-to-peak peSPL of the click. The baseline-to-peak peSPL can never be less than the peak-to-peak peSPL. If the voltages of the positive and negative phases of a click (or other transient) are equal, then the baseline-to-peak and peak-to-peak peSPL values will be numerically equal. If the click is critically damped and shows a voltage deflection in only one direction (positive or negative), then the baseline-to-peak peSPL will be 6-dB larger than the peak-to-peak peSPL. Based on the earlier discussion, the baseline-to-peak peSPL and the peak-to-peak peSPL can be

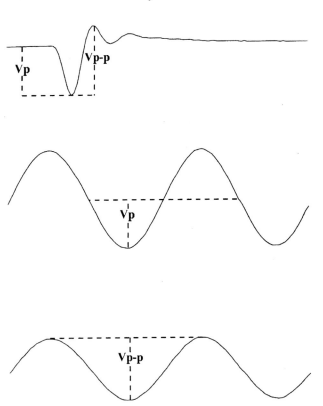

FIGURE 11.6 The procedure for obtaining peak equivalent sound pressure level (both baseline-to-peak and peak-to-peak measures) is shown. (Reprinted from Burkard R, Secor C. [2002] Overview of auditory evoked potentials. In: Katz J, ed. *Handbook of Clinical Audiology*. 5th ed. Baltimore: Lippincott Williams & Wilkins; pp 233–248, with the permission of Lippincott Williams & Wilkins.)

identical, or there can be a difference as large as 6 dB, making it imperative that you identify the measurement technique used when reporting peSPL. A fourth approach to measuring the SPL is to eliminate the sound level meter and to use the coupler, microphone, microphone conditioning amplifier, and oscilloscope. You present the click (or other transient) stimulus and measure the peak voltage on the oscilloscope. You can calibrate the microphone by using a sound source with a known SPL, or you can use the microphone sensitivity curve to convert microphone output voltage to input sound pressure (and ultimately to SPL). There are commercially available sound sources that produce known SPLs, which are known as either acoustic calibrators or pistonphones. While the manner of sound generation differs for these two sound sources, each device produces a known SPL at a known frequency, and adaptors are available to use with a variety of condenser microphone sizes. You could connect the acoustic calibrator to the microphone and measure the voltage out of the microphone conditioning amplifier. In this way, you know that a given voltage is produced when a specified SPL is present at the microphone diaphragm. Let us say your calibrator produces 114 dB SPL, and you measure 1 volt at the conditioning amplifier output. Then you place a 2-cc coupler on the microphone and mate an Etymotic ER-3A insert microphone to the coupler. You present a sine wave to the earphone, and you measure 100 mV. The SPL is: 20log(100 mV/1,000 mV) + 114 dB SPL = 94 dB SPL. The first part of the formula estimates the dB re: 114 dB SPL, which is −20 dB. You then add 114 to convert from dB re: 114 dB SPL to dB SPL.

Using the sensitivity of the microphone, you can convert the peak voltage on the oscilloscope to peak pressure (e.g., in pascals [Pa]). The sensitivity of a microphone relates the voltage out of the microphone to the sound pressure at the microphone diaphragm in, for example, mV/Pa. You then convert the pressure to SPL. For example, you measure a peak voltage of 1,000 mV. The microphone sensitivity is 10 mV/Pa. If 10 mV represents 1 Pa, then 1,000 mV represents 100 Pa. Converting to peak SPL (pSPL):
pSPL = 20log(100 Pa/0.00002 Pa) = 20log5,000,000 = 133.98.

This value should correspond to the pSPL produced by a sound level meter in peak hold mode, although if the time constant of the sound level meter is too long (say 100 μs), then the sound level meter may produce a lower value. If you record the peSPL and pSPL of the same stimuli, the baseline-to-peak peSPL value should be 3 dB less than the true pSPL value. This is because the peSPL value is actually referenced to a root mean square measure of a sine wave, rather than a peak measure. To obtain the true pSPL value, you must add 3 dB to the peSPL (using the baseline-to-peak procedure) because the crest factor (ratio of peak to root mean square) of a true sine wave is 1.414, or 3 dB (3 dB = 20log1.414).

When you calibrate an audiometer, you present tones at some number of dB above average hearing threshold, or dB HL. It is a simple matter to look up the reference equivalent threshold sound pressure levels (RETSPLs) for tones (and speech stimuli) in ANSI S3.6-2004 to see whether that particular tone is appropriately calibrated. There is, however, no national standard specifying RETSPLs for transient stimuli. For click stimuli, Stapells et al. (1982) provide threshold values for a group of normal-hearing subjects to click stimuli as presented through a TDH-39 earphone. For tone burst stimuli, there are many possible rise/fall and plateau times, as well as various gating functions and repetition rates, which makes it a challenge to obtain normative threshold values that are acceptable to most clinicians and scientists. This problem will remain until, at the very least, the audiology community can reach a consensus regarding optimal tone burst envelope parameters. What should the clinician do about this calibration problem? You should standardize the tone burst stimuli used in your clinic, and you should collect your own normative perceptual thresholds using a group of normal-hearing young adults. The threshold values contained in ANSI S3.6-2004 (the RETSPLs) were obtained for stimulus durations of greater than 100 to 200 ms. Assuming that the slope of the temporal integration function is 10 dB per decade

(Garner, 1947), then for a tone burst of approximately 5 ms in duration, we would anticipate a threshold that is approximately 15 dB higher than the RETSPL values listed in ANSI S3.6-2004.

Response Recording

In the clinic, surface (scalp) electrodes and an electrolytic paste or gel typically serve as the interface between the biologic world (your scalp) and the electrical world (the bioamplifier input). Needle electrodes can also be used; these are placed subdermally (under the skin), and the ions present in your body fluids facilitate the transfer of the electrical signal from the tissue to the electrode. Various types of electrodes, both disposable and reusable, are commercially available. Some are special purpose, but most are usable for a variety of recording situations. The locations of electrode placement on the scalp have been standardized by the development of the international 10-20 system (Jasper, 1958). For the international 10-20 system, left scalp locations are subscripted with odd numbers, while right scalp locations are subscripted with even numbers. Here, we will briefly review those scalp locations commonly used for AEP recordings. The labels for the left and right mastoid (or earlobe) are A1 and A2, respectively. Fpz is the nasion (bridge of the nose), Oz is the inion (at the external occipital protuberance), and Fz is the forehead. The vertex (Cz) is halfway between nasion and inion and midway between the ear canals.

A critical step when applying electrodes is the scalp preparation. Cleaning the scalp by abrasion and using alcohol or other skin-preparation materials remove dead skin and oils. You should measure the interelectrode impedance following electrode application, using either the impedance-testing function that comes packaged with commercially available AEP systems or using a handheld portable electrode impedance meter. Low electrode impedances are desirable (some sources state 5 kΩ or less), but it is sometimes difficult to achieve such low electrode impedances. For example, if you use a tympanic membrane electrode, it is often impossible to achieve a low electrode impedance. High electrode impedance increases the noise floor of the recording and will often result in an increase in the magnitude of the line frequency and its harmonics (60 Hz and its harmonics in the United States; 50 Hz and its harmonics in Europe). For differential recordings, which are used in most AEP applications, differences in interelectrode impedances can compromise (reduce) the elimination of common-mode noise (see below). Thus, similar impedance among electrodes is desirable.

Three electrodes are used for each recording channel when using a differential bioamplifier. The three leads are referred to as the noninverting, the inverting, and the common leads. The noninverting lead is sometimes called the positive or the active lead. The inverting lead is often referred to as the negative or the reference lead. The common lead is sometimes called the ground. In a differential amplifier, the voltage seen by the noninverting and the inverting leads are relative to common. In fact, another term for voltage is the potential difference, telling us that the voltage of one lead must be expressed relative to the voltage of a second lead. For differential amplification, the voltage from the inverting common channel is subtracted from the voltage of the noninverting common channel. Indeed, it is this subtraction (or voltage difference) that is the basis of the term "differential amplification." Following this voltage subtraction, the remainder is amplified. Differential amplification substantially reduces noise that is common to the inverting and noninverting lead. This noise, in fact, is called common mode noise. Why is this useful? Let us speculate that we are recording in a room with a lot of 60-Hz noise (e.g., from the lights). This 60-Hz line noise will often be of similar magnitude and phase at the noninverting and inverting leads. This voltage that is "common" to both of these leads will be "subtracted" prior to amplification. The common mode rejection ratio (CMRR) is a value that tells us how well "common mode" activity is eliminated. Let us say we have a bioamplifier gain (V_{out}/V_{in}) of 1,000,000. If we put 5 μV into the noninverting lead and short the inverting lead (or vice versa), we essentially eliminate the differential amplification and produce a monopolar or single-ended bioamplifier, whose output would be 5 V (5,000,000 μV). If we now apply 5 μV into the inverting and noninverting leads of a differential amplifier, due to the subtraction process used in differential amplification, the output voltage is much smaller, let us say 50 μV. To calculate the CMRR, you divide the differential voltage by the single-ended voltage, and you can convert this to a dB value by taking 20 times the base 10 logarithm of this ratio: CMRR = $20\log_{10}(5,000,000\ \mu V/50\ \mu V) = 20\log_{10}(100,000) = \sim 100$ dB. The larger the dB value is, the better the CMRR.

Anywhere from one to 256 (or more) bioamplifier channels can be used for AEP recordings. In most clinical applications, a small number of channels is used, perhaps one to four. For ABR recordings, it is common to use two recording channels, called the ipsilateral montage and the contralateral montage. For left ear stimulation, the ipsilateral channel might be vertex (noninverting), left mastoid or earlobe (inverting), and forehead (common), while the contralateral channel would be vertex (noninverting), right mastoid or earlobe (inverting), and forehead (common).

The Digital World

At the heart of evoked potential instruments is a digital microprocessor. However, the bioamplifier output (discussed earlier) is a continuous (analog) voltage. The analog voltage coming out of the bioamplifier must be converted into a digital form via a process called analog-to-digital conversion.

Figure 11.7 shows an analog representation of a sinusoid. An analog signal has a voltage value at all moments in time. For example, there is a signal at 1.5 ms and at 1.5001 ms. Also, the voltage can assume any value within a specified voltage range (e.g., ±1 V). For example, the signal can have a

voltage of 10 mV and 9.99999 mV. When our analog voltage is converted to a digital format, only a finite number of voltage values can be assumed, and we can only sample the voltage at specific time intervals. We will describe these sampling processes in a later section, but first we will describe the base 2 (or binary) number system.

BINARY NUMBER SYSTEM

In our base 10 (or decimal) number system, each place can represent 10 different values (0 through 9). In the base 2 or binary number system, each place can only represent two numbers (0 or 1). In the base 10 system, the rightmost number is multiplied by 10^0, with the exponent increasing by 1 for each number as we move to the left. The reader who is unfamiliar with exponents should refer to Speaks (1996). Although we do not think about this much, the number 94 can be described as: $94 = (9 \times 10^1) + (4 \times 10^0)$.

In a binary number system, the rules are the same, except that we can only use ones and zeroes. What is the decimal equivalent of the binary number 1100010?

$$1100010 = (1 \times 2^6) + (1 \times 2^5) + (0 \times 2^4) + (0 \times 2^3)$$
$$+ (0 \times 2^2) + (1 \times 2^1) + (0 \times 2^0)$$
$$= 64 + 32 + 0 + 0 + 0 + 2 + 0 = 98$$

As you can see, the rules of binary numbers are the same as those of decimal numbers, except that we can only use zeroes and ones. If each binary digit (called a bit) can only represent two values, then we need to use more than one bit in order to represent numbers greater than one. In our example above, the two-place number 98 in decimal is represented in binary by the seven-place number 1100010. We refer to each of these binary places as a bit, and hence, 1100010 is a seven-bit binary number. An *n*-bit binary number can assume 2^n values. Thus, a seven-bit number can assume 2^7 or 128 values. The smallest value this seven-bit number can assume is 0 (0000000), whereas the largest is 127 ($1111111 = 64 + 32 + 16 + 8 + 4 + 2 + 1 = 127$). When we need to represent a greater number of possible values in the binary system, we increase the number of bits. The number values that can be represented by a given number of bits are shown in Table 11.2 for binary numbers from one to 16 bits.

ANALOG-TO-DIGITAL CONVERSION

An analog-to-digital converter (ADC) is a device that changes the continuous activity of the real world (such as brain wave activity) into the binary coding used in the digital world. For practical reasons (it is impossible to sample an infinite sum of values), when we convert analog signals into a digital format, we cannot sample the signal at all possible times, and we must round off the amplitude values. Thus, with analog-to-digital conversion, we lose information, but we gain the versatile processing capabilities of the computer.

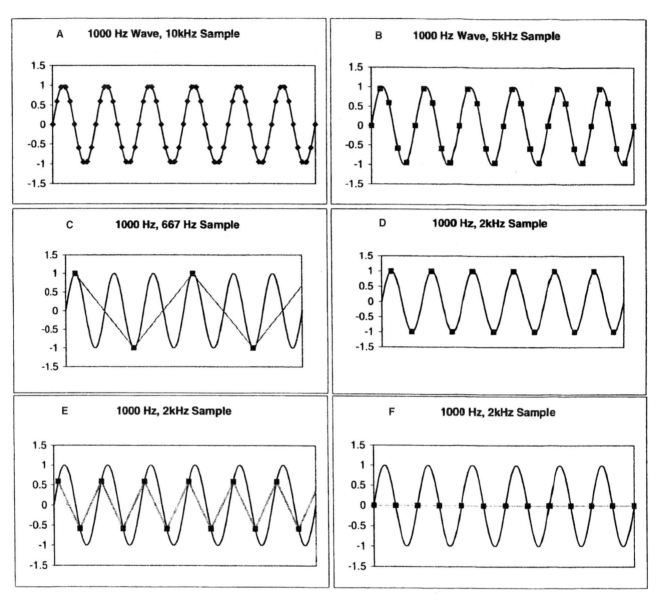

FIGURE 11.7 An analog representation of a sinusoid is shown. The time window shown represents 5 ms. Each subfigure shows an analog representation of a 1,000-Hz sinusoid, with a time scale of 5 ms. Panels **A–F** show digital representations of this sinusoid, sampled at 10,000, 5,000, 667, 2,000, 2,000, and 2,000 Hz, respectively. (Reprinted from Burkard R, Secor C. [2002] Overview of auditory evoked potentials. In: Katz J, ed. *Handbook of Clinical Audiology.* 5th ed. Baltimore: Lippincott Williams & Wilkins; pp 233–248, with the permission of Lippincott Williams & Wilkins.)

The amplitude "round off" mentioned earlier is formally known as quantization. When the amplitude of a continuous (analog) signal is rounded off in the digital world, there is often a difference between the original analog value and the digital value. This difference is called quantization error. The magnitude of this quantization error is affected by a number of factors. One of these factors is the dynamic range of the ADC. The dynamic range is the largest voltage that can be accurately digitized. A second factor in determining quantization error is the number of bits of the ADC. Let us assume that we have a ± 5-V dynamic range and a 12-bit ADC. By use of Table 11.2, we can see that a 12-bit ADC

provides 4,096 (e.g., 2^{12}) possible values. Because the total voltage range is 10 V (from −5 to +5 V) and a 12-bit ADC encodes 4,096 values, the resolution of this system is (with x = number of bits):

$$ADC \text{ resolution} = \text{Voltage range}/2^x = 10V/2^{12}$$

$$= 10V/4,096 = 0.00245V = 2.45mV$$

In this example, the resolution between two sequential points is 2.45 mV. The quantization error becomes relevant when we want to separate out amplitudes that are less than this ADC resolution. Assuming that the ADC rounds down

TABLE 11.2 The relationship between number of bits and the number of encoded values

Number of bits	Number of values (exponential)	Number of values (decimal)
1	2^1	2
2	2^2	4
3	2^3	8
4	2^4	16
5	2^5	32
6	2^6	64
7	2^7	128
8	2^8	256
9	2^9	512
10	2^{10}	1,024
11	2^{11}	2,048
12	2^{12}	4,096
13	2^{13}	8,192
14	2^{14}	16,384
15	2^{15}	32,768
16	2^{16}	65,536

Reprinted from Burkard R, Secor C. (2002) Overview of auditory evoked potentials. In: Katz J, ed. *Handbook of Clinical Audiology*. 5th ed. Baltimore: Lippincott Williams & Wilkins; pp 233–248, with the permission of Lippincott Williams & Wilkins.

to the largest value it has exceeded, the smallest non-zero amplitude this ADC can encode (called the least significant bit [LSB]) must be more negative than −2.45 mV or more positive than +2.45 mV. You are probably wondering how this might be a useful resolution because all electroencephalogram (EEG) activity is in the microvolt range and hence all EEG voltages would round off to zero (a common occurrence in Washington, DC at the present time). For example, let us assume that an off-the-scalp EEG voltage for a subject is $\pm 100\,\mu V$ (± 0.1 mV) and your evoked potential amplitude is 10 μV. How close will you estimate this value in the proposed digital system? Without amplification (as stated earlier) because 10 μV is less than the quantization range of ± 2.45 mV, you will estimate the amplitude as 0 mV. The quantization error in estimating the peak EEG amplitude in this case is 10 μV (10 μV – 0 μV) and produces a serious estimation error. How do you reduce this unacceptable error? First, we could use an ADC with more bits. Sixteen-bit ADCs are currently available for a reasonable cost. This would produce a resolution of 10 V/2^{16} = 10,000 mV/65,536 = 0.15253 mV. With this 16-bit system, 10 μV is still digitally approximated as 0 μV, again giving you a quantization error of 10 μV. In other words, this didn't help one bit (pun intended). One can get 24-bit ADCs, which provide in excess of 16 million values (16,777,216). In this case, the digital approximation is 10 V/2^{24}, with a resolution of 0.6 μV; the digital approximation in this example would be 9.6 μV, with a resulting quantization error of 0.4 μV—a much more acceptable "round-off" error.

An alternative to using a very high–resolution ADC is to provide bioamplifier gain. All commercially available evoked potential systems provide variable bioamplifier gain. With the use of a bioamplifier, we can amplify the signal of interest so that it occupies most of the ADC voltage range, and in doing so, we improve the amplitude resolution of our digital system. For our ± 5-V ADC range with 10-bit resolution, let us amplify the signal by 50,000 times. In this case, the full-scale off-the-scalp voltage that the ADC can resolve is 10 V/50,000 = 0.2 mV (note that this equals the specified EEG range of $\pm 100\,\mu V$). Because this 0.2-mV range is encoded by the 10-bit ADC (representing 1,024 values), our off-the-scalp resolution is now 0.2 mV/1,024 = 0.195 μV, and our digital estimate of the 10-μV peak amplitude is 9.75 μV, with an error of 0.25 μV. To summarize, we can reduce quantization error using several strategies: reduce the ADC voltage range, increase the number of bits of the ADC, and/or increase bioamplifier gain.

The second limitation of a digital system arises because we sample the continuous analog response at periodic time intervals. The solid line in Figure 11.7A shows a 1,000-Hz analog sine wave. The dots represent the results of digitally sampling this 1,000-Hz sine wave every 0.1 ms. This is called the sampling period. The inverse of the sampling period is the sampling frequency (1/0.1 ms = 1/0.0001 s = 10,000 Hz). Figure 11.7B shows the same 1,000-Hz sine wave, but now sampled half as often (every 0.2 ms). If we visually connect the dots, we can visualize a signal that follows the periodicity of the sine wave. If we sample even less frequently, let us say every 1.5 ms (Fig. 11.7C), we no longer adequately resolve the period of this sine wave. We now see a sine wave with a longer period (i.e., a lower frequency) than our analog 1,000-Hz sine wave. Digitally sampling an analog signal at too large a sampling period (or too low a sampling frequency) results in an inaccuracy in the estimate of the frequency of the analog signal. This inaccurate (false) frequency is referred to as an aliased frequency. The process leading to this false or inaccurate frequency is called aliasing. The Nyquist theorem can be used to avoid aliasing. According to the Nyquist theorem, in order to avoid aliasing, we must have a sampling frequency that is greater than twice the highest frequency in the analog signal that we are digitizing. The lowest digitization (sampling) frequency that can be used in order to accurately represent the frequency of a given analog signal is called the Nyquist rate. In our example, from Figure 11.7, we must sample at just above 2,000 Hz to adequately represent our 1,000-Hz sine wave. Figure 11.7D shows what might happen if we digitize at exactly 2,000 Hz (i.e., at exactly twice the frequency of the analog signal). In this case, when the sampling occurs at or near the peaks of the sine wave, we can resolve the frequency of the sine wave. Although this sine wave looks more like a triangular wave, the frequency does appear appropriate. Figure 11.7E shows the same 2,000-Hz sampling frequency, but now the sampling times are slightly shifted in time from that shown in Figure 11.7D. You can see that the frequency of the 1,000-Hz sine wave is accurate, but the peak amplitude is underestimated. Figures 11.7D and 11.7E show that sampling at exactly twice the frequency of the analog signal can adequately resolve the frequency of interest. Why, then, does the Nyquist theorem state that the sampling frequency must be just above twice the highest frequency in the analog signal? This is answered by reference to Figure 11.7F, where the 1,000-Hz sine wave is digitally sampled at 2,000 Hz, but now these sample times occur at the zero crossings and not at or near the peaks. This produces a flat line (i.e., a 0-Hz signal). Because this 0-Hz frequency is clearly different (lower than) the analog signal frequency of 1,000 Hz, this example demonstrates aliasing. To avoid aliasing, we must sample at a little more than twice the highest frequency in our signal. It is wise to sample at two times the Nyquist rate (i.e., four times the highest frequency in the analog signal of interest) just to err on the side of caution. Using an example relevant to AEP work, if we know our ABR has substantial energy from 100 to 3,000 Hz, then the Nyquist rate is just above 6,000 Hz, and this sampling rate will be adequate to prevent aliasing. If we double the Nyquist rate, then the desired sampling frequency is approximately 12,000 Hz.

Now we know that using a sampling frequency that is too low can result in aliasing. Are there any problems with using a very high sampling frequency? Using a sampling frequency that is well above that needed to prevent aliasing will result in larger data files. This is most easily understood by a numerical example. We want to obtain an ABR in an infant, and we know that we should look at a response time window (time epoch) of 20 ms. Let us also suppose that there is little energy at 1,500 Hz or above in an infant ABR. In this example, the Nyquist rate is just approximately 3,000 Hz, and if we double this to prevent aliasing, we should digitize at 6,000 Hz (a sampling period of 167 μs). If we sample every 167 μs, then we will have 120 data points in our 20-ms time window:

$$\text{response time epoch} = (\text{sampling period})$$
$$\times (\text{number of data points})$$

This can be rewritten as:

$$\text{number of data points} = (\text{response time epoch})/$$
$$(\text{sampling period})$$

Plugging our numbers from the example into this equation yields:

$$\text{number of data points} = 20 \text{ ms}/167 \ \mu s = 120 \text{ data points}$$

We would only need to store 120 data points for this ABR waveform. If we doubled the sampling frequency (i.e., four times the Nyquist rate), this would require a sampling period of 83.5 μs and a grand total of 240 data points in our memory array. Now let us sample as fast as we can. We construct a digitizer that can sample at 1 GHz (a billion samples per second). A 1-GHz sampling frequency corresponds to a sampling period of 1 nanosecond, or 0.001 μs. The number of points in our evoked potential memory array would be

20 ms = 20,000 μs/0.0001 μs = 20,000,000 data points. You would fill up a 10-gigabyte hard disk after collecting roughly 500 ABRs. If you had a busy clinic, you could fill up the hard drive quite quickly. You should digitize at a high enough rate to safely avoid aliasing, but not so fast as to have issues with data storage. Most commercial AEP units limit the number of data points that can be used to obtain a response. Let us say that your memory array is limited to 1,024 (2^{10}) words of memory. For a 20-ms time window, your sampling period is 20 ms/1,024 = 20 μs, or a sampling frequency of 50,000 Hz. In this example, aliasing is not a problem, unless you suspect that there is energy in the response that exceeds 50,000/2 = 25,000 Hz. In some instances, you will not know exactly the Nyquist frequency of the response you are measuring. In these cases, using a filter that eliminates energy at and above a frequency where aliasing could be an issue is warranted. In our example, using a filter that eliminates energy at and above 25,000 Hz would solve the problem. This type of filter is called a low-pass filter. When the purpose of a low pass is to prevent aliasing, then this low-pass filter is called an antialiasing filter.

DIGITAL-TO-ANALOG CONVERSION

In most (perhaps all) current commercially available AEP systems, the acoustic stimuli used to elicit an evoked potential are digitally generated by the computer. These digital signals are converted to analog signals by a device called a digital-to-analog converter (DAC). Aliasing can also arise with digital-to-analog conversion. In order to avoid aliasing, the output voltage of the DAC can be low-pass filtered at the appropriate frequency (i.e., less than half the digitization frequency) by a device called an anti-imaging filter. It should be noted that the earphones used for clinical AEP measures generally have low-pass cutoffs less than 10,000 Hz and that these transducers may serve as anti-imaging filters if DAC rates above 20 kHz are used.

Noise Reduction

For human recordings, AEP amplitude is typically much smaller than that of the background noise. Any unwanted electrical activity will be called noise. For AEP purposes, this noise can be comprised of both periodic and aperiodic activity and can be of both biologic and nonbiologic origin. Biologic sources of noise include muscle activity and the EEG, both of which represent aperiodic noise. Nonbiologic sources of noise include aperiodic noise arising from the bioamplifier and periodic (60-Hz, or 50-Hz for our European readers) line-power noise. The 60-Hz (or 50-Hz) noise may arise from within the AEP system itself, but often, this noise arises from the room where the AEP is being performed. The noise may be generated by overhead lights or be emitted by other electrical equipment in the room. Such 60-Hz (or 50-Hz) electrical noise is generated in the room, and the subject acts like an antenna. If this line noise is picked up by the electrodes on the subject's scalp, it is amplified (with the biologic activity). A few microvolts of line noise become a few volts if a gain of 1,000,000 is used by the bioamplifiers.

How do you reduce unwanted electrical noise? First, low electrode impedances can reduce 60-Hz (or 50-Hz) line noise. Second, making the subject comfortable and encouraging them to sleep (if that does not negatively affect the response of interest) can substantially reduce noise arising from muscle activity. Third, differential amplification (i.e., using three electrode leads per recording channel) can reduce common-mode noise. Fourth, filtering the output of the bioamplifier can reduce noise. Finally, signal averaging reduces unwanted background noise. We have previously discussed electrode application and the use of differential amplification. In the following paragraphs, we will provide more detail on the use of filtering and signal averaging to reduce unwanted noise.

Filtering involves eliminating noise that is outside the frequency range of the desired response. Most of the energy in, for example, the click-evoked ABR is in the 100- to 3,000-Hz frequency range. Selectively eliminating electrical activity below 100 Hz and above 3,000 Hz will reduce the background noise with relatively minor changes to the ABR. Figure 11.8 shows the four basic types of filter functions. A low-pass filter (Fig. 11.8A) reduces a signal above a given frequency but lets lower frequency energy pass through (i.e., lets the signals pass). A high-pass filter (Fig. 11.8B) reduces a signal below a specified frequency but passes signals above that frequency. A band-pass filter (Fig. 11.8C) passes energy between two cutoff frequencies but reduces energy above and below this frequency band. Finally, a band-reject or notch filter (Fig. 11.8D) reduces energy between two cutoff frequencies but passes energy above and below this band. The cutoff frequency (or half-power point) of a filter is the frequency at which the voltage at the filter output is reduced to 70.7% of the input (or is –3 dB). The rejection rate, or filter skirt, of a filter refers to how fast the voltage is reduced outside of the pass band. This is often reported in dB/octave. If the voltage of a signal is reduced by half (6 dB) when the

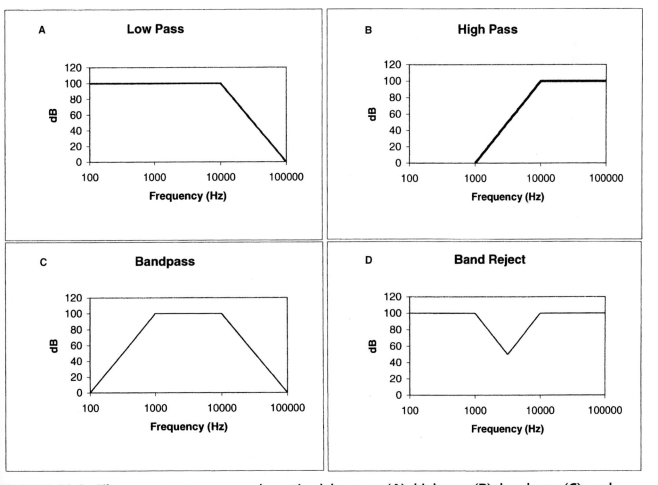

FIGURE 11.8 Filter response types are schematized: low pass (**A**), high pass (**B**), band pass (**C**), and band reject (**D**). (Reprinted from Burkard R, Secor C. [2002] Overview of auditory evoked potentials. In: Katz J, ed. *Handbook of Clinical Audiology*. 5th ed. Baltimore: Lippincott Williams & Wilkins; pp 233–248, with the permission of Lippincott Williams & Wilkins.)

frequency is doubled (one octave is a doubling of frequency), then the filter rolls off at a rate of 6 dB/octave. Many filters roll off in integer multiples of 6 dB/octave, and each of these 6 dB/octave multiples is referred to as a pole. Thus, a 48-dB/octave filter is called an eight-pole filter.

It is imperative that you know the spectrum (frequency content) of the AEP you are recording, so that when you filter, you do not throw the baby out with the bathwater (i.e., you greatly reduce the AEP while reducing the amplitude of the noise). Because most review chapters on the various AEPs will provide suggested filter settings for recording that response, determining optimal AEP filter settings should be a simple matter of following the suggestions in these chapters.

Despite our best efforts with getting the subject to relax, obtaining low and balanced electrode impedances, and using differential amplification with judicious filtering, the AEP of interest will still usually be smaller than the ongoing background electrical noise. In others words, the AEP is at a poor signal-to-noise ratio (S/N). In many instances, the response is much smaller than the amplitude of the background noise, making it difficult or impossible to identify the AEP. To improve the S/N (in order to make the AEP visible), we use time-domain signal averaging. The theory underlying signal averaging invokes several assumptions about the signal (i.e., the AEP) and the noise:

1. The AEP is the always the same in response to a constant stimulus.
2. The noise is truly random (i.e., it is different for each stimulus presentation).
3. The signal (the AEP) and the noise are independent.

For time-domain signal averaging, we present the same stimulus repeatedly while summing the response in memory. The average response is created by dividing the summed voltage at each time point in the memory array by the number of stimuli presented. Differences in the statistical properties of the signal (the AEP) and the noise lead to the improvement in the S/N. For signal averaging to work correctly, we must initiate the summation into the memory array at a constant time relative to stimulus presentation. We typically start signal averaging at the onset of the stimulus. If we do this, then, according to the first assumption above, the AEP is constant to each stimulus presentation. For example, let us say we have a 2-μV AEP that we sum over 16 stimulus presentations: $2+2+2+2+2+2+2+2+2+2+2+2+2+2+2+2 = 32 \mu$V. The average amplitude is thus 32 μV/16 sweeps = 2 μV. This is expected, as we said the stimulus is constant for each presentation. Let us say the background noise is 4 μV. The S/N = 2 μV/4 μV = 0.5. The signal is small compared to the noise, and it will be difficult to see the AEP. Let us sum together the response to 16 "noise" time epochs. In this case, because the noise segments are random, we sum these noise estimates in a manner that differs from that used for the signal. We square each value, sum these squared values, and take the square root. The interested reader is referred

TABLE 11.3	The relationship between number of sweeps and improvement in signal-to-noise ratio (S/N)
Number of sweeps	S/N Improvement
2	1.414
4	2
10	3.16
100	10
400	20
1,000	31.62
2,000	44.72
10,000	100

Reprinted from Burkard R, Secor C. (2002) Overview of auditory evoked potentials. In: Katz J, ed. *Handbook of Clinical Audiology*. 5th ed. Baltimore: Lippincott Williams & Wilkins; pp 233–248, with the permission of Lippincott Williams & Wilkins.

to Hyde (1994a) for a more detailed explanation. According to this formula: $(4^2 + 4^2 + 4^2 + 4^2 + 4^2 + 4^2 + 4^2 + 4^2 + 4^2 + 4^2 + 4^2 + 4^2 + 4^2 + 4^2 + 4^2 + 4^2)^{1/2} = 16 \mu$V. The average noise is now 16 μV/16 sweeps = 1 μV, and the S/N is now 2 μV signal/1 μV noise = 2. Thus, signal averaging over 16 sweeps changed the S/N from 0.5 to 2, a factor of 4 improvement. Under optimal conditions, the S/N increases in proportion to the square root of the number of sweeps. Table 11.3 shows the ideal S/N improvement for various numbers of sweeps.

Recommendations for the number of sweeps used clinically (in chapters that follow, and elsewhere) are based on the experimental and clinical experience of the investigators or after review of the relevant literature. These recommendations can only be considered guidelines. The number of stimulus presentations required to obtain a given response depends on response amplitude (which varies with the AEP, stimulation and recording parameters, and the particular subject), background noise amplitude (which is dependent on subject and recording factors), and the target S/N (which is dependent on your particular clinical objectives). For threshold estimation, the S/N should be on the order of 1 or more because you are really only interested in whether a response is present or not. For determination of peak latencies and amplitudes, an S/N of 2 or greater is desirable because you are trying to accurately estimate response variables, which will be influenced by poor S/N.

You might read in the literature that you should obtain 2,000 sweeps for an ABR. Such statements, however, can only be considered ballpark suggestions that will not be optimal under some circumstances. For one subject, to a lower level click stimulus, you might record a response amplitude of 0.1 μV. Let us say the subject has a 10-μV background noise. The S/N is 0.01, and this only improves by a factor of

44.7 for 2,000 sweeps (Table 11.3), and the S/N of the averaged response will still be less than 1 (0.447). In this example, the recommended number of sweeps is inadequate. In a different subject, when you present a high-level stimulus, your response might be 0.6 μV. This patient is quite relaxed and has 3 μV of noise, resulting in an S/N of 0.6/3 = 0.2. Presenting 2,000 sweeps, the S/N (under optimal conditions) is 8.94 (0.2 × 44.7), which is a better S/N than is required for most clinical purposes. You could have saved yourself some time by stopping data acquisition before the 2,000 stimuli had been presented. While guidelines of sweep numbers are of course useful, a clear understanding of the principles underlying signal averaging can lead to online protocol changes that will allow more efficient data collection, as well as reduce the incidence of stopping signal averaging before an interpretable AEP is obtained. There are techniques that allow online estimation of S/N, and stopping rules can be used that stop data acquisition when a criterion S/N (and/or probability that a response is present) is achieved or a maximum number of responses have been averaged. One such technique (called Fsp) is described in Chapter 13.

▨ NORMATIVE ASPECTS OF THE AUDITORY BRAINSTEM RESPONSE

In this section, we will review some normative aspects of the ABR. These normative aspects form the basis for the clinical applications of the ABR. This section will review the recommended recording parameters of the ABR, briefly mention several relevant subject variables, and, in more detail, review the effects of several stimulus variables on the ABR.

As shown in Figure 11.1, the ABR from a normal-hearing and neurologically intact young adult to a moderate- to high-level click stimulus is a series of five to seven positive peaks, labeled I to VII, occurring within 10 ms of click onset. The peak amplitudes are, in most instances, less than 1 μV.

Subject Variables

The ABR is not substantially influenced by attention or sleep state (Picton and Hillyard, 1974; Campbell and Bartoli, 1986; Kuk and Abbas, 1989), which makes it optimal for evaluating patients who are unable or unwilling to cooperate, such as infants or young children.

There are several subject variables that can affect the latency and the amplitude of the ABR, including core temperature, gender, and age. A decrease in core temperature results in an increase in ABR peak latencies, an increase in interwave intervals, and a decrease in peak amplitudes (Hall et al., 1988; Marshall and Donchin, 1981). It is important to monitor core temperature during intraoperative monitoring. This is because a patient's core temperature may be outside of the normal range during, for example, heart surgery

(Stockard et al., 1978), and core temperature changes can have an influence on the interpretation of the results.

Most readers will agree that sex is important. In terms of the ABR, females generally show shorter response latencies and interwave intervals, as well as larger response amplitudes, than males (Schwartz et al., 1994; Kjaer, 1979). These sex differences cannot be explained by differences in head size alone, but rather appear to be attributable, at least in part, to differences in cochlear length. Human females have shorter cochleae than their male counterparts (Sato et al., 1991). Don et al. (1993), using the high-pass subtractive masking technique, reported that shorter cochlear length results in greater traveling wave velocity, which is believed to account for some of the gender-related differences noted earlier. Finally, in regard to subject age, ABR peak latencies, interwave intervals, and amplitudes have been shown to vary with the age of a subject. Infant peak latencies and interwave intervals are longer than those seen in adults (Cox, 1985). Older subjects have ABRs that are typically reported to be longer in latency and smaller in amplitude compared with younger subjects (Schwartz et al., 1994). However, many of these older subjects have a hearing loss, which makes it difficult to separate the changes in the ABR that occur as a result of advancing age from the changes that can occur from a hearing loss.

Another issue that is not yet fully understood is how age affects the ABR interwave intervals. Rowe (1978) reported that the I to III interwave interval increased with increasing age, while the III to V interwave interval remained unchanged. In contrast, Costa et al. (1990) found that the I to II and I to III interwave intervals actually decreased with increasing age. These inconsistencies can make it challenging to interpret ABR results, especially when you take into consideration that peak latencies, as well as interwave intervals, are often used for site-of-lesion testing.

Stimulus Variables

As mentioned earlier, the ABR is sensitive to manipulations in stimulus parameters, including stimulus polarity, whether the stimuli are presented monaurally or binaurally, stimulus spectrum, level, and rate. We will review the effects of these stimulus factors on the ABR in the paragraphs that follow.

A number of studies have investigated how click polarity affects the human ABR. Hair cells are only excited by a deflection of the stereocilia in the direction of the basal body (i.e., the hair cells are depolarized by deflection of the stereocilia in one direction, and this depolarization leads to auditory nerve fiber discharge). Thus, the hair cells and eighth-nerve fibers perform a half-wave rectification of the input signal. Simple models of the auditory system suggest that the rarefaction phase of a stimulus should be the most effective (see Hall [1995], pp 143–144). Empirically, some studies have shown shorter peak latencies and larger peak amplitudes to rarefaction than to condensation clicks (Stockard et al., 1979).

However, other studies have shown that not all subjects show these trends and that polarity effects are (at best) small and variable (Schwartz et al., 1994; Borg and Lofqvist, 1981).

ABRs to monaural stimuli are smaller than to binaural stimuli (Owen and Burkard, 1991). If you collect an ABR in response to monaural stimulation from each ear and sum these monaural responses, this "summed monaural" response typically has a larger wave V amplitude than is seen when one actually binaurally stimulates the subject (Owen and Burkard, 1991). This amplitude reduction for the true binaural response, as compared to that of the "summed monaural" response, is often interpreted as evidence of binaural interaction in the ABR.

Click stimuli are broad in frequency, which results in stimulation of much of the cochlea. In order to stimulate a limited region of the cochlea, you must use a narrow-spectrum stimulus (such as a tone burst), a masking procedure, or a combination of a narrow-spectrum stimulus and maskers. Low-frequency tone bursts will typically produce longer ABR peak latencies due to the increased traveling wave delay to more apical cochlear regions. When presented at high stimulus levels, low-frequency tone bursts may actually generate an ABR that arises from the higher frequency (more basal) regions of the cochlea (Burkard and Hecox, 1983b). To reduce this basal spread of activity in response to low-frequency stimuli, several masking procedures have been developed and investigated. These masking procedures include: (1) click stimuli with notched noise (Pratt

and Bleich, 1982); (2) click stimuli and high-pass subtractive masking (Teas et al., 1962; Don and Eggermont, 1978); (3) tone burst stimuli in high-pass noise (Kileny, 1981); and (4) tone burst stimuli in notched noise (Picton et al., 1979). We will not review this literature further in this chapter. An excellent review of this topic can be found in Stapells et al. (1994).

To estimate ABR threshold, the level of the stimulus must be varied. Figure 11.9 shows ABRs across click level in one subject. At the highest click level shown, 90 dB pSPL, waves I through V are clearly seen. Peak latencies increase while peak amplitudes decrease with decreasing click level. Waves I, II, and IV are often difficult to identify at moderate click levels and below. Wave V is often the only wave that can be identified near threshold, although in some cases, wave III can also be seen at and near ABR threshold. The slope of wave V latency/intensity function (i.e., the change in wave V latency for a given increase in stimulus level) to click stimuli is typically near –40 μs/dB in normal-hearing young adults (Burkard and Hecox, 1983a; Hecox and Galambos, 1974).

Click rate also influences the ABR. Figure 11.10 shows ABRs from a normal-hearing young adult to an 85-dB normal HL (nHL) click stimulus for varying click rates. As the click rate increases from 25 to 100 Hz, peak latencies and interwave intervals increase, while peak amplitudes decrease (Burkard and Hecox, 1987). It should be noted that wave V amplitude does not always linearly decrease with increasing

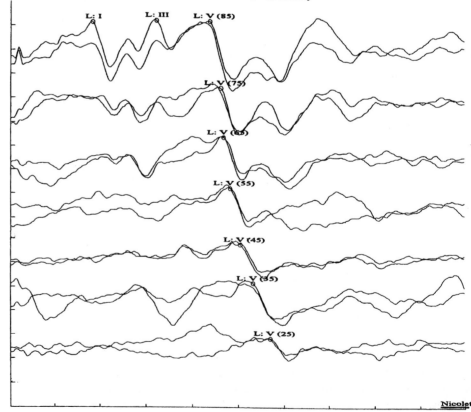

FIGURE 11.9 An auditory brainstem response click-intensity series from a normal-hearing young adult. The time window equals 15 ms, and each amplitude division represents 0.16 μV. Waves I, III, and V are indicated for the uppermost waveform, while wave V is indicated for all waveforms. The dB normal hearing level (nHL) for each waveform is indicated just to the right of wave V. (Reprinted from Burkard R, Secor C. [2002] Overview of auditory evoked potentials. In: Katz J, ed. *Handbook of Clinical Audiology*. 5th ed. Baltimore: Lippincott Williams & Wilkins; pp 233–248, with the permission of Lippincott Williams & Wilkins.)

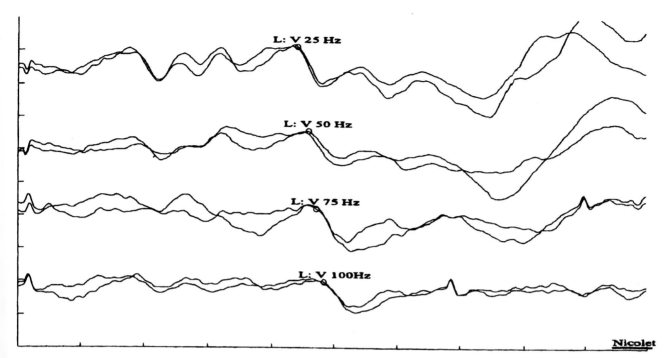

L: V 25 Hz

L: V 50 Hz

L: V 75 Hz

L: V 100Hz

Nicolet

FIGURE 11.10 An auditory brainstem response click-rate series from a normal-hearing young adult to 85 dB normal hearing level (nHL) clicks. The time window is 15 ms, and each amplitude division corresponds to 0.31 μV. (Reprinted from Burkard R, Secor C. [2002] Overview of auditory evoked potentials. In: Katz J, ed. *Handbook of Clinical Audiology.* 5th ed. Baltimore: Lippincott Williams & Wilkins; pp 233–248, with the permission of Lippincott Williams & Wilkins.)

rate. In normal-hearing young adults, Burkard and Hecox (1983a) showed a small decrease in wave V amplitude with increasing rate from 15 to 30 Hz and little amplitude change from 30 to 90 Hz. Burkard et al. (1990) used 50-dB nHL clicks in a group of normal-hearing young adults. They reported a mean wave V amplitude increase with increasing rate from 30 Hz (0.388 μV) to 90 Hz (0.409 μV). These results demonstrate that wave V amplitude to moderate-level clicks is only modestly affected by increasing rate. Because wave V is the wave most often seen at near-threshold levels, using a relatively fast stimulus repetition rate (30 to 50 Hz) is optimal for threshold estimation because this will reduce the amount of time it takes to obtain an ABR.

Let us now discuss a specific example of how stimulus presentation rate should be varied, depending on the purpose for obtaining an ABR. Let us assume that wave V amplitude changes little with increasing rate from 1 to 50 Hz. To obtain two ABRs to 2,000 click stimuli at a 1-Hz rate, it would require 66.6 minutes to obtain an ABR; at 10 Hz, it would require 6.66 minutes; and at 50 Hz, it would only take 66.6 seconds. If response amplitude changes minimally with rate, then it makes no sense to stimulate at a low click rate. However, wave I amplitude often decreases substantially for click rates above 10 Hz. If one is interested in estimating the latency or amplitude of wave I (e.g., for neurodiagnostic purposes), a click rate of 10 Hz may be optimal for identifying the latency and/or amplitude of wave I. The point of these examples is that there is

no such thing as optimal ABR stimulation parameters for all clinical (or research) applications. Parameter optimization must take into account subject age, the stimulus and recording parameters used, and the clinical purpose for the evaluation.

Recording Variables

Some suggested recording parameters (as well as stimulus parameters) for site-of lesion testing are shown in Table 11.4. For site-of-lesion testing, a higher click level (70-90 dB nHL) and lower click rate (10-20 Hz) is suggested, as this enhances the probability of observing wave I. One specific presentation level of the click is not specified, but rather a range is recommended, as presentation level might need to be increased in, e.g., those with a high frequency hearing loss, and it has been shown that changes in click level (in the moderate-to-high click level range) has rather small effects on the I-V interval (Cox, 1985). Two popular recording montages are shown (the second recording montage is in parentheses). The advantage of the first recording montage (the one not in parentheses) is that only 3 electrodes are required. However, in the case where two channels are desired (an ipsi and contra montage), the recording montage shown in parentheses is preferable. For infant testing, some people do like applying an electrode over the fontanelle near the vertex, and hence the forehead/ipsi-mastoid/contra-mastoid montage is preferable. While 1000-2000 sweeps are listed in

TABLE 11.4	Recommended auditory brainstem response stimulation and recording parameters for site-of-lesion testing
Measure	**Recommended parameter**
Click Level	70–90 dB nHL
Click Rate	10–20 Hz
Time Window	10 ms (infants: 15–20 ms)
Electrode Montage	Noninverting: Forehead (Vertex)
	Inverting: Ipsi Mastoid (Ipsi Mastoid)
	Common: Contra Mastoid (Forehead)
Number of Sweeps	1,000–2,000

nHL, normal hearing level; Ipsi, ipsilateral; Contra, contralateral.

this table, we have already discussed why this is a suggestion, and not a hard and fast rule, as we need the response to be at a favorable SNR, and hence this number may have to be adjusted accordingly. As indicated, the time window used will need to be adjusted from 10 ms to 15-20 ms when recording the ABR from infants, as the latencies of the ABR peaks are longer in infants. Recording parameters may also need to be adjusted when doing threshold estimation rather than site-of-lesion testing. For example, when determining tone burst threshold, a larger number of sweeps may be required near threshold. A time window longer than 10 ms (even in adults) might be required, especially for low-frequency tone bursts, and a rate higher than 10-20 Hz might be used (in an effort to save time). Although bioamplifier filter values are not shown in the table, often a passband of 100-3000 Hz is used for recording the click-evoked ABR. Some authors (e.g., Stapells and Picton, 1982) recommend reducing the high-pass cutoff from 100 Hz to 10 or 20 Hz when using tone burst stimuli, especially when recording responses to low-frequency tone bursts.

REFERENCES

American National Standards Institute. (2004) Specifications for Audiometers. ANSI S3.6-2004. New York: American National Standards Institute, Inc.

Borg E, Lofqvist L. (1981) Brainstem response (ABR) to rarefaction and condensation clicks in normal hearing and steep high-frequency hearing loss. *Scand Audiol.* 13 (suppl), 99–101.

Buchwald J, Huang J. (1975) Far-field acoustic response: origins in the cat. *Science.* 189, 382–384.

Burkard R. (1984) Sound pressure level measurement and spectral analysis of brief acoustic transients. *Electroencephalogr Clin Neurophysiol.* 57, 83–91.

Burkard R, Hecox K. (1983a) The effect of broadband noise on the human brainstem auditory evoked response. I. Rate and intensity effects. *J Acoust Soc Am.* 74, 1204–1213.

Burkard R, Hecox K. (1983b) The effect of broadband noise on the human brainstem auditory evoked response. II. Frequency specificity. *J Acoust Soc Am.* 74, 1214–1223.

Burkard R, Hecox K. (1987) The effect of broadband noise on the human brainstem auditory evoked response. III. Anatomic locus. *J Acoust Soc Am.* 81, 1050–1063.

Burkard R, Secor C. (2002) Overview of auditory evoked potentials. In: Katz J, ed. *Handbook of Clinical Audiology.* 5th ed. Baltimore: Lippincott Williams & Wilkins; pp 233–248.

Burkard R, Shi Y, Hecox K. (1990) A comparison of maximum length and Legendre sequences to derive BAERs at rapid rates of stimulation. *J Acoust Soc Am.* 87, 1656–1664.

Campbell K, Bartoli E. (1986) Human auditory evoked potentials during natural sleep: the early components. *Electroencephalogr Clin Neurophysiol.* 65, 142–149.

Costa P, Benna P, Bianco C, Ferrero P, Bergamasco B. (1990) Aging effects on brainstem auditory evoked potentials. *Electromyogr Clin Neurophysiol.* 30, 495–500.

Cox L. (1985) Infant assessment: developmental and age-related considerations. In: Jacobson J, ed. *The Auditory Brainstem Response.* San Diego: College-Hill Press; pp 297–316.

Dallos P. (1973) *The Auditory Periphery.* New York: Academic Press.

Davis H. (1976) Principles of electric response audiometry. *Ann Otol Rhinol Laryngol.* 25 (suppl), 1–96.

Don M, Eggermont J. (1978) Analysis of the click-evoked brainstem potentials in man using high-pass noise masking. *J Acoust Soc Am.* 63, 1084–1092.

Don M, Ponton C, Eggermont J, Masuda A. (1993) Gender differences in cochlear response time: an explanation for gender amplitude differences in the unmasked auditory brain-stem response. *J Acoust Soc Am.* 94, 2135–2148.

Garner W. (1947) The effect of frequency spectrum on temporal integration of energy in the ear. *J Acoust Soc Am.* 19, 808–815.

Hall J. (1995) *Handbook of Auditory Evoked Responses.* Boston: Allyn and Bacon.

Hall J, Bull J, Cronau L. (1988) The effect of hypo- versus hyperthermia on auditory brainstem response: two case reports. *Ear Hear.* 9, 137–143.

Hecox K, Galambos R. (1974) Brainstem auditory responses in human infants and adults. *Arch Otolaryngol.* 99, 30–33.

Hood L. (1998) Auditory neuropathy: what is it and what can we do about it? *Hear J.* 51, 10–18.

Hyde M. (1994a) Signal processing and analysis. In: Jacobson J, ed. *Principles and Applications in Auditory Evoked Potentials.* Boston: Allyn and Bacon; pp 47–83.

Hyde M. (1994b) The slow vertex potential: properties and clinical applications. In: Jacobson J, ed. *Principles and Applications in Auditory Evoked Potentials.* Boston: Allyn and Bacon; pp 179–218.

Jasper H. (1958) The ten-twenty electrode system of the international federation. *Electroencephalogr Clin Neurophysiol.* 10, 371–375.

Jewett D, Williston J. (1971) Auditory-evoked far fields averaged from the scalp of humans. *Brain.* 94, 681–696.

Kileny P. (1981) The frequency specificity of tone-pip evoked auditory brainstem responses. *Ear Hear.* 2, 270–275.

Kjaer M. (1979) Differences of latencies and amplitudes of brain stem evoked potentials in subgroups of a normal material. *Acta Neurol Scand.* 59, 72–79.

Kraus N, McGee T. (1994) Auditory event-related potentials. In: Katz J, ed. *The Handbook of Clinical Audiology.* 4th ed. Baltimore: Williams & Wilkins; pp 406–423.

Kraus N, McGee T, Stein L. (1994) The auditory middle latency response. Clinical uses, development, and generating system. In: Jacobson J, ed. *Principles and Applications in Auditory Evoked Potentials.* Boston: Allyn and Bacon; pp 155–178.

Kuk F, Abbas P. (1989) Effects of attention on the auditory evoked potentials recorded from the vertex (ABR) and the promontory (CAP) of human listeners. *Neuropsychologia.* 27, 665–673.

Marshall N, Donchin E. (1981) Circadian variation in the latency of brainstem responses and its relation to body temperature. *Science.* 212, 356–358.

Moller A. (1994) Neural generators of auditory evoked potentials. In: Jacobson J, ed. *Principles and Applications in Auditory Evoked Potentials.* Boston: Allyn and Bacon; pp 23–46.

Owen G, Burkard R. (1991) The effects of ipsilateral, contralateral and binaural broadband noise on the human BAER to click stimuli. *J Acoust Soc Am.* 89, 1760–1767.

Picton T, Hillyard S. (1974) Human auditory evoked potentials. II. Effects of attention. *Electroencephalogr Clin Neurophysiol.* 36, 191–199.

Picton T, Ouellette J, Hamel G, Smith A. (1979) Brainstem evoked potentials to tonepips in notched noise. *J Otolaryngol.* 8, 289–314.

Popper A, Fay R. (1992) *The Mammalian Auditory Pathway: Neurophysiology.* New York: Springer-Verlag.

Pratt H, Bleich N. (1982) Auditory brain stem potentials evoked by clicks in notched noise. *Electroencephalogr Clin Neurophysiol.* 53, 417–426.

Rowe J. (1978) Normal variability of the brain-stem auditory evoked response in young and old adult subjects. *Electroencephalogr Clin Neurophysiol.* 44, 459–470.

Sato H, Sando I, Takahashi H. (1991) Sexual dimorphism and development of the human cochlea. Computer 3-D measurement. *Acta Otolaryngol.* 111, 1037–1040.

Schwartz D, Morris M, Jacobson J. (1994) The normal auditory brainstem response and its variants. In: Jacobson J, ed. *Principles and Applications in Auditory Evoked Potentials.* Boston: Allyn and Bacon; pp 123–153.

Speaks C. (1996) *Introduction to Sound.* 2nd ed. San Diego: Singular.

Spoendlin H. (1972) Innervation densities of the cochlea. *Acta Otolaryngol.* 73, 235–248.

Stapells D, Picton T, Durieux-Smith A. (1994) Electrophysiologic measures of frequency-specific auditory function. In: Jacobson J, ed. *Principles and Applications in Auditory Evoked Potentials.* Boston: Allyn and Bacon; pp 251–283.

Stapells D, Picton T, Smith A. (1982) Normal hearing thresholds for clicks. *J Acoust Soc Am.* 72, 74–79.

Starr A, Picton T, Sininiger Y, Hood L, Berlin C. (1996) Auditory neuropathy. *Brain.* 119, 741–753.

Stockard J, Sharbrough F, Tinker J. (1978) Effects of hypothermia on the human brainstem auditory response. *Ann Neurol.* 3, 368–370.

Stockard J, Stockard J, Westmoreland B, Corfits J. (1979) Brainstem auditory-evoked responses: normal variation as a function of stimulus and subject characteristics. *Arch Neurol.* 36, 823–831.

Suzuki T, Horiuchi K. (1981) Rise time of pure-tone stimuli in brain stem response audiometry. *Audiology.* 20, 101–112.

Teas D, Eldredge D, Davis H. (1962) Cochlear responses to acoustic transients: an interpretation of whole-nerve action potentials. *J Acoust Soc Am.* 34, 1438–1459.

Webster D, Popper A, Fay R. (1992) *The Mammalian Auditory Pathway: Neuroanatomy.* New York: Springer-Verlag.

Yeager D, Marsh A. (1998) Sound levels and their measurement. In: Harris C, ed. *Handbook of Acoustical Measurements and Noise Control.* Woodbury, NY: Acoustic Society of America; pp 12.1–12.18.

12 Electrocochleography

Paul J. Abbas and Carolyn J. Brown

▧ INTRODUCTION

The term electrocochleography (ECoG) has been used to describe recordings of the synchronous electrical activity produced by the cochlea and auditory nerve. Surface electrodes placed on the skull in a number of different locations can be used to record such potentials, but the term electrocochleography is generally used for recordings made with electrodes placed in close proximity to the cochlea or auditory nerve. This chapter first summarizes the anatomic and the physiologic characteristics of those structures that are important contributors to the ECoG recordings. The second section describes the specific components of the ECoG and the likely source of each component. The third section provides details of procedures used to measure the ECoG. The final section focuses on clinical applications. Additionally, since measures of the electrically evoked compound action potential have become common in recent years, we have also included material relevant to the use of electrical stimulation to assess auditory function in cochlear implant recipients.

▧ ANATOMY AND PHYSIOLOGY OF THE AUDITORY PERIPHERY

Inner Ear Anatomy

The inner ear consists of a series of fluid-filled canals in the petrous portion of the temporal bone. The oval window opens into a chamber, the vestibule, and the semicircular canals, and cochlea are tubes that project from that chamber. These structures contain both the auditory (in the cochlea) and vestibular sensory organs (in the vestibule and semicircular canals) within a series of membranous canals. Figure 12.1 illustrates several important structures of the

cochlea and auditory nerve. The cochlea is essentially a coiled tube that gradually decreases in diameter from the base of the cochlea (the end closest to the vestibule) to the apex. The cochlea is approximately 35 mm in length from base to apex. A membranous cochlear duct runs most of the length of the cochlea and separates it into three fluid compartments. Figure 12.1A shows a schematic cross-section of the cochlea. The spiral of the bony cochlea surrounds the modiolus, a highly perforated bony structure in which the auditory nerve and spiral ganglion cells (cell bodies of the neurons of the auditory nerve) are located. From the modiolus, the neurons of the spiral ganglia branch out to innervate structures along the entire length of the cochlea. The central portions of these neurons form the auditory nerve, which passes through the internal auditory meatus to synapse on cells in the cochlear nucleus.

Figure 12.1B shows a cross-section of the cochlear duct. Included in this illustration is a diagram of the three fluid compartments and cellular structures contained within the cochlear duct. The three compartments, the scala vestibuli, the scala media, and the scala tympani, are bounded by the basilar membrane and Reissner's membrane. The upper compartment, the scala vestibuli, opens into the vestibule. Both the scala vestibuli and scala tympani are filled with perilymph. The scala media contains endolymph, a fluid with different ionic content. The scala media houses the organ or Corti. As illustrated in detail in Figure 12.2, the organ of Corti contains hair cells, the sensory elements responsible for the transduction of mechanical energy into electrical current. Hair cells are distinguished by the stereocilia that project from the top of the cell; these structures are a key element in the transduction process. There are two distinct hair cell types that are differentiated based on their location relative to the modiolus: inner and outer hair cells. These cell types are different in morphology, in innervation, and,

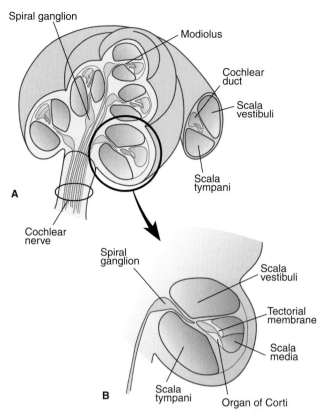

A

B

FIGURE 12.1 A. A transverse section of the cochlea showing the modiolus and the spiral cochlea duct. B. Detailed cross-section of the cochlea showing the spiral ganglion, the three scalae, and the organ of Corti. (sm, scala media; sv, scala tympani; sv, scala vestibuli). (Reprinted from Pickles JO. [1988] *An Introduction to the Physiology of Hearing.* London: Academic Press, with permission of the Academic Press.)

as discussed later, in terms of their function. Most of the approximately 30,000 afferent neurons of the auditory nerve synapse at the base of the inner hair cells peripherally and to neurons in the cochlear nucleus centrally. These neurons are called type I neurons, and each neuron connects to a single hair cell, providing point innervation in the cochlea. The remaining neurons, designated type II neurons, innervate the outer hair cells in more a distributed manner. In addition, there are efferent neurons in the auditory nerve. These neurons originate in the brainstem and synapse with outer hair cells as well as the afferent neurons at the base of the inner hair cells.

Cochlear Physiology

The stapes couples the ossicular chain to the inner ear through the oval window, an opening from the middle ear cavity into the vestibule of the inner ear. The vestibule connects directly into the scala vestibule of the cochlea. As a result, pressure changes in the fluid caused by movement of

the stapes footplate in the oval window are transmitted to the cochlea. A second opening between the cochlea and the middle ear cavity, the round window, serves as a pressure release. The pressure changes in the fluid result in movement of the membranous structures of the cochlea. A key feature of that vibration was described by von Bekesy (1960) as a traveling wave. He demonstrated that, for a specific frequency of stimulation, due to the properties of the basilar membrane, the relative amplitude and phase of vibration varied across the cochlea. The peak of that vibration was determined by the specific frequency of stimulation. This property of spectral analysis of the cochlea, such that different frequencies produce distinctive spatial patterns of excitation, is a key feature of signal processing in the auditory nervous system.

While more recent measurements of cochlear mechanical vibration have demonstrated sharper spatial tuning and highly nonlinear responses (Rhode, 1971; Sellick et al., 1982), the basic traveling wave characteristics described by Bekesy are still evident. The characteristics of the traveling wave, specifically the variation in both amplitude and phase of the response across the cochlea, are important contributors to the characteristics of the ECoG recordings, which, in some sense, integrate or sum electric potentials produced across the cochlea and auditory nerve.

Vibration of the basilar membrane results in bending or shearing of the stereocilia on the top of each hair cell, which in turn causes hair cell ion channels to open or close. The resulting ion flow into or out of the hair cell results in an electric potential, or receptor potential, within the hair cell. This receptor potential is highly nonlinear. It will have an alternating current (AC) component in response to a periodic tonal signal; however, it will also have a direct current (DC) component as well as other distortion components. This flow of current into the hair cell, in turn, triggers release of synaptic transmitter that, in turn, produces excitatory depolarization in the peripheral processes of the auditory nerve fibers. That depolarization can result in action potential generation and conduction along the length of the nerve fiber. These action potentials, generated by the neurons of the auditory nerve distributed along the length of the cochlea, carry the information essential for auditory perception. Although there are many similarities, the inner and outer hair cells perform distinct functions in the transduction process. The point innervation of the inner hair cells is consistent with a role of primary signal transmission to the central nervous system, particularly related to place information as encoded in basilar membrane mechanics. While outer hair cells clearly transduce vibration, they also have the ability to change length in response to changes in electrical potential. This motile property of the outer hair cells and the mechanical linkage between the outer hair cell and the inner hair cells results in a mechanical feedback or enhancement of the traveling wave. This mechanism produces a nonlinear basilar-membrane response, an enhanced sensitivity at low stimulus levels, and a more highly tuned response to narrowband acoustic stimulation. Another consequence of the

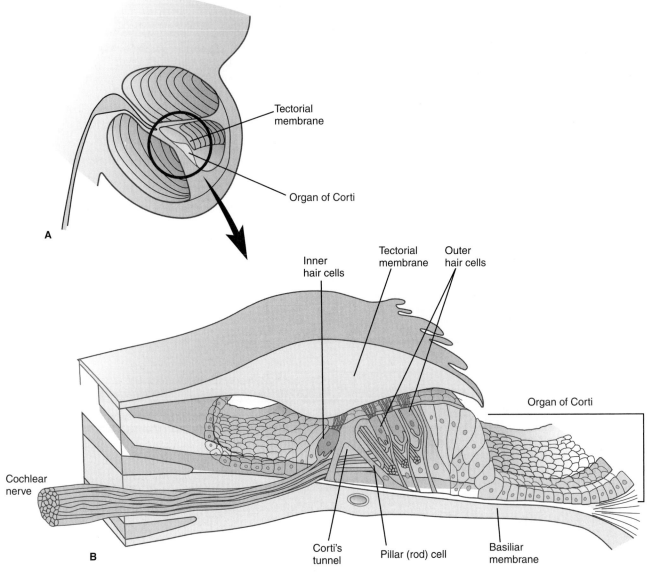

FIGURE 12.2 Detailed cross-section of the organ of Corti. (Reprinted from Lim DJ. [1980] Cochlear anatomy related to cochlear micromechanics. A review. *J Acoust Soc Am. 67*, 1686–1695, with permission of The Acoustical Society of America.)

outer hair cell motile response is the presence of otoacoustic emissions (see Chapter 22), which are conducted to the outer ear through a reverse traveling wave.

Response Properties of the Auditory Nerve

Action potentials are pulses of current that propagate along the length of an individual nerve fiber. Action potentials are used to transmit information about sound in the environment to the central nervous system. The output of the ear can be characterized by the number and timing of these action potentials. In an ear with normal sensitivity, auditory nerve fibers discharge action potentials spontaneously. Some fibers fire at relatively low rates (0.5/spikes/s or less), while others

exhibit spontaneous firing rates of up to 120 spikes/s (Liberman, 1978). This spontaneous neural activity is random and independent across fibers. The response of the auditory nerve fiber to acoustic stimulation is evident as an increase in firing rate above the spontaneous rate. The tuning properties of individual neurons generally reflect the properties of the cochlear traveling wave and inner hair cells. The driven response to acoustic stimulation is different from the spontaneous firing in that neuronal activity can be synchronized across fibers both at the onset of the stimulus as well as to the phase of a periodic stimulus.

The response of neurons to acoustic stimulation varies over time, as illustrated in the poststimulus time (PST) histogram in Figure 12.3 (Kiang et al., 1965; Westerman and Smith, 1984). This response pattern shows a large initial burst

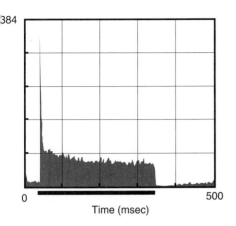

FIGURE 12.3   Typical response histogram from gerbil auditory nerve. The histogram was generated by summing 384 repetitions of a constant-intensity tone-burst stimulus, using a 1-ms bin adjusted in time to produce a maximal bin at onset. Stimulus duration is indicated by the horizontal bar. Intensity re AV threshold: 43 dB. (Reprinted from Westerman LA, Smith RL. [1984] Rapid and short-term adaptation in auditory nerve responses. *Hear Res.* 15, 249–260, with permission of Elsevier.)

measured with far-field electrodes, such as is the case when the ECoG is recorded.

The responses of auditory nerve fibers reflect the features of cochlear mechanical vibration at the place innervated by that neuron. Thus, neurons demonstrate a high degree of tuning but also show differences in latency depending upon the place along the length of the cochlea. These properties are summarized in the composite PST histogram shown in Figure 12.4 for fibers distributed along the length of the cochlea. A PST histogram, a plot of response rate as a function of time after click onset, is shown for each fiber. They are arranged along the z (depth) axis according to fiber best frequency. Because a click is broadband, it activates a wide range of the cochlea, but the latency of response varies across the length. The characteristics of the traveling wave are such that latency changes little in the base but phase (latency) changes across the apex are greater. As a result, neurons sensitive to high frequencies innervating more basal parts of the cochlea have similar latency, while those sensitive to lower frequencies have response latencies that vary across fibers. The mechanical property of the cochlea, reflected in the response of neurons, is critical to producing synchronized responses. That synchronous response, particularly in the base of the cochlea, is necessary to elicit far-field potentials such as the ECoG.

of activity that adapts rapidly and is followed by a slower rate of adaptation that is evident over the first 100 to 200 ms of stimulation. Residual effects of adaptation are evident after the tone is shut off, in that spontaneous activity is temporarily reduced, recovering to normal levels after approximately 100 ms. Not shown is a slow adaptation component that occurs over the course of several minutes if the stimulus remains on for a long period of time. The high response probability at stimulus onset is likely an important feature in producing highly synchronized responses to tone-burst stimuli as

Electrical Stimulation of the Auditory Nerve

Due in large part to the success of cochlear implants, there has been an increase in interest in how the auditory system responds to electrical stimulation. Electrodes that are surgically implanted into the cochlea stimulate auditory nerve fibers directly, bypassing nonfunctioning or absent sensory cells. The way that auditory nerve fibers respond to direct

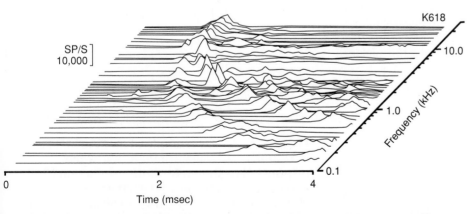

FIGURE 12.4   Poststimulus time (PST) histograms of auditory nerve fibers to click stimulus from one animal. Vertical scale is instantaneous discharge rate. Horizontal scale is time after click onset. Receding (z-axis) scale is fiber characteristic frequency (CF). (Reprinted from Kiang NYS. [1975] Figure 143-22. In: Tower DB, ed. *The Nervous System.* Volume 3. New York: Raven Press, with permission of Raven Press.)

electrical stimulation is different than how they respond to acoustic stimulation in several important ways (Kiang and Moxon, 1972; Abbas and Miller, 2004).

One important issue is frequency tuning. Since the response of auditory neurons to electrical stimulation does not depend on the mechanical properties of the cochlea, the frequency tuning properties of electrically stimulated auditory nerve fibers are very broad and do not vary across the length of the cochlea. Consequently, in cochlear implants, spatial tuning of the cochlea is generally simulated in a very gross way by stimulating with multiple electrodes placed along the length of the cochlea. Each electrode is then programmed so that it is activated by a different stimulus frequency range.

Another example of how the response of auditory neurons differs when electric as opposed to acoustic stimulation is used involves the latency of the response. When electrical stimulation is used, auditory nerve fibers are stimulated directly, and therefore, the latency of response is shorter than when these same fibers are stimulated acoustically; neither the traveling wave characteristics nor synaptic delays affect responses to electrical stimulation.

Another difference between how an auditory neuron responds to electric as opposed to acoustic stimulation is the spontaneous firing rate. Individuals with significant amounts of sensory hearing loss may not have many surviving hair cells. This will clearly be the case for most cochlear implant recipients. If that is the case, the auditory nerve fibers may show no spontaneous activity. As a result, the response to electrical stimulation is more highly synchronized across fibers.

Finally, input-output functions of electrically stimulated auditory neurons are very steep compared to those recorded in response to acoustic stimulation. Steep input-output functions result in narrow dynamic response ranges. These characteristics are at least partially the consequence of the fact that the compressive characteristics of the basilar membrane are bypassed. In addition, the nonlinear properties of the cochlea, such as distortion product generation, are not activated. Each of these properties will have significant effects on the recorded electrically evoked compound action potential (ECAP).

CHARACTERISTICS OF ELECTROCOCHLEOGRAPHY

Before techniques were developed for recording intracellular potentials from cochlear hair cells or before there were sensitive methods of measuring motion of the basilar membrane in vivo, significant insights into the mechanisms of signal transduction in the cochlea and auditory nerve were gained through study of evoked potentials recorded from electrodes placed in or near the cochlea. In many cases, placement of these electrodes was relatively noninvasive, making it possible to record these potentials from human clinical populations. These recordings form the primary components of the ECoG.

Figure 12.5 illustrates the group of potentials that form the ECoG. The responses shown in Figure 12.5 were obtained in response to a click stimulus using a needle electrode placed on the promontory of the middle ear. Each plot represents responses averaged across multiple stimulus repetitions.

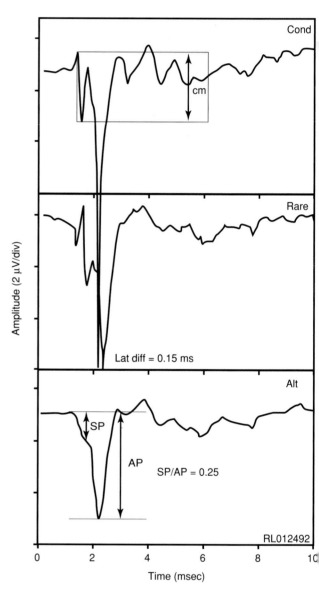

FIGURE 12.5 An example of an ECoG recording in response to a click stimulus. Averaged responses are shown for both rarefaction (RARE) and condensation click (COND) as well as for click alternating in polarity (ALT). Measurements of CM, SP, and AP amplitude are shown. (Reprinted from Levine SC, Margolis RH, Daly KA. [1998] Use of electrocochleography in the diagnosis of Ménière's disease. *Laryngoscope.* 108, 993–1000, with permission from Lippincott Williams & Wilkins.)

Averaged responses are shown to condensation clicks (COND), to rarefaction clicks (RARE), and in response to clicks that alternated in polarity (ALT) during the averaging process. The cochlear microphonic (CM) is an AC potential that is evident in the periodicity of the condensation and rarefaction traces. The CM changes polarity when the stimulus phase is inverted. As such, it is visible in response to either polarity but is minimized in the alternating polarity condition. When alternating click stimuli are used, the ECoG consists of a combination of two other potentials: the summating potential (SP) and the compound action potential (AP). The SP is a nonlinear DC component in the response (Dallos et al., 1972). In Figure 12.5, the SP evoked by a click consists of a negative shift in the baseline that has a relatively short latency and precedes the AP. Both the CM and the SP are generated in the cochlea. The AP represents synchronized activity of a large number of auditory neurons in response to a transient stimulus. Because the AP represents postsynaptic activity, the latency of the AP is approximately 1.5 ms or greater and is thus separable from the CM or the SP. The AP consists of a large negative peak (N1) followed by a smaller positive peak (P2). In some cases, a second negative peak (N2) is also recorded.

The combination of these three responses (CM, SP, and AP) makes up the ECoG as it is recorded from electrodes positioned in or near the cochlea. The following sections describe each of these potentials, as well as a potential called the endocochlear potential, in more detail.

Endocochlear Potential

The endocochlear potential (EP) is not stimulus induced, but rather, it is positive DC voltage maintained in the scala media relative to the surrounding tissue. As such, it is typically measured with electrodes placed in the scala media and can be recorded without acoustic stimulation. The source of the EP is the stria vascularis, located along the outer wall of the scala media. Since the intracellular potential of the hair cell is negative, the EP provides a large potential difference across the apical end of the hair cell, which is the driving force that allows current to flow into the hair cell. This current flow is modulated by gates in the hair cell stereocilia that are opened and closed by the motion of the basilar membrane (Hudspeth, 1989).

Cochlear Microphonic Potential

The response of the hair cell to basilar membrane vibration produces electrical changes in the surrounding tissue that are evident in the voltage measures from the surrounding scala, the round window, or the ear canal. The AC component of this potential is termed the cochlear microphonic (CM) (Wever and Bray, 1930) because it mimics the acoustic input to the ear, essentially acting as a microphone. The CM can be thought of as a summation of the receptor potentials of many individual hair cells. Many of the early recordings of the CM

were made using electrodes placed near the round window. Those recordings likely reflect primarily the activity in the basal end of the cochlea because these hair cells are closer to the recording electrode and the potentials from hair cells at the base of the cochlea respond in phase. Hair cells located in more apical regions of the cochlea will contribute less to the evoked response because they are farther away from the recording electrode. Additionally, the response from hair cells at the apex of the cochlea will tend to cancel in the average because these hair cells will exhibit greater phase differences.

In order to assess responses in different parts of the cochlea, many of the recordings of the CM in animals have used the differential electrode technique, in which electrodes are placed in both the scala tympani and scala vestibuli (Tasaki et al., 1951). The differentially amplified potential tends to accentuate sources of voltage between the electrodes, so that assessment of responses from different regions of the cochlea could be made. Those early experiments demonstrated many important traveling wave characteristics, such as compression and nonlinear growth, as well as tonal distortion products, which have become evident in more recent direct measurements of basilar membrane motion (Wever and Lawrence, 1954; Dallos et al., 1974; Dallos, 1973).

Summating Potential

The summating potential (SP) is the DC component of the response recorded and has an amplitude that is on the same order of magnitude as the CM (Dallos et al., 1972). The SP recorded in response to a tone burst differs from that recorded in response to a transient stimulus such as a click, in that the SP is sustained throughout the duration of the stimulus. The ECoG waveform illustrated in Figure 12.6 was recorded from an individual with Ménière's disease and

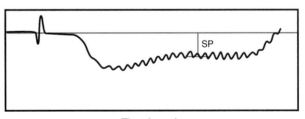

Time (msec)

FIGURE 12.6 An example of an ECoG recording in response to a tone burst in a patient with endolymphatic hydrops. Measurement of SP amplitude is shown. (Reprinted from Wuyts FL, Van de Heyning PH, Van Spaendonck MP, Molenberghs G. [1997] A review of electrocochleography: instrumentation settings and meta-analysis of criteria for diagnosis of endolymphatic hydrops. *Acta Otolaryngol.* 526 [suppl], 14–20, with permission from Taylor and Francis.)

exhibits a large SP potential. Both the CM and SP are evident throughout the tone burst; the CM is the sinusoidal component (typically measured as a peak-to-peak amplitude) that rides on top of the baseline shift that is the SP. The SP, as shown, can be measured as a shift in the average amplitude relative to a prestimulus baseline.

The SP can be modified by mechanical biasing and/or electrical polarization of the cochlear partition (Durrant and Dallos, 1972, 1974). It certainly reflects nonlinearity in the hair cell response and may be indicative of underlying asymmetries in the basilar membrane vibration (Moller, 2000). The polarity of the SP can be either positive or negative depending on a number of factors, including the frequency of stimulation and recording site (Davis et al., 1958; Dallos et al., 1972). As noted earlier, the latency of the SP is relatively short (compared to the AP) and is consequently separable from the neural response to a click stimulus. It has received a great deal of attention in clinical applications since the SP can be abnormal in individuals diagnosed with Ménière's disease.

Compound Action Potential

The output of the cochlea is basically a series of action potentials (APs) that are conducted along the 30,000 to 40,000 neurons that form the auditory nerve. The compound AP is a summation of that activity as recorded from a remote electrode. Kiang et al. (1976) used time-domain signal averaging in a unique way (i.e., they averaged activity relative to the occurrence of an AP on a particular neuron, rather than relative to presentation of a stimulus as is ordinarily done). They recorded what they termed a "unit potential" (i.e., a contribution of each fiber's AP to a recording site at the round window). Since this potential is biphasic, either random spontaneous activity or continuous stimulation with an acoustic stimulus produces APs that are randomly distributed in time, and therefore, the activity at the round window recording electrode cancels. As such, the AP requires synchronous activity so that responses are summed across a population of neurons (Goldstein and Kiang, 1958). Typically, a stimulus such as a click or tone burst is used to induce that synchronous response.

The AP, as it is recorded from the tympanic membrane (TM), the ear canal, or mastoid electrodes, is characterized by a relatively large negative peak (N1) followed by a positive peak (P2). Examples of the AP measured with a transtympanic electrode are shown in Figure 12.7A for different stimulus levels, as indicated. Figure 12.7B plots the amplitude and latency of the AP; amplitude increases and latency decreases with increasing stimulus level. In early animal experiments, Teas et al. (1962) measured the response to click stimuli presented with a background of band-pass noise in order to eliminate the contribution of specific regions of the cochlea to the AP. They demonstrated that the response to a broadband click stimulus is primarily mediated through the discharge of fibers with high characteristic

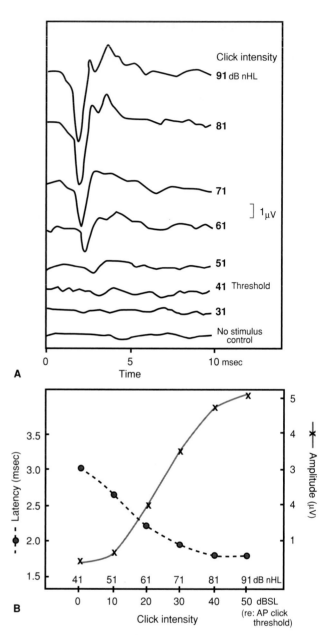

FIGURE 12.7   A. AP recorded in response to a click stimulus. Level is the parameter as indicated. B. AP latency and amplitude are plotted as a function of click level. (Reprinted from Stanton SG, Cashman MZ, Harrison RV, Nedzelski JM, Rowed DW. [1989] Cochlear nerve action potentials during cerebellopontine angle surgery: relationship of latency, amplitude, and threshold measurements to hearing. *Ear Hear.* 10, 23–28, with permission from Lippincott Williams & Wilkins.)

frequencies (CFs) that are located in the basal turn of the cochlea. This observation is consistent with observed properties of basilar membrane mechanics (i.e., a long wavelength in the basal turn of the cochlea and, consequently, a shorter latency and more synchronous firing of high-CF fibers). Thus, auditory nerve fibers at the basal end of the cochlea exhibit more cross-fiber synchrony than do fibers at the apex, resulting in an inherent "bias" in the AP to encode responses from the base of the cochlea. In human ECoG recordings, the N1 has been shown to arise from the distal portion of the auditory nerve (Moller and Janetta, 1985).

While the AP is most readily elicited using a click, it is also possible to evoke this response using tone-burst stimuli. The fast adaptation at the onset of a tone burst, evident in the PST histogram in Figure 12.4, contributes to synchrony when many neurons are activated. The APs to tone bursts or narrowband-filtered clicks show response morphologies that are similar to those recorded using broadband clicks. The latency of the N1 peak tends to increase with decreasing center frequency of the stimulus, due at least in part to traveling wave delay (Eggermont et al., 1976). The primary advantage of using tone bursts rather than clicks as stimuli is that they are more frequency specific and can be used to assess function in different regions of the cochlea. Masking experiments have demonstrated a high degree of spatial selectivity in the response (Dallos and Cheatham, 1976; Abbas and Gorga, 1981).

Electrically Evoked Compound Action Potential

Since the advent of cochlear implants, there has been interest in adapting evoked potential recording techniques to record neural responses evoked by electrical rather than acoustic stimuli. Much attention has focused on developing techniques for measuring the electrically evoked auditory brainstem response (EABR) and the electrically evoked compound AP (ECAP) measured from an intracochlear electrode and recorded in response to biphasic electrical pulses. The ECAP has general characteristics that are very similar to its acoustically evoked counterpart. There are, however, some important differences between electrically and acoustically evoked neural responses. First, presynaptic potentials (CM and SP) are not typically recorded in response to electrical stimulation. The ECAP is characterized by a single negative peak (N1) that is also followed by a less prominent positive potential (P2). The amplitude of the N1 component of the ECAP is typically larger and the latency shorter than the N1 component of the acoustically evoked AP, despite the fact that this potential is typically measured in ears with profound sensory-neural hearing loss that presumably have considerable cochlear damage. Additionally, the rate of growth of the ECAP with increasing stimulation level is particularly steep when compared with its acoustic counterpart (van den Honert and Stypulkowski, 1986; Brown et al., 1990). These differences between the acoustically and electrically evoked AP reflect the fact that single-unit APs recorded in response to electrical stimulation exhibit shorter latencies, greater across-fiber synchrony, and steeper growth characteristics compared with single-fiber responses evoked using

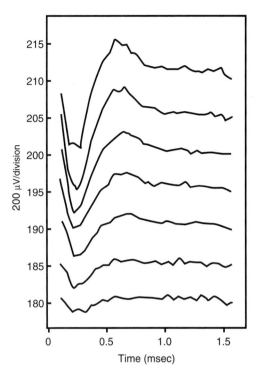

FIGURE 12.8   ECAP recordings made in an individual with a Nucleus CI24 cochlear implant. Averaged waveforms are measured in response to 25-µs/phase current pulses. Parameter is current expressed in clinical current units.

acoustic stimulation (Kiang and Moxon, 1972). Examples of an ECAP recorded in response to a single biphasic electrical pulse (25 µs/phase) are shown in Figure 12.8. An electrical artifact subtraction paradigm (see below) has been applied, and the N1 peak is typically evident at less than 0.5 ms, with amplitudes that can be as large as 2 to 3 mV in some cases.

In the early years of cochlear implant research, the possibility of using objective measures before implantation in order to predict eventual performance with the implant was investigated (Smith and Simmons, 1983). However, the limitations of promontory stimulation were quickly apparent and have constrained the utility of such measures in clinical practice (van den Honert and Stypulkowski, 1986; Nikolopoulos et al., 2000). In contrast, stimulation through the implant either at the time of surgery or postoperatively has proven to be feasible, and a number of possible applications for such measures have been and continue to be investigated. Presently, two commercial cochlear implants have built-in systems and provide software to measure the ECAP using intracochlear electrodes for both stimulation and recording. These implants have telemetry systems that allow electrical potentials measured from an intracochlear electrode to be transmitted out from the internal device. Consequently, recording the ECAP does not require additional electrodes, amplifiers, or averaging equipment.

METHODS FOR ELECTROCOCHLEOGRAPHY MEASUREMENT

Figure 12.9 illustrates a typical arrangement for acoustic stimulation and recording of the ECoG. In this case, the recording electrode is placed on the TM. A foam earplug, which contains the sound delivery tube from the earphone, is also used to fix the electrode wire against the side of the ear canal and stabilize the electrode. The following sections outline details of methods for recording ECoG, including electrode placement, stimulus and recording parameters, and data analysis.

Placement of Recording Electrode

One of the most important factors that impacts how the ECoG is recorded is the placement and the type of recording electrode that is used. In general, placing the recording electrode as close as possible to the source of the potentials will result in improved signal-to-noise ratios and more stable recordings. The trade off, however, is that positioning the recording electrode close to the cochlea can be uncomfortable for the patients. There are several options for electrode design and placement that continue to be used today. Those options are reviewed in the sections that follow.

DIRECT NERVE RECORDINGS

In animal recordings, where invasive measures can be made under general anesthesia, the auditory nerve can be exposed

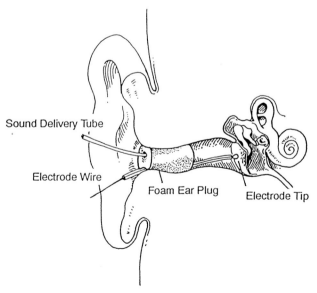

FIGURE 12.9   Schematic drawing showing typical placement of electrode tip and sound delivery in ear canal. (Reprinted from Ferraro JA. [1997] *Laboratory Exercises In Auditory Evoked Potentials.* **San Diego: Singular Publishing Group, with permission of Singular Publishing Group.)**

and an electrode can be placed directly on the auditory nerve to record AP or ECAP. While not a good site for recording the SP or the CM, the characteristics of the AP recorded in this way are similar to those recorded at the round window (Moller and Jannetta, 1981; Silverstein et al, 1985). The use of direct nerve recordings in humans, however, is limited to situations where the auditory nerve has been surgically exposed, such as during skull-base surgery. Direct nerve recordings can be particularly useful for intraoperative monitoring applications (see Chapter 17) because the favorable signal-to-noise ratio allows for response identification with very few averages.

INTRACOCHLEAR RECORDINGS

It is also possible to measure the ECoG from a recording electrode that is placed into the cochlea. In animals, electrodes can be placed into the scala and used to record the ECoG. Placing a recording electrode directly into the cochlea allows for measurement of more place-specific responses than can be recorded from an electrode in the middle ear, and it also provides for good resolution of the CM and SP (Tasaki et al., 1951, 1954). Intracochlear recording electrodes have primarily been used for research purposes with animal populations because, in most patient populations, placing a recording electrode into the cochlea would be too invasive.

Cochlear implant users represent the one population in whom it is possible to record compound APs from an intracochlear electrode. However, in this patient population, electrical rather than acoustic stimulation must be used. In 1990, Brown et al. first reported recording ECAPs from individuals who used the Ineraid cochlear implant system. This multielectrode implant allowed direct access to intracochlear electrodes through a percutaneous pedestal connector. To measure responses, one electrode pair was stimulated, and another electrode was used to record the response. The use of electrical stimulation and the close proximity of the stimulating and recording electrodes result in significant stimulus artifact problems that are described in more detail in a following section. More recently, both Cochlear Corporation and Advanced Bionics have developed methods for recording the ECAP from an electrode in the cochlea in cochlear implant systems without percutaneous connectors. The hardware/software used to record that system for patients implanted with a Nucleus cochlear implant is called neural response telemetry (NRT); details on how that system can be used to record the ECAP are found in Abbas et al. (1999). A similar system was developed by Advanced Bionics Corporation and is referred to as neural response imaging (NRI).

In addition to the obvious difference in stimulation mode, the measurement of ECAP with cochlear implants is different than acoustic ECoG recordings in that it requires no external placement of electrodes; stimulation and recording electrodes are chosen from the 16 to 22 intracochlear electrodes as well as from reference electrodes placed outside the ear. This allows for somewhat unique control of both place of stimulation along the length of the cochlea as well as the recording location. A number of studies have demonstrated that both stimulation and recording location can provide a degree of spatial specificity (Cohen et al., 2003; Abbas et al., 2004)

TRANSTYMPANIC ELECTRODES

Transtympanic electrodes have also been used successfully to record the ECoG in clinical settings. As the name implies, transtympanic electrodes are passed through the TM and positioned on either the round window or the promontory of the middle ear. A ball-tipped electrode can be placed into the middle ear through a myringotomy. Alternately, needle electrodes are available that can be used to puncture the TM. The tip of the needle electrode can then be positioned against the promontory. Either the electrode is handheld during recordings, or the foam tip of the insert earphone is used to secure the electrode within the ear canal.

Early studies demonstrated the feasibility of this approach (Aran and LeBert, 1968; Sohmer and Feinmesser, 1967; Yoshie et al., 1967). The responses that are recorded using a transtympanic electrode are large and require little signal averaging. The relative invasiveness of the procedure, however, is the largest disadvantage. Even with local anesthetic, the process of positioning a transtympanic electrode can be uncomfortable for the patient. From a practical standpoint, it also requires the services of a physician. These disadvantages have limited the routine use of transtympanic recording sites in the United States.

EXTRATYMPANIC ELECTRODES

During the 1970s and 1980s, considerable effort was put into developing less invasive methods of recording the ECoG using electrodes placed either on the TM or in the ear canal (Cullen et al., 1972; Sohmer and Feinmesser, 1967; Coats and Dickey, 1970). One type of electrode that has been used widely in clinical as well as research applications is the wick electrode, which is designed to rest against the TM. The wick electrode consists of a pliable silver wire that is insulated along its length and has a soft mesh that is connected to the active tip. That mesh is then impregnated with electrolyte before being placed into the ear canal. The tip of this electrode rests on or near the TM. The second general type of extratympanic electrode that has been widely used clinically is the TIPtrode. The TIPtrode consists of a foam tip for an insert earphone that has been covered with gold foil. When inserted into the ear canal, the foil makes contact with the ear canal, and an adapter is used to connect the foil contact to the averaging unit. The third extratympanic electrode to be commercially manufactured was originally called the Eartrode (Coats, 1974). This electrode has small "wings" of flexible plastic. A ball electrode is attached to the tip of one wing. The electrode is placed into the canal using forceps. The plastic expands to press the ball electrode gently into the wall of the ear canal. These electrodes can be placed either mid-canal or deep in the external ear canal, very close to TM. Many clinicians have manufactured their own recording electrodes. Details of making one type of TM electrode are described in Arsenault and Benitez (1991). Today, it is possible to purchase extratympanic recording electrodes directly from the companies that manufacture evoked potential recording systems.

There have been a number of studies that have compared results obtained using transtympanic, tympanic, and extratympanic electrode sites (Ruth and Lambert 1989; Stypulkowski and Staller, 1987; Ferraro et al, 1994a, 1994b; Ruth et al., 1988; Schoonhoven et al., 1995). Figure 12.10 shows the impact of recording electrode position on the amplitude of the N1 potential of the ECoG. Clearly, the amplitude of the response decreases as the recording electrode is moved away from the cochlea. Responses recorded from the ear canal are smaller and require significantly more averaging to resolve than responses recorded either from the TM or from a location in the middle ear. While the largest amplitude responses can be recorded from a transtympanic electrode, placement of that style electrode can be difficult and can cause discomfort for the patient. As a result, many clinicians have come to regard transtympanic electrodes as being overly invasive. For most applications, TM electrodes may represent a reasonable compromise between optimal electrode location, patient comfort, and ease of placement/recording.

Acoustic Electrocochleography Recording Parameters

Recording ECoG in response to acoustic stimulation can be accomplished with standard signal averaging instruments for both stimulus generation and response averaging. Most commercial instrumentation designed to measure the auditory brainstem response (ABR) can be adapted to allow for measurement of the ECoG. While some of the recording parameters used to measure the ECoG will differ from those used to measure the ABR, the similarities are strong enough that it is possible to measure a combined ECoG and ABR. This is done by using an ear canal or TM electrode as the reference in ABR recording montage, so that wave I, the peripheral auditory nerve response, is enhanced.

Table 12.1 lists typical stimulating and recording parameters. Differential amplification is typically used to record ECoG because it allows for both reduction of stimulus artifact and noise contamination in the recordings. The active (noninverting) electrode is typically placed in the ear canal, on the TM, or on the promontory of the middle ear; the reference (inverting) electrode is typically positioned on the contralateral earlobe, contralateral mastoid, or vertex; a ground (common) electrode can be placed on the forehead or other far-field surface location. With this electrode configuration, N1 of the ECoG is recorded as a negative-going peak.

The time base for recording will depend upon the stimulus used. For click stimuli, a relatively short time base of

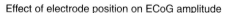

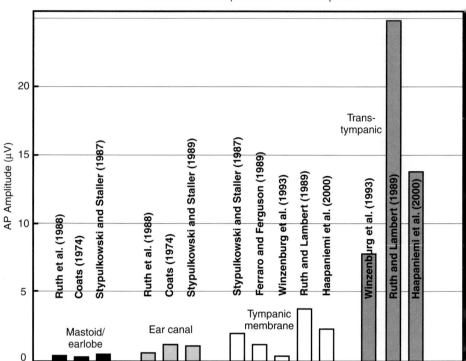

FIGURE 12.10   The effect of recording electrode position on the amplitude of the N1 component of the ECoG is shown. The measures shown were obtained from seven different studies published between 1974 and 2000. Clearly, the largest response amplitudes are obtained when transtympanic recording electrodes are used.

about 4 to 5 ms is typically more than adequate to record the ECoG. For longer tone-burst stimuli, the CM and SP potentials occur across the duration of the tone, and consequently, longer time windows would be necessary to capture those components of the response.

Amplification and the amount of signal averaging that is necessary will depend on the recording site. Those sites closer to the source of the potential (e.g., promontory) will generally produce larger amplitude responses with better signal-to-noise ratios than those recording sites farther from the source (e.g., ear canal). Consequently, greater amplification and more sweeps will be needed for more peripheral sites

(see Chapter 11). For instance 100,000 gain and 2,000 or more sweeps would be typical of an ear canal placement, whereas an order of magnitude less gain and number of sweeps are more typical for transtympanic recordings. In addition, the number of sweeps necessary will also vary with stimulus level and with degree of hearing loss, in that with smaller response amplitudes, more averaging will be needed.

The ECoG is typically recorded using band-pass filtering. The cutoff frequencies of the band-pass filter will vary depending on the stimuli used to record the response and the particular parameters of interest. The ABR is typically recorded using a band pass of 100 to 3,000 Hz. These

TABLE 12.1   Electrocochleography settings

Stimulus	Click	Tone burst
High-pass filter settings	3–5 Hz	3–5 Hz
Low-pass filter settings	3–5 kHz	3–5 kHz
Number of sweeps	500 (TT), 2,000 (ET)	500 (TT), 2,000 (ET)
Stimulus duration	100 μs	2-ms ramp, 10- to 12-ms plateau
Stimulus frequency	Broadband click	0.5, 1, 2, 4, and 8 kHz
Recording time window	5 ms	20 ms
Stimulation rate	5–12 per second	30–40 per second
Polarity	Rarefaction and condensation	Alternating
Prestimulus baseline	1–2 ms	1–2 ms
Gain	100,000 (ET)20,000–50,000 (TT)	100,000 (ET)20,000–50,000 (TT)
Artifact rejection	On	On

TT, transtympanic; ET, extratympanic.
Adapted from Wuyts et al. (1997) and Ferraro and Ruth (1994).

parameters can be used to record the N1 peak of the ECoG measured in response to click stimuli. If recording both the SP and the AP portions of the ECoG is of interest, a wider band pass must be used. That is because the SP is essentially a DC potential. High-pass filter cutoffs of approximately 3 to 5 Hz and low-pass filter cutoffs of approximately 3 to 5 kHz are typical in the literature when clicks are used to elicit the response. When filter settings as low as 3 to 5 Hz are used, slowly varying artifact or baseline shifts throughout the recording period can be more problematic. This is particularly true when tone bursts rather than click stimuli are used to record the SP (see below).

Acoustic Electrocochleography Stimulus Parameters

Sound delivery is typically accomplished using an insert earphone. For some recordings, the insert tip used to couple the sound delivery tube to the ear canal has been modified to make it part of the recording electrode. In other cases, the foam tip of the insert phone is used to hold the recording electrode in place. Since the transducer of the insert earphone is typically located close to the recording electrode leads, the stimulus artifact can be significant and problematic. Care should be taken to separate to the extent possible the transducer from the recording electrode leads and/or to use electromagnetic shielding around the transducer itself.

For many clinical applications, attempts are made to minimize both stimulus artifact and CM in the recordings in order to allow the SP and the AP to be resolved. One way to accomplish this is to use alternating polarity stimulation to make the recordings. The use of alternating polarity stimulation, however, can obscure what may be important characteristics of the response. Figure 12.5 illustrates APs measured using both condensation and rarefaction clicks. Clearly, the response latency can vary depending on the stimulus polarity. As a consequence, if alternating stimuli are used to measure the AP, the recorded waveform will have a different morphology. That is, response amplitudes recorded using an alternating stimulus will not simply be the average of the amplitudes obtained using the two different polarities. If the latency difference, or other characteristic of the response, varies among individuals or is dependent on pathology, as has been reported with Ménière's disease (Margolis et al., 1995; Levine et al., 1992), then these differences would clearly be obscured by using only alternating-polarity stimuli.

Acoustic Electrocochleography Waveform Analysis

Many, if not most, clinicians use clicks rather than tone bursts to elicit the ECoG. Clicks elicit a more synchronous response, and consequently, the AP tends to be larger than when tone bursts are used. The SP, as illustrated in Figure 12.5, is visible as a short deflection or "knee" in the waveform before the N1 peak of the AP. In some cases, the SP can be very difficult to

identify with certainty when clicks are used to elicit the ECoG. The SP in response to a tone burst has the advantage that it will be sustained and therefore can, in some cases, be more easily resolved. However, because measuring a DC potential such as the SP requires wide band-pass filter settings, slow changes in baseline activity as well as low-frequency noise can make measuring the SP a challenge, even when long-duration stimuli are used. Figure 12.11, from Levine et al. (1998), illustrates a recording with a significant change in baseline over the time course of the tone burst. The method used to overcome this problem is to linearly interpolate between the pre- and poststimulus baselines. The SP amplitude is then estimated relative to that interpolated reference and is typically measured at a point midway between the onset and offset of the tone burst.

Another method of identifying the SP when click stimuli are used has been proposed by Gibson et al. (1977) and by Coats (1981). This method takes advantage of the neural response property of adaptation; that is, the AP amplitude tends to decrease with increasing stimulus rate, while the SP, a response from the hair cells, does not. Responses are recorded using click rates of 200/s and compared with similar measures

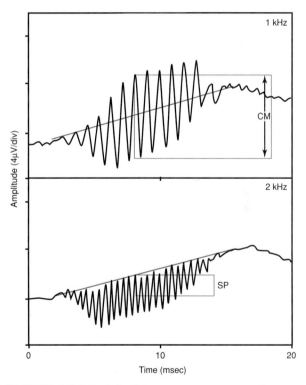

FIGURE 12.11 ECoG in response to tone-burst stimuli, illustrating the method used to determine the SP with drift in the baseline. Stimulus frequency is illustrated in each plot. (Reprinted from Levine SC, Margolis RH, Daly KA. [1998] Use of electrocochleography in the diagnosis of Ménière's disease. *Laryngoscope.* 108, 993–1000, with permission from Lippincott Williams & Wilkins.)

obtained at lower stimulation rates (8/s). The examples in Figure 12.12 illustrate how the N1 (in this case, negative is up) adapts, but the SP potential does not. This can allow for a clear identification of the SP (Gibson et al., 1977; Coats, 1981).

Also, there is not a standard convention in the literature for how to measure the amplitude of the SP and/or the AP. For instance, some investigators have reported measuring both the SP and the N1 amplitude relative to a prestimulus baseline (Coats, 1986; Ruth, 2000).Other investigators measure SP amplitude from baseline to the shoulder or "knee" point on the leading edge of the AP. The amplitude of the AP is then measured from the SP to the following negative peak (Ferraro, 2000). In other reports, the amplitude of the AP has been measured from the negative N1 peak to the following positive peak (Ferraro, 1997). Figure 12.13 illustrates how, for a typical waveform, the AP amplitude can vary considerably relative to the SP, depending on the particular method that is used. Clearly, the method of analyzing the different

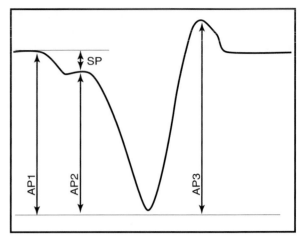

FIGURE 12.13 Schematic showing three ways for measuring the AP amplitude reported in the literature.

components of the response will yield different SP/AP ratios and impact the outcome. One method is not likely to be superior to another. The point remains, however, that care should be taken to ensure that the appropriate analysis technique is used when comparing data collected from an individual with published normative values.

Finally, some investigators have noted that the individual components of the ECoG can vary both in latency and amplitude, depending on whether or not the rarefaction or condensation clicks (or tone bursts) are used (Levine et al., 1992; Margolis et al., 1995; Sass et al., 1997).This difference can be obscured if alternating-polarity stimuli are used. This observation has led to the suggestion that separate ECoG measures be recorded in response to condensation and rarefaction clicks. Ferraro and Tibbels (1999) argued that this practice will increase test time and point out that the sensitivity of the procedure for identification of Ménière's disease has not been proven. They propose another approach where the area and/or width of the ECoG evoked using alternating-polarity click stimuli rather than peak-to-peak measures can be computed. Their technique is fast and avoids the inherent ambiguities associated with picking peaks. Results of this study show that use of this technique may result in improved sensitivity in this patient population.

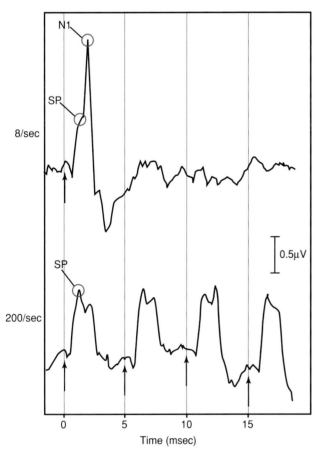

FIGURE 12.12 ECoG waveforms illustrate the effects of stimulus presentation rate on the AP and SP. Stimulus rate was 8/s for the upper trace and 200/s for the lower trace. SP and N1 levels are labeled. (Reprinted from Coats AC. [1981] The summating potential and Ménière's disease. *Arch Otolaryngol.* 104, 199–208, with permission of the American Medical Association.)

Electrical Evoked Compound Action Potential Recording Parameters

The recording of ECAP in cochlear implant users is quite different than acoustic ECoG measures. The stimulus delivery and the recording systems are incorporated into the implant. Evoked potential recording equipment is also not needed because software and interfaces to the implant can be purchased from implant manufacturers. Figure 12.14 illustrates the basic features of the Nucleus CI24 implant and the NRT system. Other implant systems are similar in principle. A computer equipped with a programming interface is used to stimulate

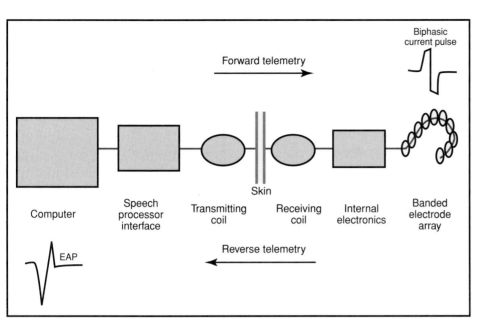

FIGURE 12.14 Schematic illustrates the elements of a cochlear implant important for recording of the electrically evoked compound action potential (EAP).

specific electrodes in the implanted array. A radiofrequency signal is transmitted across the skin to the internal receiver/stimulator. This is labeled "Forward Telemetry" in the figure. Forward telemetry is used to provide power to the internal electronics and to control stimulus generation. The CI24 device has 22 intracochlear electrodes and two extracochlear electrodes, which allow for monopolar stimulation. One extracochlear electrode is a ball electrode placed below the temporalis muscle (MP1). The second extracochlear electrode is a relatively large plate electrode located on the surface of the internal case (MP2). The internal device also has an onboard amplifier and analog-to-digital converter. This additional electronic hardware allows the voltage recorded across a specified electrode pair within the cochlea to be amplified, sampled, and transmitted back to the external coil using the "reverse telemetry system." The voltage waveform recorded from within the cochlea can then be processed, averaged, displayed, and stored on the same computer used to activate the device. This arrangement allows the ECAP to be recorded without additional averaging equipment or surface recording electrodes.

The reverse telemetry system of the CI24M device is designed to record only over a relatively short time interval (a series of 16 samples after each stimulus pulse at a maximum rate of 10 kHz, yielding a response window of 1.6 ms). Other devices presently available (Advanced Bionics CII implant and the Cochlear RE implant) have faster sampling capabilities and/or longer recording windows.

Electrical Evoked Compound Action Potential Stimulus Artifact Reduction

An important concern with electrical stimulation where the stimulus artifact has much greater amplitude than the neu-

ral response is the linearity and saturation characteristics of the internal amplifier. A number of recording parameters can be manipulated to reduce stimulus artifact. The gain of the amplifier is typically relatively low for this reason (40 or 60 dB). In the Cochlear CI24 or RE system, it is not possible to sample the stimulus waveform during the stimulus pulse. A minimum delay of 35 μs between offset of stimulation and the initiation of sampling must be specified. Nevertheless, there can be a considerable effect of the stimulus artifact still evident in the recorded potential, even after stimulus offset. Increasing the delay between stimulus onset and initiation of sampling, however, is possible and can be useful in limiting effects of stimulus artifact. At short delays, a relatively large stimulus artifact can cause amplifier saturation and a decrease in the measured response. By setting this delay long enough so that the voltage from the stimulus artifact is appropriately decayed, the amplifier is operating within its linear range when sampling begins. Finally, stimulus artifact can be affected by the choice of recording electrode. Recordings are typically made with one intracochlear electrode as the active (positive) relative to an extracochlear reference. The implants typically have 16 to 22 intracochlear electrodes; choosing a recording electrode close to the stimulating electrode typically has the effect of increasing the stimulus artifact as well as increasing the neural response. For that reason, it is advisable to choose an electrode as close as possible to the stimulating electrode but distant enough so that it does not negatively affect the recordings. A specific procedure for adjusting these parameters for the Nucleus 24 implant has been described in Abbas et al. (1999). Typically, a recording electrode adjacent to or one away from the stimulating electrode provides adequate artifact reduction.

Despite efforts such as those described in the previous paragraph, electrical stimulus artifact still significantly overlaps the neural response because of the close temporal proximity of the electrical stimulus and the neural response. Some additional stimulus artifact reduction techniques typically need to be applied to the averaged responses in order to extract the neural response from the stimulus artifact. In some recording situations, alternation of stimulus polarity can adequately cancel artifact to record the ECAP (Wilson et al., 1997). In general, however, the use of a two-pulse subtraction technique that takes advantage of the neuron's refractory properties has proven to be a more reliable recording method (Brown et al., 1990). This method is illustrated in Figure 12.15 and is incorporated into software for measuring both NRT and NRI. Typically, one measures the response to a probe pulse with and without a masker pulse preceding it. The theory behind the subtraction method is that if the masker pulse is high enough in level, then the auditory nerve fibers will fire in response to the masker pulse, and if the interpeak interval is sufficiently short, then these auditory nerve fibers will be in a refractory state and therefore unable to respond to the probe. Therefore, the probe-alone recording should contain both probe stimulus artifact and a neural response to the probe; the masker plus probe recording, however, will contain only probe stimulus artifact, and no neural response to the probe should be recorded. The subtraction of these two recordings will allow the probe stimulus artifact to be minimized without affecting the neural response to the probe.

A number of variations of this technique have been used to measure spatial selectivity in neural stimulation with intracochlear electrodes (Cohen et al., 2003; Abbas et al., 2004) and to investigate adaptation using pulse-train stimulation (Hay-McCutcheon et al., 2005).

APPLICATIONS OF ELECTROCOCHLEOGRAPHY IN CLINICAL PRACTICE

There are several applications for ECoG in clinical practice today. Over the past several decades, one of the main uses for ECoG has been to assist in the diagnosis of Ménière's disease. More recently, because it is a measure of the status of the peripheral auditory system, ECoG has also become a useful tool in the diagnosis of auditory neuropathy. It is also possible to use ECoG to assess hearing sensitivity. While this application has never gained widespread use in the United States, it is used fairly widely for this purpose in parts of Europe and Australia. ECoG has been used as a method of assessing and monitoring peripheral auditory function during skull-base surgeries (see Chapter 16). Additionally, ECAPs can be used to assist with fitting of the cochlear implant in young children. These applications are reviewed in the following sections.

Ménière's Disease

Ménière's disease is a progressive, debilitating disorder characterized by recurrent, spontaneous vertigo, fluctuating sensory-neural hearing loss, a sensation of aural fullness and tinnitus. Although Ménière's disease was first described more than a century ago (Ménière, 1861), the underlying cause of this disorder is still not well understood. The most widely accepted theory is that Ménière's disease is the result of increased endolymphatic pressure. This condition has been called endolymphatic hydrops. Unfortunately, there is

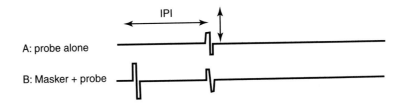

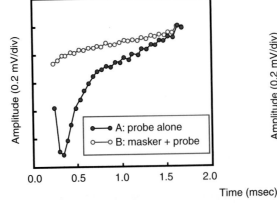
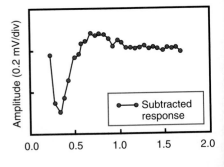

FIGURE 12.15 Illustration of the subtraction method used to reduce effects of stimulus artifact on the ECAP. Responses to conditions A and B are shown after probe presentation.

no way to confirm the presence of endolymphatic hydrops in vivo, and the diagnosis of Ménière's disease is typically made on the basis of patient history, review of the audiogram, and after other disorders with similar presenting symptoms have been ruled out. Complicating the diagnostic process is the fact that the presence and severity of the symptoms vary substantially both across patients as well as across time within an individual patient. In 1995, the Subcommittee on Equilibrium and Its Measurements of the America Academy of Otolaryngology and Head and Neck Surgery defined four levels of certainty that physicians use to describe their confidence in the diagnosis—certain, definite, probable, and possible—based on the number of symptoms the patient displays, where a diagnosis of certain Ménière's disease requires analysis of data collected postmortem. The fact that a classification system such as this is required points to the need for a better diagnostic test for the disorder. Because it reflects neural activity at both a presynaptic and a postsynaptic level, ECoG seems to have potential to fill this need.

As noted earlier, the SP can be particularly vulnerable to slow changes in the electrical and mechanical displacement of the basilar membrane and/or hair cells (Durrant and Dallos, 1972, 1974). Consistent with these observations, SP amplitudes are larger in animals with induced endolymphatic hydrops than in normal animals (Aran et al., 1984; van Deelen et al., 1987). It has been hypothesized that such changes in patients with Ménière's disease may be the result of similar changes in the cochlea (i.e., increased hydropic pressure and distention of the endolymph system), thus altering the resting position of the basilar membrane within the cochlea (Margolis et al., 1992).

In the mid-1970s, two different groups initially proposed use of ECoG measures for assisting with diagnosis of Ménière's disease (Schmidt et al., 1974; Eggermont and Odenthal, 1977; Gibson et al., 1977). Both groups noted that many individuals with classic symptoms of Ménière's disease had enlarged SPs compared to those recorded from individuals with normal hearing. Figure 12.16 shows an example of this effect. Many of these early studies relied on measurement of the cochlear potentials using transtympanic electrodes.

Over the next 10 to 15 years, as less invasive recording techniques were developed, many studies evaluated the sensitivity and specificity of the ECoG as a test for Ménière's disease and set out to define the optimal recording protocol. It quickly became apparent that methodologic factors, such as position of the recording electrode, could significantly impact the amplitude of the SP. To help control for this factor, a convention was adopted whereby the SP amplitude was expressed as a ratio relative to the amplitude of the AP. Not only did this convention help control for variance in placement of the transtympanic electrode within the middle ear, but it also allowed for the comparison across studies. Still, based on the scientific literature published between the late 1970s and the late 1980s, it is difficult to draw firm conclusions about the clinical utility of the ECoG in the diagnosis of Ménière's disease. That is partially because of small

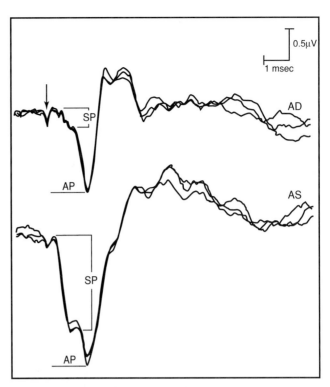

FIGURE 12.16 ECoG waveforms recorded in an individual with Ménière's symptoms in the left ear. (Reprinted from Stypulkowski PH, Staller SJ. [1987] Clinical evaluation of a new ECoG recording electrode. *Ear Hear.* 8, 304–310, with permission from Lippincott Williams & Wilkins.)

numbers of subjects but also because of differences in stimulus types, analysis methods, and recording parameters among studies.

Nevertheless, ECoG continued to be used widely over the next few years, and starting in the mid-1990s, larger retrospective studies were published that were aimed at defining the relative sensitivity and specificity of this evoked potential as a diagnostic tool. Wuyts et al. (1997) performed a meta-analysis of over 20 such studies. This review included studies with specific stimulus and recording characteristics (e.g., high-pass filter settings of 3 to 5 Hz and low-pass filter settings of 3 to 5 kHz). Figures 12.17 and 12.18 illustrate the results of separate analyses of transtympanic electrode recordings and extratympanic electrode recordings, respectively. Additionally, results obtained from studies that used clicks were analyzed separately from results obtained from studies that used tone bursts. This meta-analysis showed that, regardless of recording electrode location, most normal ears have SP/AP ratios under 0.30. Review of the data collected from patients with Ménière's disease suggested that SP/AP ratios greater than 0.35 are large enough to be considered pathologic and consistent with the presence of endolymphatic hydrops when transtympanic electrodes are used. SP/AP ratios greater than 0.42 were considered abnormally large when either TM or ear canal electrodes were used.

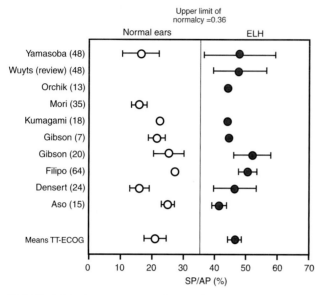

FIGURE 12.17 Meta-analysis of transtympanic (TT) ECoG SP/AP ratios obtained from a number of papers in the literature. ELH, endolymphatic hydrops. (Reprinted from Wuyts FL, Van de Heyning PH, Van Spaendonck MP, Molenberghs G. [1997] A review of electrocochleography: instrumentation settings and meta-analysis of criteria for diagnosis of endolymphatic hydrops. *Acta Otolaryngol.* **526 [suppl], 14–20, with permission from Taylor and Francis.)**

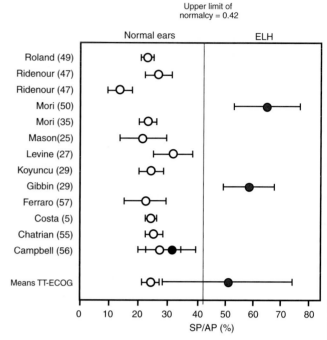

FIGURE 12.18 Meta-analysis of extratympanic (ET) ECoG SP/AP ratios obtained from a number of papers in the literature. ELH, endolymphatic hydrops. (Reprinted from Wuyts FL, Van de Heyning PH, Van Spaendonck MP, Molenberghs G. [1997] A review of electrocochleography: instrumentation settings and meta-analysis of criteria for diagnosis of endolymphatic hydrops. *Acta Otolaryngol.* **526 [suppl], 14–20, with permission from Taylor and Francis.)**

Other investigators have published fairly large-scale retrospective studies of the sensitivity of this diagnostic tool, and the results have been fairly mixed. For example, Kim et al. (2005) report results of a retrospective case review of 60 patients classified as having definite Ménière's disease and 37 patients with probable Ménière's' disease. Only 66.7% of those with definite Ménière's disease and 52.7% of those with probable Ménière's disease had abnormal ECoGs as judged by an SP/AP ratio of greater than 0.4, causing these authors to conclude that, based on its lack of sensitivity, ECoG "should not play a decisive role in determining the presence or absence of Ménière's disease" (p 128). Chung et al. (2004) report results of a similar retrospective study of the effectiveness of extratympanic ECoG in the diagnosis of Ménière's disease. This study reports on result collected from 158 patients with a medical diagnosis of Ménière's disease and 37 patients with normal hearing. An SP/AP ratio of 0.34 was used as the diagnostic criteria. Chung et al. report finding a sensitivity of only 71% and no correlation between the results of ECoG testing and the estimated stage of the disease and severity or duration of the symptoms. Ge and Shea (2002) reviewed ECoG test results obtained using a transtympanic electrode for 2,140 patients tested in the time period between 1990 and 2000. SP/AP ratios greater than 0.4 when elicited using clicks were considered enlarged in this study. These authors report finding a sensitivity rate of 76.1%. In this study, however,

the sensitivity of this procedure increased as the duration and severity of the symptoms increased. Pappas et al. (2000) reviewed results from 252 patients who had symptoms consistent with Ménière's disease. In this study, extratympanic electrodes were used to record the ECoG. A sensitivity rate of 74% was found in patients with definitive Ménière's disease. Interestingly, 42% of contralateral ears had enlarged SP/AP ratios. These investigators found no correlation between ECoG tests results and duration of symptoms.

Given that there is no gold standard for diagnosis of Ménière's disease, it is, perhaps, not surprising to find relatively low sensitivity rates (60% to 70%) for this diagnostic tool. Given these relatively low sensitivity rates, the observation of an enlarged SP/AP ratio may suggest a diagnosis of Ménière's disease; however, the finding of normal SP/AP ratio is of limited diagnostic significance. Levine et al. (1998) were particularly pessimistic, concluding that the ECoG had limited diagnostic value in the diagnosis of Ménière's disease. Ferraro (2000) has suggested that the sensitivity of this procedure may be improved if the testing is done on a day when the patient's symptoms are acute and that the sensitivity of this procedure is particularly poor for ears with hearing loss greater than 70 dB hearing level (HL).

In conclusion, the finding of an enlarged SP/AP ratio may prove helpful in the diagnosis of Ménière's disease. However, there is a great deal of evidence that a significant number of patients with confirmed Ménière's disease have normal SP/AP ratios. As a result, negative results should be interpreted with appropriate caution.

Estimation of Hearing Thresholds

Another application for the ECoG in clinical practice is as a metric for estimating hearing thresholds. The application was first proposed in 1977 (Bergholtz et al., 1977; Hooper et al., 1977; Eggermont and Odenthal, 1977). Since those early reports, a number of investigators have reported finding reasonable correlations between click-evoked ECoG thresholds and behavioral thresholds in pediatric populations (Wong et al., 1997; Schoonhoven et al., 1996, 1999; Ferron et al., 1983; Arslan et al., 1997; Bellman et al., 1984). In most cases, when ECoG is used to estimate hearing threshold, transtympanic or TM electrodes are used. This represents a significant drawback because, in most pediatric patients, the safe insertion of either electrode would likely require general anesthesia. Consequently, ABR provides an easier method of assessing hearing sensitivity in young children. Studies comparing the efficacy of both procedures have found either similar results with the two techniques (Arslan et al., 1983, 1997; Fjermedal et al., 1988; Bellman et al., 1984; Arslan et al., 1983) or have found ABR thresholds to be slightly more accurate than ECoG thresholds (Laureano et al., 1995; Dauman, 1991; Ryerson and Beagley, 1981). Based on such results, ECoG is not often used for assessing audiometric thresholds.

Enhancing Wave I of the Auditory Brainstem Response

There are often instances where it is difficult or impossible to identify wave I of the ABR. This can be particularly problematic in patients with substantial degrees of hearing loss. The absence of a clearly identifiable wave I significantly impacts the use of ABR in the identification of patients with potential retrocochlear involvement, since absence or distortion of wave I makes measurement of I-III and I-V interpeak intervals impossible (see Chapter 13). Wave I of the ABR and the N1 peak of the ECoG are identical potentials. N1 is generally recorded as a negative peak only because the electrode located closest to the cochlea/auditory nerve is typically connected to the active or noninverting input of the differential amplifier. When the ABR is recorded, the mastoid or earlobe electrode that is largely responsible for recording neural activity from the cochlea/auditory nerve is typically placed into the inverting input of the differential amplifier, resulting in a vertex-positive peak. Several investigators have demonstrated that it is possible to either record ECoG and ABR simultaneously or to record a combined ECoG/ABR by replacing the mastoid electrode used to record the ABR with either an extratympanic or transtympanic ECoG recording electrode (Ferraro and Ferguson, 1989; Ferraro and Ruth, 1994; Schlake et al., 2001). The closer the recording electrode can be placed to the cochlea, the larger wave I amplitude will be. This relatively simple technique for enhancing wave I amplitude can be useful preoperatively because it may allow for more accurate assessment of interpeak intervals than is possible using traditional ABR electrode montages. Moreover, during skull-base surgery, it is important that wave I be recorded reliably and quickly to determine whether changes observed in the ABR during surgery are due to the surgical manipulation of the auditory nerve, cochlear damage, and/or accumulation of fluid in the middle ear.

Intraoperative Monitoring

ECoG has also been used fairly widely as a tool for monitoring the status of the peripheral auditory system in the operating room. ECoG is not affected by anesthesia, a fact that makes it a potential candidate for intraoperative monitoring applications. Additionally, because the patient is generally anesthetized, it is possible to record this response using a transtympanic or tympanic electrode rather than using an electrode in the ear canal. The relatively large amplitude of ECoG also makes it an ideal candidate for intraoperative monitoring purposes because the larger the response amplitude, the more rapidly feedback about the status of the auditory system can be given to the surgeon. However, it is important to realize that ECoG should not be the sole tool for intraoperative monitoring applications. In many cases, the presence of a vestibular schwannoma will not alter the latency or amplitude of the ECoG AP or wave I of the ABR. The effect of the tumor will be to increase the I-III and I-V intervals. Although loss of the AP during the surgical procedure is strong evidence of cochlear pathology, there have been a number of cases reported in the literature where the ECoG is preserved, despite the fact that the patient has suffered a profound hearing loss. Studies have shown that the AP can be recorded in animals even when the auditory nerve is completely severed, provided that blood flow to the cochlea is not disrupted (Ruben et al., 1963; Silverstein et al., 1984).

The most common application for ECoG in the operating room is as a method of enhancing wave I of the ABR. This allows for more reliable and rapid assessment of changes in interwave intervals during the surgical procedure and allows one to distinguish changes in wave V latency caused by manipulations of the tumor or brainstem from changes that may results from the accumulation of fluid in the middle ear.

It is also possible to use an electrode positioned directly on the auditory nerve as it exits the internal auditory canal to record ECoG. This placement site will result in the largest possible response amplitudes, and often, the compound AP recorded from an electrode on the auditory nerve can be seen in the unaveraged traces, making it possible to provide the surgeon with almost real-time feedback. The electrode used for direct nerve recordings is typically a ball electrode or a cotton wick–type electrode. The major disadvantage of this procedure is that it cannot be used until the nerve is exposed, and depending on the surgical approach and the location of the tumor, it is often not possible to keep the electrode in place during the resection of the tumor from the nerve bundle.

Typically, if ECoG and ABR are both stable and do not exhibit significant latency changes during the surgical procedure, it is considered to be evidence that, at the end of the surgery, the auditory system was intact. There are a range of pathologic outcomes that can be observed including: complete loss of both ECoG AP and ABR, loss of ABR but preservation of the ECoG AP, or preservation of ECoG AP but loss or distortion of wave V of the ABR. All of these outcomes suggest that the auditory nerve and/or cochlea have been compromised and that postoperative hearing will be negatively affected.

While most surgical applications where monitoring is used have involved otoneurologic cases, there are other surgical procedures where intraoperative measurement of ECoG may be helpful. One example is in the surgical procedure to decompress or shunt the endolymphatic sac for patients with Ménière's disease. In those cases, monitoring of the SP and the AP may be useful in assessing the degree of trauma to the inner ear structures. Case studies describing results of intraoperative monitoring have been presented in the literature (Ferraro, 2000; Arenberg et al., 1993; Gibson and Arenberg, 1991; Gibson et al., 1988; Wazen, 1994). In these cases, the results of intraoperative measurement of the ECoG have been useful in predicting postoperative outcomes. Chapter 17 provides a more detailed review of intraoperative monitoring.

Auditory Neuropathy

Auditory neuropathy is a condition that is diagnosed by a finding of absent ABR in the presence of measurable otoacoustic emissions. In some cases, it is possible to measure CM and/or a compound AP in response to high-level click stimuli (Berlin et al., 1998; Starr et al., 2001). The presence of CM is consistent with the premise that an individual with auditory neuropathy has functioning outer hair cells. In most of these cases, the cochlear potentials are recorded from the mastoid electrode used to measure the ABR. Clearly, these recordings would be enhanced if a recording electrode closer to the cochlea (i.e., a TM or transtympanic electrode) were used. The primary diagnostic challenge in these cases is to rule out the possibility that the potential that is recorded is in fact CM, rather than simply stimulus artifact that is picked up on the recording electrodes.

In order to optimally record CM, relatively long tone bursts that do not alternate in polarity should be used. The CM will appear as a sinusoidal oscillation that persists while the stimulus is present. Stimulus artifact will have essentially the same characteristics. Care should be taken to separate the stimulus transducer from the recording electrodes to the extent possible. A relatively simple trick to differentiate CM from stimulus artifact is to clamp off the tube

to the insert phone and to repeat the recordings. If the response you are collecting is stimulus artifact, it should not change if you have not changed the orientation of the insert earphone transducer and the electrodes. However, clamping the tube to the insert earphone should significantly reduce the signal level and decrease or eliminate any CM.

APPLICATIONS OF ELECTRICALLY EVOKED COMPOUND ACTION POTENTIAL IN CLINICAL PRACTICE

The primary application for ECAP measures in cochlear implant users is generally in young children. It is common practice today for children as young as 10 to 12 months of age to be candidates for a cochlear implant. Early implantation presents a challenge for the programming audiologist due to limited language skills, limited listening experience, and short attention spans. Programming the implant, or developing a monophasic action potential (MAP), generally requires behavioral threshold measures for each electrode in the implanted array. As a result, the process of programming the speech processor in young children can be challenging. In these patients, it is possible to use NRT/NRI to measure the ECAP. Typically, a range of stimulus levels will be used to record the ECAP for each electrode in the array or for a subset of electrodes spread across the intracochlear electrode array. ECAP threshold is then defined as the lowest level at which a response is detectable.

Several studies have reported comparisons between ECAP thresholds and the levels used to program the speech processor in adult cochlear implant users, in whom reliable behavioral threshold measures can be made (Brown et al., 2000; Hughes et al., 2000; Mason et al., 2001; Cullington, 2000). In general, there is considerable across-subject variability, but there are significant correlations between the two measures. A number of different methods have been proposed for improving the accuracy of the MAP predictions that are based on the results of NRT/NRI testing (Brown et al., 2000; Franck and Norton, 2001; Smoorenburg et al., 2002). Nevertheless, while ECAP-based MAPs do not always predict behavioral MAPs, several investigators have reported that speech perception measures obtained using these MAPs are not significantly different from those obtained using a MAP fit using traditional behavioral programming techniques (Smoorenburg et al., 2002; Seyle and Brown 2002). That is, the performance using a physiologically based MAP is not significantly different.

A second equally important application for NRT/NRI technology is as a tool that can be used to establish that there is a neural response to electrical stimulation in cases where there is some question about device function. Although they represent the minority of patients who receive cochlear implants, there are children (or adults) who fail to respond to electrical stimulation, fail to progress as expected with their implant, or show some evidence of a decline in performance over time. The manufacturers can assist the audiologist with confirming that the device is functioning, and the presence of an ECAP can be used to confirm that the auditory nerve is responding appropriately to electrical stimulation. Such measures can be made in the operating room at the time of surgery and can also be made throughout the life of the implant. Such measures can be particularly useful if baseline measures are available; the ECAP can be used to document changes in responsiveness over time. Such information can be invaluable in trying to deal with a child who fails to progress with his/her device, in that changes in specific electrodes may be identified and, in many cases, the speech processor can be programmed to eliminate the use of those electrodes.

 ## SUMMARY

ECoG is an important tool in assessing function of the auditory system. It provides a response at the auditory periphery, whose source is the hair cells as well as the neural response from the auditory nerve. As such, ECoG can be particularly sensitive to pathologic changes in the cochlea. The recording of ECoG can, however, present particular problems that limit its utility. Transtympanic recordings provide excellent signal-to-noise ratio but are invasive. Use of extratympanic electrodes is more generally accepted, but they suffer from poorer signal-to-noise ratio as well as difficulties with artifact. These problems can be overcome, however, and several clinical applications of ECoG are presented in this chapter.

REFERENCES

Abbas PJ, Brown CJ, Shallop JK, Firszt JB, Hughes ML, Hong SH, Staller SJ. (1999) Summary of results using the Nucleus CI24M implant to record the electrically evoked compound action potential. *Ear Hear.* 20, 45–59.

Abbas PJ, Gorga MP. (1981) AP responses in forward masking paradigms and their relationship to responses of single auditory nerve fibers. *J Acoust Soc Am.* 69, 492–499.

Abbas PJ, Hughes ML, Brown CJ, Miller CA, South H. (2004) Channel interaction in cochlear implant users evaluated using the electrically evoked compound action potential. *Audiol Neurotol.* 9, 203–223.

Abbas PJ, Miller CA. (2004) Biophysics and physiology. In: Zeng FG, Fay R, Popper A, eds. *Cochlear Implants.* New York: Springer-Verlag; pp 149–212.

Aran JM, LeBert G. (1968) Les reponses nerveuseses cochleaires chez l'homnme, image du fonctionnement de l'oreille et nouveau test d'audiometrie objective. *Rev Laryngol Otol Rhinol.* 89, 361–378.

Aran JM, Rarey KE, Hawkins JE Jr. (1984) Functional and morphological changes in experimental endolymphatic hydrops. *Acta Otolaryngol.* 97, 547–557.

Arenberg IK, Kobayashi H, Obert AD, Gibson WP. (1993) Intraoperative electrocochleography of endolymphatic hydrops surgery using clicks and tone bursts. *Acta Otolaryngol.* 504 (suppl), 58–67.

Arenberg IK, Obert AD, Gibson WP. (1991) Intraoperative electrocochleographic monitoring of inner ear surgery for endolymphatic hydrops. A review of cases. *Acta Otolaryngol.* 485 (suppl), 53–64.

Arsenault MD, Benitez JT. (1991) Electrococheography: a method for making the Stupulkowski-Staller electrode and testing technique. *Ear Hear.* 12, 358–360.

Arslan E, Prosser S, Conti G, Michelini S. (1983) Electrocochleography and brainstem potentials in the diagnosis of the deaf child. *Int J Pediatr Otorhinolaryngol.* 5, 251–259.

Arslan E, Turrini M, Lupi G, Genovese E. (1997) Hearing threshold assessment with auditory brainstem response (ABR) and electrocochleography (EcochG) in uncooperative children. *Scand Audiol.* 46 (suppl), 32–37.

Bellman S, Barnard S, Beagley HA. (1984) A nine-year review of 841 children tested by transtympanic electrocochleography. *J Laryngol Otol.* 98, 1–9.

Bergholtz LM, Arlinger SD, Kylen P, Jervall LB. 91977) Electrocochleography used as a clinical hearing test in difficult-to-test children. *Acta Otolaryngol.* 84, 385–392.

Berlin CI, Bordelon J, St John P, Wilensky D, Hurley A, Kluka E, Hood LJ. (1998) Reversing click polarity may uncover auditory neuropathy in infants. *Ear Hear.* 9, 37–47.

Brown CJ, Abbas PJ, Gantz, BJ. (1990) Electrically evoked whole-nerve action potentials: data from human cochlear implant users. *J Acoust Soc Am.* 88, 1385–1391.

Brown CJ, Hughes ML, Luk B, Abbas PJ, Wolaver A, Gervais J. (2000) The relationship between EAP and EABR thresholds and levels used to program the Nucleus CI24M speech processor: data from adults. *Ear Hear.* 21, 151–163.

Chung WH, Cho DY, Choi JY, Hong SH. (2004) Clinical usefulness of extratympanic electrocochleography in the diagnosis of Ménière's disease. *Otol Neurotol.* 25, 144–149.

Coats AC. (1974) On electrocochleographic electrode design. *J Acoust Soc Am.* 56, 708–711.

Coats AC. (1981) The summating potential and Ménière's disease. *Arch Otolaryngol.* 104, 199–208.

Coats AC. (1986) Electrocochleography: recording techniques and clinical applications. *Semin Hear.* 7, 246–266.

Coats AC, Dickey JR. (1970) Nonsurgical recording of human auditory nerve action potentials and cochlear microphonics. *Ann Otol Rhinol Laryngol.* 79, 844–852.

Cohen LT, Richardson LM, Saunders E, Cowan RS. (2003) Spatial spread of neural excitation in cochlear implant recipients: comparison of improved ECAP method and psychophysical forward masking. *Hear Res.* 179, 72–87.

Cullen JK, Ellis MS, Berlin CI, et al. (1972) Human acoustic nerve action potential recordings from the tympanic membrane without anesthesia. *Acta Otolaryngol.* 74, 15–22.

Cullington H. (2000) Preliminary neural response telemetry results. *Br J Audiol.* 34, 131–140.

Dallos P. (1973) *The Auditory Periphery, Biophysics and Physiology.* New York: Academic Press.

Dallos P, Cheatham MA. (1976) Compound action potential (AP) tuning curves. *J Acoust Soc Am.* 59, 591–597.

Dallos P, Cheatham MA, Ferraro J. (1974) Cochlear mechanics, nonlinearities, and cochlear potentials. *J Acoust Soc Am.* 55, 597–605.

Dallos P, Schoeny ZG, Cheatham MA. (1972) Cochlear summating potentials: descriptive aspects. *Acta Otolaryngol.* 301 (suppl), 1–36.

Dauman R. (1991) Electrocochleography: applications and limitations in young children. *Acta Otolaryngol.* 482 (suppl), 14–26.

Davis H, Deatherage BH, Eldredge DH, Smith CA. (1958) Summating potentials of the cochlea. *Am J Physiol.* 195, 251–261.

Durrant JD, Dallos P. (1972) The effects of dc current polarization on cochlear harmonics. *J Acoust Soc Am.* 52, 1725–1728.

Durrant JD, Dallos P. (1974) Modification of DIF summating potential components by stimulus biasing. *J Acoust Soc Am.* 56, 562–570.

Eggermont JJ, Odenthal DW. (1977) Potentialities of clinical electrocochleography. *Clin Otolaryngol Allied Sci.* 2, 275–286.

Eggermont JJ, Spoor A, Odenthal DW. (1976) Frequency specificity of tone-burst electrocochleography. In: Ruben RJ, Elberling C, Salomon G, Eds. *Electrocochleography.* Baltimore: University Park Press.

Ferraro JA. (1997) *Laboratory Exercises In Auditory Evoked Potentials.* San Diego: Singular Publishing Group.

Ferraro JA. (2000) Electrocochleography. In: Roesner RJ, Valente M, Hosford-Dunn H, eds. *Audiology Diagnosis.* New York: Thieme.

Ferraro JA, Blackwell WL, Mediavilla SJ, Thedinger BS. (1994) Normal summating potential to tone bursts recorded from the tympanic membrane in humans. *J Am Acad Audiol.* 5, 17–23.

Ferraro JA, Ferguson R. (1989) Tympanic ECochG and conventional ABR: a combined approach for the identification of wave I and the I-V interwave interval. *Ear Hear.* 10, 161–166.

Ferraro JA, Ruth RA. (1994) Electrocochleography. In: Jacobson JT, ed. *Auditory Evoked Potentials: Overview and Basic Principles.* Boston: Allyn & Bacon; pp 101–122.

Ferraro JA, Thedinger BS, Mediavilla SJ, Blackwell WL. (1994) Human summating potential to tone bursts: observations on tympanic membrane versus promontory recordings in the same patients. *J Am Acad Audiol.* 5, 24–29.

Ferraro JA, Tibbels RP. (1999) SP/AP area ratio in the diagnosis of Ménière's disease. *Am J Audiol.* 8, 21–28.

Ferron P, Ouellet Y, Rouillard R, et al. (1983) Electrocochleography in the child—a 300-case study. *J Otolaryngol.* 12, 235–238.

Fjermedal O, Laukli E, Mair IW. (1988) Auditory brainstem responses and extratympanic electrocochleography. A threshold comparison in children. *Scand Audiol.* 17, 231–235.

Franck KH, Norton SJ. (2001) Estimation of psychophysical levels using the electrically evoked compound action potential measured with the neural response telemetry capabilities of Cochlear Corporation's CI24M device. *Ear Hear.* 22, 289–299.

Ge X, Shea JJ. (2002) Transtympanic electrocochleography: a 10-year experience. *Otol Neurotol.* 23, 799–805.

Gibson WPR, Arenberg IK. (1991) The scope of intraoperative electrocochleography. In: Arenberg IK, ed. *Proceedings of the Third International Symposium and Workshops on the Surgery of the Inner Ear.* Amsterdam: Kugler Publications; pp 295–303.

Gibson WPR, Arenberg IK, Best LG. (1988) Intraoperative electrocochleographic parameters following nondestructive inner ear surgery utilizing a valved shunt for hydrops and Ménière's

disease. In: Nadol JG, ed. *Proceedings of the Second International Symposium on Ménière's Disease.* Amsterdam: Kugler & Ghendini Publications; pp 170–171.

Gibson WPR, Moffat DA, Ramsden RT. (1977) Clinical electrocochleography in the diagnosis and management of Ménière's disorder. *Audiology.* 16, 389–401.

Goldstein MH, Kiang NYS. (1958) Synchrony of neural activity in electric response evoked by transient acoustic stimuli. *J Acoust Soc Am.* 30, 107–114.

Haapaniemi J, Laurikainen E, Johansson R, Karjalainen S. (2000) Transtympanic versus tympanic membrane electrocochleography in examining cochleovestibular disorders. *Acta Otolaryngol Suppl.* 543, 127–129.

Hay-McCutcheon M, Brown CJ, Abbas PJ. (2005) An analysis of the impact of auditory-nerve adaptation on behavioral measures of temporal integration in cochlear implant recipients. *J Acoust Soc Am.* 118, 1–14.

Hooper RE, Bergholtz LM, Mehta DC. (1977) Electrocochleography: a comparison of action potential and behavioral thresholds. *Scand Audiol.* 6, 99–104.

Hudspeth AJ. (1989) How the ear's works work. *Nature.* 341, 397–404.

Hughes ML, Brown CJ, Abbas PJ, et al. (2000) Comparison of EAP thresholds with MAP levels in the Nucleus 24 cochlear implant: data from children. *Ear Hear.* 21, 164–174.

Kiang NYS, Moxon EC. (1972) Physiological considerations in artificial stimulation of the inner ear. *Ann Otol.* 81, 714–730.

Kiang NYS, Moxon EC, Kahn AR. (1976) The relationship of gross potentials recorded from the cochlea to single-unit activity in the auditory nerve. In: Rubin RJ, Elberling C, Salomon G, eds. *Electrocochleography.* Baltimore: University Park Press; pp 95–115.

Kiang NYS, Watanabe T, Thomas EC, Clark LF. (1965) *Discharge Patterns of Single Auditory Nerve: Fibers in the Cat's Auditory Nerve.* Cambridge, MA: MIT Press.

Kim HH, Kumar A, Battista RA, Wiet, RJ. (2005) Electrocochleography in patients with Ménière's disease. *Am J Otol.* 26, 128–131.

Laureano AN, McGrady MD, Campbell KC. (1995) Comparison of tympanic membrane–recorded electrocochleography and the auditory brainstem response in threshold determination. *Am J Otol.* 16, 209–215.

Levine SC, Margolis RH, Daly KA. (1998) Use of electrocochleography in the diagnosis of Ménière's disease. *Laryngoscope.* 108, 993–1000.

Levine SC, Margolis RH, Fournier EM, Winzenburg SM. (1992) Tympanic electrocochleography for evaluation of endolymphatic hydrops. *Laryngoscope.* 102, 614–622.

Liberman MC. (1978) Auditory-nerve responses from cats raised in a low-noise chamber. *J Acoust Soc Am.* 63, 442.

Lim DJ. (1980) Cochlear anatomy related to cochlear micromechanics. A review. *J Acoust Soc Am.* 67, 1686–1695.

Margolis RH, Levine SM, Fournier MA, Hunter LL, Smith LL, Lilly DJ. (1992) Tympanic electrocochleography: normal and abnormal patterns of response. *Audiology.* 31, 18–24.

Margolis RH, Rieks D, Fournier EM, Levine SE. (1995) Tympanic electrocochleography for diagnosis of Ménière's disease. *Arch Otolaryngol Head Neck Surg.* 121, 44–55.

Mason SM, Cope Y, Garnham J, et al. (2001) Intra-operative recordings of electrically evoked auditory nerve action potentials in young children by use of neural response telemetry with the Nucleus CI24M cochlear implant. *Br J Audiol.* 35, 225–235.

Ménière P. (1861) Pathologic auriculaire. Memoire sur les lesions de l'oreille interne donnant lieu a des symptoms de congestion cerebrale applectiforme. *Gazzett Medicine.* 16, 88–89.

Moller A. (2000) *Hearing: Its Physiology and Pathophysiology.* San Diego: Academic Press.

Moller AR, Jannetta PJ. (1981) Compound action potentials recorded intracranially from the auditory nerve in man. *Exp Neurol.* 74, 862–874.

Moller AR, Jannetta PJ. (1985) Neural generators of the auditory brainstem response. In Jacobson JT, ed. *The Auditory Brain Stem Response.* San Diego: College-Hill Press Inc.

Nikolopoulos TP, Mason SM, Gibbin KP, O'Donoghue GM. (2000) The prognostic value of promontory electric auditory brain stem response in pediatric cochlear implantation. *Ear Hear.* 21, 236–241.

Pappas DG Jr., Pappas DG Sr., Carmichael L, Hyatt DP, Toohey LM. (2000) Extratympanic electrocochleography: diagnostic and predictive value. *Am J Otol.* 21, 81–87.

Pickles JO. (1988) *An Introduction to the Physiology of Hearing.* London: Academic Press.

Rhode WS. (1971) Observations of the vibration of the basilar membrane in squirrel monkeys using the Mossbauer technique. *J Acoust Soc Am.* 49, 1218–1231.

Ruben R, Hudson W, Chiong A. (1963) Anatomical and physiological effects of chronic section of the eighth nerve in cat. *Acta Otolaryngol.* 55, 473–484.

Ruth RA, Lambert PR. (1989) Comparison of tympanic membrane to promontory electrode recordings of electrocochleographic responses in patients with Ménière's disease. *Otolaryngol Head Neck Surg.* 100, 546–552.

Ruth RA, Lambert PR, Ferraro JA. (1988) Electrocochleography: methods and clinical applications. *Am J Otol.* 9 (suppl), 1–11.

Ruth RA, Mills JA, Ferraro JA. (1988) Use of disposable ear canal electrodes in auditory brainstem response testing. *Am J Otol.* 9, 310–315.

Ryerson SG, Beagley HA. (1981) Brainstem electric responses and electrocochleography: a comparison of threshold sensitivities in children. *Br J Audiol.* 15, 41–48.

Schlake HP, Milewski C, Goldbrunner RH, Kindgen A, Riemann R, Helms J, Roosen K. (2001) Combined intra-operative monitoring of hearing by means of auditory brainstem responses (ABR) and transtympanic electrocochleography (ECochG) during surgery of intra- and extrameatal acoustic neurinomas. *Acta Neurochir.* 143, 985–995.

Schmidt PH, Eggermont JJ, Odenthal DW. (1974) Study of Ménière's disease by electrocochleography. *Acta Otolaryngol.* 316 (suppl), 75–84.

Schoonhoven R, Fabius MA, Grote JJ. (1995) Input/output curves to tone bursts and clicks in extratympanic and transtympanic electrocochleography. *Ear Hear.* 16, 619–630.

Schoonhoven R, Lamore PJ, de Laat JA, Grote JJ. (1999) The prognostic value of electrocochleography in severely hearing-impaired infants. *Audiology.* 38, 141–154.

Schoonhoven R, Prijs VF, Grote JJ. (1996) Response thresholds in electrocochleography and their relation to the pure tone audiogram. *Ear Hear.* 17, 266–275.

Sellick PM, Patuzzi R, Johnstone BM. (1982) Measurement of basilar membrane motion in the guinea pig using the Mossbauer technique. *J Acoust Soc Am.* 72, 131–141.

Seyle K, Brown CJ. (2002) Speech perception using maps based on neural response telemetry (NRT) measures. *Ear Hear.* 23, 72S–79S.

Silverstein H, McDaniel AB, Norrell H. (1985) Hearing preservation after acoustic neuroma surgery using intraoperative direct eighth cranial nerve monitoring. *Am J Otol.* Suppl, 99–106.

Silverstein H, Wazen J, Norrell H, Hyman SM. (1984) Retro-labyrinthine vestibular neurectomy with simultaneous monitoring of VIIIth nerve action potentials and electrocochleography. *Am J Otol.* 5, 552–555.

Smith L, Simmons FB. (1983) Estimating eighth nerve survival by electrical stimulation. *Ann Otol Rhinol Laryngol.* 76, 427–435.

Smoorenburg GF, Willeboer C, van Dijk JE. (2002) Speech perception in Nucleus CI24M cochlear implant users with processor settings based on electrically evoked compound action potential thresholds. *Audiol Neurol Otol.* 7, 335–347.

Sohmer H, Feinmesser M. (1967) Cochlear action potentials recorded from the external ear in man. *Ann Otol Rhinol Laryngol.* 76, 427–436.

Stanton SG, Cashman MZ, Harrison RV, Nedzelski JM, Rowed DW. (1989) Cochlear nerve action potentials during cerebellopontine angle surgery: relationship of latency, amplitude, and threshold measurements to hearing. *Ear Hear.* 10, 23–28.

Starr A, Sininger Y, Nguyen T, Michalewski HJ, Oba S, Abdala C. (2001) Cochlear receptor (microphonic and summating potentials, otoacoustic emissions) and auditory pathway (auditory brain stem potentials) activity in auditory neuropathy. *Ear Hear.* 22, 91–99.

Stypulkowski PH, Staller SJ. (1987) Clinical evaluation of a new ECoG recording electrode. *Ear Hear.* 8, 304–310.

Tasaki I, Davis H, Eldridge DH. (1954) Exploration of cochlear potentials in guinea pig with microelectrode. *J Acoust Soc Am.* 26, 765–773.

Tasaki I, Davis H, Legouix, JP. (1951) The space-time pattern of the cochlear microphonics (guinea pig) as recorded by differential electrodes. *J Acoust Soc Am.* 24, 502–519.

Teas DC, Eldredge DH, Davis H. (1962) Cochlear response to acoustic transients: an interpretation of whole-nerve action potentials. *J Acoust Soc Am.* 34, 1438–1459.

Van Deelen GW, Ruding PR, Veldman JE, Huizing EH, Smoorenburg GF. (1987) Electrocochleographic study of experimentally induced endolymphatic hydrops. *Arch Otol Rhinol Laryngol.* 244, 167–173.

van den Honert C, Stypulkowski P. (1986) Characterization of the electrically evoked auditory brainstem response (ABR) in cats and humans. *Hear Res.* 7, 381–304.

Von Bekesy G. (1960) *Experiments in Hearing.* New York: McGraw-Hill.

Wazen JJ. (1994) Intraoperative monitoring of auditory function: experimental observation and new applications. *Laryngoscope.* 104, 446–455.

Westerman LA, Smith RL. (1984) Rapid and short-term adaptation in auditory nerve responses. *Hear Res.* 15, 249–260.

Wever EG, Bray C. (1930) Action currents in the auditory nerve response to acoustic stimulation. *Proc Natl Acad Sci USA.* 16, 344–350.

Wever EG, Lawrence M. (1954) *Physiological Acoustics.* Princeton: Princeton University Press.

Wilson BS, Finley CC, Lawson DT, Zerbi M. (1997) Temporal representations with cochlear implants. *Am J Otol.* 18, S30–S34.

Winzenburg SM, Margolis RH, Levine SC, Haines SJ, Fournier EM. (1993) Tympanic and transtympanic electrocochleography in acoustic neuroma and vestibular nerve section surgery. *Am J Otol.* 14, 63–69.

Wong SH, Gibson WP, Sanli H. (1997) Use of transtympanic round window electrocochleography for threshold estimations in children. *Am J Otol.* 18, 632–636.

Wuyts FL, Van de Heyning PH, Van Spaendonck MP, Molenberghs G. (1997) A review of electrocochleography: instrumentation settings and meta-analysis of criteria for diagnosis of endolymphatic hydrops. *Acta Otolaryngol.* 526 (suppl), 14–20.

Yoshie N, Ohashi T, Suzuki T. (1967) Non-surgical recording of auditory nerve action potentials in man. *Laryngoscope.* 177, 76–85.

13 Auditory Brainstem Response: Differential Diagnosis

Manuel Don and Betty Kwong

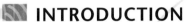 INTRODUCTION

In this chapter, we discuss how the auditory brainstem response (ABR) can be used for differential diagnosis of diseases of the eighth nerve and brainstem, as well as cochlear diseases, in particular, Ménière's disease with cochlear hydrops. In our review of the ABR as a peripheral neurodiagnostic tool, we discuss the following: (1) what an ABR represents; (2) criteria for evaluating an ABR measure; (3) current standard ABR measures; (4) recently developed ABR measures—the Stacked ABR and the cochlear hydrops analysis masking procedure (CHAMP); (5) retrocochlear and cochlear pathologies; (6) a guideline for clinical evaluation; and finally, (7) clinical cases.

WHAT AN ABR REPRESENTS

To understand how the ABR can be used for diagnosis, we need to understand its relevant underlying mechanical, physiologic, and neurophysiologic bases. As shown in earlier chapters and in Figure 13.1, the ABR is composed of several voltage deflections occurring within the first 15 ms after stimulus onset. These deflections (peaks and troughs) represent far-field synchronous activity produced by onset responses of neural elements and abrupt bends in the neural fiber tracts of the eighth nerve and the auditory brainstem pathway (Stegeman et al., 1987; Deupree and Jewett, 1988). The major measures of the ABR are the latency and amplitude of its peaks.

Peak Latencies

The most widely used ABR measure is the latency of a component peak. The latency of a peak is simply the time after stimulus onset that a given peak occurs. Figure 13.1 shows the latencies of the three major peaks (waves I, III, and V) in an ABR to a 63-dB normal-hearing level (nHL) click stimulus in a normal-hearing individual. ABR latencies are used in clinical applications because they are robust measures. In addition, latency measures are virtually unaffected by variations in the positions of the recording electrodes. However, peak latency may be difficult to determine accurately if the amount of residual noise in the average is too high. Peaks in the residual noise may add to the response peaks and alter their latencies. We address the effects of residual noise levels when we discuss amplitude measures later in this chapter.

Peak latencies are determined by a number of mechanical and physiologic processes in the cochlea, auditory nerve, and brainstem, including (1) the delay in the cochlea to the site of activation (cochlear transport time); (2) the filter impulse response time at the site of activation (cochlear filter build-up time); (3) the synaptic delay between the inner hair cells (IHCs) and the auditory nerve fibers, and finally, (4) the neural conduction time and any intervening synaptic delays to the point in the brainstem pathway responsible for the peak activity. (Don et al. [1998] discuss these processes in detail.) Thus, nearly all cochlear and retrocochlear processes affect the latency of the peak neural activity. Typically, broadband stimuli (e.g., clicks) activate the high-frequency region first. Because of the high traveling wave velocity in the basal part of the cochlea, the neural activity is strongly

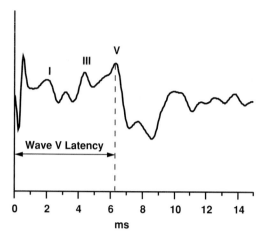

FIGURE 13.1 Wave V latency measure: A standard auditory brainstem response (ABR) response to 63-dB normal hearing level (nHL) click stimulus. The peaks of waves I, III, and V are labeled. Time on the abscissa is in milliseconds after stimulus onset. Latency of the peak of wave V is the time from the onset of the stimulus to the point of maximum deflection. The diagnostic question is whether this latency is abnormally prolonged.

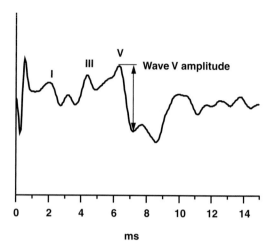

FIGURE 13.2 Wave V amplitude measure: The amplitude of wave V is the difference in magnitude between the peak of wave V and the succeeding trough (*arrow*). The diagnostic question is whether this amplitude is abnormally small. The diagnostic criterion must consider other factors (e.g., hearing loss) that can reduce the amplitude.

synchronized. This strong synchronization and early activity result in the domination of wave V peak latencies by high-frequency fibers. Although there is considerable neural activity generated from more apical, lower-frequency regions of the cochlea, it is usually phase canceled by activity from the more basal, high-frequency regions. If high-frequency regions are compromised (e.g., cochlear hearing loss), then uncanceled activity from more apical regions could dominate the response. The peak latency would then be longer, reflecting this later activation in the cochlea. Thus, the amount and configuration of hearing loss will affect latency measures.

Another major factor that determines peak latency is the level of stimulation. Peak latencies will decrease as stimulus levels increase; plots describing this relationship are referred to as latency-intensity functions. Other factors that affect latency besides the place of generation along the cochlea are age, head size, body core temperature, and gender (Don et al., 1993; Chapters 11 and 14).

Peak Amplitudes

The amplitude of an ABR component is typically measured from the peak of the component to its succeeding trough (Fig. 13.2). The amplitude depends on the amount of synchronized neural activity and varies with level of stimulation (Schwartz and Berry, 1985), hearing loss (Picton et al., 1977), neurologic pathology (Starr and Achor, 1975; Sohmer, 1983), and age (Allison et al., 1984; Psatta and Matei, 1988). These factors affect the amount of neural activity generated, the degree of synchronization among neural elements activated,

or both. In addition, as with latency measures, accurate peak amplitudes may be difficult to determine if the residual noise in the average is too high.

▨ CRITERIA FOR EVALUATING AUDITORY BRAINSTEM RESPONSE MEASURES

Defining Sensitivity and Specificity

The diagnostic value and limitation of an ABR measure for a given diagnosis can be defined quantitatively by its *sensitivity* and *specificity*. Investigations of current standard ABR measures often provide sensitivity and specificity values. However, one cannot compare these values to determine which measure is better without understanding how they were determined. Therefore, a thorough discussion of the issues of sensitivity and specificity is critical. One of the main neurodiagnostic applications of ABR measures is in the detection of eighth-nerve tumors. Therefore, we use examples of these ABR measures in our discussion of sensitivity and specificity. Note that nearly all "eighth-nerve" tumors are vestibular schwannomas arising from the vestibular nerve. However, for simplicity, throughout this chapter, we refer to these vestibular schwannomas as eighth-nerve or acoustic tumors.

We define the *sensitivity* of an ABR measure as the percentage of tumor cases detected (i.e., the true-positive rate). The *specificity* of an ABR measure is defined as the percentage of *non-tumor* cases that are correctly identified (i.e., the true-negative rate). Sensitivity and specificity depend on the diagnostic criterion and the amount of separation between the distributions of values of the ABR measure for tumor and non-tumor subjects. For a given measure, changing the diagnostic criterion to increase the sensitivity will decrease the specificity, and conversely, changing the criterion to increase the specificity will decrease the sensitivity. An ABR measure characterized by only its sensitivity without its specificity must be viewed cautiously.

In addition, a meaningful comparison of the sensitivity and specificity of ABR measures across published studies is difficult. First, there may be differences between the studies in the proportion of difficult cases (i.e., cases in which the values of the ABR measure result in false negatives or false positives) in the test populations. For example, small tumors are often missed (false-negative results) when standard ABR measures are used. Thus, for the same ABR measure and diagnostic criterion, sensitivity would be greater in a study of a test population with very few small tumors than in a study of a test population with many small tumors. Second, the criterion selected for diagnosis of a tumor may be different across studies. For example, if one study used the criterion that the value of the ABR measure must exceed the mean of the non-tumor population by one standard deviation, then sensitivity would be greater and specificity poorer than those

in another study that used a criterion of two standard deviations. Third, the medical guidelines used by the physician to decide which patients to include in the magnetic resonance imaging (MRI) test population may differ across studies. For each subject in a study's test population, the actual presence or absence of a tumor must be determined to calculate the sensitivity and specificity of the ABR measure. Because an MRI is used to make that final determination, the study's ABR test population is usually composed of patients who have been sent for an MRI. Thus, the physician's medical decisions determine the test population composition, which in turn affects the sensitivity and specificity values.

Table 13.1 illustrates how sensitivity and specificity values depend on the composition of the test population. Suppose that, of 110 individuals, five have small (≤1.0 cm) tumors, five have medium/large (>1.0 cm) tumors, and the remaining 100 have no tumors. The diagnostic criterion of the ABR measure used correctly identifies only the five larger tumors (i.e., five true-positive and five false-negative patients) and 90 of the 100 non-tumor patients (i.e., 90 true-negative and 10 false-positive patients). In Clinic X, the physicians use imaging guidelines that send all 110 patients for MRI. Clinic X would then report 50% sensitivity (only

---

TABLE 13.1   Dependence of sensitivity and specificity values on population composition

Overall Patient Population A: N = 110

Eighth-nerve Tumors: N = 10
(5 small ≤ 1.0 cm)
(5 med/large > 1.0 cm)
Non-Tumor: N = 100

Clinic X : All 110 patients sent for MRI
(Test Population for X: N = 110)

MRI - Reference for correct identification of all 110 Patients

ABR - Correctly identifies:
5 tumors > 1.0 cm = 5 true-positives
90 non-tumors = 90 true-negatives
Incorrectly identifies:
5 tumors ≤ 1.0 cm = 5 false negatives
10 non-tumor = 10 false-positives

Sensitivity: 5 of 10 tumors detected = **50%**
Specificity: 90 of 100 correctly identified = **90%**

Clinic Z : 25 patients sent for MRI; (5 med/large tumor > 1.0 cm &
20 non-tumor including 10 false positive cases)
(Test Population for Z: N = 25)

MRI - Reference for correct identification of all 25 Patients
ABR - Correctly identifies:
5 tumors > 1.0 cm = 5 true-positives
10 non-tumors = 10 true-negatives
Incorrectly identifies:
10 non-tumor = 10 false-positives

Sensitivity: 5 of 5 tumors detected = **100%**
Specificity: 10 of 20 correctly identified = **50%**

five of the 10 tumor patients sent for imaging were correctly identified by the ABR measure) and 90% specificity (90 of the 100 non-tumor patients sent for imaging were correctly identified by the ABR measure) for the ABR measure. Suppose the same 110 patients are examined in another clinical setting, Clinic Z, which uses the same ABR measure and diagnostic criterion. However, the physicians in Clinic Z use different imaging guidelines, so only the five medium/large tumor patients and 20 (including the 10 false-positive patients) of the 100 non-tumor patients are sent for imaging. Clinic Z would then report a sensitivity of 100% (all five tumor cases sent for imaging were correctly identified by the ABR measure) and a specificity of only 50% (10 of the 20 non-tumor patients sent for imaging were correctly identified by the ABR measure). For the same ABR measure, Clinic X would claim poor sensitivity but high specificity, while Clinic Z would claim excellent sensitivity but poor specificity. Thus, for the same ABR measure and the same ABR diagnostic criterion, the reported sensitivity and specificity can vary widely because the test population composition for the ABR study is determined by the physician's MRI guidelines.

░ CURRENT STANDARD AUDITORY BRAINSTEM RESPONSE MEASURES

Over the past 25 years, a large number of studies investigating the clinical applications of ABRs have been published. It is clear that retrocochlear lesions affecting the auditory pathway often show abnormalities in ABR measures.

In this section, we review the standard ABR measures that have been used for acoustic tumor detection and discuss the reasons why some of these measures have been abandoned. ABR measures are also used by neurologists to assess brainstem pathology in general, but we focus on acoustic tumors because this is the main retrocochlear problem encountered by audiologists. Most of the standard ABR measures involve abnormal latency shifts and/or reductions in peak amplitude of the components.

Latency Measures

The rationale for using latency measures is the assumption that the tumor exerts pressure on the auditory nerve, causing a change in the transmission time of neural fiber activity. This change results in poorer synchronization and delays in neural activation, leading to longer peak latencies of the combined activity of the neural fibers.

WAVE V LATENCY: COMPARISON WITH DISTRIBUTION OF NORMAL VALUES

Description
The simplest time abnormality noted in early acoustic tumor research was that the wave V latency of the ABR in tumor patients was delayed relative to the distribution of latency

values from non-tumor, normal-hearing individuals (Stephens and Thornton, 1976; Starr and Hamilton, 1976; Terkildsen et al., 1977). For a given stimulus intensity, a mean latency value and standard deviation for wave V are computed for a group of normal-hearing individuals free of neurologic disease and acoustic tumors. The value obtained in the patient is compared to this mean value, and if it exceeds the mean value by some number of standard deviations, the test result is positive for the presence of a tumor. As discussed previously, the number of standard deviations chosen as the diagnostic criterion will affect the sensitivity and specificity of the measure. The number selected usually has been empirically determined to achieve acceptable levels of sensitivity and specificity.

Limitations
Three major problems have led to the abandonment of the simple wave V latency measure in detection of acoustic tumors. First, as mentioned earlier, peripheral hearing losses can affect the latency of wave V. The effect of peripheral hearing loss on wave V latency depends on both the type and amount of loss, as well as the configuration of the hearing loss (Gorga et al., 1985; Keith and Greville, 1987; Kirsh et al., 1992; Shepard et al., 1992; Lightfoot, 1993; Watson, 1996). The underlying basis for the increase in latency of wave V in response to a simple click stimulus differs with the type of peripheral hearing loss. For conductive impairments, the increase in latency is due to a simple reduction in the amount of acoustic energy reaching the cochlea (i.e., the physical level of stimulation). The latency of wave V increases with reductions in physical stimulus levels (Hecox and Galambos, 1974).

The effect of sensory losses on wave V latency is more complex. Sensory losses, in contrast to conductive losses, do not cause a reduction of the acoustic energy reaching the cochlea. The increases in wave V latency observed with sensory impairments are related to the configuration of the hearing losses and not to a reduction in the stimulus levels. In normal-hearing individuals, the latency of wave V in the standard response to a simple high-level click stimulus is determined by neural activity initiated from the high-frequency regions of the cochlea. Not surprisingly, it has been shown that a normal latency-intensity function can be obtained from patients with low-frequency hearing loss (1 kHz and below) because of their normal higher-frequency hearing (Don et al., 1979). This domination of latency by the higher frequencies occurs because, as mentioned earlier, their earlier response activity phase cancels later activity from more apical, lower-frequency regions of the cochlea. As stimulus levels decrease, the latency becomes more influenced by middle-frequency regions of the cochlea (Eggermont and Don, 1980). In many sensory losses, there tends to be greater loss in the high frequencies. If activity from these higher frequencies no longer dominates the response, then the latency of the ABR will be greater, reflecting the shift in domination to activity from later-occurring lower frequencies.

Thus, peripheral high-frequency hearing loss can result in an apparent abnormal prolongation of the wave V latency of the standard ABR to clicks, leading to an increase in false-positive test results. Hearing loss per se does not cause true prolongation of neural activation. In fact, Don et al. (1998) demonstrated that, in an ABR initiated from a specific frequency region of the cochlea, the latency of wave V *decreases* rather than increases with hearing loss in that region.

The second problem with a simple wave V latency measure is the variability or relatively wide distribution of wave V latencies across non-tumor, normal-hearing individuals (Rowe, 1978; Chiappa et al., 1979). Some individuals have relatively short wave V latencies. If a tumor occurred in one of these individuals, it could cause a significant prolongation in latency, but the latency itself might not be abnormally long because it was initially relatively short. If the criterion latency is reduced (i.e., shorter latency) to detect these cases, then non-tumor individuals with relatively long latencies will be wrongly identified as having a tumor (false positive). Thus, because of the broad distribution of normal latency values, a latency criterion that would yield a reasonable sensitivity would have very poor specificity.

The third problem with the simple wave V latency measure is that this latency is affected by a number of other factors, such as head size, core body temperature, and gender (see review in Don et al. [1993]). Thus, this measure would require a number of other nonauditory measurements to determine the appropriate reference group for comparison.

INTERAURAL COMPARISONS OF PEAK LATENCIES

Description

This measure compares the patient's ear in which a tumor is suspected with the patient's nonsuspected ear (Selters and Brackmann, 1977; Clemis and Mitchell, 1977; Thomsen et al., 1978). This comparison, shown in Figure 13.3, is an interaural peak delay measure often referred to as the IT5 (for interaural wave V). The IT5 is computed by subtracting the wave V latency of the nonsuspected ear from the wave V latency of the suspected ear. In normal-hearing individuals free of neurologic or otologic problems, the expected difference between ears is nearly zero, that is, the latency of wave V for the two ears is essentially the same. According to Selters and Brackmann (1977), if the difference is greater than 0.2 ms after compensating for hearing loss (described later), the test result is positive for a tumor. The main advantage of this interaural measure is in detection of tumors in individuals with relatively short wave V latencies and correct identification of non-tumor individuals with relatively long wave V latencies (second problem discussed earlier). In individuals whose wave V latencies are relatively short, the tumor may cause a change in latency that is abnormally long for the individual (comparison with the non-tumor ear) but not for the population (comparison with the distribution). The IT5 would detect tumors in these individuals and have better sensitivity than the simple wave V latency measure discussed

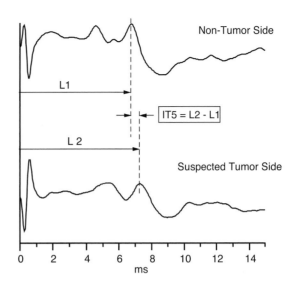

FIGURE 13.3 Interaural wave V latency comparison (IT5): The IT5 is computed by subtracting the wave V peak latency measured in the non-tumor ear from the peak latency in the ear suspected of tumor in the same individual. After correcting for hearing loss, if the IT5 is greater than 0.2 ms, then the test result is positive for an eighth-nerve tumor.

earlier. This measure would also have better specificity because non-tumor patients whose simple latencies normally exceed the requisite number of standard deviations from the mean of the normal distribution will have normal interaural delays and a correct negative diagnosis for a tumor.

As described earlier, sensory hearing loss may result in a latency increase if there is significant loss in the high frequencies. Selters and Brackmann (1977) empirically developed a formula to correct the IT5 measure for the amount of hearing loss. Based on a large number of tumor patients, they found that hearing loss at 4 kHz was critical for the IT5 measure. Since the IT5 involves a comparison between the individual's two ears, both ears must be corrected for any high-frequency loss before calculating the IT5. For each ear, they subtract 0.1 ms from the ear's wave V latency for every 10 dB of hearing loss above 50 dB of loss at 4 kHz. If the hearing loss at 4 kHz is 50 dB or less, no correction to the wave V latency is made. Then, using the corrected latencies, they calculate the IT5 (latency of suspected ear minus latency of nonsuspected ear). This correction resulted in higher sensitivity and specificity for the measure. Later in this chapter, we present some clinical cases to illustrate the use of this measure. If the corrections for hearing loss are not made, there are two possible situations that can lead to a misdiagnosis.

1. If the suspected ear has no tumor but sufficient high-frequency loss to cause a significant latency shift (>0.2 ms) and the nonsuspected ear has normal hearing, then the IT5 will be positive for a tumor. This error will reduce the specificity of the IT5 measure.

2. If the suspected ear has a tumor and the nonsuspected ear has sufficient high-frequency loss to cause a significant latency shift, then the IT5 may not exceed 0.2 ms. In this case, the latency shift caused by the tumor is offset by the latency shift in the comparison non-tumor ear caused by sensory hearing loss. This error will reduce the sensitivity of the IT5 measure.

Limitations

The IT5 appears to be one of the best standard ABR measures (Bauch et al., 1996). However, although the diagnostic criterion of IT5 >0.2 ms has been effective in detecting tumors larger than 1.0 cm, its sensitivity to smaller tumors is only about 80% (Selesnick and Jackler, 1993; Chandrasekhar et al., 1995). This major limitation is discussed on page 274. In addition, because the IT5 requires a non-tumor ear for comparison, it should not be used when bilateral tumors are suspected, as in neurofibromatosis II (NF2) patients. Furthermore, the IT5 is greatly compromised if the nonsuspected ear has a greater than moderate hearing loss resulting in absent or poorly defined ABR waveforms. Finally, the formula to correct for hearing loss assumes that the high frequencies begin to lose their domination of the latency and lower frequencies begin to dominate only when the hearing loss exceeds 50 dB at 4 kHz. In fact, even greater latency shifts may occur if there is a 50-dB loss or greater at 2 and 3 kHz as well (Eggermont and Don, 1986). Thus, this measure is most useful in detecting medium to large (>1 cm) unilateral tumors when there is relatively little impairment of the nonsuspected ear.

Interpeak Delays (I-V and I-III)

Description

Another latency abnormality noted in patients with acoustic tumors was the prolongation of the interval between peaks within a response waveform, particularly the delay between the peaks of waves I and V or I and III (Coats and Martin, 1978; Eggermont et al., 1980; Portmann et al., 1980). These early studies indicated that these interpeak intervals were prolonged in tumor patients but unaffected by conductive or cochlear hearing loss. The interpeak delay, illustrated in Figure 13.4, is presumed to reflect central conduction time up the auditory brainstem pathway. The basic assumption is that peripheral hearing problems (conductive or sensory) do not affect the neural transmission time as measured by the interpeak delay, but acoustic tumors do. Because of the location of the tumor on the eighth nerve, the specific delay is between the peaks of wave I and subsequent waves (III or V). In males, the I-V delay is normally between 4.0 and 4.2 ms, and the I-III delay is about 2.0 to 2.2 ms; in females, the delays are slightly shorter (Starr and Achor, 1975; Rowe, 1978; Chiappa et al., 1979; Elberling and Parbo, 1987). The advantage of these delay measures is that they are intra-aural; thus, the patient's nonsuspected ear is not used. If the delays are abnormally long, then the test result is positive, and a tumor is suspected. The accuracy of these measures depends on the

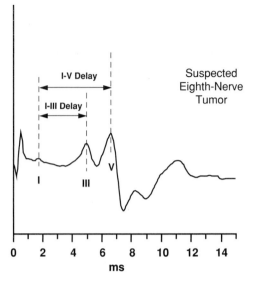

FIGURE 13.4   Wave I-V and I-III delays: The I-V and I-III delays are the latency differences between the peak of wave I and the peaks of waves V and III, respectively, in the auditory brainstem response (ABR) from the suspected ear. If either of these intervals is abnormally prolonged, then the test result is positive for an eighth-nerve tumor. (Adapted from Don M, Masuda A, Nelson RA, Brackmann DE. [1997] Successful detection of small acoustic tumors using the stacked derived-band ABR method. *Am J Otol.* 18, 608–621, with permission of the publisher.]

definition of "abnormally long." Some studies used the criterion of a specific delay, for example, a I-V delay of 4.4 ms or more (Wilson et al., 1992), whereas others used two or three standard deviations from the mean for normal-hearing subjects (Eggermont et al., 1980; Legatt et al., 1988; Grabel et al., 1991). The I-V delay is used in most clinical applications of an interpeak measure, so the following discussion focuses on the limitations of this measure.

Limitations

The first major problem with the standard I-V measure is that cochlear hearing loss in the mid-to-high frequencies often results in poor or absent wave I responses, making the I-V interval difficult or impossible to measure. The second problem, similar to the major limitation of the IT5, is its insensitivity to small tumors (Eggermont et al., 1980; Chandrasekhar et al., 1995). This lack of sensitivity is a fundamental problem with any latency measure, and we discuss this issue in depth on page 274.

The third problem is that the delay does not necessarily represent only central conduction time, as assumed earlier, when the ABRs are obtained with simple click stimuli. As described in Chapter 11, the click stimulus is a broadband signal that stimulates much of the cochlea. Therefore, the I-V delay in the standard ABR to clicks reflects not only neural conduction time, but also differences in response times (transport and filter build-up times) of the different parts of the cochlea that dominate and determine the latency of waves I and V. It has been demonstrated (Don and Eggermont, 1978; Eggermont and Don, 1986) that there is differential cochlear representation of waves I and V. Thus, it is not surprising that the I-V delay of standard ABRs is affected by stimulus level (Stockard et al., 1979) and amount and configuration of hearing loss (Coats and Martin, 1978; Sturzebecher et al., 1985; Keith and Greville, 1987; Kirsh et al., 1992; Watson, 1996). The effects of level, particularly for levels above 60 to 70 dB nHL, and hearing loss on the I-V delay appear to be relatively small (Kirsh et al., 1992). Nonetheless, the differential cochlear representation of waves I and V may, in some cases, confound the interpretation of the measured I-V delay. True neural conduction time can be estimated with waves I and V only when both waves represent activity initiated from the same place-specific region of the cochlea. A high-pass masking technique (Don and Eggermont, 1978; Parker and Thornton, 1978a) to obtain derived-band ABRs initiated from place-specific areas of the cochlea is discussed in detail later in this chapter. The I-V delay in the derived-band ABR from a place-specific region of the cochlea is largely independent of stimulus intensity (Eggermont and Don, 1980) and cochlear hearing loss (preliminary work in authors' laboratory), as well as frequency place in the cochlea (Don and Eggermont, 1978; Ponton et al., 1992). Because this true interpeak delay from cochlear place-specific ABRs is relatively independent of stimulus level and hearing loss, it avoids the problems of conductive and sensory hearing loss. Note that the I-V delay from either standard or cochlear place-specific ABRs is gender dependent (Elberling and Parbo, 1987; Sabo et al., 1992; Watson, 1996, Don et al., 1993), and reference norms for each gender must be established.

The fourth problem with the I-V standard ABR measure is that the intra-aural delay is compared to a distribution of values obtained from non-tumor individuals. As with the simple delay measure, the prolonged interpeak delay caused by a tumor may not exceed the diagnostic criterion value if a patient normally has relatively short interpeak intervals. Thus, false negatives will occur, resulting in decreased sensitivity. Similarly, non-tumor individuals with normally long I-V intervals that exceed the diagnostic criterion will be diagnosed as having a tumor, leading to false positives and decreased specificity. To address these problems, the following measure has been suggested.

INTERAURAL COMPARISON OF INTERPEAK DELAYS

Description

This is the same interpeak I-V delay described in the third measure noted earlier, except the interpeak reference is the patient's nonsuspected ear rather than the average of a group of normal-hearing individuals without tumors (Feblot and Uziel, 1982; Zollner and Eibach, 1981; Robinson and Rudge,

1983; Legatt et al., 1988; Gordon and Cohen, 1995). Note that, even though the computed difference uses the patient's nonsuspected ear, the determination of whether the difference is abnormal is still based on a distribution of the differences observed between ears for non-tumor individuals. Normally, the I-V delay is similar for both ears. This measure circumvents the problem with a patient who normally has relatively short interpeak intervals. In these patients, the I-V delay from the tumor ear may be within normal population limits but abnormally long with respect to the nonsuspected ear. Moreover, non-tumor patients with normally long I-V delays will be correctly identified because the inter-ear comparison will be normal. Thus, this I-V delay inter-ear comparison has the potential of achieving better sensitivity and specificity than comparison with the distribution of I-V delays from a population of non-tumor ears.

Limitations

The problems with this measure are the same as for the first three noted earlier for the interpeak I-V delay. In addition, the problem of an abnormal reference ear noted with the IT5 measure also applies. That is, in the rare cases involving bilateral tumors (i.e., NF2 patients), the I-V delay may be prolonged on both sides, and the interaural interpeak measure may not detect either tumor. Also, this measure requires good identification of wave I peak latencies in responses from not only one but both ears. As mentioned earlier, wave I peaks are often difficult to identify when the patients have mid- to high-frequency hearing losses.

MISCELLANEOUS LATENCY MEASURES

Other latency measures, such as latency-intensity functions (Legatt et al., 1988; Thomason et al., 1993), have also been examined. We have deliberately omitted a detailed review of these measures because they are less widely used, have not proven to be as effective as some of the latency measures discussed earlier, and are greatly affected by hearing loss. In fact, Bauch et al. (1996) claim that the best latency measures for detecting a tumor are the IT5 and the I-V delay.

GENERAL SUMMARY OF LATENCY MEASURES

The main problem with all of these latency measures is that they often fail to detect small (≤ 1.0 cm) acoustic tumors. ABR latencies are typically used in clinical applications because they are robust and fairly easy to measure. By definition, a robust measure tends to be insensitive to small perturbations. Thus, it is not too surprising that robust latency measures are insensitive to the small neural perturbations caused by small tumors. A more detailed explanation of this insensitivity to small tumors is presented later in the chapter.

Amplitude Measures

Peak amplitudes of components in an ABR depend on two equally important aspects of neural activity. First is the number of neural elements activated by the sound stimulus.

Second is the degree of synchronization of the activity of those neural elements. Thus, larger amplitudes may represent better synchronized activation of fewer elements rather than activation of larger numbers of neural elements. Amplitude measures should be very sensitive to the loss or desynchronization of eighth-nerve activity resulting from compression by an eighth-nerve tumor. The standard amplitude measures of ABR component peaks parallel those for latency measures discussed earlier.

WAVE V AMPLITUDE

Description

Similar to the simple wave V latency measure is the simple wave V amplitude measure. The amplitude is typically determined by the difference in magnitude between the peak of wave V and the succeeding trough (Fig. 13.2). The amplitude is then compared with those in a distribution of non-tumor, normal-hearing individuals to determine whether the amplitude is abnormally small. Over the years, many studies examined ABR amplitude measures in retrocochlear disease (Borg, 1982; Daly et al., 1977; Nodar and Kinney, 1980; Stephens and Thornton, 1976; Walser et al., 1982; Wielaard and Kemp, 1979; Zollner and Eibach, 1981). A special case of an amplitude measure is the absence of wave V, which often occurs when tumors are fairly large or the retrocochlear disease is extensive (Jerger et al., 1980; Cashman and Rossman, 1983; Fowler and Noffsinger, 1983; Musiek, 1982; Musiek et al., 1986; Prosser et al., 1984; Robinson and Rudge, 1983; Eggermont et al., 1980).

Limitations

In general, amplitude measures are successful in detecting large tumors that cause large reductions in wave V amplitudes. However, the overall conclusion is that because of the high variability of the simple wave V amplitude measure, it has poorer sensitivity to tumors than do latency measures. There are several reasons for the variable nature of simple amplitude measures in general.

1. *ABR electrical fields are weak.* The magnitude of the electrical activity recorded at the surface is very small, usually less than one microvolt (1 μV), because it originates from auditory brainstem structures that are deep in the skull. The amplitude or strength of an electrical field recorded at the surface of the head depends on the distance and orientation of the neural generators to the recording electrodes. Thus, individual variations in the neuroanatomy and anatomy, for example, head size (Stockard et al., 1979), skull thickness (Trune et al., 1988), and skin impedance (Beagley and Sheldrake, 1978), may affect amplitudes. In contrast, latencies are less affected by most of these individual variables.

2. *ABRs have poor signal-to-noise ratios (S/Ns).* Because the activity recorded at the surface is very small, ABRs have poor S/Ns, that is, low evoked potential amplitudes relative to the amplitude of the physiologic background

noise. Averaging a fixed number of sweeps does not guarantee that the residual noise in the average will be low enough for an accurate measure of the true amplitude of the response peak (Don and Elberling, 1994; 1996). Clinically, traces with poor S/Ns have produced major problems in identification of near-threshold responses and in reliable measurements of the components of the ABR for otoneurologic or neurologic diagnosis. Even after averaging, considerable residual noise can remain in the traces. The greater the residual noise, the more difficult it is to identify the peak and the succeeding trough for calculating the amplitude measures. In addition, peaks in the residual noise may add to the response peaks and alter their amplitudes. Thus, the uncertainties, inaccuracies, and failures that have occurred both in research and clinical applications of the ABRs may be attributed, to a large degree, to the influence of the variable residual background noise on ABR measures, particularly wave V amplitude. As discussed in previous chapters, there are several techniques to improve the S/N, such as filtering and averaging responses in the time domain. However, even with these techniques, the amount of residual noise in the ABR average is usually not controlled. In addition, the variable amount of residual noise in the average leads to variable peak amplitudes even when stimulus conditions are identical (Elberling and Don, 1984; Don and Elberling, 1994; 1996).

3. *Both the peak and trough must be identified.* Amplitude measures typically require identification of both the peak and the succeeding trough; latency measures require identification of only the peak. While identification of the peak can be difficult at times, trough identification can be equally problematic. Even when there is low residual noise in the average, identifying the peak and trough can be difficult because of great variations in waveform morphology. Therefore, amplitude measures are inherently more variable than latency measures because an additional component, a trough, must also be identified.

4. *Phase cancellation of neural elements can be significant.* The biphasic nature of the electrical neural activity means that, depending on the relative timing of activation, some neural elements can phase cancel the activity of others. In addition, a condition that causes a loss of phase-canceling neural activity could result in an increase in peak amplitude (Don et al., 1994; 1997). We mentioned earlier that, with broadband stimuli (e.g., clicks), phase cancellations of field activity from more apical regions of the cochlea occur, so that the resulting peaks in the response largely reflect activity from the most basal regions. In addition, it has been demonstrated (Don et al., 1994) that the large amplitude variations in the standard ABR to click stimuli are mainly the result of irregularities in cochlear response time (the degree of synchronization across the cochlea). Therefore, because of the variable amount of synchronization and

phase cancellation, simple amplitude measures of ABRs to clicks do not reflect the total neural response.

5. *Cochlear hearing loss complicates the interpretation of amplitude measures.* The effect of cochlear hearing loss on amplitudes of components, such as wave V, has been difficult to predict. It is obvious that the loss of activity caused by cochlear impairment should reduce the peak amplitude. However, it has been difficult to predict the amount of reduction in amplitude because of other major factors, such as synchronization and phase cancellation, that vary across individuals (Don et al., 1994; 1998).

All these limitations result in a wide distribution of wave V amplitudes in individuals without tumors. Thus, the interpretation of the amount of neural activity from simple peak amplitude measures can be difficult. It is easy to understand why peak amplitude has limited use in detecting acoustic tumors.

INTERAURAL WAVE V AMPLITUDE COMPARISON

Description

This interaural measure compares the wave V amplitude in the suspected ear to the wave V amplitude in the nonsuspected ear and is analogous to the IT5 latency comparison. As with the IT5 measure, the intent is to remove the intersubject variability by comparing results within an individual rather than with a non-tumor, normal-hearing population's distribution of values. Again, the assumption is that there is a very small difference in wave V amplitude between ears from the same individual. This intrasubject comparison may improve sensitivity by detecting tumors in subjects who normally have large wave V amplitudes and improve specificity by correctly diagnosing non-tumor subjects with small wave V amplitudes.

Limitations

The comparison between ears should help minimize amplitude variations due to subject variables and may reduce the variable effects of synchronization and phase cancellation, assuming that these factors are similar for the two ears. However, variable S/Ns and correcting or accounting for the effects of cochlear losses are still significant problems for this interaural amplitude measure. This measure is particularly limited when the nonsuspected ear has a significant cochlear loss. As with the IT5 latency measure, this interaural amplitude should not be used in cases where binaural tumors (e.g., NF2 patients) are suspected.

INTRA-AURAL WAVE V TO WAVE I AMPLITUDE RATIO

Description

This measure is the ratio of the amplitude of wave V to the amplitude of wave I, that is, the amplitude of wave V divided by the amplitude of wave I. In non-tumor patients, wave V is typically much greater than wave I. The rationale for this amplitude ratio, like that for the wave I-V delay, is the

assumption that the desynchronization or blocking of neural activity by the tumor occurs after wave I eighth-nerve activity. As a result, the amplitude of wave V should be reduced relative to wave I, and an abnormally small ratio indicates a tumor.

Limitations

Musiek et al. (1984) studied this amplitude ratio and found that normal-hearing subjects and cochlear hearing loss patients seldom had ratios less than 1. Therefore, they claimed that ratios less than 1 indicated the presence of a tumor. However, they found that only 44% of tumors were detected in this manner. In other words, while most individuals with ratios smaller than 1 had a tumor, more than half of the tumor patients had ratios greater than 1. Thus, this measure has poor sensitivity but good specificity. Other problems with this amplitude ratio are: (1) it depends on the presence of wave I, which is often absent in eighth-nerve tumor patients; (2) it may be more sensitive to variations in the audiometric configuration because the amplitude of wave I is more dependent than wave V on higher frequency regions of the cochlea (Don and Eggermont, 1978; Eggermont and Don, 1980); and (3) using a ratio of two measures that are highly variable results in an even more highly variable measure. These problems are the same ones that plague the interpeak I-V latency delay measure.

INTERAURAL WAVE V TO WAVE I AMPLITUDE RATIO

Description

This is similar to the third amplitude measure noted earlier, except the reference for the wave V to wave I amplitude ratio is the patient's nonsuspected ear instead of the distribution of values from a population of non-tumor individuals. The rationale for this measure is similar to that for the interpeak I-V latency delay comparison between ears of the same individual, discussed earlier. The interaural comparison within the same individual should improve the diagnosis of subjects who normally have much larger or much smaller wave V to wave I amplitude ratios than the mean of non-tumor individuals. While many of the tumor patients have wave V to wave I amplitude ratios greater than 1, indicating no tumor (Musiek et al., 1984), these ratios may be significantly smaller than the ratios from their non-tumor ears. Likewise, the few non-tumor subjects with low amplitude ratios in their suspected ear may have equally low amplitude ratios in their nonsuspected ear. This interaural comparison could improve both the sensitivity and specificity of the wave V to wave I amplitude ratio measure.

Limitations

While the comparison with the other ear may improve the sensitivity and specificity of this amplitude ratio measure, the other problems with the intra-aural wave V to wave I amplitude ratio noted earlier still apply and limit the value of this measure. Briefly, these are (1) the dependence on recording a measurable wave I, (2) the effect of the configuration of any cochlear sensory loss because of the differential dependence of waves I and V on different parts of the cochlea, and (3) the increased variability due to the use of a ratio of highly variable measures. One additional problem is determining how to correct for differences in sensory losses between ears.

Summary

The standard ABR measures reviewed in the previous sections are essentially the same and highly correlated. The main variation is the reference measure used for comparison. That is, we basically measure the latency of wave V and (1) compare it to the mean latency value for a population of non-tumor, normal-hearing individuals, (2) compare it to the latency of wave V of the opposite non-tumor ear, (3) subtract the latency of wave I of the same ear and compare it to the mean latency value for a population of non-tumor, normal-hearing individuals, or (4) subtract the latency of wave I and compare it to the V-I latency difference of the opposite non-tumor ear. Similarly, we measure the amplitude of wave V and (1) compare it to the mean amplitude value for a population of non-tumor, normal-hearing individuals, (2) compare it to the amplitude of wave V of the opposite non-tumor ear, (3) compute its ratio to the amplitude of wave I of the same ear and compare it to the mean ratio value for a population of non-tumor, normal-hearing individuals, or (4) compute its ratio to the amplitude of wave I and compare it to the ratio for the opposite non-tumor ear.

▨ CRITICAL EVALUATION OF STANDARD AUDITORY BRAINSTEM RESPONSE LATENCY AND AMPLITUDE MEASURES

Current Status of Standard Auditory Brainstem Response Measures

Prior to MRI, the ABR test was an important component of the clinical test battery for acoustic tumors. Early studies reported sensitivity of standard ABR measures in the 95% to 98% range (Selters and Brackmann, 1977; Barrs et al., 1985; Bauch et al., 1983; Josey et al., 1980), but these tumors were typically fairly large. Using estimates from computed tomography (CT) scans and surgical reports, Eggermont et al. (1980) examined the impact of tumor size on sensitivity and concluded that tumors smaller than 1.0 cm often go undetected by standard clinical ABR methodology. This conclusion is supported by later extensive studies comparing the sensitivity of this ABR methodology with gadolinium (Gd-DTPA)-enhanced MRI (Chandrasekhar et al., 1995; Selesnick and Jackler, 1993; Thomason et al., 1993; Kartush et al., 1992; Kotlarz et al., 1992; Wilson et al., 1992; Levine et al., 1991; Hendrix et al., 1990; Telian et al., 1989; Josey et al., 1988). These studies found that the standard

ABR latency measures discussed earlier were nearly 100% accurate in detecting all extracanalicular and intracanalicular tumors larger than 1.0 cm. However, for tumors smaller than 1.0 cm, the sensitivity of standard latency measures varied across studies from 63% to 93%, with corresponding false-negative rates ranging from 7% up to 37% (Bockenheimer et al., 1984; Dornhoffer et al., 1994). This wide range of sensitivity is probably due to the different diagnostic criteria selected (Don et al., 1997). In 1991, the National Institutes of Health Consensus Development Conference stated that the Gd-DTPA MRI is the "gold standard" for detection of a vestibular schwannoma. The Gd-DTPA MRI provides reliable identification, size, and location of tumors as small as 3.0 mm in the internal auditory canal region (House et al., 1986; Jackler et al., 1990).

Why Standard Auditory Brainstem Response Measures Cannot Detect Small Tumors

Two requirements for any ABR measure used for tumor detection are that (1) the tumor exerts sufficient pressure to desynchronize, block, or alter the conduction properties of eighth-nerve elements and (2) the tumor affects a sufficient number of those neural elements. Obviously, any ABR measure will fail if either of these two requirements is not met. However, for standard ABR latency measures such as the I-V and IT5 delays, there is an additional, third requirement: The tumor must affect the activity of those neural elements that determine the peak latency of the brainstem response to the stimulus. In other words, normal standard ABR latency measures are determined by only a subset of auditory nerve fibers. In particular, as discussed earlier, the latency of the standard ABR is determined by the high-frequency fibers. The high failure rate in detecting small intracanalicular tumors is not surprising because normal standard ABR latencies are possible if the synchronous activity of the high-frequency fibers that determine the latency is not sufficiently compromised by the tumor. Thus, even if a small tumor affected a substantial number of activated neural elements representing mid-to-low frequencies, the peak latency may not change much because the activity of these elements does not determine the peak latency of the standard ABR. If a tumor has caused a patient to seek medical attention for otologic symptoms, then it can be assumed that the tumor exerts pressure on a number of neural elements. If standard ABR latency measures detect the tumor, then a sufficient number of the neural elements that determine the peak latency have been affected. If, however, the ABR latency measures miss the tumor, then an adequate number of the appropriate neural elements was not affected. It is this possible failure to affect a sufficient number of appropriate neural elements that makes latency measures insensitive to some, but not all, small tumors. We hypothesize that the variable success of the standard ABR measures in detecting small tumors is due, in part, to the variable underlying neuroanatomic organization of eighth-nerve fibers and the variable location and encroachment of small tumors. We discuss this issue in more detail in a later section, when we review a new ABR measure that circumvents this problem. Furthermore, if cochlear hearing loss accompanies the tumor, the resulting latency decrease due to cochlear filter broadening (Don et al., 1998) may offset latency prolongation by the tumor. Thus, standard ABR latency measures may remain within normal limits. This compensatory effect of cochlear hearing loss on latency may, in some cases, account for the lack of sensitivity of the standard latency measure.

If latency is often insensitive to the effects of small tumors, what about wave V amplitude? Amplitude measures should be very sensitive to loss or desynchronization of eighth-nerve activity. As reviewed earlier in this chapter, many studies examined standard ABR amplitude measures and concluded that they are often too variable compared with latency measures. Two major contributors to this amplitude variability discussed earlier are (1) the residual noise in the average and (2) phase cancellation of activity related to progressive activation and response time variations across the cochlea. Standard ABR wave amplitude measures do not reflect all the neural activity from click stimulation because of phase cancellation. In particular, studies have shown that activity from low-frequency regions of the cochlea contributes little to the standard ABR wave V amplitude (Don et al., 1994; 1997; 2005b). Therefore, like standard latency measures, standard amplitude measures will miss tumors that do not sufficiently affect high-frequency fibers.

Any ABR test that requires a change in the standard wave V latency or amplitude will have difficulty detecting small acoustic tumors. As a result of the many studies demonstrating the inadequacy of standard ABR measures in detection of small tumors, clinical practice has shifted to using MRI to screen for acoustic tumors. Due to the low incidence of acoustic tumors, even in patients with clinically significant signs, most of the patients imaged do not have tumors. Changes in the health care delivery system now place a heavy emphasis on cost reduction and justification of expensive medical tests. The high cost, lack of availability, and other drawbacks of MRI give impetus to reconsidering less costly and more widely available methods, such as ABRs.

An ABR method capable of detecting small tumors with good specificity would be invaluable because it could (1) reduce health care costs, (2) reduce the number of patients having to endure the anxiety and discomfort of an MRI test, (3) provide a screening tool to rural communities and countries with limited access to MRIs, (4) provide an alternate test when an MRI is contraindicated, and (5) provide justification for expensive MRI testing.

The Stacked Auditory Brainstem Response: A New Measure for Detecting Small Acoustic Tumors

If a new ABR measure is to be successful at detecting small acoustic tumors, it must avoid the main shortcomings described earlier. We hypothesize that, to do so, it must be a measure of neural activity from all of the cochlea, not just the high-frequency regions. This restriction strongly suggests that any single latency measure of an ABR component, such as the wave V latency, is inadequate. We have previously cited ABR studies demonstrating that high-frequency activity dominates the latency and amplitude responses, and we hypothesized that small tumors do not always affect these fibers. Is there neuroanatomic evidence to support this hypothesis?

ANATOMIC CONSIDERATIONS

Acoustic tumors generally arise from Schwann cells in the vestibular division of the eighth nerve in the internal auditory canal and eventually extend into the cerebellopontine angle. The tumors can arise from either the superior or inferior divisions of the vestibular nerve and encroach upon the cochlear nerve. To understand the effect of a small tumor on the cochlear nerve, we need to understand the tonotopic neuroanatomic organization of the fibers in the cochlear nerve. Figure 13.5 is adapted from Spoendlin and Schrott (1989). In this transverse section of the human internal auditory canal, we see the seventh (facial) nerve (*VII; upper left*) and three divisions of the eighth (*VIII*) (auditory and vestibular) nerve.

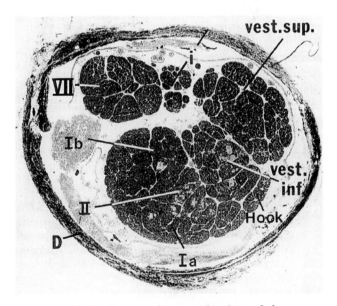

FIGURE 13.5 Tonotopic organization of the human auditory nerve. Transverse section through the internal auditory canal of an 8-year-old child, showing the position of the facial nerve (*VII*), the superior division of the vestibular nerve (*vest. sup.*), the inferior division of the vestibular nerve (*vest. inf.*), and the auditory nerve with the nerve fibers for the most basal end (*Hook*), for the lower basal turn (*Ia*), the upper basal turn (*Ib*), and the second and apical turns (*II*). (Reprinted from Spoendlin H, Schrott A. [1989] Analysis of the human auditory nerve. *Hear Res.* 43, 25–38, with permission from Elsevier Science.]

Clockwise from upper right, the divisions of the eighth nerve are as follows: first, the superior vestibular nerve; second, the inferior vestibular nerve; and third, the auditory (cochlear) nerve. In the auditory nerve, high-frequency fibers arising from the lower and upper basal turns of the cochlea lie inferiorly *(Ia)* and superiorly *(Ib),* respectively. Fibers from the second and apical turns of the cochlea lie in the medial portion of the cochlear nerve *(II),* adjacent to the inferior vestibular nerve.

This figure clearly shows that, if a tumor arose from that adjacent portion of the inferior vestibular nerve, it would affect the lower-frequency fibers in the second and apical turns first. There are tumor patients with only low-frequency or upward-sloping hearing losses (Johnson, 1977). In some of those cases, it is possible that a tumor here might be partly responsible for such hearing losses. As can be seen in this figure, depending on where the vestibular schwannoma arises, high- or low-frequency fibers can be affected first. At the House Clinic in Los Angeles, approximately half the eighth-nerve tumors originate from the superior vestibular nerve, and half originate from the inferior vestibular nerve (Dr. Fred Linthicum, 1996, personal communication). In addition, tumors do not always simply push against the nerve trunk, exerting pressure from the periphery of the trunk inward. Instead, there is strong evidence that the tumor often invades or infiltrates the nerve trunk. There have been reports of no invasion (Perre et al., 1990), but some studies have demonstrated that invasion of the cochlear nerve by solitary vestibular schwannomas is common. Neely (1985) found invasion of the nerve trunk in all 22 cases he studied; Marquet et al. (1990) and Forton et al. (1990) found invasion in over 50% of their cases; and Dr. Fred Linthicum found invasion in half of the cases in a series of 28 tumors from the House Clinic (Dr. Fred Linthicum, 1996, personal communication). In particular, NF2 tumors typically infiltrate the nerve trunk. Therefore, fibers other than those on the surface of the trunk may be affected. A measure of neural activity from all parts of the cochlea would be better in detection of the tumor than a measure confined to the high frequencies alone. Thus, an ABR measure affected by all frequencies may improve the sensitivity of the ABR in detecting small tumors.

DESCRIPTION OF THE STACKED AUDITORY BRAINSTEM RESPONSES

We mentioned earlier that amplitude measures should be able to reflect neural activity that has been desynchronized or blocked by a tumor. However, we presented several major problems with standard measures, in particular, the detrimental effect of varying S/N and the dependence of these measures on high-frequency activity because of phase cancellation of activity from lower-frequency regions. Recently, we (Don et al., 1997; 2005b) proposed a new ABR measure to circumvent these problems. This measure, the Stacked ABR amplitude, is sensitive to neural fiber activity from all frequency regions of the cochlea. Thus, the measure will reflect

the loss of synchronized neural fiber activity, no matter which fibers are compromised by a tumor, as long as the stimulus level is high enough to activate most of the neural fibers in all the frequency regions. Determining the Stacked ABR amplitude requires the derived-band and Stacked ABR techniques. A click stimulus is used to activate the whole cochlea, and the resulting response is separated into five frequency bands by using a high-pass masking and subtraction technique (Don and Eggermont, 1978; Parker and Thornton, 1978a; 1978b). The ABRs representing these five frequency bands are called derived-band ABRs and are used in constructing the Stacked ABR. Shown in Figures 13.6 to 13.8 are graphic illustrations of (1) the derived-band ABR technique and what the derived bands represent (Fig. 13.6), (2) the time-delayed cochlear activation underlying the standard ABR (Fig. 13.7), and (3) the Stacked ABR technique (Fig. 13.8).

The derived-band ABR technique requires six stimulus conditions. These six stimulus conditions are noted in the first column on the far left of Figure 13.6, and from top to bottom are the presentation of clicks alone, followed by clicks presented with simultaneous ipsilateral high-pass masking pink noise with cutoff frequencies of 8, 4, 2, 1, and 0.5 kHz. In the second column from the left are schematic representations of the cochlea with the following six frequency regions delineated: (1) above 8 kHz, (2) between 8 and 4 kHz, (3) between 4 and 2 kHz, (4) between 2 and 1 kHz, (5) between 1 and 0.5 kHz, and (6) below 0.5 kHz. If the frequency region is an area of the cochlea synchronously activated by the stimulus condition, then it is lightly shaded. In the third column is the ABR recorded to the stimulus condition. The fourth column displays five derived-band ABRs. These derived-band ABRs are obtained by subtracting two successive ABRs from column 3 (the subtraction is noted by arrows and an encircled minus sign between the two waveforms). The first derived-band ABR shown in column 4 is obtained by subtracting the ABR to clicks + 8-kHz high-pass masking noise (the second stimulus condition) from the ABR to clicks alone (the first stimulus condition). The second derived-band ABR is obtained by subtracting the ABR to clicks + 4-kHz high-pass masking noise (the third stimulus condition) from the ABR to clicks + 8-kHz high-pass masking noise (the second stimulus condition). The other derived-band ABRs in column 4 are obtained in a similar fashion from the remaining ABRs in column 3.

The lightly shaded areas of the schematic cochleae in the final column of Figure 13.6 illustrate what the derived-band ABRs in column 4 represent—isolated octave-wide regions of synchronous activity. To understand this better, look at the first derived-band ABR formed by subtracting the ABR to clicks + 8-kHz high-pass masking noise (the second stimulus condition) from the ABR to clicks alone (the first stimulus condition). As shown in the schematic representation of the cochlea in column 2, the response to clicks alone involves the sum of synchronous activity across the whole cochlea (lightly shaded areas). In the ABR to clicks + 8-kHz high-pass masking noise, the activity above 8 kHz is masked by the

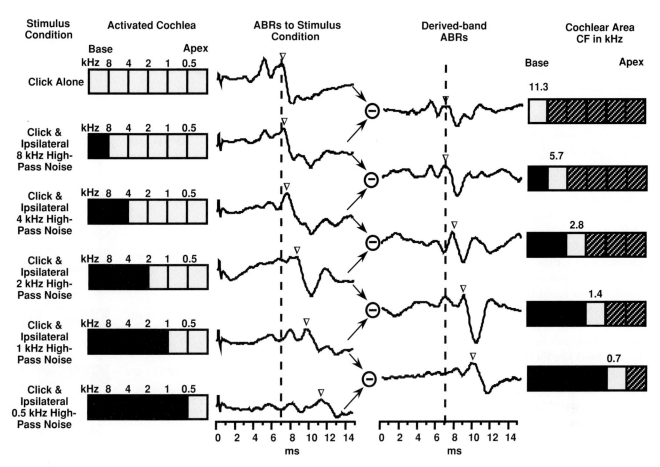

FIGURE 13.6 Schematic description of the high-pass masking and subtraction technique used to obtain derived-band auditory brainstem responses (ABRs). First column: The six stimulus conditions. Second column: Schematics of the areas of the cochlea stimulated for that condition. Third column: ABR waveforms to stimulus conditions. Fourth column: Derived-band ABR waveforms resulting from successive subtraction of conditions. Fifth column: Schematics of the octave-wide areas of the cochlea whose activity is represented in the derived-band ABRs. (See text for detailed explanation.)

noise (black area), so the response is the sum of synchronous activity from below 8 kHz (lightly shaded areas). When the ABR to clicks + 8-kHz high-pass masking noise is subtracted from the ABR to clicks alone, the activity below 8 kHz that is present in both responses is removed by the subtraction (illustrated by the hatched area of the schematic cochlea shown in column 5), leaving only the activity above 8 kHz that was present in the click alone response but masked in the clicks + 8-kHz high-pass masking noise response (lightly shaded area of schematic cochlea in column 5). As a result, in this first subtracted waveform, the first derived-band ABR, the synchronous neural activity above 8 kHz has been isolated. The process is similar for the second derived-band formed by subtracting the ABR to clicks + 4-kHz high-pass masking noise (the third stimulus condition) from the ABR to clicks + 8-kHz high-pass masking noise (the second stimulus condition). As noted earlier and seen in the schematic cochlea in column 2, in the ABR to clicks + 8-kHz high-pass masking noise, the activity above 8 kHz is masked, so the response is the sum of synchronous activity below 8 kHz.

Similarly, in the ABR to clicks + 4-kHz high-pass masking noise, the response is the sum of synchronous activity below 4 kHz (lightly shaded areas) since the activity above 4 kHz is masked by the noise (black area). When the subtraction is performed for this derived-band ABR, the activity below 4 kHz that is present in both responses is removed by the subtraction (hatched area in schematic cochlea in column 5), and the activity above 8 kHz that is masked in both responses cannot contribute (black area), leaving only the activity between 8 and 4 kHz that was present in the click + 8-kHz high-pass masking noise response but masked in the click + 4-kHz high-pass masking noise response. Thus, in this second subtracted waveform, the second derived-band ABR, the synchronous neural activity between 8 and 4 kHz has been isolated. This process is repeated by masking progressively lower frequency areas (in octave steps) of the cochlea and subtracting each resulting response from the previous one. For these successive subtractions, the common activated cochlear areas (hatched areas of schematic cochleae in column 5) are removed by the subtraction, and the common masked areas (black areas of schematic cochleae in column 5) cannot contribute any activity to the subtracted waveform. Thus, the resulting subtracted waveform, that is, the resulting derived-band ABR, reflects only the contribution from the region that was not masked in one condition but was masked in the successive condition. This subtraction procedure results in five derived-band ABRs representing activity initiated from regions of the cochlea approximately one octave wide (lightly shaded areas of schematic cochleae in column 5). The theoretical center frequencies (CFs) of these derived bands are simply and arbitrarily defined as the geometric mean of the two cutoff frequencies of the stimulus conditions involved in the subtraction. Specifically, the theoretical CF for each derived band is computed as the square root of the product of the two successive high-pass filter cutoff frequencies used for the band. For example, the derived-band ABR resulting from subtracting the response to clicks + 4-kHz high-pass masking noise from the response to clicks + 8-kHz high-pass masking noise would have a theoretical CF of about 5.7 kHz ($\sqrt{8 \times 4} \approx 5.7$). For the click alone condition, 16 kHz is used for the calculations. Thus, the theoretical derived-band CFs for the five derived-band ABRs are 11.3, 5.7, 2.8, 1.4, and 0.7 kHz.

The standard click alone ABR and the derived-band ABRs are replotted in Figure 13.7 (basically columns 4 and 5 of Fig. 13.6). The standard ABR to clicks alone (top trace) is essentially the temporally unaltered sum of activity across the entire cochlea. The derived-band ABRs plotted below the standard click alone ABR represent the responses initiated from octave-wide regions of the cochlea. Thus, the standard ABR is simply the temporally unaltered sum of the derived-band ABRs. As shown in this figure, wave V latencies are longer for each successive (lower CF) derived-band ABR. These latencies reflect the cochlear response time, composed of an apparent cochlear transport time (traveling wave delay) and a frequency-dependent synchronization time. The delay in peak activation (ΔT) from different regions of the cochlea (Fig. 13.7) demonstrates that the activity of the cochlea underlying the generation of the standard ABR is not synchronous in time but is progressively delayed as more apical cochlear regions are activated. The derived-band ABRs in the left column of Figure 13.7 clearly illustrate how activity from lower-frequency regions is phase-canceled by activity from higher-frequency regions. For example, the peak of wave V in the 0.7-kHz derived-band ABR is in phase and canceled by the trough following the peak of wave V in the 1.4-kHz derived-band ABR. Similar phase cancellation can be seen between other successive derived-band waveforms. As a result, the amplitude of the standard ABR to clicks alone does not reflect the total amount of neural activation.

Figure 13.8 illustrates the construction of the Stacked ABR from the derived-band ABRs in Figure 13.7. The Stacked ABR is constructed by (1) time shifting the derived-band waveforms so the peak latencies of wave V in each derived band coincide, and (2) adding together these shifted derived-band waveforms. The wave V peaks of the derived-band

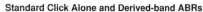

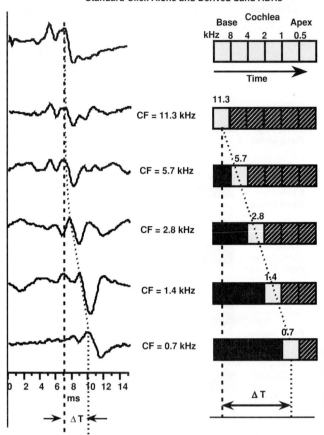

FIGURE 13.7 A series of derived-band responses on the left and schematic cochleae on the right demonstrate the time delay (ΔT) in peak activation while traversing from high- to low-frequency regions of the cochlea. This cochlear response delay is related to the apparent cochlear traveling wave delay and a frequency-dependent synchronization time. The natural sum of this activity is the standard response to clicks alone (*top waveform*). CF, center frequency.

ABRs are aligned to the wave V peak latency for the arbitrarily selected 5.7-kHz derived band. The top waveform is the Stacked ABR, the sum of the temporally aligned derived-band ABRs shown below it. By temporally aligning the peak activity initiated from each segment of the cochlea, we synchronize the total activity and minimize phase-canceling effects. Thus, compared with standard ABR amplitude measures, the amplitude of the Stacked ABR wave V reflects more directly the total amount of cochlear activity. We refer to this as the *Stacked ABR amplitude.*

Before reviewing the early results with this measure, we must discuss some important technical aspects associated with the Stacked ABR. ABRs have poor S/Ns because responses originate from deep brainstem structures located a significant distance from the surface recording electrodes.

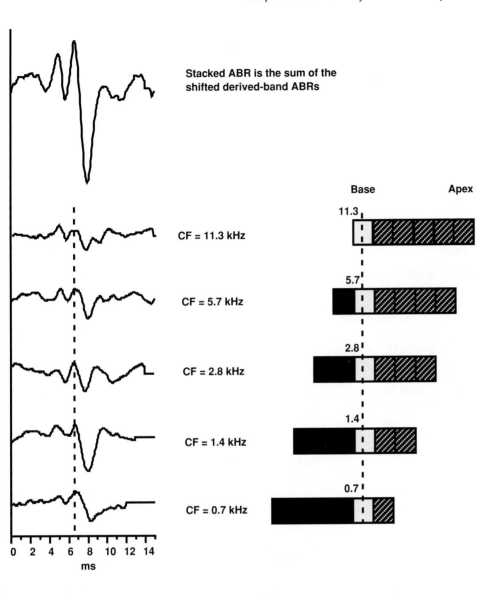

Stacked ABR is the sum of the shifted derived-band ABRs

CF = 11.3 kHz

CF = 5.7 kHz

CF = 2.8 kHz

CF = 1.4 kHz

CF = 0.7 kHz

Base   Apex

11.3
5.7
2.8
1.4
0.7

FIGURE 13.8 The Stacked auditory brainstem response (ABR) is formed by shifting the derived bands to align the wave V peaks, then adding the waveforms together. The wave V amplitude of the Stacked ABR is the new measure of interest. CF, center frequency.

Even after extensive averaging, ABRs are often still dominated by unaveraged residual background physiologic noise. In the Stacked ABR approach, it is imperative that the ABR waveforms reflect mostly neural response, not noise. Therefore, techniques for recording and processing ABRs to ensure consistently low residual noise in the averages (Elberling and Don, 1984; Don and Elberling, 1994; 1996; Chapter 14) are combined with the derived-band ABR method. In addition, we apply a Bayesian weighting approach developed by Elberling and Wahlgreen (1985) to form averages that give more weight to sweeps having less noise and to minimize the destructive effects of large episodic background noise on the ABR. Thus, the Stacked ABR method combines the derived-band ABR method with techniques that ensure low levels of residual noise and form weighted averages to minimize the destructive effects of episodic noise.

In an initial small study of 25 tumor cases, Don et al. (1997) found that five small (≤1 cm) intracanalicular tumors were missed by standard ABR latency measures (IT5 and I-V delay). However, they demonstrated that all five were detected by this new Stacked ABR method. In a larger follow-up study of 54 small tumor cases, Don et al. (2005b) demonstrated that the Stacked ABR achieved 95% sensitivity and about 88% specificity with respect to young non-tumor, normal-hearing subjects. Figure 13.9 is a plot from Don et al. (2005b) showing the cumulative percentile curves for the Stacked ABR amplitudes for non-tumor, normal-hearing (NTNH) subjects and for the small acoustic tumor (SAT) subjects. The Stacked ABR amplitudes were normalized to the mean value of adults of the same gender tested under similar testing conditions. Don et al. (2005b) established target criteria for excellent sensitivity (95%) and acceptable specificity (50%) and evaluated separately the sensitivity and specificity of these target criteria. It can be seen in Figure 13.9 that a target sensitivity of 95% yields a specificity of 88% relative to the NTNH population. Furthermore, the criterion value for a target specificity of 50% resulted in detection of all of the tumor cases in their study (100% sensitivity). Thus,

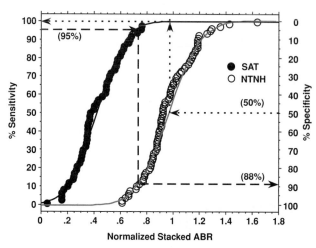

FIGURE 13.9 The cumulative distribution curves for the normalized Stacked auditory brainstem response (ABR) amplitudes for both the non-tumor, normal-hearing (NTNH) and the small acoustic tumor (SAT) populations. A criterion to achieve 95% sensitivity yields 88% specificity, and a criterion to achieve 50% specificity yields 100% sensitivity. (Reprinted from Don M, Kwong B, Tanaka C, Brackmann DE, Nelson RA. [2005b] The Stacked ABR: a sensitive and specific screening tool for detecting small acoustic tumors. *Audiol Neurotol.* 10, 274–290, with permission of the publisher, S. Karger AG, Basel.)

it appears that the Stacked ABR measure can significantly reduce the number of non-tumor patients sent for imaging, without missing a tumor.

Why is the Stacked ABR amplitude measure more sensitive to small tumors than standard latency and amplitude measures? The main reason is that temporally aligning the derived-band waveforms synchronizes the time-delayed responses across the cochlea initiated by the stimulus and summing the derived-band waveforms to form a Stacked ABR generates a stacked amplitude that reflects the total neural response. Thus, the activity of essentially all activated neural elements, rather than a subset, contributes to the stacked amplitude. Elimination of any significant amount of neural activity by the tumor will result in a significant reduction in the Stacked ABR amplitude. Thus it is more sensitive than the standard latency and amplitude measures that require compromise of specific (i.e., high-frequency) neural elements.

As described earlier, the Stacked ABR measure appears to have good specificity for normal-hearing individuals. Normal-hearing individuals made up our initial reference group because small tumors often occur in the presence of clinically normal hearing. Don et al. (2005b) noted that hearing loss can compromise the specificity because cochlear hearing losses also reduce the Stacked ABR. While a hearing loss may reduce the Stacked ABR's specificity, a hearing loss may also enhance the detection of the tumor (increase sensi-

tivity) by reducing the Stacked ABR amplitude even further. Recall that the main problem with the standard ABR measures is the lack of sensitivity for acceptable specificity. As noted by Don et al. (2005b), compensating for the hearing loss might be inappropriate because it would be compensating for the effects of the tumor. Thus, while such compensations may improve the Stacked ABR's specificity, they will compromise its sensitivity, thereby increasing the chance of missing a tumor. Missing a tumor is the greater and more serious clinical error. Further research is being undertaken to find ways to improve the specificity relative to hearing loss without compromising the desired improved sensitivity. For example, we hypothesize that cochlear loss reduces the Stacked ABR amplitude by decreasing the total neural output and that this reduction is related to the amount of hearing loss. We also hypothesize that small tumors reduce the Stacked ABR amplitude not only by decreasing the total neural output, but also by desynchronizing the neural activity. Furthermore, the amount of desynchronized neural activity is not completely reflected by changes in the audiometric thresholds. Thus, because of this additional effect of desynchronization, we expect the Stacked ABR amplitude to be reduced to a greater extent than that predicted by the audiometric hearing levels. Additional preliminary data support our hypotheses. In tumor patients, the Stacked ABR amplitude is much smaller than expected on the basis of the audiometric thresholds. Therefore, we believe that the confounding effect of cochlear hearing loss can, to a large extent, be resolved.

One current development of the Stacked ABR that should improve both its sensitivity and specificity uses interaural comparisons of the Stacked ABR. Preliminary data of interaural Stacked ABRs in non-tumor, normal-hearing individuals are shown in Figure 13.10. These data indicate that there is virtually no difference in the Stacked ABR amplitude between ears and that the standard deviation is about 10%. Recent work (Don et al., submitted for publication) suggests that interaural Stacked ABR amplitude differences greater than 10% may be diagnostic for a tumor. Other current studies of changes in the stimulus parameters that may enhance the separation of tumor and non-tumor ears may also improve the sensitivity and specificity of the Stacked ABR.

LIMITATIONS OF THE STACKED AUDITORY BRAINSTEM RESPONSE

A major limitation of the Stacked ABR is that it must be obtained with click levels no greater than 60 to 65 dB nHL (i.e., 90 to 95 dB peak equivalent sound pressure level [peSPL]). Thus, patients with average hearing losses greater than 60 dB across standard audiometric frequencies cannot be meaningfully screened with the Stacked ABR. The reason for this limitation is that higher click levels require higher masking noise levels to obtain the derived-band responses for the Stacked ABR. These higher masking noise levels would be

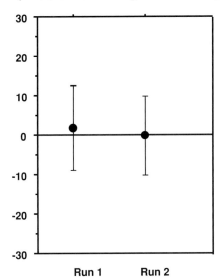

Interaural Stacked ABRs
(Difference Between Right and Left Ears)

FIGURE 13.10   Percent difference between the Stacked auditory brainstem response (ABR) amplitudes of the right and left ears for 22 non-tumor, normal-hearing subjects (12 males and 10 females). Each subject was tested twice (*Run 1* and *Run 2*). The mean difference is near 0 for both runs.

uncomfortable and unsafe for the normal-hearing subjects whose Stacked ABRs provide the diagnostic reference data. Therefore, we cannot obtain reference data for the Stacked ABR at click levels that are significantly higher than 60 to 65 dB nHL. However, this is not a critical limitation because the main use of the Stacked ABR is to detect small tumors missed by standard ABR measures. Typically, patients with small tumors do not have average hearing losses that exceed 60 dB nHL. If patients have losses that exceed 60 dB nHL due to a tumor, then the tumor is probably relatively large, and standard ABR measures will be sufficiently abnormal to preclude the need for the Stacked ABR.

Also, note that click levels less than 60 dB nHL would compromise the Stacked ABR measure because lower stimulus levels may not activate enough of the fibers compromised by the tumor. Thus, when stimulus levels are too low, a significant change in the Stacked ABR amplitude may not be observed in patients with small tumors.

Finally, as noted earlier, cochlear hearing loss will reduce the Stacked ABR amplitude. This may lead to a higher false-positive rate (lower specificity). However, current refinements aimed at resolving this confound may improve the specificity of the Stacked ABR.

Other Retrocochlear Pathologies

A number of early studies explored the effects of structural brain lesions (brainstem tumors, vascular dysfunction,

multiple sclerosis, and demyelination) on the ABR (Starr and Achor, 1975; Starr and Hamilton, 1976; Stockard and Rossiter, 1977). It is clear from these early and subsequent studies that the effects of brainstem lesions on the ABR are similar to those observed for acoustic tumors. For example, the lesions can cause prolongation of interpeak latencies (e.g., I-V delay) and abnormal peak amplitude ratios (V/I). Thus, ABR abnormalities are not specific to any retrocochlear neurologic disease. Once it is determined that the ABR abnormality is not due to either cochlear insult or the presence of an eighth-nerve tumor, the patient should be referred for neurologic investigations. In these cases, the ABR can only detect an unspecified neurologic abnormality, corroborate a suspected disease, or monitor the course of a disease. Thus, with one exception, auditory neuropathy/dyssynchrony (Starr et al., 1996), this chapter does not review the multitude of neurologic problems, such as multiple sclerosis, pontine gliomas, and vascular lesions, that may cause abnormal ABR measures. It should be emphasized that a given ABR abnormality is not specific for any one of these neurologic diseases. That is, the neurologic disease cannot be determined from the ABR abnormality. Detailed discussions of ABR abnormalities and neurologic disease can be found in the literature review in Starr and Don (1988) and the recent chapter by Musiek et al. (2007). The main reason for including a brief discussion of auditory neuropathy/auditory dyssynchrony (AN/AD) in this chapter is that ABR testing is necessary for the differential diagnosis.

Auditory Neuropathy/Auditory Dyssynchrony

Patients with AN/AD present with hearing loss for puretones, impaired word discrimination that is disproportionately poorer than the puretone loss, absent or abnormal ABRs, and normal outer hair cell function as measured by otoacoustic emissions (see Chapter 21) and cochlear microphonics (see Chapter 12) (Doyle et al., 1998). (Chapter 22 provides further discussion of AN/AD.) We review the study by Starr et al. (1996) in some detail because it provides a good characterization of this pathology. They reported on 10 young patients with hearing impairments that, by behavioral and physiologic testing, suggested a disorder of the auditory nerve. All 10 patients showed evidence of normal cochlear outer hair cell function as determined by otoacoustic emissions and cochlear microphonic testing. ABRs were absent in nine patients and severely distorted in one patient, suggesting abnormal auditory pathway function beginning with the eighth nerve. Furthermore, auditory brainstem reflexes (e.g., acoustic reflexes and crossed suppression of otoacoustic emissions) were absent in all of the tested patients. Behavioral audiometry showed mild to moderate elevations of puretone thresholds in nine patients. The configuration of the puretone loss varied across subjects: predominantly low frequency in five patients, flat in three patients, and predominantly high frequency in two patients. The extent of the hearing loss, if due solely to cochlear receptor damage, should not have resulted in the loss of ABRs.

Speech intelligibility tests were conducted in eight patients. In six of these patients, speech intelligibility was disproportionately poorer than would have been expected if the puretone losses were of cochlear origin. When the hearing impairment was first manifested, the patients were neurologically normal. Subsequently, eight of the patients developed evidence of a peripheral neuropathy. There was a hereditary basis to the neuropathy in three of the patients. Starr et al. (1996, p 741) suggested "that this type of hearing impairment is due to a disorder of auditory nerve function and may have, as one of its causes, a neuropathy of the auditory nerve, occurring either in isolation or as part of a generalized neuropathic process."

As reported by Doyle et al. (1998), cases of this rare disorder occur in pediatric populations as well. The children in this study all demonstrated absent or markedly abnormal ABRs, with normal cochlear outer hair cell function. Many also had poor word discrimination scores. AN/AD can, in rare cases, manifest itself under unusual conditions. Starr et al. (1998) reported on cases of transient deafness in three children (two siblings, ages 3 and 6, and an unrelated child, age 15) when they become febrile. More specifically, they develop a conduction block of the auditory nerves when their core body temperature rises. Extensive investigation of these children led to the conclusion that they had an auditory neuropathy. The neuropathy may be due to a demyelinating disorder of the auditory nerve and is likely to be inherited as a recessive disorder.

The diagnosis of AN/AD requires ABR tests and tests of cochlear function, such as otoacoustic emissions and cochlear microphonics. The audiologic community should be aware of this disorder because its treatment and management are different from those for sensory-neural hearing loss (Doyle et al., 1998). A thorough treatment of AN/AD can be found in a recent review chapter by Hood (2007).

We previously discussed the effects of cochlear hearing loss on ABR latency and amplitude measures. While a specific diagnosis is not possible, cochlear and retrocochlear pathologies can be distinguished on a broad scale by abnormalities in the interpeak latencies. Abnormal interpeak latencies (e.g., I-III or I-V) are usually associated with retrocochlear problems because the delay is presumably due to a problem after activation of the auditory nerve (wave I). This is only true if the measured response represents activity from a specific place in the cochlea; this is the case for derived-band ABRs. However, as discussed earlier, for the standard ABR to simple clicks, the differential cochlear representation of waves I and V (Don and Eggermont, 1978; Eggermont and Don, 1986) could lead to alterations in the I-V measure caused by stimulus levels and cochlear problems. Thus, abnormal I-V delays in standard ABRs may not be due to retrocochlear problems. In contrast, we hypothesize that abnormal I-V delays in derived-band ABRs are almost certainly due to a retrocochlear problem.

Cochlear Pathologies

Any cochlear pathology that causes hearing loss can affect ABR measures. However, like retrocochlear pathology, the nature of the abnormal ABR measure is not diagnostic for a specific disease. For example, prolongation of wave V latency can occur for a variety of cochlear and retrocochlear problems. However, ABR measures can be used to detect an unspecified abnormality, corroborate a suspected disease, or monitor the course of a disease. In general, ABR abnormalities cannot provide diagnosis of a specific cochlear pathology, with the possible exception of Ménière's disease with cochlear hydrops. A vast amount of literature documents attempts to diagnose Ménière's disease with various measures of evoked electrical activity, particularly electrocochleography (ECoG) (see Chapter 12).

The use of ABRs to diagnose Ménière's disease might seem unlikely because ABRs reflect aspects of neural synchrony rather than cochlear hair cell function. However, a reasonable assumption is that the increase in endolymphatic pressure in cochlear hydrops could increase the stiffness of the basilar membrane (Tonndorf, 1957; 1983; Flottorp, 1980). This increased stiffness could increase the speed of traveling wave propagation down the basilar membrane. Using derived-band ABR latencies obtained with high-pass noise masking and assuming a normal frequency-place map in the cochlea, Thornton and Farrell (1991) and Donaldson and Ruth (1996) calculated abnormally high traveling wave velocities in patients diagnosed with Ménière's disease. In addition, there is some single-unit evidence that such changes result in a shift of the excitation pattern along the basilar membrane toward higher frequency areas (Klis et al., 1988). This would also decrease the response time across the cochlea. Thus, short response times across the cochlea, as measured by peak latency differences between derived bands, might indicate Ménière's disease with cochlear hydrops.

Recently, Don et al. (2005a) described a method that distinguished patients diagnosed with an active case of Ménière's disease from non-Ménière's, normal-hearing subjects (NMNH). This method, referred to as the cochlear hydrops analysis masking procedure (CHAMP), involves recording ABRs to moderate-level clicks and simultaneous ipsilateral high-pass masking noise. Responses to the clicks presented alone and to clicks with masking noise high-pass filtered at 8, 4, 2, 1, and 0.5 kHz (henceforth referred to as high-pass response waveforms) are recorded. Note that the CHAMP ABR recordings are the same as those required for the Stacked ABR method described earlier. However, no derived bands are formed because there is no subtraction of the high-pass response waveforms. Instead, the unmodified high-pass response waveforms are used in the analysis. In the NMNH subjects, as in the non-tumor, normal-hearing subjects discussed previously, the latency of wave V in the ABR is observed to increase as the cutoff frequency of the high-pass masking noise is lowered (see the non-Ménière's ear data in the right panel of Fig. 13.11). Typically, the highest

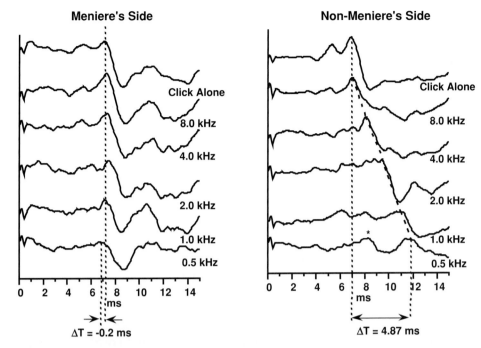

FIGURE 13.11 Auditory brainstem responses (ABRs) to clicks alone and clicks presented in the various high-pass masking noise conditions for a unilateral Ménière's disease subject. *Right panel*: ABRs from the unaffected (non-Ménière's) ear showing the large wave V latency shifts observed in the non-Ménière's, normal-hearing population. *Asterisk* indicates the peak of the undermasked component. *Left Panel*: ABRs from the diagnosed Ménière's ear showing virtually no wave V latency shifts. (Reprinted from Don M, Kwong B, Tanaka C. [2005a] A diagnostic test for Ménière's disease and cochlear hydrops: impaired high-pass noise masking of ABRs. *Otol Neurotol.* 26, 711–722, with permission of the publisher.)

unmasked frequency region dominates the latency of wave V. Therefore, as the cochlea is successively masked from 8 kHz and higher down to 0.5 kHz and higher, the peak latency of wave V increases. This increase is expected because with each lowering of the high-pass masking noise cutoff frequency, the response to the click is dominated by a lower frequency region (see column 3 of Fig. 13.6). Thus, due to factors related to the cochlear traveling wave delay, the peak latency of the response increases as the area of the unmasked cochlea is successively restricted to lower frequencies.

However, in the Ménière's disease patients, as seen in the left panel of Figure 13.11, the masking noise is insufficient such that the latency of wave V in the high-pass response waveforms is similar to that of wave V in the response to clicks alone. Our hypothesis is that the endolymphatic (cochlear) hydrops in patients with Ménière's disease alters the response characteristics of the basilar membrane such that the high-pass masking noise is less effective in masking activity from the frequency regions that are normally masked by the noise. Thus, in Ménière's disease patients, the area of the cochlea that dominates the latency of wave V in the response to clicks alone is not sufficiently masked by the noise. As a result, the observed wave V latencies in the high-

pass response waveforms are similar to those seen for the response to clicks presented alone. The undermasked wave V peak in the 0.5-kHz high-pass response waveform is referred to as the *undermasked component*. Figure 13.12 from Don et al. (2005a) plots the cumulative normal distribution for the wave V latency delay computed by subtracting the latency of wave V in the response to clicks alone from the latency of wave V in the 0.5-kHz high-pass response. It is clear that the two distributions for the NMNH and Ménière's disease populations are completely separated. A large range of latency delays (shaded area) can be selected as test criteria that will give 100% sensitivity and 100% specificity for these two study populations. Note that the NMNH data presented in Figure 13.12 use the longer latency wave V in the 0.5-kHz high-pass response. This longer latency wave V reflects synchronized activity from unmasked frequency regions of the cochlea below the 0.5-kHz high-pass masking noise. Because the intensity of the masking noise was an average determined in a previous study (Don and Eggermont, 1978), and not a level tailored to each subject in this study, the NMNH subjects requiring higher levels of masking were slightly undermasked and demonstrated an early undermasked component in addition to the normal

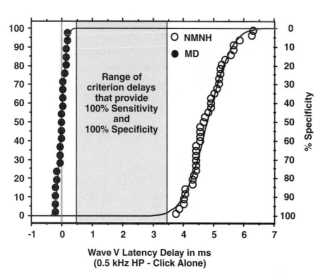

FIGURE 13.12 Plots of the cumulative normal distributions for the latency delay between wave V in the response to clicks alone and wave V in the response to clicks and 0.5-kHz high-pass (HP) masking noise for the non-Ménière's, normal-hearing (NMNH) and Ménière's disease (MD) populations. There is complete separation of these two distributions. (Reprinted from Don M, Kwong B, Tanaka C. [2005a] A diagnostic test for Ménière's disease and cochlear hydrops: impaired high-pass noise masking of ABRs. *Otol Neurotol.* 26, 711–722, with permission of the publisher.)

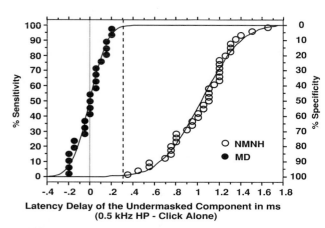

FIGURE 13.13 Cumulative normal distributions for the delay between wave V for the click alone response and the undermasked component for the 0.5-kHz high-pass (HP) for both the non-Ménière's, normal-hearing (NMNH) and Ménière's disease (MD) groups. (Reprinted from Don M, Kwong B, Tanaka C. [2005a] A diagnostic test for Ménière's disease and cochlear hydrops: impaired high-pass noise masking of ABRs. *Otol Neurotol.* 26, 711–722, with permission of the publisher.)

longer latency wave V plotted in Figure 13.12. This shorter latency undermasked component can be seen in the 0.5-kHz high-pass response of the non-Ménière's ear shown in the right panel of Figure 13.11 (marked by an asterisk). This undermasked component was also investigated. As seen in Figure 13.13, the cumulative normal distribution curves are much closer compared to those shown in Figure 13.12. However, there is still a complete separation for the two groups in this study. Thus, a criterion value of 0.3 ms (dashed line) results in 100% sensitivity and 100% specificity for the study's sample populations. In another study (Don et al., 2007), an alternative measure that uses a complex amplitude ratio to assess Ménière's disease with cochlear hydrops has been proposed. This complex amplitude ratio method is to be used when it is difficult to determine the peak latencies in the responses to clicks and 0.5-kHz high-pass masking noise. The details of this method are beyond the scope of this chapter.

Recommended Protocols

Figure 13.14 is a flowchart summary of a recommended protocol for using ABRs to screen for acoustic tumors and AN/AD.

- Perform a standard clinical ABR test. If any of the standard ABR measures (IT5, I-V, wave absence, etc.) are abnormal, send the patient for MRI testing to rule out an eighth-nerve tumor. If a tumor is found, the physician will prescribe appropriate medical treatment (e.g., surgery). If the MRI is negative, work up the patient for possible AN/AD (otoacoustic emissions, etc.) and/or refer for further neurologic testing.

- If the standard ABR measures are normal, perform the Stacked ABR using 60- to 65-dB nHL click levels. If the Stacked ABR amplitude is abnormally small, send the patient for MRI testing to rule out an eighth-nerve tumor. If a tumor is found, the physician will prescribe appropriate medical treatment (e.g., surgery). If no tumor is found, continue to observe and follow audiologically and/or refer for neurologic evalution.

- Note that the Stacked ABR should not be used for small tumor assessment in the following cases. First, a patient whose hearing loss is too severe to be tested at 60- to 65-dB nHL click levels cannot be meaningfully screened with the Stacked ABR. (See earlier discussion on the limitations of the Stacked ABR.) Second, if there is evidence of strong undermasking in the high-pass response waveforms, this may indicate the presence of Ménière's disease with cochlear hydrops, so the patient should be evaluated for Ménière's disease instead (e.g., with CHAMP). Waveforms with strong undermasking should not be used for the Stacked ABR analysis because the undermasked

ABR SCREENING PROTOCOL FOR EIGHTH NERVE TUMORS

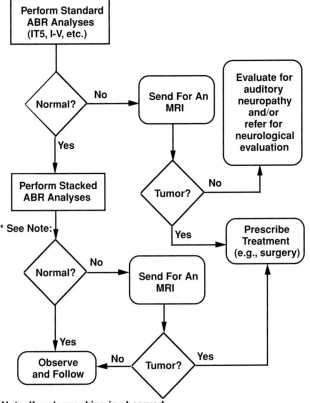

Note: If undermasking is observed in the high-pass response waveforms, do not form or use the Stacked ABR.

FIGURE 13.14 Flowchart of recommended protocol for using auditory brainstem responses (ABRs) to screen for eighth-nerve tumors. See text for explanation. MRI, magnetic resonance imaging.

responses will yield a reduced Stacked ABR amplitude that is not related to the presence of a tumor.

■ If the Stacked ABR amplitude is normal, continue to observe and follow audiologically and/or refer for neurologic evaluation.

CASE STUDIES

In this section, we present case studies that illustrate the use of ABR measures, the standard IT5 and I-V delay, and

the Stacked ABR amplitude in eighth-nerve tumor detection. All of these patients are from the House Clinic in Los Angeles. The click level used was 63 dB nHL (93 dB peSPL). The puretone average (PTA) for each patient was determined by averaging the thresholds for eight audiometric frequencies: 0.25, 0.5, 1.0, 2.0, 3.0, 4.0, 6.0, and 8.0 kHz.

Case 1: Small Tumor Detected by Standard IT5 Auditory Brainstem Response Measure

HISTORY

This 31-year-old male experienced tinnitus and sudden total hearing loss in the right ear. After about 4 days with steroid treatment, the hearing returned to normal, except for a slight 4-kHz notch that may have existed previously; a similar notch was recorded in the non-tumor left ear. After his hearing returned to normal, the only clinical symptom was fullness in the right ear. MRI with contrast (Gd-DPTA) revealed a 1-cm tumor filling the right internal auditory canal (IAC). The eighth-nerve tumor originated from the superior vestibular nerve. The tumor was removed via a midcranial fossa approach, and hearing was preserved.

AUDIOMETRIC TESTS

The patient's preoperative audiogram after recovery from the sudden hearing loss is noted in Table 13.2. The PTA was about 7 and 6 dB for the right and left ears, respectively. The speech reception threshold (SRT) was 5 dB for both ears, and the speech discrimination score (SDS) at 30 dB above SRT was 100% for both ears.

Audiometric testing in the operated ear a year after the tumor was removed revealed only about 5 dB of additional loss in the high frequencies.

ABR TESTING

The standard IT5 ABR measure obtained before surgery is shown in Figure 13.15. The IT5 was 0.9 ms. This value is well beyond the 0.2 criterion. No correction for hearing loss was necessary. This small tumor probably affected the high-frequency fibers that dominate the latency of the standard ABR.

TABLE 13.2	Case 1 pre-operative audiogram. Tumor on right side.								
Frequency	250	500	1000	2000	3000	4000	6000	8000	PTA
Right Ear	0	0	0	0	15	20	10	10	7
Left Ear	0	0	0	0	15	20	0	15	6

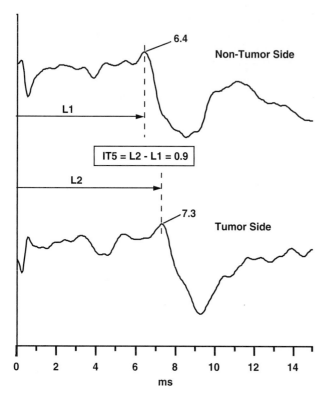

FIGURE 13.15 Case 1: Abnormal IT5. This eighth-nerve tumor patient demonstrated an abnormal IT5 (0.9 ms) with good waveform morphology. See text for case details.

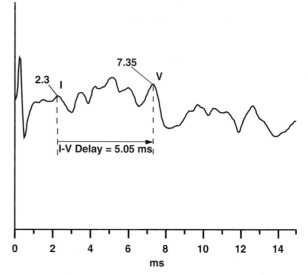

FIGURE 13.16 Case 2: Abnormal I-V delay. This eighth-nerve tumor patient demonstrated an abnormal delay (5.05 ms) between the peak of wave V and the peak of wave I. See text for case details.

Case 2: Midsize Tumor Detected by Standard I-V Auditory Brainstem Response Measure

HISTORY

This 36-year-old male noticed a progressive loss of hearing in the right ear. He then experienced mild tinnitus and a sudden loss of hearing in the right ear, which partially recovered with steroid treatment. MRI with Gd-DPTA contrast revealed a 1.5-cm eighth-nerve tumor, mainly in the IAC. The tumor was removed via a midcranial fossa approach, and some hearing was preserved.

AUDIOMETRIC TESTS

The patient's preoperative audiogram after partial recovery from the sudden hearing loss is noted in Table 13.3. The PTA was about 36 dB in the tumor ear (right) and about

14 dB in the non-tumor ear (left). The SRT was 15 and 10 dB, and the SDS at 30 dB above SRT was 76% and 96% for the tumor right ear and the non-tumor left ear, respectively. Audiometric testing a week after surgery revealed 15 to 40 dB of additional loss in the right ear and little change in the normal left ear.

ABR TESTING

The standard I-V ABR measure obtained before surgery is shown in Figure 13.16. The I-V delay was 5.05 ms, which is very abnormal. The IT5, which required no correction for hearing loss, was also very abnormal (0.9 ms) and could have been used for the diagnosis as well.

Case 3: Small Eighth-Nerve Tumor, Slight Asymmetric Hearing Loss with Puretone Average Worse in Tumor Ear, and Normal IT5 and I-V Delay

HISTORY

This 51-year-old male had a history of mild hearing loss in the right ear and some dizziness for a 6-month period. MRI with Gd-DPTA contrast revealed a 1.0-cm eighth-nerve

TABLE 13.3 Case 2 pre-operative audiogram. Tumor on right side.									
Frequency	250	500	1000	2000	3000	4000	6000	8000	PTA
Right Ear	10	10	10	25	45	40	65	80	36
Left Ear	15	10	10	10	10	25	25	10	14

TABLE 13.4 Case 3 pre-operative audiogram. Tumor on right side.									
Frequency	250	500	1000	2000	3000	4000	6000	8000	PTA
Right Ear	0	0	20	20	40	35	30	35	22
Left Ear	15	10	10	10	10	25	25	10	14

tumor in the IAC. The origin of the tumor was the inferior vestibular nerve. The tumor was removed via a midcranial fossa approach, and some hearing was preserved.

AUDIOMETRIC TESTS

The patient's preoperative audiogram is noted in Table 13.4. The PTA for the tumor ear (right) was 22 dB, and for the non-tumor ear (left), it was 14 dB. The SRT was 10 dB, and SDS at 30 dB above SRT was 100% for both ears.

ABR TESTING

The standard ABR measures obtained before surgery are shown in the upper portion of Figure 13.17. The wave V latency was actually shorter in the tumor ear. This resulted in a negative IT5 of –0.1 ms. No correction of the IT5 for hearing loss was required. Thus, the IT5 provided no hint of a tumor. The I-V delay was 4.55 ms. Although greater than the mean of a non-tumor, normal-hearing population, this delay is within 2 standard deviations of the mean. This probably would not have raised suspicion because the difference in the interaural I-V delay was only 0.2 ms. The simple wave V amplitude was about 48% smaller. However, as discussed earlier (and demonstrated in Case 4), the standard ampli-

tude measure does not always predict the tumor's presence. The Stacked ABR amplitude (lower portion of Fig. 13.17) in the tumor ear was 50% smaller than in the non-tumor ear. The 8-dB PTA difference does not account for such a reduction.

In Figure 13.18, the Stacked ABR amplitudes for both ears of this patient are plotted on the cumulative percentile curve for a group of non-tumor, normal-hearing male subjects. Although the Stacked ABR amplitude in both ears is suspiciously low (using the 20% criterion), the low value in the non-tumor ear may be due, in part, to the slight hearing loss. A clear separation is observed, and the non-tumor ear can be correctly identified (assuming this is not an NF2 case) by comparing the two ears. This demonstrates how the interaural comparison of Stacked ABR amplitudes between ears might be used to improve its specificity.

Case 4: Very Small Eighth-Nerve Tumor, Puretone Average Slightly Better in Tumor Ear, and Normal IT5 and I-V Delay

HISTORY

This 47-year-old female, at the suggestion of a psychiatrist, had an MRI with Gd-DPTA contrast scan. The results showed

FIGURE 13.17 Case 3: Small eighth-nerve tumor. Puretone average (PTA) slightly poorer in tumor ear; normal IT5 and I-V delay. Standard and Stacked auditory brainstem responses (ABRs) from a male patient whose PTA threshold was slightly poorer in the ear with a small 1.0-cm tumor. This patient demonstrated a normal IT5 (–0.1 ms) and a I-V delay that was within 2 standard deviations of the normal population. The 50% reduction in the Stacked ABR could not be accounted for by the 8-dB PTA difference.

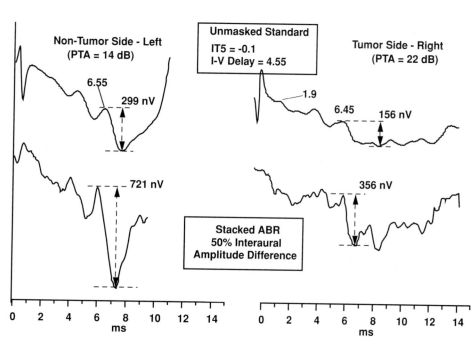

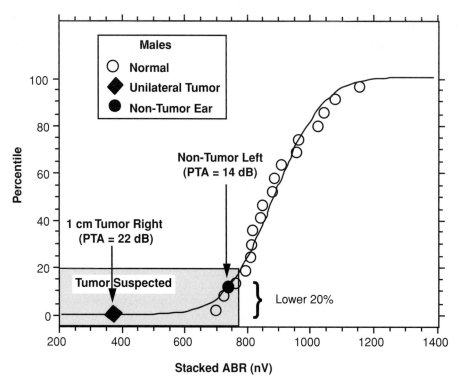

FIGURE 13.18 Stacked auditory brainstem responses (ABRs) for Case 3, shown in Figure 13.17. Stacked ABRs for both ears of the male patient shown in Figure 13.17 are plotted on the cumulative percentile curves of the Stacked ABR amplitudes for non-tumor, normal-hearing male subjects. If there was no tumor, the Stacked ABR in the suspected ear would be only slightly smaller because of the small puretone average (PTA) difference (only 8 dB). However, the Stacked ABR from the suspected ear is suspiciously lower by about 50%.

a 3- to 4-mm intracanalicular eighth-nerve tumor in the left ear. The patient had no overt symptoms, and hearing was symmetric and clinically normal. Since the patient was asymptomatic, surgery was not recommended, and the patient was simply followed. About a year later, she developed balance problems and noticed a little tinnitus that was presumably due to the tumor. Surgery was recommended because of the developing symptoms. The tumor originated from the superior vestibular nerve and had increased only slightly in size since the earlier MRI. The tumor (4 mm) was removed via a midcranial fossa approach, and hearing was preserved.

AUDIOMETRIC TESTS

The patient's preoperative audiogram is shown in Table 13.5. The PTA for the non-tumor right ear was about 22 dB, and the PTA for the ear with the tumor was about 19 dB. Note that the PTA was better in the ear with the tumor. The SRT was 15 dB for both ears, and SDS at 30 to 40 dB above SRT was 100% for both ears.

ABR TESTING

The standard ABR measures and the Stacked ABR amplitudes obtained before surgery are shown in Figure 13.19. The IT5 was 0 ms, and the I-V delay in the tumor ear was 3.75 ms. These values are completely normal. The unmasked standard wave V amplitude was 16% *larger* in the tumor ear. However, the Stacked ABR amplitude in the tumor ear was 19% *smaller* than that in the non-tumor ear. The 19% smaller amplitude is suspicious, given that hearing levels are better in the suspected ear.

In Figure 13.20, the Stacked ABR amplitudes for both ears of this patient are plotted on the cumulative percentile curve for a group of non-tumor, normal-hearing female subjects. The Stacked ABR is suspiciously low (using the 20% criterion) for the tumor ear. The suspicion of a tumor is even stronger because the lower amplitude occurred in the ear with the better PTA. Thus, even though the simple Stacked ABR amplitude would have detected this tumor, an interaural Stacked ABR amplitude comparison together with the PTA can provide additional support for a tumor diagnosis.

TABLE 13.5 Case 4 pre-operative audiogram. Tumor on left side.									
Frequency	**250**	**500**	**1000**	**2000**	**3000**	**4000**	**6000**	**8000**	**PTA**
Right Ear	20	25	25	10	10	15	45	30	22
Left Ear	15	15	15	15	10	20	35	25	19

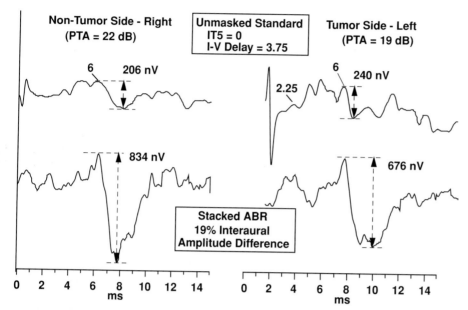

FIGURE 13.19 Case 4: Small eighth-nerve tumor. Puretone average (PTA) slightly better in tumor ear; normal IT5 and I-V delay. Standard and Stacked auditory brainstem responses (ABRs) from a female patient whose PTA threshold was slightly better in the ear with a small 4-mm tumor. The tumor ear demonstrated a completely normal IT5 (0 ms) and I-V delay (3.75 ms). In addition, the standard ABR amplitude was greater in the tumor ear by about 16%. With the indicated PTAs, if there was no tumor, the Stacked ABR amplitudes should be essentially equal, if not slightly better in the tumor (left) ear. However, despite the slightly better thresholds, the Stacked ABR amplitude was 19% smaller in the ear with the tumor.

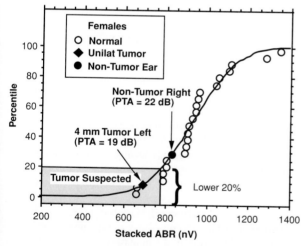

FIGURE 13.20 Stacked auditory brainstem responses (ABRs) for Case 4, shown in Figure 13.19. Stacked ABRs for both ears of the female patient shown in Figure 13.19 are plotted on the cumulative percentile curves of the Stacked ABR amplitude for non-tumor, normal-hearing female subjects. If there was no tumor, no difference in Stacked ABRs between ears would be expected because of the nearly equal hearing thresholds. However, the Stacked ABR from the suspected ear is suspiciously lower by about 19%. PTA, puretone average.

SUMMARY AND COMMENTS

In this chapter, we review applications of ABRs for differential diagnosis of diseases of the auditory nerve and brainstem, as well as cochlear diseases, in particular, Ménière's disease with cochlear hydrops. The major focus of our discussions is on the detection of acoustic tumors (vestibular schwannomas). In the past, there was heavy reliance on standard ABR measures for eighth-nerve tumor detection. However, with advancement in imaging techniques, such as MRIs with contrast, it was discovered that standard ABR measures were not sufficiently sensitive to small (≤1 cm) tumors. As a result, current practice in many clinics has shifted to using MRIs to screen for acoustic tumors. We propose some hypotheses as to why standard ABR measures often fail to detect small tumors and provide limited information on other cochlear and retrocochlear diseases. We present a new ABR measure, the Stacked ABR, which attempts to overcome the failure of standard ABRs to detect small tumors. The Stacked ABR appears promising as a more widely available, cost-effective, and objective screening tool to ensure that tumor patients are sent for MRI tests and to reduce the number of non-tumor patients sent for imaging.

In addition, we touched on an ABR method for detecting the presence of cochlear hydrops in Ménière's disease. It is hypothesized that the cochlear hydrops increases the stiffness of the basilar membrane. As a result of this change in the basilar membrane's physical properties, the normal level of pink high-pass masking noise that is sufficient to mask the response to clicks in a normal cochlea is insufficient for a patient with Ménière's disease. This test method, called CHAMP (cochlear hydrops analysis masking procedure), appears to distinguish Ménière's disease subjects with high sensitivity and specificity.

The future of ABRs in differential diagnosis depends on developing measures, such as the Stacked ABR and CHAMP, that do not have the limitations of the standard ABRs. The keys to success are (1) understanding the mechano-

neurophysiologic bases of ABRs, (2) focusing on the disease processes that affect measurable features of the ABR, and (3) using innovative stimulation and analysis techniques to develop ABR measures of these disease-related changes. Using these keys, we believe the future of ABRs can be assured.

ACKNOWLEDGMENT

We thank Ann Masuda for scheduling the patients and collecting the data presented in the clinical cases.

REFERENCES

Allison T, Hume AL, Wood CC, Goff WR. (1984) Development and aging changes in somatosensory, auditory and visual evoked potentials. *Electroencephalogr Clin Neurophysiol.* 58, 14–24.

Barrs DM, Brackmann DE, Olson JE, House WF. (1985) Changing concepts of acoustic neuroma diagnosis. *Arch Otolaryngol.* 111, 17–21.

Bauch CD, Olsen WO, Harner SG. (1983) Auditory brain-stem response and acoustic reflex test. *Arch Otolaryngol.* 109, 522–525.

Bauch CD, Olsen WO, Pool A. (1996) ABR indices: sensitivity, specificity, and tumor size. *Am J Audiol.* 5, 97–104.

Beagley HA, Sheldrake JB. (1978) Differences in brainstem response latency with age and sex. *Br J Audiol.* 12, 69–77.

Bockenheimer S, Schmidt CL, Zollner C. (1984) Neuro-otological findings in patients with small acoustic neurinomas. *Arch Otorhinolaryngol.* 239, 31–39.

Borg E. (1982) Correlation between auditory brainstem response (ABR) and speech discrimination scores in patients with acoustic neurinoma and in patients with cochlear hearing loss. *Scand Audiol.* 11, 245–248.

Cashman MZ, Rossman RN. (1983) Diagnostic features of the auditory brainstem response in identifying cerebellopontine angle tumours. *Scand Audiol.* 12, 35–41.

Chandrasekhar SS, Brackmann, DE, Devgan KK. (1995) Utility of auditory brainstem response audiometry in diagnosis of acoustic neuromas. *Am J Otol.* 16, 63–67.

Chiappa KH, Gladstone KJ, Young RR. (1979) Brainstem auditory evoked responses: studies of waveform variations in 50 normal human subjects. *Arch Neurol.* 36, 81–87.

Clemis JD, Mitchell C. (1977) Electrocochleography and brainstem responses used in the diagnosis of acoustic tumors. *J Otolaryngol.* 6, 447–459.

Coats AC, Martin JL. (1978) Human auditory nerve action potentials and brainstem evoked responses-latency-intensity functions in detection of cochlear and retrocochlear pathology. *Arch Otolaryngol.* 104, 709–717.

Daly DM, Roeser RJ, Aung MH, Daly DD. (1977) Early evoked potentials in patients with acoustic neuroma. *Electroencephalogr Clin Neurophysiol.* 43, 151–159.

Deupree DL, Jewett DL. (1988) Far-field potentials due to action potentials traversing curved nerves, reaching cut nerve ends, and crossing boundaries between cylindrical volumes. *Electroencephalogr Clin Neurophysiol.* 70, 355–362.

Don M, Eggermont JJ. (1978) Analysis of the click-evoked brainstem potentials in man using high-pass noise masking. *J Acoust Soc Am.* 63, 1084–1092.

Don M, Eggermont JJ, Brackmann DE. (1979) Reconstruction of the audiogram using brain stem responses and high-pass noise masking. *Ann Otol Rhinol Laryngol.* 88 (suppl), 1–20.

Don M, Elberling C. (1994) Evaluating residual background noise in human auditory brainstem responses. *J Acoust Soc Am.* 96, 2746–2757.

Don M, Elberling C. (1996) Use of quantitative measures of ABR peak amplitude and residual background noise in the decision to stop averaging. *J Acoust Soc Am.* 99, 491–499.

Don M, Kwong B, Tanaka C. (2005a) A diagnostic test for Ménière's disease and cochlear hydrops: impaired high-pass noise masking of ABRs. *Otol Neurotol.* 26, 711–722.

Don M, Kwong B, Tanaka C. (2007) An alternative diagnostic test for Ménière's disease and cochlear hydrops using high-pass noise masked responses: the complex amplitude ratio. *Audiol Neurotol.* 12, 359–370.

Don M, Kwong B, Tanaka C, Brackmann DE, Nelson RA. (2005b) The Stacked ABR: a sensitive and specific screening tool for detecting small acoustic tumors. *Audiol Neurotol.* 10, 274–290.

Don M, Masuda A, Nelson RA, Brackmann DE. (1997) Successful detection of small acoustic tumors using the stacked derived-band ABR method. *Am J Otol.* 18, 608–621.

Don M, Ponton CW, Eggermont JJ, Kwong B. (1998) The effects of sensory hearing loss on cochlear filter times estimated from auditory brainstem response latencies. *J Acoust Soc Am.* 104, 2280–2289.

Don M, Ponton CW, Eggermont JJ, Masuda A. (1993) Gender differences in cochlear response time: an explanation for gender amplitude differences in the unmasked auditory brain-stem response. *J Acoust Soc Am.* 94, 2135–2148.

Don M, Ponton CW, Eggermont JJ, Masuda A. (1994) Auditory brainstem response (ABR) peak amplitude variability reflects individual differences in cochlear response times. *J Acoust Soc Am.* 96, 3476–3491.

Donaldson GS, Ruth RA. (1996) Derived-band auditory brainstem response estimates of traveling wave velocity in humans. II: subjects with noise-induced hearing loss and Ménière's disease. *J Speech Hear Res.* 39, 534–545.

Dornhoffer JL, Helms J, Hoehmann DH. (1994) Presentation and diagnosis of small acoustic tumors. *Otolaryngol Head Neck Surg.* 111, 232–235.

Doyle KJ, Sininger Y, Starr A. (1998) Auditory neuropathy in childhood. *Laryngoscope.* 108, 1374–1377.

Eggermont JJ, Don M. (1980) Analysis of the click-evoked brainstem potentials in humans using high-pass noise masking: II. Effect of click intensity. *J Acoust Soc Am.* 68, 1671–1675.

Eggermont JJ, Don M. (1986) Mechanisms of central conduction time prolongation in brain-stem auditory evoked potentials. *Arch Neurol.* 43, 116–120.

Eggermont JJ, Don M, Brackmann DE. (1980) Electrocochleography and auditory brainstem electric responses in patients with pontine angle tumors. *Ann Otol Rhinol Laryngol.* 89 (suppl 75), 1–19.

Elberling C, Don M. (1984) Quality estimation of averaged auditory brainstem responses. *Scand Audiol.* 13, 187–197.

Elberling C, Parbo J. (1987) Reference data for ABRs in retrocochlear diagnosis. *Scand Audiol.* 16, 49–55.

Elberling C, Wahlgreen D. (1985) Estimation of auditory brainstem responses, ABR, by means of Bayesian reference. *Scand Audiol.* 14, 89–96.

Feblot P, Uziel A. (1982) Detection of acoustic neuromas with brainstem auditory evoked potentials: comparison between cochlear and retrocochlear abnormalities. *Adv Neurol.* 32, 169–176.

Flottorp G. (1980) Cochlear nonlinearity in Ménière's syndrome. *Hear Res.* 2, 407–409.

Forton G, Offeciers FE, Marquet J. (1990) Het acousticusneurinoma: een histopathologische studie [Acoustic neuroma: a histopathological study]. *Acta Otorhinolaryngol Belg.* 44, 399–402.

Fowler CG, Noffsinger D. (1983) Effects of stimulus repetition rate and frequency on the auditory brainstem response in normal, cochlear-impaired, and VIII nerve/brainstem-impaired subjects. *J Speech Hear Res.* 26, 560–567.

Gordon ML, Cohen NL. (1995) Efficacy of auditory brainstem response as a screening test for small acoustic neuromas. *Am J Otol.* 16, 136–139.

Gorga MP, Worthington DW, Reiland JK, Beauchaine KA, Goldgar DE. (1985) Some comparisons between auditory brain stem response thresholds, latencies, and the pure-tone audiogram. *Ear Hear.* 6, 105–112.

Grabel JC, Zappulla RA, Ryder J, Wang WJ, Malis LI. (1991) Brainstem auditory evoked responses in 56 patients with acoustic neurinoma. *J Neurosurg.* 74, 749–753.

Hecox K, Galambos R. (1974) Brain stem auditory evoked responses in human infants and adults. *Arch Otolaryngol.* 99, 30–33.

Hendrix RA, DeDio RM, Sclafani AP. (1990) The use of diagnostic testing in asymmetric sensorineural hearing loss. *Otolaryngol Head Neck Surg.* 103, 593–598.

Hood LJ. (2007) Auditory neuropathy and dys-synchrony. In: Burkard RF, Don M, Eggermont JJ, eds. *Auditory Evoked Potentials: Basic Principles and Clinical Applications.* Baltimore: Lippincott Williams & Wilkins; pp 275–290.

House JW, Waluch V, Jackler RK. (1986) Magnetic resonance imaging in acoustic neuroma diagnosis. *Ann Otol Rhinol Laryngol.* 95, 16–20.

Jackler RK, Shapiro MS, Dillon WP, Petts L, Lanser MJ. (1990) Gadolinium-DTPA enhanced magnetic resonance imaging in acoustic neuroma diagnosis and management. *Otolaryngol Head Neck Surg.* 102, 670–677.

Jerger J, Neely JG, Jerger S. (1980) Speech, impedance, and auditory brainstem response audiometry in brainstem tumors. Importance of a multiple-test strategy. *Arch Otolaryngol.* 106, 218–223.

Johnson EW. (1977) Auditory test results in 500 cases of acoustic neuroma. *Arch Otolaryngol.* 103, 152–158.

Josey AF, Glasscock ME, Musiek FE. (1988) Correlation of ABR and medical imaging in patients with cerebellopontine angle tumors. *Am J Otol.* 9 (suppl), 12–16.

Josey AF, Jackson CG, Glasscock ME. (1980) Brainstem evoked response audiometry in confirmed acoustic tumors. *Am J Otol.* 1, 285–289.

Kartush JM, Graham MD, LaRouere MJ. (1992) False-positive magnetic resonance imaging in the diagnosis of acoustic neurinomas. Letter to the editor. *Otolaryngol Head Neck Surg.* 107, 495.

Keith WJ, Greville KA. (1987) Effects of audiometric configuration on the auditory brain stem response. *Ear Hear.* 8, 49–55.

Kirsh I, Thornton A, Burkard R, Halpin C. (1992) The effect of cochlear hearing loss on auditory brain stem response latency. *Ear Hear.* 13, 233–235.

Klis JF, Prijs VF, Latour JB, Smoorenburg GF. (1988) Modulation of cochlear tuning by low-frequency sound. *Hear Res.* 36, 163–173.

Kotlarz JP, Eby TL, Borton TE. (1992) Analysis of the efficiency of retrocochlear screening. *Laryngoscope.* 102, 1108–1112.

Legatt AD, Pedley TA, Emerson RG, Stein BM, Abramson M. (1988) Normal brain-stem auditory evoked potentials with abnormal latency-intensity studies in patients with acoustic neuromas. *Arch Neurol.* 45, 1326–1330.

Levine SC, Antonelli PJ, Le CT, Haines SJ. (1991) Relative value of diagnostic tests for small acoustic neuromas. *Am J Otol.* 12, 341–346.

Lightfoot GR. (1993) Correcting for factors affecting ABR wave V latency. *Br J Audiol.* 27, 211–220.

Marquet JF, Forton GE, Offeciers FE, Moeneclaey LL. (1990) The solitary schwannoma of the eighth cranial nerve. An immunohistochemical study of the cochlear nerve-tumor interface. *Arch Otolaryngol Head Neck Surg.* 116, 1023–1025.

Musiek FE. (1982) ABR in eighth-nerve and brain-stem disorders. *Am J Otol.* 3, 243–248.

Musiek FE, Josey AF, Glasscock ME III. (1986) Auditory brain-stem response in patients with acoustic neuromas. Wave presence and absence. *Arch Otolaryngol Head Neck Surg.* 112, 186–189.

Musiek FE, Kibbe K, Rackliffe L, et al. (1984) The auditory brain stem response I-V amplitude ratio in normal, cochlear, and retrocochlear ears. *Ear Hear.* 5, 52–55.

Musiek FE, Shinn JB, Jirsa BE. (2007) The auditory brainstem response in auditory nerve and brainstem dysfunction. In: Burkard RF, Don M, Eggermont JJ, eds. *Auditory Evoked Potentials: Basic Principles and Clinical Applications.* Baltimore: Lippincott Williams & Wilkins; pp 291–312.

Neely JG. (1985) Hearing conservation surgery for acoustic tumors: a clinical-pathologic correlative study. *Am J Otol.* Suppl, 143–146.

National Institutes of Health Consensus Development Conference. (1991) Acoustic neuroma. *Consens Statement.* 9, 1–24.

Nodar RH, Kinney SE. (1980) The contralateral effects of large tumors on brain stem auditory evoked potentials. *Laryngoscope.* 90, 1762–1768.

Parker DJ, Thornton ARD. (1978a) Frequency specific components of the cochlear nerve and brainstem evoked responses of the human auditory system. *Scand Audiol.* 7, 53–60.

Parker D, Thornton ARD. (1978b) The validity of the derived cochlear nerve and brainstem evoked responses of the human auditory system. *Scand Audiol.* 7, 45–52.

Perre J, Viala P, Foncin JF. (1990) Involvement of cochlear nerve in acoustic tumors. *Acta Otolaryngol (Stockh).* 110, 245–252.

Picton TW, Woods D, Baribeau-Brown J, Healy T. (1977) Evoked potential audiometry. *J Otolaryngol.* 6, 90–119.

Ponton CW, Eggermont JJ, Coupland SG, Winkelaar R. (1992) Frequency specific maturation of the eighth nerve and brain-stem auditory pathway: evidence from derived auditory brain-stem responses (ABRs). *J Acoust Soc Am.* 91, 1576–1586.

Portmann M, Cazals Y, Negrevergne M, Aran JM. (1980) Transtympanic and surface recordings in the diagnosis of retrocochlear disorders. *Acta Otolaryngol (Stockh).* 89, 362–369.

Prosser S, Arslan E, Pastore A. (1984) Auditory brain-stem response and hearing threshold in cerebellopontine angle tumours. *Arch Otolaryngol.* 239, 183–189.

Psatta DM, Matei M. (1988) Age-dependent amplitude variation of brain-stem auditory evoked potentials. *Electroencephalogr Clin Neurophysiol.* 71, 27–32.

Robinson K, Rudge P. (1983) The differential diagnosis of cerebellopontine angle lesions. A multidisciplinary approach with special emphasis on the brainstem auditory evoked potential. *J Neurol Sci.* 60, 1–21.

Rowe JM. (1978) Normal variability of the brainstem auditory evoked response in young and old subjects. *Electroencephalogr Clin Neurophysiol.* 44, 459–470.

Sabo DL, Durrant JD, Curtin H, Boston JR, Rood S. (1992) Correlations of neuroanatomical measures to auditory brain stem response latencies. *Ear Hear.* 13, 213–222.

Schwartz DM, Berry GA. (1985) Normative aspects of the ABR. In: Jacobson JT, ed. *The Auditory Brainstem Response.* San Diego: College-Hill; pp 65–97.

Selesnick SH, Jackler RK. (1993) Atypical hearing loss in acoustic neuroma patients. *Laryngoscope.* 103, 437–441.

Selters WA, Brackmann DE. (1977) Acoustic tumor detection with brain stem electric response audiometry. *Arch Otolaryngol.* 103, 181–187.

Shepard NT, Webster JC, Baumen M, Schuck P. (1992) Effect of hearing loss of cochlear origin on the auditory brain stem response [Published erratum appears in *Ear Hear* 1992;13(5): following table of contents]. *Ear Hear.* 13, 173–180.

Sohmer H. (1983) Neurologic disorders. In: Moore EJ, ed. *Bases of Auditory Brain-Stem Evoked Responses.* New York: Grune & Stratton; pp 317–341.

Spoendlin H, Schrott A. (1989) Analysis of the human auditory nerve. *Hear Res.* 43, 25–38.

Starr A, Achor JL. (1975) Auditory brain stem responses in neurological disease. *Arch Neurol.* 32, 761–768.

Starr A, Don M. (1988) Brain potentials evoked by acoustic stimuli. In: Picton TW, ed. *Handbook of Electroencephalography and Clinical Neurophysiology: Human Event-Related Potentials, Revised Series.* Volume 3. Amsterdam: Elsevier Science Publishers; pp 97–157.

Starr A, Hamilton AE. (1976) Correlation between confirmed sites of neurological lesions and abnormalities of far-field auditory brainstem responses. *Electroencephalogr Clin Neurophysiol.* 41, 595–608.

Starr A, Picton TW, Sininger Y, Hood LJ, Berlin CI. (1996) Auditory neuropathy. *Brain.* 119, 741–753.

Starr A, Sininger Y, Winter M, Derebery MJ, Oba S, Michalewski HJ. (1998) Transient deafness due to temperature-sensitive auditory neuropathy. *Ear Hear.* 19, 169–179.

Stegeman DF, Van Oosterom A, Colon EJ. (1987) Far-field evoked potential components induced by a propagating generator: computational evidence. *Electroencephalogr Clin Neurophysiol;* 67, 176–187.

Stephens SD, Thornton AR. (1976) Subjective and electrophysiologic tests in brain-stem lesions. *Arch Otolaryngol.* 102, 608–613.

Stockard JE, Stockard JJ, Westmoreland BF, Corfits JL. (1979) Brainstem auditory-evoked responses. Normal variation as a function of stimulus and subject characteristics. *Arch Neurol.* 36, 823–831.

Stockard JJ, Rossiter VS. (1977) Clinical and pathologic correlates of brainstem auditory response abnormalities. *Neurology.* 27, 316–325.

Sturzebecher E, Kevanishvili Z, Werbs M, Meyer E, Schmidt D. (1985) Interpeak intervals of auditory brainstem response, inter-aural differences in normal-hearing subjects and patients with sensorineural hearing loss. *Scand Audiol.* 14, 83–87.

Telian SA, Kileny PR, Niparko JK, Kemink JL, Graham MD. (1989) Normal auditory brainstem response in patients with acoustic neuroma. *Laryngoscope.* 99, 10–14.

Terkildsen K, Huis in't Veld F, Osterhammel P. (1977) Auditory brain stem responses in the diagnosis of cerebellopontine angle tumours. *Scand Audiol.* 6, 43–47.

Thomason JE, Murdoch BE, Smyth V, Plath B. (1993) ABR latency-intensity function abnormality in the early detection of a cerebellopontine angle tumour: a case study. *Scand Audiol.* 22, 57–59.

Thomsen J, Terkildsen K, Osterhammel P. (1978) Auditory brain stem responses in patients with acoustic neuromas. *Scand Audiol.* 7, 179–183.

Thornton ARD, Farrell G. (1991) Apparent travelling wave velocity changes in cases of endolymphatic hydrops. *Scand Audiol.* 20, 13–18.

Tonndorf J. (1957) The mechanism of hearing loss in early cases of endolymphatic hydrops. *Ann Otol Rhinol Laryngol.* 66, 766–784.

Tonndorf J. (1983) Vestibular signs and symptoms in Ménière's disorders: mechanical considerations. *Acta Otolaryngol (Stockh).* 95, 421–430.

Trune DR, Mitchell C, Phillips DS. (1988) The relative importance of head size, gender and age on the auditory brainstem response. *Hear Res.* 32, 165–174.

Walser H, Yasargil MG, Curcic M. (1982) Auditory brainstem responses in patients with posterior fossa tumors. *Surg Neurol.* 18, 405–415.

Watson DR. (1996) The effects of cochlear hearing loss, age and sex on the auditory brainstem response. *Audiology.* 35, 246–258.

Wielaard R, Kemp B. (1979) Auditory brainstem evoked responses in brainstem compression due to posterior fossa tumors. *Clin Neurol Neurosurg.* 81, 185–193.

Wilson DF, Hodgson RS, Gustafson MF, Hogue S, Mills L. (1992) The sensitivity of auditory brainstem response testing in small acoustic neuromas. *Laryngoscope.* 102, 961–964.

Zollner C, Eibach H. (1981) Criteria for the differential diagnosis of cochlear-retrocochlear disorders with brain stem audiometry. *Arch Otolaryngol.* 230, 135–147.

Auditory Brainstem Response in Audiometric Threshold Prediction

Yvonne S. Sininger and Martyn L. Hyde

INTRODUCTION

The basic clinical tool for measurement of hearing is the puretone audiogram. The audiogram serves as the starting point for all subsequent clinical decisions regarding auditory pathology and the need for intervention. Unfortunately, providing accurate tonal thresholds is not always a simple or voluntary task for the patient. Infants and toddlers, patients with severe cognitive and/or motor deficits, and persons who would falsify their hearing loss for a variety of reasons either cannot or will not provide overt responses to sound that are sufficient for a standard audiogram. For these subjects, the audiologist requires alternative measures that can accurately predict the puretone audiogram but do not require active cooperation, task comprehension, and appropriate behavioral responses. Historically, a variety of such procedures has been used. All of them involved measuring some physiologic function that may change systematically in response to sound. Examples include heart rate, electrical resistance of the skin (galvanic skin response), rate of sucking behavior, and even generalized body movement. None of these techniques has been found to provide a practicable and accurate measure of hearing threshold, and they have largely been abandoned in favor of using auditory evoked potentials (AEPs). The most commonly used AEPs for prediction of audiometric threshold are the auditory brainstem response (ABR) and the cortical response known as N1. Most recently, the auditory steady-state response (ASSR; see Chapter 15) has been added to the armamentarium of AEP techniques for threshold prediction.

The need for objective measures to predict hearing sensitivity has grown dramatically with the advent of newborn hearing screening programs around the world. Infants who do not pass a hearing screening test, usually based on screening automated ABR, screening automated otoacoustic emissions (OAE; see Chapter 21), or some combination of the two, require a thorough, accurate, and "objective" assessment to predict hearing thresholds for a range of frequencies in each ear. It is recommended that this assessment should take place by the age of about 3 months, whenever feasible (Joint Committee on Infant Hearing, 2000). It is generally accepted that consistent behavioral responses to *threshold-level* auditory stimuli, such as a conditioned head turn response using visual reinforcement procedures, cannot be obtained until a child reaches a developmental age of 5 to 6 months (Moore et al., 1977). For babies aged 0 to 6 months, the ABR is currently the tool of choice for detailed audiometric assessment. Using ABR techniques and tone-burst stimuli, it is now feasible to obtain reasonably accurate threshold estimates for a range of frequencies, in individual ears, for most young infants. The ABR also tends to be favored as an audiometric tool for other pediatric populations who do not or cannot give appropriate behavioral responses with more conventional audiometric methods.

The cortical N1 response (Chapter 18) can also provide accurate prediction of frequency-specific audiometric thresholds, given appropriate technique and tester skills. It is most frequently used in older children and adults, especially in the context of suspected functional (nonorganic) hearing loss and in medicolegal assessments. There is a tendency for greater use of the N1 response outside the United States, for reasons that are not entirely clear (Hyde, 1997).

This chapter will provide detailed information on the underlying principles and the practice of effective and efficient techniques for threshold estimation with the ABR. It will also discuss differences among AEPs and briefly outline some strengths and weaknesses of the alternative methods, so that each can be used appropriately in the audiologic armamentarium.

PRINCIPLES OF THRESHOLD ESTIMATION USING AUDITORY EVOKED POTENTIALS

Auditory Evoked Potential Generation

AEPs are changes in bioelectrical potential, in response to controlled auditory stimulation, that are detectable using electrodes in or near the ear and on the head. Many different AEPs are associated with processing of sounds throughout the auditory system, from the cochlea through the cerebral cortex. Here, we are concerned mainly with AEPs registered via disk electrodes on the head. Such electrodes are distant from the underlying sources of AEPs and record the net, overall "far-field" potentials due to electrical events (action potentials and/or postsynaptic potentials) in neural complexes within the brain.

Each underlying neuronal event may induce a minute potential on the head, but these individual contributions are infinitesimally small and are virtually impossible to record and visualize. However, if large numbers of neuronal elements can be persuaded to generate similar electrical activity at the same time, or at least in a very short space of time, the contributions from each element can add together to yield a much larger overall net potential on the head. This is the very important concept of neural "synchrony." Most AEPs, and particularly the ABR, require a high degree of synchrony in order to register a clear potential at the scalp. Synchrony is usually induced by using transient stimuli such as clicks or brief tone bursts with short onset times; these stimuli generate a traveling wave that sweeps along the cochlear partition, exciting many primary neurons in a few milliseconds. In a normal auditory system, this barrage of neural activity then propagates rapidly up through the afferent pathways, generating synchronized neural activity at every successive neuronal level.

Synchronized electrical activity in the auditory system generates a complicated pattern of potentials on the head. The actual pattern depends on many factors, including the nature of the source potentials and the number, position, anatomical structure, and physical orientation of those sources. A crude model that may be helpful is to think of the responding neural structures as equivalent to tiny batteries, with positive and negative ends that radiate fields of electri-

cal potentials to the surface of the head. This is known as the "dipole" model of source potentials.

At any instant, the potential over the head can be visualized as a contour map, analogous to a geographical contour map of height above sea level. This three-dimensional "topography" of potential changes rapidly over time. An electrode placed on the scalp will record the evolving pattern of electrical potential at its position, as a waveform of voltage versus time. That waveform is the AEP.

Auditory Evoked Potential Recording

For an excellent review of the basic principles of electrophysiologic recordings, see Chapter 11. Principles that are specific to the ABR and threshold measurements will be emphasized here. ABR systems used for threshold estimation typically involve the use of at least three and sometimes four electrodes. A single differential pair is always accompanied by a third electrode, which is called a common or ground electrode (because this electrode does not actually go to ground, it is preferable to call this the common electrode). It is often placed on the forehead, in which case it should be at least 3 cm from any other electrode. In infants the noninverting electrode is usually on the high forehead in the midline to avoid vertex placement on hair. The inverting electrode is often placed on a mastoid process and sometimes on the earlobe or nape of the neck. If two-channel recordings (ipsilateral and contralateral to the stimulated ear) are desired (discussed later), then an inverting electrode is usually placed on both mastoids. Each mastoid electrode forms a differential recording channel with the forehead electrode. A second channel can also use an inverting electrode at the nape of the neck.

Finally, note that it is increasingly common to use disposable electrodes for infection control. However, infection control protocols differ widely across test sites.

Signal Averaging and Artifact Rejection

Appropriate electrode placement, differential amplification, and band-pass filtering are essential steps in rendering the AEP visible and measurable, but they are not sufficient. It is necessary to "extract" the AEP from the electroencephalogram (EEG) noise by averaging the recorded activity following many repetitions of the stimulus. The preamplifier output is first digitized by an analog-to-digital converter (ADC). The digitized activity is then routed to a computer. For a typical ABR, several thousand repeated stimuli may be needed, but they can be delivered rapidly because the ABR is a fast response, usually lasting less than about 25 ms after stimulus onset. Typical stimulus repetition rates for ABR recording are 10 to 50 per second. In contrast, the cortical N1 response may last several hundred milliseconds; typical stimulus rates for N1 are about one per second or two, but only about 20 to 50 stimuli are needed for averaging, because of N1's larger signal-to-noise ratio (S/N). Therefore, a typical average for either the ABR or N1 requires about 1 or 2 minutes per stimulus condition, given appropriate EEG noise conditions. Usually, the averaged response is displayed visually and inspected for typical characteristics, including amplitude, latency, and wave shape (morphology).

How much averaging is enough? That is not a simple question. For the ABR, most clinicians average between 1,000 and 4,000 sweeps. This practice has developed partly by word of mouth and partly because, empirically, about 2,000 sweeps in one or two averages per stimulus condition generally yield reasonable ABR detection results, given fairly low-noise EEG conditions. For the average observer to believe that an observed waveform is a genuine response, the peak-to-trough size of the apparent response needs to be at least about twice the size of the random fluctuations in averaged noise elsewhere in the record. Typically, this will be the case for an ABR after about 2,000 sweeps, given a quiet EEG. A problem with this fixed number of sweeps approach is that it does not take into account the stimulus level. Near threshold, the amplitude of the ABR diminishes, so, typically, at least 4,000 sweeps are needed to resolve the response. Also, the fixed N approach does not take into account the changes in EEG noise levels, both within and across subjects. Inexperienced testers can generally make fine response detection decisions when the EEG noise is low or when the response amplitude is high but may be incorrect when these conditions are not met. Testers can mistakenly identifying random fluctuations in the averaged noise that may look like a response and have the expected latency. There is also a tendency to decide that a response is absent because it does not look "right" or does not reproduce perfectly across repeated averages when the EEG noise level is so high that a real response could not be identified reliably. Insufficient averaging (excessive EEG noise) is probably the single biggest cause of inaccurate threshold predictions with the ABR.

Testers who become aware of this danger adopt various sensible strategies. They start to recognize when EEG conditions are not acceptable and when no feasible amount of averaging will yield a reliable judgment in the available test time. They become more willing to say, "Could Not Test," or more willing to insist upon maneuvers to improve the EEG (such as calming a baby, changing head position, or changing electrodes), even if it means returning another day. In less extreme conditions, experienced testers increase the number of stimuli used to generate an average response or do several repeat averages in order to increase the overall S/N.

When the EEG noise level is high or increases dramatically during an ABR test session, by far the best approach is to find out why and fix it. It could be due to subject discomfort, which increases the myogenic electrical noise; a baby waking up or fidgeting; or an electrode that has gone bad (e.g., its attachment has deteriorated, or it is almost detached from the head). Five minutes of attention to these kinds of events are worth hours of additional averaging.

Despite our best efforts, there is a range of EEG noise that will be encountered, but what is desirable is that, across this range of conditions, an averaged ABR of a given amplitude should have consistent detectability. The latest AEP equipment offers additional aids, which will be explained shortly.

Artifact rejection is an important operation that goes hand-in-hand with averaging. The ordinary rules of averaging (e.g., the square root of N law) apply strictly only when the statistical properties of the EEG noise are constant throughout the averaging process. Random signals whose statistics (mean, variance, etc.) do not change over time are called stationary processes. The EEG is not always stationary. For example, consider a sleeping baby who may have an EEG with very low amplitude and very consistent appearance. If the baby fidgets or starts to wake up, the amplitude of the EEG may increase 10-fold or even 100-fold. The high-amplitude activity may comprise a few, brief, electrical transients lasting less than 1 second, or there may be a sustained period of high amplitude, until the baby stops moving or goes back to sleep. A nice, accumulating average showing no response or even a clear response can be wrecked in seconds by these high-amplitude EEG noise artifacts. Artifact rejection systems are designed to help protect averages against these events. They do so with limited success. The protection afforded depends very much on how appropriately the rejection system is set up.

Most rejection systems are very simple. If the EEG noise reaches a certain amplitude, then the entire sweep is ignored and is not added to the accumulating average. Usually, there is a screen display of the ongoing EEG. Some systems reject sweeps only when the EEG hits the display limits. Others have the ability to set adjustable rejection limits, sometimes indicated by horizontal lines on the screen that "surround" the ongoing EEG. The latter systems are much preferred because they permit fine adjustment of the rejection levels, whereas for the "display limit" devices, the only way to change the effective rejection limits is to change the preamplifier gain, which is usually only possible in large steps.

Because efficient averaging requires stationary EEG noise, setting appropriate artifact rejection limits is an important skill that is not recognized sufficiently. A common error in clinical practice is to accumulate an average with settings such that a quiet EEG looks almost flat, with small fluctuations that occupy only a small part of the amplitude range between the artifact rejection limits. In this situation, the average can be grossly distorted in seconds by only a few artifacts that are much larger than the ongoing, quiet EEG but are still not large enough to reach the rejection level. To avoid this, rejection limits should be set such that the amplitude fluctuations in the quiet EEG occupy much of the distance between them. This can sometimes be achieved, at least approximately, by increasing the amplifier gain. In the more flexible systems, it is easily done by adjusting the rejection limits themselves.

Wherever feasible, artifact rejection limits should be set so that, even when the EEG is quiet, there are occasional rejections. A useful rule of thumb is that the rejection rate should be about 5% to 10% of the accepted sweep count in good EEG conditions. Then, any significant burst of high-amplitude EEG will cause continuous rejection, and the average will not be corrupted. The tester can pause the acquisition, address the problem, and resume the average when conditions are acceptable.

Some AEP systems include an option for what is sometimes referred to as "Bayesian" averaging (Elberling and Wahlgreen, 1985). The term refers to a Reverend Thomas Bayes, an 18th century mathematician, who derived an important formula (Bayes' Theorem) that relates probabilities of interesting events before and after the occurrence of other, associated events. An example would be the probabilities of various differential diagnoses of a disease, before and after certain diagnostic test results. The essence of Bayesian averaging is that the sweeps contributing to an average may have amplitude variance that changes over time, such as during a brief period of increased myogenic activity. In the broader field of statistics, this averaging across samples with different variances is very well known and is referred to as weighted averaging. The variances of subsets of sweeps are calculated, and more or less emphasis (weight) in the final average is given to those subsets that have lower or higher variance, respectively. Statistically, the unweighted (regular) average is the best estimator of the true mean record if the true variance of the EEG does not actually change substantially over the course of the average. However, the weighted average may be more accurate if the variance changes substantially because the influence of high-noise sweeps is reduced. The effectiveness of weighted averaging depends on the statistical and computational details, and there are many possible weighting methods.

Weighted averaging is not a substitute for correcting high-amplitude EEG problems at their source, nor is it a substitute for appropriate artifact rejection. It makes little sense to allow a grossly corrupted sweep into an average, at any weight whatsoever. "Garbage in, garbage out" is the underlying rationale for rejecting high-noise sweeps completely. However, weighted averaging may improve the stability of averages under changing EEG conditions, above and beyond that achievable by artifact rejection alone. There is a concern that weighted averaging might be overused clinically, with the presumption that it will eliminate problems of noisy EEG. It will not. The noisier the EEG, the less efficient the testing will be, regardless of the artifact rejection and/or weighting methods used. The golden rule is: Get the quietest possible EEG from the subject's head by whatever means available. Then, average with sensible artifact rejection. In addition, use weighted averaging if you find it helpful by experience.

Objective Audiometry

Audiometry with the ABR, indeed with any AEP, is often referred to as objective. In a sense, this is correct. AEP-based threshold estimates do not require an overt response to sound. In this important aspect, they are, indeed, objective,

and that is a crucial advantage of the technique. However, in most cases, the AEP threshold is determined by subjective judgment of response presence or absence in a set of averaged records. Thus the technique is not fully objective because the skills of the observer and any unconscious biases or preconceptions about threshold can affect the reported threshold estimate.

With the ABR, especially when testing very young infants, there is usually not much prior information on which to base preconceptions about thresholds. When testing older children or adults for whom other audiometric information is available, such as in cases of suspected functional hearing loss, the potential for bias is obvious. Preferably, such cases should be tested with the tester blinded to previous audiometry to the greatest extent possible.

There are several recent technical aids that have been incorporated into AEP instruments and may reduce or abolish the subjective component in ABR testing. One important aid is the computation of the residual noise level (RNL). Typically, this is an ongoing calculation as the average accumulates. It measures the variability of the noise remaining in the average record, ideally as a standard deviation (SD). For conditions of constant EEG noise, the RNL decreases according to the square root of N law. It can be used as a quantitative measure of the actual noise variability. It can also be used to set a target noise level, and averaging may be continued until the target is achieved. This can avoid unnecessary averaging for very quiet EEG, as well as adjust the amount of averaging to accommodate variations in EEG noise levels. This tool can substantially improve the accuracy and consistency of response detection judgments and will ultimately improve the accuracy of audiometric threshold predictions.

To determine reliably that a response is absent, the RNL in the average must be reduced to the point at which the response would almost certainly have been detected if it were present. When the noise level is too high, a decision that the response is absent is unreliable and gives little information about actual response presence or absence. In contrast, when a response is clearly present, it is not necessary to continue averaging until a low RNL is achieved, provided that the peak-to-peak amplitude of the so-called "response" is at least four times the size of the current RNL. For example, to decide that a response is absent, it might be considered necessary to achieve an RNL of 20 to 30 nanovolts (nV). However, if a wave of amplitude 200 nV was seen at an earlier point in the averaging, when the RNL was still about 50 nV, then the average could be stopped with fair confidence that the waveform was a genuine response.

While sensible use of the RNL can be very helpful, a significant problem with it is that the RNL estimate may be inflated by power line interference (50 or 60 Hz), but such interference may not distort the average record substantially. This can lead to a situation of apparently poor RNL despite a low level of averaged noise on visual inspection. One cause of this discrepancy is that, for any given level of power line interference in the raw EEG, the amount of distortion of the average depends strongly on the sweep repetition rate. For example, choosing a rate of exactly 30 per second would be disastrous because any 60-Hz interference would be locked in phase to the averaging and would simply summate linearly. In contrast, rates of 24 or 40 per second would cancel 60 Hz completely for every pair of sweeps, because the 60 Hz waveform would be completely out of phase from one sweep to the next. In general, effects of repetition rate on 60-Hz interference and its various harmonics are quite complicated and a detailed analysis has not been reported in the AEP literature. Seemingly peculiar rates such as 39.1 per second are often chosen, partly on the basis of clinical experience that they tend not to cause much summation of 60 Hz.

Power line interference at 60 Hz tends to be more of an issue in ABR threshold estimation in infants because the recording bandwidth may extend to frequencies as low as 30 Hz, especially for tone-burst ABR threshold measurements for low-frequency stimuli in young infants (see section on Band-Pass Filtering). One way to reduce 60-Hz interference dramatically is to use so-called "notch filters," which are a standard option in most ABR instrumentation. It is common to see recommendations to avoid or minimize use of these filters, usually on the grounds that they may cause significant distortion of the ABR (phase distortion). This issue needs careful reexamination for two reasons. First, modern notch filter techniques may not actually cause significant ABR distortion. Second, even if distortion were to occur, it may not have a substantive effect on actual ABR thresholds. It may be reasonable, therefore, to use a notch filter if there is significant and unavoidable 60-Hz interference in average records or if large RNLs occur for apparently "clean" averages. However, a greater concern with heavy reliance on notch filters is that visible 60-Hz interference in the ongoing EEG or in averages is a useful indicator of poor recording conditions, such as excessive 60-Hz radiation from power sources close to the subject, poor routing of electrode leads, asymmetric electrode impedances, and so on. The notch filter will remove these important cues. One approach is to use notch filters only when strictly necessary, after all reasonable steps to minimize 60-Hz pickup have been taken. The notch filter is not a substitute for careful recording practices.

It is also possible to compute statistical measures of the actual probability of response presence. Typically, such statistics calculate the probability that a given pattern in the average could have arisen by chance alone, when a response is truly absent, this probability is usually called alpha (the significance level). Typically, alpha might be set at 0.05 (5%), giving a 5% chance of a false-positive response detection in any single average. This type of approach is what is used in automated ABR screening systems. In that application, though, alpha is usually set much lower (0.01 or less), so that the probability of false positive response detection is very low.

Perhaps the most well-established response detection statistic is called Fsp (Don et al., 1984; Elberling and Don, 1987). The variability of the EEG noise (i.e., the variance) is calculated using the data points at a specific position from each sweep; one might choose the 50th data point in each sweep of 512 points. This is the "single point" to which the "sp" refers. The sweeps are averaged, and the variance at the single point is calculated. Call it V1. Also, the variance of all the points within a time region of interest (e.g., 10 ms across the average placed where the response is expected) is calculated; call that V2. If there is no response, V2 is just the variance of averaged noise, which has a very simple statistical relationship to the variance of the single points. In fact, statistical theory tells us that the value expected for V2 when no response is present is just V1/N (where N is the number of sweeps averaged). If a response is actually present, it will increase V2 because some points in the average, such as response peaks and troughs, will be farther from the baseline than would occur due to averaging of random EEG noise alone. But, the presence of a true response will not increase V1 because the AEP contribution is assumed to be constant at the single time point in all sweeps and so it does not contribute anything to variability. Now, consider the variance ratio N*V2/V1. On reflection, the reader will see that the value we expect for that ratio in the absence of response is unity (1.0). However, if there is response, N*V2 will tend to be greater than V1, so the ratio will be bigger than 1.0.

If we did lots of averages without any stimulus, we would get a slightly different value for the variance ratio each time, due to sampling variation of the random EEG noise. A histogram would show a statistical distribution of ratio values in the absence of response. In fact, we already know that distribution exactly, from statistical theory. It is called the Snedecor F distribution, or just F. So, if a value of Fsp is obtained for a given average, such as 2.1, for example, it can be looked up in statistical tables to see how likely it was to get a value as big as or bigger than 2.1. If that probability were less than the predetermined alpha, then something other than chance is likely to have caused such a big value, and the obvious reason is that there **was** a response, because a response increases V2.

There are many other ways of testing statistically for response presence, but the variance ratio approach is theoretically the most powerful. That is, there is no other statistical test that will detect the response as accurately in a smaller number of sweeps.

There is a bit more to Fsp than what was just described. Some numbers called degrees of freedom of V1 and V2 must be known, but we usually have a good idea what they are. Also, there is a need to be careful about how the set of points for V2 is chosen. If the response only occurs in a small part of the window, but the whole window is used to calculate V2, then the test will lose power because many of the points will just add random error to V2. This is less of a problem in screening applications, which typically use only one stimulus level, because we have a better idea of what the response will look like and when it will occur. In general threshold testing, however, the range of possible response waveforms and latencies is larger, which tends to weaken the Fsp test because a wider range of points must be included in V2. Still, even so,

Fsp can be a very useful tool for response detection, and it can be used as an aid to subjective judgment that goes beyond just the RNL. For example, if a response was judged to be present but Fsp was, say, only 1.5, then we would certainly have to think again and measure again. Typical values of Fsp that indicate alphas of 0.05 or 0.01 are about 2.5 or 3.1, respectively.

Several clues to help decide if there is a response in a given average have been mentioned earlier. Subjective methods usually take into account the size of the peaks and troughs in the averaged waveform, their latency or position in the average, and their morphology (wave shape). We may also study waveform reproducibility across two or more averages. Some experts insist on reproducibility as a minimum standard for response identification, no matter how "positive" an individual average may be, and this viewpoint is not unreasonable. If an individual average that is considered to be a response has satisfied some criterion for a low level of average noise or has a large value of Fsp, then the need to demonstrate reproducibility is reduced.

Experienced testers often make use of additional cues to response presence. For example, there is a typical trend of increasing response latency as threshold is approached. Also, genuine responses grow very gradually, not suddenly. This latter judgment requires very close attention to each average as it accumulates.

Equally important in threshold work is to make reliable decisions about response absence, that is, ruling out a response. As noted earlier, such decisions simply cannot be made reliably if the average is noisy, and it can be beneficial to make use of the RNL, if it is available. Simply showing lack of reproducibility between two averages of noisy EEG proves nothing about response absence because averaged random noise will dominate the records and is very likely to show poor reproducibility.

How do we move from response decisions at specific stimulus levels to an estimate of the ABR threshold? The usual method is to determine presence or absence over a set of stimulus levels, essentially bracketing the presumed threshold with a chain of yes/no decisions, analogous to conventional puretone audiometry. Threshold is usually defined by a clear response-negative decision at some level, coupled with a clear response-positive decision at some adjacent but higher level, typically with 5-dB or 10-dB separation. This might be called a direct threshold measurement. Other methods include some kind of extrapolation of response amplitude to zero, but extrapolation errors due to variability of measured response amplitudes are a concern, and it has not been proven that such methods offer an advantage in speed or accuracy over direct bracketing. Efficient methods of bracketing are discussed later in the context of testing strategy.

Auditory Evoked Potentials Versus Perception of Sound

It should be clear that, although AEPs and auditory perception both result from electrical activity in the auditory system, the two phenomena involve completely different processes. It follows that conventional audiometric thresholds and AEP thresholds may not be the same. Perceptual or psychophysical threshold is measured using an overt motor response, by an individual, in response to the perception of an auditory signal. In contrast, observation of an AEP constitutes measurable evidence of synchronized, neural activity in some part of the auditory system in response to controlled sounds.

For both AEPs and psychophysical measures, the threshold is judged as the lowest stimulus level that produces a reliable response. If these tests are performed in an appropriate fashion, the results of the two measurements, expressed as the threshold level of the stimulus in dB, may be highly correlated, even though the two techniques reflect very different underlying processes. This is fortunate, because it means that AEP thresholds can be used to predict or estimate psychophysical thresholds. However, it is important to realize that it is not hearing that is measured with an AEP. What is measured is simply synchronized electrical activity that is usually correlated with hearing.

There are many distinctions between AEP and psychophysical thresholds. Each varies in different ways in response to stimulus manipulations. For example, stimulus duration may have no effect on ABR threshold while significantly changing the psychophysical threshold of the same stimulus, due to temporal integration (Gorga et al., 1984). Increasing the stimulus repetition rate beyond about 10/s also increases perceptual loudness and reduces the sensory threshold but may have little or no effect on the ABR threshold (Sininger and Don, 1989).

It is important for the audiologist to understand that conventional puretone thresholds and AEP thresholds are two distinct measures that may be affected differently by specific variables. Therefore, their respective thresholds are not necessarily going to be numerically identical. It is better to start from the position that they may be very different and then to consider how best to measure and interpret ABR records to yield the most accurate prediction or estimate of the conventional threshold.

To emphasize further how AEP and psychophysical methods may yield different thresholds, consider the following scenario. Take, for example, a brief tone-burst stimulus with, say, a nominal frequency of 2 kHz, and set its level to 20 dB above the behavioral threshold for the tone burst. Shape that tone burst with a linear rise and fall envelope, and a rise-fall time of 20 ms. Such a stimulus will be easily perceptible, but it will NOT evoke a measurable ABR because a rise of 20 ms is too slow to induce the necessary underlying neural synchrony. Now change the rise-fall time to 5 ms. The sound will still be audible, although it will be fainter because psychophysically the auditory system tends to integrate the overall energy in a brief sound (temporal integration), but there will now be a detectable ABR elicited because a 5-ms rise time is fast enough to cause adequate synchrony. Clearly, the ABR threshold will be lower (better) in the second case, but the perceptual threshold will be actually be higher (poorer) in that case (because the total stimulus energy is lower). Now imagine a third situation, in which the EEG noise levels from two subjects with identical hearing thresholds are very different: Subject A has very low noise, and subject B has high noise. After a fixed amount of averaging, the ABR may be detectable for the low-noise subject but may remain undetectable for the high-noise subject, and so they will have different apparent ABR thresholds.

The bottom line is that the observed AEP threshold depends on a host of stimulus, subject, and recording variables that may not affect the perceptual threshold. In addition, poor recording conditions and inappropriate stimuli or recording methods degrade the ABR and reduce its detectability. Thus, we can expect ABR-based thresholds to approximate true perceptual thresholds only if the AEP measurements are done correctly and the EEG noise conditions are appropriate.

Differences Among Auditory Evoked Potentials

The ABR and the cortical N1 potential are generated in different regions of the brain (see Chapters 11 and 18) and consequently have different characteristics and reactions to lesions in these areas. The ABR is generated in the auditory nerve (waves I and II) and the neurons of cochlear nucleus, superior olivary complex, and lateral lemniscus of the brainstem (Moller and Jannetta, 1983). In contrast, the cortical N1 response is generated in the primary auditory cortex and association areas. For this reason, the brainstem (a site of reflexive activity) is generally impervious to cognitive state. Therefore, the ABR is unaltered by sleep state, sedation, or attention (Amandeo and Shagass, 1973), but such factors have dramatic effects on the higher level N1 response (Picton and Hillyard, 1974).

The sequential nature of processing in the auditory system implies that lesions low in the system can affect responses generated at the level of the lesion as well as higher levels that have similar stimulus/response dynamics. For example, loss of sensory cells within the cochlea may be reflected in response threshold elevation at the auditory brainstem as well as the auditory cortex. An eighth-nerve tumor may spare ABR wave I but degrade or abolish later ABR waves. A pure cortical lesion, in contrast, may influence N1 but not ABR responses. Cases of deaf patients with bilateral lesions of the auditory cortex have been described in which the ABRs were normal (Szirmai et al., 2003; Musiek et al., 2004; Kneebone and Burns, 1981). Such examples illustrate the need for caution when attempting to relate ABR results directly to hearing.

Other distinctions in the properties of various AEPs are related to the level and characteristics of their neural generators. As noted earlier, the ABR is a "fast" response that occurs early, typically within about 25 ms of the onset of the stimulus. It has a spectral composition (energy distribution) of about 50 to 1,500 Hz, which is reflected in the spacing of major peaks. In contrast, the cortical N1 response is part of the so-called N1-P2 complex, which has been referred to as the slow vertex potential (Davis, 1976). This response occurs in the range 50 to 300 ms and has a spectral composition of 1 to 10 Hz.

These two types of AEP are affected differently by disorders that cause dyssynchrony or jitter in the neural signal. Registration of a measurable ABR at the scalp requires a high degree of temporal synchrony of the very rapid underlying neural events that generate the response (action potentials and fast postsynaptic potentials). If, however, the firing patterns of individual stimulated neurons are not the same (for example, if some are delayed relative to others), then the overall activity will not sum as effectively. Rather, the scalp response will be absent or broadened, late or indistinct. Precisely this effect underlies the well-known use of the ABR in the detection of eighth-nerve tumors or other brainstem lesions that interfere with the fine timing or the volume of neural response.

The auditory nerve can suffer from axonal or demyelinating neuropathy, a disorder known collectively as auditory neuropathy/auditory dyssynchrony (AN/AD) (Starr et al., 1996). This disorder can alter the amplitude or speed of neural conduction in individual auditory neurons in unpredictable ways. Because of the stringent requirements of synchrony to produce an ABR, this response is particularly vulnerable to AN/AD. In contrast, some patients with AN/AD who have absent or severely distorted ABR will demonstrate a reasonably clear cortical N1 response, and many have no more than a mild hearing loss (Sininger and Oba, 2001). Rance et al. (2002) recorded cortical event-related potentials (ERPs) with normal amplitude and latency characteristics from approximately half of subjects with AN/AD, primarily those with fairly good speech perception ability. The cortical N1 is not only significantly larger than the ABR, but it also is generated by cortical postsynaptic potentials that have a much longer time course than the events that generate the ABR. As a result, the N1 response is much less vulnerable to short-duration jitter or lack of synchrony in auditory neurons. As the neural response ascends the auditory system, some degree of response normality may be regained even following a jittery or desynchronized response from the auditory nerve.

One must keep in mind these particular attributes of brainstem and cortical AEPs when considering their use to make judgments about a subject's audiometric profile. When a subject is sleeping or unconscious, the cortical N1 may be absent, reduced, or otherwise modified, but that is not the case with ABR. When peripheral nerve disease is present, the ABR will be unreliable as a measure of auditory sensitivity, but reasonable results may be obtained with cortical responses. Each can be used to make useful predictions but only when correctly interpreted in light of its particular characteristics (including hearing sensitivity) and understanding that there is not a one-to-one correspondence between perception of sound and registration of AEPs.

NORMATIVE ASPECTS OF THE AUDITORY BRAINSTEM RESPONSE

Appropriate use of the ABR requires an understanding of how important variables relating to subjects, stimulation, and recording methods can affect the response. ABRs are generally described on the basis of waveform morphology, including the presence and number of anticipated peaks, and by the poststimulus latency and peak-to-trough amplitude of the waves that are present. All of these parameters change up until about 2 years of age. The peaks are labeled with Roman numerals I through V and sometimes VI or VII, a convention developed by Jewett and Williston (1971).

Age

Latency for all major peaks present in the neonatal ABR (I, III, and V) shortens during the first years of life, as shown in Figure 14.1. These latency changes are attributed primarily to postnatal myelination of the brainstem pathway and to increases in synaptic density and efficiency (Salamy et al., 1994). Wave I achieves adult latency values at about 3 month of age, wave III is mature between 8 and 16 months, and wave V latency achieves adult values from 18 to 36 months of age (Salamy and McKean, 1976; Hecox and Burkard, 1982; Salamy, 1984). The I-V interpeak interval also decreases over

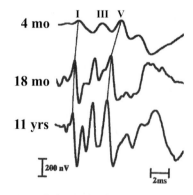

Developmental Changes in ABR
Latency, Amplitude and Spectrum

4 mo

18 mo

11 yrs

FIGURE 14.1 Click evoked auditory brainstem response (ABR) to 70-dB nHL stimulus changes character with the subject's age. Absolute and interpeak latencies decrease with age, and amplitude increases. (Adapted from Figure 6 of Sininger YS, Abdala C. [1998] Physiologic assessment of hearing. In: Lalwani AK, Grundfast KM, eds. *Pediatric Otology and Neurotology.* Philadelphia: Lippincott-Raven; pp 127–154.)

the first 2 or 3 years of life (Starr et al., 1977; Salamy et al., 1975).

ABR peak amplitudes are usually measured from the peak under consideration to the following trough. As illustrated in Figure 14.1, peak amplitudes increase during the first 1 to 2 years of life (Salamy, 1984; Jacobson et al., 1982; Durieux-Smith et al., 1985). When measured in a vertex-to-mastoid configuration, the amplitude of wave I from infants is often larger than the amplitude of wave V, but this relationship reverses over the first few years of life (Hecox and Burkard, 1982). Wave V amplitude is the parameter that is most important in determining the ABR threshold. Peak amplitude is often considered too variable to be of great clinical use (Jacobson and Hyde, 1986). However, as shown by Elberling and Don (1987), measurement of peak amplitude is highly influenced by recording noise. They demonstrated that ABR peak amplitude is reasonably stable when the level of averaged noise is controlled, as outlined earlier.

Ear and Gender

There is a general belief that the ABR is identical for stimuli presented to the left and right ears. Normative data for ABR latencies and amplitudes, for example, typically do not distinguish the ear stimulated. In fact, subtle but systematic differences can generally be found in ABRs from the two ears. When such differences are noted, ABRs recorded in response to click stimuli presented to the right ear are found to have shorter latency and larger amplitude than those elicited with stimuli to the left ear. For example, the amplitude of peak III of the ABR from adults has been shown be larger when elicited by clicks delivered to the right ear (Levine and McGaffigan, 1983; Levine et al., 1988). Eldredge and Salamy (1996) tested pre- and full-term infants and found larger peak amplitudes and shorter interpeak intervals elicited by click stimuli to the right ear than to the left. In a large-scale study of ABRs from neonates generated with 30- and 70-dB normal hearing level (nHL) clicks, wave V amplitude for both low- and high-level stimuli was found to be significantly larger and waves III and V were shorter in latency when the ABR was generated in the right ear compared with the left ear (Sininger and Cone-Wesson, 2006). Because these differences are quite small, they have no clinical significance at this time.

ABR peak amplitudes and latencies are consistently different in male and female subjects. Wave V to clicks is larger in females than males (Shepard et al., 1992; Kileny and Robertson, 1985; Michalewski et al., 1980). The latency of wave V as well as the I-V interval is also slightly shorter in females than males (McClelland and McCrea, 1979; Rosenhamer et al., 1980; Elberling and Parbo, 1987). One theory for the mechanism of sex-related differences in ABR peak latency was that the length of the brainstem pathway was shorter in women. A positive relationship does exist between head size and ABR peak latencies. However, in males and females with equal head size, females have shorter peak latencies, indicating that the mechanism for latency differences is other than brainstem length (Trune et al., 1988). Don et al. (1993) have shown conclusively that both larger amplitudes and shorter latencies of ABR peaks in females can be explained by faster traveling wave time in female cochleae, which are slightly shorter than male cochleae. In fact, the female cochlea is 13% shorter than the male cochlea (Sato et al., 1991).

Stimulus Spectrum

The ABR can be generated with a variety of stimuli but is usually elicited either with broadband clicks or with short-duration, shaped (gated) tones often referred to as tone bursts or tone pips. For some applications, a click is embedded in masking noise that has been band-reject filtered or high-pass filtered, restricting synchronous activation to specific frequency regions that are not masked. In a subject with normal hearing, the click-evoked ABR reflects activation of a wide array of hair cells and their corresponding neural elements, in response to the entire range of frequencies available through the transducer.

Short-duration (usually $\sim$100 μs) rectangular voltage pulses delivered to a broadband transducer will generate clicks that have an energy spectrum reflecting the entire frequency range of the transducer. This broadband stimulus (click) will then activate auditory regions of greatest absolute sensitivity, whether presented to a subject with normal hearing or to one with a flat audiometric configuration. The level of the click stimulus at the threshold of detection for the ABR will consequently correlate most closely to the best hearing threshold within the frequency range of the transducer. In fact, the click threshold will reflect the best threshold between about 750 and 4,000 Hz for most clinically used transducers. However, if the best hearing occurs below about 750 Hz, then the response may be difficult to discern. This may be due to phase cancellation among responses generated from various frequency regions. Band-limited masking noise may reduce this phase interference effect.

In the human, the hearing threshold curve plotted in sound pressure level (SPL) shows best sensitivity in the region of 2.5 to 4 kHz. The latency of the click-evoked ABR will most strongly reflect activation of the 2- to 4-kHz region in persons for whom the audiogram is flat. Therefore, it is not unusual to find group data indicating good correlations across subjects between hearing levels in the 2- to 4-kHz range and the ABR click threshold (Jerger and Mauldin, 1978; Moller and Blegvad, 1976; Hyde et al., 1990). However, large discrepancies can be found between the click ABR threshold and hearing sensitivity at 2 to 4 kHz in individual cases in which the configuration of the hearing loss is not flat. It follows that the click ABR threshold cannot be considered as a reliable predictor of high-frequency hearing threshold in clinical practice.

We argue that threshold measurement with clicks alone is not sufficient, despite its historical popularity. Reliance on ABR threshold measurement with clicks alone makes no more sense than reliance on behavioral audiometry with white noise bursts or speech stimuli. Clicks do not provide frequency-specific information, the very essence of audiometry. Clearly, because the click ABR threshold is just a single number, it cannot adequately describe the range of threshold values and configurations across the frequencies commonly considered to be clinically important. Moreover, a normal click ABR threshold can be observed in the presence of substantial threshold abnormality at specific frequencies. All that is required for a clear click ABR is relatively good hearing at *some* frequency in the range from about 1 to 8 kHz. Some experts have advocated the use of low-frequency tone bursts (at 500 Hz or even 250 Hz) in combination with clicks to assess higher frequencies (Gorga et al., 2006). However, getting clear ABR thresholds to 2 kHz and 4 kHz tone bursts is usually no more difficult than with a click and is significantly more informative for hearing aid fitting and for detection of high-frequency loss.

In fact, it has been established that it is possible to determine well-defined ABR thresholds using tone-burst stimuli with frequencies in the range 500 Hz to 4 kHz. It is reported that such thresholds are accurate predictors of the conventional audiometric threshold for the specific frequency (Stapells et al., 1995). When the stimulus energy spectrum is more restricted (e.g., with tone bursts), ABR amplitude tends to be reduced, and its latency will reflect the time necessary to activate the basilar membrane location associated with the primary stimulus energy peak or unmasked stimulus region (Don et al., 1979; Parker and Thornton, 1978; Kimberley et al., 1993). This is known as the traveling wave delay. Figure 14.2 demonstrates the systematic latency shifts of ABRs from an infant elicited with a series of 40-dB nHL tone bursts with center frequencies of 500 through 4,000 Hz.

Stimulus polarity can affect ABR morphology, particularly peak latency, in ways that can differ across individuals (Stockard et al., 1983; Gorga et al., 1991; Orlando and Folsom, 1995). It is often reported that a rarefaction onset phase leads to shorter latencies, but this is not a universal finding. Although phase of the stimuli (condensation and rarefaction) may have an effect on morphology of the net ABR waveform, especially with steeply sloping hearing losses, this factor was found to have no effect on threshold of the ABR in adult subjects with normal hearing, and it had no influence on wave V amplitude to low-level (25 to 30 dB nHL) clicks (Sininger and Masuda, 1990; Kevanishvili and Aphonchenko, 1981).

It is often stated that alternating stimulus phase for ABR threshold measures should be used with caution, because of the potential to reduce response amplitude or obscure waves by adding response components that are out of phase. The greatest absolute changes in ABR peak latency for condensation and rarefaction stimuli will occur with low-frequency stimuli (Orlando and Folsom, 1995; Salt and Thornton, 1984; Fowler, 1992; Don et al., 1996). The response latency differences for condensation and rarefaction stimuli often appear to roughly equal a half-period of the frequency of

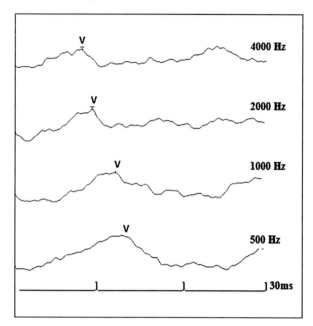

FIGURE 14.2 Auditory brainstem responses (ABRs) elicited from an infant in response to tone bursts of 40 dB nHL. As the nominal frequency of the stimulus decreases, wave V latency systematically increases, reflecting the traveling wave time along the basilar membrane.

greatest energy in the stimulus. Shifts in wave V latency for low-frequency ABRs elicited with opposite polarity stimuli could result in partial cancellation of the peak when the responses are combined. However, an argument for the use of alternating polarity is that the ABR waveform for low-frequency stimuli, especially near threshold, is much longer and slower that the typical, sharp, multipeaked waveform associated with, for example, high-level click stimuli. Consider, for example, a tone burst at 500 Hz. The half-cycle duration for this stimulus is only 1 ms. It seems at least questionable that a 1-ms difference in latency between responses for 500-Hz condensation and rarefaction onset tone bursts will cause much smearing or loss of amplitude, given a typical response that is a long, slow wave V-V' complex (V peak and its ensuing negative wave, termed V prime) lasting many milliseconds. However, stimulus alternation must be used with much caution in otoneurologic applications with click stimuli because those responses may be sharp and multipeaked, and the test depends on detailed evaluation of latency and morphology.

It should be noted that insert earphones have tubing connecting the transducer to the ear induce a small delay (typically about 0.9 ms) in stimulus arrival relative to the stimulus generation at the transducer. This situation allows the transducer to be placed further from the electrodes, reducing the size of the stimulus-induced electrical artifact, and also helps to separate the stimulus artifact from the brainstem response in time, reducing the likelihood that the two will be confused. The benefit from this effect is limited for low-frequency stimuli, for which the stimulus artifact duration may approach 10 ms or greater. Electrical stimulus artifacts are particularly common when stimulating with a bone-conduction transducer.

Stimulus Rate

For standard ABR, stimuli are presented at a fixed rate that must be equal to or less than the reciprocal of the averaging time window to avoid more than one stimulus occurring in a given window. For example, if the window was 20 ms (0.02 seconds), then stimuli could be presented at a maximum of 50/s. More sophisticated ABR techniques allow more rapid stimulation, with mathematical disentangling of overlapped ABRs, but these so-called maximum-length sequence (MLS) methods are not widely used in audiometric threshold prediction (Leung et al., 1998). In general, fast stimulus presentation rates increase ABR peak and interpeak latencies and reduce response amplitudes compared to slower rates. In adults, when using moderate stimulus levels, increasing stimulus rate above 30/s has sometimes been shown to reduce peak amplitude (Hyde et al., 1976; Suzuki et al., 1986; Don et al., 1977), but in other studies, no clear change in response amplitude was found with stimulus rates up to 80/s (Picton et al., 1981; Van Olphen et al., 1979).

In infants, more than in adults, increasing stimulus rate consistently leads to a reduction in response amplitude and/or detectability (Stockard et al., 1983; Morgan et al., 1987; Stockard et al., 1979). Lasky (1997) found larger increases in wave V latency with rate in infants than adults, but rate-related amplitude decreases were greater in adults. Klein et al. (1992) found that high stimulus rates (90/s) yielded an ABR to a 30-dB nHL click in most full-term infants but only in 50% of premature infants, indicating that very young infants may be more vulnerable to ABR amplitude reduction from high rates. For clinical applications, moderate click rates up to about 50/s should not elevate response threshold in adults or in infants, but higher rates should be used with caution (Sininger and Don, 1989; Lasky, 1991).

Minimizing test time is a *critically* important goal in evaluating infants and toddlers. High stimulus rates have the possible benefit of shortening test time because they permit more averaging in a given test time. The issue is the effect on the S/N of reduced noise due to more averaging, which is balanced against reduced response amplitude due to adaptation at high rates. Caution is needed with very high rates when the ABR is used in infants or children, especially those with fragile or underdeveloped auditory systems. Reduction in response detectability due to high stimulus rates can be confused with elevated threshold due to hearing loss.

Stimulus Level

Stimulus level has a dramatic effect on ABR amplitude and usually has a strong effect on latency. The latency of all peaks, particularly wave V, decreases with stimulus level.

The slope of the latency/intensity function for click stimuli is 33 to 35 μs/dB for infants but somewhat steeper (44 to 58 μs/dB) for adults and steeper for all subjects when the ABR is elicited with tone bursts, especially low-frequency tone bursts (Hecox and Burkard, 1982; Galambos and Hecox, 1978; Sininger et al., 1997; Jacobson et al., 1982; Schulman-Galambos and Galambos, 1975). In general, latency tends to increase most rapidly within about 10 dB of the ABR threshold. Another effect that is seen as threshold is approached is the presence of V-V' alone and diminution or disappearance of earlier waves. This reduction or absence of earlier waves and retention of only the V-V' complex is particularly prominent for low-frequency tone-burst stimuli (e.g., 500 Hz), especially near threshold, where it is not uncommon to see only a long, slow wave V, or on occasion, only a long, slow wave V' with little or no actual wave V peak (see Fig. 14.2). For these stimulus conditions, the most consistent response feature is a negative-going slope in the 15- to 20-ms region.

The fact that ABR latency tends to increase as threshold is approached is helpful in visual detection of genuine responses. For example, given an unequivocally present ABR at some stimulus level, it is extremely unlikely that a deflection that is substantially earlier in a record at a lower stimulus level is a genuine response.

ABR peak latencies may be prolonged by hearing loss, more markedly so when the hearing loss is conductive, and this information may be of some value in inferring the type of hearing loss (Picton and Durieux-Smith, 1978; Kileny, 1981). Latency information may also be useful in predicting the slope of the hearing loss (Jerger and Mauldin, 1978; Moller and Blegvad, 1976). However, latency varies with several subject, stimulus, and recording parameters, including those previously mentioned, such as age and stimulus repetition rate. Consequently, absolute ABR peak latencies are of little help in the quantitative prediction of ABR threshold. Only changes in latency with level are truly helpful in threshold determination.

Electrode Montage

ABRs are recorded with differential electrodes, so the recorded response amplitude from any given set of generators in the auditory system will be largest when the pair of electrodes on the scalp is lined up with the direction of the equivalent dipole sources in the brain. Generators for individual ABR peaks and their dipole orientation vary across peaks and, to a lesser extent, with the stimulus type and level or with the age of the subject. As mentioned, threshold applications with ABR concentrate on identification of wave V, the peak that can be most often identified at low stimulus levels. Appropriate placement of the noninverting and inverting electrodes can aid in the recording of the largest possible wave V and, consequently, in determination of the lowest possible thresholds.

Sininger and Don (1989) investigated the theoretical dipole orientation for wave V with click stimuli near threshold for adult subjects. They found the optimal orientation to be almost vertical, from just behind the vertex to the joining of the chin and throat. Assuming that the chin electrode could be simulated with linked earlobes, King and Sininger (1992) compared four electrode montages for amplitude of wave V at low sensation levels and discovered that the recording from vertex to C7 (near the nape of the neck) revealed larger wave V amplitude near threshold than electrode montages that combined the vertex or forehead with linked mastoids or a single mastoid

The optimal orientation of electrodes for recording the ABR in infants is somewhat different than seen in adults (McPherson et al., 1985; Stuart et al., 1996; Hafner et al., 1991). For audiometric purposes, it is necessary to understand the relationship between electrode montage and the threshold of the ABR. Sininger et al. (1997) determined ABR thresholds to clicks and tonal stimuli from two recording channels in neonates. The thresholds were slightly lower when recorded from the vertex to nape of the neck as compared to a vertex to mastoid. However, when 30-dB nHL click ABRs were recorded in infants from these sites and compared using a measure related to the S/N, an advantage was found for the vertex to mastoid channel (Sininger et al., 2000). The vertex to nape channel produced larger amplitude ABRs but also was contaminated by higher noise levels, probably due to cardiac noise from the torso, which is larger because of the location of the neck electrode. Both electrode montages, vertex (or high forehead) to nape and to mastoid, are excellent for threshold determination, but the nape electrode may be particularly contaminated by physiologic (cardiac) noise in infants.

Use of the high midline forehead electrode as the noninverting electrode has become popular because it avoids the issue of placing an electrode in the hair of an infant. The amplitude of wave V may be slightly reduced when the noninverting electrode is moved from the vertex to the forehead but only slightly (Kavanagh and Clark, 1989). It is common to use a two-channel recording with a single noninverting electrode on the vertex or forehead serving both channels and inverting electrodes on the mastoids ipsilateral and contralateral to the stimulation site, or with the ipsilateral mastoid and nape of the neck as inverting electrode sites. However, the ABR recorded from the mastoid contralateral to the ear stimulated is immature in preterm infants, and this recording channel is not recommended for use in threshold measurement until after about 9 months of age (Salamy et al., 1985). In summary, for threshold ABR applications in infants and young children, both the ipsilateral mastoid and central neck location are appropriate sites for the inverting electrode, and the vertex or high forehead is an appropriate site for the noninverting electrode (Stuart et al., 1996).

Band-Pass Filtering

Figure 14.1 shows the progressive changes in the waveform of the ABR with subject age. As illustrated, the spectral composition of the ABR from infants and toddlers is dominated by lower frequency energy relative to the adult ABR (Spivak, 1993). Filtering of the EEG signal reduces unwanted activity (noise), increasing the overall S/N, and this improvement in S/N is crucial for ABR threshold applications. Filtering must take the subject's age into consideration to avoid loss of energy from frequency regions contained in the infant ABR. For infants and toddlers, this means allowing more low-frequency information into the recording by reducing the low-frequency filter cutoff, relative to adult recordings.

When threshold evaluations are performed using the ABR, it is also important to consider spectral changes in the response that are caused by changes in the level and spectrum of the stimulus. The energy spectrum of the ABR shifts to lower frequency as the sensation level of the stimulus is reduced. It peaks between 500 and 1,000 Hz when high-level stimuli are used but falls below 250 Hz for near-threshold stimuli (Elberling, 1979; Malinoff and Spivak, 1990; Sininger, 1995). ABRs elicited by low-frequency stimuli also contain more low-frequency energy in comparison to those elicited by high-frequency tone bursts or by click stimuli (Hyde, 1985).

Setting the band-pass filters to include energy below 100 Hz has been shown to increase ABR amplitude when using low-level stimuli in adults (Domico and Kavanagh, 1986; Boston and Ainslie, 1980; Kavanagh et al., 1984) and particularly in infants (Hyde, 1985; Stapells, 1989; Stuart and Yang, 1994). Sininger (1995) compared 100-Hz and 30-Hz high-pass filter conditions for ABRs from infants. Setting the low end of the filter (high pass) to 30 Hz produced ABRs with greater amplitudes and better S/N, particularly when using low-frequency (500-Hz) tone bursts.

Allowing more low-frequency energy into the ABR recording, however, can also allow additional unwanted noise, including myogenic (muscle) activity, as well as 50-Hz or 60-Hz electrical interference from electrical power sources. In these conditions, the increase in response (evoked potential) can be offset by an increase in electrical noise. In clean recording conditions with low electrode impedance, little or no electrical interference, and a quiet, sleeping subject, a high-pass filter of 30 or 50 Hz should enhance the ABR amplitude for threshold measures. This is especially desirable for ABR recording with 500-Hz stimuli. If conditions are noisy, the low end of the band pass should be no higher than 100 Hz, and even that risks significant elevation of 500-Hz ABR thresholds. Filter slopes greater than 12 dB/octave are generally not recommended in order to reduce ABR waveform distortions (phase distortions) that steeply sloping analog filters may cause.

Recording Window

Special circumstances must be taken into account when determining appropriate recording windows for threshold measures using the ABR. Figure 14.2 can be used to illustrate these principles. First, in all instances of estimating

audiograms with ABR, it is important to estimate both low-frequency and high-frequency sensitivity, using tone-burst stimuli. The peak latency of the 500-Hz response is generally up to 4 ms later than the click or 4,000-Hz response, indicating the need for an extended analysis window. Inability to identify ABRs near psychophysical thresholds for 500-Hz tone bursts may be due to the use of an inadequate window length. Second, accurate response detection involves including the peak of wave V as well as the long, slow negativity that follows—what Davis termed the "slow negative potential at 10 ms" or SN10 (which is often much later than 10 ms) (Davis and Hirsh, 1979). Third, the latency of the ABR is systematically extended as the stimulus level decreases. To determine a clear ABR with low-level stimuli requires a longer recording window than is necessary for high-level responses. Finally, the latency of the ABR in infants and toddlers is significantly longer than for adults, as discussed previously. Also, to accommodate immature responses, a long recording window is needed. For threshold measurement in infants using ABR, the recording window length should be over 20 ms and ideally 25 to 30 ms.

ACCURACY OF THRESHOLD ESTIMATION WITH THE AUDITORY BRAINSTEM RESPONSE

Conceptual Model

ABRs are byproducts or "epiphenomena" of neural events that underlie hearing. Therefore, ABR thresholds should be considered statistical predictors or estimators of hearing thresholds. To clarify this concept, consider two aspects of ABR thresholds: intensity step size and the amount of averaging. ABR threshold is determined by bracketing, seeking the lowest stimulus level with a clear ABR and an adjacent lower level with no ABR. The levels are typically separated by no more than 10 dB, and the upper level is usually defined as the threshold. However, there may be ABRs present at any level between the two brackets, yet the threshold is still the upper level. The difference between the upper level and the actual point of ABR disappearance is an error ("quantization" error) due to conversion of a continuously variable threshold into a limited set of intensity levels. Over many measurements across subjects, these errors will have a range equal to the step size, and on average, the upper level (threshold) will overestimate the true ABR threshold by half the step size.

A 5-dB error may be trivial in conventional clinical audiometry, but in threshold estimation with the ABR, there are many sources of error, such as effects of EEG noise level. Because the various errors accumulate, it is important to minimize all sources of error. One approach is to use 5-dB steps for the final threshold bracket, and we recommended this if the ABR threshold is high, say above about 70 dB hearing level (HL). A 10-dB error may be significant for hearing aid prescription if the residual dynamic range is very limited.

Now consider the size of the ABR averages. If EEG noise is high, the measured ABR threshold may be way above its true value (positively biased), and its variation over repeated tests may be large. In this situation, increasing the number of sweeps will significantly reduce both the threshold bias and test-retest variability. These effects are more marked for tone-burst ABR than for click ABR, especially at low tone-burst frequencies and near-threshold levels. If, however, EEG noise levels are very low, the effects of the amount of averaging are much smaller, especially for click stimuli and at high ABR thresholds, at which ABRs may be very clear at only 5 dB above threshold, probably due to a recruitment-like effect. For a discussion of effects of residual noise on ABR click thresholds, see Don and Elberling (1996).

Given a measured ABR threshold, the next step is to infer the associated audiometric threshold. Lacking audiometric reference standards for ABR thresholds, we rely on normative data comparing ABR and behavioral thresholds in the same subjects. Caution is needed to ensure that the normative data are representative of the population and procedures for which they are applied. For example, one cannot apply adult norms to newborn and infant populations because so many variables differ in the two populations, such as transducers, EEG noise levels, ear acoustics, and ABR developmental characteristics. It is also relevant that the normative data cover an appropriate range of hearing loss types, severities, and etiologies.

For newborn and infant normative data, a limitation is that behavioral validation thresholds must be obtained when they become practicable, which may be at least 6 months after the initial ABR measurements. Hearing can change due to progression or intercurrent pathology such as middle ear disorders. If visual reinforcement audiometry (VRA) at 7 to 10 months is used, then note that VRA "thresholds" are minimum response levels (MRLs) that may be 5 to 10 dB above true thresholds. This may distort the relationship with ABR thresholds.

How should the normative data be expressed, used in clinical threshold estimation, and evaluated in terms of their implications for the accuracy of ABR-based threshold estimates?

Each normative subject gives an ABR threshold and a subsequent behavioral threshold that is assumed to be valid. These are best graphed as a scatterplot, with behavioral thresholds on the y-axis and ABR thresholds on the x-axis. The clinical task is to predict an **unknown** audiometric threshold from an **observed** ABR threshold. The normative scatterplot reveals how that prediction actually works when both thresholds are known. Some readers may recognize this as a linear regression problem. A predictive rule is derived from the normative data and then used when the behavioral threshold is not known.

Statistical simulations of this are given in Figure 14.3. In the scatterplots, each data point represents an ABR thresh-

old in early infancy and a behavioral threshold obtained at follow-up (usually by VRA). Panel A shows the simplest situation, in which the true mean behavioral thresholds equal the ABR thresholds, so the Y means fall on a line $Y = X$, which has a slope of 1.0. In that situation, if an ABR threshold of, say, 50 dB nHL were observed, the best estimate of the true behavioral threshold would be 50 dB HL. Because the mean Y always equals the corresponding value of X, the prediction can be called unbiased. Note that the values of Y are scattered about their mean, suggesting that a **range** of predicted thresholds must be considered for any given ABR threshold. Panel D is paired with panel A and shows the histogram of the distribution of differences between the ABR and behavioral thresholds, which are considered as estimation errors. In the unbiased case illustrated here, the true mean of the differences is zero, and the distribution has an SD set at 10 dB.

Panel B shows a more realistic situation, in which the mean behavioral thresholds are set at 15 dB below the ABR thresholds, so as an estimator, the ABR threshold has a constant bias of +15 dB. The solid line is the relationship $Y = X - 15$. Thus, to predict the mean behavioral threshold, 15 dB must be subtracted from any observed ABR threshold. Panel E shows the histogram of threshold errors. The mean error is 15 dB (the bias), but the distribution has the same shape and SD as for panel D. Fixed bias, after compensation by an adjustment factor, does not alter the precision of threshold estimation.

Panel C shows bias that is 15 dB at low ABR thresholds, decreasing to 0 dB as the ABR threshold increases. This is a plausible model of ABR "recruitment," with high ABR thresholds closer to true thresholds than low ABR thresholds. The difference histogram is not shown, but it would have a mean between 0 dB and 15 dB and an increased overall SD. While the SD of the scatter of Y for any single value of X is still 10 dB, the changing bias over the whole range of X increases the overall error variability.

Panel D shows an even more complicated situation that is suggested by several published datasets. Here, there is variable bias for ABR thresholds above about 30 dB, with the bias decreasing at higher ABR thresholds and even going negative at the highest levels. Below 30 dB, a different relationship holds, with very little change in ABR thresholds as the true hearing threshold declines.

In summary, the crucial point is that behavioral thresholds in dB HL and ABR thresholds in dB nHL are not necessarily identical, and there is no reason why they should be. Second, normative scatterplots of ABR and behavioral thresholds in the same subjects are the essential tool to develop prediction formulae. Third, the predictive relationship may be complicated. Fortunately, it appears that simple relationships with constant bias may be applicable to tone-pip ABR testing of infants, at least as a first approximation, for any specific tone-pip frequency. However, the bias does change across frequencies. See, for example, the important data of Stapells et al. (1995).

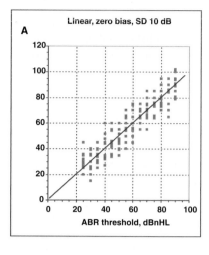

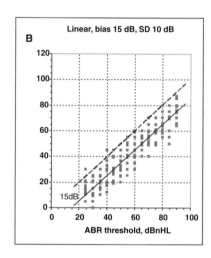

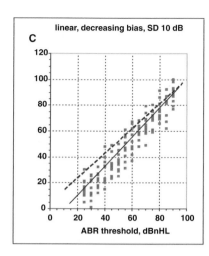

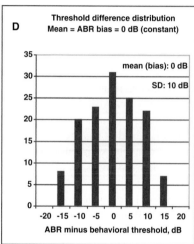

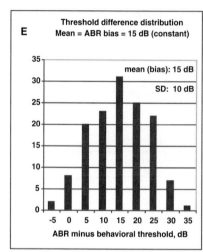

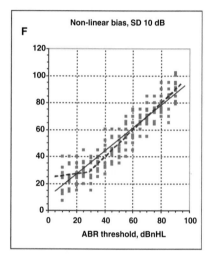

FIGURE 14.3 **Various models of normative data relating auditory brainstem response (ABR) and behavioral thresholds. (A)** A linear model with zero bias. **(B)** A linear model with 15 dB bias. **(C)** A linear model with decreasing bias at high ABR thresholds. **(D)** The error distribution from panel **A**. **(E)** The error distribution from panel **B**. **(F)** A nonlinear model. SD, standard deviation.

The predictive **accuracy** of the ABR threshold has two parts: bias and precision. Precision refers to the variability of the predicted threshold about its true value. It is reflected in the spread or scatter of estimated behavioral thresholds for any particular ABR threshold. It can be expressed as an SD of predictive error or, preferably, as a confidence interval for the predicted Y, at any value of X. The size of these confidence intervals is much more important than values of bias, because bias can be compensated, but lack of precision cannot. For example, a confidence interval of ± 15 dB for a predicted threshold implies a clinical serious limitation of predictive accuracy because it implies a plausible range of 30 dB for the true hearing level associated with any specific, observed ABR threshold. An interval of ± 10 dB is much more acceptable, and an interval of ± 5 dB is a challenging goal. Note that statements commonly found in the literature such as "70% of ABR thresholds were within 10 dB of the true audiometric threshold" are of limited value because they

do not separate bias and precision and they do not address predictive errors appropriately.

Reports that include regression formulae should be examined very critically because inappropriate or incorrect regression analysis is common. Errors include failure to recognize clear nonlinearity, inadequate sampling of the ABR threshold range, inappropriate inclusion of values at the limits of X and Y, failure to account for change in the variability of Y with increasing X, and many other errors.

Normative Data

We have just established that estimator bias can be accommodated simply by subtracting the bias from the observed ABR threshold. This type of ABR threshold adjustment is important and improves the accuracy of estimated audiometric thresholds. The only significant disadvantage of large bias is that it limits the maximum audiometric threshold that can be estimated. For example, if the highest stimulus level achievable for a particular ABR measurement was 95 dB nHL and the bias was a constant 10 dB, then it would not be possible to estimate true audiometric thresholds greater than 85 dB.

We also noted that precision of estimation, as reflected in error SDs or confidence intervals, is far more important clinically than is bias. If normative reported data give error SD values of say 10 dB, then a typical confidence interval for true threshold prediction will be at least four times the SD. It is remarkable that some published reports on ABR or ASSR accuracy claim a particular technique to be clinically successful, even with SDs greater than 10 dB!

There is a not a great deal of high-quality, normative data that relates to pediatric applications of threshold estimation by tone-burst ABR. Longitudinal, normative validation studies are extremely demanding, requiring exemplary ABR and behavioral audiometric technique, as well as large sample sizes with a full range of hearing loss types, severities, profiles, and etiologies, as well as control for delayed onset and progressive hearing loss. Even if a definitive study was reported, there would be the question of efficacy versus effectiveness. If studies are conducted by persons with extraordinary skills and experience and efficacy can be shown (it can work), then it would remain to be shown whether the procedural effectiveness works in routine clinical practice by a spectrum of practitioners with variable training and skills. This issue is especially relevant in the area of AEP-based threshold estimation, which is skill dependent to a degree that is not widely appreciated.

A good-quality study with substantial sample size reported by Stapells et al. (1995) was very informative. Tone-burst ABR thresholds (by air conduction) in infancy and childhood were compared with subsequent behavioral thresholds at corresponding audiometric frequencies for children with normal hearing and a full range of hearing losses. Careful inspection of threshold scatterplots reveals that tone-burst ABR thresholds and audiometric thresholds were approximately linearly related over an ABR threshold range from 20 to about 90 dB nHL at 500 Hz, 2 kHz, and 4 kHz. When nonlinearities at levels below 20 dB and nonresponses above 100 dB are eliminated, the data are generally consistent with a unity regression slope with a fixed bias that decreases as stimulus frequency increases. With rounding to the nearest 5 dB, the ABR threshold in dB nHL is, on average, 15, 5, and 0 dB at 500 Hz, 2 kHz, and 4 kHz, respectively.

The Stapells et al. (1995) study employed tone bursts in notch-filtered masking noise in an attempt to enhance frequency specificity. It is possible that the masking noise could have altered the characteristics of the normative data. However, Stapells, one of the pioneers of the notch-masking method, has stated that ABR thresholds to nonmasked tone bursts are "reasonably frequency specific" for hearing losses with slopes less than about 40 dB per octave (Stapells, 1998, p 18), which covers the vast majority of cases.

Stapells (2000) also reviewed and integrated tone-burst ABR studies in children and adults, including a good-quality study by Munnerley et al. (1991). Some difficulties with attempts to combine these studies are differences in techniques and calibrations, small sample sizes, and some heterogeneity of results. In general, bias values for subjects with hearing loss are larger at lower frequencies and larger in adults than in infants and children. Differences in ABR S/N as well as effects of anatomic development on stimulus SPL may contribute to these effects. Consequently, we recommend that, for threshold estimation by tone-burst ABR methods in infants, the scatterplots of Stapells et al. (1995) be used to determine threshold estimation bias, rather than the values computed from Stapells' meta-analysis (2000). This means that, for ABRs obtained with the methods and test parameters recommended by Stapells et al. (1995), the bias factors converting ABR thresholds in dB nHL to HL estimates are approximately 15, 10, 5, and 0 dB at 0.5, 1, 2, and 4 kHz, respectively.

Sininger et al. (1997) evaluated ABR threshold in normal-hearing adults and healthy neonates using clicks and tone bursts of 500, 1,500, 4,000, and 8,000 Hz. This study also used a notched-noise paradigm, and a minimum averaged background noise criterion of 40 nV was required before an average was judged to have no response. An ABR response window of 30 ms was employed, and the EEG was filtered from 30 to 1,000 Hz. Adult thresholds for 1-second duration tonal stimuli were determined psychophysically for each subject. Mean ABR thresholds for the adults were 10-, 7-, 5-, and 6-dB sensation level for 500, 1,500, 4,000, and 8,000 Hz, respectively. No behavioral assessment of hearing level was obtained from neonates, but these infants were healthy and full term and assumed to represent a normal-hearing group. For the infants, ABR thresholds using stimuli calibrated relative to average normal-hearing adults were found to be 17, 8, 6, and 0 dB nHL for 500, 1,500, 4,000, and 8,000 Hz, respectively. SDs were approximately 10 dB for all measures. These values, which represent only normal-hearing infants, are very close to those found by Stapells et al. (1995).

It is important to note that the transduction and calibration of ABR stimuli can have a major effect on reported accuracy of ABR threshold predictions. The usefulness of normative studies will depend on the audiologist's choice of stimulus level units and transducers and the manner in which calibrations are performed and how normative data are collected. Some of these issues will now be discussed.

Air-Conduction and Bone-Conduction Auditory Brainstem Response Measurements

Transducers that are currently used for ABR measurements are essentially the same as those used with audiometers. In the United States, insert transducers, specifically the Etymotic ER-3A, are favored for use with ABR over more traditional supra-aural transducers (TDH-39 or -49) for several reasons. Relative to supra-aural phones, the inserts demonstrate less stimulus artifact in the ABR recording, demonstrate greater interaural attenuation, will avoid problems of ear canal collapse often seen with supra-aural phones, and are generally more comfortable for patients. The insert transducer clips to the clothing of the patient, and the stimulus is conducted to the ear via small-diameter plastic tubing and is coupled to the ear canal with an appropriate sized pliable ear tip. The time delay of the signal transduction through the tubing will be reflected in the latency of the ABR, which is generally measured as the time following the initiation of the stimulus at the transducer. A simple correction factor (0.8 to 1 ms) that corresponds to the sound travel time via the length of the tubing can be applied to latencies of ABRs obtained using an insert earphone. Otherwise, the click ABR produced by an ER-3A insert transducer should be similar in amplitude and latency to an ABR produced by a Beyer DT-48 or close to a response from a TDH-39 or TDH-49 (Beauchaine et al., 1987; Van Campen et al., 1992).

Several bone conduction vibrators have been used successfully to provide the stimulus for ABR measurements. One difference with these transducers is that the spectrum of a broadband stimulus reportedly is considerably narrower for broadband clicks than is seen with air-conduction transducers, especially for the Radioear B-70 A (Mauldin and Jerger, 1979; Yang et al., 1987; Schwartz et al., 1985). However, the response of the B71 is quite similar to that of a standard air-conduction transducer for both broadband clicks and for a full range of frequencies of tone bursts (Gorga et al., 1993). Using a tone-burst stimulus for bone-conduction measures, with appropriate calibration in nHL, will help to avoid waveform and latency differences that may occur in click-evoked responses because of differences in the frequency responses of the transducers.

The relationship between the latency of the ABR to air- and bone-conducted stimuli can be unpredictable. In adults, Gorga found slightly longer latencies by bone conduction, even when the sensation level and spectrum of the stimuli were carefully matched (Gorga et al., 1993). In infants, the exact sensation level of a bone-conducted stimulus cannot be determined. The skull of the infant or child will have significantly different conductive properties than the skull of an adult. As evidence, Nousak and Stapells (1992) found shorter ABR latencies for 500-Hz bone-conducted tone bursts in infants compared to adults (a finding not seen by air conduction) but equivalent latencies for 2,000-Hz responses. They used a technique that restricted the frequency region of the cochlear response and concluded that the shorter latency at 500 Hz in infants was due to their greater effective stimulus level by bone conduction at that frequency. The same study provided evidence that both 500-Hz and, for the most part, 2,000-Hz tone bursts presented by bone conduction to infant skulls were stimulating the same cochlear regions as if they had been presented by air conduction. This indicates that tone-burst bone-conduction ABRs in infants can be assumed to provide comparable assessment of specific frequency regions as air-conducted stimuli.

The relationship between mode of stimulus presentation and latency in infants is unpredictable when using click stimuli. Some studies have found shorter latencies for bone- versus air-conducted stimuli in neonates, but others have shown that this could be due to transient conductive hearing loss due to fluid in the middle ear at birth, which would increase latencies of air-conducted responses (Yang et al., 1987). Stuart et al. (1994) found that the shorter latency of bone-conducted clicks disappeared about 48 hours after birth, when the latency produced by air- and bone-conducted stimuli was equivalent and, presumably, after any fluid or debris in the middle ear, related to the birthing process, had cleared.

Differences in the frequency response of air and bone transducers will also influence ABR latencies for the two measures, especially when using broadband stimuli such as clicks. In the clinical evaluation of infants, comparison of ABR thresholds for air and bone conduction will be more fruitful than comparing their latencies because of the inherent and sometimes unexplained variability in infants.

Coupling of air-conduction transducers to the ears of infants and toddlers requires only minor variations relative to their use with adults. Care must be taken to avoid ear canal collapse when using supra-aural phones. In some instances, the size of the headband cannot be reduced sufficiently, requiring the use of a foam pad or similar accommodation across the top of the head. For insert transducers, several ear tips are available in sizes to accommodate very small ear canals. On occasion, in the smallest premature infants, the tubing alone or tubing with a thin wrap of surgical tape will be all that is necessary to fit the tubing snugly in the ear canal.

Coupling of the bone-conduction transducer to the head of infants and toddlers is a much greater challenge that requires a modification of standard techniques. The bone-conduction headbands provided for adults are not only too large for infants, but also will not apply sufficient and consistent force to ensure proper coupling of the vibrator and, consequently, consistent stimulation of the infant. An excellent procedure for coupling of the bone vibrator to infants and toddlers is described by Yang and Stuart (1990), in which an elastic headband with an adjustable Velcro closure holds the bone vibrator securely on the high mastoid (i.e., on the superior-posterior part of the mastoid area of the infant). This placement has been shown to produce ABRs with the largest amplitudes and shortest latencies in infants (Yang et al., 1987). The tension on the headband can be adjusted to apply a consistent coupling force between 400 and 450 grams. The system can be calibrated using a spring scale to determine the force necessary to just lift the bone conduction vibrator away from the scalp (see picture of this setup in Fig. 14.4).

Some practitioners advocate the use of a handheld bone conductor. This technique would appear to have several disadvantages, foremost among them the inability to calibrate the pressure used. A handheld oscillator will lead to inconsistent pressure and, consequently, inconsistent stimulus level

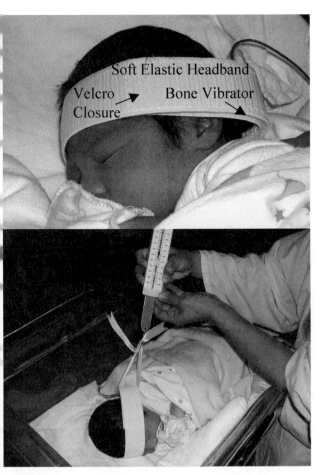

FIGURE 14.4 Bone-conduction vibrator placement on an infant subject using procedures suggested by Yang and Stuart (1990). The force applied to the bone-conduction vibrator can be calibrated using a spring scale as shown in bottom segment.

throughout and between evaluations and across clinicians. Finally, this method ties up one hand of a clinician, which could be used more effectively in performing the evaluation. Given the importance that bone-conduction threshold procedures have in the assessment of infants and toddlers, it seems desirable to strive for consistent and accurate calibration of stimuli, including the force applied to the bone vibrator. For an excellent discussion of issues related to bone conduction and calibration, see Dirks (1994).

When using ABR bone-conduction measures, the clinician will see the same drawbacks as noted with conventional audiometry and some unique issues. For example, the dynamic range of bone-conduction vibrators is dramatically reduced relative to air-conduction transducers. In infants, tympanometry is a useful additional test when no response can be obtained at the maximum output of the bone-conduction vibrator to detect conductive overlay in moderate to profound, mixed hearing losses.

Determining the ear responding to the stimulus is also a significant issue in bone-conduction ABR testing. Contralat-

eral masking can be useful, especially in cases of congenital atresia where an assessment of cochlear reserve in the affected ear is indicated. However, there are many unknowns with regard to the effect of masking noise in infant ABR testing. As an alternative to masking for bone-conducted ABRs, especially in infants and toddlers who may not be sleeping, Stapells and Ruben (1989) suggest recording from an ipsilateral and contralateral electrode montage and comparing the two. The recording side corresponding to the ear receiving maximum stimulation will generally show larger response amplitude, earlier latency, and lower threshold. This technique appears to work well in most cases, provided that the level of the stimuli used is low. Examples of this two-channel technique are shown in Figure 14.5.

Another modification of bone-conduction testing with ABR applies the principles of the sensory-neural acuity level test (Jerger and Tillman, 1960; Hicks, 1980) This technique determines the audibility of the bone-conducted signal by using a bone-conducted masker, thus avoiding some of the problems with calibration. The ability of bone-conducted noise to shift the threshold of an air-conducted ABR is related to the threshold of the bone-conducted signal. This technique was developed in adults with click stimuli but can also be used with tone-burst ABRs and can be applied to the evaluation of children (Hicks, 1980; Ysunza and Cone-Wesson, 1987; Webb and Greenberg, 1983).

Real-Ear Calibration Correction

There is much discussion regarding the need to take into consideration differences in the SPL near the eardrum of an identical stimulus delivered to an infant and an adult ear. A fixed-voltage signal delivered to an insert earphone may produce up to 30-dB higher signal levels in the newborn ear, relative to an adult ear, because of differences in the size and resonance properties of the two cavities. Such differences are taken into consideration when measuring OAEs, for example, and are especially important in fitting of amplification to children (Scollie et al., 1998).

Sininger et al. (1997) determined the SPL of stimuli with a probe-tube microphone assembly near the eardrum of infants and adults while measuring ABR thresholds. For a fixed-voltage stimulus presented via an ER-2 insert transducer, high-frequency stimuli (4,000- and 8,000-Hz tone bursts) are enhanced by about 25 dB in infants relative to adult ear canals; clicks are enhanced by about 20 dB, while 500-Hz tone bursts are nearly equal in level for the two populations (Fig. 14.6). However, the difference in SPL did not translate into lower ABR thresholds for the infants. Rather, the infants and adults have similar ABR thresholds (within 6 dB) for all stimuli when a dB nHL calibration is considered. Sininger et al. (1997) measured threshold in dB nHL (Fig. 14.7, top panel) and dB peak equivalent SPL (peSPL) from the ear canal (bottom panel) from adults and infants. The Stapells (2000) meta-analysis also noted very similar infant and adult

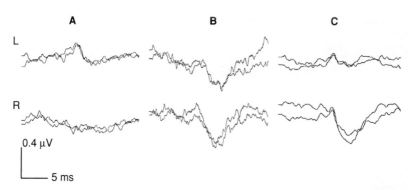

FIGURE 14.5 Bone-conduction (BC) ABR asymmetry examples in 2-channel recordings in infants under 6 months of age with unilateral sensory-neural hearing loss (SNHL). In young infants, testing is done with the bone conductor on each mastoid individually, because of transcranial transmission loss that can be substantial and differs across infants. Two recording channels are used, with the forehead referred to each mastoid. For reasons that are not entirely understood, the responding cochlea can usually be inferred as on the side for which the ABR is earlier and/or larger. In the examples, L denotes the Left mastoid channel and R the Right mastoid channel. In each case, moderate SNHL was confirmed later by Visual Reinforcement Audiometry. In column A, the stimulus is a 2kHz tonepip at 40 dBnHL in the Right ear. The response is seen only in the Left channel, consistent with a Right unilateral loss. In column B, a 30 dB 2kHz tonepip in the Right ear evokes a larger and earlier ABR in the Right channel, consistent with a Left unilateral loss. In column C, a 30 dB 2kHz tonepip in the Left ear evokes responses with identical latency in both channels, but the larger response is on the Right, consistent with a Left unilateral loss.

ABR thresholds for tone bursts *calibrated in nHL* with no correction for ear canal SPL.

The common assumption is that threshold for infants and adults is represented by a fixed SPL near the eardrum. This appears not to be the case for ABR thresholds. Most studies in which ABR and psychophysical thresholds are compared for infants and toddlers do not correct for differences in SPL at the eardrum or changes in canal resonance with age. Nevertheless, a good correspondence exists between ABR thresholds measured in nHL in adults and children of all ages (Stapells et al., 1995) . Perhaps there is a slowly changing reduction in the threshold of ABR progressing from infancy to adulthood that offsets changes in ear canal volume with growth. This is plausible, for example, on the basis of a hypothesis of improved neural synchronization as maturation progresses. Reduction in threshold might be due to changes in tympanic membrane or middle ear transduction as well. Great caution must be used before corrections for real-ear calibrations are applied to ABR measures. The data suggest that if such were assumed to be necessary, most infants would appear to have a high-frequency hearing loss (Fig. 14.7, bottom panel). More data are necessary to determine the relationship between applied stimulus levels, real-ear calibrated levels, ABR thresholds, and age. This is an important clinical question that must be answered with carefully controlled research.

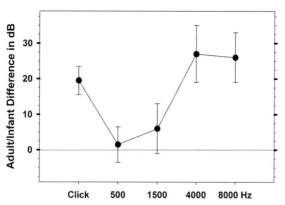

FIGURE 14.6 Difference between peak equivalent sound pressure level (peSPL) for clicks and tone bursts as measured near the eardrum of neonates and adults. Stimuli were fixed voltage presented to ER-2 insert earphones. The values measured were always higher in infant ear canal than in adults. (Adapted from Sininger YS, Abdala C, Cone-Wesson B. [1997] Auditory threshold sensitivity of the human neonate as measured by the auditory brainstem response. *Hear Res.* 104, 27–38.)

■ STRATEGY OF AUDITORY EVOKED POTENTIAL THRESHOLD TESTING

Conventional puretone audiometry in a cooperative adult is done in a standard test environment using standard equipment calibrated to well-established standards based on widely accepted normative data. The measurements,

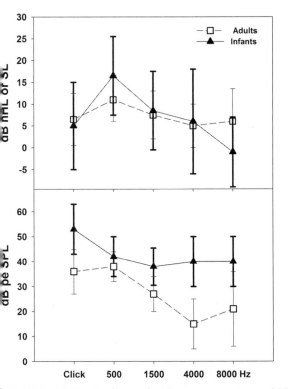

FIGURE 14.7 Auditory brainstem response (ABR) thresholds to clicks and tone bursts in infants and adults. Top panel shows values calibrated in dB normal hearing level (nHL) (sensation level [SL] for adults), and bottom panel shows the thresholds as calibrated in the ear canal of each subject in dB peak equivalent sound pressure level (peSPL). (Adapted from Sininger YS, Abdala C, Cone-Wesson B. [1997] Auditory threshold sensitivity of the human neonate as measured by the auditory brainstem response. *Hear Res.* **104, 27–38.)**

procedures, and reporting methods are all well defined. Provided the tester is appropriately trained and experienced, threats to the validity and accuracy of thresholds are few, apart from the possibility of a functional (nonorganic) hearing loss.

When carrying out an audiometric assessment of a 2-month-old infant referred from a newborn hearing screening program, there is no standard definition of "normal hearing," no standard calibration method, and no universally agreed upon procedure. There is only limited consensus on desirable components of a good test protocol, and there is no shortage of competing claims often based on studies or data that may have significant methodologic problems.

To make matters more challenging, you may be dealing with a 2-month-old infant who is not concerned about cooperating. For any useful AEP threshold testing, two things are needed: good EEG conditions and enough test time; however, both can be in short supply. Many experts advocate testing in

natural sleep, especially in the first 3 months or so, and in that situation, the child may wake at any time, and the test session may be over. Others advocate use of sedation, with different levels of sedation. But sedation is not a panacea. Some families will not accept it, some infants have poor response to common drugs, others may exhibit paradoxical excitation, the length of time of acceptable EEG results varies across infants, and local risk-management protocols for drug administration, etc., vary significantly in cost and complexity. In general, it is unusual to have both unlimited test time and good EEG conditions.

In this situation, the clinical task can be quite complicated. Decisions must be made about exactly which measurements are important and why, what stimulus and recording parameters to select, how to obtain thresholds that are acceptably accurate, and how to conduct the testing as efficiently as possible. This requires you to think on your feet, to adapt rapidly to changing circumstances, and to behave not according to a routine, but strategically. To adopt successful testing strategies consistently is a challenge, and if the challenge is embraced, it can be very rewarding clinically and professionally.

Strategic decisions may have to take into account many variables, and the decisions may need to be taken quickly and updated rapidly as conditions change or as intermediate results become available. There is a need for awareness, for engagement and adaptation, for sound clinical and technical judgment, and for substantial, practical skills. Audiometric threshold estimation with the ABR is significantly more complicated and requires greater skill than, for example, using the ABR to detect eighth-nerve tumors.

It is assumed that we are interested in ABR-based estimates of hearing thresholds from at least 500 Hz through 4 kHz. It is well established that such threshold estimates can be obtained with reasonable accuracy using tone bursts, given appropriate test protocols used by testers with appropriate training and skills. Also, some situations in which the ABR is likely to overestimate thresholds (e.g., with AN/AD) can be identified.

In essence, every ABR threshold test session is basically a collection of averages for a set of stimulus conditions, each average contributing to some decision about response presence or absence. The major exercise of strategy lies in the sequential selections of the stimulus conditions. A new choice is faced after each average, as the test progresses, and at each point, the test conditions may change (e.g., the baby may become restless), and new information about the probable threshold(s) may be inferred from the results just obtained.

For comprehensive ABR threshold estimation, we are faced immediately with choices among at least four tone-burst test frequencies (0.5, 1, 2, and 4 kHz). There is also the option of testing by air conduction or bone conduction, which is also entirely practical with the ABR. For a given tone-burst frequency and presentation route (air conduction or bone conduction), reliable response detection decisions must be made at several stimulus levels in order to bracket the response threshold with adequate precision. Moreover, several averages may be necessary for any given stimulus. For example, if subjective visual response recognition is used, it is common to require reproducibility of the averaged waveform in at least two independent averages, at least for stimulus level near the presumed threshold.

The bottom line is that, throughout this sequential procedure, each and every selection of the stimulus and recording parameters for the next average must take into account all of the information obtained to date and, to optimize efficiency, must be chosen so as to maximize the clinical information that would be obtained, given a successful next average and response decision. It is generally helpful to continually assume that the next average may be the last one available and to choose it to be maximally informative in relation to audiologic management decisions for the infant. Even if this pessimistic assumption turns out to be wrong, then all the clinical information required is likely to be obtained. However, if at any point, the assumption turns out to be correct (for example, if the child awakens or EEG conditions become irreversibly poor), then the maximum information possible in the test time will have been obtained.

The general strategy of stimulus selection depends on the key clinical question being addressed. Some examples of common questions are:

> *Is the infant's hearing within normal limits?*
> *What are the estimated audiometric thresholds at 0.5, 2, and 4 kHz?*
> *Is the estimated audiometric threshold at 2 kHz really 70 dB HL?*
> *Is there a conductive component at 500 Hz?*
> *Is there evidence of AN/AD?*

Each of these questions may be addressed most efficiently by a specific strategy of stimulus selection.

Is the Infant's Hearing Within Normal Limits?

Here, the first decision is whether one ear or both ears are included in the definition of normal. This arises in relation to whether only the referred ear should be assessed in an infant with a unilateral screening referral outcome. In some programs, even for bilateral screening referrals, if it is shown that there is one normal ear, then the assessment may be stopped, or there may be a reduced priority for follow-up effort and resource expenditure. Many clinicians would consider this approach to be inadequate. In the United States, identification of unilateral hearing loss is an accepted goal, and test results are generally expected for both ears of any infant referred from newborn hearing screening, regardless of the screening outcome. It is important to understand the local expectations of infant follow-up assessment to ensure that all appropriate testing is accomplished.

The second decision relates to the set of frequencies considered to define normal hearing. This does not necessarily mean the conventional 250 Hz through 8 kHz because, in the context of infant tone-burst ABR testing, such a range is very demanding and potentially impractical. It is legitimate to question the value of 250-Hz thresholds if 500-Hz thresholds are known and the value of thresholds above 4 kHz if the 4-kHz threshold is known. One approach to defining a more modest and practical set of frequency ranges is to ask *If I could have only one threshold, which one would it be?* Then, given that threshold, which additional threshold would add the most valuable clinical information? Then, given those two thresholds . . . , etc. At some point, a line must be drawn where the value of additional information does not justify the effort or expenditure of resources to obtain it, given that every dollar spent getting information of questionable value is a dollar not available for other audiometric or habilitation procedures.

We would argue that, in the absence of any previous audiometric information or special indications, 2 kHz is the most important single frequency. Given the 2-kHz threshold, 500 Hz might be the next most important because 1 kHz is more strongly correlated with 2 kHz and would add less new information. In fact, the choice of next most important frequency might depend on the 2-kHz threshold value obtained; for example, if 2 kHz were at 90 dB then 500 Hz might be more important than say 4 kHz because the 4-kHz threshold is not likely to be better than 2 kHz, whereas if 2 kHz were 45 dB, then 4 kHz might increase in priority, relative to 500 Hz.

Note that this type of argument relates not only to the definition of which test frequencies are indicated or not, but also to their order of execution. This line of argument does assume that a serial, adaptive choice of the next test frequency will be more efficient clinically than routine measurement across a standard set of frequencies. It remains to be seen whether new technologies such as multiple-frequency ASSR will invalidate this assumption, without incurring any countervailing disadvantage, such as loss of relative threshold sensitivity or loss of efficiency.

A third decision is to define an upper limit of threshold that will be considered normal. The absence of well-accepted standards has been discussed. Certainly, there are normative studies, but it is quite difficult to define a normal population of newborn or young infants, with there being no true gold standard measure. Normal hearing could be proven longitudinally, by long-term follow-up, or one could rely on the fact that the prevalence of permanent childhood hearing impairment (PCHI) is less than 0.5% in normative infant populations without risk indicators, but it is difficult to exclude minor conductive losses, which may exist even in nonrisk newborns with apparently normal middle ear function. Another consideration is that most infants referred for audiometric assessment in early hearing detection and intervention (EHDI) programs arise through newborn screening. ABR click screening at a nominal 35 dB nHL may well pass some newborns with thresholds of (at least) 30 dB nHL, and OAE screening may even pass some newborns with larger losses. Some would question the merit of considering a threshold of say 20 dB nHL as clinically significant in a group that has been screened at a higher effective level than that. Also, it makes some sense for the target losses for EHDI programs to be defined by the existence and desirability of useful interventions; there is some ethical concern about labeling infants as having hearing loss when there is no indicated intervention. Finally, it must be remembered that, if very low criterion levels for the presence of hearing loss are used, many more infants will be pronounced as abnormal, even though they may have only minor, transient hearing losses. A truly rational approach to defining upper limits of normality will await further investigation of the developmental impact of minimal hearing losses in infancy.

At present, some EHDI programs appear to have adopted empirical, operational definitions of the minimum target PCHI, typically believed to correspond to audiometric threshold estimates equivalent to about 30 dB HL. This points out the importance of knowing regional standards. In the United States, individual states will determine the degree of hearing loss necessary for eligibility for early intervention, but there is no national standard. If no intervention is deemed warranted for hearing loss of less than 30 dB nHL, for example, then using clinical time to discern between an ABR threshold of 10 and 15 dB makes little sense. However, there may also be instances in which it is important to find thresholds below 30 dB nHL. For example, if a sloping hearing loss is found with thresholds of 40 dB nHL at 2,000 Hz and 80 dB nHL at 4,000 Hz, it may be important to determine the 500-Hz threshold as accurately as possible to use this information for proper fitting of amplification. Certainly, in this instance, stopping at 30 dB nHL (corrected) would not be adequate given that the true threshold could be 0 or 10 dB nHL, and the true threshold would be needed to determine appropriate target gain.

Suppose that normal hearing were defined operationally as audiometric thresholds up to and including 25 dB HL at, for example, 500 Hz and 2 kHz in each ear (an argument could be made to include 4 kHz, but that does not change the strategic principles that follow). Given that ABR thresholds are known to be biased, the minimum test levels needed for ABR threshold measurements will equal the target minimum loss criteria plus the bias values or correction factor at various frequencies. The (air conduction) normative data of Stapells et al. (1995), for example, suggest bias adjustments of about 15, 5, and 0 dB for stimuli at 0.5, 2, and 4 kHz, respectively. The bias adjustments for bone-conduction stimulation may be different. Whatever the bias values adopted, the key point is that the choice of minimum stimulus levels used for ABR measurements should be governed by the degree of hearing loss considered clinically significant (target disorder). The minimum stimulus level chosen will not necessarily equal the minimum loss target dB HLs because of correction factors and may differ across frequencies and transducers.

Which frequency should be tested first, in which ear, and with what starting level? Few clinicians would dispute that 2 kHz is crucial, so testing might start there. It is reasonable to start in the referred ear for a unilateral screening referral, and for a bilateral referral, it is reasonable to start in the ear most accessible by the child's natural sleeping position, if any. As for the starting level, the rationale to start at the target minimum level is that a clear result at that level answers the normality question most efficiently. Depending on the screening protocol used, a high percentage of infants referred from screening tests, on testing, will be found to be normal and will give clear, reproducible responses at the target minimum level, provided that appropriate bias adjustments have been included. However, it is a quite common practice to start at a higher level, which may yield a clearer response, especially if initial EEG conditions are borderline. Each of the two approaches has pros and cons under specific circumstances.

We have assumed that the initial testing will be by air conduction, because even though the usual goal is to detect permanent impairment, some impairments may be due to structural conductive abnormalities and, moreover, it is clinically compelling to want to determine first whether the sensory-neural level is within normal limits.

Most clinicians are more comfortable testing air conduction first and then bone conduction if the air conduction is clearly abnormal. However, if the initial test is done at 2-kHz air conduction 30 dB nHL, and no response is seen, then what next? To ascend in 10-dB steps is potentially inefficient, all the more so in infants with severe losses. Note also that, at each stimulus level, there is a finite chance of false-positive response identification (due to random summation of EEG noise or artifact), so a lengthy sequence of tests at subthreshold levels can lead to underestimation of true thresholds, which is a serious error. Generally, a strategy of larger initial steps in stimulus level (20 or even 30 dB) increasing to the minimum necessary for resolution in the near-threshold region is more efficient and accurate. The only situation in which a 10-dB increase from the minimum test level makes much sense is when there is a possible response at the minimum level, but response confirmation is required. Conversely, starting at a high stimulus level and descending in small (e.g., 10-dB) steps is extremely inefficient because only a small proportion of screening referrals will have severe hearing losses. Also, unnecessarily high stimulus levels may awaken the child.

Note that, in general, for almost any type of threshold, adaptive procedures are more efficient than nonadaptive ones, the general principle being to focus measurement effort in the near-threshold region as quickly as possible. Since different thresholds may arise at different frequencies, it remains to be seen whether any potential efficiency advantage of multifrequency ASSR might be offset by the inefficiency of the current, typical ASSR approach of fixed stimulus levels across a set of frequencies.

Suppose now that the threshold was adequately resolved at 60 dB nHL for 2-kHz air conduction in the left ear, what next? Do you go to 500 Hz in the same ear, to bone conduction in the same ear, or to 2 kHz in the other ear? A case can be made for each choice, and the best decision may depend upon many facets of the individual child and test situation. The important point is that there should be a solid rationale for the choice you make. One consideration, especially when testing in natural sleep, is whether the desired next condition might wake up the baby. Applying a bone-conduction transducer with a Velcro headband may have that effect, as may switching test ears (unless transducers have been applied bilaterally, as is done in some centers).

If a substantial threshold elevation is seen by air conduction then a prompt move to bone-conduction testing is certainly arguable on the grounds that it is very important to confirm presence or absence of a conductive component as quickly as possible. Not only does this make a major difference in what can be reported immediately to parents, but it may also affect the follow-up effort.

If there is a conductive component, then a middle ear disorder is quite likely, in which case hearing levels may well change over time, either due to spontaneous resolution or to medical intervention. Is it appropriate to direct substantial effort in order to obtain accurate air-conduction thresholds at other frequencies in that case, or is it more important to address bone-conduction thresholds and then switch ears as soon as possible? This latter approach seems reasonable.

Turning to the strategy of averaging, it is inevitable that, in some situations, a given average will not achieve any reasonable quality target (an RNL, a subjective judgment of a clean average, or an unequivocal response) within a reasonable test time. Note that the decrease in the SD of averaged noise proceeds according to a square root of N law, so it will take four times the current N to halve the current averaged noise level, or stated differently, after twice the current number of sweeps, the noise will go down only by the square root of 2, given no change in EEG. There are no well-established guidelines about how to extract clinical inferences from potentially unreliable ABR records. A conservative approach is to consider all averages that do not achieve the target as a "could not test" (or at least highly suspect) and to merit repeat testing wherever feasible. One of the biggest issues in quality management of ABR threshold testing is reluctance to declare EEG conditions as inadequate and failure to realize that an erroneous threshold may be more harmful clinically than to provide no threshold at all.

What are the Estimated Thresholds at 0.5, 2, and 4 kHz?

The previous discussion is sufficient to cover most aspects of this question. An additional strategic point is that, on average, it will be most efficient to set the initial test level at 4 kHz at about the same level as the observed ABR threshold at 2 kHz, because the 4 kHz threshold will usually be the same or worse. The other point worth reiterating is that the highest audiometric threshold that can be estimated is the maximum

stimulus level minus the applicable bias. This means that profound hearing loss usually cannot be inferred precisely by ABR testing, except perhaps at 4 kHz where the bias may be close to zero. What can be said is that the audiometric threshold is greater than the maximum level minus the bias. The greatest restriction of estimable range will be at low frequencies, at which the bias is largest.

Is the Estimated Audiometric Threshold at 2 kHz Really 70 dB HL?

This question is answered most efficiently by more intensive measurements at those stimulus levels that will bracket a 70-dB threshold estimate, after adjustment for bias. It may be appropriate to use a 5-dB step size and to increase the number of replicated averages to increase the accuracy of the response judgments. If the clinical concern is that the threshold might be better, then a lower level should be checked, whereas if the concern is that it might be greater, then the higher level should yield a detectable response. The point is that the key test conditions are directed by the clinical question, so the strategy is different from that needed to answer an open-ended question about what the true threshold is.

Is There a Conductive Component at 500 Hz?

For typical, commercially available bone-conduction transducers, the maximum stimulus level at 500 Hz is about 55 dB nHL. Therefore, a conductive component cannot be proven if the ABR threshold for 500 Hz air conduction is greater than about 60 dB nHL and there is also no bone-conduction response at the maximum. Then, such a component can only be inferred from immittance measurements and the difference between the estimated audiometric threshold for air conduction and the bone-conduction maximum, after adjustment for bias. Of course, if the bone-conduction ABR threshold is at or less than the bone-conduction maximum, then the conductive component is estimated by subtraction. Note that because both the air-conduction and the bone-conduction audiometric threshold estimates may contain errors of perhaps 5 to 10 dB, the range of errors will be substantially larger for the estimated air-bone gap because the errors in a difference quantity may compound each other. In practice, air-bone gaps estimated by ABR measurements should be considered as very approximate.

Is there Evidence of Auditory Neuropathy/Auditory Dyssynchrony?

The most commonly quoted indicator of AN/AD is a clear OAE in the presence of absent or highly abnormal ABR waveforms. There are several issues with this definition. Quantitative criteria for OAE presence or absence are not well defined, nor are quantitative criteria for ABR depression or threshold elevation that is incompatible with the OAE records. A case

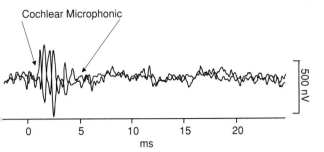

Cochlear Microphonic

500 nV

0   5   10   15   20
ms

FIGURE 14.8 This is the auditory brainstem response (ABR) from one patient with auditory neuropathy (AN). This recording shows an ABR to a rarefaction click superimposed upon a recording using a condensation click. The neural-generated portion of the ABR does not change with the click polarity, but the cochlear components will. The activity in the first few milliseconds (ms) that changes polarity with stimulus is cochlear microphonic. This is an electrical potential that is generated by the hair cells. In contrast, there is no neural component (ABR) in the recording.

of unequivocal OAE presence and no ABR at all at the highest stimulus level (usually with a click) is straightforward, but less clear situations do occur. The question of what is an unreasonable discrepancy between OAE results and an elevated ABR threshold remains problematic.

Another issue is that OAEs may be abolished by even minor middle ear abnormalities and conductive loss components, and absence of OAEs is not an uncommon finding. Of course, such patients with absent OAEs may still have AN/AD. Measurement of the cochlear microphonic potential (CM) is often helpful in such situations (see Chapter 12). It is widely accepted that a clear CM implies a functioning hair cell population and that CM is less affected by minor middle ear conditions than are OAEs. Thus, CM measurement is a routine component of AN/AD protocols. However, there are still cases that are difficult to resolve, such as those that show a small CM and a small or highly abnormal ABR waveform at the highest click levels.

The CM is usually recorded using click stimuli at a high level, with separate averages for condensation and rarefaction clicks. The CM is usually a high-frequency, oscillatory waveform at the beginning of the averaged record and may last from about 2 to 5 ms (Fig. 14.8). Unlike neural responses such as the ABR, the CM reverses polarity for the condensation and rarefaction clicks. Stimulus artifact can also appear at the beginning of the record, sometimes overlapping with the CM. Stimulus artifact, however, also reverses with stimulus polarity. With insert earphones, the 1-ms delay of ear stimulation from transducer activation (and stimulus artifact) helps to separate the artifact and the CM. A useful technique is to disconnect the tubing to the insert and average again without changing the stimulation or the recording configuration. Any initial deflection that is still present in

this condition must be due to stimulus artifact rather than CM, and any such artifact can be separated visually from the previous traces showing what is thought to be CM. Usually, the CM is longer lasting and more oscillatory than click stimulus artifact. A prominent CM in the absence of a clear or substantial ABR is indicative of AN/AD. It is also possible that the ABR may show evidence of a wave V. If the wave V is of the same magnitude or smaller than the CM component, AN/AD should be suspected.

When AN/AD is determined to be present, the absence of ABR does not necessarily imply a severe or profound audiometric threshold elevation. There is likely to be some degree of hearing loss, but its amount is undetermined by the ABR threshold if one exists. If there is a substantial ABR threshold elevation (e.g., 70 dB nHL or more) but clear OAEs, then AN/AD is a distinct possibility. The audiometric threshold estimate is then likely to be no worse than that implied by the ABR threshold but may be substantially better. It is dangerous from ABR to speculate about the degree of hearing loss when AN/AD is suspected. In these cases, behavioral measures are currently the only way to determine degree of loss. A reasonable ABR approach with consideration for AN/AD is to begin testing with an appropriate-frequency, alternating polarity tone burst such as 2,000 Hz. If no response is seen at maximum stimulus levels, switching to a high-level click stimulus and obtaining a separate average for each click polarity will give an indication of whether the original lack of response was due to severe sensory hearing loss or to AN/AD. If the patient shows signs of AN/AD, further testing with tone bursts may be of little value. In this testing protocol, it would be helpful to have OAE information prior to ABR testing, although, as previously stated, an absent OAE does not preclude AN/AD. Finally, note that a conductive hearing loss component is likely to abolish the OAE and, if large, may also abolish the CM, in which case, it is extremely difficult to determine the presence of AN/AD by ABR and CM techniques.

■ BRIEF COMMENTS ON TONE-BURST AUDITORY BRAINSTEM RESPONSE VERSUS AUDITORY STEADY-STATE RESPONSE VERSUS N1

Tone-burst ABR is currently the AEP tool of choice for estimation of the audiogram in young infants because of the vast amount of data about many aspects of response dynamics as well as the quality of existing normative threshold data. Tone-burst ABR techniques can be used in older children and in adults, and this is especially relevant to cases of possible functional hearing loss and to medicolegal situations. ABR limitations can arise from the need for very low levels of EEG noise. The EEG of even a sleeping adult generally shows a significantly higher level of myogenic activity than that of a sleeping infant, and this could lead to overestimation and increased variability of estimated audiometric thresholds. Another drawback is that, in the common testing context of suspected noise-induced hearing loss, exaggeration of hearing loss is usually most marked at low frequencies (e.g., 500 Hz), at which the tone-burst ABR is most vulnerable to myogenic noise because of its broadened waveform.

The ASSR is a very promising technique, increasingly used in infants as an alternative or adjunct to ABR. There are substantial normative threshold data for single-frequency techniques, but large-sample normative threshold data for the multifrequency approach in representative populations of young infants (with behavioral, follow-up validation) are not yet available (Rance and Rickards, 2002). Many in the clinical community have come to believe that ASSR can

quantify large hearing losses that are beyond the range of the ABR. There are several reasons to question that assumption. It is likely that much, perhaps all, of the ASSR is essentially the ABR V-V′ complex, driven at such a high stimulus rate that it resembles a sinusoidal waveform and can be detected using a simple, frequency-domain method. Why would the ASSR inherently be much more detectable than its parent phenomenon, the ABR? It is possible that ASSR methods

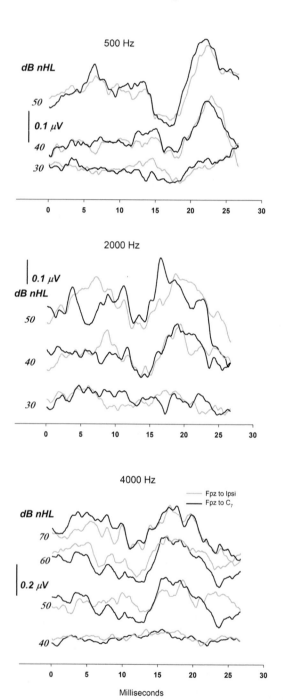

FIGURE 14.9   Auditory brainstem responses (ABRs) from one ear of an infant who failed newborn hearing screening. Both ears revealed similar results. Clear ABRs were seen with stimuli down to 20 dB normal hearing level (nHL) for 500 Hz and down to 10 or 20 dB at 4,000 Hz. This infant was judged to have normal hearing. (See text for details.)

FIGURE 14.10   Auditory brainstem responses (ABRs) from one ear of an infant who was judged to have a moderate hearing loss based on tone-burst ABR thresholds. (See text for details.)

are much more efficient than regular averaging, rendering the response easier to detect, but it is not established that this is the case when proper matching of the stimulus SPLs is imposed. A point of possible confusion is that the dB nHL reference zero for ASSR stimuli is close to 0 dB HL, whereas the dB nHL zero for typical ABR stimuli is higher because of less temporal integration. Yet, as explained earlier, changes in stimulus repetition rate may affect the ABR and psychophysical thresholds differently. Another issue is that ASSR-like responses have been reported in subjects with no useful residual hearing, and it is possible that such responses may be mediated by the vestibular system (Small and Stapells, 2004). Yet another concern is that, because the ASSR is likely a high-rate ABR, it may be depressed by neural adaptation in subjects with fragile auditory neural systems, as outlined earlier. This might cause both threshold elevation and increased variability across subjects in the difference between AEP and psychophysical thresholds. These questions, and many others, will be resolved by further, well-designed studies. It is clear that the ASSR technique offers definite advantages with respect to ease of fully objective detection methods, as well as potential advantages in efficiency.

The slow, cortical N1 response can be an accurate alternative tool for older children and adults who are awake and passively cooperative. The response is degraded in natural or sedated sleep and undergoes large maturational changes in very young children. It is not practical for widespread use as a tool for threshold estimation in infants. In adults, successful use of the N1 response requires excellent technique and considerable skills at adaptive averaging and response recognition; it is significantly more difficult to use than is the tone-burst ABR in infants. Moreover, measures such as the level

of residual noise and Fsp are much less useful than for the ABR because of the small numbers of sweeps used in averaging. However, in skilled hands, N1 has repeatedly proved to be remarkably successful, especially for assessments in compensation claimants and the medicolegal context.

CASE EXAMPLES

Two examples of ABR functions using tone bursts are shown in Figures 14.9 and 14.10. In each case, responses from only one ear and only air-conduction response are shown. Figure 14.9 shows the ABR from an infant who failed newborn hearing screening. Along with normal OAEs at the time of this diagnostic ABR test, this infant was judged to have normal hearing. In this case, testing was started with a 4,000-Hz tone burst at 50 dB nHL. Starting at this level revealed a clear response.

Note that, for both of the cases shown, the superimposed traces do not indicate replications but, instead, two channels of recording. For all recordings, an Fsp of 2.9 or greater was used to ensure the presence of response, and the absence was determined by an Fsp <2.9 after 6,144 sweeps or no obvious response by visual detection and residual noise of <18 nV. The filter settings used to gather these ABRs were 50 to 1,000 Hz (12 dB/octave).

In the first case (Fig. 14.9), a clear ABR was found in response to the 50-dB nHL 500-Hz tone burst and, subsequently, to 30 and 20 dB nHL with no clear response present to the 10-dB nHL stimulus. No correction was applied to these levels. When using the 4,000-Hz tone burst, a similar pattern was seen. Reponses both by visual and statistical detection are clear as low as 20 dB nHL. In this case, one

TABLE 14.1   Suggested stimulation and recording parameters for using tone-burst auditory brainstem response with infants and toddlers for audiometric applications

Parameter	Value	Comments
Stimulus parameters		
Type:	Windowed tone bursts: 500, 1,000, 2,000, and/or 4,000 Hz	Clicks in extreme conditions or to rule out auditory neuropathy
Rate:	<40–50/second	Coordinate with window length
Polarity:	Alternate	Eliminate cochlear microphonic and artifact
Transducers:	Insert earphones; bone-conduction vibrators	Bone conduction should not be ignored
Recording parameters		
Filters:	High pass: 30 or 100 Hz; low pass: 1,000–1,500 Hz	Shallow skirts of 12 dB/octave or less
Recording Window:	25–30 ms	Longest for 500 Hz
Electrode Placement:	Noninverting (+) at vertex or high forehead Inverting (−) at mastoid or earlobe	Second channel with inverting at nape of neck can be helpful
Averaging:	2,000–4,000 sweeps depending on noise levels; more averaging may be necessary at threshold	Online signal-to-noise ratio estimator such as Fsp is helpful; less noise will be found with sedation
Artifact Rejection:	Set to reject 5–10% of sweeps in good electroencephalogram conditions	Artifact rejection will not compensate for very noisy conditions

could argue that the response at 10 dB nHL is clear by visual detection. This level did not reach Fsp of 2.9 within 6,144 sweeps. Given that the response is well within any definition of normal hearing, no further attempts were made to determine if a true response was present at 10 dB nHL. However, if the dB levels were elevated, a replication could be helpful to determine if a response is truly present.

The second case (Fig. 14.10) illustrates 500-, 2,000-, and 4,000-Hz tone burst ABRs from an infant determined to have a moderate, high-frequency hearing loss. The thresholds for 500 and 2,000 Hz were found at 40 dB nHL, and for 4,000

Hz, the threshold was found at 50 dB. Note the importance of showing the absence of a response at levels below the judged threshold. A response was seen with the 500-Hz tone burst as low as 40 dB nHL, but no response is seen for 30 dB nHL. Applying the corrections suggested by the data of Stapells et al. (1995), we would predict audiometric thresholds of 25, 30, and 50 dB HL for 500, 2,000, and 4,000 Hz, respectively.

Suggested stimulation and recording parameters for use in audiometric assessments of infants and toddlers are found in Table 14.1.

▨ REFERENCES

Amandeo M, Shagass Ch. (1973) Brief latency click evoked potentials during waking and sleep in man. *Psychophysiology.* 10, 244–250.

Beauchaine KA, Kaminski JR, Gorga MP. (1987) Comparison of Beyer DT48 and Etymotic insert earphones: auditory brain stem response measurements. *Ear Hear.* 8, 292–297.

Boston JR, Ainslie PJ. (1980) Effects of analog and digital filtering on brain stem auditory evoked potentials. *Electroencephalogr Clin Neurophysiol.* 48, 361–364.

Davis H. (1976) Principles of electric response audiometry. *Ann Otol Rhinol Laryngol.* 85 (suppl 28), 1–96.

Davis H, Hirsh SK. (1979) A slow brain stem response for low-frequency audiometry *Audiology.* 18, 445.

Dirks DD. (1994) Bone conduction threshold testing. In: Katz J, ed. *Handbook of Clinical Audiology.* Baltimore: Williams & Wilkins; pp 132–146.

Domico WD, Kavanagh KT. (1986) Analog and zero phase-shift digital filtering of the auditory brain stem response waveform. *Ear Hear.* 7, 377–382.

Don M, Allen AR, Starr A. (1977) Effect of click rate on the latency of the auditory brainstem response in humans. *Ann Otol Rhinol Laryngol.* 86, 186–195.

Don M, Eggermont JJ, Brackmann DE. (1979) Reconstruction of the audiogram using brain stem responses and high-pass noise masking. *Ann Otol Rhinol Laryngol.* 88 (suppl 57), 1–20.

Don M, Elberling C (1996). Use of quantitative measures of auditory brain-stem response peak amplitude and residual background noise in the decision to stop averaging. *J Acoust Soc Am.* 99, 491–499.

Don M, Elberling C, Waring M. (1984) Objective detection of averaged auditory brainstem responses. *Scand Audiol.* 13, 219–228.

Don M, Ponton CW, Eggermont JJ, Masuda A. (1993) Gender differences in cochlear response time: an explanation for gender amplitude differences in the unmasked auditory brain-stem response. *J Acoust Soc Am.* 94, 2135–2148.

Don M, Vermiglio AJ, Ponton CW, Eggermont JJ, Masuda A. (1996) Variable effects of click polarity on auditory brain-stem response latencies: analyses of narrow-band ABRs suggest possible explanations. *J Acoust Soc Am.* 100, 458–472.

Durieux-Smith A, Edwards CG, Picton TW, McMurray B. (1985) Auditory brainstem responses to clicks in neonates. *J Otolaryngol.* 14 (suppl 14), 12–18.

Elberling C. (1979) Auditory electrophysiology: spectral analysis of cochlear and brainstem evoked potentials. A comment on Kevanishvili and Aphonchenko: Frequency composition of brainstem auditory evoked potentials. *Scand Audiol.* 8, 57–64.

Elberling C, Don M. (1987) Threshold characteristics of the human auditory brain stem response. *J Acoust Soc Am.* 81, 115–121.

Elberling C, Parbo J. (1987) Reference data for ABRs in retrocochlear diagnosis. *Scand Audiol.* 16, 49–55.

Elberling C, Wahlgreen D. (1985) Estimation of auditory brainstem responses (ABR) by means of Bayesian reference. *Scand Audiol.* 14, 89–96.

Eldredge L, Salamy A. (1996) Functional auditory development in preterm and full term infants. *Early Hum Dev.* 45, 215–228.

Fowler CG. (1992) Effects of stimulus phase on the normal auditory brainstem response. *J Speech Hear Res.* 35, 167–174.

Galambos R, Hecox KE. (1978) Clinical applications of the auditory brainstem response. *Otolaryngol Clin North Am.* 11, 709–722.

Gorga MP, Beauchaine KA, Reiland JK, Worthington DW, Javel E. (1984) The effects of stimulus duration on ABR and behavioral thresholds. *J Acoust Soc Am.* 76, 616–619.

Gorga MP, Johnson TA, Kaminski JR, Beauchaine KL, Garner CA, Neely ST. (2006) Using a combination of click- and tone burst-evoked auditory brain stem response measurements to estimate pure-tone thresholds. *Ear Hear.* 27, 60–74.

Gorga MP, Kaminski JR, Beauchaine KL. (1991) Effects of stimulus phase on the latency of the auditory brainstem response. *J Am Acad Audiol.* 2, 1–6.

Gorga MP, Kaminski JR, Beauchaine KL, Bergman BM. (1993) A Comparison of auditory brain stem response thresholds and latencies elicited by air- and bone-conducted stimuli. *Ear Hear.* 14, 85–94.

Hafner H, Pratt H, Joachims Z, Feinsod M, Blazer S. (1991) Development of auditory brainstem evoked potentials in newborn infants: a three-channel Lissajous' trajectory study. *Hear Res.* 51, 33–48.

Hecox K, Burkard R. (1982) Developmental dependencies of the human brainstem auditory evoked response. *Ann NY Acad Sci.* 388, 538–556.

Hicks GE. (1980) Auditory brainstem response: sensory assessment by bone conduction masking. *Arch Otolaryngol.* 106, 392–395.

Hyde ML. (1985) Frequency-specific BERA in infants. *J Otolaryngol.* 14 (suppl), 19–27.

Hyde ML. (1997) The N1 response and its applications. *Audiol Neurotol.* 2, 281–307.

Hyde ML, Riko K, Malizia K. (1990) Audiometric accuracy of the click ABR in infants at risk for hearing loss. *J Am Acad Audiol.* 1, 59–66.

Hyde ML, Stephens SDG, Thornton ARD. (1976) Stimulus repetition rate and the early brainstem responses. *Br J Audiol.* 10, 41–50.

Jacobson JT, Hyde ML. (1986) The auditory brainstem response in neonatal hearing screening. In: Swigart ET, ed. *Neonatal Hearing Screening.* San Diego: College Hill Press, Inc.; pp 67–98.

Jacobson JT, Morehouse CR, Johnson M. (1982) Strategies for infant auditory brain stem response assessment. *Ear Hear.* 3, 263–270.

Jerger J, Mauldin L. (1978) Prediction of sensorineural hearing level from the brain stem evoked response. *Arch Otolaryngol.* 104, 456–461.

Jerger J, Tillman T. (1960) A new method for the clinical determination of sensorineural acuity level (SAL). *Arch Otolaryngol.* 71, 948–955.

Jewett DL, Williston JS. (1971) Auditory-evoked far fields averaged from the scalp of humans. *Brain.* 94, 681–696.

Joint Committee on Infant Hearing. (2000). Year 2000 position statement. *Audiol Today.* 3-23.

Kavanagh KT, Clark ST. (1989) Comparison of the mastoid to vertex and mastoid to high forehead electrode arrays in recording auditory evoked potentials. *Ear Hear.* 10, 259–261.

Kavanagh KT, Harker LA, Tyler RS. (1984) Auditory brainstem and middle latency responses. I. Effects of response filtering and waveform identification. II. Threshold responses to a 500-Hz tone pip. *Ann Otol Rhinol Laryngol.* 93 (suppl 108), 2–12.

Kevanishvili Z, Aphonchenko V. (1981) Click polarity inversion effects upon the human brainstem auditory evoked potential. *Scand Audiol.* 10, 141–147.

Kileny P. (1981) The frequency specificity of tone-pip evoked auditory brain stem responses. *Ear Hear.* 2, 270–275.

Kileny P, Robertson CMT. (1985) Neurological aspects of infant hearing assessment. *J Otolaryngol.* 14 (suppl 14), 34–39.

Kimberley BP, Brown DK, Eggermont JJ. (1993) Measuring human cochlear traveling wave delay using distortion product emission phase responses. *J Acoust Soc Am.* 94, 1343–1350.

King AJ, Sininger YS. (1992) Electrode configuration for auditory brainstem response audiometry. *Am J Audiol.* 1, 63–67.

Klein AJ, Alvaqrez ED, Cowburn CA. (1992) The effects of stimulus rate on detectability of the auditory brainstem response in infants. *Ear Hear.* 13, 401–405.

Kneebone CS, Burns RJ. (1981) A case of cortical deafness. *Clin Exp Neurol.* 18, 91–97.

Lasky RE. (1991) The effects of rate and forward masking on human adult and newborn auditory evoked response thresholds. *Dev Psychobiol.* 24, 51–64.

Lasky RE. (1997) Rate and adaptation effects on the auditory evoked brainstem response in human newborns and adults. *Hear Res.* 111, 165–176.

Leung SM, Slaven A, Thornton AR, Brickley GJ. (1998) The use of high stimulus rate auditory brainstem responses in the estimation of hearing threshold. *Hear Res.* 123, 201–205.

Levine RA, Liederman J, Riley P. (1988) The brainstem auditory evoked potential asymmetry is replicable and reliable. *Neuropsychologica.* 26, 603–614.

Levine RA, McGaffigan PM. (1983) Right-left asymmetries in the human brain stem: auditory evoked potentials. *Electroencephalogr Clin Neurophysiol.* 55, 532–537.

Malinoff RL, Spivak LG. (1990) Effect of stimulus parameters on auditory brainstem response spectral analysis. *Audiology.* 29, 21–28.

Mauldin L, Jerger J. (1979) Auditory brain stem evoked responses to bone-conducted signals. *Arch Otolaryngol.* 105, 656–661.

McClelland RJ, McCrea RS. (1979) Intersubject variability of the auditory-evoked brain stem potentials. *Audiology.* 18, 462–471.

McPherson DL, Hirasugi Y, Starr A. (1985) Auditory brain stem potentials recorded at different scalp locations in neonates and adults. *Ann Otol Rhinol Laryngol.* 94, 236–243.

Michalewski HJ, Thompson LW, Patterson JV, Bowman TE, Litzelman D. (1980) Sex differences in the amplitudes and latencies of the human auditory brain stem potential. *Electroencephalogr Clin Neurophysiol.* 48, 351–356.

Moller AR, Jannetta PJ. (1983) Interpretation of brainstem auditory evoked potentials: results from intracranial recordings in humans. *Scand Audiol.* 12, 125–133.

Moller K, Blegvad B (1976). Brain stem responses in patients with sensorineural hearing loss: monaural versus binaural stimulation; the significance of audiogram configuration. *Scand Audiol.* 5, 115–127.

Moore JM, Wilson WR, Thompson G. (1977) Visual reinforcement of head-turn responses in infants under 12 months of age. *J Speech Hear Disord.* 42, 328–334.

Morgan DE, Zimmerman MC, Dubno JR. (1987) Auditory brain stem evoked response characteristics in the full-term newborn infant. *Ann Otol Rhinol Laryngol.* 96, 142–151.

Munnerley GM, Greville K, Purdy S, Keith W. (1991) Frequency-specific auditory brainstem responses: relationship to behavioural threshold in cochlear-impaired adults. *Audiology.* 30, 25–32.

Musiek FE, Charette L, Morse D, Baran JA. (2004) Central deafness associated with a midbrain lesion. *J Am Acad Audiol.* 15, 133–151.

Nousak JM, Stapells DR. (1992) Frequency specificity of the auditory brain stem response to bone-conducted tones in infants and adults. *Ear Hear.* 13, 87–95.

Orlando MS, Folsom RC. (1995) The effects of reversing the polarity of frequency-limited single-cycle stimuli on the human auditory brain stem response. *Ear Hear.* 16, 311–320.

Parker D, Thornton ARD. (1978) Cochlear traveling wave velocities calculated from the derived components of the cochlear nerve and brainstem evoked responses of the human auditory system. *Scand Audiol.* 7, 67–70.

Picton TW, Durieux-Smith A. (1978) The practice of evoked potential audiometry. *Otolaryngol Clin North Am.* 11, 263–282.

Picton TW, Hillyard SA. (1974) Human auditory evoked potentials. II. Effects of attention. *Electroencephalogr Clin Neurophysiol.* 36, 191–199.

Picton TW, Stapells DR, Campbell KB. (1981) Auditory evoked potentials from the human cochlea and brainstem. *J Otolaryngol.* 10 (suppl), 1–41.

Rance G, Cone-Wesson B, Wunderlich J, Dowell RC. (2002) Speech perception and cortical event related potentials in children with auditory neuropathy. *Ear Hear.* 23, 239–253.

Rance G, Rickards F. (2002) Prediction of hearing threshold in infants using auditory steady-state evoked potentials. *J Am Acad Audiol.* 13, 236–245.

Rosenhamer HJ, Lindstrom B, Lundborg T. (1980) On the use of click-evoked electric brainstem responses in audiological diagnosis. II. The influence of sex and age upon the normal response. *Scand Audiol.* 9, 93–100.

Salamy A. (1984) Maturation of the auditory brainstem response from birth through early childhood. *J Clin Neurophysiol.* 1, 293–329.

Salamy A, Eggermont JJ, Eldredge L. (1994) Neurodevelopment and auditory function in preterm infants. In: Jacobson JT, ed. *Principles and Applications in Auditory Evoked Potentials.* Boston: Allyn and Bacon; pp 287–312.

Salamy A, Eldredge L, Wakeley A. (1985) Maturation of contralateral brain-stem responses in preterm infants. *Electroencephalogr Clin Neurophysiol.* 62, 117–123.

Salamy A, McKean CM. (1976) Postnatal development of human brainstem potentials during the first year of life. *Electroencephalogr Clin Neurophysiol.* 40, 418–426.

Salamy A, McKean CM, Buda FB. (1975) Maturational changes in auditory transmission as reflected in human brainstem potentials. *Brain Res.* 96, 361–366.

Salt AN, Thornton ARD. (1984) The effects of stimulus rise-time and polarity on the auditory brainstem responses. *Scand Audiol.* 13, 119–127.

Sato H, Sando I, Takahashi H. (1991) Sexual dimorphism and development of the human cochlea. Computer 3-D measurement. *Acta Otolaryngol.* 111, 1037–1040.

Schulman-Galambos C, Galambos R. (1975) Brain stem auditory-evoked responses in premature infants. *J Speech Hear Res.* 18, 456–465.

Schwartz DM, Larson VD, DeChicchis AR. (1985) Spectral characteristics of air and bone conduction transducers used to record the auditory brain stem response. *Ear Hear.* 6, 274–277.

Scollie SD, Seewald RC, Cornelisse LE, Jenstad LM. (1998) Validity and repeatability of level-independent HL to SPL transforms. *Ear Hear.* 19, 407–413.

Shepard RK, Maffi CL, Hatsushika S, Javel E, Tong YC, Clark GM. (1992) Temporal and spatial coding in auditory prostheses. In: *Information Processing in Mammalian Auditory and Tactile Systems.* New York: Alan Liss Inc.; pp 281–293.

Sininger YS. (1995) Filtering and spectral characteristics of averaged auditory brain-stem response and background noise in infants. *J Acoust Soc Am.* 98, 2048–2055.

Sininger YS, Abdala C. (1998) Physiologic assessment of hearing. In: Lalwani AK, Grundfast KM, eds. *Pediatric Otology and Neurotology.* Philadelphia: Lippincott-Raven; pp 127–154.

Sininger YS, Abdala C, Cone-Wesson B. (1997) Auditory threshold sensitivity of the human neonate as measured by the auditory brainstem response. *Hear Res.* 104, 27–38.

Sininger YS, Cone-Wesson B. (2006) Lateral asymmetry in the ABR of neonates: evidence and mechanisms. *Hear Res.* 212, 203–211.

Sininger YS, Cone-Wesson B, Folsom RC, Gorga MP, Vohr BR, Widen JE, Ekelid M, Norton SJ. (2000) Identification of neonatal hearing impairment: auditory brain stem responses in the perinatal period. *Ear Hear.* 21, 383–399.

Sininger YS, Don M. (1989) Effects of click rate and electrode orientation on threshold detectability of the auditory brainstem response. *J Speech Hear Res.* 32, 880–886.

Sininger YS, Masuda A. (1990) Effect of click polarity on ABR threshold. *Ear Hear.* 11, 206–209.

Sininger YS, Oba S. (2001) Patients with auditory neuropathy: who are they and what can they hear. In: Sininger YS, Starr A, eds. *Auditory Neuropathy: A New Perspective on Hearing Disorders.* Albany, NY: Thompson Learning; pp 15–35.

Small SA, Stapells DR. (2004) Artifactual responses when recording auditory steady-state responses. *Ear Hear.* 25, 611–623.

Spivak LG. (1993) Spectral composition of infant auditory brainstem responses: implications for filtering. *Audiology.* 32, 185–194.

Stapells DR. (1989) Auditory brainstem response assessment of infants and children. *Semin Hear.* 10, 229–251.

Stapells DR. (1998) Frequency-specific evoked potential audiometry in infants. In: *Proceedings from the 1st International Conference: A Sound Foundation Through Early Amplification.* Warrenville, IL: Phonak; pp 13–30.

Stapells DR. (2000) Threshold estimation by the tone-evoked auditory brainstem response: a literature meta-analysis. *J Speech Lang Pathol Audiol.* 24, 74–83.

Stapells DR, Gravel JS, Martin BA. (1995) Thresholds for auditory brainstem responses to tones in notched noise from infants and young children with normal hearing or sensorineural hearing loss. *Ear Hear.* 16, 361–371.

Stapells DR, Ruben RJ. (1989) Auditory brain stem responses to bone-conducted tones in infants. *Ann Otol Rhinol Laryngol.* 98, 941–949.

Starr A, Amlie RN, Martin WH, Sanders S. (1977) Development of auditory function in newborn infants revealed by auditory brainstem potentials. *Pediatrics.* 60, 831–839.

Starr A, Picton TW, Sininger Y, Hood LJ, Berlin CI. (1996) Auditory neuropathy. *Brain.* 119, 741–753.

Stockard JE, Stockard JJ, Coen RW. (1983) Auditory brain stem response variability in infants. *Ear Hear.* 4, 11–23.

Stockard JE, Stockard JJ, Westmoreland BF, Corfits JL. (1979) Brainstem auditory-evoked responses: normal variation as a function of stimulus and subject characteristics. *Arch Neurol.* 36, 823–831.

Stuart A, Yang EY. (1994) Effect of high-pass filtering on the neonatal auditory brainstem response to air- and bone-conducted clicks. *J Speech Hear Res.* 37, 475–479.

Stuart A, Yang EY, Botea M. (1996) Neonatal auditory brainstem responses recorded from four electrode montages. *Commun Disord.* 29, 125–139.

Stuart A, Yang EY, Green WB. (1994) Neonatal auditory brainstem response thresholds to air- and bone-conducted clicks: 0 to 96 hours postpartum. *J Am Acad Audiol.* 5, 163–172.

Suzuki T, Kobayashi K, Takagi N. (1986) Effects of stimulus repetition rate on slow and fast components of auditory brainstem resp. *Electroencephalogr Clin Neurophysiol.* 65, 150–156.

Szirmai I, Farsang M, Csuri M. (2003) Cortical auditory disorder caused by bilateral strategic cerebral bleedings. Analysis of two cases. *Brain Lang.* 85, 159–165.

Trune DR, Mitchell C, Phillips DS. (1988) The relative importance of head size, gender and age on the auditory brainstem response. *Hear Res.* 32, 165–174.

Van Campen LE, Sammeth CA, Hall JW III, Peek BF. (1992) Comparison of Etymotic insert and TDH supra-aural earphones in auditory brainstem response measurement. *J Am Acad Audiol.* 3, 315–323.

Van Olphen AF, Rodenburg M, Vervey C. (1979) Influence of stimulus repetition rate on brainstem-evoked responses in man. *Audiology.* 18, 388–394.

Webb KC, Greenberg HJ. (1983) Bone conduction masking for threshold assessment in auditory brain stem response testing. *Ear Hear.* 4, 261–266.

Yang EY, Rupert AL, Moushegian G. (1987) A developmental study of bone conduction auditory brainstem response in infants. *Ear Hear.* 8, 244–251.

Yang EY, Stuart A. (1990) A method of auditory brainstem response testing of infants using bone-conducted clicks. *JSLPA/ROA.* 14, 69–76.

Ysunza A, Cone-Wesson B. (1987) Bone conduction masking for brainstem auditory-evoked potentials (BAEP) in pediatric audiological evaluations. Validation of the test. *Int J Pediatr Otorhinolaryngol.* 12, 291–302.

15 The Auditory Steady-State Response

Barbara Cone and Andrew Dimitrijevic

 ## OVERVIEW

Auditory steady-state responses (ASSRs) are brain potentials evoked by steady-state stimuli. They are rhythmic, electrical responses of the brain to regularly repeating stimuli. The steady-state stimuli must have a frequency or amplitude modulation, or both. The steady-state stimuli may be modulated noise or tones or trains of acoustic transients (e.g., clicks or tone bursts).

Imagine the waveform of an auditory brainstem response if two tone-burst stimuli were presented within an averaging epoch. Each tone burst would be expected to produce a response, and so the response waveform would be repeated twice, within the averaged epoch. Now, imagine a 125-ms train of 2-1-2 cycle tone bursts, say at 2,000 Hz (carrier frequency [CF]), with an interstimulus interval between each burst at 12.5 ms (80 Hz). Imagine that the response averaging epoch is also 125 ms in duration. One thousand 125-ms trains are presented, and the response to each train is averaged. There are 10 responses represented in the time-averaged waveform for the 125-ms sample. The time-averaged waveform appears as a series of peaks or a periodic wave, with 12.5-ms interpeak interval (Fig. 15.1, left panels). This is one way of conceptualizing an ASSR. The ASSR, furthermore, can be obtained for a wide range of modulation frequencies (MFs), although rates between 10 and 200 Hz have been most often investigated. For example (Fig. 15.1, right panels), the 40-Hz ASSR is obtained using clicks or tone bursts presented every 25 ms or puretones or noise amplitude modulated (AM) at 40 Hz. Because the ASSR is periodic (repeating at the same rate as the MF), it can be analyzed using frequency-domain methods. The spectrum of the response will show a statistically significant peak at the repetition rate, that is, at the MF. The latency of this periodic waveform can be expressed as a phase delay (360 degrees), relative to the onset of the start of the stimulus train, or onset modulation of tones or noise. When a response is present, the phase of the response is consistent (phase coherent) across subaverages and is "phase locked," occurring at a specific phase relative to the MF. The phase coherence/phase locking can be tested for statistical significance in addition to, or in place of, the statistical test of response spectral peak amplitude. The presence of an ASSR is dependent upon the integrity of the auditory periphery (external, middle, and inner ear, auditory nerve) for the CF, as well as the integrity of higher levels of the auditory pathway.

Since 1999, when the contribution to the previous (fifth) edition of the *Handbook of Clinical Audiology* on ASSRs was written (Sininger and Cone-Wesson, 2002), there has been a significant increase in the clinical application of ASSRs. In the summer of 1999, there were no instruments available commercially for clinicians (in the United States) to perform ASSR tests, although clinical ASSR systems produced in Australia (ERA Systems) and in Cuba (Neuronix) were available in Australia, Asia, Africa, Europe, and South America. As of 2005, there are three US companies (GSI-Nicolet, Bio-Logic, and Intelligent Hearing Systems) and two Canadian companies (MASTER, Vivosonic), in addition to the Cuban company, that have ASSR systems on the market. (ERA Systems of Australia sold the rights to their technology to GSI-Nicolet.) The ASSR has moved from the lab to the clinic during the past decade. Another change that has taken place since

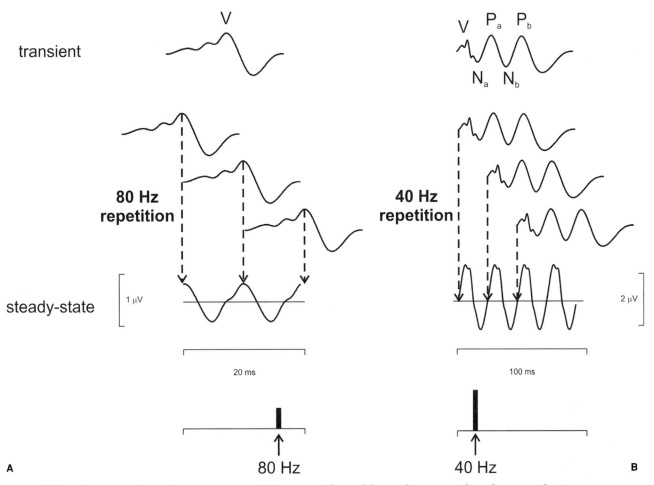

FIGURE 15.1 Examples of transient-evoked potentials and how they are related to steady-state potentials. In A, with a modulation frequency of 80 Hz, there are brainstem responses occurring every 12.5 ms, the same period as the modulated (tone) stimulus. In B, with a stimulus modulation frequency of 40 Hz, the responses occur every 25 ms, the same period as the stimulus modulation.

1999 is the nomenclature, that is, what we call this evoked potential. Previously, we wrote about "amplitude modulation following responses" (AMFR), "envelope-following response" (EFR), "steady-state evoked potentials" (SSEP), and even the "40-Hz response" (when using that MF). Because ASSRs can be obtained to amplitude or frequency modulation, AMFR was not an entirely accurate label. SSEP could be confused with the acronym for somatosensory evoked potentials. ASSR became the accepted acronym under the leadership of Terence Picton. (Some readers will remember the BAEP, BAER, BSER, and ABR acronym flurries, but a rose by any other name...)

The primary clinical application of ASSR during the past decade has been for the estimation of hearing thresholds in infants and children, and thus, this is the focus of this chapter. The ASSR is also a tool for investigating the ear and brain response to complex stimuli at supra-threshold levels. This use of ASSR may prove to be useful in estimating speech perception abilities and for evaluating audibility of complex stimuli, such as for hearing aid evaluations. These emerging applications will be highlighted in this chapter.

FUNDAMENTALS

Knowledge of neural generators, stimulus-response relationships, subject-related response factors, signal processing, and detection algorithms is necessary for interpreting ASSR results. Each of these areas will be reviewed.

Neural Generators

The generation of the ASSR at the level of the cochlea and nerve is schematized in Figure 15.2 (after Lins et al., 1995). An amplitude-modulated tone is the stimulus. The first step in sensory transduction occurs at the level of the inner hair cells. As the basilar membrane vibrates, the stereocilia on the inner hair cells move back and forth symmetrically (at low stimulus intensities), faithfully following the sound stimulation. This symmetric movement is shown in the figure as a sinusoid. Integrity of the outer and inner hair cell transduction systems is needed to obtain a normal response to the tone. The transmission of information from the inner hair cells to the auditory nerve involves the release of the

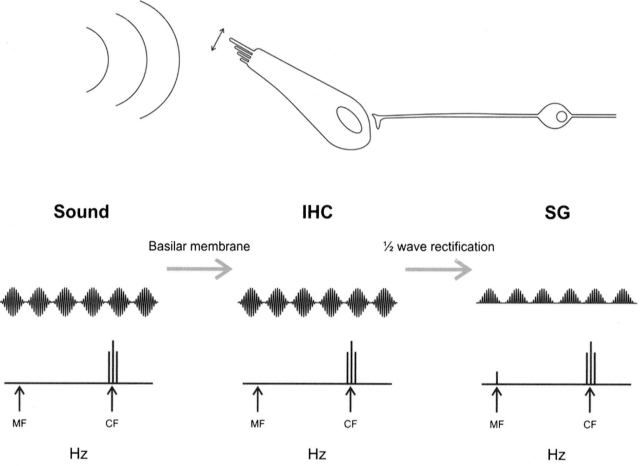

FIGURE 15.2 A model of auditory steady-state response (ASSR) generation at the level of the cochlea and eighth nerve. The modulated tone creates a basilar membrane vibration at the ''best place'' for the carrier frequency (CF). There is no energy present at the modulation frequency. Inner hair cells (IHCs) release neurotransmitters to the peripheral processes of the spiral ganglion (SG) cells. This provides a $\frac{1}{2}$ wave rectification of the stimulus, providing energy for the neural response at the modulation frequency (MF).

neurotransmitter, most likely glutamate, from the inner hair cells. Glutamate release will only occur when the stereocilia move in one direction. If there is enough glutamate uptake by the spiral ganglion cells, an action potential will occur. Because the action potentials are generated by movement of stereocilia in only one direction, the stimulus (tone) undergoes half-wave rectification. Half-wave rectification provides energy at the MF. There is no stimulus energy at the MF, yet the half-wave rectification introduces energy at the MF. It is the energy at the MF that evokes the ASSR.

Supporting evidence of this model is seen in recordings from auditory nerve made by Khanna and Teich (1989a; 1989b), who showed that presenting amplitude modulation (AM) or frequency modulation (FM) stimuli evoked responses in the auditory nerve at the MFs, in harmonics of the MFs, and at the CF.

Neurons of the eighth nerve (Ruggero, 1992), cochlear nucleus (Rhode and Greenberg, 1992), inferior colliculus (Irvine, 1992), and primary auditory cortex (Clarey et al.,

1992) are responsive to AM and FM signals, and so could be involved in the generation of the ASSR. One line of evidence that points to a relationship between MF and the underlying neural generator is that of ASSR latency. Measurement of the response phase spectrum (relative to the MF) can be used to estimate response latency. The predominant phase is used to characterize the latency of the response, and hence, the generators are assumed to be the same as those for the transient evoked response of similar latency. Modulation rates of 20 Hz or less will result in a response dominated by those generators that are responsible for the late cortical evoked potential, specifically primary auditory cortex and association areas. For modulation rates higher than 20 Hz but lower than 50 Hz, the response characteristics are similar to those found for the middle latency auditory evoked response (MLAER), with generators generally thought to be auditory midbrain, thalamus, and primary auditory cortex (Kraus et al., 1994). Modulation rates higher than 50 Hz will be dominated by evoked potentials from brainstem sites, including those for wave V and its subsequent negative trough, sometimes identified as SN-10 (Møller, 1994).

Chemical lesions of the auditory pathway were used by Kuwada et al. (2002) to determine neural generators of the ASSR. Using a rabbit model, they administered pharmacologic substances that reduced activity at selected levels of the auditory system, while recording ASSRs as MF was varied. As MF was increased, phase delay (latency) decreased. Estimated latencies for MFs <100 Hz were 27 ms, suggesting a cortical generator. At rates above 100 Hz, latencies were more consistent with brainstem generators (i.e., at ≤5 ms). When potassium chloride was administered topically to the cortex (to depress cortical activity), the ASSR for MFs <100 Hz were significantly decreased, whereas those for MFs >100 Hz were stable. It was also possible to discern two subcortical generators, based upon latency and recording site, for MFs >80 Hz. One of these subcortical generators was thought to be from a pontine-midbrain source, while the other was thought to arise from the superior olivary complex and/or cochlear nucleus. Szalda and Burkard (2005) recorded ASSRs from inferior colliculus and auditory cortex sites in awake and Nembutal-anesthetized chinchillas, as the MF of a 2,000-Hz tone was varied from 29 to 249 Hz in 20-Hz steps. Modulation rate transfer functions (MRTFs), that is, the amplitude of the ASSR plotted as a function of modulation rate, were plotted for inferior colliculus and auditory cortex sites. The inferior colliculus responses were largest at modulation rates of 109 and 170 Hz. While Nembutal anesthesia reduced the amplitude of the inferior colliculus response for modulation rates greater than 90 Hz, the peaks in the MRTF remained present. A different result was obtained from the auditory cortex. In the awake state, the auditory cortex MRTF had peaks at 29 and 70 Hz, but when anesthetized, the amplitude of the ASSR was greatly reduced, and the amplitudes were largest at 29 Hz. These results are consistent with those of Kuwada et al. (2002), in that more robust responses were found for higher modulation rates at the inferior colliculus compared to auditory cortex, whereas the cortex had more robust responses to lower modulation rates. Also, the effects of anesthesia, while reducing amplitude of all ASSRs (except low-frequency modulation rates from the inferior colliculus), had a greater effect on the cortical responses. Szalda and Burkard (2005) conclude that both the inferior colliculus and auditory cortex contribute to ASSRs obtained at MFs in the range of 70 to 100 Hz but that the effect of anesthesia significantly reduces the cortical contribution.

Studies in human subjects, using the techniques of dipole source modeling and positron emission tomography (PET), indicate both brainstem and cortical neural generators of the ASSR. Herdman et al (2002a) investigated the neural generators of ASSR for modulation rates of 12, 39, and 88 Hz in adults using dipole source modeling techniques. The results showed that the brainstem source was active for all three rates of stimulation, while the cortical sources were predominant for the two lower rates, although the ASSRs at 12 Hz were very low in amplitude. Estimated latencies of the

ASSR were also consistent with a brainstem site of generation for the 88-Hz ASSR and with cortical site(s) for the 39- and 12-Hz modulation rates. PET was used to study the generators of the 40-Hz ASSR in adults (Reyes et al., 2004). The investigators distinguished the cortical areas activated by an AM tone from those activated by a puretone. They showed that bilateral activation of primary auditory cortices, left medial geniculate, and right middle frontal gyrus, as well as the right anterior cingulate gyrus and an area of right auditory cortex, was specifically activated by the AM stimulus. The PET technique used in this study would not be sensitive to brainstem sites of activation, so these cannot be ruled out.

In summary, the ASSR has multiple generators, although the contribution of the generators varies with MF. In humans, MFs >80 Hz are thought to be generated predominantly by brainstem sites, although the contribution of cortical generators is still present. At lower MFs, the medial geniculate body, auditory radiation, and primary auditory cortex are thought to contribute to the ASSR. As for other cortical evoked responses, ASSRs at low modulation rates show laterality towards the hemisphere contralateral to the stimulated ear, although 40-Hz ASSRs show evidence of right hemispheric dominance (Ross et al., 2005).

Stimulus Factors

CARRIER FREQUENCY

Auditory sensitivity varies as a function of CF, as does ASSR threshold. The difference between ASSR and behavioral threshold also varies with CF. In general, the ASSR threshold is lowest in the mid-frequency range, at 1.5 and 2.0 kHz, in comparison to thresholds at lower or higher CFs. Response phase delays decrease systematically with CF, reflecting the tonotopic organization of the cochlea and supporting the data demonstrating that the ASSR is somewhat place specific (Herdman et al., 2002b).

Most of the data about the effect of CF on ASSR is from experiments in which ASSR threshold was measured. There is a lot of variability in methods used in these studies and, consequentially, variability in results. Some investigators report ASSR threshold in dB hearing level (HL), for which thresholds are "normalized" to an audiometric calibration, and others report thresholds in dB sound pressure level (SPL). Another consideration is that ASSR threshold is determined using algorithms based upon an estimate of the signal-to-noise ratio (S/N). Thus, longer averaging times should decrease the background noise level, thus improving the S/N and yielding lower (better) thresholds. Another consideration is that there is relatively little threshold data for those with normal hearing, with the bulk of published threshold data for those with hearing loss. Table 15.1 includes ASSR threshold data as a function of frequency in adults and infants with normal hearing. The estimation of perceptual threshold for puretones from ASSR threshold is discussed in a later section of this chapter. It should be noted that the relationship between ASSR and perceptual threshold as a function

TABLE 15.1   80-Hz auditory steady-state response (ASSR) thresholds in adults and infants with normal hearing

Study	No. of Subjects	Stimuli	Level	500 Hz	1,000 Hz	2,000 Hz	4,000 Hz
Adults							
Aoyagi et al., 1994c	20	AM	dB HL	34±15 (250 Hz)	28±14	—	30±15
Lins et al., 1996	15	AM	dB SPL	39±10	29±12	29±11	31±5
Picton et al., 1998	10	AM	dB SPL	37±10	32±15	30±7	30±7
Herdman and Stapells, 2001	10	AM	dB SPL	22±12	19±10	18±9	20±11
Perez-Abalo et al., 2001	40	AM	dB SPL	40±10	34±9	33±10	35±10
Cone-Wesson et al., 2002a	10	AM	dB SPL	52±7	—	—	23±10
Dimitrijevic et al., 2002	14	MM	dB SL	17±10	4±11	4±8	11±7
Picton et al., 2005 (short duration average)	10	MM	dB SL[a]	35±16	16±8	18±9	23±15
Picton et al., 2005 (long duration average)	10	MM	dB SL[a]	21±8	7±8	9±6	13±7
Luts and Wouters, 2005, "Master"	10	MM	dB SL[a]	24±11	17±9	14±7	21±11
Luts and Wouters, 2005, "Audera"	10	MM	dB SL[a]	48±21	40±21	33±10	30±20
Van der Werff and Brown, 2005	10	MM	dB HL	29±10	23±11	16±6	15±10
Johnson and Brown, 2005	14	AM	dB SL[a]	—	22±5[b]	14±2[b]	—
Johnson and Brown, 2005	14	MM	dB SL[a]	—	16±4[b]	14±3[b]	—
Small and Stapells, 2005[c]	10	MM	dB HL[a]	22±11	26±13	18±8	18±11
Infants							
Rickards et al., 1994 (newborns)	337	MM	dB HL[d]	41±10	—	24±9 (1,500 Hz)	35±11
Levi et al., 1995 (1 month)	35	AM	dB SPL	42±16	42±11	34±15	—
Lins et al., 1996 (<12 months)	23	AM	dB SPL	45±13	29±10	26±8	29±10
Savio et al., 2001 (newborns)	25	AM	dB nHL[e]	16±11	22±12	19±12	23±13
Savio et al., 2001 (7–12 months)	13	AM	dB nHL[e]	9±9	12±10	7±8	9±9
Cone-Wesson et al., 2002c	85	MM	dB HL[d]	39±8	34±10	26±10	39±12
Rance et al., 2005	285	MM	dB HL	32±7	32±7	24±6	28±7

The number of subjects, stimulus type and threshold level are given for each study. AM is a sinusoidally modulated puretone and MM is an amplitude and frequency modulated tone. AM modulation depth is 100% and FM modulation depth varies between 10% and 25% in various studies. There are considerable differences in ASSR recording methodology represented in these studies, with some using a single-frequency, sequential test strategy (Aoyagi, Cone-Wesson, Rance, Rickards, and Cone-Wesson) and others using multiple carriers presented simultaneously. Differences in averaging time, signal processing, and detection algorithm also vary between studies. 80-Hz ASSR refers to modulation rates in the 70- to 110-Hz range.
[a] ASSR thresholds are: ASSR threshold – pure tone threshold for that carrier frequency.
[b] Threshold and standard error estimated from bar graph.
[c] Bone-conduction stimuli.
[d] Re: adult thresholds.
[e] Re: adult thresholds. 0 dB nHL = 51, 39, 39, and 34 dB SPL at 0.5, 1.0, 2.0, and 4.0 kHz, respectively.

of frequency may be affected by sensory-neural hearing loss, with better correspondence between electrophysiologic and perceptual threshold as frequency and hearing loss severity increase.

AM AND FM MODULATION DEPTH

John et al. (2001b) evaluated the effect of amplitude and frequency modulation depth on ASSRs obtained from adults with normal hearing. A sinusoidal function at 82 Hz was used to amplitude modulate a 60-dB SPL 1,000-Hz tone at 100%, 50%, 20%, 10%, and 5%. Then, the 1.0-kHz carrier was frequency modulated (at 82 Hz) at depths of 50%, 20%, 10%, 5%, and 2%. ASSR amplitude decreased with a decrease in modulation depth by 0.5 nV/% over a 20% to 100% AM change, but the amplitude change was almost twice as steep for a change in FM depth. ASSR amplitudes in response to a 20% FM tone were larger than those for a 100% AM tone. There was no change in phase delay (latency) as modulation depth was varied. Fewer than 50% of responses reached statistical significance for AM depths less than 20% and for FM depths less than 5%.

In further experimentation, the advantage of using both AM and FM (called mixed modulation [MM]) for the same CF was demonstrated (John et al., 2001b). ASSR amplitudes were significantly larger in response to MM tones compared with responses to AM alone. Part of the reason is the spread of spectral energy for the MM signal. Sidebands for the AM will be at the CF ± MF, and sidebands for FM will be at CF ± integer multiples of the MF. The interaction of AM and FM accounts for increased MM responses. John et al. (2001b) suggest that the benefit of MM is governed by the different responses of AM and FM. An FM response maximally stimulates neurons that are slightly higher in frequency

than at the CF and therefore occur slightly earlier than the AM response (Fig. 15.3). If the FM phase is adjusted relative to the AM component, so that it is delivered slightly after the AM, then the resultant ASSR will be optimized because the "peaks" of AM and FM occur at the same time. This results in a larger ASSR response in comparison to AM or FM alone or when the phase relationships between AM and FM are not phase adjusted. John et al. (2001b) demonstrated that, when the phase of FM was varied with respect to AM, ASSR amplitude plotted as a function of FM phase delays varied in a sinusoidal fashion, with amplitude crests observed at relative phases of 0 and 270 degrees. Stimulus level and CF were also varied in this experiment, and phase delays decreased with increasing level and CF; this is homologous to the latency changes observed in ABR for changes in stimulus level and tone-burst frequency.

This parametric study showed that MM stimuli yield larger ASSR amplitudes and, hence, a greater number of responses detected, in comparison to results with pure AM stimuli. The study also showed the importance of the phase relationship between the AM and FM stimulus components in order to obtain the largest, most easily detected responses. Of course, the spectrum of the stimulus is considerably broader for an AM+FM tone than for AM alone. This would be expected to affect the frequency specificity or cochlear-place specificity of the ASSR.

MODULATION TYPE

Clicks or modulated broadband, high-pass, or low-pass noise will yield large-amplitude ASSRs with low detection thresholds. John et al. (2003) used noise and tones modulated with exponential functions to obtain ASSRs. In all cases, the ASSRs for the exponential modulations were larger than those

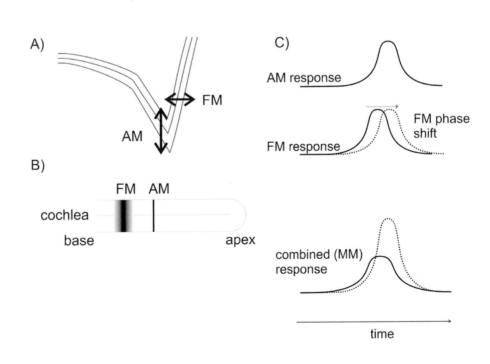

FIGURE 15.3 A model of combined amplitude modulation (AM) and frequency modulation (FM) response activation. (A) This part shows the tuning curves for auditory nerve fibers and how the AM activates the fibers slightly apical to the best frequency and how the FM activates the fibers slightly basally. **(B)** This part shows the area of the basilar membrane activated by both types of modulation. **(C)** This part indicates the time course of response to each type of modulation and the time course of the response to combined (mixed modulation [MM]) AM and FM tones.

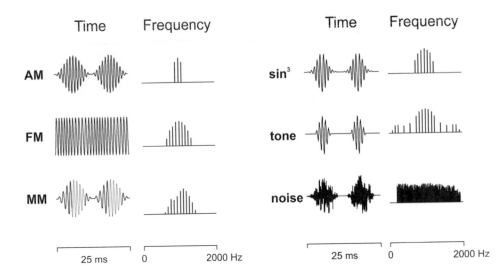

FIGURE 15.4 Time and frequency domain representation of stimuli used for auditory steady-state response (ASSR). Waveforms and spectra are shown for (sinusoidal) amplitude modulation (AM), frequency modulation (FM), mixed modulation (MM; AM+FM), exponential sine-wave modulation (sin³), tone burst (linear-ramp), and modulated noise.

for conventional, sinusoidal, and MM tones. This is predictable, given that exponential modulation results in steeper rise times that will broaden the stimulus spectra, and in fact, the shape approaches a tone burst. John et al. (2003) suggest that high-pass and low-pass modulated noise or clicks could be used to quickly estimate threshold in the low- and high-frequency ranges of hearing. This could then be followed by using frequency-specific MM tones, to make more definitive puretone threshold estimates. If threshold can be estimated quickly using less frequency-specific stimuli, then more time can be spent acquiring ASSRs for frequency-specific stimuli at levels closer to threshold. Figure 15.4 shows time- and frequency-domain representations of sinusoidal AM, FM, and MM tones, tones modulated with an exponential function, and modulated noise.

MULTIPLE MODULATION AND CARRIER FREQUENCIES

It is possible to present multiple amplitude-modulated CFs simultaneously and perform a separate analysis for each MF used in the complex stimulus. Lins and Picton (1995b) showed that it was possible to present up to four CFs in both ears. The CFs were 0.5, 1.0, 2.0, and 4.0 kHz, and there were eight different MFs, with the MF varied for ear and CF. When supra-threshold level (60 dB SPL) stimuli were used, there was no difference in response amplitude for the single tone–alone condition, four stimuli combined in one ear, or four stimuli combined in both ears. ASSR threshold was also estimated using two CF tones (500 and 2,000 Hz) in each ear. In normal ears, there does not appear to be a difference in ASSR threshold for four CFs presented simultaneously, compared to when they are presented singly, as long as the CFs are separated by an octave and the MFs (at 70 Hz or greater) are separated by 3 Hz. An illustration of this multifrequency stimulus is shown in Figure 15.5, with both time (waveforms) and frequency (spectra) domain representations of the stimulus components. Lins et al. (1996), using four simultaneously presented CFs to normal-hearing adults, showed

that the mean behavioral ASSR threshold difference was 12 dB.

Lins and Picton (1995) also showed that it was possible to measure ASSRs using the same CF (1.0 kHz) and up to four different modulation rates presented simultaneously, with modulation rates in the low (39 and 49 Hz) and high (81 and 97 Hz) range. This would appear to be a beneficial technique for testing patients who may be in a variable state of arousal, from alert to deep (stage 4) sleep, as might occur during a typical clinical test session. When adults were tested during an awake state, the amplitudes of the responses to the low MFs (presented individually) were up to three times those of the responses for high MFs (presented individually). When two different MFs were used in each ear, the responses to each MF were decreased by about 20%. In sleeping adults, when four different MFs were presented simultaneously (39, 49, 81, and 97 Hz) the amplitudes of the low MF response components decreased with sleep stage, while the amplitudes of the high MF response components remained unchanged. While only a small group of adults was tested in each of these conditions and the 1,000-Hz CF was at a supra-threshold level, the implications for a clinical test protocol are compelling. That is, if threshold estimates are needed and the patient is in an awake state, the low MF components might be best, but at the same time, high MF components can also be tested. If the patient is drifting from wakefulness to drowsiness and sleep, the stability of the high MF components will yield adequate information.

COCHLEAR PLACE SPECIFICITY

The cochlear place specificity of the ASSR evoked by MM tones, the most commonly used stimuli for ASSR tests, was evaluated by Herdman et al. (2002b) using the classic high-pass masking derived-band technique. In this method, cochlear response areas are delimited by using masking noise in which the high-pass edge of the filter is systematically lowered (e.g., from 8 to 20 kHz, to 4 to 20 kHz, and then 2 to

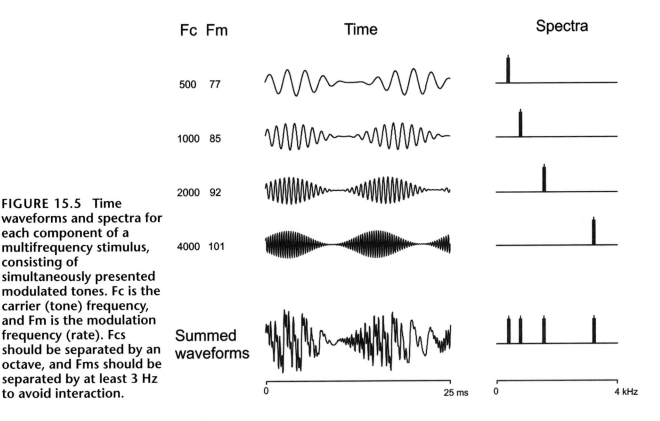

Fc Fm   Time   Spectra

500   77

1000   85

2000   92

FIGURE 15.5 Time waveforms and spectra for each component of a multifrequency stimulus, consisting of simultaneously presented modulated tones. Fc is the carrier (tone) frequency, and Fm is the modulation frequency (rate). Fcs should be separated by an octave, and Fms should be separated by at least 3 Hz to avoid interaction.

4000   101

Summed waveforms

0   25 ms   0   4 kHz

20 kHz, and so forth). An ASSR is obtained for each masker setting. Cochlear response areas are "derived" by subtracting the response obtained for adjacent masking bands (i.e., the 4 to 20 kHz ASSR from the 8 to 20 kHz condition). The derived or difference wave represents the response attributed to the 4- to 8-kHz cochlear area. Details about this technique can be found in Chapter 13. Herdman et al. (2002b) used this technique, using masker high-pass cutoffs at 0.5-octave intervals between 0.250 and 16 kHz. The derived bandwidths for cochlear place of excitation varied from 1.02 to 1.21 octaves. These results indicate slightly narrower derived bandwidths compared to those obtained when a tone burst is used to evoke the auditory brainstem response (ABR) or middle latency response (MLR). Even though the stimulus spectrum of an AM-modulated tone may have a narrower, more "frequency-specific" spectrum than does the spectrum of a tone burst, the response "place specificity" appears to be about an octave wide for modulation envelopes or tone bursts that are less than 10 ms in duration. Place specificity is better (narrowest in terms of octaves) for high-frequency CFs (>1.0 kHz) in comparison to low-frequency CFs. Picton et al. (2003) remind us that it is the cochlea that is the limiting factor for place specificity, not the stimulus. While notched-noise masking has often been recommended to improve the place specificity of tone-burst ABRs (Stapells et al., 1994), this may only be necessary in the case of steeply sloping audiometric configurations, for which spread of excitation for the tone burst or mixed-modulation tone could lead to significant discrepancies between the puretone (behavioral) and evoked potential threshold estimate. Audiogram esti-

mates derived from ASSR tests using MM stimuli appear to be accurate, even when such steep audiometric slopes exist (Herdman and Stapells, 2003), and thus, additional masking does not appear to be necessary.

Subject Factors

AGE: INFANTS

ASSR threshold decreases with age during infancy. Rickards et al. (1994) were the first to establish ASSR thresholds in newborns. ASSR threshold was estimated from the results of over 480 tests conducted at 500, 1,500, and 4,000 Hz using MFs of 72, 85, and 97 Hz, respectively. A statistical criterion of $p < 0.03$ was used to determine when a response was present, using a phase-coherence algorithm. The mean thresholds were 41, 24, and 34 dB HL (or 52.5, 30.5, and 44.5 dB SPL) for 500, 1,500, and 4,000 Hz, respectively. The Rickards et al. (1994) ASSR thresholds in newborns are elevated, when compared to ABR threshold estimates (in newborns) as determined by Sininger et al. (1997) at the same frequencies. The ASSRs in newborns show stimulus-response characteristics and derived latencies similar to those of the tone-burst evoked ABRs.

The four-CF combined MF technique was applied to testing 41 infants, ages 1 to 10 months, by Lins et al. (1996). The MFs were between 75 and 110 Hz. All infants were considered "well babies," tested during sleep, and assumed to have normal hearing. The mean ASSR thresholds found for the infants tested in a quiet room were within 10 dB of ASSR thresholds in adults and were 45 dB SPL for 500 Hz, 29 dB SPL for 1,000 Hz, 26 dB SPL for 2,000 Hz, and 29 dB SPL for 4,000 Hz. The response amplitudes and phases were also measured and compared to those of adults. On average, response amplitudes were less than 50% of those found in adults but phase measurements were similar.

Savio et al. (2001) showed that ASSR threshold decreased with age in the first year of life. In the 0- to 1-month age group, ASSR thresholds were, on average, 13 dB higher than those obtained from infants aged 7 to 12 months. John et al. (2004) measured ASSR amplitude and detectability for AM, FM, MM, and exponentially modulated tones in neonates and also in older infants (3 to 15 weeks) using stimuli at a fixed level of 50 dB HL. ASSR amplitude and detectability increased with age, suggesting that threshold might also improve with age. Reponses were largest for MM and AM tones with exponential modulations, suggesting that these stimuli would be best for testing threshold in very young infants.

Rance and Tomlin (2006) performed longitudinal ASSR threshold measures over the first 6 weeks of life in a cohort of full-term infants with normal hearing. They found an improvement in ASSR threshold of 11 dB at 0.5 kHz and 10 dB at 4.0 kHz when comparing thresholds measured in the newborn period to those measured at 6 weeks of age. These threshold differences were obtained after taking into account the level differences due to the ear canal acoustics (obtained from in situ stimulus calibration).

Unlike the ABR, there have been no large-scale parametric studies of ASSR development in infants and young children, the population most likely to undergo testing of this nature to estimate threshold. Indeed, most of the published ASSR results in infants and children concern those who have hearing loss, and it is difficult to infer normal development from results obtained in pathologic ears. ASSR tests use modulation rates much higher than tone-burst presentation rates typically used to evoke the ABR, rates at which considerable neural adaptation in both premature and full-term neonates is known to occur (Lasky, 1984). Optimization of ASSR test parameters for very young infants, particularly for threshold estimation applications, requires further research.

AGE: ADULTS

The 40-Hz ASSR does not change significantly with increasing age in adulthood (Boettcher et al., 2001; Johnson et al., 1988; Muchnik et al., 1993), although even slight to mild hearing loss among older adults may be a confounding variable. Larger amplitudes for the ASSR have been found among the elderly who have hearing levels at the "lower" end of normal (e.g., 20 to 25 dB HL), likely because of a recruitment-like phenomenon (Muchnik et al., 1993). Picton et al. (2003) report no age-related changes in the amplitude or phase of ASSRs for a 1,000-Hz puretone modulated at 3, 43, and 95 Hz in a group of normal-hearing adults aged 20 to 81 years. They do, however, report high intersubject variability in amplitude and phase measures that may have precluded finding statistically significant age-related differences.

Stimulus × Subject Interactions

MODULATION FREQUENCY × SUBJECT STATE

The MF, modulation type(s), and CF are the primary determinants of ASSR properties. There are, however, some interactive effects of subject consciousness with MF and CF on the ASSR. These were first evaluated by Cohen et al. (1991). Carrier frequencies of 250 to 4,000 Hz (octave steps) presented at 55 dB HL were used to evoke steady-state responses in awake adults at MFs of 30 to 185 Hz. MFs of 60 Hz or lower resulted in response latencies (calculated from phase delay data) in the range of 28 to 33 ms, clearly similar to the range for MLAER. For MFs at 90 Hz and above, the latencies ranged from 11.6 ms for a CF of 250 Hz to 8.9 ms for a CF of 4.0 kHz, indicating a likely homology to tone-burst evoked ABRs. In both waking and sleeping adults, for CFs at 1.0 kHz or lower, an MF of 45 Hz yielded larger ASSR S/Ns; however, this S/N advantage for a 45-Hz MF was not obvious for sleeping subjects tested with CFs at 2.0 or 4.0 kHz. At CFs of 2.0 and 4.0 kHz, MFs of 80 Hz and above yielded S/Ns that were equivalent to those at lower MFs in sleeping subjects. The Cohen et al. (1991) study established the efficacy of recording ASSR in sleeping subjects, using high (>80 Hz) MFs for CFs in the audiometric frequency range. Dobie and Wilson (1998) also determined the detectability of ASSRs in adults tested both in the awake state and during sedated sleep. MFs of 40 Hz and 90 Hz yielded peaks in the detection function for both awake and sedated sleep states for the low-frequency (640 Hz) CF presented at a moderate level, but less than 75% of the trials conducted at 38 dB SPL resulted in a detectable response, regardless of MF. Detectability was considerably reduced in the sedated sleep state compared to the awake state, particularly for MFs at 50 Hz or lower. The results obtained by Dobie and Wilson (1998) indicate that both low (40 to 50 Hz) and high (90 Hz) MFs are effective in evoking an ASSR for a CF below 1.0 kHz in awake or sleeping adults.

Adults with normal hearing were tested during natural sleep by Aoyagi et al (1994a), using CFs of 0.5, 1.0, 2.0, and 4.0 kHz presented at 50 dB HL at MFs of 20 to 120 Hz. Results were similar to those of Cohen et al. (1991), with peaks in the detectability versus MF functions found at 40 Hz and 80 Hz for CFs at 0.5 and 1.0 kHz and at 80 Hz or higher for CFs at 2.0 and 4.0 kHz. It should be noted that responses were detected at all MFs except for 20 Hz.

Lins et al. (1995) conducted a parametric study of ASSR using MFs of 67 to 111 Hz and CFs of 0.5, 1.0, and 2.0 kHz. Adult subjects were tested as they read or slept, but the effects of subject state were not evaluated as a variable. For a CF of 1.0 kHz presented at 60 dB SPL, MFs at 83 and 91 Hz yielded the largest ASSR amplitudes, significantly different from amplitudes measured at MFs of 71 and 111 Hz. Holding MF constant at 91 Hz and level constant at 60 dB SPL, they showed no significant difference in ASSR amplitude for CFs varied at 5.0, 1.0, and 2.0 kHz. Increasing the level of a 1.0-kHz (CF) tone modulated at 91 Hz from 20 to 90 dB SPL resulted in a systematic increase in amplitude and a decrease in phase that was equivalent to a 1.3-ms decrease in latency.

In summary, for CFs of ≤1.0 kHz, at near threshold levels, there may be some advantage to using MFs at approximately 40 Hz in awake or sleeping adult subjects. For higher CFs, MFs at 80 Hz or higher will be suitable. The advantage for 40-Hz MFs is not seen in sleeping infants. Empirical evidence indicates that the higher MFs are more suitable for testing infants (see following section).

STIMULUS × SUBJECT INTERACTIONS IN INFANTS AND CHILDREN

Findings of Levi et al. (1993) indicate that MFs above 40 Hz, and particularly at 80 Hz, are preferable for testing young infants with AM tones. Using AM tones at 500 and 2,000 Hz, presented at 60 dB HL (~78 dB SPL), they measured response coherence, an estimate of response power relative to overall response plus noise power, as a function of MF. The largest coherence values were obtained at 80 Hz, regardless of CF. When a 500-Hz CF was used, statistically significant responses were obtained only for MFs of 40, 50, and 80 Hz, but not at 10, 20, or 30 Hz. Using a 2,000-Hz CF, only the 80-Hz MF yielded statistically significant responses for infants. Aoyagi et al. (1994b) showed that MFs in the 80-Hz range resulted in the most stable and reliable ASSR results among normal-hearing infants and children (aged 4 months to 15 years), who were tested while sedated. Although only one CF (1,000 Hz) was used, the MF was varied from 20 to 200 Hz. Measures of phase coherence were highest for 80 Hz,

although peaks were also found at 120 and 160 Hz for infants and children less than 4 years of age; these additional peaks in the coherence functions were not clear for older children or for a group of normal-hearing adults. There was a clear advantage for the 80-Hz MF compared to the 40-Hz MF for all children, except children older than 9 years and adults.

A large-scale study of newborns completed by Rickards et al. (1994) provides compelling evidence for the efficacy of modulation rates higher that 60 Hz for obtaining responses to tones with both AM (100%) and FM (20%). CFs of 500, 1,500, and 4,000 Hz (at 55 dB HL) were used to obtain AS-SRs at MFs ranging from 35 to 185 Hz. As CF increased, so did the best MF for response detection. MFs in the 65- to 100-Hz range yielded the best detection efficiencies in sleeping newborns. In addition, latencies calculated from the response phase were in the 11- to 14-ms range, with a systematic decrease in latency with increased frequency. Both the range and the type of latency change suggest that the ASSRs recorded at high MFs in sleeping newborns are generated by the brainstem.

These studies indicate that MF should be varied with CF to get the largest amplitude responses. They further show that, for CFs <1.0 kHz, ASSRs with latency estimates in the auditory MLR range (i.e., those obtained with MFs of 30 to 50 Hz) are larger than ASSRs thought to be predominantly generated by the brainstem (i.e., at MFs >80 Hz). This may be because, at lower MFs, the modulation envelope is of longer duration, allowing greater temporal summation and thus a larger response. It is also likely due to the fact that the ASSRs from the cortex are larger than those from the brainstem. The relationship between MF and ASSR amplitude is illustrated in Figure 15.6. Although Levi et al. (1993) were able

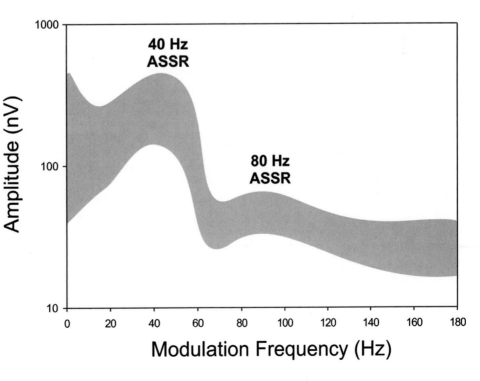

FIGURE 15.6 Auditory steady-state response (ASSR) amplitude as a function of modulation frequency (MF). Data are modeled from adults tested awake or asleep. ASSR amplitudes at 40 Hz are two to three times the amplitudes of ASSR at 80 Hz. ASSR amplitudes for MFs <20 Hz are variable in wakefulness and even more variable during sleep.

to obtain ASSRs for low-frequency MF-CF combinations in very young infants, the ASSRs for the 0.5-Hz CF at 80-Hz MFs were more consistently present and of larger amplitude than were those obtained at lower MFs. Previous research on ASSRs for 40-Hz MFs in sleeping infants and young children indicates that ASSRs are unstable at this MF (Stapells et al., 1988). This is not the case, however, for adults, in whom ASSRs for low (<1.0 kHz) CF and low (<50 Hz) MF stimuli are present during sleep and wakefulness.

Signal Processing and Acquisition Variables

FILTERING

Filtering is a crucial tool that is used in recording any type of evoked response. Filtering can be in either analog (online) or digital (offline), or a combination of both. Filtering increases the S/N by removing unwanted activity at frequencies that are not of interest and allowing focus on the frequencies at which the responses are located.

The choice of filter cutoff frequencies depends on the frequency of the intended recorded signal. If a filter's cutoff frequency is placed too close to the MF used to obtain the ASSR, then correction factors must be applied to compensate for the attenuation of the signal due to the filter. Common high-pass filter settings used in ASSR studies are 1 Hz up to 30 Hz, with low-pass filters of 300 Hz. Because the major energy of the ASSR is at the MF and the fast Fourier transformation (FFT) acts as a narrowband filter centered on the MF, the filter cutoff points are largely unimportant, unless there is a danger of saturating the bioamplifier.

ELECTRODE MONTAGE

ASSRs are readily recordable using electrode configurations similar to those used for the ABR. A number of factors contribute to the optimal placement of electrodes. Some of these include location of the ASSR generator and noise sources.

The magnitude of a scalp-recorded evoked response varies depending on the orientation of the equivalent dipole of the underlying generator. The 80-Hz ASSRs have a major component in the brainstem, most likely the ascending lateral lemniscus. The ascending "ribbon" of the lateral lemniscus acts as a vertically oriented dipole, and therefore, an electrode montage using centrally placed noninverting electrodes, such as at Cz, Fpz, or Fz, with inverting electrodes placed at mastoid, inion, or nape of neck (C7) will record large responses. The 40-Hz ASSR has neural generators that are both at the brainstem, as for the 80-Hz ASSR, and the primary auditory cortex levels. In addition to the vertical dipole (brainstem component), a radial dipole source in the primary auditory cortex (such as C3 or C4) will result in a response being recorded from laterally placed noninverting electrodes. The majority of published results in adults (from the Canadian group, led by Picton) have been obtained using a noninverting electrode at Cz, an inverting electrode at the

nape of the neck (1 to 2 cm above the hair line), and a common electrode on the clavicle. A recent study by Van der Reijden et al. (2005) evaluated the effect of electrode placement on ASSRs obtained from young infants. They recorded ASSRs from an array of 57 scalp electrodes and determined the montages that yielded the best ASSR-to-noise ratios. They showed that a Cz-Mi (vertex-ipsilateral mastoid) montage resulted in the largest ASSR-to-noise ratios. The practical result is that using the Cz-Mi montage will result in time savings during an ASSR evaluation because criterion S/Ns are reached more quickly.

Noise Sources

Every electrode placed on the scalp will have noise sources, either electrical or physiologic. Electrical noise can most often be reduced by ensuring that the contact between electrode and skin has low impedance (under 5 kΩ). Physiologic noise results from placing an electrode over a muscle. Tonic muscle activity is particularly problematic because it contains energy at frequencies (20 to 50 Hz) that are close to those of the ASSR. For example, a large amount of tonic neck muscle activity is present in an otherwise quiet subject sitting upright. If an electrode is placed at the nape of neck (C7), the recording will be contaminated with this muscle noise. In such cases, placing head supports behind the subject's neck often relieves the strain on neck muscles, ensuring less muscle activity and increased comfort for the subject.

AVERAGING

Just like every other evoked response, the ASSR becomes more easily detected through the process of averaging (see Chapter 11). By definition, an ASSR has a stable amplitude and phase. The ASSR detection algorithms (see later section) are based primarily on the S/N; that is, the ASSR signal must be significantly larger than the noise in order for the ASSR to be detected. ASSRs near threshold have very low amplitudes, and thus, we must average for a substantial time period for the averaged noise to be small enough so that the ASSR can be detected.

Another assumption of averaging and of the ASSR detection algorithms is that the background noise is stationary; however, biologic noise (e.g., coughing, sneezing, blinking, yawning, swallowing) is anything but. Invariably, when recording at near-threshold levels, the subject transiently generates muscle noise (e.g., swallowing or gross limb movements), creating a large "noise burst" that significantly alters the S/N, thus resulting in the detection algorithm indicating no response. A couple of options exist for such cases. One is to simply record for a longer period of time until the transient noise has been "averaged out." Another option is to use artifact rejection. Simply, if the voltage of an electroencephalogram (EEG) sample exceeds a predetermined value (i.e., 80 mV), then that sample is discarded. The disadvantage of artifact rejection is that the response is discarded along with the noise, so that longer test times are needed to obtain a result.

Another method to reduce the effect of the transient noise in recordings is to apply weighted averaging (Elberling and Wahlgreen, 1985; John et al., 2001a). The general concept in weighted averaging is that noisy sections of the recording (i.e., noisy EEG samples) contribute proportionally less to the overall average. Using online calculations, the "weight" of each sample can be determined by considering its variance. Noise will increase the variance of a sample. A weighted-averaging algorithm will assign the higher variance samples lesser weights and the low variance samples higher weights. Samples with large (noise) variance will contribute proportionally less to the overall average.

DETECTION METHODS

One of the major reasons that ASSRs are gaining widespread use is the fact "real-time" statistical methods may be used for response detection. It is only when an evoked response is detected using statistical methods that the technique is truly "objective."

Time and Frequency Domain Methods

Most modern techniques of ASSR detection involve transformation of the response from the time domain to the frequency domain. These transformations are usually accomplished using the Fourier transform. In the frequency domain, the ASSR can be represented as an addition of sinusoids each with its own frequency, amplitude, and phase.

The Fourier transform can be implemented in either analog or digital form. In analog form, the EEG sample is fed into a Fourier analyzer and is multiplied by the sine and cosine of the MF. After multiplication, the ASSR at the MF is observed as a sustained or direct current (DC) output, while noise yields an oscillatory or alternating current (AC) output. The Fourier analyzer output is further low-pass filtered and yields values x (from the cosine multiplication) and y (from the sine multiplication). The ASSR amplitude, a, is calculated using the following formula (Regan, 1989; Stapells et al., 1984):

$$a = (x^2 + y^2)^{0.5}$$

Response phase, θ, is calculated using the following formula:

$$\theta = \tan^{-1}(y/x)$$

The output of the Fourier transformation for a particular (modulation) frequency of interest is two dimensional, with real and imaginary components in rectangular coordinates, or as a magnitude and phase in polar coordinates (i.e., a Fourier coefficient is a complex number). These two dimensions may be graphed on a polar plot with response amplitude shown by the length of the vector and response phase (latency) as the angle of the vector in either radians (from 0 to 2π) or in degrees (from 0 to 360).

There are two general strategies for objective statistical analyses of the ASSR. One strategy involves repeated measures of ASSR phase and amplitude as obtained from the Fourier transformation. The other strategy evaluates the variability of the ASSR and adjacent noise amplitudes in the spectrum of the response.

Phase Coherence Measures

Phase coherence (PC) is related to the signal (response)-to-noise (background EEG and myogenic) ratio (S.N). The basic concept is that the phase delay of the response is measured relative to the MF. Each averaged response can be subjected to a fast Fourier transformation (FFT). For PC, the phase of the major peak at the MF frequency can be plotted in polar coordinates. The sine and cosine of the angles formed by each phase vector (for each sample) are calculated.[1] The general idea for detecting ASSRs using PC is that measurements of phase (from the Fourier transformation) are taken for a number of EEG samples. If an ASSR is indeed present, then its phase will be consistent, phase locked to the MF, across the samples. If sample phases are random, then the ASSR cannot be distinguished from background noise.

PC values vary from 0.0 to 1.0. When the sample phases are in phase with one another, there is high coherence, and the values will be closer to 1.0. When the sample phases are random, there is low coherence (values close to 0), as would be found if the samples contained only noise, with no ASSR. The statistical significance of the resulting PC value can be determined. That is, the probability that the samples come from a distribution of phase values that are randomly distributed can be tested using a variety of statistics. Usually when a significance level of $p < 0.05$ is obtained, the null hypothesis (samples of phases and sample of noise are equal) is rejected, and the samples can be considered phase locked or phase coherent, and an evoked response is deemed to be present. The amplitude or length of the phase vectors is not used in this statistical test. Very small amplitude responses that demonstrate high PC will be detected as easily as large amplitude responses with the same degree of PC.

Dobie and Wilson (Dobie and Wilson 1989a; 1989b; 1995; Dobie, 1993) have employed magnitude-squared coherence[2] (MSC) methods for detecting and defining the ASSRs. This method uses both the amplitude and phase information from the FFT. MSC (γ^2) estimates the power of the averaged response divided by the average power of the individual responses. The γ^2 will vary from 0 (no response)

---

[1] Phase coherence is:

$$PC = [(1/n\Sigma\cos\phi_I)^2 + (1/n\Sigma\sin\phi_I)^2]^{1/2},$$

where n is number of successive samples and ϕ is the phase of the Ith frequency component in the Fourier series.

[2] Magnitude squared coherence, γ^2, is:

$$MSC = \{[(1/n\Sigma A_I\phi_I)^2 + (1/n\Sigma\sin A_I\phi_I)^2]^{1/2}\}/[1/n\Sigma A_I^2],$$

where n is the number of subaverages, ϕ is phase, and A is amplitude of the Ith frequency component in a Fourier Series.

to 1 (high S/N). Since the response consists of both signal (response) and noise, the MSC can be viewed as a signal plus noise-to-noise estimate. Theoretical distributions of MSC have been determined, so it is possible to determine critical values to be used in the objective detection of an ASSR. When a critical value of MSC is exceeded by the EEG samples obtained in response to an AM tone, the null hypothesis (sample contains only noise) can be rejected, and an ASSR has been detected. Another method for determining the significance of the ASSR phase and amplitude distribution employs the Hotellings T^2 test, which is similar to a t-test, except that it calculates significance in two dimensions (amplitude and phase). Victor and Mast (1991) introduced the T^2_{circ}, which assumed equal variances in both real and imaginary dimensions. This results in confidence limits with a circular shape. Mathematically, the T^2_{circ} and γ^2 are equivalent (Dobie, 1993).

If amplitude information is ignored, that is, if all amplitude vectors are set to a value of 1, then MSC = PC^2, or PC = $(MSC)^{1/2}$. The advantage of MSC is that amplitude increases in the evoked potential will serve to increase the MSC value obtained and enhance detection as compared to methods that measure phase alone. The disadvantage of MSC is that fluctuations in background noise will have a greater effect on the MSC value compared to PC or PC^2 (PCS).

Dobie and Wilson (1995) compared MSC at two alpha levels, 0.01 and 0.10, to human visual detection of the time-domain waveform for a 40-Hz auditory evoked potential. The sensitivity and specificity of each method was determined, and a d' was calculated. Values for d' were higher for MSC at both alpha levels compared to human observers. Although thresholds were not estimated, it is clear from their data that the alpha level for MSC would have an effect on estimated threshold. In general, as the statistical criterion is relaxed, the estimated threshold decreases, but at the expense of decreased specificity (more false positives, or responses detected when there is no stimulus).

Spectral Measurements
The basis for spectral measurements of ASSR detection comes from performing an FFT on a grand averaged recording. The result is a frequency spectrum of the entire EEG. The peaks in the resulting spectrum and the amplitude and phase of the spectral peak can be measured. A steady-state response evokes activity at the MF, and therefore, the stronger the signal, the more power there is at the MF. In this measurement, the noise is defined as activity that is not at the MF. The significance of the signal is determined by comparing the power (voltage squared) of the signal to the power of the noise (a few Hz above and below the MF). An F-test can then be calculated, where the numerator is the power of the signal and the denominator is the power of the noise.

Picton et al. (2003, p 183) have described the method of spectral analysis for ASSR detection:

"The level of the background noise in a recording can be estimated by measuring the activity at frequencies in the spectrum other than that of the stimulus and response. Comparing the power of the signal to the powers at other frequencies is the basis of the F-test for hidden periodicity (Dobie and Wilson, 1996; Lins et al, 1996). The procedure calculates an F ratio of the power in the signal frequency bin (s) to the mean power in N adjacent bins:

$$F = N(x_s^2 + y_s^2)/ \sum_{\substack{j = s - N/2 \\ j \neq s}}^{s+N/2} (x_j^2 + y_j^2)$$

This is distributed as F with degrees of freedom 2 and $2N$. The F-test is essentially the same as the magnitude squared coherence when the number of individual measurements for calculating the coherence equals one less than the number of adjacent points used in the F-test, i.e., the degrees of freedom are the same (Dobie and Wilson, 1996).

The F-test has several advantages over tests based on repeated measurements of the response. First, the number of adjacent frequency-bins to which the signal response is compared can be increased beyond any easily obtained number of separate measurements of the signal response. Second, the technique can easily be adapted to omit certain frequency bins from the calculation. In this way a noise estimate can be obtained that is uncontaminated by line noise or by responses at other frequencies (if one is recording responses to multiple simultaneous stimuli)."

Figure 15.7 shows the results for PC, circular t-tests, and F-tests for trials in which responses are present compared to those in which only noise is present.

▨ CALIBRATION

Calibration of modulated tones is straightforward. The common practice is to measure the SPL of the modulated tone in the same way as for a puretone. Commercially available test instruments allow the user to select levels using dB SPL or dB HL levels. In the latter case, the 0 dB HL at each frequency would have the same SPL as a puretone at 0 dB HL (e.g., using published audiometer standards such as American National Standards Institute [ANSI] S3.6-2004 American National Standard Specification for Audiometers, or equivalent international standards [ISO-389-2, 1994; ISO-389-1, 1998]. For example, using ANSI 3.6-2004, the SPL of 2.0 kHz at 0 dB HL is 2.5 dB when presented through insert phones (calibrated in an H1A coupler).

This method of calibration is different from that used for ABR tests with clicks or tone bursts. There is no calibration standard for these transients, and recommended procedures involve the determination of a psychophysical threshold for

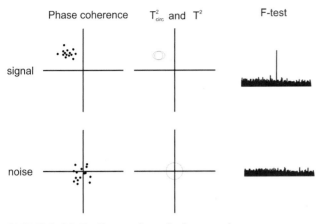

FIGURE 15.7 Examples of phase coherence, circular T^2 (T^2_{circ}) test, and F-test for a statistically significant response (''signal'') versus no response (''noise''). Each dot in the phase coherence quadrant represents the end point of a phase vector, which emanates from the 0,0 point of the vertical and horizontal axes. Similarly, the position and size of the circle drawn on the T^2 quadrant represents the presence of a statistically significant response. A result containing only noise (no response) is indicated by a circle that is at or close to the crossing of the x- and y- axes. For the F-test, the amplitude of the response spectrum peak at the modulation frequency (MF) will be significantly larger than the amplitude at adjacent frequencies.

each click and tone burst, with the average threshold being denoted as 0 dB normal HL (nHL). Determining the SPL of a transient then involves determining the peak SPL (pSPL) or peak equivalent SPL (peSPL) by measuring the SPL of a puretone that has the same amplitude as the transient (see Chapter 11).

It must be recognized that the power of a modulated tone is less than that for an unmodulated tone of the same peak amplitude. The long-term average power of a sinusoidally amplitude modulated (SAM) waveform is $(1 + m^2/2) I_0$, where I_0 is the average power when m, the modulation index, $= 0$ (Viemeister, 1979). The relative increment in power, $\Delta I/I_0$, for a modulated tone is $m^2/2$. Viemeister's classic study of temporal modulation transfer functions (1979) addressed the issue of modulation detection thresholds by measuring modulation thresholds for power-compensated wideband noise $[(1 + m\sin\omega_m t/(1 + m^2/2)^{1/2}]$ compared to those obtained with no compensation $[(1 + m\sin\omega_m t)]$. At MFs below 560 Hz, there was no effect of power compensation on modulation thresholds. Although the threshold of modulation detection is different from the threshold for a stimulus with modulation, it is worth keeping in mind that the power of modulated versus unmodulated signals is different and that there will be a discrepancy of approximately 2 to 3 dB when

psychophysical thresholds for 100% AM tones are compared to those for unmodulated tones. These differences are not compensated for when using dB HL calibration. Also, the ASSR threshold is likely dependent upon the rate of pressure change of the modulation envelope, rather than the overall pressure or power of the stimulus, but direct experimental evidence of this mechanism is scant.

■ CLINICAL APPLICATIONS OF AUDITORY STEADY-STATE RESPONSES

The primary application of ASSR in audiology is for hearing threshold estimation in those at risk for hearing loss (i.e., the prediction of the audiogram). To this end, a number of studies have compared ASSR thresholds and behavioral thresholds in infants, children, and adults with hearing loss and published regression formulae that relate ASSR threshold to puretone threshold. Alternatively, the differences between ASSR and puretone thresholds have been calculated, and these "correction" factors have been used to interpret the ASSR thresholds. In addition, ASSR thresholds to bone-conducted stimuli can be used to determine the presence and extent of a conductive impairment. The determination of a sensory versus neural hearing loss, another element of site-of-lesion evaluation, is possible under some circumstances. ASSRs have also been employed in hearing aid and cochlear implant evaluations. Recent experiments with ASSR tests employing complex and dynamic supra-threshold stimuli hold some promise for estimating psychophysical and speech perception abilities. These applications are reviewed in the following sections.

Audiogram Prediction/Hearing Threshold Estimation

A driving concept in ASSR research is the objective determination of the puretone audiogram. The goal of objectivity should be met in three ways. First, the threshold determination is based upon a physiologic response, not on a subjective perception of the subject. Second, the presence of a response is determined by the use of statistical tests, or "objective" detection algorithms. Third, the interpretation of the results is also bound by objective methods and decision-making rules.

Aoyagi et al. (1999) published an impressive set of audiograms showing examples of how they use CFs modulated at 80 Hz to predict threshold. Examples of audiogram prediction for those with both low (Fig. 15.8A) and high frequency (Fig. 15.8B) sloping losses are demonstrated. For a group of subjects with hearing losses ranging from mild to profound, correlations between the puretone audiogram and the ASSR threshold were 0.73 for 500 Hz, 0.86 for 1,000 Hz, 0.88 for 2,000 Hz, and 0.92 for 4,000 Hz.

A comprehensive study of hearing threshold prediction using ■ ASSR in a sample that included hearing-impaired

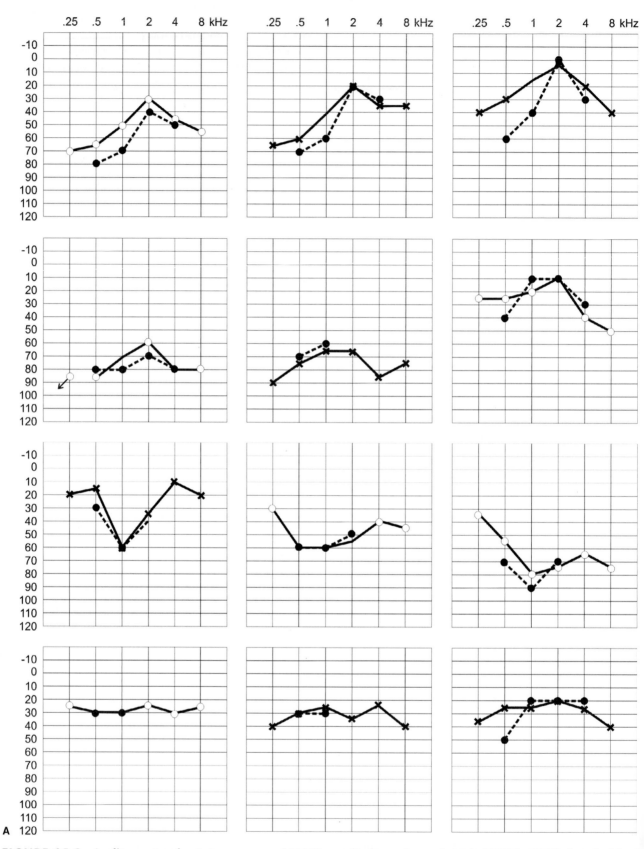

FIGURE 15.8 Auditory steady-state response (ASSR) results from Aoyagi et al. (1999). ASSR thresholds provide excellent estimates of puretone thresholds for both **(A)** low- and **(B)** high-frequency sloping audiometric configurations.

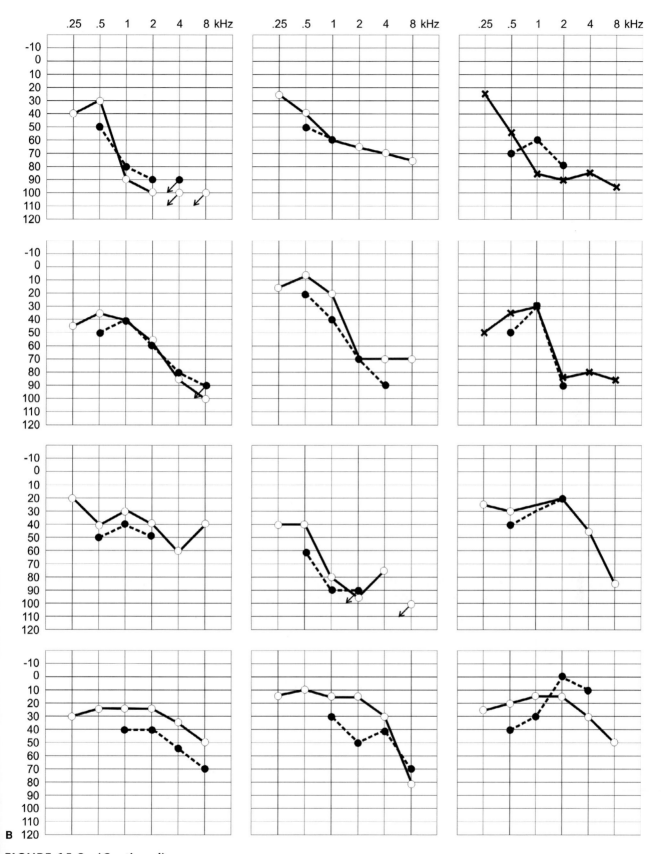

FIGURE 15.8 (*Continued*)

children and adults was reported by Rance et al. (1995). Participants had hearing losses that were moderate or worse, including some with profound hearing loss. These hearing losses were purely sensory-neural; patients with conductive loss were specifically excluded from the study. ASSR threshold estimates were made using CFs at 250, 500, 1,000, 2,000, and 4,000 Hz, all presented at an MF of 90 Hz. Pearson product-moment correlations between puretone and ASSR thresholds were at 0.96 for 250 Hz and as high as 0.99 for 2,000 and 4,000 Hz. Regression formulae were developed to predict behavioral thresholds from ASSR thresholds. Table 15.2 shows these formulae for each CF. The Y intercepts demonstrate that subjects with normal hearing (e.g., 10 dB HL) have ASSR thresholds elevated by as much as 40 dB with respect to puretone threshold in the low frequencies, whereas in mid and high frequencies, ASSR thresholds are closer to puretone thresholds. This is similar to reports of ABR thresholds to tone-burst stimuli in normal-hearing subjects (Stapells, 2000). As hearing loss increases and as CF increases, there is less discrepancy between behavioral and ASSR threshold, shown by an analysis of the standard deviations of the regressions by degree of hearing loss and by CF (Rance et al., 1995). Errors in prediction of behavioral thresholds from ASSR thresholds show standard deviations ranging from 3.6 dB for severe to profound losses at 2 kHz to 11.9 dB for mild to moderate losses at 250 Hz. These findings are very similar both qualitatively and quantitatively to the findings of Stapells et al. (1995), who developed regression formulae relating tone-burst ABR threshold to puretone threshold in infants and young children.

In a related study, the Melbourne group (Rance et al., 1998) demonstrated the advantages of using ASSRs to determine residual hearing thresholds for those infants and children from whom ABRs could not be evoked (at 100 dB nHL) using click stimuli. Again, ASSRs were obtained using CFs of 250 to 4,000 Hz with an MF of 90 Hz. In a sample of 109 children, whose hearing losses ranged from moderate to profound, the average discrepancy between ASSR and behavioral thresholds was only 3 to 6 dB (although the standard deviations were 6 to 8 dB), with larger discrepancies and standard deviations found at 250 and 500 Hz, as in the previous study. ASSR thresholds were within 20 dB of puretone threshold for 99% of the comparisons and ≤10 dB for 82% of the comparisons. The findings demonstrated the efficacy of ASSRs for estimating the audiogram in infants and children who can benefit from amplification of their residual hearing.

More recently, Rance et al. (2005) published a large series of ASSR and behavioral thresholds in infants. Clinical findings from seven audiology centers within the state of Victoria, Australia, were pooled. All centers used the GSI-Audera (GSI-Nicolet) or its predecessor, the ERA System (ERA Systems), in the collection of ASSR thresholds. Only those infants who had ASSR thresholds measured at ≤3 months of age, who subsequently yielded reliable conditioned behavioral audiometric thresholds, and who had evidence of normal middle ear function at the time of ASSR and behavioral tests were included. This sample was comprised of 575 infants (1,091 ears), whose ASSR thresholds were obtained at a mean age of 2.6 months and whose behavioral thresholds were obtained at a mean age of 9.8 months. There were 285 (of 575) infants who demonstrated normal hearing (thresholds ≤15 dB HL). The mean ASSR thresholds in this group were 32.3, 32.5, 23.3, and 28.1 dB HL for CFs at 0.5, 1.0, 2.0, and 4.0 kHz, respectively, with standard deviations ranging from 6.3 dB (2.0 kHz) to 7.5 dB (0.5 and 4.0 kHz).

TABLE 15.2   Regression formulae relating auditory steady-state response (ASSR) threshold to behavioral threshold, *Where* x = ASSR threshold

Carrier frequency	500 Hz	1,000 Hz	2,000 Hz	4,000 Hz
Cone-Wesson et al., 2002a	1.39x − 35	1.24x − 15	0.94x + 5	1.34x − 24
Dimitrijevic et al., 2002	0.88x − 9	0.92x − 1	0.89x − 0	0.99x − 8
Herdman and Stapells, 2003	0.77x − 6	0.91x − 4	0.92x − 6	1.04x − 5
Rance et al., 1995	1.30x − 40	1.18x − 26	1.05x − 19	1.19x − 24
Rance and Rickards, 2002	1.39x − 49	1.35x − 44	1.28x − 36	1.31x − 39
Rance et al., 2005	1.37x − 45	1.33x − 40	1.23x − 28	1.32x − 37
Van der Werff and Brown, 2005	1.12x − 23	1.03x − 13	1.11x − 14	1.11x − 13

(1) Cone-Wesson et al. (2002a) data based upon a sample of 51 infants, mean age 16 months, 16 with near normal or mild loss, 18 with moderate loss, and 17 with severe to profound loss; 31 had sensory-neural hearing loss (SNHL), 10 had conductive loss, and the remainder had normal hearing or mixed type loss. (2) Dimitrijevic et al. (2002) data based upon a sample of 45 adults, 31 with hearing loss and 14 with normal hearing. In the hearing loss group, there were 17 ears with mild, 19 ears with moderate, and 16 ears with severe loss. (3) Herdman and Stapells (2003) data based on a sample of 27 adults with SNHL ranging from mild to severe. (4) Rance et al. (1995) data based on a sample of 25 children with moderate to profound SNHL and 35 adults with hearing ranging from normal to profound SNHL. (5) Rance and Rickards (2002) data based upon a sample of 211 infants with a mean age of 3.2 months at the time of ASSR and a mean age of 7.9 months at the time of behavioral hearing tests. Infants with evidence of conductive or progressive losses were excluded. (6) Rance et al. (2005) data based upon 575 infants tested at a mean age of 2.6 months, with behavioral tests completed at a mean age of 9.8 months; 285 infants had normal hearing thresholds (by behavioral tests), and 271 had SNHL. (7) Van der Werff and Brown (2005) data based upon 30 subjects, 10 with normal hearing, 10 with sloping hearing losses, and 10 with flat hearing losses.

For the infants with sensory-neural hearing loss (n = 271), regression formulae were developed to relate the ASSR and behavioral thresholds. These are shown in Table 15.2 and are similar to those published by Rance et al. (1995) and Rance and Rickards (2002). In general, the slope of the regression function indicates that, as hearing loss increases in severity and CF increases in frequency, there is a closer correspondence of ASSR and behavioral threshold.

Several studies have demonstrated that ASSR thresholds have a strong relationship with puretone thresholds in adults with well-defined hearing losses. Dimitrijevic et al. (2002) tested 59 ears of 31 adults with primarily sensory-neural hearing impairments ranging in severity from mild to severe with nearly equal representation among mild, moderate, and severe degrees of loss. The ASSR thresholds showed a high correlation with the puretone thresholds, with r = 0.92 for carriers in the range of 500 to 4,000 Hz. The differences between ASSR and puretone threshold ranged from 13 ± 11 dB at 0.5 kHz and from 5 to 8 dB ± 8 to 11 dB for carriers at 1.0 to 4.0 kHz. Herdman and Stapells (2003) tested 31 male adults with sensory-neural hearing losses, some with very steep configurations, and demonstrated that the ASSR versus puretone threshold differences were, on average, 14, 8, 10, and 3 dB for CFs at 0.5, 1.0, 2.0, and 4.0 kHz, respectively. Van der Werff and Brown (2005) and Picton et al. (2005) obtained ASSRs from adults with normal hearing and those with sensory-neural hearing loss. Both studies showed that the difference between ASSR and puretone threshold was smaller in those with sensory-neural hearing loss than in the normal-hearing subjects. This is in agreement with Rance et al. (1995). Furthermore, the amplitude-growth functions were steeper in those with sensory-neural hearing loss, indicating a physiologic recruitment-like phenomenon (Picton et al., 2005). Van der Werff and Brown (2005) showed ASSR-puretone differences in the range of 8 to 18 dB HL at 0.5

and 1.0 kHz, but only 6 to 8 dB HL at 2.0 and 4.0 kHz, among adults with sensory-neural hearing losses. On the other hand, Picton et al. (2005) obtained ASSR-puretone differences of less than 5 dB HL in their group of elderly adults with sensory-neural hearing loss. One reason for these differences may be that Van der Werff and Brown (2005) averaged ASSRs for about 4 minutes, whereas Picton et al. (2005) averaged for more than 9 minutes, thus allowing resolution of responses with smaller S/Ns.

Regardless of stimulus procedure, whether it be single frequency (Rance et al., 1995) or multiple frequencies (Dimitrijevic et al., 2002; Herdman and Stapells, 2003; Picton et al., 2005; Van der Werff and Brown, 2005), or averaging time (as short as 90 seconds in Rance et al. [1995] or as long as 9 minutes in Picton et al. [2005]), it is clear that the ASSR provides a clinically useful estimate of puretone thresholds, even in sloping audiometric configurations. The largest discrepancies between ASSR and puretone threshold are obtained in those with normal cochlear function (i.e., normal or conductive hearing loss), which are on the order of 25 to 40 dB for low-frequency carriers and 10 to 20 dB for mid- and high-frequency carriers. The size of the ASSR-puretone difference is not really the issue, as this can be accounted for with a correction factor; it is the variability that is troublesome. For example, even if the ASSR-puretone difference was 45 dB at every frequency, if there was little variability (± 5 dB), then puretone threshold would be easy to estimate. What is observed, however, is that both the ASSR-puretone difference and the variability are dependent upon CF and degree of hearing loss. As the CF and degree of hearing loss increase, the ASSR-puretone difference and the variability decrease. That is, predictive error decreases with increases in severity of hearing loss and CF. Both subtractive and regression formulae methods of estimating puretone thresholds from ASSR thresholds can take this into account. Table 15.3, after

TABLE 15.3 Auditory steady-state response (ASSR) threshold–behavioral hearing threshold difference in adults, children, and infants with hearing loss

Study	No. of subjects	Stimulus	500 Hz	1,000 Hz	2,000 Hz	4,000 Hz
Van der Werff and Brown, 2005 (flat loss)	10	MM	11±5	8±4	7±5	6±5
Van der Werff and Brown, 2005 (sloping loss)	10	MM	18±8	10±7	8±6	5±4
Picton et al., 2005	10	MM	11±18	−4±9	2.5±11	5.3±12
Luts and Wouters, 2005 ("Master")	10	MM	17±12	12±8	17±8	19±12
Luts and Wouters, 2005 ("Audera")	10	MM	20±8	14±7	13±7	14±13
Herdman and Stapells, 2003	29	AM	14±13	8±9	10±10	3±10
Dimitrijevic et al., 2002	31	MM	13±11	5±8	5±9	8±11
Rance and Briggs, 2002	184	MM	6±9	6±7	4±8	3±11
Van Maanen and Stapells, 2005	23	MM	17±11	15±7	19±9	4±10

The number of subjects and stimulus type are given for each study. AM is a sinusoidally modulated puretone, and MM is an amplitude and frequency modulated tone. Rance and Briggs (2002) is the only study in which ASSR-puretone differences were published for infants and children. All other studies report differences in adults. All studies used multiple carrier frequencies presented simultaneously, except Rance and Briggs (2002) and Luts and Wouters (2005) "Audera," in which single-frequency, sequential testing was used.

Picton et al. (2003) and updated with studies published since 2003, summarizes 80-Hz ASSR threshold data from multiple clinical laboratories.

Comparison of Auditory Steady-State Response with Auditory Brainstem Response

Because a primary application of ASSR is in the estimation of threshold, it is appropriate to compare the results obtained from ASSR tests to those obtained from ABR tests using tone bursts. There are, however, a number of differences in methodology that could lead to fairly substantial differences, including stimulus spectrum, modulation envelope/tone-burst shape, rate, and response detection methods.

Aoyagi et al. (1999) directly compared tone-burst evoked ABR threshold estimates to ASSR threshold estimates, primarily in hearing impaired children tested during sedated sleep. They used a 1,000-Hz tone modulated at 80 Hz to evoke the ASSR and a 1,000-Hz tone burst (2-ms rise/fall time, 1-ms plateau) with a 53-ms interstimulus interval to evoke an ABR. Puretone thresholds ranged from 10 to 110 dB HL in the group of children tested with ABR and ASSR. The correlation of puretone threshold (in dB HL) with ABR threshold (in dB nHL) was 0.83, whereas for ASSR, the correlation with behavioral threshold was 0.86. The difference in correlation coefficients was not statistically significant. The mean difference between behavioral and ASSR thresholds was 3.8 dB (12.9 dB standard deviation), and for ABR, the difference was 6.8 dB (14.1 dB standard deviation). It is not known whether the dB nHL reference was the same for the AM tone and the tone burst.

Cone-Wesson et al. (2002a) performed a direct comparison of tone-burst evoked ABR and ASSR threshold measures in a group of 10 normal-hearing adult subjects. ABRs were evoked using 0.5- and 4.0-kHz tone bursts, with (Blackman window) onset and offset ramps of two cycles and a one-cycle plateau, presented with an interstimulus interval of 40 ms. ASSRs were evoked using carrier frequencies of 0.5 and 4.0 kHz, tested at 41 Hz, and also at 74 Hz for the 0.5-kHz CF and at 95 Hz for the 4.0-kHz CF. Sampling for each ABR trial proceeded until an Fsp criterion of 3.1 ($p < 0.01$) was met, or 6,000 artifact-free samples were obtained. Visual detection by an expert observer was used as an additional measure of ABR presence. Sixty-four 1.486-s duration samples were obtained for each ASSR trial and subjected to PC analysis using a filter centered at the MF. A response was considered present if the PC statistic reached a criterion of $p < 0.01$. Thresholds for the 46-Hz ASSR and tone burst–ABR thresholds were not statistically different. Thresholds for the 74-Hz MF–0.5-kHz CF were elevated with respect to the ABR threshold for a 0.5-kHz tone burst (and 46-Hz ASSR), but thresholds for the 95-Hz MF–4.0-kHz tone burst were 15 dB better than those for the 4.0-kHz tone burst ABR.

This study is the only one that attempted to compare threshold estimates using both ABR and ASSR methods and

that also used similar statistical criteria for judging a response to be present. There is no difference in evoked potential threshold (expressed as dB sensation level [SL]) when adults are tested with tone bursts (for ABR) or CFs modulated at 41 Hz (for ASSRs) and when both ABR and ASSR are detected using an appropriate statistical technique. These results are in agreement with Cohen et al. (1991) and Dobie and Wilson (1998), who show that a low MF (in this case, 41 Hz) is generally advantageous in testing **adults** at low CFs (1,000 Hz or lower), whereas the higher MFs (above 60 Hz) are generally better for high CF tones. In normal-hearing adults, furthermore, ABRs and ASSRs can generally be detected within 20 dB of behavioral threshold.

Van der Werff et al. (2002) obtained click and tone-burst ABR and ASSR thresholds from 32 infants and young children, all tested during sedated sleep. All of the participants in the study were being evaluated as candidates for cochlear implants, and so they were known to have significant hearing losses. They found a 0.97 correlation between click-ABR thresholds and those found for ASSRs at 2.0 and 4.0 kHz. The correlation between the 500-Hz tone burst–ABR and the 500-Hz ASSR thresholds was statistically significant but lower (0.86) than the correlations between click-ABR and high-frequency (2.0 and 4.0 kHz) ASSR. In 33% of cases, when the tone burst–ABR was absent for stimuli presented at the highest stimulus level available, an ASSR was present, albeit at elevated levels consistent with a moderately severe or greater hearing loss. Also, 58% of ears with absent click-evoked ABRs had an ASSR response. This result replicates the findings of Rance et al. (1998) and of others (Firszt et al., 2004; Luts et al., 2004; Steuve and O' Rourke, 2003; Swaenpoel and Hugo, 2004), that is, that ASSR thresholds may reveal some residual hearing when click or tone-burst ABRs are absent. This property has helped to establish ASSR as a valuable test for infants and young children undergoing evaluation for cochlear implantation.

Johnson and Brown (2005) measured ASSRs and tone-burst evoked ABRs at 1.0, 1.5, and 2.0 kHz in adults with normal hearing and those with flat or sloping sensory-neural hearing losses. ASSR thresholds were determined as the lowest level at which a statistically significant response was obtained, while ABR thresholds were determined by visual inspection of the time-domain waveforms. Overall, ABR thresholds were "closer" to behavioral thresholds than ASSRs, except in the case of steeply sloping sensory-neural hearing losses, for which ASSRs were better estimates of threshold. Both ASSR and ABR provided accurate estimates of threshold among those with sensory-neural hearing loss.

In summary, the experience of those who use the ASSR technique for predicting audiometric threshold in hearing-impaired infants and children appears to be comparable to that of those who use tone-burst evoked ABRs. Comparisons between the two techniques can be made to help formulate the most efficient and sensitive methods for this purpose. Each technique has particular strengths and limitations. An advantageous feature of the ASSR technique is that objective detection algorithms rather than visual detection methods are always used to determine presence or absence of a response. This is a particular advantage for techniques claiming to be "objective" measures.

It is difficult to determine whether or not the ASSR is detected at lower SPLs than a tone-burst evoked ABR response at the same center frequency, due to differences in stimulus calibration and response detection method. In normal-hearing subjects, visual detection of the tone-burst evoked ABRs yielded lower thresholds, although when both tone-burst ABR and ASSR were detected with automatic detection algorithms, the thresholds were equal (Cone-Wesson et al., 2002a).

40-Hz Auditory Steady-State Response Threshold Tests

The bulk of the literature concerning audiometric applications of the ASSR uses MFs of 80 Hz or higher. When it was shown that ASSR responses to 40 Hz were unstable or absent in sleeping infants and children, much of the interest in its audiometric applications diminished. Thus, there are limited data on the use of the 40-Hz ASSR for puretone threshold estimation (in adults) using the same methods for signal processing and response detection as have been used for the 80-Hz ASSR. Aoyagi et al. (1993) showed that 40-Hz ASSR was present at 11 to 18 dB above puretone threshold in normal-hearing adults and at 8 to 13 dB for adults with hearing loss. There is reason to believe that the 40-Hz ASSR threshold estimates would be as good, if not better, than those for the 80-Hz ASSR, but this has not been carefully determined. The 40-Hz ASSR has a larger amplitude

than does the 80-Hz ASSR; however, background EEG and other biologic noise is larger in that frequency region as well, so achieving a criterion S/N may require as much averaging as for a smaller amplitude response. Table 15.4 summarizes 40-Hz ASSR threshold as a function of frequency in adults.

A study by Van Maanen and Stapells (2005) performed the first comparison of 40-Hz ASSRs, 80-Hz ASSRs, and the slow cortical potential (N1/P2) in adults with normal and sensory-neural hearing loss. Their results demonstrated that multiple 40-Hz ASSRs showed the smallest difference between physiologic and behavioral thresholds compared to the other two measures. Moreover, the recording time for the 40-Hz ASSRs and the slow cortical potential were less than the recording time for the 80-Hz ASSRs. The authors concluded that the method of choice for adults was 40-Hz ASSR.

Bone Conduction

The mainstay of audiometry is the determination of puretone air-conduction (AC) and bone-conduction (BC) thresholds for the purpose of determining whether a conductive component exists and its severity. In general, an air-bone gap of >10 dB is considered indicative of a conductive hearing loss. There are a number of studies that have explored the techniques for and the results of ABR BC threshold tests (for review, see Cone-Wesson [1995]). The results of these studies are relevant to the problem of estimating BC threshold with ASSR, for which there are fewer published results. In general, there are two methods for obtaining BC thresholds. First, the stimuli used for the AC test are presented through a

TABLE 15.4 40-Hz Auditory Steady-State Response (ASSR) Threshold–Puretone Threshold Difference in Adults

Study	No. of Subjects	Stimulus	500 Hz	1,000 Hz	2,000 Hz	4,000 Hz
Klein, 1983	30 N	TB	16±10	14±7	16±7	19±7
Szyfter et al., 1984	31 N	TB	15±9	13±7	—	—
Dauman et al., 1984	30 H	TB	11±10	9±10	—	—
Lynn et al., 1984	40 H	TB	−2±12	8±11	—	—
Sammeth and Barry, 1985	16 N	TB	9±7	10±10	9±5	16±7
Kankkunen and Rosenhall, 1985	20 M	TB	8±11	5±9	4±7	3±8
Rodriguéz et al., 1986	15 N	TB	3±5	—	20±5	—
	10 H	TB	4±10	—	5±10	—
Stapells et al., 1987	6 M	TB	1±3	—	2±4	—
Milford and Birchall, 1989	22 H	TB	—	27±10	23±15	16±15
Chambers and Meyer, 1993	10 M	AM	1±5	2±5	—	—
Aoyagi et al., 1993	15 N	AM	11±10	11±11	13±10	18±12
	18 H	AM	8±7	9±6	13±8	12±6
Van Maanen and Stapells, 2005	23 M	MM	14±7	11±6	12±6	0±9

The number of subjects and their hearing status and stimulus type are given for each study. For stimulus type, TB = tone burst, AM = sinusoidally modulated puretone, and MM = amplitude and frequency modulated tone. For hearing status of subject group, N = normal hearing, H = subjects had hearing loss, and M = the group tested had members with hearing loss and normal hearing.

bone vibrator, and the difference in threshold for AC and BC test conditions is measured. The second method is to present masking noise by a bone vibrator and to determine the noise level needed to mask the response to an AC stimulus. This is known as the "sensory-neural acuity level" (SAL) technique. The level of effective BC noise needed to mask the response to the AC signal is used as the BC threshold (Ysunza and Cone-Wesson, 1987). The air-bone gap is calculated as the difference between the AC threshold and the BC effective masking level. Both techniques require careful calibration. The first requires determination of psychophysical threshold for the stimuli used for the BC test. Presumably, if a psychophysical air-bone gap exists, this will also be apparent in the difference between AC and BC ASSR threshold. The SAL technique requires physiologic calibration of the BC noise masker for a panel of normal-hearing listeners. White noise or band-passed noise may be used, but it is crucial to determine effective masking levels for each CF X noise-masker combination. (White noise effective masking levels would be higher than those for band-passed noise.) The level of noise needed to mask a response at 5 or 10 dB SL (re: ASSR threshold) should be determined. The level of BC noise needed to mask the response to a 5-dB SL AC stimulus equals 5 dB of effective masking. The BC effective masking levels are used as the estimate of the BC threshold. The difference between the AC threshold and the BC effective masking level (for a stimulus presented at 5 dB above AC ASSR threshold) is the measure of the air-bone gap. The BC effective masking level equals the BC threshold for that frequency.

Both conventional BC thresholds (Dimitrijevic et al., 2002; Lins et al., 1996; Small and Stapells, 2005) and the SAL technique (Cone-Wesson et al., 2002c) have been used to estimate air-bone gaps from ASSR threshold tests. The advantage of the first "direct" method is that the procedure mimics that which is typically done during behavioral testing and so has the comfort of face validity. A disadvantage of obtaining ASSRs to BC stimuli is that electromechanical artifact of the BC stimulus is "steady state," and is present during the entire recording and thus can obscure the neural response, or, worse, cause the detection algorithm to return a "false-positive" (i.e., an artifactual) response (Small and Stapells, 2004). An artifactual response may arise if the sampling rate of the signal is a harmonic of the CF. There are two methods for reducing or eliminating this artifact: (1) change the digital-to-analog conversion rate so that it is not a harmonic of the CF; or (2) use a steep antialiasing (low-pass) filter (Picton and John, 2004; Small and Stapells, 2005). Some commercially available instrumentation may not allow these procedures, in which case the chance of artifact during BC testing is very high.

The advantage of the SAL method is that the stimulus for both the AC and BC threshold test is the same (i.e., the AC stimulus). There is no difference in transducer. Also, the artifact produced by the BC oscillator is noise and thus should not be mistaken for the response. The level of the artifact would be expected to diminish with averaging. The disadvantage is that the effective masking levels must be measured physiologically, not psychophysically.

The real conundrum in BC ASSR (or ABR) tests is not really the stimulus or masker, but the fact that the skulls of infants less than 1 year of age transduce BC stimuli much differently than in adults. Studies (Cone-Wesson and Ramirez, 1997; Foxe and Stapells, 1993; Stapells and Ruben, 1989; Stuart et al., 1990; Yang et al; 1987) have shown that the immature skull appears to "focus" the BC signal at the temporal bone, leading to higher effective stimulus levels than in an adult. Thus, infants exhibit very low ABR thresholds compared to adults, and air-bone gaps exceeding 10 to 15 dB are not uncommon. A huge problem is that psychophysical thresholds for BC stimuli have not been determined in infants <1 year old. When adult threshold norms are used (i.e., dB HL or dB nHL), all infants appear to have an air-bone gap.

Hearing Aid Fitting and Cochlear Implant Mapping

There is considerable interest in using "objective" measures to fit and demonstrate benefit from amplification, particularly in preverbal infants and toddlers. It is possible to measure ASSR thresholds in the unaided and then aided condition (Dimitrijevic et al., 2004; Picton et al., 1998) and demonstrate functional gain. One advantage of using ASSRs for this purpose, compared to ABR, is that the AM (or MM) tones appear to be transduced by hearing aid microphones and circuitry more accurately than are click or tone-burst stimuli, at least when used in a linear mode. It is still necessary, however, to measure the fidelity of this transduction and to calibrate the sound field prior to making this type of measurement. At the present time, measures of functional gain, using either behavioral or electrophysiologic measures, are not recommended (Scollie and Seewald, 2002). Rather, the careful determination of threshold as a function of frequency and verification of target gains (based upon the threshold data) using in situ electroacoustic measures are preferred. The ASSR test, then, has a role in hearing aid fitting by providing an accurate estimate of threshold upon which hearing aid targets can be based. Yet, to quote Picton et al. (2003, p 211), "...demonstrating that the hearing aid is causing sounds to activate responses in the brain at intensities where there was no response without the aid is an important confirmation of the benefit of the aid. This is essential in patients who do not have clear or reliable thresholds (either behavioral or physiologic) without aids." ASSR methods for the estimation of the loudness discomfort levels, another crucial variable in hearing aid fitting, have not yet been developed.

ASSRs may be present at higher stimulus levels (when tone-burst evoked ABRs are absent at the upper limits of the instrumentation) and thus can more accurately indicate the severity of a hearing loss and residual hearing levels. This is always a consideration when cochlear implantation is being considered. As in the case of hearing aids, the ASSR provides the audiometric data upon which implantation decisions can be made.

In the past several years, the major cochlear implant companies have developed hardware and software for recording eighth-nerve action potentials in response to electrical stimulation, using the electrode and signal processor of the implant. The lowest current level needed to elicit an electronically evoked eighth-nerve action potential (E-AP) is used in an implant "mapping" algorithm. The levels for threshold and uncomfortable stimulus levels must be programmed. (Abbas et al., 1999; Seyle and Brown, 2002; see Chapter 12). The E-AP threshold rarely coincides with perceptual threshold, although there seems to be a consistent offset of E-AP threshold with perceptual threshold across the electrode array (Franck, 2002; Firszt et al., 2002). There has been some research in the use of the electrically evoked ASSR for the same purpose, that is, to estimate electrical stimulation threshold (Menard et al., 2004). Based upon previous experience with E-AP and electrically evoked ABR (Brown et al., 2000), it is likely that the E-ASSR thresholds will not be obtained at perceptual threshold levels. Like the E-AP methods, there may be a consistent offset (for an individual) between his/her E-ASSR threshold and his/her perceptual threshold, so that it may only be necessary to obtain a few perceptual thresholds, and the rest of the map could be determined on the basis of the E-ASSR threshold. At the present time, there appears to be no particular advantage for using an E-ASSR threshold procedure over an E-AP measurement. In fact, the E-ASSR measurement is technically challenging because of the steady-state nature of the electrical stimulus artifact.

Differential Diagnosis of Sensory versus Neural Losses

There is still limited information on the effect of neurologic compromise on the 80-Hz ASSR. The only conditions for which there are published data are for auditory neuropathy (Rance et al, 1999; 2005) and neurologic compromise due to prematurity (Cone-Wesson et al., 2002b). A summary of ASSR findings in 19 children with auditory neuropathy showed that there is no correspondence between behavioral hearing sensitivity and ASSR threshold (Rance et al., 2005). Puretone sensitivity was widely distributed between normal hearing and profound hearing loss, but the average ASSR threshold, regardless of CF, was around 85 to 90 dB HL. Correlations between puretone and ASSR thresholds averaged 0.51 in the group with auditory neuropathy, compared to an average of 0.97 in the group with normal hearing or sensory-neural hearing loss. ASSRs cannot be used to estimate the puretone sensitivity of those with auditory neuropathy. One problem that may occur, however, is in the case of an infant with auditory neuropathy for whom evoked otoacoustic emissions are absent. Unless one specifically tested for the presence of the cochlear microphonic, the absence of acoustic reflexes and an absent ABR might be interpreted

as a severe to profound sensory-neural hearing loss. Because ASSRs are known to be present in cases of severe to profound sensory-neural hearing loss when ABRs are absent (Van der Werff et al., 2002), the presence of ASSR at elevated levels could be mistaken for a sensory-neural hearing loss[3].

A discrepancy between behavioral thresholds and ASSR thresholds may be used as an indicator of neurologic dysfunction. Shinn (2005) obtained 40-Hz ASSR thresholds in a group of patients with well-defined brain lesions. They showed that the discrepancy between behavioral threshold and ASSR threshold was greater in the patient group when compared to a control group of adults with normal neurologic status. This is qualitatively similar to the results of Rance et al. (2005), who also show large discrepancies between behavioral and ASSR threshold in the patients with auditory neuropathy.

It is unwise to use ASSR thresholds to estimate perceptual thresholds when the status of the central auditory system is unknown. It should be possible, though, to use ABR in conjunction with ASSRs to help determine the impact of neural hearing loss. ABR wave I-V interwave intervals and/or abnormal waveform morphology (i.e., missing components, abnormal amplitude and latency of components) are useful for determining the presence of brainstem dysfunction (see Chapter 13). The combination of a supra-threshold click-evoked ABR along with ASSR threshold may be a rational way to approach an electrophysiologic assessment of the brainstem auditory system.

Supra-threshold Auditory Steady-State Response and Perceptual Correlates

Dimitrijevic et al. (2001) demonstrated a correlation between the ASSRs for independent amplitude- and frequency-modulated tones and word recognition scores in normal-hearing adults. Specifically, they measured word recognition across stimulus level and compared the scores across level to the number of ASSRs present for an eight-tone complex composed of four CFs, with each CF amplitude and frequency modulated at different rates. The number of ASSR components detected at each stimulus level was significantly correlated with the word recognition score at a similar level. This approach was used in hearing-impaired (as well as normal-hearing) subjects by Dimitrijevic et al. (2004). They obtained ASSRs to stimuli with carrier frequencies, levels, and modulation depths designed to have similar characteristics to speech. Word recognition abilities were also determined using standardized monosyllabic word lists (Auditec recordings of W-22 and NU-6). There were strong correlations between the word recognition score and the number of ASSR components present for young adults with normal hearing, for

---

[3] It is also possible to evoke a response from the vestibular system when high-level modulated stimuli are used. These may be mistaken for auditory responses unless steps to rule out other sources of artifact are undertaken (Gorga et al., 2004).

elderly adults with normal hearing, and for elderly adults with hearing loss. These investigators suggest that ASSRs for multiple modulated tones correlate with word recognition scores because both speech and multiple modulated tones contain information that varies rapidly in intensity and frequency. The ASSR "score" (i.e., the number of response components present for the eight-component stimulus) was modeled as an indicator of how much acoustic information was available to the listener. The more information available in the speech frequency range and for which the auditory system can process rapidly changing intensity and frequency cues, the better are the word recognition (speech discrimination) capabilities.

ASSRs in response to supra-threshold modulated noise have been correlated with temporal gap detection and the detection of modulation (Purcell et al., 2004). Young and old adult listeners had ASSRs recorded for modulated noise, in which the frequency of modulation was swept across the range of 20 to 600 Hz. They also underwent psychophysical tests of gap detection and modulation detection. First, the highest MF at which an ASSR was detected (using a 25% modulation depth) was significantly correlated ($r = 0.72$) with the modulation detection threshold. Second, the amplitude and phase (latency) of the ASSRs in several ranges of modulation were also correlated with modulation detection. Third, several of the ASSR response parameters were also correlated with gap detection. Because temporal processing is crucial for speech understanding, it is appropriate to develop electrophysiologic methods by which temporal processing may be assessed. The ASSR may provide a way of doing so.

Proposed Auditory Steady-State Response Threshold Estimation Protocol

There are several ways to optimize ASSR threshold estimation tests. These take into account stimulus, acquisition, and patient factors that would be expected to influence the results.

STIMULUS

For adults, MFs may be at 40 Hz ± 5 Hz. Because the effects of MM stimuli have not been formally evaluated at 40 Hz, sinusoidal AM tones are recommended for 40-Hz ASSRs. For infants and children, the modulation rates should be ≥ 80 Hz and ≤ 120 Hz, MM should be used, and the MF should increase with increasing CF. If more than one CF is presented at a time, then the MFs for each CF should be separated by at least 3 Hz. The threshold for modulated noise should be determined prior to that for modulated tones. The threshold for modulated noise can be used to determine the level for initiating a threshold search for specific CFs. A 5-dB step size should be used for ASSR threshold searching with puretones, although a 10-dB step size may be useful for initial testing with modulated noise.

ACQUISITION

Filter settings should be at 1 to 300 or 30 to 300 Hz. The analog-to-digital conversion rate should be at 1,000 Hz or higher (but most commercial instruments do not allow choice of an analog-to-digital conversion rate). Artifact rejection, if available, should be employed. The electrode montage for infants and young children should be Cz (vertex) to Mi (ipsilateral mastoid), with the common electrode on the opposite mastoid or forehead. For adults, an Fpz (high forehead) to Oz (inion) may be used.

PATIENT

Infants and young children should be in quiet sleep during the estimation of thresholds. A sedative or light anesthesia may be needed if the infant is not able to maintain quiet sleep for the duration of a complete test (40 to 60 minutes). Adults may be awake but should be encouraged to recline in a comfortable chair, relax, and be still.

TEST METHOD

Testing should not be initiated until the patient is sufficiently quiet. This can usually be determined by observing the patient and the ongoing EEG. Threshold is determined by decreasing the stimulus by 10 dB for each level at which the response criterion is met (i.e., the detection algorithm returns a result that meets the $p < 0.05$ level) and increasing by 5 dB when no response is detected. How many averages does it take to determine that a response is *not* present? Some decisions must be made a priori regarding the amplitude of the response that is to be detected. This decision, then, determines the amount of averaging needed because it is the averaging process that allows the response to be resolved out of the background noise, as noise decreases with increased averaging. For example, detection of a response of 15 nV would require averaged noise levels to be lower than 10 nV. Depending on how "noisy" the recording is, it may take 10 to 12 minutes to obtain such fine resolution. A 10-nV "noise" criterion has been recommended as a stopping rule for terminating a trial averaging (Picton et al., 2003). Averaging should then proceed for as long as it takes to meet this criterion or until a response is detected, whichever comes first. If the noise criterion is not met and a response is not detected, then this should be reported as a failure to achieve the a priori criterion. In such cases, a "threshold" cannot be determined. Raising the noise criterion will mean that ASSR thresholds are elevated in comparison to published norms for which the noise criterion was met.

There are other rules that may be employed at the discretion of the clinician, however, when application of these rules would be expected to affect threshold. For example, following the custom of "repeating" a trial as for ABR, some would require that a response be present for two independent trials given at the same level. This means that the criterion that a response is present has been made stricter. Using a stricter criterion will result in elevated thresholds in comparison to the more lax criterion. To avoid spurious "false-positive" responses, some require that the ASSR also be present at 10 dB above the lowest level for which a response is detected (to the same stimulus). False positives are sometimes seen when using a multifrequency technique wherein the ASSR thresholds vary as a function of frequency. For example, the threshold for a 500-Hz CF may be at 35 dB HL, and the threshold for a 2,000-Hz CF may be at 15 dB HL. In testing the 2,000-Hz response to threshold, a "response" to the 500-Hz CF may be detected at 15 dB HL, but not at 20, 25, or 30 dB HL. Thus, the "response" obtained at 15 dB HL is not considered valid.

INTERPRETATION OF THRESHOLDS

The ASSR thresholds should be interpreted with respect to published data that have established the relationship between ASSR and puretone threshold. This may involve the use of regression formulae (see Table 15.2) or correction factors (see Table 15.3). An important aspect of interpreting ASSR thresholds in this way is to acknowledge the sample characteristics upon which they were based, such as the age (infants, children, or adults), the type of hearing losses (conductive, sensory-neural, or mixed), and the range of hearing losses represented.

Case Study

Some of these principles are illustrated in the following case (Fig. 15.9). The response spectra are shown in the left panel,

with *open triangles* denoting responses for tones presented to the right ear, and *filled triangles* denoting responses for tones presented to the left ear. The audiograms are shown on the right, with *open circles* denoting behavioral thresholds and *filled squares* indicating the ASSR thresholds. For the right ear, ASSRs at 500 Hz and 1.0 kHz are present at 40 dB HL; at 2.0 and 4.0 kHz, ASSRs are present at 60 and 70 dB HL, respectively. For the left ear, a response to 500 Hz is seen at 70 and 50 dB HL, but not at 60 dB HL. The response at 1.0 kHz is present at 40 dB HL, and the response at 2.0 kHz is present at 50 dB HL. The ASSR threshold at 4.0 kHz is 80 dB HL. Is ASSR threshold at 0.5 kHz at 70 dB HL or 50 dB HL? A steep upward slope to the audiogram between 0.5 and 1.0 kHz is not unheard of but not likely, given the overall configuration of the audiogram. Other information, such as tympanometry and acoustic reflex thresholds may also be used to interpret ASSR thresholds. Finally, the 0.5-kHz response is absent at 40 and 30 dB HL, suggesting that 50 dB HL is the threshold. However, if one adopted a conservative criterion, requiring the response to be present at 10 dB above the lowest level detected, then the threshold would be judged to be 70 dB HL.

Using ASSR-puretone threshold differences determined from a study of adults with sensory-neural hearing loss (Herdman and Stapells, 2003), the right ear puretone thresholds would be estimated to be 26, 32, 50, and 67 dB HL for octave frequencies at 0.5, 1.0, 2.0, and 4.0 kHz, respectively, and left ear thresholds would be estimated at 36, 32, 40, and 77 dB, respectively, for the same frequencies. A mild to severe,

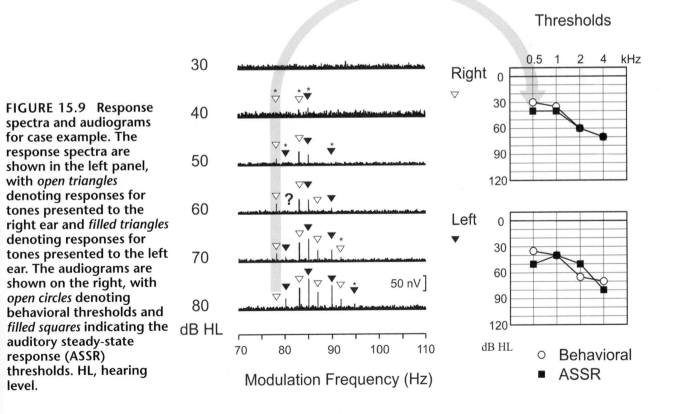

FIGURE 15.9 Response spectra and audiograms for case example. The response spectra are shown in the left panel, with *open triangles* denoting responses for tones presented to the right ear and *filled triangles* denoting responses for tones presented to the left ear. The audiograms are shown on the right, with *open circles* denoting behavioral thresholds and *filled squares* indicating the auditory steady-state response (ASSR) thresholds. HL, hearing level.

TABLE 15.5	Test results as a function of level			
	Carrier Frequency (Hz)			
Level (dB HL)	**500**	**1,000**	**2,000**	**4,000**
10	0	0	X	0
0	X	X	0	0
10	0	0	0	0
20	X	X	0	0
30	X	0	0	0
40	X	X	X	0
50	X	X	X	X
60	X	X	X	0

X refers to a significant response, and 0 refers to a nonsignificant response. See text for a discussion of threshold determination given these patterns of response/no response.

sloping bilateral loss is indicated. Comparing the estimated puretone thresholds to the true puretone thresholds, some discrepancies are obvious, but none exceed 10 dB.

Threshold Rules for Auditory Steady-State Response Tests

Consider the threshold test findings in Table 15.5. This case is riddled with many problems. At 500 Hz, significant responses are obtained at 0 and 20 dB HL but not at 10 dB HL. Is threshold at 0 or 20 dB HL? At 1,000 Hz, responses are present at 0, 20, and 40 dB HL but not at 10 or 30 dB HL. Where is the threshold? The significant responses at 0 dB may be false positives (with a statistical criterion of $p > 0.05$, there is a 5% probability of a false positive). On the other hand, the nonsignificant response at 10 dB may be a false negative. In these types of scenarios, it is essential to establish rules for ASSR threshold determination prior to the interpretation of the results. These rules should be reported in the results.

EXAMPLES OF RULES

1. If there is one nonsignificant response at a stimulus level greater than the level at which a significant response was observed and significant responses are obtained at all higher stimulus levels, then it is assumed that the nonsignificant response is a false negative. In the example given in Table 15.5, the threshold for 500 Hz is 0 dB HL because the 10-dB HL result is assumed to be a false negative. At 1,000 Hz, the threshold is at 20 dB HL because the 30-dB HL response is considered a false negative. The 0-dB HL response is a false positive.
2. A significant response must be obtained at 20 dB above the lowest level at which there is a significant response. This is important to rule out any potential false positives. In the example above, the threshold for 2,000 Hz would be 40 dB HL, and the 4,000-Hz threshold is unknown

because the significant response at 50 dB HL could be a false positive.
3. When in doubt, repeat tests at levels for which there are questionable responses.

STOPPING RULES FOR AUDITORY STEADY-STATE RESPONSE TESTS

For those who use instrumentation that allows the user to increase the number of sweeps for an average, the decision to stop recording must also be rule bound. The problem is the determination of no response. Specifically, if there is no response, how would we know if sampling for another 5 to 10 minutes might have resulted in a significant response? Usually, a "low-noise" and/or "time" rule can be used. Some potential stopping rules include:

1. Stop after 3 to 5 minutes when responses are significant (i.e., statistical significance must be maintained over a 3- to 5-minute period).
2. Stop after 12 to 15 minutes when no responses are significant.
3. Stop when averaged residual noise levels are at 10 to 15 nV (for 80-Hz ASSR) or 60 to 90 nV (for 40-Hz ASSRs).
4. Stop after 12 minutes or when averaged residual noise levels are 10 nV, whichever comes first.

As in the case of threshold rules, it is imperative to report the stopping rules used.

▨ SUMMARY AND CONCLUSION

The clinical application of ASSRs, especially for threshold estimation in infants and young children, has increased tremendously during the past decade. This is reflected in the steady flow of published studies ($n > 75$) since 2000, the existence of several commercially available systems for recording ASSRs, and the number of workshops and continuing education programs provided by professional organizations on the integration of ASSRs into clinical practice.

ASSRs provide an excellent estimate of hearing threshold across the audiometric range (250 to 8,000 Hz), particularly for those with moderate and greater degrees of hearing loss. Threshold tests can be completed in an objective fashion, due to the detection algorithms indicating statistically significant responses. Results can also be interpreted objectively using regression formulae or correction factors for conversion of ASSR thresholds to (behavioral) puretone threshold estimates. Thresholds can be estimated for both AC and BC stimuli. Beyond threshold tests, ASSRs have been shown to be correlated with some aspects of supra-threshold hearing, particularly word recognition ability.

No single audiometric test stands alone as a diagnostic measure, including the ASSR. ASSRs should be used in conjunction with tests of middle ear function (tympanometry and acoustic reflex tests), cochlear function (evoked otoacoustic emissions) and other evoked potentials (ABR), and, when possible, behavioral hearing tests. Tympanometry and acoustic reflex tests will aid in the interpretation of elevated ASSR thresholds, especially in the case of young infants with conductive hearing losses. The presence of otoacoustic emissions when ASSRs indicate significantly elevated thresholds is an indicator of auditory neuropathy. Click-evoked ABR tests provide important information about neural synchrony and brainstem integrity through the absolute and relative latencies of their constituent peaks; this information is not yet available from phase measurements of ASSRs. Although ASSRs are often used to estimate threshold in those too young or disabled to yield reliable behavioral thresholds, there should also be systematic attempts to document the patient's response to sound.

The goal is always to obtain the most information possible about the patient's hearing ability. ASSRs contribute a substantial amount towards that goal.

REFERENCES

Abbas PJ, Brown CJ, Shallop JK, Firszt JB, Hughes ML, Hong SH, Staller SJ. (1999) Summary of results using the nucleus CI24M implant to record the electrically evoked compound action potential. *Ear Hear.* 20, 45-59.

Aoyagi M, Furuse H, Yokota M, Kiren T, Suzuki Y, Koike Y. (1994a) Detectability of amplitude-modulation following response at different carrier frequencies. *Acta Otolaryngol.* 511 (suppl), 23–27.

Aoyagi M, Kiren T, Furuse H, Fuse T, Suzuki Y, Yokota M, Koike Y. (1994b) Effects of aging on amplitude modulation-following response. *Acta Otolaryngol.* 511 (suppl), 15–22.

Aoyagi M, Kiren T, Furase H, Fuse T, Suzuki Y, Yokota M, Koike Y. (1994c) Pure-tone threshold prediction by 80-Hz amplitude-modulation following responses. *Acta Otolaryngol Suppl.* 511 (abstract), 7–19.

Aoyagi M, Kiren T, Kim Y, Suzuki Y, Fuse T, Koike Y. (1993) Frequency specificity of amplitude-modulation-following response detected by phase spectral analysis. *Audiology.* 32, 293–301.

Aoyagi M, Suzuki Y, Yokota M, Furuse H, Watanabe T, Ito T. (1999) Reliability of 80-Hz amplitude modulation-following response detected by phase coherence. *Audiol Neuro-otol.* 4, 28–37.

Boettcher FA, Poth EA, Mills JH, Dubno JR. (2001) The amplitude-modulation following response in young and aged human subjects. *Hear Res.* 153, 32–42.

Brown CJ, Hughes ML, Luk B, Abbas PJ, Wolaver A, Gervais J. (2000) The relationship between EAP and EABR thresholds and levels used to program the nucleus 24 speech processor: data from adults. *Ear Hear.* 21, 151–163.

Chambers RD, Meyer TA. (1993) Reliability of threshold estimation in hearing-impaired adults using the AMFR. *J Am Acad Audiol.* 4, 22–32.

Clarey JC, Barone P, Imig TJ. (1992) Physiology of thalamus and cortex. In: Popper AN, Fay RR, eds. *The Mammalian Auditory Pathway: Neurophysiology.* New York: Springer-Verlag.

Cohen LT, Rickards FW, Clark GM. (1991) A comparison of steady state evoked potentials to modulated tones in awake and sleeping humans. *J Acoust Soc Am.* 90, 2467–2479.

Cone-Wesson B. (1995) Bone-conduction ABR tests. *Am J Audiol.* 4, 14–19.

Cone-Wesson B, Dowell RC, Tomlin D, Rance G, Ming WJ. (2002a) The auditory steady-state response: comparisons with the auditory brainstem response. *J Am Acad Audiol.* 13, 173–187.

Cone-Wesson B, Parker J, Swiderski N, Rickards FW. (2002b) The auditory steady-state response: full term and premature neonates. *J Am Acad Audiol.* 13, 260–269.

Cone-Wesson B, Ramirez GM. (1997) Hearing sensitivity in newborns estimated from ABRs to bone-conducted sounds. *J Am Acad Audiol.* 8, 299–307.

Cone-Wesson B, Rickards FW, Poulis C, Parker J, Tan L, Pollard J. (2002c) The auditory steady-state response: clinical observations and applications in infants and children. *J Am Acad Audiol.* 13, 270–282.

Dauman R, Szyfter W, Charlet de Sauvage R, Cazals Y. (1984) Low frequency thresholds assessed with 40 Hz MLR in adults with impaired hearing. *Arch Otorhinolaryngol.* 240, 85–89.

Dimitrijevic A, John MS, Picton TW. (2004) Auditory steady-state responses and word recognition scores in normal hearing and hearing-impaired adults. *Ear Hear.* 25, 68–84.

Dimitrijevic A, John MS, Van Roon P, Picton TW. (2001) Human auditory steady-state responses to tones independently modulated in both frequency and amplitude. *Ear Hear.* 22, 100–111.

Dimitrijevic A, John MS, Van Roon P, Purcell DW, Adamonis J, Ostroff J, Nedleski JM, Picton TW. (2002) Estimating the audiogram using multiple auditory steady-state responses. *J Am Acad Audiol.* 13, 205–224.

Dobie RA. (1993) Objective response detection. *Ear Hear.* 14, 31–35.

Dobie RA, Wilson MJ. (1989a) Analysis of auditory evoked potentials by magnitude-squared coherence. *Ear Hear.* 10, 2–13.

Dobie RA, Wilson MJ. (1989b) Objective response detection in the frequency domain. *Electroencephalogr Clin Neurophysiol.* 88, 516–524.

Dobie RA, Wilson MJ. (1993) Objective response detection in the frequency domain. *Electroencephalogr Clin Neurophysiol.* 88, 516–524.

Dobie RA, Wilson MJ. (1995) Objective versus human observer detection of 40-Hz auditory-evoked potentials. *J Acoust Soc Am.* 97, 3042–3050.

Dobie RA, Wilson MJ. (1996) A comparison of the t-test, F-test and coherence methods of detecting steady-state auditory-evoked potentials, distortion product otoacoustic emissions or other sinusoids. *J Acoust Soc Am.* 100, 2234–2246.

Dobie RA, Wilson MJ. (1998) Low-level steady-state auditory evoked potentials: effects of rate and sedation on detectability. *J Acoust Soc Am.* 104, 3482–3488.

Elberling C, Wahlgreen O. (1985) Estimation of auditory brainstem response, ABR, by means of Bayesian inference. *Scand Audiol.* 14, 89–96.

Firszt JB, Chambers RD, Kraus N, Reeder RM. (2002) Neurophysiology of cochlear implant users I: effects of stimulus current level and electrode site on the electrical ABR, MLR, and N1-P2 response. *Ear Hear.* 23, 502–515.

Firszt JB, Gaggl W, Runge-Samuelson CL, Burg LS, Wackym PA. (2004) Auditory sensitivity in children using the auditory steady-state response. *Arch Otolaryngol Head Neck Surg.* 130, 536–540.

Foxe JJ, Stapells DR. (1993) Normal infant and adult auditory brainstem responses to bone-conducted stimuli. *Ear Hear.* 14, 85–93.

Franck KH. (2002) A model of a nucleus 24 cochlear implant fitting protocol based on the electrically evoked whole nerve action potential. *Ear Hear.* 23 (suppl), 67S–71S.

Gorga MP, Neely ST, Hoover BM, Dierking DM, Beauchaine KL, Manning C. (2004) Determining the upper limits of stimulation for auditory steady-state response measurements. *Ear Hear.* 25, 302–307.

Herdman AT, Lins O, Van Roon P, Stapells DR, Scherg M, Picton TW. (2002a) Intracerebral sources of human auditory steady-state responses. *Brain Topogr.* 15, 69–86.

Herdman AT, Picton TW, Stapells DR. (2002b) Place specificity of multiple auditory steady-state responses. *J Acoust Soc Am.* 112, 1569–1582.

Herdman AT, Stapells DR. (2001) Thresholds determined using the monotic and dichotic multiple steady-state response technique in normal-hearing subjects. *Scand Audiol.* 30, 41–49.

Herdman AT, Stapells DR. (2003) Auditory steady state response thresholds of adults with sensorineural hearing impairment. *Int J Audiol.* 42, 237–248.

Irvine D. (1992) Physiology of the auditory brainstem. In: Popper AN, Fay RR, eds. *The Mammalian Auditory Pathway: Neurophysiology.* New York: Springer-Verlag.

John MS, Brown DK, Muir PJ, Picton TW. (2004) Recording auditory steady-state responses in young infants. *Ear Hear.* 25, 539–553.

John MS, Dimitrijevic A, Picton TW. (2001a) Weighted averaging of steady-state responses. *Clin Neurophysiol.* 112, 555–562.

John MS, Dimitrijevic A, Picton TW. (2003) Efficient stimuli for evoking auditory steady-state responses. *Ear Hear.* 24, 406–423.

John MS, Dimitrijevic A, Van Roon P, Picton TW. (2001b) Multiple auditory steady-state responses to AM and FM stimuli. *Audiol Neurootol.* 6, 12–27.

Johnson BW, Weinberg H, Ribary U, Cheyne DO, Ancill R. (1988) Topographic distribution of the 40 Hz auditory evoked-related potential in normal and aged subjects. *Brain Topogr.* 1, 117–121.

Johnson TA, Brown CJ. (2005) Threshold prediction using the auditory steady-state response and the toneburst auditory brainstem response: a within-subject comparison. *Ear Hear.* 26, 559–576.

Kankkunen A, Rosenhall U. (1985) Comparison between thresholds obtained with pure-tone audiometry and the 40-Hz middle latency response. *Scand Audiol.* 14, 99–104.

Khanna SM, Teich MC. (1989a) Spectral characteristics of the responses of primary auditory-nerve fibers to amplitude-modulated signals. *Hear Res.* 39, 143–157.

Khanna SM, Teich MC. (1989b) Spectral characteristics of the responses of primary auditory nerve fibers to frequency-modulated signals. *Hear Res.* 39, 159–175.

Klein AJ. (1983) Properties of the brain-stem response slow-wave component. I. Latency, amplitude and threshold sensitivity. *Arch Otolaryngol.* 109, 6–12.

Kraus N, McGee T, Stein L. (1994) The auditory middle latency response. In: Jacobsen JT, ed. *Principles and Applications in Auditory Evoked Potentials.* Boston: Allyn and Bacon; pp 123–154.

Kuwada S, Anderson JS, Batra R, Fitzpatrick DC, Teissier N, D'Angelo WR. (2002) Sources of the scalp-recorded amplitude-modulation following response. *J Am Acad Audiol.* 13, 188–204.

Lasky RE. (1984) A developmental study on the effect of stimulus rate on the auditory evoked brain-stem response. *Electroencephalogr Clin Neurophysiol.* 59, 411–419.

Levi EC, Folsom RC, Dobie RA. (1993) Amplitude-modulation following response (AMFR): effects of modulation rate, carrier frequency, age and state. *Hear Res.* 68, 42–52.

Levi EC, Folsom RC, Dobie RA. (1995) Coherence analysis of envelope-following responses (EFRs) and frequency-following responses (FFRs) in infants and adults. *Hear Res.* 89, 21–27.

Lins OG, Picton P, Picton TW. (1995) Auditory steady-state responses to tones amplitude-modulated at 80-110 Hz. *J Acoust Soc Am.* 97, 3051–3063.

Lins OG, Picton TW. (1995) Auditory steady-state responses to multiple simultaneous stimuli. *Electroencephalogr Clin Neurophysiol.* 96, 420–432.

Lins OG, Picton TW, Boucher BL, Durieux-Smith A, Champagne SC, Moran LM, Perez-Abalo MC, Martin V, Savio G. (1996) Frequency specific audiometry using steady-state responses. *Ear Hear.* 17, 81–96.

Luts H, Desloovere C, Kumar A, Vandermeersch E, Wouters J. (2004) Objective assessment of frequency-specific hearing thresholds in babies. *Int J Pediatr Otorhinolaryngol.* 68, 915–926.

Luts H, Wouters J. (2005) Comparison of MASTER and AUDERA for measurement of auditory steady-state responses. *Int J Audiol.* 44, 244–253.

Lynn JM, Lesner SA, Sandridge SA, Daddario CC. (1984) Threshold prediction from the auditory 40-Hz evoked potential. *Ear Hear.* 5, 366–370.

Menard M, Galleyo S, Truy E, Berger-Vachon C, Durrant JD, Collet L. (2004) Auditory steady-state response evaluation of auditory thresholds in cochlear implant patients. *Int J Audiol.* 43 (suppl 1), S39–S43.

Milford CA, Birchall JP. (1989) Steady-state auditory evoked potentials to amplitude-modulated tones in hearing-impaired subjects. *Br J Audiol.* 23, 137–142.

Møller AR. (1994) Neural generators of auditory evoked potentials. In: Jacobsen JT, ed. *Principles and Applications in Auditory Evoked Potentials.* Boston: Allyn and Bacon; pp 23–46.

Muchnik C, Katz-Putter H, Rubinstein M, Hildesheimer M. (1993) Normative data for 40-Hz event-related potentials to 500-Hz tonal stimuli in young and elderly subjects. *Audiology.* 32, 27–35.

Perez-Abalo MC, Savio G, Torres A, Martin V, Rodriguez E, Galan L. (2001) Steady-state responses to multiple amplitude-modulated tones: an optimized method to test frequency-specific thresholds in hearing-impaired children and normal-hearing subjects. *Ear Hear.* 22, 200–211.

Picton TW, Dimitrijevic A, Perez-Aballo M-C, Van Roon P. (2005) Estimating audiometric thresholds using auditory steady-state responses. *J Am Acad Audiol.* 16, 140–156.

Picton TW, Durieux-Smith A, Champagne SC, Whittingham J, Moran LM, Giguere C, Beauregard Y. (1998) Objective evaluation of aided thresholds using auditory steady-state responses. *J Am Acad Audiol.* 9, 315–331.

Picton TW, John MS. (2004) Avoiding electromagnetic artifacts when recording auditory steady-state responses. *J Am Acad Audiol.* 15, 541–554.

Picton TW, John MS, Dimitrijevic A, Purcell D. (2003) Human auditory steady-state responses. *Int J Audiol.* 42, 177–219.

Purcell DW, John SM, Schneider BA, Picton TW. (2004) Human temporal auditory acuity as assessed by envelope following responses. *J Acoust Soc Am.* 116, 3581–3593.

Rance G, Beer DE, Cone-Wesson B, Shepherd RK, Dowell RC, King AM, Rickards FW, Clark GM. (1999) Clinical findings for a group of infants and young children with auditory neuropathy. *Ear Hear.* 20, 238–252.

Rance G, Briggs RJS. (2002) Assessment of hearing in infants with moderate to profound impairment: the Melbourne experience with auditory steady-state evoked potential testing. *Ann Otol Rhinol Laryngol.* 111, 22–28.

Rance G, Dowell RC, Rickards FW, Beer DE, Clark GM. (1998) Steady-state evoked potential and behavioral hearing thresholds in a group of children with absent click-auditory brain stem response. *Ear Hear.* 19, 48–61.

Rance G, Rickards FW. (2002) Prediction of hearing threshold in infants using auditory steady-state evoked potentials. *J Am Acad Audiol.* 13, 236–245.

Rance G, Rickards FW, Cohen LT, DeVidi S, Clark GM. (1995) The automated prediction of hearing thresholds in sleeping subjects using auditory steady state evoked potentials. *Ear Hear.* 16, 499–507.

Rance G, Roper R, Symons L, Moody LJ, Poulis C, Dourlay M, Kelly T. (2005) Hearing threshold estimation in infants using auditory steady-state responses. *J Am Acad Audiol.* 16, 291–300.

Rance G, Tomlin D. (2006) Maturation of auditory steady-state responses in normal babies. *Ear Hear.* 27, 20–39.

Regan D. (1989) Human brain electrophysiology. In: *Evoked Potentials and Evoked Magnetic Fields in Science and Medicine.* New York: Elsevier.

Reyes SA, Salvi RJ, Burkard RF, Coad ML, Wack DS, Galantowicz PJ, Lockwood AH. (2004) PET imaging of the 40 Hz auditory steady state response. *Hear Res.* 194, 73–80.

Rhode WS, Greenberg S. (1992). Physiology of the cochlear nuclei. In: Popper AN, Fay RR, eds. *The Mammalian Auditory Pathway: Neurophysiology.* New York: Springer-Verlag.

Rickards FW, Tan LE, Cohen LT, Wilson OJ, Drew JH, Clark GM. (1994) Auditory steady-state evoked potential in newborns. *Br J Audiol.* 28, 327–337.

Rodriguez R, Picton T, Linden D, Hamel G, Laframboise G. (1986) Human auditory steady state responses: effects of intensity and frequency. *Ear Hear.* 7, 300–313.

Ross B, Herdman AT, Pantev C. (2005) Right hemispheric laterality of human 40 Hz auditory steady-state responses. *Cerebr Cortex.* 15, 2029–2039.

Ruggero MA. (1992) Physiology and coding of sound in the auditory nerve. In: Popper AN, Fay RR, eds. *The Mammalian Auditory Pathway: Neurophysiology.* New York: Springer-Verlag.

Sammeth CA, Barry SJ. (1985) The 40-Hz event-related potential as a measure of auditory sensitivity in normals. *Scand Audiol.* 14, 51–55.

Savio G, Cardenas J, Perez-Abalo M, Gonzalez A, Valdes J. (2001) The low and high frequency auditory steady state responses mature at different rates. *Audiol Neurootol.* 6, 279–287.

Scollie SD, Seewald RC. (2002) Evaluation of electroacoustic test signals. I: comparison with amplified speech. *Ear Hear.* 23, 477–487.

Seyle K, Brown CJ. (2002) Speech perception using maps based on neural response telemetry measures. *Ear Hear.* 23 (Suppl), 72S–79S.

Shinn JB. (2005) The auditory steady state response in individuals with neurological insult of the central auditory nervous system. Unpublished doctoral dissertation. Storrs, CT: University of Connecticut.

Sininger YS, Abdala C, Cone-Wesson B. (1997) Auditory threshold sensitivity of the human neonate as measured by the auditory brainstem response. *Hear Res.* 104, 27–38.

Sininger YS, Cone-Wesson B. (2002) Threshold prediction using auditory brainstem response and steady-state evoked potentials with infants and young children. In: Katz J, ed. *Handbook of Clinical Audiology.* 5th ed. Philadelphia: Lippincott Williams & Wilkins.

Small SA, Stapells DR. (2004) Stimulus artifact issues when recording auditory steady-state responses. *Ear Hear.* 25, 611–623.

Small SA, Stapells DR. (2005) Multiple auditory steady-state responses to bone-conduction stimuli in adults with normal hearing. *J Am Acad Audiol.* 16, 172–183.

Stapells DR. (2000) Threshold estimation by the tone-evoked auditory brainstem response: a literature meta-analysis. *J Speech Lang Pathol Audiol.* 24, 74–83.

Stapells DR, Galambos R, Costello JA, Makeig S. (1988) Inconsistency of auditory middle latency and steady-state responses in infants. *Electroencephalogr Clin Neurophysiol.* 71, 289–295.

Stapells DR, Gravel JS, Martin BA. (1995) Thresholds for auditory brainstem responses to tones in notched noise from infants and young children with normal hearing or sensorineural hearing loss. *Ear Hear.* 16, 361–371.

Stapells DR, Linden D, Suffield JB, Hamel G, Picton TW. (1984) Human auditory steady state potentials. *Ear Hear.* 5, 105–113.

Stapells DR, Makeig S, Galambos R. (1987) Auditory steady-state responses: threshold prediction using phase coherence. *Electroencephalogr Clin Neurophysiol.* 67, 260–270.

Stapells DR, Picton TW, Durieux-Smith A. (1994) Electrophysiologic measures of frequency-specific auditory function. In: Jacobson JT, ed. *Principles and Applications in Auditory Evoked Potentials.* Boston: Allyn & Bacon; pp 251–283.

Stapells DR, Ruben RJ. (1989) Auditory brain stem responses to bone-conducted tones in infants. *Ann Otol Rhinol Laryngol.* 98, 941–949.

Steuve MP, O'Rourke C. (2003) Estimation of hearing loss in children: comparison of auditory steady-state response, auditory brainstem response, and behavioral test methods. *Am J Audiol.* 12, 125–136.

Stuart A, Yang EY, Stenstrom R. (1990) Effect of temporal area bone vibrator placement on auditory brain stem response in newborn infants. *Ear Hear.* 11, 363–369.

Swanpoel D, Hugo R. (2004) Estimations of auditory sensitivity for young cochlear implant candidates using the ASSR: preliminary results. *Int J Audiol.* 43, 377–382.

Szalda K, Burkard R. (2005) The effects of Nembutal anesthesia on the auditory steady-state response (ASSR) from the inferior colliculus and auditory cortex of the chinchilla. *Hear Res.* 203, 32–44.

Szyfter W, Dauman R, de Sauvage RC. (1984) 40 Hz middle latency responses to low frequency tone pips in normally hearing adults. J *Otolaryngol.* 13, 275–280.

Van der Reijden CS, Mens LHM, Snik AdFM. (2005) EEG derivations providing auditory steady-state responses with high signal-to-noise ratios in infants. *Ear Hear.* 26, 299–309.

Van Maanen A, Stapells DR. (2005) Comparison of multiple auditory steady-state responses (80 vs 40 Hz) and slow cortical potentials for threshold estimation in hearing-impaired adults. *Int J Audiol.* 44, 613–624.

Vander Werff KR, Brown CJ. (2005) The effect of audiometric configuration on threshold and suprathreshold auditory steady-state responses. *Ear Hear.* 26, 310–326.

Vander Werff KR, Brown CJ, Gienapp BA, Clay KMS. (2002) Comparison of auditory steady-state response and auditory brainstem response thresholds in children. *J Am Acad Audiol.* 13, 227–235.

Victor JD, Mast J. (1991) A new statistic for steady-state evoked potentials. *Electroencephalogr Clin Neurophysiol.* 78, 378–388.

Viemeister NF. (1979) Temporal modulation transfer functions based upon modulation thresholds. *J Acoust Soc Am.* 66, 1364–1380.

Yang EY, Rupert AL, Moushegian G. (1987). A developmental study of bone conduction auditory brainstem response in infants. *Ear Hear.* 8, 244–251.

Ysunza A, Cone-Wesson B. (1987). Bone conduction masking for brainstem auditory-evoked potentials (BAEP) in pediatric audiological evaluations. Validation of the test. *Int J Pediatr Otorhinolaryngol.* 12, 291–302.

CHAPTER

16 Intraoperative Neurophysiology: Monitoring Auditory Evoked Potentials

William Hal Martin and Yongbing Shi

INTRODUCTION: INTRAOPERATIVE MONITORING OF AUDITORY EVOKED POTENTIALS

Whenever a surgical team considers neural structures and pathways to be *at risk* for damage due to the nature of the surgical approach, the state of the disease, or the complexity of the procedure, intraoperative neurophysiologic monitoring should be performed.

The auditory pathway and hearing function are often *at risk* during procedures involving access to the cerebellopontine angle (CPA). Injury may occur in the cochlea, along the auditory nerve, or at higher levels along the auditory pathway. Damage may be caused by mechanical (compression, avulsion, cutting, and stretching), ischemic (vasospasm of the acoustic artery), and thermal (heat damage from electrocautery) bases. The auditory nerve is particularly sensitive to mechanical manipulation and is easily damaged. The intracranial segment of this nerve is covered by central myelin (oligodendrocytes) and has no perineurium, making it vulnerable to physical contact. The internal auditory artery, a branch of the basilar artery, supplies the entire membranous labyrinth and can go into vasospasm with manipulation, resulting in permanent hearing loss. Early detection of changes in auditory pathway function allows the surgical team to modify their procedure and is the key to reducing or eliminating permanent damage during surgery. Intraoperative monitoring of auditory evoked potentials can provide the surgical team with early warnings and enable them to avert

damage to the auditory pathway and reduce the likelihood of causing hearing loss.

Procedures that place the auditory nerve at risk include resection of vestibular schwannomas; vestibular nerve section; microvascular decompression of cranial nerves V, VII, VIII, and IX; resection of other CPA and fourth ventricle tumors; repair of CPA arteriovenous malformations; and aneurysm repair. Neuromonitoring of auditory evoked potentials from the cochlea through the midbrain reduces the risk of hearing loss or other neural damage in all of these procedures.

BACKGROUND

Jewett and colleagues (Jewett, 1970; Jewett et al., 1970; Jewett and Williston, 1971) were the first to conclusively demonstrate that a series of scalp-recorded potentials was generated by the ascending activation of the auditory pathway. In their earliest papers, they noted the great potential for this method in diagnostic medicine. The activity was called the auditory brainstem response (ABR; Fig. 16.1). Other investigators demonstrated strong relationships between abnormalities of the ABR and neurologic disorders (Starr and Achor, 1975; Starr and Hamilton, 1976; Starr, 1976; Stockard and Rossiter, 1977). In the late 1970s, clinicians realized the possibility of helping surgeons reduce what was an expected hearing loss after CPA surgery and began exploring the use of ABRs for monitoring. The pioneers of ABR monitoring (Levine et al., 1978; Levine, 1980; Hashimoto et al., 1980; Raudzens and Shetter, 1981; Grundy et al., 1981) indicated

Auditory Brainstem Response

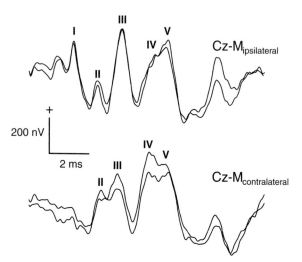

FIGURE 16.1 Auditory brainstem response (ABR) recorded from an adult in response to 75 dB nHL click stimuli presented at 24.1/s. The upper recording was made with electrodes at the vertex and mastoid ipsilateral to the ear stimulated. The lower recording was made contralateral to the ear stimulated. Waves I through V are marked.

that intraoperative monitoring during resection of vestibular schwannomas was technically feasible and probably helpful in reducing morbidity.

Based on experience and experimentation, clinicians found that other auditory evoked potentials could be monitored simultaneously with the ABR. Electrocochleography (ECoG), using electrodes placed in the ear canal, on the tympanic membrane, or on the cochlear promontory, provided information about the most distal section of the auditory nerve and verified blood supply to the cochlea (Fig. 16.2).

Electrocochleogram

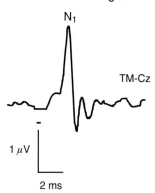

FIGURE 16.2 Electrocochleogram recorded from an adult in response to an alternating polarity, 75 dB nHL click stimuli presented at 24.1/s. An electrode was placed on the tympanic membrane (TM) on the side of the stimulated ear. The electrocochleography compound action potential is noted as N1.

Compound Action Potential

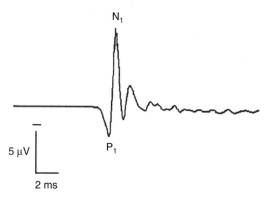

FIGURE 16.3 Auditory nerve compound action potential (AN-CAP) recorded using a wick electrode placed at the root entry zone of the eighth cranial nerve into the brainstem to 75 dB nHL click stimuli presented at 24.1/s. P1 and N1 of the AN-CAP are identified.

Direct recording of the auditory nerve compound action potential (AN-CAP; Fig. 16.3) added the most valuable information—a nearly real-time measure of auditory nerve function. Simultaneous recording with the three techniques gave the opportunity to monitor multiple levels of auditory pathway function at the same time. ECoG evaluated cochlear and distal auditory nerve function. The AN-CAP could be recorded proximal to the tumor site, giving continuous information about the status of the entire auditory nerve. The ABR gave an overview of the activity of the entire auditory pathway from the distal auditory nerve through the midbrain. Changes in brainstem function resulting from compression or ischemia could be monitored. Currently, auditory evoked potentials are monitored for a wide range of surgical procedures involving brainstem structures.

Several manufacturers offer evoked potentials systems that are capable of simultaneous recording of ECoG, AN-CAPs, and ABRs. Interleaving right and left ear stimuli and averaging responses from both sides in parallel allows rapid data acquisition from both sides of the auditory pathway. This method provides an excellent combination of large amplitude responses with very short averaging times (ECoG and AN-CAP) to evaluate immediate changes in auditory nerve function, with the scalp-recorded ABR providing a slower but more global picture of brainstem function. Hearing preservation during CPA surgery was once nearly impossible to achieve. Now, it has become a common outcome, thanks to the information provided by intraoperative auditory evoked potential monitoring.

DESCRIPTION OF RESPONSES

The ABR is differentially recorded from two electrodes placed on the scalp, one near the vertex and one near the stimulated ear. The resulting waveform is a series of between five and seven vertex-positive peaks that were designated by Roman numerals by Jewett (1970) (Fig. 16.1). The peaks that are useful for clinical purposes are waves I, III, and V due to their stability within and across subjects. The latency of each peak is determined as the time from the onset of the stimulus to the peak of the response and is measured in milliseconds. For higher level click stimuli, the normal wave I has a typical latency of ≤ 2 ms. Waves II through V are each present at approximately 1-ms intervals after wave I. Since the responses are recorded from the scalp, they are considered far-field responses and have low amplitudes (wave V is typically $<0.5\ \mu V$). Due to the small amplitude relative to the background electrical noise, a considerable amount of preacquisition filtering and signal averaging must be performed in order to record the responses. More details about the ABR can be found in Chapters 11, 13, and 14.

ECoG consists of three responses. The cochlear microphonic (CM) and summating potential (SP) are potentials generated in response to cochlear activation by an acoustic stimulus. They are not typically monitored during surgery, although the presence of an SP indicates that blood flow to the cochlea has not been disrupted by the surgical procedure. The initial activation of the myelinated segment of the auditory nerve results in a compound action potential (CAP) recorded in the ECoG (Fig. 16.2). It is referred to as the N1, but it is identical to wave I of the ABR. ECoG responses are optimally recorded from an electrode placed as close to the cochlea as possible, typically either on the tympanic membrane or directly on the basal turn of the cochlea (promontory). Due to the proximity of the electrode to the source of the response, the amplitude of this near-field response is relatively large (2 to 20 μV), and less signal averaging must be performed to acquire a reliable response. This considerably reduces the time it takes to interpret the response. The reader is referred to Chapter 12 for a more complete treatment of ECoG.

The CAP may also be recorded directly from an electrode placed on the auditory nerve (AN-CAP; Fig. 16.3). The N1 peak of this near-field response occurs at about the same latency as the ABR wave II, although it is not wave II and has a different mechanism of generation, as will later be described. Immediately before the N1 is a peak of opposite polarity noted as P1. The P1-N1 of the AN-CAP requires little averaging because it is often large in amplitude (up to 50 μV).

ANATOMY AND PHYSIOLOGY

Intact peripheral hearing is essential for intraoperative monitoring of the auditory pathway. We can consider the ear like a window to the brain. If the window is dirty, we have great difficulty getting a clear picture of the brain. So it is with a hearing loss. If the preoperative hearing loss, regardless of etiology, diminishes the ability to record a reliable ABR, then monitoring during surgery is not possible. It is important to

verify that an ABR can be recorded preoperatively and to determine the patient's preoperative puretone thresholds and speech recognition capabilities.

Increasing the stimulus level can compensate for a conductive hearing loss. A cochlear or retrocochlear hearing loss may provide a more difficult problem. It is important to understand that the earliest waves of the ABR are predominately generated by synchronous discharges of fibers from the basal, high-frequency end of the cochlea. A high-frequency sensory-neural hearing loss may decrease the amplitude of the ABR waves, making it difficult or impossible to monitor. It should also be noted that the tonotopic distribution of frequency along the basilar membrane (base to apex, high to low frequency) is maintained along the auditory pathway. Axons from the low-frequency apex of the cochlea are at the center of the auditory nerve. Axons carrying increasingly higher frequency information are twisted around and on top of the low-frequency core. The highest frequency fibers are on the outer surface of the auditory nerve bundle and are, therefore, most vulnerable to damage from tumors, surgical manipulation, and tumor resection.

Generators of the Auditory Evoked Potentials

The auditory pathway begins in the modiolus of the cochlea, where the myelinated dendrites of the auditory nerve pass into and through the spiral ganglia en route to forming a nerve bundle in the internal auditory canal. The acoustic and vestibular sections of the auditory nerve merge within the temporal bone and align with the intracranial section of the facial nerve. Together, they exit the internal auditory canal and connect to the brainstem (Figs. 16.4 and 16.5). All auditory nerve fibers synapse at either the posterior ventral cochlear nucleus (PVCN) or the anterior ventral cochlear nucleus (AVCN). Fibers that synapse at the PVCN also have connections with the dorsal cochlear nucleus (DCN). From the cochlear nucleus onward, there are several pathways and combinations of pathways. The vast majority of fibers cross the brainstem to the opposite side via the trapezoid body (TB). Some synapse in either the medial or lateral superior olivary nuclei (MSO, LSO). Others pass through the lateral lemniscus (LL) en route to the inferior colliculus (called posterior colliculus and labeled PC in this figure). All ascending fibers synapse at the inferior colliculus before ascending to the medial geniculate body at the level of the thalamus and then on to the primary auditory cortex.

As mentioned earlier, EcoG N1 is equivalent to wave I of the ABR. Both are generated within the internal auditory canal by the most distal section of the myelinated auditory nerve. ABR wave II occurs at about the same latency as N1 of the AN-CAP, when the electrode is placed at the auditory nerve root entry zone adjacent to the brainstem (Møller and Jannetta, 1982; Møller et al., 1988). N1 of the AN-CAP is generated as the action potential passes across the recording electrode. N1 is thus a good indicator of all activity distal

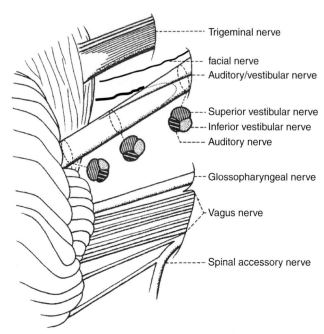

Trigeminal nerve

facial nerve

Auditory/vestibular nerve

Superior vestibular nerve
Inferior vestibular nerve
Auditory nerve

Glossopharyngeal nerve

Vagus nerve

Spinal accessory nerve

FIGURE 16.4   The eighth cranial nerve (schematic) as viewed from a dorsal approach. Cross-sections of the auditory/vestibular nerve are identified at three locations along the nerve. Note that the acoustic and vestibular sections of the nerve change position around the axis of the nerve as it passes from the internal auditory canal to the brainstem (right to left). (Reproduced with permission from Lang J. [1985] Anatomy of the brainstem and the lower cranial nerves, vessels, and surrounding structures. *Am J Otol.* **November [suppl], 1–19.)**

to the point of its recording. However, Martin et al. (1995) demonstrated that there was no relationship between the near-field recorded N1 of the AN-CAP and the far-field wave II of the ABR. Wave II and the negative peak between waves I and II (i.e., I_n) are stationary potentials. A stationary potential is recorded in the far field when the electrical fields surrounding a nerve carrying an action potential are distorted. This can occur when the medium surrounding the nerve changes in shape or conductivity or when the nerve makes a sharp change in direction (Kimura et al., 1984; 1986; Jewett and Deupree, 1989; Deupree and Jewett, 1988, Jewett et al., 1990; Nakinishi, 1982; 1983; Stegeman et al., 1987). Martin et al. (1995) found that the latency of wave II was dependent on the fluid level surrounding the intracranial section of the auditory nerve during CPA surgery. When the nerve was completely submerged in fluid, the latencies of waves I, III, and V were stable. When the fluid was suctioned off the nerve and the nerve was suspended in air, the latency of wave II decreased significantly, but the latencies of waves I, III, and V remained unchanged. Based on the conductivity differences between bone (surrounding the nerve in the internal auditory canal), cerebrospinal fluid (CSF; surrounding

the nerve between the exit of the canal and the attachment to the brainstem), and brain tissue (of the brainstem), Martin et al. (1995) determined that the normal wave II was generated as the propagating action potential passed from the highly conductive CSF to the poorly conducting tissue of the brainstem. Wave I_n was generated as the propagating action potential passed from the poorly conducting bone of the internal auditory canal into the highly conductive CSF within the cranium.

The idea that stationary potentials can generate far-field responses is not new. It has been used to explain the results of somatosensory evoked potential studies (Kimura, et al., 1984; 1986). However, the work of Martin et al. (1995) demonstrated that conditions exist along the auditory pathways that are sufficient to generate stationary potentials. CAPs generated in a large-volume conductor (e.g., the head) are not recorded well in the far field. In contrast, stationary potentials are readily recorded from the surface of a large-volume conductor. These results mandate a new look at the generation mechanisms underlying the scalp-recorded ABR. The currently proposed generators of ABR waves have been based on comparisons of near-field and far-field recordings. Although it is possible to find near-field activity that coincides with a scalp-recorded peak, there may be no relationship between the two events at all.

Scalp-recorded wave III has been recorded at the same time as near-field activity in the cochlear nucleus (Møller and Jannetta, 1983). However, other recordings from the area of the cochlear nucleus in the lateral recess of the fourth ventricle indicate activity that coincides with wave III_n (the negative peak between III and IV) (Møller et al., 1994; 1995). Other results indicate that the auditory nerve may continue to be active during the generation of scalp-recorded waves III and IV (Møller and Jho, 1991).

Several areas of the auditory pathway are active at the same time that wave IV can be recorded from the scalp, including the cochlear nucleus, superior olivary complex, lateral lemniscus, and, possibly, trapezoid body (Møller, 1995). Wave IV also appears to be generated by events contralateral to the stimulated ear.

It has been suggested that the sharp peak of wave V is generated by the lateral lemniscus as it terminates into the inferior colliculus and that the activity of the inferior colliculus is responsible for the generation of the relatively slow and large negativity following the peak of V. This has also been called the SN10 potential (Møller, 1995). However, there is evidence that all activity at or beyond the peak of wave IV could be generated by the inferior colliculus contralateral to the stimulus. Durrant et al. (1994) recorded three-channel Lissajous trajectories (3-CLTs) of the ABR from a woman who had previously undergone gamma knife obliteration of the right inferior colliculus. A 3-CLT is a three-dimensional view of the ABR revealing dipole orientation and magnitude for the activity of waves I-V (Williston et al., 1981; Pratt et al., 1985; Martin et al., 1987a; 1987b). The responses to right ear stimulation were completely normal for activity

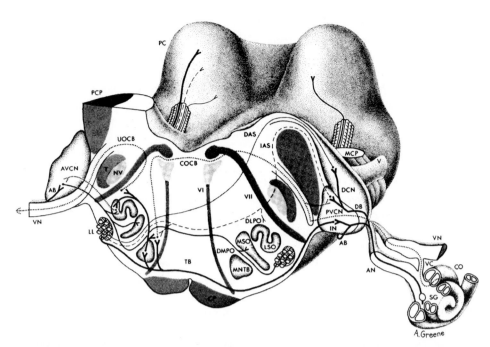

FIGURE 16.5   Schematic of the connections within the human auditory pathway. Represented are: AB, ascending branch of the eighth nerve; AN, eighth nerve; AVCN, anteroventral cochlear nucleus; CO, cochlea; COCB, crossed olivocochlear bundle; CP, cerebral peduncle; DAS dorsal acoustic stria; DB, descending branch of the eighth nerve; DCN dorsal cochlear nucleus; DLPO, dorsal periolivary region; DMPO, dorsomedial periolivary nucleus; IAS, intermediate acoustic stria; IN, posteroventral AVCN (interstitial nucleus); LL, lateral lemniscus; LSO, lateral superior olive; MCP, middle cerebellar peduncle; MNTB, medial nucleus of the trapezoid body; MSO, medial superior olive; PC, posterior colliculus; PCP, posterior cerebellar peduncle; PVCN, posteroventral cochlear nucleus; SG, spiral ganglion; TB, trapezoid body; TNV, descending trigeminal tract and nucleus; UOCB, uncrossed olivocochlear bundle; VC, vestibulo-cochlear anastomosis; VN, vestibular nerve; VI, abducens nerve root and nucleus; VII, facial nerve and root. (Reproduced with permission from Morest DK. [1975] Structural organization of the auditory pathways. In: Tower D, ed. *The Nervous System; Human Communication and Its Disorders.* **New York: Raven Press; p 22.)**

corresponding to waves I-V. The same was true for activity corresponding with waves I through the peak of IV to left ear stimulation. However, all activity beyond the peak of wave IV to left ear stimulation was absent. This suggests two things: first, that all of the activity contributing to the scalp-recorded wave V comes from the side of the brainstem contralateral to the stimulus, and second, that the structure of the inferior colliculus must be intact for the generation of waves V and V_n. Although no degeneration below the inferior colliculus could be identified using magnetic resonance imaging (MRI), it is possible that the synaptic connections between the lateral lemniscus and the inferior colliculus had been damaged. This would support the hypothesis that the peak of wave V could be generated by events at that junction.

It would be nice to have a one-to-one correspondence between specific nuclei along the auditory pathway and the positive peaks of the ABR. However, this is only true for wave I. Beyond wave I, the generation of the ABR becomes relatively complex and is attributed to either physical phenomena such as stationary potentials or to complex interactions between multiple, simultaneously active generators. It is important to realize that just because activity can be recorded at a given point in time in the near field, it does not directly follow that the same activity is represented by a positive or negative peak on the scalp. This makes the interpretation of changes in the ABR difficult. Despite the continuing discussions about the exact mechanisms underlying the generation of the scalp-recorded ABR, clinical evidence has demonstrated that it is a highly sensitive indicator of auditory pathway disorders and of *alterations in function* such as those induced by surgical manipulations. As such, the ABR remains a valuable tool for neuromonitoring. Using only ABR, we cannot assign waveform changes to specific structures. However, it is safe to use changes in the ABR as direct evidence of a change in function along the pathway that may warrant the immediate attention of the surgical team.

METHODS

Stimulus Parameters

A stimulus of adequate sound pressure level must be used in order to evoke a clear, large-amplitude response throughout the entire duration of the surgical procedure. In other clinical settings, the clinician can check the placement of headphones if there appears to be a problem. During surgery, the stimulating system must be placed correctly and securely at the beginning of the surgery because the sterile field cannot be violated during the procedure. Stimulus parameters must be selected that will guarantee the largest amplitude, most reliable response in the shortest amount of time.

PLACING THE TRANSDUCERS

The placement of the stimulating transducer is important to ensure that consistent stimulus delivery is maintained throughout the procedure. The type of transducer that can be used is limited by the nature of the surgical approach. Typically, the pinna of the operated ear is either sutured or taped forward, towards the face and out of the way of the surgical exposure. This precludes the use of any standard supra-aural audiometric headphones. Insert earphones are invaluable for intraoperative monitoring. The insert earphone has a disposable, foam rubber tip with a tube that allows the stimulus to pass through the "ear plug" aspect of the tip. The tube in the foam rubber tip is attached to another tube connecting the plug with a small plastic box enclosing the transducer. This permits the transducer to be out of the surgical site while the tube passes under the forward-folded pinna, into the ear canal. Insert earphones are available with nearly every commercially available evoked potential system.

The timing of earphone placement must be negotiated with the other surgical partners, including the anesthesia staff, nursing staff, medical residents preparing and positioning the patient, and of course, the surgeon. It is often practical to place the insert earphones in the ear after the patient has been anesthetized but prior to the final positioning of the head, especially if the head will go into a clamp for stability. If the area behind the ear is to be shaved, that should be done before placement of the earphone. The earphone can be placed in the canal, along with an electrode to record the ECoG if needed, after shaving but before the final sterile draping and cleansing of the operative site. It is important to examine the ear canal with an otoscope prior to placing the earphone and any electrodes in the ear canal. Earwax may occlude the stimulus delivery tube, making monitoring impossible. Once the patient is prepped and in position, it is possible, but extremely difficult and disruptive, to replace an earphone. The earphone can be secured along with any electrodes in the area by covering them with bioclusive patches. These patches are available in several sizes and can be used to hold the pinna forward, secure the insert earphone in place, secure electrodes near the ear, and seal the stimulus delivery system and electrodes from liquids. The ear on the surgical side is often exposed to liquid soap, blood, CSF, and saline during the surgery. If the ear is not sealed, fluid may leak into the ear canal, creating a conductive hearing loss and artificially delaying the responses. In addition, fluid can come in contact with recording electrodes, shorting them together or serving as a recording antenna and increasing the amount of electrical noise in the recordings. All of these technical problems can be avoided by carefully sealing the ear during placement of the headphone. When folding the ear forward, make sure that there is minimal blanching of the skin on the pinna. If the pinna is folded too sharply or compressed too firmly, blood supply to the cartilage will be compromised causing postoperative problems.

Depending on the procedure, it may be necessary to place earphones in both ear canals. The nonsurgical ear will not need to be folded forward, but a bioclusive patch may still be used to secure the earphone and any electrodes at that ear. It is prudent to monitor responses from both surgical and nonsurgical sides whenever possible. If there is a technical problem with the evoked potentials system, the nonsurgical side may serve as a control recording. If alternate stimulation of the two ears (also called interleaved stimulation) is not available, it is more important to spend time monitoring the surgical side. Occasional recordings of the nonsurgical side can be made during noncritical periods during the procedure. In cases where the tumor is particularly large or wrapped around the brainstem or when the brainstem in general is in jeopardy, responses from the nonsurgical side may be helpful to the surgical team.

Once the insert earphones are secured and in place, the transducers may be fixed to the patient, the table, or the head clamp. It is important to locate the transducers as far from the recording electrodes as possible to reduce stimulus artifact. It is even more important that the transducers are located in a place where they will not get wet or be dislodged by anyone moving the patient or adjusting other devices or cables connected to the patient. Wires from the transducers to the evoked potential monitoring system should be secured firmly and routed in a course that will decrease the risk of them being pulled by activities in the operating room, ranging from moving X-ray equipment to staff walking through the room.

STIMULUS TYPE, LEVEL, AND RATE

Brief-duration tone bursts have been used (Møller, 1995), but 100-μs click stimuli are used by most clinicians. A click provides a broad-spectrum stimulus activating much of the basilar membrane. The transient stimulus serves to synchronize the response of the auditory nerve fibers, resulting in well-defined peaks in the ABR. Clicks are not frequency specific and thus are not optimal for audiometric purposes. However, they are the stimulus of choice for neurodiagnostic purposes and for intraoperative neuromonitoring.

The stimulus level will be based on the individual's preoperative hearing thresholds, the preoperative ABR results, and the recording conditions within the operating room. It is important to stimulate at a high enough level to obtain maximum amplitude responses. Normally, this would be at or above 70 dB normal hearing level (nHL). However, it is also important to not stimulate for prolonged periods of time using excessively intense stimuli that could cause cochlear trauma.

The stimulus presentation rate should be as high as the recording situation permits. The faster an average can be acquired, the sooner the monitoring clinician can interpret the responses and communicate that information to the surgical team. The limiting factor is often the limitations of the evoked potential monitoring system. Several systems can present stimuli at rates up to 100 per second. However, the data acquisition rate is often much less than that. The acquisition rate of the system is the rate at which individual sweeps are stored and averaged by the processor. Each evoked potential system requires a set amount of time to digitize each data point of a sweep, average those values with the previously acquired data, store them, and display them. We could call this administrative overhead, and it is determined by the computational speed of the computer and/or the efficiency of the data acquisition software. This may not be obvious to the user. It can be determined by measuring the amount of time it takes to acquire a predetermined number of sweeps (including the number of artifact rejected sweeps). If it takes 60 seconds to acquire 3,000 sweeps (e.g., when presenting stimuli at 100 stimuli per second), then the system is acquiring data at a rate of 50 sweeps per second. In that case, it would be a waste to stimulate at a faster rate because data would be being continually lost and the signal (ABR response) would be needlessly degraded by using a higher stimulus rate. The manufacturer should be able to provide the acquisition speed of the system. If not, one can determine it manually as described earlier.

The stimulus presentation rate may also be limited if you are presenting interleaved stimuli to both ears. Some evoked potential systems allow the user to stimulate each ear alternately and permit averaging responses to each stimulus in separate memories. This is an excellent way to continuously monitor both sides of the auditory pathway simultaneously and avoid gaps in the information available to the surgical team. However, the rate of stimulation may have to be slower to accommodate the duration of sweeps to both the right and left ears during acquisition. Stimulus rates of 30 to 50 Hz will permit nearly instantaneous recording of near-field potentials, such as the ECoG-CAP and AN-CAP, and will acquire an adequate ABR in less than 1 minute.

Recording Parameters

The two keys to successful intraoperative neuromonitoring are speed and signal-to-noise ratio. As with stimulation parameters, all recording parameters must be selected and implemented with the goal of producing the most reliable responses as quickly as possible. Electrodes must be secure and in locations that will provide large-amplitude, consistent signals. The recording devices must process the incoming signal efficiently and without adding unwanted artifacts or distortion. The system must be able to display the results in a manner that facilitates interpretation and comparison to baseline recordings.

ELECTRODES

Auditory Brainstem Response

The standard electrode montage for recording the ABR is with the noninverting (+) electrode located at the vertex (Cz) or high forehead and the inverting electrode (–) on the mastoid or ear lobe. It is unlikely that the mastoid will be available on the surgical side during a procedure, so the inverting electrode may be placed in the skin immediately anterior to the earlobe or tragus. This location will provide an ABR equivalent to that recorded using the more conventional montage. Alternative montages may be used, depending upon the number of recording channels available. A vertex (Cz) to contralateral (nonsurgical) ear channel is useful for peak identification and can be used as an ipsilateral channel if the nonsurgical side is to be monitored. Vertex (Cz) to a noncephalic site (e.g., shoulder) recorded simultaneously with an ear-to-ear channel has also been recommended.

Standard electroencephalogram (EEG) cup electrodes may be used for recording ABRs intraoperatively, but the application process is time consuming and must be done prior to the patient entering the room. Disposable "snap on" electrodes, like those used for electrocardiographic recordings, also may be used. These electrodes may be purchased in several sizes, some small enough to be practical for ABR monitoring. Skin preparation is still required to reach low electrode-skin impedances appropriate for recording, and this takes time. Standard EEG needle electrodes can be quickly applied and secured, take up little area on the patient, and can be disposable or reused given careful precautions. Needle electrodes provide consistent, stable electrode-skin impedances without skin preparation. Care must be given to avoid burns related to improper grounding of electrocautery equipment (Møller, 1995).

If needle electrodes are to be reused, they should be carefully inspected before each application and discarded if there is any sign of having bending or metal fatigue. Many needle electrodes are made of a brittle metal (platinum) that will snap if bent repeatedly. Needle electrodes may be inadvertently bent if the lead wires are tugged or strained. If a needle tip breaks off in a patient, immediately circle the entry point with some form of marking pen. Notify the surgeon. Do not attempt to remove it by probing the skin with forceps looking for the tail (broken) end of the needle.

Electrocochleography

An electrode placed on the promontory or the tympanic membrane can be used to record the ECoG. The inverting electrode is placed near the cochlea, and the noninverting electrode is placed on the opposite ear. A method for transtympanic ECoG was described by Hall (1992) in which the tip of a standard EEG needle electrode is passed through the tympanic membrane and placed on the promontory. The wire lead from the electrode passes out of the external auditory canal to the biological preamplifier. A physician should place the transtympanic electrode. This may alter the flow of setting up the patient on the operating room table. The wire and needle are held in place by the insertion of the foam plug of an insert earphone. Tape or bioclusive secures the entire system. Similarly, a tympanic membrane electrode developed by Stypulkowski and Staller (1987) can be secured in the ear canal. Premade tympanic membrane electrodes are commercially available. A tympanic membrane electrode can be safely placed by a trained nonphysician and provides a large enough signal to make signal averaging time negligible. The electrode can be inserted in the ear canal after the patient has been anesthetized. A nasal speculum can be used to open the ear canal, and the tympanic membrane will typically be seen if the overhead light is directed down the canal. The tympanic membrane electrode can be slid into the canal to the point that it makes contact with the membrane. Another alternative is to insert the tip of the needle electrode into the ear canal close to the tympanic membrane and secure it in place with the foam tip of the insert earphone. Transtympanic electrodes provide the largest signal of the three options, followed by the tympanic membrane electrode and then the canal recording.

Auditory Nerve Compound Action Potential

The AN-CAP recording electrode must be placed on the auditory nerve by the surgeon. It should be placed as soon as possible following opening of the dura and exposure of the auditory nerve in order to identify changes in function related to exposure and retraction of the cerebellum. There are at least two commercially available electrodes that are appropriate for recording CAPs from the auditory nerve (Fig. 16.6). One is a small, single contact strip electrode connected to a delicate lead wire. The strip is placed on the most proximal portion of the nerve. A cotton surgical pad may be placed over the lead wire to secure it against the cerebellum or brain-

stem and to keep it out of the way of the surgeon's field of work. An alternative is a Cueva, C-shaped self-retaining electrode (Cueva et al., 1998). This electrode is approximately 6 mm in diameter and is attached to the root entry section of the auditory nerve using an applicator. If the lead wire is pulled, the electrode is designed to detach from the nerve without causing injury. The lead from the electrode placed on the nerve is connected to the inverting input on the amplifier. The noninverting input can be connected to a sterile needle electrode placed in an exposed muscle flap in the surgical field. Either of these options will provide stable conditions for recording the AN-CAP, but the described applications are limited to suboccipital or retrosigmoid surgical approaches. If a middle cranial approach is necessary, the plate electrode may be placed between the floor of the internal auditory canal and the cochlear nerve, outside the dura as described by Roberson et al. (1996). Møller (1995) has also noted that a small wick electrode (equivalent in size to the plate electrode) can be placed in the lateral recess of the fourth ventricle to perform near-field monitoring if the CPA tumor is of sufficient size that it precludes placing an electrode on the auditory nerve.

Direct brainstem recording has been described, in which the recording electrode is attached to a retractor that is placed at the cerebellomedullary junction (Matthies and Samii, 1997a). It is claimed that ABRs recorded using this technique are 10 times greater in amplitude than those recorded using conventional methods and take only 5 to 15 seconds to average. The greater amplitude and shorter recording time have potential benefits in intraoperative monitoring. This approach makes it possible to monitor ABRs with poor morphology, enhances interpretation of ABR amplitude changes, and improves monitoring results updates.

AMPLIFICATION AND FILTERING

Biologic amplifiers that are used in the operating room must meet stricter standards than those used in the clinic. They must be optically isolated to eliminate the possibility of electrocution of the patient. The amplifiers must have an exceptionally fast recovery from saturation after an electrical overload. Electrocautery with both monopolar and bipolar cautery units will cause an amplifier to saturate or overload. During this condition, the amplifier produces no output and does not faithfully replicate the electrophysiologic activity. The recovery times of biologic preamplifiers range from a few milliseconds to several minutes. Monitoring cannot proceed during the time when the amplifier remains "blocked." Some manufacturers give specifications for amplifier recovery time, but most often, the system has to be tested under actual conditions in the operating room. For this and many other reasons, it is important to test an evoked potential monitoring system in the operating room(s) in which it will be used before buying it.

Biologic amplifiers also filter the incoming signal. Signal detection is enhanced when activity not relevant to the

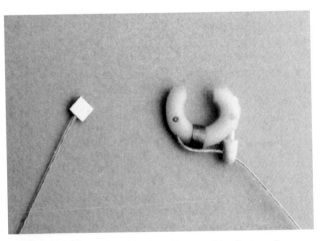

FIGURE 16.6   A single contact strip electrode (*left*) and Cueva C electrode (*right*), which can be placed directly on the eighth nerve following surgical exposure for the purpose of recording AN-CAP. (Photo provided by AD-TECH Medical Instrument Corp., Racine, WI.)

signal of interest is reduced. The ABR has spectral energy from 50 Hz to 1,000 Hz; however, in clinical practice, the lower frequency components below 100 Hz are often attenuated using high-pass filtering. This dramatically reduces the 60-Hz interference without degrading the ABR waveform. High- and low-pass filter cutoff values of 100 Hz and 2,000 Hz, respectively, are adequate for intraoperative monitoring. The slope of the high-pass filter should be 6 dB/octave. The slope of the low-pass filter may be steeper, up to 24 dB/octave. Zero phase-shift digital filtering has been described by Møller (1995) and can enhance waveforms. Unfortunately, these filters are not available on most commercially available systems.

The biologic amplifier should have exceptional common mode rejection capabilities (120 dB) in order to assist in reducing competing electrical noise found in the operating room. The input impedance of the amplifier should be high (100 MΩ), and the amplifier should be able to tolerate up to ± 1 V of direct current (DC) offset before saturating. These technical specifications will improve signal detection and reduce the possibility of errors in the amplification process.

The gain of the amplifier should be set at the highest level possible that will not produce continual artifact rejection during normal recording (i.e., not during cautery). This may differ for each type of neural activity recorded. The ABR is the smallest signal and will require the highest gain. AN-CAP activity is so large that it is often visualized in the unaveraged, raw EEG activity. To prevent amplifier overload and peak clipping of the response, a lower gain may be needed. If the patient has a pre-existing hearing loss, the amplitude of responses may be diminished. Hearing loss may decrease the amplitude of the ABR more than that of the ECoG, and therefore, the amplifier gain must be adjusted accordingly.

SIGNAL RECORDING

The duration of the sweep (also known as epoch or recording window) should be appropriate to give an accurate and easily measured picture of the response. ECoG and AN-CAP are short-latency responses that occur well within the first 10 ms following the stimulus. The ABR typically falls within that same time frame but may be prolonged due to pathology. Therefore, it is preferable to use a longer sweep duration of 15 to 20 ms for ABR recordings. Some systems permit setting the sweep duration of each recording channel. Others require one sweep duration for all channels. In the case of the latter, the selection must be made to accommodate the longest response of interest.

Artifact rejection may be employed during intraoperative monitoring as it is in other clinical settings. Some systems permit artifact rejection functions to act independently for each recording channel. This option should be used whenever possible in order to prevent a single noisy channel (having many sweeps rejected) from slowing down the averaging process for the rest of the acquisition channels. The primary cause of artifact will be electrocautery. Some systems provide the user with a sensing device that can be connected to the

cautery units. Whenever they are activated, amplifiers are automatically grounded, and averaging ceases temporarily. Averaging is the process most responsible for increasing the signal-to-noise ratio of the response. The actual acquisition and averaging of individual sweeps occurs at a rate determined by the computational speed of the computer and the efficiency of the acquisition program. It may or may not be equivalent to the stimulus rate (as discussed in some detail earlier).

The marked difference in signal size between the different auditory evoked potential components means that a different number of sweeps may need to be averaged for each. The AN-CAP is by far the largest signal and will require as few as 5 or 10 sweeps to obtain an average. That takes less than 1 second. The ECoG-CAP is also relatively large and, depending on the patient's preoperative hearing ability, may take from 1 to 20 seconds to obtain an adequate averaged response. The ABR, by comparison, is much smaller and will require from 10 seconds to 2 minutes to obtain an average. As a result, there may be times of critical surgical activity in which the monitoring emphasis will be placed upon the AN-CAP and ECoG-CAP. By monitoring these two responses, rapid, nearly real-time information can be provided to the surgical team.

Response Measurement and Clinical Interpretation

In clinical diagnostic electrophysiology, measures of waveform latencies and amplitudes are compared with appropriate normative values. The interpretation is based on the variation of the patient's response from the normal range. However, during intraoperative monitoring, each patient serves as his or her own control, and comparisons are made between baseline recordings and measures taken at later times during the procedure. The measures used in both situations are often very similar. However, repeated measures are made during monitoring, and interpretation is made in terms of the changes that are observed during the course of the operation.

By itself, ECoG is not helpful for neuromonitoring because it only evaluates the most distal end of the auditory pathway. All surgical interventions will take place rostral to the generator of the ECoG-CAP, making it of little value for tracking the effects of surgical procedures. However, it remains useful as a stable and readily recorded reference point from which interpeak intervals to later waves may be measured.

Useful measures for the ABR during monitoring include the latencies of waves I, III, and V; however, some waves may not be present due to pre-existing pathology. The I-III, I-V, and III-V interpeak intervals as well as the wave V amplitude are also useful if present. In cases of pre-existing hearing loss, wave I of the ABR may be too low in amplitude to be readily recorded. In this case, the N1 of the ECoG-CAP is an excellent alternative and reference point for measuring interpeak intervals. It is important to have wave I latency as a reference point for interpeak measures. Absolute latencies may be affected by a change in stimulus level due to technical problems (e.g., displaced transducer, blood in the ear canal). Wave I serves as the anchor and reference point to account for peripheral events. The interpeak intervals serve as indicators of neural conduction time. If increases are noted in the III-V interval, this suggests that there are changes in function of the structure rostral to the generators of wave III. In these cases, Møller (1995) suggests that systemic changes, such as changes in cerebral circulation, could be occurring and that the anesthesiologist should be notified. If wave III can be recorded, changes in the I-III interpeak interval can be used to identify changes in auditory nerve function. Matthies and Samii (1997b) reported that the disappearance of wave III was the earliest and most sensitive measure and highly predictive of postoperative deafness and, therefore, recommend that special attention be paid to deterioration of wave III. They also noted that wave III was particularly sensitive to specific surgical maneuvers during eighth-nerve tumor resection. Specifically, pulling of the tumor-nerve bundle down or laterally, drilling, and direct nerve manipulation caused deterioration of wave III, which was correlated with postoperative hearing loss. The loss of wave V was the most definite indicator of postoperative deafness, but it did not predict whether the loss would be permanent or temporary. The loss of V was the least helpful sign because it typically followed earlier warning signs, the loss of waves I and/or III. In general, the ABR shows high sensitivity but poor specificity (high false-positive rate) for predicting postoperative hearing loss (Colletti et al., 1998).

The latency of the N1 of the AN-CAP and the P1-N1 amplitude are valuable measures, and the morphology of the AN-CAP is also very informative. The amplitude of the AN-CAP is directly proportional to the number of active auditory nerve fibers. If fibers are damaged, asynchronous firing or conduction blocks will decrease the amplitude of the AN-CAP. Stretching of the auditory nerve (e.g., during cerebellar retraction) will increase the latency of the AN-CAP N1 but not necessarily decrease the amplitude. A nearly total conduction block of the auditory nerve will eliminate only the negativity (N1) of the normally triphasic waveform, leaving only a positive (P1) peak (Fig. 16.7) (Møller, 1988; 1995). Normally, the initial positive peak in the AN-CAP is likely generated as the depolarizing front of the auditory nerve action potential approaches the recording electrode and the negative peak generated as the action potential passes over the electrode. If the nerve is damaged just distal to the electrode, the depolarizing front approaches, but never passes, the electrode. Changes in the AN-CAP are the most responsive indicators of trauma to the auditory nerve that currently can be monitored (Colletti et al., 1998).

Many evoked potential monitoring systems today permit the "trending" of data over time. That is, repeated measurement (e.g., I-III interpeak intervals) can be tracked and displayed automatically in graphical form. This data reduc-

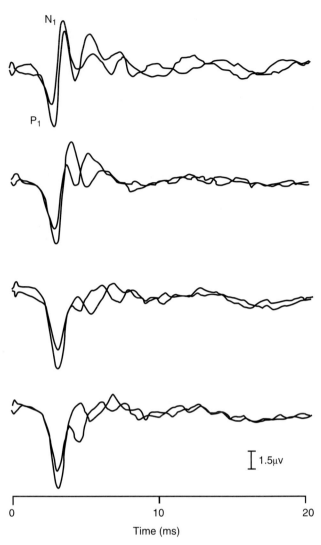

FIGURE 16.7 Auditory nerve compound action potential (AN-CAP) recorded sequentially (top to bottom) during a microvascular decompression of the trigeminal nerve. The initial triphasic waveform was reduced to a single positive peak (P1) indicating a total conduction block. (Reprinted with permission from Møller AR. [1995] *Intraoperative Neurophysiologic Monitoring.* Luxembourg: Harwood Academic Publishers; p 98.)

tion is helpful but should not replace actual inspection of the averaged waveforms. Changes in morphology of the AN-CAP may not translate directly into trending values. It is advisable to display a cascade view of sequentially recorded waveforms (e.g., Figs. 16.8, 16.9, 16.11, and 16.15) for continuous visual evaluation.

Documentation of services and results is very important. A "paper trail" must be in place for billing and audit purposes to demonstrate that the service was provided. This can be in the form of notes in the patient's chart at the time of surgery, a hard copy of waveform measures taken during the procedure, data storage of the individual waveforms, and the final report of the results delivered to the surgeon and patient's chart. The record should include times of recordings, times and comments about anesthesia levels, blood pressure and temperature, and notation of any comments made to the surgeons. These documents become essential if there should be any unfortunate outcomes that lead to litigation.

Anesthesia and Temperature Effects

The ECoG-CAP and AN-CAP are extremely resistant to the effects of anesthesia. The ABR is not affected by barbiturates, benzodiazepines, ketamine, nitrous oxide, propofol, and muscle relaxants. Halogenated agents probably have a mild effect on ABR latency and amplitude that is proportional to the administered dosage (Nuwer, 1986). There is active research on using AEPs in monitoring depth of general anesthesia. While AEPs by themselves do not show high degrees of accuracy in predicting anesthesia levels (46%), when combined with other monitoring modalities (e.g., EEG), they are shown to improve predicting capabilities to 90% or better (Jeleazcov et al., 2006). AEP and EEG parameters have also been used to determine consciousness during surgery (Schneider et al., 2005). Some studies have concluded that AEP monitoring can help titrate the volatile anesthetic and lead to a significant reduction in the anesthetic requirement (Recart et al., 2003).

ABR latency and amplitude are systematically affected by core body temperature. As temperature is decreased below 35°C, there is a prolongation of latencies and interpeak intervals and a decrease in the amplitude of all waves (Stockard et al., 1978).

Criteria for Warning

Some clinicians support an arbitrary warning criterion of a 50% decrease in amplitude and/or a 10% increase in latency for any evoked potential being monitored. These are not unreasonable criteria, but they have not been demonstrated to be predictive of postoperative function for monitoring of the auditory system. It is preferable to report any change in the response beyond the test-retest variability permitted by the conditions that cannot be accounted for by the effects of anesthesia or other technical factors.

A strategy for communication must be established between the neuromonitoring clinician and the surgical team prior to the surgery. The surgeon and monitoring staff should discuss the case prior to the surgery to determine what structures are at risk and what monitoring will be appropriate. During the procedure, communication must be bidirectional: the monitoring team providing the surgeons with relevant information as needed and the surgeons informing the monitoring group of actions that may warrant special attention. The monitoring team may also need to communicate with the anesthesia staff to gain information about blood pressure, temperature, and the type and level of anes-

thetic agents employed. Each surgeon will have his or her own preference for how changes in responses are communicated to him or her. It is also helpful if the entire operating room staff is familiar with the neuromonitoring process and importance.

STRATEGIES FOR INTRAOPERATIVE AUDITORY EVOKED POTENTIAL MONITORING

Hearing Preservation

The most common application of auditory evoked potential intraoperative monitoring will be for the purposes of hearing preservation. If a relatively small tumor is to be resected (<2 cm in diameter), it will often be possible to monitor the ECoG-CAP, AN-CAP, and ABR on the surgical side. The same applies for removal of other CPA tumors; microvascular decompression procedures of cranial nerves VII, VIII, and IX; and vestibular nerve sections. As tumor size increases, it is less likely that an electrode can be placed to record the AN-CAP. In those cases, ECoG-CAP and ABR on the operated side should be monitored along with ABR on the nonoperated side.

CASE 1

Figure 16.8 illustrates changes of the AN-CAP during resection of a 1.9-cm vestibular schwannoma from a 33-year-old man (Colletti and Fiorino, 1998). His preoperative puretone average (PTA) was 26 dB hearing level (HL), and speech recognition was 90%. There were some changes in the waveform during tumor resection, but the AN-CAP was present (at a lower than original amplitude) at closing. The postoperative PTA was 47 dB HL, and the speech discrimination was 70%.

CASE 2

A 39-year-old man, with a 2-cm diameter vestibular schwannoma on the right side, presented with vertigo and a sense of fullness and tinnitus on the right but with normal puretone thresholds, word recognition, and ABR. Hearing preservation was a high priority. ECoG, AN-CAP, and ABR were all simultaneously monitored and are presented in Figures 16.9A and 16.9B. The nerve and tumor were exposed with little deterioration of the various responses. In some cases, recordings of the ECoG and AN-CAP were stored before an adequate average of the ABR could be obtained (Fig. 16.9A). Small changes in the AN-CAP N1 during drilling of the canal were reported to the surgeon who interrupted the procedure long enough for the responses to recover before proceeding. The first marked change in response occurred when the vestibular nerve was sectioned in order to remove the tumor (Fig. 16.9B; AN-CAP waveforms; transition between the first

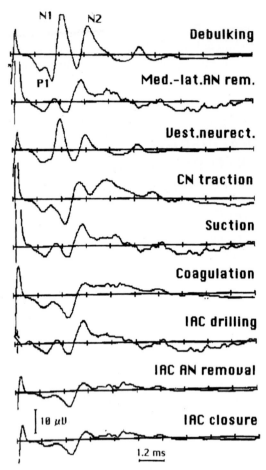

FIGURE 16.8 Sequence of auditory nerve compound action potential (AN-CAP) recorded during a retrosigmoid-transmeatal removal of a 1.9-cm vestibular schwannoma from a 33-year-old man for the purposes of hearing preservation (Case 1). The most significant change in the waveform accompanied sectioning of the vestibular nerve. AN, auditory nerve; Vest. neurect., vestibular neurectomy; CN, cranial nerve; IAC, internal auditory canal. (Reprinted with permission from Colletti V, Fiorino FG. [1998] Advances in monitoring of seventh and eighth cranial nerve function during posterior fossa surgery. *Am J Otol.* 19, 506.)

and second waveforms from the top). The ABR showed significant deterioration during the latter stages of the tumor resection but partially recovered during closing (Fig. 16.9B; last record). Pre- and postoperative audiometric results are shown in Figures 16.10A and 16.10B, respectively. Normal hearing was preserved through 4 kHz, as was word recognition.

Case 3

A 62-year-old woman with a 1.5-cm vestibular schwannoma located within the left internal auditory canal presented with vertigo, unilateral tinnitus, and a mild unilateral left, high-

frequency hearing loss but with normal word recognition and normal ABR results. Hearing preservation was a high priority. Simultaneous, multilevel monitoring was performed (Fig. 16.11). It became apparent in the early stages of resection that the tumor was integrated into both the vestibular and acoustic sections of the eighth nerve. Despite a cautious approach by the surgeon, including breaks when changes in the AN-CAP were identified, the responses deteriorated during tumor resection. Note the deterioration of the AN-CAP N1 and corresponding deterioration of the ABR while the ECoG N1 remains unchanged. A total conduction block of the auditory nerve is indicated by the presence of the AN-CAP P1 with an absent N1 (Fig. 16.11; fourth AN-CAP recording from the top). Note the corresponding absence of an ABR during the same recording period. No hearing was present after the procedure.

In some cases, multilevel monitoring may fail to preserve hearing but remains beneficial to the surgeon by providing instructional information about surgical maneuvers that result in damage to the auditory pathway. Two examples follow.

Case 4

A 66-year-old woman with a 2.5-cm vestibular schwannoma located in the right CPA presented with vertigo; unilateral tinnitus; a mild to severe, sloping, high-frequency hearing loss; impaired word recognition; and increased ABR I-III and I-V interpeak intervals. Hearing preservation was attempted. Despite the tumor size and location, an electrode was placed upon the root entry zone of the eighth nerve into the brainstem, and multilevel monitoring was performed. Figure 16.12 presents results of the AN-CAP monitoring and shows that the responses abruptly disappeared during tumor resection. No postoperative hearing was present. A review of the procedure, including a video, and the time sequence of the AN-CAP recordings revealed that the responses disappeared as the tumor was peeled off the nerve in a medial direction. The conclusion was that the eighth nerve was avulsed from the temporal bone during the peeling due to medially directed pressure on the nerve.

Case 5

A 44-year-old woman with a 1.5-cm left vestibular schwannoma located completely within the internal auditory canal presented with unilateral tinnitus, a sense of fullness, a moderate left high-frequency hearing loss, impaired word recognition, and prolonged ABR I-III and I-V interpeak intervals. Hearing preservation was attempted using multilevel monitoring. Figure 16.13 presents the results of ECoG monitoring and shows that the tumor was exposed without change of the ECoG-CAP. While drilling the bone of the internal auditory canal to expose the tumor, the ECoG-CAP, as well as the AN-CAP and ABR, abruptly disappeared. Only a low-amplitude, broad peak remained in the ECoG recording, which is believed to be the SP. The tumor was completely resected, and

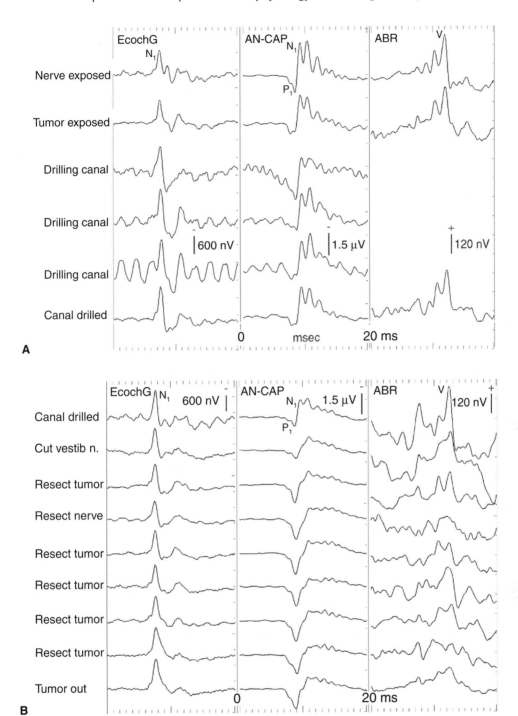

FIGURE 16.9 (A) Simultaneous, multilevel monitoring of electrocochleography (ECoG), auditory nerve compound action potential (AN-CAP), and auditory brainstem response (ABR) during removal of a 2-cm diameter vestibular schwannoma on the right side in a successful attempt to preserve hearing in a 39-year-old man (Case 2). The surgical team was notified of each small shift in latency of the AN-CAP N1 (the first large upward peak). The surgical team responded by letting the nerve recover to baseline values before proceeding. **(B)** Continuation of recordings from the same case as shown in Figure 16.9A (Case 2). Cutting the vestibular nerve had a marked effect on the AN-CAP N1 and the ABR. Responses remained stable throughout the tumor resection, and hearing was preserved. Note the relatively noisy quality of the ABR recordings compared to the ECoG and AN-CAP recordings.

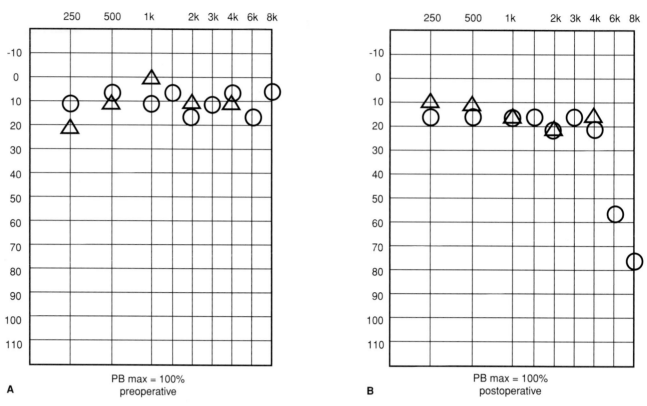

FIGURE 16.10 (A) Pre- and **(B)** postoperative audiometric and speech results from the case illustrated in Figures 16.9A and 16.9B (Case 2). Note that hearing function below 4 kHz and word recognition were both preserved following tumor resection.

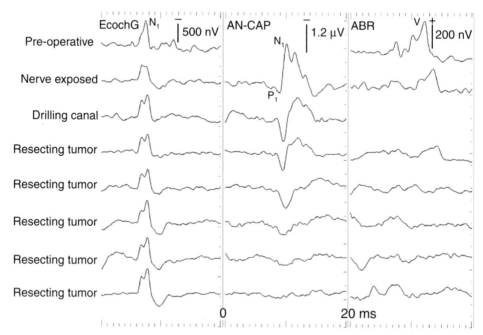

FIGURE 16.11 Simultaneous, multilevel monitoring of electrocochleography (ECoG), auditory nerve compound action potential (AN-CAP), and auditory brainstem response (ABR) during removal of a 1.5-cm diameter vestibular schwannoma on the left side in an unsuccessful attempt to preserve hearing in a 62-year-old woman (Case 3). The tumor was involved in both the vestibular and acoustic divisions of the eighth nerve. As a consequence, tumor resection resulted in a total conduction block of the CAP, producing only a P1 in the AN-CAP recordings and eliminating the ABR (fourth waveforms from the bottom). Note that the ECoG-CAP, distal to the procedure, remained stable.

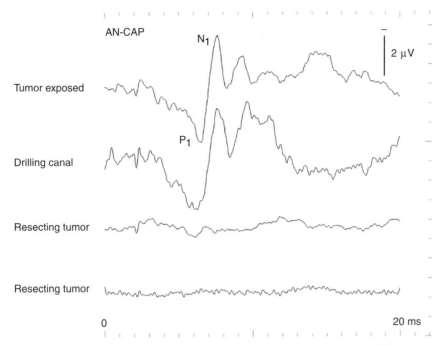

FIGURE 16.12   Auditory nerve compound action potential (AN-CAP) recorded from the eighth nerve at the root entry zone from a 66-year-old woman during resection of a 2.5-cm vestibular schwannoma located on the right side (Case 4). The responses abruptly disappeared during tumor resection. It was concluded that medial tension on the nerve caused avulsion from the temporal bone. Hearing was not preserved.

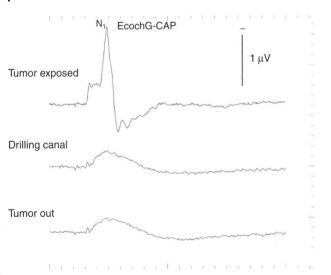

FIGURE 16.13   Electrocochleography (ECoG) compound action potential (CAP) recorded from the tympanic membrane of a 44-year-old woman during resection of a 1.5-cm left vestibular schwannoma located completely within the internal auditory canal (Case 5). During tumor exposure by drilling, the ECoG-CAP, as well as the auditory nerve compound action potential (AN-CAP) and auditory brainstem response (ABR), abruptly disappeared. A low-amplitude, broad peak remained in the ECoG recording, which is probably the summating potential. Hearing was not preserved. It was concluded that the blood supply to the cochlea was lost during drilling, most probably due to vasospasm.

the eighth nerve remained anatomically intact. No postoperative hearing was present. It was concluded that the blood supply to the cochlea was lost during drilling, most probably due to vasospasm.

Hearing Restoration

A second, far less frequent application of auditory evoked potential monitoring is for hearing restoration. Hearing may be temporarily compromised by pressure exerted by a CPA tumor or cyst on the auditory nerve. Removal of the offending growth can restore some or all hearing function. Monitoring during these procedures can track improvements, providing the surgical team with information about the positive consequences of their efforts, and help the team from injuring auditory structures directly.

CASE 6

Kileny et al. (1998) present an interesting report on a patient discovered to have a 2.5-cm diameter meningioma in the right CPA. The patient had a mild to profound right-side sensory-neural hearing loss with no measurable word recognition. The preoperative ABR on the right was severely abnormal, with only wave I reliably identified (Fig. 16.14). In contrast, transient evoked otoacoustic emissions from the right cochlea were essentially normal. This indicated that cochlear function was intact and suggested the possibility of hearing restoration. ABRs were monitored during the surgery (Fig. 16.15). This provided documentation of recovery and protection of restored function. The ABR

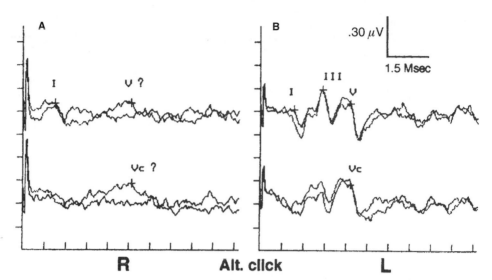

FIGURE 16.14 Preoperative auditory brainstem responses (ABRs) recorded prior to resection of a 2.5-cm diameter meningioma in the right cerebellopontine angle (CPA; Case 6, Figs. 16.14 to 16.17). Ipsilateral recordings are in the top records, and contralateral recordings are below. **(A)** Recordings from the tumor side (right ear). The patient had a mild to profound, right-side sensory-neural hearing loss with no measurable word recognition. Transient evoked otoacoustic emissions from the right cochlea were essentially normal. **(B)** Recordings from the nontumor side (left ear). R, right; L, left. (Reprinted with permission from Kileny PR, Edwards BM, Disher MJ, Telian SA. [1998] Hearing improvement after resection of cerebellopontine angle meningioma: case study of the preoperative role of transient evoked otoacoustic emissions. *J Am Acad Audiol.* 9, 252.)

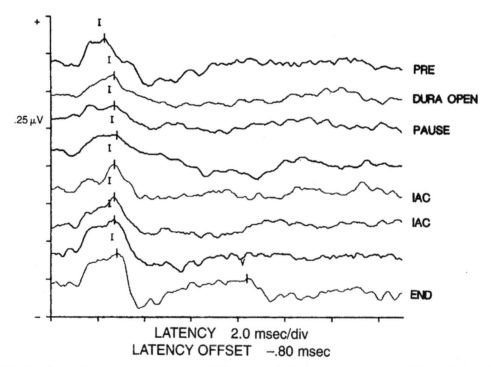

FIGURE 16.15 Auditory brainstem responses (ABRs) recorded on the surgical side (right ear) during the tumor resection described in Case 6. The ABR recovered slightly during the procedure and was present but abnormal at the end of surgery. IAC, internal auditory canal. (Reprinted with permission from Kileny PR, Edwards BM, Disher MJ, Telian SA. [1998] Hearing improvement after resection of cerebellopontine angle meningioma: case study of the preoperative role of transient evoked otoacoustic emissions. *J Am Acad Audiol.* 9, 253.)

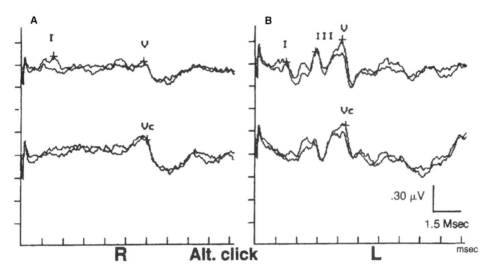

FIGURE 16.16   Postoperative auditory brainstem responses (ABRs) from Case 6 at 3 months after tumor resection. Ipsilateral recordings are in the top records, and contralateral recordings are below. **(A)** Results from the surgical side. The I-V interpeak interval is prolonged; however, wave V is clearly present. **(B)** Recordings from the nonsurgical side. R, right; L, left. (Reprinted with permission from Kileny PR, Edwards BM, Disher MJ, Telian SA. [1998] Hearing improvement after resection of cerebellopontine angle meningioma: case study of the preoperative role of transient evoked otoacoustic emissions. *J Am Acad Audiol.* 9, 254.)

recovered slightly during the procedure and was present, but still abnormal, after the surgery (Fig. 16.16). Hearing function recovered to normal and remained so at last report, 3 years after the procedure (Figs. 16.17A and 16.17B). Others have reported hearing restoration following removal of small eighth-nerve tumors assisted by intraoperative neuromonitoring (Fischer et al., 1980).

Life Preservation

In cases having very large brainstem tumors (>3 to 4 cm in diameter), it is unlikely that preoperative hearing will be present on the tumor side. In such cases, it still may be useful to monitor ABR function for the purpose of life preservation. In these cases, the ABR contralateral to the surgical

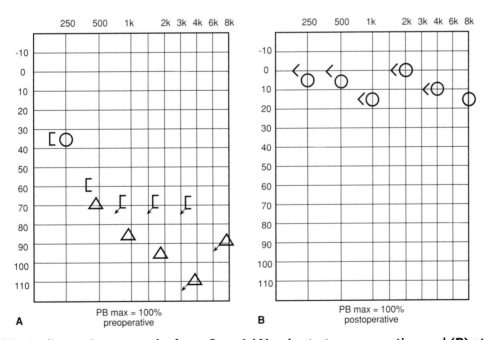

FIGURE 16.17   Audiometric test results from Case 6 **(A)** prior to tumor resection and **(B)** at 3 months after the procedure. Note the significant improvement in hearing at all frequencies. (Reprinted with permission from Kileny PR, Edwards BM, Disher MJ, Telian SA. [1998] Hearing improvement after resection of cerebellopontine angle meningioma: case study of the preoperative role of transient evoked otoacoustic emissions. *J Am Acad Audiol.* 9, 252–253.)

side may be monitored. Changes in wave V will represent changes in function of the pons to midbrain region of the surgical side and may assist the surgical team in evaluating the consequences of their efforts. It has been reported that changes in the ABR contralateral to the tumor preceded changes in blood pressure as a result of pressure on the brainstem (Møller, 1995). The ABR is therefore useful to assist the surgical team in determining the safe limits of tumor.

▚ EFFICACY

The literature regarding the effectiveness of auditory evoked potential monitoring in hearing preservation during CPA surgery is muddled by the myriad of factors that can influence outcomes. Problems with comparing studies result from the following unresolved differences:

1. The number of surgeons involved in the study, their skill levels, and, more importantly, their personal philosophies regarding hearing preservation and utilizing monitoring.
2. Different surgical approaches that may or may not be related to the location of the tumor.
3. Mixing several pathologies into one study.
4. The type of monitoring applied in the study, ranging from using one (ECoG-CAP, AN-CAP, or ABR) to using all three.
5. Different criteria for what was considered a critical change in the evoked potential response.
6. A different criterion for what was considered hearing preservation. Some studies used a 50 dB PTA/50% word recognition criterion, others used 70 dB PTA/15% recognition, and others used any hearing versus no hearing.

It is not too surprising that, using such varied experimental conditions and criteria, the results of the studies should conflict.

Two studies contend that auditory evoked monitoring did not improve hearing preservation (Cohen et al., 1993; Kveton, 1990). In contrast, at least 10 studies state that the monitoring did improve hearing preservation (Fischer et al., 1980; Jannetta et al., 1984; Radtke et al., 1989; Slavit et al., 1991; Fischer et al., 1992; Harper et al., 1992; Kurokawa et al., 1992; Matthies and Samii, 1997b; Colletti and Fiorino, 1998; Colletti et al., 1998). Of particular interest was a report by Colletti and Fiorino (1998) in which outcomes of cases monitored by just ABR or ABR and AN-CAP were compared. Both groups were matched for preoperative audiometric PTAs (500 Hz to 3 kHz). Postoperatively, the ABR-only group had significantly poorer PTAs (82.5 dB) than did the ABR and AN-CAP monitored group (54.1 dB).

Recent studies indicate that the type of surgery should be taken into consideration when interpreting how ABR changes during surgery may predict postoperative hearing outcomes. It seems that, for non-CPA tumor surgeries, such as microvascular decompressions, hearing loss usually oc-

curs only with permanent loss of wave V, whereas much smaller changes in wave V may be indicative of severe hearing impairment in CPA tumor surgeries (James and Husain, 2005).

The need to use a standard hearing outcome rating has been emphasized (Hardy, 2000). A number of studies have reported their results using the Gardner-Robertson Scale, which defines postoperative hearing in five categories: I (excellent) – average PTA at 30 dB HL or better with speech discrimination (SD) at 70% or better; II (serviceable) – PTA between 31 and 50 dB HL with SD between 50% and 69%; III (not serviceable) – PTA between 51 and 90 dB HL with SD between 5% and 49%; IV (poor) – PTA greater than 90 dB HL with SD below 5%; and V (deaf) – no hearing. It has been suggested that a Gardner-Robertson Scale rating of I should be used as the gold standard for good hearing preservation outcome in surgeries involving risks to auditory function.

It is becoming increasingly evident that multilevel monitoring, whenever possible, affords the most opportunity for hearing preservation. Monitoring with the ABR alone should be done only in cases of large tumors, with no ipsilateral hearing, and when the contralateral ABR is to be monitored. Otherwise, ECoG-CAP should be used to ensure the presence of a reliable wave I as a reference for interpeak measures. AN-CAP recordings are the most rapidly recorded and sensitive to changes in auditory nerve function and are to be used whenever it is technically feasible.

Special Techniques

The previously described methods of recording AN-CAP used monopolar recording techniques. It is also possible to use a bipolar recording electrode, which has some distinct advantages and provides alternative methods of nerve identification. Rosenberg et al. (1993) developed a bipolar electrode recording probe (BERP) and a technique for identifying the cochlear and vestibular divisions of the eighth cranial nerve. In roughly 25% of cases, it is difficult or impossible to visually identify the cleavage plane between the cochlear and vestibular divisions of the nerve, significantly increasing the risk for hearing loss during vestibular neurectomy. The two tips of the bipolar electrode served as the noninverting and inverting recording electrodes. The tips of the BERP touched lengthwise along the exposed eighth nerve during recording (Fig. 16.18). A response during stimulation with click stimuli indicates that the probe is contacting the cochlear division of the nerve. No response indicates that the probe is touching the vestibular division (Fig. 16.19). The nerve can be mapped and the cleavage plane identified prior to nerve sectioning. Click stimuli were presented at a level of ≤25 dB sensation level (SL; above the patient's threshold for the click). Higher level stimuli resulted in current spread of the signal to the vestibular division of the nerve and decreased the specificity of the response. Very low–level stimulation increased specificity but required a longer averaging time, making multiple, repeated tests impractical.

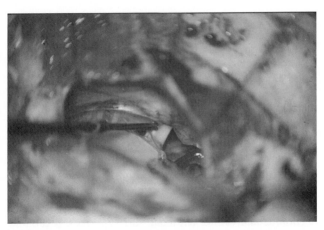

FIGURE 16.18   Bipolar electrode recording probe placed on the exposed eighth nerve prior to a vestibular nerve section. The probe is on the cochlear division, near the cleavage plane between the cochlear and vestibular divisions of the nerve. The probe tips must be placed along the longitudinal axis of the nerve during recording. The cochlear division is slightly brighter than the vestibular division in this case, making visual differentiation between the divisions relatively easy. (Reprinted with permission from Rosenberg SI, Martin WH, Pratt H, Schwegler JW. [1993] Bipolar cochlear nerve recording technique: a preliminary report. *Am J Otol.* 14, 364.)

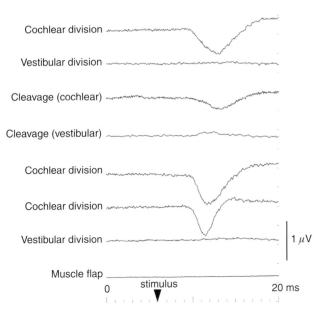

FIGURE 16.19   Recordings of eighth-nerve activity made with a bipolar electrode recording probe prior to sectioning the vestibular nerve in a 41-year-old woman with a history of treatment-resistant vertigo and right classic Ménière's disease (Case 7). Click stimuli presented at 25 dB SL produced well-defined responses when the probe tips were placed on the cochlear division. When the probe tips were placed on the vestibular division, no response could be recorded. A control recording from the muscle flap also yielded no response. (Reprinted with permission from Rosenberg SI, Martin WH, Pratt H, Schwegler JW. [1993] Bipolar cochlear nerve recording technique: a preliminary report. *Am J Otol.* 14, 364.)

CASE 7

A 41-year-old woman with a history of treatment-resistant vertigo and right classic Ménière's disease underwent a vestibular nerve section (adapted from Rosenberg et al., 1993). The cleavage plane was visually identified and

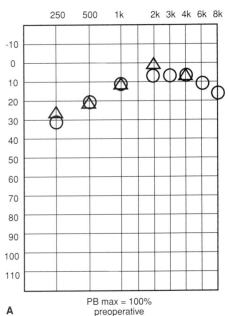

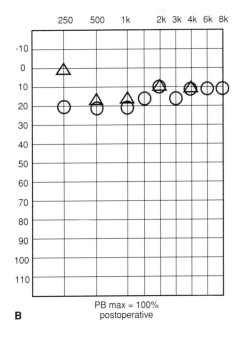

FIGURE 16.20 Audiometric and word recognition test results (A) prior to and (B) following vestibular nerve section in Case 7 (see Fig. 16.19). Hearing function was preserved.

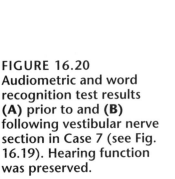

confirmed electrophysiologically by recording eighth-nerve activity using the BERP in response to 25-dB SL click stimuli (Fig. 16.19). Pre- and postoperative audiometric puretone and word recognition scores indicated no deterioration of auditory function as a result of the procedure (Figs. 16.20A and 16.20B).

Colletti and Fiorino (1998) demonstrated the same principle applied to differentiating between the auditory nerve and an eighth-nerve tumor. Responses were obtained from nerve tissue but not from tumor. This information is particularly useful when a surgeon has exposed the tumor and is developing a strategy for tumor resection with hearing preservation. Butler et al. (1995) also used a bipolar recording electrode for identifying auditory nerve tissue to improve hearing preservation during vestibular schwannoma resection. Instead of using click stimuli and averaging the AN-CAP, a 500-Hz tone is presented continually via headphone to the patient. The unaveraged signal recorded from the bipolar recording probe is amplified and routed to a speaker so the surgical team can hear the activity. When the recording probe is in contact with audi-tory nerve tissue, a 500-Hz tone is immediately broadcast from the speaker. This method provides real-time identification of nerve tissue in a way similar to that of broadcasting facial electromyography following direct facial nerve stimulation.

CONCLUSIONS

Intraoperative neurophysiologic monitoring of the auditory system is a useful tool to the surgeon when he or she anticipates the possibility of damage to auditory structures during a surgical procedure. Monitoring cannot compensate for poor technique and cannot eliminate surgical errors. It can and does reduce postoperative morbidity by providing the surgeon with additional information about the functional status of the structures involved that would not be available otherwise. In the hands of a trained neuromonitoring clinician and an informed surgeon, appropriate, multilevel auditory evoked potential monitoring will surely benefit the patient.

REFERENCES

Butler S, Coakham H, Maw R, Morgan H. (1995) Physiological identification of the auditory nerve during surgery for acoustic neuroma. *Clin Otolaryngol.* 20, 312–317.

Cohen NL, Lewis WS, Ransohoff J. (1993) Hearing preservation in cerebellopontine angle tumor surgery: the NYU experience 1974-1991. *Am J Otol.* 14, 423–433.

Colletti V, Fiorino FG. (1998) Advances in monitoring of seventh and eighth cranial nerve function during posterior fossa surgery. *Am J Otol.* 19, 503–512.

Colletti V, Fiorino FG, Mocella S, Policante Z. (1998) ECochG, CNAP and ABR monitoring during vestibular schwannoma surgery. *Audiology.* 37, 27–37.

Cueva RA, Morris GF, Prioleau GR. (1998) Direct cochlear nerve monitoring: first report on a new atraumatic, self-retaining electrode. *Am J Otol.* 19, 202–207.

Deupree DL, Jewett DL. (1988) Far-field potentials due to action potentials traversing curved axon, reaching cut nerve ends, and crossing boundaries between cylindrical volumes. *Electroencephalogr Clin Neurophysiol.* 70, 355–362.

Durrant JD, Martin WH, Hirsh B, Schwegler JW. (1994) 3CLT ABR analyses in human subject with unilateral extirpation of the inferior colliculus. *Hear Res.* 72, 99–107.

Fischer G, Costantini JL, Mercier P. (1980) Improvement of hearing after microsurgical removal of acoustic neuroma. *Neurosurgery.* 7, 154–159.

Fischer G, Fischer C, Remond J. (1992) Hearing preservation in acoustic neurinoma. *J Neurosurg.* 76, 910–917.

Grundy BL, Lina A, Procopio PT, Jannetta PJ. (1981) Reversible evoked potential changes with retraction of the eighth cranial nerve. *Anesth Analg.* 60, 835–838.

Hall JW III. (1992) Intraoperative monitoring. In: *Handbook of Auditory Evoked Responses.* Needham Heights, MA: Allyn and Bacon; p 521.

Hardy DG. (2000) Acoustic neuroma surgery as an interdisciplinary approach. *J Neurol Neurosurg Psychiatry.* 69, 147–148.

Harper CM, Harner SG, Slavit DL, et al. (1992) Effect of BAEP monitoring on hearing preservation during acoustic neuroma resection. *Neurology.* 42, 1551–1553.

Hashimoto I, Ishiyama Y, Totsuka G, Mizutani H. (1980) Monitoring brainstem function during posterior fossa surgery with brainstem auditory evoked potentials. In: Barber C, ed. *Evoked Potentials.* Lancaster, United Kingdom: MTP Press Limited; pp 377–390.

James ML, Husain AM. (2005) Brainstem auditory evoked potential monitoring: when is change in wave V significant? *Neurology.* 65, 1551–1555.

Jannetta PJ, Møller AR, Møller MB. (1984) Technique of hearing preservation in small acoustic neuromas. *Ann Surg.* 200, 513–523.

Jeleazcov C, Schneider G, et al. (2006) The discriminant power of simultaneous monitoring of spontaneous electroencephalogram and evoked potentials as a predictor of different clinical states of general anesthesia. *Anesth Analg.* 103, 894–901.

Jewett DL. (1970) Volume conducted potentials in response to auditory stimuli as detected by averaging from the cat. *Electroencephalogr Clin Neurophysiol.* 28, 609–618.

Jewett DL, Deupree DL. (1989) Far-field potentials recorded from action potentials and from a tripole in a hemicylindrical volume. *Electroencephalogr Clin Neurophysiol.* 72, 439–449.

Jewett DL, Deupree DL, Bommannan D. (1990) Far-field potentials generated by action potentials of isolated sciatic nerves in a spherical volume. *Electroencephalogr Clin Neurophysiol.* 57, 105–117.

Jewett DL, Romano MN, Williston JS. (1970) Human auditory evoked potentials: possible brain stem components detected on the scalp. *Science.* 167, 1517–1518.

Jewett DL, Williston JS. (1971) Auditory-evoked far fields averaged from the scalp of humans. *Brain*. 94, 681–696.

Kileny PR, Edwards BM, Disher MJ, Telian SA. (1998) Hearing improvement after resection of cerebellopontine angle meningioma: case study of the preoperative role of transient evoked otoacoustic emissions. *J Am Acad Audiol*. 9, 251–256.

Kimura J, Kimura A, Ishida T, Kudo Y, Suzuki S, Machida M, Matsuoka H, Yamada T. (1986) What determines the latency and amplitude of stationary peaks in far-field recordings? *Ann Neurol*. 19, 479–486.

Kimura J, Mitsudojme A, Yamada T, Dickins QS. (1984) Stationary peaks from a moving source in far-field recording. *Electroencephalogr Clin Neurophysiol*. 58, 351–361.

Kurokawa Y, Uede T, Hashi K. (1992) Functional results of preservation of cranial nerves in removal of acoustic neurinoma. *No Shinkei Geka*. 10, 139–145.

Kveton JF. (1990) The efficacy of brainstem auditory evoked potentials in acoustic tumor surgery. *Laryngoscope*. 100, 1171–1173.

Lang J. (1985) Anatomy of the brainstem and the lower cranial nerves, vessels, and surrounding structures. *Am J Otol*. November (suppl), 1–19.

Levine RA. (1980) Monitoring auditory evoked potentials during acoustic neuroma surgery. In: Silverstein H, Norell H, eds. *Neurological Surgery of the Ear*. Eugene, OR: Aesculapius Publishing Co; pp 287–293.

Levine RA, Montgomery WW, Ojemann RG, Pringer MFB. (1978) Evoked potential detection of hearing loss during acoustic neuroma surgery. *Neurology*. 28, 339.

Martin WH, Jewett DL, Williston JS, Gardi JN. (1987a) The 3-channel Lissajous' trajectory of the auditory brainstem response. III. Formation, analysis and reliability of planar segments in the cat. *Electroencephalogr Clin Neurophysiol*; 68:333-340.

Martin WH, Pratt H, Schwegler JW. (1995) The origin of the human auditory brainstem response wave II. *Electroencephalogr Clin Neurophysiol*. 96, 357–370.

Martin WH, Sininger YS, Jewett DL, Gardi JN, Morris JH III. (1987b) The 3-channel Lissajous' trajectory of the auditory brainstem response. II. Methodology. *Electroencephalogr Clin Neurophysiol*. 68, 327–332.

Matthies C, Samii M. (1997a) Direct brainstem recording of auditory evoked potentials during vestibular schwannoma resection: nuclear BAEP recording. Technical note and preliminary results. *J Neurosurg*. 86, 1057–1062.

Matthies C, Samii M. (1997b) Management of vestibular schwannomas (acoustic neuromas): the value of neurophysiology for intraoperative monitoring of auditory function in 200 cases. *Neurosurgery*. 40, 459–468.

Møller AR. (1988) *Evoked Potentials in Intraoperative Monitoring*. Baltimore: Williams & Wilkins.

Møller AR. (1995) *Intraoperative Neurophysiologic Monitoring*. Luxembourg: Harwood Academic Publishers; pp 45–126.

Møller AR, Jannetta PJ. (1982) Compound action potentials recorded intracranially from the auditory nerve in man. *Neurology*. 78, 144–157.

Møller AR, Jannetta PJ. (1983) Auditory evoked potentials recorded from the cochlear nucleus and its vicinity in man. *J Neurosurg*. 59, 1013–1018.

Møller AR, Jannetta PJ, Jho HD. (1994) Click-evoked response from the cochlear nucleus: a study in humans. *Electroencephalogr Clin Neurophysiol*. 92, 215–224.

Møller AR, Jannetta PJ, Sekhar LN. (1988) Contributions from the auditory nerve to the brainstem auditory evoked potentials (BAEPs): results of intracranial recording in man. *Electroencephalogr Clin Neurophysiol*. 71, 198–211.

Møller AR, Jho HD. (1991) Compound action potentials recorded from the intracranial portion of the auditory nerve in man: effects of stimulus intensity and polarity. *Audiology*. 30, 142–163.

Møller AR, Jho HD, Yokota M, Jannetta PJ. (1995) Contribution from crossed and uncrossed brainstem structures to the brainstem auditory evoked potentials (BAEP): a study in humans. *Laryngoscope*. 105, 596–605.

Morest DK. (1975) Structural organization of the auditory pathways. In: Tower D, ed. *The Nervous System; Human Communication and Its Disorders*. New York: Raven Press; p 22.

Nakinishi T. (1982) Action potentials recorded by fluid electrodes. *Electroencephalogr Clin Neurophysiol*. 53, 343–345.

Nakinishi T. (1983) Origin of action potentials recorded by fluid electrodes. *Electroencephalogr Clin Neurophysiol*. 55, 114–115.

Nuwer MR. (1986) Brainstem auditory monitoring and related techniques. In: *Evoked Potential Monitoring in the Operating Room*. New York: Raven Press; pp 158–161.

Pratt H, Bleich N, Martin WH. (1985) Three-channel Lissajous' trajectories of the human auditory brain-stem evoked potentials. I. Normative measures. *Electroencephalogr Clin Neurophysiol*. 61, 530–538.

Radtke RA, Erwin CW, Wilkins RH. (1989) Intraoperative brainstem auditory evoked potentials: significant decrease in postoperative morbidity. *Neurology*. 39, 187–191.

Raudzens P, Shetter A. (1981) Intraoperative brain stem potentials. Presented at the 50th Annual Meeting of the American Association of Neurological Surgeons, Boston, MA, April 5–9.

Recart A, Gasanova I, et al. (2003) The effect of cerebral monitoring on recovery after general anesthesia: a comparison of the auditory evoked potential and bispectral index devices with standard clinical practice. *Anesth Analg*. 97, 1667–1674.

Roberson J, Senne A, Brackmann D, Hitselberger WE, Saunders J. (1996) Direct cochlear nerve action potentials as an aid to hearing preservation in middle cranial fossa acoustic tumor resection. *Am J Otol*. 17, 653–657.

Rosenberg SI, Martin WH, Pratt H, Schwegler JW. (1993) Bipolar cochlear nerve recording technique: a preliminary report. *Am J Otol*. 14, 362–368.

Schneider G, Hollweck R, et al. (2005) Detection of consciousness by electroencephalogram and auditory evoked potentials. *Anesthesiology* 103, 934–943.

Slavit DH, Harner SG, Harper CM Jr, Beatty CW. (1991) Auditory monitoring during acoustic neuroma removal. *Arch Otolaryngol Head Neck Surg*. 117, 1153–1157.

Starr A. (1976) Auditory brain stem response in brain death. *Brain*. 99, 543–554.

Starr A, Achor LJ. (1975) Auditory brainstem responses in neurological disease. *Arch Neurol*. 32, 761–768.

Starr A, Hamilton AE. (1976) Correlation between confirmed sites of neurological lesions and abnormalities of far-field auditory brain stem responses. *Electroencephalogr Clin Neurophysiol*. 41, 595–608.

Stegeman DF, Van Oosterom A, Colon EJ. (1987) Far-field evoked potential components induced by a propagating generator: computational evidence. *Electroencephalogr Clin Neurophysiol*. 67, 176–187.

Stockard JJ, Rossiter K. (1977) Clinical and pathologic correlates of brainstem auditory evoked response abnormality. *Neurology.* 27, 316–325.

Stockard JJ, Sharbrough F, Tinker J. (1978) Effects of hypothermia on the human brain stem auditory response. *Ann Neurol.* 3, 368–370.

Stypulkowski PH, Staller SJ. (1987) Clinical evaluation of a new ECoG recording electrode. *Ear Hear.* 8, 304–310.

Williston JS, Jewett DL, Martin WH. (1981) Planar curve analysis of the three-channel auditory brainstem response: a preliminary report. *Brain Res.* 223, 181–184.

17 Middle Latency Auditory Evoked Potentials: Update

Anthony T. Cacace and Dennis J. McFarland

INTRODUCTION

Middle latency auditory evoked potentials (MLAEPs) occur in a time frame from approximately 15 to 70 ms. Over the years, this class of evoked potentials has been alluring to researchers, relevant for students, and potentially important for clinicians based on its presumed value in estimating auditory thresholds and in assessing higher order auditory processes. Herein, we update information on this topic focusing on anatomy and generator sites, theoretical and practical recording considerations, and topics relevant to clinical concerns. Our review on this topic is illustrative but not exhaustive.

ANATOMIC FRAME OF REFERENCE

Knowledge of thalamic and cortical anatomy is necessary to understand MLAEPs. In this regard, the auditory thalamus (medial geniculate nucleus [MGN]) is an integral component of the subcortical auditory pathways (Fig. 17.1). On route to the cerebral cortex, ascending thalamocortical fibers course through the sublenticular portion of the internal capsule (Truex and Carpenter, 1964) whereby the ventral division of MGN projects to the core or primary-like areas of auditory cortex located on the superior aspect of the temporal lobe; the dorsal division of MGN projects more diffusely (Rauschecker et al., 1997; Rauschecker, 1998). The ventral MGN sends direct projections in parallel to primary and rostral areas of auditory cortex, which have a propensity to be highly responsive to puretone stimuli. The dorsal medial

and other aspects of the MGN send direct inputs to caudal-medial aspects of auditory cortex. These caudal-medial areas of auditory cortex respond preferentially to more complex broadband stimuli. Auditory cortical regions also project back to the medial geniculate regions from which they receive projections (Pandya et al., 1994). Thus, both feedforward and feedback neural projections coexist. These reciprocal relationships allow thalamocortical circuits to be interactive with the environment, thus allowing spectral and/or temporal transformations of stimulus representations to dynamically modify perception and behavior. In this regard, the classical view of the thalamus as being merely a "passive relay area" requires modification and updating (Winer et al., 2005).

The auditory cortex consists of a core area on the superior temporal plane (including Heschl's gyrus) (Fig. 17.2A). The core contains three cochleotopically organized fields that are highly responsive to puretone stimuli (Kaas et al., 1999). The core area is surrounded by a belt of association areas, which in turn are surrounded by parabelt association areas, extending to the lateral surface of the superior temporal gyrus. The belt also receives afferent input from the core area and dorsal divisions of the medial geniculate complex, with minor projections from ventral and medial geniculate areas. The parabelt has strong connections with the belt area and minimal connections with the core and receives thalamic inputs in parallel with belt inputs across its subdivisions. Additionally, the belt and parabelt zones consist of several regions that are distinct in terms of cyto-architecture and connections (Hackett et al., 1999). A block diagram from Kaas et al. (1999) summarizes known neuroanatomic relationships relevant to higher level thalamocortical processing

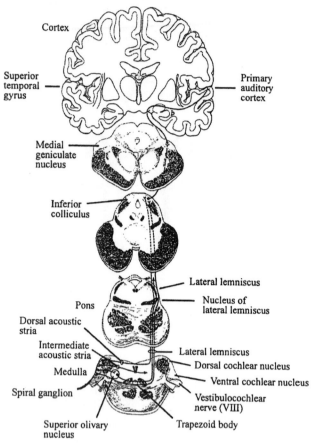

Cortex

Superior
temporal
gyrus

Primary
auditory
cortex

Medial
geniculate
nucleus

Inferior
colliculus

Lateral lemniscus

Pons

Nucleus of
lateral lemniscus

Dorsal acoustic
stria

Intermediate
acoustic stria

Lateral lemniscus

Medulla

Dorsal cochlear nucleus

Ventral cochlear nucleus

Spiral ganglion

Vestibulocochlear
nerve (VIII)

Superior olivary
nucleus

Trapezoid body

FIGURE 17.1 Diagram of the central auditory system emphasizing subcortical pathways from cochlear nucleus to primary auditory cortex. Of particular interest is the medial geniculate nucleus of the thalamus. From this level, thalamocortical axons course through the sublenticular process of the internal capsule and terminate in superior temporal gyrus. (Adapted from Kelly JP. [1985] Auditory system. In: Kandel ER, Schwartz JR, eds. *Principles of Neural Science.* 2nd ed. New York: Elsevier; pp 396–408, with permission.)

(Fig. 17.2B) described earlier. There is also speculation and some support for the view that these various auditory association areas may be specialized for processing distinct auditory features, such as temporal and spatial information, in a manner analogous to what has been described in visual cortical areas (Rauschecker et al., 1997). Polysensory regions of the temporal, parietal, and frontal cortices also receive input from auditory cortex (Pandya, 1995). Thus, there are both feedforward and feedback connections within and between subregions, including connections with multimodal insula and the superior temporal sulcus and long association connections with amygdala and prefrontal cortex. Indeed, these complex connections within auditory cortex, various multimodal association areas, and other regions in the mesial temporal lobe fall within the framework of contemporary neuroanatomic investigation. Whereas much of

the empirical information described herein is derived from studies of the macaque monkey and cat, contemporary neuroanatomic staining methods and various imaging-related activation studies suggest that human auditory cortex can be subdivided into at least eight different putative regions (Rivier and Clarke, 1997). Human investigations continue to be elaborated upon by the increased use of functional neuroimaging methodology (Melcher et al., 1999; Schönwiesner et al., 2002; Rao and Talavage, 2005).

GENERAL CONCEPTUAL FRAMEWORK OF AUDITORY EVOKED POTENTIALS

For students embarking in the area of electrophysiologic investigation, the neuroanatomic and biophysical underpinnings of these responses are particularly important. Because of known complexities of structure and function, a degree of sophistication and background training is necessary to proceed in a competent manner. However, a degree of caution is also required when it comes to interpreting these data. This is understandable because electrical activity measured from scalp electrodes in response to sensory stimulation represents the sum (superposition) of the electrical fields projected by all active sites at any given point in time. These include thalamic nuclei, the ascending thalamocortical fibers, primary auditory and auditory association areas, polysensory association areas, and inter- and intracortical fiber tracts. The polarity, spatial distribution, and whether or not electrical potentials generated from brainstem or from within the brain can even be detected at the scalp by surface electrodes depend, in large part, on the underlying geometry (organizational matrix) of active cell populations. To emphasize this point, idealized and highly schematic examples of the spatial organization of different cell patterns and the resultant electric field distributions from these populations of cells are shown in Figure 17.3. This schema, based on the work of Lorente de Nó (1947), forms the basis of the transformation of electric activity from near-field (intracranial) to far-field potentials detectable at the scalp. Therefore, one needs to be cognizant of this information when considering generator sources as well as the limitations of surface recordings. In this context, populations of neurons (cell bodies and their respective dendrites) can be regarded as sources of electrical current with a positive charge at one location and negative charge at another (so-called stationary dipoles). For different populations of neurons in the central nervous system (CNS), the electric field distributions have been classified as closed (Figs. 17.3A and 17.3B), open (Fig. 17.3C), and open-closed fields (Fig. 17.3D). In an open field configuration, if all dendrites from these populations of cells are orientated in the same general direction, then in theory, the far-field potentials will be large and easily detectable at the scalp. The morphologic polarization of pyramidal cells with long and

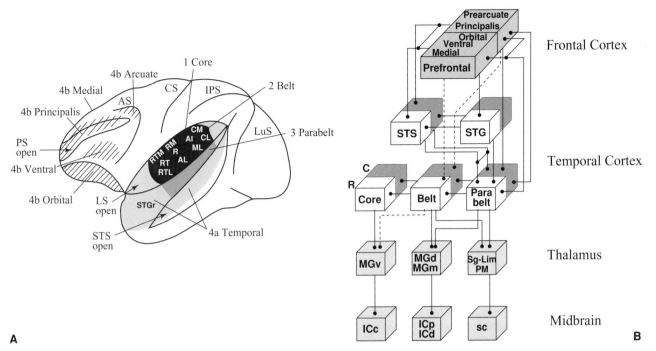

FIGURE 17.2 (A) Schemata of contemporary auditory cortical neuroanatomy based on levels and regions of processing. In this representation, the lateral sulcus (LS) is opened to show auditory areas of the lower bank, and the superior temporal sulcus (STS) has been opened to show the extension of auditory-related cortex in this sulcus. Level 1 represents the core (darkest shading); level 2 represents the belt (moderate shading); level 3 represents the parabelt (light shading); level 4a represents the temporal region (dense hatching); and level 4b represents the frontal region (sparse hatching). In this diagram, the following abbreviations are used: AL, anterolateral; AS, arcuate sulcus; CL, caudolateral; CS, central sulcus; IPS, intraparietal sulcus; LuS, lunate sulcus; ML, middle lateral; PS, principle sulcus; RM, rostromedial; RTL, lateral rostrotemporal; RTM, medial rostrotemporal; STGr, rostral superior temporal gyrus. **(B)** Block diagram providing details of known connections and levels of processing to the primate auditory cortex. The *solid lines* represent major connections, and the *dashed lines* represent minor connections. According to this framework, the main stream of processing involves the central nucleus of the inferior colliculus (ICc), the ventral nucleus of the medial geniculate complex (MGv), and the core areas of the auditory cortex. A parallel stream involves the dorsal (ICd) and pericentral (ICp) divisions of the inferior colliculus, the dorsal (MGd) and medial (MGm) divisions of the medial geniculate complex, and the belt cortex. The superior colliculus (SC) projects to parts of the medial pulvinar (PM), suprageniculate (Sg), and limitans (Lim) nuclei, as a possible third source of input to the parabelt cortex. Additional levels of processing include cortex of the superior temporal gyrus (STG), adjoining belt and parabelt regions, superior temporal sulcus (STS), and prefrontal cortex. The preferential connections of rostral (R) and caudal (C) sectors of cortex are indicated. (Both the anatomic representation and block diagram are taken from Kaas JH, Hackett TA, Tramo MJ. [1999] Auditory processing in primate cerebral cortex. *Curr Opin Neurosci.* 9, 164–170, with permission.)

vertically directed apical dendrites that terminate in the most superficial layers of cortex (gyral crests) can be characterized in this manner. Such cell populations, which line the walls of sulci, can generate both strong electric and extracranial magnetic fields (Lewine and Orrison, 1999). In neocortical tissue, which is composed of characteristic cell layers, the polarity of the sources and resultant fields are thought to be at a right angle to the plane of the surface and are consistent with this notion of cell distribution (Nunez, 1995).

However, in populations of neurons in which the cell bodies are positioned in the center with dendrites projecting in all directions (so-called closed fields or open-closed field configurations; Figs. 17.3A, 17.3B, and 17.3D),

the amplitudes of the resultant far-field electric potentials will be much smaller. In fact, they may not be detectable at the scalp at all. This observation results from the fact that various components of these electric fields can cancel each other. Complications for surface recordings from human auditory cortex also arise from the inherent convoluted nature and complex three-dimensional geometry of the superior temporal plane. Galaburda and Sanides (1980, p 603) report that the superior temporal plane is "one of the most highly folded in the human brain." Furthermore, individual differences complicate matters further by introducing additional variability between hemispheres and brains.

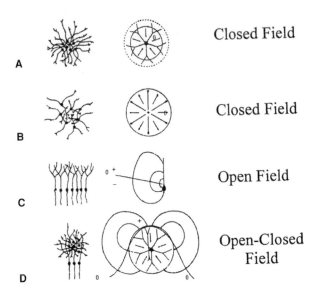

FIGURE 17.3 Examples of (**A and B**) closed, (**C**) open, and (**D**) open-closed fields for different populations of neurons in the central nervous system (CNS). The left column represents different populations of neurons; the right column represents activated neuronal populations together with arrows representing the lines of current flow at the instant when the impulse has invaded the cell bodies. The zero (0) indicates the isopotential line. In A, the schematic depicts the oculomotor nucleus with dendrites oriented radially outward. The isopotential lines are circles with current flowing entirely within the nucleus. This results in a closed field with all points outside the nucleus remaining at zero potential. In B, the schematic depicts the neurons of the superior olive having dendrites oriented radially inward. Here also, the currents result in a closed field. In C, the accessory olive is represented by single neurons and associated long dendritic processes. In this arrangement, the sources and sinks permit the spread of current in the volume of the brain, and this results in an open-field configuration. In D, two structures mixed together generate an open-closed field. (Adapted from Lopes da Silva F, Van Rotterdam A. [1999] Biophysical aspects of EEG and magnetoencephalogram generation. In: Niedermeyer E, Lopes da Silva, eds. Electroencephalography: Basic Principals, Clinical Applications and Related Fields. 4th ed. Baltimore: Williams & Wilkins; pp 93–109, based on the work of Lorente de No [1947], with permission.)

Given the spatial geometry of active cell populations in both the thalamus and on the superior temporal plane, the resultant electric fields in response to acoustic stimulation should project toward the top of the head and be maximum at medial-central and/or anterior-central locations. Moreover, these potentials, which are localized at central scalp locations, should be diffuse because, in theory, their sources are at

a distance. In these circumstances, electric-field projections should be broader with greater distance from the generator source. This is in contrast to the projections from auditory association areas on the lateral surface of the temporal lobe, which in theory should produce more focal and lateralized scalp distributions because the generators are closer to the scalp. Recent evidence and other supporting data show that there is considerable divergence in the auditory thalamocortical pathway (Winer et al., 2005), and consequently, this results in more complex radial and tangential cell orientations, as previously reported (Cetas et al., 1999). Thus, based on empirical evidence and results from modeling experiments, we assume that multiple sources are simultaneously active in the middle (approximately 15 to 70 ms) and longer (>70 and <256 ms) latency range and that there is considerable overlap in both their temporal and spatial distributions. This should be kept in mind when considering the issue of spatial sampling (i.e., the number of electrodes necessary to delineate MLAEPs) and the complexities involved in component waveform identification and recovery.

■ RECORDING CONSIDERATIONS

In audiology clinics, auditory evoked potential (AEP) studies generally use surface electrodes. Electrode placement on the surface of the scalp is based on specific conventions. This allows for standardization that enables comparisons to be made between different laboratories and countries (Jasper, 1958; Sharbrough et al., 1991).

Generally, middle latency recordings are based on single-channel recordings (Thornton et al., 1977; Musiek et al., 1984), from linear arrays (Cohen, 1982; Scherg and von Cramon, 1986a), or from more comprehensive matrix designs (Wood and Wolpaw, 1982; Jacobson and Grayson, 1988; Cacace et al., 1990; Yvert et al., 2001).

A restrictive set of MLAEPs may be recorded from a single channel, with electrodes placed, for example, at the vertex (noninverting electrode), a known reference site (inverting electrode), and ground (common). Evoked potentials recorded from just two electrodes (active and reference) can be compared to sampling the waveform with only two points in time (Lopes da Silva, 1999). Auditory brainstem responses (ABRs) are far-field potentials that produce broadly distributed responses from peripheral and brainstem auditory pathways (Møller, 1988); however, MLAEPs originate from sources closer to the surface of the scalp. As a result, MLAEPs show more variation with electrode position, and consequently, some degree of spatial sampling appears necessary. Most early MLAEP studies were limited to single-channel recordings (Mendel, 1985).

The electrical potential recorded at any electrode, at any point in time, can be regarded as the signal of interest corrupted with unwanted noise. If the noise is random and uncorrelated with the signal, then averaging of multiple samples can improve the signal-to-noise ratio proportional to the square root of N, where *N* is the number of samples in the average (Lopes da Silva, 1999; see Chapter 11). In theory, by averaging many poststimulus epochs of an electroencephalogram (EEG), the noise component decreases toward zero, and the AEP waveform can be extracted from the noise. This is the most common analytical strategy for capturing the reactivity of "synchronized" EEG to a sensory stimulus (Dawson, 1951; 1954). This processing technique and its underlying assumptions fall under the heading of the "additive model." The additive model assumes that data from the individual trials are composed of a linear combination of stimulus (or time-locked activity) and background noise. However, a shortcoming of the additive model is the way in which non–stimulus-locked activity (i.e., induced, emergent, or unlocked activity) is handled (Baar and Bullock, 1992; Ohl et al., 2003; McFarland and Cacace, 2004). The unlocked activity involves two additional types of signals that are embedded in the ongoing background EEG. These signals include: (1) EEG that is *reactive* to the stimulus but *not* locked to the event, and (2) unwanted noise. This distinction is important because the additive model treats all EEG activity not time locked to the stimulus as noise. As a result, unlocked, induced, or emergent activity is eliminated from the time-domain average by phase cancellation. Unlocked activity is largely rhythmic or oscillatory in nature, and therefore, it does not have a fixed waveform. In this context, the unlocked component represents those frequency-dependent changes in EEG rhythmicities that are modulated by sensory stimulation. The point is that these oscillatory dynamics thought to underlie EEG reactivity cannot be captured by signal averaging in the time domain, and therefore, alternative methods such as frequency-domain analysis are needed (Cacace and McFarland, 2006). Precisely how important this is for MLAEPs is not entirely known, although unlocked oscillatory activity is a rich source of information about brain function in perceptual, cognitive, and motor paradigms (Baar and Bullock, 1992; Snyder and Large, 2005). With more complex tasks used to elicit longer latency AEPs (i.e., oddball or other cognitive-related paradigms; see Chapter 18), research has shown that unlocked EEG spectral power is associated with attended targets during a frequency discrimination task (McFarland and Cacace, 2004). Additionally, Kruglikov and Schiff (2003) have shown that MLAEPs vary with the phase of the background EEG. They suggest that a new conceptualization is needed to account for their findings. Phase resetting may also have important implications related to perception (Ross et al., 2004a; 2005).

Ultimately, the more effective the clinician/researcher is in isolating and removing sources of noise contamination during data acquisition, the better the recordings will be. Noise sources can be picked up by induction, including extracranial electrical fields such as the 60-Hz noise from nearby power lines (50 Hz in Europe) and electrical potentials resulting from the movement of the wires connecting the electrodes to the amplifying system. Other intracranial

TABLE 17.1	Middle latency electromyographic (EMG) potentials
Reflex	**Description**
Postauricular muscle	Variable from subject to subject and even within subjects. Large negative peak at 11.8 ± 0.8 ms and positive peak at 16.4 ± 0.7 ms.
Temporalis muscle	Very easily recordable from subjects with clenched teeth. Large negative peak at 17.2 ± 1.9 ms and positive peak at 22.8 ± 2.8 ms.
Neck muscles	Recordable from the inion. Begins as early as 7.4 ms. Has multiple components: negative waves at 11.3 + 0.2 and 24.6 ± 1.5 ms and positive waves at 16.8 + 2.4 and 33.8 ± 0.5 ms.
Frontalis muscle	Highly variable response. There is usually a distinct positive component at approximately 30 ms.

Adapted from Picton TW, Hillyard SA, Krausz HI, Galamabos R. (1974) Human auditory evoked potentials: I. Evaluation of components. *Electroencephalogr Clin Neurophysiol.* 36, 179–190.

nonauditory noise sources include low-frequency potentials induced by lateral eye movements, higher frequency fields resulting from vertical eye movements (blinks), and broadband signals resulting from electromyographic (EMG) activity. Distinguishing true "*neurogenic*" from "*myogenic*" activity has complicated the interpretation of MLAEPs for some time (Cacace and McFarland, 2002). Sources of EMG contamination are provided in Table 17.1. Moreover, if the underlying noise (lateral eye movements, eye blinks, EMG) is in-phase (i.e., time-locked) with stimulus presentation rate (e.g., 50 to 60 Hz or a harmonic thereof), then the signal averaging strategy discussed earlier will not be successful. In summary, to improve the quality of the recorded potentials, it is generally considered advisable to minimize and/or control as best as possible exogenous and endogenous artifacts and sources of contamination.

Bandwidth is another important consideration in recording MLAEPs. Scherg (1982) has reported that MLAEPs are readily detectable with averaging over a relatively wide bandwidth (1.0 Hz to 5,000 Hz). Campbell and Leandri (1984) have demonstrated that filtering can introduce temporal and amplitude distortions and artifacts that may not be distinguishable from true potentials. With available technology, it is possible to design an optimal filter for detecting middle latency components, but this requires knowledge of relevant signal-processing issues. Alternative signal-processing methods, such as correcting for latency jitter (Lopes da Silva, 1999), may also prove useful for improving signal-to-noise ratio. In the audiologic literature, technical considerations related to temporal and amplitude distortions have been discussed (Kraus et al., 1994). The issue of filter bandwidth is also related to the context in which MLAEPs are recorded. For example, it has been suggested that combining ABR and MLAEP recording can enhance threshold estimation for frequencies <1,000 Hz (Musiek and Geurkink, 1981; Scherg, 1982; Kavanaugh et al., 1984). In this context, the filter's passband needs to be relatively broad to accommodate both ABR and MLAEP spectra. The digital signal-processing strategy of Scherg (1982), including dual artifact rejection algorithms and broad bandwidth (1.0 to 5,000 Hz), appears optimal for these types of recordings. However, the variability of MLAEP detection during different stages of sleep complicates broad bandwidth recordings, particularly when estimating frequency-specific thresholds in infants and young children. In contrast to combining ABRs and middle latency responses (MLRs), others have focused on the simultaneous recording of middle and longer latency AEPs (Cacace et al., 1990; Wood and Wolpaw, 1982; Knight et al., 1988). In this context, the low-pass cutoff frequency can be more restrictive, and the passband of 1.0 to 300 Hz is adequate.

The middle latency waveform has been characterized by the amplitude and latency of individual components, by means of area under the curve, or by spectral analysis. Various authors describe different numbers of middle latency potentials. Musiek et al. (1984) identify four positive and three negative waves at the vertex, which they label as Po, Na, Pa, Nb, Pb, Nc, and Pc, similar to the nomenclature used by Thornton et al. (1977). Celesia and Brigell (1999) describe three negative and two positive middle latency waves, while Scherg (1982) identifies a single negative and positive peak. Pynchon et al. (1998) describe a procedure involving baseline correction, rectification, and integration of the vertex waveform across an interval determined by the latency of Na and Nb. The rational for this method is based on the premise that it "is believed to represent the total amount of neural energy contributing to the evoked response" (Pynchon et al., 1998, p 1). As noted earlier, because the potential recorded at the scalp evoked by acoustic stimulation is the superposition of electrical fields projected by all active underlying neural sources and because sources may cancel, the net projection will vary with the point on the scalp being considered. Thus, it is unlikely that an integration of the scalp waveform at a single point on the scalp represents the total amount of neural energy contributing to the evoked potential.

While standardized electrode placements are important for continuity and comparison of results between laboratories, the site of the reference (inverting) electrode is particularly important in recordings that are limited to a single channel or when a few channels are used during data acquisition.

Reference (Noninverting) Electrode

An electrical potential on the scalp, or any other place for that matter, is always recorded between two points. Although some recording montages are referred to as being monopolar, they are in fact recordings between two electrodes: an electrode of interest and a shared reference (or common, when truly a monopolar recording). The potential waveform recorded at any noninverting electrode varies with the reference electrode site used (Gencer et al., 1996). If sources are modeled as dipoles, then a given component will be larger when it is close to the electrode in question and parallel in orientation to a line drawn between the electrode and the reference.

Wolpaw and Wood (1982) suggest that the optimal site for a reference electrode is the place on the head or body where the potential field is most stable. This ensures that changes in the evoked potential field over time reflect changes in the vicinity of the recording electrode(s) and not a complex combination of changes at both reference and recording electrode locations. The balanced noncephalic sternovertebral reference of Stephenson and Gibbs (1951) is an optimal choice for AEP recordings. Chen et al. (1997) have shown that MLAEPs are larger with a balanced noncephalic reference as compared to linked earlobes. Importantly, if hemispheric asymmetries exist, as seen in longer latency AEPs (Wolpaw and Penry, 1975; Cacace et al., 1988), then the balanced noncephalic reference is preferred over other sites.

If clinicians are sampling from many electrodes sites on the scalp, then "reference-free derivations," such as the common average reference or the Laplacian method, can be used and may be preferred to alternative possibilities. The common average reference assumes that if one samples the time/voltage waveform at electrode locations all around the skull, the average voltage value of all points would sum to zero. In theory, this approach would provide a reference that would not favor any one electrode over another and presumably would not distort the "*true*" response. However, this assumption depends on the number of sites sampled. Rarely could one sample all locations around the skull, and as a result, significant biases can occur with this method. The Laplacian method (McFarland et al., 1997) may be used to improve the distinctiveness of the various evoked potential components. This relatively underused but powerful method is useful in helping to identify middle and long latency responses.

Defining Auditory Evoked Potential Components: Analysis Strategy

Electrode placements for clinical studies need to be based on detailed topographic studies in the time frame of interest. Figure 17.4 shows the waveforms at several recording sites (central, Cz, and temporal, T3 and T4) and detailed topographic maps in the middle latency range for two individual subjects, which are representative of average data (Cacace et al., 1990). In the middle latency range (approximately 15 to 70 ms), three components were dominant: two centered at or near the vertex (Pa [P30] and Pb [P50 or P1]) and one

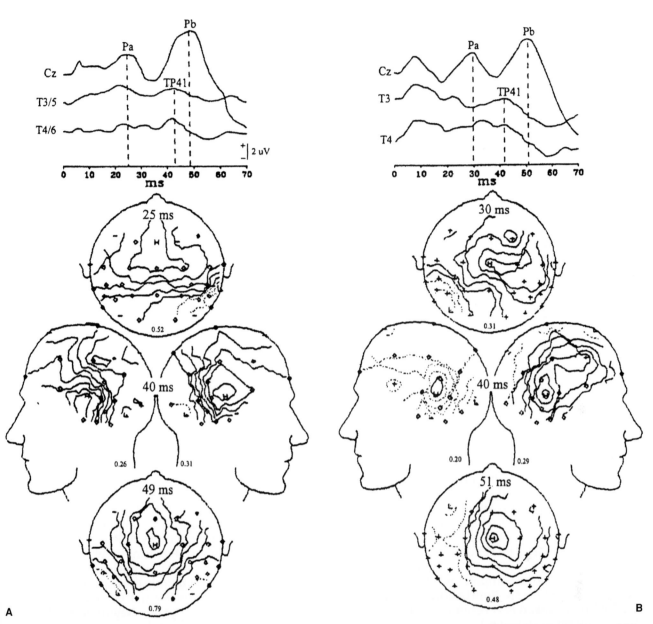

FIGURE 17.4 Middle latency waveforms and corresponding topographies for two individuals **(A and B)** at central scalp locations (Cz) and over auditory cortex on the lateral surfaces of the temporal lobes (T3/5 or T3 and T4/6 or T4). Data represented are in response to binaural clicks. Middle latency components Pa and Pb are seen in the vertex waveforms, and TP41 is seen in the temporal waveforms. The central and lateral view topographies are designated at times when components Pa, Pb, and TP41 are maximum. *Solid lines* represent positive voltages, *dashed lines* represent negative voltages; H = high point; L = low point. (Reprinted from Cacace AT, Satya-Murti S, Wolpaw JR. [1990] Middle latency auditory evoked potentials: vertex and temporal components. *Electroencephalogr Clin Neurophysiol. 77,* 6-18, with permission.)

centered over the posterior lateral surface of each temporal area (i.e., over auditory cortex [TP41]). Law et al. (1993) show that the Laplacian results enhance the temporal components of the middle and long latency response compared to the standard recordings (Fig. 17.5). The spatiotemporal dipole model of Scherg and von Cramon (1986a) also identify a radial source potential in the middle latency range that is consistent with TP41.

Møller (1994) suggests that intracerebral recordings can clarify the origin of scalp potentials, but coincidence in latencies does not necessarily constitute proof that near-field potentials are the sources of far-field potentials recorded at the scalp. For example, early cortical potentials in the middle latency range (approximately 13 ms) are small and can only be recorded from a limited area of the posterior aspect of Heschl's gyrus. Subsequent potentials recorded at 30 ms are

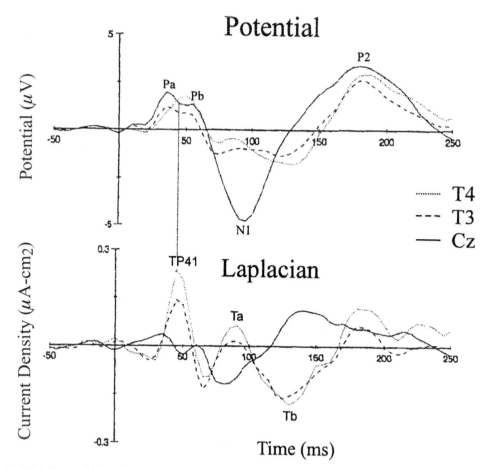

FIGURE 17.5 Middle and long latency auditory evoked potential (AEP) waveforms are compared in the standard (*top*) potential versus Lapacian derivation (*bottom*), at central (Cz) and right and left temporal lobe sites (T4, T3). Data are in response to mid-frequency tone pips presented at 50 dB sensation level (SL). The electrodes were based on 19 recording sites, referenced to a balanced sternovertebral lead. The top waveform, designated as potential, shows well-known middle and long latency AEP components at Cz (Pa, Pb, N1, P2). The temporal middle latency AEP (MLAEP) component TP41 is not well observed, and T-complex components (Ta and Tb) are obscured. However, with the Laplacian derivation (*bottom*), the MLAEP temporal component TP41 and T-complex are clearly enhanced by this transformation. (Adapted from Law SK, Rohrbaugh JW, Adams CM, Eckardt MJ. [1993] Improving spatial and temporal resolution in evoked EEG responses using surface Laplacians. *Electroencephalogr Clin Neurophysiol.* 88, 309–322, with permission.)

much larger. Liegeos-Chauvel et al. (1994) note that the response of the planum temporale is more diffuse and extended than Heschl's gyrus and, therefore, is more capable of being propagated to the surface. Hashimoto (1982) used intraventricular electrodes and found that the No-Po-Na complex appeared largest in the vicinity of the inferior colliculus. In addition, it was argued that thalamic contributions to surface recordings are minimal due to the closed-field structure of thalamic cells. Thus, the initial response of the primary auditory area is not clearly associated with a reliable scalp potential, a view that has been noted by others (Goff et al., 1977). Using evoked magnetic field recordings, Kuriki et al. (1995) observed distinct AEP components at latencies of 11 ms, 19 ms, and 33 ms in four subjects.

Middle Latency Component Pa: Evidence for Neural Origin

Human pial surface recordings demonstrate a positive peak of Pa latency over temporal and parietal lobes (Chatrian et al., 1960; Ruhm et al., 1967; Celesia, 1976; Lee et al., 1984). Human neuromagnetic recordings show a positive peak at approximately 30 ms (Pelizzone et al., 1987). A positive peak of approximately 30 ms was reported from within the brain (Goff et al., 1977). Furthermore, neuromuscular blockers do not eliminate Pa (Harker et al., 1977; Kileny et al., 1983). Multielectrode probe measures at depths above and below Heschl's gyrus failed to show a Pa phase reversal (Goff et al., 1977) (Fig. 17.6), as would occur if Pa were generated at this

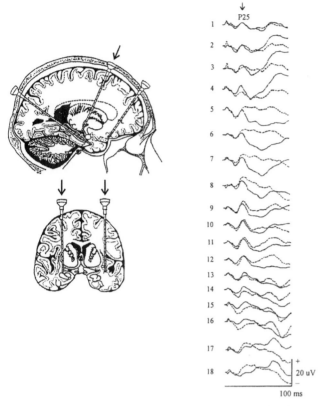

FIGURE 17.6 Middle latency auditory evoked potentials recorded from bilateral frontotemporal probes from within the human brain. *Arrows* indicate the approximate location of the probe. Each probe has 18 contact points (electrodes), with electrode 1 at the most superficial location and electrode 18 at the deepest location. Individual waveforms are grand averages, shown at the right side of the figure. Waveforms represented by *solid lines* are from the right-sided probe; *dashed lines* are from the left-sided probe. Middle latency component Pa is clearly seen at a latency approximating 25 ms. As shown in the graph (*right panel*), Pa amplitude remains relatively constant across recording locations. No phase reversal for Pa is noted at depths above and below Heschl's gyrus. (Adapted from Goff WR, Allison T, Lyons W, Fisher TC, Conte R. [1977] Origins of short latency auditory evoked potentials in man. In: Desmedt JE, ed. *Auditory Evoked Potentials in Man. Psychopharmacology Correlates of Evoked Potentials.* Karger: Basel; pp 30–44, with permission.)

site. Neuromagnetic recordings show that the supratemporal auditory cortex is active during Pa and a change in waveform morphology occurs in the anterior-posterior plane (Pelizzone et al., 1987). Pial surface recordings show a similarly oriented change (Lee et al., 1984).

Pa is unaffected by sleep apnea (i.e., ancillary evidence of a noncortical origin) (Pratt et al., 1984; Mosko et al., 1984).

Recent modeling studies suggest that Pa is produced by tangentially oriented dipole sources in auditory cortex (Scherg and von Cramon, 1986a) but could be from similarly oriented subcortical sources.

Middle Latency Component Pb: Evidence for a Neural Origin

Recordings from the pial surface in humans demonstrate a positive peak at Pb latency over temporal and parietal lobes (Chatrian et al., 1960). Human neuromagnetic recordings show a positive peak at approximately 50 ms (Farrell et al., 1980; Pantev et al., 1986; Hari et al., 1987; Pelizzone et al., 1987). A positive peak at approximately 50 ms was reported from within the brain but was less prominent than Pa (Goff et al., 1977). Pb is altered by stage of sleep (Erwin and Buchwald, 1986) and in patients with Alzheimer's disease (Buchwald et al., 1989).

MIDDLE LATENCY AUDITORY EVOKED POTENTIAL PB SOURCE

Multielectrode probe measures from within the human brain at depths above and below Heschl's gyrus failed to show a Pb phase reversal (Goff et al., 1977; Goff, 1978). Neuromagnetic recordings show that the supratemporal auditory cortex is also active during Pb and that a change in waveform morphology occurs in the anterior-posterior plane (Pellizone et al., 1987). Reite et al. (1988) suggests that the source is the planum temporale. Goff (1978) reports a positive peak comparable in latency at a depth and location corresponding to the hippocampus, and it has been shown that Pb disappears with large lesions to the hippocampus (Woods et al., 1987). Because depth recordings do not show a phase reversal across Heschl's gyrus and since Pb depends on stage of sleep, Pb may not originate in auditory cortex but in subcortical structures.

Middle Latency Auditory Evoked Potential TP41: A New Component

Because early studies have used relatively few electrodes and concentrated on central and not temporal scalp areas, the temporal middle latency component was not identified. In addition, most studies used ear or mastoid reference electrodes. Whereas these active reference electrode sites distort but do not obscure Pa and Pb, they markedly obscure and even eliminate TP41. However, it is noteworthy that the appearance of TP41 may require long interstimulus intervals (ISIs) (1 s: Knight et al., 1988; 3.3 s: Cacace et al., 1990) or pseudo-random intervals (Scherg and von Cramon, 1986a). Furthermore, TP41 may habituate to large numbers of stimuli. Nevertheless, detailed topographic analysis shows that TP41 is highly localized over lateral temporal scalp locations of each hemisphere in response to left, right, and binaural click stimulation.

TP41: EVIDENCE FOR A NEURAL ORIGIN

TP41 is undoubtedly neural in origin. In our experience, subjects were relaxed, and online monitoring of temporal channels did not show overt EMG activity. The postauricular muscle reflex is seen more anteriorly with induced muscle tension, and this component has a much shorter latency (Picton et al., 1974; Streletz et al., 1977). A positive peak of comparable latency has been seen in human pial surface recordings over lateral temporal and perisylvian regions (Ruhm et al., 1967; Celesia, 1976). Also, TP41 matches the P39 radial dipole source potentials in the left and right hemispheres hypothesized by Scherg and von Cramon (1986a) in their spatiotemporal dipole model.

▨ SUBJECT AND STATE VARIABLES

Age and Gender Effects

The middle latency components can be affected by age. McGee and Kraus (1996) have reviewed many relevant issues that are important towards understanding the complexity of maturational changes in infants and young children, which continue through the first decade of life. In adults, Kelly-Ballweber and Dobie (1984) and Woods and Clayworth (1986) found that Pa latency and amplitude increased with age throughout the life span. Gender effects were not found in the Woods and Clayworth (1986) study, and Kelly-Ballweber and Dobie (1984) only studied males. In a study limited to females, Chambers and Griffiths (1991) showed that Pa amplitude grows linearly with age, although interpretation can be complicated by changes in hearing sensitivity. In partial contrast, Erwin and Buchwald (1986) found a significant increase in Pa amplitude but not latency with age. Data of Newman and Moushegian (1989) also report larger MLAEP amplitudes in older subjects at higher stimulation rates. Amenedo and Diaz (1998) showed a positive relationship between Na-Pa amplitude and age for individuals between 20 and 86 years old.

Pfeifferbaum et al. (1979) reported that Pb (P1 or P50) amplitudes increased with age in women. However, their data are difficult to compare with other studies because they combined Pa and Pb in their data analysis. Chambers (1992) also found larger Pb amplitudes in older individuals. Using a paired-stimulus paradigm and binaural stimulation, Papanicolaou et al. (1984) showed differential recovery cycle effects on P1-N1 amplitude, characterized by a more rapid recovery in young versus older individuals. Recovery cycle effects for P1 latency, however, were not significant, and gender effects were not evaluated. With binaural stimulation, Erwin and Buchwald (1986) found longer Pb latencies in older women. They speculated that menopausal-related hormonal instability might have contributed to this finding. Spink et al. (1979) also failed to find age-related changes in Pb latency, although their sample size was small. Amenedo and Diaz

(1998) showed a positive relationship between Nb-Pb amplitude and age for individuals between 20 and 86 years old.

The middle latency component Pb is thought to be abnormal in individuals with Alzheimer's disease (AD) (Buchwald et al., 1989). In subjects with AD, Pa latencies and amplitudes were normal, but a significant decrease in Pb amplitude was found. Based on experimental animal work and human studies, Buchwald and colleagues propose that Pb is generated by cells in thalamic nuclei that receive input from cholinergic cells of the midbrain reticular activating system. They suggest that the abnormality observed with Pb in patients with AD is attributed to dysfunction in cholinergic cells in the midbrain.

With respect to AD, current interest is focused on developing physiologic biomarkers that are capable of delineating prodromal states that precede disease onset from those associated with normal aging. It is becoming established that, in the earliest phases, AD produces a relatively pure impairment in episodic memory, also known as minimal cognitive impairment (MCI). The pathophysiology of AD begins within the mesial temporal lobe, where alterations of synaptic efficacy within the hippocampus occur prior to overt neuronal degeneration (Selkoe, 2002). Early symptoms appear to correlate with dysfunction of chlolinergic and glutamatergic synapses (Small et al., 2001). Additionally, quantitative morphometric studies of biopsies obtained from temporal and frontal cortices within 2 to 4 years of onset revealed over a 25% to 35% decrease in the density of synapses per cortical neuron (Davies et al., 1987). Correlations of postmortem cytopathology with premortem cognitive deficits indicate that synapse loss is more robustly correlated with disease onset than are numbers of plaques or tangles, degree of neuronal perikaria loss, or extent of cortical gliosis (Terry et al., 1991).

Using relatively low stimulation rates, Irimajiri et al. (2005) found that the middle latency P50 (Pb) component had larger amplitudes and longer latencies in patients with AD than in age-matched controls, although there was still a modest overlap between groups. Several other studies have questioned whether Pb abnormalities can be used as a reliable marker of CNS dysfunction in AD and suggest that this abnormality is not a primary deficit (Fein et al., 1994; Phillips et al., 1997).

In patients with Parkinson's disease, an initial abnormal Pb (absence of response or prolonged latencies) was normalized following posterior ansa-pallidotomy. The restoration of Pb correlated with improvements in other areas (e.g., rigidity, tremors, and gait) and overall improvement in the Unified Parkinson's Disease Rating Scale (Mohamed et al., 1996). Using magnetoencephalography (MEG), others have also documented a Pb abnormality in Parkinson's disease (Pekkonen et al., 1998). These observations have led to studies investigating neurobiochemical differences of MLAEP generators in humans. For example, by blocking postsynaptic muscarinic receptors with scopolamine, Buchwald et al. (1991) showed that the scalp-recorded Pb is eliminated but reappears after the administration of physostigmine, a cholinergic agonist.

It is suggested that Pb depends on cholinergic mechanisms "most likely with the brainstem-thalamic component of the ascending reticular activating system" (Buchwald et al., 1991, p 308). Additionally, there was also an enhancement of Pa amplitude following scopolamine administration and a reduction in amplitude after physostigmine administration. Jääskeläinen et al. (1999) evaluated the effects of scopolamine on middle latency magnetic fields in humans with the intent of determining the role of the transmitter acetylcholine in modulating the cortical generators of Pa and Nb. Scopolamine had the effect of significantly increasing Pa amplitude.

Extremely large amplitude MLR components have been reported in individuals with problematic tinnitus (Gerken et al., 2001), an effect that may be related to alterations in inhibitory mechanisms (Gerken et al., 1996). Enhancement of steady-state magnetic fields have also been reported in patients with tinnitus problems (Diesch et al., 2004); in this study, variations in component amplitude were not observed in the normal-hearing and hearing loss groups. Whereas MLAEP amplitudes reportedly increase with age, very large amplitudes were less common in the elderly group than in the younger group with problematic tinnitus. Because increased amplitude MLAEPs have been associated with elderly individuals with MCI and with individuals with problem tinnitus, larger MLAEPs may not be pathognomonic of any particular dysfunction and may result from different underlying mechanisms.

Handedness

Hood et al. (1990) found that Pb varies with handedness, being 4 ms longer in left-handed adults. Stewart et al. (1993) also found a progressive increase in the latency of the MLAEP components in left-handed individuals, with the greatest effect being on Pb.

State Variables

Whereas MLAEPs are generally unaffected by attention (Picton and Hillyard, 1974), attention-related effects have been shown for amplitude-modulated steady-state responses (Tiitinen et al., 1997; Ross et al., 2004b). Short latency AEPs (i.e., electrocochleography and ABR) have been used in the operating room for purposes of monitoring auditory function during otologic or otoneurologic surgery (Møller, 1988). Middle latency AEPs have also been applied successfully to issues of importance to anesthesiologists (i.e., Thornton and Sharpe, 1998), such as monitoring depth of anesthesia, in the development of adaptive controllers to deliver anesthesia (Huang et al., 1999; Nayak and Roy, 1999), and in the assessment of different hypnotic states in infants and young children (Weber et al., 2004). Knowledge of anesthesia-related issues is important to audiologic testing in the operating room when assessing electrically evoked responses during cochlear implant surgery. Kileny et al. (1983) showed that MLAEPs are not affected by nitrous oxide and narcotic analgesics.

■ STIMULUS CONSIDERATIONS IN MIDDLE LATENCY RESPONSES

Middle latency responses can be affected by changes in various stimulus parameters, including frequency, level, duration, rise-fall time, monaural versus binaural presentation, and spectral complexity (McFarland et al., 1977; Thornton et al., 1977; Kodera et al., 1977; Mendel, 1980; Burrows and Barry, 1990; McPherson and Starr, 1993; Chen et al., 1997). For example, increases in stimulus rise time have the general effect of significantly increasing latency and decreasing peak amplitudes of Na, Pa, and P1 or Pb (Kodera et al., 1979). Vivion et al. (1980) similarly found that the latencies of five middle latency components (Pa, Nb, Pb, Nc, and Pc) increased and their amplitudes decreased as rise time increased from 3 to 10 ms or as the equivalent duration increased from 10 to 30 ms. Thornton et al. (1977) and McFarland et al. (1977) performed parametric studies on MLAEPs in normal-hearing adults using tone bursts varying in frequency and level. Thornton et al. (1977) used linearly gated tone bursts centered at 250, 1,000, and 4,000 Hz and evaluated amplitude and latency components Na, Pa, Nb, and Nc over a broad range of levels (no stimulus, 10 to 80 dB hearing level [HL], in 10-dB steps). An inverse relationship was found between latency and frequency, but latency was only slightly affected by changes in stimulus level. Input/output functions varied with frequency and depended on the specific middle latency component studied. Using somewhat different frequencies (500, 1,000, and 3,000 Hz) and levels (0, 10, 20, 35, and 50 dB normal HL [nHL]), McFarland et al. (1977) found small reductions in latency with increases in stimulus frequency and level.

Because of time-domain considerations (i.e., onset latency of components of interest and recording epoch necessary to capture component responses), stimulus duration and rise-fall times are constrained to avoid overlap of middle latency components. Thus, stimulus generation trade-offs are necessary, and these physical limitations have their greatest impact when choosing stimuli for audiometric purposes. In behavioral audiometry, relatively long-duration puretone stimuli (>200 ms) and slow (>20 ms) rise times are used to obtain frequency-specific thresholds. Long-duration stimuli with associated slow rise-fall times are advantageous because energy is present only at the nominal frequency and onset and offset transients (unwanted spread of energy) are avoided. If we assume normal middle ear integrity, then the goal of the audiogram is to selectively sample different areas on the basilar membrane to evaluate for auditory system integrity, where higher thresholds are correlated with greater damage to the auditory periphery.

Audiogram reconstruction is an ambitious goal using evoked potentials because the degree of frequency specificity is influenced by temporal constraints. Therefore, the type of windowing function used (e.g., linear vs. nonlinear [e.g., cosine^2, Dolph-Chebychev, Blackman, etc.]) (Harris, 1978) is thought to be important because nonlinear windowing functions influence how energy is distributed by frequency. Issues of cochlear place and frequency specificity are ongoing concerns in electrophysiologic assessment. How they are dealt with depends on the philosophy of the examiner as well as available instrumentation. For example, when stimuli are presented in isolation, the same limitations apply as in the behavioral puretone audiometry (high-frequency stimuli have better frequency selectivity and neural synchrony than low-frequency stimuli); depending on stimulus level and based on basilar membrane traveling wave characteristics, low-frequency stimuli have poorer frequency selectivity and poorer synchrony, and therefore, one is less confident in the precision of frequency-dependent thresholds, particularly if hearing loss exists. Alternatively, stimuli can be presented in the presence of various types of masking noise (e.g., high-pass, notched, broadband) in order to restrict the spread of excitation in the cochlea and, in this way, to improve the place specificity of the response. The first option is relatively straightforward to apply with current computer technology. The masking option is much more complex and more difficult to implement, particularly in the clinical setting, and the results can have more complex rather than simpler interpretations (Halpern and Dallos, 1986; Margolis et al., 1981).

The results of recent studies can help clinicians to select the appropriate stimuli for AEP testing. The degree of frequency and place specificity was studied in normal-hearing subjects by comparing brainstem and MLAEPs to short-duration, linear rise-fall, and Blackman-windowed (500 and 3,000 Hz) stimuli presented at a moderate level (Oates and Stapells, 1997a; 1997b). The stimuli with linear rise-fall times were constructed based on a 2-1-2 design (two cycles of rise time, two cycles of fall time, and one cycle of plateau). The Blackman-windowed stimuli were five cycles in total duration, with no plateau (50% rise/50% fall times). Stimuli were either presented alone or in the presence of high-pass noise at various high-pass cutoff frequencies (Oates and Stapells, 1997a). Subtracting the response obtained at one high-pass masker cutoff frequency from the response obtained at a higher frequency high-pass cutoff, Oates and Stapells (1997b) evaluated the place specificity of these derived responses (see Chapter 13). The results from both studies showed that, at moderate input levels (52 to 53 dB nHL), few or no differences exist in the place specificity under these various stimulus conditions and that either linear or Blackman-windowed stimuli presented in isolation were appropriate.

These findings must be tempered in patients with steeply sloping high-frequency hearing loss in whom higher stimulus levels are needed to elicit a response. Here, side-lobe energy contamination to lower frequencies becomes more of an issue, and the windowing function takes on greater importance, particularly if masking is not used. Conse-

quently, the result of such side-band energy contamination would be to underestimate the magnitude of high-frequency hearing loss. However, in the case of low-frequency hearing loss, spread of excitation to higher stimulus frequencies, as stimulus level is increased, is potentially a much greater concern. In this instance, stimulus shaping alone may be insufficient to guarantee frequency and place specificity. Based on thresholds derived from psychoacoustic studies, special masking procedures in conjunction with click or tone-burst stimuli may be needed to ensure more accurate thresholds (Halpin et al., 1994; Turner et al., 1983; Thornton and Abbas, 1980).

Erwin and Buchwald (1986) studied recovery cycle effects for middle latency components Pa and Pb (P1) in part to assess whether these components may arise from different generator systems. They showed that increasing stimulus presentation rate (0.5, 1, 5, 8, and 10/s) differentially affected peak-to-peak amplitudes of Pb but not Pa. They suggest that this evidence supports the existence of separate neural generators for Pa and Pb. Using a noncephalic reference, Nelson et al. (1997) reported a rate effect for Pb, showing that this component is largest at slower rates and for lower frequencies (500 Hz vs. 4,000 Hz). Using MEG, Onitsuka et al. (2003) also found a rate effect for P50m but not P30m. These findings are in partial contrast to those of McFarland et al. (1975), in which rates as high as 8/s had little effect on the middle latency waveform.

Recent interest has focused on stimulus-evoked and -induced oscillatory activity, particularly in the gamma (40 Hz) range (Jacobson and Fitzgerald, 1997; Tallon-Baudry and Bertrand, 1999). This response may be related to the 40-Hz steady-state potential identified by Galambos et al. (1981) (see Clinical Use of Middle Latency Potentials on page 385). Evoked oscillatory activity is phase-locked to the stimulus and can be seen in the averaged waveforms. Induced activity is not phase-locked and requires spectral analysis or some related technique. There has been speculation that gamma rhythms are neural correlates of various perceptual processes (Tallon-Baudry and Bertrand, 1999).

▨ CLINICAL USE OF MIDDLE LATENCY POTENTIALS

Threshold Estimation

EFFECTS OF HEARING LOSS ON MIDDLE LATENCY AUDITORY EVOKED POTENTIALS

Initially, it was felt that MLAEPs could serve as a means of threshold estimation in the lower frequency range for audiometric purposes. This view came about since MLAEPs are less dependent on temporal synchrony than ABRs and because frequency-specific ABRs are less reliable below 1,000 Hz than above this frequency (Gorga et al., 1988). Clearly, this type of application is important in the assessment of hearing sensitivity in infants and young children. Xu et al. (1995a; 1995b; 1996) used the cross-correlation of two MLAEP waveforms to ensure response identification and found agreement between evoked potential and behavioral thresholds in individuals with moderate hearing loss based on a stimulus format of 4-2-4 (4-ms rise-fall times, 2-ms plateau; presumed linear window; at 500, 1,000, and 2,000 Hz). Hausler et al. (1991) also reported good agreement between MLAEPs and behavioral responses in infants and developmentally delayed children. However, others have expressed caution in estimating low-frequency (500-Hz) thresholds with MLAEPs, particularly in children (Barajas et al., 1988a; 1988b).

Galambos et al. (1981) described a steady-state auditory potential elicited by a continuous 40-Hz tone. Initial studies in normal-hearing and hearing-impaired adults showed promise at threshold estimation in both the low- and high-frequency range with this technique (Galambos et al., 1981; Stapells et al., 1988; Dauman et al., 1984; Lynn et al., 1984; Lenarz et al., 1986). As noted earlier, since the response could be detected near threshold and because the amplitude of the response varied with stimulus level, there was interest in developing this technique for hearing assessment. Kileny and Shea (1986) reported that the steady-state response was sensitive to brainstem and midbrain lesions but was unaffected by cortical lesions. However, interest in transient or steady-state MLAEPs waned when they were found to be absent in infants and were affected by sleep, particularly stages II and III, sedation, and anesthesia (Linden et al., 1985; Plourde and Picton, 1990; Shallop, 1993; Stapells et al., 1988; Osterhammel et al., 1985; Picton et al., 1987; Kraus et al., 1989). Because different stages of sleep differentially affect MLAEP response detection, particularly in children, having instrumentation to quantify sleep stage becomes an important consideration. Because most clinical audiologists are not trained in this procedure and available clinical instrumentation is not geared for sleep-stage analysis, this area should be approached with caution. Furthermore, MLAEPs are more variable in young children and in response to low-level clicks (Kavanaugh et al., 1988). Other steady-state procedures, however, may prove valuable, such as the use of an 80-Hz amplitude modulated response (see Chapter 15; Aoyagi et al., 1994), particularly when thresholds are assessed during sleep (Cohen et al., 1991).

Presently, there is a resurgence of interest in human steady-state responses. For example, recent work has shown that multiple frequencies and both ears can be tested simultaneously, and in adults, relatively good agreement has been obtained with behavioral thresholds using high rate amplitude-modulated tones (Dimitrijevic et al., 2002). However, artifactual responses have been reported to both air- and bone-conduction stimuli at suprathreshold levels (Small and Stapells, 2004; Gorga et al., 2004; Jeng et al., 2004). This is noteworthy because spurious data pose a serious problem when testing infants with significant hearing loss. Picton et al. (2003) provide a current review of this evolving literature.

Potentially, MLAEPs could be used to detect either peripheral hearing loss or central auditory processing disorders. Because MLAEPs are less dependent on neural synchrony than ABRs, suggested applications include threshold assessment in the low-frequency range (<1,000 Hz), particularly when neurologic damage may affect neural synchrony, making threshold detection with ABRs difficult or impossible (Kraus and McGee, 1990; McGee and Kraus, 1996). However, the most important clinical need for AEPs, such as early identification of peripheral hearing loss in infants and young children, involves the settings in which MLAEP variability is highest. As noted earlier, sleep and anesthesia affect MLAEPs, and as a result, they may not be useful in patients who cannot or will not cooperate with the examiner. Based on various studies (Mackersie et al., 1993; Wu and Stapells, 1994; Oates and Stapells, 1997a; 1997b), the frequency specificities of MLAEPs and ABRs at low (500 Hz) and high frequencies (2,000 Hz) were found to be relatively similar. Therefore, because of the general robustness of the ABR response and its independence from state variables, the need to use MLAEPs for low-frequency threshold detection on a routine basis, at least at 500 Hz, is questionable. It appears more pragmatic in most instances to use ABRs in assessing low-frequency thresholds (Kodera et al., 1977).

Site-of-Lesion Testing

An analysis of the effects of cerebral lesions on MLAEPs can provide information about underlying neural generators. In addition, correlation of evoked potential results with perceptual disturbances provides a means of establishing the validity of various components as indices of central auditory processing. Woods et al. (1984) examined a case of bitemporal lesions associated with cortical deafness, in which they observed a positive wave at 57 ms and a negative wave at 98 ms that had normal topographies, latencies, and amplitudes. They suggested that one possible explanation of these results is that middle latency vertex potentials are produced by polysensory cortex in the vicinity of auditory areas. In a subsequent study, Knight et al. (1988) reported reduced amplitudes of temporal and vertex middle latency peaks in a group of patients with lesions of the superior temporal gyrus. In contrast, lesions of the inferior parietal lobe produced minimal effects. They concluded that the superior temporal gyrus played a critical role in the generation of these potentials. Scherg and von Cramon (1986b; 1990) suggest that there are three types of AEP alterations resulting from unilateral lesions to central auditory pathways: an "acoustic radiation" type, with unilateral reduction in middle latency dipole source potentials and preserved tangential and radial dipole source potentials; a "primary auditory cortex" type, with unilateral reduction of both middle and long latency radial and tangential dipole source potentials; and an "auditory association" type, showing normal MLAEPs with a localized reduction of long latency radial N150 and preserved tangential long latency dipole source potentials.

As we noted earlier, the issue of number of electrodes (i.e., spatial sampling of MLAEPs) becomes crucial in attempting to determine the effects of CNS lesions (space-occupying tumors or vascular insults) on these potentials. For example, initial studies have limited electrode placements to central scalp locations and, therefore, are limited in scope. In fact, many studies evaluating the effect of brain lesions in the middle latency range have not even placed recording electrodes over temporal lobe sites or have used reference electrode sites that make the data uninterpretable! Parving et al. (1980) recorded MLAEPs in a patient with auditory agnosia. In this case, computed tomography (CT), regional blood flow measures, and scintinography documented the lesion. A normal Pa response was found. Although they concluded that Pa was neurogenic in origin (an important issue at that time), they also argued that MLAEPs cannot be regarded as being generated exclusively, if at all, in primary auditory cortex. Özdamar et al. (1982) report a case of cortical deafness with preserved ABRs but absent middle latency peak Pa. Based on CT studies, Özdamar and colleagues concluded that the absence of the MLAEP component Pa was due to hematomas and infarcts of the left and right temporal lobes. However, as noted below, this interpretation has been challenged, suggesting that secondary changes due to retrograde degeneration of subcortical structures were not ruled out as a cause for this abnormality. In 19 patients with temporal lobe lesions studied by Kraus et al. (1982), it was found that Na-Pa was reduced over the involved hemisphere. According to these authors, normal intersubject amplitude variability and the occasional myogenic contamination of the response make it difficult to establish reliable diagnostic criteria that could be used clinically for diagnosis of patients with temporal lobe lesions. In two patients with central deafness resulting from bilateral localized vascular lesions at the level of the putamen, Tanaka et al. (1991) reported auditory thresholds in the moderately severe to profound range, intact ABRs (waves I-VI), and complete absence of middle latency component Pa bilaterally. Interestingly, the long latency AEP (N1P2 complex) was preserved in both cases. In a review of other bilateral auditory cortex lesion cases that did not produce cortical deafness, Woods et al. (1984) were unable to support the view that the primary generators of middle and long latency AEPs reside exclusively in auditory cortex. They suggest that abnormalities found in MLAEPs are associated with subcortical lesions or cortical lesions extensive enough to denervate thalamic projection nuclei. They also suggest that abnormalities of the long latency N1 component recorded from central scalp reflect lesion extensions into multimodal areas of the inferior parietal lobe. Woods et al. (1987) reported a case of cortical deafness in an 82-year-old woman, resulting from successive strokes of the right and left temporal lobes secondary to bilateral occlusion of the posterior temporal branch of the middle cerebral arteries. Middle and long latency AEPs (P1, N1, P2) were preserved despite moderate to profound puretone behavioral thresholds and absence of auditory discriminations. According to the authors, this case is an example of dissociated perception from the generation of MLAEPs and long latency AEPs. Based on a three- or four-electrode array in the coronal plane (Cz, C6, C5, T3, T4), Kileny et al. (1987) showed that Pa was reduced over the involved hemisphere but remained intact over the contralateral hemisphere in individuals with unilateral lesions of the temporal lobe. In this study, the ABRs, particularly wave V latency, were normal regardless of the site of lesion. However, no mention was made of TP41. In comparing conventional MLAEPs with those obtained using the maximum-length-sequence technique in controls and individuals with CNS lesions, no advantage was observed using the more sophisticated technique (Musiek and Lee, 1997). In a study that used both magnetic and electric AEPs, Leinonen and Joutsiniemi (1989) examined four patients with temporal lobe infarcts and recorded AEPs in the 40- to 200-ms range. Responses were abnormal in all four patients and missing in two. In one individual, responses were of abnormally high amplitude, and in another, parts of the response sequence were missing. Electric AEPs were in accordance with the magnetic field measures, although magnetic recordings are *insensitive* in evaluating radially oriented dipoles (Lewine and Orrison, 1999) and therefore cannot delineate the TP41 or later T-complex waveforms. In 12 patients with intractable seizures, Jacobson et al. (1990) found that Pa was unaffected by anterior temporal lobectomy, while Na latency and Na/Pa amplitude showed significant increases after surgery. They suggest that changes in Na and Na/Pa amplitude reflect a loss of the modulating influence of the cortex on the subcortical generators of Na. In 24 patients with primarily temporal lobe lesions (i.e., by CT documentation), Na and Pa obtained over vertex were normal, whereas MLAEPs over the coronal plane showed Pa amplitude to be attenuated or absent over the damaged temporal lobe, relative to the vertex or intact hemisphere (Shehata-Dieler et al., 1991). Again, no mention was made of abnormalities to the temporal component, TP41. Vizioli et al. (1993) suggested that Na and Pa have different generator sites, based on findings from three individuals with brain lesions (two craniopharyngiomas and one left cystic astrocytoma). Toyoda et al. (1998) suggest that large-vessel vascular disease, including Moyamoya-like vasculopathy, significantly affects auditory evoked MEG fields and dipole source localization in the middle latency range. Toyoda and colleagues also correlated MEG abnormalities with changes in blood flow based on positron emission tomography (PET) and showed that reduced perfusion in areas encompassing both the auditory radiations and auditory cortex correlated with the deficits in the auditory evoked magnetic fields. Setzen et al. (1999) found absent MLAEPs and long latency AEPs but normal transient evoked and distortion product otoacoustic emissions and ABRs in a child with Moyamoya disease with central deafness. In this case, digital subtraction angiography showed that the middle cerebral artery was absent on the right side and almost completely occluded on the left side, except for a prominent angular/parietal branch. However, the lesions in this case were more diffuse, including subcortical and cortical ischemic damage and focal lesions in frontal, parietal, and temporal lobes. The absence and occlusion of the vessels noted earlier are significant because they supply blood to the lateral two thirds of each hemisphere (motor, tactile, and auditory areas) as well as to adjacent subcortical sites (Taveras, 1996). Additionally, unilateral lesions of the superior temporal gyrus abolish TP41 over the lesioned hemisphere. No change in either latency or amplitude of TP41 is observed with inferior parietal lobe lesions (Knight et al., 1988).

Stach et al. (1994) showed a selective alteration of middle and long latency AEP components in Rett's syndrome (cerebroatrophic hyperammonemia), with preserved brainstem function. The progressive and gender-specific nature of this disease primarily affects gray matter of the brain, and characteristics of these individuals include autistic behavior, ataxia, dementia, seizures, cerebral atrophy, and biochemical abnormalities. The implication of these findings is that various AEP components may help delineate gray matter (cortical) from subcortical involvement and may be valuable in tracking disease progression. In individuals with partial epilepsy, brainstem and middle latency responses were found to be unaffected, whereas alterations in later cortical responses (N1/P2) were noted (Japaridze et al., 1997). Along these lines, the T-complex hemispheric latency difference has been shown to be very sensitive to both acute and chronic antiepilepic drug effects (Wolpaw and Penry, 1978).

Cochlear Implants

The use of MLAEPs has been suggested for the evaluation of cochlear implant candidates (Gardi, 1985; Miyamoto, 1986; Kileny and Kemink, 1987; Kileny et al., 1989). These authors have generally found that MLAEPs evoked by electrical pulses are similar to those evoked by acoustic stimulation. In adults, electrically evoked MLAEP thresholds correlated positively with acoustic thresholds obtained using the implanted device. Furthermore, in postlingually deafened adults, MLAEP variations in amplitude and latency were related to specific speech perception abilities. In contrast to electrically evoked ABRs, studies using MLAEPs have additional advantages: they are not influenced by electrically induced stimulus artifacts; longer stimulus pulse trains can be used, which results in lower levels of stimulation; and a greater proportion of the auditory pathway is activated, which may correlate better with outcome. When P1 (P50 or Pb) is used as a marker of auditory system maturation, its latency becomes adult-like by 15 years of age (Eggermont et al., 1997). The P1 peak latency was found to mature at the same rate in normal-hearing and implanted children, and it was found that the time to maturity in implanted subjects is delayed by an amount approximately equal to the duration of deafness. Such experimental data provide important information on the effect of acoustic deprivation on auditory system maturation. Kelly et al. (2005) studied middle and long latency AEPs in experienced adult cochlear implant users and compared them to speech perception measures. Electrode sites were limited to central scalp locations. For middle latency component Pa, similar latencies and amplitudes were found in normal-hearing and cochlear implant groups. The authors

noted considerable intersubject variability and found no relation between MLAEPs and cochlear implant performance for sentences and word lists. Gordon et al. (2005) evaluated the electrically evoked middle latency response in children receiving cochlear implants. Except for testing that was performed at the time of surgery, recordings were made when individuals were awake using a standard central recording location and recording epoch (80 ms). Middle latency AEP detection increased dramatically over a 5-year period (from poor detection at the time of surgery in the operating room to near 100% detection after 5 years of use). These results suggest that electrically evoked MLAEPs are not useful clinically for predicting optimum stimulation levels or assessing cochlear implant function at early stages of device use. Whereas MLAEPs were not found to be particularly useful during early stages of cochlear implant usage, they may be a valuable tool to track activity in thalamocortical pathways in cochlear implant use over time.

Central Auditory Processing Disorders

It has been suggested that MLAEPs may be valuable indices of central auditory processing disorders (Musiek and Baran, 1987; Pasman et al., 1997). Numerous authors have reported abnormalities for various components of the MLAEP waveform over central scalp locations in individuals with multiple sclerosis. The frequency of reported abnormalities, which ranged from 45% to 73%, depended in part on the statistical criteria used to define these abnormalities (Versino et al., 1992; Celebisoy, 1996; Robinson and Rudge, 1977). Interestingly, in the series reported by Celebisoy (1996), none of the patients with abnormalities of middle latency component Pa had cortical lesions. The fact that all individuals had subcortical white matter lesions argues for a subcortical generator of Pa, a position that has been articulated by others. Furthermore, combining electrophysiologic and imaging studies with sensitive perceptual measures may also help to demonstrate that Pa does not have a cortical origin (Hendler et al., 1990; Rappaport et al., 1994).

Other related applications to sensory processing have been in the area of psychiatric research concerned with the neurobiology of schizophrenia. It has been hypothesized that schizophrenics have a sensory disturbance described as an "inability" to filter out extraneous noise stimuli from meaningful sensory inputs (Freedman et al., 1987; Boutros and Belger, 1999). Schizophrenics do not show the normal attenuation of the response to the second stimulus of a pair of acoustic stimuli. This has been interpreted as an inability of the schizophrenic brain to inhibit or gate its response to specific stimuli. With MLAEPs, the P50 response to the second stimulus is larger than normal, and this has been interpreted as a deficit in P50 response suppression. As a potential marker for sensory gating, a considerable literature now exists linking a disturbance in this phenomenon to brain neurobiochemical abnormalities and developmental and genetic influences (Freedman et al., 1995; Myles-Worsley et al., 1999; Adler et al., 1998; Clementz et al., 1998; Light et al.,

1999). Reduced suppression of the P50 to the second click in a pair has also been found in patients with posttraumatic stress disorder (Karl et al., 2006). As noted previously, many issues in this area remain to be fully explored.

Understanding the neurobiologic basis of why MLAEPs could be abnormal in various forms of learning disabilities is another challenging area that is incompletely understood. Abnormal MLAEPs have been reported in specific children or selected groups with learning disabilities or other handicaps (Kileny and Berry, 1983; Jerger et al., 1987; Arehole et al., 1995). However, other studies in children with a wide range of cognitive, neurologic, speech, and language disorders have failed to find MLAEP abnormalities between control children and those from various diagnostic categories (Mason and Mellor, 1984; Kraus et al., 1985).

Additionally, comprehensive case studies can be useful in illuminating how structural and functional abnormalities may differentially affect MLAEP waveforms. For example, Ali and Jerger (1992) found that phase coherence in middle latency steady-state responses distinguished groups of elderly subjects matched for hearing loss but differing in speech understanding. They suggest that this measure may be a useful predictor for early identification of central auditory processing disorder. Experimental studies designed to explore binaural processing in the middle latency range reflect a range of topics of importance in electrophysiologic measurement (McPherson and Starr, 1993). In neonates, binaural processing as assessed by the binaural interaction component is thought to be immature (Cone-Wesson et al., 1997). In four cases, Jerger et al. (1993) show a binaural interference effect in elderly hearing-impaired individuals, where performance on selected behavioral speech tests and responses of MLAEPs (reduced Pa amplitudes) to both behavioral and electrophysiologic measures were abnormal on tasks of binaural processing. The mechanism or mechanisms of this interference effect are not known, although comparisons have been made with binocular rivalry, a well-known phenomenon in the visual system.

Are Middle Latency Auditory Evoked Potentials Modality Specific?

As noted in our discussion of the literature, several authors have suggested that polysensory areas contribute to the generation of AEPs. Of primary concern here is the extent to which alterations in AEPs are influenced by pathology in pansensory or supramodal brain areas. This topic has been the concern of investigations using other AEP components, such as the mismatch negativity. For example, Alho et al. (1994) report that lesions to the frontal cortex can impair the generation of this response.

We have previously discussed the issue of modality specificity in the context of behavioral measures used for evaluating central auditory processing disorders (Cacace and McFarland, 1998; McFarland and Cacace, 1995; Cacace and McFarland, 2005). It would be logical to expect that those with central auditory processing disorders would have more difficulty with tasks involving acoustic input than with tasks involving other sensory modalities. With behavioral measures, this requires multimodal perceptual testing. With evoked potentials, there are two possible strategies for establishing modality specificity of evoked potential effects. The first involves demonstrating that AEPs are abnormal and that potentials evoked by stimulation of other sensory modalities are normal. The second strategy would examine the extent to which MLAEPs serve as predictors of conditions that have been documented to be auditory specific by behavioral measures. This latter approach is most important because, ultimately, the significance of electrophysiologic measures must be validated by their behavioral (functional) correlates. A third potential strategy would be to quantify multimodal interactions of evoked potentials. To date, neither of these approaches has been investigated extensively. Thus, the clinical use of MLAEPs as tests of central auditory processing disorders must await further research.

░ CONCLUSION

MLAEPs have intrigued individuals for well over half a century. Based on this overview, it is evident that MLAEPs have been applied to virtually all areas of auditory research, and one cannot escape the conclusion that these potentials have more theoretical than practical value. As an audiometric tool for threshold determination in infants, MLAEPs have not been particularly reliable. In general, routine clinical applications are limited, although sophisticated research studies continue to add to the literature on this topic (Rupp et al., 2004).

░ REFERENCES

Adler LE, Olincy A, Waldo M, Harris JG, Griffith J, Stevens K, Flach K, Nagamoto H, Bickford P, Leonard S, Freedman R. (1998) Schizophrenia, sensory gating, and nicotinic receptors. *Schizophr Bull.* 24, 189–202.

Alho K, Woods DL, Algaza A, Knight RT, Näätänen R. (1994) Lesions of frontal cortex diminish the auditory mismatch negativity. *Electroencephalogr Clin Neurophysiol.* 91, 353–362.

Ali AA, Jerger J. (1992) Phase coherence of the middle latency response in the elderly. *Scand Audiol.* 21, 187–194.

Amenedo E, Diaz F. (1998) Effects of aging in middle latency evoked potentials: a cross-sectional study. *Biol Psychiatry.* 43, 210–219.

Aoyagi M, Kiren T, Furuse H, Fuse T, Suzuki Y, Yokota M, Koike Y. (1994) Pure-tone threshold prediction by 80-Hz amplitude-modulation following response. *Acta Otolaryngol.* 511 (suppl), 7–14.

Arehole S, Augustine LE, Simhadri R. (1995) Middle latency response in children with learning disabiloties: preliminary findings. *J Commun Dis.* 28, 21–38.

Barajas JJ, Exposito M, Fernandez R, Marin LJ. (1988a) Middle latency response to a 400 Hz tone pip in normal-hearing and hearing impaired subjects. *Scand Audiol.* 17, 21–26.

Barajas JJ, Fernandez R, Bernal MR. (1988b) Middle latency and 40 Hz auditory evoked responses in normal hearing children: 500 Hz thresholds. *Scand Audiol Suppl.* 30, 99–104.

Başar E, Bullock TH. (1992) *Induced Rhythms in the Brain.* Boston: Birkhauser; 1992.

Boutros NN, Belger A. (1999) Midlatency evoked potentials attenuation and augmentation reflect different aspects of sensory gating. *Biol Psychiatry.* 45, 917–922.

Blaettner U, Scherg M, von Cramon D. (1989) Diagnosis of unilateral telencephalic hearing disorders: evaluation of a simple psychoacoustic pattern discrimination test. *Brain.* 112, 177–195.

Buchwald JS, Erwin RJ, Read S, Van Lancker D, Cummings JL. (1989) Midlatency auditory evoked responses: differential abnormality of P1 in Alzheimer's disease. *Electroencephalogr Clin Neurophysiol.* 74, 378–384.

Buchwald JS, Rubinstein EH, Schwafel J, Strandburg RJ. (1991) Midlatency auditory evoked responses: differential effects of cholinergic agonist and antagonist. *Electroencephalogr Clin Neurophysiol.* 80, 303–309.

Burrows DL, Barry SJ. (1990) Electrophysiological evidence for the critical band in humans: middle latency responses. *J Acoust Soc Am.* 88, 180–184.

Cacace AT, Dowman R, Wolpaw JR. (1988) T complex hemispheric asymmetries: effects of stimulus intensity. *Hear Res.* 34, 225–232.

Cacace AT, McFarland DJ. (1998) Central auditory processing disorder in school-age children: a critical review. *J Speech Lang Hear Res.* 41, 355–373.

Cacace AT, McFarland DJ. (2002) Middle-latency auditory evoked potentials: basic issues and potential applications. In: Katz J, ed. *Handbook of Clinical Audiology.* 5th ed. Philadelphia: Lippincott Williams & Wilkins; pp 349–377.

Cacace AT, McFarland DJ. (2005) The importance of modality specificity in diagnosing central auditory processing disorder. *Am J Audiol.* 14, 112–123.

Cacace AT, McFarland DJ. (2006) Frequency domain analysis of event related potentials and oscillations. In: Burkard RF, Don M, Eggermont JJ, eds. *Auditory Evoked Potentials: Basic Principles and Clinical Application.* Baltimore: Lippincott Williams & Wilkins; pp 124–137.

Cacace AT, Satya-Murti S, Wolpaw JR. (1990) Middle latency auditory evoked potentials: vertex and temporal components. *Electroencephalogr Clin Neurophysiol.* 77, 6–18.

Campbell JA, Leandri M. (1984) The effects of high pass filters on computer-reconstructed evoked potentials. *Electroencephalogr Clin Neurophysiol.* 57, 99–101.

Celebisoy N. (1996) Middle latency auditory evoked potentials (MLAEPs) in (MS). *Acta Neurol Scand.* 93, 318–321.

Celesia GG. (1976) Organization of auditory cortical areas in man. *Brain.* 99, 403–414.

Celesia GG, Brigell M. (1999) Auditory evoked potentials. In: Niedermeyer E, Lopes da Silva F, eds. *Electroencephalography: Basic Principals, Clinical Applications and Related Fields.* 3rd ed. Baltimore: Williams and Wilkins; pp 994–1013.

Cetas JS, de Venecia, McMullen NT. (1999) Thalamocortical afferents of Lorente de Nó: medical geniculate axons that project to primary auditory cortex have collateral branches to layer. *Brain Res.* 830, 203–208.

Chambers RD. (1992) Differential age effects for components of the adult auditory middle latency response. *Hear Res.* 58, 123–131.

Chambers RD, Griffiths SK. (1991) Effects of age on the adult auditory middle latency response. *Hear Res.* 51, 1–10.

Chatrian GE, Petersen MC, Lazarte JA. (1960) Responses to clicks from human brain: some depth electrographic observations. *Electroencephalogr Clin Neurophysiol.* 12, 479–489.

Chen C, Ninomiya H, Onitsuka T. (1997) Influence of reference electrodes, stimulation characteristics and task paradigms on auditory P50. *Psychiatry Clin Neurosci.* 51, 139–143.

Clementz BA, Geyer MA, Braff DL. (1998) Multiple site evaluation of P50 suppression among schizophrenia and normal comparison subjects. *Schizophr Res.* 30, 71–80.

Cohen LT, Rickards FW, Clark GM. (1991) A comparison of steady-state evoked potentials to modulated tones in awake and sleeping humans. *J Acoust Soc Am.* 90, 2467–2479.

Cohen MM. (1982) Coronal topography of the middle latency auditory evoked potentials (MLAEPs) in man. *Electroencephalogr Clin Neurophysiol.* 53, 231–236.

Cone-Wesson B, Ma E, Fowler CG. (1997) Effect of stimulus level and frequency on ABR and MLR bunaural interaction in human neonates. *Hear Res.* 106, 163–178.

Dauman R, Szyfter W, Charlet de Sauvage R, Cazals Y. (1984) Low frequency thresholds assessed with 40 Hz MLR in adults with impaired hearing. *Arch Otorhinolaryngol.* 240, 85–89.

Davies CA, Mann DM, Sumpter PQ, Yates PO. (1987) A quantitative morphometric analysis of the neuronal and synaptic content of the frontal and temporal cortex in patients with Alzheimer's disease. *J Neurol Sci.* 2, 151–164.

Dawson GD. (1951) A summating technique for detecting small signals in a large irregular background. *J Neurophysiol.* 115, 2–3.

Dawson GD. (1954) A summation technique for the detection of small evoked potentials. *Electroencephalogr Clin Neurophysiol.* 6, 65–84.

Diesch E, Struve M, Rupp A, Ritter S, Hulse M, Flor H. (2004) Enhancement of steady-state auditory evoked magnetic fields in tinnitus. *Eur J Neurosci.* 19, 1093–1104.

Dimitrijevic A, John MS, Van Roon P, Purcell DW, Adamonis J, Ostroff J, Nedzelski JM, Picton TW. (2002) Estimating the audiogram using multiple auditory steady-state responses. *J Am Acad Audiol.* 4, 205–224.

Eggermont JJ, Ponton CW, Don M, Waring MD, Kwong B. (1997) Maturational delays in cortical evoked potentials in cochlear implant users. *Acta Otolaryngol.* 117, 161–163.

Erwin R, Buchwald J. (1986) Midlatency auditory evoked responses: differential recovery cycle characteristics of sleep in humans. *Electroencephalogr Clin Neurophysiol.* 65, 383–392.

Farrell DE, Tripp JH, Norge R, Teyler TJ. (1980) A study of the auditory evoked magnetic field of the human brain. *Electroencephalogr Clin Neurophysiol.* 49, 31–37.

Fein G, Biggins C, van Dyke C. (1994) The auditory P50 response is normal in Alzheimer's disease when measured via a paired click paradigm. *Electroencephalogr Clin Neurophysiol.* 92, 536–545.

Freedman R, Adler LE, Gerhardt GA, Waldo M, Baker N, Rose GM, Drebling C, Nagamoto H, Bickford-Wimer P, Franks R. (1987)

Neurobiological studies of sensory gating in schizophrenia. *Schizophr Bull.* 13, 669–678.

Freedman R, Hall M, Adler LE, Leonard S. (1995) Evidence in postmortem brain tissue for decreased numbers of hippocampal nicotinic receptors in schizophrenia. *Biol Psychiatry.* 38, 22–33.

Galaburda A, Sanides F. (1980) Cytoarchitectonic organization of the human auditory cortex. *J Comp Neurol.* 190, 597–610.

Galambos R, Makeig S, Talmachoff PJ. (1981) A 40-Hz auditory potential recorded from the human scalp. *Proc Natl Acad Sci.* 78, 2643–2647.

Gardi JN. (1985) Human brainstem and middle latency responses to electrical stimulation. Preliminary observations. In: Schindler RA, Merzenich M, eds. *Cochlear Implants.* New York: Raven Press; pp 351–363.

Gencer NG, Williamson SJ, Gueziec A, Hummel R. (1996) Optimal reference electrode selection for electrical source imaging. *Electroencephalogr Clin Neurophysiol.* 99, 163–173.

Gerken GM. (1996) Central tinnitus and lateral inhibition: an auditory brainstem model. *Hear Res.* 97, 75–83.

Gerken GM, Hesse PS, Wiorkowski JJ. (2001) Auditory evoked responses in control subjects and in patients with problem tinnitus. *Hear Res.* 157, 52–64.

Goff WR. (1978) The scalp distribution of auditory evoked potentials. In: Naunton RF, Fernandez C, eds. *Evoked Electrical Activity in the Auditory Nervous System.* New York: Academic Press; pp 505–524.

Goff WR, Allison T, Lyons W, Fisher TC, Conte R. (1977) Origins of short latency auditory evoked potentials in man. In: Desmedt JE, ed. *Auditory Evoked Potentials in Man. Psychopharmacology Correlates of Evoked Potentials.* Karger: Basel; pp 30–44.

Gordon KA, Papsin BC, Harrison RV. (2005) Effects of cochlear implant use on the electrically evoked middle latency response in children. *Hear Res.* 204, 78–89.

Gorga MP, Kaminski JR, Beauchaine KA, Jesteadt W. (1988) Auditory brainstem responses to tone bursts in normally hearing subjects. *J Speech Hear Res.* 31, 87–97.

Gorga MP, Neely ST, Hoover BM, Diekering DM, Beuachaine ML, Manning C. (2004) Determining the upper limits of stimulation for auditory steady-state response measurements. *Ear Hear.* 25, 302–307.

Hackett TA, Stepniewska I, Kaas JH. (1999) Callosal connections of the parabelt auditory cortex in macaque monkeys. *Eur J Neurosci.* 11, 856–866.

Halpern DL, Dallos P. (1986) Auditory filter shapes in the chinchilla. *J Acoust Soc Am.* 80, 765–775.

Halpin C, Thornton A, Hasso M. (1994) Low-frequency sensorineural loss: clinical evaluation and implication for hearing aid fitting. *Ear Hear.* 15, 71–81.

Hari R, Pelissone M, Makela JP, Hallstrom J, Leionen L, Lounaasmaa OV. (1987) Neuromagnetic responses of the human auditory cortex to on- and offsets of noise bursts. *Audiology.* 26, 31–43.

Harker LA, Hosick E, Voots RJ, Mendel MI. (1977) Influence of succinylcholine on middle component auditory evoked potentials. *Arch Otolaryngol.* 103, 133–137.

Harris FJ. (1978) On the use of windows for harmonic analysis with the discrete Fourier transform. *Proc IEEE.* 66, 51–83.

Hashimoto I. (1982) Auditory evoked potentials from the human midbrain: slow brain stem responses. *Electroencephalogr Clin Neurophysiol.* 53, 652–657.

Hausler R, Cao M, Magnin C, Mulette O. (1991) Low frequency hearing threshold determination in newborns, infants, and mentally retarded children by middle latency responses. *Acta Otolaryngol Suppl.* 482, 58–71.

Hendler T, Squires NK, Emmerich DS. (1990) Psychophysical measures of central auditory dysfunction in multiple sclerosis: neurophysiological and neuroanatomical correlates. *Ear Hear.* 11, 403–416.

Hood LJ, Martin DA, Berlin CI. (1990) Auditory evoked potentials differ at 50 milliseconds in right- and left-handed listeners. *Hear Res.* 45, 115–122.

Huang JW, Ying-Ying L, Nayak A, Roy RJ. (1999) Depth of anesthesia estimation and control. *IEEE Trans Biomed Eng.* 46, 71–81.

Irimajiri R, Golob EG, Starr A. (2005) Auditory brain-stem, middle-and long-latency evoked potentials in mild cognitive impairment. *Clin Neurophysiol.* 116, 1918–1929.

Jääskeläinen IP, Hirvonen J, Huttunen J, Kaakkola S, Pekkonen E. (1999) Scopolamine enhances middle-latency auditory evoked magnetic fields. *Neurosci Lett.* 259, 41–44.

Jacobson GP, Fitzgerald MB. (1997) Auditory evoked gamma band potential in normal subjects. *J Am Acad Audiol.* 8, 44–52.

Jacobson GP, Grayson AS. (1988) The normal scalp topography of the middle latency auditory evoked potential Pa component following monaural click stimulation. *Brain Topogr.* 1, 29–36.

Jacobson GP, Privitera M, Neils JR, Grayson AS, Yeh HS. (1990) The effects of anterior temporal lobectomy (ATL) on the middle-latency auditory evoked potential (MLAEP). *Electroencephalogr Clin Neurophysiol.* 75, 230–241.

Japaridze G, Kvernadze D, Geladze D, Kevanishvili Z. (1997) Auditory brainstem response, middle-latency response, and slow cortical potential in patients with partial epilepsy. *Seizure.* 6, 449–456.

Jasper HH. (1958) The ten-twenty electrode system of the International Federation. *Electroencephalogr Clin Neurophysiol.* 10, 371–375.

Jeng FC, Brown CJ, Johnson TA, Vander Werff KR. (2004) Estimating air-bone gaps using auditory steady-state responses. *J Am Acad Audiol.* 15, 67–78.

Jerger S, Martin RC, Jerger J. (1987) Specific auditory perceptual dysfunction in a learning disabled child. *Ear Hear.* 8, 78–86.

Jerger J, Silman S, Lew HL, Chmiel R. (1993) Case studies in binaural interference: converging evidence from behavioral and electrophysiologic measures. *J Am Acad Audiol.* 4, 122–131.

Kaas JH, Hackett TA, Tramo MJ. (1999) Auditory processing in primate cerebral cortex. *Curr Opin Neurosci.* 9, 164–170.

Karl A, Malta LS, Maercker A. (2006) Meta-analytic review of event-related potential studies in post-traumatic stress disorder. *Biol Psychol.* 71, 123–147.

Kavanaugh KT, Domico WD, Crews PL, McCormick VA. (1988) Comparison of the intrasubject repeatability of auditory brainstem and middle latency responses elicited in young children *Ann Otol Rhinol Laryngol.* 97, 264–271.

Kavanaugh KT, Harker LA, Tyler RS. (1984) Auditory brainstem and middle latency responses. I. Effects of response filtering and waveform identification. II. Threshold responses to a 500-Hz tone pip. *Acta Otolaryngol.* 108, 1–12.

Kelly AS, Purdy SC, Thorne PR. (2005) Electrophysiological and speech perception measures of auditory processing in experienced adult cochlear implant users. *Clin Neurophysiol.* 116, 1235–1246.

Kelly JP. (1985) Auditory system. In: Kandel ER, Schwartz JR, eds. *Principles of Neural Science*. 2nd ed. New York: Elsevier; pp 396–408.

Kelly-Ballweber D, Dobie RA. (1984) Binaural interaction measured behaviorally and electrophysiologically in young and old adults. *Audiology*. 23, 181–194.

Kileny PR, Berry BA. (1983) Selective impairment of late vertex and middle latency auditory evoked responses. In: Mencher G, Gerber S, eds. *The Multiply Handicapped Hearing Impaired Child*. New York: Grune & Stratton.

Kileny PR, Dobson D, Gelfand ET. (1983) Middle latency auditory evoked responses during open heart surgery with hypothermia. *Electroencephalogr Clin Neurophysiol*. 55, 268–276.

Kileny PR, Kemink JL. (1987) Electrically evoked middle-latency auditory evoked potentials in cochlear implant candidates. *Arch Otolaryngol*. 113, 1072–1077.

Kileny PR, Kemink JL, Miller JM. (1989) An intrasubject comparison of electric and acoustic middle latency responses. *Am J Otol*. 10, 23–27.

Kileny PR, Paccioretti D, Wilson AF. (1987) Effects of cortical lesions on middle-latency auditory evoked responses (MLR). *Electroencephalogr Clin Neurophysiol*. 66, 108–120.

Kileny PR, Shea SL. (1986) Middle-latency and 40-Hz auditory evoked responses in normal-hearing subjects: click and 500-Hz thresholds. *J Speech Hear Res*. 29, 20–28.

Knight RT, Scabini D, Woods DL, Clayworth C. (1988) The effects of lesions of the superior temporal gyrus and inferior parietal lobe on temporal and vertex components of the human AEP. *Electroencephalogr Clin Neurophysiol*. 70, 499–509.

Kodera K, Yamane H, Yamada O, Suzuki J. (1977) Brainstem response audiometry at speech frequencies. *Audiology*. 16, 469–479.

Kraus N, Kileny P, McGee T. (1994) Middle latency auditory evoked potentials. In: Katz J, ed. *Handbook of Clinical Audiology*. 4th ed. Baltimore: Williams & Wilkins; pp 387–405.

Kraus N, McGee T. (1990) Clinical applications of the middle latency response. *J Am Acad Audiol*. 1, 130–133.

Kraus N, McGee T, Comperatore C. (1989) MLRs in children are consistently present during wakefulness, Stage I, and REM sleep. *Ear Hear*. 10, 339–345.

Kraus N, Ozdamar O, Hier D, Stein L. (1982). Auditory middle latency responses (MLRs) in patients with cortical lesions. *Electroencephalogr Clin Neurophysiol*. 54, 275–287.

Kraus N, Smith D, Reed N, Stein L, Cartee C. (1985) Auditory middle latency responses in children: effect of age and diagnostic category. *Electroencephalogr Clin Neurophysiol*. 62, 343–351.

Kruglikov SY, Schiff SJ. (2003) Interplay of electroencephalogram phase and auditory-evoked neural activity. *J Neurosci*. 23, 10122–10127.

Kuriki S, Nogai T, Hirata Y. (1995) Cortical sources of middle latency responses of auditory evoked magnetic field. *Hear Res*. 92, 47–51.

Law SK, Rohrbaugh JW, Adams CM, Eckardt MJ. (1993) Improving spatial and temporal resolution in evoked EEG responses using surface Laplacians. *Electroencephalogr Clin Neurophysiol*. 88, 309–322.

Lee YS, Leuders DS, Dinner RP, Lesser J, Hahn J, Klem G. (1984) Recording of auditory evoked potentials in man using chronic subdural electrodes. *Brain*. 107, 115–131.

Leinonen L, Joutsiniemi SL. (1989) Auditory evoked potentials and magnetic fields in patients with lesions of the auditory cortex. *Acta Neurol Scand*. 79, 316–325.

Lenarz T, Gulzow J, Grozinger M, Hoth S. (1986) Clinical evaluation of 40-Hz middle-latency responses in adults: frequency specific threshold estimation and suprathreshold amplitude characteristics. *J Otorhinolaryngol Relat Spec*. 48, 24–32.

Lewine JD, Orrison WW. (1999) Magnetic source imaging: integration of magnetoencephalography and magnetic resonance imaging. In: Stark DD, Bradley WG, eds. *Magnetic Resonance Imaging*. Vol III. 3rd ed. St. Louis: Mosby; pp 1575–1593.

Liegeos-Chauvel C, Musolino A, Badier JM, Marquis P, Chauvel P. (1994) Evoked potentials recorded from the auditory cortex in man: evaluation and topography of the middle latency components. *Electroencephalogr Clin Neurophysiol*. 92, 204–214.

Light GA, Malaspina D, Geyer MA, Luber BM, Coleman EA, Sackeim HA, Braff DL. (1999) Amphetamine disrupts P50 suppression in normal subjects. *Biol Psychiatry*. 46, 990–996.

Linden R, Campbell KB, Hamel G, Picton TW. (1985) Human auditory steady state evoked potentials during sleep. *Ear Hear*. 6, 167–174.

Lopes da Silva F. (1999) Event-related potentials: methodology and quantification. In: Niedermeyer E, Lopes da Silva F, eds. *Electroencephalography: Basic Principals, Clinical Applications and Related Fields*. 4th ed. Baltimore: Williams & Wilkins; pp 947–957.

Lopes da Silva F, Van Rotterdam A. (1999) Biophysical aspects of EEG and magnetoencephalogram generation. In: Niedermeyer E, Lopes da Silva, eds. *Electroencephalography: Basic Principals, Clinical Applications and Related Fields*. 4th ed. Baltimore: Williams & Wilkins; pp 93–109.

Lorente de No R. (1947) Analysis of the distribution of action currents of nerve in volume conductors. *Stud Rockefeller Inst Med Res*. 132, 384–482.

Lynn JM, Lesner SA, Sandridge SA, Daddario CC. (1984) Threshold prediction from the auditory 40-Hz evoked potential. *Ear Hear*. 5, 366–370.

Mackersie C, Down KE, Stapells DR. (1993) Pure-tone masking profiles for human auditory brainstem and middle latency responses. *Hear Res*. 65, 61–68.

Margolis RH, Dubno JR, Hunt SM. (1981) Detection of tones in band-reject noise. *J Speech Hear Res*. 24, 336–344.

Mason SM, Mellor DH. (1984) Brainstem, middle latency, and late cortical potentials in children with speech and language disorder. *Electroencephalogr Clin Neurophysiol*. 59, 297–307.

McFarland DJ, Cacace AT. (1995) Modality specificity as a criterion for diagnosing central auditory processing disorders. *Am J Audiol*. 4, 36–48.

McFarland DJ, Cacace AT. (2004) Separating stimulus-locked and unlocked components of the auditory event related potential. *Hear Res*. 193, 111–120.

McFarland DJ, McCane LM, David SV, Wolpaw JR. (1997) Spatial filter selection for EEG-based communication. *Electroencephalogr Clin Neurophysiol*. 103, 386–394.

McFarland WH, Vivion MC, Goldstein R. (1977) Middle components of the auditory evoked response to tone-pips in normal-hearing and hearing-impaired subjects. *J Speech Hear Res*. 20, 781–798.

McFarland WH, Vivion MC, Wolf KE, Goldstein R. (1975) Reexamination of the effects of stimulus rate and number on middle components of the averaged electroencephalic response. *Audiology*. 14, 456–465.

McGee T, Kraus N. (1996) Auditory development reflected by middle latency response. *Ear Hear*. 17, 419–429.

McPherson DL, Starr A. (1993) Binaural interaction in auditory evoked potentials: brainstem middle- and long-latency components. *Hear Res*. 66, 91–98.

Melcher JR, Talavage TM, Harms MP. (1999) Functional MRI of the auditory system. In: Moonen CTW, Bandettini P, eds. *Medical Radiology: Diagnostic Imaging and Radiation Oncology*. New York: Springer-Verlag; pp 393–406.

Mendel MI. (1980) Clinical use of primary cortical responses. *Audiology*. 19, 1–15.

Mendel MI. (1985) Middle and late auditory evoked potentials. In: Katz J, ed. *Handbook of Clinical Audiology*. 3rd ed. Baltimore: Williams & Wilkins; pp 565–581.

Miyamoto RT. (1986) Electrically evoked potentials in cochlear implant subjects. *Laryngoscope*. 96, 178–185.

Mohamed AS, Iacono RP, Yamada S. (1996) Normalization of middle latency auditory P1 potential following posterior ansapalladotomy in idiopathic Parkinson's disease. *Neurol Res*. 18, 515–520.

Møller AR. (1988) *Evoked Potentials in Intraoperative Monitoring*. Baltimore: Williams & Wilkins.

Møller AR. (1994) Neural generators of auditory evoked potentials. In: Jacobson JT, ed. *Principles and Applications in Auditory Evoked Potentials*. Boston: Allyn and Bacon.

Mosko SS, Knipher KF, Sassin JF, Donnelly J. (1984) Middle latency evoked potential in sleep apneics during waking and as a function of arterial oxygen saturation during apneas. *Sleep*. 7, 239–246.

Musiek FE, Baran J. (1987) Central auditory assessment: thirty years of challenge and change. *Ear Hear*. 8, 22–35.

Musiek FE, Geurkink NA. (1981) Auditory brainstem and middle latency evoked response sensitivity near threshold. *Ann Otol Rhinol Laryngol*. 90, 236–240.

Musiek FE, Geurkink NA, Weider DJ, Donnelly K. (1984) Past, present, and future applications of the auditory middle latency response. *Laryngoscope*. 94, 1545–1553.

Musiek FE, Lee WW. (1997) Conventional and maximum length sequences middle latency response in patients with central nervous system lesions. *J Am Acad Audiol*. 8, 173–180.

Myles-Worley M, Coon H, McDowell J, Byerley W. (1999) Linkage of a composite inhibitory phenotype to a chromosome 22q locus in eight Utah families. *Am J Med Genet*. 88, 544–550.

Nayak A, Roy RJ. (1999) Anesthesia control using midlatency auditory evoked potentials. *IEEE Trans Biomed Eng*. 45, 409–421.

Nelson MD, Jall JW III, Jacobson GP. (1997) Factors affecting the recordability of auditory evoked response components Pb (P1). *J Am Acad Audiol*. 8, 89–99.

Newman J, Moushegian G. (1989) Comparison of rate effects on the auditory middle latency response (MLR) in young and elderly adults. *J Acoust Soc Am*. 85, S38.

Oates P, Stapells DR. (1997a) Frequency specificity of the human auditory brainstem and middle latency responses to brief tones. I. High-pass noise masking. *J Acoust Soc Am*. 102, 3597–3608.

Oates P, Stapells DR. (1997b) Frequency specificity of the human auditory brainstem and middle latency responses to brief tones. II. Derived response analyses. *J Acoust Soc Am*. 102, 3609–3619.

Ohl FW, Deliano M, Scheich H, Freeman W. (2003) Analysis of evoked and emergent patterns of stimulus-evoked auditory cortical activity. *Rev Neurosci*. 14, 35–42.

Onitsuka T, Ninomiya H, Sato E, Yamamoto T, Tashiro N. (2003) Differential characteristics of the middle latency auditory evoked magnetic responses to interstimulus intervals. *Clin Neurophysiol*. 114, 1513–1520.

Osterhammel PA, Shallop JK, Terkildsen K. (1985) The effect of sleep on the auditory brainstem response (ABR) and the middle latency response (MLR). *Scand Audiol*. 14, 47–50.

Özdamar Ö, Kraus N, Curry F. (1982) Auditory brain stem and middle latency responses in a patient with cortical deafness. *Electroencephalogr Clin Neurophysiol*. 53, 224–230.

Pandya DN. (1995) Anatomy of the auditory cortex. *Rev Neurol*. 151, 486–494.

Pandya DN, Rosene DL, Doolittle AM. (1994) Corticothalamic connections of auditory-related areas of the temporal lobe in the rhesus monkey. *J Comp Neurol*. 345, 447–471.

Pantev C, Lutkenhoner B, Hoke M, Lehnertz K. (1986) Comparison between simultaneous recorded auditory evoked magnetic fields and potentials elicited by ipsilateral, contralateral, and binaural tone burst stimulation. *Audiology*. 25, 54–61.

Papanicolaou AC, Loring DW, Eisenberg HM. (1984) Age-related differences in recovery cycle of auditory evoked potentials. *Neurobiol Aging*. 5, 291–295.

Parving A, Salomon G, Elberling C, Larsen B, Lassen NA. (1980) Middle components of the auditory evoked response in bilateral temporal lobe lesions. Report on a patient with auditory agnosia. *Scand Audiol*. 9, 161–170.

Pasman J, Rotteveel J, Maasen B, Graaf R, Visco Y. (1997) Diagnostic and predictive value of auditory evoked responses in preterm infants. II. Auditory evoked responses. *Pediatr Res*. 42, 670–677.

Pekkonen E, Ahveninen J, Virtanan J, Teravanainen H. (1998) Parkinson's disease selectively impairs preattentive auditory processing: an MEG study. *NeuroReport*. 9, 2949–2952.

Pellizone M, Hari R, Makela JP, Huttunen J, Ahlfors S, Hamalainen M. (1987) Cortical origin of middle-latency auditory evoked responses in man. *Neurosci Lett*. 82, 303–307.

Pfeifferbaum A, Ford JM, Roth WT, Hopkins WF, Kopell BS. (1979) Event-related potential changes in healthy aged females. *Electroencephalogr Clin Neurophysiol*. 46, 81–86.

Phillips NA, Connolly JF, Matecole CC, Gray J. (1997) Individual differences in auditory middle latency responses in elderly adults and in patients with Alzheimer's disease. *Int J Psychophysiol*. 27, 125–136.

Picton TW, Dimitrijevic A, John MS. (2002) Multiple auditory steady-state responses. *Ann Otol Rhinol Laryngol Suppl*. 189, 16–21.

Picton TW, Hillyard SA. (1974) Human auditory evoked potentials. II. Effects of attention. *Electroencephalogr Clin Neurophysiol*. 36, 191–199.

Picton TW, Hillyard SA, Krausz HI, Galamabos R. (1974) Human auditory evoked potentials: I. Evaluation of components. *Electroencephalogr Clin Neurophysiol*. 36, 179–190.

Picton TW, John MS, Dimitrijevic A, Purcell D. (2003) Human auditory steady-state responses. *Int J Audiol*. 42, 177–219.

Picton TW, Vajsar J, Rodrigues R, Campbell KB. (1987) Reliability estimates for steady-state evoked potentials. *Electroencephalogr Clin Neurophysiol*. 68, 119–131.

Plourde G, Picton TW. (1990) Human auditory steady-state responses during general anesthesia. *Anesth Analg.* 71, 460–468.

Pratt H, Peled R, Scharf B, Lavie P. (1984) Auditory middle latency evoked potentials during sleep apnea. *Isr J Med Sci.* 20, 593–597.

Pynchon KA, Tucker DA, Ruth RA, Barrett KA, Herr DG. (1998) Area-under-the-curve measure of the auditory middle latency response (AMLR) from birth to early adulthood. *Am J Audiol.* 7, 1–5.

Rao AA, Talavage TM. (2005) Reliability of phase-encode mapping in the presence of spatial non-stationarity of response latency. *Neuroimage.* 28, 563–578.

Rappaport JM, Gulliver JM, Phillips DP, Van Dorp RA, Mazner CE, Bhan V. (1994) Auditory temporal resolution in multiple sclerosis. *J Otolaryngol.* 23, 307–324.

Rauschecker JP. (1998) Parallel processing in the auditory cortex of primates. *Audiol Neurootol.* 3, 86–103.

Rauschecker JP, Tian B, Pons T, Mishkin M. (1997) Serial and parallel processing in rhesus monkey auditory cortex. *J Comp Neurol.* 382, 89–103.

Reite M, Teale P, Zimmerman J, Davis K, Whalen J. (1988) Source location of a 50 msec latency auditory evoked field component. *Electroencephalogr Clin Neurophysiol.* 70, 490–498.

Rivier F, Clarke S. (1997) Cytochrome oxidase, acetylcholinesterase, and NADPH-diaphorase staining for human supratemporal and insular cortex: evidence for multiple auditory areas. *Neuroimage.* 6, 288–304.

Robinson K, Rudge P. (1977) Abnormalities of the auditory evoked potentials in patients with multiple sclerosis. *Brain.* 100, 19–40.

Ross B, Herdman AT, Pantev C. (2004a) Stimulus induced reset of 40-Hz auditory steady-state responses. *Neurol Clin Neurophysiol.* 30, 21.

Ross B, Herdman AT, Pantev C. (2005) Stimulus induced desynchronization of human auditory 40-Hz steady-state responses. *J Neurophysiol.* 94, 4082–4093.

Ross B, Picton TW, Herdman AT, Hillyard SA, Pantev C. (2004b) The effect of attention on the auditory steady state response. *Neurol Clin Neurophysiol.* 22, 1–4.

Ruhm H, Walker E Jr, Flanigin H. (1967) Acoustically evoked potentials in man: mediation of early components. *Laryngoscope.* 77, 806–822.

Rupp A, Gutschalk A, Uppencamp S, Scherg S. (2004) Middle latency auditory-evoked fields reflect psychoacoustic gap detection thresholds in human listeners. *J Neurophysiol.* 92, 2239–2247.

Scherg M. (1982) Simultaneous recording and separation of early and middle latency auditory evoked potentials. *Electroencephalogr Clin Neurophysiol.* 54, 339–341.

Scherg M, von Cramon D. (1986a) Evoked dipole source potentials of the human auditory cortex. *Electroencephalogr Clin Neurophysiol.* 65, 344–360.

Scherg M, von Cramon D. (1986b) Psychoacoustic and electrophysiologic correlates of central hearing disorders in man. *Eur Arch Psychiatry Neurol Sci.* 236, 56–60.

Scherg M, von Cramon D. (1990) Dipole source potentials of the auditory cortex in normal subjects and in patients with temporal lobe lesions. In: Grandori F, Hoke M, Romani GL, eds. *Auditory Evoked Magnetic Fields and Electric Potentials.* Basel: Karger; pp 165–193.

Schönwiesner M, von Cramon DY, Rübsamen R. (2002) Is it tonotopy after all? *Neuroimage.* 17, 1144–1161.

Selkoe DJ. (2002) Alzheimer's disease is a synaptic failure. *Science.* 298, 789–791.

Setzen G, Cacace AT, Eames F, Riback P, Lava N, McFarland DJ, Artino LA, Kerwood J. (1999) Central deafness in a young child with moyamoya disease: paternal linkage in a Caucasian family. Two case reports and a review of the literature. *Int J Pediatr Otorhinolaryngol.* 48, 53–76.

Shallop JK. (1993) Electric response audiometry: the morphology of normal responses. *Adv Oto-Rhino-Laryngol.* 29, 124–139.

Sharbrough F, Chatrian G-E, Lesser RP, Lüders H, Nuwer M, Picton TW. (1991) American electroencephalographic society guidelines for standard electrode position nomenclature. *J Clin Neurophysiol.* 8, 200–202.

Shehata-Dieler W, Shimizu H, Soliman SM, Tusa RJ. (1991) Middle latency auditory evoked potentials in temporal lobe disorders. *Ear Hear.* 12, 377–388.

Small DH, Mok SS, Bornstein JC. (2001) Alzheimer's disease and A-beta toxicity: from top to bottom. *Nat Rev Neurosci.* 8, 595–598.

Small SA, Stapells DR. (2004) Artifactual responses when recording auditory steady-state responses. *Ear Hear.* 25, 611–623.

Snyder JS, Large EW. (2005) Gamma-band activity reflects the metric structure of rhythmic tone sequences. *Brain Res Cogn Brain Res.* 24, 117–126.

Spink U, Johannsen HS, Pirsig W. (1979) Acoustically evoked potential: dependence on age. *Scand Audiol.* 8, 11–14.

Stach BA, Stoner WR, Smith SL, Jerger JF. (1994) Auditory evoked potentials in Rett syndrome. *J Am Acad Audiol.* 3, 226–230.

Stapells DR, Galambos R, Costello JA, Makeig S. (1988) Inconsistency of auditory middle latency and steady-state responses in infants. *Electroencephalogr Clin Neurophysiol.* 71, 289–295.

Stephenson WA, Gibbs FA. (1951) A balanced noncephalic reference electrode. *Electroencephalogr Clin Neurophysiol.* 3, 237–240.

Stewart MG, Jerger J, Lew HL. (1993) Effect of handedness on the middle latency auditory evoked potential. *Am J Otol.* 14, 595–600.

Streletz LJ, Katz L, Hohenberger M, Cracco R. (1977) Scalp recorded auditory evoked potentials and sensorimotor responses: an evaluation of components and recording techniques. *Electroencephalogr Clin Neurophysiol.* 43, 192–206.

Tallon-Baudry C, Bertrand O. (1999) Oscillatory gamma activity in humans and its role in object representation. *Trends Cogn Sci.* 4, 151–162.

Tanaka Y, Kamo T, Yoshida M, Yamadori A. (1991) "So-called" cortical deafness. *Brain.* 114, 2385–2410.

Taveras JM. (1996) *Neuroradiology.* 3rd edition. Baltimore: Williams & Wilkins.

Terry RD, Masliah E, Salmon DP, Butters N, DeTeresa R, Hill R, Hansen LA, Katzman R. (1991) Physical basis of cognitive alterations in Alzheimer's disease: synapse loss is the major correlate of cognitive impairment. *Ann Neurol.* 4, 572–580.

Thornton AR, Abbas PJ. (1980) Low-frequency hearing loss: perception of filtered speech, psychophysical tuning curves, and masking. *J Acoust Soc Am.* 67, 638–643.

Thornton AR, Mendel MI, Anderson CV. (1977) Effects of stimulus frequency and intensity on the middle components of the averaged auditory electroencephalic response. *J Speech Hear Res.* 20, 81–94.

Thornton C, Sharpe RM. (1998) Evoked responses in anaesthesia. *Br J Anaesth.* 81, 771–781.

Tiitinen T, May P, Naatanen R. (1997) The transient 40-Hz response, mismatch negativity, and attentional processes in humans. *Prog Neuropsychopharmacol Biol Psychiatry.* 21, 751–771.

Toyoda K, Ibayashi S, Yamamoto T, Kuwabara Y, Fujishima M. (1998) Auditory evoked magnetic response in cerebrovascular disease: a preliminary study. *J Neurol Neurosurg Psychiatry.* 64, 777–784.

Truex RC, Carpenter MB. (1964) *Human Neuroanatomy.* Baltimore: Williams & Wilkins.

Turner C, Burns EM, Nelson DA. (1983) Pure tone pitch perception and low-frequency hearing loss. *J Acoust Soc Am.* 73, 966–975.

Versino M, Bergamaschi R, Romani A, Banfi P, Callieco R, Citterio A, Gerosa E, Cosi V. (1992) Middle latency auditory evoked potentials improve detection of abnormalities along auditory pathways in multiple sclerosis patients. *Electroencephalogr Clin Neurophysiol.* 84, 296–299.

Vivion MC, Hirsch JE, Frye-Osier JL, Goldstein R. (1980) Effects of rise-fall time and equivalent duration on middle components of AER. *Scand Audiol.* 9, 223–232.

Vizioli L, Bucciero A, Quaglietta P, Mosca F. (1993) Auditory middle latency responses in patients with intracranial space-occupying lesions. *J Neurosurg Sci.* 37, 77–81.

Weber F, Bein T, Hobbhahn J, Taeger K. (2004) Evaluation of the Alaris auditory evoked potential index as an indicator of anesthetic depth in preschool children during induction of anesthesia with sevoflurane and remifemanil. *Anesthesiology.* 101, 294–298.

Winer JA, Miller LM, Lee CC, Schreiner CE. (2005) Auditory thalamocortical transformation: structure and function. *Trends Neurosci.* 28, 255–263.

Wolpaw JR, Penry K. (1975) A temporal component of the auditory evoked potential. *Electroencephalogr Clin Neurophysiol.* 39, 609–620.

Wolpaw JR, Penry K. (1978) Acute and chronic antiepileptic drug effect on the T complex interhemispheric latency difference. *Epilepsia.* 19, 99–107.

Wood CC, Wolpaw JR. (1982) Scalp distribution of human auditory evoked potentials. II. Evidence for overlapping sources and involvement of auditory cortex. *Electroencephalogr Clin Neurol.* 54, 25–38.

Woods DL, Clayworth CC. (1986) Age-related changes in human middle latency auditory evoked potentials. *Electroencephalogr Clin Neurophysiol.* 65, 297–303.

Woods DL, Clayworth CC, Knight RT, Simpson GV, Naeser MA. (1987) Generators of middle- and long-latency auditory evoked potentials: implications from studies of patients with bitemporal lesions. *Electroencephalogr Clin Neurophysiol.* 68, 132–148.

Woods DL, Knight RT, Neville HJ. (1984) Bitemporal lesions dissociate auditory evoked potentials and perception. *Electroencephalogr Clin Neurophysiol.* 57, 208–220.

Wu C, Stapells DR. (1994) Pure-tone masking profiles for human brainstem and middle latency responses to 500-Hz tones. *Hear Res.* 78, 169–174.

Xu Z-M, De Vel E, Vinck B, Van Cauwenberge P. (1995a) Selecting the best tone-pip stimulus-envelope time for estimating an objective middle-latency response threshold for low- and middle-tone sensorineural hearing losses. *Eur Arch Otorhinolaryngol.* 252, 275–279.

Xu Z-M, De Vel E, Vinck B, Van Cauwenberge P. (1995b) Application of cross-correlation function in the evaluation of objective MLR thresholds in the low and middle frequencies. *Scan Audiol.* 24, 231–236.

Xu Z-M, De Vel E, Vinck B, Van Cauwenberge P. (1996) Middle latency responses to assess objective thresholds in patients with noise-induced hearing losses and Ménière's disease. *Eur Arch Otorhinolaryngol.* 253, 222–226.

Yvert B, Crouziex A, Bertrand O, Seither-Preisler A, Pantev C. (2001) Multiple supratemporal sources of magnetic and electric auditory evoked middle latency components in humans. *Cereb Cortex.* 11, 411–423.

Cortical Event-Related Potentials to Auditory Stimuli

David R. Stapells

⬛ INTRODUCTION

This chapter concerns the "slow" and "late" cortical event-related potentials (ERPs) that may be recorded in response to auditory stimuli. Occurring at least 50 ms following stimulus onset, these responses follow the cochlear and eighth-nerve responses (Chapter 12), the auditory brainstem responses (ABRs; Chapters 13 and 14), and the early cortical middle latency auditory evoked potentials (MLAEPs; Chapter 17), as indicated in Table 18.1. In contrast to the earlier responses, the slow and, especially, the late ERPs are closely linked to perceptual processes such as discrimination and may be elicited by almost any type of auditory stimuli, from simple tonal stimuli, to speech stimuli, to full sentences. Although often considered together as the "late" auditory evoked potentials (AEPs), the present chapter maintains the original "slow" and "late" classifications (Davis, 1976; Picton et al., 1985) because of differences in their functional significance. When combined with the earlier auditory ERPs, one can obtain measures of the timing, strength, and anatomic location—ranging from cochlea, brainstem, auditory cortical, and tertiary cortical areas—of processes underlying auditory perception. Recordings of ERPs to auditory stimuli thus provide a spatiotemporal window into the brain processes underlying the sensory and perceptual processes of the auditory system.

Cortical ERPs, especially the slow cortical P1-N1-P2 sequence and the mismatch negativity (MMN), have provided insight into brain processes that underlie many aspects of auditory perception, including frequency, intensity, and duration discrimination (Giard et al., 1995; Joutsiniemi et al., 1998; Näätanen et al., 1987a; Sams et al., 1985; Stapells and

So, 1998); gap detection (Bertoli et al., 2001; Desjardins et al., 1999; Heinrich et al., 2004; Stapells et al., 2002); temporal integration (Yabe et al., 1998; Tervaniemi et al., 1994); auditory scene analysis (Alain et al., 2005; Ritter et al., 2000; Sussman, 2005); processes related to the precedence effect (Damaschke et al., 2005; Dimitrijevic and Stapells, 2006; Stapells and Wu, 2000); music perception and training (Trainor et al., 1999; 2003); audiovisual integration (Besle et al., 2004; Pettigrew et al., 2004); categorical speech perception (Aaltonen et al., 1987; Maiste et al., 1995; Sharma et al., 1993; Tsui et al., 2000); and effects of training and brain plasticity (Kraus, McGee, Carrell, King et al., 1995; Tremblay et al., 1997; 1998; Tremblay and Kraus, 2002), to name a few. Furthermore, these responses are being used to study maturation of auditory processing (Cheour et al., 1998a; Gomes et al., 1999; Martin et al., 2003; Morr et al., 2002; Ponton et al., 1996b; Wang et al., 2005; Wunderlich et al., 2006; Molholm et al., 2004), auditory aging (Alain and Woods, 1999; Anderer et al., 1998; Cooper et al., 2005; Friedman et al., 1998; Goodin et al., 1978; Harkrider et al., 2005; Jerger and Martin, 2005; Pekkonen et al., 1996; Tremblay et al., 2003), and processing in clinical populations, such as those with sensory-neural hearing loss (SNHL) and hearing aids (Korczak et al., 2005; Oates et al., 2002; Ponton et al., 2001), cochlear implants (Beynon et al., 2005; Gordon et al., 2005; Kelly et al., 2005; Kraus et al., 1993c; Lonka et al., 2004; Micco et al., 1995; Pelizzone et al., 1987; Ponton et al., 1998; Sharma et al., 2002; Singh et al., 2004), auditory processing disorder (Gravel and Stapells, 1993; Jirsa, 1992; Jirsa and Clontz, 1990; Klein et al., 1995; Kraus et al., 1993b; Liasis et al., 2003; Yencer, 1998), and language impairment (Hagoort and Kutas, 1995; Klein et al., 1995; Leppänen and

TABLE 18.1 Classification of human auditory evoked potentials

Function	Anatomy	Latency	Relationship to stimulus		
			Transient	**Steady-state**	**Sustained**
Sensory	Cochlear and eighth nerve Brainstem Early cortical Cortical	First *(0–5 ms)* Fast *(2–20 ms)* Middle *(10–100 ms)* Slow *(50–300 ms)*	Eighth nerve CAP ABR waves I and II ABR (waves III, IV, and V) MLAEP (Na, Pa, Nb) **Slow "vertex" potential** (P1, **N1**, P2, N2)	Cochlear microphonic FFR, >60-Hz ASSR ~ 40-Hz ASSR <20-Hz ASSR	Summating potential Pedestal of FFR Cortical Sustained Potential
Processing-Contingent Potentials	Cortical	Late *(150–1,000 ms)*	**Mismatch negativity (MMN)** Processing negativity (Nd) **N2b** **P3a,P3b** LAN, **N400**, P600		CNV

CAP, compound action potential; ABR, auditory brainstem response; MLAEP, middle latency auditory evoked potential; FFR, frequency following response; ASSR, auditory steady-state response; LAN, left anterior negativity; CNV, contingent negative variation.

Lyytinen, 1997; Neville et al., 1993; Shafer et al., 2005; Uwer et al., 2002). Finally, work has focused on possible use of the cortical ERPs to add to the clinical assessment of individuals with these disorders as well as other problems. To date, success has been somewhat limited, with the exception of the slow cortical P1-N1-P2 sequence, which currently has unquestionable clinical applications.

This chapter provides an introduction to several cortical ERPs, specifically, the slow cortical P1-N1-P2, MMN, N2b-P3b, and the N400 (shown in bold in Table 18.1), as well as some current clinical data and applications. There are literally hundreds of papers published considering the cortical ERPs to auditory stimuli. While several groups of researchers in audiology and hearing sciences have contributed significantly to this work, most of the work in the area has been carried out by researchers within the domains of psychology, psychophysiology, cognitive neuroscience, and neurophysiology, and the great majority of these papers are published in journals representing these fields. The vastness of this literature makes it impossible for the present chapter to provide more than an introduction to these responses. Within each section of the present chapter, readers are referred to papers providing more comprehensive reviews of the response(s) in question. To become knowledgeable of the cortical auditory ERPs, audiologists must become familiar with the extensive literature that exists outside of the audiologic literature. Readers are also referred to the large number of excellent general reviews of ERPs (Cone-Wesson and Wunderlich, 2003; Burkard et al., 2007; Hill-yard and Picton, 1987; Näätänen, 1992; Picton and Hillyard, 1988; Polich, 2004; Polich and Criado, 2006; Rugg and Coles, 1995a).

The ERP nomenclature that is most common within the (current) literature has been adopted for this chapter. Thus, "N1" is used for the vertex-negative slow cortical wave, rather than "N100," and "P3a" and "P3b" are used for the late positive component "P3," rather than "P300." (One problem with latency-based nomenclature is that, depending upon the stimuli and/or task, the waves very often are not near the designated latency!) The exception to this is the use of "N400." Readers of this chapter will also note that the various waveform figures are plotted such that negativity is plotted upwards, which reflects the fact that most of the cortical ERP literature present the waveforms "negative-up," although this appears to be changing.

CLASSIFICATION OF AUDITORY EVENT-RELATED POTENTIALS

AEPs are brain responses "evoked" by the presentation of auditory stimuli. Brain responses, however, often reflect more than just activity evoked by a sensory stimulus, hence the term "event-related potential" (Coles and Rugg, 1995). ERPs are brain responses that are time-locked to some specified event. The "event" may occur within a sensory modality or across modalities. The "event" may be a physical stimulus (such as an auditory tone), a change in a train of stimuli (such as a series of 1,000-Hz tones briefly changing to 2,000-Hz tones), a missing stimulus (such as a tone omitted from a sequence of tones), or a stimulus that has been designated as a "target" stimulus. Indeed, the "event" may be the result of the psychological demands of the situation (Donchin et al., 1978) and little related to the specific sensory stimuli. The AEPs are a subset of the ERPs.

As outlined in Table 18.1, there are many ERPs that may be recorded in response to auditory events, and there are several methods to classify them. These ERPs can be divided into two major categories: sensory (auditory) evoked potentials (EPs) and processing-contingent potentials (PCPs) (Steinschneider et al., 1992). Sensory EPs are mainly "obligatory" brain responses to the physical properties of the stimuli. The auditory ERPs may be classified according to their presumed site of generation, their latency relative to stimulus onset, or their relationship to the stimulus (Table 18.1) (Picton, 1990). The present chapter focuses on the transient auditory sensory EPs and PCPs originating within cortical structures.

Auditory sensory EPs reflect activation of the auditory pathways, from the cochlea to the cortex. They occur as early as stimulus onset and extend to as late as 300 ms poststimulus. The AEPs of cortical origin are affected by arousal level and attention; those that are subcortical in origin are essentially unaffected by attention and state (Steinschneider et al., 1992). The "processing-contingent potentials are associated with further processing of sensory stimuli, beyond that driven by the physical properties of the stimulus.... [PCPs] are associated with both active, attention-dependent, perceptual or cognitive processes, and with automatic processing that is not under volitional control, as when a novel or unexpected change in a stimulus characteristic occurs" (Coles and Rugg, 1995, p 16).

Often called "endogenous," PCPs represent processing beyond obligatory sensory processing stages (Steinschneider et al., 1992). In contrast, the sensory EPs are often called "exogenous," in that they represent obligatory sensory processing, are dependent on the presence of the stimuli, and are sensitive to changes in the physical characteristics of the stimuli. However, as Steinschneider et al. (1992) have pointed out, all ERPs are endogenous by virtue of their generation within the brain, and none of the ERPs are entirely endogenous, in the sense of being independent of sensory input. Furthermore, some so-called exogenous ERPs are altered by endogenous processes. For example, N1 of the slow cortical AEP, a sensory EP that is generally considered as being exogenous, is nonetheless affected by endogenous processes such as attention. The MMN, generally considered an endogenous PCP related to change detection, is highly dependent on the physical characteristics of the differences between auditory stimuli. Coles and Rugg (1995) point out that the exogenous-endogenous distinction is an oversimplification and that it is more accurate to conceive "of an exogenous-endogenous *dimension* that is roughly coextensive with time" (Steinschneider et al., 1992, p 16). In this author's view, strict adherence to the dichotomy implied by these terms will almost certainly result in misinterpretation of ERP results.

▨ GENERAL TECHNICAL ISSUES FOR EVENT-RELATED POTENTIALS

Stimulation Techniques

With the exception of recordings of the slow cortical response for threshold estimation purposes, the cortical ERPs require special, and often complex, stimulation techniques. The simplest of these techniques, often called the "oddball" technique, requires two different "events," which may be two different stimuli, a stimulus and an omitted stimulus, or the same stimulus but presented at a different intensity, ear, etc. Typically, one event called the "standard" is presented for the majority of the trials (e.g., with a probability of 0.8 to 0.95), and the other event, called the "deviant," is presented for the remainder of the trials (i.e., with a probability of 0.2 to 0.05). Most often, the standards and deviants are presented in a pseudorandom order. Depending on the ERP being recorded and the purpose of the study, the subject may either ignore the stimuli (such as for MMN recordings, where subjects often watch a closed-captioned video) or be attending to and responding to the deviants (such as for P3 recordings, where subjects often push a button to, or count, the deviants). The computer averaging the brain's responses must be capable of calculating separate averages to the standard and deviant stimuli. The response to the deviants is then typically compared to the response to the standards (see below).

From the simple oddball paradigm described earlier, stimulation paradigms (and subsequent analyses) may become very complex. Stimuli differing on one or more dimensions may be used, as might more complex stimuli such as speech. For example, it is quite common to include multiple deviant stimuli, especially for MMN studies (Deacon et al., 1998; Giard et al., 1995; Näätänen et al., 2004; Ritter et al., 1995; Schroger, 1996), allowing one to assess the brain's differential response to changes of differing degree, etc. Other variations include multiple "target" deviant stimuli, including "novel" stimuli, where the subject may have to respond differentially to the different stimuli; and presentation of a series of stimuli, such as words in a sentence, where recordings are obtained for the whole sentence, with event markings for each word in the sentence. The computer analyzing these results must be capable of keeping track of responses to each stimulus, as well as the subject's different responses to them. In most cases, averaging and analyses of these results are carried out offline, after the subject has left. Unfortunately, most current clinical audiology equipment does not allow one to make up and/or use stimuli other than tones simply differing in frequency (and these are usually at least a half-octave apart) or level, and most clinical equipment is not capable of keeping track of responses to more than two stimuli or of keeping track of subject's behavioral response accuracy and reaction times. As noted below, it is likely that, with the exception of slow cortical response for threshold estimation, application of the cortical ERPs for clinical audiology will require increasingly complex stimulation and recording capabilities.

Artifact Issues

Electrical potentials generated by eye movements and blinks are a major problem when recording cortical ERPs; one must pay careful attention to ocular artifact for all cortical ERPs, except recordings of the slow cortical response, for the purpose of threshold estimation. These ocular potentials are large—often larger than the ERP of interest—and are easily entrained by the stimulus sequences used to evoke cortical ERPs such as the MMN, P3, or N400 (Picton, 1992). There are a number of approaches to this problem, and all require one or two electroencephalogram (EEG) analysis channels that preferentially record the electro-oculogram (EOG). At a minimum, the EOG is monitored using electrodes above and below the eyes (for vertical eye movements and blinks). (A second EOG channel for horizontal eye movements may also be monitored by placing electrodes on the outer canthi.) Trials containing potentials in the EOG channel(s) exceeding some criterion (usually ± 100 μV) are then rejected *for all recording channels*.[1] The EOG must still be recorded and averaged with the EEG to ensure that small eye movements and blinks (those that are within ± 100 μV) do not become time-locked to the stimuli (Picton, 1992).

Multiple recording channels are essential when evaluating ocular artifacts. Comparison of the average waveform in the EOG channel and of the anterior-posterior scalp distribution of a response will aid in determining whether a response may be contaminated by EOG; for example, a positive response at electrode Pz (e.g., P3b) that decreases in amplitude for more anterior electrodes (Cz, Fz) is unlikely to be largely EOG. If the opposite is true, however, or if there is little change in amplitude, one cannot say whether the wave is neural or ocular in origin, at least not without a vertical EOG channel.

A large drawback of rejection of trials with EOG artifact is that, for some subjects, few trials may remain after rejection. To decrease the number of rejections, subjects are typically instructed to limit their blinks and eye movements during a recording block. This can be very difficult for some individuals and impossible for longer periods. Furthermore, by dividing their attention between their eyes and the stimuli, the resulting brain response may be altered (Picton, 1992; Verleger, 1991). Alternative methods to deal with eye blinks and movements involve techniques to record and correct for ocular artifacts rather than reject them (Gratton et al., 1983); most recent methods use multichannel recordings and either source localization or spatial filters to remove ocular artifact (Berg and Scherg, 1991; Ille et al., 2002; Scarff et al., 2004).

Although not perfect and available only on more sophisticated equipment, these methods usually provide more accepted and less contaminated trials, particularly in patient populations.

Electromagnetic potentials from stimulus transducers are another source of artifact that may be a problem for recording, analysis, and interpretation of cortical ERPs. These are particularly a problem when longer duration stimuli such as speech are used, especially when recording responses in cochlear implant users to acoustic stimuli, where radiofrequency pulses appear in the electrodes surrounding the implant magnet (Boothroyd, 2005; Martin et al., 2007). Even with such artifact, multichannel recordings often allow one to analyze responses in channels not affected by the artifact. Electromagnetic artifact can be high enough to saturate EEG amplifiers, in which case the amplifiers must be "blocked" during the stimulus. One approach to the stimulus-artifact problem is to use very brief stimuli and directly stimulate the intracochlear electrodes and to bypass the processing unit (i.e., not use acoustic stimuli) (Ponton et al., 1993). Use of brief stimuli (< 10 to 20 ms) may solve many problems. Nevertheless, there is interest in cortical ERPs to acoustic speech stimuli in cochlear implant users, and successful recordings have recently been reported (Beynon et al., 2005; Gordon et al., 2005; Kelly et al., 2005; Lonka et al., 2004; Singh et al., 2004).

Multiple-Channel Recordings

In contrast to recordings of the auditory brainstem or middle latency responses, cortical ERP recordings require the acquisition of multiple EOG/EEG channels. (Again, the exception to this is the recording, for threshold purposes, of the slow cortical P1-N1-P2 response.) An individual reviewing the nonaudiology cortical ERP literature will quickly see that most studies over the past 10 years obtain recordings for at least eight to 16 EOG/EEG channels and that recent studies now obtain recordings for 32, 64, or 128 channels. Studies using 32 or more channels typically use special electrode "caps" that speed electrode application and location accuracy. There are several purposes for multiple-channel recordings; in addition to detecting and correcting/removing artifacts (discussed earlier), it determines the minimum number of channels required.

ERP waveform identification (Is that MMN? Is that P3b?) requires an indication of the general scalp distribution of the wave and evidence that it is not due to ocular artifact. For example, P3b is a parietocentral positive deflection. That is, it should be largest at Pz and decrease in amplitude from Pz to Cz to Fz. If the waveform does not show this distribution, it may be EOG artifact (requiring at least a vertical EOG channel), it may be P3a or some other wave, or it may be noise. Thus, for the waveform identification that might be used in clinical testing, a *minimum of four* appropriately placed electrode channels (one EOG and three EEG) is required, although more channels are desirable.

---

[1] Users should ensure that their clinical evoked potential system is capable of this all-channel ("linked") rejection. Although standard on most equipment, one major manufacturer's popular clinical evoked potential system is not currently capable of this all-channel artifact rejection.

Investigation of the scalp topography ("mapping": the distribution of amplitudes across the head) and/or the location(s) of the intracranial source(s) (the "generators") of a cortical ERP wave requires substantially more electrode channels (Picton et al., 1995). Again, the number required depends on the purpose; reasonable scalp topography "maps" and source analyses are possible using only 16 scalp electrodes, providing that one understands and accepts the limits on the spatial accuracy placed by level of noise in the ERP recordings and errors in the measuring electrode locations (as a rule of thumb, for noise-free data, spatial accuracy is approximately half the distance between electrodes). Provided that data are noise free, increased spatial accuracy may be obtained with use of an increasing number of electrodes; however, with increasing number of electrodes, the effects of position noise (inaccuracy in measuring electrode locations) and model noise (errors in the model of the head) cause additional problems, including adding "ghost" sources to the analyses. A practical upper limit is about 64 electrodes (Bertrand et al., 1998; Yvert et al., 1997).

It is important for readers to realize that (1) responses recorded at the scalp typically represent the activities of multiple overlapping generator sources, and (2) responses recorded at a particular electrode do not necessarily arise from brain regions close to that electrode—indeed, they likely do not. Along the same line, the maximal amplitude of an ERP is not necessarily recorded at the scalp electrodes closest to its source. Topographic maps of ERP amplitudes by themselves do not, therefore, indicate the number or location of generator(s) underlying the ERP. Significant differences in topographies of the waves, however, do suggest different sources. To unravel the underlying sources and to determine the location(s) of these sources, the topographic data must be further analyzed using source analysis software (such as BESA or LORETA) (Anderer et al., 1998; Pascual-Marqui et al., 1994; Picton et al., 1995; Scherg and von Cramon, 1986a). Source analyses are highly complicated and require knowledge of assumptions and procedures of these analyses as well as knowledge of the underlying anatomy and physiologic processes in order to place appropriate constraints on the source model (Picton et al., 1995). It is quite likely that future clinical applications in audiology will involve abnormalities involving comparison of waves at different electrodes or abnormalities concerning the scalp distribution and/or sources of ERPs, all of which will require more sophisticated capabilities than what is available with most equipment currently used clinically.

Cortical Event-Related Potential Measures

The analysis of cortical ERP waves involves procedures and measures different from simply obtaining the latency and peak-to-peak amplitudes used for ABR and MLAEP analyses. Latency measures are similar to ABR/MLAEP measures, although "onset" and "offset" latency measures are also sometimes obtained. In contrast to the ABR/MLAEP, amplitude measures are almost always obtained for cortical ERPs, with several possible methods. With the exception of the threshold slow cortical response, where N1-P2 peak-to-peak amplitudes are typically measured, the amplitudes of cortical ERP peaks are almost always measured relative to a prestimulus baseline. This baseline is usually the average amplitude over the 50 to 100 ms preceding the stimulus. Equipment must therefore be able to begin recording prior to stimulus presentation, obtain the average amplitude over the prestimulus baseline, and "baseline correct" the averages based on this baseline. Once this baseline correction is completed, amplitude measures are typically obtained by measuring the mean voltage over a predetermined window (usually 25 to 100 ms in duration) or by measuring the peak voltage (i.e., the maximum voltage). Other, less common measures are the duration and the "area" of a response (essentially, the amplitude X duration). Latency and amplitude measures may be reported for one electrode site, several electrode sites, or a large number of sites (as in "mapping"), depending on the purpose of the study.

Additional waveform manipulations are often performed prior to obtaining latency and amplitude measures. Some sort of waveform subtraction is commonly performed, particularly for studies of the MMN, Nd, and N2b, giving a "difference wave." The most common subtraction procedure is to subtract the response to the standards from the response to the deviants, giving a difference wave presumably reflecting the brain's response to the change in stimuli and/or task. However, it is important to realize that waves in the resulting difference wave may reflect latency/amplitude differences between the obligatory (sensory) responses to the different stimuli, or stimulus-specific refractoriness, rather than a task-dependent or change-detection process. This issue is particularly of concern for ERPs in the latency range of N1, especially the MMN. There are a number of stimulus/recording procedures devised to attempt to control these issues: (1) reduce stimulus-related difference waves by avoiding large stimulus changes; (2) maintain stimulus constancy by counterbalancing the stimuli, such that, in separate blocks, each is presented as a deviant and standard, then subtract the waveform recorded when a stimulus was a standard from the waveform when the same stimulus was a deviant (sometimes called the "flip-flop" control); or (3) maintain stimulus constancy by recording a control recording to each stimulus alone, with the same interstimulus interval (ISI) as in the standard-deviant sequence, and subtract the control waveform from the deviant waveform to the same stimulus ("control alone"). All of these procedures have disadvantages: the flip-flop is time consuming; and the control alone does not have the standard-deviant context, and there is uncertainty about which stimulus interval to use (interstimulus or interdeviant). Neither method controls for stimulus rate issues. One approach that avoids some of these issues is to use a very fast ISI (e.g., 50 to 100 ms) that attenuates P1-N1-P2 and leaves MMN (Javitt et al., 1998); this method, unfortunately, makes recording of P1-N1-P2 impossible, and MMN must be interpreted with caution as rate and acoustic issues (such as the "N1 effect," see below) may not have been accounted for (Martin et al., 2007). Some recent studies have concluded that the flip-flop method is not required (Jacobsen and Schroger, 2003; Sharma et al., 2004). As yet, however, there is no general consensus about which of these procedures is best.

DESCRIPTION OF RESPONSES

Slow Cortical Response (P1-N1-P2)

Recorded at the vertex, the slow cortical response is comprised of a positive wave at about 50 ms (P1), a large negative wave at about 80 to 100 ms (N1), and a subsequent positive wave at about 180 to 200 ms (P2). As shown in the waveforms of Figure 18.1, N1 is recorded maximally from frontocentral electrodes, such as the vertex. It is slightly larger (~10%) from frontocentral electrodes that are contralateral to the stimulated ear. Näätänen and Picton (1987) and Hyde (1997) have published comprehensive reviews of the auditory N1 response.

Originally, the auditory evoked P1-N1-P2 sequence was considered part of a larger class of "vertex" potentials that were maximum in amplitude near the vertex for different modalities and, thus, believed to represent a nonspecific cerebral process. The subject of much controversy, Vaughan and Ritter (1970) originally proposed that the auditory

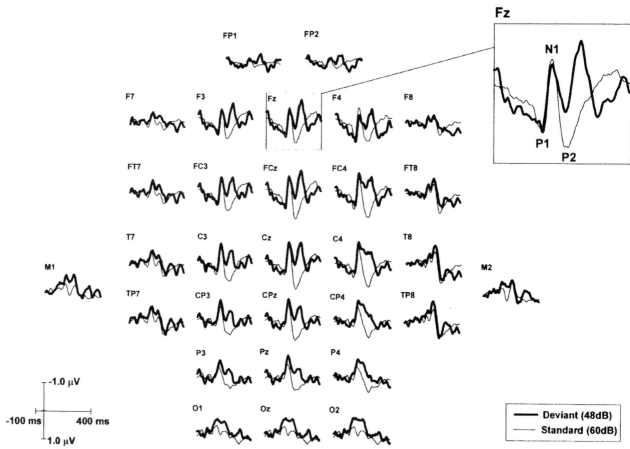

FIGURE 18.1   Scalp distribution of the cortical event-related potentials (ERPs) to standard and deviant 1,000-Hz tones. Shown are responses to 1,000-Hz tone bursts presented at 80 dB normal hearing level (nHL; standards, 0.9 probability) and 68 dB nHL (deviants, 0.1 probability), with an onset-to-onset interstimulus interval of 600 ms. Recordings, obtained from 100 ms prestimulus to 400 ms poststimulus, are referenced to an electrode on the tip on the nose. Standard waves: Slow cortical responses P1, N1 (peaking at about 120 ms), and P2 are labelled for the zoomed-in channel Fz (*box, upper right*). N1 decreases in amplitude (becomes less negative relative to prestimulus baseline) going from frontal-central electrodes (Fz, FCz, Cz) to posterior (CPz, Pz, Oz) electrodes. The response at the temporal electrodes (T7, T8) shows a double-peaked waveform (the T-complex) in the N1 latency region. At the mastoids (M1, M2), N1 inverts in polarity (becomes positive), reflecting its origin in the auditory cortex. Deviant waves: In addition to the slow cortical P1-N1-P2 waves, the response to the 12-dB lower deviants contains an additional negativity beginning, in these waveforms, after N1 and peaking at about 200 to 225 ms. This is the mismatch negativity, which is best visualized in the deviant-minus-standard difference waves (see Fig. 18.4). In this and all subsequent figures, negativity is represented by an upwards deflection.

vertex response was actually generated in the auditory cortex bilaterally on the superior aspect of the temporal lobe and not within areas nonspecific to the auditory modality. To a large extent, Vaughan and Ritter have been shown to be correct, and the term "vertex" potential is no longer thought to be appropriate or helpful (Näätänen and Picton, 1987). The N1, however, is not a unitary component, and thus, the generators are not singular.

GENERATORS

The scalp distribution of the auditory N1, the magnetic fields recorded at the same latency as the N1, and the effects of cerebral lesions on the N1 suggest three different components contributing to the scalp-recorded wave, two of which are generated within the auditory cortex bilaterally. The generation site of third component is still unclear but appears to be in modality nonspecific areas (Näätänen and Picton, 1987). The first component is a frontocentral negativity (N1b at 80 to 100 ms) generated by bilateral vertically oriented dipoles in (and, likely, around) the primary auditory cortices, as originally proposed by Vaughan and Ritter (1970). It is, therefore, best recorded near the vertex and typically inverts in polarity at electrodes below the level of the auditory cortex (e.g., at the mastoids) when a nose reference is used (Vaughan and Ritter, 1970). Studies measuring N1 using an electrode on or near the vertex and using a relatively short (i.e., ≤3 seconds) ISI will be primarily measuring this first component. The second component is the biphasic T-complex, originally described by Wolpaw and Penry (1975), with a positive wave at 100 ms and a negative wave at 150 ms. This complex, best recorded using midtemporal electrodes, probably originates bilaterally in auditory association cortex in the superior temporal gyrus. This component has a radially-oriented generator. The third component is one that corresponds best with early notions of a nonspecific response. It is a vertex-negative wave at about 100 ms, the generator of which is possibly within frontal motor and/or premotor cortex, under the influence of reticular formation and the ventral lateral nucleus of the thalamus (Näätänen and Picton, 1987). ISIs of less than 4 seconds reduce the amplitude of this component. There may also be other subcomponents of the N1 (Näätänen, 1992; Picton et al., 1995; Scherg et al., 1989).

N1 FUNCTIONAL SIGNIFICANCE

As pointed out by Näätänen and Picton (1987), all three N1 components respond to a steep change in physical energy that has remained constant at least for a short time. Thus, a stimulus onset from a quiet background or a continuous tone that occasionally changes its frequency is usually associated with an N1 wave (Picton et al., 2000). N1 thus seems to reflect auditory cortex mechanisms sensitive to change (Näätänen and Picton, 1987). Alain et al. (1997) note, however, that N1 probably not only indexes change, but also cortical activity that occurs throughout the sensation of sounds. The N1 generators—at least component 1—may reflect the result of some sort of "attention-triggering" process, representing the initial readout of information from sensory analyzers

(Näätänen and Picton, 1987). N1 may also reflect the formation of a memory trace for the eliciting stimulus to be used in subsequent trace comparison processes (see following "Mismatch Negativity" section). Thus, the presence of N1 to a stimulus provides physiologic evidence of the arrival at the auditory cortex of sensory information. N1, therefore, reflects the presence of "audible" stimuli. Although necessary for discrimination, the presence of N1 does not, by itself, indicate discrimination (Martin and Boothroyd, 2000; Martin et al., 1999; Martin et al., 1997; Martin and Stapells, 2005; Martin et al., 2007; Whiting et al., 1998) [see following "Mismatch Negativity" and "Late Attention-Related Waves (N2b-P3a/P3b)" sections]. Nevertheless, N1 does provide proof of the arrival of "potentially discriminable" information to the auditory cortex and, thus, likely has clinical importance (Martin and Boothroyd, 1999; Martin et al., 2007). It is quite likely that the different subcomponents underlying the scalp-recorded N1 will have different functional significance and, hence, be affected differently by dysfunction (Klein et al., 1995).

STIMULUS EFFECTS

The N1 may be elicited by a change in amplitude of an auditory stimulus, by a change in its frequency, by a change in its spatial location, and by speech stimuli. The P1-N1-P2 can be recorded in response to changes in ongoing sounds, such as changes in spectrum, amplitude, and periodicity cues in consonant-vowel stimuli or formant-frequency changes in an ongoing vowel. Such stimuli, often containing multiple acoustic changes, result in multiple and sometimes overlapping P1-N1-P2 complexes; Martin and colleagues have termed these the "acoustic change complex" (ACC) (Martin and Boothroyd, 1999; 2000; Ostroff et al., 1998). The ACC may be useful in exploring the neural detection of time-varying acoustic cues in individuals with impaired speech detection (Martin et al., 2007).

Stimulus Frequency

There is no major effect of stimulus frequency on N1 amplitude. At higher stimulus levels, N1 amplitudes are greater in response to 250- to 1,000-Hz stimuli than 2,000- to 4,000-Hz stimuli; these differences decrease or disappear near threshold or if the stimuli are equated in loudness (for review, see Hyde [1997]).

Stimulus Rise-Fall and Duration

The N1 wave is evoked by relatively abrupt changes in energy that has remained constant for at least a short time. N1 latency and amplitude are determined by the slope of the change. N1 amplitude increases with stimulus duration increase up to about 30 ms (Alain et al., 1997; Onishi and Davis, 1968) and decreases with rise-fall times longer than 50 ms (Onishi and Davis, 1968). Stimuli with very slow onsets do not elicit N1 (500 ms or more, depending upon the stimulus type, intensity, etc.). Sustained stimuli elicit N1 at their onset and, if the stimulus has been on for at least 0.5 seconds, at their offset (Näätänen, 1992). (A different response, the cortical sustained potential, is seen following N1 with stimuli of long duration.) It is likely that the onset dependency of N1 is a true onset response, rather than some artifact of neural synchronization (Näätänen and Picton, 1987). N1 thus seems to reflect auditory cortex mechanisms sensitive to change.

Interstimulus Interval

The ISI or rate of stimulus presentation has substantial effects on N1-P2 amplitude. N1-P2 amplitude increases as ISI is increased from <1 second until at least 10 seconds. The most efficient ISI (i.e., the ISI to obtain the best signal-to-noise ratio within a given time) is between 1 and 2 seconds (Picton et al., 1977). The effect of ISI on N1 amplitude is smaller for stimuli of lower intensity (Näätänen and Picton, 1987). Much of the decrease in N1 amplitude with stimulus repetition is due to generator refractoriness. In studies where responses to trains of stimuli were investigated, the largest decrease in N1 amplitude was seen to occur by the second stimulus (Näätänen and Picton, 1987). Of considerable importance, if the stimulus is changed (e.g., in frequency), N1 amplitude substantially recovers. These effects have been interpreted in terms of the degree of overlap between the neuronal populations activated by the two stimuli (Butler, 1968; Näätänen and Picton, 1987); stimuli that deviate considerably from

the ongoing stimuli activate "fresh" elements and thus elicit a larger N1 (Näätänen and Picton, 1987). Often referred to as the "Butler effect" or "N1 effect," this recovery of N1 with change in stimulus can be mistaken as MMN (see below).

Stimulus Intensity

With increasing stimulus intensity, N1 latency decreases, and its amplitude increases. With ISIs <3 seconds, the N1 amplitude tends to saturate at high levels. However, with longer ISIs, N1 amplitude shows less saturation. It is likely that the lack of saturation at long ISIs reflects the nonspecific non–auditory cortex generator (Näätänen and Picton, 1987). With optimal subject, stimulus, and recording characteristics, N1 is visible to within 5 to 10 dB of behavioral threshold. Thus, the P1-N1-P2 slow cortical response has important uses for the clinical evaluation of threshold (Hyde, 1997; Lightfoot and Kennedy, 2006; Tsui et al., 2002; Van Maanen and Stapells, 2005).

RECORDING PARAMETERS

Table 18.2 summarizes stimulus, recording, and waveform measure parameters for recording P1-N1-P2 of the slow cortical response for threshold estimation purposes. Readers should note that these parameters would be different when recording N1 for purposes other than threshold estimation. Typically, the latter require multiple-channel

---

TABLE 18.2   Parameters for slow cortical response (P1-N1-P2) thresholds

Population:	*Best:* Awake, alert, eyes open, adults or children age 6 years or older (reading book or watching closed-caption TV) *Possible:* Children under age 6 years who are awake and quiet *Difficult:* Sleeping infants and children; "noisy" adults
Stimuli:	250- to 4,000-Hz tone bursts Rise-fall times: 20 ms Plateau time: 20 ms Rate: 1 per 2 seconds (i.e., 0.5/s rate)

Recording:	Electrodes: 1 channel:
	     Inverting: Cz (vertex) or Fz[a]
	     Noninverting: ipsilateral OR contralateral mastoid (not linked)
	     (switching mastoids when switching ears not required)
	 1- to 30-Hz or 1- to 15-Hz EEG filters
	 Sensitivity/artifact reject: ±100 μV (Gain = 10,000–20,000)
	 Analysis time: –500 to +1,000 ms (i.e., 500-ms prestimulus)
	 # trials per average: 25–50
	 # replications: 2 (often 3, especially if <6 years or asleep)
	 "Control" (no stimulus) runs <u>not</u> required – use prestimulus time

Wave measures:	Waveform *must* be repeatable and 2–3 times larger than average amplitude of prestimulus *Awake/alert ≥6 years:* N1 latency and N1-P2 amplitude (P1 latency and amplitude <10 years) *Asleep or <6 years:* variable; repeatability of poststimulus tracing (i.e., presence/absence of a response) is most important. Sleeping adults often show very large N2. Awake young children often show large positive wave P1.

EEG, electroencephalogram.
[a] Connecting Cz or Fz electrode to "inverting" (often labelled as "–") will result in a "negative up" recording (with the N1 wave pointing upwards). "Negative-up" (as depicted in this chapter) versus "positive-up" is a matter of choice; either is correct.

recordings (including EOG) and different waveform measures (typically, baseline-to-peak amplitude measures, as well as peak latencies) and may involve considerably more complex stimuli and stimulation paradigms. Recordings of the N2b-P3b complex to auditory stimuli almost always contain clear N1 waves, as do most MMN stimulation and recording paradigms (provided that the ISI is at least 500 ms). Parameters for obtaining these later waves are provided in subsequent sections.

SUBJECT FACTORS

Attention

N1 amplitude is larger (i.e., more negative) when a subject pays attention to the stimuli. The exact nature of auditory selective attention on the N1 is a matter of some debate. Specifically, one view holds that the attention-related larger amplitude is a selective enhancement of N1 (Hillyard et al., 1973), whereas the other view holds that the enhanced N1 amplitude is the result of a "processing negativity" superimposed on, but different from, the N1 (Näätänen, 1982). It is possible that both views are correct (Näätänen and Picton, 1987).

Alertness and Sleep

N1 amplitude evoked by unattended auditory stimuli is greater the higher the level of alertness, although this may be due primarily to the nonspecific N1 component (Näätänen, 1992). The waveforms in the latency range of the slow response undergo large and complex changes with sleep. Most striking is the emergence of a large negativity at about 300 ms, sometimes called "N2" (not to be confused with N2b of the N2b-P3b complex; see below). Figure 18.2 shows these changes in the slow response with drowsiness (Picton et al., 1976). The changes appear to be different for different sleep stages (Näätänen, 1992), which likely explains much of the variability of N1 and N1 thresholds in earlier studies without formal sleep-staging procedures.

Maturation

The slow cortical response undergoes substantial changes during maturation, and these changes appear to continue into teenage years. These changes are not simple changes in latency or amplitude; rather, they are complex changes in the appearance, morphology, scalp distribution, amplitude, and latency of the P1-N1-P2 waves of the slow cortical

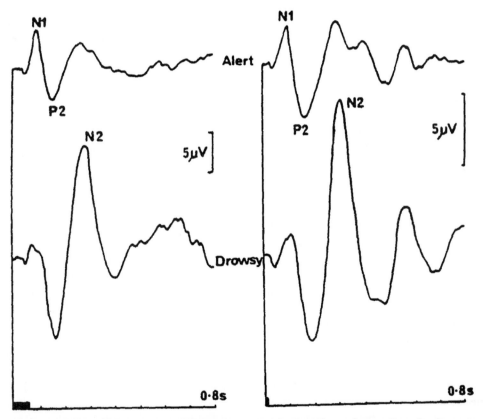

FIGURE 18.2 Modification of the slow cortical response during drowsiness. Results from two subjects are shown in response to 60- to 70-dB normal hearing level (nHL) 1,000-Hz tone bursts. The responses recorded while alert/awake (*top*) show the typical N1-P2 response. In contrast, when drowsy or asleep (*bottom*), the slow response shows a different morphology, with a large N2 wave at about 300 ms. (Reprinted from Picton TW, Hillyard SA, Galambos R. [1976] Habituation and attention in the auditory system. In: Keidel WD, Neff WD, eds. *Handbook of Sensory Physiology. Volume V, Auditory System, Part 3: Clinical and Special Topics*. Berlin: Springer-Verlag; pp 343–389, with permission from Springer-Verlag GmbH & Co. KG.)

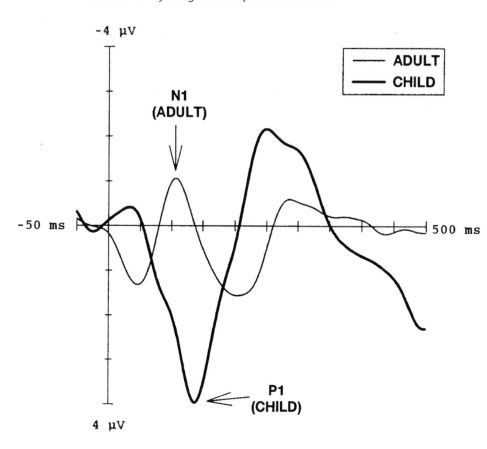

FIGURE 18.3 Slow cortical responses in an adult and a 7-year-old child. Shown are the responses at electrode Cz, recorded in response to the speech stimulus /ba/ (natural token from female speaker, edited to 150-ms duration) presented via a loudspeaker at 80 dB sound pressure level (SPL), using an onset-to-onset interstimulus interval of 627 ms. The adult response shows the P1-N1-P2 complex, with N1 at about 100 ms. In contrast, the child's response shows a large-amplitude positive peak at about 140 ms, followed by a negativity at about 250 ms. (These recordings were obtained in association with Peggy Oates-Korczak and Diane Kurtzberg.)

response. It is quite likely that the three or more underlying subcomponents of the N1 wave, as well as P1, show different developmental courses. Kurtzberg et al. (1984) have demonstrated the importance of multiple-channel recordings when investigating the maturation of the slow cortical ERP. Wunderlich and Cone-Wesson (2006) provide a comprehensive review of the maturation of P1-N1-P2.

A number of investigators have studied the development of P1-N1-P2. Kurtzberg and colleagues have investigated the slow cortical response to tonal and speech stimuli in premature and full-term newborns, in infants during the first 2 years of life, and in older children (Gomes et al., 2001; Kurtzberg, 1989; Kurtzberg et al., 1984; Novak et al., 1989; Steinschneider et al., 1992; Vaughan and Kurtzberg, 1989). They have developed a five-stage classification of the newborn's slow cortical ERP maturation level based on comparison of responses recorded in midline-central (e.g., Fz or Cz) and lateral-temporal (T4/T4 or halfway between C3/C4 and the mastoids) electrode sites. Presumably, these sites reflect maturation of the auditory cortex on the superior surface of the superior temporal gyrus versus that of secondary auditory cortex on the lateral surface of the superior temporal gyrus. At birth, most normal infants show either a positive wave at the midline-central electrode and a negative wave in the lateral electrode or positive waves at both electrodes. By age 3 months, 90% of normal infants show this latter pattern. Maturational changes then continue, with the lat-

eral response exhibiting a maturational sequence that lags behind the midline-central response (Kurtzberg et al., 1984; Steinschneider et al., 1992). Wunderlich et al. (2006) and Ponton et al. (1996b) have further delineated the maturational changes in P1-N1-P2. Neville and colleagues have also reported on scalp distribution changes with maturation of the slow cortical response (for review, see Neville [1995]). As shown in Figure 18.3, the slow cortical response of childhood is characterized by a relatively large P1 wave, which may (Sharma et al., 1997; Wunderlich et al., 2006) or may not (Ponton et al., 1996b) be followed by a clear N1 wave. Latencies of these waves decrease with maturation until the later teens, by which time N1 has become the more prominent wave of adulthood (Wunderlich et al., 2006).

Mismatch Negativity

Originally discovered in 1978 by Näätänen et al. (1978), the MMN is elicited by infrequent changes (i.e., deviant stimuli) in a sequence of a repetitive (i.e., standard) auditory stimulus or features of the auditory stimulus (Näätänen et al., 2005; Winkler et al., 1997). As shown in the waveforms of Figures 18.1 and 18.4, this frontocentral-negative ERP wave is usually seen as an increased negativity in the latency region following the peak of N1 and during P2. Usually peaking 100 to 300 ms after stimulus onset, it may be seen as an enlarged N1, a second negative peak, or an attenuation of the P2 wave

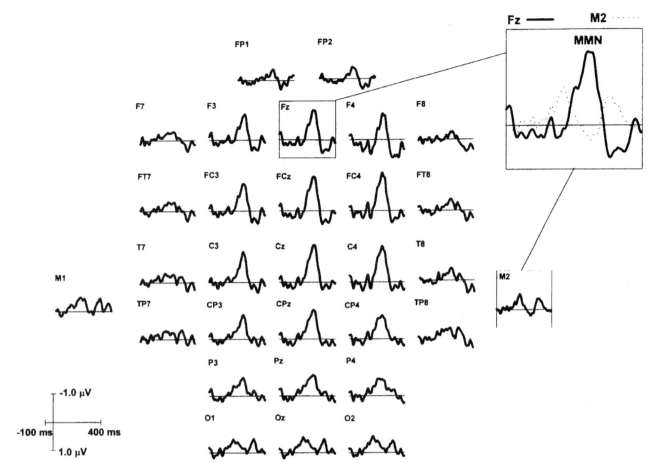

FIGURE 18.4 Scalp distribution of the mismatch negativity (MMN) to 12-dB intensity decrements. Shown are the deviant-minus-standard difference waves from the waveforms shown in Figure 18.1. The MMN, peaking at about 200 to 225 ms, is labelled for the zoomed-in channel Fz (*box, upper right*), which also shows waveform recorded at the right mastoid (M2). The MMN is larger (more negative) in frontal-central electrodes, especially at F4 (right frontal), decreases in amplitude (becomes less negative) at posterior electrodes, and inverts in polarity at the mastoids. The initial positivity at 100 ms (Fz) reflects an N1 effect due to N1 being smaller in amplitude to the 68- versus 80-dB normal hearing level (nHL) tone bursts.

(Picton, 1990).[2] The MMN is usually best visualized in the difference waveform (Fig. 18.4).

The MMN reflects a central code of stimulus change. According to Näätänen et al. (2005, p 25), it is "generated by an automatic change-detection process in which a disconcordance is found between the input from the deviant auditory event and the sensory-memory representation of the regular aspects of the preceding auditory stimulation." MMN amplitude and latency are related to the degree the deviant stimulus differs from the standards, not the absolute levels of the deviant/standard stimuli. Although the subject of recent dispute (Jaaskelainen et al., 2004; Näätänen et al.,

2005), the MMN does not appear to be generated by the deviant stimulus activating new afferent sensory elements per se—the basis of the "N1 effect"—as clearly demonstrated by MMNs elicited by stimuli where no "fresh afferents" would be activated, such as a decrease in intensity (Näätänen and Picton, 1987; Stapells and So, 1998) or a shortening in duration (Jacobsen and Schroger, 2003; Joutsiniemi et al., 1998), or by the occasional too-early stimulus in a stimulus sequence (Näätänen et al., 1993a). The presence of a memory representation of the standard is required to elicit the MMN (Näätänen et al., 2005), and only when a stimulus differs from one that occurred previously *but not adjacently in time* does one obtain an MMN (Picton et al., 2000).

Although Picton originally classified the MMN as being within the "slow" cortical response category (Picton et al., 1985), he subsequently moved it into the "late" ERP category (Picton, 1990). This latter classification is more appropriate, considering the later and more complex processing reflected by the MMN (see below). Reviews of the MMN

---

[2] Stimulus "onset," for mismatch negativity, is the minimum time required by the brain to determine if a stimulus or stimulus feature has changed. For example, if standards are 75 ms in duration and deviants are the same stimuli except that they are 50 ms in duration, then "onset" time begins at 50 ms. A response to this stimulus change could not be initiated until at least 50 ms, the end of the deviant stimuli.

have been published by Näätänen and colleagues (Näätänen, 1992; 1995; 2000; Näätänen and Alho, 1995; 1997; Näätänen and Picton, 1987) and by Picton et al. (2000).

GENERATORS

Scalp current density analyses of MMN scalp distribution (Giard et al., 1990), dipole source analyses (Maiste et al., 1995; Scherg et al., 1989), findings in brain-damaged patients (Alho et al., 1994), human intracranial recordings (Kropotov et al., 2000), and magnetoencephalographic recordings (Csépe et al., 1992; Hari et al., 1984; Tiitinen et al., 1993) have all contributed to our current understanding of the intracranial sources of the MMN. These studies point to two subcomponents of the human MMN, as originally suggested by Näätänen and Michie (1979): (1) one subcomponent with bilateral generators in the supratemporal plane (auditory cortex), and (2) a second subcomponent in the frontal cortex. The specific location of the frontal generators is unknown (Giard et al., 1998). Studies in animals have also suggested subcortical MMN generators, such as the thalamus (Kraus et al., 1994a; 1994); however, there is no evidence that, in humans, the MMN generators are also located within subcortical structures (Alho, 1995; Giard et al., 1998; Picton, 1995). Interestingly, the exact location of the MMN generators within the auditory cortices appears to depend upon which sensory feature (e.g., intensity, frequency, duration, etc.) of sound is being processed (Giard et al., 1998).

MISMATCH NEGATIVITY FUNCTIONAL SIGNIFICANCE

The MMN reflects a preattentive central code—originating in auditory and possibly frontal cortices—of stimulus change. As discussed earlier, the MMN does not reflect stimulation of "new afferents," although without careful consideration of stimuli, such refractory processes can contaminate the MMN (Cranford et al., 2003; Jacobsen and Schroger, 2003). The MMN is believed to reflect the deviation of the incoming stimulus from the auditory sensory memory trace of the frequently presented auditory stimulus or stimulus feature (Näätänen et al., 2005; Winkler et al., 1997).[3] Some data suggest that the MMN reflects separate, independent processing of different auditory features (Deacon et al., 1998; Giard et al., 1995; Molholm et al., 2004; Ritter et al., 1995). Just what the "deviant" stimulus is may be quite complex. For example, the "deviant" may be a feature (e.g., duration) among otherwise different standard stimuli that changes only with the improbable deviant stimuli, or it may be a change in a pattern of stimuli (Picton et al., 2000). The presence of the MMN indicates that the change-detection system at the level of the auditory cortex has discriminated the standard/deviant stimuli. The MMN is highly correlated with behavioral discrimination of stimuli, and thus, its presence likely indicates that an individual is able to discriminate the stimuli.

However, presence of the MMN does not, by itself, indicate conscious perception of the change, which requires activation of attention-triggering mechanisms (Näätänen and Alho, 1997).

STIMULUS EFFECTS

The MMN is elicited by any discriminable change in auditory stimulation, such as changes in frequency, intensity, duration, or rise time or when a constant ISI is occasionally shortened.[4] An MMN is also elicited by changes in more complex stimuli, such as speech stimuli, rhythmic patterns, and complex spectrotemporal patterns (for reviews, see Näätänen [1992], Näätänen and Alho [1997], Näätänen and Picton [1987], and Picton et al. [2000]). Generally, the larger the acoustic difference(s), the earlier and larger is the MMN, although there may be ceiling effects in amplitude with large differences (Picton et al., 2000). With the appropriate stimulus and recording parameters (see Table 18.3), MMNs have been reported for changes (to 1,000-Hz standards) in frequency as small as 0.5% to 2% (Sams et al., 1985) and for decreases in intensity as small as 2 to 3 dB (Näätänen et al., 1987b; Stapells and So, 1998).

Because the MMN often occurs in the N1 latency range, it is important to not mistake changes that occur to N1 with stimulus change with the MMN (see above). For example, if the N1 to a 1,000-Hz tone occurs earlier (but with the same amplitude) as the N1 to a 500-Hz tone, the resulting 1,000-Hz ERP minus 500-Hz ERP difference wave would show a negativity based simply on the latency differences (it cannot be a "change" detector within the brain because the tones were presented alone). The same result could be obtained if these two tones were presented as deviants and standards and mistakenly measured as an MMN. Additionally, when the N1 is refractory to repeated stimuli, a deviant stimulus with too large a change will cause a large increase in N1 amplitude because new, nonrefractory neural elements are stimulated (the N1 effect) (Butler, 1968). Although the resulting difference wave indicates that the brain has the information to detect a change in the stimulus (a necessary precursor to a change detector mechanism), it does not represent the actual *detection* of the change (Martin and Boothroyd, 1999; Martin et al., 2007).[5] As discussed earlier, there are a number of controls for the N1 effect involving which waveform to subtract from the deviant waveform (Jacobsen and Schroger, 2003).

---

[3] Although once believed to be only elicited by auditory stimuli, there appears to be MMN analogs in other sensory systems, such as the somatosensory (Akatsuka et al., 2005; Kekoni et al., 1997) and visual (Maekawa et al., 2005) systems.

[4] According to current theory, any change in a stimulus feature, perceptible or not, gives rise to an MMN by the MMN generator system. Whether it is recordable at the scalp, however, depends upon various signal-to-noise issues. That is, the MMN to a very small change may be too small to pick up at the scalp and/or too small to recognize in background electrical (EEG) noise (Näätänen and Alho, 1997).

[5] According to Näätänen and Alho (1997, p 343), "in order to be able to demonstrate a discriminative process at the physiological level, the data should contain...a code of the stimulus difference. It is by no means sufficient to show that two consecutive afferent responses differ from one another, for it may be that the difference between the two responses is not detected at any higher level of processing." Thus, the fact that the N1s elicited by two different stimuli differ and thus produce an N1 effect does not mean the change has been detected at a higher level. Näätänen et al. (2005) recently reviewed this issue.

Additional controls are to (1) avoid large stimulus differences (which, in addition to large N1 effects, may result in a P3a wave, discussed below) and (2) employ stimulus differences that most likely involve the same neuronal populations in the generation of the N1 (for example, deviants such as decreases in intensity or duration of the same stimulus). As Lang et al. (1995) point out, if the stimulus deviance in the passive/ignore condition causes a P3a wave to be elicited, then the deviance is likely too large (i.e., will also elicit a large N1 effect).

Stimulus Duration, Rise, and Fall Times
Little information exists concerning the effects of these parameters on the MMN. The MMN has been elicited by brief stimuli (e.g., clicks), relatively long stimuli (speech stimuli of 200 to 300 ms in duration), and everything in between.

Probability of Occurrence of Deviant Stimuli
The MMN is typically elicited using single- or multiple-deviant oddball paradigms (see earlier discussion). In contrast to the later N2b-P3b series of waves (see below), however, the predictability of the oddball sequence does not appear to have an effect on the MMN (Scherg et al., 1989).Thus, the standard/deviant oddball paradigms may be pseudorandom or nonrandom (e.g., every 10th stimulus is a deviant) (Scherg et al., 1989; Stapells and So, 1998; Stapells et al., 2002; Tsui et al., 2000).

The lower the probability of the deviant stimuli, the greater is the MMN amplitude; for example, a much larger MMN is recorded when the deviant probability is 0.02 compared to 0.10 (Näätänen et al., 1987b; 1983). It appears that probability is a larger determinant of MMN amplitude than either ISI or interdeviant interval (IDI) (Javitt et al., 1998). Deviant stimulus probabilities of 0.1 or lower are typically used.

Of considerable importance is the fact that the amplitude of the MMN strongly depends on the probability of the immediately preceding stimuli—often called their "local probability" (Näätänen, 1992). That is, as the number of standard stimuli before a deviant increases, the representation of the standard increases, so that a greater "mismatch" occurs and, thus, a larger amplitude MMN when the deviant stimulus is presented. If two deviants are presented in a row, the MMN will be smaller to the second deviant. Furthermore, the standard stimulus after presentation of a deviant actually elicits a small MMN (Näätänen, 1992). Thus, in practice, the final average MMN will be enhanced if (1) deviants do not occur together and (2) averaging of the response to the standard stimuli *excludes* the response to each standard following a deviant (Lang et al., 1995).

Interstimulus Interval
The MMN is hypothesized to be generated by a process that registers a change from the memory representation of the standard stimulus ("sensory memory"). Thus, with longer intervals between stimuli, one would predict the memory trace for the standards to decay and, thus, MMN amplitude to decrease (Näätänen, 1992). Indeed, longer ISIs do appear to result in smaller MMNs, and little or no MMN is seen with ISIs longer than 10 seconds (Mäntysalo and Näätänen, 1987). The close relationship between MMN and "sensory memory" is of great interest to cognitive psychologists, and a large and expanding literature concerning this topic exists. Through ISI manipulations, there may be clinical applications of the MMN due to its relationship to memory.

To date, studies of the MMN have shown good success with ISIs (time *between* stimuli) of about 300 to 500 ms (Lang et al., 1995). There are data, however, that would support the use of much shorter ISIs, at least when using short stimuli and lower deviant probabilities. For example, Javitt et al. (1998) reported largest amplitudes using an ISI of 150 ms (50-ms tones, 0.05 probability), and Näätänen and colleagues have reported MMN with onset-to-onset ISIs as low as 60 ms (for review, see Näätänen [1992]). Näätänen and colleagues recently showed much-reduced amplitude MMNs using a 300-ms ISI compared to a 500-ms ISI (Näätänen et al., 2004). Readers are further cautioned that the data are, as yet, still not clear as to optimal ISIs for speech (Kraus et al., 1995b) or other complex stimuli or for younger subjects.

Stimulus Intensity
If the degree of deviance (in dB) is held constant, MMN amplitudes decrease and latencies increase as stimulus level is lowered (Schroger, 1996; Stapells and So, 1998). This is likely the result of fewer cortical neurons overall being involved in the responses to the two stimuli when intensity is decreased. Increasing the degree of deviance for these lower intensity stimuli, however, restores the MMN amplitude and latency (Stapells and So, 1998).[6]

Speech Stimuli
Many studies have demonstrated the MMN to speech stimuli, including vowel (Aaltonen et al., 1987; Cheour-Luhtanen et al., 1995) and consonant-vowel syllables (Dehaene-Lambertz et al., 2000; Kelly et al., 2005; Kraus et al., 1995b; 1992; Maiste et al., 1995; Martin et al., 1999; Rivera-Gaxiola et al., 2000; Sams et al., 1990; Sharma et al., 1993; Sharma et al., 2004; Tsui et al., 2000). The literature concerning the phonetic sensitivity of MMN is somewhat contradictory, with some studies indicating the MMN reflects acoustic rather than phonetic differences (Maiste et al., 1995; Sams et al., 1990; Sharma et al., 1993; Tsui et al., 2000), whereas others have shown effects of language environment for phonetic contrasts that are native versus nonnative to an individual's language (Dehaene-Lambertz et al., 2000; Näätänen et al., 1997; Rivera-Gaxiola et al., 2000). Phillips (2001) provides a comprehensive review of this topic. Further research is required.

RECORDING PARAMETERS
Table 18.3 summarizes stimulus, recording, and waveform measure parameters for recording the MMN to standard/

---

[6] The fact that MMN amplitude increases even though the intensities of the standards and deviants are *lower* (such as when one lowers the levels of both *and* increases the deviance by lowering the deviant even further) provides further evidence that the MMN is a response to the change, and not differences in afferent (i.e., N1) responses (Näätänen et al., 2005).

TABLE 18.3   Sample parameters for mismatch negativity

Subject:	Awake, alert, eyes open (reading book or watching closed-caption TV)
Total number of stimuli (standards + deviants):	2,000–4,000 (broken up into subblocks)
Standard/deviant probabilities (single deviant):	Standards: 0.9; deviants: 0.1
Onset-to-onset interstimulus interval	300–600 ms (tonal stimuli) 600–1,000 ms (speech stimuli; depends upon stimulus)
Stimuli: Frequency-MMN (60–80 dB SPL):	*(Control for N1 effect must be done if deviance is large; see text)* Standard stimuli: 1,000-Hz tones Rise-fall times: 20 ms; Plateau time: 20 ms Deviant stimuli: 1,020-1,100 Hz tones Rise-fall times: 20 ms; Plateau time: 20 ms
Stimuli: Intensity-MMN (1,000-Hz tones; Rise-fall times: 20 ms; Plateau time: 20 ms):	*(Control for N1 effect <u>not</u> required; see text)* Standard stimuli: 80 dB SPL Deviant stimuli: 65–70 dB SPL (10- to 15-dB *decrement*)
Stimuli: Duration-MMN (1,000-Hz tones; 60–80 dB SPL):	*(Control for N1 effect <u>not</u> required; see text)* Standard stimuli: 75-ms total duration (5-ms rise-fall; 65-ms plateau) Deviant stimuli: 25-ms total duration (5-ms rise-fall; 15-ms plateau)
Stimuli: Speech-MMN (65–80 dB SPL; CV stimuli; 150-ms duration):	*(Control for N1 effect <u>required</u>; see text)* Standard/deviant stimuli: /ba/ vs. /da/ for place of articulation; /da/ vs. /ta/ for voice onset timing
Stimuli: Multiple deviants (e.g., stimuli differing in frequency, duration, intensity, etc):	Complicated but possible; may be more efficient; requires advanced equipment. For details, see Deacon et al., 1998; Näätänen et al., 2004.
Recording:	Minimum (4 channels): Vertical EOG; Fz; Pz; mastoid; *Reference:* Tip of nose Additional channels: Cz, F3, F4, other mastoid, T7, T8 (8 or more channels preferred) EEG filters: 0.1–30 Hz (Offline: digital low-pass filter: 15 Hz) Sensitivity/artifact reject: ±100 μV (Gain = 10,000–20,000) Analysis time: −50 to +500 ms (longer for longer speech stimuli)
Wave measures:	Responses to standards: N1 peak latency and baseline-to-peak amplitude MMN presence/absence: Assess scalp distribution and EOG Statistical analyses *(see text)* Group data: paired t-test of subjects' difference waves Individual data: PC1 analysis of subblocks of difference waves Integrated MMN (MMNi) Difference waves (amp/lat): Mean-MMN amplitude: Obtain mean amplitude over 50-ms window (usually at Fz), window center determined from group or normal grand mean waveform MMN peak latency (i.e., at maximum amplitude; usually at Fz) MMN peak amplitude (i.e., at maximum amplitude, usually at Fz)
Other measures:	MMN "area" and/or MMN duration (onset/offset difficult to determine)

CV, consonant-vowel.

deviant stimuli differing in frequency, intensity, duration, or speech syllable. Readers should note that parameters, such as degree of deviance, number of trials to record, etc, may be changed based on the purpose of the recordings, as well as initial experiences with MMN.

Number of Trials

The poor signal-to-noise ratio of the MMN is likely the most serious problem facing any clinical application of the MMN. The number of standard/deviant trials required to successfully record and measure the MMN depends on the response's signal-to-noise ratio. The noise level of the difference wave is determined primarily by the noise levels in the response to the deviants (due to its fewer number of trials). MMN amplitude is typically less than 2 μV, compared to the 0.5 to 1 μV amplitude of ABR wave V. EEG noise levels for MMN, however, are about two to four times those of the ABR. The subtraction procedure (to obtain the difference wave) also adds noise (about 1.4 times). Therefore, one must record one-quarter to one-half the number of trials (number of deviants) when recording the MMN as one does when recording the ABR (Picton et al., 1995). Thus, one must record between 250 and 2,000 deviant responses for the MMN (assuming one typically records 1,000 to 4,000 trials for the ABR) (Picton et al., 1983). Even with 250 to 400 deviants, the MMN may not be detectable in some normal individuals, although one might be able to detect the MMN in the grand mean waveform across a group of individuals. Due to the long test times required to obtain these numbers, the MMN may be impractical for clinical application. Use of shorter ISIs thus helps to shorten test time, provided that MMN amplitude is not too reduced (Näätänen et al., 2004). Future research using the scalp distribution and/or sources of the MMN may act as a spatial filter to improve the signal-to-noise ratio of the response (Picton et al., 1995), whereas shorter ISIs may increase the number of trials one can record within a given time.

Detection of the Mismatch Negativity/Response Measures

The preceding section indicates that difficulty often exists with detecting the MMN in the background EEG noise. Researchers experienced with MMN use visual observation of the morphology, latency, and, importantly, the scalp distribution of the MMN when determining whether it is present or absent. Unfortunately, when responses are small and/or when waveforms are noisy, even experts have difficulty correctly detecting the MMN from individuals (McGee et al., 1997). Research is currently focused on developing and assessing statistical measures to detect the MMN. Analyses using point-by-point t-tests of an individual's response are problematic (due to the problem of determining degrees of freedom) and do not appear to be useful (McGee et al., 1997). The "integrated MMN" (MMNi) measure developed by Ponton et al. (1997) may aid in detecting the MMN, although it may also miss responses (McGee et al., 1997) and may not work when large stimulus deviances elicit a P3a following the

MMN (Picton et al., 2000; Sharma et al., 2004). Taking a different approach, Achim (1995) developed a measure ("PC1") based on principle components analysis of subaverages of the difference wave (Picton, 1998). No ideal objective measure of the MMN has yet been established. Clinical application of the MMN, however, will require a reliable statistical measure of MMN presence/absence; much work remains.

Detecting and measuring the MMN in group data (e.g., eight to 10 individuals) is far less problematic. First, the signal-to-noise ratio is much better, making the response and its scalp distribution easier to visualize. Second, point-by-point t-test analyses on waveforms from groups are appropriate, so determination of MMN presence/absence for a group or of differences between groups is feasible. Third, using the grand mean waveform to determine the appropriate window (typically 25 to 100 ms wide), one can then obtain amplitude and latency at the point of maximum amplitude within the window or calculate the mean amplitude within the window. These measures do not require an observer to decide whether a response is present or absent. Statistical tests can then be used to determine whether the MMN measures differ between conditions and/or groups.

Peak latency and the mean amplitude within a predetermined window are the most common MMN measures in the literature. MMN peak amplitude is next most common. Less common are measures such as MMN onset/offset latency, duration, and area. MMN "area" has been suggested to be useful (McGee et al., 1997; Sharma et al., 2004); however, this measure requires determination of the onset and offset of the MMN, which are measures that are quite difficult with the low signal-to-noise waveforms obtained from single subjects. Furthermore, measures involving the early portion of the MMN waveform (e.g., onset latency, duration, area) are likely confounded by an N1 effect (Picton et al., 1995; Scherg et al., 1989). The optimal MMN measures for different populations and/or different deviants have not yet been determined.

SUBJECT FACTORS

Discrimination Accuracy and Effects of Training

Under most circumstances, the presence, latency, and amplitude of the MMN are highly correlated with behavioral discrimination of simple (e.g., frequency [Sams et al., 1985]; intensity [Stapells and So, 1998]; duration [Bertoli et al., 2001; Heinrich et al., 2004; Joutsiniemi et al., 1998; Stapells et al., 2002]) and complex (e.g., nonspeech [Näätänen et al., 1993b; Winkler et al., 1997]; speech [Martin et al., 1999; Martin and Stapells, 2005; Oates et al., 2002]) stimuli. Thus, stimuli that cannot be discriminated show no MMN; stimuli that are poorly discriminated elicit smaller and later MMNs; those that are easier to discriminate elicit large, earlier MMNs. The MMN also appears to reflect individual differences in discrimination performance. Finally, the MMN appears to reflect learning effects that are seen with nonspeech (Alho et al., 1993; Näätänen et al., 1993a) and speech (Kraus et al.,

1995a; Tremblay et al., 1998; Winkler et al., 1999) discrimination training. The close relationship between the MMN and discrimination and its reflection of training effects suggest both interesting and important clinical applications in audiology. It must be noted, however, that the MMN is not always strongly correlated with discrimination performance, and changes in MMN amplitude/latency have been disassociated from perceptual discrimination for both nonspeech and speech stimuli (Dalebout and Stack, 1999; Kumar and Jayaram, 2005; Maiste et al., 1995; Sharma et al., 1993; Stapells and So, 1998; Tsui et al., 2000).

Attention

Of considerable importance, especially for possible clinical applications or studies of infants, is the fact that the MMN can be elicited *independent* of attention. That is, the MMN does not require subjects to pay attention to the stimuli, a fact further emphasized by the presence of MMN in comatose patients (Fischer et al., 1999; Kane et al., 1996; Naccache et al., 2005). Although the withdrawal of attention does not abolish the MMN, MMN amplitude can be changed by some selective attention conditions (Alain and Woods, 1997; Näätänen, 1991; Woldorff et al., 1998). Indeed, because of unwanted and confusing overlapping components that occur with attention, the preferred MMN paradigm is to ensure the subject does not pay attention to the stimuli (e.g., watching a closed-captioned video).

Alertness and Sleep

The MMN has been recorded during sleep, albeit with difficulty. In addition to comatose patients (Fischer et al., 1999; Kane et al., 1996; Naccache et al., 2005), the MMN has been recorded in sleeping infants (Alho et al., 1990; Cheour et al., 1998b; Cheour-Luhtanen et al., 1995; 1996; Kurtzberg et al., 1995) and sleeping adults (Campbell et al., 1991; Loewy et al., 1996). Campbell and coworkers, however, reported the sleep MMN to be quite small in amplitude, only recordable during stage 2 and REM sleep, and difficult to record in the early portion of the night (Campbell et al., 1991; Loewy et al., 1996; Sabri et al., 2000). Small standard-deviant differences that elicit a clear MMN when awake may not elicit MMN during sleep (Sabri et al., 2003). Lang et al. (1995) report MMN amplitude decreases with increased sleepiness in adult subjects. Thus, the few data available indicate that the MMN is difficult to record in sleeping adults but may be present in sleeping infants. Further research is needed. Interestingly, the presence of the MMN during coma appears to be a predictor of good clinical outcome (Butler et al., 1998; Fischer et al., 1999; Kane et al., 1996; Naccache et al., 2005).

Maturation

In contrast to the slow P1-N1-P2 cortical response, the data to date indicate far less of a maturational effect on the MMN. Ponton et al. (1998) report that the MMN to duration changes appears adult-like by age 5 to 6 years, with some studies showing small decreases in latency during infancy (Morr et al., 2002; Ponton et al., 2000; Shafer et al., 2000). Other studies have shown somewhat different results. Kraus

et al. (1993a) report that the MMNs to speech stimuli in 7- to 11-year-old children have the same latency but are larger in amplitude than those of adults. Kurtzberg et al. (1995) report that the grand mean MMNs to frequency deviants were adult-like in a group of 25 newborns and another group of 8-year-old children. Contrasting these studies, other studies of MMN in newborns and infants show responses that, although negative, do not resemble those from adults (Alho et al., 1990; Cheour-Luhtanen et al., 1995; 1996). Martin et al. (2003) have shown that the scalp distribution of the MMN changes with maturation through at least 11 years of age. There is a clear need to obtain maturational MMN data specific to each type of deviant using consistent scalp recording locations.

One aspect of the developmental MMN studies that seems clear is that the MMN is more difficult to obtain in normal infants and children (i.e., many cases do not show an MMN), and when obtained, it shows greater intersubject variability than that seen in adults (Uwer and von Suchodoletz, 2000). This is especially the case in infants (Alho et al., 1990; Cheour-Luhtanen et al., 1995; 1996; Kurtzberg et al., 1995; Lang et al., 1995). Currently, it is not possible to interpret the meaning of an absent MMN. This has major implications for any clinical application of the MMN.

Inter- and Intraindividual Variability

Lang et al. (1995) report that one third of a group of 139 healthy adults failed to show a clear MMN to changes in stimulus frequency. Dalebout and Fox (2001) found that only 29% of their adult group showed MMNs to easily discriminated speech stimuli. Kurtzberg et al. (1995) report that no indication of an MMN was evident in 25% of a group of 25 healthy newborns or in 20% of a group of 10 school-age children. Joutsiniemi et al. (1998) report that 39 of 40 adult subjects showed MMN to 50-ms decrements in duration, but only 32 of 40 subjects show a MMN to 25-ms decrements. Wunderlich and Cone-Wesson (2006) report that only about 30% of their subjects showed MMN to speech stimuli. More recently, Sharma et al. (2006) found that MMN was only present in approximately 50% of their child subjects, including normal controls. Thus, using current methods, the MMN is not always visible in normal subjects, even though the stimulus contrasts are clearly discriminable.

When responses are present, the MMN shows considerable intrasubject variability, much more than the slow P1-N1-P2 responses (for review, see Martin et al. [2007]). Studies of the MMN elicited by frequency (Escera et al., 1998; Pekkonen et al., 1995; Tervaniemi et al., 1999), duration (Joutsiniemi et al., 1998; Pekkonen et al., 1995; Tervaniemi et al., 1999), intensity (Stapells et al., 1999; Tervaniemi et al., 1999), or speech (Dalebout and Fox, 2001; Uwer and von Suchodoletz, 2000) deviants indicate that the repeatability across sessions for individual subjects is only fair to poor, with typical test-retest correlation coefficients at about 0.5 to 0.6. Somewhat better results have been reported for the MMN to duration decrements (Pekkonen et al., 1995; Tervaniemi et al., 1999). In contrast to the poor repeatability of the MMN at the individual level, repeatability across sessions for results from groups of subjects appears to be very good (Escera et al., 1998; Joutsiniemi et al., 1998; Pekkonen et al., 1995; Stapells et al., 1999). These results suggest that MMN is ready for clinically-oriented studies of *groups* but it is not yet appropriate for assessment of individuals in the clinic.

Late Attention-Related Waves (N2b-P3a/P3b)

When subjects are ignoring standard and deviant stimuli and when the magnitude of deviation is quite large (e.g., 1,000-Hz vs. 2,000-Hz tones), the MMN is often followed by a positive wave occurring 200 to 300 ms after the stimulus change that is largest in the frontal-central electrodes. This wave, designated P3a (Squires et al., 1975) likely reflects that the stimulus was noticed (i.e., an attention switch) (Näätänen, 1992; Picton, 1992). When attention is introduced and the subject is instructed to detect the deviant stimuli, the picture becomes much more complex (Näätänen, 1992). In addition to the MMN and P3a, the response to the deviants contains a central-negative wave, N2b, and a prominent positive wave, P3b, that is largest in the centroparietal region.[7] N2b likely represents the perceptual registration of the stimulus change (Picton, 1992). N2b usually occurs in attend conditions and is almost always followed by P3a (Näätänen, 1992). The most conspicuous wave, P3b, was first described in 1965 by Sutton et al. As Näätänen (1992) has suggested, this wave, also called P3 or P300, is probably the first ERP wave that reflects both stimulus deviation and recognition that the stimulus is a target. These waves are shown in Figure 18.5. Some stimulus paradigms introduce a third stimulus—a "novel" or "distractor" stimulus—resulting in a clearer P3a (see reviews by Polich [2004] and Polich and Criado [2006]). Extensive reviews of the various P3 waves have been published by Hillyard and Picton (1987), Näätänen (1992), Picton (1992), Polich (2004), and Pritchard (1981). N2b has been reviewed by Näätänen and colleagues (Näätänen, 1992; Näätänen and Gaillard, 1983).

GENERATORS

The intracranial sources of N2b, P3a, and P3b are complicated, multiple, and poorly understood. The different scalp distributions of these three waves indicate that they are not generated by identical sources (although there is likely partial overlap). These waves are not modality specific (i.e., they may be elicited by stimuli in any sensory modality or by combinations of sensory modalities), thus their generators are not restricted to modality-specific cerebral regions. N2b scalp topographies imply generators within secondary visual and auditory cortical regions, which extend beyond the areas activated in P1-N1-P2 responses. It is thought that N2b "represents activation of rather extensive brain systems that

are involved in intramodal discriminative processing" (Steinschneider et al., 1992, p 280). The scalp distribution of the various P3 waves varies across experiments, and it is likely that widespread but possibly focal regions contribute to the P3 waves, including hippocampal, sensory-specific cortex, centroparietal cortex, and frontal cortex (Picton, 1992). Both the frontal lobe and the hippocampus have been suggested as necessary for P3a generation, whereas the temporoparietal pathway contributes to P3b (Polich, 2004).

N2B-P3B FUNCTIONAL SIGNIFICANCE

As indicated earlier, the presence of frontal P3a likely reflects that the stimulus was noticed by some attention-triggering mechanism and perhaps reflects a redirection of attention monitoring (Polich, 2004). It does not necessarily indicate "conscious" perception of the change; it is a matter of debate whether P3a reflects a top-down attention switching or bottom-up control over responses to distractors (Polich and Criado, 2006). N2b likely represents the preconscious perceptual registration of the stimulus change and possibly the early stages of stimulus evaluation and classification processes (Hillyard and Picton, 1987; Novak et al., 1990). The parietal P3b indicates conscious recognition that the stimulus is a target. P3b latency is generally independent (although related) to response selection time; it typically occurs later than reaction time, and thus, it has been suggested to reflect the postdecision evaluation of the deviant stimulus within a series of standard stimuli and, possibly, to reflect a process of closure (Hillyard and Picton, 1987; Picton, 1992; Verleger, 1997). P3b latency can be used to provide a measure of the relative timing of the stimulus classification/evaluation process (including discrimination, recognition, and classification) (Coles et al., 1995; Kutas et al., 1977). P3b latency is often associated with "cognitive efficiency" (Polich and Criado, 2006).

The complex sequence of N2b-P3a/P3b waves is apparently triggered by the earlier cerebral processes generating first the N1 wave, then the MMN. The MMN "appears to represent the first, preconscious, step in discriminating stimulus deviation and to trigger the chain of further cerebral processes, which lead to conscious discrimination of stimulus deviation" (Näätänen, 1992, p 246). These processes apparently generate the post-MMN endogenous components.

STIMULUS EFFECTS

Types of Stimuli

The N2b-P3b sequence can be elicited by stimuli within any sensory modality as well as across modalities and to missing stimuli. Speech- and language-based stimuli, such as syllables and words, presented visually or as auditory stimuli also may be used to elicit P3b. To better elicit P3a, an infrequent and distinct stimulus such as a white-noise "distractor" may be used (see reviews by Hillyard and Picton [1987], Näätänen [1992], Picton [1992], and Polich [2004]).

---

[7] MMN was originally referred to as N2a (Näätänen et al., 1982), although the N2a of other modalities is not the MMN (Näätänen, 1992).

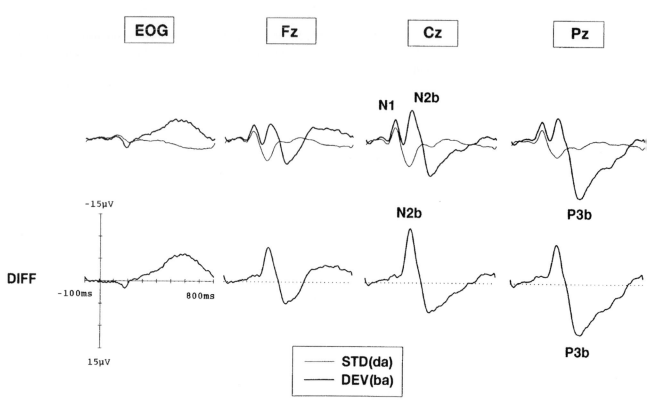

FIGURE 18.5   Event-related potentials (ERPs) obtained in an active discrimination condition. Shown are the standard (STD) and deviant (DEV) responses recorded at electrode sites Fz, Cz, and Pz as well as a vertical electro-oculogram (EOG) channel. The difference waves (DIFF) were obtained by subtracting the standard from the deviant waves. Stimuli were /da/ presented as the standard (pseudorandom probability = 0.9) stimuli and /ba/ presented as the deviant (pseudorandom probability = 0.1) stimuli, using an onset-to-onset interstimulus interval of 1,100 ms, and presented at 65 dB sound pressure level (SPL) via a loudspeaker. Subjects (adults) pushed a button whenever the deviant stimulus was presented. Standard waves: Slow cortical responses P1, N1, and P2 are present (N1 labelled at 125 ms), with N1 amplitude largest at electrode Cz. Deviant waves: Slow cortical responses P1, N1, and P2 are present. N1 is larger in amplitude to the deviants compared to the N1 to the standards due to the stimulus change and the longer interval between deviants compared to standards. This results in less refractory generators and, thus, a larger N1 (the N1 effect). Additional waves present in response to the deviants are N2b and P3b. At 230 ms, ERP N2b is largest at electrode Cz; at 380 ms, ERP P3b is largest at electrode Pz. Difference waves: ERP N2b is best visualized in the difference waves. The ERPs in the scalp electrodes are larger than deflections in the EOG channel, indicating that they are not ocular artifacts. (These recordings were obtained in association with Peggy Oates-Korczak and Diane Kurtzberg.)

Stimulus Intensity

P3b is generally viewed as an "endogenous" potential that is relatively immune to stimulus factors, especially those that do not change perception. However, significant increases in P3b latency and decreases in P3b amplitude have been shown with relatively small decreases in intensity (Covington and Polich, 1996), even though behavioral measures show no change (Martin et al., 1997; Martin and Stapells, 2005).

Task Difficulty

As the difficulty of a task (e.g., stimulus discrimination) increases, the latency of P3b increases, and its amplitude decreases (Picton, 1992), as seen, for example, with the effects of noise masking or hearing loss on responses to speech stimuli (Martin et al., 1997; Martin and Stapells, 2005; Oates et al., 2002; Whiting et al., 1998).

Probability of Occurrence of Deviant Stimuli and Interstimulus Interval

ISI and temporal probability covary. The P3b wave is larger when the deviant stimulus is more improbable, with amplitudes increasing with decreasing temporal probability until reaching a maximum at about one deviant in 10 seconds (Picton, 1992). Typical probabilities of the deviant stimuli that are employed range between 0.05 and 0.20.

RECORDING PARAMETERS

Table 18.4 summarizes stimulation and recording parameters as well as waveform measures for recording the N2b-P3b waves using simple "active" oddball paradigms. Three-stimulus "distractor" paradigms and passive paradigms,

TABLE 18.4   Sample parameters for N2b-P3b

Subject:	Awake, alert, eyes open, adults or children age 6 years or older
Active task:	Push button for deviants (preferred; allows calculation of reaction time) OR count deviants (vary number of deviants)
Total number of stimuli (standards + deviants):	100–200 or more (broken up into subblocks)
Single-deviant paradigm: Standard/deviant probabilities:	Standards: 0.8; Deviants: 0.2
3-stimulus distractor paradigm: Probabilities:	Standards: 0.8; Deviants: 0.1; Distractor: 0.1
Onset-to-onset interstimulus interval (ms):	1,100–2,000 (longer for more difficult contrasts or for children)
Stimuli:	Stimulus contrasts may be tonal (differing in frequency, intensity, duration, location), complex tonal, or speech (consonant-vowel syllables or words). Difficulty may be manipulated by making differences smaller, by adding masking noise, etc. **Distractor stimulus should be distinctly different (such as noise burst).** Sample contrasts can be found in the MMN parameters of Table 18.3. Controls for N1 effect are only needed if difference response in N1 latency region to be analyzed (i.e., for MMN in active condition).
Recording:	Minimum (4 channels): Vertical EOG; Fz; Cz; Pz. *Reference:* Mastoid (not linked) or tip of nose Additional Channels: For N1 and MMN: Mastoids (using tip of nose as reference), T7, T8 (8 or more channels preferred) EEG filters: 0.1–30 Hz (Offline: digital low-pass filter: 15 Hz) Sensitivity/artifact reject: $\pm100\ \mu$V (Gain = 10,000–20,000) Analysis time: −100 to +600 ms (longer for speech stimuli)
Wave measures:	
P3a & P3b presence/absence:	Assess scalp distribution and EOG
Responses to standards:	N1 peak latency and baseline-to-peak amplitude (at Cz or Fz)
Responses to deviants:	P3b peak latency and baseline-to-peak amplitude (at Pz)
Difference wave:	N2b peak latency and baseline-to-peak amplitude (at Cz)
Responses to distractor:	P3a peak latency and baseline-to-peak amplitude (at Fz)
Other measures:	If mastoid (with nose reference) available: Difference wave: MMN amplitude and latency at M1 and M2 (see Table 18.3). MMN, *when visible at mastoid,* will be positive at mastoid using nose tip reference. This differentiates it from N2b, which does not invert at the mastoids.

both designed to elicit P3a, which usually require large stimulus deviances, are reviewed by Polich (1989; 2004).

Number of Trials

The amplitude of P3b is quite large, often about 10 μV; hence, fewer trials (deviants) are required compared to the MMN. In some subjects, the P3b wave may even be recognized in single trials. Typical numbers of trials range from 25 to 200 deviants, with more being required for subjects with smaller responses or who are noisy or for more difficult tasks where P3b amplitude is small.

Detection of the N2b-P3b/Response Measures

The scalp distribution plays a large role in identifying N2b and P3b (see above). Measures for N2b are usually made at Cz in the difference wave. N2b does not invert at the mastoid (when using a nose reference), differentiating it from MMN. P3a measures are usually made on the distractor/novel waveform in the frontal (Fz) electrodes. Measures for P3b are usually made on the deviant waveform at Pz (sometimes at Cz). P3b amplitude and latency are usually measured at the maximum positive amplitude between 250 ms and 400 to 800 ms, depending on task difficulty. Offline digital low-pass filtering (3- to 6-Hz cutoff) of the response may aid in the measurement of P3b (Martin et al., 1997; Picton, 1992). Both N2b and P3b amplitudes may also be measured by calculating the mean amplitude within predetermined windows. Some measure of response reliability, such as replicated waveforms, should probably be available if these waves are to be measured in individual clinical subjects.

SUBJECT FACTORS

Attention

The N2b-P3b complex generally only occurs in response to task-relevant stimuli to which a subject is paying attention (Picton, 1992). Thus, elicitation of this response complex typically requires subject cooperation (Picton et al., 1985). The frontal P3a can be elicited without attention using large stimulus deviances and/or distractor/novel stimuli (Coles and Rugg, 1995; Courchesne et al., 1975; Näätänen, 1992; Polich, 1989; 2004; Squires et al., 1975).

Maturation and Aging

The N2b-P3b waves undergo major changes with maturation, although they are very difficult to study in infants and children due to (1) different scalp distributions and morphologies from adults and (2) difficulties with attention and artifacts (Picton, 1992; Taylor, 1988). The scalp distribution of P3b changes significantly with maturation. A large frontocentral negative wave (Nc), elicited by novel stimuli or, in children, by simple oddball stimuli, may overlap the P3b (Courchesne, 1978; Picton, 1992). The relationship of the late parietal positivity in children to the adult P3b is uncertain (Picton, 1992). This parietal positive wave is present during oddball paradigms for children aged 5 years and older. It decreases in latency with increasing age, especially between the ages of 5 and 12 years (Martin et al., 1988; Taylor, 1988). In very young infants, the response to deviants elicits a late frontal-negative response at approximately 700 to 800 ms. This negativity, called the cortical discriminative response (CDR) by Kurtzberg and colleagues (Kurtzberg, 1989; Kurtzberg et al., 1988; Steinschneider et al., 1992), has been suggested to be the infant analog of the adult MMN (Näätänen, 1992), although it is much later in latency. The fact that it is only seen in the waking state in infants makes this interpretation questionable (Kurtzberg et al., 1995).

After about the age of 18 years, the latency of P3b increases (with a slope of about 1.3 ms per year) and amplitudes decrease (Goodin et al., 1978; Picton, 1992). The scalp distribution of P3b also changes with aging, being smaller at the vertex in aged subjects (Picton, 1992).

Late Language-Related Waves (N400, LAN, P600)

There are a number of later ERP waves that appear to be specific to language comprehension.[8] The literature concerning these waves is relatively new and growing quickly. In the present chapter, only a brief introduction to these responses is presented. Comprehensive reviews of the ERPs related to linguistic stimuli have been published by Hillyard and Picton (1987), Kutas and colleagues (Hagoort and Kutas, 1995;

Kutas, 1997), Osterhout and Holcomb (1995), Phillips (2001), and, more recently, Friederici (2004).

The N400 was first described in the seminal study by Kutas and Hillyard in 1980. These authors reported that semantically inappropriate words (e.g., "He spread the warm bread with socks") elicited a large-amplitude negative wave with a latency of about 400 ms, relative to the waves elicited by semantically appropriate words (e.g., "It was his first day at work"). Words that are semantically appropriate but physically aberrant (e.g., words printed in larger font or spoken words presented at a higher sound pressure level [SPL]) elicit a positive-going potential. Most words in a sentence elicit an N400, the amplitude of which is sensitive to semantic aspects of sentence context. Largest N400s are elicited by semantically anomalous words; anomalies related in meaning to words expected but not presented in a context produce smaller N400s (Hagoort and Kutas, 1995; Osterhout and Holcomb, 1995). The scalp distribution of the N400 is fairly broad but tends to be larger posteriorly and slightly larger over the right hemisphere (Kutas et al., 1988). Little is known of the intracranial generators of the N400.

ERPs have also been associated with syntactic violations within sentences. The P600 (Osterhout and Holcomb, 1995) is a widely-distributed positive wave beginning at about 500 ms following a syntactically anomalous word within a sentence, with a typical peak latency of about 600 ms. This P600 appears to be quite distinct from the N400 elicited by semantically anomalous words (Hagoort and Kutas, 1995; Kutas, 1997; Osterhout and Holcomb, 1995). Violations of phrase structure, apparent subcategorization violations, and violations of subjacency have all been associated with the P600 (Osterhout and Holcomb, 1995). The cognitive events underlying the P600 are not yet known, and there is little evidence that this response is a direct manifestation of sentence comprehension. Indeed, the P600 may be a member of the P3 family of waves, although recent evidence suggests otherwise (Osterhout and Holcomb, 1995). Preceding the P600 is the N280, also termed the LAN (left anterior negativity), which has been proposed by Neville et al. (1991) as being sensitive to violations of syntax, such as phrase structure or grammatical word category violations (e.g., "The professor disagreed with the student's of description the problem"). The LAN (N280) is a negative peak largest at frontal sites over the left hemisphere. In contrast, the ERPs to open-class words showed an N400 over posterior sites and not the frontal N280 (Neville et al., 1992).[9] Recently, researchers have begun to use these language-related ERPs to study normal and impaired development of language processing (Mills et al., 2004; Neville et al., 1993; Neville and Bavelier, 2002). Although they would seem clearly relevant to the field, the later language-related ERPs have not yet received attention from researchers in audiology or speech-language pathology.

---

[8] Here, "language-specific" is used for responses apparently specific to linguistic stimuli, including words and sentences.

[9] See Kutas (1997) for a contrasting view of the N280-N400 relationship.

CLINICAL APPLICATIONS OF AUDITORY CORTICAL EVENT-RELATED POTENTIALS

Prior to considering the "clinical" applications of cortical ERPs, one must first determine the purpose of such measures. In general, there are two ways cortical ERPs may (or may not) be of importance for clinical work. First, the cortical ERPs might be used clinically for the purpose of diagnosis, management, etc, of an individual patient. In this first purpose, many issues must be considered before the cortical ERP measure is no longer "experimental" in nature, including the sensitivity and specificity of the measure for detecting and diagnosing dysfunction (and correctly identifying normal results), the time the test requires, and whether there is an equally good or better test available that may be faster and/or less expensive (i.e., the test's cost-benefit ratio). Use of cortical ERPs for this first purpose is strongly dependent on the ease and accuracy of detecting a response (and rejecting a "no response"), between- and especially within-subject variability, and repeatability. Table 18.5 lists the current status of use of the cortical ERPs to auditory stimuli for individual clinical patients. As suggested by Table 18.5, with one notable exception, the auditory cortical ERPs *currently* have very limited use for the application to individual clinical patients in audiology. The exception to this is the use of the slow cortical P1-N1-P2 response, especially for threshold estimation purposes.

In the second purpose, recordings of cortical ERPs (usually with other measures such as behavioral measures) obtained from *groups* (or subgroups) of clinical populations may help us understand the brain processes underlying the dysfunction of a particular group, as compared to a normal or other control group. Such information may lead to new therapeutic interventions (or changes to existing ones) and may also help us to better understand normal function. ERP recordings for this latter purpose are better classified as "clinical research" (that is, they are not involved in the diagnosis or treatment of an individual patient). They often do not require identification of responses or abnormalities within an *individual's* waves; rather, they depend on group-level results. As such, their utility is less affected by responses that are difficult to detect within individuals, between- and within-subject variability, and repeatability issues, etc. Auditory cortical ERPs provide a unique dynamic spatiotemporal window into brain processes underlying auditory processing and perception—a window that is far more temporally precise than current functional imaging techniques, such as functional magnetic resonance imaging (MRI) (Rugg and Coles, 1995b; Steinschneider et al., 1992). They have provided, and are likely to provide even further, interesting and useful information concerning clinical groups. It is likely that more complicated, more sensitive, and importantly, more specific stimulation paradigms will be required to determine the presence of dysfunction within groups or individuals.

That is, tests should be adjusted so that they evaluate a specific hypothesis about a disorder or a patient (Picton, 1992). The ubiquitous frequency-deviant oddball paradigm (e.g., 1,000 Hz vs. 2,000 Hz) is likely to be insensitive to many disorders. Thus, when evaluating a patient or group suspected of having disorders of central auditory processing, one should use a stimulus paradigm that taps into features known to depend on this processing. For example, the slow P1-N1-P2 has been evoked by changes in the lateralization of sounds, a process requiring intact central auditory processing (McEvoy et al., 1990; Picton et al., 1991). Similarly, patient groups with language disorders should be tested using paradigms involving different levels of speech-language processing (Neville and Bavelier, 2002; Steinschneider et al., 1992). It is also likely that multielectrode, generator source analysis techniques will provide new information concerning auditory dysfunction arising within central structures (Scherg and von Cramon, 1986b).

Finally, detection of a response in an individual patient typically requires some estimate of the signal-to-noise ratio in the waveform. Most studies of the cortical ERPs have studied these responses in groups and have not required response detection in individuals. Identification of specific ERPs is substantially aided by evaluation of scalp distribution, requiring the observer to have the required background and experience with the responses; however, some measure of response signal-to-noise ratio should also be employed. This is particularly important for waves with low signal-to-noise ratios, such as the MMN. Visual observation of replicated waveforms provides one possible signal-to-noise ratio measure; other measures include a correlation coefficient between replications (Picton et al., 1983), integrated MMN (MMNi) (Ponton et al., 1997), or principle component analysis of subaverages (PC1) (Achim, 1995).

Clinical Applications of P1-N1-P2

INDIVIDUAL LEVEL

The slow P1-N1-P2 cortical ERP is the measure of choice when an electrophysiologic estimate of hearing threshold is required for any patient who is likely to be passively (or actively) cooperative[10] and alert (Hyde, 1997; Hyde, 1988; 1994; Hyde et al., 1986; Lightfoot and Kennedy, 2006; Rickards et al., 1996; Tsui et al., 2002; Van Maanen and Stapells, 2005). Thus, it is the measure of choice for most older children and adults, and it has been especially useful for medicolegal and compensation cases. Figure 18.6 shows waveforms and thresholds for slow cortical P1-N1-P2 results obtained from a 12-year-old child with a high-frequency SNHL. The P1-N1-P2 and behavioral thresholds are within 10 dB of each other. The threshold estimation accuracy of the slow P1-N1-P2 cortical potentials is shown in Figure 18.7, which presents results from two studies carried out in

---

10 "Passively cooperative" includes watching TV, reading a book, or even quiet play or distraction by a toy or cartoon video.

TABLE 18.5   Audiologic applications of cortical auditory event-related potentials (ERPs)

Response	Clinical purpose	Current clinical status (2006)	2010
Slow P1-N1-P2	Frequency-specific threshold estimation	**Excellent** in alert/awake and passively cooperative adults and children **Possible** in quiet, awake infants with hearing loss, hearing aids, or auditory neuropathy	* * * *
		Possible but questionable in any drowsy/asleep individual; ***only present response helpful***; absent response nondiagnostic (minimum response level, not threshold)	
	Demonstrate cortical responsivity to specific sound(s) especially when ABR/MLAEP is absent or abnormal	**Excellent** in alert/awake and passively cooperative adults and children	* * * *
		Possible in any drowsy/asleep individual; ***only present response helpful***; absent response nondiagnostic (minimum response level, not threshold)	* * *
MMN	Demonstrate auditory cortex detection of stimulus change	**Questionable** in *any* population; ***only present response helpful***; absent response nondiagnostic	**
	Demonstrate effect of intervention/therapy	**Questionable/doubtful** in *any* population. With perhaps the exception of the MMN to duration decrements, MMN currently does not demonstrate acceptable within-subject repeatability.	?
N2b-P3b	Demonstrate conscious perception of stimulus	**Good** in alert/awake cooperative adults and children (≥6 years) *Probably only of use in compensation/medicolegal context (use behavioral measures for other contexts)*	* * *
		Questionable in any drowsy/asleep individual or infant/young child; ***only present response helpful***; Absent response nondiagnostic (minimum response level, not threshold)	
	Determine discrimination capabilities	**Questionable** in any population, especially if drowsy/asleep individual, or infant/young child; ***only present response helpful***; absent response nondiagnostic (minimum response level, not threshold); *probably only of use in compensation/medicolegal context (use behavioral measures for other purposes)*	?
	Demonstrate effect of intervention	**Questionable/doubtful** in *any* population; *behavioral measures likely more sensitive, reliable, and easier to obtain*	?
N400	Investigate language processing	**Questionable/doubtful** in *any* population; data in individuals currently too limited	?

****, Excellent likelihood of clinical utility within 5 years; ***, good likelihood of clinical utility within 5 years; **, fair likelihood of clinical utility within 5 years; ?, likelihood of clinical utility within 5 years unknown (and possibly low).

our labs, one in the 1980s and the other one in the past few years. Even though they were obtained two decades apart, these results shows remarkable similarity and indicate that the P1-N1-P2 provides reasonably accurate estimates of the audiogram.

It is unfortunate, especially in the United States, that the P1-N1-P2 slow cortical response is underused, having been replaced by the ABR. P1-N1-P2, however, may be elicited by longer duration, more frequency-specific stimuli compared with the ABR; the response is more resilient to electrophysiologic noise arising from small movements than is the ABR; and P1-N1-P2 represents a more complete picture of the auditory system. Threshold estimation is as accurate as or more accurate than that of the ABR or 80-Hz auditory

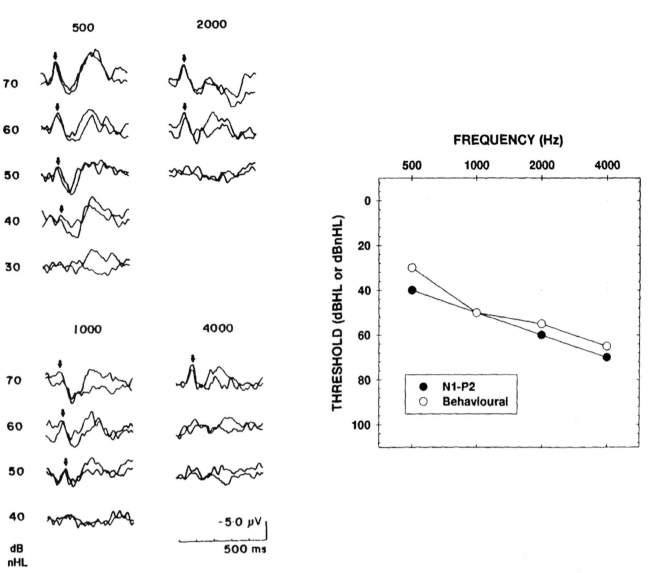

FIGURE 18.6 Slow cortical response thresholds in a 12-year-old with sensory-neural hearing loss (SNHL). Stimuli are 60-ms tone bursts presented via earphones at a rate of 1 per second. *Left,* waveforms with responses present are identified by *downward arrows,* which indicate the location of the N1 wave. *Right,* the audiogram shows the puretone behavioral and slow cortical N1-P2 thresholds. Thresholds for the two measures are within 10 dB of each other. (Data were obtained in association with Terry Picton and Andrée Durieux-Smith.)

steady-state response (Hyde, 1997; Stapells, 1984; Van Maanen and Stapells, 2005), and thresholds are obtained more quickly (Van Maanen and Stapells, 2005). Finally, in contrast to the ABR or MLAEP, the P1-N1-P2 response can be elicited by complex stimuli, such as speech stimuli, and may be used to assess cortical discrimination *capacity* to detect changes within these stimuli (Martin and Boothroyd, 1999; Martin et al., 2007). These speech stimuli may be presented while the patient is using their hearing aids, thus providing functional measures of hearing aid benefit (Gravel et al., 1989; Korczak et al., 2005; Kurtzberg, 1989). Dillon (2005) and Purdy et al. (2005) have recently shown favorable results using the slow cortical potentials in infants with hearing aids.

The slow cortical response is also very useful in demonstrating higher level (cortical) responsivity to sound when earlier, lower level responses (e.g., ABR or otoacoustic emissions) suggest neuropathy (Gravel and Stapells, 1993; Michalewski et al., 2005; Rance et al., 2002; Starr et al., 1996) (see Case 2 presented later in this chapter). Recordings of slow cortical responses in children with auditory neuropathy can predict perceptual skills in these young subjects (Rance et al., 2002). Furthermore, the absence or abnormality of slow cortical responses in the presence of intact earlier responses may be used to suggest higher level ("central") dysfunction (Gravel et al., 1989; Klein et al., 1995; Kurtzberg et al., 1988; Stapells and Kurtzberg, 1991). In the latter case, it is important to obtain recordings in the appropriate state, which is typically awake but quiet; absent cortical responses in a sleeping child are usually noncontributory.

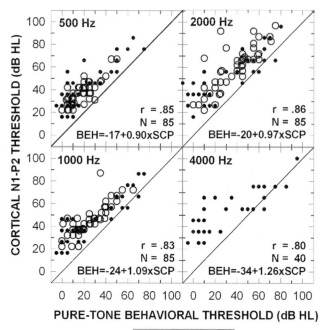

FIGURE 18.7 Estimation of behavioral puretone thresholds using the slow cortical N1-P2 responses. Results from two studies in adults with normal hearing or sensory-neural hearing loss showing good threshold estimation accuracy of the slow cortical responses. In addition to thresholds, each panel shows the overall correlation coefficient, number of subjects, and regression equation for the data across both studies. Results shown by *filled circles* are replotted from: Stapells DR. (1984) Studies in evoked potential audiometry. Unpublished Doctoral dissertation, University of Ottawa, Ottawa, Ontario Canada. Results shown by *open circles* are replotted from: Van Maanen A, Stapells DR. (2005) Comparison of multiple auditory steady-state responses (80 vs 40 Hz) and slow cortical potentials for threshold estimation in hearing-impaired adults. *Int J Audiol.* 44, 613–624.

GROUP LEVEL

The P1-N1-P2 sequence has been investigated in various groups with dysfunction, including neurologic disease, language dysfunction, and central auditory processing disorder (for review, see Cone-Wesson and Wunderlich [2003], Leppänen and Lyytinen [1997], Martin et al. [2007], and Steinschneider et al. [1992]). Some work suggests that the slow cortical responses in children with auditory processing disorder differ significantly from controls (Liasis et al., 2003); work on much larger groups is required. Young adults with verbal auditory agnosia have shown significantly delayed N1 latencies for temporal electrodes (although normal at Cz) (Klein et al., 1995). N1 latencies increase and amplitudes decrease with SNHL or with noise masking that simulates

hearing loss. The changes are not as large as those seen with the later ERPs (MMN, N2b, P3b). N1 remains present even when stimuli are audible but not discriminable (Korczak et al., 2005; Martin et al., 1999; 1997; Martin and Stapells, 2005; Oates et al., 2002; Whiting et al., 1998). Extensive work by Ponton and colleagues has provided interesting insights into differences (and similarities) between auditory system maturation in normal-hearing children and hearing-impaired children with cochlear implants (Ponton et al., 1996a; 1996b; 2000). Although currently not a diagnostic tool for individual patients with specific disorders (other than hearing loss), much has and will be learned from this response about normal and dysfunctional auditory processing. Future studies taking a hypothesis-driven approach to a particular dysfunction and using more complex stimuli and multiple electrodes are likely to be fruitful.

CASE 1: SLOW CORTICAL RESPONSE IN ADULT COMPENSATION CASE

KJ is a male aged 47 years who reports speaking little English. He presented with complaints of hearing difficulty, balance problems, and back pain, after having been involved in a motor vehicle accident a few weeks previously. Puretone audiometry showed bilateral SNHL with a flat configuration of 70 to 80 dB hearing level (HL). Reliability of these thresholds was rated as poor. Immittance results were normal, and acoustic reflex thresholds were 90 to 95 dB HL. Speech recognition thresholds, obtained using live voice with digits, were 25 dB HL bilaterally. Despite limitations of such testing, the inconsistency with the puretone thresholds is clear. Speech recognition scores were not obtainable due to nonresponse.

The patient was tested with slow cortical potentials by an audiologist who was blind to the previous audiometric results. The slow cortical potential protocol at Mt. Sinai Hospital (Toronto, Canada) is oriented towards determination of behavioral threshold reliability, as distinct from obtaining estimates of all puretone thresholds. If a discrepancy with volunteered thresholds is clear, attempts are made to reinstruct the patient and obtain a reasonable set of behavioral thresholds. Only in the situation of intractable discrepancy are management decisions based on the slow cortical threshold estimates (Hyde, 1988). A nonorganic loss component is typically overlaid on a genuine loss, with this nonorganic component usually maximal at low frequencies (Hyde, 1997; 1988; Hyde et al., 1986).

KJ's right ear slow cortical potential results for 500-Hz tone bursts are shown in Figure 18.8. The moderately high levels of alpha activity (~8 Hz) shown in this patient's waveforms are probably the greatest practical problem when undertaking this test, requiring experience and skill to interpret these waveforms. The waveforms in Figure 18.8 show a threshold of 40 dB HL. Based on large-sample normative data (Hyde et al., 1986), this yields an estimated behavioral threshold of 30 dB HL. Left ear results, not shown, yielded an estimated threshold of 25 dB HL.

Following comparison of the slow cortical potential and behavioral thresholds, the patient was retested by an

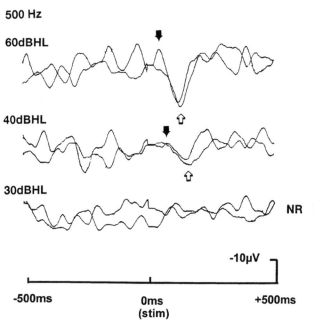

500 Hz

60dBHL

40dBHL

30dBHL

NR

-10μV

-500ms   0ms   +500ms
(stim)

FIGURE 18.8   Case 1: Slow cortical response in an adult compensation case. KJ's responses to 500-Hz tone bursts, presented at a rate of 0.6 per second. Waveforms with responses present are identified by the *arrows*, with N1 indicated by the *downward filled arrows* and P2 indicated by the *upward open arrows*. Note the prominent alpha activity (~8 Hz), making response determination more difficult. The N1-P2 threshold was determined to be 40 dB hearing level (HL), which, based on a larger sample, results in a behavioral threshold estimate of 30 dB HL. Following this electrophysiologic testing, behavioral retesting ultimately obtained a threshold of 35 dB HL. (Data were provided by Martyn Hyde.) NR, no response.

audiologist experienced with nonorganic hearing loss. After repeated reinstruction, the patient yielded behavioral pure-tone thresholds showing a bilateral SNHL sloping from mild at 500 Hz to moderate at 8,000 Hz, within 5 dB of the slow cortical potential estimates.[11]

CASE 2: SLOW CORTICAL POTENTIALS IN INFANT WITH AUDITORY NEUROPATHY

NA is a 2.5-year-old infant with severe cerebral palsy. He was born in south Asia with very high bilirubin levels requiring exchange transfusions. He was seen for ABR audiometry after behavioral audiologic testing proved inconclusive. NA was sedated and slept quietly for over 2 hours during the testing. Immittance testing, completed prior to the physiologic testing while NA was asleep, revealed normal tympanograms bilaterally with absent ipsilateral reflexes. ABR testing began with low-level, 2,000-Hz, air-conducted brief tones but, due to nonresponses, quickly proceeded to maximum intensi-

ties. No responses were seen to 500-, 2,000-, or 4,000-Hz air-conducted brief tones (90 to 100 dB normal hearing level [nHL]) or to bone-conducted 500- and 2,000-Hz brief tones (45 to 60 dB nHL). ABR recordings to 100 dB nHL rarefaction air-conducted clicks, shown in the center of Figure 18.9, also failed to show a response, although a cochlear microphonic early in the waveforms may be present. Similar results were seen for condensation clicks. Based on these ABR results, which considered alone suggest a severe/profound impairment bilaterally, we next attempted to record transient-evoked otoacoustic emissions (TEOAEs). Shown in the left of Figure 18.9, clear and unequivocal click-evoked TEOAEs are present bilaterally. This pattern of ABR/TEOAE results is known as auditory neuropathy/auditory dyssynchrony and suggests dysfunction at the inner hair cell/eighth-nerve synapse and/or eighth nerve/brainstem, with possibly normal outer hair cell function (Berlin et al., 1998; Kraus et al., 2000; Starr et al., 1996; see Chapter 22). Individuals with auditory neuropathy may have normal, mildly elevated, or severely elevated behavioral thresholds, although their suprathreshold abilities, especially those involving temporal processing, are typically quite impaired (Hood, 1998; Kumar and Jayaram, 2005; Michalewski et al., 2005; Rance et al., 2002; Starr et al., 1996; Zeng et al., 1999). Thus, an important question with each auditory neuropathy case concerns what information is reaching the cortex and what are the behavioral thresholds. In NA's case, we attempted to record slow cortical responses to binaural clicks while he remained asleep. The slow cortical potentials, shown on the right of Figure 18.9, demonstrated clear and highly replicable to 80- and 60-dB nHL binaural clicks (lower intensities were not tested). These results indicated that peripheral thresholds are significantly better than the severe-profound thresholds suggested by the ABR results. Because the slow cortical potentials reflect higher level (compared to the ABR) processes that are typically well correlated to behavioral thresholds, these results suggested that NA's behavioral thresholds were likely no worse than 50 dB HL.

These results show the utility of obtaining slow cortical potentials in individuals with auditory neuropathy and other neurophysiologic disorders, especially when behavioral thresholds are unreliable or not available (Rance et al., 2002). In NA's case, behavioral minimum response levels (MRLs; likely not thresholds) obtained in the sound field several months later indicate MRLs of 30 to 40 dB HL at 500 to 1,000 Hz and 50 dB HL at 4,000 Hz. MRLs to speech were 50 dB HL. There is currently much interest in using cortical ERPs to more complex stimuli to assess suprathreshold abilities in individuals with auditory neuropathy (e.g., gap detection) (Michalewski et al., 2005).

Clinical Applications of Mismatch Negativity

INDIVIDUAL LEVEL

At the time of writing this chapter (2006), the *current* use of the MMN for clinical assessment of individual patients

---

[11] This case was provided by Dr. Martyn Hyde (Mt. Sinai Hospital, Toronto, Canada).

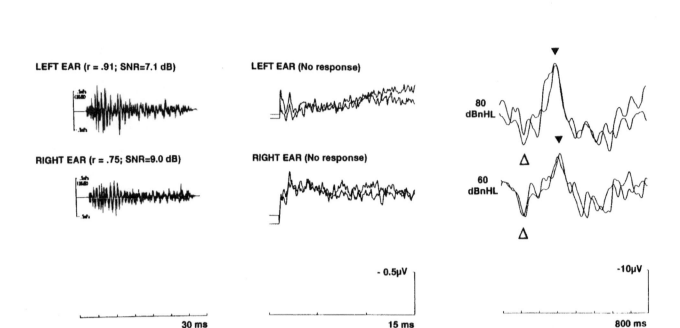

FIGURE 18.9   Case 2: Slow cortical response in infant with auditory neuropathy. Shown are NA's click-evoked otoacoustic emissions for each ear (*left*), his auditory brainstem responses to 100-dB normal hearing level (nHL) rarefaction clicks for each ear (*center*), and his slow cortical responses to clicks presented binaurally (*right*). Otoacoustic emissions are clearly present for both ears. In contrast, his brainstem response recordings show no neural components (i.e., waves I to V) in response to clicks or to brief tones presented at maximum intensities. Early in the click-evoked waves, there may be a cochlear microphonic present, which reversed polarity when stimulus polarity was reversed. NA's click-evoked slow cortical responses show a large-amplitude, highly replicable negative wave at about 300 ms (*filled triangles*) in response to 80- and 60-dB nHL clicks. There is also an earlier positive wave at about 100 ms (*open triangles*), which may be P1. Lower intensities were not tested. The slow cortical response and cochlear (transient-evoked otoacoustic emission) results indicate that perceptual thresholds are much better than indicated by the brainstem response results, a fact later confirmed by behavioral audiometry. SNR, signal-to-noise ratio.

is at best doubtful (see Table 18.5) and likely inappropriate, especially in infants and children (Dalebout and Fox, 2001; Dalebout and Stack, 1999; Martin et al., 2007; Oates et al., 2002; Picton et al., 2000; Sharma et al., 2006; Uwer and von Suchodoletz, 2000). As discussed in the earlier MMN section, much research is still required before the MMN can be applied clinically. Optimal stimulation, recording, and measurement parameters are not yet agreed upon. Repeatability of the MMN is too poor to monitor therapy. Even more important, the literature indicates that the MMN is frequently not recordable to easily perceptible contrasts in some normal individuals.

The problems with the MMN in individuals severely restrict the type of clinical judgments that currently may be made from MMN results. For example, if an MMN is clearly present to a specific contrast, one can suggest that the patient's auditory cortex was able to discriminate the contrast. Although the MMN is highly correlated with perception, the MMN does not represent conscious processing (Picton et al., 2000). If an MMN is not present, no statement (negative or positive) of the patient's capabilities is possible. Furthermore, if the MMN appears, disappears, or changes amplitude/latency on subsequent testing, no statement about a *change* in processing capability is currently warranted. Finally, these issues notwithstanding, there are practical limitations concerning the long test times required to obtain the MMN to even a single contrast.

As indicated in Table 18.5, however, it is possible that, within a few years, the MMN will be applicable to individual patients, at least for some stimulus types and some patient populations. Much research has been carried out on the MMN in clinical populations since the last version of this chapter (2000). Nevertheless, use of the MMN for individual patients still requires much research. As a result of the difficulties and uncertainties with MMN, the initial excitement by audiologists about the MMN has faded, and some researchers have turned their attention to the slow cortical potentials. The future may see, however, clinical applications for the MMN, such as (1) the assessment of auditory discrimination capabilities in patients with hearing loss and hearing aids (Korczak et al., 2005; Oates et al., 2002) and (2) the prediction of outcome for comatose patients (Fischer et al., 1999; Kane et al., 1996; Naccache et al., 2005). Figure 18.10 shows the slow cortical response and

MMN results obtained from a hearing-impaired child with and without her hearing aids. The slow cortical response (P1) clearly shows the improvement using her hearing aids; the MMN results are not as clear but do suggest that her brain is able to discriminate the speech sounds. Compared to the MMN, the slow cortical response's much better response signal-to-noise ratio may make it a better candidate for such assessments (Cone-Wesson and Wunderlich, 2003; Martin and Boothroyd, 1999; Martin et al., 2007; Picton et al., 2000).

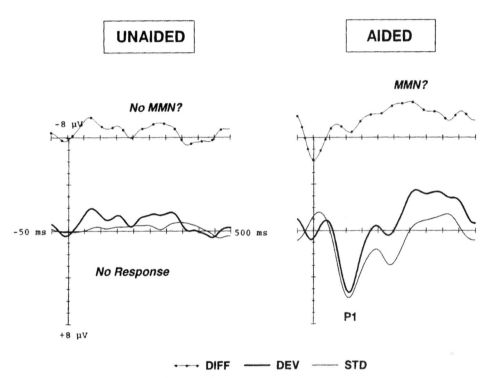

FIGURE 18.10 Slow cortical response and mismatch negativity (MMN) results obtained from a 7-year-old child with moderate to severe sensory-neural hearing loss recorded as part of her participation in a research study. This child's audiogram shows best-ear thresholds of 45, 70, 75, 65, 55, and 75 dB hearing level (HL) for 250, 500, 1,000, 2,000, 4,000, and 8,000 Hz, respectively. She had worn personal hearing aids (Unitron UM60-PP) binaurally since the age of 3 years. *Bottom,* her responses to the standard (STD; /ba/, 0.9 probability) and deviant (DEV; /da/, 0.1 probability) stimuli presented through a loudspeaker at 65 dB sound pressure level (SPL). *Left,* waveforms obtained without her hearing aids. *Right,* waveforms obtained while she wore both hearing aids set at their usual setting. *Top,* the difference (DIFF) waves resulting from the subtraction of the standard waves from the deviant waves. No slow cortical response is seen in the unaided condition. The small and inconsistent negativity in the unaided difference wave is, likely, noise. In contrast, in the aided condition, a clear P1 wave of the slow cortical response is seen in both the response to the standards and the response to the deviants. Furthermore, the response to the deviants in the aided condition is more negative following P1. The difference wave better shows this negativity. Although it is likely the MMN, this MMN is equivocal, as it did not show an inversion at the mastoids and its scalp distribution was broader than typically seen for the MMN. This may be due to the age of the child, the use of speech stimuli, and/or noise in the data. Behaviorally, this child found the /ba-da/ discrimination quite difficult in the unaided and the aided conditions. The MMN results, however, suggest that her brain is able to discriminate these stimuli when she wears her hearing aids, although the results are not clear. In contrast, the slow cortical responses (P1) very clearly show the improvement using her hearing aids. Compared with the MMN, the slow cortical response's much better response signal-to-noise ratio may make it a better candidate for such assessments. (These recordings were obtained in association with Peggy Oates-Korczak and Diane Kurtzberg.)

GROUP LEVEL

Over recent years, the MMN has been the subject of intense research in many patient populations. In particular, studies of the MMN in patients with cochlear implants, central auditory processing disorders, language disorders, learning disabilities, and neurologic disorders are providing insight into the processes underlying these disorders and will likely lead to the eventual application of the MMN to assessment of individual patients. Several reviews of these clinical group studies have been published (Cone-Wesson and Wunderlich, 2003; Csépe and Molnár, 1997; Leppänen and Lyytinen, 1997; Martin et al., 2007; Picton, 1998; Picton et al., 2000). As with the slow cortical potentials, studies using hypothesis-driven (concerning a particular clinical population) stimulus paradigms are likely to provide the most useful information.

Of particular relevance to audiologists, interest exists in using MMN to assess discrimination in individuals with SNHL and to assess changes occurring with use of hearing aids. Reports in the literature have mostly been of single cases (Kraus and McGee, 1994). Simulating hearing loss in a group of normal listeners using noise masking, we have shown increased MMN latencies and decreased MMN amplitudes with decreased audibility (Martin et al., 1999; Martin and Stapells, 2005). We have also recently studied a group of adults with SNHL and have reported that, similar to noise masking, SNHL results in later MMN latencies and smaller MMN amplitudes (Oates et al., 2002); with hearing aids, responses improved (Korczak et al., 2005).

Clinical Application of N2-P3, N400, LAN, and P600

INDIVIDUAL LEVEL

At present, only P3b of these later ERPs has any, albeit limited, clinical application at the individual level for clinical audiology. The uncertainty of the cerebral origin of P3b and its exact role in cognitive processing make the clinical utility of this ERP quite limited (Picton, 1992). Furthermore, because of the wide limits of normal variability of P3b amplitude and latency, P3b measurements cannot provide specific diagnostic information (Picton, 1992). As indicated in Table 18.5, the presence of the centroparietal P3b may be used to infer conscious perception of an auditory stimulus. The greatest utility would be for those patients seen for medicolegal/functional assessment. When told to push a button when they detect the deviant stimuli, individuals who exaggerate thresholds may demonstrate a large P3b to a stimulus even though they failed to press the button for stimuli below their presumed thresholds. The P3b indicates that they perceived the stimulus (Picton and Durieux-Smith, 1978). This use of P3b is less useful in other populations because active cooperation of the patient is required. Future research may indicate a clinical use of the P3a to unattended stimulus

sequences that contain large deviances or are novel (Polich, 2004; Polich and Criado, 2006).

Few data exist for N400, LAN, or P600 for clinical populations, especially at the individual level, and it is not possible to predict their use in the future. Their relationship to language processing should make them of great interest for audiology and speech-language pathology.

GROUP LEVEL

There is a large literature concerning P3b in many clinical populations (for reviews, see Hagoort and Kutas [1995], Leppänen and Lyytinen [1997], Picton [1992], and Polich [2004]). Of particular interest to audiologists, P3b latency has been reported to be delayed in 14 of 18 children with central auditory processing disorders (12 of 18 children showed delayed N1 latency), and changes in P3b reflected behavioral changes with therapeutic intervention (Jirsa, 1992; Jirsa and Clontz, 1990). It must be noted that (1) not all children produced a P3b, (2) nearly one quarter of the children with central auditory processing disorder showed P3b within the normal range, and (3) behavioral testing alone was able to demonstrate the deficits and the improvement. Finally, a subsequent study failed to demonstrate these P3b differences (Yencer, 1998). It is possible that, as with N1 and MMN, P3b stimulation parameters that specifically tap into central auditory processing may prove more fruitful. As discussed earlier, the slow cortical P1-N1-P2 sequence shows some promise for assessment of central auditory processing disorder. Uncertainty concerning the cerebral origin and role of P3b, the fact that this is not an "auditory" response, and the fact that behavioral testing can demonstrate the deficits make the audiologic clinical utility of the P3b ERP quite limited (Picton, 1992).

Our laboratory has investigated the use of P3b to assess discrimination in individuals with SNHL and to assess changes occurring with use of hearing aids. Our noise-masking studies simulating hearing loss have shown increased latencies and decreased amplitudes with decreased audibility. Furthermore, P3b latency increases may occur before any change in behavioral percent-correct performance (Martin et al., 1997; Martin and Stapells, 2005; Whiting et al., 1998). As with MMN, SNHL also results in later P3b latencies and smaller P3b amplitudes (Oates et al., 2002); with hearing aids, responses improved (Korczak et al., 2005).

There are few studies of the N400, LAN, and/or P600 in clinical populations, and most of these are to visually presented words (for reviews, see Hagoort and Kutas [1995], Mills et al. [2004], Neville et al. [1993], and Neville and Bavelier [2002]). As researchers studying patient populations in audiology and speech-language pathology learn more about these language-related ERPs, N400 and P600 will undoubtedly be used to provide insight into brain processing underlying normal and impaired language processes.

ACKNOWLEDGEMENTS

Funding for preparation of this article was obtained from the Natural Sciences and Engineering Research Council of Canada. Martyn Hyde generously provided the results and information concerning Case 1. I thank those individuals with whom I have had the good fortune to collaborate on cortical ERPs. These individuals include my former students Brett Martin and Peggy Oates-Korczak. In particular, I thank Terence Picton, Martyn Hyde, Diane Kurtzberg, and Herbert G. Vaughan Jr, who have been mentors and teachers in this area and who are now friends and colleagues.

REFERENCES

Aaltonen O, Niemi P, Nyrke T, Tuhkanen M. (1987) Event-related brain potentials and the perception of a phonetic continuum. *Biol Psychol.* 24, 197–207.

Achim A. (1995) Signal detection in averaged evoked potentials: Monte Carlo comparison of the sensitivity of different methods. *Electroencephalogr Clin Neurophysiol.* 96, 574–584.

Akatsuka K, Wasaka T, Nakata H, Inui K, Hoshiyama M, Kakigi R. (2005) Mismatch responses related to temporal discrimination of somatosensory stimulation. *Clin Neurophysiol.* 116, 1930–1937.

Alain C, Reinke K, He Y, Wang C, Lobaugh N. (2005) Hearing two things at once: neurophysiological indices of speech segregation and identification. *J Cogn Neurosci.* 17, 811–818.

Alain C, Woods DL. (1997) Attention modulates auditory pattern memory as indexed by event-related brain potentials. *Psychophysiology.* 34, 534–546.

Alain C, Woods DL. (1999) Age-related changes in processing auditory stimuli during visual attention: evidence for deficits in inhibitory control and sensory memory. *Psychol Aging.* 14, 507–519.

Alain C, Woods DL, Covarrubias D. (1997) Activation of duration-sensitive auditory cortical fields in humans. *Electroencephalogr Clin Neurophysiol.* 104, 531–539.

Alho K. (1995) Cerebral generators of mismatch negativity (MMN) and its magnetic counterpart (MMNm) elicited by sound changes. *Ear Hear.* 16, 38–50.

Alho K, Huotilainen M, Tiitinen H, Ilmoniemi RJ, Knuutila J, Näätänen R. (1993) Memory-related processing of complex sound patterns in human auditory cortex. An MEG study. *Neuroreport.* 4, 391–394.

Alho K, Sainio K, Sajaniemi N, Reinikainen K, Näätänen R. (1990) Event-related brain potential of human newborns to pitch change of an acoustic stimulus. *Electroencephalogr Clin Neurophysiol.* 77, 151–155.

Alho K, Woods DL, Algazi A, Knight RT, Näätänen R. (1994) Lesions of the frontal cortex diminish the auditory mismatch negativity. *Electroencephalogr Clin Neurophysiol.* 91, 353–362.

Anderer P, Pascual-Marqui R, Semlitsch H, Saletu B. (1998) Differential effects of normal aging on sources of standard N1, target N1 and target P300 auditory event-related brain potentials revealed by low resolution electromagnetic tomography (LORETA) *Electroencephalogr Clin Neurophysiol.* 108, 160–174.

Berg P, Scherg M. (1991) Dipole models of eye movements and blinks. *Electroencephalogr Clin Neurophysiol.* 79, 36–44.

Berlin CI, Bordelon J, St. John P, Wilensky D, Hurley EK, Hood LJ. (1998) Reversing click polarity may uncover auditory neuropathy in infants. *Ear Hear.* 19, 37–47.

Bertoli S, Heimberg S, Smurzynski J, Probst R. (2001) Mismatch negativity and psychoacoustic measures of gap detection in normally hearing subjects. *Psychophysiology.* 38, 334–342.

Bertrand O, Yvert B, Giard MH, Pernier J. (1998) Precautions in ERP mapping and source identification. Paper presented at the First International Workshop on Mismatch Negativity and Its Clinical Applications, Helsinki, Finland, October 16–18, 1998.

Besle J, Fort A, Delpuech C, Giard MH. (2004) Bimodal speech: early suppressive visual effects in human auditory cortex. *Eur J Neurosci.* 20, 2225–2234.

Beynon A, Snik A, Stegeman D, van den Broek P. (2005) Discrimination of speech sound contrasts determined with behavioral tests and event-related potentials in cochlear implant recipients. *J Am Acad Audiol.* 16, 42–53.

Boothroyd A. (2005) Measuring auditory speech perception capacity in young children. In: Seewald RC, Bamford JM, eds. *A Sound Foundation through Early Amplification 2004.* Basel: Phonak AG; pp 129–140.

Burkard R, Don M, Eggermont JJ. (2007) *Auditory Evoked Potentials: Basic Principles and Clinical Application.* Baltimore: Lippincott Williams & Wilkins.

Butler RA. (1968) Effect of changes in stimulus frequency and intensity on habituation of the human vertex potential. *J Acoust Soc Am.* 44, 945–950.

Butler SR, Simpson TP, Manara AR, Kane NM, Rowlands CA, Barton RL. (1998) Prognostic value of auditory mismatch negativity in coma. Paper presented at the First International Workshop on Mismatch Negativity and Its Clinical Applications, Helsinki, Finland, October 16–18, 1998.

Campbell K, Bell I, Bastien C. (1991) Evoked potential measures of information processing during natural sleep. In: Broughton R, Ogilvie R, eds. *Sleep, Arousal and Performance.* Cambridge, MA: Birkhauser; pp 88–116.

Cheour M, Alho K, Ceponiené R, Reinikainen K, Sainio K, Pohjavuori M, et al. (1998a) Maturation of mismatch negativity in infants. *Int J Psychophysiol.* 29, 217–226.

Cheour M, Ceponiene R, Lehtokoski A, Luuk A, Allik J, Alho K, et al. (1998b) Development of language-specific phoneme representations in the infant brain. *Nat Neurosci.* 1, 351–353.

Cheour-Luhtanen M, Alho K, Kujala T, Sainio K, Reinikainen K, Renlund M, et al. (1995) Mismatch negativity indicates vowel discrimination in newborns. *Hear Res.* 82, 53–58.

Cheour-Luhtanen M, Alho K, Sainio K, Rinne T, Reinikainen K, Pohjavouri M, et al. (1996) The ontogenetically earliest discriminitive response of the human brain. *Psychophysiology.* 33, 478–481.

Coles MGH, Rugg MD. (1995) Event-related potentials: an introduction. In: Coles MGH, Rugg MD, eds. *Electrophysiology of Mind. Event-Related Potentials and Cognition.* Oxford, England: Oxford University Press; pp 1–26.

Coles MGH, Smid HGOM, Scheffers MK, Otten LJ. (1995) Mental chronometry and the study of human information processing. In: Coles MGH, Rugg MD, eds. *Electrophysiology of Mind. Event-Related Potentials and Cognition.* Oxford, England: Oxford University Press; pp 86–131.

Cone-Wesson B, Wunderlich J. (2003) Auditory evoked potentials from the cortex: audiology applications. *Curr Opin Otolaryngol Head Neck Surg.* 11, 372–377.

Cooper RJ, Todd J, McGill K, Michie PT. (2006) Auditory sensory memory and the aging brain: a mismatch negativity study. *Neurobiol Aging.* 27, 752–762.

Courchesne E. (1978) Neurophysiological correlates of cognitive development: changes in long-latency event-related potentials from childhood to adulthood. *Electroencephalogr Clin Neurophysiol.* 45, 468–482.

Courchesne E, Hillyard SA, Galambos R. (1975) Stimulus novelty, task relevance, and the visual evoked potential in man. *Electroencephalogr Clin Neurophysiol.* 39, 131–143.

Covington JW, Polich J. (1996) P300, stimulus intensity, and modality. *Electroencephalogr Clin Neurophysiol.* 100, 579–584.

Cranford JL, Walker LJ, Stuart A, Elangovan S, Pravica D. (2003) Potential contamination effects of neuronal refractoriness on the speech-evoked mismatch negativity response. *J Am Acad Audiol.* 14, 251–259.

Csépe V, Molnár M. (1997) Towards the possible clinical application of the mismatch negativity component of event-related potentials. *Audiol Neurootol.* 2, 354–269.

Csépe V, Pantev C, Hoke M, Hampson S, Ross B. (1992) Evoked magnetic responses of the human auditory cortex to minor pitch changes: localization of the mismatch field. *Electroencephalogr Clin Neurophysiol.* 48, 538–548.

Dalebout SD, Fox LG. (2001) Reliability of the mismatch negativity in the responses of individual listeners. *J Am Acad Audiol.* 12, 245–253.

Dalebout SD, Stack JW. (1999) Mismatch negativity to acoustic differences not differentiated behaviorally. *J Am Acad Audiol.* 10, 388–399.

Damaschke J, Riedel H, Kollmeier B. (2005) Neural correlates of the precedence effect in auditory evoked potentials. *Hear Res.* 205, 157–171.

Davis H. (1976) Principles of electric response audiometry. *Ann Otol Rhinol Laryngol.* 85, 1–96.

Deacon D, Nousak J-M, Pilotti M, Ritter W, Yang C-M. (1998) Automatic change detection: does the auditory system use representations of individual stimulus features or gestalts? *Psychophysiology.* 35, 413–419.

Dehaene-Lambertz G, Dupoux E, Gout A. (2000) Electrophysiological correlates of phonological processing: a cross-linguistic study. *J Cogn Neurosci.* 12, 635–647.

Desjardins RN, Trainor LJ, Hevenor SJ, Polak CP. (1999) Using mismatch negativity to measure auditory temporal resolution thresholds. *Neuroreport.* 10, 2079–2082.

Dillon H. (2005) So, baby, how does it sound? Cortical assessment of infants with hearing aids. *Hear J.* 58, 10–17.

Dimitrijevic A, Stapells DR. (2006) Human electrophysiological examination of buildup of the precedence effect. *Neuroreport.* 17, 1133–1137.

Donchin E, Ritter W, McCallum WC. (1978) Cognitive psychophysiology: the endogenous components of the ERP. In: Calloway E, Tueting P, Koslow SH, eds. *Event-Related Brain Potentials in Man.* New York: Academic Press; pp 349–441.

Escera C, Alho K, Winkler I, Näätänen R. (1998) Neural mechanisms of involuntary attention to acoustic novelty and change. *J Cogn Neurosci.* 10, 590–604.

Fischer C, Morlet D, Bouchet P, Luaute J, Jourdan C, Salord F. (1999) Mismatch negativity and late auditory evoked potentials in comatose patients. *Clin Neurophysiol.* 110, 1601–1610.

Friederici AD. (2004) Event-related brain potential studies in language. *Curr Neurol Neurosci Rep.* 4, 466–470.

Friedman D, Kazmerski VA, Cycowicz YM. (1998) Effects of aging on the novelty P3 during attend and ignore oddball tasks. *Psychophysiology.* 35, 508–520.

Giard MH, Lavikainen J, Reinikainen K, Perrin F, Bertrand OM, Pernier J, et al. (1995) Separate representation of stimulus frequency, intensity and duration in auditory sensory memory: an event-related potential and dipole model analysis. *J Cogn Neurosci.* 7, 133–143.

Giard MH, Perrin F, Pernier J, Bouchet P. (1990) Brain generators implicated in processing of auditory stimulus deviance: a topographic event-related potential study. *Psychophysiology.* 27, 627–640.

Giard MH, Yvert B, Bertrand O, Pernier J. (1998) Sources of the electrical MMN. Paper presented at the First International Workshop on Mismatch Negativity and Its Clinical Applications, Helsinki, Finland, October 16–18, 1998.

Gomes H, Dunn M, Ritter W, Kurtzberg D, Brattson A, Kreuzer JA, et al. (2001) Spatiotemporal maturation of the central and lateral N1 components to tones. *Dev Brain Res.* 129, 147–155.

Gomes H, Sussman E, Ritter W, Kurtzberg D, Cowan N, Vaughan HG Jr. (1999) Electrophysiological evidence of developmental changes in the duration of auditory sensory memory. *Dev Psychol.* 35, 294–302.

Goodin DS, Squires KC, Henderson BH, Starr A. (1978) Age-related variations in evoked potentials to auditory stimuli in normal human subjects. *Electroencephalogr Clin Neurophysiol.* 44, 447–458.

Gordon KA, Tanaka S, Papsin BC. (2005) Atypical cortical responses underlie poor speech perception in children using cochlear implants. *Neuroreport.* 16, 2041–2045.

Gratton G, Coles MGH, Donchin E. (1983) A new method for off-line removal of ocular artifact. *Electroencephalogr Clin Neurophysiol.* 55, 468–484.

Gravel JS, Kurtzberg D, Stapells DR, Vaughan HGJ, Wallace IF. (1989) Case studies. *Semin Hear.* 10, 272–287.

Gravel JS, Stapells DR. (1993) Behavioral, electrophysiologic and otoacoustic measures from a child with auditory processing dysfunction. *J Am Acad Audiol.* 4, 412–419.

Hagoort P, Kutas M. (1995) Electrophysiological insights into language deficits. In: Johnston RJ, Baron JC, eds. *Handbook of Neuropsychology.* Vol. 10. Amsterdam: Elsevier; pp 105–133.

Hari R, Hämäläinen M, Ilmoniemi R, Kaukoranta E, Reinikainen K, Salminen J, et al. (1984) Responses of the primary auditory cortex to pitch changes in a sequence of tone pips: neuromagnetic recordings in man. *Neurosci Lett.* 50, 127–132.

Harkrider AW, Plyler PN, Hedrick MS. (2005) Effects of age and spectral shaping on perception and neural representation of stop consonant stimuli. *Clin Neurophysiol.* 116, 2153–2164.

Heinrich A, Alain C, Schneider B. (2004) Within- and between-channel gap detection in the human auditory cortex. *Neuroreport.* 15, 2051–2056.

Hillyard SA, Hink RF, Schwent VL, Picton TW. (1973) Electrical signs of selective attention in the human brain. *Science.* 182, 177–180.

Hillyard SA, Picton TW. (1987) Electrophysiology of cognition. In: Plum F, ed. *Handbook of Physiology, Section 1: The Nervous System—Higher Functions of the Nervous System.* Vol. V. Bethesda, MD: American Physiological Society; pp 519–584.

Hood LJ. (1998) Auditory neuropathy: what is it and what can we do about it? *Hear J.* 51, 10–18.

Hyde ML. (1988) Auditory evoked potentials. In: Alberti PW, Ruben RJ, eds. *Otologic Medicine and Surgery.* Vol. 1. New York: Churchill Livingstone; pp 443–485.

Hyde ML. (1994) The slow vertex potential: properties and clinical applications. In: Jacobson JT, eds. *Principles and Applications in Auditory Evoked Potentials.* Needham Heights, MA: Allyn and Bacon; pp 179–218.

Hyde ML. (1997) The N1 response and its applications. *Audiol Neurootol.* 2, 281–307.

Hyde ML, Alberti PW, Matsumoto N, Li Y. (1986) Auditory evoked potentials in audiometric assessment of compensation and medicolegal patients. *Ann Otol Rhinol Laryngol.* 95, 514–519.

Ille N, Berg P, Scherg M. (2002) Artifact correction of the ongoing EEG using spatial filters based on artifact and brain signal topographies. *J Clin Neurophysiol.* 19, 113–124.

Jaaskelainen IP, Ahveninen J, Bonmassar G, Dale AM, Ilmoniemi RJ, Levanen S, et al. (2004) Human posterior auditory cortex gates novel sounds to consciousness. *Proc Natl Acad Sci USA.* 101, 6809–6814.

Jacobsen T, Schroger E. (2003) Measuring duration mismatch negativity. *Clin Neurophysiol.* 114, 1133–1143.

Javitt DC, Grochowski S, Shelley A-M, Ritter W. (1998) Impaired mismatch negativity (MMN) generation in schizophrenia as a function of stimulus deviance, probability, and interstimulus/interdeviant interval. *Electroencephalogr Clin Neurophysiol.* 108, 143–153.

Jerger JJ, Martin J. (2005) Some effects of aging on event-related potentials during a linguistic monitoring task. *Int J Audiol.* 44, 321–330.

Jirsa RE. (1992) The clinical utility of P3 AERP in children with auditory processing disorders. *J Speech Hear Res.* 35, 903–912.

Jirsa RE, Clontz KB. (1990) Long latency auditory event-related potentials from children with auditory processing disorders. *Ear Hear.* 11, 222–232.

Joutsiniemi S-L, Ilvonen T, Sinkkonen J, Huotilainen M, Tervaniemi M, Lehtokoski K, et al. (1998) The mismatch negativity for duration decrement of auditory stimuli in healthy subjects. *Electroencephalogr Clin Neurophysiol.* 108, 154–159.

Kane NM, Curry SH, Rowlands CA, Manara AR, Lewis T, Moss T, et al. (1996) Event-related potentials—neurophysiologic tools for predicting emergence and early outcome from traumatic coma. *Intensive Care Med.* 22, 39–46.

Kekoni J, Hämäläinen H, Saarinen M, Gröhn J, Reinikainen K, Lehtokoski A, et al. (1997) Rate effect and mismatch responses in the somatosensory system: ERP recordings in humans. *Biol Psychol.* 46, 125–142.

Kelly AS, Purdy SC, Thorne PR. (2005) Electrophysiological and speech perception measures of auditory processing in experienced adult cochlear implant users. *Clin Neurophysiol.* 116, 1235–1246.

Klein SK, Kurtzberg D, Brattson A, Kreuzer JA, Stapells DR, Dunn MA, et al. (1995) Electrophysiologic manifestations of impaired temporal lobe auditory processing in verbal auditory agnosia. *Brain Lang.* 51, 383–405.

Korczak PA, Kurtzberg D, Stapells DR. (2005) Effects of sensorineural hearing loss and personal hearing aids on cortical event-related potential and behavioral measures of speech-sound processing. *Ear Hear.* 26, 165–185.

Kraus N, Bradlow AR, Cheatham MA, Cunningham J, King CD, Koch DB, et al. (2000) Consequences of neural asynchrony: a case of auditory neuropathy. *J Assoc Res Otolaryngol.* 1, 33–45.

Kraus N, McGee N. (1994) Auditory event-related potentials. In: Katz J, Gabbay WL, eds. *Handbook of Clinical Audiology.* 4th ed. Baltimore: Williams & Wilkins; pp 406–423.

Kraus N, McGee T, Carrell T, King C, Littman T, Nicol T. (1994a) Discrimination of speech-like contrasts in the auditory thalamus and cortex. *J Acoust Soc Am.* 96, 2758–2768.

Kraus N, McGee T, Carrell T, King C, Tremblay K, Nicol T. (1995a) Central auditory system plasticity associated with speech discrimination training. *J Cogn Neurosci.* 7, 25–32.

Kraus N, McGee T, Carrell T, Sharma A. (1995b) Neurophysiologic bases of speech discrimination. *Ear Hear.* 16, 19–37.

Kraus N, McGee T, Carrell T, Sharma A, Micco A, Nicol T. (1993a) Speech-evoked cortical potentials in children. *J Am Acad Audiol.* 4, 238–248.

Kraus N, McGee T, Ferre J, Hoeppner J, Carrell T, Sharma A, et al. (1993b) Mismatch negativity in the neurophysiologic/behavioral evaluation of auditory processing deficits: a case study. *Ear Hear.* 14, 223–234.

Kraus N, McGee T, Littman T, Nicol T, King C. (1994b) Nonprimary auditory thalamic representation of acoustic change. *J Neurophysiol.* 72, 1270–1277.

Kraus N, McGee T, Sharma A, Carrell T, Nicol T. (1992) Mismatch negativity event-related potential elicited by speech stimuli. *Ear Hear.* 13, 158–164.

Kraus N, Micco AG, Koch DB, McGee T, Carrell T, Sharma A, et al. (1993c) The mismatch negativity cortical evoked potential elicited by speech in cochlear-implant users. *Hear Res.* 65, 118–124.

Kropotov JD, Alho K, Näätänen R, Ponomarev VA, Kropotova OV, Anichkov AD, et al. (2000) Human auditory-cortex mechanisms of preattentive sound discrimination. *Neurosci Lett.* 280, 87–90.

Kumar A, Jayaram M. (2005) Auditory processing in individuals with auditory neuropathy. *Behav Brain Funct.* Available at: http://www.behavioralandbrainfunctions.com/content/1/1/21.

Kurtzberg D. (1989) Cortical event-related potential assessment of auditory system function. *Semin Hear.* 10, 252–261.

Kurtzberg D, Hilpert PL, Kreuzer JA, Vaughan HG. (1984) Differential maturation of cortical auditory evoked potentials to speech sounds in normal full-term and very low-birthweight infants. *Dev Med Child Neurol.* 26, 466–475.

Kurtzberg D, Stapells DR, Wallace IF. (1988) Event-related potential assessment of auditory system integrity: implications for language development. In: Vietze PM, Vaughan HGJ, eds. *Early Identification of Infants with Developmental Disabilities.* Philadelphia: Grune Stratton; pp 160–180.

Kurtzberg D, Vaughan HG, Kreuzer JA, Fleigler KZ. (1995) Developmental studies and clinical application of mismatch negativity: problems and prospects. *Ear Hear.* 16, 104–116.

Kutas M. (1997) Views on how the electrical activity that the brain generates reflects the functions of different language structures. *Psychophysiology.* 34, 383–398.

Kutas M, Hillyard SA. (1980) Reading senseless sentences: brain potentials reflect semantic incongruity. *Science.* 207, 203–205.

Kutas M, McCarthy G, Donchin E. (1977) Augmenting mental chronometry: the P300 as a measure of stimulus evaluation time. *Science.* 197, 792–795.

Kutas M, Van Petten C, Besson M. (1988) Event-related potential asymmetries during the reading of sentences. *Electroencephalogr Clin Neurophysiol.* 69, 218–233.

Lang AH, Eerola O, Korpilahti P, Holopainen I, Salo S, Aaltonen O. (1995) Practical issues in the clinical application of mismatch negativity. *Ear Hear.* 16, 117–129.

Leppänen PHT, Lyytinen H. (1997) Auditory event-related potentials in the study of developmental language-related disorders. *Audiol Neurootol.* 2, 308–240.

Liasis A, Bamiou D-E, Campbell P, Sirimanna T, Boyd S, Towell A. (2003) Auditory event-related potentials in the assessment of auditory processing disorders: a pilot study. *Neuropediatrics.* 34, 23–29.

Lightfoot G, Kennedy V. (2006) Cortical electric response audiometry hearing threshold estimation: accuracy, speed and the effects of stimulus presentation features. *Ear Hear.* 27, 443–456.

Loewy DH, Campbell KB, Bastien C. (1996) The mismatch negativity to frequency deviant stimuli during natural sleep. *Electroencephalogr Clin Neurophysiol.* 98, 493–501.

Lonka E, Kujala T, Lehtokoski A, Johansson R, Rimmanen S, Alho K, et al. (2004) Mismatch negativity brain response as an index of speech perception recovery in cochlear-implant recipients. *Audiol Neurootol.* 9, 160–162.

Maekawa T, Goto Y, Kinukawa N, Taniwaki T, Kanba S, Tobimatsu S. (2005) Functional characterization of mismatch negativity to a visual stimulus. *Clin Neurophysiol.* 116, 2392–2402.

Maiste A, Wiens AS, Hunt MJ, Scherg M, Picton TW. (1995) Event-related potentials and the categorical perception of speech sounds. *Ear Hear.* 16, 68–90.

Mäntysalo S, Näätänen R. (1987) The duration of a neuronal trace of an auditory stimulus as indicated by event-related potentials. *Biol Psychol.* 24, 183–195.

Martin BA, Boothroyd A. (1999) Cortical, auditory, event-related potentials in response to periodic and aperiodic stimuli with the same spectral envelope. *Ear Hear.* 20, 33–44.

Martin BA, Boothroyd A. (2000) Cortical, auditory, evoked potentials in response to changes of spectrum and amplitude. *J Acoust Soc Am.* 107, 2155–2161.

Martin BA, Kurtzberg D, Stapells DR. (1999) The effects of decreased audibility produced by high-pass noise masking on N1 and the mismatch negativity to speech sounds /ba/ and /da/. *J Speech Lang Hear Res.* 42, 271–286.

Martin BA, Shafer V, Morr M, Kreuzer J, Kurtzberg D. (2003) Maturation of mismatch negativity: a scalp current density analysis. *Ear Hear.* 24, 463–471.

Martin BA, Sigal A, Kurtzberg D, Stapells DR. (1997) The effects of decreased audibility produced by high-pass noise masking on cortical event-related potentials to speech sounds /ba/ and /da/. *J Acoust Soc Am.* 101, 1585–1599.

Martin BA, Stapells DR. (2005) Effects of low-pass noise masking on auditory event-related potentials to speech. *Ear Hear.* 26, 195–213.

Martin BA, Tremblay KL, Stapells DR. (2007) Principles and applications of cortical auditory evoked potentials. In: Burkard R, Don M, Eggermont J, eds. *Auditory Evoked Potentials: From Basic Principles and Clinical Application.* Baltimore: Lippincott Williams & Wilkins; pp 482–507.

Martin L, Barajas J, Fernandez R, Torres E. (1988) Auditory event-related potentials in well-characterized groups of children. *Electroencephalogr Clin Neurophysiol.* 71, 375–381.

McEvoy LK, Picton TW, Champagne SC, Kellett AJ, Kelly JB. (1990) Human evoked potentials to shifts in the lateralization of a noise. *Audiology.* 29, 163–180.

McGee T, Kraus N, Nicol T. (1997) Is it really a mismatch negativity? An assessment of methods for determining response validity in individual subjects. *Electroencephalogr Clin Neurophysiol.* 104, 359–368.

Micco AG, Kraus N, Koch DB, McGee TJ, Carrell TD, Sharma A, et al. (1995) Speech-evoked cognitive P300 potentials in cochlear implant recipients. *Am J Otol.* 16, 1–7.

Michalewski HJ, Starr A, Nguyen TT, Kong Y-Y, Zeng F-G. (2005) Auditory temporal processes in normal-hearing individuals and in patients with auditory neuropathy. *Clin Neurophysiol.* 116, 669–680.

Mills DL, Prat C, Zangl R, Stager CL, Neville HJ, Werker JF. (2004) Language experience and the organization of brain activity to phonetically similar words: ERP evidence from 14- and 20-month-olds. *J Cogn Neurosci.* 16, 1452–1464.

Molholm S, Gomes H, Lobosco J, Deacon D, Ritter W. (2004) Feature versus gestalt representation of stimuli in the mismatch negativity system of 7- to 9-year-old children. *Psychophysiology.* 41, 385–393.

Morr ML, Shafer VL, Kreuzer JA, Kurtzberg D. (2002) Maturation of mismatch negativity in typically developing infants and preschool children. *Ear Hear.* 23, 118–136.

Näätänen R. (1982) Processing negativity—evoked potential reflection of selective attention. *Psychol Bull.* 92, 605–640.

Näätänen R. (1991) Mismatch negativity outside strong attentional focus: a commentary on Woldorff et al. (1991) *Psychophysiology.* 28, 478–484.

Näätänen R. (1992) *Attention and Brain Function.* Hillsdale, NJ: Lawrence Erlbaum Associates.

Näätänen R. (1995) The mismatch negativity: a powerful tool for cognitive neuroscience. *Ear Hear.* 16, 6–18.

Näätänen R. (2000) Mismatch negativity (MMN) perspectives for application. *Int J Psychophysiol.* 37, 3–10.

Näätänen R, Alho K. (1995) Mismatch negativity: a unique measure of sensory processing in audition. *Int J Neurosci.* 80, 317–337.

Näätänen R, Alho K. (1997) Mismatch negativity: the measure for central sound representation accuracy. *Audiol Neurootol.* 2, 341–353.

Näätänen R, Gaillard AWK. (1983) The N2 deflection of ERP and the orienting reflex. In: Gaillard AWK, Ritter W, eds. *EEG Correlates of Information Processing: Theoretical Issues.* Amsterdam: North Holland; pp 119–141.

Näätänen R, Gaillard AWK, Mäntysalo S. (1978) Early selective attention effect on evoked potential reinterpreted. *Acta Psychol.* 42, 313–329.

Näätänen R, Jacobsen T, Winkler I. (2005) Memory-based or afferent processes in mismatch negativity (MMN): a review of the evidence. *Psychophysiology.* 42, 25–32.

Näätänen R, Jiang D, Lavikainen J, Reinikainen K, Paavilainen P. (1993a) Event-related potentials reveal a memory trace for temporal features. *Neuroreport.* 5, 310–312.

Näätänen R, Michie PT. (1979) Early selective attention effects on the evoked potential. A critical review and reinterpretation. *Biol Psychol.* 8, 81–136.

Näätänen R, Paavilainen P, Alho K, Reinikainen K, Sams M. (1987a) Interstimulus interval and the mismatch negativity. In: Barber C, Blum T, eds. *Evoked Potentials III.* London: Butterworths; pp 392–397.

Näätänen R, Paavilainen P, Alho K, Reinikainen K, Sams M. (1987b) The mismatch negativity to intensity changes in an auditory stimulus sequence. In: Johnson RJ, Rohrbaugh JW, Parasuraman R, eds. *Current Trends in Event-Related Potential Research.* New York: Elsevier; pp 125–131.

Näätänen R, Pakarinen S, Rinne T, Takegata R. (2004) The mismatch negativity (MMN): towards the optimal paradigm. *Clin Neurophysiol.* 115, 140–144.

Näätänen R, Picton T. (1987) The N1 wave of the human electric and magnetic response to sound: a review and an analysis of the component structure. *Psychophysiology.* 24, 375–424.

Näätänen R, Sams M, Järvilehto T, Soininen K. (1983) Probability of deviant stimulus and even-related brain potentials. In: Sinz R, Rosenzwieg MR, eds. *Psychophysiology.* Amsterdam: Elsevier Biomedical Press; pp 397–405.

Näätänen R, Schröger E, Karakas S, Tervaniemi M, Paavilainen P. (1993b) Development of a memory trace for a complex sound in the human brain. *Neuroreport.* 4, 503–506.

Näätänen R, Simpson M, Loveless NE. (1982) Stimulus deviance and evoked potentials. *Biol Psychol.* 14, 53–98.

Naccache L, Puybasset L, Gaillard RI, Serve E, Willer J-C. (2005) Auditory mismatch negativity is a good predictor of awakening in comatose patients: a fast and reliable procedure. *Clin Neurophysiol.* 1601–1610)

Neville HJ. (1995) Developmental specificity in neurocognitive development in humans. In: Gazzaniga MS, ed. *The Cognitive Neurosciences.* Cambridge, MA: The MIT Press; pp 219–231.

Neville HJ, Bavelier D. (2002) Human brain plasticity: evidence from sensory deprivation and altered language experience. *Prog Brain Res.* 138, 177–188.

Neville HJ, Coffey SA, Holcomb PJ, Tallal P. (1993) The neurobiology of sensory and language processing in language-impaired children. *J Cogn Neurosci.* 5, 235–253.

Neville HJ, Mills DL, Lawson DS. (1992) Fractionating language: different neural subsystems with different sensitive periods. *Cortex.* 2, 244–258.

Neville HJ, Nicol JL, Barss A, Forster KI, Garrett M. (1991) Syntactically based sentence processing classes: evidence from event-related brain potentials. *J Cogn Neurosci.* 3, 151–165.

Novak GP, Kurtzberg D, Kreuzer JA, Vaughan HG. (1989) Cortical responses to speech sounds and their formants in normal infants: maturational sequence and spatiotemporal analysis. *Electroencephalogr Clin Neurophysiol.* 73, 295–305.

Novak GP, Ritter W, Vaughan HG, Wiznitzer ML. (1990) Differentiation of negative event-related potentials in an auditory discrimination task. *Electroencephalogr Clin Neurophysiol.* 75, 255–275.

Oates PA, Kurtzberg D, Stapells DR. (2002) Effects of sensorineural hearing loss on cortical event-related potential and behavioural measures of speech-sound processing. *Ear Hear.* 23, 399–415.

Onishi S, Davis H. (1968) Effects of duration and rise time of tone bursts on evoked V potentials. *J Acoust Soc Am.* 44, 582–591.

Osterhout L, Holcomb PJ. (1995) Event-related potentials and language comprehension. In: Coles MGH, Rugg MD, eds. *Electrophysiology of Mind. Event-Related Potentials and Cognition.* Oxford, England: Oxford University Press; pp 171–215.

Ostroff JM, Martin BA, Boothroyd A. (1998) Cortical evoked response to acoustic change within a syllable. *Ear Hear.* 19, 290–297.

Pascual-Marqui R, Michel C, Lehmann, D. (1994) Low resolution electromagnetic tomography: a new method for localizing electrical activity in the brain. *Int J Psychophysiol.* 18, 49–65.

Pekkonen E, Rinne T, Näätänen R. (1995) Variability and replicability of the mismatch negativity. *Electroencephalogr Clin Neurophysiol.* 96, 546–554.

Pekkonen E, Rinne T, Reinikainen K, Kujala T, Alho K, Näätänen R. (1996) Aging effects on auditory processing: an event-related potential study. *Exp Aging Res.* 22, 171–184.

Pelizzone M, Hari R, Makela J, Kaukoranta E, Montandon P. (1987) Cortical activity evoked by a multichannel cochlear prosthesis. *Acta Otolaryngol.* 103, 632–636.

Pettigrew CM, Murdoch BE, Ponton CW, Kei J, Chenery HJ, Alkut P. (2004) Subtitled videos and mismatch negativity (MMN) investigations of spoken word processing. *J Am Acad Audiol.* 15, 469–485.

Phillips C. (2001) Levels of representation in the electrophysiology of speech perception. *Cognitive Science: A Multidisciplinary Journal.* 25, 711–731.

Picton TW. (1990) Auditory evoked potentials. In: Daly DD, Pedley TA, eds. *Current Practice of Clinical Electroencephalography.* 2nd ed. New York: Raven Press; pp 625–678.

Picton TW. (1992) The P300 wave of the human event-related potential. *J Clin Neurophysiol.* 9, 456–479.

Picton TW. (1995) The neurophysiological evaluation of auditory discrimination. *Ear Hear.* 16, 1–5.

Picton TW. (1998) Mismatch negativity: the normal, the deviant and the useful. Paper presented at the First International Workshop on Mismatch Negativity and its Clinical Applications, Helsinki, Finland, October 16–18, 1998.

Picton TW, Alain C, Otten L, Ritter W, Achim A. (2000) Mismatch negativity: different water in the same river. *Audiol Neurootol.* 5, 111–139.

Picton TW, Durieux-Smith A. (1978) The practice of evoked potential audiometry. *Otolaryngol Clin North Am.* 11, 263–282.

Picton TW, Hillyard SA. (1988) Endogenous event-related potentials. In: Picton TW, ed. *Handbook of Electroencephalography and Clinical Neurophysiology. Vol. 3. Human Event-Related Potentials.* Amsterdam: Elsevier; pp 361–426.

Picton TW, Hillyard SA, Galambos R. (1976) Habituation and attention in the auditory system. In: Keidel WD, Neff WD, eds. *Handbook of Sensory Physiology. Volume V, Auditory System, Part 3: Clinical and Special Topics.* Berlin: Springer-Verlag; pp 343–389.

Picton TW, Linden RD, Hamel G, Maru JT. (1983) Aspects of averaging. *Semin Hear.* 4, 327–341.

Picton TW, Lins OG, Scherg M. (1995) The recording and analysis of event-related potentials. In: Boller F, Grafman J, eds. *Handbook of Neuropsychology.* New York: Elsevier Science; pp 3–73.

Picton TW, McEvoy LK, Champagne SC. (1991) Human evoked potentials and the lateralization of a sound. *Acta Otolaryngol.* 491 (suppl), 139–143.

Picton TW, Rodriguez RT, Linden RD, Maiste AC. (1985) The neurophysiology of human hearing. *Hum Commun Can.* 9, 127–136.

Picton TW, Woods DL, Baribeau-Bräun J, Healey TMG. (1977) Evoked potential audiometry. *J Otolaryngol.* 6, 90–119.

Polich J. (1989) P300 from a passive auditory paradigm. *Electroencephalogr Clin Neurophysiol.* 74, 312–320.

Polich J. (2004) Clinical application of the P300 event-related brain potential. *Phys Med Rehabil Clin North Am.* 15, 133–161.

Polich J, Criado JR. (2006) Neuropsychology and neuropharmacology of P3a and P3b. *Int J Psychophysiol.* 60, 172–185.

Ponton CW, Don M, Eggermont JJ, Kwong B. (1997) Integrated mismatch negativity (MMNi): a noise-free representation of evoked responses allowing single-point distribution-free statistical tests. *Electroencephalogr Clin Neurophysiol.* 104, 143–150.

Ponton CW, Don M, Eggermont JJ, Waring MD, Kwong B. (1998) Maturation of the mismatch negativity (MMN): effects of profound deafness and cochlear implant use. Paper presented at the First International Workshop on Mismatch Negativity and its Clinical Applications, Helsinki, Finland, October 16–18, 1998.

Ponton CW, Don M, Eggermont JJ, Waring MD, Kwong B, Masuda A. (1996a) Auditory system plasticity in children after long periods of complete deafness. *Neuroreport.* 8, 61–65.

Ponton CW, Don M, Eggermont JJ, Waring MD, Masuda A. (1996b) Maturation of human cortical auditory function: differences between normal-hearing children and children with cochlear implants. *Ear Hear.* 17, 430–437.

Ponton CW, Don M, Waring MD, Eggermont JJ, Masuda A. (1993) Spatio-temporal source modeling of evoked potentials to acoustic and cochlear implant stimulation. *Electroencephalogr Clin Neurophysiol.* 88, 478–493.

Ponton CW, Eggermont JJ, Don M, Waring MD, Kwong B, Cunningham J, et al. (2000) Maturation of the mismatch negativity: effects of profound deafness and cochlear implant use. *Audiol Neurootol.* 5, 167–185.

Ponton CW, Vasama JP, Tremblay K, Khosla D, Kwong B, Don M. (2001) Plasticity in the adult human central auditory system: evidence from late-onset unilateral deafness. *Hear Res.* 154, 32–44.

Pritchard WS. (1981) Psychophysiology of P300. *Psychol Bull.* 89, 506–540.

Purdy SC, Katsch R, Dillon H, Storey L, Sharma M, Agung K. (2005) Aided cortical auditory evoked potentials for hearing instrument evaluation in infants. In: Seewald RC, Bamford JM, eds. *A Sound Foundation Through Early Amplification 2004.* Basel: Phonak AG; pp 115–127.

Rance G, Cone-Wesson B, Wunderlich J, Dowell R. (2002) Speech perception and cortical event related potentials in children with auditory neuropathy. *Ear Hear.* 23, 239–253.

Rickards FW, deVidi S, McMahon DS. (1996) Cortical evoked response audiometry in noise induced hearing loss claims. *Aust J Otolaryngol.* 2, 237–241.

Ritter W, Deacon D, Gomes H, Javitt DC, Vaughan HGJ. (1995) The mismatch negativity of event-related potentials as a probe of transient auditory memory: a review. *Ear Hear.* 16, 52–67.

Ritter W, Sussman E, Molholm S. (2000) Evidence that the mismatch negativity system works on the basis of objects. *Neuroreport.* 11, 61–63.

Rivera-Gaxiola M, Csibra G, Johnson M, Karmiloff-Smith A. (2000) Electrophysiological correlates of cross-linguistic speech perception in native English speakers. *Behav Brain Res.* 111, 13–23.

Rugg MD, Coles MGH, eds. (1995a) *Electrophysiology of Mind. Event-Related Potentials and Cognition.* Oxford, England: Oxford University Press.

Rugg MD, Coles MGH. (1995b) The ERP and cognitive psychology: conceptual issues. In: Coles MGH, Rugg MD, eds. *Electrophysiology of Mind. Event-Related Potentials and Cognition.* Oxford, England: Oxford University Press; pp 27–39.

Sabri M, De Lugt DR, Campbell KB. (2000) The mismatch negativity to frequency deviants during the transition from wakefulness to sleep. *Can J Exp Psychol.* 4, 230–242.

Sabri M, Labelle S, Gosselin A, Campbell KB. (2003) Effects of sleep onset on the mismatch negativity (MMN) to frequency deviants using a rapid rate of presentation. *Cogn Brain Res.* 17, 164–176.

Sams M, Aulanko R, Aaltonen O, Näätänen R. (1990) Event-related potentials to infrequent changes in synthesized stimuli. *J Cogn Neurosci.* 2, 344–357.

Sams M, Paavilainen P, Alho K, Näätanen R. (1985) Auditory frequency discrimination and event-related potentials. *Electroencephalogr Clin Neurophysiol.* 62, 437–448.

Scarff C, Reynolds A, Goodyear B, Ponton C, Dort J, Eggermont J. (2004) Simultaneous 3-T fMRI and high-density recording of human auditory evoked potentials. *Neuroimage.* 23, 1129–1142.

Scherg M, Vajsar J, Picton T. (1989) A source analysis for the late human auditory evoked potentials. *J Cogn Neurosci.* 1, 336–355.

Scherg M, von Cramon D. (1986a) Evoked dipole source potentials of the human auditory cortex. *Electroencephalogr Clin Neurophysiol.* 65, 344–360.

Scherg M, von Cramon D. (1986b) Psychoacoustic and electrophysiologic correlates of central hearing disorders in man. *Eur Arch Psychiatry Neurol Sci.* 236, 56–60.

Schroger E. (1996) Interaural time and level differences: integrated or separated processing? *Hear Res.* 96, 191–198.

Shafer VL, Morr ML, Datta H, Kurtzberg D, Schwartz RG. (2005) Neurophysiological indexes of speech processing deficits in children with specific language impairment. *J Cogn Neurosci.* 17, 1168–1180.

Shafer VL, Morr ML, Kreuzer JA, Kurtzberg D. (2000) Maturation of mismatch negativity in school-age children. *Ear Hear.* 21, 242–251.

Sharma A, Dorman MF, Spahr AJ. (2002) A sensitive period for the development of the central auditory system in children with cochlear implants: implications for age of implantation. *Ear Hear.* 23, 532–539.

Sharma A, Kraus N, McGee T, Carrell T, Nicol T. (1993) Acoustic versus phonetic representation of speech as reflected by the mismatch negativity event-related potential. *Electroencephalogr Clin Neurophysiol.* 88, 64–71.

Sharma A, Kraus N, McGee T, Nicol T. (1997) Developmental changes in P1 and N1 central auditory responses elicited by consonant-vowel syllables. *Electroencephalogr Clin Neurohysiol.* 104, 540–545.

Sharma M, Purdy SC, Newall P, Wheldall K, Beaman R, Dillon H. (2004) Effects of identification technique, extraction method, and stimulus type on mismatch negativity in adults and children. *J Am Acad Audiol.* 15, 616–632.

Sharma M, Purdy SC, Newall P, Wheldall K, Beaman R, Dillon H. (2006) Electrophysiological and behavioral evidence of auditory processing deficits in children with reading disorder. *Clin Neurophysiol.* 117, 1130–1144.

Singh S, Liasis A, Rajput K, Towell A, Luxon L. (2004) Event-related potentials in pediatric cochlear implant patients. *Ear Hear.* 25, 598–610.

Squires NK, Squires KC, Hillyard SA. (1975) Two varieties of long-latency positive waves evoked by unpredictable auditory stimuli in man. *Electroencephalogr Clin Neurophysiol.* 38, 387–401.

Stapells DR. (1984) Studies in evoked potential audiometry. Unpublished Doctoral dissertation, University of Ottawa, Ottawa, Ontario Canada.

Stapells DR, Hirayama M, So MR. (1999) Inter- and intra-subject variability of the intensity-MMN. Paper presented at the XVI Biennial Symposium of the International Evoked Response Audiometry Study Group, Tromsø, Norway, May 30–June 3, 1999.

Stapells DR, Kurtzberg D. (1991) Evoked potential assessment of auditory system integrity in infants. *Clin Perinatol.* 18, 497–518.

Stapells DR, So MR. (1998) Intensity-MMN disassociated from behavioural perception by changing base intensity of standards. Paper presented at the First International Workshop on Mismatch Negativity and its Clinical Applications, Helsinki, Finland, October 16–18, 1998.

Stapells DR, Tremblay LA, Yee W. (2002) Mismatch negativity cortical erp measures of "central" auditory gap detection. Poster presented to the Midwinter meeting of the Association for Research in Otolaryngology. St. Petersburg Beach, FL, February, 2002. Available at: http://www.aro.org/archives/2002/2002556.html.

Stapells DR, Wu C-Y. (2000) The role of auditory cortical processing in the "Franssen" auditory illusion: a mismatch negativity ERP investigation. Poster presented at the Midwinter Meeting of the Association for Research in Otolaryngology, St. Petersburg Beach, FL, February, 2000. Available at: http://www.aro.org/archives/2000/5757.html.

Starr A, Picton TW, Sininger Y, Hood LJ, Berlin CI. (1996) Auditory neuropathy. *Brain.* 119, 741–753.

Steinschneider M, Kurtzberg D, Vaughan HGJ. (1992) Event-related potentials in developmental psychology. In: Rapin I, Segalowitz SJ, eds. *Child Neuropsychology.* Vol. 6. Amsterdam: Elsevier; pp 239–299.

Sussman ES. (2005) Integration and segregation in auditory scene analysis. *J Acoust Soc Am.* 117, 1285–1298.

Sutton S, Braren M, Zubin J. (1965) Evoked potential correlates of stimulus uncertainty. *Science.* 150, 1187–1188.

Taylor MJ. (1988) Developmental changes in ERPs to visual language stimuli. *Biol Psychol.* 26, 321–328.

Tervaniemi M, Lehtokoski A, Sinkkonen J, Virtanen J, Ilmoniemi RJ, Näätänen R. (1999) Test-retest reliability of mismatch negativity for duration, frequency, and intensity changes. *Clin Neurophysiol.* 110, 1388–1393.

Tiitinen H, Alho K, Huotilainen M, Ilmoniemi J, Simola J, Näätanen R. (1993) Tonotopic auditory cortex and the magnetoencephalographic (MEG) equivalent of the mismatch negativity. *Psychophysiology.* 30, 537–540.

Trainor LJ, Desjardins RN, Rockel C. (1999) A comparison of contour and interval processing in musicians and nonmu-

sicians using event-related potentials. *Aust J Psychol.* 51, 147–153.

Trainor LJ, Shahin A, Roberts LE. (2003) Effects of musical training on the auditory cortex in children. *Ann NY Acad Sci.* 999, 506–513.

Tremblay KL, Kraus N. (2002) Auditory training induces asymmetrical changes in cortical neural activity. *J Speech Lang Hear Res.* 45, 564–572.

Tremblay KL, Kraus K, McGee T. (1998) The time course of auditory perceptual learning: neurophysiological changes during speech-sound training. *Neuroreport.* 16, 3557–3560.

Tremblay KL, Kraus N, Carrell T, McGee TD. (1997) Central auditory system plasticity: generalization to novel stimuli following listening training. *J Acoust Soc Am.* 102, 3762–3773.

Tremblay KL, Piskosz M, Souza P. (2003) Effects of age and age-related hearing loss on the neural representation of speech cues. *Clin Neurophysiol.* 114, 1332–1343.

Tsui B, Wong LL, Wong EC. (2002) Accuracy of cortical evoked response audiometry in the identification of non-organic hearing loss. *Int J Audiol.* 41, 330–333.

Tsui V, Shi R, Werker J, Stapells D. (2000) MMN measures of categorical perception of native and non-native consonant contrasts. Poster presented at the 2nd International Congress on Mismatch Negativity and its Clinical Applications, Barcelona, Spain, June 15–18, 2000. Available at: http://www.ub.es/congres/mmn2000/Abstracts/Tsui.htm.

Uwer R, Albrecht R, von Suchodoletz W. (2002) Automatic processing of tones and speech stimuli in children with specific language impairment. *Dev Med Child Neurol.* 44, 527–532.

Uwer R, von Suchodoletz W. (2000) Stability of mismatch negativities in children. *Clin Neurophysiol.* 111, 45–52.

Van Maanen A, Stapells DR. (2005) Comparison of multiple auditory steady-state responses (80 vs 40 Hz) and slow cortical potentials for threshold estimation in hearing-impaired adults. *Int J Audiol.* 44, 613–624.

Vaughan HG, Kurtzberg D. (1989) Electrophysiologic indices of normal and aberrant cortical maturation. In: Kellaway P, Noebels JL, eds. *Problems and Concepts in Developmental Neurophysiology.* Baltimore: The Johns Hopkins University Press; pp 263–287.

Vaughan HG, Ritter W. (1970) The sources of auditory evoked responses recorded from the human scalp. *Electroencephalogr Clin Neurophysiol.* 28, 360–367.

Verleger R. (1991) The instruction to refrain from blinking affects auditory P3 and N1 amplitudes. *Electroencepahlogr Clin Neurophysiol.* 78, 240–251.

Verleger R. (1997) On the utility of P3 as an index of mental chronometry. *Psychophysiology.* 34, 131–156.

Wang W, Datta H, Sussman E. (2005) The development of the length of the temporal window of integration for rapidly presented auditory information as indexed by MMN. *Clin Neurophysiol.* 116, 1695–1706.

Whiting KA, Martin BA, Stapells DR. (1998) The effects of broadband noise masking on cortical event-related potentials to speech sounds /ba/ and /da/. *Ear Hear.* 19, 218–231.

Winkler I, Kujala T, Tiitinen HPS, Alku P, Lehtokoski A, et al. (1999) Brain responses reveal the learning of foreign language phonemes. *Psychophysiology.* 36, 638–642.

Winkler I, Tervaniemi M, Näätänen R. (1997) Two separate codes for missing-fundamental pitch in the human auditory cortex. *J Acoust Soc Am*. 102, 1072–1082.

Woldorff MG, Hillyard SA, Gallen CC, Hampson SR, Bloom FE. (1998) Magnetoencephalographic recordings demonstrate attentional modulation of mismatch-related neural activity in human auditory cortex. *Psychophysiology*. 35, 283–292.

Wolpaw JR, Penry JK. (1975) A temporal component of the auditory evoked response. *Electroencephalogr Clin Neurophysiol*. 39, 609–620.

Wunderlich JL, Cone-Wesson B. (2006) Maturation of CAEP in infants and children: a review. *Hear Res*. 212, 212–223.

Wunderlich JL, Cone-Wesson BK, Shepherd R. (2006) Maturation of the cortical auditory evoked potential in infants and young children. *Hear Res*. 212, 185–202.

Yabe H, Tervaniemi M, Sinkkonen J, Huotilainen M, Ilmoniemi RJ, Näätänen R. (1998) Temporal window of integration of auditory information in the human brain. *Psychophysiology*. 35, 615–619.

Yencer KA. (1998) The effects of auditory integration training for children with central auditory processing disorders. *Am J Audiol*. 7, 1–13.

Yvert B, Bertrand O, Thevenet M, Echallier JF, Pernier J. (1997) A systematic evaluation of the spherical model accuracy in EEG dipole localization. *Electroencephalogr Clin Neurophysiol*. 102, 452–459.

Zeng F-G, Oba S, Garde S, Sininger Y, Starr A. (1999) Temporal and speech processing deficits in auditory neuropathy. *Neuroreport*. 10, 3429–3435.

CHAPTER 19

Clinical Neurophysiology of the Vestibular System

Kamran Barin

OVERVIEW

Vestibular function tests are an important part of the clinical assessment and management of patients with dizziness and other balance disorders (Goebel, 2001). Laboratory evaluation of human vestibular pathways, however, is hampered by the fact that there is no direct access to the responses of the vestibular end organ. One must rely solely on secondary motor responses to assess the vestibular pathways. Therefore, accurate interpretation of the vestibular tests and development of proper diagnosis and management plans are critically dependent on understanding the neurophysiology of the vestibular system (Shepard, 2001a; 2001b). This chapter describes the structure and function of the vestibular system in healthy individuals and examines how different abnormalities affect the vestibular pathways. The focus of this chapter is on topics that have clinical relevance, including clinical manifestations and findings in vestibular function tests during various stages of vestibular abnormalities.

Role of Vestibular Pathways

The vestibular system provides the central nervous system (CNS) with sensory information regarding the orientation and movement of the head in space (Hain et al., 2000). Head movements possess six degrees of freedom, including linear motion along three dimensions and rotation about three axes. Therefore, the vestibular end organ consists of multiple receptors, with each receptor responsible for detection and neural encoding of one type of head motion (Baloh and Honrubia, 2001).

The vestibular system contributes to at least two important reflexes—the vestibulo-spinal reflex (VSR) and the vestibulo-ocular reflex (VOR). The vestibular system has a peripheral component consisting of the labyrinth and the vestibular nerve and a central component consisting of the vestibular nuclei (Wilson and Melvill-Jones, 1979). For both reflexes, the peripheral vestibular system passes the information about the orientation and movements of the head to the motor centers, such as the spinal cord or the oculomotor nuclei, via the central vestibular pathways. Figure 19.1 represents a schematic diagram of these two reflexes.

VESTIBULO-SPINAL REFLEX

The VSR is one of the motor control mechanisms that contribute to postural stability during routine tasks such as upright standing or walking and during more complex tasks such as running or jumping. To accomplish this goal, the VSR must constantly receive sensory information about the orientation of all body segments, including the head, neck, torso, and legs. In addition to the vestibular system, at least two other sensory systems, proprioception and vision, supply the VSR with sensory input regarding the orientation of different body segments (Horak and Shupert, 2000). Proprioceptive receptors lie within the muscles and joints and provide information about the relative orientation of two adjacent body segments. The visual system provides information about the relative orientation of the body with respect to the external environment. There are other sensory mechanisms that participate in postural stability, but their contributions are not well understood at this time.

If we impose restrictions on the type and speed of body movements, for example standing quietly on a solid surface

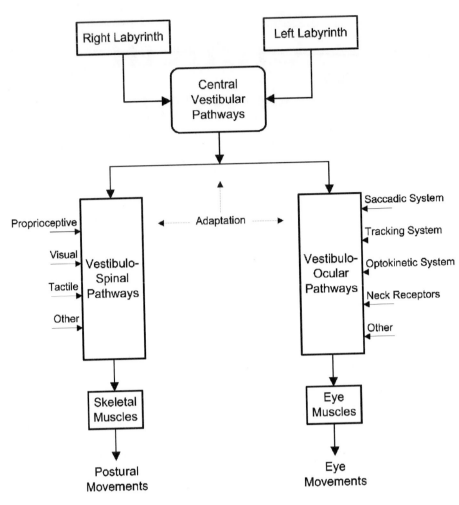

FIGURE 19.1
Vestibulo-ocular and vestibulo-spinal pathways and their interactions with other sensory mechanisms.

with eyes open, there will be an overlap of the sensory inputs from the vestibular, proprioceptive, and visual systems. Even then, the overlap is limited to a narrow frequency range of body motion. Indeed, these sensory mechanisms are by no means redundant because their operational frequency ranges are, for the most part, distinct. For example, the visual system is best suited for low-frequency movements, typically less than 1 Hz, because of the inherently large delays within the visual neural pathways (Howard, 1982). The reaction time for the proprioceptive receptors is around 100 ms or less, which makes them more effective for fast, high-frequency (~10 Hz and higher) movements (Shepard and Telian, 1996). The operational range of the vestibular system is somewhere between those of the visual and proprioceptive systems and covers frequencies of about 0.1 to 3 Hz (Baloh and Honrubia, 2001).

To maintain postural stability, the VSR pathways must detect spatial orientation of all body segments with respect to an earth-fixed reference frame. The visual and proprioceptive systems, however, provide orientation information relative to a reference frame that itself may vary with respect to an earth-fixed reference frame. For example, if we stand on a solid surface, proprioceptive receptors from the ankle joint can determine the orientation of the lower legs with respect

to the support surface (Nashner, 2001). If the orientation of the support surface is known with respect to an earth-fixed reference frame, then the orientation of the body segment can be inferred from the proprioceptive inputs. Otherwise, as may be the case for moving or compliant support surfaces, the proprioceptive cues do not provide accurate orientation information with respect to an earth-fixed reference frame (Allum and Shepard, 1999).

Similarly, the visual system can provide accurate orientation information only when there is an object in the field of view with known orientation with respect to an earth-fixed reference frame. For example, during the takeoff phase of a plane, one must first look out of the window and determine the orientation of the plane with respect to an object on the ground. Only then can the visual input provide the orientation of the body with respect to an earth-fixed reference frame (Redfern et al., 2001).

On earth and in the presence of gravity, the vestibular system is the only sensory mechanism that provides orientation information with respect to an earth-fixed reference frame. This unique aspect of the vestibular system plays an important role as the sensory inputs from multiple receptors are weighed and integrated to determine the body orientation. When there is ambiguity among the sensory inputs, the

VSR pathways use the information from the vestibular system to maintain postural stability (Nashner and McCollum, 1985).

How does a total loss of vestibular input affect the VSR function? Postural stability will not be significantly affected in conditions where either visual or proprioceptive inputs can provide accurate orientation information with respect to an earth-fixed reference frame. An example of such a condition is standing on a solid surface with eyes open. On the other hand, postural stability of a patient with total loss of vestibular function will severely deteriorate when standing on a compliant surface in total darkness or with eyes closed (Nashner, 2001). Under such conditions, neither the visual nor the proprioceptive system provides spatially accurate orientation information, and consequently, the patient is likely to fall.

The loss of proprioceptive input has a far more devastating effect on postural stability. Even when the vestibular and visual systems provide accurate information about the orientation of the head, the proprioceptive system is needed to transmit that information from one body segment to another until the orientation of all body segments is established (Allum et al., 1993). As a result, patients with total loss of proprioceptive cues will be unable to stand or walk unassisted. Conversely, loss of the visual system should have a minimal effect on postural stability as long as the vestibular system is intact. Under normal conditions, the visual and vestibular systems provide overlapping orientation information. Therefore, the visual input is crucial for postural stability only if there is damage to the vestibular receptors.

VESTIBULO-OCULAR REFLEX

The VOR is one of the eye movement control mechanisms that contribute to gaze stabilization during head motion. Gaze stabilization is necessary because images must stay long enough on the retina to be encoded into neural signals (Leigh and Zee, 1991). Otherwise, everything will appear blurry during head motion, and we would be unable to have clear vision. To achieve a steady retinal image during head motion, the information from the peripheral vestibular system is passed to the oculomotor pathways, where compensatory eye movements are generated by moving the eyes with the same velocity but in the opposite direction of head movements. This VOR function is the foundation of many vestibular function tests such as caloric and rotation tests.

There are other oculomotor control systems that interact with the VOR. As mentioned earlier, the vestibular system works best for the so-called *natural* head movements (i.e., brief head movements that fall within the frequency range of about 0.1 to 3 Hz). Therefore, vestibular control of gaze stabilization during natural head movements is nearly perfect. However, for sustained head movements where the frequency is below 0.1 Hz, the vestibular system does not provide accurate information regarding the head velocity. An example of one such movement is rotating at a constant velocity for a

long period of time. For these types of low-frequency head movements, the vestibular function is supplanted by a visual subsystem called the *optokinetic system*. The optokinetic reflex is activated by the movement of an image across the retina and then attempts to stabilize the image by moving the eyes in the same direction (van Die and Collewijn, 1982). By integrating the inputs from both vestibular and optokinetic reflexes, the CNS achieves gaze stabilization over a wide frequency range of head motion (Howard, 1993).

Saccadic and *tracking* mechanisms are other visual subsystems that also contribute to gaze stabilization in humans and other *foveate* animals. The fovea is the most sensitive part of the retina and is densely packed with neural receptors. Thus, the images on the fovea can be seen in far better detail than the images on the rest of the retina. The saccadic system quickly brings the image of a new object of interest onto the fovea (Westheimer, 1954). Eye velocities during saccadic eye movements can exceed 400 degrees per second, making them the fastest type of eye movements (Baloh and Honrubia, 2001). These high velocities are necessary because vision is impaired during saccades. Another role of the saccadic system is to rapidly move the eyes toward the center, as the vestibular- and optokinetic-mediated reflexive eye movements drive the eyes toward the orbital periphery (Cohen and Henn, 1972).

The tracking system, also known as the smooth pursuit system, keeps the image of a moving object on the fovea. The movement of images on the fovea, called *foveal slip*, triggers the tracking mechanisms, which try to match the eye velocity to the object velocity (Pola and Wyatt, 1980). One would expect the eyes to follow the object but never catch it because of the inherent delay in the visual pathway. However, when the movement of the object is predictable, the tracking system can quickly estimate its properties and drive the eyes such that the image of the moving object remains on the fovea at all times. This feature of the tracking system works well as long as the frequency of motion is less than 1 Hz (Leigh and Zee, 1991).

The tracking system interacts with the vestibular system when one is asked to fixate on a stationary object during vestibular stimulation. As the VOR moves the eyes, the image of the object moves across the fovea, thus triggering the tracking mechanisms (Chambers and Gresty, 1982). The eye movements generated by the tracking system oppose and override the eye movements generated by the vestibular system and lead to *fixation suppression* (Halmagyi and Gresty, 1979). There is disagreement as to whether the tracking system is the only contributor to the fixation suppression or whether another system, *vestibular cancellation*, also participates in this task (Tomlinson and Robinson, 1981). Although this discussion is beyond the scope of this chapter, it is clear that the tracking system has a major role in fixation suppression.

Vestibular function tests attempt to evaluate different types of eye movements. However, the optokinetic test in the vestibular test battery is usually a test of the tracking system and not a true test of the optokinetic system. Although the tracking and optokinetic mechanisms both originate from the visual system, there are distinct differences between the two (Leigh and Zee, 1991). Optokinetic eye movements are reflexive, whereas tracking eye movements are voluntary. Stimulation of the optokinetic system generates a strong sensation of self-motion, which is not a feature of the tracking system stimulation. The optokinetic stimulation originates from the retina and requires motion of the full visual field. In contrast, the tracking stimulus must be small enough to fit on the fovea. Most laboratory tests use a small target as the stimulus for both tracking and optokinetic tests, which precludes stimulation of the optokinetic system. Some of the newer test devices do use full-field visual stimulation, but even then, one cannot eliminate the contribution of the tracking system because the stimulus covers both the retina and fovea. Instructing the subjects to avoid fixating on any part of the visual surround can reduce the contribution of the tracking system, but this is a difficult task for most subjects. The only true test of the optokinetic system is based on moving the visual surround for an extended period of time and then turning the room light off and measuring the eye movements in total darkness. This is called the *optokinetic after-nystagmus* test, but most laboratories are not equipped to perform it (Leigh and Zee, 1991). Therefore, one should recognize the limitations of testing the optokinetic system.

The proprioceptive receptors of the neck also contribute to gaze stabilization through the cervico-ocular reflex (Peterson et al., 1985). This reflex can be activated by moving the torso while holding the head stationary in space. However, the cervico-ocular reflex does not seem to play a prominent role in gaze stabilization as long as vestibular receptors are intact.

How does a total loss of vestibular function affect the VOR function? Since the vestibular system keeps a stationary image of objects on the retina during head motion, total loss of vestibular function will cause the sensation that stationary objects are moving during head motion. This symptom, called *oscillopsia*, is indeed common in patients with bilateral vestibular loss (Brandt, 1996). In addition, loss of vestibular function can lead to the deterioration of visual acuity during head motion.

Damage to the other gaze-stabilization mechanisms can cause different eye movement abnormalities and visual disturbances. The exact type of abnormality depends on the site and nature of the damage, but it usually indicates a CNS lesion. This topic is discussed in more detail in Chapter 20.

Adaptation of Vestibular Pathways

The vestibular pathways are often exposed to environmental and developmental changes such as aging. These pathways possess a high degree of plasticity to overcome the effects of these natural changes, as well as those caused by disease and trauma (Zee, 2000). When dealing with natural changes, the process is referred to as *adaptation*, whereas the process after

a vestibular loss is called *compensation*. Both adaptation and compensation mechanisms employ very similar strategies. They range from modifying the gain and the baseline firing of the vestibular neural pathways to completely substituting those pathways with other sensory mechanisms.

The exact nature of vestibular adaptation or compensation is not fully understood, but it seems to originate from the cerebellum. The adaptive mechanisms appear to be activated when neural responses from the vestibular system do not match our anticipated head movements. For example, natural head movements generate brief high-frequency neural changes. If changes in the neural activity do not subside after a short period of time, such as in the case of an astronaut during extended space flight or a patient with a labyrinthine lesion, the assumption is that the vestibular pathways are not operating optimally and adaptive changes are necessary (Curthoys and Halmagyi, 2000).

Management plans for patients following a vestibular lesion are influenced by the extent and timing of the vestibular compensation process. Ideally, tests of vestibular function should provide information not only about the presence of a vestibular lesion, but also about the level of compensation. However, determining the compensation level from the available diagnostic tests is not trivial and requires a complete understanding of the vestibular compensation process. This and other neurophysiologic properties of the vestibular pathways will be discussed in the remainder of this chapter.

ORGANIZATION OF THE VESTIBULAR SYSTEM

The vestibular end organ resides next to the cochlea within the inner ear in a chamber called the bony labyrinth (Fig. 19.2). The membranous labyrinth, which houses the vestibular receptors, is suspended within the bony labyrinth. The inner ear space is filled with two types of fluid with distinct chemical compositions. The bony labyrinth contains *perilymph*, which is similar to the cerebrospinal fluid in its chemical composition and has a higher sodium-to-potassium concentration ratio (Salt and Konishi, 1986). The membranous labyrinth contains *endolymph*, which is similar to the intracellular fluid in its chemical composition and has a higher potassium-to-sodium concentration ratio. In a normal labyrinth, the endolymphatic and perilymphatic fluids never come into contact with each other.

The vestibular receptors are embedded in five different areas of the membranous labyrinth (Fig. 19.3). Three of these receptors are located in the enlarged portion of each semicircular canal, called the *ampulla*. The *cristae ampullaris* within each ampulla contains the vestibular sensory cells. The openings of the three semicircular canals converge in a cavity, called the *vestibule*. The *maculae* of the *utricle* and *saccule* reside in the vestibule and contain the remaining two vestibular receptors. The organization of the sensory cells within the

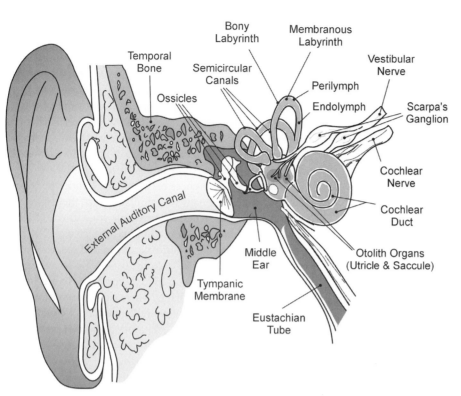

FIGURE 19.2 Bony and membranous labyrinths and the adjacent structures within the temporal bone.

membranous labyrinth allows the vestibular system to detect different types of head movements.

Structure of Hair Cells

The vestibular receptors are packed with specialized sensory cells called hair cells. The hair cells transduce mechanical energy generated by the forces applied to the head into neural activity (Carey and Della Santina, 2005). These forces, which are either due to head motion or to gravity, cause the inner ear fluids to move and lead to the displacement of the hair cells.

Figure 19.4 shows the structure of a hair cell. Each cell consists of three functional components: the cilia or hairs, the cell body, and the afferent and efferent nerve endings. The cilia form a relatively rigid bundle on top of the cell body. One long thick hair, called the *kinocilium*, resides on one side, and approximately 70 shorter hairs, called *stereocilia*, reside next to it. The length of the stereocilia decreases with increasing distance from the kinocilium.

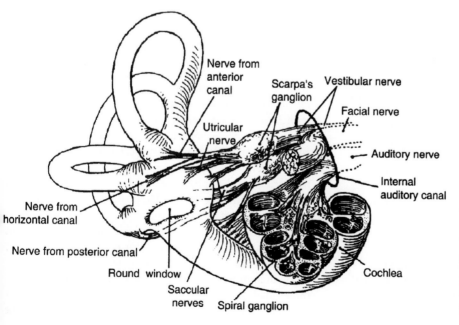

FIGURE 19.3 Vestibular receptors. (Reprinted from Baloh RW, Honrubia V. [2001] *Clinical Neurophysiology of the Vestibular System.* New York: Oxford University Press, with permission of Oxford University Press, Inc.)

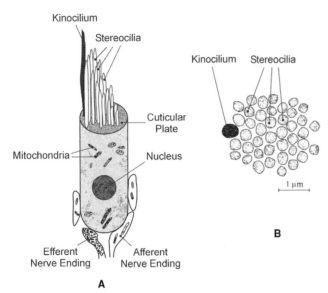

FIGURE 19.4   Structure of a hair cell. (A) Side view. (B) Top view. (Reprinted with permission from Canalis RF, Lambert PR, eds. [2000] *The Ear: Comprehensive Otology.* **Philadelphia: Lippincott Williams & Wilkins.)**

There are two types of hair cells (Fig. 19.5). The cell body in *type I* hair cells is shaped like a flask, which is wider in the midsection and narrower at the apex and the base. The cell body is almost completely encased by a large afferent nerve ending called *chalice* or *calyx*. The efferent nerve endings do not directly contact the cell body. Instead, they are attached to the calyx. The cell body in *type II* hair cells is shaped like

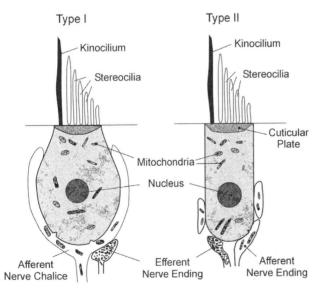

FIGURE 19.5   Type I and type II hair cells. (Reprinted with permission from Canalis RF, Lambert, PR, eds. [2000] *The Ear: Comprehensive Otology.* **Philadelphia: Lippincott Williams & Wilkins.)**

a cylinder. There are multiple afferent and efferent nerve endings, and both are attached directly to the cell body.

The ratio of type I to type II hair cells is different in different species. Even in the same species, this ratio varies from one receptor area to another. A detailed discussion of the differences in the morphology and distribution of type I and type II hair cells is beyond the scope of this chapter. However, the differences in the attachment of the afferent and efferent nerve endings seem to primarily affect the adaptation of the two cell types (Baloh and Honrubia, 2001).

Despite the differences between type I and type II hair cells, they are functionally very similar. In fact, they share two important features. First, they generate spontaneous neural activity in the absence of any stimulus (Fig. 19.6A). The rate of this tonic neural firing varies across animal species, but in mammals, the average rate is about 70 to 90 spikes per second (Goldberg and Fernandez, 1971). Second, the hair cells are directionally polarized. That is, when the stereocilia are bent toward the kinocilium, the neural firing rate of the afferent nerve fiber increases and an excitatory response is generated (Fig. 19.6B). Conversely, when the stereocilia are bent away from the kinocilium, the neural firing rate decreases and an inhibitory response is generated (Fig. 19.6C). The excitatory and inhibitory responses of the afferent nerve fibers are not symmetrical. The excitatory neural activities can increase from the tonic level to as high as 400 spikes per second. On the other hand, the maximum range of inhibitory responses is from the tonic firing rate down to the disappearance of neural activity.

The excitatory and inhibitory responses are generated only when the hair cells bend in their plane of polarization, that is, in a plane that passes through the kinocilium and divides the stereocilia in two approximately equal halves (Fig. 19.6). The neural firing rate does not change if the hair cells bend in a plane that is perpendicular to the plane of polarization or when they are subjected to forces that compress the stereocilia.

Structure of Semicircular Canals

Each labyrinth contains three semicircular canals that are arranged in three mutually perpendicular planes. They are *lateral* (or *horizontal*), *anterior* (or *superior*), and *posterior* semicircular canals. When the head is upright, the lateral canals reside in a plane that makes an upward angle of approximately 30 degrees with respect to the horizontal plane (Fig. 19.7A). The anterior canals reside in vertical planes that are turned approximately 45 degrees forward from the frontal plane (Fig. 19.7B). The posterior canals also reside in vertical planes but are turned approximately 45 degrees backward from the frontal plane. This unique arrangement of the semicircular canals allows for each canal in the right ear to be paired with a canal in the left ear, such that they reside in approximately parallel planes. The planes of these three canal pairs form a three-dimensional coordinate system. The canal pairs are: right and left lateral canals, right

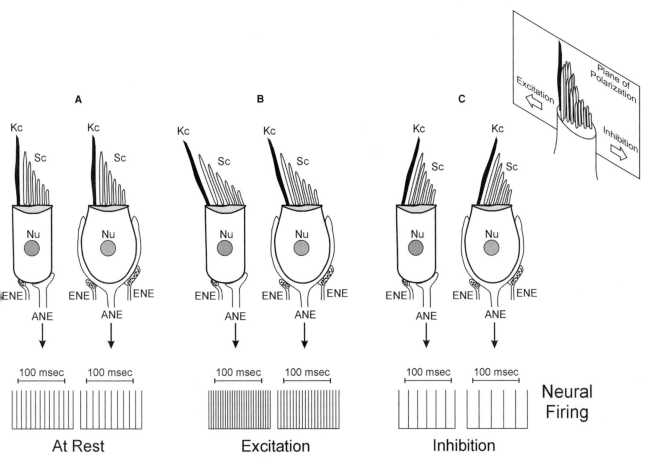

FIGURE 19.6   Firing rate of the primary afferent neurons as a function of the stereocilia displacement. (A) At rest. **(B)** Depolarization as a result of bending toward the kinocilium (excitatory response). **(C)** Hyperpolarization as a result of bending away from the kinocilium (inhibitory response). Kc, kinocilium; Sc, stereocilia; ANE, afferent nerve ending; ENE, efferent nerve ending; Nu, nucleus. (Reprinted with permission from Canalis RF, Lambert, PR, eds. [2000] *The Ear: Comprehensive Otology*. Philadelphia: Lippincott Williams & Wilkins.)

anterior and left posterior canals, and right posterior and left anterior canals.

Each semicircular canal consists of a partially circular duct attached to a shared cavity within the utricular sac of the vestibule. This forms a closed ring that is filled with endolymph. The semicircular canal duct enlarges near its opening at the vestibule to form the ampulla (Lysakowski, 2005). The crista ampullaris that covers the base of the ampulla is packed with approximately 7,000 hair cells (Fig. 19.8). The nerve endings that make synaptic contact with the hair cells merge to form the primary afferent nerve fiber of each semicircular canal. The cilia from the hair cells are embedded in the *cupula*, a gelatinous mass that rises from the base of the crista and completely seals the ampulla. The cupula functions as a plug that divides the semicircular canal into two compartments.

All of the hair cells in each crista have the same orientation. As a result, when the cupula bends, all of the hair cells undergo identical polarization and generate simultaneous excitation or inhibition. Although the orientation of the hair cells is identical within each semicircular canal, such is not the case for different canals. In the lateral canals, the hair cells are all oriented with their kinocilia pointing toward the utricular sac. Therefore, when the cupula bends toward the utricular sac (*ampullopetal*), it generates an excitatory response, and when the cupula bends away from the utricular sac (*ampullofugal*), it generates an inhibitory response. The orientation of the hair cells in the anterior and posterior semicircular canals is the opposite of the orientation of the hair cells in the lateral canal. Consequently, ampullopetal deflection of the cupula generates inhibitory responses, and ampullofugal deflection of the cupula generates excitatory responses, in the anterior and posterior canals.

The density of the cupula is identical to that of the surrounding endolymph (Baloh and Honrubia, 2001). When the semicircular canal is motionless, the cupula floats within the endolymph, and the embedded hair cells remain at their neutral position. At rest, the rate of neural firing in the afferent nerve fibers from each semicircular canal is equal to the sum of tonic neural activity of the individual hair cells.

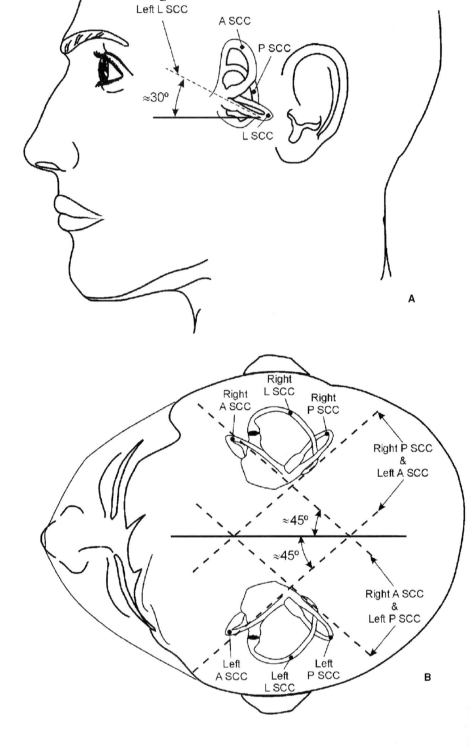

FIGURE 19.7 Orientation of the semicircular canals. **(A)** Side view. **(B)** Top view. A SCC, anterior semicircular canal; L SCC, lateral semicircular canal; P SCC, posterior semicircular canal. (Reprinted with permission from Canalis RF, Lambert, PR, eds. [2000] *The Ear: Comprehensive Otology.* Philadelphia: Lippincott Williams & Wilkins.)

Sudden head rotation in the plane of the canal generates relative motion of the endolymph with respect to the canal wall (Fig. 19.8). The viscosity of the endolymph causes the fluid to lag behind, thus creating a force across the cupula that is in the opposite direction of rotation. As a result, the cupula and stereocilia embedded in it deflect and, depending on the direction of rotation, generate either a sudden increase or decrease in the neural firing rate of the afferent neurons (Fernandez and Goldberg, 1971).

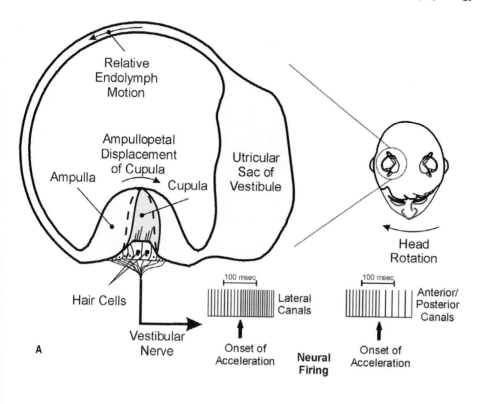

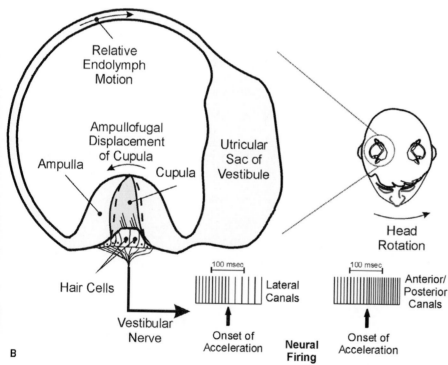

FIGURE 19.8 Structure and neural firing of semicircular canals in response to head rotations in the plane of the canal. (A) Ampullopetal displacement of cupula. **(B)** Ampullofugal displacement of cupula. *Solid arrows* indicate the onset of head rotation. **(Based on Canalis RF, Lambert PR, eds. [2000]** *The Ear: Comprehensive Otology.* **Philadelphia: Lippincott Williams & Wilkins.)**

The neural firing rate will eventually return to its tonic level if the rotation continues at a constant velocity for an extended period of time. In humans, during an approximately 20-second period of constant-velocity rotation, the difference between the endolymph and canal wall velocities will gradually decrease, and the force across the cupula will accordingly diminish. If the rotation suddenly ends, the endolymph flow and the cupula deflection will be in the opposite direction. The neural firing rate in this case is the same as if the canal was rotated in the opposite direction of the initial rotation.

Many of the physiologic functions of the semicircular canals can be explained by their structural properties. First, because the specific gravities of the cupula and endolymph are the same, semicircular canals, for the most part, are not responsive to gravity and other linear forces.

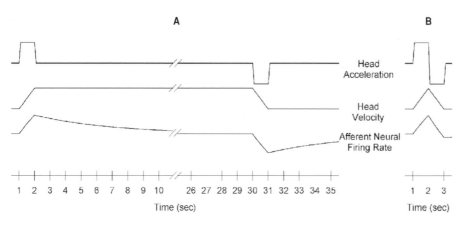

Head
Acceleration

Head
Velocity

Afferent Neural
Firing Rate

Time (sec)

FIGURE 19.9 Neural responses of a semicircular canal following head rotation. **(A)** Prolonged head rotation. **(B)** Brief head rotation. (Reprinted with permission from Canalis RF, Lambert, PR, eds. [2000] *The Ear: Comprehensive Otology.* Philadelphia: Lippincott Williams & Wilkins.)

Second, the canals respond to *changes* in the angular head velocity, in other words, the angular head acceleration. However, the afferent neural firing rate does not match the output of an ideal accelerometer (Barber and Stockwell, 1980). Figure 19.9A shows that the afferent neural firing rate is a damped version of the head acceleration because of the endolymph viscosity and the cupula mass. For natural head movements that are represented by brief and relatively fast movements, the afferent neural firing rate represents the head velocity (Fig. 19.9B). For these head movements, the head velocity information can be used directly by the VOR pathways to generate compensatory eye movements. This explains why the canals operate optimally for natural head movements and are not very sensitive to low-frequency head motion.

Finally, the afferent neural firing rate of the semicircular canals deviates from the output of an ideal accelerometer in one other way. As noted before, the excitatory response of a hair cell has a greater dynamic range than the inhibitory response. Therefore, the canal responses can saturate more

quickly when the head rotates in a direction that generates inhibitory responses than when the head rotates in a direction that generates excitatory responses (Fernandez and Goldberg, 1971). This is the basis of *Ewald's second law*, which states that the excitatory responses from the semicircular canals are stronger than the inhibitory responses. However, this asymmetry can be observed only for high-frequency, large-amplitude head movements that are not commonly encountered in our normal daily activities.

Structure of Otolith Organs

The utricle and saccule, also known as the otolith organs, are housed in two cavities within the vestibule. Both cavities are filled with endolymph, which allows the utricle and saccule to interact without a direct connection. Neither the utricle nor the saccule is entirely planar (Lindeman, 1969). The utricle is an oval-shaped structure with its average plane approximately parallel to the plane of the lateral semicircular canal (Fig. 19.10). The average plane of the saccule is

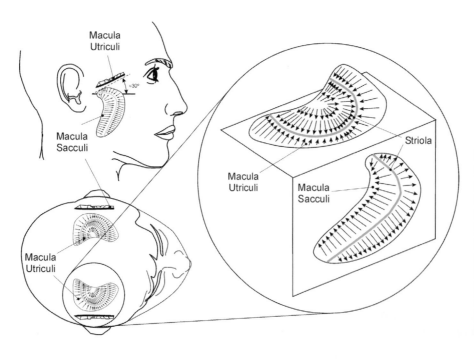

FIGURE 19.10 Orientation of the utricle and saccule. The direction for the excitatory responses of the hair cells is indicated by the *arrows*. (Reprinted with permission from Canalis RF, Lambert, PR, eds. [2000] *The Ear: Comprehensive Otology.* Philadelphia: Lippincott Williams & Wilkins.)

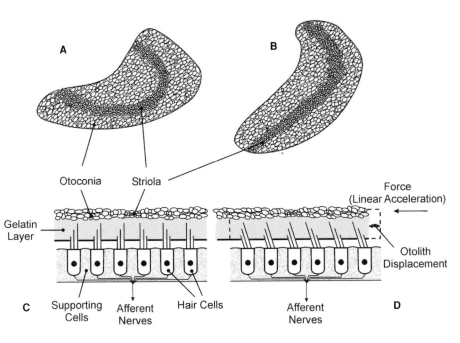

FIGURE 19.11 Structure and neural responses of the otolith organs. (A) Macula of utricle. (B) Macula of saccule. (C) Macula at rest. (D) Macula in response to linear acceleration of the head. (Reprinted with permission from Canalis RF, Lambert, PR, eds. [2000] *The Ear: Comprehensive Otology.* **Philadelphia: Lippincott Williams & Wilkins.)**

approximately perpendicular to the plane of the utricle and parallel to the sagittal plane.

The surfaces of both otolith organs are covered by a sensory neuroepithelium called the *macula* (Fig. 19.11). The macula is packed with hair cells, with their cilia embedded in the *otolithic membrane* (Lim, 1984). The function of the otolithic membrane is similar to that of the cupula in the crista. It contains a gelatinous layer topped by calcium carbonate crystals (*calcite*). These crystals are called *otoconia* or *otoliths*. The size of otoconia on the macula is not uniform. Both maculae of utricle and saccule have a narrow band in the middle, called the *striola*, where the otoconia are smaller. The striola divides the macula into regions, with each region having its own distinct hair cell arrangement. Unlike the crista, the hair cells in the macula are not all polarized in the same direction. In the utricle, the hair cells on both sides of the striola are arranged with their kinocilium facing the striola. In the saccule, the hair cell arrangement is reversed, with the kinocilium facing away from the striola.

The density of the macula is almost three times higher than that of the surrounding endolymph. Therefore, linear translation of the head generates forces that displace the otolithic membrane. Any arbitrary force applied to the head can be divided into two components, with one component parallel to and the other component perpendicular to the plane of the macula (Goldberg and Fernandez, 1976). The perpendicular component generates a compressive force across the otolithic membrane and does not change the firing rate of the embedded hair cells. The parallel component, however, generates a shear force, moves the otoconia and the underlying gelatinous layer, and causes deflection of the embedded cilia (Fig. 19.11D). Depending on

the direction of the shear force, some hair cells generate an increase in the afferent neural firing rate, some generate a decrease, and yet others remain at their tonic level. Since the utricle and saccule are approximately perpendicular, the component of a force that is compressive to the hair cells in one macula will act as a shear force to the hair cells in the other macula. Therefore, the direction and magnitude of a force applied to the head can be determined by summing its two components, which are decoded by the utricle and saccule.

It is reasonable to assume that the stimulus to the otolith organs is the linear acceleration of the head. However, the afferent neural responses from the otolith organs do not resemble the responses of a simple linear accelerometer. Instead, encoding of linear head acceleration into neural signals is a far more complex process that includes both the magnitude and pattern of hair cell excitation or inhibition. For example, identical head accelerations in the anterior-posterior and lateral directions produce distinct patterns of hair cell excitation and inhibition in the otolith organs. This explains how a mostly two-dimensional structure consisting of the utricle and saccule can detect linear movements of the head in three dimensions (Hain et al., 2000).

The most important function of the otolith organs on earth is detecting the direction of gravity. Like any other linear acceleration applied to the head, gravity affects the neural activity of the otolith organs. But unlike other types of accelerations, the direction and magnitude of gravity remain constant, which allows the vestibular receptors to detect the head orientation with respect to an absolute earth-fixed reference frame. As noted earlier, this feature of the vestibular system distinguishes it from other sensory mechanisms. In fact, the otolith organs can detect static head tilts in three dimensions by identifying the relative distribution of the gravity vector on utricle and saccule of each ear.

Blood Supply to Labyrinth

The membranous labyrinth receives its blood supply from the labyrinthine artery (Fig. 19.12). The labyrinthine artery originates either directly from the basilar artery or more commonly from the anterior inferior cerebellar artery (Lysakowski, 2005). The anterior vestibular artery is a branch of the labyrinthine artery that supplies blood to the ampullae of lateral and anterior canals, the utricle, and the superior portion of the saccule. The other branch of the labyrinthine artery is the common cochlear artery, which itself divides into the main cochlear artery and the vestibular-cochlear artery. The posterior vestibular artery is a branch of the vestibular-cochlear artery that supplies blood to the ampulla of the posterior canal as well as the inferior portion of the saccule.

The labyrinthine arteries lack collateral anastomotic connections with other major arteries. As a result, the peripheral vestibular structures are highly susceptible to ischemic events. A 15-second interruption of blood supply can impair the vestibular receptors, and after prolonged ischemia, the damage may become irreversible. Because the blood supply to the labyrinth is provided by multiple independent arterial branches, ischemic events can cause a focal lesion in one area of the labyrinth without affecting other areas.

Vestibular Nerve and Central Vestibular Pathways

The sensory information from the labyrinth is sent to the CNS via the vestibular portion of the eighth nerve. The vestibular nerve consists of bipolar neurons with their peripheral synapses on the hair cells and their central synapses on the *vestibular nuclei* (Brodal, 1974). The cell bodies of the neurons are located in *Scarpa's (vestibular) ganglion* (Fig. 19.3). Scarpa's ganglion is divided into a superior portion and an inferior portion. The latter is connected to the nerve fibers from the crista of the posterior canal and the macula of the saccule. The nerve fibers from the cristae of the lateral and anterior canals, the macula of the utricle, and a branch of the saccular nerve converge on the superior portion of Scarpa's ganglion. The vestibular nerve maintains two branches as it leaves the superior and inferior ganglia and merges with the auditory nerve to form the eighth (vestibulocochlear) cranial nerve.

The eighth nerve travels through the internal auditory canal and enters the brainstem lateral to the cerebellopontine angle. Most of the vestibular nerve fibers connect to the vestibular nuclei, but some branches innervate the cerebellum directly. The vestibular nuclei process information from the peripheral vestibular system and provide the initial integration of the sensory inputs before passing the signal on to the motor centers (Precht, 1979). The role of the cerebellum is to monitor the vestibular responses and initiate adaptive mechanisms when necessary (Robinson, 1976).

The vestibular nuclei are groups of neurons that reside in the pons and extend to the medulla. Two sets of nuclei are located in the brainstem, one on each side of the brain. Each set contains more than 10 separate neural structures. Four of them, the superior, medial, lateral, and descending nuclei, play an important role in processing the vestibular signal.

The vestibular nerve from each ear connects directly to the ipsilateral vestibular nuclei (Fig. 19.13). However, there is an indirect connection to the contralateral vestibular nuclei through the considerable number of interconnecting neurons between the right and left sides. The vestibular nuclei receive afferent input from other structures, including the cerebellum, the reticular formation, the spinal cord, and the cervical junction. The efferent nerve fibers from the vestibular nuclei project back to the same areas.

Figure 19.13 is a simplified representation of the VOR and VSR pathways. The signals from the vestibular nuclei are sent to the oculomotor nuclei either directly via the medial longitudinal fasciculus or indirectly through the reticular formation. The neural structures that innervate the eye muscles reside in three oculomotor nuclei: *the third (oculomotor) nucleus, the fourth (trochlear) nucleus, and the sixth (abducens) nucleus.* Each nucleus is composed of two sets of neural cell bodies, each residing on one side of the midbrain. Excitatory responses from one side are usually coupled with equal and precisely timed inhibitory responses from the other side, so that the resulting eye movements are conjugate.

The vestibular nuclei are not the only structures that send neural commands to the oculomotor nuclei. In fact, the oculomotor nuclei serve as the final common pathway for all types of eye movements, including saccadic, tracking, and optokinetic eye movements. Eye movements

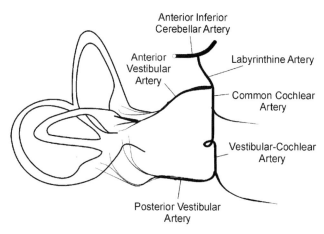

FIGURE 19.12 Arterial blood supply to the vestibular system. (Based on Cummings CW, et al., eds. [2005] *Otolaryngology—Head & Neck Surgery.* **Philadelphia: Elsevier Mosby.)**

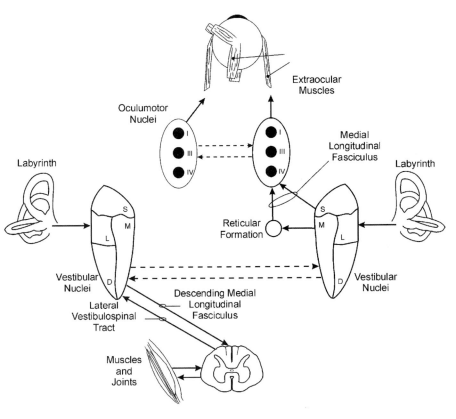

FIGURE 19.13 Central vestibular pathways. S, superior vestibular nucleus; M, medial vestibular nucleus; L, lateral vestibular nucleus; D, descending vestibular nucleus. (Based on Canalis RF, Lambert, PR, eds. [2000] *The Ear: Comprehensive Otology.* **Philadelphia: Lippincott Williams & Wilkins.)**

are controlled by six extraocular muscles. Each muscle is paired with another muscle such that the contraction of one muscle (*agonist*) occurs simultaneously with the relaxation of its muscle pair (*antagonist*). The muscle pairs move the eyes in three planes that coincide approximately with the planes of the semicircular canals (Table 19.1). This arrangement simplifies the task of generating compensatory eye movements by allowing one pair of the semicircular canals to drive one pair of eye muscles (Baloh and Honrubia, 2001).

Unlike the VOR, the VSR pathways must control the activities of many more muscles and joints. In fact, the VSR is not a single reflex. Rather, it is composed of a series of context-sensitive motor commands that are initiated based on the available sensory inputs and the required task (Brooks, 1986). The motor neurons in the spinal cord that control the activities of the skeletal muscles are connected to the vestibu-

lar nuclei via three primary pathways. The lateral and medial vestibulo-spinal tracts originate directly from the secondary vestibular neurons. The reticulospinal tract is connected to the vestibular nuclei indirectly through the reticular formation. For a more in depth discussion of VSR, see Chapter 20.

NORMAL VESTIBULAR RESPONSES

The structure of the individual vestibular receptors and their central connections were described in the previous section. In this section, the normal function of the peripheral and central vestibular pathways and their responses to different stimuli will be considered. The focus of this section is on the eye movement responses because most of the vestibular function tests are based on the assessment of the VOR pathways.

Semicircular Canal Responses to Head Rotation

Figure 19.7 shows that the hair cells in the cupulae of the two lateral semicircular canals are oriented in opposite directions. That means when the head is rotated in the plane of these canals, the hair cells in one canal will bend in one direction and generate excitatory responses, while the hair cells in the other canal will bend in the opposite direction and generate inhibitory responses. The hair cells in the other

TABLE 19.1	The extraocular muscle pairs and their plane of action when the eye is at center gaze
Muscle pair	**Plane of action**
Lateral rectus and medial rectus	Horizontal
Superior rectus and inferior rectus	Vertical 23° lateral
Superior oblique and inferior oblique	Vertical 51° medial

paired canals are oriented in a similar manner. In essence, any head motion that causes an increase in neural firing from one canal is always coupled with a decrease in neural firing from its paired canal in the other ear. This type of arrangement, called a *push-pull* arrangement, accomplishes a number of objectives that are important to the VOR function (Hain et al., 2000). First, the push-pull arrangement prevents the system from responding to changes in the afferent neural firing that are not generated by head motion. For example, changes in the body temperature or chemical composition of the inner ear fluids may affect the tonic activity of the afferent neurons. However, as long as these changes are identical in both labyrinths, they are not falsely interpreted as head movements. Second, the push-pull arrangement effectively neutralizes the asymmetry between the excitatory and inhibitory responses of the canal. As mentioned before, the inhibitory responses of the canals saturate at much lower head accelerations than the excitatory responses do. High-acceleration head motion to one direction that causes saturation of inhibitory responses from one side will produce a similar saturation of the response from the paired canal when the head is accelerated in the opposite direction. As a result, the difference between the neural firing rates from the two labyrinths will be the same regardless of the direction of head motion. Lastly, the push-pull arrangement increases the resolution and signal-to-noise ratio of the overall system by providing neural firing rates that are twice as large as those produced from a single canal.

Figure 19.14 demonstrates changes in the afferent neural firing rate of the labyrinths in response to both brief and sustained head rotations in the plane of the lateral canals. When the head is at rest, neural firings from the right and left ears are equal (Cohen, 1974). Acceleration of the head increases the neural firing from the leading ear (the left ear, in this example) and decreases it from the opposite side. For natural head movements, neural firing rates are proportional to the head velocity. If the excitatory and inhibitory neural firings are transmitted to the appropriate eye muscles, then the eyes will move in the opposite direction of the head motion, with a velocity that matches the head velocity. Once the head stops, the neural firing rates in both labyrinths return to their tonic level and the eyes also stop moving. That is essentially a simplified description of how the VOR operates.

For sustained head rotations, the asymmetry between the excitatory and inhibitory responses lasts much longer. Immediately after the onset of the head rotation, the eyes will slowly drift in the opposite direction of the head acceleration. When the eyes approach their orbital limit, they jump quickly in the opposite direction of the slow drift. This rhythmic to-and-fro pattern of eye movements, known as *nystagmus*, will continue as long as there is an asymmetry between the excitatory and inhibitory neural firings. However, the velocity of the slow component of the nystagmus, which defines the nystagmus intensity, gradually declines as the magnitude of the asymmetry between the right and left neural firing rates decreases.

Nystagmus that is provoked by head motion is known as vestibular nystagmus because its slow component is mediated by the VOR. Other processes, both physiologic and pathologic, can also generate the slow component of nystagmus. The fast component, however, is always generated by the saccadic system (Ron et al., 1972). Nystagmus has historically been identified by the direction of its fast phase. To avoid confusion when describing nystagmus, one must specifically state which component of nystagmus is being identified. This is usually done by adding the term *beat* or *beating* after the direction to signify the fast phase of nystagmus. For example, in Figure 19.14, nystagmus is left-beating because, when it is generated by head motion, nystagmus beats in the direction of head acceleration.

Vestibular nystagmus has a number of unique characteristics (Baloh and Honrubia, 2001). First, vestibular nystagmus is strongly suppressed by visual fixation because the neural pathways from the tracking system project to the vestibular nuclei and prevent the VOR from generating the slow phase of vestibular nystagmus. Second, the slow phase of vestibular nystagmus is usually linear. That is, the slow-phase eye velocity is approximately constant during each beat of nystagmus. Third, the intensity of vestibular nystagmus is increased when gaze is directed toward the fast phase of nystagmus. This is known as *Alexander's law* (Robinson et al., 1984). Finally, mental alertness affects the presence and perhaps the intensity of vestibular nystagmus (Davis and Mann, 1987). The slow phase of vestibular nystagmus does not appear to be affected by alertness, since it can be provoked even in comatose individuals. However, the eyes remain deviated to one side once they reach the orbital limit (Kasper et al., 1992). Therefore, alertness seems to affect the fast phase of nystagmus, which requires higher cortical level intervention.

Vestibular nystagmus that is generated by head motion reveals an important property of the VOR pathways. As noted earlier, the afferent neural firing from the semicircular canals eventually returns to its tonic level once the cupula returns to the neutral position after a prolonged constant-velocity head rotation. Typically, this occurs 15 to 20 seconds after the onset of the rotation. However, the nystagmus lasts about three times longer (Fig. 19.15A). The increase in the duration of nystagmus is because the neural activity from the peripheral vestibular system is not directly fed to the oculomotor system. Instead, central vestibular pathways act as a *velocity storage mechanism* that essentially slows the flow of neural activity from the peripheral vestibular system (Raphan et al., 1979). Mathematically, this is equivalent to a leaky neural integrator that extends the low-frequency response of the VOR. Figure 19.15B shows the frequency response of the slow-phase eye velocity versus head velocity both with and without the velocity storage mechanism. When the VOR generates perfectly compensatory eye movements, the amplitudes of slow-phase eye velocity and head velocity are equal but in the opposite directions. For these eye movements, the gain (ratio of slow-phase eye velocity to head velocity) is equal to 1, and the phase (time difference of slow-phase eye velocity to head

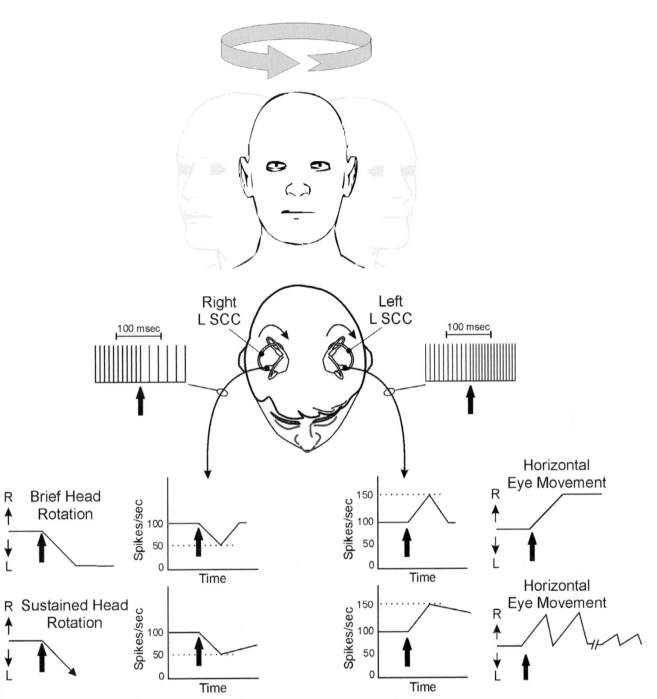

FIGURE 19.14 Changes in the neural firing and the resulting eye movements following brief and sustained head rotations in the plane of the lateral canals. *Solid arrows* indicate the onset of head rotation. L SCC, lateral semicircular canal; R, right; L, left. (Based on Canalis RF, Lambert, PR, eds. [2000] *The Ear: Comprehensive Otology.* Philadelphia: Lippincott Williams & Wilkins.)

velocity) is equal to 180 degrees. In Figure 19.15B, the phase is shown after a 180-degree correction so that, for compensatory eye movements, the phase is equal to zero. Without the velocity storage mechanism, compensatory eye movements are limited to approximately 0.15 to 10 Hz. The addition of the velocity storage mechanism extends the low-frequency response to 0.05 Hz without significantly affecting the high-frequency response. As we will see later, the velocity storage mechanism is sensitive to various lesions of the VOR pathways.

So far, the discussion of eye movement responses to head rotation has been limited to the stimulation of lateral semicircular canals. Head movements in the planes of the other two canal pairs also generate compensatory eye movements (Raphan and Cohen, 2002). For example, the right anterior canal and the left posterior canal can be stimulated by

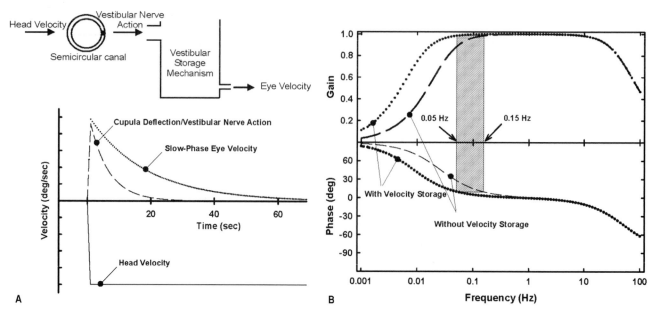

FIGURE 19.15 Velocity storage mechanism. **(A)** Changes in the vestibular neural activity and slow-phase eye velocity in response to a sudden change in the head velocity. **(B)** Frequency responses (gain and phase) of the slow-phase eye velocity versus head velocity both with and without the velocity storage mechanism. (Based on Canalis RF, Lambert, PR, eds. [2000] *The Ear: Comprehensive Otology.* Philadelphia: Lippincott Williams & Wilkins.)

turning the head 45 degrees to the left and moving the head up or down in the sagittal plane (Fig. 19.16A). In this case, downward head motion increases the neural activity from the right anterior canal and decreases it from the left posterior canal. Consequently, the eyes slowly drift upward and, in the case of sustained rotation, downbeat nystagmus is generated. In addition to the vertical component, the nystagmus also has a torsional component (rotation of the eye about the visual axis) with the fast phases of torsion directed toward the stimulated ear (toward the right ear or counterclockwise in this case). The torsional component of the nystagmus seems to be necessary because the plane of head rotation and eye movements do not coincide as they do in the case of lateral canal stimulations. This notion is supported by the fact that the torsional component of the nystagmus is decreased when gaze is directed parallel to the plane of the canal pairs and is increased when gaze is directed perpendicular to the canal pairs (Epley, 2001). Figure 19.16B shows the head motion and the resulting eye movements when the head rotates in the plane of the left anterior and right posterior canals.

Semicircular Canal Responses to Temperature Gradients

Although head movements are the natural way of stimulating the vestibular receptors, nonphysiologic stimuli are more common in the clinical evaluation of the vestibular function. In the caloric test, which is considered the most important part of the electronystagmography (ENG) test battery,

temperature changes are used to induce endolymph flow and generate vestibular stimulation (Hart, 1984). Unlike head movements that always stimulate both labyrinths simultaneously, caloric stimuli can be used to provoke responses from each labyrinth independently.

In caloric testing, the patient is placed in the supine position with the head or upper body raised about 30 degrees (Fig. 19.17A). In this position, both lateral semicircular canals reside in the vertical plane and are affected by gravity. However, the cupulae of the lateral canals usually remain in their neutral positions because their densities are equal to the surrounding endolymph. In the caloric test, the external auditory canal in one ear is irrigated by a medium (water or air) that has a significantly different temperature compared to the body temperature (O'Neill, 1987). As a result, the density of the fluid in the area of the canal that is closest to the site of irrigation changes, and the endolymph moves within the canal due to the effect of gravity. For example, warm irrigations in the standard caloric position cause the endolymph to become lighter and rise. In the lateral canals, this generates an ampullopetal flow and leads to an excitatory response from the afferent neurons of the irrigated ear. Since the neural activity from the nonirrigated ear remains at its tonic level, an asymmetry between the neural firings from the two lateral canals develops as if the head was being accelerated horizontally toward the irrigated ear. Consequently, the VOR generates vestibular nystagmus to counteract the perceived head rotation with its fast phase beating toward the irrigated ear. This nystagmus has the exact same characteristics as those described in the previous section.

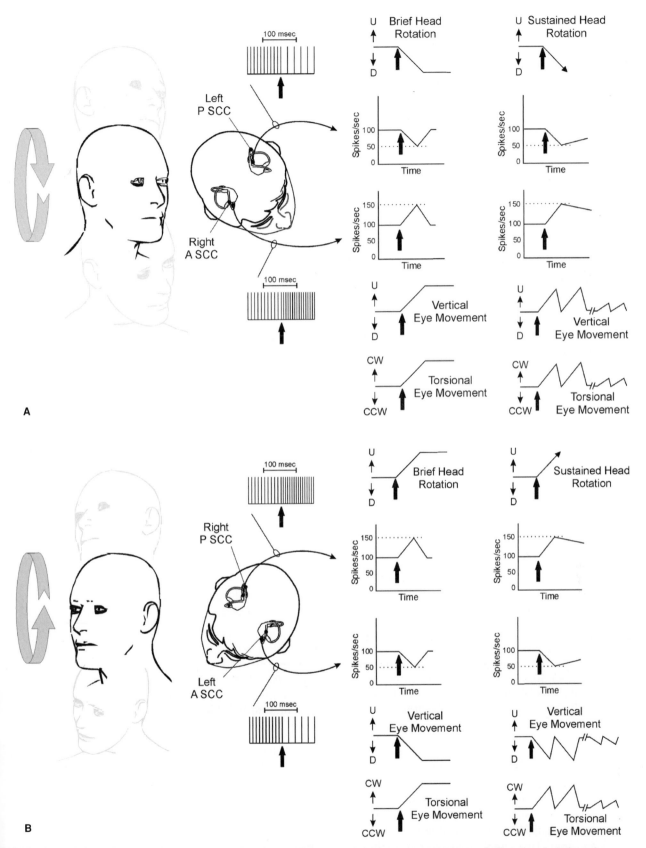

FIGURE 19.16   Changes in the neural firing and the resulting eye movements following brief and sustained head rotations in the vertical plane. (A) Head rotation in the plane of right anterior and left posterior canals. **(B)** Head rotation in the plane of left anterior and right posterior canals. *Solid arrows* indicate the onset of head rotation. A SCC, anterior semicircular canal; L SCC, lateral semicircular canal; P SCC, posterior semicircular canal; U, up; D, down; CW, clockwise; CCW, counter-clockwise.

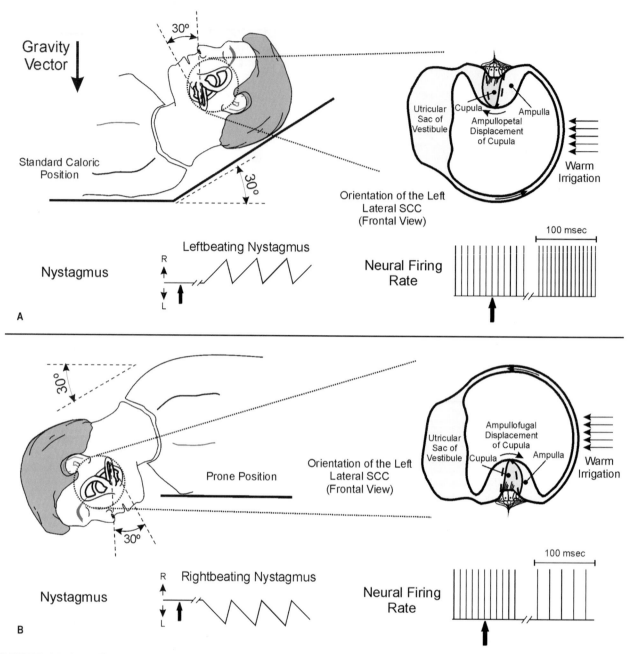

FIGURE 19.17 Changes in the neural firing and the resulting eye movements during caloric stimulation. (A) Supine with the head tilted up 30 degrees. **(B)** Prone with the head tilted down 30 degrees. *Solid arrows* indicate the onset of irrigation. SCC, semicircular canal. (Based on Canalis RF, Lambert, PR, eds. [2000] *The Ear: Comprehensive Otology.* Philadelphia: Lippincott Williams & Wilkins.)

Cold irrigations in the standard caloric test position cause the endolymph to become heavier and sink. This generates an inhibitory response from the irrigated ear and results in an asymmetry as if the head was accelerating away from the irrigated ear. An acronym, COWS (cold opposite, warm same), is used to quickly identify the direction of caloric-induced nystagmus. For example, cold irrigation of the right ear or warm irrigation of the left ear generates left-beating nystagmus exactly as if the head was being accelerated toward the left ear.

The mechanism for the caloric nystagmus was initially proposed by Barany over a century ago (Hood, 1989). Based on this theory, caloric responses are dependent on the presence of gravity. However, experiments aboard the space shuttle initially cast doubts on this theory when caloric responses were observed in the absence of gravity. It is now believed that gravity is still the main mechanism for generating caloric responses. However, warm and cool temperatures can also directly affect the vestibular nerve and generate changes in the neural firing rate. This effect accounts for a small component of the caloric response (about 10%) and apparently was the reason for the observed nystagmus in the absence of gravity. There is compelling evidence in support of this explanation. Figure 19.17B shows the orientation of the lateral canal when the patient is placed in a prone position with the head tilted down about 30 degrees. Warm irrigations in this head position generate ampullofugal endolymph flow and cause inhibitory responses from the irrigated ear (Lee, 1969). Based on the earlier explanation, the direction of nystagmus should change if the patient is moved from the supine to prone position during the caloric stimulation. Furthermore, the nystagmus intensity in the prone position is expected to be slightly lower than the nystagmus intensity in the supine position because, in the prone position, the component of the caloric response generated by direct vestibular nerve stimulation is subtracted from the component of caloric response generated by gravity. In the supine position, these two components of the caloric response are added, making the overall response slightly stronger. Experimental data exactly match these predictions and lend strong support to the theory of how caloric responses are generated (Coates and Smith, 1967). Caloric testing in the prone position has a clinical application, where ice-water calorics are performed in the supine and prone positions to determine if there is a residual response from an ear that is not responsive to the standard caloric stimulation.

Caloric responses originate primarily from the stimulation of the lateral semicircular canals. Theoretically, it is possible to generate caloric responses from the anterior and posterior semicircular canals (Fetter et al., 1998). In practice, however, the anatomic organization of the semicircular canals prevents the temperature gradient from reaching the vertical canals because they are too distant from the external auditory canal. As a result, caloric responses are dominated by the lateral canal stimulation. Nonetheless, in many individuals, caloric irrigations induce vertical and torsional eye movements, indicating partial stimulation of the anterior and posterior canals (Aw et al., 1998).

Responses to Otolith Stimulation

Methods for both stimulation of the otolith organs and measurement of the responses are far more complicated than those of the semicircular canals. As noted earlier, the otolith organs respond to dynamic changes in linear velocity and static changes in the head orientation. It is reasonable to assume that the synergetic relationship between the right-left semicircular canals also exists between the right-left otolith organs. Because of the complex pattern of hair cell activation in the otolith organs, however, the push-pull arrangement might be confined to distinct areas of the macula on each side, instead of involving the entire saccule or utricle.

As expected, stimulation of the otolith organs produces compensatory eye movements to keep images steady on the retina (Paige, 2002). The mechanism that mediates this function is called the *linear vestibulo-ocular reflex (LVOR)*. The characteristics of the otolith-driven compensatory eye movements depend on the type of stimulation.

Electrical stimulation of the nerve fibers from the utricle or saccule, as well as direct stimulation of the macular regions, produces steady eye deviations (Curthoys, 1987). The direction and the plane of these deviations are related to the area of hair cell activation on the macula. Nystagmus has also been reported, but it was not possible to rule out inadvertent stimulation of the nerve fibers from the semicircular canals (Niven et al., 1966).

When head tilts are used to produce otolith stimulation, the resulting eye movements can be torsional or oblique (include both horizontal and vertical components). Lateral head tilts in humans generate torsional eye movements called *ocular counter-rolling* (Markham and Diamond, 2003). The direction of these eye movements is in the opposite direction of head tilts, but the amplitude is typically much smaller (Paige, 1991). Head tilts in the pitch plane produce vertical eye movements, but one cannot rule out the role of the anterior and posterior canals in generating these eye movements.

Linear head accelerations have been used to generate otolith stimulation, but there are a number of controversies regarding the eye movement responses. First, purely based on the principles of physics, one would assume the effect of linear head accelerations to be the same as the effect of gravity during static head tilts. This assumption is not supported by experimental data (Paige, 2002). The otolith organs appear to differentiate between gravity and other linear accelerations by designating low-frequency stimuli as static head tilts and high-frequency stimuli as dynamic head movements. This is logical because the role of the vestibular system is to complement the visual system. That can be best achieved when gravity is treated differently than other linear accelerations that induce head motion (Merfeld et al., 1999). Second, the role of semicircular canals and other visual systems (such as the tracking mechanism) cannot be overlooked in contributing to the eye movements generated during linear head accelerations. Finally, eye movements during linear head movements are highly dependent on the distance of the target being viewed (Paige, 1991). For these reasons, as well as the complexity of the instrumentation, the use of linear head accelerations has not become widespread in clinical testing of the otolith organs.

A few recent developments appear to be promising for clinical testing of otolith function. First, eccentric rotation (rotation about an axis that is parallel to the vertical axis of the head) appears to produce robust otolith stimulation (Furman and Baloh, 1992). When the patient is seated with the head bent forward about 30 degrees from the upright position, the centripetal and tangential forces generated during eccentric rotation provide the linear acceleration needed to stimulate the utricles. Furthermore, different areas of the utricle can be stimulated by changing the orientation of the subject with respect to the rotation axis (e.g., facing toward or away from the rotation axis and all other angles in between). The saccules can also be tested by changing the head orientation to place them in the plane of the centripetal and tangential forces (Paige, 2002).

The second development in this area is related to the assessment of the otolith responses. Otolith-mediated eye movements are usually three dimensional, covering horizontal, vertical, and torsional directions. The measurement of these eye movements, especially the torsional ones, poses technical challenges. An indirect method of assessing the otolith responses, the *subjective visual vertical (SVV)* test, provides a much simpler alternative to the direct measurement of torsional eye movements (Clarke et al., 2001). The patient is seated upright in a completely darkened room and then asked to align a dimly-lit light bar in the vertical (or horizontal) plane. Normal individuals in the absence of otolith stimulation can set the bar within 2 degrees of the true vertical. In the presence of otolith stimulation, such as stimulations produced by eccentric rotation, or in the case of otolith lesions, the subjects tend to align the bar off-vertical, according to their perceived level of head tilt (Clement et al., 2002). This method is currently being standardized for clinical testing.

Another emerging method for clinical testing of otolith function is *vestibular-evoked myogenic potentials (VEMP)*. Loud monaural acoustic clicks or tone bursts evoke short-latency electromyogram (EMG) responses from the neck (i.e., sternocleidomastoid) muscles (Welgampola and Colebatch, 2005). These responses originate from the labyrinth, most likely the saccule. The ipsilateral responses are much larger than contralateral ones. Currently, the sound intensity for which the VEMPs are initiated and the latency of the muscle responses are used to evaluate the saccule and the inferior vestibular nerve (Zhou and Cox, 2004).

EFFECTS OF LESIONS ON VESTIBULAR PATHWAYS

Diseases of the vestibular receptors and their neural pathways are among the most common causes of dizziness and other balance disorders (Furman and Cass, 1996). This section describes how different vestibular lesions affect VOR and VSR function. Manifestations of these lesions on vestibular function tests during various stages of vestibular compensation are also discussed.

Effects of Unilateral Peripheral Vestibular Lesions

Some peripheral vestibular lesions reduce or obliterate the tonic activity of the vestibular nerve from one labyrinth. These lesions either damage the hair cells or disrupt the vestibular nerve function. Figure 19.18 shows the eye movements after an *acute* lesion in each of the vestibular receptors as well as a lesion of the vestibular nerve (Curthoys and Halmagyi, 2000). A unilateral decrease in the tonic neural activity results in an asymmetry identical to that produced by actual head movements. The patient perceives the head

rotating toward the intact ear in the plane of the damaged canal. This illusion of motion, called *vertigo*, is the hallmark of vestibular lesions. The conflict between the sensory information from the vestibular receptors and information from other sensory modalities causes the patient to experience nausea, vomiting, and other vegetative symptoms.

Figure 19.18A shows the effect of a sudden lesion in the right lateral canal. The asymmetry in the right-left neural firing is similar to that produced by head movements in Figure 19.14. That is, the patient perceives that the head is being accelerated toward the left ear in the plane of the lateral canals. The resulting nystagmus is horizontal with the fast phase beating away from the side of the lesion.

The effect of a sudden lesion in the right anterior canal is shown in Figure 19.18B (Halmagyi et al., 1992). The patient perceives that the head is being accelerated upward in the plane of right anterior–left posterior canals. The resulting compensatory eye movements have both a vertical component beating upward and a torsional component with the fast phase directed away from the damaged ear (in this case, clockwise). The vertical component of the nystagmus is more prominent in the ipsilateral eye, and the torsional component is more prominent in the contralateral eye.

Figure 19.18C shows the effect of a sudden lesion in the right posterior canal. The patient perceives that the head is being accelerated downward in the plane of right posterior–left anterior canals. This nystagmus also has vertical and torsional components, with the torsional component beating in the same direction and the vertical component beating in the opposite direction of that in Figure 19.18B.

Sudden loss of the utricle or saccule is perceived by the patient as a static head tilt toward the intact side (Curthoys et al., 1991). In animals, loss of otolith function causes postural abnormalities, including actual head tilt toward the damaged ear to counteract the perceived head tilt. In humans, actual head tilts are rare, but loss of otolith function is manifested by a static torsion of the eyes toward the damaged side (Fig. 19.18D).

The effect of a sudden loss of the entire labyrinth or the vestibular nerve is shown in Figure 19.18E. The resulting eye movements are a combination of all of the eye movements generated by the loss of each receptor. They consist of horizontal and torsional nystagmus, both beating away from the side of lesion. However, the nystagmus does not have a vertical component because the vertical components generated by the loss of tonic neural activities from the anterior and posterior canals are in opposite directions and cancel out. Consistent with the observed eye movements, these patients often describe a sensation of rotation that is predominantly in the horizontal plane.

Vestibular Compensation after Unilateral Peripheral Vestibular Lesions

As discussed earlier, natural vestibular stimuli, such as head movements, generate neural activity that usually lasts a short

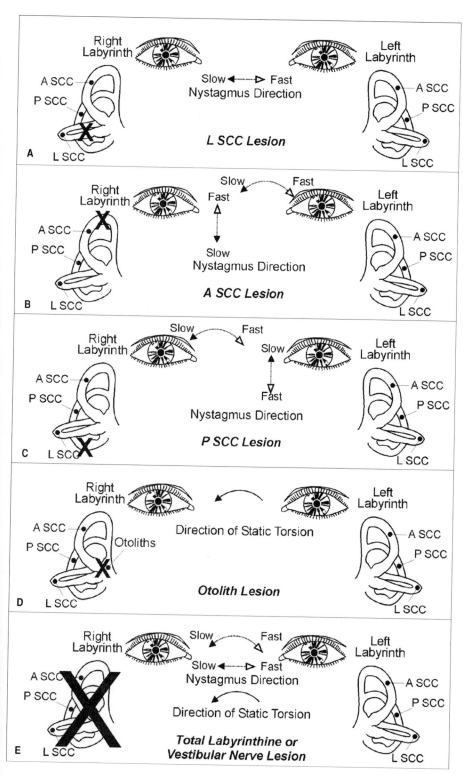

FIGURE 19.18
Nystagmus and other eye movements after an acute lesion in each of the vestibular receptors. **(A)** Lateral canal lesion. **(B)** Anterior canal lesion. **(C)** Posterior canal lesions. **(D)** Otolith lesions. **(E)** Total labyrinthine or vestibular nerve lesion. A SCC, anterior semicircular canal; L SCC, lateral semicircular canal; P SCC, posterior semicircular canal.

period of time. Prolonged vestibular stimulation activates adaptive control mechanisms that are responsible for making adjustments to the vestibular pathways to improve their performance (Zee, 2000). In the case of excessive vestibular stimulation, the adaptive mechanisms will attempt to reduce the sensitivity of the VOR. For example, nystagmus intensity declines after repeated exposure to head rotations or

after applying caloric irrigations for an extended period of time. These adaptive mechanisms are part of a more global compensation system that is responsible for recovery after vestibular damage.

The effects of a unilateral peripheral vestibular lesion described in the previous section can be seen only during the acute phase of the lesion. Persistent asymmetry in the firing rate of the vestibular neurons signals a possible malfunction and activates the vestibular compensation mechanisms (Curthoys, 2000). In the case of a unilateral vestibular loss, vestibular compensation consists of two distinct processes. The first part is *static compensation*, in which the static balance between the tonic neural activity is restored and the neural asymmetry is eliminated or at least substantially reduced. The second part is *dynamic compensation*, in which the properties of vestibular pathways are modified to account for the fact that one labyrinth no longer produces adequate neural activity in response to head motion.

Figure 19.19 shows the steps that lead to static compensation after a unilateral peripheral vestibular lesion. It should be noted that this is a functional representation of a complex process and may not exactly match the physiologic events. For example, the compensation mechanism is shown for horizontal eye movements only, but the process is also applicable to nystagmus in other planes (Curthoys and Halmagyi, 2000). Figure 19.19A shows the neural activity and the resulting compensatory eye movements immediately after the head is rotated in the horizontal plane toward the left ear (counterclockwise). For simplicity, neural firing rates are shown for one afferent nerve fiber, with the tonic level set arbitrarily at 100 spikes per second. Furthermore, the change in the neural firing rate for the given head acceleration is set (hypothetically) at 50 spikes per second. Since both labyrinths are intact in Figure 19.19A, a total neural asymmetry of 100 spikes per second (50 spikes per second from excitatory responses and 50 spikes per second from inhibitory responses) is generated for the given head motion. The slow phase of the resulting nystagmus is in the opposite direction of head motion, and its velocity approximately matches the head velocity.

Figure 19.19B shows the neural asymmetry and the resulting nystagmus immediately following a total unilateral vestibular loss. Since the asymmetry is the same as in Figure 19.19A, the nystagmus direction and intensity are also the same as those in Figure 19.19A. This pathologic nystagmus, commonly referred to as *spontaneous nystagmus*, is a form of vestibular nystagmus and will be discussed in more detail later in this chapter. Vestibular function tests at this stage are likely to show a significant unilateral caloric weakness in the damaged ear and strong spontaneous nystagmus in the absence of fixation. Residual nystagmus is likely to be present with fixation too, and it should follow Alexander's law.

Persistent asymmetry in the neural activity triggers vestibular compensation mechanisms. The first step in the compensation process is the reduction of neural asymmetry by *clamping* the neural activity of the intact labyrinth (Fig. 19.19C). This step begins within hours after the onset of the lesion, and its effect is similar to that of antivertigo medications that suppress the vestibular neural activity at the brainstem level. Vestibular function tests at this stage are likely to show a significant unilateral caloric weakness and spontaneous nystagmus in the absence of fixation. Residual nystagmus may still be present with fixation. The reduction

in the neural asymmetry results in the reduction of the nystagmus intensity as well as the patient's symptoms. Instead of a unilateral weakness, caloric testing may show a bilateral weakness if the clamping effect is strong enough. If so, rotation testing is likely to reveal that the loss of bilateral function (gain reduction) is limited to low frequencies.

Within a few days after the onset of the clamping stage, neural activity appears in the vestibular nuclei at the site innervated by the vestibular nerve from the damaged side (Fig. 19.19D). This neural activity does not come from the labyrinth. It originates from the vestibular-compensation centers that are most likely located within the cerebellum. At the same time, the clamping effect is reduced, and the tonic neural activity in the vestibular nuclei of the intact side is increased. This leads to continued improvement of the patient's symptoms and further decrease of the spontaneous nystagmus intensity. Vestibular function tests at this stage continue to show a significant unilateral caloric weakness and spontaneous nystagmus in the absence of fixation, but nystagmus with fixation is likely to diminish.

After a few weeks, the neural activity is restored at the vestibular nuclei of the damaged side, and the clamping of the tonic neural firing from the intact site is completely removed (Fig. 19.19E). Restoration of symmetry to the tonic neural activity abolishes the pathologic nystagmus and indicates the completion of static compensation. Vestibular function tests continue to show a significant unilateral caloric weakness after static compensation, but spontaneous nystagmus will be either minimal or absent altogether.

Several features of static compensation are noteworthy because it represents a significant milestone in the process of recovery after a peripheral vestibular lesion. First, animal studies show that static compensation can be delayed or eliminated if the animal is immobilized and vision deprived (Zee, 2000). However, in the absence of other confounding abnormalities, humans can achieve static compensation spontaneously by maintaining their normal daily activity level. Second, static compensation takes place regardless of whether the unilateral lesion is sudden or gradual. In the case of a gradual loss, such as in a patient with a vestibular schwannoma, the compensation process takes place gradually and in small increments (Jenkins, 1985). As a result, the patient may have a significant loss of unilateral vestibular function and not experience the kind of severe vertigo and other symptoms that are associated with a sudden loss of peripheral vestibular function. Third, the push-pull arrangement of the labyrinths that neutralizes the inherent asymmetry between the excitatory and inhibitory responses from one semicircular canal is no longer possible after a unilateral loss of peripheral vestibular function. Therefore, nystagmus intensity caused by head rotation toward the side of lesion is expected to be significantly lower than that caused by head rotation toward the intact side (Baloh and Honrubia, 2001). The latter generates inhibitory responses, while the former generates excitatory responses from the remaining labyrinth. In practice, this type of asymmetry is typically observed

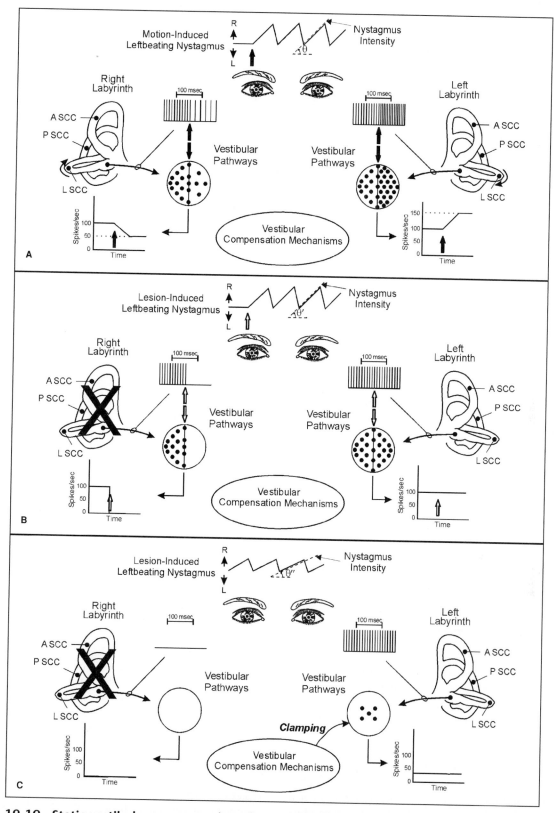

FIGURE 19.19   Static vestibular compensation after a unilateral vestibular lesion. See the text for the description of compensation steps. *Solid arrows* identify the onset of the head acceleration. *Hollow arrows* identify the onset of the lesion. θ, θ', and θ'' represent slow-phase nystagmus intensities. The density of dots represents the level of neural firing. A SCC, anterior semicircular canal; L SCC, lateral semicircular canal; P SCC, posterior semicircular canal. (Based on Canalis RF, Lambert, PR, eds. [2000] *The Ear: Comprehensive Otology.* Philadelphia: Lippincott Williams & Wilkins.)

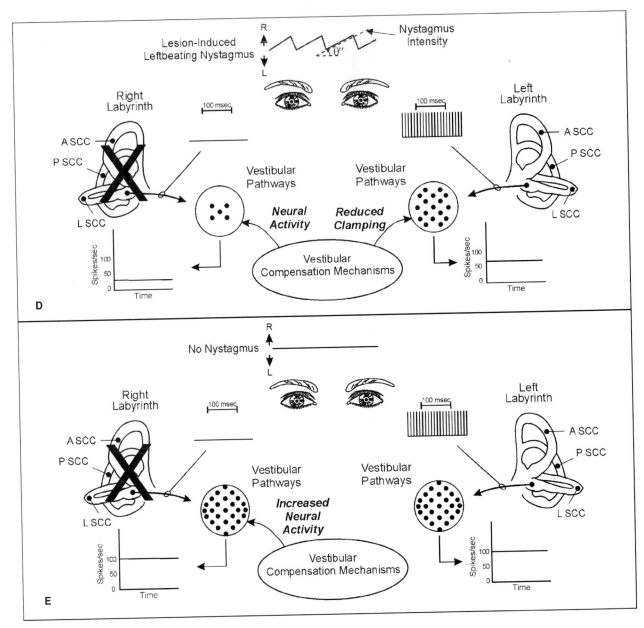

FIGURE 19.19 (*Continued*)

during the early stages of compensation in which there is strong clamping of the neural activity. In these stages, the inhibitory responses from the intact labyrinth saturate quickly during head rotations toward the side of lesion, but the excitatory responses during head rotations toward the intact side can increase significantly more. After the completion of static compensation, the response asymmetry can only be seen for high-acceleration head movements. The phenomenon of asymmetric eye movement responses after a unilateral vestibular loss is used in a bedside test of vestibular function called *head thrust* (Halmagyi et al., 2001). The examiner moves the patient's head briskly to one side while the patient is fixating on a target. In patients with a severe loss of vestibular function, the eye velocity does not match the head velocity when the head is accelerated toward the side of

lesion. As a result, the examiner looks for evidence that the eyes are falling behind, and the patient must use *corrective saccades* to refocus on the target. Finally, static compensation is most effective for stable lesions. Fluctuations in the tonic neural activity of the affected labyrinth, as in the case of a patient with Ménière's disease, disrupt the compensation process and may prolong the symptoms. If function is restored to the diseased labyrinth during the compensation stages in which the neural activity of the intact labyrinth is clamped, the asymmetry between the right-left neural activities will suddenly be reversed (Fig. 19.20). Consequently, the nystagmus direction will also be reversed with the fast phase now beating *toward* the diseased labyrinth (Jacobson et al., 1998). This type of nystagmus, called *recovery nystagmus*, is sometimes seen in patients with Ménière's disease

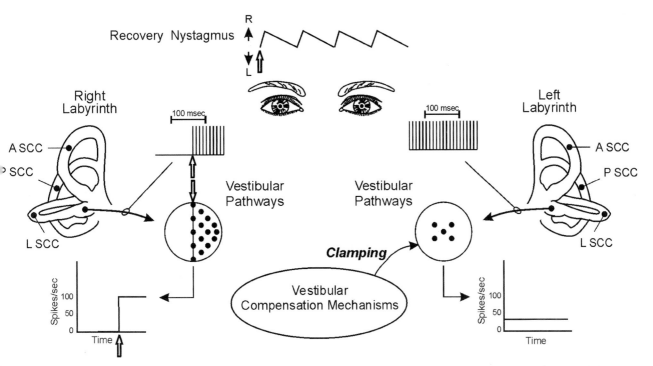

FIGURE 19.20 Recovery nystagmus. *Hollow arrows* identify the onset of restoration of neural activity after the lesion. Abbreviations and other symbols are defined in Figure 19.19.

(McClure et al., 1981). The reversal of asymmetry triggers a secondary compensation process and, in effect, prolongs the symptoms. As a result, frequent fluctuations may lead to deactivation of the compensation mechanisms. This forms the basis for one of the more common treatment methods for Ménière's disease, which involves making the vestibular lesion permanent. In the past, this was done surgically by removing the labyrinth or cutting the vestibular nerve (Hillman et al., 2004). Currently, a more effective method is injecting a vestibulotoxic agent, such as gentamicin, into the middle ear space.

Static compensation is effective in reducing the symptoms only as long as the head remains stationary. Figure 19.21 shows the neural activity and the resulting eye movements in response to the same head rotation as in Figure 19.19A. The magnitude of neural asymmetry in this case is only half of that generated by two functioning labyrinths for the same head rotation (Fig. 19.21A). Since the intensity of compensatory eye movements is also half of what it should be, the images will not remain stationary on the retina, and the patient will not have clear vision during head movements. To achieve dynamic compensation, the VOR pathways must be reprogrammed to generate eye movements that fully compensate for head movements as they did before the lesion (Zee, 2000). It would seem that changing the gain of the pathway and doubling the neural activity from the vestibular nerve would accomplish this task in the above example (Fig. 19.21B). However, such a change will also affect the frequency response of the VOR. For example, one way of increasing

VOR gain is by increasing the flow rate of the velocity storage mechanism in Figure 19.15. Although this action increases the gain, it also reduces the storage capacity of the velocity storage mechanism. If the storage capacity of the velocity storage mechanism is gradually reduced, the low-frequency performance of the VOR will be degraded (Hain and Zee, 1992). This prediction has been confirmed by rotation tests that show a decrease in the gain and an increase in the phase of VOR for low-frequency head movements in patients following a unilateral peripheral vestibular lesion (Fig. 19.15B) (Stockwell and Bojrab, 1997). The process of dynamic compensation is perhaps more complex than a simple change in the VOR gain. Most likely, the vestibular signals have to be remapped to ensure proper integration of the orientation information from all sensory inputs.

Currently, ENG testing is not capable of measuring the level of dynamic compensation because the test results before and after dynamic compensation are the same. Other vestibular tests, such as dynamic visual acuity test or posturography, attempt to quantify the level of dynamic compensation (Herdman et al., 1998; Nashner, 2001). However, these methods are functional and indirect ways of assessing this process.

Understanding the physiology of dynamic compensation helps with identifying methods that can promote and expedite the process. For example, head-eye coordination exercises in the plane of different semicircular canals are ideal for this purpose. Head movements can start at low frequencies and gradually increase to cover the entire frequency range

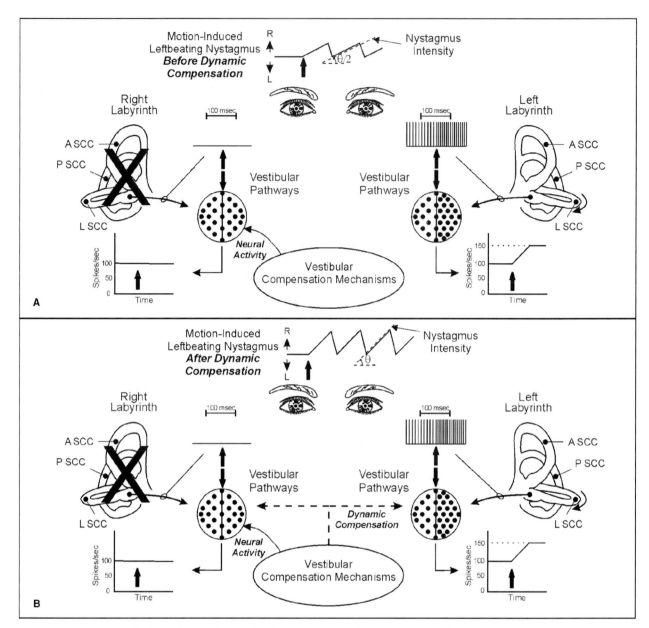

FIGURE 19.21 **(A)** Before dynamic vestibular compensation. **(B)** After dynamic vestibular compensation. See the text for the description of compensation steps. Abbreviations and other symbols are defined in Figure 19.19. (Based on Canalis RF, Lambert, PR, eds. [2000] *The Ear: Comprehensive Otology.* Philadelphia: Lippincott Williams & Wilkins.)

of the VOR. The difficulty of the task can be varied by asking the patient to start the exercises while sitting and progress to walking (Shepard and Telian, 1996).

Effects of Central Vestibular Lesions

The vestibular nuclei receive information from the peripheral vestibular system via the primary vestibular neurons and transmit the information to the motor centers via the secondary vestibular neurons. There are at least two ways that the function of the central vestibular pathways may become disrupted. First, tonic neural activity of the secondary

vestibular neurons can be reduced or abolished, just as they are in the primary vestibular neurons (Fig. 19.22). In the case of a unilateral central vestibular lesion, the neural asymmetry and the resulting nystagmus are virtually identical and indistinguishable from those generated as a result of a peripheral lesion (Baloh and Honrubia, 2001). Vestibular function tests for this type of lesion are likely to show spontaneous nystagmus but no caloric weakness.

A second type of central vestibular lesion spares the tonic neural activity but affects the gain of the secondary vestibular neurons. This type of lesion was first described by Halmagyi et al. (2000), who identified 1% of their patients

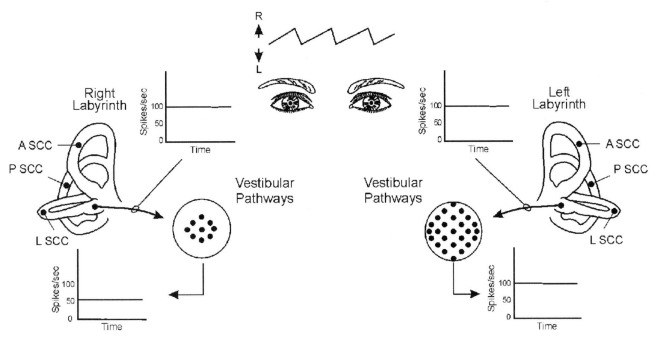

FIGURE 19.22 Nystagmus generated by static asymmetry of the secondary vestibular neurons within the vestibular nuclei. Abbreviations and other symbols are defined in Figure 19.19.

with an uncommon type of directional preponderance in the caloric test. Significant directional preponderance indicates that the intensity of caloric-induced nystagmus to one direction (right-beating or left-beating) is much larger than the nystagmus intensity to the opposite direction. Typically, directional preponderance signifies the presence of spontaneous nystagmus, which causes the caloric responses to be stronger for irrigations where spontaneous and caloric nystagmus directions coincide. In this case, however, significant directional preponderance was present without any spontaneous nystagmus or unilateral caloric weakness. Halmagyi et al. (2000, p 559) postulated that "an isolated directional preponderance reflects a gain asymmetry between neurons in the medial vestibular nucleus on either side." This is an extremely rare condition and must be interpreted cautiously.

There are other lesions that can affect the central vestibular pathways. For example, *periodic alternating nystagmus* is most likely caused by cyclical modulation of tonic neural activities of the secondary vestibular neurons (Furman et al., 1990). This unusual type of nystagmus is manifested as a nystagmus that, in a *single head position*, changes direction every few minutes. More detailed discussion of central vestibular lesions is beyond the scope of this chapter, but additional information on this topic can be found in Baloh and Honrubia (2001) and Leigh and Zee (1991).

Pathologic Vestibular Nystagmus

Spontaneous nystagmus refers to nystagmus that is present in the absence of visual and vestibular stimuli. It indicates an imbalance in the VOR pathways, which includes peripheral vestibular, central vestibular, and higher level oculomotor

structures in the CNS (Baloh and Honrubia, 2001). Is it possible to localize the source of imbalance within the VOR? To answer this question, it is necessary to examine the characteristics of the nystagmus that originates from each of the above structures. The focus of this discussion is on *horizontal* spontaneous nystagmus. Although spontaneous nystagmus with vertical and torsional components is possible, the clinical significance of those findings is not as clear at this time.

First, it should be noted that spontaneous nystagmus does not always signify pathology. Mild spontaneous nystagmus is present in some healthy asymptomatic individuals, indicating that some level of asymmetry is tolerable (Levo et al., 2004). Similarly, many patients, after compensation following a unilateral vestibular lesion, continue to have residual nystagmus, even though they are no longer symptomatic. As a result, it is generally accepted that the intensity of spontaneous nystagmus must exceed 6 degrees per second before it is considered pathologic (Isaacson and Rubin, 2001).

Peripheral vestibular lesions cause nystagmus that subsides over time due to the compensation process. In the acute phase, the nystagmus typically beats away from the side of the lesion. However, the direction of the nystagmus is not always a reliable indicator of the side of lesion because, in some cases, the nystagmus can beat in the opposite direction (e.g., recovery nystagmus). The characteristics of nystagmus following a peripheral vestibular lesion are identical to those of the vestibular nystagmus generated by head rotation. That is, the nystagmus has linear slow phases, follows Alexander's law, and, most importantly, is suppressed by visual fixation. In contrast, visual fixation does not suppress nystagmus generated by nonvestibular pathways in the CNS.

Nystagmus originating from the central vestibular pathways is more difficult to differentiate from nystagmus originating from the peripheral vestibular pathways. The characteristics of nystagmus due to a static imbalance within the central vestibular pathways appear to be the same as those of nystagmus originating from the peripheral vestibular pathways (Baloh and Honrubia, 2001). As a result, spontaneous nystagmus that is suppressed by fixation is considered to be a nonlocalizing vestibular nystagmus originating from either peripheral or central pathways.

Spontaneous nystagmus is manifested in the static position test as nystagmus that remains intensity- and direction-fixed in different head positions. *Positional nystagmus*, on the other hand, can change intensity or direction in *different* head positions (Barber and Stockwell, 1980). For example, nystagmus that beats in one direction in sitting and supine positions may beat right when the head is positioned with the right ear down and beat left when the head is positioned with the left ear down. This is referred to as *geotropic* nystagmus because the nystagmus beats toward earth in both head positions. *Ageotropic* or *apogeotropic* nystagmus refers to nystagmus that is left-beating with the right ear down and right-beating with the left ear down.

It would be tempting to assume that peripheral vestibular lesions could not generate direction-changing positional nystagmus. However, that is not the case. An example of a peripheral vestibular process that can generate direction-changing nystagmus in different head positions is *positional alcohol nystagmus (PAN)* (Oosterveld, 1973). Typically, the endolymph and cupula have the same specific gravity. Therefore, when the head is turned right or left in the supine position, the cupulae remain floating in the canals and do not deflect in response to gravity (Fig. 19.23A). When a person ingests a sufficient amount of alcohol, the alcohol reaches the cupula before it reaches the endolymph. Since the specific gravity of alcohol is less than that of the endolymph, the cupulae become lighter than the surrounding endolymph. Now when the head is turned right or left, the cupulae deflect upward in both head positions (Fig. 19.23B). This causes excitation of the undermost ear and inhibition of the uppermost ear in both head positions and generates geotropic nystagmus. Conversely, alcohol leaves the cupulae before it

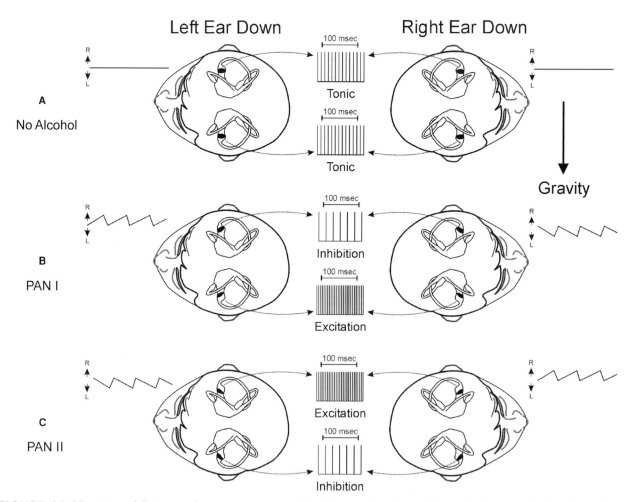

FIGURE 19.23 Neural firing and eye movements in different head positions before and after ingesting alcohol. (A) Before ingesting alcohol. **(B)** Two hours after ingesting alcohol (positional alcohol nystagmus [PAN] I). **(C)** Twelve hours after ingesting alcohol (PAN II).

leaves the endolymph, causing downward deflection of the cupulae in head right and head left positions (Fig. 19.23C). This causes excitation of the uppermost ear and inhibition of the undermost ear in both head positions and generates ageotropic nystagmus. The geotropic part of the nystagmus, called *PAN I*, begins approximately 2 hours after ingesting alcohol and lasts about 4 hours. The nystagmus disappears once alcohol diffuses into both the cupula and endolymph. The ageotropic part of the nystagmus, called *PAN II*, begins approximately 12 hours after ingesting alcohol and lasts up to 48 hours. The opposite of this phenomenon occurs when patients ingest a substance that has a higher specific gravity than the endolymph, such as "heavy water" or glycerol (Brandt, 1990).

Based on the above example, it is possible for certain metabolic disorders to change the chemical composition and specific gravity of the cupula or endolymph and cause direction-changing nystagmus in head right and left positions. There is another possibility. The afferent neural pathways from the semicircular canals merge with the neural pathways from the utricle and saccule to form the vestibular nerve. Although the semicircular canals themselves are not sensitive to gravity, their neural output can be modulated by the head position through the shared neural pathways with the otolith organs.

In summary, the intensity of horizontal nystagmus without fixation must be greater than 6 degrees per second to be considered abnormal. When abnormal, positional nystagmus and all of its variations (including spontaneous, geotropic, and ageotropic nystagmus) are considered nonlocalizing findings that can originate from either peripheral or central vestibular pathways.

Effects of Bilateral Peripheral Vestibular Lesions

Total loss of bilateral vestibular function impairs both the VOR and VSR (Sargent et al., 1997). The loss of VSR function causes varying degrees of disequilibrium that is aggravated in the absence of vision. The loss of VOR function causes oscillopsia and other visual disturbances during head motion. These symptoms have long-term consequences that are far more serious than those experienced after a unilateral loss of vestibular function. Ironically, after a bilateral lesion, patients do not experience vertigo, nausea, vomiting, and other debilitating symptoms that are common immediately after a unilateral vestibular lesion. Those symptoms are caused by an asymmetry in the vestibular pathways, which does not occur in bilateral lesions.

Bilateral vestibular lesions are relatively infrequent compared to unilateral ones. The most common cause of bilateral peripheral lesions is vestibulotoxicity. However, central lesions that block the transmission of neural activity from both labyrinths can also cause bilateral vestibular loss (Baloh and Honrubia, 2001). In many cases, bilateral loss of function is partial. For example, in the case of vestibulotoxicity, the loss of function is initially confined to low-frequency head movements (Furman and Kamerer, 1989). High-frequency responses are usually preserved unless vestibulotoxicity continues and the loss becomes complete.

Recovery after a bilateral loss of vestibular function is limited. In the case of complete lesions, there is no vestibular-mediated system to facilitate compensation. Instead, inputs from other receptors, such as visual and neck receptors, have to be substituted for the vestibular system. The contribution of these receptors to postural and gaze stability increases substantially in patients with bilateral lesions. However, the compensation process is not as effective because the operational frequency range for the visual and neck receptors is different from the frequency range of the vestibular receptors (Brown et al., 2001).

A bilateral vestibular lesion is manifested in the vestibular function tests as a bilateral caloric weakness. The caloric test, however, cannot differentiate between complete and partial vestibular lesions. Some form of rotation testing is required for that purpose. Caloric testing yields bilaterally reduced responses for both types of lesions because caloric irrigations are considered to be very low-frequency vestibular stimuli ($\sim$0.003 Hz). Rotation tests can also distinguish true bilateral vestibular lesions from poor caloric irrigations (Furman and Kamerer, 1989).

Pathophysiology of Benign Paroxysmal Positional Vertigo

Benign paroxysmal positional vertigo (BPPV) is one of the most common vestibular disorders (Furman and Cass, 1999). It is characterized by a severe but brief bout of dizziness and perhaps nausea when the head is moved to a critical position. Diagnosis of BPPV is based on the *Dix-Hallpike maneuver* (Solomon, 2000). In this maneuver, the patient sits on an exam table with the head turned about 45 degrees toward one ear. The examiner moves the patient rapidly from a sitting to supine position, with the head hanging slightly over the edge. Healthy individuals with no BPPV may have a beat or two of nystagmus immediately after the movement, but patients with BPPV have a characteristic nystagmus accompanied by vertigo and possible nausea. The nystagmus and the symptoms typically appear after a few seconds of delay and dissipate in about a minute. The nystagmus has both torsional and vertical components. In 90% of the cases, the torsional component beats toward the undermost ear, and the vertical component beats upward. After the response subsides, the examiner returns the patient to the sitting position and repeats the maneuver with the head turned toward the opposite ear. Some patients generate a milder response when they are returned to the sitting position, but the nystagmus directions are opposite of those generated when moving the patient from a sitting to a supine position. BPPV-type responses are fatigable. That is, if the maneuver is repeated for the affected side, the response declines in intensity and may not be present at all.

An underlying mechanism of BPPV was first offered by Schuknecht (1969). He proposed that particles, most likely otoconia from the otolith organs, adhered to the cupula of the posterior semicircular canal and made it sensitive to gravity. This type of BPPV, called *cupulolithiasis*, does exist but is rare. It is now generally accepted that a far more common type of BPPV is caused by the free-floating particles, called canaliths, within the semicircular canal (Hall et al., 1979). This type is called *canalithiasis*. Although BPPV of posterior canal origin accounts for 90% of the cases, we now know that BPPV can originate from other canals as well (Epley, 2001).

Figure 19.24 shows the orientation of the right posterior canal during different phases of a right Dix-Hallpike maneuver. When the head is turned toward the right ear, the right posterior and left anterior canals are placed in the plane of motion. Thus, the Dix-Hallpike maneuver in a normal individual generates a momentary response from these canal pairs. In patients with canalithiasis of the posterior canal, the particles gather at the lowest point of the canal in the

upright head position. At the completion of head motion, gravity causes the canaliths to sink because they are heavier than the surrounding endolymph. It should be noted that canaliths are not separate marble-shaped particles as shown here (Parnes and McClure, 1992). Instead, the particles form a sticky cluster resembling a floating "blob" in a lava lamp. As a result, it takes a few seconds before the particles gather enough momentum and begin to sink. This explains why BPPV responses have a delayed onset. Movement of the canaliths causes an ampullofugal flow of the endolymph, which generates excitatory responses from the posterior canal. The direction of nystagmus in the most common form of BPPV indicates excitation of the posterior canal (see Fig. 19.16). Once the maneuver is complete, the canaliths gather again in the lowest point of the canal, and the endolymph flow ceases. This explains why BPPV responses are transient. When the patient is returned to the sitting position, the particles move in the opposite direction and cause eye movements consistent with inhibitory responses from the posterior canal.

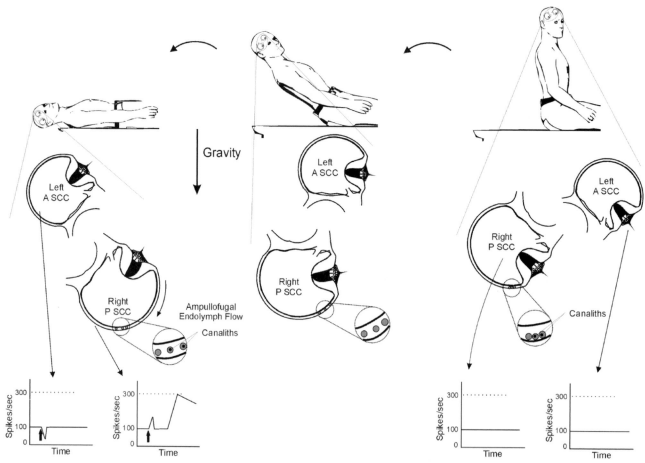

FIGURE 19.24 **Changes in the neural firing during different phases of a right Dix-Hallpike maneuver in a patient with benign paroxysmal positional vertigo involving canalithiasis of the right posterior canal.** *Solid arrows* indicate the onset of the maneuver. The initial change in the neural firing is due to the head movement, and the subsequent change is due to the movement of the canaliths. A SCC, anterior semicircular canal; P SCC, posterior semicircular canal. **(Based on Honrubia V, Baloh RW, Harris MR, Jacobson KM. [1999] Paroxysmal positional vertigo syndrome.** *Am J Otol.* **20, 465–470.)**

Fatigability of the response in BPPV is usually attributed to the central compensation mechanisms. However, there may be another explanation. Because of their composition, canaliths may disperse along the canal and not be able to generate adequate momentum if the procedure is repeated immediately. This view is supported by the observation that, if the maneuver is repeated after waiting several minutes, the response is as strong as the initial one. Perhaps fatigability is due to both separation of the particles and central compensation mechanisms.

Figure 19.24 also suggests a treatment method for posterior canal BPPV. If the head continues to rotate in the plane of the posterior canal for a total of 360 degrees, the canaliths will eventually move out of the canal and into the vestibule, where they can no longer generate BPPV symptoms. Although this exact procedure has been attempted, a more common approach is to move the head 180 degrees in a way that inverts the canal with respect to gravity (Furman et al., 1998; Li and Epley, 2006). The

particles can then fall out of the canal by the gravitational force. This is the basis of the *canalith repositioning therapy*, which is the most common treatment approach to BPPV (Epley, 2001).

BPPV of anterior canal origin is more controversial. The incidence of this entity was very high in initial reports (Herdman et al., 1994), but subsequent studies show anterior canal BPPV constitutes only 2% of the total BPPV cases (Honrubia et al., 1999; Korres et al., 2002). Figure 19.25 shows the orientation of the left anterior canal during a right Dix-Hallpike maneuver. The anatomic orientation of the anterior canal prevents the canaliths from gathering at the lowest point of the canal as they do in the case of posterior canal BPPV. The only likely place for the canaliths is above the anterior canal cupula. Therefore, the Dix-Hallpike maneuver will cause the particles to crash against the cupula and generate inhibitory responses. This is the opposite of what is expected for anterior canal BPPV and cannot be distinguished from posterior canal BPPV. The head movement has to be strong

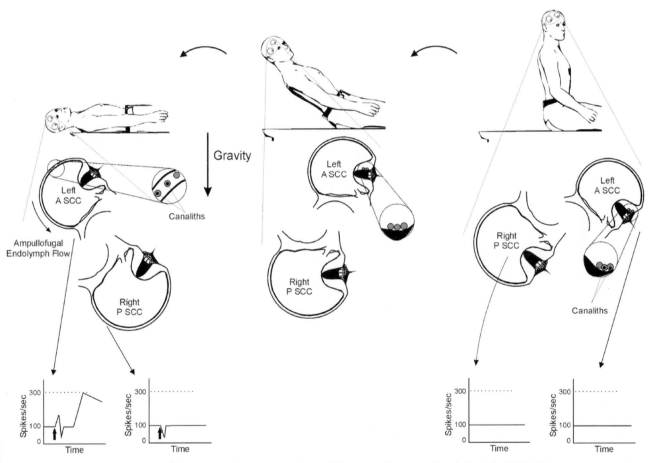

FIGURE 19.25 Changes in the neural firing during different phases of a right Dix-Hallpike maneuver in a patient with benign paroxysmal positional vertigo involving canalithiasis of the left anterior canal. *Solid arrows* indicate the onset of the maneuver. The initial change in the neural firing is due to the head movement, and the subsequent change is due to the movement of the canaliths. A SCC, anterior semicircular canal; P SCC, posterior semicircular canal. (Based on Honrubia V, Baloh RW, Harris MR, Jacobson KM. [1999] Paroxysmal positional vertigo syndrome. *Am J Otol.* 20, 465–470.)

enough to push the canaliths back into the canal and generate excitatory responses as expected. Even if one accepts this explanation for the mechanism of anterior canal BPPV, there is still another issue. As is obvious in Figure 19.25, simply moving the patient back to the sitting position will push the canaliths out of the anterior canal and resolve the condition. This may explain why the incidence of anterior canal BPPV is so low. Some investigators propose that a right Dix-Hallpike maneuver can produce responses from the *right* anterior canal. This is unlikely because the right anterior canal is perpendicular to the plane of rotation. However, since the canals are not perfectly orthogonal, it is possible that a small response from the right anterior canal can be produced by a right Dix-Hallpike maneuver. In that case, a left Dix-Hallpike maneuver is expected to produce a much stronger response because the right anterior canal is in the plane of head rotation.

So far, only cases of canalithiasis have been discussed, mainly because there is no definitive way of distinguishing them from anterior or posterior canal cupulolithiasis. The only differences seem to be much shorter delay in onset and longer duration of nystagmus for cupulolithiasis. Treatment methods are also the same, except that the particles adher-

ing to the cupula first have to be dislodged, for example by using a bone oscillator, before proceeding with the therapy (Li, 1995).

BPPV can also originate from the lateral semicircular canals (McClure, 1985). The diagnosis is made by the *roll maneuver* (Epley, 2001). Figure 19.26 shows the mechanism of a right lateral canal BPPV. In the roll maneuver, the lateral canals are first placed in the vertical plane by moving the patient to the supine position with the head bent forward by 30 degrees. Now the head is turned briskly toward the right ear. Patients with lateral canal BPPV will generate strong horizontal nystagmus that beats toward the undermost ear. When the maneuver is repeated toward the opposite ear, again horizontal nystagmus is generated that beats toward the undermost ear, but the response is not as intense as when the head is turned toward the affected ear. Figure 19.26A shows why this happens. Head rotation toward the canal with BPPV causes the canaliths to move and generates an ampullopetal endolymph flow in the affected ear. This causes excitation of the undermost canal and generates horizontal nystagmus beating toward that ear. When the head is turned away from the affected side, canalith movements result in ampullofugal endolymph flow. This causes inhibition

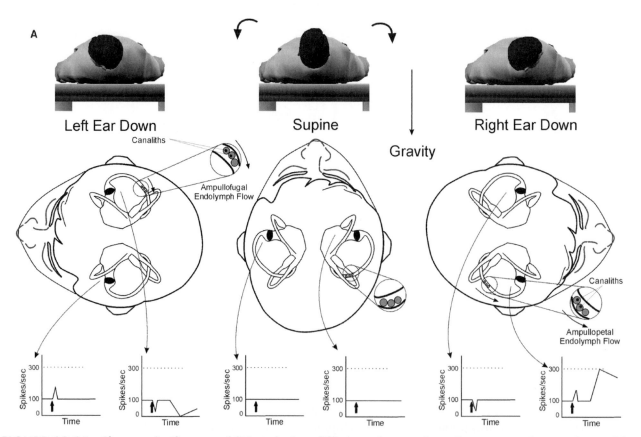

FIGURE 19.26   Changes in the neural firing during different phases of a roll maneuver in a patient with benign paroxysmal positional vertigo involving the right lateral canal. (A) Canalithiasis. **(B)** Cupulolithiasis. *Solid arrows* indicate the onset of the maneuver. The initial change in the neural firing is due to the head movement, and the subsequent change is due to the movement of the canaliths.

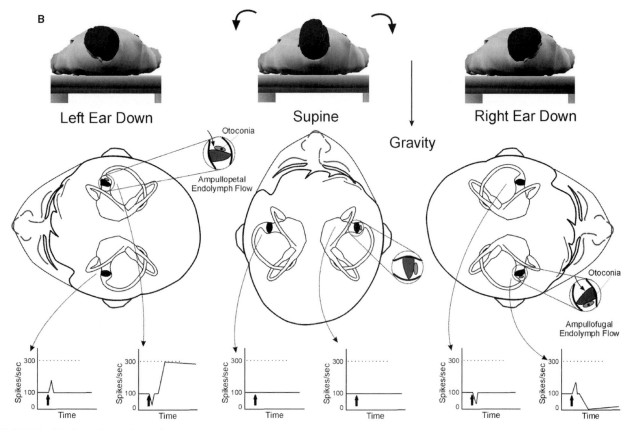

FIGURE 19.26   *(Continued)*

of the affected ear. Because of the asymmetry between the excitatory and inhibitory responses, the nystagmus intensity when the head is turned toward the affected ear is stronger than the nystagmus intensity when the head is turned away. In the case of lateral canal cupulolithiasis (Fig. 19.26B), the roll maneuver causes ageotropic nystagmus with the stronger response generated for head rotation toward the intact ear (Honrubia et al., 1999).

In the case of lateral canal canalithiasis, the treatment involves rotating the patient 360 degrees in the plane of the lateral canals in order to move the particles out of the canal (Epley, 2001). The same is true for lateral canal cupulolithiasis except that, again, the particles should be dislodged from the cupula before proceeding with the therapy.

SUMMARY

The vestibular receptors provide the CNS with sensory information about the orientation and movement of the head in space. This information is critical for postural control and gaze stabilization. Abnormalities within the vestibular system and its pathways are common in patients who suffer from dizziness and other balance problems. A comprehensive knowledge of the neurophysiology of the vestibular pathways is essential for identifying and differentiating different types of abnormalities. It is also important to recognize that the vestibular pathways possess a high degree of plasticity, which changes the clinical manifestation of vestibular abnormalities.

REFERENCES

Allum JH, Honegger F, Schicks H. (1993) Vestibular and proprioceptive modulation of postural synergies in normal subjects. *J Vestib Res.* 3, 59–85.

Allum JH, Shepard NT. (1999) An overview of the clinical use of dynamic posturography in the differential diagnosis of balance disorders. *J Vestib Res.* 9, 223–252.

Aw ST, Haslwanter T, Fetter M, Heimberger J, Todd MJ. (1998) Contribution of the vertical semicircular canals to the caloric nystagmus. *Acta Otolaryngol.* 118, 618–627.

Baloh RW, Honrubia V. (2001) *Clinical Neurophysiology of the Vestibular System.* New York: Oxford University Press.

Barber HO, Stockwell CW. (1980) *Manual of Electronystagmography.* St. Louis: CV Mosby.

Barin K, Durrant JD. (2000) Applied physiology of the vestibular system. In: Canalis RF, Lambert PR, eds. *The Ear: Comprehensive Otology.* Philadelphia: Lippincott Williams & Wilkins, pp 113–140.

Brandt T. (1990) Positional and positioning vertigo and nystagmus. *J Neurol Sci.* 95, 3–28.

Brandt T. (1996) Bilateral vestibulopathy revisited. *Eur J Med Res.* 1, 361–368.

Brodal A. (1974) Anatomy of the vestibular nuclei and their connections. In: Kornhuber HH, ed. *Handbook of Sensory Physiology: The Vestibular System.* Berlin: Springer-Verlag, pp 239-352.

Brooks VB. (1986) *The Neural Basis of Motor Control.* New York: Oxford University Press.

Brown KE, Whitney SL, Wrisley DM, Furman JM. (2001) Physical therapy outcomes for persons with bilateral vestibular loss. *Laryngoscope.* 111, 1812–1817.

Carey JP, Della Santina C. (2005) Principles of applied vestibular physiology. In: Cummings CW et al., eds. *Otolaryngology—Head & Neck Surgery.* Philadelphia: Elsevier Mosby; pp 3115–3159.

Chambers BR, Gresty MA. (1983) The relationship between disordered pursuit and vestibulo-ocular reflex suppression. *J Neurol Neurosurg Psychiatr.* 46, 61–66.

Clarke AH, Schonfeld U, Hamann C, Scherer H. (2001) Measuring unilateral otolith function via the otolith-ocular response and the subjective visual vertical. *Acta Otolaryngol Suppl.* 545, 84–87.

Clement G, Maciel F, Deguine O. (2002) Perception of tilt and ocular torsion of normal human subjects during eccentric rotation. *Otol Neurotol.* 23, 958–966.

Coats AC, Smith SY. (1967) Body position and the intensity of caloric nystagmus. *Acta Otolaryngol.* 63, 515–532.

Cohen B (1974). The vestibulo-ocular reflex arc. In: Kornhuber HH, ed. *Handbook of Sensory Physiology: The Vestibular System.* Berlin: Springer-Verlag; pp 477–540.

Cohen B, Henn V. (1972) The origin of quick phases of nystagmus in the horizontal plane. *Bibl Ophthalmol.* 82, 36–55.

Curthoys IS. (1987) Eye movements produced by utricular and saccular stimulation. *Aviat Space Environ Med.* 58, A192–A197.

Curthoys IS. (2000) Vestibular compensation and substitution. *Curr Opin Neurol.* 13, 27–30.

Curthoys IS, Dai MJ, Halmagyi GM. (1991) Human ocular torsional position before and after unilateral vestibular neurectomy. *Exp Brain Res.* 85, 218–225.

Curthoys IS, Halmagyi GM. (2000) Clinical changes in vestibular function with time after unilateral vestibular loss. In: Herdman SJ, ed. *Vestibular Rehabilitation.* Philadelphia: FA Davis Co.; pp 172–194.

Davis RI, Mann RC. (1987) The effects of alerting tasks on caloric induced vestibular nystagmus. *Ear Hear.* 8, 58–60.

Epley JM. (2001) Human experience with canalith repositioning maneuvers. *Ann NY Acad Sci.* 942, 179–191.

Fernandez C, Goldberg JM. (1971) Physiology of peripheral neurons innervating semicircular canals of the squirrel monkey. II. Response to sinusoidal stimulation and dynamics of peripheral vestibular system. *J Neurophysiol.* 34, 661–675.

Fetter M, Aw S, Haslwanter T, Heimberger J, Dichgans J. (1998) Three-dimensional eye movement analysis during caloric stimulation used to test vertical semicircular canal function. *Am J Otol.* 19, 180–187.

Furman JM, Baloh RW. (1992) Otolith-ocular testing in human subjects. *Ann NY Acad Sci.* 656, 431–451.

Furman JM, Cass SP. (1996) *Balance Disorders: A Case Study Approach.* Philadelphia: FA Davis.

Furman JM, Cass SP. (1999) Benign paroxysmal positional vertigo. *N Engl J Med.* 341, 1590–1596.

Furman JM, Cass SP, Briggs BC. (1998) Treatment of benign positional vertigo using heels-over-head rotation. *Ann Otol Rhinol Laryngol.* 107, 1046–1053.

Furman JM, Kamerer DB. (1989) Rotational responses in patients with bilateral caloric reduction. *Acta Otolaryngol.* 108, 355–361.

Furman JM, Wall C 3rd, Pang DL. (1990) Vestibular function in periodic alternating nystagmus. *Brain.* 113, 1425–1439.

Goebel JA. (2001) *Practical Management of the Dizzy Patient.* Philadelphia: Lippincott Williams & Wilkins.

Goldberg JM, Fernandez C. (1971) Physiology of peripheral neurons innervating semicircular canals of the squirrel monkey. I. Resting discharge and response to constant angular accelerations. *J Neurophysiol.* 34, 635–660.

Goldberg JM, Fernandez C. (1976) Physiology of peripheral neurons innervating otolith organs of the squirrel monkey. II. Directional selectivity and force-response relations. *J Neurophysiol.* 39, 985–995.

Hain TC, Ramaswamy TS, Hillman MA. (2000) Anatomy and physiology of the normal vestibular system. In: Herdman SJ, ed. *Vestibular Rehabilitation.* Philadelphia: FA Davis Co.; pp 3–24.

Hain TC, Zee DS. (1992) Velocity storage in labyrinthine disorders. *Ann NY Acad Sci.* 656, 297–304.

Hall SF, Ruby RR, McClure JA. (1979) The mechanics of benign paroxysmal vertigo. *J Otolaryngol.* 8:151–158.

Halmagyi GM, Aw ST, Cremer PD, Curthoys IS, Todd MJ. (2001) Impulsive testing of individual semicircular canal function. *Ann NY Acad Sci.* 942, 192–200.

Halmagyi GM, Aw ST, Cremer PD, Todd MJ, Curthoys IS. (1992) The human vertical vestibuloocular reflex in response to high-acceleration stimulation after unilateral vestibular neurectomy. *Ann NY Acad Sci.* 656, 732–738.

Halmagyi GM, Cremer PD, Anderson J, Murofushi T, Curthoys IS. (2000) Isolated directional preponderance of caloric nystagmus: I. Clinical significance. *Am J Otol.* 21, 559–567.

Halmagyi GM, Gresty MA. (1979) Clinical signs of visual-vestibular interaction. *J Neurol Neurosurg Psychiatr.* 42, 934–939.

Hart CW. (1984) Caloric tests. *Otolaryngol Head Neck Surg.* 92, 662–70.

Herdman SJ, Tusa RJ, Blatt P, Suzuki A, Venuto PJ, Roberts D. (1998) Computerized dynamic visual acuity test in the assessment of vestibular deficits. *Am J Otol.* 19, 790–796.

Herdman SJ, Tusa RJ, Clendaniel RA. (1994) Eye movement signs in vertical canal benign paroxysmal positional vertigo. In: Fuchs AF, Brandt T, Buttner U, Zee D, eds. *Contemporary Ocular Motor and Vestibular Research.* Stuttgart: Thieme; pp 385–387.

Hillman TA, Chen DA, Arriaga MA. (2004) Vestibular nerve section versus intratympanic gentamicin for Meniere's disease. *Laryngoscope.* 114, 216–222.

Honrubia V, Baloh RW, Harris MR, Jacobson KM. (1999) Paroxysmal positional vertigo syndrome. *Am J Otol.* 20, 465–470.

Hood JD. (1989) Evidence of direct thermal action upon the vestibular receptors in the caloric test. A re-interpretation of the data of Coats and Smith. *Acta Otolaryngol.* 107, 161–165.

Horak FB, Shupert C. (2000) Role of the vestibular system in postural control. In: Herdman SJ, ed. *Vestibular Rehabilitation.* Philadelphia: FA Davis Co.; pp 25–51.

Howard IP. (1982) *Human Visual Orientation.* New York: John Wiley & Sons.

Howard IP. (1993) The optokinetic system. In: Sharpe JA, Barber HO, eds. *The Vestibulo-Ocular Reflex and Vertigo.* New York: Raven Press; pp 163–184.

Isaacson JE, Rubin AM. (2001) Performing the physical exam: detecting spontaneous and gaze-evoked nystagmus. In: Goebel JA, ed. *Practical Management of the Dizzy Patient.* Philadelphia: Lippincott Williams & Wilkins; pp 61–71.

Jacobson GP, Pearlstein R, Henderson J, Calder JH, Rock J. (1998) Recovery nystagmus revisited. *J Am Acad Audiol.* 9, 263–271.

Jenkins HA. (1985) Long-term adaptive changes of the vestibuloocular reflex in patients following acoustic neuroma surgery. *Laryngoscope.* 95, 1224–1234.

Kasper J, Diefenhardt A, Mackert A, Thoden U. (1992) The vestibuloocular response during transient arousal shifts in man. *Acta Otolaryngol.* 112, 1–6.

Korres S, Balatsouras DG, Kaberos A, Economou C, Kandiloros D, Ferekidis E. (2002) Occurrence of semicircular canal involvement in benign paroxysmal positional vertigo. *Otol Neurotol.* 23, 926–932.

Lee MD. (1969) The caloric test in the supine and prone positions. *J Laryngol Otol.* 83, 797–801.

Leigh RJ, Zee DS. (1991) *The Neurology of Eye Movements.* Philadelphia: FA Davis Co.

Levo H, Aalto H, Petteri Hirvonen T. (2004) Nystagmus measured with video-oculography: methodological aspects and normative data. *ORL.* 66, 101–104.

Li JC. (1995) Mastoid oscillation: a critical factor for success in canalith repositioning procedure. *Otolaryngol Head Neck Surg.* 112, 670–675.

Li JC, Epley J. (2006) The 360-degree maneuver for treatment of benign positional vertigo. *Otol Neurotol.* 27, 71–77.

Lim DJ. (1984) The development and structure of the otoconia. In: Friedmann I, Ballantyne J, eds. *Ultrastructural Atlas of the Inner Ear.* London: Butterworths; pp 245–269.

Lindeman HH. (1969) Studies on the morphology of the sensory regions of the vestibular apparatus. *Adv Anat Embryol Cell Biol.* 42, 1–113.

Lysakowski A. (2005) Anatomy of vestibular end organs and neural pathways. In: Cummings CW, et al., eds. *Otolaryngology—Head & Neck Surgery.* Philadelphia: Elsevier Mosby; pp 3089–3114.

Markham CH, Diamond SG. (2003) Ocular counterrolling in response to static and dynamic tilting: implications for human otolith function. *J Vestib Res.* 12, 127–134.

McClure JA. (1985) Horizontal canal BPV. *J Otolaryngol.* 14, 30–35.

McClure JA, Copp JC, Lycett P. (1981) Recovery nystagmus in Ménière's disease. *Laryngoscope.* 91, 1727–1737.

Merfeld DM, Zupan L, Peterka RJ. (1999) Humans use internal models to estimate gravity and linear acceleration. *Nature.* 398, 615–618.

Nashner LM. (2001) Computerized dynamic posturography. In: Goebel JA, ed. *Practical Management of the Dizzy Patient.* Philadelphia: Lippincott Williams & Wilkins; pp 143–170.

Nashner LM, McCollum G. (1985) The organization of human postural movements: a formal basis and experimental synthesis. *Behav Brain Sci.* 8, 135–172.

Niven JI, Hixson WC, Correia MJ. (1966) Elicitation of horizontal nystagmus by periodic linear acceleration. *Acta Otolaryngol.* 62, 429–441.

O'Neill G. (1987) The caloric stimulus. Temperature generation within the temporal bone. *Acta Otolaryngol.* 103, 266–272.

Oosterveld WJ. (1973) On the origin of positional alcohol nystagmus. *Acta Otolaryngol.* 75, 252–258.

Paige GD. (1991) Linear vestibuloocular reflex (LVOR) and modulation by vergence. *Acta Otolaryngol.* 481 (suppl), 282–286.

Paige GD. (2002) Otolith function: basis for modern testing. *Ann NY Acad Sci.* 956, 314–323.

Parnes LS, McClure JA. (1992) Free-floating endolymph particles: a new operative finding during posterior semicircular canal occlusion. *Laryngoscope.* 102, 988–992.

Peterson BW, Goldberg J, Bilotto G, Fuller JH. (1985) Cervicocollic reflex: its dynamic properties and interaction with vestibular reflexes. *J Neurophysiol.* 54, 90–109.

Pola J, Wyatt HJ. (1980) Target position and velocity: the stimuli for smooth pursuit eye movements. *Vision Res.* 20, 523–534.

Precht W. (1979) Labyrinthine influences on the vestibular nuclei. *Prog Brain Res.* 50, 369–381.

Raphan T, Cohen B. (2002) The vestibuloocular reflex in three dimensions. *Exp Brain Res.* 145, 1–27.

Raphan T, Matsuo V, Cohen B. (1979) Velocity storage in the vestibuloocular reflex arc (VOR). *Exp Brain Res.* 35, 229–248.

Redfern MS, Yardley L, Bronstein AM. (2001) Visual influences on balance. *J Anxiety Dis.* 15, 81–94.

Robinson DA. (1976) Adaptive gain control of the vestibuloocular reflex by the cerebellum. *J Neurophysiol.* 39, 954–969.

Robinson DA, Zee DS, Hain TC, Holmes A, Rosenberg LF. (1984) Alexander's law: its behavior and origin in the human vestibuloocular reflex. *Ann Neurol.* 16, 714–722.

Ron S, Robinson DA, Skavenski AA. (1972) Saccades and the quick phase of nystagmus. *Vision Res.* 12, 2015–2022.

Salt AN, Konishi T. (1986) The cochlear fluids: perilymph and endolymph. In: Altschuler RA, Hoffman DW, Bobbin RP, eds. *Neurobiology of Hearing: The Cochlea.* New York: Raven Press; pp 109–122.

Sargent EW, Goebel JA, Hanson JM, Beck DL. (1997) Idiopathic bilateral vestibular loss. *Otolaryngol Head Neck Surg.* 116, 157–162.

Schuknecht HF. (1969) Cupulolithiasis. *Arch Otolaryngol.* 90, 765–778.

Shepard NT. (2001a) Electronystagmography (ENG) testing. In: Goebel JA, ed. *Practical Management of the Dizzy Patient.* Philadelphia: Lippincott Williams & Wilkins; pp 113–127.

Shepard NT. (2001b) Rotational chair testing. In: Goebel JA, ed. *Practical Management of the Dizzy Patient.* Philadelphia: Lippincott Williams & Wilkins; pp 129–141.

Shepard NT, Telian SA. (1996) *Practical Management of the Balance Disorder Patient.* San Diego: Singular Publishing Group, Inc.

Solomon D. (2000) Benign paroxysmal positional vertigo. *Curr Treat Opt Neurol.* 2, 417–427.

Stockwell CW, Bojrab DJ. (1997) Interpretation and usefulness of rotational testing. In: Jacobson GP, Newman CW, Kartush JM, eds. *Handbook of Balance Function Testing.* St. Louis: Mosby Year Book; pp 249–260.

Tomlinson RD, Robinson DA. (1981) Is the vestibulo-ocular reflex cancelled by smooth pursuit? In: Fuchs A, Becker W, eds.

Progress in Oculomotor Research. New York: Elsevier/North-Holland; pp 533–539.

van Die G, Collewijn H. (1982) Optokinetic nystagmus in man: role of central and peripheral retina and occurrence of asymmetries. *Hum Neurobiol.* 1, 111–119.

Welgampola MS, Colebatch JG. (2005) Characteristics and clinical applications of vestibular-evoked myogenic potentials. *Neurology.* 64, 1682–1688.

Westheimer G. (1954) Mechanism of saccadic eye movements. *AMA Arch Ophthalmol.* 52, 710–724.

Wilson VJ, Melvill Jones G. (1979) *Mammalian Vestibular Physiology.* New York: Plenum Press.

Zee DS. (2000) Vestibular adaptation. In: Herdman SJ, ed. *Vestibular Rehabilitation.* Philadelphia: FA Davis Co.; pp 77–90.

Zhou G, Cox LC. (2004) Vestibular evoked myogenic potentials: history and overview. *Am J Audiol.* 13, 135–143.

20 Evaluation of the Patient with Dizziness and Balance Disorders

Neil T. Shepard

▨ INTRODUCTION

The majority of patients afflicted with an acute balance disorder recover spontaneously with only symptomatic treatment from the medical community (Igarashi, 1984; Pfaltz, 1983; Curthoys and Halmagyi, 1995). For reasons that are poorly understood, some of these patients develop chronic balance system problems requiring significant investments from a variety of medical and surgical specialists to evaluate and manage their disorder.

Vertigo and balance disorders constitute a significant public health problem in the United States and elsewhere (Yardley, et al 1998b). Estimates of the number of persons in this country seeking medical care for disequilibrium or vertigo range as high as 7 million per year. Approximately 30% of the US population has experienced episodes of dizziness by age 65 (Roydhouse, 1974). There are no indications that the problem of balance disorders is diminishing, particularly as the population ages (Herdman, 1994; Kroenke and Mangelsdorff, 1989). Another compelling issue relates to the increased incidence of falls with aging. Balance disorders and dizziness are important risk factors for falls in the elderly. Since it can be inferred from epidemiologic studies that balance disorders increase the probability of an injurious fall, the management of balance disorders in the elderly population becomes a critical issue (Blake et al., 1988; Tinetti et al., 1988; Herdman et al., 2000; Hall et al., 2004). It is estimated that 30% of those over 65 years of age experience at least one fall per year. Although less than 10% of these result in fractures, 20% require formal attention by the medical establishment (Gillespie et al., 2003). The introduction of numerous fall prevention programs has provided the opportunity to evaluate their effectiveness in reducing the rate of falls in those at risk for falls. In a Cochrane systematic review of 62 randomized controlled studies involving over 21,000 subjects, the authors concluded that effective programs to reduce the risk for and rate of falls in the elderly are available (Gillespie et al., 2003). Results of this type further emphasize the need to have effective and efficient techniques for the assessment and overall management of those persons of any age who are presenting with symptoms of imbalance, vertigo, or falling, or other symptoms that fall under the general descriptor of dizziness.

This chapter is the clinical companion to the preceding chapter (Chapter 19, Clinical Neurophysiology of the Vestibular System). A clear understanding of those concepts and principles is vital to the appreciation of the information presented herein. The anatomy and physiology of the vestibular and balance systems form the basis against which interpretations of patients presenting history, signs, symptoms, and laboratory test results are developed. A word about nomenclature is important at this juncture. The term dizziness typically has little informational value when patients use it to describe their problem. It is an all inclusive term that is taken to mean symptoms ranging from true vertigo (perception of the world spinning around the patient or the patient spinning within their environment) to near syncopal events (fainting or lightheadedness) to complaints of being off-balance or unsteady when standing and/or walking. Dizziness can also imply combinations of all of the above. Therefore, when discussing the presenting history with a patient, attempts are made to avoid the use of the term. However, "dizziness" or "the dizzy patient" phrasing can be useful as a general descriptor and will be used throughout this chapter to collectively imply the broad-ranging symptoms and functional problems encountered by patients. When needed, the specific symptom descriptors will be used.

OVERVIEW OF THE MANAGEMENT OF THE DIZZY AND BALANCE-DISORDER PATIENT

Priority of Management

While the goal of establishing a working diagnosis and beginning management is a common theme, the tools used and the complexity of the treatment plan are different for the acute versus the chronic dizzy patient. When evaluating a patient with the acute onset of vertigo for the first time, establishing a preliminary diagnosis and ruling out life-threatening causes of a neurologic or cardiovascular nature are of primary importance. This is typically accomplished by use of history, clinical examinations, perhaps an emergency computed tomography (CT) scan, and screening cardiovascular testing. It is unlikely that vestibular testing would be needed in this process. If auditory symptoms are reported, the patient should get a thorough audiometric evaluation and radiographic studies to rule out a cerebellar pontine angle (CPA) lesion, for which balance testing would not be required. In certain cases where eye movement abnormalities on the clinical examination suggest central involvement, use of videonystagmography (VNG)/electronystagmography (ENG) with extensive ocular-motor evaluation would be a reasonable follow-up study. When managing the acute onset of vertigo or imbalance, after significant neurologic and cardiovascular causes have been ruled out, the judicious use of medications to control symptoms is appropriate. This should be accompanied with the recommendation of returning to routine daily activities as soon as these can be tolerated and not avoiding provocative movement activities. This will help to promote early use of the central vestibular compensation system. Since the majority of first-onset events of vertigo represent stationary peripheral lesions, the central compensation process will be critical to the patient's recovery.

The chronic (symptoms continuing beyond 12 weeks) dizzy patient is managed somewhat differently, assuming the previous acute evaluation has been performed. In the vast majority of cases, the unstated question being asked is: Why hasn't the central vestibular compensation process (see Chapter 19) controlled the current patient's symptoms? Reassessment of the preliminary diagnosis and determination of the factors preventing recovery now must be addressed. This lack of improvement could involve a progressive or unstable peripheral or central system lesion (a lesion with a fluctuating locus of damage) or a stable lesion (fixed locus of tissue damage) with poor central compensation. Determin-

ing which of these situations exists requires detailed historical information, assisted by results from the various laboratory studies. Perhaps more important than the actual diagnosis is the determination of which of these situations is responsible for the continued symptoms. This determination strongly influences the formulation of the diagnostic and treatment plan. This plan may involve a medical, surgical, or vestibular and balance rehabilitation therapy (VBRT) program. Combinations of these interventional strategies are also used in various types of patients, such as those with Ménière's disease, mass lesions of the CPA, migraine-associated dizziness (MAD), or traumatic brain injury and patients with psychological causes or exacerbations of their conditions. The use of a vestibular rehabilitation program is by far the most common form of treatment for the chronic patient. In general, less than 10% of chronic, dizzy patients are candidates for surgical procedures.

Medical versus Surgical Management

For most chronic vestibular disorders (peripheral or central in origin) or nonvestibular disorders resulting in complaints of dizziness, no disease-specific pharmacologic treatment is available. Stimulant medications such as caffeine and amphetamines have not generally been used in the clinical setting, despite animal research suggesting that they may enhance vestibular compensation. The use of medications in the treatment of balance-disorder patients falls into three major categories: (1) general suppression of vestibular symptoms; (2) pharmacologic treatment of specific conditions that are suspected to cause vestibular symptoms, such as Ménière's disease or migraine variants; and (3) treatment of the patient who has a clinical anxiety or depressive disorder that may be the primary cause of the dizziness or secondary to an intractable peripheral or central vestibular disorder.

The agents typically prescribed for symptomatic relief of dizziness include benzodiazepines, antihistamines, and anticholinergic agents (Zee, 1985). In general, these medications are ineffective in preventing acute vertiginous spells, yet they may be quite effective in reducing the intensity of a spell and controlling the associated nausea and vomiting. A variety of medications can be used in the situation of psychological causes or exacerbations, typically in the benzodiazepine and selective serotonin reuptake inhibitor (SSRI) categories (Staab, 2000; Staab et al., 2002a; 2002b). However, the physician must remember that all of these agents are centrally sedating. Active head and eye movements produce sensory error signals that trigger compensation mechanisms in the central nervous system after injuries to the peripheral and central vestibular system. It is almost certain that vestibular suppressants for dizziness inhibit the brain's ability to properly apprehend the sensory conflicts in the balance system, retarding (probably not preventing) central compensation (Peppard, 1986). Thus, although vestibular suppressants are appropriate for the short-term control of acute symptoms, they may be counterproductive with respect to the eventual desired outcome. This is particularly true in the setting of a fixed unilateral lesion, such as is seen after an episode of acute labyrinthitis or vestibular neuritis. Some patients with longstanding vestibular complaints after a peripheral injury may improve simply by weaning them from their vestibular suppressants.

It is not unusual to encounter patients with intense episodes of vertigo who have already seen several physicians and tried multiple medical treatments without success. Those who are disabled by their symptoms are often desperate for relief. While it is proper to consider surgical treatment in this setting, the physician must recognize that unsuccessful surgery may greatly aggravate the patient's discouragement with his or her disease and the medical profession. The astute clinician recognizes the vulnerability of this patient population and seeks to guide them toward rational and effective surgical options when available, while sheltering them from invalidated treatment practices. It is beyond the scope of this chapter to discuss the technical aspects of the surgical procedures that are available for the treatment of vertigo. These are available in standard reference materials (Jackler and Brackmann, 1994).

In most cases, the process of central vestibular compensation reliably relieves dizziness resulting from insults to the peripheral vestibular system, provided that the lesion is either stable or produces only an insidious progressive deterioration (e.g., vestibular schwannoma). On the other hand, if the lesion is unstable or rapidly progressive, compensation is not possible unless the lesion can be stabilized by medical or surgical treatment. Ménière's disease is the prototypical disorder in this latter category, wherein the ear may fluctuate between normal labyrinthine function and dramatic cochleovestibular symptoms. Vestibular system surgery seeks to stabilize inner ear function in the setting of an unstable system, whether by correcting a defect that underlies the disorder or by ablating function in the pathologic ear.

Certain surgical procedures are applicable only to a particular diagnosis. Some of these are widely accepted as both rational and effective, such as posterior semicircular canal occlusion for intractable benign paroxysmal positional vertigo (Parnes and McClure, 1991) or the middle fossa approach to repair superior semicircular canal dehiscence (Minor, 2005; Minor et al., 1998). Other disease-specific operations, such as endolymphatic sac surgery for Ménière's disease, repair of round or oval window perilymphatic fistula, and microvascular decompression of the eighth nerve, continue to generate controversy. These operations are enthusiastically embraced by some practitioners, while others have abandoned their use. All of the operations in this group have as their unifying feature the desirable goal of correcting a pathologic process that is unique to the particular diagnosis, while preserving any portion of inner ear function that is unaffected by the disease process. Success in this setting obviously hinges on making an exact diagnosis and selecting operations with proven efficacy.

On the other hand, procedures designed to ablate unilateral vestibular function, such as labyrinthectomy and vestibular nerve section, may be applied to any peripheral vestibular disorder where the lesion site is confined to the labyrinth. In this setting, an exact etiologic diagnosis is less critical. Instead, the physician must be certain that the problem is attributable to peripheral system dysfunction and that the pathologic ear has been correctly identified. In addition, it should be clear that the peripheral labyrinthine disorder is fluctuating or rapidly progressive in nature, rather than simply a failure of central compensation for a stable lesion. On the other hand, if the ongoing vertigo represents poor initial central vestibular compensation or recent decompensation following a stable vestibular lesion, ablative surgery is not likely to be necessary or particularly effective. A good summary of the current state of medical and surgical treatments for dizziness is available by Telian and Wyatt (2008a and 2008b).

Vestibular and Balance Rehabilitation Programs in Management

Vertigo or disequilibrium may persist due to poor central nervous system compensation after any acute injury to the vestibular system, even if there is no ongoing labyrinthine dysfunction. In addition, some patients will develop maladaptive postural-control strategies that are destabilizing or bothersome in certain settings. These patients often benefit from a program of vestibular rehabilitation. Such programs are most effective when customized to the needs of the individual patient and supervised by an appropriately trained physical therapist (Shepard and Telian, 1995; 2005; Hall et al., 2004; Whitney and Rossi, 2000; Shepard et al., 1993b; Shumway-Cook and Horak, 1990; Yardley et al., 1998a).

Current knowledge about the process of central compensation for vestibular lesions suggests that avoidance of movements and body positions that provoke vertigo, as well as the traditional practice of prescribing vestibular suppressants for these patients, may be counterproductive. The stimulus for recovery from an acute vestibular lesion seems to be repeated exposure to the sensory conflicts produced by movement. Therefore, once the severe symptoms are resolved, the patient's medications should be discontinued, and an informal program of increased activities that promote recovery should be encouraged. For most individuals, recovery will be rapid and nearly complete. For some, the symptoms of vestibular dysfunction may persist. These chronic patients are candidates for formal programs of vestibular rehabilitation. In general, vestibular rehabilitation programs are symptom-driven activities. The key elements in deciding whether a patient is appropriate for such a management technique are based primarily on the patient's presenting symptoms. Table 20.1 is a summary of those patients who would be appropriate to be considered for a vestibular and balance rehabilitation program and those who would be inappropriate. The volume of literature describing the clinic efficacy of

---

TABLE 20.1   Vestibular and Balance Rehabilitation

Appropriate

- Patients with head or visual motion-provoked symptoms.
- Symptoms that are continuous with motion exacerbation.
- Evaluations revealing balance or gait dysfunction with or without either of the traits listed above.
- History and testing information supports a stable peripheral or central lesion site.
- Age is not a determining factor.

Inappropriate

- Symptoms of only spontaneous events that are more frequent than one time every 6 to 8 weeks and that last longer than 15 minutes at a time.
- No provocative activity or balance dysfunction can be realized during the therapy evaluation; therefore, nothing is found on which to base exercise activities.
- Progressive central lesions involving gait and balance have not been shown to respond to therapy for balance and gait. These patients may benefit from exercises to reduce eye and head movement sensitivity and safety with ambulation-oriented goals.

---

this form of management as a primary form of treatment or in conjunction with medical/surgical approaches has grown significantly in the last decade. An article summarizing this literature is available (Whitney and Rossi, 2000). As a general statement, vestibular and balance rehabilitation programs provide significantly improved management for a large percentage (estimated as high as 70%) of patients with complaints of balance and dizziness for whom other methods of treatment have been unsuccessful. A more detailed discussion of this management option is beyond the scope of this chapter. The interested reader is referred to other sources for extensive coverage of this topic (Herdman, 2000; 2007; Shepard and Telian, 2005).

▨ LABORATORY STUDIES OF BALANCE SYSTEM FUNCTION

In considering the evaluation of the patient with complaints of vertigo, lightheadedness, imbalance, or a combination of these descriptors, one must look beyond just the peripheral and central vestibular system with its ocular motor connections. The various pathways involved in postural control, only part of which have direct or indirect vestibular input, should be kept in mind during an evaluation. Additionally, significant variations in symptoms and test findings can be generated by migraine disorders (Shepard, 2006; Furman et al., 2003; 2005; Neuhauser et al., 2001; Tusa, 2000a) and/or

anxiety disorders (Furman et al., 2005; Staab and Ruckenstein, 2003; Staab, 2000; Tusa, 2000b; Yardley, 2000), yet these are diagnosed primarily by case history and require a specific line of questioning.

The evaluation of the dizzy patient should be guided by what information is needed to make initial and subsequent management decisions. Tests considered extent- and site-of-lesion studies, ENG, rotational chair, otolith function tests, and specific protocols in postural control assessment (motor control test and postural evoked potentials) give results that are unable to be used to predict symptom type or magnitude or level of disability of an individual patient. Conversely, patient complaints cannot be used to predict, in detail, the outcomes of these tests. In a limited manner, more functionally oriented evaluation tools, such as computerized dynamic posturography (CDP) using the sensory organization protocol and dynamic visual acuity testing (Herdman et al., 1998) provide for some correlation between results, patient symptoms, and functional limitations. If specific or general health inventories like the Dizziness Handicap Inventory (Jacobson and Newman, 1990) are added to the testing, predictive assessment of disability is improved but remains limited. It is hypothesized that the reason for this dichotomy in test results versus functional disability and symptom complaints is the inadequacy of the laboratory tests to fully characterize the status of the central vestibular compensation process (Jacobson et al., 1991; Shepard and Telian, 1996; Zee, 2000). It is the exception, not the rule, that vestibular and balance laboratory tests return results that would drive management of the dizzy patient. It would be extremely rare if these studies returned a diagnosis. Therefore, the routine use of these tools to determine how to proceed with the management of a dizzy patient is a false line of reasoning and not productive in the majority of the patients.

The role of the major laboratory studies of ENG, rotary chair, otolith testing, and postural control assessment varies with the subtests found within each of these major groupings. Determination of extent and site of lesion within the peripheral and central vestibular ocular-motor control systems is a primary focus of these studies. The characterization of functional limitations in static and dynamic postural control (this may relate directly to gait abnormalities) is a second primary focus. Lastly, together with the characterization of the symptoms, the use of the laboratory studies aids in determining the utilization of a VBRT program. In this later purpose, the primary information is that given in Table 20.1, the symptom presentation. Aspects of postural control may be helpful in the design and monitoring of the VBRT, whereas the extent- and site-of-lesion studies do not contribute to determination of the appropriateness of such a program of management, nor are they of use in monitoring program effectiveness. VOR tests of caloric or rotational chair can be used to support the application of a specific type of therapy exercise (adaptation) in vestibular and balance rehabilitation programs.

Overall, the use of the laboratory information is in the confirmation of the suspected site of lesion and the diagnosis that has been derived from the patient's history and physical examination with the office vestibular evaluation. This does not imply a prioritized order to the testing versus the office visit. With chronic dizzy patients, it can be very useful to triage them to at least core laboratory evaluations (to be discussed later) prior to the office visit. A detailed discussion of the overall utility of laboratory tests in assisting in the diagnosis and management of the dizzy patient is presented elsewhere and is beyond the scope of this chapter (Shepard, 2007; Shepard et al., 2003).

The use of laboratory studies to provide for the initial management decisions as to treatment path requires the use of a full clinical history to provide a context for interpretation of the laboratory tests. These are the initial management decisions that involve determination of a diagnosis and whether the patient should be approached with medication, surgical procedures, VBRT program, or a combination of these options. Once this first decision is made, then the isolated test findings from the vestibular and balance studies may well be useful in helping to design the specifics of the treatment path selected and in monitoring progress along that path.

In summary, the following are required elements to make management decisions for the chronic dizzy patient: detailed neurotologic history, office vestibular and physical examination, and formal audiometric testing, given the inescapable anatomic relationship between the auditory and vestibular peripheral systems. The following are considered important but less likely to directly drive the management in the typical case: laboratory vestibular and balance function studies, neuroradiographic evaluations, and serologic tests. It is important to realize that there will be patients for whom unexpected findings on any one of these latter studies will either alter the complete course of the management or add dimensions to the management not originally considered. Therefore, while less likely to directly drive management, the vestibular and balance function studies, radiologic and serologic evaluations are of significant importance. But, for the majority of patients, the vestibular and balance tests will be confirmatory in nature.

Additionally, certain protocols within the balance function studies are very useful in monitoring the natural history of a disorder or the effects of particular medical or surgical treatments (Shepard and Telian, 1996). Each of the major groupings of tests (ENG, rotary chair, otolith function evaluation, and CDP) will be discussed in turn. The purpose of these discussions is to describe the utility of the test(s), not the specifics of how they are performed or detailed interpretations, for which the reader is referred elsewhere (Jacobson et al., 1993; Shepard and Telian, 1996; Baloh and Honrubia, 1990; Leigh and Zee, 1999; Baloh and Halmagyi, 1996; Furman and Cass, 1996; Bronstein et al., 1996; Goebel, 2000b; Jacobson and Shepard, 2008; Shepard and Solomon, 2000).

Neurotologic History

Before consideration of the actual laboratory tests, some discussion of the neurotologic history is needed. Given the various tools for assessment, the history is the single most important factor in determining the course of management and therefore requires some discussion (Jacobson et al., 1993; Shepard and Telian, 1996; Baloh and Honrubia, 1990; Leigh and Zee, 1999; Baloh and Halmagyi, 1996; Furman and Cass, 1996; Bronstein et al., 1996; Rosenberg and Gizzi, 2000; Goebel, 2000a). The differentiation between the various peripheral vestibular disorders is particularly dependent on historical information and the conclusions that the physician draws from the interview. Most vestibular disorders cannot be distinguished from one another simply by vestibular testing or other diagnostic interventions. Failure to properly discriminate these disorders on historical grounds may be the source of considerable ongoing distress for the patient and may lead to improper management by the physician. Since subsequent treatment decisions will be based on the clinical diagnosis, it is particularly appropriate to spend additional time during the history to clarify important features. In addition, balance function study results are best interpreted in light of a proper clinical history. The main reason that the patient is seeking medical attention for his or her balance disturbance should be identified. Although little specific diagnostic information may be gained, it is often helpful to hear an account of the patient's perception of his or her illness prior to pursuing more specific questions. One can often gain a sense for how much functional disability the vestibular symptoms have produced. The psychosocial impact of the illness may also become clear in the patient's initial comments. Sometimes patients will volunteer that their symptoms are trivial or have resolved completely, but they simply want to make sure that they have not suffered a stroke or developed a brain tumor. If the patient is not permitted to share this information freely, important aspects of the individual's care may be overlooked.

Once the patient has shared the main concerns raised by his or her condition, the first specific questions should be phrased to gain information regarding the initial onset of symptoms. The characteristics and intensity of the balance disturbance at that time provide useful insight for the differential diagnosis. If the patient can recount specifics surrounding the symptom onset, such as date and time of day, along with the activity interrupted by intense vertigo, the examiner can be reasonably certain that the patient has suffered a significant peripheral labyrinthine insult. Surprisingly, if the professional does not specifically inquire, patients who are preoccupied with recent symptoms and disability may neglect to report a very profound vestibular crisis that occurred initially. If the onset was more insidious and the patient is unable to provide any account of an initial event, an acute peripheral disorder is less likely. Other important issues to discuss at this stage of the interview include the association of physical trauma, barotrauma, or an intercurrent illness prior to the onset of vertigo. Patients should also be asked about previous remote episodes of vertigo.

It is very important to question the patient regarding the association of a hearing loss or other auditory symptoms with the onset of vertigo. A complete audiometric assessment should be performed early in the evaluation. The presence of an associated sensory-neural hearing loss, whether stable, progressive, or fluctuating, is the single strongest incriminating factor in identifying a pathologic labyrinth (Shonel et al., 1991). The presence of other otologic symptoms such as aural fullness and tinnitus may also be helpful in lateralization. A history of previous otologic surgery or familial hearing loss is also important.

Most patients with acute vertigo will improve with supportive, expectant management. When this is not the case, they may present for evaluation after several months or years of dizziness. The patient should be asked to describe the progression of symptoms over time, along with the nature and duration of typical spells. Specifically, one wishes to know whether the spells are continuous or occur in discrete episodes. If the symptoms are episodic, it is extremely important to distinguish whether they are spontaneous or motion-provoked. If the symptoms are brief and predictably produced by head movements or body position changes, the patient most likely has a stable vestibular lesion but has not yet completed central nervous system compensation. Those who describe these symptoms sometimes also note a chronic underlying sense of disequilibrium or lightheadedness. The chronic symptoms may be quite troublesome, but any intense vertigo should be primarily motion-provoked. These patients are suitable candidates for vestibular rehabilitation. It is important to point out that historical information is essential in deciding who might benefit from rehabilitation therapy.

If the episodic spells described by the patient are longer periods of intense vertigo that occur spontaneously and without warning, this is probably progressive or unstable peripheral dysfunction. One must also suspect a progressive labyrinthine lesion if the vertigo is accompanied by fluctuating or progressive sensory-neural hearing loss. Such patients are managed with medical therapy, and if this fails, they constitute the best candidates for surgical intervention. Such patients are not candidates for vestibular rehabilitation, except as an adjunctive modality.

Additional history regarding current or prior use of medications should be elicited. Many patients are under the mistaken impression that vestibular suppressants will prevent spells of vertigo and take them habitually. Because oversedation from these centrally acting drugs may retard central nervous system compensation for vestibular lesions, one should consider tapering or discontinuing these medications whenever possible. Medications that must be continued should be directed toward particular symptoms that specifically interfere with the patient's recovery process.

Other psychosocial aspects can be important in understanding the patient's situation. Complicating features of anxiety, depression, or excessive dependence on psychotropic medications should be identified. It is desirable to understand the degree of functional disability produced by the patients' vestibular complaints, especially with respect to their professional and favorite social activities. The stability and commitment of their psychological support system should also be evaluated. The reader is referred to two summary articles that discuss the area of psychological impact and the management techniques available to deal with this important area (Yardley, 2000; Staab, 2000).

As discussed earlier, two of the critical elements in developing a differential diagnosis involve the determination of spontaneous versus visual or head movement provocation and the temporal characteristics of the symptoms. These two features play such a major role in the development of the working diagnosis that a more detailed discussion is appropriate. Table 20.2, which is not intended to be exhaustive, suggests the use of these two aspects of the patient history and the possible sources to consider in the diagnosis. To further differentiate between the diagnostic options, the other historical information and auditory function can be immediately useful. Baloh and Halmagyi (1996) and Furman and Cass (1996) contain detailed descriptions of specific disorders by history and test findings.

Electronystagmography/ Videonystagmography

Traditional ENG (Shepard, 2000a), using electro-oculography for eye movement recordings, is a process that indirectly estimates the position of the eye as a function of time. The estimates are reliable whether recorded with eyes open or closed and in a darkened or well-lit environment. Changes in eye position are indicated by the polarity of the corneal-retinal potential (dipole) relative to each electrode placed near the eye (Fig. 20.1). These electrodes are typically placed at each lateral canthus and above and below at least one eye with a common electrode on the forehead (Fig. 20.2). Since the primary purpose of the vestibular apparatus is to control eye movements when the head is in motion, the movements of the eyes may be used to infer the activity of the peripheral vestibular end organs and their central vestibulo-ocular pathways. More recently, the technique of infrared video-oculography (VNG) has begun to replace the standard electro-oculography. This technique has the advantage of providing a direct estimate of the eye position as a function of time and a reduction in electrical artifacts. It is very important to recognize that both the ENG and VNG techniques are two-dimensional recording systems. They both produce permanent recording of eye movements in the horizontal (yaw) plane and the vertical (pitch or sagittal) plane. Therefore, even though the video systems allow for visualization of three-dimensional eye movements (in the yaw, pitch, and roll planes), the quantification via the after-test traces is the same for both techniques, only representing yaw and pitch movements. In neither technique are the torsional movements (eye movements in the roll plane) quantified. The VNG systems do allow for the qualitative description of torsional eye movements that were observed during the testing. This qualitative observation of eye movements and the

TABLE 20.2   Suggested differential diagnostic entries based on temporal course and symptom characteristics

Temporal course of symptoms	"Dizziness" characteristics	Auditory characteristics	Differential to consider
Episodic – seconds	HM-HP provoked	Normal	BPPV; uncompensated stable peripheral lesion; VBI
Episodic – seconds-minutes <60	Spontaneous	Normal or mild fluctuations	Migraine; TIA; anxiety disorders; Ménière's (spells over 20 min)
Episodic – minutes-hours <24	HM-HP provoked	Normal	Uncompensated stable peripheral lesion; migraine
Episodic – minutes-hours <24	Spontaneous	Fluctuant + progressive	Labyrinthine disorders (e.g., Ménière's and autoimmune)
Episodic – minutes-hours <24	Spontaneous	Normal or mild fluctuations	Migraine; anxiety disorders; cardiovascular
Days	Spontaneous resolving in 1–3 days to HM-HP Provoked	Normal	Vestibular neuritis; vascular event
Days	Spontaneous resolving in 1–3 days to HM-HP provoked	Sudden loss at time of vertigo onset	Labyrinthitis; PICA or AICA distribution stroke
Days typically <7	Spontaneous or HM-HP provoked relatively constant overall	Normal or mild fluctuation	Migraine
Continuous	May or may not be exacerbated by HM-HP	Normal	Central vestibular system disorders; anxiety disorders; nonvestibular disorders such as sensory or motor neuropathy of lower limbs

HM, head movement; HP, head position; BPPV, benign paroxysmal positional vertigo; VBI, vertebrobasilar insufficiency; TIA, transient ischemic attack; PICA, posterior inferior cerebellar artery; AICA, anterior inferior cerebellar artery.

lower noise trace are the primary benefits of a VNG system versus an ENG system.

In consideration of which system will serve for the evaluations being performed, it is important to realize that, although video can be used on the majority of patients, electrode techniques are still required for certain groups of patients. The more consistent types of patients for whom electrode techniques are required are: (1) patients with claustrophobia who will not tolerate the goggle systems during vision-removed testing; (2) patients with dark areas on the lids or around the eye (e.g., permanent eye makeup, dark areas on the sclera from hemorrhage or injury) that confuse the video system, which makes a distinction between the dark pupil-iris area and the lighter sclera in order to track the eye movements; and (3) children under age 6 who often do not tolerate the goggles with vision removed (also, the goggle systems are difficult if not impossible to fit on the face of a child age 5 or under, since they are designed primarily for the adult). Another practical consideration that is independent of video or electrode techniques is that, when setting up a testing laboratory, it is imperative to have, at a minimum, two recording channels: one for horizontal eye movements and one for vertical eye movements. The interpretation of horizontal movements (especially when

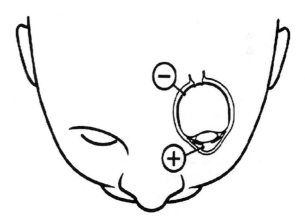

FIGURE 20.1   Shown schematically is the corneal-retinal potential that forms the basis for electro-oculography as an indirect recording technique for eye movement position as a function of time. Electrodes placed around the eyes (see Fig. 20.2) detect changes in electric field potential as the eyes move. (Reprinted with permission from Shepard NT, Telian SA. [1996] *Practical Management of the Balance Disorder Patient.* **San Diego: Singular Publishing Group).**

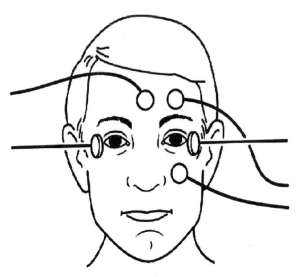

FIGURE 20.2 Typical electrode montage for monitoring eye position as a function of time in both the lateral and vertical dimensions. Note that given the dipole nature of the eyes shown in Figure 20.1 and the use of electrodes lateral and vertical to the anterior-posterior axis of the eye, this type of configuration is not responsive to torsional movements of the eyes. The torsional movements have, as their axis of rotation, the central anterior-posterior axis. (Reprinted with permission from Shepard NT, Telian SA. [1996] *Practical Management of the Balance Disorder Patient.* **San Diego: Singular Publishing Group).**

using electrodes) may require a vertical trace to differentiate between true nystagmus and artifactual events from eye blinks. In addition to recognition of vertical nystagmus, eye movements that can occur in diagonal directions require both horizontal and vertical traces for characterization.

A typical horizontal ENG trace of right-beating nystagmus (could be from either electrodes or video techniques) is shown in Figure 20.3. In this figure, a rapid upward deflection of the trace (fast or saccade component of the nystagmus) is seen, followed in each case by a slower downward drift of the trace (slow component of the nystagmus). The convention in the recordings is that the upward trace deflections represent rightward (horizontal trace) or upward (vertical trace) eye movements. Conversely, downward deflections of the trace represent leftward and downward eye movements. The convention for the description of torsional eye movements is to refer to the superior pole of the eye and describe the nystagmus (as with horizontal and vertical) by the direction of the beat of the nystagmus by the patient's right and left. It is confusing to the reader of a clinical report to use clockwise/counterclockwise notations. Therefore, a patient described to have a right-beating and right-torsional nystagmus would have eye movements with the fast component of the nystagmus beating horizontally to the patient's right, together with the superior pole of the eye beating also to the

patient's right in the roll plane. Calculation of the principle parameter used in the analysis of horizontal and vertical nystagmus for ENG/VNG slow-component eye velocity is illustrated in Figure 20.4.

The ENG/VNG evaluation is a series of subtests performed to assess portions of the peripheral and central vestibular systems. It is important to understand that peripheral vestibular system assessment with ENG/VNG is significantly limited, typically reflecting function of the horizontal semicircular canal, with restricted information from vertical canals and otolith organs. With the use of computerized ENG/VNG systems, which afford significant visual stimulus control and quantitative analysis, evaluation of the central vestibulo-ocular pathways can be quite thorough.

The ENG/VNG consists of the following groups of subtests: ocular-motor evaluation, typically with smooth pursuit tracking, saccade analysis, gaze fixation, and optokinetic stimulation; spontaneous nystagmus; rapid positioning (Dix-Hallpike maneuver); positional nystagmus; and caloric irrigations. The slow-component eye velocity of the nystagmus (Fig. 20.4) is the measurement of interest because it reflects the portion of the nystagmus that is generated by the vestibulo-ocular reflex (VOR). The Hallpike maneuver should be analyzed by direct examination because a two-dimensional quantification recording of the usual eye movement is misleading. The Hallpike test should not be analyzed post hoc by two-dimensional recorded eye movements. The ocular-motor tests are quantified according to the eye movements generated during the task and analyzed by comparison to established normative data.

OCULAR-MOTOR TESTS

Just as the eyes serve as the window for investigating the function of the peripheral vestibular system, they also provide a means to investigate the ocular-motor pathways in the brainstem and cerebellum that are required for the function of the VOR.

There are a variety of testing paradigms that can assist in identifying abnormalities in the central ocular-motor control systems that may produce the patient's complaints. Smooth pursuit tests the ability to track a moving object with smooth eye movements and head still. Smooth pursuit is the most sensitive of the ocular-motor tests but provides poor lesion site localization within the multiple pathways involved in pursuit generation (Shepard and Telian, 1996; Leigh and Zee, 1999). Abnormalities with pursuit are typically taken as an indication of possible vestibulocerebellar region involvement because this is the area common to all of the pursuit pathways. Saccade testing evaluates rapid movement of the eye in order to place an object of interest on that portion of the retina providing for best visual acuity, the fovea. Saccade testing is not as sensitive as pursuit testing but can provide information that helps in the identification of brainstem versus posterior cerebellar vermis involvement. Suggestions for possible frontal or parietal lobe involvement can also be

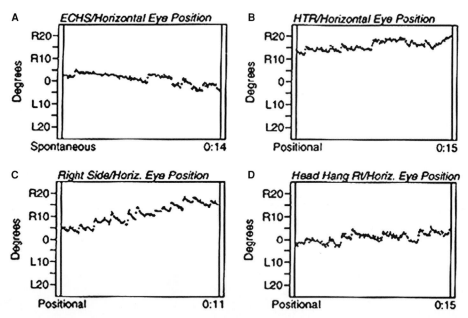

FIGURE 20.3 Panels **A–D** plot horizontal eye position in degrees as a function of time, each showing right-beating nystagmus. The time in the lower right corner of each panel is the total elapse time in seconds for that recording, not the total time shown. Each panel represents 7 seconds of tracing. **(A)** ECHS—eyes closed head straight, spontaneous. **(B)** HTR—eyes closed head turned right, sitting position.**(C)** Eyes closed, lying on the right side (right decubitus position). **(D)** Eyes closed, hyperextension of the neck (by approximately 30 degrees) with the head turned to the right. These are four of a total of 11 positions tested on this patient. (Reprinted with permission from Shepard NT, Telian SA. [1996] *Practical Management of the Balance Disorder Patient.* San Diego: Singular Publishing Group).

obtained from saccade testing via additional paradigms (anti- and remembered saccades) (Leigh and Zee, 1999). Gaze fixation evaluates the ability to hold the eyes in a fixed direction of gaze without drifting off the target, typically straight ahead, to the right and left, and up and down. Gaze fixation provides general suggestions of brainstem/cerebellar involvement in most instances of abnormal results. More specific indications for particular nuclei involvement in the brainstem can be made with certain types of abnormalities.

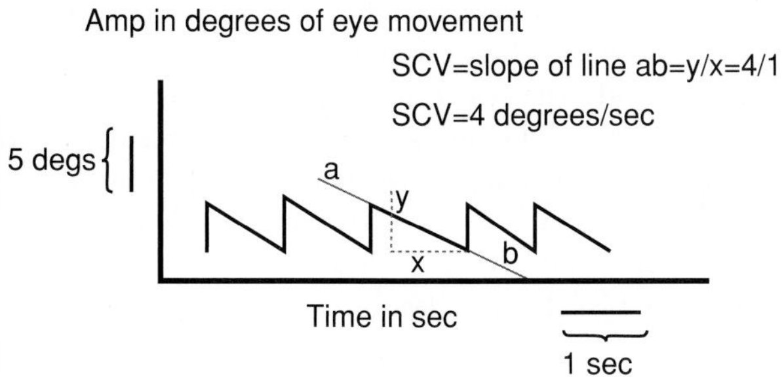

Specific abnormalities of fixation, referred to as saccade intrusions, can be indicative of a variety of possible brainstem and cerebellar disorders (Leigh and Zee, 1999). Optokinetic stimulation measures jerk nystagmus eye movements created by repeated objects moving across the subject's visual field and filling at least 80% of the visual field. Optokinetic stimulation is the least sensitive, probably due to the combination of both smooth pursuit and saccade systems allowing the optokinetic nystagmus to be generated by a combination of foveal and peripheral retinal stimulation. At present, it best serves as a cross check, with significant abnormalities seen during pursuit or saccade testing. Be aware that, with a typical light bar stimulus for optokinetic testing, most of the time it amounts to another form of smooth pursuit testing (foveal optokinetic task) and not true optokinetic testing. Typical recordings and analysis of smooth pursuit and reactionary saccade testing are illustrated in Figures 20.5 and 20.6.

FIGURE 20.4 Right-beating nystagmus is illustrated along with the calculation of slow-component eye velocity (SCV), the slope of the line (ab). As discussed in the text, upward trace deflections represent rightward eye movement with downward indicating leftward eye movement.

SPONTANEOUS NYSTAGMUS

This test is performed with the patient sitting with head straight and eyes closed. The purpose is to record eye movements when visual fixation is removed, without any provocative head movements or positions. Jerk nystagmus is the principal abnormality of interest in most situations. Other forms of abnormal eye movements, such as pendular nystagmus

FIGURE 20.5 Shown is an example of smooth pursuit eye movement recording with the target at 0.71 Hz. Shown in the top panel is a plot of horizontal eye position as a function of time (500 msec time mark shown) for sinusoidal tracking (*dotted trace*). In the same plot (*smooth line*) the target position in degrees as a function of time is given. The panel below the eye and target position plots gives the value of velocity gain as a function of frequency of target movement. The shaded region represents abnormal performance.

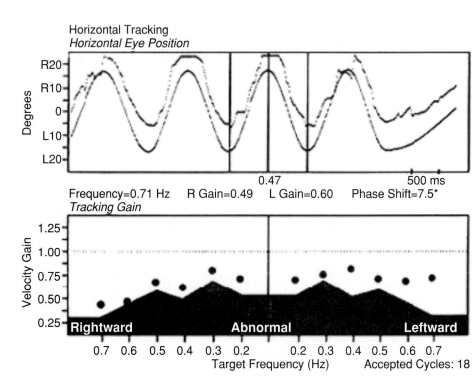

Horizontal Tracking
Horizontal Eye Position

Frequency=0.71 Hz   R Gain=0.49   L Gain=0.60   Phase Shift=7.5*
Tracking Gain

Target Frequency (Hz)   Accepted Cycles: 18

(sinusoidal horizontal repeating eye movements, no distinguishable slow and fast components), may be seen. Clinically significant, direction-fixed nystagmus is interpreted to indicate possible pathology within the peripheral vestibular system if the ocular motor evaluation is normal (Fig. 20.3 A). Care in interpretation is needed because spontaneous nystagmus can also be seen in migraine and anxiety disorders (Furman et al., 2005).

HEAD SHAKE NYSTAGMUS

This protocol is commonly associated with the direct office examination but can be usefully incorporated as part of the ENG/VNG (Walker and Zee, 2000). This is performed by the use of reciprocal horizontal head movements at 3 to 4 Hz for 10 seconds with fixation removed. When the head is brought to a stop, recording of eye movements is continued long enough to capture nystagmus that had been provoked or no nystagmus if the test is negative. The presence of three or more horizontal nystagmus beats is suggestive of a peripheral asymmetry. In most cases, the direction of the fast component of the nystagmus is way from a paretic lesion; however, this is not always the case, and the nystagmus may beat toward the lesion side. Vertical nystagmus resulting from the horizontal head shake is a positive sign for brainstem and/or cerebellar involvement and is referred to as cross-coupling nystagmus. Although the sensitivity for identification of peripheral involvement is reported to be only fair, the ease of the test and its short time for execution make it very reasonable to add to the ENG battery (Jacobson et al., 1990).

HYPERVENTILATION NYSTAGMUS

Another of the office examination tools that can be easily and effectively used during an ENG/VNG protocol is the hyperventilation nystagmus test. The use of hyperventilation testing has a dual purpose. First, the identification of this type of nystagmus is suggestive of eighth cranial nerve involvement on the side to which the fast component of the

Slope of this part of the
eye trace = Velocity of Saccade

Target   Eye movement

B   A

Latency to onset

$$Accuracy = 100 \times \frac{A}{B}$$

FIGURE 20.6 Schematic of eye and target position in degrees, as a function of time, demonstrating the calculations of velocity, latency, and accuracy of the saccade eye movement for analysis. The three parameters of velocity, latency, and accuracy are then used to characterize the patient's performance. (Reprinted with permission from Shepard NT, Telian SA. [1996] *Practical Management of the Balance Disorder Patient.* San Diego: Singular Publishing Group).

nystagmus is directed. The nystagmus (recovery nystagmus) results from the absence of myelin from a section of the nerve. Often, this is secondary to a demyelination process from disease or a mass lesion (Minor et al., 1999). The second use is to identify an individual more likely to be experiencing an anxiety disorder. This is recognized by the production of symptoms of lightheadedness/imbalance within 30 seconds of starting the hyperventilation, with no nystagmus visualized by the completion of 1 minute of hyperventilation. Hyperventilation is more likely to provoke dizziness, lightheadedness, autonomic symptoms, and acute anxiety attacks in patients with certain anxiety disorders than in the general population (Papp et al., 1993). It also may provoke lightheadedness and autonomic arousal without significant anxiety in patients with autonomic dysfunction (e.g., hyperventilation syndrome) (Han et al., 1998). Anxiety disorders or dysautonomia should be suspected in patients who experience a marked reproduction of their symptoms, without nystagmus, during hyperventilation (Staab et al., 2002a).

DIX-HALLPIKE MANEUVER

This well-known test is used primarily to elicit evidence for benign paroxysmal positional vertigo (BPPV). Because BPPV typically involves a single canal at a time, the description of the nystagmus is critical to identification of the canal involved. Each canal has an individual and unique eye movement signature that can be used to recognize which canal is causing this disorder (Herdman and Tusa, 2000). In the variants of BPPV, only the horizontal canal variant does not have torsional eye movement; all others involve torsional movements and, therefore, cannot be accurately recorded with standard electro-oculography or video-oculography systems, as both are two dimensional in the printed output (see earlier discussion).

The Dix-Hallpike maneuver (Fig. 20.7) is also typically part of the standard ENG/VNG protocol. Classically, positive Dix-Hallpike responses produce a complex nystagmus with torsional (roll plane) and vertical components as dominant. There is also a minor yaw plane component in the majority of the classic posterior canal responses. The fast component of the torsional aspect of the nystagmus is directed toward the involved ear (left torsional for left ear and right torsional for right ear, from the patient's perspective, relative to the superior pole of the eye; this may not always be the underneath ear). To adequately detect this action, the movements must be viewed by the examiner (directly or with video equipment), and not reviewed after the fact by two-dimensional recordings from standard surface electrode or standard video-recording techniques. This may require the examiner to turn on the lights and visualize the patient's eyes during the maneuver when using the ENG technique. Fixation suppression in this situation is not a problem because the central nervous system does not have a fixation-suppression system for torsional nystagmus and the fixation-suppression system is not effective on sudden bursts of pitch or yaw plane

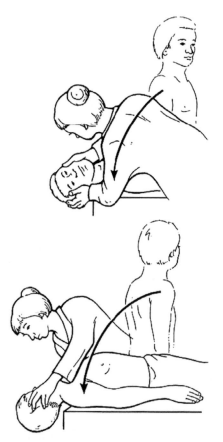

FIGURE 20.7 Illustrations of the technique for the Dix-Hallpike maneuver, for right side (*top*) and left side (*bottom*). Note that the patient's eyes are open and fixating on the examiner. (Reprinted with permission from Shepard NT, Telian SA. [1996] *Practical Management of the Balance Disorder Patient*. San Diego: Singular Publishing Group).

nystagmus (Leigh and Zee, 1999). Therefore, the eyes can be viewed directly when Frenzel lenses or video recording equipment is not available.

POSITIONAL NYSTAGMUS

Positional nystagmus is the most common abnormality noted with ENG evaluation. In this study, the patient is moved slowly into stationary positions. The eye movements are monitored as in the spontaneous nystagmus test and should be done without visual fixation (Fig. 20.3, B–D). The more common positions include: sitting head turned right, sitting head turned left, supine, supine head turned left, supine head turned right, right decubitus (right side), left decubitus (left side), and preirrigation position (head and shoulders elevated by 30 degrees up from the horizontal plane). In cases where no cervical region injuries or active pathologies are reported, use of head hanging (neck hyperextended) straight, right, and left adds three additional positions for testing prior to the preirrigation position. The purpose of this subtest is to investigate the effect of different head positions within the gravitational field. Positional nystagmus is typically classified by the direction of the fast component of the nystagmus but measured by the velocity of the slow component. It may be either direction-fixed (always beating in the same direction) or direction-changing (both right- and left-beating nystagmus observed during the exam). Direction-changing nystagmus may be subclassified, when appropriate, into geotropic (toward the pull of gravity, toward the underneath ear) or ageotropic (away from the pull of gravity, away from the underneath ear).

The clinical interpretation of positional nystagmus is taken as indicative of peripheral system involvement (with two notable exceptions), as long as the ocular-motor studies, done in a thorough manner (i.e., requiring a computerized system) are normal. The exceptions to this situation are: (1) when the direction-changing nystagmus is observed while the patient remains in one head position, that is, without a change in gravitational orientation; and (2) if persistent down-beating vertical nystagmus is noted with no horizontal component. These are typically interpreted as indicative of central pathway involvement (usually low posterior fossa), independent of the ocular motor results, unless an alternative explanation is apparent. If spontaneous, direction-fixed nystagmus is present and no significant change in that nystagmus (average slow-component velocity) is noted, then the nystagmus in the positions is taken as a reflection of the spontaneous findings and not considered as positional. This situation would suggest little or no influence of the otolith organs in the modulation or generation of the nystagmus but would not otherwise alter the general interpretation of peripheral system involvement, assuming normal ocular motor studies.

Since positional nystagmus can be produced by central or peripheral lesions, the presence of abnormal ocular motor studies (the most sensitive test indication of central nervous system involvement) precludes the use of positional nystagmus as an indicator of peripheral system lesion. Clinical significance of the positional nystagmus is typically determined by a combination of the number of positions in which it is present and the velocity range of the slow component of the nystagmus. One suggested set of criteria based on studies of presence of positional nystagmus in a normal population is listed below (Barber and Stockwell, 1980).

- Slow-component eye velocity (SCV) >5 degrees/second
- SCV <6 degrees/second—persistent nystagmus in four or more of the 8 to 11 positions
- SCV <6 degrees/second—sporadic in all positions tested
- Direction-changing within a given head position

Two other conditions that can produce positional nystagmus without ocular-motor abnormalities must be considered before peripheral system involvement is suggested. Migraine headache conditions can produce these findings, in addition to mild caloric asymmetries (Cutrer and Baloh,

1992; Johnson, 1998; Furman et al., 2003). No particular patterns of positional nystagmus are indicative of migraine. Since migraines and dizziness related to migraine are diagnoses of exclusion, it is important to keep this in mind if the total presentation of the patient is not convincing for peripheral system involvement. Anxiety disorders are somewhat less well documented in producing positional eye movement abnormalities. The most commonly recognized eye movements associated with anxiety, especially related to the testing process causing symptoms, are macro-square wave jerks (square waves of 5- to 15-degree subtended arc with normal intersaccade intervals) (Leigh and Zee, 1999). This type of intrusion saccade is noted only with fixation removed. Classic positional jerk nystagmus of a direction-fixed or direction-changing nature can also be provoked by anxiety disorders (Papp et al., 1993).

CALORIC IRRIGATIONS

The caloric test is the study that is most likely to lateralize a peripheral lesion with objective, repeatable eye movement data. The stimulus employed is nonphysiologic compared to the normal function of the system during head motion, where one side is stimulated and the other is simultaneously inhibited. Nevertheless, the caloric test is the only portion of the test battery that provides a measure of unilateral labyrinthine function but does so only for the horizontal canal.

The three primary delivery methods for caloric irrigations are: closed-loop water (circulates water in a thin latex balloon that expands in the external auditory canal); open-loop water (water runs into the external auditory canal and drains out); or air flow. During any of the methods, the fluid or air is set at temperatures above or below that of the body; typically, temperatures of 44°C for warm and 30°C for cool are used for the open-loop water systems. All are reasonably reliable when the tympanic membrane is intact. When tympanic perforations or short ventilation tubes are present, the closed-loop water irrigation method is preferable. Summarizing studies in both terrestrial and weightless environments, there appear to be at least two mechanisms operating to produce the caloric VOR response to the temperature changes. The one that seems to predominate in routine testing involves gravity and the density changes that occur in the endolymph of the horizontal canal when it is heated or cooled (density decreased or increased, respectively). The head is positioned so that the horizontal canal is oriented parallel to the gravitational vector, with the nose of the patient upward and the head tilted 30 degrees upward from the horizontal plane. During a warm irrigation, the less dense fluid of the horizontal canal endolymphatic space attempts to rise upward. Since the fluid cannot flow around the canal secondary to the cupula, the change in fluid density results in a pressure differential across the cupula that produces a deviation of the cupula toward the utricle, causing stimulation of the horizontal canal. The reverse action

TABLE 20.3   Formulas for the calculation of reduced vestibular response and directional

Preponderance

Reduced Vestibular Response (RVR) = {[(RW + RC) – (LW + LC)]/(RW + RC + LW + LC)} × 100%

Directional Preponderance (DP) = {[(RW + LC) – (LW + RC)]/(RW + RC + LW + LC)} × 100%

RW, right warm; RC, right cool; LW, left warm; LC, left cool.

occurs for the more dense area of cooled fluid, causing inhibition. These reactions result in the well-known mnemonic "COWS," which refers to the direction of the fast component of the nystagmus: Cold Opposite, Warm Same (relative to the side of irrigation).

The traditional interpretation of caloric stimulation uses a relative comparison of maximum, average slow-component eye velocity on the right versus the left (see Table 20.3 for Jongkee's formulas) (Fitzgerald and Hallpike, 1942). These values are used to provide a percent comparison of response magnitude (reduced vestibular response) and direction bias of eye movement (directional preponderance) (Fig. 20.8). Although four irrigations are typical, there are

situations where "ice water" (4°C) is used and other situations where only two irrigations of either warm or cool are sufficient (Shepard and Telian, 1996; Jacobson et al., 1995). Directional preponderance is interpreted as a bias in the central system, making it easier to produce nystagmus in one direction than another. This bias most often is a result of asymmetrical peripheral function, for which the central compensation process is incomplete, and less likely a result of a central system lesion.

Since the peripheral vestibular system functions across a frequency range, it is reasonable to question what portion of that range a caloric response occupies. The equivalent angular acceleration response falls in the lower frequency range

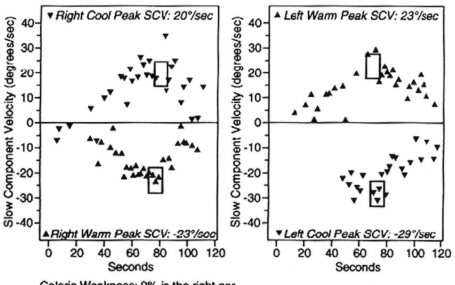

Caloric Weakness: 9% in the right ear
Directional Preponderance: 9% to the right

FIGURE 20.8 Plots of slow-component eye velocity (SCV) from nystagmus provoked by open-loop water irrigations as a function of time. Each *triangle* represents one SCV movement of the eye from the nystagmus trace. Responses for the right ear are shown on the left, those for the left ear are shown on the right. The orientation of the triangles represent either cool (30°C), ▼, or warm (44°C), ▲, irrigations. The plots are arranged so that right-beating nystagmus SCVs are on the bottom (right warm, left cool) and left beating nystagmus SCVs are on the top (right cool, left warm). The velocity values given in the top or bottom of each plot represent the average maximum SCV calculated for the nystagmus beats within the rectangle shown on each plot. These maximum, average SCV values were used to calculate the caloric weakness and directional preponderance values shown at the bottom of the figure. Nine percent in the right ear means a 9% weaker response on the right compared to the left. Nine percent to the right means a 9% greater response for right-beating nystagmus compared to left-beating nystagmus. For purposes of calculation, rightward SCVs are assigned a negative number, and leftward SCVs are assigned a positive number. (Reprinted with permission from Shepard NT, Telian SA. [1996] *Practical Management of the Balance Disorder Patient.* San Diego: Singular Publishing Group).

of response of the system (0.002 to 0.004 Hz). Therefore, absence of a caloric response to warm, cool, or ice water irrigations cannot be taken as an indication of complete lack of function. Testing by rotational chair evaluation is the tool needed to help define the true extent of a bilateral peripheral vestibular system lesion.

Rotational Chair–Sinusoidal Harmonic Acceleration

Rotary chair testing has been used to expand the evaluation of the peripheral vestibular system. As with the ENG/VNG findings, the rotational chair evaluation can assist in site-of-lesion determination, counseling the patient, and confirmation of clinical suspicion of diagnosis and lesion site, but it is not likely to significantly alter or have an impact on the course of patient management, except in the bilateral peripheral weakness patient (discussed below).

Suggested criteria for when chair testing may be of clinical use is given below (Shepard and Telian, 1996; Ruckenstein and Shepard, 2000).

- When the ENG is normal and ocular-motor results are either normal or observed abnormalities would not invalidate rotational chair results. Chair testing is used here to expand the investigation of peripheral system involvement and compensation status.
- When the ENG suggests a well-compensated status (no spontaneous or positional nystagmus), despite the presence of a clinically significant unilateral caloric weakness and ongoing symptom complaints. Chair testing is used here to expand the investigation of compensation in a patient with a known lesion site and complaints suggesting poor compensation.
- When warm and cool caloric irrigations are below 10°/s bilaterally, when caloric irrigations cannot be performed, or when results in the two ears may not be compared reliably due to anatomic variability. Chair testing is used in these cases to verify and define the extent of a bilateral weakness or to further investigate the relative responsiveness of the peripheral vestibular apparatus in each ear when caloric studies are unreliable or unavailable.
- When a baseline is needed to follow the natural history of the patient's disorder (such as possible early Ménière's disease) or for assessing the effectiveness of a particular treatment, like that of chemical ablation of one or both peripheral vestibular systems.

A review of 2,266 patients (Shepard and Telian, 1996) was used to investigate the clinical utility of rotary chair testing in the evaluation of the peripheral vestibular system. Among this group of patients, 16% had completely normal ENG studies. Among those with normal ENG results, rotary chair testing indicated abnormalities suggesting peripheral system involvement in 80% of the cases. Patients with only positional nystagmus were reviewed, with greater than 80%

having abnormalities from rotary chair testing supporting peripheral system involvement. In all cases of bilateral caloric weakness, the chair findings confirmed the bilateral reduction in peripheral system function. The test further defined the extent of the lesion as mild in half of these patients and moderate to severe in the other half. This additional information plays an important role in designing a vestibular rehabilitation program for these patients. It is in the bilateral patient that rotational chair testing can have a direct impact on the management course in a rehabilitation program. There are also patients who, for reasons other than vestibular dysfunction, have mildly reduced caloric responses. Of these patients, greater than 90% had normal rotary chair responses, suggesting that indications of bilateral paresis were false-positive findings or that the extent of the bilateral lesions was mild and restricted to only the very low frequency range of function. Rotational chair is the only tool currently available for defining the extent of a suspected bilateral peripheral lesion.

Patients diagnosed with Ménière's disease, labyrinthitis, or vestibular neuritis by clinical presentation and hearing test results, independent of balance function test results, numbered 311 during the period of this study (Shepard and Telian, 1996). Of this group, ENG was abnormal in 90%, suggesting a test sensitivity of this value. Rotary chair had a sensitivity suggesting peripheral system involvement of only 66%. However, it is important to note that the 66% of patients identified by chair testing did not completely overlap with those identified by ENG, as the combination of ENG and chair testing had a sensitivity of 100% in this group. Since there is no objective gold standard for identification of balance system lesions, there is currently no way to develop specificity figures, that is, the percentage of patients who do not have peripheral or central system abnormalities who will have normal test results. There is also no good means for developing accurate sensitivity figures. Therefore, the above group of 311 patients was well advanced in their respective disorders, and clearly the use of ENG and rotary chair together does not have a sensitivity of 100%. A better estimate would be in the 80% range based on the clinical diagnosis breakdown of the 2,266 patients.

From this discussion, there appears to be good support for obtaining, in a subgroup of patients, the adjunctive information available from total-body, low-frequency rotary chair testing in the investigation of peripheral vestibular system function.

As with the ENG/VNG test, the protocols for rotational chair testing are not new, and some have been used for well over a century. When considering the use of the chair protocols, it is important to remember that the peripheral vestibular systems have a "push-pull" arrangement, such that if one side is stimulated with angular or linear acceleration, the opposite side is inhibited in its neural activity. Therefore, the chair is not a tool that can be used to isolate one peripheral system from the other for evaluation, as each stimulus affects both sides simultaneously.

Electro-oculography or video-oculography can be used to monitor and record the outcome measure of interest—jerk nystagmus that is generated in response to the angular chair acceleration stimulus. The VOR is the slow component of the jerk nystagmus and, as with ENG/VNG, is the portion of the eye movement for which velocity is calculated for analysis.

It must be remembered that, with total body rotational testing, the stimulus is being delivered to the head via movement of the whole body. Thus, the head must be secured to the chair with a restraint system (Fig. 20.9). To make analysis as simple as possible, it is assumed that, whenever the chair moves, the head is also making the same movement. Because of the potential for movement of the skin relative to the skull, this assumption becomes faulty at frequencies greater than 1 Hz. Because of this, most commercial systems and clinical research have restricted test frequencies to 1 Hz or less. Shown in Figure 20.9 is a generic chair system, consisting of a chair on a computer-controlled electric torque motor. The head is held firmly to the chair, and the system is in an enclosure to allow for testing in darkness with the eyes open.

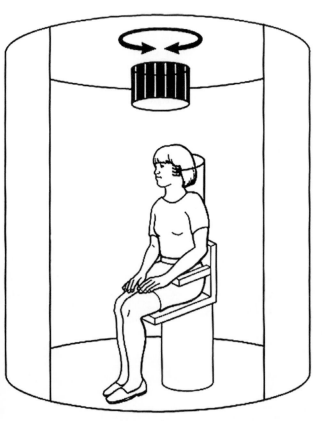

FIGURE 20.9 Generic rotational chair setup. The chair is on a computer-controlled motor within an enclosure and can be rotated in either direction. A device for holding the head to the chair is shown. A means for producing optokinetic stimulation is shown as the drum in the ceiling. (Reprinted with permission from Shepard NT, Telian SA. [1996] *Practical Management of the Balance Disorder Patient.* **San Diego: Singular Publishing Group).**

Means for providing visual stimuli, such as an optokinetic stimulus, are standard.

SINUSOIDAL ROTATION

Typically, starting with the lower frequencies, the chair is stimulated with sinusoidal waveforms at a specific frequency from 0.01 to 1 Hz. Signal averaging is used in order to improve the signal-to-noise ratio and thereby improve the reliability and validity of the analysis. Multiple cycles of a given frequency are delivered, stimulating repetitive to-and-fro movement of the chair in a sinusoidal harmonic acceleration paradigm. The slow-component eye velocity response from each cycle of stimulation is added to subsequent responses and divided by the number of cycles used, providing an average response for the test frequency. The frequency is then changed, and the process is repeated. Ideally, the more cycles that can be averaged, the more reliable the signal is. Pragmatically, the number of cycles needs to be considered in light of the period (length of time for a single cycle) of the stimulus. Because the period at 0.01 Hz is 100 seconds, to do more than three cycles becomes prohibitive. Unfortunately, the very low frequencies (<0.08 Hz) produce the weakest response from the VOR and, therefore, have the poorest signal-to-noise ratio. In general, the very low frequencies are also most likely to produce unpleasant neurovegetative symptoms such as nausea. The frequencies from 0.16 Hz and above can be completed quickly, allowing responses from as many as 10 cycles to be averaged. For all frequencies tested, the peak chair velocity is typically fixed at 50 to 60°/s. Therefore, as the frequency is increased, the subject experiences increasing acceleration with decreasing excursion of the chair.

Three parameters are measured during rotational chair testing to characterize the function of the VOR and thereby evaluate the function of the peripheral vestibular system. These parameters are phase, gain, and asymmetry. Figure 20.10 shows a schematized version of an averaged slow-component velocity response from multiple cycles of stimulation at a single frequency. The chair velocity is also shown, which correlates to head velocity, assuming the head is properly stabilized. The parameters that characterize VOR function are developed by comparing the slow-component eye velocity profile to the head velocity profile.

Phase

This parameter of the VOR is the least intuitive of the three but has the greatest clinical significance due to its ability to indicate peripheral system dysfunction. Phase measurements objectify the timing relationship between head movement and reflex eye movement. Figure 20.10 illustrates findings expected from a normally functioning VOR system at test frequencies below 0.16 Hz. Under these circumstances, the compensatory eye movements can lead the head movement, as shown in Figure 20.10. The amount of this phase lead is called the phase angle and is typically measured in degrees. The center panel of Figure 20.11 shows a plot of phase angle

SINUSOIDAL HARMONIC ACCELERATION TESTING

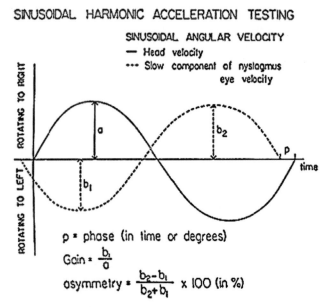

FIGURE 20.10 This figure shows pictorial and formulated definitions of the three major parameters used for analyzing sinusoidal harmonic acceleration testing. See text for further details.

versus frequency of rotation in a patient with normal rotary chair findings. The phase results can be used to calculate the system time constant from any frequency tested; however, assumptions can be applied that significantly simplify the calculations if the frequencies are restricted to 0.04 Hz and below (Baloh and Honrubia, 1990). In general, in this restricted frequency range, the relationship between phase angle and time constant is an inverse proportion. As phase angle increases, time constant decreases.

As seen in the center panel of Figure 20.11, the normal range for phase (based on two standard deviations above and below the mean) is indicated by the clear area. An increase in the phase lead outside this range implies an abnormally low time constant. From experimental studies of the velocity storage integrator (vestibular nucleus region) that regulates the VOR system time constant, we know that damage to the labyrinth or the vestibular portion of the eighth cranial nerve causes a decrease in the time constant. Hence, increased phase lead, implying an abnormally low time constant, strongly suggests pathology in the peripheral system. One caution in this interpretation is that damage in the vestibular nuclei within the brainstem may also result in an abnormally low time constant. Therefore, other clinical information is needed to help localize the lesion to the labyrinth or eighth nerve. The significance of an abnormally low phase lead (abnormally high time constant) may suggest a lesion in the nodulus region of the cerebellum, an area that influences the velocity storage integrator in the brainstem (Waespe et al., 1985).

Gain

The second parameter of the VOR measured in rotary chair testing is gain (eye velocity divided by head velocity; Fig. 20.10). Gain measures give an indication of the overall responsiveness of the system. Unilateral peripheral weaknesses can cause a mild reduction in gain, especially at the lowest frequencies. However, the principle clinical use of gain measures is to define the extent of a bilateral reduction in peripheral system responsiveness. The gain value and the magnitude of the phase lead help to verify that severely reduced or absent responses to caloric irrigations accurately reflect a bilateral weakness and do not result from an artifact of alertness or

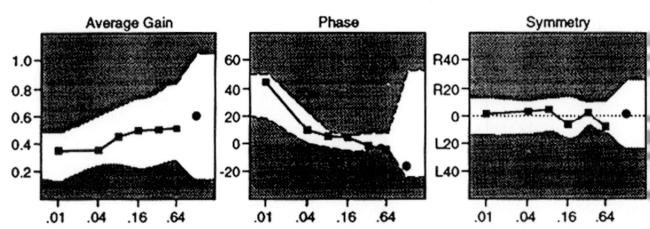

FIGURE 20.11 Normal rotary chair results from a patient. The plot on the left shows gain (eye velocity divided by head velocity) as a function of frequency of chair sinusoidal stimulation. The center plot shows phase angle in degrees as a function of frequency, and the plot to the right gives symmetry data in percentage as a function of frequency. The darkened areas represent the abnormal performance based on a two standard deviation above and below the mean. (Reprinted with permission from Shepard NT, Telian SA. [1996] *Practical Management of the Balance Disorder Patient.* San Diego: Singular Publishing Group).

some other test pitfall. The panel on the left in Figure 20.11 shows normal results for gain as a function of sinusoidal frequency stimulation.

Asymmetry

In Figure 20.10, the schematic representation of asymmetry involves a comparison between the slow-component eye velocity to the right (positive values) compared to the left (negative values). It is important to recognize that these values are calculated and named by the direction of the eye movement that is produced by the VOR, that is, the slow component. The situation is reversed when discussing directional preponderance from caloric irrigations. Directional preponderance values are calculated by slow-component velocity but, by convention, are named by the direction of the fast component of the nystagmus. Therefore, a patient who exhibits a right-beating directional preponderance (left slow-component velocity greater than right slow-component velocity) may show a left asymmetry on rotational chair testing, indicating that, during chair testing, left slow-component velocity was greater than right slow-component velocity. These results are consistent with the directional preponderance. Directional preponderance and asymmetry from chair testing will not always both be abnormal. Both directional preponderance (caloric testing) and asymmetry (rotary chair testing) give an indication of bias within the system, favoring larger slow-component velocities in one direction versus the other. A bias usually results from a peripheral lesion with incomplete dynamic compensation in the central nervous system. Less commonly, it may indicate the presence of an uncompensated lesion in the central pathways. Whenever a VOR asymmetry is noted on rotary chair testing, the finding may be due to abnormalities in either peripheral system, either a peripheral weakness on the side of the stronger slow-component velocity response or an irritative lesion on the opposite side. For example, a patient with an uncompensated right peripheral weakness will generally demonstrate a right greater than left slow-component velocity asymmetry. This is due to an ability to produce a greater rightward compensatory eye movement when rotated toward the intact left side and a less intense leftward compensatory eye movement response after rotation toward the weaker right side. The right panel in Figure 20.11 shows a normal result for the asymmetry measurement.

STEP TEST

This protocol is performed, as in the sinusoidal case, with the test booth in total darkness. A fixed chair velocity between 60 and 240°/sec is achieved by applying an acceleration impulse with a magnitude near 100°/s^2. Once the desired velocity is reached, the acceleration is returned to 0°/s^2, and the patient continues at the desired velocity. The VOR response to the initial acceleration stimulus is known as per-rotary nystagmus. The slow-component eye velocity intensity decays over time if the chair velocity is constant, and the subject

falsely perceives that the chair is slowing down. The decay in slow-component eye velocity over time can be utilized to estimate the system's "time constant," a parameter that characterizes the timing relationship between the head movement and subsequent eye movement response (see interpretation below). After 45 to 60 seconds of fixed-velocity rotation, a second impulse is applied to the chair. This is a deceleration step, usually of equal magnitude to the initial acceleration, bringing the chair to a rapid stop. Although the chair is now stationary, the subject will perceive motion in the opposite direction. The VOR response will produce nystagmus beating in the direction opposite to that produced by the initial acceleration, known as postrotary nystagmus. The decay of the slow-component eye velocity over time should be similar to that seen after the acceleration impulse, and ideally, both should give similar estimates of the system's time constant. The entire procedure is then repeated with the initial rotation in the opposite direction. Realize that, if the initial acceleration is clockwise, then the right horizontal canal is stimulated and the left is inhibited for the per-rotary response. When the sudden deceleration is applied for the sudden stop, the left horizontal canal is stimulated and the right is inhibited. This entire situation would then reverse when the initial rotation is counterclockwise.

The information about gain and asymmetry obtained from this protocol is available for constant velocity steps at low velocities (60°/s) and high velocities (240°/s). In the uncompensated peripheral lesion, both the low- and high-velocity steps may demonstrate asymmetry in gain values. In the case of the compensated unilateral hypofunction case, only the high-velocity step usually results in gain asymmetries. For estimating the time constant, the most reliable value is that obtained from the low-velocity step. At the high-velocity step, the time constant is typically a lower estimate. The results of either the low- or high-velocity step are heavily influenced by the noise in both the recording and physiologic systems and by the arousal of the patient prior to the acceleration, as averaging is not used in this paradigm. As a result, there will be patients for whom the estimates of time constant from the two protocols do not agree. Ideally, the step test and the sinusoidal acceleration tests can be used in parallel to increase the accuracy of estimates of the system time constant, individual periphery gains from the step procedure, and overall gain from the sinusoidal protocol, with possible asymmetrical peripheral responsiveness. For further detailed descriptions of the chair test, the reader is referred to previously published literature (Wall, 1990; Baloh and Honrubia, 1990; Stockwell and Bojarb, 1993a; 1993b; Shepard, 2000b).

Otolith Function Testing

Only recently have tools for the investigation of the otolithic organs, the utricle and saccule, begun to appear in more frequent clinical use. As with ENG/VNG, rotational chair, and postural control assessment (see below), a full discussion of this area is beyond the scope of the chapter. Therefore, the reader is referred to other existing literature for a more detailed discussion of techniques and possible clinical uses (see references in following sections discussing the utricle and saccule). Since this area of investigation is relatively new for routine clinical use, the full extent of clinical utilization is still not clearly established. For organizational simplicity, the two otolith organs will be considered separately.

UTRICULAR EVALUATION

The primary technique for attempting to assess the function of the utricle is a test of subjective visual vertical (SVV). The principle underlying this test is that a subject's ability to set a projected line to true vertical is due to the detection of the pull of gravity, primarily via the utricles. If a pathologic insult disrupts the peripheral functioning of the utricular organ or the central utricular pathways, a resulting change in the position of the eye in regards to the true horizontal occurs, along with a static ocular counter roll. In the acute interval (2 to 8 weeks) following disruption to the utricle or its central pathways, the individual will set the line off vertical, tilted in the direction of the ocular counter roll. However, as the acute phase of the lesion passes, the individual's performance returns to normal (Vibert et al., 1999). Attempts at the use of rotational chair paradigms and conflicting visual backgrounds to defeat the quick return to normal and allow for a longer term investigation of the utricular system have been investigated. The interested reader is referred to literature providing descriptions of the various techniques and investigations on patients (Bohmer and Mast, 1999; Vibert et al., 1999; Clark et al., 2003; Pavlou et al., 2003).

SACCULAR EVALUATION

The vestibular evoked myogenic potential (VEMP) test takes advantage of the saccule being responsive to pressure waves, like the auditory system, in addition to linear acceleration. The ability to stimulate this receptor organ with sound allows for investigation of the saccule via the vestibulocolic pathways (reflexive activity of cervical region musculature in response to stimulation of the vestibular system with angular or linear stimulation; see Chapter 19). The technique allows for individual investigation of the each saccule by monitoring the electromyographic (EMG) activity of the ipsilateral sternocleidomastoid (SCM) muscle. It is important to know that the response being recorded in response to a brief intense acoustic stimulus is a release from contraction of the SCM. In general, the technique uses surface electrodes, one over the central area of the SCM referenced commonly to the manubrium of the sternum, with a common on the forehead. The SCM ipsilateral to the saccule to be stimulated is placed into contraction by positioning of the head or head movement against resistance, and a click or low-frequency (<1 kHz) tone burst is delivered to the ear at sound levels at or above 85 dB normal hearing level (nHL). Using averaging, as in the auditory brainstem response (see Chapter 11), a biphasic electrical response representing a release from con-

traction, temporally synchronized to the acoustic presentation, is developed with 75 to 150 acoustic presentations. This technique has many variations in stimuli and contraction methodology, without an accepted standard procedure at the time of this writing (Cheng et al., 2003; Colbatch and Halmagyi, 1992; Halmagyi and Colbatch, 1995; Li et al., 1999).

A number of investigative reports have been published within the last 5 years that provide for a wide range of clinical uses. Given the involvement of the saccule in Ménière's disease (or the more general category of endolymphatic hydrops), some of the current investigative work has focused on the use of the VEMP in relationship to Ménière's (Rauch et al., 2004). Additionally, a major use of the VEMP has been in the identification of superior semicircular canal dehiscence. A characteristic, abnormally low threshold for the VEMP response has been consistently found in this form of perilymphatic fistula, which can be used as diagnostic criteria (in addition to a low-frequency conductive hearing loss that is not of middle ear origin) to proceed on to the definitive special high-resolution CT investigation (Streubel et al., 2001).

Although investigations continue to better define the clinical uses of the VEMP, what is clear is that it represents an independent measure of a portion of the vestibular labyrinth separate from that of the caloric test. It also provides for the only specific, clinically routine test of the inferior division of the vestibular portion of the eighth cranial nerve. A significant body of literature is developing around the use of the VEMP test, in addition to the few salient references provided in this section, to which the interested reader is referred.

Postural Control Assessment

Just as all patients who are being evaluated in the laboratory need tests for peripheral and central vestibulo-ocular pathway involvement, they also require some assessment of postural control ability. However, just as in the use of ENG and rotational chair, not all patients need high-tech, formal postural control assessment. There are several different general approaches to formal postural control testing, each with specific technical equipment requirements and goals for the testing (Shepard and Telian, 1996; Monsell et al., 1997; Allum and Shepard, 1999; Jacobson and Shephard, 2008). To reduce the scope of this discussion, comments will be restricted to the most common formal assessment tool used in the United States, which is CDP as formulated in the EquiTest equipment described in detail elsewhere (Shepard et al., 1993a; Nashner, 1993a; 1993b; 1993c). Briefly, the equipment detects vertical and horizontal forces from the feet by two independent force plates upon which the subject stands. The force plates can be made to translate forward or backward and rotate toes up or down to provoke movement of the subject's center of mass. The rotation movements can also be stimulated by the subject's own movements to create information from the ankle that is inaccurate. The visual surround can also be made to move, stimulated by the subject's movements or independent of subject activity. Two principle testing protocols (discussed later) are used in patient evaluation. The first is the sensory organization test (SOT), using patient-stimulated floor and visual surround movements. The second, using the translation and rotations of the support surface to cause subject movements, is called the motor control test (MCT).

As with rotational chair testing, suggested guidelines can and have been developed to decide for a given patient when full CDP would be most clinically useful. The decision to use CDP is based on the same core set of studies used in deciding about the rotational chair, with the addition of a postural control screening test that approximates the SOT protocol of the CDP. The screening test, called the Clinical Test of Sensory Interaction in Balance (CTSIB) (Shumway-Cook and Horak, 1986), has been shown to accurately screen for those patients who have the highest probability of showing abnormalities on SOT (El-Kashlan et al., 1998). The current modified CTSIB used for this purpose is described in detail elsewhere (Shepard and Telian, 1996). Briefly, the CTSIB uses time as an outcome measure and approximates SOT conditions 1, 2, 4, and 5 (conditions of the SOT test are described in Fig. 20.12) by the use of a foam

cushion to disrupt foot support surface cues. Therefore, based on the results of the CTSIB and the patient's full neurotologic history, CDP would be called for under the following conditions:

- If the CTSIB was abnormal with a fall reaction, significantly increased sway, or a sudden change of strategy for maintaining stance during a trial. Based on the comparison between CTSIB and dynamic posturography, we know that the patient who can perform CTSIB in the normal range is very unlikely to fail the sensory organization portion of dynamic posturography. On the other hand, dynamic posturography is needed to further delineate postural control difficulties when abnormal performance is noted on the CTSIB.
- If the patient has a major complaint involving unsteadiness when standing or walking, independent of the CTSIB results. Dynamic posturography, especially the MCT, is used in this case to further investigate postural control. This patient would also be a candidate for postural evoked response testing, a third special protocol that can be used with CDP in conjunction with lower limb EMG recording, described later.
- If the patient had a history of known pathology involving the postural control pathways that may influence the patient's overall performance, even though unsteadiness is not a major complaint.

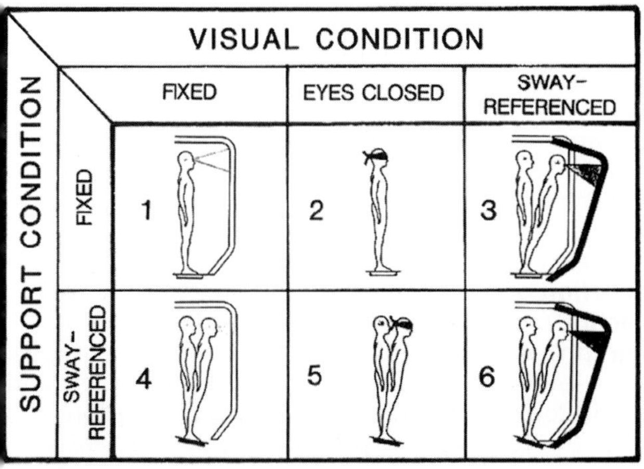

FIGURE 20.12   Six test conditions for the sensory organization portion of dynamic posturography. In the first three conditions, accurate foot somatosensory cues are available to the patient in all of the tests. The first and second conditions are simply eyes open and eyes closed. Condition 3 provides for orientationally inaccurate visual information in that, if the patient sways anterior/posterior, the visual surround moves with the patient (sway referenced). In conditions 4, 5, and 6, inaccurate foot somatosensory cues are provided by tilting the platform equal to the patient's sway in the sagittal plane (sway referenced). Then, for each of these latter three conditions, eyes open, eyes closed, and sway referenced visual surround are presented, respectively. (From NeuroCom Int., Inc. Instruction Manual, with permission.)

The survey of 2,266 consecutive balance disorder patients introduced in the chair discussion can again be used to assess the percentage of patients with abnormalities on dynamic posturography (EquiTest) and to study the types of patients most likely to have abnormal posturography results. In general, when all patients with indications of peripheral system involvement are considered, only 30% to 35% show abnormalities on formal CDP. However, there was a group of 4% to 5% of this total population of 2,266 patients for whom CDP was the only abnormal finding across all the tests of ENG and rotational chair. This group was primarily over 65 years of age, with the chief complaint of unsteadiness with standing and walking. These patients had no complaints when sitting or lying and no perceptions of vertigo or other abnormal movements. These statistics played a principle role in the development of the earlier discussed criteria for when to proceed for full CDP.

The protocols for EquiTest assess various aspects of quiet and dynamic postural control abilities. Although certain aspects of postural control are prerequisites for gait activities and certain abnormalities of postural control may cause ambulation problems, posturography cannot be used in isolation to evaluate gait deficits. Gait evaluation has its own complete set of parameters that must be tested under a completely different set of conditions.

SENSORY ORGANIZATION TEST

Briefly, the SOT measures the ability to perform volitional, quiet stance during a series of six specific conditions (Fig. 20.12). The first three provide for uninterrupted, accurate foot support surface information on a surface with adequate friction that is larger than the foot size. Condition 1 has eyes open, while in Condition 2, the eyes are closed. Under Condition 3, the visual surround moves in a pattern that is stimulated by the anterior/posterior sway movements of the patient. Conditions 1 and 2 are a modified Romberg test (a qualitative clinical test of patient stability when standing with feet together, arms folded, and eyes opened or closed), as the feet are at their normal separation rather than close together. Condition 3 presents a situation of visual conflict, where visually accurate information is provided that is of no significant help in maintaining quiet stance. Condition 3 presents misleading optokinetic and foveal visual cues about the position of the body in space. Conditions 4, 5, and 6 use the same sequence of the three visual conditions but with the foot support surface giving misleading information. As with the movement of the visual surround in Condition 3, when testing under Conditions 4, 5, and 6, sway movements of the patient in the sagittal (anterior/posterior) plane drive the movement of the support surface in a rotational manner about an axis parallel to the ankle joint. In this way, somatosensory and proprioceptive information is not removed in Conditions 4, 5, and 6, but this information is of limited use in maintaining upright stance in that there is a disrupted relationship between body position and the ankle angle (that angle made between the upper surface of the foot and the anterior portion of the lower leg). Typically, after the simpler Conditions 1 and 2, three trials are given for each of the more challenging conditions. The average performance is taken as representative of the patient's postural control ability under that sensory condition.

The equilibrium score is a percentage representing the magnitude of sway in the sagittal plane for each trial of each condition. Details of how this score is obtained will not be repeated here (Shepard et al., 1993a; Nashner, 1993a; 1993b). However, it is important to realize that this score is based on a normal value of 12.5 degrees of anterior/posterior sway about the ankle joint, typically 8 degrees forward and 4.5 degrees backward. It is assumed that this range of sway is available to patients during the test. Some patients may not have this normal range because of physical restrictions at the ankle or because of limits of sway patients have adopted secondary to their sense of imbalance and fear of a potential fall. It is important to recognize the patient who has a reduction in limits of sway. If the limits of sway are reduced more than 50%, the interpretation of the patient's results may be inaccurate (Shepard and Telian, 1996). Figure 20.13A shows an example of the graphical representation of these results in a patient with normal CDP findings.

As with the overall balance system evaluation, this study is also interpreted using pattern recognition. The

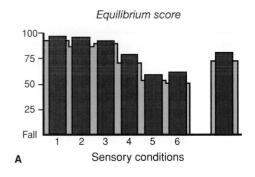

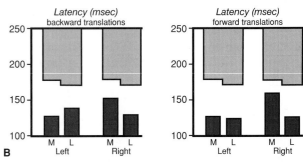

FIGURE 20.13 Results of dynamic posturography testing in a patient with all results interpreted as normal. (A) Bar graph at the top plots a percent equilibrium score for each of the six sensory organization test conditions (see Fig. 20.12). A score of 100 indicates no sway in the sagittal plane with "Fall" indicating that sway reached a magnitude equal to the theoretical limits of sway for the patient in the sagittal plane. The composite graph is a numerical average of the scores from the other six conditions. (B) Bar graphs in the bottom row (from movement coordination portion of the testing) plot latency to onset of active recovery to induced forward sway (left graph) and induced backward sway (right graph). The latencies are given in milliseconds for left and right leg for two sizes of platform translations. See the text for interpretation of these results.

combinations of the six conditions that are abnormal are used to define a pattern of abnormality that can then be functionally interpreted. Table 20.4 presents the most common patterns and a commonly used nomenclature. By far, the most common pattern is the vestibular dysfunction pattern, comprising approximately 45% of all abnormalities on this test in my experience. The most important aspect of interpretation for the SOT is that it provides information as to which input system cues the patient is unable to utilize for performing the task of maintaining postural control. In other words, it provides a relative measure of the patient's ability to utilize the sensory input cues of vision, vestibular, and proprioceptive/somatosensory to maintain quiet upright stance. The test does NOT provide relative information as to which of the sensory systems has lesions,

TABLE 20.4 Abnormalities of sensory organization testing

- Vestibular dysfunction pattern: Abnormal on conditions 5 and 6 (alternatively condition 5 alone).
- Vestibular dysfunction pattern indicates the patient's difficulty in using vestibular information alone for maintenance of stance. When provided with accurate visual and/or foot somatosensory information, stance is within a normal range.
- Visual vestibular dysfunction pattern: Abnormal on conditions 4, 5, and 6.
- Visual and vestibular dysfunction pattern indicates the patient's difficulty in using accurate visual information with vestibular information or vestibular information alone for maintenance of stance. When provided with accurate foot support surface cues, stance is within a normal range.
- Visual preference pattern: Abnormal on conditions 3 and 6 (alternatively condition 6 alone).
- Visual preference pattern indicates the patient's abnormal reliance on visual information, even when inaccurate. When provided with accurate foot support surface information together with accurate or absent visual cues or absent vision and vestibular information alone, stance is within a normal range.
- Visual preference/vestibular dysfunction pattern: abnormal on Conditions 3, 5, and 6.
- Visual preference and vestibular dysfunction pattern indicates the patient's difficulty in using vestibular information alone and the patient's abnormal reliance on visual information, even when inaccurate. When provided with accurate foot support surface information together with accurate or absent visual cues, stance is within a normal range.
- Somatosensory/vestibular dysfunction pattern: abnormal on conditions 2, 3, 5, and 6.
- Somatosensory and vestibular dysfunction pattern indicates the patient's difficulty in using foot support surface information with vestibular information or vestibular information alone for maintenance of stance. When provided with accurate visual information, stance is within a normal range.
- Severe dysfunction pattern: Abnormal on four or more conditions not covered in the above descriptions, for example, conditions 3, 4, 5, and 6; or 2, 3, 4, 5, and 6; or 1, 2, 3, 4, 5, and 6.
- Severe dysfunction pattern indicates the patient's difficulty with stance independent of the sensory information (vestibular, visual, and/or somatosensory) provided. Note that these situations many times involve a dominant feature such as significantly abnormal conditions 5 and 6 or they may involve equally distributed difficulties on all conditions affected.
- Inconsistent pattern: abnormal on conditions 1, 2, 3, or 4, or any combination and normal on conditions 5 and 6.
- Inconsistent pattern indicates that performance of the patient is difficult to explain with normal or typical pathophysiologic conditions and could imply volitional or nonvolitional exaggerated results.

causing postural control abnormalities. Therefore, SOT of CDP provides no site-of-lesion information; it is strictly a test of functional ability. The test in no way implies that there is a central or peripheral vestibular system lesion, nor does it imply central or peripheral pathway lesions in the visual or somatosensory/proprioceptive systems. The information should be interpreted only to reflect which input information the patient is able (or conversely, unable) to use for the task at hand.

Dynamic posturography is useful for identification of patients who may be exaggerating their condition. Work by several investigators (not all with EquiTest) has attempted to quantify the use of this tool to identify these patients and a list of qualitative factors that would raise questions in this dimension (Allum et al., 1994; Cevette et al., 1995; Goebel et al., 1997).

MOTOR CONTROL TEST

Information about patients' ability to react to unexpected perturbations in their center of mass position is obtained with the motor control protocol. The center of mass perturbations are created by abrupt anterior or posterior horizontal translations of the support surface. Typically, three increasingly large translations in both directions are administered.

The increase in size of the translation creates a stimulus intensity series. The profile of the surface movement is varied for each patient based on height, so that all translations are normalized to a 6-foot tall person (Shepard et al., 1993a). This allows for direct comparison of results across patients. After the three posterior and the three anterior translations, unexpected rotations about the ankle are used (adaptation test). Contrary to the horizontal translations, the typical muscle response that is mapped to the stimulus provoked by rotary stimuli is destabilizing. The patient must then be able to adapt to the new stimulus on repeated trials. Five randomly timed toes up or toes down rotations provide relative information about the patient's ability to adapt to this familiar but destabilizing stimulus. For this protocol, as with the SOT, floor reaction force detected by the force plates in the support surface is measured. The principal output parameter is the latency to onset of active recovery from the unexpected translations (Fig. 20.13B). Other information obtained from the protocol includes weight distribution onto right or left leg and a relative measure of strength as a function of the size of the perturbation (Shepard et al., 1993a).

This study is used less as a functional evaluation than the SOT, and more to evaluate the long-loop pathway. This pathway begins with inputs from the ankle region (tendon and muscle stretch receptors), then projects to the motor cortex and back to the various muscles of postural control, including upper and lower body. When an abnormal latency to onset of active recovery from induced sway is noted, then problems in the long-loop pathway should be considered. The explanation may be as simple as ongoing joint or back pain, a congenital condition of the back or lower limbs, or an acquired lesion involving the neural pathways of the tracts on either the afferent or efferent side. Therefore, abnormalities of the movement coordination test related to latency are nonspecific indicators of potential problems in the long tracts or the musculoskeletal system needed to coordinate recovery from unexpectedly induced sway in the sagittal plane. Other abnormalities from this portion of the testing include inappropriate weight bearing or an inability to properly scale the strength of the response to the increasing size of the perturbations. Such findings may provide information that helps explain the patient's complaints of disequilibrium. These abnormalities are unlikely to directly implicate neurologic involvement if the latency findings are normal. In many cases, the weight shift or scaling problems may be maladaptive behaviors developed in response to the initial symptoms of the vestibular disorder (for specific patient examples of this and other MCT/SOT abnormalities, see Shepard and Telian [1996]). A detailed discussion of the interpretations of this protocol and that of the postural evoked responses (PERs; see following section) are beyond the scope of this chapter, but such reviews are provided elsewhere (Shepard, 2000c; Nashner, 1993b).

POSTURAL EVOKED RESPONSES

Details of the testing protocol used are given elsewhere and will only be reviewed briefly here (Shepard, 2000c; Lawson et al., 1994; Nashner, 1993c). Muscle activity from the distal lower extremities is stimulated by sudden toe up rotations of the support surface (the force plate platform of EquiTest). The muscle activity stimulated by this dorsiflexion movement at the ankle is recorded with surface EMG electrodes. In the paradigm used for the patients presented here, the response from the medial gastrocnemius and the anterior tibialis is recorded. To improve the signal-to-noise ratio of the evoked EMG activity, the rotation is repeated, with random interstimulus intervals, and the EMG responses are rectified and averaged over 15 to 20 responses. This allows for clearer identification of onset and offset times of muscle contraction following the stimulus. There are three specific responses obtained, as illustrated in Figure 20.14. The short latency (SL) and medium latency (ML) responses are seen from the contraction of the gastrocnemius shown in traces from channels 1 and 3 (CH1 and CH3) of Figure 20.14. The third response is the long latency (LL) response obtained from the contraction of the anterior tibialis, shown in channels 2 and 4 (CH2 and CH4) of Figure 20.14.

The EMG patterns for contraction from the gastrocnemius and the anterior tibialis muscles are compared to those that have been associated with specific pathologies, such as multiple sclerosis, Parkinson's disease, or specific neurologic lesions. Patterns have been described for lesions in the anterior cerebellum and the basal ganglia, as well as for spinal cord compression. When the contraction pattern is unrecognized, the interpretation is based upon knowledge of the underlying neural pathways considered responsible for the specific muscle activity. In general, these involve mediation of the SL response via the spinal cord (H-reflex). The ML response is primarily controlled via the spinal cord, with amplitude size determined by the brainstem and basal ganglia. The functional stretch reflex, the LL response, involves brainstem and cortical activity. Defined patterns of muscle response have been associated with specific lesion sites and disease classifications (Dichgans and Diener, 1987). Normative results for the paradigm have been developed across age and have been shown to have sensitivity and specificity of 68% and 87%, respectively, for identifying the specific disease entities reflected by the defined patterns of abnormal responses (Lawson et al., 1994; Shepard et al., 1994). As with the MCT, the EMG evaluation does not distinguish afferent from efferent disruptions that may underlie the abnormal muscle responses. With additional clinical investigations of sensitivity in the lower limbs and/or the use of lower limb somatosensory evoked responses, pathology affecting sensory input can be distinguished from motor output abnormalities.

THE CLINICAL UTILITY OF COMPUTERIZED DYNAMIC POSTUROGRAPHY

The CDP tests described earlier can provide data ranging from purely functional information to that of specific site-of-lesion, postural-control pathways by changing the protocol and the output parameters. Therefore, for the classic peripheral vestibular lesion patient, the utility of CDP lies in the use of SOT for functional information related to functional dimensions of compensation not available from the extent- and site-of-lesion studies of ENG and chair. For the patient with a less well-defined lesion site or evidence of central system involvement, the functional information is then supplemented with data that approach a more specific evaluation of the central and peripheral postural control pathways. Additionally, CDP can serve to help in the design and monitoring of vestibular and balance rehabilitation programs, primarily the SOT protocol with the emphasis on functional performance.

▨ OFFICE "BEDSIDE" EVALUATIONS OF THE BALANCE SYSTEM

A variety of test procedures may be used in the office setting to assess the balance disorder patient. These, like the laboratory studies, assist in the identification of the extent and site of the lesion. These straightforward clinical tests are

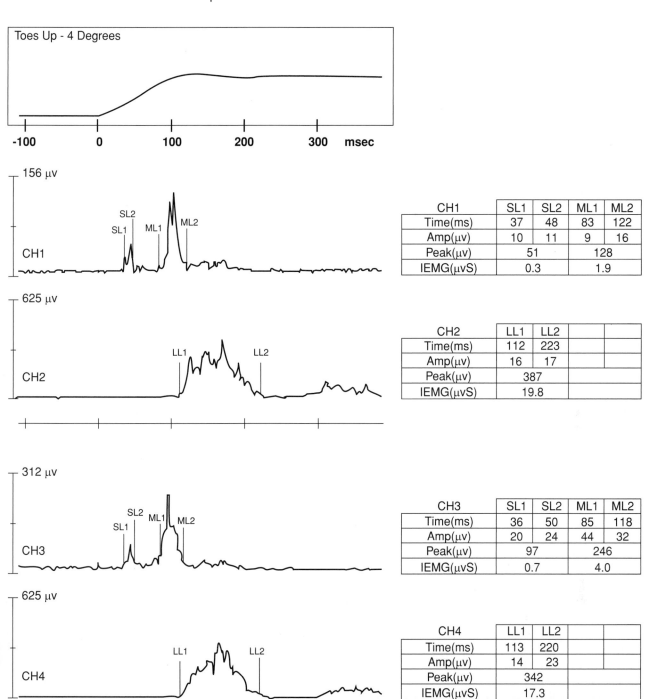

FIGURE 20.14 Postural evoked response results for a normal subject. The plot at the top shows the position profile of the rotation of the surface the subject is standing on, as a function of time. Deflection upward indicates toe up rotation. The four plots on the left give the averaged, rectified surface electromyographic (EMG) responses in amplitude of contraction (in microvolts) as a function of time. Channels 1 and 3 (CH1 and 3) are results from the left and right gastrocnemius muscles, respectively. Channels 2 and 4 (CH2 and 4) are the results from the left and right anterior tibialis muscles, respectively. The short latency (SL), medium latency (ML), and long latency (LL) responses are indicated at onset with a number 1 and at offset with a number 2. The tables at the right give the numerical values for each response, indicating onset and offset times and amplitudes, peak amplitude contraction, and integrated amplitude (IEMG).(Reprinted with permission from Shepard NT, Telian SA. [1996] *Practical Management of the Balance Disorder Patient.* San Diego: Singular Publishing Group).

essentially variations of the related laboratory studies but have less ability to quantify the outcomes. The theoretical basis behind many of these tests is well founded in the physiologic considerations discussed earlier. Due to the subjective nature of these tools, the validity and reliability of these tests are reduced compared to the formal laboratory studies. Unfortunately, little clinical research exists to define the sensitivity/specificity and test reliability for these procedures. The interested reader is referred to work by Baloh and Honrubia (1990), Leigh and Zee (1999), Shumway-Cook and Horak (1986), Halmagyi and Curthoys (1988), Shepard and Telian (1996), Beynon et al. (1998), Jacobson et al. (1990), and Schubert et al. (2004). These references describe a variety of these procedures, how they are performed, and what performance measures are available. The most recent summary article on this topic is from Walker and Zee (2000).

While the bedside vestibular and balance evaluation cannot be described in the limited scope of this chapter, it is important that the person evaluating the dizzy patient be aware that simple tools do exist that provide for an evaluation that, in the majority of patients, produces the same impressions as the extensive laboratory studies discussed earlier. These tools are, however, not as sensitive to mild anomalies as the laboratory studies. It is also important to recognize that the bedside chair study and the CTSIB study of balance can both be used with the ENG to expand the laboratory investigation when formal equipment, such as rotational chair and posturography, are not readily available.

For the formal balance laboratory, the main clinical utility of the office procedures is their use just prior to performing the ENG. Tests of ocular motor control (ocular range of motion, smooth pursuit, and saccades) give a quick indication of the patient's control of volitional eye movements and cue the examiner to possible overt indications of possible central nervous system involvement. The head thrust examination (Halmagyi and Curthoys, 1988) gives an immediate indication of unilateral or bilateral peripheral hypofunction of significance and possible prediction related to caloric testing (Beynon et al., 1998; Shepard, 1998; Perez and Rama-Lopez, 2003).

▨ VESTIBULAR AND BALANCE REHABILITATION

The general principles of designing vestibular rehabilitation programs involve exposing the patient to the stimuli that provoke vertigo, cause slippage of the visual signal on the retina, and challenge areas of deficiency in postural control. First, the therapist must identify those activities or environmental situations that provoke symptoms. Second, the patient's functional deficits regarding balance and gait must be identified. These may be caused by the vestibular symptoms or by maladaptive behavior that has developed in response to the symptoms. Lastly, it is desirable to challenge the sedentary lifestyle that the vestibular disorder patient often adopts. An active lifestyle including regular exercise that accounts for age and other health constraints will serve as a maintenance program once active therapy is completed. Therefore, in the development of any customized therapy exercise program, four areas should always be given consideration:

1. Adaptation exercises—activities with the goal of improving the gain of the VOR, thereby reducing the slippage of visual images on the retina with head movement.
2. Habituation exercises—the use of repeated head and visual movement activities to facilitate a reduction in the symptoms provoked by a specific movement.
3. Balance and gait exercises—these activities are targeted at improvement in both static and dynamic balance abilities together with overall improvement in gait under a variety of environmental conditions. The exercises in this group may well incorporate both adaptation and habituation activities simultaneously with balance and gait.
4. General conditioning exercises—the activities in this group may represent part of the active therapy program, such as a walking program or Tai Chi, that can be continued indefinitely at the end of the formal therapy interval. These activities are used to maintain the accomplishments of the active therapy program and continue to challenge the patient's maintenance of the compensation process.

The specific details of the physical therapy evaluation needed to arrive at a customized plan for treatment have certain consistent features, despite individual variations on the theme. Detailed literature exists describing this evaluation process (Herdman, 2000; 2007; Shumway-Cook and Horak, 1990; Smith-Wheelock et al., 1991; Shepard and Telian, 1995; 2005).

What is considered the role of the audiologist in the process of vestibular and balance rehabilitation? Position statements from various professional societies, including American Speech-Language and Hearing Association (Shepard et al., 1999), state that the audiologist should, with additional training, consider the area of BPPV as within their scope of practice. Additionally, the audiologist is an important member of a team of professionals working on the assessment and overall treatment of the patient with chronic balance and dizziness complaints. However, the remainder of the aspects of vestibular and balance rehabilitation should fall to the physical and occupational therapists with specialized postgraduate training in this area.

▨ CASE STUDIES

The following two cases provide an integration of the earlier discussions by presenting patients with increasing complexity. The first is typical of cases seen in otolaryngology practices. The second case could easily present to an otology practice, on referral from a neurologist, seeking information about a possible peripheral system involvement.

Case 1

A 77-year-old female had symptoms of vertigo that began with an acute vestibular crisis lasting continuously for 36 hours that improved over time to unsteadiness provoked only by head movement. She denied any changes in hearing or auditory symptoms at the time of the event. She had been bothered by the motion-provoked unsteadiness for several years at the time of evaluation. Audiometric testing indicated bilateral high-frequency sensory-neural hearing loss, worse on the left than the right, with excellent speech recognition bilaterally. Magnetic resonance imaging (MRI) results were normal for her age. She presented to the ENG with ventilation tubes with long shafts in place bilaterally, preventing use of open- or closed-loop caloric irrigation. (Air caloric testing could have been used but was unavailable.) Mild right-beating positional nystagmus was noted with slow

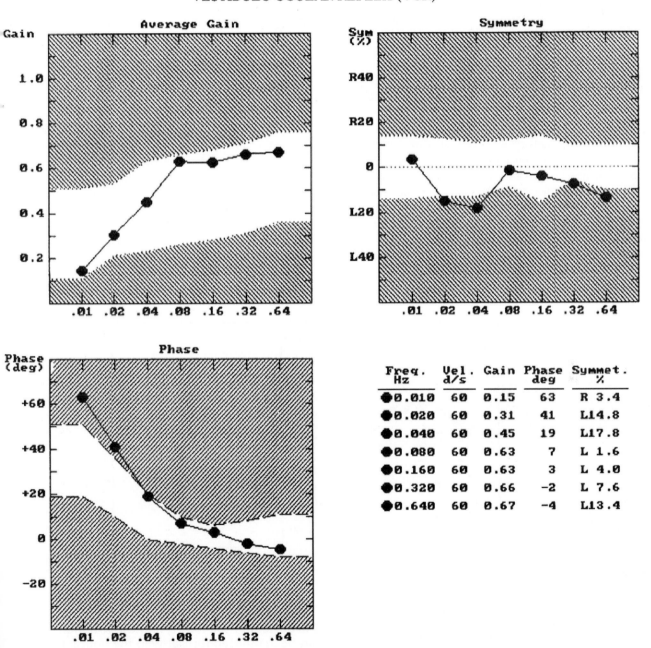

Freq. Hz	Vel. d/s	Gain	Phase deg	Symmet. %
0.010	60	0.15	63	R 3.4
0.020	60	0.31	41	L14.8
0.040	60	0.45	19	L17.8
0.080	60	0.63	7	L 1.6
0.160	60	0.63	3	L 4.0
0.320	60	0.66	-2	L 7.6
0.640	60	0.67	-4	L13.4

FIGURE 20.15 Chair results for Case 1. The figure gives the results for sinusoidal stimulation. The panels give the results for gain, asymmetry, and phase as indicated above each panel. To the right of the panel that graphically depicts the phase results is a tabular representation of the results.

component velocity of 6°/s in six of 11 positions. The remainder of her ENG was normal with normal ocular motor results. Her office examination was also normal for ocular motor evaluation, with an inconsistently positive head thrust to the left. Her SOT was abnormal with a vestibular dysfunction pattern with repeated falls on conditions 5 and 6 (three trials of each).

The results of the ENG suggested possible peripheral system involvement, either left paresis or right irritative lesion given the positional, direction-fixed, right-beating nystagmus and normal ocular motor results. The left paretic lesion was felt to be more likely given the head thrust results and the greater loss of hearing on the left by puretone findings. She was considered to have a lack of physiologic compensation (given the clinically significant positional nystagmus) and functional compensation (given the abnormal postural control result). The lack of caloric results prevented developing further support for or against dysfunction within the peripheral vestibular system as suggested by the other results. In this case, rotary chair results, shown in Figure 20.15, gave strong indications of peripheral system involvement, with abnormal time constant (as indicated from an abnormal phase lead, normal gain, and a left greater than right slow-component velocity asymmetrical response to the rotational stimuli). These objective findings supporting peripheral system involvement demonstrate the usefulness of the information obtained from rotary chair evaluation. In this case, the abnormal phase lead was a strong indication of peripheral system involvement, with the asymmetry suggesting a

finding consistent with lack of central system compensation. The direction of the asymmetry plus the greater loss of hearing on the left, the positive head thrust test on the left, and the positional right-beating nystagmus were consistent and suggestive that the left side was more likely to be involved.

This patient was diagnosed with a viral insult (vestibular neuritis), probably on the left, as the most likely etiology. She was treated with a vestibular rehabilitation home program using habituation, adaptation, and balance and gait exercises, with complete resolution of residual symptoms within a 12-week course of treatment. Her postural control abilities, as tested by SOT, returned to a normal range.

Case 2

A 65-year-old male presented with sudden onset of disequilibrium and nausea after heart catheterization in the fall of 1989. Brainstem stroke was suspected, but neuroradiographic studies at the time were negative. Current symptoms were constant unsteadiness and lightheadedness with sudden pulling or pushing (pulsion) sensation spontaneously two to three times per week lasting several seconds. His constant symptoms were exacerbated by head movements. The patient had a past history of significant cardiac disease, requiring a triple coronary artery bypass operation in 1980. Bilateral tinnitus and aural fullness were reported with a mild, high-frequency, bilateral sensory-neural hearing loss.

ENG revealed left-beating spontaneous and positional nystagmus with slow-component eye velocity of 4 to 6°/s.

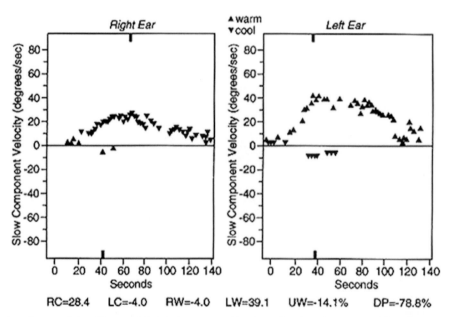

RC=28.4   LC=-4.0   RW=-4.0   LW=39.1   UW=-14.1%   DP=-78.8%

FIGURE 20.16   See legend for Figure 20.8. These are the results for Case 2. In this figure, the maximum, average slow-component velocity values are given at the bottom of the figure, and the rectangle showing the 10-second interval used for the average has been omitted for clarity in the figure. RC, right cool; LC, left cool; RW, right warm; LW, left warm; UW, unilateral weakness (14.1% in the right ear); DP, directional preponderance (78.8% to the left). (Reprinted with permission from Shepard NT, Telian SA. [1996] *Practical Management of the Balance Disorder Patient.* **San Diego: Singular Publishing Group).**

Bithermal, alternating caloric irrigations produced only left-beating nystagmus. However, as can be seen in Figure 20.16, the average values for slow-component eye velocity were significantly lower than the spontaneous value for right warm and left cool (irrigations normally resulting in right beats) and increased compared to spontaneous for the right cool and left warm (those causing left beats). This results in no unilateral weakness but a significant (79%) left directional preponderance. In this case, the ocular-motor results were significantly abnormal, with saccadic disruptions in smooth pursuit but, more importantly, with a pattern that suggested a specific lesion of the left lateral medullary region of the brainstem. This is what had been suspected at the onset of his symptoms, but there were no objective indications to verify that lesion until these findings were observed and recorded. Figure 20.17 demonstrates a condition called ocular-lateral pulsion, a key finding in Wallenberg's syndrome (Waespe and

Wichmann, 1990), implicating the medullary region stroke. Shown are the traces obtained with the eyes open, when fixation was removed by turning the lights off. In both the upper and lower panels of horizontal eye movement, deviation to the left when visual fixation was removed is apparent. The vertical movements are not of great importance and show typical eye blinks. These traces represent the primary finding leading to a diagnosis of lateral medullary infarct. This finding occurs with a lesion in the medulla that is lateralized by the direction that the eyes deviate toward when visual fixation is removed. It is recognizable in the ENG recordings with electrodes (when using direct current coupling,

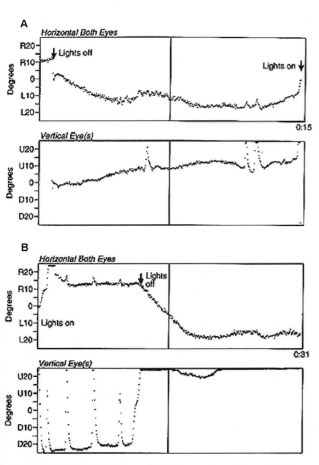

FIGURE 20.17 Plots of horizontal and vertical eye positions as a function of time. For both **A** and **B**, eyes are open, and the *arrows* indicate times of lighted and darkened room. Panel **B** is a continuation of the trace in panel **A**. For both **A** and **B**, the patient is sitting, with head straight. (Reprinted with permission from Shepard NT, Telian SA. [1996] *Practical Management of the Balance Disorder Patient.* San Diego: Singular Publishing Group).

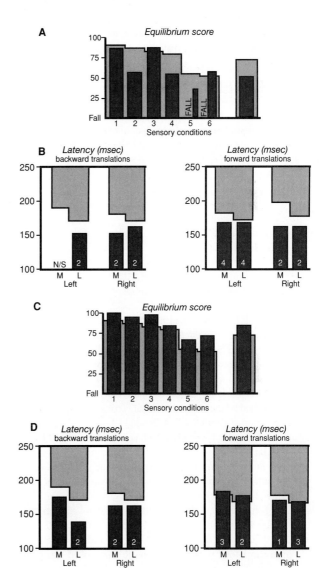

FIGURE 20.18 (A, B) Sensory organization test and latency results before therapy, respectively. **(C, D)** Sensory organization test and latency results after therapy for Case 2, respectively. (Reprinted with permission from Shepard NT, Telian SA. [1996] *Practical Management of the Balance Disorder Patient.* San Diego: Singular Publishing Group).

an amplifier filtering technique that does not distort the recorded signal; Jacobson et al., 1993), or with VNG direct visualization, and recording as the eyes repeatedly have to be recentered from a lateral position whenever fixation is returned. This finding, although of great significance in the diagnosis of the brainstem lesion in this patient, is also the most likely explanation for his persistent left-beating nystagmus and the left directional preponderance. This helps reduce any suspicion of peripheral system involvement.

This case also presents an example of the use of dynamic posturography to help rule out significant long-loop, automatic pathway coordination problems. The presence of such abnormalities would have altered the approach to his vestibular rehabilitation program. As it stands, his abnormalities reflect balance difficulties related to sensory input abnormalities, probably secondary to a central vestibular system lesion in the medulla, not motor control abnormalities. Figures 20.18A and 20.18B shows the SOT and latency results of movement coordination testing for this patient prior to his vestibular rehabilitation program. These results, together with clinical evaluations showing dysmetria and other indicators of cerebellar, pyramidal, or extrapyramidal tract involvement, demonstrate that the unsteadiness and mild gait ataxia may be related only to sensory input integration. This patient's difficulty with absent visual information and the use of accurate visual information when present, together with gait activities, constituted a major part of his vestibular rehabilitation program. The results after therapy are given in Figures 20.18C and 20.18D. Although he reported mild symptoms remaining, he had major subjective improvement together with the improvement demonstrated on objective testing.

▨ REFERENCES

Allum JHJ, Huwiler M, Honegger F. (1994) Objective measures of non-organic vertigo using dynamic posturography. In: Taguchi K, Igarashi M, Mori S, eds. *Vestibular and Neural Front: Proceedings of the 12th International Symposium on Posture and Gait.* Amsterdam: Elsevier; pp 51–55.

Allum JHJ, Shepard NT. (1999) An overview of the clinical use of dynamic posturography in the differential diagnosis of balance disorders. *J Vestib Res.* 9, 223–252.

Baloh RW, Halmagyi GM, eds. (1996) *Disorders of the Vestibular System.* New York: Oxford University Press.

Baloh R, Honrubia V. (1990) *Clinical Neurophysiology of the Vestibular System.* 2nd ed. Philadelphia: F.A. Davis.

Barber HO, Stockwell CW. (1980). *Manual of Electronystagmography.* 2nd ed. St. Louis: C.V. Mosby.

Beynon GJ, Jani P, Baguley DM. (1998) A clinical evaluation of head impulse testing. *Clin Otolaryngol.* 23, 117–122.

Blake AJ, Morgan K, Bendall MJ, et al. (1988) Falls by elderly people at home: prevalence and associated factors. *Age Aging.* 17, 365–372.

Bohmer A, Mast F. (1999) Chronic unilateral loss of otolith function revealed by the subjective visual vertical during off center yaw rotation. *J Vestib Res.* 9, 413–422.

Bronstein AM, Brandt T, Woollacott M, eds. (1996) *Clinical Disorders of Balance, Posture and Gait.* London: Arnold.

Cevette MJ, Puetz B, Marion MS, Wertz ML, Muenter MD. (1995) A physiologic performance on dynamic posturography. *Otolaryngol Head Neck Surg.* 112, 676–688.

Clarke AH, Schonfeld U, Helling K. (2003) Unilateral examination of utricle and saccule function. *J Vestib Res.* 13, 215–225.

Cheng PW, Huang TW, Young YH. (2003) The influence of clicks versus short tone bursts on the vestibular evoked myogenic potentials. *Ear Hear.* 24, 195–197.

Colebatch JG, Halmagyi GM. (1992) Vestibular evoked potentials in human neck muscles before and after unilateral vestibular deafferentation. *Neurology.* 42, 1635–1636.

Curthoys IS, Halmagyi GM. (1995) Vestibular compensation: a review of the oculomotor, neural, and clinical consequences of unilateral vestibular loss. *J Vestib Res.* 5, 67–107.

Cutrer FM, Baloh RW. (1992) Migraine-associated dizziness. *Headache.* 32, 300–304.

Dichgans J, Diener HC. (1987) The use of short- and long-latency reflex testing in leg muscles of neurological patients. In: Struppler A, Weindl A, eds. *Clinical Aspects of Sensory-Motor Integration: Implications for Neurological Patients.* New York: Springer-Verlag; pp 165–175.

El-Kashlan HK, Shepard NT, Asher A, et al. (1998) Evaluation of clinical measures of equilibrium. *Laryngoscope.* 108, 311–319.

Fitzgerald G, Hallpike CS. (1942) Studies in human vestibular function: I. Observations of the directional preponderance of caloric nystagmus resulting from cerebral lesions. *Brain.* 65, 115.

Furman JM, Balaban CD, Jacob RG, Marcus DA. (2005) Migraine-anxiety related dizziness (MARD): a new disorder? *J Neurol Neurosurg Psychiatry.* 76, 1–8.

Furman JM, Cass SP. (1996) *Balance Disorders: A Case-Study Approach.* Philadelphia: FA Davis Co.

Furman JM, Marcus DA, Balaban CD. (2003) Migrainous vertigo: development of a pathogenetic model and structured diagnostic interview. *Curr Opin Neurol.* 16, 5–13.

Gillespie LD, Gillespie WJ, Robertson MC, Lamb SE, Cumming RG, Rowe BH. (2003) Interventions for preventing falls in elderly people. *Cochrane Database Syst Rev.* 4, CD000340.

Goebel J. (2000a) Management options for acute versus chronic vertigo. In: Shepard NT, Solomon D, eds. *The Otolaryngologic Clinics of North America.* Philadelphia: WB Saunders; pp 471–482.

Goebel J, ed. (2000b) *Practical Management of the Dizzy Patient.* Philadelphia: Lippincott Williams & Wilkins.

Goebel J, Sataloff RT, Hanson JM, et al (1997) Posturographic evidence of nonorganic sway patterns in normal subjects, patients and suspected malingerers. *Otolaryngol Head Neck Surg.* 117, 293–302.

Hall CD, Schubert MC, Herdman SJ. (2004) Prediction of fall risk reduction as measured by dynamic gait index in individuals with unilateral vestibular hypofunction. *Otol Neurotol.* 25, 746–751.

Halmagyi GM, Colebatch JG. (1995) Vestibular evoked myogenic potentials in the sternomastoid muscle are not of lateral canal origin. *Acta Otolaryngol.* 520, 1–3.

Halmagyi GM, Curthoys IS. (1988). A clinical sign of canal paresis. *Arch Neurol.* 45, 737–739.

Han JN, Stegen K, Schepers R, Van den Bergh O, Van de Woestijne KP. (1998) Subjective symptoms and breathing pattern at rest and following hyperventilation in anxiety and somatoform disorders. *J Psychosom Res.* 45, 519–532.

Herdman SJ. (1994) Preface. In: Herdman SJ, ed. *Vestibular Rehabilitation.* Philadelphia: FA Davis; pp ix–x.

Herdman SJ, ed. (2000) *Vestibular Rehabilitation.* 2nd ed. Philadelphia: FA Davis.

Herdman SJ, ed. (2007) *Vestibular Rehabilitation.* 3rd ed. Philadelphia: FA Davis.

Herdman SJ, Blatt P, Schubert MC, Tusa RJ. (2000) Falls in patients with vestibular deficits. *Am J Otol.* 21, 847–851.

Herdman SJ, Tusa RJ. (2000) Assessment and treatment of patients with benign paroxysmal positional vertigo. In: Herdman SJ, ed. *Vestibular Rehabilitation.* 2nd ed. Philadelphia: FA Davis.

Herdman SJ, Tusa RJ, Blatt P, Suzuki A, Venuto VJ, Roberts D. (1998) Computerized dynamic visual acuity test in the assessment of vestibular deficits. *Am J Otol.* 19, 790–796.

Horak FB, Diener HC, Nashner LM. (1989) Influence of central set on human postural responses. *J Neurophysiol.* 62, 841–853.

Igarashi M. (1984) Vestibular compensation: an overview. *Acta Otolaryngol.* 406, 78–82.

Jackler RK, Brackmann D, eds. (1994) *Textbook of Neurotology.* Philadelphia: Mosby.

Jacobson GP, Calder JA, Shepherd VA, Rupp KA, Newman GW. (1995) Reappraisal of the monothermal warm caloric screening test. *Ann Otol Rhinol Laryngol.* 104, 942–945.

Jacobson GP, Newman CW. (1990) The development of the dizziness handicap inventory. *Arch Otolaryngol Head Neck Surg.* 116, 424–427.

Jacobson GP, Newman CW, Hunter L, Balzer G. (1991) Balance function test correlates of the Dizziness Handicap Inventory. *J Am Acad Audiol.* 2, 253–260.

Jacobson GP, Newman CW, Kartush JM, eds. (1993). *Handbook of Balance Function Testing.* St. Louis: Mosby Year Book, Inc.

Jacobson GP, Newman CW, Safadi I. (1990) Sensitivity and specificity of the head-shaking test for detecting vestibular system abnormalities. *Ann Otol Rhinol Laryngol.* 99, 539–542.

Jacobson GP, Shephard NT (Eds.) (2008) *Balance Function Assessment and Management.* San Diego: Plural Publishing Group.

Johnson GD. (1998) Medical management of migraine-related dizziness and vertigo. *Laryngoscope.* 108 (suppl 85), 1–30.

Kroenke K, Mangelsdorff AG. (1989) Common symptoms in ambulatory care: incidence, evaluation, therapy and outcome. *Am J Med.* 86, 262–266.

Lawson GD, Shepard NT, Oviatt DL, Wang Y. (1994) Electromyographic responses of lower leg muscles to upward toe tilts as a function of age. *J Vestib Res.* 4, 203–214.

Leigh RJ, Zee DS. (1999) *The Neurology of Eye Movements.* 3rd ed. Philadelphia: FA Davis.

Li MW, Houlden D, Tomlinson RD. (1999) Click evoked EMG responses in sternocleidomastoid muscles: characteristics in normal subjects. *J Vestib Res.* 9, 327–334.

Minor LB. (2005) Clinical manifestations of superior semicircular canal dehiscence. *Laryngoscope.* 115, 1717–1727.

Minor LB, Haslwanter T, Straumann D, Zee DS. (1999) Hyperventilation-induced nystagmus in patients with vestibular schwannoma. *Neurology.* 53, 2158–2167.

Minor LB, Solomon D, Zinreich JS, Zee DS. (1998) Sound- and/or pressure-induced vertigo due to bone dehiscence of the superior semicircular canal. *Arch Otolaryngol Head Neck Surg.* 124, 249–258.

Monsell EM, Furman JM, Herdman SJ, Konrad HR, Shepard NT. (1997) Technology assessment: computerized dynamic platform posturography. *Otolaryngol Head Neck Surg.* 117, 394–398.

Nashner LM (1993a) Practical biomechanics and physiology of balance. In Jacobson GP, Newman CW, Kartush JM, eds. *Handbook of Balance Function Testing.* St. Louis: Mosby Year Book; pp 280–307.

Nashner LM. (1993b) Computerized dynamic posturography. In: Jacobson GP, Newman CW, Kartush JM, eds. *Handbook of Balance Function Testing.* St. Louis: Mosby Year Book; pp 280–307.

Nashner LM. (1993c) Computerized dynamic posturography: clinical applications. In: Jacobson GP, Newman CW, Kartush JM, eds. *Handbook of Balance Function Testing.* St. Louis: Mosby Year Book; pp 280–307.

Neuhauser H, Leopold M, von Brevem M, Arnold G, Lempert T. (2001) The interrelations of migraine, vertigo, and migrainous vertigo. *Neurology.* 56, 436–441.

Papp LA, Klein DF, Gorman JM. (1993) Carbon dioxide hypersensitivity, hyperventilation, and panic disorder. *Am J Psychiatry.* 150, 1149–1157.

Parnes LS, McCLure JA. (1991) Posterior semicircular canal occlusion in the normal hearing ear. *Otolaryngol Head Neck Surg.* 104, 52–57.

Pavlou M, Wijnberg N, Faldon ME, Bronstein AM. (2003) Effect of semicircular canal stimulation on the perception of the visual vertical. *J Neurophysiol.* 90, 622–630.

Peppard SB. (1986) Effect of drug therapy on compensation from vestibular injury. *Laryngoscope.* 96, 878–898.

Perez N, Rama-Lopez I. (2003) Head-impulse and caloric tests in patients with dizziness. *Otol Neurotol.* 24, 913–917.

Pfaltz CR. (1983) Vestibular compensation: physiological and clinical aspects. *Acta Otolaryngol.* 9, 402–406.

Rauch SD, Zhou G, Kujawa SG, Guinan JJ, Herrmann BS. (2004) Vestibular evoked myogenic potentials show altered tuning in patients with Ménière's disease. *Otol Neurotol.* 25, 333–338.

Rosenberg ML, Gizzi M. (2000) Neuro-otologic history. In: Shepard NT, Solomon D, eds. *The Otolaryngologic Clinics of North America.* Philadelphia: WB Saunders; pp 471–482.

Roydhouse N. (1974) Vertigo and its treatment. *Drug.* 7, 297–309.

Ruckenstein M, Shepard NT. (2000) Balance function testing: a rationale approach. In: Shepard NT, Solomon D, eds. *The Otolaryngologic Clinics of North America.* Philadelphia: WB Saunders.

Schubert MC, Tusa RJ, Grine LE, Herdman SJ. (2004) Optimizing the sensitivity of the head thrust test for identifying vestibular hypofunction. *Phys Ther.* 84, 151–158.

Shepard NT. (1998) Caloric weakness needed to achieve a positive head thrust test. XX Barany Society Meeting, Wuerzburg, Germany, September 12–15, 1998.

Shepard NT. (2000a) Lab tests—electronystagmography (ENG) testing. In: Goebel J, ed. *Practical Management of the Dizzy Patient.* Philadelphia: Lippincott Williams & Wilkins.

Shepard NT. (2000b) Lab tests—rotational chair testing. In: Goebel J, ed. *Practical Management of the Dizzy Patient.* Philadelphia: Lippincott Williams & Wilkins.

Shepard NT. (2007) *Clinical Utility of the Motor Control Test (MCT) and Postural Evoked Responses (PER).* Clackamas, OR: NeuroCom Publication; pp 1–20.

Shepard NT. (2006) Differentiation of Ménière's disease and migraine associated dizziness: a review. *J Am Acad Audiol.* 17, 69–80.

Shepard NT. (2007) *Management of the Patient with Chronic Complaints of Dizziness: An Overview of Laboratory Studies.* Clackamas, OR: NeuroCom Publication.

Shepard NT, Garrus NP, Hecker EB, Henry KG, Herdman S, Stockwell CW. (1999) Role of audiologists in vestibular and balance rehabilitation: position statement, guidelines, and technical report. *ASHA.* 19, 13–22.

Shepard NT, Lawson GD, Boismier T, Oviatt DL, Wang Y. (1994) Surface EMG response from lower leg muscles in the assessment of balance disorder patients. Abstract from the XIIth International Symposium on Posture and Gait, Vestibular and Neural Front, Matsumoto, Japan.

Shepard NT, Schultz A, Alexander NB, Gu MJ, Boismier T. (1993a) Postural control in young and elderly adults when stance is challenged: clinical versus laboratory measurements. *Ann Otol Rhinol Laryngol.* 102, 508–517.

Shepard NT, Solomon D, eds. (2000) Practical issues in the management of the dizzy and balance disorder patients. *The Otolaryngologic Clinics of North America.* Philadelphia: WB Saunders.

Shepard NT, Solomon D, Ruckenstein M, Staab J. (2003) Evaluation of the vestibular (balance) system. In: Ballenger JJ, Snow JB, eds. *Otorhinolaryngology Head and Neck Surgery.* 16th ed. San Diego: Singular Publishing Group; pp 161–194.

Shepard NT, Telian SA. (1995) Programmatic vestibular rehabilitation. *Otolaryngol Head Neck Surg.* 112, 173–182.

Shepard NT, Telian SA. (1996) *Practical Management of the Balance Disorder Patient.* San Diego: Singular Publishing Group.

Shepard NT, Telian SA. (2005) Vestibular and balance rehabilitation: program essentials. In: *Otolaryngology – Head and Neck Surgery.* 4th edition. Philadelphia: Elsevier.

Shepard NT, Telian SA, Smith-Wheelock M, Raj A. (1993b) Vestibular and balance rehabilitation therapy. *Ann Otol Rhinol Laryngol.* 102, 198–205.

Shonel G, Kemink JL, Telian SA. (1991) Prognostic significance of hearing loss as a lateralising indicator in the surgical treatment of vertigo. *J Layngol Otol.* 105, 18–20.

Shumway-Cook A, Horak FB. (1986) Assessing the influence of sensory interaction on balance. Suggestion from the field. *J Am Phys Ther.* 66, 1548–1550.

Shumway-Cook A, Horak FB. (1990) Rehabilitation strategies for patients with vestibular deficits. *Neurol Clin.* 8, 441–457.

Smith-Wheelock M, Shepard NT, Telian SA. (1991) Physical therapy program for vestibular rehabilitation. *Am J Otol.* 12, 218–225.

Staab JP. (2000) Treatment of psychological issues in patients with dizziness and balance disorders. In: Shepard NT, Solomon D, eds. *Otolaryngologic Clinics of North America.* Philadelphia: WB Saunders.

Staab JP, Ruckenstein MJ. (2003) Which comes first: psychogenic dizziness versus otogenic anxiety. *Laryngoscope.* 113, 1714–1718.

Staab JP, Ruckenstein MJ, Solomon D, Shepard NT. (2002a) Exertional dizziness and autonomic dysregulation. *Laryngoscope.* 112, 1346–1350.

Staab JP, Ruckenstein MJ, Solomon D, Shepard NT. (2002b) Serotonin reuptake inhibitors for dizziness with psychiatric symptoms. *Arch Otolaryngol Head Neck Surg.* 128, 554–560.

Stockwell CW, Bojrab DI. (1993a) Background and technique of rotational testing. In: Jacobson GP, Newman CW, Kartush JM, eds. *Handbook of Balance Function Testing.* St. Louis: Mosby Year Book; pp 237–248.

Stockwell CW, Bojrab DI. (1993b) Interpretation and usefulness of rotational testing. In: Jacobson GP, Newman CW, Kartush JM, eds. *Handbook of Balance Function Testing.* St. Louis: Mosby Year Book; pp 249–260.

Streubel SO, Cremer PD, Carey JP, Weg N, Minor LB. (2001) Vestibular-evoked myogenic potentials in the diagnosis of superior canal dehiscence syndrome. *Acta Otolaryngol.* 545, 41–49.

Telian SA, Wiet RM. (2008a) Medical treatment of vertigo that is otologic in origin. In Jacobson GP and Shepard NT (Eds.) *Balance Function Assessment and Management.* San Diego: Plural Publishing Group, pp 469–478.

Telian SA, Wiet RM. (2008b) Surgical treatment of vertigo that is otologic in origin. In Jacobson GP and Shepard NT (Eds.) *Balance Function Assessment and Management.* San Diego: Plural Publishing Group, pp 479–497.

Tinetti ME, Speechley M, Ginter SF. (1988) Risk factors for falls among elderly persons living in the community. *N Engl J Med.* 319, 1701–1707.

Tusa RJ. (2000a) Diagnosis and management of neuro-otological disorders due to migraine. In: Herdman SJ, ed. *Vestibular Rehabilitation.* Philadelphia: FA Davis; pp 298–315.

Tusa RJ. (2000b) Psychological problems and the dizzy patient. In: Herdman SJ, ed. *Vestibular Rehabilitation.* Philadelphia: FA Davis; pp 316–330.

Vibert D, Hausler R, Safran AB. (1999) Subjective visual vertical in peripheral unilateral vestibular diseases. *J Vestib Res.* 9, 145–152.

Waespe W, Cohen B, Raphan T. (1985) Dynamic modification of the vestibulo–ocular reflex by the nodulus and uvula. *Science.* 228, 199–202.

Waespe W, Wichmann W. (1990) Oculomotor disturbances during visual-vestibular interaction in Wallenberg's lateral medullary syndrome. *Brain.* 113, 821–846.

Walker MF, Zee DS. (2000) Bedside vestibular examination. In: Shepard NT, Solomon D, eds. *Otolaryngologic Clinics of North America.* Philadelphia: WB Saunders.

Wall C. (1990) The sinusoidal harmonic acceleration rotary chair test: theoretical and clinical basis. *Neurol Clin.* 8, 269–285.

Whitney SL, Rossi MM. (2000) Efficacy of vestibular rehabilitation. In: Shepard NT, Solomon D, eds. *Otolaryngologic Clinics of North America.* Philadelphia: WB Saunders.

Yardley L. (2000) Overview of psychological effects of chronic dizziness and balance disorders. In: Shepard NT, Solomon D, eds. *Otolaryngologic Clinics of North America.* Philadelphia: WB Saunders.

Yardley L, Beech S, Zander L, Evans T, Weinman J. (1998a) A randomized controlled trial of exercise therapy for dizziness and vertigo in primary care. *Br J Gen Pract.* 48, 1136–1140.

Yardley L, Owen N, Nazareth I, Luxon L. (1998b) Prevalence and presentation of dizziness in a general practice community sample of working age people. Br J Gen Pract. 48, 1131–1135.

Zee DS. (1985) Perspectives on the disorder of vertigo. *Arch Otolaryngol.* 111, 609–612.

Zee DS. (2000) Vestibular adaptation. In: Herdman S, ed. *Vestibular Rehabilitation.* 2nd ed. Philadelphia: FA Davis; pp 77–90.

HAPTER
21 Otoacoustic Emissions

Beth Prieve and Tracy Fitzgerald

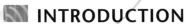

INTRODUCTION

Otoacoustic emissions (OAEs) are a fascinating auditory phenomenon of interest to both auditory scientists and clinicians alike. OAEs are sounds that originate in the cochlea and propagate through the middle ear and into the ear canal where they can be measured using a sensitive microphone. OAEs were first described by David Kemp in 1978, and by 1980, he published a series of articles describing OAEs evoked by various types of stimuli in normal-hearing and hearing-impaired ears. Since that time, an extensive body of research has been produced examining many aspects of OAEs and their relation to auditory functioning. The goal of this chapter is to introduce students and clinicians to the theories underlying OAE generation, the types of OAEs, and their measurement and clinical use.

HYPOTHESES OF OTOACOUSTIC EMISSION GENERATION AND THEIR RELATIONSHIP TO AUDITORY FUNCTION

The Traveling Wave and the Cochlear Amplifier

In order to understand how OAEs are generated, we will start with a brief review of the physiologic processes in the cochlea during the mechanical-to-electrical transduction of a sound. The process begins when the stapes footplate moves in and out of the oval window. This movement results in pressure variations in the fluids of the cochlea that displace the flexible cochlear partition (composed of the basilar membrane,

organ of Corti, and tectorial membrane). The displacement takes the form of a wave pattern, referred to as the "traveling wave," which moves from the base of the cochlea to the apex (Bekesy, 1949). The amplitude of the displacement increases as the traveling wave moves towards the apex, at some point reaching a maximum followed by a rapid decrease in amplitude. The location along the cochlear partition where the maximum displacement or "peak" of the traveling wave occurs is dependent upon the frequency of the incoming signal. High-frequency stimuli peak close to the base of the cochlea, while progressively lower frequencies peak progressively closer to the apex.

A healthy, living cochlea demonstrates nonlinear behavior and refined frequency specificity at low stimulus levels, similar to the characteristics demonstrated by individual hair cells and auditory nerve fibers (Rhode, 1971; Ruggero and Rich, 1991). Basilar membrane responses measured at the peak of the traveling wave grow linearly at low stimulus levels but grow at progressively smaller rates at moderate to high stimulus levels (Ruggero et al., 1997). Active biologic mechanisms, often referred to as the "cochlear amplifier," are believed to be responsible for the nonlinear characteristics of cochlear responses, as well as the exceptional sensitivity and frequency selectivity seen in a healthy cochlea as compared to a damaged or dead cochlea (Dallos, 1988; Dallos, 1992; Davis, 1983). The cochlear amplifier is hypothesized to contribute additional energy that enhances the vibration of the basilar membrane at the peak of the traveling wave, particularly at low stimulus levels (Davis, 1983). Precisely how the cochlear amplifier "boosts" the responses is not known. Current evidence indicates that outer hair cells (OHCs) contribute to this process. Numerous investigators have reported reduced auditory sensitivity, broader tuning, and abnormal response growth when OHCs are damaged or missing (Dallos and Harris, 1978; Dallos and Wang, 1974; Harrison and Evans, 1979; Khanna and Leonard, 1986a; 1986b; Liberman and Dodds, 1984a; 1984b; Ryan and Dallos, 1975).

Otoacoustic Emissions and Outer Hair Cells

OAEs are a preneural phenomenon. They can be measured even when the eighth nerve has been severed (Siegel and Kim, 1982a) or when eighth-nerve activity is blocked chemically (Arts et al., 1990). Unlike neural responses, OAEs are unaffected by stimulus rate (Grandori, 1985; Kemp, 1982; Kemp and Chum, 1980) and reverse polarity along with the stimulus (Schmiedt and Adams, 1981). In addition, OAEs, particularly those evoked using low stimulus levels, are vulnerable to such agents as acoustic trauma (Hamernik et al., 1996; Mills, 2003; Schmiedt, 1986; Zurek et al., 1982), hypoxia (Rebillard and Lavigne-Rebillard, 1992), and ototoxic medications (Brown et al., 1989; Henley et al., 1996), which cause hearing loss and damage to OHCs (Dallos and Harris, 1978; Ryan and Dallos, 1975). OAEs do not appear to be vulnerable to selective loss of inner hair cells (IHCs) (Liberman et al., 1997).

Two hypotheses regarding the role of OHCs in the cochlear amplifier have been explored: somatic motility of OHCs and nonlinear mechanics of the OHC stereocilia bundle. OHCs demonstrate rapid changes in length in response to electrical stimulation (Ashmore, 1987; Brownell et al., 1985). When a large number of OHCs are stimulated in an isolated cochlear preparation, basilar membrane motion can be observed (Mammano and Ashmore, 1993). "Prestin" is thought to be the molecular motor responsible for somatic OHC motility (Santos-Sacchi et al., 2001; Zheng et al., 2000). Reduced OHC length, absence of OHC motility, and IHC and OHC loss in the basal portion of the cochlea were observed in mice when the prestin gene was deleted (Liberman et al., 2002). The mutant mice had thresholds elevated by 35 to 60 dB when measured by auditory brainstem responses and OAE thresholds (Liberman et al., 2002) or compound action potentials (Liberman et al., 2004).

It seems unlikely that somatic motility of OHCs is the sole source of cochlear amplifier energy and OAEs. OAEs have been measured from species that do not have OHCs (Manley et al., 1996; 1987; Stewart and Hudspeth, 2000; Taschenberger and Manley, 1997). OAEs measured in nonmammalian species, whose hair cells are not capable of somatic motility, have been attributed to active hair bundle movements of the hair cell stereocilia (Ricci et al., 2000). Hair cell stereocilia bundles demonstrate frequency selectivity, can provide amplification, and have a force-generating component, which are all properties needed for the cochlear amplifier.[1]

Liberman et al. (2004) presented evidence that both OHC somatic motility and stereocilia may contribute to the

production of OAEs in mammals and that their contributions may be stimulus level dependent. Liberman et al. (2004) reported that one type of OAE, distortion product otoacoustic emissions (DPOAEs; see "Distortion Product Otoacoustic Emissions" section later in this chapter for further descriptions), was measurable in mutant mice lacking the prestin gene but only at high stimulus levels. Liberman et al. argued that the presence of these DPOAEs in the mutant mice indicates that OHC somatic motility is not necessary for their production at high stimulus levels. They hypothesized that the OHC stereocilia generate mechanical distortions, and because stereocilia are directly coupled to the organ of Corti, hair bundle movements could contribute to basilar membrane motion.

One final note regarding OAEs and OHCs is that OHCs receive the majority of the ear's efferent innervation (Spoendlin, 1973; Warr et al., 1986), which may act as a regulatory system that allows higher neurologic centers to exert control over cochlear processes such as OHC motility. Direct electrical stimulation of efferent fibers has been shown to reduce or enhance OAE responses (Guinan, 1986; Mountain, 1980; Siegel and Kim, 1982b). Indirect stimulation of the efferent system by means of ipsilateral, contralateral, or binaural stimulation has also been shown to alter OAE levels (Berlin et al., 1993; 1995; Brown, 1988; Collet et al., 1990; Kujawa et al., 1992; 1993; 1994).

Two Otoacoustic Emission Generation Mechanisms

For many years, all OAEs were thought to arise from the same mechanism, that is, nonlinear electromechanical distortion within the cochlea resulting, at least in part, from OHC somatic motility (Allen and Neely, 1992; de Boer, 1983; Kemp and Brown, 1983). More recently, the theory that OAEs arise from two different mechanisms has changed the way researchers talk about the sources of OAEs and OAE classification (Shera and Guinan, 1999; Talmadge et al., 1999). In early work, Kemp et al. studied phase changes as a function of stimulus frequency for different types of OAEs and found two distinct patterns (Kemp, 1986; Kemp and Brown, 1983). Shera and Guinan later attributed the two patterns to different mechanisms: nonlinear distortion and linear coherent reflection. Nonlinear distortion emissions are attributed directly to the action of OHCs. The source of nonlinear distortion, or "wave-fixed," emissions is believed to follow the traveling wave envelope of the stimulus (Shera and Guinan, 1999). Therefore, because the shape of the traveling wave does not change significantly as the stimulus is swept in frequency, the phase at any point moving with the traveling wave envelope will not change significantly, as schematized in the left panel of Figure 21.1. Thus, nonlinear distortion emissions are characterized by gradual phase changes as the stimulus frequencies are increased.

Reflection, or "place-fixed," emissions are characterized by phase that rotates rapidly with changes in stimulus

---

[1] For a review of the specific data from hair cell stereocilia providing support for their role in cochlear amplification, the reader is referred to Ricci (2003).

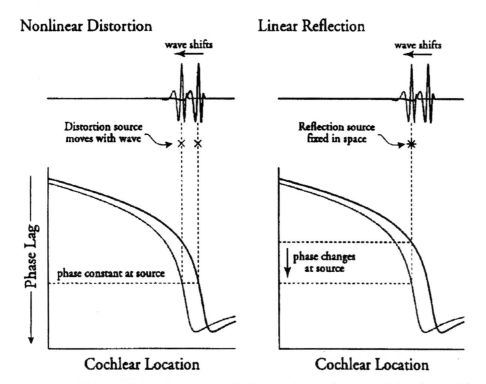

FIGURE 21.1 Schematic illustrations of the phase behavior for emissions arising from either nonlinear distortion (*left panel*) or coherent linear reflection (*right panel*) mechanisms. In either panel, the f2 traveling wave at two frequencies is shown, one peaking at a more apical location than the other (*top*) along with the corresponding phase lag versus the distance along the basilar membrane (*bottom*). The phase lag function for the more apical wave lies above that for the more basal wave. For ease of viewing, the f2 traveling waves have been exaggerated relative to the size of the stapes, the f1 traveling waves are not shown, and the distortion and reflection sources are idealized as single points (*asterisks*). As seen in the panel on the left, as f2 is changed to a higher frequency (more basal), the distortion source moves with the wave; therefore, the phase of the wave at the source remains constant as frequency is increased. In the right panel, as f2 is changed to a higher frequency, the reflection source remains fixed; therefore, the phase at the source changes rapidly as frequency is increased. (Reprinted with permission from Kalluri R, Shera C. [2001] Distortion-product source unmixing: s test of the two-mechanism model for DPOAE generation. *J Acoust Soc Am.* 25, 86–97; ©2001 by American Institute of Physics.)

frequency, as shown by a schematic diagram in the right panel of Figure 21.1. These emissions are proposed to be the result of the incoming traveling waves scattering off of random impedance perturbations in the mechanics of the cochlea or impedance mismatches present at or near the largest displacement of the traveling wave (Shera and Guinan, 1999). The source of the impedance perturbations is not known, but hypotheses include variations in OHC cell arrangement or variations in OHCs at the cellular level (Shera, 2004). Shera and Guinan (1999) explain the nonlinear behavior of reflection emissions, such as compressive growth functions, as the result of level-dependent amplification of the forward and reverse traveling waves due to action of the cochlear amplifier. In this way, reflection emissions, although not generated by the action of OHCs, would be acted upon by these forces and would, therefore, still be vulnerable to changes in OHC function.

OAEs measured in the ear canal are likely a combination of energy from both mechanisms (Knight and Kemp, 1999;

2000; 2001; Shera and Guinan, 1999; Yates and Withnell, 1999). At this time, it is not known whether emissions arising from the two mechanisms might be used differently to provide information about cochlear function. Shera (2004) and others have suggested that, by "unmixing" the energy from the two mechanisms and examining each separately, diagnostic and screening tests with OAEs might be improved. Additional research is necessary to determine whether the two mechanisms may be used to improve OAE clinical applications.

■ MEASUREMENT OF OTOACOUSTIC EMISSIONS

A general recording setup for measuring OAEs includes a sensitive, miniature microphone that fits in the ear canal. Typically, the microphone is housed in a small probe that is coupled to the ear with a foam or rubber tip. The probe contains one or two speakers that allow for presentation of sound stimuli. The microphone measures the OAE coming from the ear and, in the case of some OAEs, also measures the stimuli presented to the ear. The output of the microphone is then amplified. Typically, the amplified output is sampled via an analog-to-digital converter, either housed in a computer or in a stand-alone piece of equipment. The output is then appropriately analyzed for the type of OAE.

Because all OAEs are low-level signals, the recording technique of signal averaging must be used. In this technique, the energy in the ear canal is viewed over a particular time period. Many pieces of equipment use time-synchronous averaging. Each time the stimulus is presented, the sound in the ear canal is sampled, and the start of the sample is synchronized with the onset of the stimulus. The stimulus is presented hundreds of times, and each sample is averaged with the previous samples. Signal averaging relies on two assumptions. The first assumption is that, with each stimulus presentation, the OAE response will be the same and will be synchronized or time-locked to the stimulus. The second assumption is that any noise or artifact will be random and not synchronized to the signal. Averaging should, therefore, reduce the level of the noise while preserving the OAE, thus improving the signal-to-noise ratio.[2]

Averaging can also be accomplished in the frequency domain. There are two methods of frequency domain averaging. In one method, only the magnitude of the signal is taken into consideration. With multiple stimulus presentations, the variance of the noise is reduced, but the level of the noise remains constant. In the second method, which is preferable, both the magnitude and phase of the signal are taken into consideration. With this type of averaging, the residual noise in the trace is reduced, similar to that observed in time-synchronous averaging.

The noise level arising from a combination of environmental and internal sources has a significant effect on OAE recordings. High noise levels can obscure low-level OAEs. When high noise levels are present, the number of averages collected must be increased, thereby increasing the test time necessary to obtain a clear OAE recording. Several factors can aid in reducing the effects of noise. First, it is essential to minimize the amount of environmental noise by choosing a quiet or, if possible, sound-treated room as the location for testing. Nonessential equipment, such as fans, should be turned off. Second, the state of the patient being tested must be assessed and addressed. The high noise levels produced by an infant or child that is crying, talking, or generally restless will make testing impossible or extremely difficult. Instructing parents ahead of time as to the nature of the test and that an infant should be asleep during testing can be extremely helpful. Adult patients and older children should be given clear instructions to remain still and quiet during testing. Finally, the importance of an adequate probe fit cannot be

overemphasized. A snug and secure probe fit will generally reduce the effects of environmental noise, as well as prevent the loss of low-frequency stimulus energy.

TYPES OF OTOACOUSTIC EMISSIONS

Before the recent classification of OAEs based on generation mechanism (Shera and Guinan, 1999), OAEs were classified into two types, spontaneous and evoked. As the name suggests, spontaneous otoacoustic emissions (SOAEs) are recorded in the absence of any external stimulation. Evoked otoacoustic emissions (EOAEs) are measured during or following presentation of an acoustic stimulus to the ear. EOAEs are further subcategorized by the type of stimulus used and related measurement procedure. The clinical literature continues to use this traditional taxonomy; therefore, we will use it here for description of OAEs and their clinical applications.

Spontaneous Otoacoustic Emissions

Spontaneous otoacoustic emissions (SOAEs) are measured in the absence of external stimulation. They can be measured by viewing what is recorded by the microphone in the frequency domain. As Figure 21.2 illustrates, SOAEs appear as puretone-like signals coming from the ear. This ear has multiple SOAEs, that is, SOAEs at more than one frequency.

SOAEs are measurable in approximately 50% of normal-hearing children and adults. The actual estimates range from 40% (Strickland et al., 1985) to as high as 72% (Talmadge et al., 1993). The wide range of estimates could be due to small sample sizes and recording systems with different noise

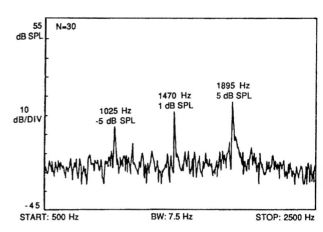

FIGURE 21.2 An example of spontaneous otoacoustic emissions (SOAEs) measured from a normal-hearing human. Three SOAEs are measurable. (Modified and used with permission from Lonsbury-Martin BL, Whitehead ML, Martin GK. [1991] Clinical applications of otoacoustic emissions. *J Speech Hear Res.* 34, 964–981; ©1991 by American Speech-Language-Hearing Association.)

---

[2] For more detailed information regarding principles of averaging, see Chapter 11 and Hyde (1994).

floors. Statistical analyses based on grouped data indicate that the prevalence of SOAEs is higher in females than in males and in right ears than in left ears. Having an SOAE in one ear increases the likelihood that an SOAE will be present in the other ear (Bilger et al., 1990). Research on the prevalence of SOAEs in neonates and infants compared to older children and adults has produced mixed results. While some data suggest that the prevalence of SOAEs is higher in neonates than it is in adults (Kok et al., 1993a), other studies have found no significant differences between neonates and adults (Burns et al., 1992; Strickland et al., 1985).

The typical frequencies and levels of SOAEs measured from adults differ from those measured in infants. The majority of SOAEs measured from adults have frequencies between 1,000 and 2,000 Hz (Bright, 2002). These are the frequencies that coincide with the most sensitive behavioral thresholds in human ears and may reflect the band-pass characteristics of the middle ear. The majority of SOAEs from neonate and infant ears are between the frequencies of 2,000 and 5,000 Hz (Burns et al., 1992; Prieve and Huta, 1999). The higher frequency SOAEs recorded from neonates and infants may be due to differences in middle ear or ear canal size. The average SOAE level for neonates is 8.5 dB sound pressure level (SPL), which is significantly higher than the average SOAE level of −2.6 dB SPL found in adults (Burns et al., 1992). Prieve and Huta (1999) reported that infants have higher SOAE levels than children aged 4 to 8 years of age, teenagers, and adults. Prevalence of SOAEs tends to decrease in the elderly population; however, many older individuals also have less sensitive hearing thresholds. Therefore, it is difficult to determine whether the finding of fewer SOAEs in the elderly is linked with old age or the elevated thresholds (Bonfils, 1989; Mazelova et al., 2003).

SOAEs can be measured in ears having hearing loss no greater than 25 to 30 dB hearing level (HL) (Bonfils, 1989; Bright and Glattke, 1986). Because they can be measured in only 50% of normal-hearing ears, they are not a useful clinical test. For example, if an individual does not have SOAEs, the clinician cannot distinguish whether that ear has normal-hearing or hearing loss. However, EOAEs from ears with measurable SOAEs are different than EOAEs from ears with no measurable SOAEs (Prieve et al., 1997a; 1997b; Probst et al., 1986; Zwicker, 1983). The presence of SOAEs is considered evidence of an "active" element in the cochlea (Kim, 1986).

Spontaneous Otoacoustic Emissions and Tinnitus

Following Kemp's (1979) first report of SOAEs, speculation arose that they might be an objective correlate of at least some forms of tinnitus. Investigators hypothesized that the active processes of the cochlea might in some cases cause "self-oscillation" that is perceived as tinnitus (Moller, 1989). Studies examining the connection between SOAEs and tinnitus have generally reported that the two phenomena appear to be independent events (Bonfils, 1989; Hazell, 1984;

Penner, 1990; Penner and Burns, 1987; Probst et al., 1987; Tyler and Conrad-Ames, 1981; Zurek, 1981). Reports of a possible causative relationship between SOAEs and tinnitus have been limited to a few case studies of patients who had normal-hearing sensitivity in at least some frequency regions (Penner, 1988; 1989a; 1989b; Wilson and Sutton, 1981).

Most early studies examining SOAEs and tinnitus focused on pitch matching, that is, whether the frequency of a tone judged to match the pitch of the tinnitus was close to the frequency of an SOAE. Penner and Burns (1987) proposed that pitch matching alone is not sufficient evidence to suggest that an SOAE can be considered the cause of tinnitus. They proposed two additional measures. First, the tinnitus should become inaudible when the SOAE is suppressed by an external stimulus. Second, the iso-masking contours[3] for the tinnitus should not be flat. Using the above criteria to evaluate a group of 121 tinnitus sufferers, Penner (1990) concluded that only 2.42% of the group had tinnitus apparently caused by an SOAE. She estimated that SOAEs were responsible in only about 1% to 9% of tinnitus cases.

Stimulus Frequency Otoacoustic Emissions

Stimulus frequency otoacoustic emissions (SFOAEs) occur at the same frequency and at the same time as a continuous puretone applied to the ear. The microphone in the ear canal records the combination of the puretone being presented to the ear and the SFOAE evoked by the puretone. Because the stimulus and SFOAE are occurring at the same time and at the same frequency, specialized measurement techniques must be used to extract the SFOAE from the evoking stimulus. Common techniques involve introducing a second stimulus differing in intensity or frequency that takes advantage of the nonlinear properties of the SFOAE (Brass and Kemp, 1991; Schairer et al., 2003: Schairer and Keefe, 2005; Shera and Guinan, 1999). For example, using a tone that is slightly higher or lower in frequency than the evoking stimulus suppresses the SFOAE. A vector subtraction can be made between the SPL in the ear canal when the tone is presented alone (tone plus SFOAE) and the SPL when the tone is presented in the presence of the suppressor (tone alone). The difference between the two conditions is attributed to the SFOAE or, depending on the specifics of the second tone, the portion of the SFOAE that remains unsuppressed by the second tone (Shera and Guinan, 1999). Other methods employing three or four condition intervals have also been used and produce similar results (Brass and Kemp, 1991; Schairer et al., 2003; Schairer and Keefe, 2005).

Averaged SFOAE levels generally grow linearly for low stimulus levels and then saturate for high stimulus levels. According to the two-mechanism model of OAE generation, SFOAEs are considered linear coherent reflection emissions

---

[3] Iso-masking contours for tinnitus are produced by presenting an individual with tones of different frequencies and plotting the level at each frequency required to mask the person's tinnitus. The iso-masking contours for tinnitus are typically flat (Penner and Burns, 1987).

(Shera and Guinan, 1999; Talmadge et al., 1999). However, evidence suggests that they are a reflection-type emission close to threshold but include distortion-type generation at mid to high levels (Goodman et al., 2003; Schairer et al., 2003; Schairer and Keefe, 2005).

SFOAEs are not used clinically because their characteristics in ears with normal hearing and hearing loss have not been extensively studied. In addition, there are no commercial devices designed to record SFOAEs. However, a recent laboratory experiment in 85 ears showed that SFOAEs identified hearing loss as well as other EOAEs at 1,000 and 2,000 Hz. At 500 Hz, they were superior to other EOAEs in identifying hearing loss (Ellison and Keefe, 2005). Further research on SFOAEs under clinical conditions will elucidate their possible use in general clinical settings.

Transient-Evoked Otoacoustic Emissions

Transient-evoked otoacoustic emissions (TEOAEs) were the first type of OAE reported in the literature (Kemp, 1978). As their name suggests, TEOAEs are measured after the presentation of a transient or brief stimulus. A click or tone burst is presented to the ear, and the response occurs after a brief time delay. Measurement of TEOAEs is accomplished using time-synchronous averaging. Although the averaging reduces the amount of noise in the trace, it does not remove the stimulus artifact at the start of the recording. The stimulus artifact under typical recording conditions is much larger than the recorded TEOAE. The energy from the stimulus may also persist in the ear canal long enough to obscure the onset of the TEOAE response. Therefore, the first few milliseconds of the trace are usually eliminated from the final averaged waveform to remove energy due to the stimulus.

Figure 21.3 is an example of a typical click-evoked otoacoustic emission (COAE) waveform recorded from an adult

ear. This example was obtained using Otodynamics ILO88 software and accompanying hardware, the first commercially available program for recording TEOAEs. The waveform of the click stimulus is located in the upper left-hand corner of the display. The amplitude spectrum of the click is displayed in the box under the heading "Stim = 80.0 dB." The click used to evoke the COAE was 80 dB peak SPL (pSPL). The largest portion of the display in the lower right contains the waveform of the COAE in the time domain. Notice that the first 2.5 ms have been eliminated to remove the stimulus artifact. If you look closely, you can see that the response is actually comprised of two waveforms that have been superimposed. During testing, TEOAE measurement software alternately stores an averaged response in each of two separate buffers, resulting in two averaged traces (labeled "A" and "B" in Fig. 21.3). Comparison of these two waveforms allows the software to determine several TEOAE parameters. For instance, the software calculates the difference between the two waveforms and reports this as the noise level in dB SPL, displayed next to "A-B" in the right-hand column (1.8 dB SPL). The cross power spectrum of the two waveforms is also calculated and displayed. The cross power spectrum can be seen in the upper right portion of the display under the heading "Response FFT" (Response Fast Fourier Transform). TEOAE levels are indicated by the dark-shaded regions, while the noise levels are indicated by the superimposed lighter shaded regions.[4]

TEOAEs are often evaluated in terms of level, percent reproducibility, and TEOAE/noise (sometimes called signal-to-noise ratio [S/N or SNR]). The level of the TEOAE is usually expressed in dB SPL. The level in the example is 10.7 dB SPL and can be found next to the term "Response" in the right-hand column. Below the heading "Band Repro% SNR dB," the percentage reproducibility of the TEOAE in each of the linear frequency bands beginning at 1,000, 2,000, 3,000, 4,000, and 5,000 Hz is listed. Percent reproducibility in this case refers to a how well the two TEOAE traces correlate with one another. The software computes interwaveform correlations in each frequency band, as well as for the broadband waveform, and displays them as percentages. TEOAE/noise or S/N is a ratio of the level of the TEOAE (the "signal") to the level of the noise expressed in dB. TEOAE/noise may be given for the overall TEOAE response or in separate frequency bands. TEOAE/noise levels in Figure 21.3 are listed for the same linear frequency bands under the percent reproducibility.

TEOAEs initially received the most attention as a possible clinical tool. Early studies established that TEOAEs were measurable in nearly all ears with normal sensitivity and middle-ear function (Bonfils et al., 1988b; Grandori, 1985; Johnson and Elberling, 1982; Kemp, 1978; Kemp et al., 1986; Norton and Neely, 1987; Probst et al., 1986). In contrast, TEOAEs were absent in almost all ears with sensory-neural

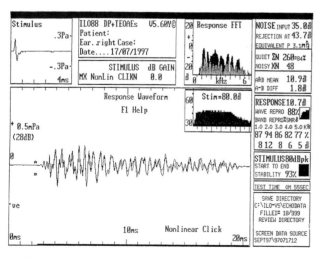

FIGURE 21.3   An example of a click-evoked otoacoustic emission (COAE) recorded from the ear canal of an adult using the Otodynamics ILO88 system.

---

[4] For more detailed information regarding the technical aspects of the Otodynamics ILO88 system and its display properties, see Bray (1989).

hearing loss that exceeded 30 to 50 dB HL (Bonfils et al., 1988b; Collet et al., 1993b; Kemp, 1978; Probst et al., 1987; Robinette, 1992; Stevens, 1988).

BASIC CHARACTERISTICS OF TRANSIENT-EVOKED OTOACOUSTIC EMISSIONS AND THE EFFECTS OF STIMULUS AND RECORDING PARAMETERS

Kemp (1978) noted in his initial report on TEOAEs that the different frequency components of the evoked responses emerge at different times. Kemp called this phenomenon "frequency dispersion" (Kemp, 1978, p 1387). The dominant period of oscillation changes over time, such that higher frequency components of the response appear first, followed by lower frequency components. Typically this phenomenon is described in terms of "latency"; higher frequency components have shorter latencies, whereas lower frequency components have longer latencies (Grandori, 1985; Kemp, 1978; Wilson, 1980; Wit and Ritsma, 1980). Although the measured latencies vary across individuals, the pattern of increasing latency with decreasing frequency remains constant across individuals (Grandori, 1985; Kemp, 1978).

The spectrum of a TEOAE is dependent upon several factors related to the stimulus and recording parameters. One such factor is the spectrum of the evoking stimulus. Broadband click stimuli generally evoke broadband responses. Tone burst–evoked OAEs (TBOAEs) are more frequency specific and typically limited to the frequency range of the narrowband stimuli used to evoke them (Norton and Neely, 1987; Probst et al., 1986; Stover and Norton, 1993). Figure 21.4 displays TBOAEs evoked by tone bursts with carrier frequencies at 1,000 (Fig 21.4A) and 4,000 Hz (Fig. 24.1B) that were measured with the Otodynamics ILO88 system. The features of the display are identical to those in Figure 21.3. The spectrum of TBOAE energy is narrower than that of the broadband COAE response shown in Figure 21.3.

TEOAE spectra are also influenced by the filter setting and recording time window. As mentioned previously, the stimulus artifact must be removed from the start of the averaged trace. Unfortunately, the removal of the first few milliseconds from the trace may also result in the loss of some high-frequency components of the response. The greater the number of milliseconds eliminated from the start of the trace, the greater the amount of high-frequency energy that is potentially eliminated. Conversely, reducing the length of the response time window can result in the loss of some low-frequency energy. The exact TEOAE spectrum and the latency of the different frequency components measured are unique to each individual (Kemp, 1978; Norton and Neely, 1987). These individual TEOAE features are stable within a given ear over time, barring changes in hearing sensitivity (Antonelli and Grandori, 1986; Grandori, 1985; Kemp, 1978, 1982; Kemp et al., 1986; Wilson, 1980).

TEOAE level varies with stimulus level. TEOAE level displays nonlinear growth characteristics in the majority of ears. An example of a TEOAE growth or input/output (I/O)

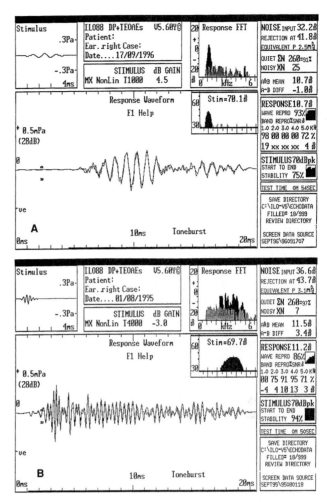

FIGURE 21.4 Examples of tone burst–evoked otoacoustic emissions (TBOAEs) recorded from adults using tone bursts centered at (A) 1,000 Hz and (B) 4,000 Hz. The recordings were obtained using the Otodynamics ILO88 system.

function can be seen in Figure 21.5. At low to moderate stimulus levels, growth is fairly linear. However, at higher levels of stimulation, typically between 50 and 80 dB pSPL depending on the type of stimulus used, growth functions show saturation (Grandori, 1985; Stover and Norton, 1993; Wilson, 1980; Zwicker, 1983). As the stimulus level is increased at these high levels, little or no growth in the TEOAE level is noted. The growth function in Figure 21.5 shows saturation between click levels of 60 and 70 dB pSPL.

TEOAE level also varies widely across individuals. For example, Robinette (1992) reported COAE levels for a group of 265 normal-hearing adults that ranged from 0.1 to 22.3 dB SPL in response to clicks presented at a mean level of 81 dB pSPL (standard deviation [SD] = 2.7 dB). Results from studies in our laboratory have indicated that the SD for COAE levels recorded at click levels from 40 to 80 dB pSPL is approximately 5 dB (Prieve and Falter, 1995; Prieve et al., 1997a).

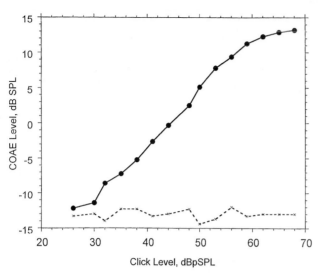

FIGURE 21.5 A click-evoked otoacoustic emission (COAE) growth function recorded from an adult. The *filled circles* indicate COAE levels in dB sound pressure level (SPL). The small Xs connected by dotted lines (*X*-----*X*) indicate the corresponding noise floor levels in dB SPL. The COAE level grows linearly with increases in stimulus levels at low to moderate levels of stimulation; however, the COAE level begins to saturate at higher levels of stimulation (60–70 dB peak SPL [pSPL]).

It is important to keep in mind the spectrum of the stimulus when examining TEOAE growth functions and, in particular, when making comparisons between COAEs and TBOAEs. Although a tone burst and click may have the same overall peak level, the energy from the click is distributed across a much broader range of frequencies. This will result in a lower spectrum level at any given frequency for the click. When click and tone-burst stimuli are equated for spectrum level, levels and growth behavior of TEOAEs evoked by the two stimuli are similar (Prieve et al., 1996).

The presence of SOAEs affects both the spectrum and the level of TEOAEs. SOAEs can synchronize to the evoking stimulus, resulting in peaks at those frequencies in the TEOAE spectrum (Kulawiec and Orlando, 1995). Probst et al. (1986) reported a greater number of peaks in the COAE spectra of persons with SOAEs than in the spectra evoked from ears in persons without any measurable SOAEs. Group data have also indicated that TEOAE levels are higher and TEOAE thresholds are lower in ears with SOAEs compared to ears without any measurable SOAEs (Moulin et al., 1993; Osterhammel et al., 1996; Prieve and Falter, 1995; Prieve et al., 1997a; Probst et al., 1986).

Distortion Product Otoacoustic Emissions

Distortion product otoacoustic emissions (DPOAEs), which are sometimes called acoustic distortion products (ADPs), are measured simultaneously with the presentation of two

puretone stimuli, called "primaries," to the ear. The frequencies of the primaries are conventionally designated as "f1" and "f2" (f1 < f2), and the corresponding levels of the primaries are designated as "L1" and "L2." When f1 and f2 are reasonably close in frequency, interaction of the two primaries on the basilar membrane results in the output of energy by the cochlea at other discrete frequencies that are arithmetically related to the frequencies of the primaries (e.g., f2-f1, 2f1-f2, 3f1-2f2, 2f2-f1). DPOAEs can therefore be measured using narrowband filtering centered at the frequency of interest. The spectrum in Figure 21.6 displays the primaries and DPOAEs measured in the ear canal of a 16-month-old child (using the Otodynamics ILO92 software). Notice that DPOAEs are present at frequencies both lower (e.g., 2f1-f2, 3f1-f2) and higher (e.g., 2f2-f1) than the primaries. DPOAEs are thought to be a combination of energy from a nonlinear distortion component originating at the region of overlap between the primaries and a reflection component originating from the region of the DPOAE frequency (Shera and Guinan, 1999). The mechanism that dominates the response seems to depend on which DPOAE is being measured, as well as the primary levels and the frequency relationships between the primaries (Knight and Kemp, 2000; 2001).

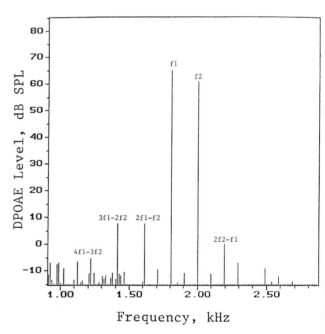

FIGURE 21.6 A spectrum showing two input primaries (f1 = 1.807 kHz, f2 = 2.002 kHz, L1 = 65 dB sound pressure level [SPL], and L2 = 60 dB SPL) and the resulting distortion product otoacoustic emissions (DPOAEs) from the ear of a 16-month-old child. Several DPOAEs occurring at frequencies below the primaries (4f1-3f2 = 1.222 kHz, 3f1-2f2 = 1.417 kHz, and 2f1-f2 = 1.612 kHz) and above the primaries (2f2-f1 = 2.197 kHz) are labeled.

DPOAE measurement systems typically provide a measure of both the DPOAE and surrounding noise level. The noise level is most often determined by averaging the levels in several frequency bins on either side of the DPOAE of interest. The presence of a particular DPOAE is determined by comparing the level measured within its frequency bin with the noise levels in the surrounding frequency bins and employing some difference criterion. For instance, the DPOAE might be considered present if its level is 3 dB or more above the level of the surrounding noise floor or if its level exceeds two SDs above the mean noise level.

DPOAEs, like TEOAEs, can be measured in nearly all ears with normal hearing and normal middle ear function and are stable within a given ear over time (Lonsbury-Martin et al., 1990a; 1990b). On average, the 2f1-f2 DPOAE has the largest level in human and other mammalian ears compared to other DPOAEs (Gaskill and Brown, 1990). As a result, 2f1-f2 is the DPOAE that has been the most extensively investigated, particularly for clinical purposes (Gorga et al., 1997). The 2f1-f2 DPOAE has sometimes been referred to as the cubic difference tone (CDT). Unless otherwise specified, the use of the term DPOAE will henceforth refer to 2f1-f2.

BASIC CHARACTERISTICS OF THE 2F1-F2 DISTORTION PRODUCT OTOACOUSTIC EMISSION AND THE EFFECTS OF STIMULUS AND RECORDING PARAMETERS

DPOAE levels vary widely across individual ears. Typical DPOAE levels reported for adults range from 45 to 75 dB below the level of equal-level primaries (Lonsbury-Martin et al., 1990a; Vinck et al., 1996). As with TEOAEs, DPOAE levels are generally larger in ears with measurable SOAEs compared to ears without any measurable SOAEs (Cianfrone et al., 1990; Moulin et al., 1993; Prieve et al., 1997b; Wier et al., 1988).

Early studies revealed that 2f1-f2 level is highly dependent upon various parameters of the primaries, including their frequency, frequency separation, level separation, and overall level (Gaskill and Brown, 1990; Harris et al., 1989). A large body of literature has been devoted to determining the "optimal" stimulus parameters that will yield the largest DPOAE levels in normal-hearing persons.

The frequency separation of the two primaries, generally described as the f2/f1 ratio, influences the DPOAE level that will be measured. Figure 21.7 displays DPOAE level as a function of f2/f1 as measured from an individual adult ear for f2 = 4,000 Hz and L2 levels of 40, 50, and 60 dB SPL when L1 − L2 = 15 dB. As f2/f1 is decreased from larger values (∼1.5) to progressively smaller values, DPOAE level increases to a broad maximum and then progressively decreases. The exact shape of the function and the f2/f1 that produces the maximum DPOAE level vary across individuals, stimulus levels, and frequencies (Neely et al., 2005). However, when data are averaged across many persons, the largest DPOAE levels have repeatedly been obtained with an f2/f1 of approximately 1.2 (Abdala, 1996; Brown and Gaskill, 1990a; 1990b;

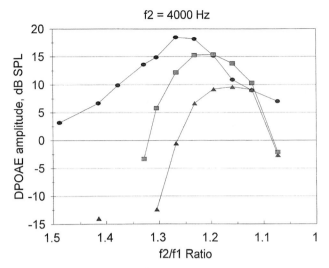

FIGURE 21.7 A graph of distortion product otoacoustic emission (DPOAE) level as a function of f2/f1 ratio from an adult ear at three different stimulus levels (f2 = 4,000 Hz). The primary levels used to evoke the DPOAEs were L1 = 75 and L2 = 60 dB sound pressure level (SPL) (*circles*), L1 = 65 and L2 = 50 dB SPL (*squares*), and L1 = 55 and L2 = 40 dB SPL (*triangles*). As the f2/f1 ratio is decreased from a value of approximately 1.5, the DPOAE level increases to a broad maximum at ratios of 1.2 to 1.3 and then declines as the ratio is further decreased. The band-pass–shaped function is typical in both infants and adults.

Brown et al., 1994; 1995; Gaskill and Brown, 1990; Harris et al., 1989; Lasky, 1998; Smurzynski et al., 1990).

The general shape and features of f2/f1 functions appear to be the same for neonates, infants, and adults (Abdala, 1996; Brown et al., 1995; Fitzgerald and Prieve, 1999; Lasky, 1998), although subtle differences have been found between genders and among preterm newborn infants and adults (Vento et al., 2004).

The decrease in level at large ratios (i.e., when the two primary frequencies are widely separated) is not surprising. The farther apart the primaries are from one another, the less the interaction of their respective traveling waves on the basilar membrane. Several theories were initially offered to explain the decrease in DPOAE level at small ratios, including a filtering mechanism within the cochlea (Allen and Fahey, 1993; Brown and Gaskill, 1990a), suppression of the DPOAE by the primaries and of the primaries by one another (Kanis and de Boer, 1997), or the interaction of waves from two or more sources within the cochlea results in cancellation of some energy (Harris et al., 1989; Kemp, 1986). Stover et al. (1999) presented data that support the third hypothesis. Ratio functions with the expected band-pass shape were obtained from participants with normal hearing at both the 2f1-f2 frequency and at the primary frequencies and from participants with normal hearing at the 2f1-f2 frequency but mild hearing loss in the region of the primary frequencies (who still produced measurable DPOAEs). However, in the cases where hearing was normal at the f2 frequency but impaired at the 2f1-f2 frequency, the ratio functions had what the authors called a "high-pass shape." Stover et al. (1999) posited that the second source at the DPOAE place (reflection emission) was no longer contributing to the overall DPOAE because of the hearing loss in that frequency region. In any event, clinical studies have generally fixed f2/f1 to values approximating 1.2 in order to evoke maximal DPOAE levels in the greatest number of persons (Gorga et al., 1997).

When DPOAEs are measured in small frequency steps (<50 Hz), large variations in the DPOAE level, termed "fine structure," are evident (He and Schmiedt, 1993). An example of DPOAE fine structure recorded from an adult is shown in Figure 21.8. DPOAE levels were measured using primaries stepped across frequency in 12.5-Hz steps. Measurements were made with f2 levels ranging from 40 to 69 dB SPL. As primary levels increase, the fine structure pattern shifts to lower frequencies, and the level differences between peaks and troughs become less pronounced.

Fine structure is believed to result from the interaction of energy from the nonlinear distortion and reflection components. Depending on the phases of these two sources, they may combine constructively, such that a higher DPOAE level is measured in the ear canal (peaks), or destructively, such that a lower level is measured (dips). Support for this theory comes from studies that have attempted to reduce/eliminate the second source from the DPOAE region either through suppression or selective hearing loss. Heitmann et al. (1998) demonstrated that fine structure was eliminated when a suppressor tone was presented at 25 Hz above the 2f1-f2 frequency. Mauermann et al. (1999) reported that fine structure was not present for participants with normal hearing in the region of the primary frequencies but hearing loss in the region of the 2f1-f2 frequency. In their participants with normal hearing in the DPOAE frequency region, fine structure was preserved as long as DPOAEs were present.

The level difference between the two primaries (L1 vs. L2) also affects the measured DPOAE level. Although most of the early work on DPOAEs was done using equal-level primaries (Lonsbury-Martin et al., 1990a), the level difference that produces the largest DPOAE levels depends on overall primary levels (Gaskill and Brown, 1990; Harris et al., 1989; Whitehead et al., 1995). Equal-level primaries produce the largest DPOAEs at high levels of stimulus presentation; however, the level difference between the two primaries that produces the largest DPOAEs increases (L1 > L2) as the overall level of the primaries decreases (Gaskill and Brown, 1990; Harris et al., 1989; Hauser and Probst, 1991; Kummer et al., 1998; Rasmussen et al., 1993; Whitehead et al., 1995). The level difference between the two primaries that produces the highest DPOAE levels varies across individuals (Neely et al., 2005); however, using conventional measurement techniques, it would not be feasible to determine the best separations for each individual prior to actual testing in a clinical setting. Kummer et al. (1998) suggested using the

equation L1 = 0.4*L2 + 39 dB (for L2 <65 dB SPL) to set the primary levels in order to generate maximal DPOAE levels. The equation was based on earlier data (Gaskill and Brown, 1990) and designed to allow for level-dependent changes in the overlap between the two primaries at the f2 place. The same equation was recommended for use regardless of f2 frequency (Kummer et al., 2000). Later work by Neely and colleagues indicated that larger DPOAE levels could be measured if the L1 and L2 relationship varied with f2 frequency as well as with L2 level (Johnson et al., 2006; Neely et al., 2005). These authors recommended that both L1 and f2/f1 should vary with L2 and f2 to obtain maximum DPOAE levels (Johnson et al., 2006).

As would be expected, changes in the overall levels of the primaries also affect DPOAE level. As with TEOAEs, the effects of overall primary levels on DPOAE level are usually graphed as a growth function. With the primaries fixed at a specific pair of frequencies, the DPOAE level is recorded as the levels of the primaries are increased. In general, DPOAE level increases as the levels of the primaries increase. Growth functions that include data averaged across a group of persons usually display growth similar to that seen for TEOAEs (Lonsbury-Martin et al., 1990a). However, individual growth functions have a variety of shapes (Nelson and Kimberley, 1992; Stover and Norton, 1993). Figure 21.8 illustrates three examples of DPOAE growth functions, including growth with changes in slope and complex patterns with dips or decreases in DPOAE level with increases in overall stimulus level. The patterns seen in the growth functions can be attributed to the individuals' underlying fine structure. Examination of growth functions can facilitate determination of DPOAE threshold, that is, the lowest primary levels that evoke a detectable DPOAE.

Transient-Evoked Otoacoustic Emissions, Distortion Product Otoacoustic Emissions, and Patient Characteristics

Whenever a measurement tool is proposed for clinical use, an important step is to determine normative values. One part of this process is to determine whether measured differences can be explained by patient characteristics such as age or gender. TEOAE levels change with development from infancy to adulthood; however, the exact time course remains uncertain. Early group data established that COAE levels in neonates (infants <1 month of age) are larger than in adults (Collet et al., 1993a; Kok et al., 1992; 1993b; Norton, 1993) and in older children (Bergman et al., 1995; Norton, 1994). Other data suggest that COAE levels are significantly larger in those under 1 year of age compared to other age groups (Prieve et al., 1997a) and that COAE levels in children are larger than those in adults (Norton and Widen, 1990; Prieve et al., 1997a; Spektor et al., 1991). Differences in COAE level with development appear to be frequency dependent. When COAE levels were analyzed in separate frequency bands, analysis of variance (ANOVA) indicated significant differences in

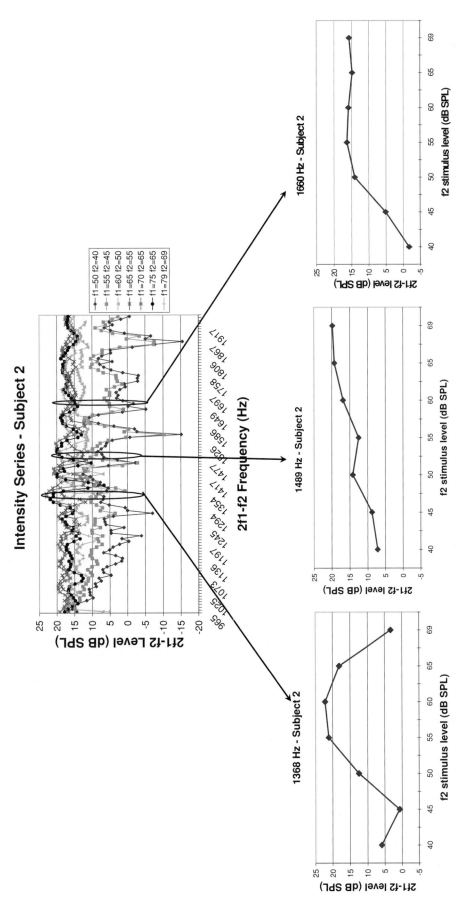

FIGURE 21.8 The top panel depicts distortion product otoacoustic emission (DPOAE) level as a function of DPOAE frequency in an individual for increasing primary levels. The primaries were increased in 12.5-Hz steps, allowing observation of DPOAE microstructure. Microstructure is most pronounced for low-level primaries, and the pattern changes with increasing primary levels. The three lower panels each depict DPOAE level for a particular frequency as primary levels are increased. The shape of DPOAE input/output (I/O) functions vary depending on the underlying fine structure patterns at that frequency.

COAE level between age groups for mid to high frequencies but not for 1,000 Hz and below (Prieve et al., 1997a). COAE level differences between the age groups appear independent of stimulus level or the presence/absence of SOAEs (Prieve et al., 1997a). Prieve et al. (1997a) reported that differences in COAE level between infants and all other age groups were statistically significant at the three click levels that were tested (40, 60, and 80 dB pSPL), suggesting that COAE growth functions do not differ markedly between infants and adults in terms of shape or slope.

DPOAE levels also change with development. Neonates have higher DPOAE levels compared to adults, but the details of how they differed varied across studies (Lafreniere et al., 1991; Lasky et al., 1992; Smurzynski et al., 1993). A few studies have indicated that DPOAE levels in neonates and older infants are higher than those in adults across a broad range of frequencies (Abdala and Sininger, 1996; Bergman et al., 1995; Brown et al., 1994; Prieve et al., 1997b). Prieve et al. (1997b) examined DPOAE levels in infants, children, and adults ranging from 4 weeks to 29 years of age. As with their study of COAEs, they found significant differences in DPOAE level with age that were frequency dependent but that were independent of stimulus level or SOAE status. Infants under 1 year of age had higher DPOAE levels than teens and adults for f2 frequencies from 1,500 to 5,000 Hz. Additionally, infant DPOAE levels were higher than those from all other age groups for f2 frequencies of 2,000 and 3,000 Hz. Children aged 1 to 3 years had higher mean DPOAE levels than adults at 3,000, 5,000, and 6,000 Hz. Overall, these results were similar to those for COAE levels across age groups (Prieve et al., 1997b).

The differences in EOAE levels across age groups have most often been attributed to anatomic changes in the outer or middle ear systems that occur with development. Ear canal diameter and length increase with development, as does middle ear volume (see Keefe et al. [1993] for review). Studies of middle ear admittance using tympanometry and acoustic reflectance also indicate developmental changes (Holte et al., 1991; Keefe et al., 1993). Whatever the causes, developmental differences in EOAE levels have definite clinical implications. Separate norms may be necessary for children under 6 years of age, regardless of stimulus level (Prieve et al., 1997a; 1997b).

The effect of increased age on EOAEs has been more difficult to study because behavioral thresholds tend to worsen with increasing age, creating a confounding factor. Several early studies reported decreasing COAE levels with increasing age; however, they did not control for auditory threshold (Bonfils et al., 1988a; Collet et al., 1990; Robinette, 1992) or report a significant effect of age on audiometric thresholds (Bonfils et al., 1988a; Collet et al., 1990; Robinette, 1992). The results of later studies that attempted to control for behavioral thresholds indicated no aging effects on TEOAEs (Castor et al., 1994; Prieve and Falter, 1995; Stenklev and Laukli, 2003; Stover and Norton, 1993). Stenklev and Laukli (2003) and Stover and Norton (1993) used statistical means

to compensate for the effects of varying auditory threshold and found no significant difference in TEOAE level or threshold due to aging itself. Prieve and Falter (1995) examined the effects of age on COAEs in normal-hearing young adults versus middle-aged adults who were closely matched for hearing thresholds (15 dB HL or better at all audiometric test frequencies). They found no significant differences in COAE level or threshold between groups.

Researchers examining the effects of advanced age on DPOAE levels have also encountered the confounding factor of elevated auditory thresholds in older adults. Not surprisingly, when no attempt was made to compensate statistically for decreased thresholds or when thresholds were not matched across age groups, decreased DPOAE levels and DPOAE thresholds with increasing age have been reported (Gates et al., 2002; Mazelova et al., 2003). Several studies that strictly controlled for hearing thresholds or used statistical compensation found no significant differences in DPOAE level with age (Karzon et al., 1994; Stover and Norton, 1993; Strouse et al., 1996). Cilento et al. (2003) used multivariate linear regression analyses to assess the effects of both hearing thresholds and age on DPOAE levels measured from a large sample of adults. They reported no significant effect of increased age for the male participants; decreases in DPOAE level were attributed to increases in hearing thresholds with age. Decreases in DPOAE levels for females, however, were attributed both to increasing hearing levels and to increasing age.

Still other studies have reported a frequency-dependent aging effect on DPOAE levels. Kimberley et al. (1994) and Whitehead et al. (1994) noted reduced DPOAE levels at high frequencies for older persons with normal hearing. Dorn et al. (1998) also presented evidence of a possible aging effect using multivariate regression analysis to simultaneously examine the effects of aging, threshold, and frequency on DPOAE level. All participants included in the analyses at a particular f2 frequency were required to have normal-hearing thresholds at that frequency, although not necessarily at all frequencies tested. Significant effects of age, threshold, and frequency on DPOAE level were found in their large group of participants aged 5 to 79 years. DPOAE levels were lower as age, threshold, and f2 increased. Interestingly, an age-by-frequency interaction was reported, but not an age-by-threshold interaction. These data suggest that, although there were no significant differences in threshold across the age groups, older persons had lower level, high-frequency DPOAEs. The authors reported that the small but significant differences occurred at only 6,000 and 8,000 Hz and were unlikely to be clinically significant or to require the use of correction factors in clinical interpretation of DPOAEs.

There are small but significant differences in EOAE levels depending on ear and gender. Females, on average, have larger TEOAEs than males (Aidan et al., 1997; Kulawiec and Orlando, 1995; Moulin et al., 1993; Robinette, 1992), and right ears, on average, have larger TEOAEs than left ears

(Aidan et al., 1997; Robinette, 1992) in both adults and neonates. The exact reasons for these differences are unknown, although investigators hypothesize that the smaller size of the female ear canal on average compared to the male ear canal may result in the higher TEOAE levels measured in female ears (Robinette, 1992). The greater number of SOAEs measured in right ears as compared to left ears and in females as compared to males (Penner et al., 1993) may also contribute to the noted TEOAE level differences (Kulawiec and Orlando, 1995; Moulin et al., 1993).

Conflicting results have been reported regarding differences in DPOAEs measured from females versus males. Some researchers have found that DPOAE levels are larger in females than in males (Cacace et al., 1996; Gaskill and Brown, 1990). Others have reported significant differences between the sexes at only select frequencies. Moulin et al. (1993) reported significantly larger DPOAE levels in female ears versus male ears only when 2f1-f2 equaled 2,000 Hz at primary levels of 50, 60, and 70 dB SPL. No significant gender differences were noted at any stimulus level when 2f1-f2 equaled 500, 1,000, 4,000, or 5,000 Hz. Lonsbury-Martin et al. (1997) reported higher DPOAE levels from female ears compared to male ears when the geometric mean of f1 and f2 was higher than 2,000 Hz, but the differences were statistically significant only for geometric mean primary frequencies in the 5,000-Hz range. Lonsbury-Martin et al. (1997) reported no significant differences in DPOAE levels between the right and left ears.

CLINICAL APPLICATIONS

Before beginning a discussion of clinical applications of EOAEs, it should be noted that middle ear status has an effect on EOAE measurements. Stimuli used to evoke the EOAE must pass through the middle ear to stimulate the cochlea, and the EOAE energy must pass through the middle ear in order for it to be detected in the ear canal. Middle ear pathology may reduce OAE amplitude or eliminate the ability to measure OAEs entirely, depending on the type and severity of the pathology (Owens et al., 1992; 1993; Rossi et al., 1989; Trine et al., 1993; Wiederhold, 1990). Most of the clinical research studies of OAEs have attempted to include only ears free of middle ear pathology, usually confirmed by routine immittance testing and/or the absence of any air-bone gaps on the audiogram. When possible, obtaining standard immittance measures to elucidate middle ear function will aid in interpretation of OAE results, particularly when using OAEs for differential diagnosis.

Identification of Hearing Loss

It has been known since the earliest research on OAEs that individuals with substantial cochlear hearing loss have no measurable EOAEs. In his original report, Kemp (1978) demonstrated that individuals with moderate hearing loss

had no TEOAEs for low-level stimuli. Shortly thereafter, others began investigating the extent to which EOAEs were altered in hearing-impaired ears. Generally, these early reports tested relatively small numbers of participants (~50). The results from these studies indicated that EOAEs either were not measurable from persons with hearing loss (Avan and Bonfils, 1991; Bonfils and Uziel, 1989; Probst et al., 1987; Stevens, 1988) or were substantially reduced in level relative to normal-hearing individuals (Harris, 1990; Martin et al., 1990; Smurzynski et al., 1990). These studies found that the minimum hearing level required for measurable EOAEs ranged from 25 to 40 dB HL. Studies also suggested that EOAEs could be "frequency specific," that is, they were generally present at frequencies where hearing was normal and not measurable at frequencies where there was hearing loss (Lonsbury-Martin et al., 1991; Smurzynski et al., 1990). These experiments fueled later research addressing the accuracy to which EOAEs could detect hearing loss.

For audiologists, the critical questions are as follows: Given an EOAE test result, what is the expected hearing loss, and what is the range of error? The first step in addressing these questions is to view distributions of EOAEs in normal-hearing and hearing-impaired populations. The goal is to select appropriate criteria that will classify a person as either normal or hearing impaired. Figure 21.9 illustrates

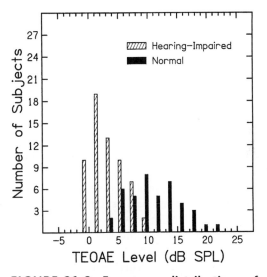

FIGURE 21.9 Frequency distributions of transient-evoked otoacoustic emission (TEOAE) level (dB sound pressure level [SPL]) evoked by 80-dB peak equivalent SPL (peSPL) clicks (nonlinear recording mode) for normal-hearing ears (*solid bars*) and hearing-impaired ears (*striped bars*). (Modified and reprinted with permission from Prieve BA, Gorga MP, Schmidt A, Neely ST, Peters J, Schultes L, Jesteadt W. [1993] Analysis of transient-evoked otoacoustic emissions in normal hearing and hearing impaired ears. *J Acoust Soc Am.* 93, 3308–3319; ©1993, Acoustical Society of America.)

histograms for TEOAE level evoked by 80-dB pSPL clicks from normal-hearing participants (solid bars) and hearing-impaired participants (striped bars). Normal-hearing participants tend to have TEOAEs with higher levels (bars farther to the right on the x-axis), and hearing-impaired participants tend to have TEOAEs with lower levels (farther to the left on the x-axis). However, some overlap exists between the two groups of participants; that is, there are some normal-hearing and hearing-impaired participants who have similar TEOAE levels. Unfortunately, this overlap means that it will not be possible to separate the two groups with complete accuracy using EOAEs as they are currently measured, although test performance, as we will see, is still fairly good.

STATISTICAL DECISION THEORY AND RELATIVE OPERATING CHARACTERISTIC CURVES

One way to evaluate how well EOAE levels identify hearing status as normal or impaired is to use statistical decision theory. This theory underlies signal detection theory (Green and Swets, 1974) and clinical decision analysis (Hyde et al., 1991; Weinstein and Fineberg, 1980). To complete these analyses, data must be collected on a large group of participants for whom hearing status is known. Audiometric threshold is used as the "gold standard" against which the EOAE results are compared. First, an audiometric criterion is used to classify each person as normal hearing or hearing impaired. A typical audiometric criterion is 20 dB HL (Gorga et al., 1997). Those with audiometric thresholds of 20 dB HL or better would be classified as having normal hearing. If their thresholds were higher than 20 dB HL, they would be classified as having hearing impairment. Second, an EOAE criterion is used to classify each person as normal hearing or hearing impaired. For example, the EOAE criterion might be a level of 1 dB SPL. Any person with an EOAE level of 1 dB SPL or higher would be classified as normal hearing, and any person with an EOAE level below 1 dB SPL would be classified as hearing impaired. Finally, two-by-two tables are constructed to compare how well the classification of hearing status (normal or impaired) using EOAEs compared with actual status as defined by audiometric thresholds. Figure 21.10 illustrates such a table. Continuing our example, if the person had an EOAE level lower than the criterion for that two-by-two table and was hearing impaired, it would be considered a "hit," and the count would increase by one in the cell labeled "A." If the EOAE level was higher than the criterion and the person were hearing impaired, it would be considered a "miss," and the count in cell "C" would increase by one. If the EOAE level was higher than the criterion and the person had normal hearing, it would be considered a "correct rejection" (cell "D"). If the EOAE level were lower than the criterion but the person had normal hearing, it would be considered a "false alarm" (cell "B").

Two-by-two tables are constructed for various EOAE parameters (e.g., EOAE level, EOAE/noise, percent repro-

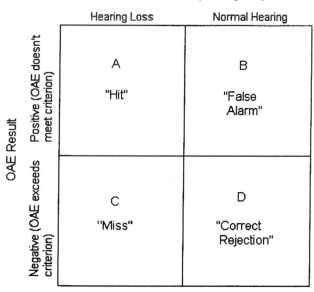

FIGURE 21.10 Example of a two-by-two decision matrix used to determine the percentage of hits, false alarms, etc., for a particular criterion of a selected evoked otoacoustic emission (EOAE) parameter.

ducibility) and criteria (e.g., range of EOAE levels in dB SPL, range of EOAE/noise, range of percent reproducibility). For each parameter, different EOAE criteria are systematically used. Our earlier example began with a criterion of EOAE level = 1 dB SPL. Next, the criterion could be increased to 2 dB SPL, and another table would be constructed in the same manner. The criterion would be systematically raised until many two-by-two tables were constructed. The percentage of hits ("hit rate") can be plotted as a function of the percentage of false alarms from all of the two-by-two tables, resulting in a relative operating characteristic (ROC) curve. Example ROC curves from Prieve et al. (1993) for overall TEOAE level (squares), TEOAE/noise (circles), and percent reproducibility (triangles) are shown in Figure 21.11. The dotted lines illustrate theoretical ROC curves and their corresponding d', which is a measure of the distance between two means of populations having equal-variance, Gaussian distributions.[5]

The less overlap there is between the two populations, the more accurately the test will identify members of the two groups and the more the data in the ROC curve will be located in the upper left-hand corner of the plot. One way to measure the accuracy of the test is to measure the area under the ROC curve, notated as P(A). The area under the curve provides an approximation of the hit rate averaged across all false alarm rates. A perfect test that completely separates the two groups would yield a P(A) of 1.0 (hit rate rises

---

[5] For detailed information regarding statistical decision theory, see Green and Swets (1974).

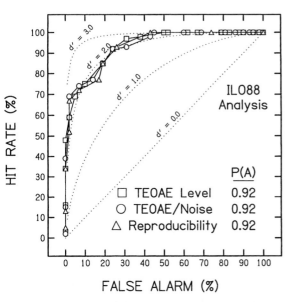

FIGURE 21.11 Relative operating characteristic (ROC) curves for broadband responses from the ILO88. Transient-evoked otoacoustic emission (TEOAE) level, TEOAE/noise, and percent reproducibility are represented by different symbols. (Modified and reprinted with permission from Prieve BA, Gorga MP, Schmidt A, Neely ST, Peters J, Schultes L, Jesteadt W. [1993] Analysis of transient-evoked otoacoustic emissions in normal hearing and hearing impaired ears. *J Acoust Soc Am.* 93, 3308–3319; ©1993, Acoustical Society of America.)

to 1.0, while false alarm rate remains at 0), whereas a test that separates the two groups no better than chance would yield a P(A) of 0.5 (equal hit and false alarm rates for the various criteria).

TRANSIENT-EVOKED OTOACOUSTIC EMISSIONS

For broadband TEOAEs, the ability to separate normal and hearing-impaired ears is good and equally so for the three different TEOAE parameters analyzed. The areas under the ROC curves shown in Figure 21.11 are all 0.92. For this analysis, the broadband TEOAE data were compared to the worst threshold at 500, 1,000, 2,000 or 4,000 Hz. To determine if reduction or absence of TEOAEs in a particular frequency band could predict hearing loss at the corresponding audiometric frequency, the broadband TEOAE was parsed into 1-octave bands. The ROC curves for each of the bands are shown in Figure 21.12. Again, all three TEOAE parameters perform almost equally well for separating normal-hearing from hearing-impaired ears. Identification of hearing loss is excellent at 2,000 and 4,000 Hz, indicated by the fact that the ROC curves fall into the upper left-hand corner of the plots and the P(A) values are high. Identification of hearing loss is fair at 1,000 Hz, and there is virtually no separation in the responses from normal-hearing and hearing-impaired ears at 500 Hz. These results suggest that TEOAEs evoked by 80-dB pSPL clicks parsed into frequency bands identify hearing loss well at 2,000 and 4,000 Hz but not at lower frequencies. Prieve et al. (1993) also found that ROC curves were best when using audiometric criteria of 20 or 25 dB HL to separate normal-hearing and hearing-impaired ears.

Subsequent studies have expanded on this early research to determine if improvement in identification of hearing loss can be obtained when different stimulus parameters and analyses are performed. One stimulus parameter that

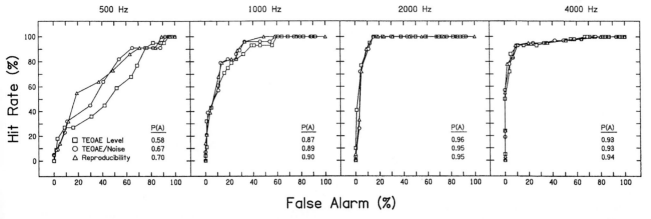

FIGURE 21.12 Relative operating characteristic (ROC) curves for octave bands centered at 500, 1,000, 2,000, and 4,000 Hz. Bands were analyzed from the broadband transient-evoked otoacoustic emission (TEOAE) response. (Modified and reprinted with permission from Prieve BA, Gorga MP, Schmidt A, Neely ST, Peters J, Schultes L, Jesteadt W. [1993] Analysis of transient-evoked otoacoustic emissions in normal hearing and hearing impaired ears. *J Acoust Soc Am.* 93, 3308–3319; ©1993, Acoustical Society of America.)

has been investigated is stimulus type. Several studies have used tone bursts instead of clicks to evoke TEOAEs, with the thought that a greater concentration of energy in a limited spectral region may enhance identification of hearing loss. The results have been mixed as to whether tone bursts are superior to clicks for identifying hearing loss. One research team has found that tone bursts centered at 500 Hz provide better separation of normal and hearing-impaired ears than using a 500-Hz band analyzed from a wideband, click-evoked TEOAE (Lichtenstein and Stapells, 1996). Another research team found this also to be true if using the same set of criteria for TEOAE "presence" but not to be true using a different set of criteria (Harrison and Norton, 1999). Both Lichtenstein and Stapells (1996) and Harrison and Norton (1999) found that a 2,000-Hz band analyzed from a click-evoked TEOAE identified hearing loss better than a tone burst centered at 2,000 Hz. Finally, another group of investigators found that tone burst–evoked TEOAEs were more highly correlated with hearing loss than were click-evoked TEOAEs analyzed into bands centered at 500, 1,000, 2,000, and 4,000 Hz (Vinck et al., 1998).

Stimulus level has also been varied. Harrison and Norton (1999) reported that the hit rate for identification of hearing loss given a 5% false-positive rate is higher for 80-dB peak equivalent SPL (peSPL) clicks than for 86-dB peSPL clicks. Another study has also shown that TEOAEs evoked by 86-dB peSPL clicks have a lower hit rate but higher correct rejection rate than those evoked by 65-dB peSPL clicks (Vinck et al., 1998). Based on these results, it appears that mid-level clicks (65 to 80 dB pSPL) may be best for identification of hearing loss.

Investigators have performed multivariate analyses to determine whether using several different TEOAE parameters (such as TEOAE level and the surrounding noise) for various frequencies can identify hearing loss better than using a single parameter to identify hearing loss at the corresponding frequency. The assumption is that a multivariate approach may take advantage of any interactions across frequency and result in an improvement of identification of hearing loss. Hussain et al. (1998) measured TEOAEs over a 12.5-ms window evoked by 80-dB pSPL clicks in participants having normal hearing and hearing loss. They used two types of multivariate analysis, discriminant analysis and logistic regression, to analyze TEOAE and noise levels in octave bands centered at 1,000, 2,000, and 4,000 Hz. The areas under the ROC curves were calculated, and univariate results (TEOAE level and TEOAE/noise) were compared to multivariate results (those obtained using discriminant analysis and logistic regression). Hussain et al. (1998) found significant improvement in identification of hearing loss at 1,000 Hz using multivariate analysis.

Vinck et al. (1998) used two stimulus levels (86 and 65 dB pSPL) and two stimulus types (tone bursts and clicks) to determine if these combinations would result in better identification of hearing loss. Using discriminant functions, they found that hearing status at 4,000 and 8,000 Hz could

be classified into three groups (<20 dB HL, 20 to 35 dB HL, and >35 dB HL) with 100% accuracy by using two click levels and four tone bursts presented at two levels. The studies using multivariate analyses suggest that, in the future, combinations of OAEs at more than one frequency will predict auditory status with the greatest accuracy.

DISTORTION PRODUCT OTOACOUSTIC EMISSIONS

For clinical purposes, DPOAE levels are usually examined as a function of primary tone frequency. The primary tone levels, level difference, and frequency ratio are held constant while the primaries are changed in frequency. The resulting graph of DPOAE level as a function of frequency has been called a "DP-gram." Figure 21.13 is an example of a DP-gram from an adult ear. Most commonly, DPOAE level is graphed as a function of $f2$ frequency. This convention is a result of evidence suggesting that the principal source of DPOAEs was the nonlinear distortion component originating in the region of overlap between the primaries. Animal studies have indicated that $2f1$-$f2$ output is reversibly reduced following presentation of a puretone-fatiguing stimuli in the region of the primaries (Kim et al., 1980). Maximal suppression of $2f1$-$f2$ occurs when the suppressor tone is in the region of the primary frequencies, particularly $f2$, in both animals (Brown and Kemp, 1984; Faulstich et al., 1996; Kemp and Brown, 1983; Koppl and Manley, 1993; Martin

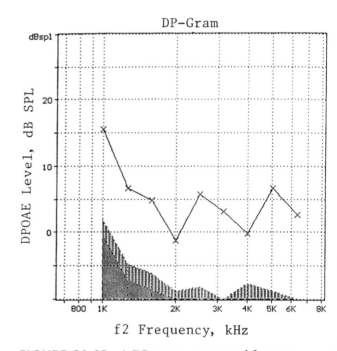

FIGURE 21.13 A DP-gram measured from an adult. The distortion product otoacoustic emission (DPOAE) level in dB sound pressure level (SPL), indicated by the *X's*, is graphed as a function of f2 frequency. The *shaded areas* indicate noise levels in dB SPL. (Adapted from the output of the Otodynamics ILO92 system.)

et al., 1987) and humans (Abdala and Sininger, 1996; Abdala et al., 1996; Gaskill and Brown, 1996; Harris et al., 1992; Kummer et al., 1995). As a result, most clinical studies have assumed that a given 2f1-f2 measure will reflect the hearing sensitivity at the f2 frequency (Gorga et al., 1997) or, in some cases, at the frequency equal to the geometric mean of the primaries (Lonsbury-Martin and Martin, 1990). The current, two-mechanisms theory (Shera and Guinan, 1999; Talmadge et al., 1999) suggests that the 2f1-f2 place may not be the primary source of DPOAEs for every frequency, but methods to extract each component separately for identification of hearing loss have not been reported for large clinical populations.

Considerable effort has been made to determine how well DPOAEs identify hearing loss. One of the first questions to be addressed was the most appropriate stimulus parameters to use for accurate identification of hearing loss. Based on prior research, most clinicians have adopted an f2/f1 of approximately 1.22 because, on average, it evokes the largest 2f1-f2. With regard to the choice of primary levels when using DPOAEs for clinical purposes, the use of the highest stimulus levels appears to be inappropriate. Recording systems themselves generate distortion products at high levels, and DPOAEs have been recorded using high-level primaries (75 dB SPL and higher) from animals that have dead or damaged cochleae (Lonsbury-Martin et al., 1987; Rosowski et al., 1984; Zurek et al., 1982). Such a finding would suggest that low- to moderate-level primaries would be preferable for clinical purposes (Moulin et al., 1994).

Early animal research indicated that DPOAEs evoked by low-level stimuli more accurately reflected changes in the "active" mechanism of the cochlea (Schmiedt and Adams, 1981). Simultaneously, other emerging research suggested that 2f1-f2 DPOAE levels evoked by low- and mid-level stimuli were greatest when unequal-level primaries were presented (Gaskill and Brown, 1990). With these previous studies in mind, Whitehead et al. (1995) showed, in individual case studies, that DPOAEs evoked by low-level, unequal-level stimuli were more sensitive to hearing loss than those evoked by high-level, equal-level stimuli. Sun et al. (1996) directly tested this notion in a larger group of normal-hearing and hearing-impaired ears. They found that area under the ROC curve was greater when unequal-level stimuli (L1 = 65 dB SPL; L2 = 50 dB SPL), rather than equal-level stimuli (L1 = L2 = 65 dB SPL), were used.

Later work by Stover et al. (1996) used unequal-level stimuli (L1 = L2 + 10 dB) at nine different frequencies and 12 different L2 levels to evoke DPOAEs in a group of normal-hearing and hearing-impaired participants. They found that areas under the ROC curves were greatest for L2 levels of 55 dB SPL, regardless of the frequency. In addition, using several different L2 levels did not improve the accuracy of identification of hearing loss. DPOAEs identified hearing loss best at frequencies above 500 Hz.

Based on this preliminary work by Stover et al. (1996), Gorga et al. (1997) tested 1,267 ears using primary levels of

L1 = 65 dB SPL and L2 = 55 dB SPL in a clinical setting. The data were analyzed in many ways to determine the best way to use DPOAEs to diagnose hearing loss. Gorga et al. (1997) reported how well hearing loss could be identified at a particular audiometric frequency by using the DPOAE evoked by an f2 of the same frequency. ROC curves indicated that identification of hearing loss was best at 4,000 and 6,000 Hz, with good identification at 1,500, 2,000, 3,000, and 8,000 Hz. They found that DPOAE/noise, rather than DPOAE level, was marginally superior at identifying hearing loss for most frequencies. To make the data more clinically applicable, they plotted cumulative distributions of DPOAE/noise for each frequency. Figure 21.14 illustrates the cumulative distributions at 4,000 Hz. In this plotting scheme, the percentage of persons having a DPOAE/noise value equal to or less than that shown on the x-axis is plotted. Data from normal-hearing participants are represented by solid lines, and data from hearing-impaired participants are represented by dotted lines. By plotting data in this manner, the value that represents the lowest 5% of DPOAE/noise from normal-hearing ears and the DPOAE/noise that represents the highest 5% from hearing-impaired ears can be determined. The panel for 4,000 Hz illustrates how these cumulative distributions can be used. The 95th percentile for

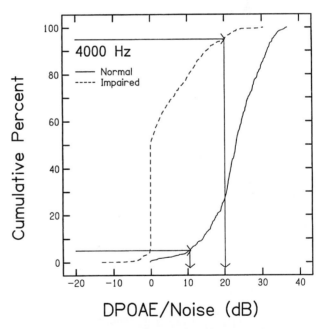

FIGURE 21.14 Cumulative distributions for distortion product otoacoustic emission (DPOAE)/noise from normal-hearing ears (*solid line*) and hearing-impaired ears (*dotted line*) for f2 = 4,000 Hz. (Modified and used with permission from Gorga MP, Neely ST, Ohlrich B, Hoover B, Redner J, Peters J. [1997] From laboratory to clinic: a large scale study of distortion product otoacoustic emissions in ears with normal hearing and ears with hearing loss. *Ear Hear.* 18, 440–455; ©1997, Lippincott Williams & Wilkins.)

hearing-impaired persons (read from the y-axis) is at 20.0 dB (read from the x-axis). The 5th percentile for the normal-hearing persons is at 10.5 dB.

Gorga et al. incorporated the 5th and 10th percentiles from normal-hearing ears and the 90th and 95th percentiles from hearing-impaired ears into a plot that can be used clinically and is shown in Figure 21.15. The top panel represents data for DPOAE level, and the bottom panel represents data for DPOAE/noise. In the top panel, the top solid line represents the 95th percentile of DPOAE level for the hearing-impaired ears. The top of the darkened area is the 90th percentile of DPOAE level from the hearing-impaired ears. The lowest solid line represents the 5th percentile of DPOAE level from the normal-hearing ears, and the bottom of the solid portion represents the 10th percentile of DPOAE level from the normal-hearing ears. The solid area represents DPOAE level from the 10th percentile from the normal-hearing ears to the 90th percentile for the hearing-impaired ears. When testing an individual, if his/her DPOAE level falls above the top line, the audiologist can be confident that the ear is normal hearing. If the patient's data fall below the lowest solid line, the audiologist can be confident that the ear is hearing impaired. The solid area is the "area of uncertainty." If an individual's data fall in that range, the clinician cannot be sure whether the ear is impaired or normal hearing. If DPOAE/noise is the parameter used, comparisons are made to the chart in the bottom panel. These charts illustrate how one can compare individual data to a large group of normal and hearing-impaired ears. However, these charts cannot be used "as is" unless the exact recording parameters are the same as those used by Gorga and colleagues.

To further their investigation, this research group tried to improve identification of hearing loss by using two types of multivariate analyses. Discriminant function analysis and logistic regression were used to probe whether DPOAE status at other frequencies could aid in the prediction of hearing loss at a chosen frequency. After performing the multivariate analyses, they found that the logistic regression analyses provided the best identification of hearing loss and reduced the "area of uncertainty" compared to that of their former univariate analysis (a single DPOAE parameter at a single frequency). The results of the multivariate analysis suggest that taking into account DPOAE level and S/N at various frequencies can improve DPOAE test performance at a given audiometric frequency (Dorn et al., 1999).

Finally, Gorga et al. (1999) performed an analysis on the a priori DPOAE criteria of 3, 6, and 9 dB DPOAE/noise ratios for various combinations of audiometric data. They found that using logistic regression gave them the best identification of hearing loss. They also found that using even the most stringent of the criteria, 9 dB, the sensitivity of DPOAEs (the ability of DPOAEs to accurately identify a hearing-impaired ear) was never more than 90%. Most errors were made when hearing loss ranged between 21 and 40 dB HL, with sensitivity approaching 100% for hearing loss greater than 40 dB HL (Gorga et al., 1999).

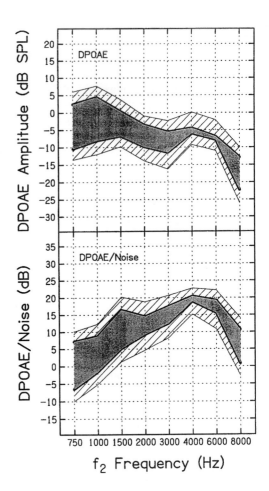

FIGURE 21.15 Distortion product otoacoustic emission (DPOAE) level (*top panel*) and DPOAE/noise (*bottom panel*) plotted as a function of f2 frequency. The top-most solid line represents the 95th percentile of responses from hearing-impaired ears. The bottom-most solid line represents the 5th percentile of responses from normal-hearing ears. The area with diagonal lines on the bottom of the darkened area represents the 5th to 10th percentile of responses from normal-hearing ears. The area with diagonal lines at the top of the darkened area represents the 90th to 95th percentile of responses from hearing-impaired ears. (Modified and used with permission from Gorga MP, Neely ST, Ohlrich B, Hoover B, Redner J, Peters J. [1997] From laboratory to clinic: a large scale study of distortion product otoacoustic emissions in ears with normal hearing and ears with hearing loss. *Ear Hear.* 18, 440–455; ©1997, Lippincott Williams & Wilkins.)

In 2005, Gorga et al. published a follow-up study that confirmed and expanded on the earlier data set published between 1997 and 1999. DPOAEs were collected from 345 ears of 187 participants. Their ages ranged from 2 to 86 years, with a median age of 29.7 years. Data were collected using the same paradigm as the previous studies; however, a commercially available system was used (Bio-logic Scout 3.45) instead of the custom system used in the previous studies. DPOAE test performance, measured by P(A) areas under ROC curves that matched an f2 frequency with an audiometric frequency, was similar to their previous report (Gorga et al., 1997). They used the coefficient constants generated by the Logit functions (LF) from the logistic regression analyses performed on data from their previous work (Dorn et al., 1999) and applied them to the current data. The resulting DPOAEs that were transformed to LF scores provided similar P(A) and percent failure results to their previous study, confirming that the equations could be generalized to new data sets. They found that calculating the LF scores resulted in improved identification of hearing loss, especially for lower frequency primaries, and that many participants with mild hearing loss met passing criteria, similar to their previous work. Using an a priori criterion of 6 dB S/N to diagnose hearing loss based on all four audiometric frequencies of 2,000, 3,000, 4,000, and 6,000 Hz, identification of severe and profound hearing loss was 100%, and the identification of moderate hearing loss was close to 100%. Only slight improvements were noted using the LF scores. Most interesting in this study was the way they transformed LF scores to probability that an ear was normal, denoted as P(N). This allowed data from individual patients to be converted to a probability that the results were from a normal ear.[6]

In summary, the results from the studies on the 2f1-f2 DPOAE indicate that it is an excellent, but not perfect, tool for identifying hearing loss. Identification of hearing loss is better at mid to high frequencies than at lower ($\leq$1,000 Hz) and higher (8,000 Hz) frequencies. Taking into account DPOAE parameters at frequencies other than the frequency of interest improves identification of hearing loss.

A few researchers have investigated use of another DPOAE, 2f2-f1, for clinical testing. Results indicated that 2f1-f2 predicted hearing status (normal vs. impaired) better than 2f2-f1 at all test frequencies (Fitzgerald and Prieve, 2005; Gorga et al., 2000a), even when stimulus parameters were set to obtain the most robust 2f2-f1 levels (Fitzgerald and Prieve, 2005). Combining information from both 2f1-f2 and 2f2-f1 using multivariate analyses improved prediction of hearing status, but the improvements were very slight compared to the performance of 2f1-f2 alone (Fitzgerald and Prieve, 2005; Gorga et al., 2000).

Prediction of Hearing Threshold

EOAE levels, EOAE/noise, and EOAE thresholds have all been examined for their ability to allow clinicians to predict behavioral thresholds. Early work in this area did not provide compelling evidence to indicate that EOAEs could be used for this purpose. Work continues in this area with

more encouraging results for the use of EOAEs to predict thresholds; however, predictions have a wide range of variability.

TRANSIENT-EVOKED OTOACOUSTIC EMISSIONS

Many studies have examined the correlations between audiometric thresholds and various TEOAE measures. Collet et al. (1991) measured COAEs evoked by 80-dB pSPL clicks and analyzed the power spectrum in 200-Hz bands between 500 and 5,300 Hz for comparison with audiometric thresholds. They reported significant correlations between behavioral thresholds at the audiometric frequencies between 250 and 8,000 Hz and COAE spectrum levels in the 200-Hz bands. However, a given behavioral test frequency correlated significantly with a broad range of COAE frequency bands. In addition, many of the COAE frequency bands correlated significantly with more than one behavioral threshold frequency. Collet et al. (1991) concluded that the relationship between the two measures was too complex to allow for prediction of behavioral thresholds using COAE levels.

The results of studies examining the correlations between COAE thresholds and hearing thresholds have been similarly discouraging. Comparisons of broadband COAE thresholds and audiometric thresholds have yielded low correlations, with the strongest relationships occurring in the mid frequencies (1,000 or 2,000 Hz) (Avan et al., 1991; Collet et al., 1989). Fitzgerald (1995) compared COAE thresholds measured in one-third octave bands with psychophysical thresholds measured at the corresponding center frequency of each one-third octave band. Statistically significant correlations between the two thresholds were obtained in the range from 1,000 to 2,500 Hz, but none of the correlations were high enough to suggest a predictive relationship. Fitzgerald (1995) suggested that the range of COAE threshold values measured for any given behavioral threshold is too large to allow prediction of behavioral sensitivity with COAE thresholds.

There is some evidence that greater accuracy can be obtained in predicting behavioral thresholds if a variety of transient stimuli presented at two levels are used. Vinck et al. (1998) used tone bursts centered at 500, 1,000, 2,000, and 4,000 Hz and clicks, each presented at 86 and 65 dB pSPL, to determine whether hearing threshold could be predicted from TEOAE results. They analyzed 120 variables from these five stimuli presented at two levels using multiple regression. Vinck et al. found that using all tone bursts and clicks at the two levels produced R^2 values of 0.88 for prediction of pure-tone audiometric thresholds at 500, 1,000, 2,000, and 4,000 Hz. Prediction of mean thresholds at 4,000 and 8,000 Hz was accurate within $\pm$ 10 dB.

DISTORTION PRODUCT OTOACOUSTIC EMISSIONS

DPOAE level tends to increase and DPOAE threshold tends to decrease as audiometric thresholds decrease (as thresholds improve) (Lonsbury-Martin and Martin, 1990;

---

[6] Detailed information on the calculation and use of P(N) and LF scores can be found in Gorga et al. (2005).

Martin et al., 1990; Nelson and Kimberley, 1992). Although strong relationships exist between DPOAE level and auditory threshold, the variability in DPOAE measures across individuals limit the usefulness of using DPOAE to predict audiometric threshold.

Gorga et al. (1993) examined the relationship between audiometric thresholds at 4,000 and 8,000 Hz and DPOAE/noise for the corresponding f2 frequencies in a group of patients with both normal hearing and hearing impairment. The frequencies 500, 1,000, and 2,000 Hz were not examined due to a lack of any apparent relationship when DPOAE levels were plotted as a function of audiometric threshold. Correlations between the two measures were −0.85 and −0.71 at 4,000 and 8,000 Hz, respectively, indicating that DPOAE/noise increased as audiometric threshold decreased (as threshold improved) (Gorga et al., 1993). Although a strong relationship between the two measures undoubtedly exists at these frequencies, examination of the data indicates that, as with DPOAE level and threshold, the range of DPOAE/noise levels for a given audiometric threshold is quite large. For instance, at 4,000 Hz, patients with an audiometric threshold of 0 dB HL had DPOAE/noise levels that ranged from approximately 7 to 40 dB (Gorga et al., 1993). Such variability across persons would make accurate prediction of one threshold by another extremely difficult.

Janssen and colleagues have advocated the use of DPOAE thresholds calculated from 2f1-f2 DPOAE growth functions to estimate hearing thresholds (Boege and Janssen, 2002; Janssen et al., 2005). In their original paper, Boege and Janssen (2002) measured growth functions from participants with normal hearing and with sensory-neural hearing loss for frequencies between 488 and 8,008 Hz using $L2 = 20 - 65$ dB SPL with L1 level set using the equation $L1 = 0.4*L2 + 39$ dB described earlier (Kummer et al., 2000). DPOAE threshold estimation was only performed on those growth functions in which three or more data points met or exceeded a 6-dB DPOAE/noise criteria. The DPOAE data were converted to pressure values (μPa), and a linear regression analysis was performed on the pressure growth functions. The DPOAE threshold was calculated from the regression line as the value of L2 at which the pressure equaled 0 μPa. Puretone thresholds were measured at corresponding f2 frequencies using a computer-controlled method of adjustment. The authors reported a mean difference of 2.2 dB between the estimated DPOAE threshold and the puretone threshold (SD = 12.7 dB). When detailed criteria to accept the fit of the regression line were used, approximately 70% of the measured growth functions met the criteria. The mean difference between the DPOAE and puretone thresholds was 2.5 dB (SD = 10. 9 dB) when only those growth functions that met the criteria were considered.

Janssen et al. (2005) applied this procedure to neonates and reported that threshold estimation using the linear regression criteria was possible in only 33.1% to 74.6% of the growth functions across frequency, with the highest percentages for mid-high test frequencies. On average, hearing threshold estimation was possible at about two thirds of the test frequencies for a given single neonate ear. They attributed the differences from results in adults (Boege and Janssen, 2002) to the poor test conditions (hospital or home settings) for the neonates and resulting higher noise floors.

Gorga et al. (2003) replicated the work of Boege and Janssen (2002) using their 6-dB S/N and linear regression criteria. They noted that the correlations between the estimated DPOAE threshold and audiometric thresholds were highest for mid-high f2 frequencies (2,000 to 4,000 Hz) and poorest for the lowest f2 frequencies tested (500 and 750 Hz). The authors reported that only 37.4% of the growth functions from their sample of 227 participants met the criteria for threshold estimation analysis, as compared with the 70% reported by Boege and Jannsen (2002). Gorga et al. (2003) noted that the majority of ears whose growth functions failed to meet the 6-dB S/N criteria had hearing thresholds of 30 dB HL or poorer. However, about 81% of the growth functions that were rejected because they did not meet the linear regression criteria were recorded from ears with normal hearing thresholds. This translated to a false-positive rate of 19.3% for their sample. Gorga et al. (2003) suggested that increasing the range of primary levels tested up to 85 dB SPL and changing the linear regression criteria for inclusion might increase the number of growth functions that could be accepted for further threshold estimation. To summarize these studies, the number of growth functions that do not meet linear regression criteria is of great concern using this technique, and at this time, the estimation of behavioral thresholds from DPOAE threshold or levels is not clinically feasible.

Clinical Questions

WHICH SHOULD I USE: TRANSIENT-EVOKED OTOACOUSTIC EMISSIONS OR DISTORTION PRODUCT OTOACOUSTIC EMISSIONS?

Based on the current literature, either type of EOAE can identify hearing loss well. Gorga et al. (1993) directly compared TEOAEs and DPOAEs in a group of normal-hearing and hearing-impaired participants. They found that TEOAEs were slightly better at identifying hearing loss at 500 and 1,000 Hz, that DPOAEs were better at identifying hearing loss at 4,000 Hz, and that both identified hearing loss with the same accuracy at 2,000 Hz. Both types of EOAEs are "frequency specific," meaning that either can provide information about hearing loss in a specific frequency region. One advantage of DPOAEs is that, with current instrumentation, frequencies higher than 5,000 Hz can be tested. With improvements in equipment, it may be possible to test higher frequency TEOAEs in the future. DPOAEs are different from TEOAEs in that they can be measured in ears with greater hearing loss (Harris and Probst, 2002). Perhaps further investigation will determine how this aspect can be used for clinical advantage. Additionally, the two-source theory of OAE generation suggests that examining the nonlinear distortion and linear coherent reflection components separately may enhance the clinical use of OAEs (Shera and Guinan, 1999; Talmadge et al., 1999). No data are available at this time to verify this possibility.

CRITERIA

Although excellent research substantiating the ability of EOAEs to determine auditory status is available, there are no studies that provide definitive EOAE criteria for clinical use. TEOAE/noise (Hussain et al., 1998; Harrison and Norton, 1999) and percent reproducibility (Prieve et al., 1993; Glattke et al., 1995) appear to be the parameters that identify hearing loss with the greatest accuracy. For evaluating broadband TEOAEs, an overall level of 6 dB SPL or an overall reproducibility of >70% seems to be reasonable (Hurley and Musiek, 1994; Prieve et al., 1993). Harrison and Norton (1999) suggest using a 3-dB S/N for a frequency band taken from a broadband TEOAE from data collected on children. Clinicians cannot directly use the data presented by Hussain et al. (1998) because analysis of TEOAE into bands was done using a custom program and it is uncertain how its output relates to that from other commercial manufacturers. Multivariate analysis appears promising for improved accuracy in the identification of hearing loss, especially at 1,000 Hz. At this time, the software to use this technique clinically is not available.

A thorough investigation of the estimation of hearing loss using DPOAEs in a clinical setting has been conducted by Gorga and colleagues. DPOAE/noise appears to be the most sensitive parameter if using a univariate approach; however, clinicians should also pay attention to absolute level (Gorga et al., 2005). A clinically useful chart is shown in Figure 21.15. In order to use this chart, one must make sure that the audiologist's own piece of equipment provides similar DPOAE levels when using the same stimulus parameters. Only the DPOAE level chart may be able to be used clinically because recording parameters greatly affect the DPOAE/noise. If stimulus and recording conditions are similar to those described in Gorga et al. (2005), LF scores can be calculated using the LF coefficients and constants from Dorn et al. (1999). The calculation of the probability that an ear is normal based on LF scores, as described in Gorga et al. (2005), could be extremely useful.

Ultimately, the specific EOAE criteria clinicians should use to identify a person as hearing impaired depends on how many "false alarms" (over-referrals) can be dealt with in an economic manner. For this reason, the prevalence of hearing loss in the population that is being tested is of utmost importance. Different criteria may be chosen depending on whether EOAEs are being used in a hearing clinic, where the prevalence of hearing loss is quite high, as opposed to a hearing screening, where the prevalence of hearing loss may be much lower.

NEWBORN HEARING SCREENING

The Joint Committee on Infant Hearing (JCIH, 2007) recommends universal newborn hearing screening, meaning that all newborn infants should be screened for hearing loss. As of 2007, 45 states in the United States are conducting universal newborn hearing screening. The JCIH has recommended that newborns cared for in a well-baby nursery be screened with either EOAEs or auditory brainstem responses (ABRs) (JCIH, 2007). EOAEs have been widely used in large-scale screening programs that included both high-risk and large-scale universal newborn hearing screening programs (Finitzo et al., 1998; Maxon et al., 1997; Prieve and Stevens, 2000; Spivak et al., 2000; Vohr et al., 1998). When used as a screening tool, the program directors chose EOAE criteria that each ear must meet. If the criteria were met, then an infant was said to "pass" the newborn hearing screening. If the criteria were not met, the infant was considered to have "failed" the in-hospital screening and either returned at a later time for a rescreening or was referred for further diagnostic testing. The referral rates for outpatient retesting reported by these programs range between 3% and 10%. These screening programs provide evidence that universal newborn hearing screening is feasible using OAEs.

A large-scale study funded by the National Institutes of Health (NIH) directly compared the screening tools of DPOAEs, TEOAEs, and screening ABR (SABR). The NIH study was conducted on 4,478 infants cared for in the neonatal intensive care unit, 353 well-babies with risk indicators for hearing loss based on the JCIH 1994 Position Statement (JCIH, 1995), and 2,348 infants cared for in the well-baby nursery with no risk indicators for hearing loss at seven different institutions across the United States. TEOAEs, DPOAEs evoked by two different primary level pairs, and ABRs evoked by 30-dB nHL clicks were measured in random order from both ears of each infant using a computerized test program that included passing criteria, response filtering, noise/artifact rejection, and minimum, maximum, and low-noise stopping rules specifically chosen for each measure (Gorga at al., 2000b; Norton et al., 2000a; Sininger et al., 2000). One of the important findings from the NIH study is that the percentage of infant passes was similar for SABRs, TEOAEs, and DPOAEs (L1 = 65 and L2 = 50 dB SPL). The percentages of passes increased if the criteria specified passing either an EOAE or an ABR.

In order to determine the sensitivity and specificity of each screening tool, 4,911 infants were tracked for follow-up behavioral hearing testing at 8 to 12 months corrected age. Sixty-four percent of infants targeted for follow-up returned for audiometric testing, and of those, 95.6% could be reliably tested using visual reinforcement audiometry with insert earphones. Minimal response levels (MRLs) were determined using frequency-modulated tones at frequencies of 1,000, 2,000, and 4,000 Hz, and speech awareness threshold (SAT) was determined using speech presented by live voice through a microphone. MRLs higher than 20 dB HL indicated hearing loss, and infant responses at 20 dB HL were considered normal (Widen et al., 2000). ROC curves were constructed for SABR, TEOAEs, and DPOAEs using an MRL at 1, 2, or 4 kHz; the SAT or puretone average (PTA) of 2 and 4 kHz; or a PTA including 1, 2, and 4 kHz of ≤20 as "normal" (Norton et al., 2000b). The areas under the ROC curves for all four tests ranged from 0.70 to 0.94 and were similar to each other for most measures, indicating that each test identified hearing loss well. None of the areas were 1.0, indicating that no test identified hearing loss with 100% accuracy. There were slight differences among the measures. ROC curves for DPOAEs evoked by equal primary levels of 75 dB SPL had lower areas than those for DPOAEs evoked by primary levels of L1 = 65 and L2 = 50 dB SPL, indicating that DPOAEs evoked by higher level primaries were not as good at identifying hearing loss as those evoked by mid-level primaries. TEOAEs, DPOAEs at 65/50 dB SPL, and SABR performed similarly for MRLs of 2 and 4 kHz, PTA including 2 and 4 kHz, and SAT. TEOAEs and DPOAEs at 65/50 dB SPL

outperformed SABR slightly for most of these measures. Finally, SABR outperformed TEOAEs and DPOAEs for an MRL at 1,000 Hz and was slightly better for a PTA that includes 1,000 Hz. An analysis of failure rate based on severity of hearing loss was performed for a hit rate of 80%. The majority of moderate, severe, and profound hearing losses were identified at a rate at or close to 100% using any of the measures. Mild hearing loss was the severity most incorrectly identified, with 40% to 50% of ears with mild hearing loss meeting the screening criteria (Norton et al., 2000b). An extensive set of data is provided by this study and can help guide clinicians in understanding EOAE and ABR tools as newborn hearing screening tools. Additionally, clinicians should be aware that ABR and OAE screening are equally effective at identifying moderate, severe, and profound hearing loss.

▨ DIFFERENTIAL DIAGNOSIS

EOAEs are an excellent tool in the audiometric test battery for cases of differential diagnosis. Because EOAEs are generated in the cochlea independent of afferent fiber activation, they allow us to test for a "mechanical" versus an inner hair cell or neural hearing loss. One type of auditory disorder that can now be identified is auditory neuropathy. In these

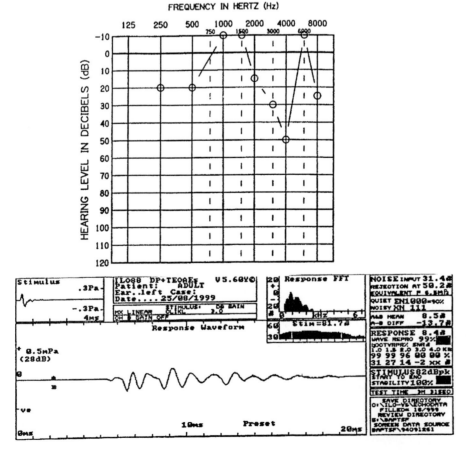

FIGURE 21.16 Audiogram and transient-evoked otoacoustic emissions (TEOAEs) for Case Study 1: TEOAEs in an adult.

cases, the EOAEs are normal, ABRs and acoustic reflexes are abnormal or absent, and hearing thresholds range from mild to profound in severity.

The addition of EOAEs to the test battery for patients with vestibular schwannoma is also an important consideration. Although most patients having tumors also do not have EOAEs, which is thought to be due to interrupted blood supply to the cochlea, there is a small number of patients who have EOAEs despite poor behavioral thresholds. In these cases, the audiologist could recommend that a surgical procedure that preserves the cochlea be performed so that any residual hearing may be saved (Robinette et al., 2002).

Other auditory conditions for which EOAEs may prove to be valuable are under investigation. For example, EOAEs are being studied for monitoring of hearing loss due to ototoxic drugs (Yardley et al., 1998) and susceptibility to and monitoring of hearing loss due to noise exposure (Lapsley Miller et al., 2004; Lucertini et al., 2002; Marshal et al., 2001; Marshall and Heller, 1998; Seixas et al., 2004; Sliwinska-Kowalska and Kotylo, 2002; Veuillet et al., 2001; Vinck et al., 1999). Some researchers are investigating the possibility that EOAEs are altered in unique ways in individuals with Ménière's disease (Kusuki et al., 1998; Sakashita et al., 1998).

CASE STUDIES

Case Study 1: Adult Click-Evoked Otoacoustic Emissions

Patient 1 is an 18-year-old adult male with bilateral high-frequency sensory-neural hearing loss. The patient reported that he had been hearing-impaired since birth but that the etiology of the hearing loss was unknown. A hearing evaluation revealed a unique pattern of thresholds with two frequency regions of extremely low thresholds in the right ear. The top half of Figure 21.16 is the patient's audiogram for the right ear. Hearing levels improved from borderline normal at 250 to 500 Hz to extremely low values (−10 dB HL) at 1,000 and 1,500 Hz and back to 15 dB HL at 2,000 Hz. His hearing levels then sloped to a mild to moderate hearing loss from 3,000 to 4,000 Hz, followed by another rise to −10 dB HL at 6,000 Hz and a borderline normal value of 25 dB HL at 8,000 Hz.

A TEOAE was measured from the right ear using clicks presented at approximately 82 dB pSPL. The display from the ILO88 system is shown in the bottom half of Figure 21.16, with the COAE analyzed into half-octave bands. COAEs were present in the half-octave bands from 1,000 to 2,000 Hz, where hearing levels were within normal limits. As expected, no COAE energy was present in the 3,000- to 4,000-Hz bands where hearing loss is indicated on the audiogram. The COAE screening does not yield information above 4,000 Hz for comparison with the normal and borderline normal thresholds obtained in this patient at higher frequencies. However,

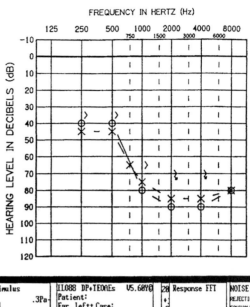

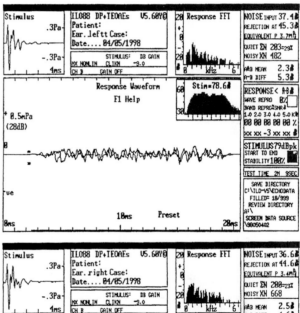

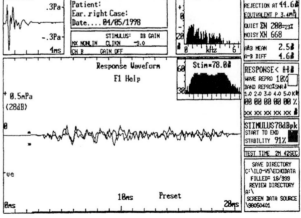

FIGURE 21.17 Audiogram and transient-evoked otoacoustic emissions (TEOAEs) for Case Study 2: TEOAEs in a child.

this case does illustrate good correspondence between the presence/absence of COAEs and the measured hearing levels from 1,000 to 4,000 Hz. Also of note are the excellent probe fit and low noise level that are typically easy to obtain in a cooperative adult.

Case Study 2: Transient-Evoked Otoacoustic Emissions from a Child

Patient 2 was referred to us when he was 3:3 (years : months). His parents had first suspected he had a hearing loss by the time he was 1:0. He was taken to an ear, nose, and throat (ENT) specialist, who inserted ventilating tubes into his eardrums when the child was 1:6. At 2:1, this patient had a hearing evaluation, which revealed a moderate to severe mixed hearing loss bilaterally. Expressive and receptive language and phonologic skills were significantly reduced. At that time, the patient underwent a second surgery for pressure equalization (PE) tubes and, afterwards, was fit with binaural hearing aids. Because the patient did not seem to be responding well to hearing aids and was difficult to test behaviorally, he was seen for hearing and OAE testing.

The top panel in Figure 21.17 illustrates the patient's audiogram, which was obtained after several visits. Patient 2 has a mild, sloping to profound sensory-neural hearing loss bilaterally. Because the patient was not responding well to hearing aids, it was important to rule out auditory neuropathy. The middle panel in Figure 21.17 illustrates the TEOAEs measured from the left ear, and the bottom panel illustrates the TEOAEs from the right ear. Click stimuli presented at approximately 80 dB pSPL were used. No TEOAEs are present, consistent with outer hair cell pathology. Notice the unusual

click stimulus waveform, a typical finding when open ventilating tubes are present. Because of the absence of TEOAEs in the presence of a mild to profound sensory-neural hearing loss, it was felt that this child's hearing loss contained a cochlear component and that amplification was an appropriate method of rehabilitation. As the child matured, became adjusted to his hearing aids, and received special services, the child became more verbal and compliant in behavior.

Case Study 3: Sensory-Neural Hearing Loss in an Infant

Patient 3 was referred because she failed a newborn hearing screening before hospital discharge. She was seen at 8 months of age, after having audiologic evaluations done at other facilities on three different occasions. Figure 21.18 shows estimates of behavioral thresholds, depicted by triangles, based on ABRs evoked by tone bursts collected during natural sleep. Figure 22.18A shows data for the right ear, and Figure 22.18B shows data for the left ear. ABR thresholds estimate a mild to severe sensory-neural hearing loss in the left ear and a mild hearing loss in the right ear at 4,000 Hz. Tympanometry was within normal limits for both ears. TEOAEs and DPOAEs were absent in the left ear. In the right ear, TEOAEs were present in 2,000-Hz and 3,000-Hz half-octave bands but were absent in the 4,000-Hz band. DPOAEs were higher than two

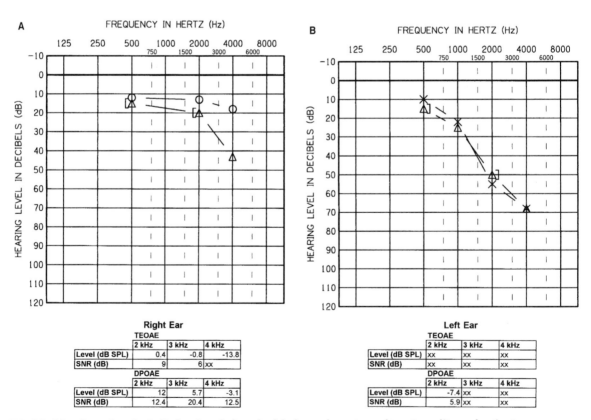

Right Ear

TEOAE	2 kHz	3 kHz	4 kHz
Level (dB SPL)	0.4	-0.8	-13.8
SNR (dB)	9	6	xx

DPOAE	2 kHz	3 kHz	4 kHz
Level (dB SPL)	12	5.7	-3.1
SNR (dB)	12.4	20.4	12.5

Left Ear

TEOAE	2 kHz	3 kHz	4 kHz
Level (dB SPL)	xx	xx	xx
SNR (dB)	xx	xx	xx

DPOAE	2 kHz	3 kHz	4 kHz
Level (dB SPL)	-7.4	xx	xx
SNR (dB)	5.9	xx	xx

FIGURE 21.18   Case Study 3. Behavioral thresholds based on tone-burst auditory brainstem response, behavioral thresholds measured with visual reinforcement audiometry at 8 months of age, and transient-evoked otoacoustic emissions (TEOAEs) and distortion product otoacoustic emissions (DPOAEs) measured at 3 months of age.

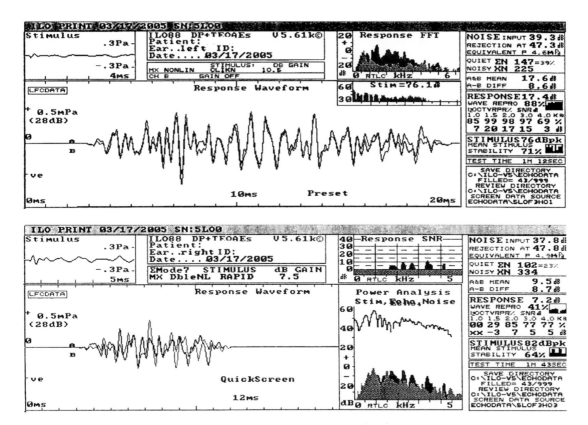

FIGURE 21.19 Case Study 4. Transient-evoked otoacoustic emissions (TEOAEs) for an infant aged 3 months with middle ear dysfunction in both ears. Middle ear effusion was confirmed surgically 1 week after audiologic measures were obtained.

standard deviations above the noise floor between 1,500 and 4,000 Hz. Behavioral thresholds obtained using visual reinforcement audiometry are shown on the audiograms using typical conventions (x for left ear, circle for right ear). ABR estimates of behavioral thresholds were in good agreement with actual behavioral thresholds except for 4,000 Hz in the right ear. The behavioral threshold was 20 dB HL, which is a slight, rather than mild, hearing loss, as suggested by ABR threshold estimates. Lack of TEOAEs in the 4,000-Hz band was consistent with the slightly higher thresholds.

Case Study 4: Conductive Hearing Loss in an Infant

Patient 4 is a 4-month-old baby who passed his newborn hearing screening at birth but who developed middle ear effusions due to a congenital disorder. Based on ABR

thresholds, it appeared that patient 4 had a conductive hearing loss in the right ear at 500 Hz. A tympanogram using a 1,000-Hz probe tone was flat. Figure 21.19 shows that TEOAEs in the right ear (lower panel of Fig. 21.19) were low level but had greater than 4-dB OAE-to-noise ratio from 2,000 to 4,000 Hz. Patient 4 underwent a myringotomy 1 week after testing. The pediatric otolaryngologist noted effusion in the right ear. Although one might expect that middle ear pathology would eliminate EOAEs, TEOAEs were present in this infant despite an air-bone gap based on tone burst ABR, a flat tympanogram, and confirmed effusion.

■ ACKNOWLEDGEMENTS

The authors thank Lea Georgantas and Lisa Lahtinen for technical assistance.

■ REFERENCES

Abdala C. (1996) Distortion product otoacoustic emission (2f1-f2) amplitude as a function of f2/f1 frequency ratio and primary tone level separation in human adults and neonates. *J Acoust Soc Am.* 100, 3726–3740.

Abdala C, Sininger, Y. (1996) The development of cochlear frequency resolution in the human auditory system. *Ear Hear.* 17, 374–385.

Abdala C, Sininger YS, Ekelid M, Zeng FG. (1996) Distortion product otoacoustic emission suppression tuning curves in human adults and neonates. *Hear Res.* 98, 38–53.

Aidan D, Lestang P, Avan P, Bonfils P. (1997) Characteristics of transient-evoked otoacoustic emissions (TEOEs) in neonates. *Acta Otolaryngol (Stockh).* 117, 25–30.

Allen JB, Fahey PF. (1993) A second cochlear-frequency map that correlates distortion product and neural tuning mechanisms. *J Acoust Soc Am.* 94, 809–816.

Allen JB, Neely ST. (1992) Micromechanical models of the cochlea. *Phys Today.* 45, 40–47.

Antonelli A, Grandori F. (1986) Long term stability, influence of the head position and modelling considerations for evoked otoacoustic emissions. *Scand Audiol.* 25 (suppl), 97–108.

Arts HA, Norton SJ, Rubel EW. (1990) Influence of perilymphatic tetrodotoxin and calcium concentration on hair cell function. *Abstr Midwtr Mtg Assoc Res Otolaryngol.* 13, 194.

Ashmore JF. (1987) A fast motile response in guinea-pig outer hair cells: the cellular basis of the cochlear amplifier. *J Physiol.* 388, 323–347.

Avan P, Bonfils P. (1991) Frequency specificity of human distortion product otoacoustic emissions. *Audiology.* 32, 12–26.

Avan P, Bonfils P, Loth D, Narcy P, Trotoux J. (1991) Quantitative assessment of human cochlear function by evoked otoacoustic emissions. *Hear Res.* 52, 99–112.

Bekesy GV. (1949) The vibration of the cochlear partition in anatomical preparation and in models of the inner ear. *J Acoust Soc Am.* 21, 233–245.

Bergman BM, Gorga MP, Neely ST, Kaminiski JR, Beauchaine KL, Peters J. (1995) Preliminary descriptions of transient-evoked and distortion-product otoacoustic emissions from graduates of an intensive care nursery. *J Am Acad Audiol.* 6, 150–162.

Berlin CI, Hood LJ, Hurley AE, Wen H, Kemp DT. (1995) Binaural noise suppresses linear click-evoked otoacoustic emissions more than ipsilateral or contralateral noise. *Hear Res.* 87, 96–103.

Berlin CI, Hood LJ, Wen H, Szabo P, Cecola RP, Rigby P, Jackson DR. (1993) Contralateral suppression of non-linear click-evoked otoacoustic emissions. *Hear Res.* 71, 1–11.

Bilger RC, Matthies ML, Hammel DR, Demorest ME. (1990) Genetic implications of gender differences in the prevalence of spontaneous otoacoustic emissions. *J Speech Hear Res.* 33, 418–432.

Boege P, Janssen T. (2002) Pure-tone threshold estimation from extrapolated distortion product otoacoustic emission I/O-functions in normal and cochlear hearing loss ears. *J Acoust Soc Am.* 111, 1810–1818.

Bonfils P. (1989) Spontaneous otoacoustic emissions: clinical interest. *Laryngoscope.* 99, 752–756.

Bonfils P, Bertrand Y, Uziel A. (1988a) Evoked otoacoustic emissions: normative data and presbycusis. *Audiology.* 27, 27–35.

Bonfils P, Piron J-P, Uziel A, Pujol R. (1988b) A correlative study of evoked otoacoustic emission properties and audiometric thresholds. *Arch Otorhinolaryngol.* 245, 53–56.

Bonfils P, Uziel A. (1989) Clinical application of evoked acoustic emissions: results in normally hearing and hearing impaired subjects. *Ann Otol Rhinol Laryngol.* 98, 326–331.

Brass D, Kemp DT. (1991) Time-domain observation of otoacoustic emissions during constant tone stimulation. *J Acoust Soc Am.* 90, 2415–2427.

Bray PJ. (1989) Click evoked otoacoustic emissions and the development of a clinical otoacoustic hearing test instrument. Doctoral dissertation. University of London, London, United Kingdom.

Bright KE. (2002) Spontaneous otoacoustic emissions. In: Robinette MS, Glattke TJ, eds. *Otoacoustic Emissions.* New York: Thieme; pp 74–94.

Bright KE, Glattke TJ. (1986) Spontaneous otoacoustic emissions in normal ears. In: Collins MJ, Glattke TJ, Harker LA, eds. *Sensorineural Hearing Loss.* Iowa City: University of Iowa Press; pp 201–208.

Brown AM. (1988) Continuous low level sound alters cochlear mechanics: an efferent effect? *Hear Res.* 34, 27–35.

Brown AM, Gaskill SA. (1990a) Can basilar membrane tuning be inferred from distortion measurement? In: Dallos P, Geisler CD, Matthews JW, Ruggero MA, Steele CR, eds. *Mechanics and Biophysics of Hearing.* New York: Springer-Verlag; pp 164–169.

Brown AM, Gaskill SA. (1990b) Measurement of acoustic distortion reveals underlying similarities between human and rodent mechanical responses. *J Acoust Soc Am.* 88, 840–849.

Brown AM, Kemp DT. (1984) Suppressibility of the 2f1-f2 stimulated acoustic emissions in gerbil and man. *Hear Res.* 13, 29–37.

Brown AM, McDowell B, Forge A. (1989) Acoustic distortion products can be used to monitor the effects of chronic gentamicin treatment. *Hear Res.* 42, 143–156.

Brown AM, Sheppard SL, Russell PT. (1994) Acoustic distortion products (ADP) from the ears of term infants and young adults using low stimulus levels. *Br J Audiol.* 28, 273–280.

Brown AM, Sheppard SL, Russell PT. (1995) Differences between neonate and adult cochlear mechanical responses. *Auditory Neurosci.* 1, 169–181.

Brownell WE, Bader CR, Betrand D, de Ribaupierre Y. (1985) Evoked mechanical responses of isolated cochlear outer hair cells. *Science.* 227, 194–196.

Burns EM, Arehart KH, Campbell SL. (1992) Prevalence of spontaneous otoacoustic emissions in neonates. *J Acoust Soc Am.* 91, 1571–1575.

Cacace AT, McClelland WA, Weiner J, McFarland DJ. (1996) Individual differences and the reliability of 2f1-f2 distortion-product otoacoustic emissions: effects of time-of-day, stimulus variables, and gender. *J Speech Hear Res.* 39, 1138–1148.

Castor X, Veuillet E, Morgon A, Collet L. (1994) Influence of aging on active cochlear micromechanical properties and on the medial olivocochlear system in humans. *Hear Res.* 77, 1–8.

Cianfrone M, Mattia M, Altissimi G, Turchetta R (1990) Distortion product otoacoustic emissions and spontaneous otoacoustic emission suppression in humans. In: Grandori F, Cianfrone G, Kemp DT, eds. *Cochlear Mechanisms and Otoacoustic Emissions.* Basel: Karger; pp 126–138.

Cilento BW, Norton SJ, Gates GA. (2003) The effects of aging and hearing loss on distortion product otoacoustic emissions. *Otolaryngol Head Neck Surg.* 129, 382–389.

Collet L, Gartner L, Veuillet E, Moulin A, Morgon A. (1993a) Evoked and spontaneous otoacoustic emissions: a comparison of neonates and adults. *Brain Dev.* 15, 249–252.

Collet L, Gartner M, Moulin A, Kauffmann I, Disant F, Morgon A. (1989) Evoked otoacoustic emissions and sensorineural hearing loss. *Arch Otolaryngol Head Neck Surg.* 115, 1060–1062.

Collet L, Kemp DT, Veuillet E, Duclaux R, Moulin A, Morgon A. (1990) Effect of contralateral auditory stimuli on active cochlear micromechanical properties in human subjects. *Hear Res.* 43, 251–262.

Collet L, Levy V, Veuillet E, Truy E, Morgon A. (1993b) Click-evoked otoacoustic emissions and hearing threshold in sensorineural hearing loss. *Ear Hear.* 14, 141–143.

Collet L, Veuillet E, Chanal JM, Morgan A. (1991) Evoked otoacoustic emissions: correlates between spectrum analysis and audiogram. *Audiology.* 30, 164–172.

Dallos P (1988) Cochlear neurobiology: Some key experiments and concepts of the past two decades. In: Edelman GM, Gall WE, Cowan WM, eds. *Auditory Function–Neurobiological Bases of Hearing.* New York: Wiley; pp 153–188.

Dallos P. (1992) The active cochlea. *J Neurosci.* 12, 4575–4585.

Dallos P, Harris D. (1978) Properties of auditory nerve responses in absence of outer hair cells. *J Neurophysiol.* 41, 365–383.

Dallos P, Wang C-Y. (1974) Bioelectric correlates of kanamycin intoxication. *Audiology.* 13, 277–289.

Davis H. (1983) An active process in cochlear mechanics. *Hear Res.* 9, 79–90.

de Boer E. (1983) Wave reflection in active and passive cochlea models. In: *Mechanics of Hearing.* New York: Springer; pp 135–142.

Dorn PA, Piskorski P, Gorga MP, Neely ST, Keffe DH. (1999) Predicting audiometric status from distortion product otoacoustic emissions using multivariate analyses. *Ear Hear.* 20, 149–163.

Dorn PA, Piskorski P, Keefe DH, Neely ST, Gorga MP. (1998) On the existence of an age/threshold/frequency interaction in distortion product otoacoustic emissions. *J Acoust Soc Am.* 104, 964–971.

Ellison JC, Keefe DH. (2005) Audiometric predictions using SFOAE and middle-ear measurements. *Ear Hear.* 26, 487–503.

Faulstich BM, Kossl M, Reimer K. (1996) Analysis of non-linear cochlear mechanics in the marsupial *Monodelphis domestica*: ancestral and modern mammalian features. *Hear Res.* 94, 47–53.

Finitzo T, Albright K, O'Neal J. (1998) The newborn with hearing loss: detection in the nursery. *Pediatrics.* 102, 1452–1460.

Fitzgerald TS. (1995) Comparison of click-evoked otoacoustic emission thresholds measured in one-third octave bands with psychophysical thresholds. Research Apprenticeship. Syracuse University, Syracuse, NY.

Fitzgerald TS, Prieve BA. (1999) DPOAE frequency ratio functions in infants and adults. *Abstr Midwtr Mtg Assoc Res Otolaryngol.* 22, 92.

Fitzgerald TS, Prieve BA. (2005) Detection of hearing loss using 2f2-f1 and 2f1-f2 distortion product otoacoustic emissions. *J Speech Hear Res.* 48, 1165–1186.

Gaskill SA, Brown AM. (1990) The behavior of the acoustic distortion product, 2f1-f2, from the human ear and its relation to auditory sensitivity. *J Acoust Soc Am.* 88, 821–839.

Gaskill SA, Brown AM. (1996) Suppression of human acoustic distortion product: dual origin of 2f1-f2. *J Acoust Soc Am.* 100, 3260–3274.

Gates GA, Mills D, Nam B-H, D'Agostino R, Rubel EW. (2002) Effects of age on the distortion product otoacoustic emission growth functions. *Hear Res.* 163, 53–60.

Glattke TJ, Pafitis IA, Cummiskey C, Herrer GR. (1995) Identification of hearing loss in children using measures of transient otoacoustic emission reproducibility. *Am J Audiol.* 4, 71–86.

Goodman SS, Withnell RH, Shera C. (2003) The origin of SFOAE microstructure in the guinea pig. *Hear Res.* 183, 7–17.

Gorga MP, Dierking DM, Johnson TA, Beauchaine KL, Garner CA, Neely ST. (2005) A validation and potential clinical applica-tion of multivariate analyses of distortion-product otoacoustic emission data. *Ear Hear.* 26, 593–607.

Gorga MP, Neely ST, Bergman BM, Beauchaine KL, Kaminski JR, Peters J, Jesteadt W. (1993) Otoacoustic emissions from normal-hearing and hearing-impaired subjects: distortion product responses. *J Acoust Soc Am.* 93, 2050–2060.

Gorga MP, Neely ST, Dorn PA. (1999) DPOAE test performance for a priori criteria and for multifrequency audiometric standards. *Ear Hear.* 20, 345–362.

Gorga MP, Neely ST, Dorn PA, Hoover B. (2003). Further efforts to predict pure tone thresholds from distortion product emissions input/output functions. *J Acoust Soc Am.* 113, 3275–3284.

Gorga MP, Neely ST, Ohlrich B, Hoover B, Redner J, Peters J. (1997) From laboratory to clinic: a large scale study of distortion product otoacoustic emissions in ears with normal hearing and ears with hearing loss. *Ear Hear.* 18, 440–455.

Gorga MP, Nelson K, Davis T, Dorn PA, Neely ST. (2000a) Distortion product otoacoustic emission test performance when 2f1-f2 and 2f2-f1 are used to predict auditory status. *J Acoust Soc Am.* 107, 2128–2135.

Gorga MP, Norton SJ, Sininger YS, Cone-Wesson B, Folsom RC, Vohr BR, Widen JE, Neely ST. (2000b) Identification of neonatal hearing impairment: distortion product otoacoustic emissions during the perinatal period. *Ear Hear.* 21, 400–424.

Grandori F. (1985) Nonlinear phenomenon in click- and tone-burst-evoked otoacoustic emissions from human ears. *Audiology.* 24, 71–80.

Green DM, Swets JA. (1974) *Signal Detection Theory and Psychophysics.* New York: Wiley.

Guinan JJ. (1986) Effect of efferent neural activity on cochlear mechanics. In: Grandore IGCF, ed. *Cochlear Mechanics and Otoacoustic Emissions. Scand Audiol.* (suppl 25), 53–62.

Hammernik RP, Ahroon WA, Lei SF. (1996) The cubic distortion product otoacoustic emissions from the normal and noise-damaged chinchilla cochlea. *J Acoust Soc Am.* 100, 1003–1012.

Harris FP. (1990) Distortion-product otoacoustic emissions in humans with high-frequency sensorineural hearing loss. *J Speech Hear Res.* 33, 594–600.

Harris FP, Lonsbury-Martin BL, Stagner BB, Coats AC, Martin GK. (1989) Acoustic distortion products in humans: systematic changes in amplitude as a function of f2/f1 ratio. *J Acoust Soc Am.* 85, 220–229.

Harris FP, Probst R. (2002) Otoacoustic emissions and audiometric outcomes. In: Robinette MS, Glattke TJ, ed. *Otoacoustic Emissions.* 2nd ed. New York: Thieme; pp 213–242.

Harris FP, Probst R, Xu L. (1992) Suppression of the 2f1-f2 otoacoustic emission in humans. *Hear Res.* 64, 133–141.

Harrison RV, Evans EF. (1979) Cochlear fibre responses in guinea pigs with well defined cochlear lesions. *Scand Audiol Suppl.* 9, 83–92.

Harrison WA, Norton SJ. (1999) Characteristics of transient evoked otoacoustic emissions in normal-hearing and hearing impaired children. *Ear Hear.* 20, 75–86.

Hauser R, Probst R. (1991) The influence of systematic primary-tone level variation L2-L1 on the acoustic distortion product emission 2f1-f2 in normal human ears. *J Acoust Soc Am.* 89, 280–286.

Hazell JWP. (1984) Spontaneous cochlear acoustic emissions and tinnitus. Clinical experience and the tinnitus patient. *Laryngol Otol (London).* 9 (suppl), 106–110.

He N-J, Schmiedt RA. (1993) Fine structure of the 2f1-f2 acoustic distortion product: changes with primary level. *J Acoust Soc Am.* 94, 2659–2669.

Heitmann J, Waldmann B, Schnitzler HU, Plinkert PK, Zenner HP. (1998) Suppression of distortion product otoacoustic emissions (DPOAE) near 2f1-f2 removes DP-gram fine structure: evidence for a secondary generator. *J Acoust Soc Am.* 103, 1527–1531.

Henley CM, Weatherly RA, Martin GK, Lonsbury-Martin B. (1996) Sensitive developmental periods for kanamycin ototoxic effects on distortion-product otoacoustic emissions. *Hear Res.* 98, 93–103.

Holte L, Margolis R, Cavanagh R. (1991) Developmental changes in multifrequency tympanograms. *Audiology.* 30, 1–24.

Hurley RM, Musiek FE. (1994) Effectiveness of transient-evoked otoacoustic emissions (TEOAEs) in predicting hearing level. *J Am Acad Audiol.* 5, 195–203.

Hussain DM, Gorga MP, Neely ST, Keefe DH, Peters J. (1998) Transient evoked otoacoustic emissions in patients with normal hearing and in patients with hearing loss. *Ear Hear.* 19, 434–449.

Hyde ML. (1994) Signal processing and analysis. In: Jacobson JT, ed. *Principles and Applications in Auditory Evoked Potentials.* Boston: Allyn and Bacon; pp 47–83.

Hyde ML, Davidson MJ, Alberti PW. (1991) Auditory test strategy. In: Jacobson JT, Northern JL, eds. *Diagnostic Audiology.* Austin: Pro-Ed; pp 295–322.

Janssen T, Gehr DD, Klein A, Müller J. (2005) Distortion product otoacoustic emissions for hearing threshold estimation and differentiation between middle-ear and cochlear disorders in neonates. *J Acoust Soc Am.* 117, 2969–2979.

Johnson NJ, Elberling C. (1982) Evoked otoacoustic emissions from the human ear. I. Equipment and response parameters. *Scand Audiol.* 11, 3–12.

Johnson TA, Neely ST, Garner C, Gorga MP. (2006) Influence of primary-level and primary frequency ratios on human distortion product otoacoustic emissions. *J Acoust Soc Am.* 119, 418–428.

Joint Committee on Infant Hearing. (1995) 1994 Position statement. *Pediatrics.* 95, 152–156.

Joint Committee on Infant Hearing. (2007) Year 2007 position statement: principles and guidelines for early hearing detection. *Pediatrics.* 20, 898–921.

Kanis LJ, de Boer E. (1997) Frequency dependence of acoustic distortion products in a locally active model of the cochlea. *J Acoust Soc Am.* 101, 1527–1531.

Karzon RK, Garcia P, Peterein JL, Gates GA. (1994) Distortion product otoacoustic emissions in the elderly. *Am J Otol.* 5, 596–605.

Keefe DH, Bulen JC, Arehart KH, Burns EM. (1993) Ear-canal impedance and reflection coefficient in human infants and adults. *J Acoust Soc Am.* 94, 2617–2638.

Kemp DT. (1978) Stimulated acoustic emissions from within the human auditory system. *J Acoust Soc Am.* 64, 1386–1391.

Kemp DT. (1979) Evidence of mechanical nonlinearity and frequency selective wave amplification in the cochlea. *Arch Otorhinolaryngol.* 224, 37–45.

Kemp DT. (1982) Cochlear echoes: implications for noise-induced hearing loss. In: Hamernik RP, Henderson D, Salvi R, eds. *New Perspectives on Noise-Induced Hearing Loss.* New York: Raven Press; pp 189–207.

Kemp DT. (1986) Otoacoustic emissions, traveling waves and cochlear mechanisms. *Hear Res.* 22, 95–104.

Kemp DT, Bray P, Alexander L, Brown AM. (1986) Acoustic emission cochleography—practical aspects. *Scand Audiol.* 25 (suppl), 71–94.

Kemp DT, Brown AM. (1983) A comparison of mechanical nonlinearities in the cochleae of man and gerbil from ear canal measurements. In: Klinke R, Hartmann R, eds. *Hearing: Physiological Bases and Psychophysics.* Berlin: Springer-Verlag; pp 82–88.

Kemp DT, Chum R. (1980) Observations on the generator mechanism of stimulus frequency emissions-two tone suppression. In: van den Brink G, Bilsen FA, eds. *Psychophysical, Physiological, and Behavioral Studies in Hearing.* Delft, The Netherlands: Delft University Press; pp 34–42.

Khanna SM, Leonard DG. (1986a) Measurement of basilar membrane vibrations and evaluation of cochlear condition. *Hear Res.* 23, 37–53.

Khanna SM, Leonard DG. (1986b) Relationship between basilar membrane tuning and hair cell condition. *Hear Res.* 23, 55–70.

Kim DO. (1986) Active and nonlinear cochlear biomenchanics and the role of outer-hair-cell subsystem in the mamallian auditory system. *Hear Res.* 22, 105–114.

Kim DO, Molnar CE, Matthews JW. (1980) Cochlear mechanics: nonlinear behavior in two-tone responses as reflected in cochlear-nerve-fiber responses and in ear-canal sound pressure. *J Acoust Soc Am.* 67, 1704–1721.

Kimberley BP, Hernadi I, Lee AM, Brown DK. (1994) Predicting pure tone thresholds in normal and hearing-impaired ears with distortion product emissions and age. *Ear Hear.* 15, 199–209.

Knight RD, Kemp DT. (1999). Relationships between DPOAE and TEOAE amplitude and phase characteristics. *J Acoust Soc Am.* 106, 1420–1435.

Knight RD, Kemp DT. (2000) Indications of different distortion product otoacoustic emission mechanisms from a detailed f1, f2 area study. *J Acoust Soc Am.* 107, 457–473.

Knight RD, Kemp DT. (2001) Wave and place fixed DPOAE maps of the human ear. *J Acoust Soc Am.* 109, 1513–1525.

Kok MR, van Zanten GA, Brocaar MP. (1992) Growth of evoked otoacoustic emissions during the first days postpartum. *Audiology.* 31, 140–149.

Kok MR, van Zanten GA, Brocaar MP. (1993a) Aspects of spontaneous otoacoustic emissions in healthy newborns. *Hear Res.* 69, 115–123.

Kok MR, van Zanten GA, Brocaar MP, Wallenburg HCS. (1993b) Click-evoked otoacoustic emissions in 1036 ears of healthy newborns. *Audiology.* 21, 213–224.

Koppl C, Manley GA. (1993) Distortion-product otoacoustic emissions in the bobtail lizard. II. Suppression tuning characteristics. *J Acoust Soc Am.* 93, 2834–2844.

Kujawa SG, Glattke TJ, Fallon M, Bobbin RP. (1992) Intracochlear application of acetylcholine alters sound-induced mechanical events within the cochlear partition. *Hear Res.* 61, 106–116.

Kujawa SG, Glattke TJ, Fallon M, Bobbin RP. (1993) Contralateral sound suppresses distortion product otoacoustic emissions through cholinergic mechanisms. *Hear Res.* 68, 97–106.

Kujawa SG, Glattke TJ, Fallon M, Bobbin RP. (1994) A nicotinic-like receptor mediates suppression of distortion product otoacoustic emissions by contralateral sound. *Hear Res.* 74, 122–134.

Kulawiec JT, Orlando MS. (1995) The contribution of spontaneous otoacoustic emissions to the click evoked otoacoustic emissions. *Ear Hear.* 16, 515–520.

Kummer P, Janssen T, Arnold W. (1995) Suppression tuning characteristics of the 2f1-f2 distortion product otoacoustic emission in humans. *J Acoust Soc Am.* 98, 197–210.

Kummer P, Janssen T, Arnold W. (1998) The level and growth behavior of the 2f1-f2 distortion product otoacoustic emission and its relationship to auditory sensitivity in normal hearing and cochlear hearing loss. *J Acoust Soc Am.* 103, 3431–3444.

Kummer P, Janssen T, Hulin P, Arnold W. (2000) Optimal L1–L2 primary tone level separation remains independent of test frequency in humans. *Hear Res.* 146, 47–56.

Kusuki M, Sakashita T, Kubo T, Kyunai K, Ueno K, Hikawa H, Wada T, Nakai Y. (1998) Changes in distortion product emissions from ears with Meniere's Disease. *Acta Otolarngol (Stockh).* 538 (suppl), 78–89.

Lafreniere D, Jung JD, Smurzynski J, Leonard G, Kim DO, Sasek J. (1991) Distortion-product and click-evoked otoacoustic emissions in healthy newborns. *Arch Otolaryngol Head Neck Surg.* 117, 1382–1389.

Lapsley Miller JA, Marshall L, Heller LM. (2004) A longitudinal study of changes in evoked otoacoustic emissions and pure-tone thresholds as measured in a hearing conservation program. *Int J Audiol.* 43, 307–322.

Lasky RE. (1998) Distortion product otoacoustic emissions in human newborns and adults. I. Frequency effects. *J Acoust Soc Am.* 103, 981–991.

Lasky RE, Perlman J, Hecox K. (1992) Distortion-product otoacoustic emissions in human newborns and adults. *Ear Hear.* 13, 430–441.

Liberman MC, Chesney CP, Kujawa SG. (1997) Effects of selective inner hair cell loss on DPOAE and CAP in carboplatin-treated chinchillas. *Auditory Neurosci.* 3, 255–268.

Liberman MC, Dodds LW. (1984a) Single neuron labeling and chronic cochlear pathology. II. Stereocilia damage and alterations of spontaneous discharge rates. *Hear Res.* 16, 43–53.

Liberman MC, Dodds LW. (1984b) Single-neuron labeling and chronic cochlear pathology. III. Stereocilia damage and alterations of threshold tuning curves. *Hear Res.* 16, 55–74.

Liberman MC, Gao J, He DZ, Wu X, Jia S, Zuo J. (2002) Prestin is required for electromotility of the outer hair cell and for the cochlear amplifier. *Nature.* 419, 300–304.

Liberman MC, Zuo J, Guinan JJ. (2004) Otoacoustic emissions without somatic motility: can stereocilia mechanics drive the mammalian cochlea? *J Acoust Soc Am.* 116, 1649–1655.

Lichtenstein V, Stapells DR. (1996) Frequency-specific identification of hearing loss using transient-evoked otoacoustic emissions to clicks and tones. *Hear Res.* 98, 125–136.

Lonsbury-Martin BL, Harris FP, Stagner BB, Hawkins MD, Martin GK. (1990a) Distortion product emissions in humans. I. Basic properties in normally hearing subjects. *Ann Otol Rhinol Laryngol.* 99, 3–14.

Lonsbury-Martin BL, Harris FP, Stagner BB, Hawkins MD, Martin GK. (1990b) Distortion-product otoacoustic emissions in humans. II. Relations to acoustic immittance and stimulus frequency and spontaneous otoacoustic emission in normally hearing subjects. *Ann Otolaryngol.* 236 (suppl), 14–28.

Lonsbury-Martin BL, Martin GK. (1990) The clinical utility of distortion-product otoacoustic emissions. *Ear Hear.* 11, 144–154.

Lonsbury-Martin BL, Martin GK, Probst R, Coats AC. (1987) Acoustic distortion products in rabbit ear canal. I. Basic features and physiological vulnerability. *Hear Res.* 28, 173–189.

Lonsbury-Martin BL, Martin GK, Whitehead ML. (1997) Distortion product otoacoustic emissions. In: Robinette MS, Glattke TJ eds. *Otoacoustic Emissions: Clinical Applications.* New York: Thieme; pp 83–109.

Lonsbury-Martin BL, Whitehead ML, Martin GK. (1991) Clinical applications of otoacoustic emissions. *J Speech Hear Res.* 34, 964–981.

Lucertini M, Moleti A, Sisto R. (2002) On the detection of early cochlear damage by otoacoustic emission analysis. *J Acoust Soc Am.* 111, 972–978.

Mammano F, Ashmore JF. (1993) Reverse transduction measured in the isolated cochlea by laser Michelson interferometry. *Nature.* 365, 838–841.

Manley GA, Gallo L, Koppl C. (1996) Spontaneous otoacoustic emissions in two gecko species, *Gekko gecko* and *Eublepharis macularius. J Acoust Soc Am.* 99, 1588–1603.

Manley GA, Schulze M, Oeckinghaus H. (1987) Otoacoustic emissions in a song bird. *Hear Res.* 26, 257–266.

Marshall L, Heller LM. (1998) Transient-evoked otoacoustic emissions as a measure of noise induced threshold shift. *J Speech Lang Hear Res.* 41, 1319–1334.

Marshall L, Lapsley Miller JA, Heller LM. (2001) Distortion-product otoacoustic emissions as a screening tool for noise-induced hearing loss. *Noise Health.* 3, 43–60.

Martin GK, Lonsbury-Martin BL, Probst R, Scheinin SA, Coats AC. (1987) Acoustic distortion products in rabbit ear canal. II. Sites of origin revealed by suppression contours and pure-tone exposures. *Hear Res.* 28, 191–208.

Martin GK, Ohlms LA, Franklin DJ, Harris FP, Lonsbury-Martin BL. (1990) Distortion-product emissions in humans. III. Influence of sensorineural hearing loss. *Ann Otolaryngol Rhinol Laryngol.* 99, 30–42.

Mauermann M, Uppenkamp S, van Hengel PWJ, Kollmeier B. (1999) Evidence for the distortion product frequency place as a source of distortion product otoacoustic emission (DPOAE) fine structure in humans. II. Fine structure for different shapes of cochlear hearing loss. *J Acoust Soc Am.* 106, 3484–3491.

Maxon AB, White KR, Culpepper B, Vohr BR. (1997) Maintaining acceptably low referral rates in TEOAE-based newborn hearing screening programs. *J Commun Disord.* 30, 457–475.

Mazelova J, Popelar J, Syka J. (2003) Auditory function in presbycusis: peripheral vs. central changes. *Exp Gerontol.* 38, 87–94.

Mills DM. (2003) Differential responses to acoustic damage and furosemide in auditory brainstem and otoacoustic emission measures. *J Acoust Soc Am.* 113, 914–924.

Moller AR. (1989) Possible mechanisms for tinnitus. *Hear J.* 42, 68–76.

Moulin A, Bera JC, Collet L. (1994) Acoustic distortion products and sensorineural hearing loss. *Audiology.* 33, 305–326.

Moulin A, Collet L, Veuillet E, Morgon A. (1993) Interrelations between transiently evoked otoacoustic emissions, spontaneous otoacoustic emissions and acoustic distortion products in normally hearing subjects. *Hear Res.* 65, 216–233.

Mountain DC. (1980) Changes in endolymphatic potential and crossed olivocochlear bundle stimulation alter cochlear mechanics. *Science.* 210, 71–72.

Neely ST, Johnson TA, Gorga MP. (2005) Distortion-product otoacoustic emission measured with continuously varying stimuli. *J Acoust Soc Am.* 117, 1248–1259.

Nelson DA, Kimberley BP. (1992) Distortion-product emissions and auditory sensitivity in human ears with normal hearing and cochlear hearing loss. *J Speech Hear Res.* 35, 1142–1159.

Norton SJ. (1993) Application of transient evoked otoacoustic emissions to pediatric populations. *Ear Hear.* 14, 65–73.

Norton SJ. (1994) Emerging role of evoked otoacoustic emissions in neonatal hearing screening. *Am J Otol.* 15 (suppl 1), 4–12.

Norton SJ, Gorga MP, Widen JE, Folsom RC, Sininger Y, Cone-Wesson B, Vohr BR, Mascher K, Fletcher K. (2000a) Identification of neonatal hearing impairment: evaluation of transient evoked otoacoustic emission, distortion product otoacoustic emission, and auditory brainstem response test performance. *Ear Hear.* 21, 508–528.

Norton SJ, Gorga MP, Widen JE, Vohr BR, Folsom RC, Sininger YS, Cone-Wesson B, Fletcher KA. (2000b) Identification of neonatal hearing impairment: transient evoked otoacoustic emissions during the perinatal period. *Ear Hear.* 21, 425–442.

Norton SJ, Neely ST. (1987) Tone-burst evoked otoacoustic emissions from normal-hearing subjects. *J Acoust Soc Am.* 81, 1860–1872.

Norton SJ, Widen JE. (1990) Evoked otoacoustic emission in normal-hearing infants and children: emerging data and issues. *Ear Hear.* 11, 121–127.

Osterhammel PA, Rasmussen AN, Olsen SO, Nielsen LH. (1996) The influence of spontaneous otoacoustic emissions on the amplitude of transient-evoked emissions. *Scand Audiol.* 25, 187–192.

Owens JJ, McCoy MJ, Lonesbury-Martin BL, Martin GK. (1992) Influence of otitis media on evoked otoacoustic emission in children. *Semin Hear.* 13, 53–65.

Owens, JJ, McCoy MJ, Lonesbury-Martin BL, Martin GK. (1993) Otoacoustic emissions in children with normal ears, middle ear dysfunction, and ventilating tubes. *Am J Otol.* 14, 34–40.

Penner MJ. (1988) Audible and annoying spontaneous otoacoustic emissions. *Arch Otolaryngol Head Neck Surg.* 114, 150–153.

Penner MJ. (1989a) Aspirin abolishes tinnitus caused by spontaneous otoacoustic emission. *Arch Otolaryngol Head Neck Surg.* 115, 871–875.

Penner MJ. (1989b) Empirical tests demonstrating two coexisting sources of tinnitus: a case study. *J Speech Hear Res.* 32, 458–462.

Penner MJ. (1990) An estimate of the prevalence of tinnitus caused by spontaneous otoacoustic emissions. *Arch Otolaryngol Head Neck Surg.* 116, 418–423.

Penner MJ, Burns EM. (1987) The dissociation of SOAEs and tinnitus. *J Speech Hear Res.* 30, 396–403.

Penner MJ, Glotzbach L, Huang T. (1993) Spontaneous otoacoustic emissions: measurement and data. *Hear Res.* 68, 229–237.

Prieve BA, Falter SR. (1995) COAEs and SSOAEs in adults with increased age. *Ear Hear.* 16, 521–528.

Prieve BA, Fitzgerald TS, Schulte LE. (1997a) Basic characteristics of click-evoked otoacoustic emissions in infants and children. *J Acoust Soc Am.* 102, 2860–2880.

Prieve BA, Fitzgerald TS, Schulte LE, Kemp DT. (1997b) Basic characteristics of distortion product otoacoustic emissions in infants and children. *J Acoust Soc Am.* 102, 2871–2879.

Prieve BA, Gorga MP, Neely ST. (1996) Click- and tone-burst-evoked otoacoustic emissions in normal-hearing and hearing-impaired ears. *J Acoust Soc Am.* 99, 3077–3086.

Prieve BA, Gorga MP, Schmidt A, Neely ST, Peters J, Schultes L, Jesteadt W. (1993) Analysis of transient-evoked otoacoustic emissions in normal hearing and hearing impaired ears. *J Acoust Soc Am.* 93, 3308–3319.

Prieve B, Huta H. (1999) SOAE's in infants and children. Presented to the American Auditory Society, Scottsdale, AZ.

Prieve B, Stevens F. (2000) The New York State Universal Newborn Hearing Screening Demonstration Project: introduction and overview. *Ear Hear.* 21, 85–91.

Probst R, Coats AC, Martin GK, Lonsbury-Martin BL. (1986) Spontaneous, click-, and tonebust-evoked otoacoustic emissions from normal ears. *Hear Res.* 21, 261–275.

Probst R, Lonsbury-Martin BL, Martin GK, Coats AC. (1987) Otoacoustic emissions in ears with hearing loss. *Am J Otolaryngol.* 8, 73–81.

Rasmussen AN, Popelka GR, Osterhammel PA, Nielsen LH. (1993) Clinical significance of relative probe-tone levels on distortion product otoacoustic emissions. *Scand Audiol.* 22, 223–229.

Rebillard G, Lavigne-Rebillard M. (1992) Effect of reversible hypoxia on the compared time courses of endocochlear potential and 2f1-f2 distortion products. *Hear Res.* 62, 142–148.

Rhode WW. (1971) Observations of the vibrations of the basilar membrane in squirrel monkeys using the Mossbauer technique. *J Acoust Soc Am.* 49, 1218–1231.

Ricci A. (2003) Active hair bundle movements and the cochlear amplifier. *J Am Acad Audiol.* 14, 325–338.

Ricci AJ, Crawford AC, Fettiplace R. (2000) Active hair bundle motion linked to fast transducer adaptation in auditory hair cells. *J Neurosci.* 20, 7131–7142.

Robinette MS. (1992) Clinical observations with transient evoked otoacoustic emissions with adults. *Semin Hear.* 13, 23–36.

Robinette MS, Cevette, MJ, Webb TM. (2002) Otoacoustic emissions in differential diagnosis. In: Robinette MS, Glattke TJ, eds. *Otoacoustic Emissions.* 2nd ed. New York: Thieme; pp 297–324.

Rosowski JJ, Peake WT, White JR. (1984) Cochlear nonlinearities inferred from two-tone distortion products in the ear canal of the alligator lizard. *Hear Res.* 13, 141–158.

Rossi G, Solero P, Rolando M, Olina M. (1989) Are delayed oto-acoustic emissions (DEOE) solely the outcome of an active intracochlear mechanism? *Scand Audiol.* 18, 99–104.

Ruggero MA, Rich NC. (1991) Application of a commercially manufactured Doppler shift laser velocimeter to the measurement of basilar membrane vibration. *Hear Res.* 51, 215–230.

Ruggero MA, Rich NC, Recio A, Narayan SS, Robles L. (1997) Basilar-membrane responses to tones at the base of the chinchilla cochlea. *J Acoust Soc Am.* 101, 2151–2163.

Ryan A, Dallos P. (1975) Effect of absence of cochlear outer hair cells on behavioral auditory threshold. *Nature.* 253, 44–46.

Sakashita T, Takeshi K, Kusuki M, Kynai K, Ueno K, Hikawa C, Wada T, Shibata T, Nakai Y. (1998) Patterns of change in growth function of distortion product otoacoustic emissions in Ménière's disease. *Acta Otolaryngol (Stockh).* 538 (suppl), 70–77.

Santos-Sacchi J, Shen W, Zheng J, Dallos P. (2001) Effects of membrane potential and tension on prestin, the outer hair cell lateral membrane motor protein. *J Physiol.* 531, 661–666.

Schairer KS, Fitzpatrick D, Keefe DH. (2003) Input-output functions for stimulus-frequency otoacoustic emissions in normal-hearing adult ears. *J Acoust Soc Am*. 114, 944–966.

Schairer KS, Keefe DH. (2005) Simultaneous recording of stimulus-frequency and distortion-product otoacoustic emission input-output functions in human ears. *J Acoust Soc Am*. 117, 818–832.

Schmiedt RA. (1986) Acoustic distortion in the ear canal. I. Cubic difference tones: effects of acute noise injury. *J Acoust Soc Am*. 79, 1481–1490.

Schmiedt RA, Adams JC. (1981) Stimulated acoustic emissions in the ear canal of the gerbil. *Hear Res*. 5, 295–305.

Seixas NS, Kujawa SG, Norton S, Sheppard L, Neitzel R, Slee A. (2004) Predictors of hearing threshold levels and distortion product otoacoustic emissions among noise exposed young adults. *Occup Environ Med*. 61, 899–907.

Shera CA. (2004) Mechanisms of mammalian otoacoustic emission and their implications for the clinical utility of otoacoustic emissions. *Ear Hear*. 25, 86–97.

Shera CA, Guinan JJ. (1999) Evoked otoacoustic emissions arise by two fundamentally different mechanisms: a taxonomy for mammalian OAEs. *J Acoust Soc Am*. 105, 782–798.

Siegel JH, Kim DO. (1982a) Cochlear biomechanics: vulnerability to acoustic trauma and other alterations as seen in neural responses and ear-canal sound pressure. In: Hamernik D, Henderson D, Salvi R, eds. *New Perspectives on Noise-Induced Hearing Loss*. New York: Raven Press; pp 137–151.

Siegel JH, Kim DO. (1982b) Efferent control of cochlear mechanics? Olivocochlear bundle stimulation affects cochlear biomechanical nonlinearity. *Hear Res*. 6, 171–182.

Sininger YS, Cone-Wesson B, Folsom RC, Gorga MP, Vohr BR, Widen JE, Ekelid M, Norton SJ. (2000) Identification of neonatal hearing impairment: auditory brain stem responses in the perinatal period. *Ear Hear*. 21, 383–399.

Sliwinska-Kowalska M, Kotylo P. (2002) Occupational exposure to noise decreases otoacoustic emission efferent suppression. *Int J Audiol*. 41, 113–119.

Smurzynski J, Jung MD, Lafreniere D, Kim DO, Kamath MV, Rowe JC, Holman MC, Leonard G. (1993) Distortion-product and click-evoked otoacoustic emissions of preterm and full-term infants. *Ear Hear*. 14, 258–274.

Smurzynski J, Leonard G, Kim DO, Lafreniere DC, Jung MD. (1990) Distortion product otoacoustic emissions in normal and impaired adult ears. *Arch Otolaryngol Head Neck Surg*. 116, 1309–1316.

Spektor Z, Leonard G, Kim DO, Jung MD, Smurzynski J. (1991) Otoacoustic emissions in normal and hearing-impaired children and normal adults. *Laryngoscope*. 101, 965–976.

Spivak L, Dalzell L, Berg A, Bradley M, Cacace A, Campbell D, DeCristofaro J, Greenberg E, Gross S, Orlando M, Pinhiero J, Regan J, Stevens F, Prieve B. (2000). The New York State Universal Newborn Hearing Screening Demonstration Project: inpatient outcome measures. *Ear Hear*. 21, 92–103.

Spoendlin H. (1973) The innervation of the cochlear receptor. In: Moller A, ed. *Basic Mechanisms of Hearing*. New York: Academic Press; pp 185–234.

Stenklev NC, Laukli E. (2003) Transient evoked otoacoustic emissions in the elderly. *Int J Audiol*. 42, 132–139.

Stevens JC. (1988) Click-evoked oto-acoustic emissions in normal and hearing-impaired adults. *Br J Audiol*. 2, 45–49.

Stewart CE, Hudspeth AJ. (2000) Effects of salicylates and aminoglycosides on spontaneous otoacoustic emissions in the Tokay gecko. *Proc Natl Acad Sci USA*. 97, 454–459.

Stover L, Gorga MP, Neely ST, Montoya D. (1996) Toward optimizing the clinical utility of distortion product otoacoustic emission measurements. *J Acoust Soc Am*. 100, 956–967.

Stover L, Neely ST, Gorga MP. (1999) Cochlear generation of intermodulation distortion revealed by DPOAE frequency functions in normal and impaired ears. *J Acoust Soc Am*. 106, 2669–2678.

Stover L, Norton SJ. (1993) The effects of aging on otoacoustic emissions. *J Acoust Soc Am*. 94, 2670–2681.

Strickland AE, Burns EM, Tubis A. (1985) Incidence of spontaneous otoacoustic emissions in infants and children. *J Acoust Soc Am*. 78, 931–935.

Strouse AL, Ochs MT, Hall JW. (1996) Evidence against the influence of aging on distortion-product otoacoustic emissions. *J Am Acad Audiol*. 7, 339–345.

Sun XM, Kim DO, Jung MD, Randolph KJ. (1996) Distortion product otoacoustic emission test of sensorineural hearing loss in humans: comparison of unequal- and equal-level stimuli. *Ann Otol Rhinol Laryngol*. 105, 982–990.

Talmadge CL, Long GR, Murphy WJ, Tubis A. (1993) New off-line method for detecting spontaneous otoacoustic emissions in human subjects. *Hear Res*. 71, 170–182.

Talmadge CL, Long GR, Tubis A, Dhar S. (1999) Experimental confirmation of the two-source interference model for the fine structure of distortion product otoacoustic emissions. *J Acoust Soc Am*. 105, 275–292.

Taschenberger G, Manley GA. (1997) Spontaneous otoacoustic emissions in the barn owl. *Hear Res*. 110, 61–76.

Trine MB, Hirsch JE, Margolis RH. (1993) The effect of middle ear pressure on transient evoked otoacoustic emissions. *Ear Hear*. 14, 401–407.

Tyler RS, Conrad-Ames D. (1981) Spontaneous acoustic cochlear emissions and sensorineural tinnitus. *Br J Audiol*. 16, 193–194.

Vento B, Durrant J, Sabo D, Boston J. (2004) Development of f2/f1 ratio functions in humans. *J Acoust Soc Am*. 115, 2138–2147.

Veuillet E, Martin V, Suc B, Vesson JF, Morgon A, Collet L. (2001) Otoacoustic emissions and medial olivocochlear suppression during auditory recovery from acoustic trauma in humans. *Acta Otolaryngol*. 121, 278–283.

Vinck BM, De Vel E, Xu ZM, Van Cauwenberge PB. (1996) Distortion product otoacoustic emissions: a normative study. *Audiology*. 35, 231–245.

Vinck BM, Van Cauwenberge PB, Corthals P, De Vel E. (1998) Multivariant analysis of otoacoustic emissions and estimation of hearing thresholds: transient evoked otoacoustic emissions. *Audiology*. 37, 315–334.

Vinck BM, Van Cauwenberge PB, Leroy L, Corthals P. (1999) Sensitivity of transient evoked and distortion product otoacoustic emissions to the direct effects of noise on the human cochlea. *Audiology*. 38, 44–52.

Vohr BR, Carty LM, Moore PE, Letourneau K. (1998) The Rhode Island hearing assessment program: experience with statewide hearing screening. *J Pediatr*. 133, 353–359.

Warr WB, Guinan JJ, White JS. (1986) Organization of the efferent fibers: the lateral and medial olivocochlear systems. In: Altschuler RA, Hoffman DW, Bobbin RP, eds. *Neurobiology of Hearing: The Cochlea*. New York: Raven Press; pp 333–348.

Weinstein MC, Fineberg HV. (1980) *Clinical Decision Analysis.* Philadelphia: Saunders.

Whitehead ML, McCoy MJ, Lonsbury-Martin BL, Martin GK. (1995) Dependence of distortion product otoacoustic emissions on primary levels in normal and impaired ears. I. Effects of decreasing L2 below L1. *J Acoust Soc Am.* 97, 2346–2358.

Whitehead ML, Stagner BB, Lonsbury-Martin BL, Martin GK. (1994) Measurement of otoacoustic emissions for hearing assessment. *IEEE Eng Med Biol Mag.* April/May, 210–226.

Widen JE, Folsom RC, Cone-Wesson B, et al. (2000) Identification of neonatal hearing impairment: hearing status at 8 to 12 months corrected age using a visual reinforcement audiometry protocol. *Ear Hear.* 21, 471–487.

Wiederhold ML. (1990) Effects of tympanic membrane modification on distortion product otoacoustic emissions in the cat ear canal. In: Dallos P, Geisler CD, Matthews JW, Ruggero MA, Steele CR, eds. *Mechanics and Biophysics of Hearing.* New York: Springer-Verlag; pp 251–258.

Wier CC, Pasanen EG, McFadden D. (1988) Partial dissociation of spontaneous otoacoustic emissions and distortion product during aspirin use in humans. *J Acoust Soc Am.* 84, 230–237.

Wilson JP. (1980) Evidence for a cochlear origin for acoustic re-emissions, threshold fine structure, and tonal tinnitus. *Hear Res.* 2, 233–252.

Wilson JP, Sutton GJ. (1981) Acoustic correlates of tonal tinnitus. In: Evered D, Lawrenson G, eds. *Tinnitus (CIBA Foundation Symposium).* London: Pitman Books Ltd; pp 82–107.

Wit HP, Ritsma RJ. (1980) Evoked acoustical responses from the human ear: some experimental results. *Hear Res.* 2, 253–261.

Yardley MPJ, Davies CM, Stevens JC. (1998) Use of transient evoked otoacoustic emissions to detect and monitor cochlear damage by platinum containing drugs. *Br Soc Audiol.* 32, 305–316.

Yates GK, Withnell RH. (1999). The role of intermodulation distortion in transient-evoked otoacoustic emissions. *Hear Res.* 136, 49–64.

Zheng J, Shen W, He DZ, Long KB, Madison LD, Dallos P. (2000) Prestin is the motor protein of cochlear outer hair cells. *Nature (London).* 405, 149–155.

Zurek PM. (1981) Spontaneous narrowband acoustic signals emitted by human ears. *J Acoust Soc Am.* 69, 514–523.

Zurek PM, Clark WW, Kim DO. (1982) The behavior of acoustic distortion products in the ear canals of chinchillas with normal or damaged ears. *J Acoust Soc Am.* 7, 774–780.

Zwicker E. (1983) Delayed evoked otoacoustic emissions and their suppression by Gaussian-shaped pressure impulses. *Hear Res.* 11, 359–371.

22 Current Physiologic Bases of Audiologic Interpretation and Management

Charles I. Berlin and Linda J. Hood

▨ INTRODUCTION

The premises of this chapter depend on the reader being aware of the following research-based principles:

1. Audiologists are capable of separating outer from inner hair cell function.

2. This differentiation is essential because the hair cells have vastly different functions that are NOT always reflected in the audiogram. Outer hair cells are nature's wide dynamic amplifier (Ruggero, 1992 cited in Berlin et al., 1996), and when they are present, hearing aids are usually, but not always, contraindicated.[1]

3. Thus someone can appear to be severely impaired by behavioral audiogram, have no auditory brainstem response (ABR), and appear to be deaf physiologically but have normal otoacoustic emissions, creating a conflict that we will discuss in great length in the body of the chapter. See also Berlin et al. (2002).

4. Outer hair cell function is measured with two tests: otoacoustic emissions and cochlear microphonics (CM). (See body of chapter for measurements of CM.) When we see normal emissions, we also acquire indirect data on the mechanical status of the middle ear because if the middle ear is obstructed, the emissions will be attenuated or blocked. However, normal emissions do not guarantee normal or near-normal audiograms despite conventional wisdom to the contrary (Bonfils and Uziel, 1989).

5. CM come from any hair cell and reflect the electrical fields around the hair cells. They can be measured during ABR by reversing click polarity and observing the reversal of the waves that will *only* occur if the waves come from hair cells rather than nerve fibers (Berlin et al., 1998).

6. Inner hair cells, which are the primary driving force of the eighth nerve (Spoendlin, 1979), can be measured with five different tests, one of which includes middle ear muscle reflexes. The reflexes are *not* normal and not present in auditory neuropathy/auditory dyssynchrony (AN/AD) (Berlin et al., 2005). Thus, normal emissions and *absent* reflexes are a hallmark of AN/AD and can also be used to rule out central auditory processing disorder (CAPD) in the presence of normal audiograms. The audiogram alone, no matter how mild or severe, cannot be relied on to reveal the underlying physiologic state of the inner ear and brainstem. For example, we found that more than 10% of children in a school for the deaf had unexpectedly normal emissions (Cheng et al., 2005).

7. In this chapter, we are advising our colleagues to pretest the physiology with tympanometry, reflexes, and emissions before accepting the audiogram at face value, not only for the differential diagnosis of AN/AD but also for uncovering measurement errors (misplaced earphones, collapsed canals, functional hearing loss, out of calibration systems, etc.). More rationale is found in Berlin et al. (2002).

---

[1] Only five of our 260 patients with auditory neuropathy/auditory dyssynchrony (AN/AD) have benefited from hearing aids (In preparation, 2008). None of Rance's (2005) adult patients and only about half of their children with AN/AD report benefit from hearing aids. Deltenre et al. (1999) report some hearing aid success once emissions have disappeared. (See Berlin et al. [2007].)

■ HISTORICAL OVERVIEW: HOW AND WHY INTERPRETING HEARING FROM THE PURETONE AUDIOGRAM MAY MISS CRITICAL PHYSIOLOGIC UNDERPINNINGS

Before the electronic age, physicists and students of hearing used methods such as whistles (Urbantschitsch, 1881), tuning forks, and monochords (Guild, 1956) to outline human hearing abilities in frequency, intensity, and temporal dimensions. However, these tools provided only rudimentary qualitative assessments because of limitations in quantifying the stimuli. Electronic assessment of hearing sensitivity began well before the official beginnings of "audiology" in the Army's 1940 to 1955 Aural Rehabilitation programs. It was part of a design initiative by electrical engineers and physicists to develop commercially feasible telephones. In order to accomplish that, quantifying the frequency, intensity, and temporal range of human hearing was essential. In response to this need, the engineers developed the Western Electric 1-A audiometer and worked with psychophysicists like Fletcher, Boring, Stevens, and Davis (Fletcher, 1929; Stevens and Davis, 1938) to outline what became the core of speech communication psychophysics and engineering in those decades.

In what may have been among the first medical uses of the device for people with hearing loss, Stacey Guild and his associates rolled that very same Western Electric 1-A battery-operated device from ward to ward at the Johns Hopkins Hospital to test the puretone sensitivity of dying patients. When the patients died, Guild, an anatomist, quickly harvested and processed their temporal bones using a technique of embedding, decalcifying, and serial sectioning that is still in use today (Guild, 1956; Schuknecht and Gulya, 1986). Guild and his colleagues then published a landmark paper on the importance of the basal turn of the cochlea to high-frequency hearing (Guild, 1956). At about the same time, von Békésy published his work on the traveling wave (reviewed in von Békésy [1970]), which shed serious doubts on the then-dominant Helmhotz theory of hearing (Wever, 1959). Through this developmental period of the scientific bases of our profession, hearing and hearing loss were referenced to the puretone audiogram, and to this day, hearing loss is quantified and codified by legal and educational groups in terms of puretone hearing loss (see, for example, the American Academy of Otolaryngology–Head and Neck Surgery tables (1979) for percentage of hearing loss, various educational programs on quantification of hearing loss, and this text).

Carhart and Tillman (1972), Jerger et al. (1959), and others in Europe began to use speech audiometry, also developed by psychologists and telephone engineers, in innovative ways to refine the diagnosis and management of hearing loss. The hearing aid industry, of course, made major contributions to that technology for its own purposes, but even

today, in medicolegal and health insurance circles, the "gold standard" for the quantification of hearing loss remains the puretone audiogram.

Much of what we have taught and been taught as cardinal rules of audiology in the past 40 years might have to be recast in light of new findings. For example, it is only relatively recently that the active process of outer hair cell (OHC) micromechanics and the cochlear amplifier have been introduced (Brownell et al., 1985). Intact OHCs lead to normal otoacoustic emissions (OAEs). Because the OHC is part of nature's wide dynamic range compression amplifier (cochlear amplifier) (Davis, 1983; Ruggero, 1992), generally hearing aids are not physiologically appropriate when emissions are present, regardless of the audiogram. Similarly, the long-standing practice of fitting hearing aids to an audiogram presumes intact inner hair cells (IHC), which we now know are the key element in depolarizing primary auditory neurons (Spoendlin, 1979). If the IHCs are not present or not functioning (e.g., in dead zones) (Moore et al., 2000) or if the neurons themselves are either inaccessible or dysfunctional (Amatuzzi, 2001; Starr et al., 2003), then hearing aids will usually be of limited value. These two conditions actually cover most of the underlying causes of what has come to be called auditory neuropathy/auditory dyssynchrony (AN/AD). Thus "treating the audiogram" without regard to the underlying physiology, a common practice for many years, continues to this day in practices in which air, bone, and speech audiometry are the sole tests offered. The reviews in this chapter and the sample patients that follow address the importance of adding physiologic tests such as OAEs, middle ear muscle reflex (MEMR) testing, and, if emissions are or were present and reflexes are absent, an ABR to every intake battery. These procedures are of little value directly to surgeons, who generally focus on medical and mechanical pathologies of the auditory system; our profession requires that we manage the patient nonmedically, and therefore, we need data that guide us with respect to intervention strategies. As you read the following pages, imagine how the patient care displayed here would change if we had only air, bone, and speech audiometry and required the permission of a medical or health maintenance organization (HMO) gatekeeper to perform tests that would only offer surgical and medical direction.

Beginning in the late 1930s, some of the physiologic mysteries of the ear were being unraveled, and discoveries were being reported that did not fit the model of the puretone audiogram threshold sensitivity being traceable to a particular event in the cochlea. The CM and the eighth-nerve compound action potential (CAP) (Wever et al., 1949; Wever, 1959), the endocochlear potential (EP) (von Békésy, 1960; Konishi, 1979), the summating potential (SP) (see Chapter 12), and later on OAEs (see Chapter 21; Eggermont, 1979; Kemp, 1978; Spoendlin, 1979) kept warning us that these physiologic tests should not be expected to match "hearing sensitivity" and that the audiogram could not yet be objectified or predicted, not even by neural single-unit population studies (Kiang, 1965). Then major differences between IHC and OHC function (Spoendlin, 1979) were reported but did not reach widespread audiologic application for years (e.g., dead zones, AN/AD). What is more distressing is that hearing losses were identified that disagreed with our incomplete notion of physiology, and physiologic and psychophysical findings were discovered that disagreed with von Békésy's predictions based on a linear inner ear (Kemp, 1978; Berlin et al., 1978). These articles faced difficulties in being published because they flew in the face of conventional wisdom and the persistent belief in the linearity of the inner ear in life as well as postmortem.

When we found normal behavioral audiograms despite very poor clinical measures of hearing (such as speech perception in noise for example), we imagined that there must be a "central disorder" or a problem with the "second filter" (neural processing central to the cochlea). The active processes, based on such factors as hair cell motility and OHC tuning, were not clearly understood, and the ear was viewed by most of us as a linear organ that, when properly understood, would lead us to the ultimate goal of "the objective audiogram." To this day, some colleagues are pursuing the tone-burst ABR and the auditory steady-state response (ASSR) as tools for this purpose. However, to date, astute researchers like Gorga et al. (2006) recognize that audiograms of patients with AN/AD cannot be interpreted in the way they would be for people with primarily missing OHCs and normal IHCs; in addition, neither the tone-burst ABR nor the ASSR generates reliable audiograms for such patients.

Auditory Physiology and Audiograms Fail to Agree in Some Auditory Disorders

This chapter will review current advances in physiology to show how using the puretone audiogram alone to gauge hearing may have serious limitations in the presence of AN/AD and similar temporal auditory disorders (Starr et al., 1996). Two salient examples of data that were misinterpreted because of failure to support conventional versions of auditory physiology follow.

First, in the early 1970s, one of us (C.I.B.) reported on a series of patients with little or no hearing below 8 kHz but islands of normal sensitivity above 10 kHz. The papers were rejected for publication in part because the reviewers thought there must have been a technical error in our earphones, oscillators, or switching mechanisms. Normal hearing sensitivity at 10 kHz with little usable hearing at lower frequencies was theoretically impossible according to traveling wave theory and what was then known of tuning in the (postmortem) cochlea (von Békésy, 1960; Berlin et al., 1978). We know now that interaction of OHC active processes and IHC depolarization can produce very sharp tuning in the high frequencies with little behavioral sensitivity in the low frequencies and without invoking a central or second filter. We built a hearing aid that shifted lower frequency information to higher frequencies (an upward-shifting translating

hearing aid) for that condition, which, until recently, was the only usable tool to help such patients (Berlin et al., 1978).

A second example is the failure to test or use MEMR in routine diagnostic intake evaluations (see Chapter 10). We have seen many patients sent to us from other clinics who had all the signs of a central auditory processing disorder (CAPD), including a virtually normal puretone audiogram, poor hearing in noise, poor dichotic listening, poor Staggered Spondaic Word scores, and degraded performance on pitch pattern tests, as well as some language and speech delay. However, on intake, we noted that MEMRs had not been tested and were presumed to be normal because of the normal audiogram. When we found that MEMRs were absent in many "normal-hearing" patients, we subsequently performed ABRs and found abnormalities (see Chapters 11, 13, and 14). Seeing AN/AD in the ABR, we realized that finding absent MEMRs at intake would have saved all concerned many hours of time and frustration, as well as avoided misdirection (Berlin et al., 2002). Clearly the "normal puretone audiogram" reflected neither the underlying physiology nor the patients' true hearing limitations.

The Importance of a Test Battery Intake Screen

This chapter stresses the importance of a test battery screen on intake (Jerger and Hayes, 1976; Hannley et al., 1983), including tympanometry, MEMRs, and OAEs, that is completed before any behavioral audiometry. The advantages are many beyond correctly identifying AN/AD. With this preliminary triage, the audiologist will not waste time and energy pursuing misleading data. For example, a patient with normal OAEs, MEMRs, and tympanometry should not show a significant puretone loss, but if hearing loss is seen on the very first puretone test, then the audiologist can stop and seek out the source of the discrepancy. In this case, the discrepancy could result from a variety of sources, including a patient with functional hearing loss, the audiologist failing to put the earphones on or in the patient's ear, a collapsed ear canal, or a cerumen-obstructed insert earphone. These and many other sources of error (such as disconnected earphones, misrouting of signals, or equipment malfunction), which are usually caught well after considerable time has been wasted collecting misleading or inaccurate data from the patient, could be pre-empted by this preliminary sorting procedure.

HOW WE CAN NOW INTERPRET THE AUDIOGRAM THROUGH THE PHYSIOLOGY?

There are now five well-studied electrophysiologic/electroacoustic phenomena in the ear that reveal much of the underlying physiology and allow us to follow a careful audiologic strategy in clarifying audiologic diagnosis for all new patients. These five phenomena are described here.

1. The *endocochlear potential* (EP) is an 80-mV direct current (DC) potential composed of 140 mV of aerobic potential and –60 mV of anaerobic potential. It is the cochlea's battery, and without it, none of the other potentials can be recorded from the outside. The most common genetic defect in hearing, a *GJB2* (connexin 26) mutation, blocks the flow of ions in parts of the cochlea and can often strike first at the EP. The resultant loss of the battery makes the ear appear "dead" but leaves the hair cells and nerve fibers intact, for awhile. Thus, what appears to be a sensory-neural loss, implying loss of nerve fibers or hair cells, is in fact a loss of the driving force behind them, and the critical structures are still intact. This is the one potential that currently eludes measurement in humans, and once we learn how to record it through future research, we will gain many more diagnostic insights.

2. The *cochlear microphonic* (CM) or cochlear potential (Wever et al., 1949) is an alternating current (AC) potential reflecting the mechanical deformation and current flow around both OHCs and IHCs when they are activated. It is recordable during electrocochleography (ECoG) or ABR and is identifiable by its salient characteristic of polarity inversion when the stimulus polarity is inverted (Fig. 22.1). This characteristic is not exhibited by the eighth-nerve CAP.

3. The *compound action potential* (CAP) represents the synchronous discharge of many eighth-nerve single units in response to a pulsatile stimulus (Kiang, 1965). The CAP is also seen as wave I in the ABR.

4. The *summating potential* (SP) is a DC offset potential whose source is still controversial (Offner et al., 1987) but whose size relative to the CAP is often used as an index of Ménière's disease (Ferraro and Durrant, 2006).

5. *Otoacoustic emissions* (OAEs) are sounds that are associated with function of the OHCs of the cochlea, which, if seen, confirm the integrity of:
   a. The OHCs
   b. The middle and outer ear pathways for the sounds to reach the recording microphone placed in the external canal
   c. The endocochlear potential, without whose presence there would be little recordable electrical activity from the cochlea

Figure 22.2, from the classic work of Konishi (1979), shows the effect of oxygen and hemoglobin deprivation on the SP, EP, and N1 and N2 components of the CAP. Note that when the EP falls, all of the other recorded potentials drop sharply and then they return when the EP returns. The loss of oxygen alone could account for all of the potentials disappearing. However, subsequent studies (Honrubia and Ward, 1969) have shown that biasing the cochlea by applying a DC current, while maintaining oxygen flow, also seriously affects other potentials.

HOW THIS TRIAGE STRATEGY ALLOWS YOU TO KNOW WHAT THE BEHAVIORAL RESULTS SHOULD BE BEFORE YOU GET THEM

Recording normal tympanometry, normal MEMRs, and normal OAEs from new patients on intake should predict normal or nearly normal speech reception thresholds (SRTs) and normal or nearly normal puretone sensitivity at the corresponding frequencies. Once behavioral responses to either speech or puretones begin to be collected, if they differ from "normal" or "nearly normal" in any way, the tests should be aborted, and a search should be made for technical errors (e.g., misplaced earphones, broken connections, malfunctioning audiometer) or functional hearing loss. Table 22.1 shows the expected audiologic results for various combinations of tympanograms, MEMRs, OAEs, and ABRs. We suggest to our beginning students that they copy this template and keep it as a desk reference until the principles become ingrained.

Is This Triage Procedure Cost Effective?

One might argue that performing immittance, reflexes, and emissions on every new patient before audiometry is not cost

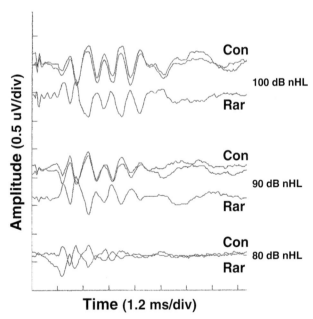

FIGURE 22.1 Auditory brainstem response (ABR) with complete inversion of all waves when the polarity of the clicks are inverted and a complete average is taken for each polarity. This result (obtained from patient 5 described later in the chapter) is consistent with a picture of cochlear microphonics, rather than neural synchrony and a normal ABR. nHL, normal hearing level; Con, condensation click; Rar, rarefaction click.

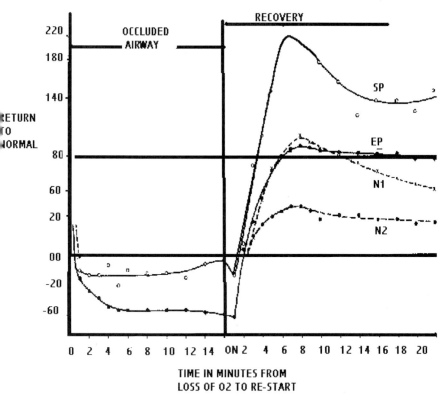

FIGURE 22.2 Effect of oxygen deprivation on the summating potential (SP), endocochlear potential (EP), and compound action potential (CAP) N1 and N2. (Reprinted, with permission of publisher, from Konishi T. [1979]. Some observations on negative endocochlear potential during anoxia. *Acta Otolaryngol.* 87, 506–516.)

effective. Our data suggest just the reverse. First, one must accept that managing patients by their puretone audiogram information alone, when they really have normal OHCs and compromised IHCs or nerve fibers, is likely to be ineffective. We would be managing the audiogram and not responding to the underlying physiology.

Reports of AN/AD in schools for the deaf and other reports (Cheng et al., 2005) suggest that between 10% and 15% of patients with diagnoses of hearing loss in fact have normal OHCs, as evidenced by present OAEs. This may be an underestimation because only now are universal hearing screening programs using ABR, and thus uncovering many patients who would otherwise not have been identified. Screening programs that use OAEs only will not identify AN/AD patients unless reflexes are added to the mix (Berlin et al., 2005). The combination of OAEs and MEMRs reduces this type of error to nearly zero. Although the fiscal cost is considerable, the human cost is enormous.

The cost of discarding tests for which charges have been made and collected, having to redo many of the tests without reimbursement, and recommending and charging for hearing aids that are not useful all result in a set of problems that could have been avoided by a preaudiometric validation procedure. Before we collect audiometric data, shouldn't we have a basis to determine whether the results are credible and proper for use in making rehabilitation decisions or whether there is a need to study the patient more deeply than the audiogram suggests?

Later in this chapter, we cite a case in which a child was misdiagnosed as having a CAPD and sent to language-training schools when he really had AN/AD. We have seen separate cases where a sharply *upward* sloping cochlear hearing loss, with predictably normal emissions but *present* reflexes, led to a misdiagnosis of CAPD based solely on the misinterpretation that normal OAEs always mean a normal puretone audiogram.

It is clear that we have an obligation to reduce testing error in our patients. At present, we know of no other procedure that minimizes potential errors, saves retesting time, and reduces hearing aid fitting errors more than the triage of tympanometry, MEMRs, and OAEs.

NINE PATIENTS WITH COMMON AUDIOGRAMS BUT VASTLY DIFFERENT PHYSIOLOGIC UNDERPINNINGS CLARIFIED BY THE TRIAGE

We will present four "corner audiograms" representing six patients: two siblings with *GJB2* mutations (connexin 26) with severe deafness; two siblings with AN/AD with normal OAEs, absent MEMRs, and no ABR; a posttraumatic beating patient who demonstrates inverting ABRs and no MEMRs and who was mislabeled as "hysterical" because she generated a corner audiogram but had normal OAEs (the original clinicians who made the diagnosis failed to evaluate MEMRs and never did an ABR); and finally, a truly hysterical patient with normal ABR, MEMRs, and OAEs but a corner puretone audiogram.

Then we will discuss two patients with nearly normal puretone audiograms, one of whom one of the authors

TABLE 22.1 Outline of generally expected audiologic results roughly predicted by tympanograms, middle ear muscle reflexes (MEMRs), and otoacoustic emissions (OAEs) (TREO)

Test procedure	Normal hearing	Primarily outer hair cell loss	Inner hair cell and/or auditory nerve	Conductive	Functional or nonorganic
Tympanometry	Type A most commonly expected	Type A most commonly expected	Type A most commonly expected	Type B or C occasionally; type A in otosclerosis	Type A most commonly expected
MEMR	Present at or below 90 dB HL	Present at or below 90 dB HL	Absent or above 95 dB despite normal emissions	Absent or elevated by hearing loss	Normal
OAE	Normal and robust, S/N > 6 dB	Absent or compromised because of hair cell loss	Normal and robust, S/N > 6 dB	Absent or obscured	Same as normal hearing, unless there is an organic overlay
Speech perception in quiet and noise (if recordable)	Follows Articulation Index (AI)[a] rules	Follows AI rules	Does NOT follow AI rules; speech in noise inordinately poor	Follows AI rules with correction for hearing loss	Often SRT much better than puretone sensitivity
ABR (not for tumor assessment but for synchrony) using one total average to a positive and one average to a negative (not alternating) polarity click	Normal latencies and latency-intensity function	Normal or steep-sloped latency-intensity functions until stimuli are below audibility; absolute latencies unaffected by puretone loss	Absent synchrony, no latency-intensity function, large cochlear microphonics sometimes lasting 4–6 ms	Latencies shifted to the right proportional to the amount of hearing loss	Same as normal unless there is a functional overlay

HL, hearing level; S/N, signal-to-noise ratio; SRT, speech recognition threshold; ABR, auditory brainstem response.
Note that combinations of any finding can occur and the ultimate *absence* of OAEs, which was seen in about one third of our auditory neuropathy/auditory dyssynchrony patients, does not cure the patient of the desynchronization; this must be factored into the management.
[a] See French and Steinberg (1947) and Kamm et al. (1985).

(C.I.B.) initially misdiagnosed as having CAPD but who had no MEMRs and no ABR and ultimately was shown to have AN/AD as part of his Charcot-Marie-Tooth disease. The second patient's near-normal puretone audiogram almost prevented her from getting a cochlear implant, which ultimately habilitated her. Finally, we will discuss a patient with a normal puretone audiogram who had been treated for 4 years with a diagnosis of CAPD in a program for "language-disordered children." He was ultimately shown to have no MEMRs, normal OAEs, and no ABR and showed AN/AD rather than CAPD.

We suggest that many old patients with CAPD may show AN/AD upon re-examination, especially patients who show severe CAPD based on SCAN (Screening Test for Auditory Processing Disorders in Children) or similar procedures. Because cochlear implantation is a viable management option for AN/AD patients, differentiating CAPD from AN/AD has serious consequences. This difference can be screened for easily and inexpensively by evaluating MEMRs and OAEs in the same patient. If the OAEs are present and/or the audiogram is normal and the MEMRs are elevated or absent, then an ABR is strongly recommended, with separate responses obtained for positive- and negative-polarity clicks to evaluate whether the response is dominated by a large CM (Berlin et al., 1998).

Patients 1 and 2: *GJB2* (Connexin 26) Deafness in a Pair of Siblings

The older of these two boys was correctly diagnosed as profoundly deaf at 9 months of age by ABR (OAEs were not clinically available at the time) and aided within 2 weeks. He was raised in a strict auditory verbal environment. When his younger brother was born, the mother called one of us (C.I.B.) with the concern that her newborn might also be deaf. There were no screening programs in place at the time, so we rolled a (not-so) portable ABR unit to the hospital area and confirmed the deafness when we found that there was no ABR. Again, OAEs were unavailable, and we did not feel the need to run any more tests at the time. Although that was adequate for these two patients, we will show how it is nowadays a risky practice (Berlin et al., 2002). The ultimate clarification occurred when we performed molecular genetic testing and found that these boys were both homozygous for a 35delG mutation in the *GJB2* gene (connexin 26) (Keats and Berlin, 1999).

Patients 3 and 4: AN/AD Traceable to an *OTOF* (Otoferlin) Mutation in Patients Who Were Early Users of Cued Speech, which Supported Their Ultimate Language and Speech Successes with Cochlear Implants

These siblings (the elder a female), who were 2 years apart in age, showed corner audiograms, normal OAEs, absent

MEMRs, and no ABRs. They were ultimately shown to have *OTOF* gene mutations related to otoferlin (Varga et al., 2003), which presumably affected their IHC function. (Note: Neonatal anoxia can also lead to spotty or even complete IHC loss while maintaining OHC function [Amatuzzi et al., 2001] and a diagnosis of AN/AD.) Both patients were implanted with great language success. Part of their language success may be traceable to their early and continued use of Cued Speech as a language-acquisition tool (Cornett and Daisey, 1992). This tool allows the normal-hearing parents full access to their own language and vocabulary and allows the children to eavesdrop on the syntax, morphology, and phonology of their home language. Then when hearing was restored following cochlear implantation, a natural transition to spoken language was quite fluid (Smith, 2004). Because the development of language is so unpredictable in AN/AD patients (7% of the patients in our sample needed no intervention), we now recommend Cued Speech as a language-acquisition tool to parents to allow them to watch and wait to see whether their AN/AD children will need any surgical or hearing aid assistance. After implantation, despite the fact that auditory-verbal training is the most powerful of the methods invoked, we do *not* ask that cueing be terminated but recommend that the parents use it as needed. It is, after all, a tool to facilitate communication, and the patient is still deaf when the implant is not working.

Patient 5: A Posttraumatic Adult-Onset AN/AD Patient

This patient was sent to us for an electrophysiologic evaluation for a possible functional overlay to a physical hearing loss. She was seen in September 1999 for delayed auditory feedback testing (Chase, 1958) and ABR, OAE, MEMR, and OAE suppression testing (medial olivocochlear reflex) (Collet et al., 1990; Berlin et al., 1993). The referring audiologist was able to obtain OAEs but felt they were inconsistent with her deaf voice and deaf behavior. His clinical instincts were correct here, but not because she had a functional or nonorganic overlay, but rather because of the paradoxical coexistence of normal OAEs and an absent ABR. We also found that she had normal OAEs but an absent ABR with large CMs and absent MEMRs, which were all consistent with a diagnosis of AN/AD rather than functional hearing loss, as was originally suspected.

History

Patient 5 was 21 years old at the time of the exam, reportedly finished 10th grade, and, at around age 18 years, was beaten severely by her then husband whose name was not offered. No police report or criminal charges were filed, and there is no legal record of the incident according to the informants. Soon thereafter, she was said to have gone deaf over the space of a few weeks.

OBSERVATIONS

She showed no effect of delayed auditory feedback, thus reducing the likelihood of functional overlays. Her voice was deaf sounding and metallic and reflected hearing much like what is postulated for adventitiously deaf patients who have developed normal language pretraumatically.

TEST RESULTS

OAEs were unusually robust (Fig. 22.3), and the ABR to positive- and negative-polarity clicks showed CM but no evidence of neural responses (Fig. 22.1). Her delayed auditory feedback was unaffected (Chase, 1958), and her MEMRs were absent. She was also studied with efferent suppression of OAEs by putting a suppressor stimulus (broadband noise) in one or both ears and looking for the OAEs to reduce in size. She showed no suppression, which is an observation also consistent with AN/AD (Berlin et al., 1993; Hood et al., 2003).

MANAGEMENT

Cochlear implantation was recommended after completion of psychiatric and psychological testing, but she has not yet accepted that recommendation.

Patient 6: A Truly Hysterical Patient with Functional Hearing Loss

This patient, too, presented with a corner audiogram, ostensibly after dental anesthesia. Her OAEs were normal, but her

MEMRs were present at 75 to 85 dB hearing level (HL) in both ears, and her ABR showed a normal latency-intensity function (Fig. 22.4). Thus, in contrast to the previous patient who was suspected of having a functional hearing loss because of the normal OAEs in the presence of a corner audiogram, this patient actually *had* a functional hearing loss. This was confirmed by the other tests in the battery (MEMRs and OAEs), emphasizing that results of a single test in these conditions may be misleading (Jerger and Hayes, 1976).

Patient 7: A Patient Misdiagnosed as Having CAPD Based on a Nearly Normal Audiogram but Very Poor Speech Perception in Noise

This young man was first seen at age 12 years and misdiagnosed as having CAPD based on the seemingly incongruous findings of a nearly normal audiogram, predictably normal OAEs, and complaints of very poor hearing in noise plus failure on virtually all of the recommended CAPD tests of the time (Keith, 2000). It was not until we found absent MEMRs that we considered looking past his failures on all of the behavioral CAPD tests and performing an ABR. The results (Fig. 22.5) were startling and ultimately led to a diagnosis of Charcot-Marie-Tooth disease, a hereditary motor sensory neuropathy that often also involves AN/AD.

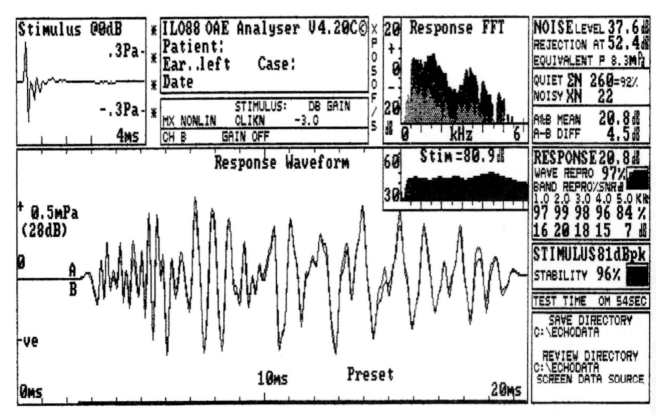

FIGURE 22.3 Normal otoacoustic emissions in the presence of a "corner audiogram" misinterpreted by referring agents as proof of a hysterical hearing loss (patient 5).

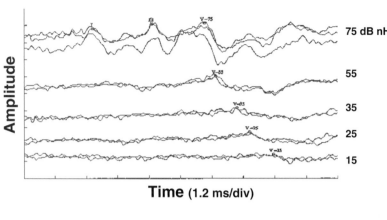

FIGURE 22.4 Normal auditory brainstem response (ABR) latency-intensity function in patient 6 in the presence of a "corner audiogram" with normal emissions and normal reflexes. nHL, normal hearing level.

This young man, now in his late 20s, shows:

1. Fluctuating puretone audiograms (Fig. 22.6), which started out in the grey zone and migrated all over the audiogram
2. Dependence on lip reading for daily communication
3. No ability to use the phone
4. That he now requires Computer Aided Texting to manage in his college degree program

He was offered a cochlear implant but has so far declined.

Patient 8: Initially Denied a Cochlear Implant Because Her Audiogram Was "Too Good"

Patient 8 and her father both presented with a unique form of AN/AD. They both had nearly normal audiograms in the high frequencies and quite poor speech understanding on the phone, in background noise, and, of course, without lip reading. When the daughter began to go blind because of Leber's disease, she was implanted, and her success was remarkable, being able to talk on the phone and generate 70% discrimination in noise (+10 signal-to-noise ratio), when preoperatively her discrimination was less than 10% in quiet and 0% in noise. The audiogram and the results speak for themselves (Fig. 22.7).

Patient 9: Managed Incorrectly as a CAPD Patient in a School for Language-Impaired Children When He Had AN/AD

Patient 9 (born January 16, 1995) was seen for auditory evaluation in June 2001. He was being educated as a child with CAPD. His birth was normal (full-term, long labor); he

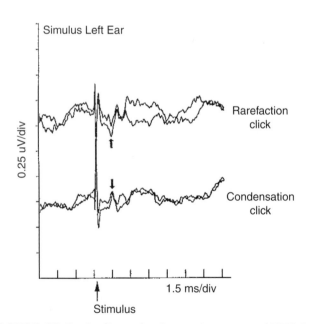

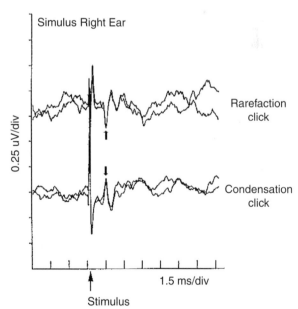

FIGURE 22.5 Auditory brainstem response (ABR) in the presence of a nearly normal audiogram (see grey zone in Fig. 22.6). (Adapted from Hood LJ. [1998] *Clinical Applications of the Auditory Brainstem Response.* San Diego: Singular Publishing Group.)

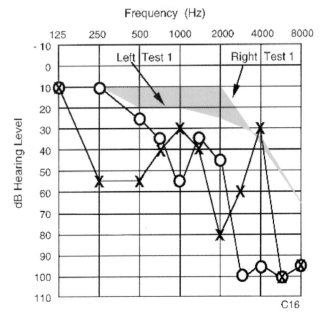

PURE TONE THRESHOLDS

MIDDLE EAR MUSCLE REFLEXES

	Stimulus Right					Stimulus Left			
	500	1k	2k	4k		500	1k	2k	4k
Contra	Ab	Ab	Ab	Ab	Contra	Ab	Ab	Ab	Ab
Ipsi	Ab	Ab	Ab	Ab	Ipsi	Ab	Ab	Ab	Ab

SPEECH AUDIOMETRY

Test Condition	Right Ear	Left Ear
Words in Quiet (PB Max)	84% at 50 HL	48% at 80 HL
Words in Noise (PB Max)	0% at 50 HL	0% at 80 HL

FIGURE 22.6 Inconsistent audiogram of patient 7 that was initially recorded in the grey zone listed as Left Test 1 and Right Test 1. Note absent middle ear muscle reflexes and inordinately poor speech in noise. (Adapted from Hood LJ. [1998] *Clinical Applications of the Auditory Brainstem Response.* San Diego: Singular Publishing Group.)

weighed over 9 lb but had *no* jaundice. However, he needed an intravenous line because of a *Staphylococcus* infection, and he received gentamicin and vancomycin. He started babbling at 7 or 8 months, pointed and grunted a lot, and began single words by the end of his first year. However, by the end of his second year, his mother noticed that he was falling behind. He had middle ear infections for the first 2 years of his life, but he outgrew those. He has had no real problems with ear infections since then. Although he never complained about pain, he was found to have an active middle ear infection at around age 4 years.

Between 3.5 and 4 years, while he was being managed as a child with CAPD, his mother started "the mission" to find out why he was so auditorily handicapped. She had been told he had normal hearing based on normal OAEs. We did the following tests and included the following information in the report.

TYMPANOMETRY AND MEMRS

These evaluated the mechanics of his middle ear and reflex arc of the middle ear muscles. The tympanometry and mechanics test results were normal; however, his MEMRs were absent.

OAEs

These evaluate OHC function, cochlear battery function, and middle ear function. All of these were normal.

ABR WITH BOTH POSITIVE- AND NEGATIVE-POLARITY CLICKS

This separates neural from hair cell responses. The patient's hair cell responses dominated the tracings.

DIAGNOSIS

The results support a diagnosis of AN/AD.

RECOMMENDATIONS

Patient 9 has AN/AD and *not* a CAPD-based language disorder. This misdiagnosis could have been completely avoided had MEMRs been added to the intake diagnostic battery. The absence of the reflex would have signaled the need for an ABR. We made the following recommendations to the family after we showed them what AN/AD sounds like:

■ Make sure when you talk to patient 9 that you are facing him and have his attention.
■ Consider adopting Cued Speech as a visual language tool in your family to improve patient 9's access to vocabulary and language visually.
■ If you desire a cochlear implant, auditory verbal and oral techniques should dominate after the implant, although cues need not be abandoned unless you so desire.
■ We also recommended that patient 9's mother contact a list serve for parents of children with AN/AD at www.auditoryneuropathy@yahoo.com.

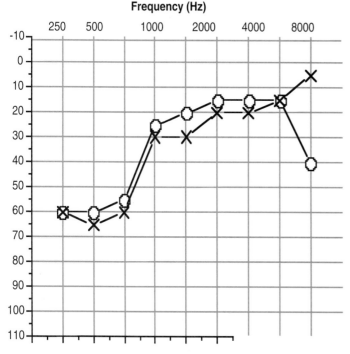

Immittance	Right Ear	Left Ear
Tympanogram	Type _A_	Type _A_
Peak Pressure	-20 mmH20	-80 mmH20
Static Compliance	1.1 cc	1.3 cc

ACOUSTIC REFLEXES

	Stimulus Right					Stimulus Left			
	500	1 K	2 K	4K		500	1 K	2 K	4K
R. Ipsi	NR	→			L. Ipsi	NR	→		
R.Contra	NR	→			L.Contra	NR	→		
Reflex Decay					Reflex Decay				

Speech Threshold (SRT)
R: 20, L: 25 dB HL

Recognition in Quiet
R: 8%, L: 10% at MCL

Recognition in Noise
R & L: 0% at +10 S/N

Post-Cochlear Implant
74% in noise at +10 S/N for sentences (Pre-CI=0%)

FIGURE 22.7 Patient 8 with auditory neuropathy/auditory dyssynchrony who demonstrated markedly improved performance with implant despite nearly normal audiogram in the high frequencies.

DISCUSSION AND CONCLUSIONS

The material on which this chapter has been based could easily have been entitled "Fifty Years of My (C.I.B.) Audiologic Mistakes and How to Avoid Them." With the advent of OAEs and MEMRs and our increased understanding of auditory physiology and genetics, it is time we stepped out from behind the puretone audiogram as an inviolable gold standard for hearing and recognized its limitations. Without physiologic validation, an audiogram can be an obstacle rather than an aid to patient management in general and to hearing aid fitting in particular (Spoendlin, 1979; Moore et al., 2000; Hogan and Turner, 1998; Berlin et al., 2002; Rance, 2005). We strongly urge our colleagues to adopt a triage of tympanometry, MEMRs, and OAEs on every new patient before puretone audiometry is performed; these precautions may save time and money, as well as prevent many common management errors. This will also allow a validation stamp to be impressed on the audiogram to tell the audiologists when the results can be trusted and/or used for habilitation.

REFERENCES

American Academy of Otolaryngology–Head and Neck Surgery. Guide for the evaluation of hearing handicap. *JAMA.* 241, 2055–2059.

Amatuzzi MA, Northrup CL, et al. (2001) Selective inner hair cell loss in premature infants and cochlear pathological patterns from neonatal intensive care unit autopsies. *Arch Otolaryngol Head Neck Surg.* 127, 629–636.

Berlin CI, Bordelon J, St. John P, Wilensky D, Hurley A, Kluka E, Hood LJ. (1998) Reversing click polarity may uncover auditory neuropathy in infants. *Ear Hear.* 19, 37–47.

Berlin CI, Hood LJ, Cecola RP, Jackson DF, Szabo P. (1993) Does type I afferent neuron dysfunction reveal itself through lack of efferent suppression? *Hear Res.* 65, 40–50.

Berlin CI, Hood LJ, Hurley A, Wen H. (1996) Hearing aids only for hearing-impaired patients with abnormal otoacoustic emissions. In: Berlin C, ed. *Hair Cells and Hearing Aids*. San Diego: Singular Publishing Group.

Berlin CI, Hood LJ, Jeanfreau J, Morlet T, Brashears S, Keats BJB. (2002) The physiological basis of audiological management. In: Berlin CI, Ricci A, Hood LJ, eds. *Hair Cells Micromechanics and Otoacoustic Emissions*. San Diego: Delmar-Thompson.

Berlin CI, Hood LJ, Morlet T, Wilensky D, St. John P, Montgomery E, Thibodeaux M. (2005) Absent or elevated middle ear muscle reflexes in the presence of normal otoacoustic emissions: a universal finding in 136 cases of auditory neuropathy/dys-synchrony. *J Am Acad Audiol.* 16, 546–553.

Berlin CI, Keats BJB, Hood LJ, Gregory P, Rance G. (2007) Auditory neuropathy/dys-synchrony (AN/AD). In: Schwartz S, ed. *Choices in Deafness: A Parents' Guide to Communication Options*. 3rd ed. Bethesda, MD: Woodbine House.

Berlin CI, Wexler KF, Jerger JF, Halperin HR, Smith S. (1978) Superior ultra-audiometric hearing: a new type of hearing loss which correlates highly with unusually good speech in the "profoundly deaf." *Otolaryngology.* 86, ORL/111–ORL/116.

Bonfils P, Uziel A. (1989) Clinical applications of evoked acoustic emissions: results in normally hearing and hearing-impaired subjects. *Ann Otol Rhinol Laryngol.* 98, 326–331.

Brownell WE, Bader CR, Bertrand D, de Ribaupierre Y. (1985) Evoked mechanical responses of isolated cochlear outer hair cells. *Science.* 227, 194–196.

Carhart R, Tillman TW. (1972) Individual consistency of hearing for speech across diverse listening conditions. *J Speech Hear Res.* 15, 105–113.

Chase RA. (1958) Effect of delayed auditory feedback on the repetition of speech sounds. *J Speech Hear Disord.* 23, 583–590.

Cheng X, Li L, Brashears S, Morlet T, Ng SS, Berlin C, Hood L, Keats B. (2005) Connexin 26 variants and auditory neuropathy/dys-synchrony among children in schools for the deaf. *Am J Med Genet A.* 139, 13–18.

Collet L, Kemp DT, Veuillet E, Duclaux R, Moulin A, Morgon A. (1990) Effect of contralateral auditory stimuli on active cochlear micro-mechanical properties in human subjects. *Hear Res.* 43, 251–262.

Cornett RO, Daisey ME. (1992) *The Cued Speech Resource Book for Parents of Deaf Children*. Raleigh, NC: National Cued Speech Association.

Davis H. (1983) An active process in cochlear mechanics. *Hear Res.* 9, 79–90.

Deltenre P, Mansbach AL, Bozet C, Christiaens F, Barthelemy P, Paulissen D, Renglet T. (1999) Auditory neuropathy with preserved cochlear microphonics and secondary loss of otoacoustic emissions. *Audiology.* 38, 187–195.

Eggermont JJ. (1979) Summating potentials in Ménière's disease. *Arch Otorhinolaryngol.* 222, 63–75.

Ferraro JA, Durrant JD. (2006) Electrocochleography in the evaluation of patients with Ménière's disease/endolymphatic hydrops. *J Am Acad Audiol.* 17, 45–68.

Fletcher H. (1929) *Speech and Hearing*. New York: Van Nostrand.

French NR, Steinberg JC. (1947) Factors governing the intelligibility of speech sounds. *J Acoust Soc Am.* 19, 90–119.

Gorga MP, Johnson TA, Kaminski JR Beauchaine KL, Garner CA, Neely ST. (2006) Using a combination of click- and tone burst-evoked auditory brain stem response measurements to estimate pure-tone thresholds. *Ear Hear.* 27, 60–74.

Guild SR. (1956) Hearing. *Ann Otol Rhinol Laryngol.* 65, 507–510.

Hannley M, Jerger JF, Rivera VM. (1983) Relationships among auditory brain stem responses, masking level differences and the acoustic reflex in multiple sclerosis *Audiology.* 22, 20–33.

Hogan CA, Turner CW. (1998) High-frequency audibility: benefits for hearing-impaired listeners. *J Acoust Soc Am.* 104, 432–441.

Honrubia V, Ward PH. (1969) Cochlear potentials inside the cochlear duct at the level of the round window. *Ann Otol Rhinol Laryngol.* 78, 1189–1200.

Hood LJ. (1998) *Clinical Applications of the Auditory Brainstem Response*. San Diego: Singular Publishing Group.

Hood LJ, Berlin CI, Bordelon J, Rose K. (2003) Patients with auditory neuropathy/dys-synchrony lack efferent suppression of transient evoked otoacoustic emissions. *J Am Acad Audiol.* 14, 302–313.

Jerger JF, Carhart R, Tillman TW, Peterson JL. (1959) Some relations between normal hearing for pure tones and for speech. *J Speech Hear Res.* 2, 126–140.

Jerger JF, Hayes D. (1976) The cross-check principle in pediatric audiometry. *Arch Otolaryngol.* 102, 614–620.

Kamm CA, Dirks DD, Bell TS. (1985) Speech recognition and the Articulation Index for normal and hearing-impaired listeners. *J Acoust Soc Am.* 77, 281–288.

Keats BJB, Berlin CI. (1999) Genomics and hearing impairment. *Genome Res.* 9, 7–16.

Keith RW. (2000) Development and standardization of SCAN-C test for auditory processing disorders in children. *J Am Acad Audiol.* 11, 438–445.

Kemp DT. (1978) Stimulated acoustic emissions from within the human auditory system. *J Acoust Soc Am.* 64, 1386–1391.

Kiang NYS. (1965) Discharge patterns of single fibers in the cat's auditory nerve. Special technical report, no. 13. Cambridge, MA: MIT Press.

Konishi T. (1979) Some observations on negative endocochlear potential during anoxia. *Acta Otolaryngol.* 87, 506–516.

Moore BC, Huss M, Vickers DA, Glasberg BR, Alcántara JI. (2000) A test for the diagnosis of dead regions in the cochlea. *Br J Audiol.* 34, 205–224.

Offner FF, Dallos P, Cheatham MA. (1987) Positive endocochlear potential: mechanism of production by marginal cells of stria vascularis. *Hear Res.* 29, 117–124.

Rance G. (2005) Auditory neuropathy/dys-synchrony and its perceptual consequences. *Trends Amplif.* 9, 1–43.

Ruggero M. (1992) Responses to sound of the basilar membrane of mammalian cochlea. *Curr Opin Neurobiol.* 2, 449–456.

Schuknecht HF, Gulya AJ. (1986) *Anatomy of the Temporal Bone with Surgical Implications*. Philadelphia: Lea & Febiger.

Smith J. (2004) Cued speech and cochlear implants: a view from two decades. *On Cue.* 1, 17.

Spoendlin H. (1979) Sensory neural organization of the cochlea. *J Laryngol Otol.* 93, 853–877.

Starr A, Michalewski HJ, Zeng FG, Fujikawa-Brooks S, Linthicum F, Kim CS, Winnier D, Keats BJB. (2003) Pathology and physiology of auditory neuropathy with a novel mutation in the MPZ gene. *Brain.* 126, 1604–1619.

Starr A, Picton TW, Sininger Y, Hood LJ, Berlin CI. (1996) Auditory neuropathy. *Brain*, 741–753.

Stevens SS, Davis H. (1938) *Hearing, Its Psychology and Physiology.* New York: J. Wiley & Sons, Inc.

Urbantschitsch V. (1881) Zur Lehre von der Schallempfindung. *Arch Gesch Physiol.* 24, 574–595.

Varga R, Kelley PM, Keats BJ, Starr A, Leal SM, Cohn E, Kimberling WJ. (2003) Non-syndromic recessive auditory neuropathy is the result of mutations in the otoferlin (OTOF) gene. *J Med Genet.* 40, 45–50.

von Békésy G. (1960) *Experiments in Hearing.* New York: McGraw-Hill.

von Békésy G. (1970) Travelling waves as frequency analyzers in the cochlea. *Nature.* 225, 1207–1209.

Wever EG, Lawrence M, et al. (1949) Effects of oxygen deprivation upon the cochlear potentials. *Am J Physiol.* 159, 199–208.

Wever EG. (1959) The cochlear potentials and their relation to hearing. *Ann Otol Rhinol Laryngol.* 68, 974–989.

SECTION III

SPECIAL POPULATIONS

Assessment of Hearing Loss in Children

Allan O. Diefendorf

INTRODUCTION

The current trend in public health and primary health care practice is to view infants and young children suspected of or at risk for hearing loss (see Appendix 23.1) as a high priority for diagnostic evaluation and confirmation of hearing status. This emphasis in hearing health care represents a standard of service delivery that has evolved over the past 35 years of advocacy by the Joint Committee on Infant Hearing (JCIH 1972; 1982; 1991; 1994; 2000; 2007). Specifically, the JCIH has advocated that universal detection has as its goal that 100% of infants with significant congenital hearing loss shall be identified by 3 months of age and shall have appropriate intervention initiated by 6 months of age.

To achieve beneficial outcomes for children who are hard of hearing and deaf, an audiologist must provide comprehensive diagnostic evaluation of hearing status within weeks of referral. The diagnostic evaluation provides the first opportunity for developing a relationship with the family and for initiating audiologic care (diagnosis, counseling, intervention, and ongoing care coordination). The interaction with the family during the diagnostic evaluation is critical because the support, guidance, and education a family receives at this time help to facilitate smooth transitions between referral source and early intervention programs in a timely manner for the family and lead to higher rates of compliance with audiologic recommendations.

During the diagnostic process, the integrity of the auditory system is evaluated for each ear, and the status of hearing sensitivity across the speech frequency range is described, as is the type (nature) of hearing loss. In turn, these data provide essential information for medical management when indicated, as well as the data required to initiate amplification protocols. Finally, these data are further used as a baseline for continued audiologic monitoring.

The purpose of this chapter is to focus on the audiologic assessment and diagnosis of infants and young children with hearing loss. Additionally, this chapter is developed with an emphasis on the following premise: audiologic procedures must be age appropriate, outcome based, and cost effective, and all procedures must have demonstrated validity and reliability.

JUSTIFICATION FOR EARLY DETECTION OF HEARING LOSS

Undetected hearing loss in infants and young children compromises optimal language development and personal achievement. Without appropriate opportunities to learn language, children will fall behind their hearing peers in language, cognition, social-emotional development, and academic achievement. However, research demonstrates that when hearing loss is identified early (prior to 6 months of age) and followed immediately (within 2 months) with appropriate intervention services, the outcomes in language development, speech development, and social-emotional development will be significantly better when compared with children with later identified congenital hearing loss (Yoshinaga-Itano et al., 1998; Carney and Moeller, 1998; Moeller, 2000). Moreover, when the same identification and intervention benchmarks are achieved (prior to 6 months of age), children perform as much as 20 to 40 percentile points higher on school-related measures (reading, arithmetic, vocabulary, articulation, intelligibility, social adjustment, and behavior) (Yoshinaga-Itano, 1995; 2003; Yoshinaga-Itano and Sedey, 2000). Therefore, early detection of hearing loss in infants and young children is justifiable as a priority in public health in general, with the specific responsibility placed on the health care subspecialty of audiology.

REFERRAL PATTERNS IN PEDIATRIC HEARING HEALTH CARE

The early identification of hearing loss and follow-up diagnostics assessment are currently carried out through referrals from a variety of sources. These sources include state-mandated newborn hearing screening programs and early intervention agencies, primary care providers who coordinate regular medical home visits, and other medical specialists (e.g., otolaryngologists, developmental pediatricians, neurologists) involved with infants and young children. This early referral has been advocated based on the mounting evidence that the earlier confirmation of hearing loss occurs, the earlier intervention can begin, thereby increasing the likelihood of optimizing a child's potential in all developmental areas.

Early Hearing Detection and Intervention Program Referrals

In recent years, the emphasis on universal early detection of hearing loss in infants has grown considerably. For example, in 1993, only 11 hospitals were screening more than 90% of their newborns. By 2005, every state had implemented a newborn hearing screening program, and data suggest that about 95% of newborn infants in the United States are screened for hearing loss prior to hospital discharge (National Center for Hearing Assessment and Management [NCHAM], 2007). During this same time period, it became clear that screening is only the first step in a "*process*" necessary to identify infants and young children with hearing loss. The next step is to provide these children and their families with timely access to diagnostic follow-up and, when necessary, referral to appropriate, culturally sensitive, and family-centered intervention services. It should be noted that all professional groups involved in the early detection of hearing loss have replaced the phrase "universal newborn hearing screening (UNHS) programs" with the term "early hearing detection and intervention (EHDI) programs." This conceptual change was introduced when it became apparent that screening was just a critical first step. Experience has shown that, in order to successfully identify and serve infants and young children with hearing loss and help their families, professionals must go beyond screening. To be successful, all elements of follow-up need to be included to meet and serve the child's and family's complex needs.

To successfully serve infants and young children with hearing loss, an agency within the EHDI program (usually the State Department of Health) has the responsibility of tracking and initiating referrals. To achieve optimal follow-up benchmarks, State Departments of Health and state Part C programs should be working closely together. Part C of the Individuals with Disabilities Education Act (IDEA) mandates responsibility for Child Find and intervention for children with disabilities, and requires all states to provide appropriate early intervention programs for all infants and young children meeting the disability criteria. As such, systematic communication is required between State Departments of Health and Part C programs to facilitate referrals to audiologists. This is achieved when a hospital's newborn hearing screening outcomes are communicated in parallel to State Departments of Health and state Part C programs. In turn, audiologic referrals can and should be made as soon as possible by Part C program coordinators. Clearly, well-coordinated tracking and surveillance systems must be developed by states to achieve the desired outcomes. Optimally, within the limits of confidentiality, each service provider within the EHDI system (e.g., hospital, practitioner, public health agency, public and private education agencies) participates in information management to track elements of care to each infant and family.

The Child's Medical Home

It is clear that services for infants and young children suspected of or at risk for hearing loss would be optimal if they were connected soon after birth to a primary care physician who is familiar with the children's circumstances, is knowledgeable about the consequences of hearing loss, is an advocate/facilitator for early referral, and is known and trusted by the family. To this end, primary care physicians, working in partnership with parents and other health care professionals including audiologists, make up the infant's "medical home." A *medical home* is defined as an approach to providing health care services where care is accessible, family-centered, continuous, comprehensive, coordinated, compassionate, and culturally competent. The primary care physician acts in partnership with parents in a medical home to identify and access services needed in developing a global plan of appropriate and necessary health and habilitative care for infants identified with hearing loss (American Academy of Pediatrics, 2002; Tonniges and Palfrey, 2004). Thus, the medical home serves as an important link between families, all service providers, and the state early intervention agency.

As newborn hearing screening programs have reached the benchmark of screening a minimum of 95% of newborns, the goal of 95% of those referred achieving follow-up has been difficult. The State of Colorado reports that 76% of infants achieved follow-up audiologic evaluations to confirm or exclude congenital hearing loss (Mehl and Thomson, 1998). In a 1999 review of the Texas screening program, 97% of newborns were screened, yet only 64% returned for follow-up (Finitzo and Crumley, 1999). These numbers indicate the challenge of continuity of care from screening to audiologic follow-up and confirmation of hearing loss. As such, the medical home is part of a system responsible for assuring that a child is referred *and* scheduled for audiologic follow-up in a timely manner. The physician has the opportunity to articulate to parents the importance of

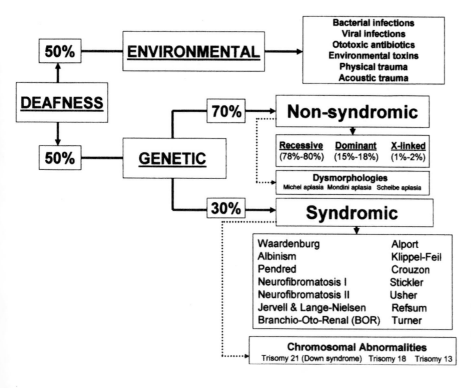

FIGURE 23.1 The distribution of hearing loss etiology into "genetic" causes and "environmental" causes.

audiologic follow-up and to actively demonstrate the importance by facilitating early referrals to audiologists. Moreover, the child's medical home ensures that children and families enter the health care and early intervention system with minimal obstacles and that they attend appointments.

Other Medical Specialists

The most effective approach to the early detection of and intervention for hearing loss involves a multidisciplinary team working individually and collectively to assess a patient. As such, early referrals to appropriate professionals are essential to facilitate accurate diagnosis and, in turn, result in efficient and effective patient care plans.

A wide array of health care providers (e.g., primary care physicians, audiologists, otolaryngologists, ophthalmologists, geneticists, developmental pediatricians) and education service providers (e.g., speech-language pathologists, educators of children who are deaf or hard of hearing, early intervention professionals involved in delivering EHDI services) is essential given the complexity of hearing loss. Hearing loss can exist as a single entity, or it may be one aspect of multiple anomalies. Figure 23.1 details the distributions of etiologies relative to hearing loss, providing information on the biologic complexity of individuals with hearing loss. As such, early referrals between and among specific service providers are essential for a thorough assessment of the individual suspected of hearing loss.

With the current focus on *early* detection of hearing loss, referrals to audiologists are occurring at earlier and earlier ages. The importance of audiologic diagnosis of hearing loss cannot be overstated; often the identification of hearing loss

may be the first indication of a compromised sensory system. In turn, the medical workup of the patient may lead to additional findings of other sensory system or body system involvement.

In concert with audiologic care coordination by the audiologist, every infant with a confirmed hearing loss must be evaluated by an otolaryngologist with pediatric expertise and have at least one exam by an ophthalmologist experienced in evaluating infants. Additionally, Figure 23.1 clearly suggests that families should be offered a genetics consultation. This evaluation can provide families with information on etiology of hearing loss, prognosis for progression, associated disorders (e.g., renal, vision, cardiac), and likelihood of recurrence in future offspring.

Finally, the success of EHDI programs depends on families working in partnership with professionals as a well-coordinated team. The roles and responsibilities of each team member should be well defined and clearly understood.

ESTABLISHING THE ETIOLOGY OF HEARING LOSS

As with all disorders, early detection enables early intervention and improves prognosis. In the case of hearing loss, early detection can influence the type of educational programming for the child and the need for family counseling. After a hearing loss is confirmed, at the same time as early intervention is begun, consideration should be given to identify the etiology of the hearing loss.

As greater numbers of children with hearing loss are identified early through newborn hearing screening, more evidence regarding the distribution of different etiologies may provide additional insights. However, long-standing data on profound hearing loss in infancy indicates that 50% of congenital hearing loss is thought to be due to environmental factors and 50% is hereditary (Fig. 23.1) (Gorlin et al., 1995; Morton, 1999). Hearing loss is a feature in over 600 syndromes (usually named after an individual or individuals [e.g., Waardenburg syndrome, Down syndrome] or the prominent features of the condition [e.g., brachio-oto-renal syndrome]) where the affected individual has other characteristics *in addition* to hearing loss (Nance, 2003). Conversely, nonsyndromic hearing loss is named according to the following scheme (DFN = deafness):

- DFNA: autosomal dominant disorders
- DFNB: autosomal recessive disorders
- DFN: X-linked disorders

A genetic trait determined by its own pair of genes can be inherited in one of these three modes. It is the trait itself (and not the gene) that is dominant, recessive, or X-linked. However, for simplification, genes are often referred to as "dominant," "recessive," or "X-linked." A dominant trait is expressed when *one* copy of the gene pair codes for the trait. In autosomal recessive genetic disorders, a person inherits two copies of an autosomal gene with a change (mutation) in *both* copies. In X-linked inheritance, genes are located on the X chromosome and can be "recessive" or "dominant." Over 120 genes associated with hearing loss have been identified, and this number grows annually (Nance, 2003). In addition, remarkably, a single gene called *GBJ2* that codes for a protein named connexin 26 gives rise to more than half of the genetic cases of hearing loss in the United States (Genetic Evaluation of Congenital Hearing Loss Expert Panel, 2002). As the widespread use of newly developed vaccines decreases the prevalence of etiologies such as measles, mumps, rubella, and childhood meningitis, the percentage of early-onset hearing loss attributable to genetic etiologies should increase. For these reasons and because family planning for subsequent children may be under consideration by the family, the multidisciplinary team, whether formally developed or informally constituted by the primary care physician in the medical home, should depend on the geneticist to establish the etiologic basis for hearing loss.

■ AGE-APPROPRIATE ASSESSMENT

The use of age-appropriate techniques in diagnostic audiology is vital in the evaluation of infants and young children. It requires clinicians to select differential diagnostic techniques that are within the child's developmental capabilities. Because children undergo rapid sensory, motor, and cognitive development and because some children will present with multiple developmental problems, it is vital that assessment tools are appropriate for the neurodevelopmental status of the young child. Factors (physical and cognitive)

that can influence developmental status must be considered prior to the selection of an assessment strategy. Some problems may be relatively easy to identify (e.g., cerebral palsy). Others (e.g., learning disabilities, Asperger syndrome, or others on the autism spectrum) are more difficult to identify. Of course, knowledge of the handicapping conditions will enable the audiologist to plan effective diagnostic strategies. The audiologist must investigate the factors involved in each individual by use of interviews, case histories, assessments by other professionals, and close observation. Provision of appropriate services depends on a thorough knowledge of the individual to be served and his or her family background.

■ COMPREHENSIVE AUDIOLOGIC ASSESSMENT

The goal of the initial diagnostic assessment of infants and young children is to confirm or rule out hearing loss, to quantify the magnitude and configuration of hearing loss, and to assess the integrity of the auditory system. Additionally, comprehensive assessment should be provided for each ear even if only one ear was in question from the newborn hearing screening.

A *comprehensive audiologic assessment* must be viewed as a "process" and not an isolated clinical visit. Serial evaluations may be necessary to develop reliable profiles of hearing status and developmental abilities. It is not uncommon for an audiologist to formulate a working diagnosis of the child's audiologic status in parallel with developing initial management options. Thus, ongoing assessment is an integral part of the management process. After the initial audiologic assessment is completed, frequent follow-up visits are essential in order to monitor infants' overall auditory status, their development of auditory skills, and their functional use of hearing. Moreover, it must be recognized that single-point assessment does not adequately address the issue of fluctuating and/or progressive hearing loss.

The Test Battery Approach

The initial audiologic test battery to confirm hearing loss must include physiologic measures and, when developmentally appropriate, behavioral methods. The use of any test alone for assessing children's hearing sensitivity is discouraged. The desirability of using multiple tests in clinical practice is based on the complex nature of the auditory mechanism and the fact that auditory dysfunction may result from pathology at one or more levels of the auditory system. In test battery selection, the audiologist should use test procedures that are outcome based and cost effective, and greater weight should be given to the results of those tests for which validity and reliability are highest. If test results are not in agreement, the reason for the discrepancy must be explored before arriving at an audiologic diagnosis.

Jerger and Hayes (1976) promoted the concept of a test battery approach so that a single test is not interpreted in solation but, instead, various tests act as cross-checks of the inal outcome. Hanley (1986) noted that cross-checks not only establish what the auditory disorder is, but also clearly establish what the auditory disorder is not. Thus, audiologists benefit by having a battery of tests appropriate for the diagnosis of hearing loss in infants and young children. As pointed out by Turner (2003), the purpose of multiple tests is to increase the accuracy of audiologic diagnosis. This is accomplished when appropriate diagnostic tests are selected for the *individual's* "test battery." Subsequently, tests must be carefully administered and data appropriately interpreted, followed by a clinical decision based on the entire test battery. After weighing the agreement/disagreement between tests, the audiologist can reach a confident diagnosis. Clinical decision involves not only test selection, but also determining the number of tests administered during a single session, interpreting individual test data, and then drawing conclusions based on the performance of the entire test battery.

PEDIATRIC AUDIOLOGIC ASSESSMENT PROCEDURES

Audiologic assessment of infants and young children includes a thorough case history, otoscopic inspection, and both physiologic and behavioral measures. As stated earlier, the need for a battery of tests in pediatric assessment is essential in order to optimally plan for and meet the diverse needs of the pediatric population (e.g., age, physical status, developmental level, neuromaturational level).

Case History

The case history is a component of the audiologic assessment that guides the audiologist in constructing an initial "developmental profile" based on the child's physical, developmental, and behavioral performance. It also can serve as the first cross-check on the audiologic test outcome.

Some background health-related and developmental information (American Speech-Language-Hearing Association [ASHA], 2004) can be obtained prior to the initial evaluation (by telephone and/or mail). However, the majority of information is generally obtained at the time of the evaluation in a face-to-face interaction with the child and family. Face-to-face interaction provides the opportunity for posing questions based on observations, initial impressions, and interactions with the child. Moreover, this is an excellent time to establish rapport with the child and parent(s)/caregivers. The outcome of the case history is particularly important because it will often guide the strategy for the audiologic assessment and for making subsequent recommendations and referrals.

Otoscopic Inspection

Otoscopy is intended as a general inspection of the external ear and tympanic membrane for obvious signs of disease,

malformations, or blockage from atresia, stenosis, foreign bodies, cerumen, or other debris. Moreover, because several audiologic assessment procedures require the insertion of a probe into the external auditory canal, the visual inspection serves to verify that there is no contraindication to placing a probe in the ear canal.

AUDIOLOGIC TEST BATTERY: BIRTH TO 6 MONTHS OF AGE

Ear-specific assessment is the goal for both behavioral and physiologic procedures because a unilateral hearing loss, even in the presence of one normal-hearing ear, may place a child at significant developmental and/or educational risk (Bess, 1982; Bess et al., 1988; 1998; Bovo et al., 1988; Oyler et al., 1988). Therefore, determining hearing sensitivity for each ear facilitates medical/surgical diagnosis and treatment, selecting and fitting amplification when appropriate, establishing baseline function, and monitoring auditory status when progressive, fluctuating, or late-onset hearing loss is suspected.

To be developmentally appropriate, the audiologic test battery for young infants, birth through 6 months, consists primarily of physiologic measures. These measures currently include the auditory brainstem response (ABR) as the gold standard, the auditory steady-state response (ASSR) to supplement/augment ABR findings, distortion product or transient-evoked otoacoustic emissions, and acoustic immittance. (For a more complete discussion of these procedures, see Chapters 14 and 15.)

Measurement of auditory evoked potentials, especially the ABR, can provide accurate estimates of threshold sensitivity in young infants. To maximize reliable electrophysiologic measurements in infants, an adequate signal-to-noise ratio (S/N) must be maintained, and an extended recording window must be used to identify threshold responses. The number of signals averaged may vary according to the amount of background noise, the response amplitude, and the presence of hearing loss. In addition, for stimulus conditions close to threshold and for frequency-specific stimuli, especially low-frequency stimuli, a 20- to 25-ms recording window is essential.

The ABR protocol with infants should include frequency-specific stimuli using insert earphones, unless contraindicated, for air-conduction testing. For these measurements, short-duration, rapid-onset tone bursts are used. Knowledge of the spectra of these stimuli is needed because they are affected by various stimulus parameters. When air-conduction thresholds obtained by ABR are found to be abnormal, estimates of bone-conduction sensitivity should be completed as well. Bone-conduction ABR is important for quantifying the degree of the conductive component when hearing loss is present. It is important when doing bone-conduction ABRs that attention is paid to ensure adequate pressure of the bone vibrator on the mastoid (Yang and Stewart, 1990). Additionally, because of stimulus artifact concerns, care must be taken to separate the bone vibrator from the electrode due to electromagnetic leakage.

At a minimum, responses to low- and high-frequency stimuli should be obtained for each ear to estimate audiometric configuration. High-frequency assessment should use 2,000-Hz tone bursts (The Pediatric Working Group, 1996), and the low-frequency assessment should use 250- or 500-Hz tone bursts (Stapells et al., 1995; Stapells and Oates, 1997). These data not only strengthen behavioral estimates of hearing loss, but they also facilitate the selection and fitting of amplification (hearing aids and frequency modulation [FM] systems). Hearing aid fitting protocols for use with infants that are based on frequency-specific information are now available (American Academy of Audiology, 2003; The Pediatric Working Group, 1996; Seewald et al., 1997; Stelmachowicz, 2000).

Although the use of click stimuli alone is not sufficient for the estimation of audiometric configuration, a click stimulus can provide useful information regarding neural integrity. Assessment of interwave latencies, ear asymmetries, and morphology relative to age-appropriate norms may be completed as part of the ABR assessment and used along with other clinical and/or medical findings.

If there are risk indicators for neural hearing loss (auditory neuropathy/auditory dyssynchrony [AN/AD]) such as hyperbilirubinemia or anoxia (although some AN/AD patients have no risk factors and are found in the well-baby nursery [e.g., nonsyndromic recessive AN/AD such as that related to otoferlin-based AN/AD]), then audiologic assessment should include click-evoked ABR. When recording a high-level (80 to 90 dB normal hearing level [nHL]) click ABR, responses should be measured separately for condensation and rarefaction single-polarity stimuli, and responses should be displayed in such a way as to identify the cochlear microphonic (CM) (i.e., superimposing averages to identify out-of-phase components). In these instances, precautions must be taken to distinguish the CM from a stimulus artifact.

Many children in this age group can be tested during natural sleep, without sedation, using sleep deprivation with nap and feeding times coordinated around the test session. However, active or older infants may require sedation to allow adequate time for acquisition of high-quality recordings and sufficient frequency-specific information.

The ASSR is a synchronized brain response to modulated tones with emerging clinical applications. The ASSR uses a continuous frequency-specific stimulus that is modulated (i.e., frequency and/or amplitude modulated) and presented at a given frequency. The recorded response is generated in the electroencephalogram (EEG) response rather than specifically in the auditory brainstem pathway, as is the case with the ABR. Whereas the ABR response is determined through the identification of peaks and troughs in the time domain, the presence or absence of the ASSR is determined through statistical algorithms in the frequency domain. Clearly, the ASSR holds promise as a method of estimating frequency-specific hearing sensitivity in individuals; however, more data are needed regarding the predictive accuracy of the ASSR as a function of age, stimulus type, recording time, and the magnitude of hearing loss. Because of its recent development, the ASSR does not have the evidence-based underpinnings with diverse clinical populations to recommend it as the *sole* measure of auditory status in the infant and young child populations. For example, issues related to threshold estimation within the first three months of life have been reported (John, et al., (2004) and some concerns about recording artifact under certain stimulus conditions have been expressed (Small and Stapells, 2004; Gorga, et al., 2004). Research in this area is ongoing, and improvements/recommendations in methodology are expected.

Otoacoustic emissions (OAEs) expand the pediatric audiology test battery by providing a physiologic means of assessing preneural auditory function (Gorga et al., 1993; Kemp et al., 1990; Norton and Widen, 1990). That is, OAEs are most likely generated by the outer hair cells in the cochlea and serve as an indirect measure of these hair cells. OAEs are not, in and of themselves, necessary for hearing, nor are they a mechanism of hearing, but rather, they reflect the status of structures that are necessary for hearing.

Evoked OAEs occur in response to an external auditory stimulus and are present in nearly all normal-hearing individuals. Thus, the presence of OAEs is consistent with normal or near-normal hearing thresholds in a given frequency region. Moreover, measuring OAEs clinically permits the differentiation between sensory and neural components of the sensory-neural hearing loss (Lonsbury-Martin et al., 1993). Used in conjunction with ABR, OAEs are useful not only in the differential diagnosis of cochlear hearing loss but also in the identification of infants and young children with neurologic dysfunction.

Transient-evoked OAEs (TEOAEs) are elicited following a transient (click) stimulus at approximately 80 dB peak sound pressure level (SPL). Although the transient click stimulus is a broadband stimulus that is not frequency specific, the response is analyzed in the frequency domain, thus providing information across frequencies from 500 to 5,000 Hz, although test performance is best for mid to high frequencies. Distortion product OAEs (DPOAEs) are elicited following stimulation with two tones. DPOAEs are measured in response to two tones (primaries) that interact to produce nonlinear distortions in the cochlea. The two tones typically are selected so that the frequency ratio between the tones (f2/f1) is 1.22, which is known to produce the largest distortion product at most test frequencies in humans.

Response criteria typically include S/N and/or have a response reproducibility of greater than an established percentage at defined frequencies (see Chapter 21 for further details). Schemes for trying to determine the degree of hearing loss and/or predicting thresholds using OAEs have been investigated (Martin et al., 1990; Boege and Janssen, 2002; Dorn et al., 2001; Gorga et al., 1996; 2002; 2003). Although some strategies have met with success, variability is such that threshold predictions should be viewed cautiously.

Because of their remarkable stability over time within the same ear, OAEs also are useful for monitoring the status of disease conditions that are progressive, including certain genetic disorders such as Usher syndrome (Meredith et al., 1992). In addition, over shorter time courses, OAEs are advantageous for monitoring the effects of treatments that are potentially damaging to the ear, like those involving such ototoxic antibiotics as tobramycin (Katbamna et al., 1999) or such antitumor agents as cisplatin (Ress et al., 1999).

Acoustic immittance measures are an integral part of the pediatric assessment battery. Clinical decisions should be made on a quantitative assessment of the tympanogram, including consideration of equivalent ear canal volume, peak compensated static acoustic admittance, tympanometric width or gradient, and tympanometric peak pressure (see Chapters 8 to 10 for a detailed description of the components of the acoustic immittance test battery).

Under the age of approximately 4 months, interpretation of tympanograms may be compromised when a conventional low-frequency (220- or 226-Hz) probe tone is used (Paradise et al., 1976; Purdy and Williams, 2000). As such, a higher probe-tone frequency (e.g., 1,000 Hz) is recommended for identifying middle ear disorders in infants less than 4 months of age, and normative data for 1,000-Hz tympanometry are now available for neonates and young infants (Margolis et al., 2003). Once a child reaches the age of 7 months, a low-frequency (226-Hz) probe tone is appropriate. Between 5 and 7 months of age, however, there is still a possibility of false-negative tympanograms in ears with middle ear effusion. Therefore, use of a 1,000-Hz probe tone for tympanometry in this subset of infants is recommended when attempting to identify middle ear effusion.

When a quantitative assessment of a tympanogram is used, care must be taken to ensure that there is correspondence between the graphic representation of the tympanogram and the absolute quantities indicated. With the pediatric population, sometimes there are irregularities in the tympanogram shape (due to movement artifact, crying, or vocalizing) that may be mistaken for a tympanogram peak by the instrument and may provide misleading absolute values.

In addition to providing confirmation of middle ear status, acoustic reflex measurement is useful in the interpretation of other components in the audiologic test battery. That is, the acoustic reflex may provide supplemental information relevant to the functional status of the middle ear, cochlea, and brainstem pathway (see Chapters 10 and 22). For example, acoustic reflexes are absent when AN/AD exists (Starr et al., 1996). Although there are insufficient data for routine use of acoustic reflex measurements in the initial diagnostic assessment under the age of 4 months, the acoustic reflex should be used to supplement the test battery at older ages. Together, these measures are fundamental components of the pediatric audiology test battery.

AUDIOLOGIC TEST BATTERY: INFANTS 6 MONTHS OF AGE AND OLDER

For newborns and young infants (<6 months), a physiologic measure is the approach of choice when attempting to define an individual's auditory sensitivity. However, as valuable as physiologic procedures are in the early confirmation of hearing loss, the audiologist inevitably returns to behavioral testing to substantiate test results and monitor a child's hearing longitudinally. Therefore, assessing auditory sensitivity in older infants and children (>6 months) can be completed efficiently and effectively with both behavioral and physiologic measures.

The audiologic test battery for infants age 6 months of age and older includes conditioned behavioral audiometry (either visual reinforcement audiometry [VRA] or conditioned play audiometry [CPA]), OAEs, acoustic immittance, and speech detection and/or recognition measures. ABR should be performed, as necessary, when behavioral measures are not sufficiently reliable to provide ear-specific estimates of type, degree, and configuration of hearing loss or when additional physiologic data are necessary to support other clinical questions (e.g., neurologic status). Moreover, the desire for behavioral hearing test results should not delay the selection and fitting of amplification when valid and reliable frequency-specific threshold information is available by physiologic measurement.

Behavioral Observation Audiometry

It is now known that unconditioned behavioral observation techniques with infants and young children are confounded by poor test-retest reliability and high inter- and intrasubject variability (Weber, 1969; Thompson and Weber, 1974). This places limitations on the use of behavioral observation audiometry (BOA) for determining auditory sensitivity. Therefore, BOA is no longer recommended for assessing frequency-specific threshold sensitivity in newborns, young infants (<5 months), or those children whose developmental disabilities preclude them from learning operant conditioning procedures. However, another goal in pediatric assessment is to examine auditory *function*. Although ABR can quantify auditory sensitivity in infants with compromised cognitive function, BOA can provide useful insight into the quality of the child's auditory responsiveness. Moreover, BOA can provide an estimate of functional capabilities useful in planning intervention for these children. That is, the audiologist can predict potential difficulties in auditory development and recommend aural habilitation strategies intended to improve the child's functional use of sound.

PROCEDURAL GUIDELINES

Infants under a developmental age of 5 months generally display a variety of reflexive and orienting responses to external stimuli. The accurate judgment of these behaviors, however, may require the use of multiple examiners. One examiner can present auditory stimuli, while one or more examiners monitor state changes and cues signal presentations when the child's listening state is appropriate. Multiple examiners also may be necessary to judge response behaviors in order to reduce two common errors of observation: (1) judging that a response occurred when, in reality, there was no response and (2) judging that no response occurred when, in reality, a response did occur.

Because so many behaviors are monitored (e.g., head or limb reflex, increased motion, decreased motion, whole-body startle, eye widening, nonnutritive sucking, searching, eye blink or flutter, localization, smiling, laughing, pointing), it is important to minimize false-positive responses of the observers. To minimize the examiner's expectations of the outcome of the test, the observer(s) should not be informed about the child's developmental status, previous test results, or medical status. Therefore, examiners should have minimal information about each patient before testing.

Response behaviors seen during BOA can be separated into those that are attentive-type, orienting behaviors (e.g., increased and decreased motion, eye widening, searching, localization, smiling, laughing, pointing) and those considered reflexive (e.g., head or limb reflex, whole-body startle, sucking, eye blink or flutter). Analyzing response behaviors may provide useful information in determining how youngsters attach meaning to sound. If response behavior is reflexive from a child known to have near-normal hearing, it may indicate a child who does not attach much functional meaning to sound. On the other hand, children who show orienting responses to sound are likely demonstrating a higher level of cortical functioning.

Operant Conditioning

It is possible to approach the assessment of infants and young children behaviorally through operant conditioning paradigms, specifically through an operant discrimination procedure. In an operant discrimination procedure, a stimulus is used to cue the child that a response results in reinforcement. That is, the stimulus serves as a cue to perform a specified behavior (i.e., a behavioral response). In turn, operant behavior (the response) is increased by the application of positive reinforcement. Reinforcement is used to strengthen an easily monitored single response and keep the child in an aroused and motivated state. If the reinforcement is sufficiently powerful, the response will be continued over repeated presentations of the stimulus. As demonstrated by Moore et al. (1975; 1977), audiometric signals (e.g., pure-tones or warble tones) have limited reinforcing properties. Consequently, a positive reinforcement having high interest value (appealing to the infant) must be used to reinforce the response behavior.

Maintaining motivation and a high response probability through the use of age-appropriate reinforcement allows

audiologists to investigate, over time, an infant's or young child's auditory response behavior. This allows more precise estimation of ability (i.e., hearing sensitivity) and reduces the habituation found in behavioral assessment without reinforcement (i.e., BOA).

Conditioned behavioral audiometry is an efficient and cost-effective approach for clinical use. However, this requires knowledge of potential pitfalls, as well as use of procedural modifications/enhancements that increase reliability and validity (Diefendorf and Gravel, 1996; Renshaw and Diefendorf, 1998). For example, potential pitfalls include the overactive child, controlling and minimizing false responses, and the timeliness and proper use of reinforcement. As such, conditioned behavioral audiometry requires knowledge of operant conditioning, the proper use of distraction, the proper use of reinforcement, and the importance of developmental age on successful outcomes. Beyond the time, cost, and ease of administration, the most important advantage of behavioral tests is that they allow infants and young children to demonstrate actively what they perceive. In turn, this fosters a valid description of their functional hearing abilities.

Visual Reinforcement Audiometry

Normally developing infants make head turns toward a sound source in the first few months of life. This neuromotor response undergirds the behavioral approach audiologists use to investigate auditory behavior. Indeed, by the time an infant has reached a chronologic/developmental age of 5 to 6 months, operant conditioning coupled with this behavioral response enables audiologists to implement VRA.

The success of VRA is related to the fact that the response (a head turn; Fig. 23.2) and reinforcer (three-dimensional visual animation that is seen when the head is turned toward it) are well suited to the developmental level of children

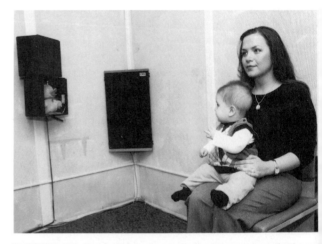

FIGURE 23.2   A "head turn" response coupled with visual reinforcement (a three-dimensional, mechanical toy housed in a smoked Plexiglas enclosure).

between 6 months and 2 1/2 years of age. Once the child is under stimulus control, he or she will continue to respond at low sensation levels long enough to provide an accurate estimate of threshold.

In VRA, conditioned head turns are reinforced by an attractive three-dimensional animated toy that is activated near the source of the sound that is presented. Visual stimuli containing movement, color, and contour appear to be more effective reinforcement than less complex visual stimuli. Complex visual reinforcement, such as three-dimensional animated toys, is critical for maintaining response behaviors over repeated trials (Moore et al., 1975). The visual reinforcement is frequently housed in a smoked Plexiglas enclosure. Activation of the visual reinforcement results in lighting the enclosure and animation of the toy (Fig. 23.2).

The success of VRA also is related to the developmental status of the child being examined. Developmental issues that must be recognized include the impact of corrected age (corrected age is determined by subtracting the estimated weeks of prematurity from the infant's chronologic age) on VRA performance and the impact of mental age on VRA performance. Moore et al. (1992) concluded that VRA performance is related to corrected age. They studied 60 premature infants (36 weeks of gestation or less) at corrected ages of 4 to 9 months. Their results imply that premature infants with a corrected age of 8 or 9 months are likely to perform acceptably in response to VRA (can be conditioned and respond with high success before habituation to task); that premature infants with a corrected age of 6 or 7 months may perform but with less success (can be conditioned but have limited responses before habituation to the task); and that premature infants with a corrected age of 4 or 5 months are not likely to respond to the VRA procedure. A comparison of these data to results of previous studies on full-term infants demonstrates that although full-term infants are likely to respond with high clinical success to VRA by a chronologic age of 6 months (Moore et al., 1977), premature infants are not likely to respond to VRA with good clinical success until approximately a corrected age of 8 months.

Widen (1990) evaluated VRA as a function of developmental age in premature, high-risk babies. Clearly, the developmentally mature babies were more often tested successfully (the ability to be conditioned and provide threshold for at least one stimulus). The data from Moore et al. (1992) and Widen (1990) are highly consistent; that is, both reports indicate that VRA success with premature infants is related to corrected age and that VRA success with these infants is greater as they approach 8 to 9 months of corrected age.

Why is it that premature infants, even after prematurity is corrected for, lag several months behind normally developing, full-term infants? Premature infants have been shown to display significantly poorer performance on standardized measures of mental ability (Bayley Scales of Infant Development [BSIDs]) when compared to full-term infants of the same postpartum age (Rubin et al., 1973; Goldstein et al., 1976). Moreover, Kopp (1974) concluded that the quality and quantity of cognitive exploration, which preterm infants engage in less when compared with full-term infants, also may account for reduced motor development.

Several studies have reported on the use of VRA in children with Down syndrome and other developmental disabilities. Greenberg et al. (1978) reported on the use of VRA in 46 individuals with Down syndrome between the ages of 6 months and 6 years. As would be expected, the proportion of successful tests increased as age increased. Because it is expected that chronologic age would be a very poor predictor of success with the VRA procedure in these children, the BSIDs (Bayley, 1969) were used to provide an estimate of developmental level. If children with Down syndrome are considered on the basis of their developmental age, in contrast to chronologic age, it would be logical to assume that results might be similar to those found with normally developing infants. However, whereas Wilson et al. (1976) found that normally developing infants 6 months of age and older accomplished the VRA procedure with a high rate of success, Greenberg et al. (1978) found that individuals with Down syndrome did not achieve a high rate until 10 to 12 months BSID mental age equivalent. These investigators further pointed out that when one is predicting potential success with the VRA procedure for children with Down syndrome, the BSID mental age equivalent score provides the most distinct distribution between successful and unsuccessful tests, with the dividing point being a BSID mental age equivalent of at least 10 months. Similarly, Wilson et al. (1983) reported that 80% of the children with Down syndrome, in their study, were testable by 12 months of age using VRA.

For the child with special needs, Thompson et al. (1979) indicated that VRA was an effective test procedure for 88% of the low-functioning children in their study, if all children under a developmental age of 9 months were excluded. One challenge facing the audiologist using VRA for the child with special needs is that the child may often be older than ideal for this type of operant procedure. Gravel and Traquina (1992) noted that younger infants (6 to 18 months) were easier to assess than older toddlers (18 to 24 months), and children ages 21 to 24 months were less tolerant of earphones, more distractible, and less interested in the reinforcers.

In summary, when VRA is considered in clinical protocols (Fig. 23.3), audiologists must consider: (1) corrected age adjusted for prematurity rather than chronologic age or (2) mental age/developmental age when disparities exist between corrected age and the child's developmental status. Of the two predictors of VRA performance (corrected age and mental age), corrected age may be the more practical one to use in most cases because it can be obtained from parental report, case history information, and/or hospital records and does not require tests necessary to determine mental age.

TEST ROOM ARRANGEMENT

Figure 23.4 presents the room arrangement most commonly used for VRA. The audiologist in the control room has full

**Age Considerations
For Optimizing Success in VRA**

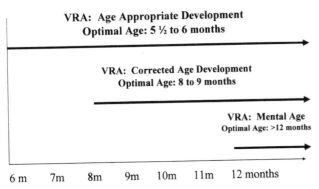

FIGURE 23.3 Age considerations for optimizing success in visual reinforcement audiometry (VRA).

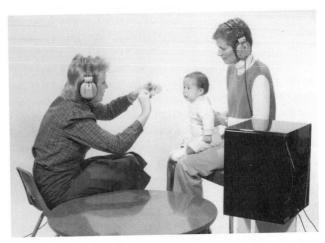

FIGURE 23.5 A second examiner maintaining the interest of an infant in a midline position.

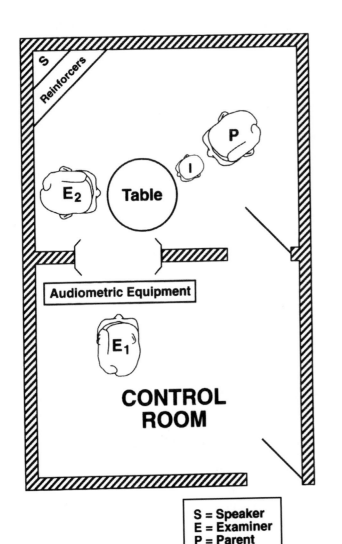

FIGURE 23.4 Test room arrangement commonly used in visual reinforcement audiometry (VRA).

view of the testing situation. The ability to selectively darken only the audiologist's side of the test booth can be helpful. The infant, parent, and a second examiner are located within the test suite. The second examiner, seated at the infant's side, maintains the infant's head in a midline position by quietly encouraging the child to observe passively or to play with colorful, nonnoisy toys (Fig. 23.5). An appealing toy is manipulated by the examiner in front of the infant as a distractor. The examiner's role is to maintain the infant's attention at midline and return the infant to this position once a response is made and reinforcement is completed. The audiologist must be creative in keeping the child alert and in a listening posture without the child becoming so focused on the activity. The toys used for this purpose should be appealing but not so attractive as to overly occupy the infant's attention. The closer the audiologist is to the child, the more easily the child is engaged in the activity. If the infant under test shows too much interest in the colorful, nonnoisy toys, then the potential exists for no response during a signal trial or for elevated response levels due to decreased attention. Conversely, if the examiner and toys are not sufficiently interesting, the likelihood of false alarms (random looking toward the visual reinforcer) will be high.

Often a touch of the hand on a child's shoe or leg will quietly redirect the child to a midline position. Actually sitting on the floor in front of the child allows for a totally unobstructed view of the child for the control room audiologist and being located slightly below the level of the child is a nonthreatening position. Obviously, it is difficult to balance entertaining the child without totally consuming the child's attention.

A single examiner in the control room can use a mechanical "centering toy" positioned at midline in the test room for maintaining a child's midline distraction. While the use of a "centering toy" is an alternative to the more traditional approach of using two examiners, this approach distances the single examiner (in the control room) from the infant (in the exam room). Although a single examiner may be more cost effective and clinically practical in busy settings, it also reduces the flexibility of maintaining the infant at midline with a second examiner and multiple distraction toys. That is, the centering toy is always the same toy, is somewhat noisy, and may be too much distraction for some infants. Additionally, the centering toy may compete with the actual visual reinforcers because they are so much alike. The fact that the centering toy is not housed in a dark Plexiglas box raises the concern that the constant viewing of the animated toy may result in less interest with the visual reinforcers. When only one examiner is used for assessment, the use of computer-assisted test procedures can overcome some of the disadvantages described above. That is, a microcomputer interfaced with a clinical audiometer can be controlled from the test room, allowing the examiner to maintain a closer position to the infant in the exam room.

Depending on the child's acceptance and responses, insert earphones or headphones can be used, rather than the sound field speakers, to obtain ear-specific information during VRA testing. The preferable transducers are insert earphones. Inserts are useful for a number of reasons, including their comfort and light weight, their increased interaural attenuation compared to conventional earphones, and the reduced risk of ear canal collapse.

CONDITIONING IN VISUAL REINFORCEMENT AUDIOMETRY

In clinical assessment, the first phase of VRA is the conditioning process. Response shaping is critical to the success of the operant procedure. Two different approaches that can be attempted in the first phase are (1) pairing a supra-threshold auditory stimulus with the visual reinforcer or (2) presenting a supra-threshold auditory stimulus and observing a spontaneous response from the infant, followed by activation of the reinforcer. Evidence suggests that different signals (e.g., tones, filtered noise, speech) are equally effective during the conditioning phase (Thompson and Folsom, 1984; Primus and Thompson, 1985). Successful completion of the training phase is the achievement of a pre-established criterion of consecutive head turn responses. If the criterion is not reached (usually two or three responses following two or three conditioning trials), phase 1 retraining is necessary until the criterion is met. The number of training trials needed before phase 2 trials begin varies, but the training phase is usually brief.

A key to response shaping is the presentation of a supra-threshold stimulus. For most infants, supra-threshold will be 30, 50, or 70 dB. However, some children, particularly those children with moderately severe to severe hearing loss, may require 90 dB or higher to qualify as a supra-threshold stimulus. Because hearing status is unknown, supra-threshold estimates also are unknown. Therefore, the possibility exists that the stimulus selected to shape the response behavior might be inaudible. Given that most infants can be expected

to have normal hearing, the most efficient test is one that uses a low starting level, approximately 30 dB. However, failure to condition rapidly should alert the audiologist to a potential equipment/calibration problem or a child who requires a greater starting intensity for conditioning. Attention to either issue must be immediate for a successful outcome.

A further clinical variation of this basic procedure is used for situations when the infant's head turn is not being shaped by the auditory stimulus at high-intensity levels. A bone oscillator is placed on the infant's mastoid on the side of the reinforcer. If necessary, the bone oscillator can be removed from the headband and held in the child's hand or rested against the child's arm to use as a vibrotactile stimulus. The traditional conditioning procedure is initiated, that is, pairing the stimulus with the reinforcement. The stimulus usually selected for bone-conducted conditioning is a 250-Hz narrowband noise presented at 60 dB hearing level (HL). An infant with severe or profound hearing loss with no other developmental disabilities will show appropriate behavioral responses as long as the stimulus is salient (can be felt, even if not heard). Responses are obtained in this manner; subsequently, earphone or insert phone presentations follow with starting intensity levels dependent on the bone-conduction responses. If the youngster under test fails to display conditioned responding, other issues such as compromised physical status, developmental delay, or immaturity are raised. For example, Condon (1991) noted several cognitive attainments that are necessary for a child to be assessed reliably using VRA. The child must be developing object permanence (i.e., knowing that objects exist in space and time, even when the child can no longer see them or act on them) and the ability to anticipate the reappearance of at least partially hidden objects, discover simple causality (i.e., an event or behavior is dependent on the other for its occurrence) and means-end relationships (i.e., behaviors that result in anticipated outcomes), and use simple schemes to explore toys.

Successful completion of training occurs when the infant is making appropriate responses and random head turning is at a minimum. Subsequently, the test phase of VRA begins. Signal intensity is attenuated after every "yes" response or increased after every "no" response. Using a conventional staircase (up-down) procedure, signal intensity is raised and lowered by 10 dB. Testing is continued until a stopping criterion (ascending and descending until four reversals points have been achieved; refer to Fig. 23.6) is met. Threshold (minimum response level) is then defined as the mean of the reversal points.

PROCEDURAL GUIDELINES

The key to implementing valid and reliable behavioral techniques is to use procedures supported by clinical research. That is, many aspects of VRA have been reported in the literature that, taken together, provide the guidelines for clinical approaches.

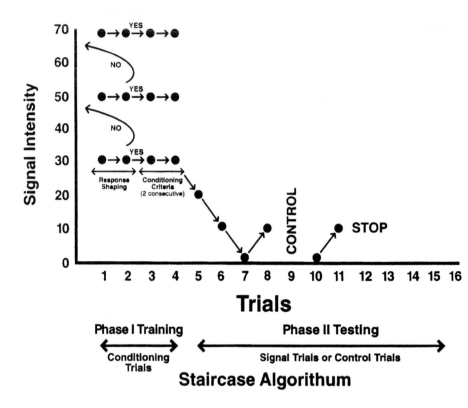

FIGURE 23.6 Algorithm commonly used in visual reinforcement audiometry (VRA).

The recommended trial duration (incorporating the signal and response interval) is approximately 4 seconds (Primus, 1992). That is, the signal duration is approximately 4 seconds, and this 4-second interval also defines the period of time during which a response is judged to be present or not. Responses outside of the 4-second period are not interpreted as valid responses.

Visual reinforcement is provided only for correct responses that occur during signal trials. It is sometimes helpful to use the light initially, eventually adding the light plus animation. The novelty of the task may be preserved longer by introducing the more complex reinforcement as the testing progresses. Moreover, by starting with the light only, the audiologist can gauge any potential for a fearful response to the reinforcement. The novelty of VRA also may be strengthened with older children by using moving images generated by a digital video disc (DVD) player/monitor. Schmida et al. (2003) used digital video with 19- to 24-month-old children. Their results demonstrated a greater number of head turn responses before habituation when viewing video reinforcement than when viewing conventional animated toy reinforcement. These results support the hypothesis that the complex and dynamic nature of the video reinforcement would be more effective in achieving a greater number of responses than the conventional toy reinforcer prior to habituation in the 2-year-old age group.

In general, a 100% reinforcement schedule (reinforcement for every correct response) results in more rapid conditioning, yet more rapid habituation. Conversely, an intermittent reinforcement schedule produces slower conditioning but also a slower rate of habituation. Consequently, most clinicians recommend a protocol that begins with a 100% reinforcement schedule and then gradually shifts to an intermittent reinforcement schedule.

Primus and Thompson (1985) compared a 100% reinforcement schedule to an intermittent reinforcement schedule with 2-year-old children. The two reinforcement schedules resulted in no differences in the infants' rate of habituation or the number of infant responses to stimulus trials. These findings provide an excellent guideline for delivering reinforcement. Since Primus and Thompson's data suggest that withholding reinforcement should not affect the amount of response behavior, reinforcement should not be provided if the audiologist is at all uncertain about the validity of an infant's head turn response (Diefendorf and Gravel, 1996). The risk of reinforcing a random head turn is that it may lead to confusion for a child during the test session and increase the child's rate of false responding. Failure to reinforce a correct head turn, however, does not degrade performance. In this situation, withholding reinforcement for a correct but ambiguous response is viewed as intermittent reinforcement, which will not interfere with subsequent infant behavior.

Reinforcement duration also is a factor influencing response outcome from children around the age of 2 years (Culpepper and Thompson, 1994). Decreasing the duration of a child's exposure to the visual reinforcer (e.g., 4 seconds to 0.5 second) results in an increase in response behavior and a decrease in habituation. Audiologists may increase the amount of audiometric information obtained from children by decreasing their exposure to the visual reinforcer. For the child with special needs who may have a slower response, the visual reinforcer should be activated for a sufficient length of time for the child to very briefly observe it, but prolonged visual reinforcement should be avoided.

Ensuring valid VRA outcomes depends on separating true responses from false responses (false positives) during threshold acquisition. Based on normal response behavior from adults, the assumption is made that infants also produce a number of incorrect responses during the testing phase of VRA.

Throughout testing, two types of trials are presented: signal trials that contain a stimulus and control trials that do not. Reinforcement is provided only for correct responses during signal trials. False-positive responses are monitored by inserting control trials in the staircase algorithm (see Fig. 23.6). A response observed during a control trial (and never reinforced) is evidence of false responding. Thus, it is possible to systematically estimate errors or chance responding (false responses during signal trials) by calculating the number of responses during control trials. Moore (1995) recommended that one out of four presentations should be a control trial and that test results are questionable if the false-positive rate exceeds 25%. Eilers et al. (1991a) suggest that a false alarm rate of 30% to 40% is acceptable and adopting such a rate as acceptable does not compromise the accuracy of thresholds for clinical assessment. Clearly, high false alarm rates (>50%) require the audiologist to further consider that test results may be inaccurate.

Excessive false responses suggest that the infant is not under stimulus control. As such, audiologists should focus on two factors to rectify clinical outcomes: (1) reinstituting phase 1 shaping and conditioning, and (2) increasing the entertainment level of the activity to engage the child's interest at a midline position before starting a test trial. When in the test room, an examiner must be able to choose from a variety of toys available and judge when a toy change in either direction (enhanced novelty and thus more entertaining, or simpler/less novel and thus less entertaining) is necessary to maintain the child's midline focus and optimum response state. Occasionally, overactive parents can bias their children to respond, thereby resulting in excessive false responses. Therefore, parents may need to wear headphones through which "masking" music or noise is delivered.

Threshold determination in audiometry is based on the lowest intensity level where responses are obtained approximately 50% of the time. In VRA, as the staircase algorithm proceeds, how many reversals should be required before identifying the hearing threshold? Too few may sacrifice response accuracy. However, too many will increase test time, in turn reducing the number of stimulus presentations that could be spent obtaining thresholds to other stimuli. Testing of one stimulus may be stopped once the infant has exhibited between three and four response reversals (Eilers et al., 1991a; 1991b). Eilers and her colleagues found that using

six rather than three response reversals before discontinuing the threshold search had minimal effect on threshold. Yet tests with a three-reversal stopping rule were significantly shorter than those with six reversals. As stopping rules are increased from three to six, there is about a 50% increase in the number of test trials, with no improvement in response accuracy. These results suggest that, by using relatively few reversals to estimate threshold, a staircase algorithm may be shortened to increase efficiency without sacrificing accuracy. Thus, there is no need to continue testing beyond three or four reversals since the results obtained are not substantially better because of it.

Audiologists must proceed as if the next piece of information from the youngster under test will be their last. This strategy dictates air versus bone conduction, another frequency versus speech, or switching ears. If the second ear is tested and the child turns in the wrong direction, the reinforcer display is activated regardless. The light and animation from the reinforcer will attract the child's attention back to the reinforcer. Obviously, two reinforcers, one on each side of a test room, alleviate this concern, and although desirable, they are not necessary for successful assessment outcomes.

Thresholds obtained with the VRA procedure for infants 6 to 12 months of age have been shown to be within 10 to 15 dB of those obtained from older children and adults (Gravel and Wallace, 1998; Nozza and Wilson, 1984). In addition, VRA thresholds are similar across the age span (6 to 24 months) and show good reliability when compared to thresholds obtained from the same child at older ages (Diefendorf, 1988).

CONDITIONED PLAY AUDIOMETRY

Operant conditioning of behavioral responses to sound continues to be an effective approach for older children. What changes as children age, however, are the response behavior and the reinforcement that is used. Like the operant head-turn procedure, play audiometry uses positive reinforcement to support response behavior. In CPA, children learn to engage in an activity (e.g., putting rings on a spindle, dropping or stacking blocks, putting together simple puzzles) each time they hear the test signal. These activities are assumed to be interesting to children, are within their motor capability, and represent a specific behavior that is used to denote a response to a stimulus.

For youngsters with limited gross motor/fine motor skills, a variety of responses (e.g., finger swing, hand motion, arm motion, eye motion, visual gaze) can be used to trigger an electronic switch, in turn activating a computer screen programmed for appropriate visual reinforcement. The goal is to select the most appropriate task and the most interesting reinforcement while at the same time recognizing the physical limitations that may compromise the child's success. If the physical demands are too great, then the task will detract from maintaining a listening posture. If the task is too simple, the child will have less motivation to participate and will tire of the task. The critical decision for the audiologist is to select a specific behavior that is used to denote a specific response to a stimulus.

CPA follows the traditional operant conditioning paradigm of stimulus → response → reinforcement, in which the play activity/motor activity is the response behavior and social praise/another reward is the reinforcement. Three challenges exist in play audiometry that require a skillful audiologist who is comfortable with children. First, the audiologist must select a response behavior that the child is capable of performing. The second challenge is teaching the child to wait, listen, and only respond with the motor behavior when the auditory signal is presented. The third challenge is that the audiologist also must be skilled in delivering social reinforcement that is natural and rewarding at the appropriate time and interval.

Separation of response behavior and reinforcement is essential in CPA. While the play activity is fun for the child, it is not the reinforcement. A separate reinforcement is essential to minimize habituation and maximize repeated response behavior. In addition to social praise, other forms of reinforcement have been suggested. Tokens that can be traded for small toys at the end of the test session, unsweetened cereal, and a changing computer display screen all have been used successfully with play audiometry.

Audiologic literature suggests that CPA is widely accepted among clinicians who practice pediatric audiology (Thompson et al., 1989). It is generally recognized that most 3-year-olds can be tested using play audiometry. Yet, how young can children be to still achieve successful audiologic outcomes? Thompson and Weber (1974) demonstrated that the rate of success in obtaining detailed information with CPA is limited for children under the age of 30 months. However, some 2-year-olds can be conditioned to play audiometry (Thompson et al., 1989). In addition, when 2-year-olds are proficient with CPA, there is a greater likelihood that they will provide more responses before habituation than they would if tested by VRA. Because overlap exists between VRA and CPA as suitable techniques with children in this age range, the successful evaluation of a younger child with CPA ultimately depends on the following: the audiologist's observational skills of the child's developmental/maturational level, the interpersonal skills established between the audiologist and child, and the experience/comfort level of the audiologist with young children.

Experience with CPA indicates that reliable threshold responses can be obtained when conditioning has been established and response criterion is maintained. Results from a clinical study (Diefendorf, 1981) of 40 preschoolers, aged 30 to 48 months, revealed thresholds at an audiometric level of 10 dB HL or better. These findings were in close agreement with other 4-year-old children (Gerwin and Glorig, 1974).

Striving to improve behavioral testing techniques is important because behavioral tests will continue to be the foundation of the audiologist's test battery. Moreover, behavioral tests provide the critical link between electrophysiologic measures and the child's daily use of audition.

OTHER AUDIOMETRIC PROCEDURES FOR CHILDREN

Because language and vocabulary are emerging in infants and young children, it may not be feasible to establish a traditional speech reception threshold (SRT). An alternative approach is the determination of a speech detection threshold (SDT).

The SRT and SDT represent different criteria (intelligibility vs. detectability). The SRT is recognized as the intensity at which an individual is able to identify simple speech materials approximately 50% of the time. The SDT may be defined as the level at which a listener may just detect the presence of an ongoing speech signal (e.g., bai-bai-bai presented with an overall duration of approximately 2 seconds). Naturally, for a given individual, the threshold values will not be the same. Speech can be detected at intensity levels lower than it can be understood. This difference is on the order of 8 to 12 dB.

Once the audiologist has determined that the child is successful with a play audiometry task, obtaining an SRT for each ear may be useful (see Chapter 5 for a more detailed discussion of speech audiometry). This testing can be accomplished with headphones or insert earphones, if tolerated, or through the sound field speakers.

The child who is ready for play audiometry typically has a communication strategy to express needs and wants at a more sophisticated level, whether with oral speech, signs, or a communication board. Family members often describe various communication skills that the child possesses, such as following commands, pointing to body parts or pictures in a storybook, or identifying colors. The audiologist is then able to expand the test battery to include an SRT rather than an SDT.

A spondee picture board can be very helpful in obtaining an SRT from the child with special needs who may be reluctant to respond in an unfamiliar test situation. If the child uses a communication board, then items from the communication board can be selected to use for the SRT. Identification of body parts also can be used to obtain an SRT.

Regardless of the test materials used, it is recommended that a preliminary step in determining an SRT for young children is first to familiarize the child with the test stimuli through both auditory and visual modalities and to eliminate those words that are not within the child's receptive vocabulary. The use of either picture or object pointing rather than a verbal response will require that the number of items be limited to 12 or less (Olsen and Matkin, 1979). Otherwise, the visual scanning task and the demands placed on memory and attention become contaminating variables. When obtaining an SRT, Northern and Downs (2002) suggest the use of a carrier phrase. They recommend a procedure in which the phrase "show me" is uttered and the hearing level is dropped quickly by 10 to 15 dB for the test word. These authors suggest that the utilization of the carrier phrase, such as "point to" or "show me," will often serve to focus the child's attention to the auditory task at hand. Finally, since a child's attention span is limited and test time can be a factor, it is often more expedient to work in 10-dB rather than 5-dB steps when establishing an SRT.

The bone-conducted SRT can be extremely useful in obtaining additional data from children, and although it is typically underused, it is readily available to audiologists. Once a hearing loss is identified or suspected, any information that can be obtained regarding the type of hearing loss (conductive or sensory-neural) is helpful in the management of the child. Some children with special needs will be much less consistent for tonal stimuli, thereby compromising traditional bone-conducted puretone testing. However, the bone oscillator will deliver clear speech stimuli without any need for additional correction or modification. Dolan and Morris (1990) confirmed that the functions relating the percentage of correctly identified W-1 spondees to stimulus level and the slope of these functions were comparable for TDH-39 headphones and KH80 and B-72 bone vibrators.

A bone-conducted SRT can offer valuable information in a very short period of time. Often the child will tolerate the bone oscillator during the more entertaining speech reception task but will not tolerate it for tonal testing. A frequently asked question regarding the use of the bone oscillator for speech reception testing relates to the potential for a false threshold that results in a vibratory response rather than a hearing response. It is true that the bone oscillator will vibrate for a speech stimulus, as well as low-frequency tonal stimuli, as the maximum output of the bone oscillator is approached. However, an important distinction must be made. A child will not be able to select the appropriate picture or item on the basis of a tactile sensation alone. If the child can complete the SRT, then a true hearing threshold by bone conduction has been obtained, and concerns regarding simply a vibratory response can be eliminated.

The value of the bone-conducted SRT becomes even greater with the introduction of masking. Many youngsters become confused when masking is introduced during puretone testing. With the bone-conducted SRT, it is relatively easy to introduce masking into the nontest ear without interruption of the SRT procedure. Confirmation of a bilateral conductive component to a hearing loss is possible for many children who will not cooperate for masked puretone testing. Similarly, a unilateral sensory-neural or conductive hearing loss can be confirmed.

The measurement of speech perception with the pediatric population must consider a number of variables that can confound test outcome. The selection of test materials within a child's receptive vocabulary competency, the designation of an appropriate response task, the utilization of reinforcement, and the reduction or alleviation of memory load are important factors that affect the reliability and validity of pediatric measurement.

Haskins (1949) developed phonetically balance (PB) lists composed of monosyllabic words selected from the spoken vocabulary of kindergartners (PBK). The PBK lists of 50 words each have been widely used in working with children. Yet the receptive vocabulary level of the particular child under audiologic study is often not ascertained before administering these materials. Consequently, the PBK-50 scores may be depressed in that they reflect vocabulary deficits as well as problems in speech perception. Clinicians must exercise caution in administering this test unless there is a relatively good assurance that the receptive vocabulary age of the child approaches at least that of a normal-hearing kindergartner. To bypass this problem, Ross and Lerman (1970) developed the Word Intelligibility by Picture Identification (WIPI) test. The WIPI test includes picture plates with six illustrations per plate. Four of the illustrations have words that rhyme, and the other two illustrations are presented as foils to decrease the probability of a correct guess. The use of WIPI materials is appropriate for those children with receptive vocabulary ages of 4 years and greater.

There are differences between the PBK words and WIPI test approach to speech perception testing besides the evident fact that the latter is pictorially represented. PBK words represent an open response paradigm in which the child is forced to give a response from an unlimited set of possibilities, whereas the WIPI is a closed response set with the child's response being a forced choice (Kirk et al., 1997). As such, the use of the WIPI as a closed-set test improves the discrimination scores by about 10%.

The Northwestern University-Children's Perception of Speech (NU-CHIPS) test by Elliott and Katz (1980) was developed as a speech perception test appropriate for younger children. Test materials are limited to monosyllabic words that are documented to be in the recognition vocabulary of children with normal hearing as young as age 3 years. Additionally, the authors report that children with hearing loss and a receptive language age of a least 2.6 years (as measured by the Peabody Picture Vocabulary Test; Dunn and Dunn, 1981) demonstrate familiarity with the words and pictures of the test.

Continued surveillance for hearing impairment that may interfere with communication, development, health, or future academic performance must continue for preschool children. For this age group (3 to 5 years), screening for hearing impairment is a pass-refer procedure to identify individuals who require further audiologic evaluation or other assessments. Hearing impairment is defined as unilateral or bilateral sensory-neural and/or conductive hearing loss greater than 20 dB HL in the frequency region from 1,000 to 4,000 Hz.

Unlike the newborn and school-age populations, when nearly all children are accessible in hospitals and schools, preschoolers are generally not available in large, organized groups that lend themselves to universal screening for hearing impairment. As such, an interdisciplinary, collaborative effort is particularly important for this age group. Physicians and other professionals who make up the child's medical home and other professionals who specialize in child development should be included in the planning and implementation of the hearing screening program to maximize the likelihood of prompt referral of children at risk of hearing impairment.

SUMMARY

Reaching the goal of early detection of hearing loss is facilitated by vigilant follow-up of infants and young children at risk for or suspected of having hearing loss. Furthermore, early detection of hearing loss is optimized by audiologists providing detailed audiologic assessment in a timely manner for those children referred from the screening process, early intervention lead agencies, the child's medical home, and other medical specialists. The accuracy and precision of our audiologic test battery also are critical in monitoring children with hearing loss and following children for delayed-onset hearing loss. Important and fundamental decisions in management and intervention depend on the audiometric outcomes and diagnosis provided by audiologists. If the development of this information is not accurate, precise, timely, and cost effective, we diminish the quality of services provided and compromise the credibility of our discipline. When these standards are met, audiologists positively impact the patients they serve and their families and are important members of the early multidisciplinary health care team.

the**Point**

Additional text material for this chapter can be found at http://thepoint.lww.com/Katz6e

REFERENCES

American Academy of Audiology. (2003) Pediatric amplification protocol. Available at: http://www.audiology.org/NR/rdonlyres/53D26792-E321-41AF-850F-CC253310F9DB/0/pedamp.pdf.

American Academy of Pediatrics. (2002) The medical home. *Pediatrics.* 110, 184–186.

American Speech-Language-Hearing Association. (2004) Guidelines for the audiologic assessment of children from birth to 5 years of age. Available at: http://www.asha.org/members/deskref-journals/deskref/default

Bayley N. (1969) *Bayley Scales of Infant Development: Birth to Two Years.* San Antonio, TX: Psychological Corp.

Bess FH. (1982) Children with unilateral hearing loss. *J Acad Rehabil Audiol.* 15, 131–144.

Bess FH, Dodd-Murphy J, Parker RA. (1998) Children with minimal sensorineural hearing loss: prevalence, educational performance, and functional status. *Ear Hear.* 19, 339–354.

Bess FH, Klee T, Culbertson J. (1988) Identification, assessment and management of children with unilateral sensorineural hearing loss. *Ear Hear.* 7, 43–51.

Boege P, Janssen T. (2002) Pure-tone threshold estimation from extrapolated distortion product otoacoustic emission I/O functions in normal and cochlear hearing loss ears. *J Acoust Soc Am.* 111, 1810–1818.

Bovo R, Martini A, Agnoletto M, Beghi A, Carmignoto D, Milani M, Sangaglia AM. (1988) Auditory and academic performance of children with unilateral hearing loss. *Scand Audiol.* 30 (suppl), 71–74.

Carney A, Moeller MP. (1998) Treatment efficacy: hearing loss in children. *J Speech Hear Res.* 41, S61–S84.

Condon MC. (1991) Unique challenges: children with multiple handicaps. In: Feigin J, Stelmachowicz P, eds. *Pediatric Amplification.* Omaha NE: Boys Town National Research Hospital.

Culpepper B, Thompson G. (1994) Effects of reinforcer duration on the response behavior of preterm 2-year olds in visual reinforcement audiometry. *Ear Hear.* 15, 161–167.

Diefendorf AO. (1981). The effect of a pre-play period on play audiometry. Paper presented at Tennessee Speech and Hearing Association convention, Memphis, TN.

Diefendorf AO. (1988) Behavioral evaluation of hearing-impaired children. In: Bess FH, ed. *Children with Hearing Loss: Contemporary Trends.* Nashville: Bill Wilkerson Center Press; pp 71–81.

Diefendorf AO, Gravel JS. (1996) Visual reinforcement and behavioral observation audiometry. In: Gerber SE, ed. *Handbook of Pediatric Audiology.* Washington, DC: Gallaudet University Press; pp 55–83.

Dolan TG, Morris SG. (1990) Administering audiometric speech tests via bone conduction: a comparison of transducers. *Ear Hear.* 11, 446–449.

Dorn PA, Konrad-Martin D, Neely ST, Keefe DH, Cry E, Gorga MP. (2001) Distortion product otoacoustic emission input/output functions in normal-hearing and hearing-impaired human ears. *J Acoust Soc Am.* 110, 3119–3131.

Dunn L, Dunn L. (1981) *Peabody Picture Vocabulary Test—Revised.* Circle Pines, MN: American Guidance Service.

Eilers RE, Miskiel E, Ozdamar O, Urbano R, Widen J. (1991a) Optimization of automated hearing test algorithms: simulations using an infant response model. *Ear Hear.* 12, 191–198.

Eilers RE, Widen J, Urbano R, Hudson TM, Gonzales L. (1991b) Optimization of automated hearing test algorithms: a comparison of data from simulations and young children. *Ear Hear.* 12, 199–204.

Elliott LL, Katz D. (1980) *Development of a New Children's Test of Speech Discrimination (Technical Manual).* St Louis, MO: Auditec.

Finitzo T, Crumley WG. (1999) The role of the pediatrician in hearing loss from detection to connection. *Pediatr Clin North Am.* 46, 15–34.

Genetic Evaluation of Congenital Hearing Loss Expert Panel. (2002) Genetics evaluation guidelines for the etiologic diagnosis of congenital hearing loss. *Genet Med.* 4, 162–171.

Gerwin KS, Glorig A, eds. (1974) *Detection of Hearing Loss and Ear Disease in Children.* Springfield, IL: Charles C. Thomas.

Goldstein K, Caputo D, Taub H. (1976) The affects of prenatal and perinatal complications on development at one year of age. *Child Dev.* 47, 613–621.

Gorga MP, Neely ST, Bergman B, Beauchaine K, Kaminski J, Peters J, Jesteadt W. (1993) Otoacoustic emissions from normal-hearing and hearing-impaired subjects: distortion product responses. *J Acoust Soc Am.* 93, 2050–2060.

Gorga MP, Neely ST, Dierking DM, Dorn PA, Hoover BM, Fitzpatrick D. (2003) Distortion product otoacoustic emission tuning curves in normal-hearing and hearing-impaired human ears. *J Acoust Soc Am.* 114, 262–278.

Gorga MP, Neely ST, Dorn PA. (2002) Distortion product otoacoustic emissions in relation to hearing loss. In: Robinette MS, Glattke TJ, eds. *Otoacoustic Emissions: Clinical Applications.* 2nd ed. New York: Thieme Medical; pp 243–272.

Gorga MP, Stover LT, Neely ST. (1996) The use of cumulative distributions to determine critical values and levels of confidence for clinical distortion product otoacoustic emission measurements. *J Acoust Soc Am.* 100, 968–977.

Gorlin RJ, Toriello HV, Cohen MM. (1995) *Hereditary Hearing Loss and Its Syndromes.* New York: Oxford University Press.

Gravel JS, Traquina DN. (1992) Experience with the audiological assessment of infants and toddlers. *Int J Pediatr Otolaryngol.* 23, 59–71.

Gravel JS, Wallace IF. (1999) Otitis media and communication during pre-school years. Paper presented at ICIS2000 Doctorial Consortium, Brisbane, Australia.

Greenburg D, Wilson WR, Moore JM, Thompson G. (1978) Visual reinforcement audiometry (VRA) with young Down syndrome children. *J Speech Hear Dis.* 43, 448–458.

Hanley M. (1986) *Basic Principles of Auditory Assessment.* San Diego: College Hill Press.

Haskins H. (1949) A phonetically balanced test of speech discrimination for children. Master's thesis, Northwestern University, Evanston, IL.

Jerger J, Hayes D. (1976) The cross-check principle in pediatric audiometry. *Arch Otolaryngol.* 102, 614–620.

John MS, Brown DK, Muir PJ, Picton TW. (2004) Recording auditory steady-state responses in young infants. *Ear Hear.* 25, 536–553.

Joint Committee on Infant Hearing (JCIH). (1972) Supplementary statement on infant hearing screening. *ASHA.* 16, 160.

Joint Committee on Infant Hearing (JCIH). (1982) 1982 position statement. *ASHA.* 24, 1017–1018.

Joint Committee on Infant Hearing (JCIH). (1991) 1990 position statement. *ASHA.* 33, 3–6.

Joint Committee on Infant Hearing (JCIH). (1994) Position statement. *ASHA.* 36, 38–41.

Joint Committee on Infant Hearing (JCIH). (2000) Year 2000 position statement: principles and guidelines for early hearing detection and intervention programs. *Am J Audiol.* 9, 9–29.

Joint Committee on Infant Hearing (JCIH). (2007) Year 2007 position statement: principles and guidelines for early hearing detection and intervention programs. *Pediatrics.* 120, 898–921.

Katbamna B, Homnick DN, Marks JH. (1999) Effects of chronic tobramycin treatment on distortion product otoacoustic emissions. *Ear Hear.* 20, 393–402.

Kemp DT, Ryan S, Bray P. (1990) A guide to the effective use of otoacoustic emissions. *Ear Hear.* 11, 93–105.

Kirk KI, Diefendorf AO, Pisoni DB, Robbins AM. (1997) Assessing Speech Perception in Children. In: Mendel LL, Danhauer JL, eds. *Audiologic Evaluation and Management and Speech Perception Assessment.* San Diego: Singular Publishing Group, 101–132.

Kopp C. (1974) Fine motor abilities of infants. *Dev Med Child Neurol.* 16, 629–636.

Lonsbury-Martin BL, McCoy MJ, Whitehead ML, Martin GK. (1993) Clinical testing of distortion-product otoacoustic emissions. *Ear Hear.* 14, 11–22.

Margolis RH, Bass-Ringdahl S, Hanks WD, Holte K, Zapala DA. (2003) Tympanometry in newborn infants—1 kHz norms. *J Am Acad Audiol.* 14, 383–392.

Martin GK, Ohlms LA, Franklin DJ, Harris FP, Lonsbury-Martin BL. (1990) Distortion product emissions in humans III. Influence of sensorineural hearing loss. *Ann Otol Rhinol Laryngol Suppl.* 147, 30–42.

Mehl AL, Thomson V. (1998) Newborn hearing screening: the great omission. *Pediatrics.* 101. E4.

Meredith R, Stephens D, Sirimanna T, Meyer-Bisch C, Reardon W. (1992) Audiometric detection of carrier of Usher's syndrome type II. *J Audiol Med.* 1, 11–19.

Moeller MP. (2000) Early intervention and language outcomes in children who are deaf and hard of hearing. *Pediatrics.* 106, 1–9.

Moore JM. (1995) Behavioral assessment procedures based on conditioned head-turn responses for auditory detection and discrimination with low-functioning children. *Scan Audiol Suppl.* 41, 36–42.

Moore JM, Thompson G, Folsom R. (1992). Auditory responsiveness of premature infants utilizing visual reinforcement audiometry (VRA). *Ear Hear.* 13, 187–194.

Moore JM, Thompson G, Thompson M. (1975) Auditory localization of infants as a function of reinforcement conditions. *J Speech Hear Disord.* 40, 29–34.

Moore JM, Wilson WR, Thompson G. (1977) Visual reinforcement of head-turn responses in infants under 12 months of age. *J Speech Hear Disord.* 40, 29–34.

Morton C. (1999) The NIDCD Working Group on genetic testing for deafness and other communication disorders: considerations for developing and implementing testing. Presented at Workshop on the Genetics of Congenital Hearing Impairment, Centers for Disease Control and Prevention and Gallaudet University, June 7, 1999, Atlanta, GA.

Nance WE. (2003) The genetics of deafness. *Ment Retard Dev Disabil Res Rev.* 9, 109–119.

National Center for Hearing Assessment and Management. (2007) EDHI legislation. Available at: http://www.infanthearing.org/legislative/index.html.

Northern JL, Downs MP. (2002) *Hearing in Children.* Baltimore: Lippincott Williams & Wilkins.

Norton SJ, Widen JE. (1990) Evoked otoacoustic emissions in normal-hearing infants and children: emerging data and issues. *Ear Hear.* 11, 121–127.

Nozza R, Wilson WR. (1984) Masked and unmasked pure tone thresholds of infants and adults: development of auditory frequency selectivity and sensitivity. *J Speech Hear Res.* 27, 613–622.

Olsen WO, Matkin ND. (1979) Speech audiometry. In: Rintelmann WF, ed. *Hearing Assessment.* Baltimore: University Park Press.

Oyler R, Oyler A, Matkin ND. (1988) Demographics and educational impact. *Lang Speech Hear Services Schools.* 19, 201–209.

Paradise J, Smith DG, Bluestone CD. (1976) Tympanometric detection of middle ear effusion in infants and young children. *Pediatrics.* 58, 198–210.

Primus M. (1992) Operant response in infants as a function of time interval following signal onset. *J Speech Hear Res.* 35, 1422–1425.

Primus M, Thompson G. (1985) Response strength of young children in operant audiometry. *J Speech Hear Res.* 18, 539–547.

Purdy SC, Williams MJ. (2000) High frequency tympanometry: a valid and reliable immittance test protocol for young infants? *N Z Audiol Soc Bull.* 10, 12–21.

Renshaw JJ, Diefendorf AO. (1998) Adapting the test battery for the child with special needs. In: Bess FH, ed. *Children with Hearing Impairment.* Nashville, TN: Vanderbilt Bill Wilkerson Press; pp 83–103.

Ress BD, Sridhar KS, Balkany TJ, Waxman GM, Stagner BB, Lonsbury-Martin BL. (1999) Effects of cis-platinum chemotherapy on otoacoustic emissions. The development of an objective screening protocol. *Otolaryngol Head Neck Surg.* 121, 693–701.

Ross M, Lerman J. (1979) Picture identification test for hearing-impaired children. *J Speech Hear Res.* 13, 44–53.

Rubin R, Rosenblatt C, Balow B. (1973) Psychological and educational sequelae of prematurity. *Pediatrics.* 52, 352–363.

Schmida MJ, Peterson HJ, Tharpe AM. (2003) Visual reinforcement audiometry using digital video disc and conventional reinforcers. *Am J Audiol.* 12, 35–40.

Seewald RC, Cornelisse LE, Ramji KV, Sinclair ST, Moodie SK, Jamieson DG. (1997) *DSL v4.1 for Windows: A Software Implementation of the Desired Sensation Level (DSL[i/o]) Method for Fitting Linear Gain and Wide-Dynamic-Range Compression Hearing Instruments.* User's manual. London, Ontario, Canada: University of Western Ontario.

Stapells DR, Gravel JS, Martin BA. (1995) Thresholds for auditory brainstem responses to tones in notched noise from infants and young children with normal hearing or sensorineural hearing loss. *Ear Hear.* 16, 361–371.

Stapells DR, Oates P. (1997) Estimation of the pure-tone audiogram by the auditory brainstem response: a review. *Audiol Neurootol.* 2, 257–280.

Starr A, Picton TW, Sininger Y, Hood LJ, Berlin CI. (1996) Auditory neuropathy. *Brain.* 119, 741–753.

Stelmachowicz PG. (2000) How do we know we've got it right? Electroacoustic and audiometric measures. In: Seewald R, ed. *A Sound Foundation through Early Amplification: Proceedings of an International Conference.* Stafa, Switzerland: PHONAK AG.

The Pediatric Working Group. (1996) *Amplification for Infants and Children with Hearing Loss.* Nashville, TN: Vanderbilt Bill Wilkerson Press.

Thompson G, Folsom RC. (1984) A comparison of two conditioning procedures in the use of visual reinforcement audiometry (VRA). *J Speech Hear Disord.* 49, 241–245.

Thompson G, Weber B. (1974) Responses of infants and young children to behavioral observation audiometry (BOA). *J Speech Hear Disord.* 39, 140–147.

Thompson G, Wilson WR, Moore JM. (1979) Application of visual reinforcement audiometry (VRA) to low-functioning children. *J Speech Hear Disord.* 54, 174–179.

Thompson MD, Thompson G, Vethivelu S. (1989) A comparison of audiometric test thresholds for 2-year-old children. *J Speech Hear Disord.* 54, 174–179.

Tonniges TF, Palfrey JS. (2004) The medical home. *Pediatrics.* 113, 1471–1548.

Turner RG. (2003) Double checking the cross-check principle. *J Am Acad Audiol.* 14, 269–277.

US Department of Health and Human Services. (2000) *Healthy People 2010.* 2nd ed. Washington, DC: US Government Printing Office.

Weber BA. (1969) Validation of observer judgments in behavior observation audiometry. *J Speech Hear Disord.* 34, 350–354.

Widen JD. (1990) Behavioral screening of high-risk infants using visual reinforcement audiometry. *Semin Hear.* 11, 342–356.

Wilson WR, Folsom RC, Widen JE. (1983) Hearing impairment in Down's syndrome children. In: Mencher G, Gerber S, eds. *The Multiply Handicapped Hearing Impaired Child.* New York: Grune & Stratton.

Wilson WR, Moore J, Thompson G. (1976) Sound-field auditory thresholds of infants utilizing visual reinforcement audiometry (VRA). Paper presented at the ASHA Annual Convention, November 20–23, 1976, Houston, TX.

Yang EY, Stewart A. (1990) A method of auditory brain stem response to bone conducted clicks in testing infants. *J Speech Lang Pathol Audiol.* 14, 69–76.

Yoshinaga-Itano C. (1995) Efficacy of early identification and intervention. *Semin Hear.* 16, 115–120.

Yoshinaga-Itano C. (2003). From screening to early identification and intervention: discovering predictors to successful outcomes for children with significant hearing loss. *J Deaf Stud Deaf Educ.* 8, 11–30.

Yoshinaga-Itano C, Sedey A. (2000) Development of audition and speech: implications for early intervention with infants who are deaf or hard of hearing. In: Yoshinaga-Itano C, Sedey AL, eds. Language, Speech and Social-Emotional Development of Children Who Are Deaf and Hard of Hearing: The Early Years. *Volta Rev.* 100, 213–234.

Yoshinaga-Itano C, Sedey A, Coulter DK, Mehl AL. (1998) Language of early and later identified children with hearing loss. *Pediatrics.* 102, 1161–1171.

APPENDIX 23.1

Risk Indicators Associated with Permanent Early-Onset and/or Late Progressive Hearing Loss in Children (Joint Committee on Infant Hearing, 2007)

1. Caregiver concern* regarding hearing, speech, language, or developmental delay
2. Family history* of permanent childhood hearing loss
3. Neonatal intensive care of >5 days, assisted ventilation ≥10 days, prolonged exposure to ototoxic medications ≥7 days (gentamicin and tobramycin) or loop diuretics (furosemide/Lasix), hyperbilirubinemia requiring exchange transfusion and extracorporeal membrane oxygenation* (ECMO)
4. In utero infections such as cytomegalovirus,* herpes, rubella, syphilis, and toxoplasmosis
5. Craniofacial anomalies, including those involving the pinna and ear canal, ear tags, ear pits, and temporal bone anomalies
6. Physical findings such as white forelock, associated with a syndrome known to include a sensory-neural or permanent conductive hearing loss
7. Syndromes associated with progressive hearing loss* such as neurofibromatosis, osteopetrosis, and Usher syndrome
8. Neurodegenerative disorders,* such as Hunter syndrome, or sensory motor neuropathies, such as Friedreich's ataxia and Charcot-Marie-Tooth syndrome
9. Culture-positive postnatal infections associated with sensory-neural hearing loss,* including confirmed bacterial and viral (especially herpes viruses and varicella) meningitis
10. Head trauma, especially basal skull/temporal bone fracture,* requiring hospitalization
11. Chemotherapy

*Risk indicators that are of greater concern for delayed-onset hearing loss.

24 Educational Audiology

Cheryl DeConde Johnson

INTRODUCTION

Audiology services in schools have been clearly defined in the Individuals with Disabilities Education Act (IDEA) since the law was first implemented in 1975. The most recent update, IDEA 2004 (US Department of Education, 2006), contains the most significant changes in policy since the inception of the law. This chapter will address educational audiology services, focusing on the roles and responsibilities as defined in IDEA as well as models for service delivery, caseload guidelines, licensure considerations, participation on the Individual Education Program team, program development and evaluation, and ethics and conduct considerations.

EDUCATIONAL AUDIOLOGY SERVICES ACCORDING TO THE INDIVIDUALS WITH DISABILITIES EDUCATION ACT

Audiology is considered a related educational service under IDEA along with other services such as speech-language pathology and occupational therapy. There is one definition of audiology for Part B, which pertains to children 3 to 21 years old, and another for Part C, which pertains to infants and toddlers from birth to age 3 years. These definitions are as follows (as taken directly from the act; http://idea.ed.gov/):

Part B—Definition of Audiology 34CFR300.34(c)(1)
Audiology includes:

(i) *Identification of children with hearing loss;*
(ii) *Determination of the range, nature, and degree of hearing loss, including referral for medical or other professional attention for the habilitation of hearing;*
(iii) *Provision of habilitation activities, such as language habilitation, auditory training, speech reading, (lipreading), hearing evaluation, and speech conservation;*
(iv) *Creation and administration of programs for prevention of hearing loss;*
(v) *Counseling and guidance of children, parents, and teachers regarding hearing loss; and*
(vi) *Determination of children's needs for group and individual amplification, selecting and fitting an appropriate aid, and evaluating the effectiveness of amplification.*

Part C—Definition of Audiology 34CFR303.12(d)
Audiology includes:

(i) *Identification of children with auditory impairments, using at risk criteria and appropriate audiological screening techniques;*
(ii) *Determination of the range, nature, and degree of hearing loss and communication functions, by use of audiologic evaluation procedures;*
(iii) *Referral for medical and other services necessary for the habilitation or rehabilitation of children with auditory impairment;*
(iv) *Provision of auditory training, aural rehabilitation, speech reading and listening device orientation and training, and other services;*
(v) *Provision of services for the prevention of hearing loss; and*
(vi) *Determination of the child's need for individual amplification, including selecting, fitting, and dispensing of appropriate listening and vibrotactile devices, and evaluating the effectiveness of those devices.*

There are some slight differences between these definitions. These include:

- **Agency Responsibility**. Part B is the responsibility of the education system, while Part C responsibility depends on the identified lead agency within each state. Common agencies for Part C are education, health, or human services. Provision of services within the Part C definition depends on a variety of variables including income, the family's insurance, Medicaid and other state insurance programs, state agency services such as those provided through a state school for the deaf, and available services in the family's community. However, under Part C, a family should never be denied services due to inability to pay; ultimately, the community and state-lead agency must provide funding for the necessary services.

- **Identification.** Part C specifies use of appropriate screening techniques as part of identification; Part B does not.
- **Assessment**. Assessment of communication function as determined by use of audiologic procedures has been added to Part C.
- **Habilitation**. Assistive listening device orientation is included as part of habilitation in Part C; it is not mentioned in the Part B definition.
- **Prevention**. Part C provides for direct provision of services, whereas Part B calls for creation and administration of programs to prevent hearing loss. Direct services include monitoring children at risk of developing late-onset hearing loss.
- **Counseling.** Counseling services are absent in the Part C definition.
- **Amplification**. Part C adds "dispensing" in addition to selecting, fitting, and evaluating the effectiveness of the device.

There are several provisions in IDEA 2004 that pertain to audiology and other services to children and youth who are deaf or hard of hearing. These include definitions, assistive technology devices and services, monitoring of hearing aids and cochlear implants, use of assistive technology outside of school, interpreting, and consideration of special factors. Appendix 24.1 contains the specific regulations for these areas. The following sections will discuss each of the areas within the audiology definition.

IDENTIFICATION

Identification of children with hearing loss suggests several roles for audiologists. Identification does not explicitly mean screening of all children, but rather screening as a step in the process toward identification of hearing loss. Resources and regulations in each state generally dictate the level of involvement of the audiologist at this stage. States that have mandated hearing screening of children in schools usually have the associated regulations within health or education agencies that direct those services. Because these procedures apply to all children, basic screening is considered a population-based event that should be completed by nurses, health aides,

volunteers, or other individuals designated by the responsible agency, rather than an activity under the umbrella of special education.

Audiologists, however, do have a significant role in hearing screening programs. They should work with the appropriate state agencies to establish screening procedures, referral criteria, and follow-up activities as well as provide training for those individuals who conduct the screening. Screening procedures should include measures to target specific populations of students. For example, acoustic immittance may be part of a screening protocol for young children to identify middle ear problems, whereas the addition of 6,000 and/or 8,000 Hz to a puretone protocol for middle and high school–age students might identify potential noise-induced hearing loss. Audiologists may also assist with establishing databases to ensure that all students are screened and that follow-up is completed.

Children who are very young or unable to respond with traditional puretone screening methods may require special procedures as well as the expertise of an audiologist to conduct the screening. Fortunately, the development of otoacoustic emissions as a screening procedure has enabled more widespread screening of children who are young and difficult to assess by nonaudiologists. With effective training and supervision, audiologists can manage these screening programs, leaving time for follow-up screening, audiologic assessment, and other audiologic activities. A summary of appropriate school screening roles for audiologists is as follows:

- Facilitate multiagency and community cooperation for hearing identification and referral.
- Coordinate efforts with nurses, local deaf/hard of hearing services teams, and relevant community resources to implement hearing identification, assessment, and referral procedures.
- Manage required preschool, school-age, and Child Find screenings following state policies and procedures. Screening may be conducted by trained paraprofessionals or volunteers under the supervision of the school nurse or educational audiologist.
- Provide technical support to the screening team including training; perform screenings for difficult to assess children/students.
- Conduct follow-up activities to ensure that those referred have received the prescribed service.

Audiologists from a variety of work settings may be involved in newborn hearing screening programs. Educational audiologists have an instrumental role in that they provide nonbiased information about available community services as well as serve as a link between early intervention and educational programs and services. The Educational Audiology Association (EAA) position statement (2002) on the roles of educational audiologists in newborn hearing screening outlines examples of specific involvement (Table 24.1).

TABLE 24.1   Early detection and intervention of hearing loss: roles and responsibilities for educational audiologists

IDEA Part C: role of audiologist [300.12(d)(2)]	Examples of activities provided by the educational audiologist
1. *Identification of children with hearing loss, using at-risk criteria and appropriate audiologic screening techniques*	■ Attend equipment trainings at hospitals ■ Review (score) screening results when automated scoring is not available ■ Provide screening in-service ■ Assist with data tracking and management ■ Provide screening rechecks prior to referral for diagnostic evaluation ■ Track referrals from screening to rescreening to assessment ■ Provide information to families about the screening/rescreening process and necessary follow-up steps for assessment where appropriate ■ Participate as a resource provider for the community ■ Refer to Part C point of entry within 2 days of rescreening to initiate referral process for possible service coordination and IFSP services (Note: In some communities, this step may not be completed until a hearing loss is actually diagnosed; however, if the family needs support and assistance to obtain a hearing evaluation, the Part C referral should be initiated)
2. *Determination of the range, nature, and degree of hearing loss and communication functions, by use of audiologic evaluation procedures*	■ Refer for initial diagnostic evaluation, assisting the family in locating appropriate pediatric audiologic testing facilities (following rescreen) ■ Refer to confirm diagnosis if necessary (Note: In some settings, the educational audiologist may be the diagnostic evaluator) ■ Contact the Part C point of entry within 2 days of hearing loss confirmation to initiate the IFSP process ■ Begin IFSP process with family and appropriate infant and toddler community agencies and supports (Note: All referral steps must be delineated in the IFSP, especially to justify insurance and other third-party payor commitments; the evaluation and assessment process must be completed within 45 calendar days from the referral) ■ Offer written materials about the evaluation and assessment process or procedures used
3. *Referral for medical and other services necessary for the habilitation or rehabilitation of children with hearing loss*	■ Assist family in understanding diagnostic information (e.g., medical, genetics) ■ Assist family in identifying appropriate medical or other services ■ Provide unbiased information to families ■ Act as liaison between medical providers, family, and other IFSP team members
4. *Provision of auditory training, aural rehabilitation, speechreading and listening device orientation and training, and other services*	■ Participate with the multidisciplinary IFSP team to plan services ■ Assist IFSP team in developing functional outcomes around the priorities the family has identified ■ Provide parents with information about their service agency options considering necessary service provider qualifications (Note: In some settings, the educational audiologist may be the direct service provider) ■ Assist family in transition from Part C to Part B (school) services
5. *Provision of services for prevention of hearing loss*	■ Provide hearing screening services as available through local Part C and Part B (Child Find) agencies ■ Conduct ongoing monitoring of "at-risk" children ■ Provide information on genetic counseling

TABLE 24.1 *(Continued)*

IDEA Part C: role of audiologist [300.12(d)(2)]	Examples of activities provided by the educational audiologist
6. *Determination of the child's need for individual amplification, including selecting, fitting, and dispensing appropriate listening and vibrotactile devices, and evaluating the effectiveness of those devices*	■ Refer for hearing instrumentation (Note: In some settings, the educational audiologist may be the direct service provider for selecting and fitting of amplification) ■ Assist family in identifying financial resources for amplification
7. *Counseling and guidance of children, parents, and teachers regarding hearing loss (proposed 9/2000 IDEA Part C regulations)*	■ Identify needs of parents through the IFSP process and assist family in identifying appropriate service providers ■ Organize parent support groups ■ Provide unbiased descriptions of communication, amplification, and education options ■ Locate appropriate service providers for family's choice of communication, amplification, and education options

IFSP, Individualized Family Service Plan.
From the Educational Audiology Association. (2002) Early detection and intervention of hearing loss: roles and responsibilities for educational audiologists. Available at: http:// www.edaud.org.

ASSESSMENT

Audiologic assessment with an educational perspective provides a slightly different focus than the traditional clinical evaluation. The goal in the educational setting is not only to define the parameters of the hearing loss, including the necessary referrals for diagnosis, treatment, and hearing instrument fittings, but also to determine the educational implications of the hearing loss for the individual. To address this additional need, audiologic assessment includes evaluations that consider communication function, listening skill development, hearing loss adjustment, and environmental factors such as classroom acoustics and classroom communication patterns. Table 24.2 summarizes these individual and environmental assessment areas and recommended procedures.

Hearing Assessment

Audiologic assessment for hearing loss includes standard measures as well as additional ones to yield a comprehensive profile of a child's auditory abilities. Assessment should include speech recognition tests that address the variety of listening situations encountered in the learning environment such as the ability to understand soft speech and speech in noise. When possible, audiologists should include procedures that provide more detailed information regarding speech perception including ones that analyze suprasegmental (e.g., duration, loudness, pitch) and phonetic features of speech, phonemes, words, sentences, and discourse. The added information gained from knowing the auditory perception capabilities of these components assists speech-language pathologists and deaf education teachers in speech

development, planning, and intervention. Otoacoustic emissions are available in most educational audiology settings and should be used when additional information is needed about the integrity of a child's auditory system or used with children who are low functioning or difficult to assess. Assessment should also include testing with the child's personal amplification to assure that it is providing the intended benefit. Educational audiologists and private audiologists should work collaboratively to ensure that the comprehensive assessment is completed without duplication of effort.

Communication Assessment

Assessment in the area of communication provides the audiologist information on how children are communicating in their classroom and school environments with teachers and peers (normal hearing and deaf or hard of hearing). A self-assessment protocol such as the Classroom Participation Questionnaire (Antia et al., 2007) is useful in identifying preferred communication patterns and determining how well the child is able to understand and be understood by peers and teachers. The protocol also includes information about the children's feelings (positive and negative) regarding their ability to communicate. The audiologist can use this information to adjust hearing assistance technology, and it can also serve as a counseling tool to help students determine strategies they might employ to improve or remediate poor communication situations. The information may also be informative regarding the appropriateness of placement decisions, particularly components under consideration [34CFR300.324(2)(iv)] in the development of the Individual Education Program (IEP) in IDEA.

TABLE 24.2 Educational audiology assessment for individuals with hearing loss

Individual measures	Environment measures

1. Hearing
  ■ Case history
  ■ Otoscopic
  ■ Air and bone conduction
  ■ Speech reception (unaided/aided)
  ■ Acoustic immittance
  ■ OAEs (as appropriate)
  ■ MCL/UCL (unaided/aided)
  ■ Word recognition at soft and average hearing levels and in noise (unaided/aided)
  ■ Aided verification procedures for hearing assistance technology (probe microphone)
  ■ Aided validation procedures for hearing assistance technology
2. Communication
  ■ Classroom Participation Questionnaire (Antia et al., 2007)
3. Listening
  ■ Functional listening measures
4. Hearing loss adjustment
  ■ Self-Assessment of Communication–Adolescents (Elkayam and English, 2003)
  ■ Significant Other Assessment of Communication–Adolescents (Elkayam and English, 2003)
5. Self-Advocacy
  ■ Listening Development Profile (Johnson et al., 1997)
	1. Classroom acoustics
	  ■ Noise measurements
	  ■ Reverberation measurements
	2. Classroom communication
	  ■ Classroom observation/teacher interview
	3. Instruction
	  ■ Classroom observation/teacher interview
	4. Administrative support
	  ■ Teacher/administrator interview

OAEs, otoacoustic emissions; MCL, most comfortable loudness; UCL, uncomfortable loudness.

Listening Assessment

Listening skills assessment is an essential component in the evaluation of children with hearing loss. Functional assessments such as the Functional Listening Evaluation (FLE) (Johnson et al., 1997); observation tools such as the Early Listening Function (ELF) (Anderson, 2002), the Children's Home Inventory for Listening Difficulties (CHILD) (Anderson, 2000), the Listening Inventory for Education (LIFE) (Anderson and Smaldino, 1998), the Children's Auditory Performance Scale (CHAPS) (Smoski et al., 1998), and the Functional Auditory Performance Indicators (FAPI) (Stredler-Brown and Johnson, 2004); as well as self-assessments such as the student component of the LIFE provide critical information about the development of listening and communication skills. These findings support needed accommodations, document benefits of those accommodations, and identify areas of skill development for the IEP.

Hearing Loss Adjustment and Self-Advocacy

Classroom performance is often affected by one's level of friendship development, self-esteem, and confidence.

Including measures in the assessment process, such as English's (2002) Children's Peer Relationship Scale (CPR) (Note: the CPR is a set of discussion points, not a test) and the Self-Assessment of Communication–Adolescents (SAC-A) and Significant Other Assessment of Communication–Adolescents (SOAC-A) by Elkayam and English (2003), identifies levels of self-identification and adjustment to hearing loss and issues associated with lack of adjustment. The reader is referred to Kris English's chapter on audiologic counseling (Chapter 43) for an in-depth discussion on these topics.

The audiologist should also determine how well a student is able to self-advocate for his or her communication needs. The Listening Development Profile (Johnson et al., 1997) defines four levels of listening development in which a sophisticated listener is characterized with the following self-advocacy skills:

■ Demonstrates knowledge of audiograms
■ Is knowledgeable regarding amplification options and assistive devices
■ Uses amplification systems appropriately including troubleshooting
■ Advocates for services including communication/listening environment accommodations

- Utilizes professionals and agencies
- Educates others about hearing loss and its implications

Instruments such as those mentioned earlier often translate to counseling opportunities. The audiologist should be prepared to address issues that are identified by the student during the assessment or interview process. Sufficient time should be scheduled during the assessment period or shortly thereafter to give students the opportunity to at least briefly talk about their problems and for the audiologist to begin to skillfully guide them through a problem-solving process. Anytime a student divulges sensitive information, it deserves at least acknowledgement and a response, even if brief. Time for more in-depth counseling can be scheduled once the "door has opened" (English, 2002).

Classroom Acoustics

Assessment includes conducting classroom noise and reverberation measurements and making recommendations for improvement of the listening environment. Depending on the sophistication of the equipment used by the audiologist and the problems identified, the noise measurements may be sufficient for determining the need for acoustic treatment. The measurements may also be considered a screening that can be used as a basis for referral to an acoustic engineer. American National Standards Institute (ANSI) classroom noise standards (ANSI, 2002) provide the impetus for making acoustic modifications. These standards specify that, for typical classrooms (under 10,000 cubic feet), unoccupied noise levels should not exceed 35 dBA and reverberation levels should be less than 0.6 second. Crandell et al. (2005) recommend that a better goal would be 30 to 35 dBA. Recent emphasis on educational outcomes for all students has highlighted the importance of the learning environment. Furthermore, it has been shown that poor classroom acoustics can also lead to voice fatigue and, subsequently, increased absences by teachers (Allen, 1995).

Classroom acoustics should be addressed prior to the implementation of hearing assistance technology. Rooms with high reverberation levels may preclude the use of sound distribution systems (sound field amplification systems) because amplification of highly reverberant areas can exacerbate speech intelligibility problems.

Audiologists need a sound level meter that can measure down to, at least, 35 dBA in order to complete noise measurements. Reverberation levels can be estimated using known sound absorption coefficients of typical materials used in school construction. Software programs such as the Reverberation Analysis Software Program (E.A. Acoustical Engineering, Inc., 2004) provide a direct means for audiologists to determine reverberation characteristics and estimate improvements resulting from various acoustic treatments.

Classroom Communication, Instruction, and Administrative Support

Interviews and observation provide important information about the appropriateness of the classroom context (e.g., general classroom physical environment, communication patterns, instructional style, the teacher's ability and flexibility in addressing the individual learning styles of students, and classroom management). These variables require careful attention when determining the classroom placement for a child as well as when making a recommendation for hearing assistance technology. Administrative support is also critical in ensuring that the needs of the students are consistently met. School principals and special education administrators set the tone for their school's acceptance of students with diverse learning needs. Evidence to look for includes:

- School administration and teacher support for students with disabilities
- School administration and teacher knowledge about hearing loss
- School administration and teacher commitment to making the required accommodations for children with hearing loss
- School administration and teacher willingness to use and support assistive technology
- School administration and teacher willingness to work with specialists
- Opportunities for individualized attention in the classroom

Auditory Processing Disorder Assessment

Another component of audiologic assessment is the evaluation of auditory processing abilities, an area of audition that should not be overlooked. The individual's ability to understand what the ear hears is essential to the development of communication skills and for learning in school. The school setting is a common environment for identifying children with learning difficulties that may be auditory in nature. Educational audiologists should establish a multidisciplinary process with speech-language pathologists, school psychologists, and learning disabilities specialists to consider children who may have auditory processing problems. The process should include screening and diagnostic procedures as well as intervention and treatment options. For more information on this topic, the reader is referred to Chapters 25 to 28 of this text.

Assessment Considerations for Eligibility for Services

To be eligible for special education, IDEA requires that there be an adverse impact of the disability on learning. Analysis of the findings must show that, without special education and related services, the child is unable to reasonably benefit from a free and appropriate public education (FAPE). Therefore, audiologic assessment must include the procedures required by individual states for eligibility determination. For example, one of the Colorado eligibility criteria is unaided word recognition of 80% or less in quiet at typical conversation levels. As a result, this procedure is completed for all children with hearing loss. Assessments are required for initial eligibility and triennial evaluations. Because audiologic assessment for children and youth are typically completed annually in order to monitor hearing thresholds, use and performance of hearing technologies, and functional performance, the audiologist may need to include annual hearing evaluations in the child's IEP.

When children with hearing loss are not eligible for special education services, their hearing and educational performance should be monitored at least annually to ensure that they do not become eligible at some time in the future. This monitoring can be accomplished by the audiologist under a 504 Plan or as part of new provisions under IDEA 2004, Early Intervening Services or Response to Intervention. Audiologists should be aware of their options for these procedures according to their state regulations.

Interpretation of test results and recommendations should be detailed in a written report. It is helpful to include background information, test results, implications, and recommendations. Including a specific section on recommendations for the teacher and other school professionals often helps to highlight the most critical components and accommodations they need to know. Reviewing the report information in person provides a forum for discussion about the student as well as an opportunity for reinforcement of the issues, challenges, and necessary accommodations. Teachers appreciate when information is distilled to the essential elements they need to know. Therefore, including a short list of accommodations on a 4 × 6 card can be very helpful. Getting the student involved in developing his or her own list of accommodations has an even greater impact.

SUMMARY OF AUDIOLOGIC ASSESSMENT ROLES

A summary of appropriate assessment roles for educational audiologists include:

- Conduct audiologic evaluations on all children/students referred by the screening program.
- Conduct annual audiologic evaluations for all children/students with known educationally significant hearing loss (ESHL) (ESHL is generally considered to be one that has at least a 20-dB puretone average [PTA] of 500, 1,000, and 2000 Hz or 1,000, 2,000, and 4,000 Hz in the better ear or a unilateral hearing loss).
- Assess the range and nature of the hearing impairment and resulting communication functions, including evaluation of the effectiveness of hearing aids

and hearing assistance technology when prescribed and interpretation of the results for specific communication and educational implications.

- Annually monitor the hearing thresholds of children/students with hearing losses that are not in the range typically considered to be educationally significant and therefore have not been deemed to impact their access to their educational programs (thus, if any changes in hearing occur to an extent that they meet state criteria, these children will be able to be referred for a consideration of special education and related services in an expeditious manner).
- Make recommendations for amplification and hearing assistance technology.
- Refer all children with ESHL to the teacher of the deaf/hard of hearing (ToD) for consideration of special education and related services. With the ToD:
  ○ Conduct performance reviews (e.g., Screening Instrument for Targeting Educational Risk [S.I.F.T.E.R.], available from www.edaud.org; or grade checks) on students with newly identified ESHL.
  ○ Schedule building-level child study conferences on students referred with ESHL to discuss hearing impairment, associated communication and learning implications, student performance, and recommendations for accommodations and instructional modifications.
  ○ Refer students who exhibit associated communication and educational concerns (e.g., a child with auditory processing disorder [APD]) who may require special education and related services or 504 services to benefit from their educational program.
  ○ Conduct annual performance reviews (e.g., S.I.F.T.E.R., grade checks) to monitor performance for children/students with known hearing losses who have not been eligible for special education services due to lack of evidence of the adverse effect of that hearing loss on learning.

■ AMPLIFICATION

One of the primary roles of audiologists in the school setting is the provision of services related to amplification. IDEA provides significant regulation about providing amplification devices and monitoring the function of amplification including personal devices, such as hearing aids and cochlear implants, and assistive technology:

- *Determination of children's needs for group and individual amplification, selecting and fitting an appropriate aid, and evaluating the effectiveness of amplification [34CFR300.34(c)(1)(iv)]*

- *Routine checking of hearing aids and external components of surgically implanted medical devices (34CFR300.113)*
  - (a) *Hearing aids. Each public agency must ensure that hearing aids worn in school by children with hearing impairments, including deafness, are functioning properly.*
  - (b) *External components of surgically implanted medical devices.*
    - (1) *Subject to paragraph (b)(2) of this section, each public agency must ensure that the external components of surgically implanted medical devices are functioning properly.*
    - (2) *For a child with a surgically implanted medical device who is receiving special education and related services under this part, a public agency is not responsible for the post-surgical maintenance, programming, or replacement of the medical device that has been surgically implanted (or of an external component of the surgically implanted medical device).*
- *Assistive Technology (34CFR300.5-.6)*
  Assistive technology device means any item, piece of equipment, or product system, whether acquired commercially off the shelf, modified, or customized, that is used to increase, maintain, or improve the functional capabilities of children with disabilities. The term does not include a medical device that is surgically implanted, or the replacement of such device.
  Assistive technology service means any service that directly assists a child with a disability in the selection, acquisition, or use of an assistive technology device. The term includes:
  - (a) *The evaluation of the needs of a child with a disability, including a functional evaluation of the child in the child's customary environment;*
  - (b) *Purchasing, leasing, or otherwise providing for the acquisition of assistive technology devices by children with disabilities;*
  - (c) *Selecting, designing, fitting, customizing, adapting, applying, maintaining, repairing, or replacing assistive technology devices;*
  - (d) *Coordinating and using other therapies, interventions, or services with assistive technology devices, such as those associated with existing education and rehabilitation plans and programs;*
  - (e) *Training or technical assistance for a child with a disability or, if appropriate, that child's family; and*
  - (f) *Training or technical assistance for professionals (including individuals providing education or rehabilitation services), employers, or other*

individuals who provide services to, employ, or are otherwise substantially involved in the major life functions of children with disabilities.

The exclusion for cochlear implants was added in IDEA 2004 to limit the growing demands on schools for cochlear implant programming. IDEA 2004 also strengthened the responsibility of schools to monitor device function. As a result, schools should always include a monitoring plan that specifies who monitors the device, when it is conducted, the procedures used, and what will happen if a problem is identified. It is recommended that this plan be included in the IEP. A sample amplification monitoring plan is provided in Appendix 24.2.

Hearing assistance technology, also known as assistive listening devices, that is required for the child to receive FAPE must be designated in the IEP and provided by the school as well as the accompanying services that are indicated. These services begin with a functional assessment in the child's classroom or other "customary" environment. Tools such as functional listening evaluations, observation checklists, and self-assessments provide this essential information. These same tools are also used to validate the effectiveness of recommended assistive technology devices to assure that they provide the desired benefit. Fitting of the hearing assistance technology should be conducted using accepted probe microphone procedures (American Speech-Language-Hearing Association [ASHA], 1999) with the specific goal of enhancing audibility of the desired speech signal (usually the teacher's voice), while maintaining access to the discourse of classmates. Educational audiologists must have access to appropriate hardware and software to complete these fittings. Device selection considerations are based on environmental, individual, and technologic factors such as conditions within the learning environment, the age of the student, developmental abilities, device wearability and ease of use, compatibility with other technologies, and potential interference issues. Audiologists must also plan and implement orientation and education programs to assure realistic expectations and to improve the acceptance of, adjustment to, and benefit from hearing assistance technology as well as from hearing aids and cochlear implants. These programs should include the student, the student's classmates, relevant teachers, and school support staff, as well as the parents when devices are used at home. To summarize, selecting and fitting hearing assistance technology should include the following steps:

- Determination of candidacy for hearing assistance technology
- Considerations of device options and device selection
- Fitting and verification procedures
- Orientation and training activities
- Validation procedures
- Monitoring procedures

HABILITATION

Educational audiologists provide a wide range of habilitation services depending on their specific responsibilities in the schools. Even though audiologists usually receive more graduate preparation in auditory skill development than speech-language pathologists or deaf educators, they are often the least likely to provide these services. Regardless of the specific services delivered, the educational audiologist should support and advocate for appropriate intervention methods that include the following:

- Auditory skill development and listening skill training
- Speech skill development, including phonology, voice, and rhythm
- Visual communication systems and strategies, including speechreading, manual communication, and cued speech
- Language development (expressive and receptive) of oral, signed, cued, and/or written language, including pragmatics
- Selection and use of appropriate instructional materials and media
- Use of assistive technologies, such as those necessary to access radio, television, and telephones, as well as pagers and alerting devices
- Case management and care coordination with family/parent/guardian, school, and medical and community services
- Habilitative and compensatory skill training to reduce academic deficits as related to, but not limited to, reading and writing

- Social skills, self-esteem, and self-advocacy support and training
- The transition between, but not limited to, levels, schools, programs, and agencies
- Support for a variety of education options for children/students with hearing loss and/or APD

To provide input regarding the associated communication and educational implications of the impairment and the needed services, the audiologist must attend all annual and triennial IEP meetings for students with ESHL. Specific habilitation activities that are the responsibility of the audiologist are identified in Table 24.3, along with suggested ways to document them in the IEP. Since the IEP is the contract that assures services, they must be included in the IEP, along with the frequency with which they are provided and who provides them.

COUNSELING

Counseling services might include the student, the student's family, as well as school staff. Counseling students about their hearing loss provides information, emotional support, and the opportunity to develop self-advocacy skills in students who are deaf and hard of hearing. Students need to be able to describe their hearing loss and the necessary accommodations they need in various learning and communication situations. As discussed earlier in the chapter, the Listening Development Profile (Johnson et al., 1997) suggests a framework for addressing some of these self-advocacy skills, while English (1997) provides a curriculum for self-advocacy activities. Audiologists should work with the school hearing team (school psychologist, speech-language pathologist,

TABLE 24.3 Audiology individual education program (IEP) services and suggestions for where to include them in the IEP

Service	Where to Include Service in the IEP
Training students regarding use of their hearing aids, cochlear implants, and hearing assistance technology	■ IEP goals and objectives — counseling, assistive technology services
Counseling and training for students regarding self-advocacy skills	■ IEP goals and objectives — counseling
Recommending acoustic modifications based on classroom acoustic evaluations that structure or modify the learning environment	■ Accommodations
Educating and training teachers, other school personnel, and parents, when necessary, about the student's hearing loss, communication access needs, amplification, and classroom and instructional accommodations and modifications	■ Related services – counseling ■ Related services – parent counseling and training ■ Assistive technology needs and services
Monitoring the functioning of hearing aids, cochlear implants, and hearing assistance technology (by who, how often, where, procedures used to monitor, and what will occur when a problem is identified)	■ Related services ■ Monitoring plan addendum

educational interpreter, and deaf education teachers as well as the students' classroom teachers) to assure that goals are consistently supported and developing skills are reinforced.

The incidence of emotional disturbance in students with hearing loss is reported to be 1.9% by the 2004–2005 Gallaudet Annual Survey (Gallaudet Research Institute, 2005). Whenever students exhibit significant problems, audiologists should also refer and defer to the school counselor or school psychologist; preferably, this professional has expertise with children who are deaf and hard of hearing. When providing counseling services, the audiologist should:

- Assure that parents/guardians receive comprehensive, unbiased information regarding hearing loss, communication options, educational programming, and amplification options, including cochlear implants in cases of severe to profound hearing loss
- Demonstrate sensitivity to cultural diversity and other differences in characteristics, including those found among individuals and within family/guardian systems (including deaf culture)
- Demonstrate effective interpersonal communication skills

Parent counseling and training is a separate, related service in IDEA. The law specifies that support should be provided to families if it is needed for their children to meet their IEP goals and to receive FAPE. Parents can choose whether or not they desire the support. Unfortunately, this service is underused and can be difficult to implement due to confusion about how to include the service in the IEP, how to provide the service, and how to promote and monitor parent compliance. IDEA states the following:

34CFR300.24(c)(8)

  (i) *Parent counseling and training means assisting parents in understanding the special needs of their child*
  (ii) *Providing parents with information about their child's development*
  (iii) *Helping parents to acquire the necessary skills that will allow them to support the implementation of their child's IEP or IFSP.*

Counseling for school staff is focused on information that teachers and others need in order to understand the implications of hearing loss and implement appropriate accommodations. Ongoing services should be included in the child's IEP as discussed in the previous section on habilitation.

PREVENTION

Noise-induced hearing loss in children is a growing problem. Based on the results of the Third National Health and Nutrition Examination Survey (NHANES III), Niskar et al. (2001) estimated that 12.5% of children 6 to 19 years old have noise-induced hearing threshold shifts in one or both ears. An earlier study by Blair et al. (1996) found that 97% of the 273 third graders surveyed in their study were exposed to high levels of noise. In recognition of this evidence, the US Department of Health and Human Services (2005) in its Healthy People 2010 report includes the following objective related to hearing loss prevention: "Objective #28-17: Noise-induced hearing loss in adolescents. Reduce the proportion of adolescents who have elevated hearing thresholds, or audiometric notches, in high frequencies (3, 4, or 6 kHz) in both ears, signifying noise-induced hearing loss." Prevention of hearing loss, even though required under IDEA, usually receives the least emphasis of all of the audiology services in school audiology practices. Concern in this area is growing based on some of the following issues:

- Schools, as government entities, are exempt from the US Occupational Safety and Health Administration's (OSHA) standards unless there are state OSHA-like requirements. Yet, shop class noise levels have been reported to range from 85 to 115 dB (Langford and West, 1993).
- Noise regulations that do exist in schools apply primarily to classified staff (e.g., grounds, facility, print shop, cooking staff).
- Insurance companies for schools have limited knowledge of noise exposure hazards.
- School hearing screening is not mandated in all states; thus, a mechanism to identify children with potential noise-induced hearing loss is not consistently available; when screening programs do exist, they generally are not designed to identify students with noise induced hearing loss.

Although there are many resources available that provide hearing loss prevention education (e.g., Dangerous Decibels, www.dangerousdecibels.org; Crank it Down, www.hearingconservation.org; Wise Ears, www.nidcd.nih.gov/health/wise/index.htm), the difficulty lies in coordinating efforts for implementing a systematic hearing loss prevention education program within the curriculum. With the required effort that is necessary to address this area for all students, it is imperative this service be part of a larger agenda shared by health and general education services. Hearing prevention education needs a national focus as a preventable health condition. Educational audiologists should support such an effort by promoting the following activities:

- Noise education activities that are embedded within the school health and science curriculums at multiple grade levels
- Identification of "at risk" and "dangerous" noise sources

- Mandatory noise safety instruction for classes with potentially hazardous noise exposure, including strategies to minimize noise exposure in those settings
- Mandatory use of hearing protection for all individuals who work in noise hazard areas
- Mandatory monitoring of hearing levels of classified employees and teachers who work in noise hazard areas
- Training for school employees in hearing loss prevention, proper use of ear protection, noise control strategies, and interpretation of hearing test results
- School policies to limit decibel levels and exposure time at school-sanctioned events
- Required hearing screening of students that includes protocols targeted to identification of noise-induced hearing loss

MODELS OF SERVICE PROVISION, CASELOADS, AND LICENSURE

Models of Service Provision

There are two methods that schools may use to deliver audiology services: (1) employment directly by the local education agency (LEA) responsible for providing special education and related services, or (2) through a contract with an individual, organization, or agency for specified audiology services. The LEA is either the local school district or a consortium established by the state that provides special education services for a group of school districts. These state consortiums are usually referred to as Boards of Cooperative Educational Services (BOCES), intermediate units (IU), or school districts, and they are structured under the respective state department of education to provide special education services.

Although both models can be effective, the model of educational audiologists hired by LEAs usually results in more comprehensive services. As employees of the education agency, educational audiologists are accepted as peers of the teachers and other staff and may be more effective as agents working within the system. Their schedules may also be designed around the school day, resulting in more availability and flexibility for meeting student needs and providing teacher support. Contracted services are often more limited because they are restricted to the specific services that are negotiated. School districts usually prioritize these services to the minimum necessary to provide follow-up to screenings, audiologic assessment, and hearing assistive technology management. Contracts must assure that services are in compliance with state and federal requirements and that timelines are met. One of the most significant challenges with contracted services is supervision. In these situations, the school administrator providing oversight often has little

knowledge of the roles and responsibilities of audiologists, and it is not uncommon for these audiologists to be less familiar with the scope of practice in the schools when they are from private practice or other noneducational settings.

Another employment setting that carries unique responsibilities for the educational audiologist is schools for the deaf. In this environment, the audiology role must support the communication systems that are used by the students. Still, it is the audiologist who bears much of the responsibility to assure auditory communication access to those students who use their hearing and listening abilities whether as a primary means of communication or to supplement or accompany visual systems (e.g., sign language). It often requires a slightly different approach, one that is sensitive to the wishes of the child, his or her family, and the culture of the school.

Caseloads

Caseloads for audiologists are recommended at one audiologist for every 10,000 students (ASHA, 2002; Colorado Department of Education [CDE], 2004). This ratio assumes a caseload of children with hearing loss and auditory processing problems based on prevailing prevalence rates. Factors that may influence this ratio for a school system include the following:

- The geographic area and travel time, such as within a BOCES or intermediate school district
- The number of students with hearing loss served by the administrative unit
- The quantity and diversity of frequency modulated (FM) and other hearing assistive technologies (e.g., personal, auditory trainers, classroom sound field FM systems)
- The quantity of special tests that are performed such as speechreading, auditory skill development, and auditory processing
- The amount of in-house equipment calibration, test-check, and maintenance activities that are performed
- Involvement with local newborn and early childhood screening and follow-up

When direct services to students are provided by the audiologist, the ratio must be further adjusted using caseload guidelines for consultant and itinerant teacher service delivery models.

Licensure

Audiologists who provide services in the schools must adhere to state licensing requirements. Several states have specific certification or licensure for audiologists who are employed in school settings that are often administered through the state department of education. Some states, such as Colorado, also require a school-based practicum in audiology. Appendix 24.3 contains the knowledge and skills that are required by the CDE for audiology licensure (CDE, 1994). Audiology graduate programs in Colorado must demonstrate that their programs fulfill these standards in their curricula so that the graduates are eligible for state department of education licensure in audiology.

ROLE ON THE INDIVIDUAL EDUCATION PROGRAM TEAM

Special education eligibility and IEP development require input from the educational audiologist to ensure that information about the implications of the child's auditory, listening, and communication skills is understood. To assist in planning for the learning and communication of children with hearing loss, the audiologist uses data from a variety of sources (e.g., teacher, student, and parent interviews; observations; informal and formal assessments; classroom acoustic evaluations), explains the implications of hearing and listening on the child's ability to communicate and learn, and recommends appropriate hearing assistance technology.

After a comprehensive profile of a child is developed, the educational audiologist is a resource for planning and implementing evidence-based interventions to increase academic, communication, and social performance. Ultimately, the audiologist's goal as an IEP team member is to collaborate with educators, parents, and other related service professionals to create supportive, communication-accessible learning environments for all students.

PROGRAM DEVELOPMENT AND EVALUATION

An effective educational audiology program undergoes continuous evaluation to determine whether the services continue to meet the needs of the students, staff, and others it serves. Mechanisms for identifying program gaps and updating technology and services require systematic review and, in turn, help to prioritize future needs. The Self Assessment: Effectiveness Indicators for Audiology Services in the Schools (Johnson et al., 1997) is an example of an assessment tool designed for audiologists to document the status of their programs and services for their administrators. The self-assessment can be supported with any available data from publications, national data sources, professional standards, needs assessments, and surveys. Together, this data can be very powerful for affecting change. Some suggested applications of this process include the following:

1. Prioritize what you can currently do within the confines of your resources. Decide if you will focus on quantity (e.g., more services but less comprehensive) or quality (e.g., fewer services but more comprehensive).

2. Look for other ways to accomplish the services that students require. For example, if you are unable to provide habilitation services, consider a speech-language pathologist or deaf education teacher who might be able to provide the services with your consultative support.

3. Meet with your administration to identify services that will not be able to be provided and how they will be covered. Make it an administrative decision rather than your personal one. Then, if parents or teachers complain that something is not being done (e.g., you are unable to attend IEP meetings), then they can address the problem with your administrator.

4. Develop a 1- to 3-year plan for improving existing services or developing new services that you would like to add in the future. Include assistive technology and audiologic equipment in this plan as well as additional staff resources, if necessary.

5. Work with your state department of education, state professional organizations, and parents to elicit support for improving and expanding services.

ETHICS AND CONDUCT IN EDUCATION SETTINGS

The ethical responsibility for implementing the audiology requirements of IDEA based on the scope of practice discussed in this chapter can be challenging. Given the resource limitations that exist, educational audiologists frequently struggle with doing the right thing. The following questions are just some examples of the ethical dilemmas faced daily by educational audiologists.

- Are you able to evaluate students as often as best practices recommend?
- Are you able to conduct comprehensive assessment procedures that evaluate the functional aspects of hearing ability such as speech in noise, soft speech, speech with and without visual cues, and listening skills?
- Do you have access to current technology for conducting hearing evaluations and providing habilitation?
- Are you able to provide hearing assistive technology to *all* students who would benefit?
- Are you able to recommend the hearing technology that best suits a child's hearing needs?
- Are you able to meet with teachers and staff to discuss the results of each student's audiologic assessment and describe the implications of the loss on hearing and learning?
- Are you able to attend all initial and triennial IEP meetings for students with hearing loss?
- Are you able to consult or teach students about the effects of noise exposure and requirements for hearing protection?

■ Are you able to advocate for appropriate classroom acoustics?

Educational audiologists are often in a position of trying to balance the services they should provide with the resources (mostly time) available to do them. As a result, they often have to make decisions regarding which services continue and which services need to be cut or modified. Reconciling the responsibility for providing "adequate" services versus what is often referred to as "the Cadillac model" can be challenging. Audiologists should be prepared to justify all of their activities under the scope of audiology that is mandated by IDEA to avoid the issue of their administrators perceiving that they are doing more than the law requires. The ethical issue that is faced is, "How does one balance providing the necessary range and quality of audiologic services so that children get what they need and are entitled to with what individual school settings allow?" Given the emphasis on accountability that is currently present in the education system, every audiologist should have an ongoing evaluation process for their program that provides data on student numbers, types of services, use of amplification, and student performance, coupled with a plan for addressing unmet needs. Sufficient evidence is needed before a special education director can justify supporting an audiologist's request for additional funds, time, or resources. Even with all of the challenges that audiologists face working in the schools, the sense of gratification that is experienced when a student successfully graduates makes all of these efforts worthwhile.

REFERENCES

Allen L. (1995) The effect of sound-field amplification on teacher vocal abuse problems. Paper presented at the Educational Audiology Association Conference, Lake Lure, NC.

American National Standards Institute. (2002) Acoustical Performance Criteria, Design Requirements, and Guidelines for Schools. ANSI S12.60-2002. Melville, NY: Acoustical Society of America.

American Speech-Language-Hearing Association. (1999) Guidelines for fitting and monitoring FM systems. Available at: http://www.asha.org/NR/rdonlyres/9C8083C1-8D35-4B4A-84A6-A3B04B709E32/0/18866_1.pdf.

American Speech-Language-Hearing Association. (2002) Audiology service provision in and for schools. Avialable at: http://www.asha.org/docs/pdf/GL2002-00005.pdf.

Anderson K. (2000). Children's Home Inventory of Listening Difficulties. Available at: http://www.hear2learn.com.

Anderson K. (2002) Early Listening Function. Available at: http://www.hear2learn.com.

Anderson K, Smaldino J. (1998) Listening Inventory for Education. Available at: http://www.hear2learn.com.

Antia S, Sabers D, Stinson M. (2007) Validity and reliability of the Classroom Participation Questionnaire with deaf and hard of hearing students in public schools. *J Deaf Stud Deaf Educ.* 12, 158–171.

Blair J, Benson P, Hardegree D. (1996) Necessity and effectiveness of a hearing conservation program for elementary students. *Educ Audiol Assoc Monogr.* 4, 12–15.

Colorado Department of Education. (1994) Rules for the Administration of the Educator Licensing Act of 1991, Special Services Endorsement: School Audiologist (Sec 2260.5-R-11.01). Denver: Colorado Department of Education.

Colorado Department of Education. (2004) Standards of Practice for Audiology Services in the Schools. Denver: Colorado Department of Education.

Crandell C, Smaldino J, Flexer C. (2005) *Sound Field Amplification: Applications to Speech Perception and Classroom Acoustics.* Clifton Park, NJ: Thompson Delmar Learning.

E.A. Acoustical Engineering, Inc. (2004) Reverberation Analysis Software Program, V1.0. Plymouth, MN: E.A. Acoustical Engineering, Inc.

Educational Audiology Association. (2002) Early detection and intervention of hearing loss: roles and responsibilities for educational audiologists. Available at: http:// www.edaud.org.

Elkayam J, English K. (2003) Counseling adolescents with hearing loss with the use of self-assessment/significant other questionnaires. *J Am Acad Audiol.* 14, 485–499.

English K. (1997) *Self Advocacy for Students Who Are Deaf or Hard of Hearing.* Austin: Pro-Ed.

English K. (2002) The Children's Peer Relationship Scale. In: *Counseling Children with Hearing Impairment and Their Families.* Boston: Allyn & Bacon; p 58.

Gallaudet Research Institute. (2005) *Regional and national summary report of data from the 2004–2005 Annual Survey of Deaf and Hard of Hearing Children and Youth.* Washington, DC: Gallaudet Research Institute, Gallaudet University.

Johnson CD, Benson PV, Seaton J. (1997) *Educational Audiology Handbook.* San Diego: Singular Publishing Group.

Langford J, West D. (1993) A study of noise exposure and hearing sensitivity in a high school woodworking class. *Lang Speech Hear Serv Sch.* 24, 167–173.

Niskar S, Kieszak S, Holmes A, Esteban E, Rubin C, Brody D. (2001) Estimated prevalence of noise-induced hearing threshold shifts among children 6 to 19 years of age: The Third National Health and Nutrition Examination Survey, 1988-1994, United States. *Pediatrics.* 108, 40–43.

Smoski W, Brunt M, Tannahill C. (1998) Children's Auditory Performance Scale. Available at: http://www.edaud.org.

Stredler-Brown A, Johnson CD. (2004) Functional auditory performance indicators. Available at: http://www.cde.state.co.us/cdesped/sd-hearing.asp.

US Department of Education. (2006) Assistance to States for the Education of Children with Disabilities and Preschool Grants for Children with Disabilities; Final Rule, 34 CFR Parts 300 and 301, August 14, 2006.

US Department of Health and Human Services. (2005) Healthy People 2010. Objective #28-17. Washington, DC: US Department of Health and Human Services.

APPENDIX 24.1

IDEA 2004 Key Regulations Pertaining to Deaf Education and Audiology

PART B RELATED SERVICES 34CFR300.34(b)

Exception; services that apply to children with surgically implanted devices, including cochlear implants.

[1] Related services do not include a medical device that is surgically implanted, the optimization of that device's functioning (e.g., mapping), maintenance of that device, or the replacement of that device.

[2] Nothing in paragraph (b)(1) of this section—

   (i) Limits the right of a child with a surgically implanted device (e.g., cochlear implant) to receive related services (as listed in paragraph (a) of this section) that are determined by the IEP Team to be necessary for the child to receive FAPE.

   (ii) Limits the responsibility of a public agency to appropriately monitor and maintain medical devices that are needed to maintain the health and safety of the child, including breathing, nutrition, or operation of other bodily functions, while the child is transported to and from school or is at school; or

   (iii) Prevents the routine checking of an external component of a surgically-implanted device to make sure it is functioning properly, as required in §300.113(b).

PART B — DEFINITION OF AUDIOLOGY 34CFR300.34(c)(1)

Audiology includes:

   (i) Identification of children with hearing loss;

   (ii) Determination of the range, nature, and degree of hearing loss, including referral for medical or other professional attention for the habilitation of hearing;

   (iii) Provision of habilitation activities, such as language habilitation, auditory training, speech reading, (lipreading), hearing evaluation, and speech conservation;

   (iv) Creation and administration of programs for prevention of hearing loss;

   (v) Counseling and guidance of children, parents, and teachers regarding hearing loss; and

   (vi) Determination of children's needs for group and individual amplification, selecting and fitting an appropriate aid, and evaluating the effectiveness of amplification.

PART C — DEFINITION OF AUDIOLOGY 34CFR303.12(d)

Audiology includes:

   (i) Identification of children with impairments, using at risk criteria and appropriate audiological screening techniques;

   (ii) Determination of the range, nature, and degree of hearing loss and communication functions, by use of audiologic evaluation procedures;

   (iii) Referral for medical and other services necessary for the habilitation or rehabilitation of children with auditory impairment;

   (iv) Provision of auditory training, aural rehabilitation, speech reading and listening device orientation and training, and other services;

   (v) Provision of services for the prevention of hearing loss; and

   (vi) Determination of the child's need for individual amplification, including selecting, fitting, and dispensing of appropriate listening and vibrotactile devices, and evaluating the effectiveness of those devices.

PART B INTERPRETING SERVICES 34CFR300.34(c)(4)

Interpreting services includes:

(i) The following when used with respect to children who are deaf or hard of hearing: oral transliteration services, cued language transliteration services, and sign language transliteration and interpreting services, and transcription services, such as communication access real-time translation (CART), C-Print, and TypeWell; and

(ii) Special interpreting services for children who are deaf-blind.

PART B ASSISTIVE TECHNOLOGY 300.105(a)(2)

On a case-by-case basis, the use of school-purchased assistive technology devices in a child's home or in other settings is required if the child's IEP Team determines that the child needs access to those devices in order to receive FAPE.

PART B ROUTINE CHECKING OF HEARING AIDS AND EXTERNAL COMPONENTS OF SURGICALLY IMPLANTED MEDICAL DEVICES 34CFR300.113

(a) *Hearing aids.* Each public agency must ensure that hearing aids worn in school by children with hearing impairments, including deafness, are functioning properly.

(b) *External components of surgically implanted medical devices.*

   (1) Subject to paragraph (b)(2) of this section, each public agency must ensure that the external components of surgically implanted medical devices are functioning properly.

   (2) For a child with a surgically implanted medical device who is receiving special education and related services under this part, a public agency is not responsible for the post-surgical maintenance, programming, or replacement of the medical device that has been surgically implanted (or of an external component of the surgically implanted medical device).

PART B DEVELOPMENT, REVIEW, AND REVISION OF IEP, CONSIDERATION OF SPECIAL FACTORS 34CFR300.324(2)(iv)

The IEP Team **must-**

(iv.) Consider the communication needs of the child, and in the case of a child who is deaf or hard of hearing, consider the child's language and communication needs, opportunities for direct communications with peers and professional personnel in the child's language and communication mode, academic level, and full range of needs, including opportunities for direct instruction in the child's language and communication mode;

ASSISTIVE TECHNOLOGY; PART B 34CFR300.5-.6 & C: 34CFR303.12

Assistive technology device means any item, piece of equipment, or product system, whether acquired commercially off the shelf, modified, or customized, that is used to increase, maintain, or improve the functional capabilities of children with disabilities. The term does not include a medical device that is surgically implanted, or the replacement of such device.

Assistive technology service means any service that directly assists a child with a disability in the selection, acquisition, or use of an assistive technology device. The term includes-

(a) The evaluation of the needs of a child with a disability, including a functional evaluation of the child in the child's customary environment;

(b) Purchasing, leasing, or otherwise providing for the acquisition of assistive technology devices by children with disabilities;

(c) Selecting, designing, fitting, customizing, adapting, applying, maintaining, repairing, or replacing assistive technology devices;

(d) Coordinating and using other therapies, interventions, or services with assistive technology devices, such as those associated with existing education and rehabilitation plans and programs;

(e) Training or technical assistance for a child with a disability or, if appropriate, that child's family; and

(f) Training or technical assistance for professionals (including individuals providing education or rehabilitation services), employers, or other individuals who provide services to, employ, or are otherwise substantially involved in the major life functions of children with disabilities.

PART B DEFINITIONS 34CFR300.8(b)

[2] *Deaf-blindness* means concomitant hearing and visual impairments, the combination of which causes such severe communication and other developmental and educational needs that they cannot be accommodated in special education programs solely for children with deafness or children with blindness.

[2] *Deafness* means a hearing impairment that is so severe that the child is impaired in processing linguistic information through hearing, with or without amplification that adversely affects a child's educational performance.

[5] *Hearing impairment* means an impairment in hearing, whether permanent or fluctuating, that adversely affects a child's educational performance but that is not included under the definition of deafness in this section.

APPENDIX 24.2
Sample Personal Amplification Monitoring Plan

Student's Name: _Aiden Hears_ Date: _August 15, 2006_

Teacher: _Mrs. Nice_ Grade: _2_

Hearing Aid Brand/Model: RE _Phonak Supero 411_ LE _Phonak Supero 411_

Cochlear Implant: _____ ❏RE ❏LE

Hearing Assistance Device: Brand/Model: _Phonak Campus SX/MLxS_

1. Individual responsible for basic monitoring of device(s):

   ❏Teacher:_____ ❏Nurse:_____
   ☒Aide:_ _Mrs. Health Aide_ ❏Audiology Asst:_____
   ☒Self-monitoring by student: _check battery_

2. Where will device(s) be monitored? ❏General education classroom ❏Special education classroom ☒Nurseís office ❏Other: _____

3. When will device(s) be monitored (daily/weekly and time of day)? _Daily at beginning of school day_

4. Procedures used to monitor device(s):

   Basic Check:
   By: _Mrs. Health Aide_

1. Verify that HA/FM is turned on and working.
2. Conduct Ling 6 sounds test.

   Troubleshooting
   Strategies:
   By: _Mrs. Health Aide_

Hearing Aid check: battery, earmold, tubing, intermittency and static
FM system check: battery, FM connection and channel, intermittency and static

   Advanced Check:
   By: _Dr. Audiology_

1. Verify status using basic troubleshooting strategies.
2. Conduct electroacoustic check.

5. What will occur if device is malfunctioning? _Audiologist will send hearing aid home with note indicating problem so that parents can take it to their dispensing audiologist for repair; school will continue to provide amplification access with FM system by adding a school-owned receiver._

Parent Approval of Plan:

   ❏ I agree with amplification monitoring plan. Initials_____Date_____

APPENDIX 24.3
Knowledge and Skills for Audiologists Employed in School Settings

1. The school audiologist is knowledgeable about the procedures necessary to identify hearing loss in children/students, including, but not limited to the following, and is able to:
   (a) perform identification audiometric procedures, including puretone audiometric screening, immittance measurements, otoacoustic emissions, and other electrophysiological measurements.
   (b) establish, administer, and coordinate hearing and/or auditory processing disorders (APD) identification programs.
   (c) train and supervise audiology support, or other personnel, as appropriate to screening for hearing loss and/or APD.
   (d) maintain accurate and accountable records for referral and follow-up of hearing screenings.

2. The school audiologist is knowledgeable about and is able to effectively implement the procedures necessary to assess hearing loss in children/students, including, but not limited to:
   (a) performing comprehensive audiologic evaluations, including puretone air and bone conduction measures; speech reception and word recognition measures, such as situational functional hearing measures; immittance measures; otoscopy and other tests, including interpretation of electrophysiological measures; and differential determination of auditory disorders, and/or APD, to determine the range, nature, and degree of hearing loss (or processing related difficulties) and communication function.
   (b) performing comprehensive educationally and developmentally relevant audiologic assessments of children/students, ages birth to 21, using bias-free procedures, and appropriate to receptive and expressive ability, and behavioral functioning.
   (c) providing recommendations for appropriate medical, educational, and community referrals for other services, as necessary, for the identification and management of children/students with hearing loss and/or APD, and their families/guardians.
   (d) interpreting, in writing and verbally, audiologic assessment results, functional implications, and management recommendations, to educational personnel, parents/guardians, and other appropriate individuals, including physicians and professionals, as part of a multidisciplinary process.
   (e) selecting, maintaining, and calibrating audiologic equipment.
   (f) providing access to assessment information, through interpreters/translators when needed.

3. The school audiologist is knowledgeable about procedures of evaluation and provision of amplification instrumentation to children/students in school, and is able to:
   (a) determine children's/students' needs for, and the appropriateness of, hearing aids, cochlear implants, and other hearing-assistance technology.
   (b) perform the appropriate selection, verification, and maintenance of hearing-assistance technology, including ear mold impressions and modifications.
   (c) evaluate situational functional communication performance, to validate amplified or electrically-stimulated hearing ability.
   (d) plan and implement orientation and education programs, to assure realistic expectations, and to improve acceptance of, adjustment to, and benefit from hearing aids, cochlear implants, and hearing-assistance technology.

(e) assess whether hearing aids, cochlear implants, and other hearing-assistance technology, as used in school, are functioning properly.

(f) notify parents/guardian when a repair, and/or maintenance, of personal hearing-assistance devices is required.

4. The school audiologist shall be knowledgeable about, and is able to:

(a) identify appropriate intervention methods, necessary levels of service, and vocational and work-study programming, as part of a multidisciplinary team process, integrating:

   (i) auditory skill development, aural rehabilitation, and listening-device orientation and training;

   (ii) speech skill development, including phonology, voice, and rhythm;

   (iii) visual communication systems and strategies, including speech-reading, manual communication, and cued speech;

   (iv) language development, i.e. expressive and receptive oral, signed, cued and/or written language, including pragmatics;

   (v) the selection and use of appropriate instructional materials and media;

   (vi) the structuring of learning environments, including acoustic modifications;

   (vii) case management and care coordination with family/parent/guardian, school, and medical and community services;

   (viii) habilitative and compensatory skill training, to reduce academic deficits, as related to, but not limited to, reading and writing;

   (ix) social skills, self-esteem, and self-advocacy support and training;

   (x) the transition between, but not limited to levels, schools, programs, and agencies;

   (xi) support for a variety of education options, for children/students with hearing loss and/or auditory processing disorders.

(b) develop and implement treatment plans that facilitate communication competence, which may include, but not be limited to, speech-reading; auditory/aural development; communication strategies; and visual-communication systems and strategies.

(c) provide and/or make recommendations with regard to assistive technology, such as, but not limited to hearing aids and hearing-assistance technology, to include radio/television, telephone, pager, and alerting convenience.

(d) provide developmentally-appropriate aural (re)habilitation services, including, but not limited to programming in the child's natural environment, if appropriate, in the areas of speech-reading, listening, communication strategies, use and care of hearing aids, cochlear implants, hearing-assistance technology, and self-management of hearing needs.

(e) provide information and training to teachers, administrators, children/students, parents/guardians, and other appropriate professionals and individuals, regarding hearing and auditory development; hearing loss and/or APD, and implications for communication, learning, psychosocial development, and the setting and meeting of vocational goals; hearing aids, cochlear implants, and hearing assistance devices; effective communication strategies; effects of poor classroom acoustics and other environmental barriers to learning; and EHDI (early hearing detection and intervention) programs and resources.

(f) apply appropriate instructional modifications and classroom accommodations to curricula delivery and academic methodology, materials, and facilities.

(g) conduct analyses of classroom acoustics, and make recommendations for improvement of the listening environment, utilizing principles of classroom acoustics, acoustical measurement, and acoustical modifications.

5. The school audiologist is knowledgeable about the parameters of information counseling and advocacy, and is able to:

(a) counsel families/guardians, and children/students with hearing loss and/or APD, to provide emotional support; information about hearing loss and the implications thereof; and strategies to maximize communication, academic success, and psychosocial development.

(b) assure that parents/guardians receive comprehensive, unbiased information regarding hearing loss; communication options; educational programming; and amplification options, including cochlear implants, in cases of severe to profound hearing loss.

(c) demonstrate sensitivity to cultural diversity and other differences in characteristics, including those found among individuals, and within family/guardian systems, and including deaf culture.

(d) demonstrate effective interpersonal communication skills, in a variety of settings, for a variety of circumstances.

6. The school audiologist is knowledgeable about the parameters associated with hearing conservation, and is able to:

(a) develop, implement, and/or manage programs for the prevention of hearing loss.

(b) provide education, when appropriate, as related to, and regarding access to, hearing protection devices.

7. The school audiologist is knowledgeable about ethical conduct, and is able to:

(a) comply with federal and state laws, regulations, and policies, including local district and school policies, and relevant case law, regarding referral, assessment, placement, related processes, and the delivery of service(s).

(b) effectively articulate the role of the school audiologist, as part of the special education team, within the learning community.

(c) incorporate knowledge of school systems, multidisciplinary teams, and community, national, and professional resources, into planning.

(d) effectively collaborate with teachers, parents and related personnel, in case management, with flexibility, and in a professional manner.

(e) utilize a range of interpersonal communication skills, such as, but not limited to consultation, collaboration, counseling, listening, interviewing, and teaming, as appropriate, in the identification of, prevention of harm to, assessment of, and/or intervention with children/students suspected of, or identified as, having auditory disabilities.

(f) mentor and supervise audiology support personnel, so that the auditory needs of children/students are effectively addressed.

(g) maintain accurate records and data, as relevant to the planning, management, and evaluation of programs.

(h) educate other professionals and the community about implications of hearing loss.

(i) initiate requests, or network, to acquire support when needed.

Taken from: Colorado Department of Education. (1994) Rules for the Administration of the Educator Licensing Act of 1991, Special Services Endorsement: School Audiologist (Sec 2260.5-R-11.01). Denver: Colorado Department of Education.

25 Mechanisms Underlying Central Auditory Processing

Larry Medwetsky

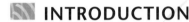

INTRODUCTION

It has been 50 years since Helmer Mykelbust first postulated a disorder of auditory perception in children that resembled hearing loss, yet in whom no hearing loss was present (Mykelbust, 1954). He described these difficulties as auditory perception deficits, which, over time, has come to be referred to as central auditory processing deficits. However, even after all this time, there still remains a lack of consensus of what underlies central auditory processing as well as what aspects should be evaluated by audiologists. This chapter will attempt to address many of these issues as well as describe a model of central auditory processing that can serve as the basis for evaluating and addressing the needs of those with suspected central auditory processing disorders (CAPDs).

BACKGROUND

Berry and Eisenson (1956) stated that children with auditory perceptual disorders can hear sounds but are unable to recognize the sounds they hear. At about this time, Bocca et al. (1954; 1955) published what are often considered as the seminal papers on site-of-lesion testing. These researchers surmised that, for many of their patients, puretone testing and conventional speech audiometry (i.e., word recognition scores) did not sufficiently task higher order auditory regions and thus were not sensitive in identifying these perceptual impairments. To challenge the central auditory nervous system (CANS) sufficiently, Bocca and his associates "sensitized" speech materials through low-pass filtering. They demonstrated that temporal lobe tumors could be lo-

calized using difficult-speech tests through a reduction of word recognition in the ear contralateral to the damaged hemisphere, despite normal hearing for puretones. This initial work spurred many other investigators to develop new test procedures for assessing the integrity of and determining specific sites of lesions of the CANS for adult patients presenting with a variety of neurologic disorders (Matzker, 1959; Katz, 1962; Smith and Resnick, 1972; Jerger and Jerger, 1974).

As interest grew in site-of-lesion testing, a number of professionals became interested in examining processing-related difficulties as they pertained to children. A committee, sponsored by the National Institutes of Health, was formed in 1963 and culminated in the first publication that focused on processing-related difficulties in children, of which auditory dysfunction was identified as one of the central processing dysfunctions (Chalfant and Scheffelin, 1969). The work of this committee inspired other professionals to adapt tests that had been originally developed for site-of-lesion testing for use in the assessment of central auditory processing capabilities in children, such as the application of the Staggered Spondaic Word (SSW) test (Katz and Ilmer, 1972). In 1977, a number of researchers gathered together at the first Central Auditory Dysfunction Symposium in Cincinnati, Ohio (Keith, 1977). Much of the focus of the conference was on children with language-based disabilities. Central auditory dysfunction was conceptualized as a disorder in taking in and using auditory information and, in turn, can result in children having learning disabilities and language disorders. In 1985, Willeford and Burleigh (1985) published the *Handbook of Central Auditory Processing Disorders in Children*, in which they described CAPD as a specific learning disability. Lucker (2007, p 11) points out that

Willeford and Burleigh cited PL94-192 as support for CAPD as being one manifestation of a specific learning disability, which stated "a disorder in one or more of the basic psychological processes involved in understanding or in using language, spoken or written, which may manifest itself in an imperfect ability to listen, think, speak, read, write, spell, or do mathematical calculations."

However, there were others who disagreed with the concept that central auditory processing difficulties were the basis of these children's difficulties and who questioned whether, in fact, it actually exists. Rees (1973; 1981) questioned whether auditory processing disorder was a meaningful concept and suggested that difficulties in articulation, language development, or reading acquisition could not be explained simply on the basis of underlying auditory processing disorders. Rees questioned whether CAPD was an actual disorder or merely a reflection of a language disorder that was manifested when stimuli were presented auditorily. In general, language processing proponents contend that most information about language exists in the mind and that very little information is actually gleaned from the acoustic signal; that is, most language processing, even for auditorily processed signals, involves using higher level linguistic and cognitive knowledge and applying it to the incoming acoustic signal (Duchan and Katz, 1983; Nittrouer, 2002; Kamhi, 2004).

On the other hand, there are those who propose that central auditory processing auditory mechanisms/disorders do exist and can be isolated (Keith, 1981; Jerger, 1998; Kraus and Nichol, 2005; Rawool, 2006a; 2006b). Jerger suggested that there were three lines of converging evidence in support of a relatively pure auditory perceptual disorder. First, there is significant audiologic evidence from children and adults with known lesions of the central auditory system; in turn, when similar symptomatology is observed in children with listening problems, a problem in central auditory processing in the brain is at least suspect. Second, there have been many in-depth studies of children and adults in which the only complaint is an apparent inability to hear well in difficult listening situations (and from what we can infer, the children exhibited no concomitant speech/language deficits). And third, the unique listening problems of elderly persons, may, in at least some cases, be related to age-related changes in the central auditory system (Frisina and Frisina, 1997; Kim et al., 2002).

Because of the lack of a clear definition of what constituted CAPD, the American Speech-Language-Hearing Association (ASHA) convened a task force in 1995 to develop a consensus statement regarding a definition of CAPD and establishing best practice principles related to the diagnosis and management of children with CAPD (ASHA, 1996). The task force defined *central auditory processes* as the *auditory system mechanisms and processes* responsible for the following behavioral phenomena:

- Sound localization and lateralization
- Auditory discrimination

- Auditory pattern recognition
- Temporal aspects of audition, including:
  - Temporal resolution
  - Temporal masking
  - Temporal integration
  - Temporal ordering
- Auditory performance decrements with competing acoustic signals
- Auditory performance decrements with degraded acoustic signals

The consensus group indicated that these mechanisms are presumed to apply to nonverbal as well as verbal signals and to affect many areas of function, including speech and language. Many neurocognitive mechanisms and processes are also engaged; some are specifically dedicated to acoustic signals, whereas others (e.g., attentional processes, long-term language representations) are not. With respect to these nondedicated mechanisms and processes, the term central auditory processes refers specifically to their deployment in the service of acoustic signal processing.

The consensus group furthermore defined "A Central Auditory Processing Disorder (CAPD) as an observed deficiency in one or more of the above-listed behaviors. For some, CAPD is presumed to result from the dysfunction of processes and mechanisms dedicated to audition; for others, CAPD may stem from some more general dysfunction, such as an attention deficit or neural timing deficit, that affects performance across modalities. It is also possible for CAPD to reflect coexisting dysfunctions of both sorts" (ASHA, 1996, p 43). Although the consensus task force was a worthy endeavor, there were significant problems with this consensus statement. As Jerger (1998) stated, the problem with this consensus statement is that the task force simply listed all of the deficits described in the literature. Furthermore, he stated that the difficulty with this kind of definition is that it does not provide much of a conceptual framework for understanding the phenomenon.

In 2000, a gathering of 14 scientists and clinicians met to reach a consensus on the problem of diagnosing auditory processing disorders in school-aged children (i.e., the Bruton Conference). In addition to proposing a name change from CAPD to auditory processing disorders (APD), this group broadly defined APD as a deficit in the processing of information that is specific to the auditory modality (Jerger and Musiek, 2000). This focus of auditory processing being specific to the auditory system is reflected in the work by Cacace and McFarland (2005) who suggested that one can only truly examine auditory processing and APD via modality specificity (i.e., isolating what processes are truly due to auditory processing mechanisms from processes that may engage more global, cognitive mechanisms). However, these approaches to conceptualizing and examining auditory processing mechanisms have been criticized by a number of researchers and clinicians as being too narrow in focus and impractical clinically (Katz et al., 2002; Katz and

Tillery, 2005). Modality specificity was also criticized by ASHA's Working Group on Auditory Processing Disorders (2005) in that the requirement of "modality specificity" as a diagnostic criterion for (C)APD is not consistent with how processing actually occurs in the central nervous system (CNS). The ASHA working group concluded that basic cognitive neuroscience has shown that there are few, if any, entirely compartmentalized areas in the brain that are solely responsible for a single sensory modality.

The most recent attempt to achieve a consensus regarding auditory processing mechanisms was through a second task force convened by ASHA in 2005 (ASHA, 2005). The committee in many ways maintained the same definition of this disorder as the 1995 group; however, it attempted to reconcile the importance/prominence of auditory processing with the recognition that complete modality specificity as a diagnostic criterion is neurophysiologically untenable. In diagnosing APDs, the group stated that one should expect the sensory processing perceptual deficit in (C)APD to be more pronounced, in at least some individuals, when processing acoustic information. An APD was to be best viewed as a deficit in neural processing of auditory stimuli that may coexist with, but is not the result of dysfunction in other modalities. The committee also recognized the work of the Bruton group and considered the term APD; however, because of the confusion and controversy regarding the use of the new term, particularly because most definitions of the disorder focus on the *central* auditory nervous system (CANS), the members of the ASHA working group agreed to use the term *(central) auditory processing disorder [(C)APD]* for the purpose of the report, with the understanding that the terms *APD* and *(C)APD* are to be considered synonymous.

In reviewing the aforementioned document, one of the main accomplishments of the second ASHA task force was in recognizing that a unitary view of auditory processing of speech was too simplistic and narrow in scope because this process likely engages both higher order auditory processing skills as well as more generalized cognitive processing/language skills. For example, Woldoff and Hillyard (1991) and Woldorff et al. (1993), in assessing the neural mechanisms of selective attention through the use of event-related potentials, found that the flow of auditory sensory information can be altered by attention at a relatively early stage of processing, with an enhancement of a positive wave in the interval 20 to 50 ms after onset (origin arising from an anatomic locus of the thalamus and/or auditory cortex) as well an enhanced negative wave at approximately 100 ms after onset (with likely origins from multiples sources including the auditory cortex as well as frontal cortical regions). These findings indicate that higher order cognitive influences on auditory processing can begin as early as 20 ms after onset.

Recently, Tampas et al. (2005) compared mismatch negativity (MMN) responses for neurophysiologic representations of nonspeech, frequency glide representations to acoustically similar within-category consonant-vowel (CV) speech stimuli. The MMN is a frontocentrally negative component of the auditory event-related potential that usually peaks at 100 to 250 seconds from stimulus onset and is elicited by any discriminable change in some repetitive aspect of the ongoing stimulation without regard to the subject's attention or task (Naatanen, 1999; see Chapter 26 by Abrams and Kraus for more information on MMN). Tampas et al. (2005) found more discriminability to changes for the nonspeech, frequency glide presentations and greater differences across categorical boundaries versus within boundaries. These findings indicate that: (1) speech is processed differently than other acoustic stimuli; (2) categorical perception is present as early as the level of MMN generators; and (3) parallel processing of both acoustic (sensory) and phonetic (categorical) information occurs at the level of the MMN generators.

Naatanen (1999) reviewed the MMN literature involving the perception of speech sounds by the human brain as reflected by MMN and its magnetic equivalent. Some of the key areas covered were the perception of nonlinguistic acoustic stimuli versus speech sounds as well as the development of language-specific phoneme traces. Research from a number of sources (Naatanen, 1999; Dehaene-Lambertz, 1997; Sharma and Dorman, 1999) was consistent with the existence of language-specific phonetic memory traces whose activation is independent from more generalized, nonlinguistic acoustic stimuli. That is, the MMN results suggest two parallel processes. Both speech and nonspeech sounds are mapped continuously into auditory perception, but in addition, speech sounds are preperceptually classified into different phonetic categories. It is the development/distinctiveness of these long-term memory (LTM) phonemic traces that accounts for categorical perception (i.e., an inability to perceive within-category differences). It is the LTM phonemic traces that result in individuals being unable to discriminate between different phonetic representations within a phonemic category but able to accurately discriminate across phonemic boundaries. In addition, the research shows that the development of these language-specific memory traces generally emerge between 6 and 12 months, but some phonemes emerge by 3 months (Dehaene-Lambertz and Baillet, 1998). It is likely that the LTM phonetic traces engage only those neurons that simultaneously process and become activated by specific attributes of the incoming signal, whereas there are other types of neurons that respond only to nonlinguistic changes (or to specific phonetic features, rather than to the entire phonemic/acoustic aspects) and are activated by various attributes such as onset/offset, duration, frequency, or amplitudinal changes.

To obtain the P300 electrophysiologic response, higher order cognitive functions are required. The P300 response depends on attention to and discrimination of stimulus differences and is elicited using an oddball paradigm in which a frequent (expected) stimulus is presented in a series with occasional rare (unexpected) stimuli. The subject is asked to count the number of rare events (Kraus and McGee, 1994). Most commonly, the auditory P300 is elicited by tones, but other stimuli including speech can be used. P300 has even been elicited by presenting words with one semantic attribute interspersed with words from a different category. Picton and Hillyard (1988) stated that attention, auditory discrimination, memory, and semantic expectancy appear to be underlying features of P300 responses.

In summary, one can see the impact of higher cognitive influences such as attention as early as 20 ms after onset, and by as early as 170 ms after onset, one can see the intertwining of linguistic (phonetic) and sensory (auditory) processing. By 300 ms after onset, the acoustic information has not only been transformed to phonemic representations, but has also activated lexical (word) representations, thus allowing for semantic categorizations and expectancies.

To further illustrate the limitations of a unitary view to processing, the following examples are provided:

1. Although puretone threshold testing is often thought to be an auditory task, signal detection theory teaches us that thresholds not only are dependent on the "true threshold," but are also heavily influenced by other factors, such as attention, motivation, fatigue, etc. It is because of these other factors that we do not consider a threshold to be significantly different from ones previously obtained unless it exceeds 5 dB. Hence, behavioral and cognitive processing skills influence even the most basic of auditory behavioral measurements (Gelfand, 1998).

2. For word recognition scores, students and clinicians are always warned about a foreign language influence, word frequency effects, etc. If word recognition (not even taking into account comprehension) was solely an auditory processing skill, then we would not be concerned with these other factors.

3. In the speech and hearing sciences, difficulties in speech-in-noise are often attributed to poor temporal or frequency resolution or to an inability to binaurally separate signals (ASHA, 1995; Musiek and Chermak, 1995). Yet, in the cognitive psychology domain, speech-in-noise difficulties are often attributed to backward/forward masking relative to a weakly stored memory trace of the target stimulus (Massaro, 1976) or to a limited processing capacity (Windsor and Hwang, 1999). It is likely that speech-in-noise difficulties may be due to any or a combination of these factors depending on the individual and particular listening demands.

4. One of the basic auditory skills listed in both the 1996 and 2005 ASHA Working Group documents is that of auditory localization. However, in actual realization in everyday life, localization involves not only the auditory aspect, but also a development/conception of the physical environment; auditory factors alone will not result in accurate localization and orientation of sounds. It is for this reason that individuals who are blind from birth must undergo orientation/mobility training in order to ascertain sound origins.

This research highlights the difficulties in espousing a purely auditory processing approach to the delineation of specific difficulties encountered in the processing of spoken language. On the other hand, what about the language processing views espoused by individuals such as Norma Rees, who questioned the existence of CAPDs? Rawool (2006a; 2006b) compiled a list of articles demonstrating age-related changes within the aging auditory system that impact on individuals' ability to process speech effectively. These changes are independent of any cognitive changes that may also be present and are demonstrated by: (1) anatomic changes in various CANS locations; (2) compromised processing as examined via functional magnetic resonance imaging (MRI); and (3) slower neurotransmission in the neural auditory pathways as reflected in electrophysiologic measures, such as the auditory brainstem response (ABR), auditory middle latency response, auditory late response, P300, and even the acoustic reflex pathways.

In addition to the work on aging systems, others have used speech-evoked ABR (specifically the plosive /d/) to examine the CANS capabilities of learning disabled and normally functioning children (Warrier et al., 2004; Wible et al., 2005). The investigators have found that approximately one third of learning-disabled children reveal abnormal ABR responses to the acoustic transients of speech (occurring within the region of 20 to 50 ms after onset), such as abnormally late responses for negative onset peak A and a significantly smaller slope between onset peaks V and A; these responses were especially impacted by the presence of background noise. It is likely that this difficulty results in the development of impoverished phonemic templates in LTM for many of these children and, in turn, poorly developed language skills and phonologic awareness/phonics difficulties.

Therefore, even in the most basic of behavioral auditory or speech-language tasks, it appears that auditory processing and other higher order cognitive processing skills are intimately intertwined and cannot easily be separated to their distinct components. This has been neatly summarized by Kent (1992), who stated that a substantial amount of evidence points to the conclusion that speech is perceived both on (1) the basis of the acoustic signal and (2) predictions based on its context and familiarity. Analysis of the acoustic signal (bottom-up processing) is based on the selection of cues from a continuously flowing pattern in which there are no distinct segments but yet can be extracted by the listener into discrete units (phonemes, syllables, words, etc.). Predictability of the spoken message (top-down processing) is based on the situational context, semantic-syntactic cues, and the cognitive resources of the listener. These different sources of information result in the inherent richness and redundancy of the spoken signal and allow most listeners to perceive the spoken message even when confronted with poor listening situations and/or competing stimuli.

In summary, there is clear evidence that some aspects of the processing of spoken language can be isolated as a purely auditory processing deficit; however, it is also clear that, except for the earliest stages of speech processing, subsequent processing engages both cognitive and linguistic processes. Therefore, we need to ascertain our goal when examining an individual who comes to us with difficulty in the accurate processing of speech. We can limit ourselves to delineating only those processes that can be attributed only to or almost exclusively to auditory processing (which would entail using only those procedures up to the level of the MMN generators). Or, if our goal as clinicians is to determine why individuals break down in everyday life (where both central auditory system processes and higher order cognitive processes are continually engaged/intertwined), then we should not limit ourselves to a narrow view to central auditory processing, but rather, we should adopt a view that considers all of the factors that may be involved in the normal processing of acoustic stimuli, primarily speech. We should recall that the primary reason why most individuals come to audiologists for central auditory processing testing is because they are experiencing some form of listening difficulty that is impacting them in school, work, home, or recreational endeavors. Their hope is that we will be able to determine whether they have some underlying processing deficit and, if so, the specific nature of these deficits and, in turn, give them appropriate recommendations/strategies that will help them overcome these deficits. Therefore, any approach to assisting these individuals should be one that is pragmatic, with the primary goal being to help these individuals address their needs in their everyday listening environments.

This has led to the model that I first proposed in the fifth edition of this handbook (Medwetsky, 2002) and further delineated when I was asked to write for the *ASHA Leader* in 2006 (Medwetsky, 2006). That is, rather than an auditory processing approach, I advocate one that examines the auditory processing of spoken language (i.e., Spoken-Language Processing [S-LP] model). Although I recognize the critical role of the speech pathologist in examining specific breakdowns in the various language processes, audiologists have testing tools that allow us to identify the impact of higher order language processing difficulties on S-LP, even in individuals who have been identified with good speech and language skills through traditional speech and language measures. Thus, as part of an interdisciplinary team, we can alert the speech-language pathologist to administer some higher order language tests that can corroborate and expand upon our findings. In addition, we can help psychologists become better aware of how various cognitive processes (such as attentional allocation and sequencing) may be impacting on S-LP and, in turn, learning. I even believe that the S-LP model can help to better delineate individuals with attention deficit/hyperactivity disorder (ADHD) from those who may have an S-LP disorder that is not due to any attentional allocation deficits. Thus, I strongly feel that to focus solely on an auditory processing approach limits what we can offer as professionals.

▨ CONCEPTUALIZATION OF AUDITORY PROCESSING OF SPOKEN LANGUAGE

I will not cover all aspects related to the processing of spoken language. To do so would probably entail a separate handbook. However, I will cover what I feel to be those aspects most relevant to S-LP testing and its management (as well as to contrasting ADHD and S-LP disorders [S-LPDs]). In addition, some of what will be covered will be theoretical suppositions by this author, based on the literature and my own research, that will hopefully be resolved by future research efforts.

Transduction of the Acoustic Signal

The acoustic stimulus undergoes a number of transformations before it can exist in a form that can be used by the CANS. The acoustic stimulus is transformed mechanically, hydraulically, and electrically, via the middle ear, cochlea, and central auditory nervous system (including the eighth nerve). Until the level of the superior olivary nucleus, in the medullary tegmentum, all impulses are relayed ipsilaterally. Subsequently, from the superior olivary nucleus and higher in the CANS, there are a number of decussation points (i.e., locations where fibers cross-over). These decussation points allow for the comparison of stimulus features from both cochleas (Bhatnagar and Korabic, 2006; Phillips, 2007).

Neuroelectric representations of spatial, temporal, and intensity information are extracted from the input and maintained faithfully throughout all levels of the CANS (Philips, 1998; 2007). There are least 20 regions in which tonotopic organization is maintained at the level of the cortex, which, in turn, allows for significant interaction between processing regions for attenuating and enhancing signal representations. In addition, this allows for an extremely important phenomenon known as auditory coherence to occur, more recently referred to as auditory scene analysis (ASA). ASA is concerned with how acoustic streams are maintained and segregated from each other. In everyday life, sounds can momentarily mask each other, yet somehow we are able to separate the competing sound sources. Our ability to do so has been attributed by some researchers to ASA (Bregman, 1978; 1994; Green et al., 1995; Cusak et al., 2004). These researchers feel that ASA underlies the individual's ability to localize or to separate sounds; the latter, in turn, underlies the ability by which an individual can selectively attend to a target message in the face of a competing message.

Bregman (1978), in summarizing the major findings on ASA, wrote the following:

1. Stimuli originating from the same spatial source will be grouped together.
2. Elements will be grouped together if they are similar (e.g., spectral composition).

3. Elements changing at a similar rate will tend to be grouped into the same acoustic stream. Smooth and regular change suggests signals arising from the same source, while large discontinuities in frequency and intensity suggest a change in the source (or originating from a different source).

4. Stimuli undergoing the same kinds of change at the same time are grouped as part of the same event. That is, it is likely that many frequency components arising from an acoustic source will (a) come on and go off at more or less the same time and (b) glide up and down in pitch together (be amplitude-modulated together, etc.).

5. The organization of perceptual events and subsequent decomposition of acoustic stream(s) have also been shown to be affected by the observer's goals, memories, and skills. An example of this is the ability of individuals, listening to a familiar language, to break up the acoustic stream into separate words.

These suppositions by Bregman help to explain a number of phenomena. First, elements that are grouped together into the same acoustic stream allow the listener to perceive the stream as originating from one source. Hence, this allows the listener to localize sound sources, the variables determining location dependent on the relative intensity, and phase relationships at the ears. Second, the ASA principle allows us to better understand the factors underlying binaural separation. Signals originating from two or more sources (i.e., distinguished on the basis of position in auditory space, spectral composition, and differences in the rate of change regarding amplitude, frequency, etc.) will be grouped into separate streams. This, in turn, allows the listener to separate the signals perceptually, facilitating selective/divided auditory attention, etc.

Third, ASA allows for the segmentation of acoustic signals into a number of distinguishing components. Those frequency changes that occur slowly in time and perceived to be from the same acoustic stream (e.g., low-amplitude modulation rate) are analyzed and interpreted for their suprasegmental aspects (fundamental frequency—pitch; variations in fundamental frequency contours—intonation; simultaneous variation in frequency, amplitude, and duration—stress), whereas those frequency changes that occur rapidly in time (and perceived to be from the same acoustic stream) are analyzed for their spectral features. Naatanen (1999) reported that stimulus patterns imitating the rapid-transition acoustic features of consonant-vowel-consonant (CVC) syllables had no clear hemisphere lateralization, but if temporally stretched, magnetic MMN became right-hemisphere predominant (thus suggesting that suprasegmental features of speech are best analyzed in the right hemisphere), while the MMN responses to speech stimuli were best localized to the left posterotemporal region corresponding to Wernicke's area (auditory cortex).

The ability to process and ultimately segment acoustic streams into their more fundamental components is dependent on a number of physical attributes. These include:

1. Audibility of the acoustic features contained in the stimulus.

2. Normal temporal resolution/processing abilities. Temporal resolution refers to the minimum time interval required to segregate or resolve acoustic events. Temporal resolution has been most popularly measured by gap-detection tasks in which listeners have to detect the presence of a temporal gap in a burst of noise; that is, the smaller the gap that can be detected, the better the temporal resolution. Studies of auditory gap detection have direct bearing on examining the mechanisms involved in the detection and discrimination of changes in streams of sounds across time (Phillips, 1998). Many speech sounds are distinguished on the basis of very rapid spectral components. One example is identifying the place of articulation for initial stop consonants; research shows that the key information is contained in the plosive burst (interval lasting approximately 20 ms) and in the rapid formant transition to the following vowel. Another example of an acoustic cue of extremely short duration is that of voice onset time (VOT). The VOT allows us to distinguish initial voiced from voiceless stop consonants (e.g., /b/ vs. /p/, /t/ vs. /d/, /k/vs. /g/) based on whether we perceive a period of silence between the initial stop consonant and subsequent vowel. If a gap is detected, then a voiceless stop consonant is perceived; otherwise, a voiced stop consonant is perceived. VOTs vary from approximately 20 to 45 ms depending on the particular stop consonants produced. Individuals whose time resolution is very poor (e.g., longer than 100 ms) will have great difficulty perceiving many speech sounds on the basis of their rapidly changing temporal components.

3. Normal frequency resolution. Frequency resolution refers to an individual's ability to discriminate successive sounds on the basis of frequency, which, in turn, allows the person to perceive the frequency of the different formants (peak energy bands) of vowels and frequency peaks in consonant sounds. The threshold limen for frequency (i.e., the frequency difference that must exist before an individual can distinguish that the sounds are, in fact, different) is typically larger for listeners who have a hearing loss than those who have normal hearing. Frequency resolution may also be impaired in some individuals with S-LPD.

4. Normal amplitude resolution. Amplitude resolution refers to an individual's ability to discriminate successive (identical) sounds on the basis of amplitude differences. Amplitude resolution plays a key role in (a) allowing the listener to perceive amplitude modulations as conveyed in the overall amplitude envelope (one key component of overall suprasegmental transmission) and syllabic stress, and (b) consonant-vowel intensity relationships,

which also allow the listener to perceive the number of syllables within words. Amplitude resolution is usually not impaired in most listeners, even in those who have a significant hearing loss.

Higher Order Cognitive Processing of the Acoustic Stimulus

After the transduction of the acoustic stimulus into its neurologic representation at the level of the auditory nerve, it undergoes a number of subsequent transformations at the various levels of the CANS. Various types of neurons become engaged and, depending on their properties, extract/enhance different acoustic features. By the level of the auditory cortex, not only are there neurons that can detect/discriminate specific features, but there also appear to be specific neuronal populations that do not respond to any single frequencies or their combinations, but rather to the ratio of their formant frequencies, such as f2/f1 ratios (Naatanen, 1999). The central function of these neurons and the phonetic traces that are created is presumably to act as recognition templates in speech perception, enabling one to correctly perceive the speech sounds uttered. Each phonemic input probably activates its closest phonemic trace, the one best corresponding to it. There are likely many phonemic trace alternatives for the same phoneme category, but the end result is that the ultimate conscious perception of the phoneme is categorically based. That is, although there may be many phonetic feature variations, the brain ultimately develops quite specific phonemic boundaries for which any variation within the boundary is perceived as one phoneme and any acoustic variation across the categorical boundary is perceived as belonging to another phonemic category. These neuronal populations appear to reside in Wernicke's area (a region encircling the auditory cortex). Syllables and words also appear to have their own recognition patterns or traces, whereby the phonologic representations are combined. In the literature, these syllabic/word phonemic representations have come to be known as the phonologic lexemes, which, in turn, activate their respective semantic representation, known as the lemma (Caramazza, 1997; Levelt, 2001). Note that suprasegmental features, such as syllabic stress, pauses, etc., and syntactical features somehow interact with phonologic decoding to ultimately determine the lemma that is activated. Examples of this interaction include:

- Per'-mit (stress on first syllable) is a noun and means a license, whereas per-mit' (stress on the second syllable) is a verb and means to allow.
- "That's an airplane" (with falling intonation) is a statement, whereas "That's an airplane?" (with rising intonation) is a question.
- The word "watch" has different meanings, such as "to watch" (verb; stress on *watch*), and "new watch" (noun; stress on the preceding word *new*).

The process of matching the lexical (i.e., word) representation with its acoustic input is known as lexical decoding, and the speed with which this occurs is known as lexical decoding speed. Another way to define lexical decoding speed is the speed and accuracy with which one can decode the incoming speech stimuli into their corresponding words. Lexical decoding speed depends on a number of features, including:

- An individual's neurologic representation of phonemic templates. The more disorganized/inaccurately represented, the more inaccurate speech perception will be and/or the longer it will take to activate the corresponding lemma.
- Semantic organization/clustering. The more organized the neuronal pathways are regarding the characterization of various semantic attributes (e.g., animate/inanimate, large/small, motile/immobile, shape, etc.), the faster the speed is in which the phonologic representation can activate its corresponding lemma (i.e., conceptual representation).
- Spread of activation. When a concept is activated, neuronal excitation spreads to other neuronal regions to which it has become associated. For example, upon hearing the word "animal" in a sentence, all neuronal regions representing concepts associated with animal become activated to some extent, although, those animals that have been most frequently encountered through various exposures (such as television, reading, or actual encounter) will have the strongest activations.
- Priming is a specific aspect related to the spread of activation, whereby syntactic, semantic, and even phonologic information ultimately restricts the neuronal region of highest activation to a limited number of choices for information that has yet to be presented. For example, in the sentence "My mother baked a "/k/…,"" when the word "baked" is uttered, this results in the neuronal regions most associated with baking to be activated. When "a" is uttered, this indicates that the following word will be an object, negating any baking utensils as being possible choices, and it will be of a singular form. Last, when the initial phoneme /k/ of the incomplete word is heard, this eliminates the word pie, and thus the only choices left are cake and quiche. Although quiche is a possible choice, the word cake has a greater likelihood of occurrence with baking and thus is more strongly connected and consequently has a lower activation threshold in this context.

Although not usually characterized as lexical decoding speed, the intertwining of linguistic and auditory processing (as well as a number of cognitive mechanisms that will be discussed in the upcoming sections) is what allows one to easily understand conversations on the telephone, even though acoustic information below 300 Hz and above 3,000 Hz is not available through most telephone lines. It is only when someone says an unfamiliar name/street address or term that a normal-hearing/processing listener encounters any difficulty. At that point, the talker may need to spell out the word (but even then, the talker may need to identify the word begun by that speech sound, such as /f/ for frank or /s/ for Spanish, since many of these speech sounds rely on acoustic energy being present above 3,000 Hz). Thus, it is the presence of the linguistic/situational context redundancies that allow the listener to process the information so easily, but in the absence of any key contextual information, it is only then that the listener becomes "hard of hearing."

When discussing the processing of spoken language, I will focus on those situations where previously presented information has corresponding concepts stored in LTM, that is, not entailing any mechanisms involved in learning new lexicon. In the left hemisphere, this refers to the language processing region (e.g., phonetic templates, semantic concepts represented by lemma and syntactic rules), whereas in the right hemisphere, this entails the processing of the various prosodic aspects that help one to process speech more easily/efficiently. Please note that LTM refers to stored neuronal templates, residing in a resting state. This information is not readily accessible to us, that is, it resides in our subconsciousness. It is only when a specific cluster of neurons have been activated and are firing with sufficient strength that we become aware of the concept that these neurons represent. Activation of these stored concepts depends on a number of factors:

- Activation threshold for a particular concept. This depends on (1) the frequency with which a concept has been activated in the past (i.e., frequently activated concepts have stronger neuronal connections and thus are more easily triggered) and (2) the emotional importance of the concept to that individual, such as one's name) (Kahneman, 1973; Klatzky, 1984). The activation threshold likely relates to limbic and hippocampal influences resulting in lowered activation thresholds that result in easy activation (Cartling, 1995).
- Individual's expectations, which depend highly on the topic and situational context.
- Linguistic context (such as any preceding syntactic, semantic, and phonologic information) as well as world knowledge. For example, in the sentence "My mother baked a /k/...," the individual uses the preceding linguistic information as well as world knowledge about the topic to complete the sentence without ever hearing the word "cake."
- Amount of attentional allocation given to that particular stimulus (i.e., attentional mechanisms excite and temporarily lower the activating thresholds for those stored concepts corresponding to the target stimulus).
- Strength and discriminability of the target stimulus. Strength refers to stimulus intensity; stimuli with

strength sufficiently greater than the concept's activation thresholds are more likely to activate it from LTM. Discriminability refers to the presence or absence of salient features within a stimulus. That is, there is a greater likelihood that a stimulus will be processed accurately if its featural content is complete. Stimulus saliency is affected by both extrinsic and intrinsic factors. Extrinsic factors include the presence of competing noise (possibly masking certain acoustic features), limited signal bandwidth (e.g., transmitted signals across telephone lines), and distorted speech productions, whereas intrinsic factors include the degree to which outer/inner hair cells are intact, sharpness of tuning curves, and effectiveness of various CANS neuronal regions to accurately extract acoustic features.

INTEGRATION

Integration is defined here as the ability to combine information from different sensory sources into unified concepts. One form of integration involves the integration of acoustic or linguistic information from different processing regions. A second form is the degree to which one can integrate information across modalities (e.g., integrating acoustic with visual information, such as in lipreading). One example of integration in the broadest sense is localization. As mentioned earlier, the localization of a sound in space is a binaural phenomenon, whereby interaural differences in both intensity and phase relations allow the listener to determine the origin of a particular sound source. Because this process requires an internal fusion of the signals reaching both ears, localization is an example of binaural fusion or integration. Difficulties in localization would be manifested by a decreased ability to locate respective sound sources and, in turn, likely impact binaural separation. The latter would result in a decreased ability to attend to the target source in competing message situations (i.e., a poorer ability to function in noisy settings).

Another example of integration is the efficient transfer of information between hemispheres across the corpus callosum. As mentioned earlier, suprasegmental information (such as syllabic demarcation, prosody, stress, overall pitch contours) is processed by most individuals in the right hemisphere, whereas linguistic information (such as segmental cues, lexicon, semantic and syntactic relations) is processed in the left hemisphere. On dichotic tests involving spoken language (i.e., where the stimuli presented to one ear are different than those presented to the other ear), young children typically show a right ear advantage. This right ear advantage is due to the neural transmission pathways as well as corpus callosum development. The strongest neurologic connections between the ears and cortical processing regions are those that involve the contralateral pathways. Subsequently, information presented to the right ear is transmitted most effectively via the contralateral pathway to the speech/language processing (left) hemisphere, whereas information presented to the left ear is transmitted most effectively to the right hemisphere. However, because speech is processed primarily in the left hemisphere, the information must be relayed across the corpus callosum (i.e., the largest tract of fibers connecting the two hemispheres) to the left hemisphere. Since the corpus callosum does not fully mature until 11 to 12 years of age, younger children typically reveal a right ear advantage in dichotic listening situations (e.g., in a party, younger children will likely hear the main talker better in the right ear). In addition to this normal age effect, there are individuals who, on dichotic tasks, reveal a much greater difference between ears than would be expected. That is, they show a disparate level of performance between ears, with right ear performance being significantly better for speech stimuli; on nonverbal tasks, the opposite may occur with left ear performance being significantly superior.

As mentioned earlier, the processing of speech entails the processing of not only the linguistic aspects (segmental aspects of speech), but also the suprasegmental (prosodic) aspects. That is, at the same time the phonetic aspects of speech are being analyzed, the individual is also processing the prosodic aspects of speech as well. For most individuals, suprasegmental information is thought to be processed in the right hemisphere, in parallel to the segmental, lexical information being processed in the left hemisphere. The work of Meyer and colleagues (Meyer et al., 2005; Zaehle et al., 2004) has shown that the left hemisphere preferentially extracts rapid information from short integration windows, whereas the right hemisphere is more adept at extracting slow information from long integrations windows; these attributes are undoubtedly due to the response characteristics of the neuronal regions located in the auditory cortical regions within each hemisphere. The ability of the right posterior temporal gyrus (encompassing right Heschl's gyrus and surrounding neuronal regions) to process the slower changing amplitude modulations and frequency contours allows it to contribute to speech processing by effectively determining the overall sentence prosody. Recently, Abrams et al. (2008), using electrophysiologic measures, determined that right-hemisphere auditory cortex is dominant for coding syllable patterns in speech (i.e., syllabic demarcation). The efficient, accurate processing of speech, therefore, entails auditory-linguistic integration of the various components carried in the speech signal across different processing regions in both hemispheres. How the different cues come to be integrated as a unitary concept and where this occurs anatomically/physiologically is not known at the present time. The presence of suprasegmental information has been shown to improve listener accuracy, especially in difficult listening situations (Collier and Hart, 1975; Wingfield, 1996). These researchers found that that the presence of suprasegmental cues, in conjunction with syntactical markers, helps the listener to divide spoken language into its component phrase structures (i.e., various suprasegmental cues, such as rhythm and pauses, have been found to

coincide with clausal boundaries). This helps the listener to derive the intended semantic content as well as process more information per chunk, which allows the individual to process longer sentences. Prosodic information also allows the listener to perceive yes/no questions ("That's a car?") on the basis of a rising fundamental frequency contour and even the affective (emotional) aspects conveyed by the overall intonation patterns (Wildgruber et al., 2005; Ethofer et al., 2006). On the other hand, some aspects of suprasegmental features, specifically the aspect of syllabic stress, have been determined to occur within the left hemisphere (Arciuli and Slowiaczek, 2007). When one considers that syllabic stress is determined by frequency, durational, and amplitudinal aspects of short duration, Ariculli and Slowiaczek's findings make much sense. Syllabic stress also plays a vital role in the determination of the specific conceptual realization of the word; for example, in most two syllable words, when the stress is on the first word, it is a noun, and when it present on the second syllable, it is a verb (as illustrated earlier by per'-mit [noun] vs. per-mit' [verb]). Last, suprasegmental markers have been shown to help the listener segregate competing voices from one another, thus enabling the listener to attend to and process the target talker more effectively in difficult listening situations.

▧ SHORT-TERM MEMORY

The active, conscious awareness of concepts is known as short-term memory (STM). STM is limited, both in capacity and time. The duration of STM has been estimated from being as short as 2 seconds to as long as 30 seconds; however, these time variations are likely due to different experimental paradigms. For example, the absence of any continued processing of a concept or the presence of any factors interfering with subsequent attention to that concept results in an individual being unable to recall the concept after approximately 2 seconds. However, this does not mean that the neuronal region is still not in a primed state; it is just not strong enough for the person to recall without assistance. However, if the examiner were to provide a number of alternatives as to what the concept might have been, most individuals will be able to correctly choose the correct item as long as not too much time has passed.

Information can be maintained in STM for longer durations if the individual engages some aspect of attentional allocation (e.g., subauditorization, visualization, analysis of content). Processes such as these result in the neurons firing over and over again, thus maintaining a firing level that is above its activation threshold and allowing the trace to remain in conscious memory. Therefore, the critical variable in maintaining information in STM is some aspect of attention. Attention is defined here as the neurophysiologic process whereby the targeted neuronal regions have temporarily adjusted (i.e., lowered the activation thresholds) in order to remain in a heightened state with ongoing neural firing. In the absence of sufficient attention, there is a cessation of firing, and the percept fades from STM; thus, it may not enter more permanent forms of memory (such as intermediate-term memory or LTM). Therefore, attention is critical for remembering information. Who has not forgotten where they have put their keys? It is not because of a memory problem that we forgot, but rather, it is due to not having allocated sufficient attention in the first place (i.e., we may have been thinking about something else and thus did not allocate sufficient attention to form strong enough neuronal linkages to allow any longer term memory traces to develop).

Before we leave this topic, it would be well to discuss the differences between STM and working memory. These terms are sometimes used interchangeably. However, it appears that most researchers now use these terms differently and differentiate them on the type of processing that might be engaged on a particular task. STM generally refers to the passive maintenance of information such as entailed on a straightforward digit span task (e.g., *repeat these numbers*). Working memory entails the notion of the manipulation of information (Fuster, 1997). In general, working memory involves: (1) attentional allocation and inhibitory processes; (2) phonologic (verbal material) and visuospatial (nonlinguistic information) representations; and (3) various processing mechanisms to manipulate the various sensory aspects that have been activated.

Short-Term Memory Span

There is a limit to how much can actually be held in STM or working memory at any one point in time, known as the span of apprehension. Initially, Miller (1956) proposed that, on average, humans could hold seven elements (chunks) of information in STM, regardless of the type of stimuli (e.g., digits, letters, words, etc.). Later research has revealed that the memory span does indeed depend on the category of chunks used (e.g., span is around seven for digits, six for letters, and five for words) and even on specific features within a category; for example, STM span is lower for long words (i.e., with more syllables) than for short words.

Cowan (2001) has recently proposed that STM actually has a capacity of about four chunks in young adults. It appears that the maximum number of neuronal regions that can maximally fire at any one time is four. It is not clear whether attentional allocation can be allocated to more than one region at a time or it is shifted rapidly from one region or another, thus maintaining a neuronal trace in an active state. Yet, it does appear that there is a limit to how many traces can be maintained in an active state (i.e., four neuronal regions). Any attempt to exceed this capacity would be self-defeating because one would not be able to shift attention to more than four regions without one region fading from an active state. Thus, time is the key element. This does not mean that one cannot recall more than four items at a time. For example, there are individuals who can recall up to 80 digits at a time. However, the means by which they do so is by using

encoding strategies whereby the digits in a list are grouped (usually in groups of three to five), which, in turn, can be associated/grouped further (Ericsson and Kintsch, 1995). It is important to note that practicing skills such as these does not expand general working memory capacity. For example, in an individual who can recall 80 digits, when it comes to the recall of random words (where grouping is much more difficult), the individual may not recall any more than five to six words. Another example of increasing the number of items recalled (but still limited by the number of neuronal regions that can be actively maintained in working memory) is when a linguistically/contextually redundant sentence is presented. As mentioned earlier, young adults may recall five randomly presented words. However, many adults will not have trouble recalling verbatim the following sentence: "My mother and father went to the store, bought some milk and cookies, came home by car, and went to bed." This sentence is comprised of a total of 21 words, yet a person may not have difficulty recalling any of the words. The reason is that the syntactic structure, semantic relations, use of suprasegmental inflection and pausing (coinciding with grammatical clauses), and world knowledge all act in concert to allow the individual to process this sentence in five chunks, that is, within the working memory capacity of the individual.

There are several hypotheses about the nature of the capacity limit. One is that there is a limited pool of cognitive resources available to keep representations active and thereby available for processing (Just and Carpenter, 1992). Another theory is that memory traces in STM decay within a few seconds unless refreshed through rehearsal, and because the speed of rehearsal is limited, we can maintain only a limited amount of information (Towse et al., 2000). Another theory is that representations in STM can interfere with each other (Waugh and Norman, 1965), such as through (1) content interference (the more similar the content, the greater the interference) or (2) verbal rehearsal (be it vocal or subvocal), which then interferes with the maintenance of other items being held in STM. It is likely that STM (or working memory) span is influenced by the combination of all of these factors.

In general, the STM span for verbal content depends strongly on the amount of time it takes for the individual to speak the content aloud (or via subvocalizations) and on the lexical status of the contents (i.e., the familiarity/utilization frequency of the words for that individual; in turn, this impacts on the organization of neural connectivity, firing rates, etc.). Thus, the more familiar the content of an item, the faster that item can activate its corresponding neuronal region and the stronger the memory trace is. As mentioned earlier, maintenance of memory traces in STM over time is highly dependent on the amount of attentional allocation to maintain neuronal firing.

Last, the content in STM or working memory appears to involve neuronal representations within the frontal lobe and prefrontal cortex (i.e., after initial processing within the sensory regions and the traces are in recurrent maintenance in STM).

SEQUENCING

Not only does information have to be maintained in STM or working memory, but somehow the information must also be tagged regarding its order of occurrence. In reviewing the literature, it is clear that the lateral prefrontal cortex (LPFC) is involved in formulating and carrying out plans and sequences of action (Romine and Reynolds, 2004). This includes the representation and construction of sequences of spoken and written language (Fuster, 2001), with one role being to consciously represent sequences of speech or behaviors and the other role being to initiate and execute them in an orderly fashion. Because of its vital role in working memory, it is likely that this same region is also involved in the receptive aspects of ordering phonologic information to derive its lexical representations and lexical storage/sequencing. Recent work by Gelfand and Bookheimer (2003) supports this contention in that their data indicated that left prefrontal cortex (PFC) areas appear to mediate the processes underlying phonologic processing. Their data also suggested a role of the posterior portion of Broca's area in subvocal articulation, which also contributes to the ability to maintain phonologic sequence within phonologic working memory. At the heart of phonologic working memory is an articulatory control process (i.e., rehearsal) that acts to refresh and maintain phonologic material in the memory store for a short period. That is, an individual can form and hold in phonologic storage a sequentially accurate phonologic representation of incoming speech, thus permitting the listener to process the input, especially input for which sequential order is important to comprehension, such as directions (Montgomery, 2002). Subsequent recall of information, such as entailed on a memory recall task, requires also that there must be some mechanism available for recording sequential information. That is, the memory trace must contain information about the occurrence of events in relationship to each other (Gillam et al., 1995). For example, on serial recall tasks, these ordered item presentations presumably entail intermittent reactivations in rehearsal processes at some point in recall (Baddeley, 1986). On the other hand, Lee and Estes (1981) proposed that individuals form a mental representation that consists essentially of the words in order, with mental markers for their serial positions.

ATTENTIONAL ALLOCATION

Because the human listener has a limited capacity for processing incoming stimuli (Miller, 1956; Kahneman, 1973; Windsor and Hwang, 1999), it has been proposed that the importance of attentional allocation is to limit the amount of information processed at any one time (Kahneman, 1973). Attentional allocation, under the control of the central executor (to be discussed later), allows the individual to focus selectively on a limited amount of information (and, in competing noise situations, to block out irrelevant stimuli), thereby maximizing the extent to which target in-

formation is processed and stored. There appear to be various stages in which attentional allocation can be effectively implemented in S-LP. The earliest impact of attentional allocation appears to occur within 20 to 50 ms after stimulus onset and appears to be a gating mechanism that is implemented at the levels of the thalamus and lateral Heschl's gyrus (Frank et al., 2001; Petkov et al., 2004). After consciously selecting the acoustic information of interest, the PFC, via the cortical-thalamic loop, gates incoming acoustic information by filtering the "undesired" spectrotemporal and auditory location information, while allowing the target acoustic information to pass through for further processing. At the level of the sensory memory stage (~200 to 250 ms), attentional allocation (i.e., neuronal stimulation) allows for the increased likelihood that the stored corresponding information in LTM will become activated and thus enter an individual's STM. Subsequently, attentional allocation plays an important role in the maintenance of information in STM and ultimately a role in transferring the information to LTM (by altering the strength of neural connectivity as well as organizational architecture); that is, one component of attentional allocation—elaborative rehearsal—seems to be required for effective LTM storage. Elaborative rehearsal requires significant cognitive effort and involves either (1) rote memorization for stimuli with minimal or no contextual cues present (e.g., the rote memorization of information, either auditory alone or combined with other senses, such as in memorizing a list of numbers whereby the individual repeats or even visualizes the string of numbers) or (2) active processing of information in which much contextual information is present (i.e. thinking about the meaning of the new information while attempting to relate it to information already in LTM; this may also engage visualization). Anything that interferes with the active processing of the signal will impact on the subsequent retention of the information processed.

Terms such as attention deficit disorder may imply that attention is a unitary process; however, individuals who use such terms classify attention on the basis of observable behaviors (e.g., *Diagnostic and Statistical Manual of Mental Disorders, 4th Edition* characterization of ADHD symptoms; Barkley, 1998) rather than the underlying cognitive processes. In fact, attention can be allocated in many ways depending on the task. These include:

1. Preparatory attention: the decision process whereby the listener chooses which stimuli to attend to prior to the presentation.
2. Active processing: the ability to repeat (rote-memory span task) or elaborate on the information processed (such as thinking about and analyzing contextually presented information as would occur in most everyday listening situations). This process maintains and slows down the rate of decay of items stored in STM/working memory as well as enhances transfer of information into LTM.
3. Focused attention: the ability to attend to a signal in quiet or in noise.

4. Selective attention: the ability to attend to a target stimulus in the face of one or more competing stimuli.
5. Divided attention: the ability to share attention among two or more competing target stimuli.
6. Sustained attention: the ability to maintain attention to target stimuli over a sustained period of time.
7. Vigilance: the ability to maintain preparedness for response to an intermittent signal (such as a mother of a newborn who is able to ignore essentially all stimuli while sleeping but will jump to her feet the instant she perceives her baby to be crying).

As mentioned earlier, it appears that human beings are able to shift attentional allocation among a maximum of three to five active neuronal firing regions (Cowan, 2001). The limiting factor appears to be the extent to which the PFC can shift attentional focus and maintain neuronal firing among the different neuronal regions. That is, there is a time constraint in which reactivation of a neuronal region must occur before neuronal decay begins to take place, and once the limit of three to five neuronal regions has been reached, any more information results in overloading the attentional allocation system and subsequent forgetting of information.

Neurophysiologic Underpinnings of Attentional Allocation

The following is my best consolidation of information of a very complex system that involves great interconnectivity and parallel systems between many cortical and subcortical regions. Relevant articles are listed at the end of this section, and Figures 25.1 and 25.2 provide a framework for locating a number of the key brain areas that will be described in this chapter.

At the core is the PFC. The PFC has often been referred to as the central executive system (or internal gatekeeper) and is responsible for regulating behaviors and inhibiting irrelevant stimuli/responses (Barkley, 1998). The PFC is actually comprised of a number of closely related but distinct physiologic substrates that direct and integrate functions across various processing regions. The PFC is responsible for a number of critical functions, such as self-directed actions, organization of behavior across time, and goal-directed, future-oriented, purposeful action. One of its most important roles (localized to the dorsolateral PFC) is that of attentional allocation (i.e., determining the stimuli/behaviors to which resources will be focused/allocated at any point in time); thus, it plays a large role in controlling our overall behavior. The PFC has both efferent and afferent connections to the anterior cingulate cortex (ACC) and the striatum (consisting of the putamen, caudate nucleus, and the nucleus accumbens). The dorsal region of the ACC (dACC) appears to play an evaluative role in the attentional decision-making process by assessing the stimulus features that best match the intended PFC actions, thereby allotting greater attention to behaviorally relevant stimuli, while limiting the processing of distracting events. For example, when distracting voices intrude upon a conversation at a noisy social gathering, we must concentrate more attention on the speakers of interest to better comprehend their speech. It appears that the dACC ascertains and boosts attentional resources toward the behaviorally relevant stimuli by narrowing the neurons' receptive field, such that their activity is driven mainly by the attended stimulus. Thus, the dACC biases processing resources to

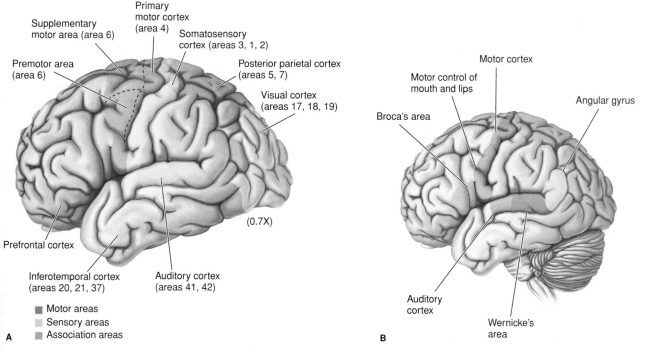

FIGURE 25.1   A, Surface anatomy of the brain. B, Key components of the language system.

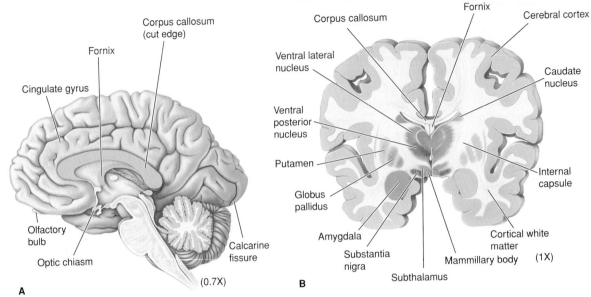

FIGURE 25.2   A, Medial view of the brain. B, Cross-sectional anatomy of the brain.

task-relevant dimensions. There is also a feedback component; on a moment-by-moment basis, in which the particular dimension that has been processed is compared with what is anticipated in working memory (i.e., fed back to the PFC), if the information is congruent, those particular stimulus features are maintained in working memory, and if not, a change in attentional focus occurs within the dACC (thus the dACC plays a critical evaluative role in conflict management). As mentioned, there are also efferent/afferent connections from the PFC to the striatum. The PFC modulates striatal synaptic function so that the incoming stimulus features best matching the targeted dimensions will be the most likely to activate subsequent neuronal synapses and be processed at the level of the PFC. Thus, the striatum plays more of a role as a relay station, whereby different weightings are applied to neuronal synapses subsequent to PFC and dACC actions.

The striatum, in turn, has afferent/efferent fibers to the basal ganglia (BG), which in turn, has afferent/efferent fibers to the thalamus. In the past, the BG (globus pallidus and substantia nigra) was often thought to just be linked to efficient motor movements, and when damaged in people with Parkinson's disease, tremors would often be displayed. Recently, the BG has been determined to also play a key role in attentional allocation and sequencing, be it of motoric movements or thought processes. The striatal projections to the BG exhibit an inhibitory function, whereas the BG structures exhibit an inhibitory function on the thalamic structures. The BG nuclei are predominantly in an active firing state (i.e., in the absence of any striatal activation, they serve to inhibit thalamic neurons from firing). Therefore, when the striatal neurons fire, they serve as a brake on the BG neurons, which serves to disinhibit the thalamic neurons. It is the striatal weightings that determine which acoustic features will receive attention and which will be disinhibited or ignored.

It is this gating or breaking action on stimuli transmitted to the thalamus and, in turn, to the sensory areas of the cortex that allows for coherent transmission of "targeted" stimulus features in the presence of distracting "irrelevant" features. Finally, parallel loops between the cortical sensory areas and the PFC allow for further processing of designated sensory input and ultimately activation of the corresponding LTM neuronal representations.

One last mechanism that should be mentioned regarding attentional allocation is the reticular activating system, which is a set of subcortical structures that underlies arousal level. Arousal level modulates the degree to which the PFC is able to function and allocate attention effectively. Thus, significant under- or overarousal greatly hinders effective PFC functioning, and it is only at moderate arousal levels that the PFC performs its executive functions in its most efficacious manner.

To obtain a greater understanding of the anatomic regions and neurophysiologic processes that subserve attention, the reader is referred to the following: Portas et al. (1998), Frank et al. (2001), Petkov et al. (2004), Weissman et al. (2005), Gruber et al. (2006), Chang et al. (2007), Hazy et al. (2007), http://en.wikipedia.org/wiki/Anterior_cingulate_cortex, and http://en.wikipedia.org/wiki/Striatum.

Selective Attention

Processing in noise versus quiet presents significantly different challenges to the listener. Selective attention can be defined as the ability to selectively focus on one stream of information while ignoring or blocking out competing, "irrelevant stimuli." The ability to attend, process, and accurately identify target acoustic stimuli in the presence of competing stimuli depends on at least three factors:

1. Neurophysiologic ability to derive/separate acoustic streams and, in turn, selectively attend to the designated acoustic stream of information
2. Strength/fidelity of the CANS neurologic firing patterns (i.e., how faithfully, cohesively, and strongly the CANS system neurons transmit the incoming auditory information) impacts on the strength of the resulting memory traces; for example, in someone with a hearing loss, the CANS neurons would transmit at least some aspects of the incoming auditory information that was either of less intensity or even absent to higher cortical areas and, in turn, would result in weaker memory traces.
3. Mental load of the task relative to listener's processing capacity.

The following sections elaborate on the functional processes used in selective attention to provide an understanding of the many ways selective attention can break down in everyday life.

AUDITORY SCENE ANALYSIS

As discussed earlier, the sounds that arrive at a listener's ear are often a mixture of stimuli arising from different sources. The human auditory system takes advantage of the regularities in sounds we hear to perceptually separate competing stimuli into different acoustic streams, each of which ideally corresponds to a single source. This ability, known as ASA, uses probabilities of co-occurrences in sounds that allow acoustic elements to be grouped into streams and, once formed, allow the listener to select one (or more) streams and reject others. Medwetsky (1994) studied the effectiveness of different acoustic cues in selective attention by examining the listeners' ability to selectively attend/recall target sentences in the presence of competing sentences. The target and competing sentences were presented under headphones and presented to either the same or separate ears. Both target and competing sentences were presented by the same female talker, or one sentence was spoken by the female talker and the other by a male talker. Medwetsky found that spatial location was the most effective cue, but even in the absence of spatial cues (i.e., sentences were presented in the same headphone), gender differences (e.g., fundamental frequency) allowed listeners to perform nearly as well as when spatial cues were present. Note that even when neither spatial nor talker cues were present, when provided the topics of both sentences beforehand (for short sentences), listeners were able to recall the target sentence with a fair degree of accuracy. They likely were able to do so based on the short-term spectral coherence and linguistic information present in the sentences, although they could not perform the task with the same precision as when spatial and fundamental frequency cues were present. That is, even though both sentences were presented by the same talker, within each sentence, the transition from one speech element to another exhibited a cohesive spectral transition that was different from the other sentence; in addition, the different linguistic content in each sentence allowed

the listener to ascertain which of the competing words made most sense to include in each sentence relative to the specific sentence topic.

Speech-in-Noise

Speech-in-noise refers to the ability of a listener to filter speech that is embedded in a nonlinguistic noise; in general, this type of masking is referred to as energetic or peripheral masking. One important component of speech-in-noise processing involves frequency resolution/tuning curves for initial speech-to-noise enhancement. That is, the sharper the tuning curves, the more easily extraneous frequency components can be rejected from interfering with speech perception. However, in individuals with hearing loss (and likely in some individuals with normal hearing with processing-related disorders), the tuning curves tend to be wider and allow for more extraneous stimuli to be processed.

Another aspect that can affect speech-in-noise perception is poor temporal resolution. Temporal resolution is typically measured by the ability to detect brief silent gaps between two short identical sounds (single-channel gap detection is typically in the range of 2 to 11 ms in adults) or to detect silent gaps delineated by spectrally disparate spectral markers (i.e., where the stimulus component[s] prior to the gap is of a different frequency region than that following the gap [between-channel gap detection]). Between-channel gaps are typically in the range of 10 to 20 ms or longer depending on the stimuli and are more typical of what happens in the actual perception of complex stimuli, such as unvoiced stop consonants /p/ and /t/ (Smith et al., 2006). Stuart (2005) examined one aspect of temporal resolution for word recognition in continuous and interrupted noise in children. Stuart indicated that adult listeners typically experience a perceptual advantage (i.e., a release from masking) when interrupted noise is used compared with continuous noise at equivalent signal-to-noise ratios, which is evidence of the benefits of good temporal resolving power. Northwestern University–Children's Perception of Speech (NU-CHIPS) words were used for subjects 6 and 16 years of age with continuous or interrupted background noise (signal-to-noise ratios ranging from 10 to –20 dB). Stuart (2005) found that performance:

1. Was better in the interrupted noise
2. Improved in either condition with age
3. Did not reach adult-like performance until 11 years of age

Stuart concluded that these changes reflected maturation of the CANS.

Warrier et al. (2004) compared speech-evoked cortical responses in background noise or in quiet for normal control children and children with learning disabilities (LD). Timing differences between the electrophysiologic responses were obtained in quiet and in background noise. The results indicated that 23% of those with LD exhibited cortical neural timing abnormalities such that their neurophysiologic representations of speech sounds became significantly more distorted in the presence of background noise as compared to their normal peers. A number of these LD children also participated in a commercial training program that included the training of phoneme perception in the presence of background noise. Results not only showed improved phonologic perception, but also improved cortical timing.

The aforementioned studies show that the integrity of transmission within the auditory nervous system is important in processing speech in the presence of noise and that this physiologic ability improves with age. However, the Warrier et al. (2004) study showed that only 23% of their LD children exhibited abnormal cortical responses in the presence of noise, which is not surprising considering the heterogeneity of this population. The following two studies demonstrate that neurophysiologic transmission in the CANS is not the only factor that impacts on speech perception in noise.

Bell and Wilson (2001) developed sentence material that varied in frequency of word use and phonetic confusability. Each sentence contained three key words (seven to nine syllables), with each word characterized as high or low use frequency and high or low confusability (based on the number of other phonemically similar words). The results indicated that, in both quiet and noise listening conditions, high-use words were more intelligible than low-use words and there was an advantage for phonetically unique words. These results indicate that significant nonacoustic sources of variation can impact spoken word recognition in the presence of noise.

Bradlow and Alexander (2007) indicated that previous research on speech recognition had shown that differences can be demonstrated under less than optimal listening conditions between native and proficient nonnative listeners. This is primarily because nonnative listeners appear to be less effective in using compensatory information at higher levels of processing to recover from information loss at the phoneme recognition level (i.e., nonnative speakers have less developed phonemic representations for their nonnative language in LTM). These authors investigated whether this disadvantage could be overcome in the presence of background noise by manipulation of (1) sentences that varied in degree of last word predictability and (2) how the productions were spoken (ordinary vs. clear speech). While native listeners were able to benefit from either source of enhancement, nonnative listeners' speech-in-noise performance improved only when both sources of enhancement were present (i.e., high predictability and use of clear speech). The authors concluded that (1) speech-in-noise recognition performance can be impacted at processing levels higher than just acoustic transmission within the CANS (be it at the level of phonemic representations or the semantic/syntactic level) and (2) nonnative listeners and, presumably by extension, individuals with S-LP disorders can take advantage of acoustic enhancements in the speech signal as well; however, they require more sources of enhancement to improve performance.

Last, although backward and forward masking have sometimes been attributed to being lower order CANS phenomena, it appears that they are dependent on both lower order and higher ordering processing mechanisms (note that in background masking tasks, a stimulus is presented immediately before a masker of different acoustic attributes, such as a tone presented immediately prior to a shower-type noise, whereas in forward masking tasks, the stimulus is presented immediately after the masker). That is, the strength/fidelity of CANS neurologic firing patterns impact on the strength of ensuing memory traces. Weak and/or distorted acoustic/neurologic transmission results in weak memory traces that are easily susceptible to the effects of forward/backward masking and thus can result in a reduced ability to perceive signals in noise.

In summary, the evidence indicates that speech-in-noise performance is affected by multiple mechanisms. This has important implications for diagnostic assessment and subsequent management for those with such difficulties. Although the use of FM systems improves listening performance in the presence of background noise, by itself, it may not result in long-term neurologic changes to enable the listener to process speech better in the absence of such systems. By determining the specific underlying cause for the speech-in-noise difficulties, the clinician can initiate a therapeutic process that may address the core of this difficulty and thus ultimately overcome the speech-in-noise deficit.

Binaural Separation

Binaural separation refers to listening situations in which a listener is exposed to acoustic stimuli originating from different locations in space and the ability of the listener to use acoustic cues reaching both ears. Research has shown that spatial cues are the most effective in enabling individuals to selectively attend to "target" stimuli while ignoring competing "irrelevant" stimuli originating from other locations (Medwetsky, 1994). Kidd et al. (1998) examined the release from masking due to spatial separation of sources and found that identification performance improved with increasing separation of signal and masker. Much larger improvements were found for spatial separation of the signal and an informational masker (i.e., similar content as signal) than for a speech signal and an energetic masker (i.e., random spectral noise such as white or speech-shaped noise). This finding suggests that in listening situations where there are multiple talkers (e.g., cocktail party), binaural separation cues play a key role in allowing the listener to selectively attend to the target talker and ignore the competing "irrelevant" talkers, whereas in situations involving a talker surrounded by nonlinguistic noises, the overall signal-to-noise energy ratio is the crucial factor. It appears that spatial location is accurately tracked by human auditory sensory memory (as evidenced in MMN studies) and multiple auditory streams can be derived that enable the listener to attend to a selected stream (Nager et al., 2003). Nager et al. (2003) found that the greater the separation, the stronger the MMN component that is elicited. This is likely due to the ease with which neuronal attentional direction can be implemented.

Selective attention involving binaural separation is typically assessed clinically using headphones via the presentation of dichotic stimuli, whereby the listener is directed to attend to and recall stimuli presented to one of the ears, while ignoring competing stimuli originating from the other ear. In dichotic tasks, stimuli are best transmitted to the cortices via the contralateral pathways. The ear to which the listener is told to recall stimuli guides "automatic attentional direction." In the case of dichotic-selective attention tasks, attentional direction (1) increases the likelihood of neural firing in the auditory receptive areas in the hemisphere contralateral to the designated ear and (2) engages inhibitory processes in the opposite hemisphere (Nager et al., 2003; Petkov et al., 2004). If an individual is told to recall stimuli presented to the right ear, he or she would automatically (subconsciously) direct attention to the left hemisphere, and vice versa if told to recall stimuli from the left ear.

Selective Auditory Attention Associated with Capacity and Load

According to Limited Resource Theory (Kahneman, 1973; Windsor and Hwang, 1999), individuals are limited in the amount of resources they can allocate to a task. An individual's ability to complete a task successfully can be reduced to the relationship between two variables: capacity and load. Capacity is defined as the total reservoir of energy that an individual has available to expend on a particular task, while load refers to the amount of energy that must be expended. Figure 25.3 summarizes this relationship. The outer circle represents capacity, while the inner circle represents the load. The arrows indicate that both capacity and load can increase or decrease. As long as the load is less than the capacity, an individual can complete the task successfully; however, if the load exceeds capacity, then difficulty and failure on that task would likely result. Note that if the

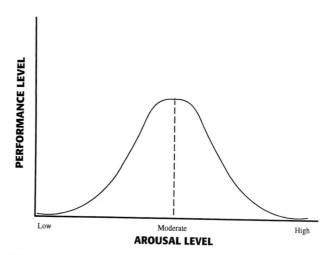

FIGURE 25.4 **Relationship between performance level and arousal level.**

load lessens relative to capacity, then an individual will have a greater amount of residual resources to do concurrent tasks.

An individual's capacity for a particular task at any point in time is determined by three variables: (1) inherent physical attributes, (2) environmental influences (such as achieved through training), and (3) arousal level. To help illustrate these three concepts, the following example is provided. In weightlifting, the weight is the load, and the task required is the lifting of the weight. A person brings inherent physical attributes (muscle size and mass) to the task. However, through weightlifting training, the person can increase his muscle mass and therefore his capacity for lifting the weight. Arousal levels can also impact performance significantly; that is, individuals tend to perform at optimum levels if refreshed and not fatigued or stressed. Figure 25.4 illustrates the relationship between performance level and arousal level. As expected, individuals achieve their optimum performance levels at moderate arousal levels, that is, when they are refreshed and relaxed. However, when individuals are fatigued or bored (arousal levels are significantly decreased) or are significantly stressed (arousal levels are significantly increased), performance levels subsequently decrease.

The load required by a particular task can also change over time. For example, when a person first learns to drive, the task is so new that the individual must pay attention to many variables (such as the steering wheel, brakes, rearview mirror, etc.). This results in the load being very high, so much so that there are few mental resources left to allocate to other tasks, such as talking to passengers. However, over time, through many repetitions, the task of driving becomes more automatic, resulting in a significant reduction of the mental load, with the person possibly arriving at a destination without being able to recall which roads he took to get there. This example illustrates how the conscious effort of allocating attention to a task is important for later recall, such as remembering where you put your keys. If you consciously paid attention to the act of placing your keys down,

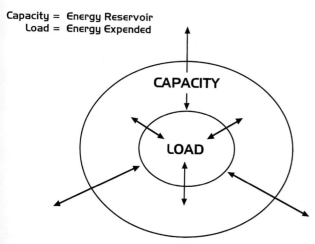

Capacity = Energy Reservoir
Load = Energy Expended

CAPACITY

LOAD

FIGURE 25.3 **Relationship between capacity and load.**

you will most likely remember where you have placed them. However, if your mind is "elsewhere" or you just drop your keys down, you may find yourself spending hours looking for them.

When load is discussed in the context of S-LP, one typically refers to an individual's mental workload expended on a task (Kahneman, 1973; Gopher and Donchin, 1986). Numerous factors determine the amount of mental expenditure on an auditory S-LP task, including: (1) the discriminability of the stimuli; (2) the amount of information that must be processed over a specific time frame; (3) the presence of any competing noise/reverberant sound energy and, in turn, the effective signal-to-noise ratio; and (4) the location of the target source relative to competing sources. The factors that impact on a person's capacity on such a task include the listener's: (1) hearing threshold profile; (2) temporal, frequency, amplitude, and phase resolution; (3) phonologic, lexical, semantic, syntactic, and prosodic representation/organization; (4) auditory integration capacity/speed; and (5) sequencing and attentional allocation abilities. Hence, the extent to which mental energy must be expended relative to the perceiver's capacity to process the information quickly and effectively determines whether the listener will be able to process spoken language successfully. For example, an individual with an S-LPD may be able to recall sentences in quiet with 100% accuracy; however, it may be taking all of his or her mental resources to do so. If a competing noise is introduced, the listener must divert some of his or her attentional mechanisms to block out the "irrelevant" stimuli and, by doing so, may not leave enough resources to process the target stimuli. In the listening situation in which competing stimuli are presented in a dichotic listening task (i.e., the target sentences are presented under one earphone, while the competing "irrelevant" sentence stimuli are presented in the other earphone), any difficulty in processing the target stimuli cannot be due to peripheral masking but to other sources. These sources include (1) possible difficulties in allocating attention to targeted neuronal regions; (2) perceptual separation distances may be less in some individuals with processing disorders (i.e., in individuals with poorer auditory coherence abilities); and (3) the mental effort required is greater than the total mental resources available.

Divided and Sustained Auditory Attention

As mentioned earlier, divided attention refers to the processing of two or more acoustic streams. In dichotic listening tasks, this entails allocating attention to two incoming streams of information, thus twice the amount of information must be processed per unit of time. It is easy to understand that if there are any underlying processing deficits of consequence, divided attention will suffer.

Sustained attention refers to the ability of maintaining attention to a single source of information for an unbroken period of time. Any factor that increases the mental load of a task will hinder one's ability to maintain mental effort over any sustained period of time. This will be discussed in further detail later on in the section related to ADHD.

▧ CENTRAL EXECUTIVE SYSTEM

The central executive system (CES) is a theorized cognitive system that integrates, organizes, coordinates, and executes key cognitive functions. The executive processes have been implicated in complex cognition tasks such as problem solving, modifying behavior as appropriate in response to changes in the environment, inhibiting prepotent responses (i.e., those responses that have the greatest likelihood of being triggered due to previous learning), and implementing schemas (underlying organizational pattern or conceptual frameworks) that organize behavior over time. The CES was traditionally prescribed to lie in the region of the PFC, but with its significant afferent/efferent connections to subcortical and cortical association areas, most researchers now consider the CES to include not only the PFC but also the ACC, striatum, BG, thalamus, reticular activating system (RAS), and limbic system. Neurophysiologically, it appears to rely on the accurate deployment/uptake of a number of key neuronal transmitters—dopamine, norepinephrine, and serotonin (Hunt, 2006; Volkow et al., 2001; http://www.sciencedaily.com/releases/2006/11/061129151028.htm; http://www.drugdigest.org/DD/HC/Causes/0,4045,550286,00 html).

Key to the PFC's ability to coordinate all of the various functions is an appropriately set arousal level system. That is, the RAS is key to regulating PFC function by optimizing dopaminergic release and optimal CES function (Riccio et al., 1993; Nadeau, 1995; Wagner, 2000). The lower the level of norepinephrine in the RAS, the less able this system is to excite the PFC neurons (Faraone and Biederman, 1998). In turn, when PFC dopamine is at abnormally low levels, the PFC exhibits less ability in regulating the various other regions in which it interfaces.

The CES plays a number of key roles relative to S-LP. First, as discussed earlier, it is key to attentional allocation, be it at (1) a preattentive (gating) level, (2) alteration of activation thresholds of concepts stored in LTM (i.e., impacting on the likelihood that sensory-acoustic traces will activate corresponding LTM representations into conscious concepts), or (3) recurrent attention (key to maintaining neuronal firing, thus allowing concepts to be maintained in STM). A second, key function is the ability of the CES to maintain the sequential organization/representation of events over time. For example, on a memory task that requires the recall of a series of items (be it a serial recall memory task for a list of items or the correct order of words recalled such as on the SSW test), some kind of mechanism must be available for recording sequential information; that is, the memory trace must contain information about the time of occurrence of events in relationship to each other (Gillam et al., 1995). As pointed out earlier in the section on sequencing, ordered item representations presumably are intermittently reactivated in rehearsal processes at some point in recall, with mental markers for their serial positions. This ability to sequence events over time is believed to be mediated by the lateral PFC (Romine and Reynolds, 2004).

SUMMARIZING THE PROCESSES ENGAGED IN SPOKEN-LANGUAGE PROCESSING

The following is a summary of the key stages in which incoming acoustic stimuli are transformed into neurologic representations and ultimately reach the level of consciousness, be it in quiet or in the presence of distractors:

- Incoming stimuli undergo a number of transductions and are ultimately converted to neurologic representations.
- Preattentive mechanisms determine which stimulus attributes are allowed to pass through and which are inhibited at the level of the thalamus and Heschl's gyrus; that is, individuals often must listen in the presence of competing noise and in order to attend to the "target" stimuli in noise, the brain directs attention to those neurons corresponding to the stimuli of interest, while ignoring/inhibiting the neurons corresponding to the "competing" stimuli.
- The neurologic representations are compared to patterns stored in LTM; if there is a match and sufficient attention is paid to the signal, then the LTM representation is activated into consciousness (this activated state is called STM). This matching and activation process, known as decoding, must be done quickly and accurately.
- Information can reside in STM for a very short period of time, unless attention is devoted to maintaining this information (e.g., rehearsal or active processing—thinking about what has been presented).
- For most individuals, linguistic information is processed in the left hemisphere, while suprasegmental information is processed in the right hemisphere; these are somehow integrated "on the fly."
- The processed information must be retained in the same order as presented.
- There is a limit to how many neuronal regions can be attended to at any one point in time; if it involves the processing of simultaneous acoustic streams, then even two acoustic streams poses a great mental load, but if it requires the memorization of sequential stimuli, then it appears that a typical adult can shift at-

tention (allow for recurrent activation) of four to five neuronal regions.

- A separate process in the early years involves the establishment of individual sound families (phonemes) and their symbolic representations, which is reliant on normal temporal, frequency, and amplitude resolution.

This conceptualization of the underlying processes is illustrated in Figure 25.5.

SPOKEN-LANGUAGE PROCESSING DISORDERS

Having a conceptual framework of the processes underlying normal auditory S-LP allows us to better understand the consequences of different underlying deficits. As described in the following sections, S-LP disorder (S-LPD) is not a unitary disorder, and if we are to implement appropriate management techniques, we must be able to ascertain the specific nature of these deficits. This entails using a test battery approach that seeks to assess the various auditory-linguistic processing skills (various test battery approaches to diagnostic intervention are described in Chapter 27).

Deficits in Acoustic Feature Extraction

Any deficiencies in hearing sensitivity or in temporal, frequency, amplitude, or phase resolution can impact significantly on accurate feature extraction and thus on the ultimate processing and resolution of the intended target message(s). A number of important consequences result from incomplete feature extraction. First, individuals will have difficulty (1) establishing accurate phonemic boundaries and thus phonemic representations in LTM; (2) understanding and learning to manipulate the sounds that make up the words of their language (i.e., phonologic awareness); and consequently, (3) learning to represent these sounds by letters (i.e., sound-symbol association or the more commonly used term "phonics"). Phonologic awareness and sound-symbol association difficulties impact negatively on learning how to read and spell, especially for words that are novel or infrequently used. In addition, because of the greater allocation of mental resources that will have to be expended to decode words, phonologic awareness/phonics difficulties will impact on one's lexical decoding speed (be it for auditory processing or when reading), comprehension, and ultimate retention of the overall material.

Second, Tallal and colleagues (Tallal et al., 1996; Merzenich et al., 1996) have proposed that deficiency in temporal resolution is the major component underlying language learning deficits in many children. Although Tallal's assumption is a subject of much debate, it does suggest that an inability to derive stable/accurate phonetic features

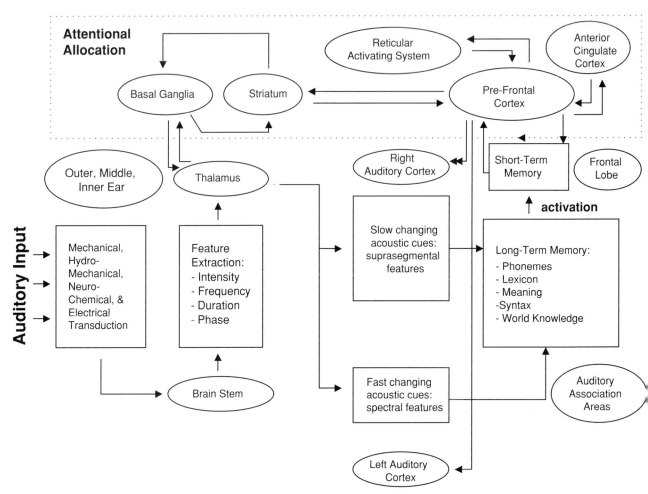

FIGURE 25.5 Key processes engaged in the auditory processing of spoken language and their corresponding anatomic regions. The processes are listed in the *boxes*, while the anatomic regions are indicated in the *circles*.

impacts negatively on an individual's ability to learn the linguistic code of his or her language.

Third, impoverished stimuli are at greater risk to the effects of masking (Pickett et al., 1983). Thus, individuals who are unable to derive acoustic cues accurately from spoken stimuli are at greater risk for experiencing difficulty in background noise. This difficulty likely arises from either filtering difficulties in simultaneous masking tasks or weak sensory memory traces that are subject to the effects of forward/backward masking.

Lexical Decoding Speed Deficits

Lexical (i.e., word) decoding deficits refer to difficulties that individuals encounter in processing the words of a language, be it in the verbal or written form. The nature of these difficulties may lie in accuracy, speed, or a combination of both. For example, individuals with lexical decoding difficulties (due to an actual processing disorder, hearing loss, or unfamiliarity with a language or topic area) may experience significant difficulty keeping up with the material presented

by a talker. Initially, these individuals may get the gist of what is being presented, but with the continued presentation of material, they may fall behind as they continue to work on the earlier presented material. This results in gaps of information being processed and consequently impacts on comprehension. In addition, because of the greater mental expenditure they must exert to process the information, they may fatigue quickly. Subsequently, they may "tune out" after a while and no longer be able to "attend" to the talker. The persistence of these behaviors may lead others to speculate the presence of an attention deficit disorder–inattentive type when, in fact, the disorder is due to an underlying processing deficit.

Lexical decoding speed deficits may be due to a number of underlying causes. First, if an individual has poor acoustic feature extraction skills (such as an individual with hearing loss or an individual with normal hearing sensitivity but deficiencies in temporal, frequency, and/or amplitude resolution), this may result in an inability to derive accurate neural firing patterns with which to compare with prototypes in LTM. This will result in either inaccurate perception or prolonged processing time (as the individual tries to resolve the intended message). Second, if over time an individual has not been able to store information in LTM in an organized/systematic fashion (including rules governing semantic relations, semantic categories, syntax, etc.), it will take longer for that individual to match the acoustic trace with its counterpart in LTM. The corollary also holds true. When the same individual must initiate a response, it will take longer to retrieve words from LTM since the same language region in LTM must be accessed; therefore, the individual may exhibit delayed responses or stumble in trying to get out the response.

Deficits in Auditory Attention

Deficits in auditory attention are often described on the basis of observable behaviors such as reflected in the comment, "Johnny has trouble paying attention in class" or by professionals using the American Psychiatric Association DSM-IV guidelines to examine possible symptomatology/manifestations of an attention deficit disorder. As discussed earlier, I defined attention as an underlying cognitive process that allows the listener to focus selectively on stimuli of interest, while ignoring or blocking out irrelevant competing stimuli, thereby limiting the amount of information processed to resolution. Using this definition as a guide requires us to assess an individual's underlying attentional skills rather than focusing on observable behaviors. This is a productive approach since, in many cases, the same behaviors can be observed even though the underlying cause may be quite different. This is illustrated in the following three examples:

1. Jack is a "gifted" child who is functioning many grade levels above his classmates, yet his teacher teaches to the average student in his class. Consequently, Jack is often bored, and thus, he daydreams, is fidgety, does not seem to be "listening," and has difficulty sustaining attention, etc.
2. Jill, on the other hand, has underlying processing deficits and finds it hard to keep up with the teacher and process the information presented. She often becomes fatigued and "tunes out" as a result. Consequently, Jill often daydreams, is fidgety, does not seem to be "listening," and has difficulty sustaining attention, etc.
3. Larry is an adult who is attending a seminar with which he has little background knowledge; no overheads are being used, and the topic matter is presented quickly. He tries to keep up with the information, but he is struggling with the concepts being presented. Eventually, he becomes so fatigued and discouraged that he starts to daydream, becomes fidgety, does not seem to be "listening," and has difficulty sustaining attention, etc.

These three examples show clearly that, by examining only the observable behaviors, one might not be able to ascertain the actual underlying cause of these difficulties. Therefore,

it is important to determine the true nature of an individual's difficulty if one is to adopt appropriate management strategies.

As discussed earlier under the rubric of ASA, competing sounds can be categorized as coming from different sources based on the auditory coherence within each signal on the basis of frequency, phase, and intensity relationships. This allows the listener to separate perceptually the two or more competing signals and, in turn, allows the individual to accurately/efficiently devote attentional resources to target stimuli and block out competing stimuli. Hence, any individual who is unable to use the underlying acoustic cues to maintain auditory coherence of incoming stimuli will be at significantly greater risk in noisy situations.

If a listener errs in how attention is directed initially (i.e., preparatory attention), all subsequent processing will be for naught. Hence, the child who is unable to direct his attention correctly/consistently to the designated talker will have significant difficulty at home and at school. If ADHD has been ruled out, then management approaches must focus on metacognitive approaches that assist the child in being able to direct his attention appropriately.

Selective attention, the process whereby the listener selects a target source and ignores all competing stimuli, is critical when listening in the presence of background noise. Significant findings on speech-in-noise and selective attention tasks, may be due to attentional allocation and/or underlying processing deficits. Examples of how underlying processing deficits can impact on selective attention include the following:

1. *Acoustic feature extraction.* Incomplete neuroelectrical representations of target stimuli leave them vulnerable to the effects of forward and backward masking by competing stimuli. In addition, the mental expenditure entailed in matching incoming stimuli with stored prototypes in LTM may use up much of an individual's capacity on the task, leaving little residual capacity. Thus, in a quiet listening condition, the listener may be able to process the incoming stimuli, although with much effort. If competing noise/messages are introduced, this may leave the listener without sufficient resources to process the target stimuli, while simultaneously blocking out the competing stimuli. Consequently, this individual experiences significant difficulty in processing target stimuli in the competing noise situation.
2. *Lexical decoding speed.* An individual who has poorly organized neuronal networks (thus impacting on the speed in which incoming information can be matched with prototypes in LTM) would be expected to exhibit significantly increased mental expenditure during the processing of target stimuli. If competing noise is introduced, the ability to access the relevant information while blocking out the competing noise may exceed the listener's processing capacity and cause him or her to falter in this listening situation.

3. *ASA.* Deficits in the ability to maintain and segregate acoustic streams would obviously impact on an individual's ability to process and focus on the target acoustic stream, while ignoring the irrelevant acoustic stream.

4. *Auditory-linguistic integration (ALI).* Collier and Hart (1975) compared performance by normal adults using sentence stimuli in both quiet and in noise. The stimuli were presented using either natural speech (i.e., with normal inflections, rhythms, etc.) or robotic speech, whereby the speech was presented in a flat, mono-tone voice. They found a slight advantage for natural speech in quiet but a 30% difference in favor of natural speech in the speech-in-noise condition. This suggests that individuals who have difficulty integrating suprasegmental with linguistic information (i.e., lexicon, semantic, and syntactic derivations) are likely to encounter difficulty in speech-in-noise situations. One reason may be due to the impact of poor integration, which reduces auditory coherence, making it more difficult to separate two or more acoustic streams. A second reason may be reduced effectiveness in using suprasegmental information to divide sentences into smaller chunks that otherwise could overload one's processing/memory span abilities (i.e., when suprasegmental cues coincide with grammatical clauses, they allow us to process/retain smaller units). In addition, ALI deficits would also result in the right ear dominant effects noted earlier in the chapter; that is, these individuals would exhibit greater processing difficulties in the left versus the right ear in situations involving competing spoken messages.

Divided attention to two or more competing messages requires the listener to process and retain at least twice the amount of information as on the selective attention task. Therefore, any processing difficulties affecting selective attention will exert an even greater impact on divided attention. An example of a divided attention task in which individuals with S-LPD often have great difficulty is that of note taking. When an individual takes notes, such as in a lecture, he/she must write down what the presenter has already said and must also continue to listen to what the presenter is presently saying. Therefore, two streams of information must be processed at the same time. Consequently, an individual with an underlying processing deficit (entailing increased mental load) would be at increased risk for difficulties on this task.

Sustained attention requires an individual to process information over a prolonged period of time. Examples of sustained attention include listening to a teacher during class or a presenter in a seminar. This skill is not often assessed in the clinic setting; that is, many speech-in-noise tests use individual words or sentence materials, thus resulting in breaks between presentations. An exception is to use continuous performance tests (such as the Auditory Continuous Per-formance Test by Keith [1994]). It is possible that an individual, especially an older child or adult, with an underlying processing deficit may be able to perform within age norms on tasks involving words or sentence materials but, when required to sustain attention over a long period of time, may show a decrement in performance over time. That is, the mental expenditure required over time may eventually exceed the individual's capacity and result in diminished performance.

Fading Memory

Fading memory is characterized by difficulty in retaining and recalling earlier presented information (Medwetsky, 2005). I believe that fading memory is the consequence of an attentional allocation deficit that involves the need for recurrent activation of neuronal regions, that is, the maintenance of information in passive STM or active working memory (e.g., in problem-solving tasks). Recall that the ability to direct attention to target stimuli allows for retention in STM and, ultimately, in LTM if sufficient attention is directed to maintaining this information in STM (e.g., through elaborative rehearsal), whereas irrelevant stimuli that are not attended to fade rapidly from memory. A logical extension from this postulate is that individuals with fading memory are unable to direct their attention effectively toward the processing and retention of target stimuli. Therefore, any management strategy addressing fading memory must include metacognitive strategies that improve an individual's ability to allocate attention appropriately and effectively.

Individuals with fading memory not only have difficulty retaining earlier presented information (resulting in a reduced STM/working memory span), but they may also exhibit difficulties in the presence of background noise. The latter is likely due to two causes. First, if the underlying cause of fading memory put forth by this author is correct, then an individual with fading memory likely has difficulty allocating attention effectively; hence, that individual will be less capable of focusing attention on the target stimuli while blocking out competing stimuli. Second, if individuals with fading memory are able to retain information for less time in STM (as compared to peers), then any factor that increases the amount of time in which stimuli need to be processed will reduce the amount of information that can be retained in STM. Because competing noise can mask acoustic features in the target signal, it will likely result in increased processing time and resources to match the target stimulus with the prototype in LTM.

Auditory Integration Deficits

Integration deficits can be manifested in a number of different ways. In the broadest sense, if we consider the ability to binaurally integrate the temporal/amplitude cues as involved in localization, then any deficit in the latter will impact not only localization but also possibly selective attention tasks involving binaural separation of competing talkers. A second type of integration deficit and one that is often observed in individuals with S-LPD involves an inability of the corpus callosum to effectively transfer information between the hemispheres. The impact of such corpus callosum deficiencies will be reflected by:

1. A right ear advantage in group settings; hence, in these situations, the talker should be on the listener's right side.

2. Increased difficulty integrating the nonlinguistic, suprasegmental information (processed in the right hemisphere) with the linguistic information processed in the left hemisphere. In turn, this will impact the ease with which the listener can:

   ■ Distinguish declaratives from yes/no sentences, even though the wording is the same (e.g., "That's an airplane!" vs. "That's an airplane?")

   ■ Determine the meaning in ambiguous sentences based on the particular stress, pausing, etc. (e.g., "The farmer **out standing** in the field" vs. "The farmer **outstanding** in the field")

   ■ Integrate the prosodic information (right hemispheric function) and sociolinguistic information/context (important in pragmatics; e.g., telling the difference between happy/sad); in the most extreme case with autism, individuals may exhibit flat voicing patterns and be very literal in how they interpret linguistic information

3. The ease/speed with which information is integrated across processing regions; this can impact reading/writing speed, reading comprehension, organization of written material, and problem solving tasks, depending on the abstractness of the concepts etc.

4. Difficulty integrating auditory-visual information between the hemispheres. Examples include (a) forming sound (phoneme)–symbol (alphabet letter) associations, (b) integrating acoustic input with speechreading cues, and (c) integrating the perception of facial features (right hemispheric function) with linguistic information (important in pragmatics). The latter may also be one of the reasons why autistic individuals find it so difficult to listen and look at a talker's face at the same time; that is, they exhibit an inability to effectively integrate the two streams of information, which results in sensory overload.

Sequencing Deficits

Individuals often present in the clinic setting with a case history including: (1) an inability to follow directions, (2) being disorganized, and (3) poor spelling (exhibited by letter reversals). These behaviors are often corroborated in testing by the listener's response patterns during S-LP testing. That is, these individuals will often recall the stimuli correctly

but repeat them out of sequence. In confirmed site-of-lesion cases, Katz and Pack (1975) found that, in adults with sequencing deficits, in the Rolandic region and the region anterior to it were most likely involved. Evidence in support of Katz's findings come from Luria (1966) and research on ADHD (Barkley, 1998). One of the primary deficits entailed with ADHD involves poor sequencing/imitation, organization, and planning; neurophysiologic evidence points to a deficit in the PFC. Recent research also indicates a role of the BG, with the BG interfacing with the PFC to not only allocate attention but also maintain the correct sequencing of stimuli (Frank et al., 2001).

It should be noted that a number of researchers have suggested that sequencing insufficiencies are due to poor temporal resolution/patterning and that, by increasing the interstimulus interval or by increasing the individual's temporal resolving ability, sequencing skills can be improved (Tallal et al., 1996). However, this contention has been countered by Philips (1998), whose research indicates that the inability of these subjects to recall items in the correct order during testing is not due to poor temporal patterning, but rather these individuals are unable to discriminate and identify the stimuli in the first place.

Deficits Involving the Central Executor and Arousal Level System

As mentioned earlier, the central executor is believed to be key to self-regulation, planning/organization, and working memory (Barkley, 1998). It is believed that the central executor accomplishes the aforementioned by allocating attention to and integrating information across the various processing regions. When it is unable to do so effectively, individuals exhibit behaviors consistent with ADHD. CES deficiencies can arise from a number of underlying causes, such as:

1. A deficit in the dopaminergic release/uptake system due to: (1) an underproduction of dopamine in the PFC; (2) deficient PFC dopamine receptor sites in the PFC or BG; and/or (3) or an oversupply of dopamine transporters, resulting in overremoval of extracellular dopamine (Teicher et al., 2000; Volkow et al., 2001; Krause et al., 2002; Spencer et al., 2007)

2. A modulation deficit involving the arousal level system (mediated by the RAS), which in many of these individuals is in a state of underarousal.

Underarousal of the central executor (through the mediation of the PFC-striatal network) results in an underproduction of dopamine in the PFC, the consequence being that the central executor is not able to mediate the functions for which it is thought to exert control, primarily behavioral self-regulation and monitoring and interference control.

Individuals with ineffective CESs may exhibit difficulties such as:

1. Difficulty initiating and regulating attentional allocation
2. An inability to analyze tasks to their basic components as well as difficulty with organizing these components to formulate goals and plans. In turn, these difficulties impact goal-directed behavior and persistence on tasks.
3. Impulsivity and distractibility
4. Difficulty with STM/working memory due to a poorer ability to initiate reflection, less effective generation of metacognitive strategies/rules and self-questioning, and an inability to hold events in mind

Relative to S-LP, deficits of the CES can impact on attentional allocation and sequencing, depending on the particular CES structures involved. Deficits in attentional allocation may negatively impact on S-LP in a number of different ways, including:

1. Preattentive, gating mechanisms at the level of the thalamus and Heschl's gyrus, thus impacting on speech-in-noise
2. The ease with which LTM representations are activated, thus impacting on lexical decoding speed
3. Recurrent attentional mechanisms, thus reducing the ease with which items can be held in STM and, in turn, decreasing working memory span (on serial recall tasks, this reduces the ability with which earlier presented items will be recalled, leading to fading memory)
4. The ability to maintain sustained attention to targeted stimuli and inhibitory actions against "irrelevant" stimuli; in a certain segment of the population, CES deficits have been shown to result in individuals responding to the most reinforcing stimuli present, thus resulting in impulsive responses and an inability to stay on task when rewards are delayed
5. Sequencing; that is, individuals may recall all items presented but in the wrong order (usually entailing adjacent items)

Audiologists who do central auditory processing testing often assess individuals with suspected ADHD and are asked to provide their best clinical judgment as to whether that individual has clinical signs that support the presence of ADHD and/or a processing disorder. Depending on the specific PFC regions involved, ADHD can be manifested by various behaviors from the most obvious (e.g., hyperactivity/impulsivity) to more subtle behaviors (e.g., inattentiveness, inability to sustain attention, or a reduced working memory span). I believe the diagnostic information that we can obtain during testing can provide much useful information relative to this issue. Based on my readings, observations, and analyses of the empirical data, if one truly has some aspect of ADHD, then that individual will most likely exhibit a fading memory sign; this supposition is supported by the findings obtained by Tillery et al. (2000), who found that fading memory was the most prominent processing sign of individuals with ADHD. This is because attentional allocation is critical to maintaining earlier presented information. Psychologists have known for many years that when individuals are asked to do a serial recall task involving a long string of items, subjects tend to recall the earlier (primacy effect) and later (recency effect) items the best, while items in the middle tend to be forgotten most easily (Gillam et al., 1995). Early item recall enhancement appears to be due to applying various forms of rehearsal strategies (i.e., attentional allocation). If rehearsal is somehow interfered with (i.e., attentional allocation is not directed to maintaining these items in STM), then the primacy effect is diminished or eliminated. By extension, any individual who is unable to allocate attention effectively would likely exhibit difficulties in recalling earlier presented items, thus exhibiting fading memory. Of course, individuals with ADHD may exhibit other processing-related difficulties. However, in the absence of any fading-memory signs, it is unlikely that ADHD is a contributing factor to an individual's processing-related difficulties. Also, if a sequencing deficit is noted, this is another supporting sign that a CES deficit is present, although it may not necessarily be accompanied by inattentiveness, hyperactivity, or impulsivity, since the deficit may involve only a specific region of the PFC.

Please note that, although there are various tests of continuous performance (e.g., the Auditory Continuous Performance Test [ACPT]) (Keith, 1994), it is not always the case that someone who exhibits sustained attention difficulties on these tasks has ADHD. The ACPT is used to assess auditory attention and vigilance over a sustained period of time—approximately 10 minutes. The test consists of a simple word identification task, whereby the listener listens to a list of words (repeated six times) and is requested to raise his or her thumb every time the word "dog" is heard and ignore occurrences of any other words. In scoring results on the ACPT, one determines the number of inattentive errors (thumb is not raised for the word *dog*) as well as impulsive errors (thumb is raised for words other than *dog*). I not only analyze the number of errors obtained over the course of the test, but also the ratio of inattentive to impulsive errors. If almost all of the errors are of the inattentive type (and especially if there are a number of delayed responses, i.e., the listener raises his/her thumb two or three words later), then I generally attribute this sustained difficulty to poor lexical decoding speed, rather than to ADHD. This is especially the case if the SSW findings indicate the presence of lexical decoding speed difficulty and no presence of any fading memory signs.

Thus, if individuals have significant CES deficits, they will indeed display S-LP–related deficits. The nature of these deficits will be related to some aspect of CES function involving attentional allocation and/or sequencing. Thus, if someone has ADHD, one would not expect only receptive deficits (e.g., phonologic awareness, lexical decoding speed, and/or integration), but at minimum, a fading memory sign would also have to be present, possibly accompanied by a sequencing deficit.

CONCLUDING REMARKS

This chapter presented an integrative approach to understanding S-LP as it occurs in everyday life. In this model, CANS mechanisms as well as underlying language/cognitive processes play key roles in the processing of spoken language. By understanding how spoken language is transformed from the acoustic signal and ultimately processed/retained in conscious memory, be it in quiet or in competing noise, one can then understand how S-LPDs can be produced, depending on where the specific breakdowns occur. This is not a trivial concern because management strategies will be most effective when they address the individual's specific difficulties. It is clear that if we are to lessen the difficulties of individuals with S-LP deficits, we must (1) be aware of the various components involved in normal S-LP, (2) recognize how breakdowns in any of the processing stages can result in specific deficits, (3) use a comprehensive test battery approach that allows us to determine if and what types of deficits are present, and (4) recommend and/or implement management strategies that will address the specific problems. For an in-depth discussion on S-LP (also known as central auditory processing) evaluation and management, the reader is referred to Chapters 27 and 28 as well as to other publications on these topics (Bellis, 2003; Parthasarathy, 2006; Chermak and Musiek, 2007; Geffner and Ross-Swain, 2007).

In addition to the discussion on S-LPD, this chapter has presented information on ADHD. It is important that we understand and recognize the manifestations of ADHD on S-LP, how we can differentiate other processing deficits from those that may be caused by ADHD, and in turn, how we can assist in the appropriate management of the affected individual.

In summary, we have the opportunity to make a great difference in the lives of individuals who are referred to us with suspected S-LPD/CAPD by impacting on academic performance and/or quality of life. With the information presented in this and in subsequent chapters, it is our hope that the reader will have a better understanding of the underlying causes of S-LPD and its manifestations, as well as a greater awareness of the approaches used in identifying and addressing the specific deficits encountered.

REFERENCES

Abrams DA, Nichol T, Zecker S, Kraus N. (2008) Right-hemisphere auditory cortex is dominant for coding syllable patterns in speech. *J Neurosci.* 28, 3958–3965.

American Speech-Language-Hearing Association. (1996) A Task Force on Central Auditory Processing Consensus Development: central auditory processing: current status of research and implications for clinical practice. *Am J Audiol.* 5, 41–54.

American Speech-Language-Hearing Association. (2005) (Central) auditory processing disorders. Technical report: Working Group on Auditory Processing Disorders. Rockville, MD: American Speech-Language Hearing Association.

Arciuli J, Slowiaczek LM. (2007) The where and when of linguistic word-level prosody. *Neuropsychologia.* 45, 2638–2642.

Baddeley AD. (1986) *Working Memory.* Oxford, England: Oxford University Press.

Barkley RA. (1998) *ADHD and the Nature of Self-Control.* New York: The Guilford Press.

Bell TS, Wilson RH. (2001) Sentence recognition materials based on frequency of word use and lexical confusability. *J Am Acad Audiol.* 12, 514–522.

Bellis TJ. (2003) *Assessment and Management of Auditory Processing Disorders in the Educational Setting: From Science to Practice.* 2nd ed. Clifton Park, NY: Thomson Delmar Learning.

Berry MF, Eisenson J. (1956) *Speech Disorders: Principles and Practices of Therapy.* New York: Appleton-Century-Crofts.

Bhatnagar SC, Korabic EW. (2006) Neuroanatomy and neurophysiology of the central auditory pathways. In: Parthasarathy TK, ed. *An Introduction to Auditory Processing Disorders in Children.* Mahwah, NJ: Lawrence Erlbaum Associates.

Bocca E, Calearo C, Cassinari V. (1954) A new method for testing hearing in temporal lobe tumors. *Acta Otolaryngol.* 44, 219–221.

Bocca E, Calearo C, Cassinari V, Migliavacca F. (1955) Testing cortical hearing in temporal lobe tumors. *Acta Otolaryngol.* 45, 289–304.

Bradlow AR, Alexander JA. (2007) Semantic and phonetic enhancements for speech-in-noise recognition by native and non-native listeners. *J Acoust Soc Am.* 121, 2339–2349.

Bregman AS. (1978) The formation of auditory streams. In: Requin J, ed. *Attention and Performance VII.* Hillsdale, NJ: Lawrence Erlbaum Associates.

Bregman AS. (1994) *Auditory Scene Analysis: The Perceptual Organization of Sound.* Cambridge, MA: MIT Press.

Cacace AT, McFarland DJ. (2005) The importance of modality specificity in diagnosing central auditory processing disorder. *Am J Audiol.* 14, 112–123.

Caramazza A. (1997) How many levels of processing are there in lexical access? *Cogn Psychol.* 14, 177–208.

Cartling B. (1995) A generalized neuronal activation function derived from ion-channel characteristics. *Network Computation Neural Syst.* 6, 389–401.

Chalfant JC, Scheffelin MA. (1969) Central processing dysfunctions in children: a review of the research. Bethesda, MD: National Institute of Neurological Diseases and Stroke, National Institutes of Health, US Department of Health, Education, and Welfare, Monograph No. 9.

Chang C, Crotazz-Herbette S, Menon V. (2007) Temporal dynamics of basal ganglia response and connectivity during verbal working memory. *Neuroimage.* 34, 1253–1269.

Chermak GD, Musiek FE. (2007) *Handbook of (Central) Auditory Processing Disorder: Comprehensive Intervention.* Volume II. San Diego: Plural Publishing.

Collier R, Hart J. (1975) The role of intonation in speech perception. In: Cohen A, Nooteboom SG, eds. *Structure and*

Process in Speech Perception. Heidelberg, Germany: Springer Verlag.

Cowan N. (2001) The magical number 4 in short-term memory: a reconsideration of mental storage capacity. *Behav Brain Sci.* 24, 87–115.

Cusak R, Deeks J, Aikman G, Carlyon RP. (2004) Effects of location, frequency region, and time course of selective attention on auditory scene analysis. *J Exp Psychol Hum Percept Perform.* 30, 643–656.

Dehaene-Lambertz G. (1997) Electrophysiologic correlates of categorical phoneme perception in adults. *Neuroreport.* 8, 919–924.

Dehaene-Lambertz G, Baillet S. (1998) A phonological representation in the infant brain. *Neuroreport.* 9, 1885–1888.

Duchan J, Katz J. (1983) Language and auditory processing: top down plus bottom up. In: Lasky E, Katz J, eds. *Central Auditory Processing Disorders: Problems of Speech, Language, and Learning.* Baltimore: University Park Press; pp 31–45.

Ericsson KA, Kintsch W. (1995) Long-term memory. *Psychol Rev.* 102, 211–245.

Ethofer T, Anders S, Erb M, Herbert C, Wiethoff S, Kissler J, Grodd W, Wildgruber D. (2006) Cerebral pathways in processing of affective prosody: a dynamic causal modeling study. *Neuroimage.* 30, 580–587.

Faraone SV, Biederman J. (1998) Neurobiology of attention-deficit hyperactivity disorder. *Biol Psychiatry.* 44, 951–958.

Frank MJ, Loughry B, O'Reilly RC. (2001) Interactions between frontal cortex and basal ganglia in working memory: a computational model. *Cogn Affect Behav Neurosci.* 1, 137–160.

Frisina DR, Frisina RD. (1997) Speech recognition in noise and presbycusis: relations to possible neural mechanisms. *Hear Res.* 106, 95–104.

Fuster JM. (1997) *The Prefrontal Cortex: Anatomy, Physiology, and Neuropsychology of the Frontal Lobe.* 2nd ed. Philadelphia: Lippincott Williams & Wilkins.

Fuster JM. (2001) The prefrontal cortex—an update: time is the essence. *Neuron.* 30, 319–333.

Geffner D, Ross-Swain D. (2007) *Auditory Processing Disorders: Assessment, Management, and Treatment.* San Diego: Plural Publishing.

Gelfand JR, Bookheimer SY. (2003) Dissociating neural mechanisms of temporal sequencing and processing phonemes. *Neuron.* 38, 831–842.

Gelfand SA. (1998) *Hearing: An Introduction to Psychological and Physiological Acoustics.* New York: Marcel Dekker.

Gillam RB, Cowan N, Day LS. (1995) Sequential Memory in Children with or without language impairment. *J Speech Hear Res.* 38, 393–402.

Gopher D, Donchin E. (1986) Workload: an examination of the concept. In: Boff KR, Kaufman L, Thomas JP, eds. *Handbook of Perception and Human Performance. Volume II: Cognitive Processes and Performance.* New York: John Wiley & Sons.

Green PD, Cooke MP, Crawford MD. (1995) Auditory scene analysis and hidden Markov model recognition of speech in noise. *Proceedings from the 1995 IEEE Conference on Acoustics, Speech, and Signal Processing;* pp 401–404.

Gruber AJ, Dayan P, Gutkin BS, Solla SA. (2006) Dopamine modulation in the basal ganglia locks the gate to working memory. *J Comput Neurosci.* 20, 153–166.

Hazy T, Frank MJ, O'Reilly RC. (2007) Toward an executive without a homunculus: computational model of the prefrontal/basal ganglia system. *Philosoph Transact R Soc B.* 362, 1601–1613.

Hunt RD. (2006) Functional roles of norepinephrine and dopamine in ADHD. Available at: http://www.medscape.com/viewarticle/523–887.

Jerger J. (1998) Controversial issues in central auditory processing disorders. *Semin Hear.* 19, 393–397.

Jerger J, Jerger S. (1974) Auditory findings in brainstem disorders. *Arch Otolaryngol.* 93, 573–580.

Jerger J, Musiek F. (2002) Report on the consensus conference on the diagnosis of auditory processing disorders in school-aged children. *J Am Acad Audiol.* 11, 467–474.

Just MA, Carpenter PA. (1992) A capacity theory of comprehension: individual differences in working memory. *Psychol Rev.* 63, 122–149.

Kahneman D. (1973) *Attention and Effort.* Englewood Cliffs, NJ: Prentice Hall.

Kamhi AG. (2004) A meme's eye view of speech-language pathology. *Lang Speech Hear Serv Sch.* 35, 105–111.

Katz J. (1962) The use of staggered spondaic words for assessing the integrity of the central auditory nervous system. *J Aud Res.* 2, 327–337.

Katz J, Ilmer R. (1972) Auditory perception in children with learning disabilities. In: Katz J, ed. *Handbook of Clinical Audiology.* Baltimore: William and Wilkins.

Katz J, Johnson C, Bradner S, Delagrange T, Ferre J, King J, Krossover D, Lucker J, Medwetsky L, Rosenberg G, Saul R, Stecker N, Tillery KL. (2002) Clinical and research concerns seen in Jerger and Musiek (2000) APD recommendations. *Audiol Today.* 14, 14–17.

Katz J, Pack G. (1975) New developments in differential diagnosis using the SSW test. In: Sullivan MD, ed. *Proceedings of a Symposium on Central Auditory Processing Disorders.* Omaha, NE: University of Nebraska Medical Center.

Katz J, Tillery KL. (2005) Can APD tests resist supramodal influences? *Am J Audiol.* 14, 124–127.

Keith RW. (1977) *Central Auditory Dysfunction.* New York: Grune & Stratton.

Keith RW. (1981) Audiological and auditory language tests of central auditory function. In: Keith RW, ed. *Central Auditory and Language Disorders in Children.* Houston: College-Hill Press.

Keith RW. (1994) *ACPT: Auditory Continuous Performance Test.* San Antonio: The Psychological Corporation.

Kent R. (1992) Auditory processing of speech. In: Katz J, Stecker NA, Henderson D, eds. *Central Auditory Processing: A Transdisciplinary View.* St. Louis: Mosby.

Kidd G Jr, Mason CR, Rohtla TL, Deliwala PS. (1998) Release from masking due to spatial separation of sources to the identification of nonspeech auditory patterns. *J Acoust Soc Am.* 104, 422–431.

Kim S, Frisina DR, Frisina RD. (2002) Effects of age on contralateral suppression of distortion product otoacoustic emissions in human listeners with normal hearing. *Audiol Neurotol.* 7, 348–357.

Klatzky RL. (1984) *Memory and Awareness: An Information Processing Perspective.* New York: W.H. Freeman and Company.

Kraus N, McGee T. (1994) Mismatch negativity in the assessment of central auditory function. *Am J Audiol.* 3, 139–151.

Kraus N, Nicol T. (2005) Brainstem origins for cortical 'what' and 'where' pathways in the auditory system. *Trends Neurosci.* 28, 176–181.

Krause K-H, Dresel S, Krause J, Kung HF, Tatsch K, Lochmuller H. (2002) Elevated striatal dopamine transporter in a drug naïve patient with Tourette syndrome and attention deficit/hyperactivity disorder: positive effect of methylphenidate. *J Neurol.* 249, 1116–1118.

Lee CL, Estes WK. (1981) Order and position in primary memory for letter strings. *J Verb Learn Verb Behav.* 16, 395–418.

Levelt WJM. (2001) Spoken word production: a theory of lexical access. *Proc Natl Acad Sci USA.* 98, 13464–13471.

Lucker JR. (2007) History of auditory processing and its disorders in children. In: Geffner D, Ross-Swain D, eds. *Auditory Processing Disorders: Assessment, Management, and Treatment.* San Diego: Plural Publishing; pp 3–24.

Luria AR. (1966) *Higher Cortical Functions in Man.* New York: Basic Books; pp 106–108.

Massaro DW. (1976) Auditory information processing. In: Estes WK, ed. *Handbook of Learning and Cognitive Processes. Volume IV: Attention and Memory.* Hillsdale, NJ: Lawrence Erlbaum Associates; pp 275–320.

Matzker J. (1959) Two new methods for the assessment of central auditory function in cases of brain disease. *Ann Otol Rhinol Laryngol.* 68, 1185–1196.

Medwetsky L. (1994) The importance of spatial and talker cues in competing sentence recall. Unpublished doctoral dissertation. New York: Graduate Center, City University of New York.

Medwetsky L. (2002) Central auditory processing. In: Katz J, ed. *Handbook of Clinical Audiology.* 5th ed. Philadelphia: Lippincott Williams & Wilkins; pp 495–509.

Medwetsky L. (2005) SSW reports: APD or CAPD or SLPD? FYI-Tidbits. *SSW Rep.* 27, 1–6.

Medwetsky L. (2006) Spoken language processing: a convergent approach to conceptualizing (central) auditory processing. *ASHA Leader.* 11, 13–17.

Merzenich MM, Jenkins WM, Johnston P, Schreiner C, Miller SL, Tallal P. (1996) Temporal processing deficits of language-learning impaired children ameliorated by training. *Science.* 271, 77–81.

Meyer M, Zaehle T, Gountouna VE, Barron A, Jancke L, Turk A. (2005) Spectro-temporal processing during speech perception involves left posterior auditory cortex. *Neuroreport.* 16, 1985–1989.

Miller GA. (1956) The magical number seven, plus-or-minus two: some limits in our capacity for processing information. *Psychol Rev.* 63, 81–97.

Montgomery JW. (2002) Understanding the language difficulties of children with specific language impairments: does verbal working memory matter? *Am J Speech Lang Pathol.* 11, 77–91.

Musiek FE, Chermak GD. (1995) Three commonly asked questions about central auditory processing disorders: management. *Am J Audiol.* 4, 15–18.

Mykelbust HR. (1954) *Auditory Disorders in Children: A Manual for Differential Diagnosis.* New York: Grune & Stratton.

Naatanen R. (1999) The perception of speech sounds by the human brain as reflected by the mismatch negativity (MMN) and its magnetic equivalent (MMNm). *Psychophysiology.* 38, 1–21.

Nager W, Teder-Salejarvi W, Kunze S, Munte TF. (2003) Pre-attentive evaluation of multiple perceptual streams in human audition. *Neuroreport.* 14, 871–874.

Nittrouer S. (2002) A perspective on what clinicians need to understand about speech perception and language processing. *Lang Speech Hear Serv Sch.* 33, 237–252.

Parthasarathy TK. (2006) *An Introduction to Auditory Processing Disorders in Children.* Mahwah, NJ: Lawrence Erlbaum Associates.

Petkov CI, Kang X, Ahlo K, Bertrand O, Yund EW, Woods DL. (2004) Attentional modulation of human auditory cortex. *Nat Neurosci.* 7, 658–663.

Phillips DP. (1998) Sensory representations, the auditory cortex, and speech perception. *Semin Hear.* 19, 319–332.

Phillips DP. (2007) An introduction to central auditory neuroscience. In: Musiek FE, Chermak GD, eds. *Handbook of (Central) Auditory Processing Disorder: Auditory Neuroscience and Diagnosis.* Volume 1. San Diego: Plural Publishing; pp 53–88.

Pickett JM, Revoile SG, Danaher EM. (1983) Speech cue measures on impaired hearing. *Hear Res Theory.* 2, 57–92.

Picton TW, Hillyard SA. (1988) Endogenous event-related potentials. In Picton TW, ed. *Human Event-Related Potentials: Volume 3. EEG Handbook.* New York: Elsevier; pp 361–426.

Portas CM, Roos G, Howsemann AM, Josephs O, Turner R, Frith CD. (1998) A specific role for the thalamus in mediating the interaction between attention and arousal in humans. *J Neurosci.* 18, 8979–8989.

Rawool VW. (2006a) A temporal processing primer. *Hear Rev.* 13, 30–34.

Rawool VW. (2006b) The effects of hearing loss on temporal processing. Part 2: looking beyond simple audition. *Hear Rev.* 13, 32, 34, 39.

Rees NS. (1973) Auditory processing factors in language disorders: the view from Procrustes bed. *J Speech Hear Disord.* 38, 304–315.

Rees NS. (1981) Saying more than we know: is auditory processing disorder a meaningful concept? In: Keith RW, ed. *Central Auditory and Language Disorders in Children.* Houston: College-Hill Press.

Riccio CA, Hynd GW, Cohen MJ, Gonzalez JJ. (1993) Neurological basis of attention deficit hyperactivity disorder. *Except Child.* 60, 118–124.

Romine CB, Reynolds CR. (2004) Sequential memory: a developmental perspective on its relation to frontal lobe functioning. *Neuropsychol Rev.* 14, 43–64.

Sharma A, Dorman MF. (1999) Cortical auditory evoked potential correlates of categorical perception of voice-onset time. *J Acoust Soc Am.* 106, 1078–1083.

Smith B, Resnick D. (1972) An auditory test for assessing brainstem integrity: preliminary report. *Laryngology.* 82, 414–424.

Smith NA, Trainor LJ, Shore DI. (2006) The development of temporal resolution: between-channel gap detection in infants and adults. *J Speech Lang Hear Res.* 49, 1104–1113.

Spencer TJ, Biederman J, Madras BK, Dougherty DD, Bonab AA, Livni E, Meltzer PC, Martin J, Rauch S, Fischman AJ. (2007) Further evidence of dopamine transporter dysregulation in ADHD: a controlled PET imaging study using Altropane. *Biol Psychiatry.* 62, 1059–1061.

Stuart A. (2005) Development of auditory temporal resolution in school-age children revealed by word recognition in continuous and interrupted noise. *Ear Hear.* 26, 78–88.

Tallal P, Miller SL, Bedi G, Byma G, Wang X, Nagarajan SS, Schreiner C, Jenkins WM, Merzenich MM. (1996) Language comprehension in language-learning impaired children improved with acoustically modified speech. *Science.* 271, 81–84.

Tampas JW, Hardicker AW, Hedrick MS. (2005) Neurophysiological indices of speech and nonspeech stimulus processing. *J Speech Lang Hear Res.* 48, 1147–1164.

Teicher MH, Anderson CM, Polcari A, Glod CA, Maas LC, Renshaw PF. (2000) Functional deficits in basal ganglia of children with attention-deficit/hyperactivity disorder shown with functional magnetic resonance imaging relaxometry. *Nat Med.* 6, 470–473.

Tillery KL, Katz J, Keller W. (2000) Effects of methylphenidate (Ritalin) on auditory performance in children with attention and auditory processing disorders. *J Speech Lang Hear Res.* 43, 893–901.

Towse JN, Hitch GJ, Hutton U. (2000) On the interpretation of working memory span in adults. *Psychol Rev.* 99, 122–149.

Volkow ND, Wang G-J, Fowler JS, Logan J, Gerasimov M, Maynard L, Ding Y-S, Gatley SJ, Gifford A, Franceschi D. (2001) Therapeutic doses of oral Methylphenidate significantly increases extracellular Dopamine in the human brain. *J Neurosci.* 21, RC121:1–5.

Wagner BJ. (2000) Attention deficit hyperactivity disorder: current concepts and underlying mechanisms. *J Child Adolesc Psychiatr Nurs.* 13, 113–124.

Warrier CM, Johnson KL, Hayes EA, Nicol T, Kraus N. (2004) Learning impaired children exhibit timing deficits and training-related improvements in auditory cortical responses to speech-in-noise. *Exp Brain Res.* 157, 431–441.

Waugh NC, Norman DA. (1965) Primary memory. *Psychol Rev.* 72, 89–104.

Weissman DH, Gopalakrishnan A, Hazlett CJ, Woldorff MG. (2005) Dorsal anterior cingulate cortex resolves conflict from distracting stimuli by boosting attention toward relevant events. *Cereb Cortex.* 15, 229–237.

Wible B, Nicol T, Kraus N. (2005) Correlation between brainstem and cortical auditory processes in normal and language-impaired children. *Brain.* 128, 417–423.

Wildgruber D, Riecker A, Hertrich A, Erb M, Grodd W, Ethifer T, Ackermann H. (2005) Identification of emotional intonation by fMRI. *Neuroimage.* 24, 1233–1241.

Willeford J, Burleigh J. (1985) *Handbook of Central Auditory Processing Disorders in Children.* Orlando, FL: Grune and Stratton; pp 49–86.

Windsor J, Hwang M. (1999) Children's auditory lexical decisions: a limited processing approach capacity account of language impairment. *J Speech-Lang-Hear Res.* 42, 990–1002.

Wingfield A. (1996) Cognitive factors in auditory performance: context, speed of processing, and constraints of memory. *J Am Acad Audiol.* 7, 175–182.

Woldorff MG, Gallen CG, Hampson SA, Hillyard SA, Pantev C, Sobel D, Bloom FE. (1993) Modulation of early sensory processing in human auditory cortex during selective auditory attention. *Proc Natl Acad Sci USA.* 90, 8722–8726.

Woldorff MG, Hillyard SA. (1991) Modulation of early auditory processing during selective listening to rapidly presented tones. *Electroencephalogr Clin Neurophysiol.* 79, 170–191.

Zaehle T, Wüstenberg T, Meyer M, Jäncke L. (2004) Evidence for rapid auditory perception as the foundation of speech processing: a sparse temporal sampling fMRI study. *Eur J Neurosci.* 20, 2447–2456.

▨ WEBSITES

Anterior Cingulate Cortex. (2007) http://en.wikipedia.org/wiki/Anterior_cingulate_cortex Striatum. (2007) http://en.wikipedia.org/wiki/Striatum.

High Dopamine Transporter Levels Not Correlated with ADHD. (2006) www.sciencedaily.com/releases/2006/11/061129151028.htm.

Attention Deficit–Hyperactivity Disorder: What Causes It? (2007) Available at: www.drugdigest.org/DD/HC/Causes/0,4045,550286,00.html.

Reticular Activating System. (2007) www.newideas.net/adhd/neurology/reticular-activating-system.

26 Auditory Pathway Representations of Speech Sounds in Humans

Daniel A. Abrams and Nina Kraus

▨ INTRODUCTION

An essential function of the central auditory system is the neural encoding of speech sounds. The ability of the brain to translate the acoustic events in the speech signal into meaningful linguistic constructs relies in part on the representation of the acoustic structure of speech by the central nervous system. Consequently, an understanding of how the nervous system accomplishes this task would provide important insight into the basis of language perception and cognitive function.

One of the challenges faced by researchers interested in this subject is that speech is a complex acoustic signal that is rich in both spectral and temporal features. In everyday listening situations, the abundance of acoustic cues in the speech signal provides enormous perceptual benefits to listeners. For example, it has been shown that listeners are able to shift their attention between different acoustic cues when perceiving speech from different talkers to compensate for the inherent variability in the acoustic properties of speech between individuals (Nusbaum and Morin, 1992).

There are two basic approaches that researchers have adopted for conducting experiments on speech perception and underlying physiology. One approach uses "simple" acoustic stimuli, such as tones and clicks, as a means to control for the complexity of the speech signal. While simple stimuli enable researchers to reduce the acoustics of speech to its most basic elements, the auditory system is nonlinear (Sachs and Young, 1979; Sachs et al., 1983; Rauschecker, 1997; Nagarajan et al., 2002), and therefore, responses to simple stimuli generally do not accurately predict responses

to actual speech sounds. A second approach uses speech and speech-like stimuli (Galbraith et al., 2004; Kraus and Nicol, 2005; Krishnan, 2005; Musacchia et al., 2008; Banai and Kraus, in press). There are many advantages to this approach. First, these stimuli are more ecologically valid than simple stimuli. Second, a complete description of how the auditory system responds to speech can only be obtained by using speech stimuli, given the nonlinearity of the auditory system. Third, long-term exposure to speech sounds and the subsequent use of these speech sounds in linguistic contexts induces plastic changes in the auditory pathway, which may alter neural representation of speech in a manner that cannot be predicted by simple stimuli. Fourth, when speech stimuli are chosen carefully, the acoustic properties of the signal can still be well controlled.

This chapter reviews the literature that has begun to elucidate how the human auditory system encodes acoustic features of speech. This chapter is organized into five sections, with each section describing what is currently known about how the brain represents a particular acoustic feature present in speech (Table 26.1). These acoustic features of speech were chosen because of their essential roles in normal speech perception. Each section contains a description of the acoustic feature and an elaboration of its relevance to speech perception, followed by a review and assessment of the data for that acoustic feature. An important consideration is that the acoustic features described in this chapter are not mutually exclusive. For example, one section of this chapter describes the neural encoding of "periodicity," which refers to acoustic events that occur at regular time intervals. Many features in the speech signal are periodic; however,

TABLE 26.1   Acoustic features in speech and neurophysiologic representation

Acoustic features in speech	Feature's role in the speech signal	Brainstem measure	Cortical measure
1. Periodicity	Temporal cue for the fundamental frequency and low formant frequencies (50–500 Hz)	Frequency following response	N100m source location and amplitude; non-primary auditory cortex activity patterns (fMRI)
2. Formant structure	Ubiquitous in vowels, approximants, and nasals; essential for vowel perception	Frequency following response	N100m source location; STS activity (fMRI)
3. Frequency transitions	Consonant identification; signal the presence of diphthongs and glides; linguistic pitch	Frequency following response	Left vs. right STG activity (fMRI)
4. Acoustic onsets	Phoneme identification	ABR onset complex	N100m source location; N100 latency
5. Speech envelope	Syllable and low frequency (<50 Hz) patterns in speech	N/A	N100m phase-locking

STS, superior temporal sulcus; fMRI, functional magnetic resonance imaging; STG, superior temporal gyrus; ABR, auditory brainstem response; N/A, not applicable.

describing the neurophysiologic encoding of all of the periodic features that are processed simultaneously in the speech stimulus in a study of the auditory system would be experimentally unwieldy. Consequently, for the sake of simplicity and to reflect the manner in which they have been investigated in the auditory neuroscience literature, some related acoustic features will be discussed in separate sections. Efforts will be made throughout the chapter to identify when there is overlap among acoustic features.

▨ THE SIGNAL: BASIC SPEECH ACOUSTICS

The speech signal can be described according to a number of basic physical attributes (Johnson, 1997). An understanding of these acoustic attributes is essential to any discussion of how the auditory system encodes speech. The linguistic roles of these acoustic features are described separately within each section of the chapter.

Fundamental frequency. The fundamental frequency is a low-frequency component of speech that results from the periodic beating of the vocal folds. In Figure 26.1A, the frequency content of the naturally produced speech sentence "The young boy left home" is plotted as a function of time; greater amounts of energy at a given frequency are represented with red lines, while smaller amounts of energy are depicted in blue. The fundamental frequency can be seen as the horizontal band of energy in Figure 26.1A that is closest to the x-axis (i.e., lowest in frequency). The fundamental frequency is notated F0 and contributes to the perceived pitch of an individual's voice.

Harmonic structure. An acoustic phenomenon that is related to the fundamental frequency of speech is known as the harmonic structure of speech. Harmonics, which are integer multiples of the fundamental frequency, are present in ongoing speech. The harmonic structure of speech is displayed in Figure 26.1A as the regularly spaced horizontal bands of energy seen throughout the sentence.

Formant structure. Another essential acoustic feature of speech is the formant structure. Formant structure describes a series of discrete peaks in the frequency spectrum of speech that are the result of an interaction between the frequency of vibration of the vocal folds and the resonances within a speaker's vocal tract. The frequencies of these peaks, as well as the relative frequency separations between peaks, varies for different speech sounds. The formant structure of speech interacts with the harmonic structure of speech; the harmonic structure is represented by integer multiples of the fundamental frequency, and harmonics that are close to a resonant frequency of the vocal tract are formants. In Figure 26.1, the formant structure of speech is represented by the series of horizontal and occasionally diagonal red lines that run through most of the speech utterance. The word "left" has been enlarged in Figure 26.1B to better illustrate this phenomenon. The broad and dark patches seen in this figure represent the peaks in the frequency spectrum of speech that are the result of an interaction between the frequency of vibration of the vocal folds and the resonances of a speaker's vocal tract. The frequency of these peaks, as well as the relative frequency between peaks, varies for different speech sounds within the sentence. The lowest frequency formant is known as the first formant and is notated F1, while subsequent formants are notated F2, F3, etc.

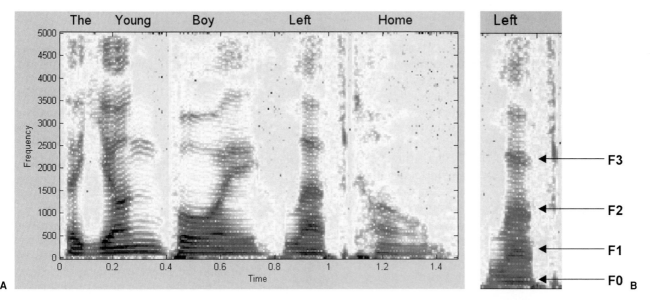

FIGURE 26.1 Spectrogram for the naturally produced speech sentence "The young boy left home." (A) The complete sentence; **(B)** the word "left" is enlarged to illustrate the frequency structure; the fundamental frequency (F0) and formants (F1-F3) are represented in the spectrogram by broader dark band regions of energy.

THE MEASURES OF BRAIN ACTIVITY

We begin by describing the neurophysiologic measures that have been used to probe auditory responses to speech and speech-like stimuli; comprehensive descriptions of these measures can be found elsewhere (Sato, 1990; Hall, 1992; Jezzard et al., 2001) as well as in various chapters in this text. Historically, the basic research on the neurophysiology of speech perception has borrowed a number of clinical tools to assess auditory system function.

Brainstem Responses

The auditory brainstem response (ABR) consists of small voltages originating from auditory structures in the brainstem in response to sound. Although these responses do not pinpoint the specific origin of auditory activity among the auditory brainstem nuclei, the great strength of the ABR (and auditory potentials in general) is that they precisely reflect the time-course of neural activity at the microsecond level. The ABR is typically measured with a single active electrode referenced to the earlobe or nose. Clinical evaluations using the ABR typically use brief acoustic stimuli, such as clicks and tones, to elicit brainstem activity. The ABR is unique among the auditory evoked potentials (AEPs) because of the remarkable reliability of this response, both within and across subjects. In the clinic, the ABR is used to assess the integrity of the auditory periphery and lower brainstem (Hall, 1992). The response consists of a number of peaks, with wave V being the most clinically reliable. Deviations on the order of microseconds are deemed "abnormal" in the clinic and are associated with some form of peripheral hearing damage or with retrocochlear pathologies. Research using the ABR to probe acoustic processing of speech uses similar recording procedures but different acoustic stimuli.

Cortical Responses

CORTICAL EVOKED POTENTIALS AND FIELDS

Cortical evoked responses are used as a research tool to probe auditory function in normal and clinical populations. Cortical evoked potentials are small voltages originating from auditory structures in the cortex in response to sound. These potentials are typically measured with multiple electrodes, often referenced to a "common reference," which is the average response measured across all electrodes. Cortical evoked "fields" are the magnetic counterpart to cortical evoked potentials; however, instead of measuring voltage across the scalp, the magnetic fields produced by brain activity are measured. Electroencephalography (EEG) is the technique by which evoked potentials are measured, and magnetoencephalography (MEG) is the technique by which evoked fields are measured. Similar to the ABR, the strength of assessing cortical evoked potentials and fields is that they provide detailed information about the time-course of activation and how sound is encoded by temporal response properties of large populations of auditory neurons, although these techniques are limited in their spatial resolution. Due to large inter- and intrasubject variability in cortical responses, they are not generally used clinically. Results from these two methodologies are generally compatible, despite some differences in the neural generators that contribute to each of these responses. Studies using both EEG and MEG are described interchangeably throughout this chapter despite the subtle differences between the measures. The nomenclature of waveform peaks is similar for EEG and MEG and typically involves an N or P, depicting a negative or positive deflection, followed by a number indicating the approximate latency of the peak. Finally, the letter "m" follows the latency for MEG results. For example, N100 and N100m are the labels for a negative deflection at 100 ms as measured by EEG and MEG, respectively.

Functional Imaging

Functional imaging of the auditory system is another often-used technique to quantify auditory activity in the brain. The technology that is used to measure these responses, as well as the results they yield, is considerably different from the previously described techniques. The primary difference is that functional imaging is an indirect measure of neural activity; that is, instead of measuring voltages or fields resulting from activity in auditory neurons, functional imaging measures hemodynamics, a term used to describe changes in metabolism as a result of changes in brain activity. The data produced by these measures produce a three-dimensional map of activity within the brain as a result of a given stimulus. The strong correlation between actual neural activity and blood flow to the same areas of the brain (Smith et al., 2002a) has made functional imaging a valuable investigative tool to measure auditory activity in the brain. The two methods of functional imaging described here are functional magnetic resonance imaging (fMRI) and positron emission tomography (PET). The difference between these two techniques is that fMRI measures natural levels of oxygen in the brain because oxygen is consumed by neurons when they become active. PET, however, requires the injection of a radioactive isotope into a subject. The isotope emits positrons, which can be detected by a scanner, as it circulates in the subject's bloodstream. Increases in neural activity draw more blood and, consequently, more of the radioactive isotope to a given region of the brain. The main advantage that functional imaging offers relative to evoked potentials and evoked fields is that it provides extremely accurate spatial information regarding the origin of neural activity in the brain. A disadvantage is the poor resolution in the temporal domain; neural activity is often integrated over the course of seconds, which is considered extremely slow given that speech tokens are as brief as 30 ms. Although recent work using functional imaging has begun describing activity in subcortical regions, the work described here will only cover studies of the temporal cortex.

ACOUSTIC FEATURES OF SPEECH

Periodicity

DEFINITION AND ROLE IN THE PERCEPTION OF SPEECH

Periodicity, as defined by Rosen, refers to temporal fluctuations in the speech signal between 50 and 500 Hz (Rosen, 1992). Important aspects of the speech signal that contain periodic acoustic information include the fundamental frequency and low-frequency components of the formant structure (note that encoding of the formant structure of speech is covered in a later section). The acoustic information provided by periodicity conveys both phonetic information as well as prosodic cues, such as intonation and stress, in the speech signal. As stated in Rosen's paper, this category of temporal information represents both the periodic features in speech and the distinction between the periodic and aperiodic portions of the signal, which fluctuate at much faster rates.

This section will review studies describing the neural representation of relatively stationary periodic components in the speech signal, most notably the fundamental frequency. An understanding of the mechanism for encoding a simple periodic feature of the speech signal, the F0, will facilitate descriptions of complex periodic features of the speech signal, such as the formant structure and frequency modulations.

PHYSIOLOGIC REPRESENTATION OF THE PERIODICITY IN THE HUMAN BRAIN

Auditory Brainstem

The short-latency frequency-following response (FFR) is an electrophysiologic measure of phase-locked neural activity originating from brainstem nuclei that represents responses to periodic acoustic stimuli up to approximately 1,000 Hz (Smith et al., 1975; Stillman et al., 1978; Gardi et al., 1979; Galbraith et al., 2000). Based on the frequency range that can be measured with the FFR, a representation of the fundamental frequency can be measured using this methodology (Cunningham et al., 2001; King et al., 2002; Krishnan et al., 2004; 2005; Musacchia et al., 2007; Russo et al., 2004; 2005; 2008; Song et al. (in press); Wible et al., 2004; Johnson et al., 2005; Wong et al., 2007), as well as the F1 in some instances (encoding of F1 is discussed in detail in the Formant Structure section).

A number of studies have shown that F0 is represented within the steady-state portion of the brainstem response (i.e., FFR) according to a series of negative peaks that are temporally spaced in correspondence to the wavelength of the fundamental frequency. An example of F0 representation in the FFR can be seen in Figure 26.2, which shows the waveform of the speech stimulus /da/ (top), an experimental stimulus that has been studied in great detail, as well as the brainstem response to this speech sound (bottom). A

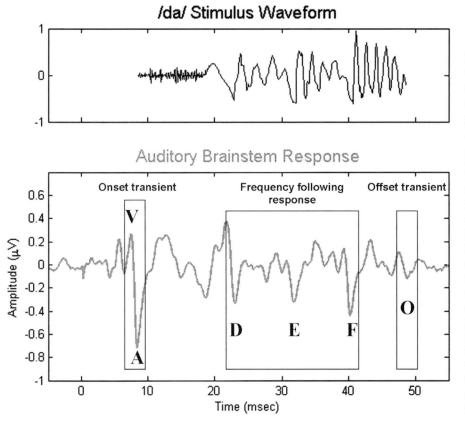

/da/ Stimulus Waveform

Auditory Brainstem Response

Onset transient

Frequency following response

Offset transient

V

A

D E F

O

Time (msec)

FIGURE 26.2 Acoustic waveform of the synthesized speech stimulus /da/ (*above*) and grand average auditory brainstem responses to /da/ (*below*). The stimulus has been moved forward in time to the latency of onset responses (peak V) to enable direct comparisons with brainstem responses. Peaks V and A reflect the onset of the speech sound, and peak O reflects stimulus offset. Peaks D, E, and F represent a phase-locked representation to the fundamental frequency of the speech stimulus, and the peaks between D, E, and F occur at the F1 frequency.

cursory inspection of this figure shows that the primary periodic features of the speech waveform provided by the F0 are clearly represented in peaks D, E, and F of the FFR brainstem response. Importantly, it has been shown that the FFR is highly sensitive to F0 frequency; this aspect of the brainstem response accurately "tracks" modulations in frequency (Krishnan et al., 2004), a topic that is discussed in depth in the Frequency Transitions section of this chapter.

A hypothesis regarding the brainstem's encoding of different aspects of the speech signal has been proposed in a recent paper (Kraus and Nicol, 2005). Specifically, it is proposed that the source (referring to vocal fold vibration) and filter aspects (vocal musculature in the production of speech) of a speech signal show dissociation in their acoustic representation in the auditory brainstem. The source portion of the brainstem's response to speech is the representation of the F0, while the filter refers to all other features, including speech onset, offset, and the representation of formant frequencies. For example, it has been demonstrated that brainstem responses are correlated within source and filter classes but are not correlated between classes (Russo et al., 2004). Moreover, in a study of children with language-learning disabilities whose behavioral deficits may be attributable to central auditory processing disorders, it has been shown that source representation in the auditory brainstem is normal, while filter class representation is impaired (Cunningham et al., 2001; King et al., 2002; Hayes et al., 2003; Wible et al., 2004; 2005). An interesting note is that a recent study showed

that source cues (F0) are abnormally represented in many children with autism spectrum disorder, which has important implications for some of their behavioral deficits (Russo et al., 2008). These data suggest that the acoustic representations of source and filter aspects of a given speech signal are differentially processed and provide evidence for neural specialization at the level of the brainstem. Additionally, it is proposed that this scheme may constitute brainstem origins for cortical "what," "where" pathways (Kraus and Nicol, 2005).

Cortex

It has been shown that neurons in the auditory cortex respond robustly with time-locked responses to slow rates of stimulation ($< \sim25$ Hz) and generally do not phase-lock to frequencies greater than approximately 100 Hz (Creutzfeldt et al., 1980; Eggermont, 1991; Steinschneider et al., 1998; Lu et al., 2001). Therefore, cortical phase-locking to the fundamental frequency of speech, which is greater than 100 Hz, is poor, and it is generally thought that the brainstem's phase-locked (i.e., temporal) representation of F0 is transformed at the level of cortex to a more abstract representation. For example, it has been shown that cortical neurons produce sustained, nonsynchronized discharges throughout a high-frequency (>50 Hz) stimulus (Lu et al., 2001), resulting in a more abstract representation of the stimulus frequency compared to time-locked neural activation.

An important aspect of F0 perception is that listeners native to a particular language are able to perceive a given speech sound as invariant regardless of the speaker's F0, which varies considerably among men (F0 = ~100 Hz), women (F0 = ~200 Hz), and children (F0 = up to 400 Hz). For example, the speech sound "dog" is categorized by a listener to mean the exact same thing regardless of whether an adult or a child produces the vocalization, even though there is a considerable difference in the acoustic properties of the adult's and child's vocalization with respect to the fundamental frequency. To address how auditory cortical responses reflect relatively large variations in F0 between speakers, N100m cortical responses were measured with MEG for a set of Finnish vowel and vowel-like stimuli that varied in F0, while keeping all other formant information (F1-F4) constant (Makela et al., 2002). Results indicated that N100m responses were extremely similar in spatial activation pattern and amplitude for all vowel and vowel-like stimuli, irrespective of the F0. This is a particularly intriguing finding given that N100m responses differed when 100-, 200-, and 400-Hz puretone stimuli were presented to the same subjects in a control condition. The similarity of the speech-evoked brain responses, which were independent of the F0 frequency, suggests that variances in F0 may be filtered out of the neural representation by the time it reaches the cortex. The authors suggest that the insensitivity of cortical responses to variations in the F0 may facilitate the semantic categorization of the speech sound. An alternative interpretation of this finding is that the representation of F0 has been transformed at the level of cortex in a manner that was not reflected in these particular spatial activation measures. For example, it is plausible that the F0 is transformed to a rate-based code at the level of cortex as opposed to a place code. If this were the case, then the F0 would not be expected to be reflected in the spatial maps described in this study.

In summary, periodicity of the fundamental frequency is robustly represented in the FFR of the ABR. Moreover, the representation of the fundamental frequency is normal in learning-disabled children despite the abnormal representations of speech-sound onset and first formant frequency. This disparity in the learning-disabled auditory system provides evidence that different features of speech sounds may be served by different neural mechanisms and/or populations and first formant frequency in a certain segment of the learning disabled population. In the cortex, MEG results suggest that the spatial organization of cortical responses are relatively insensitive to changes in the fundamental frequency of speech, however it remains a possibility that F0 is coded in cortex in another manner.

Formant Structure

ROLE IN THE PERCEPTION OF SPEECH

Formant structure describes a series of discrete peaks in the frequency spectrum of speech that are the result of an interaction between vibration of the vocal folds and the resonances within a speaker's vocal tract (see introduction of this chapter for a more complete acoustic description of the formant structure). The formant structure is a dominant acoustic feature of sonorants, a class of speech sounds that includes vowels, approximants, and nasals. The formant structure has a special role in the perception of vowels in that formant frequencies, particularly the relationship between F1 and F2 (Peterson and Barney, 1952), are the primary phonetic determinants of vowels. For example, the essential acoustic difference between /u/ and /i/ is a positive shift in F2 frequency (Peterson and Barney, 1952). Due to the special role of formants for vowel perception, much of the research regarding the formant structure of speech uses vowel stimuli.

PHYSIOLOGIC REPRESENTATION OF FORMANT STRUCTURE IN THE HUMAN BRAIN

Auditory Brainstem

The question of how the human auditory brainstem represents important components of the formant structure was addressed in a study by Krishnan (2002). In this study, brainstem (FFR) responses to three steady-state vowels were measured, and the spectral content of the responses were compared to that of the vowel stimuli. All three of the stimuli had approximately the same fundamental frequency; however, the first two formant frequencies were different in each of the vowel stimuli. Results indicate that at higher stimulus intensities, the brainstem FFR accurately represents F1 and F2; however, the representation of F1 has an increased representation relative to F2. The author indicates the similarity between this finding and a similar result in a classic study of vowel representation in the auditory nerve of anesthetized cats (Sachs and Young, 1979) in which the predominance of the representation to F1 was also demonstrated. These data provide evidence that phase-locking serves as a mechanism for encoding critical components of the formant structure not only in the auditory nerve, but also in the auditory brainstem.

Auditory Cortex

A number of studies have described the representation of formant structure in the human cortex as a means of investigating whether a cortical map of phonemes, termed the "phonemotopic" map, exists in the human brain. Specifically, researchers want to know if the phonemotopic map is independent of the tonotopic map or, alternatively, whether phonemes are more simply represented according to their frequency content along the tonotopic gradient in auditory cortex. To this end, investigators have measured cortical responses to vowel stimuli, a class of speech sounds that differ acoustically from one another according to the distribution of F1-F2 formant frequencies. Vowel stimuli also offer the advantage of exhibiting no temporal structure beyond the periodicity of the formants.

The method that has been used to investigate the relationship between the tonotopic map in human auditory cortex and the representation of formant structure has been to compare cortical source locations for tones and specific speech sounds with similar frequency components. For example, in one study (Diesch and Luce, 1997), N100m source location was measured in response to separately presented 600-Hz and 2,100-Hz puretones, as well as a two-tone composite signal comprising the component puretones (i.e., simultaneous presentation of the 600-Hz and 2,100-Hz puretones). These responses were compared to isolated formants, defined as the first and second formant frequencies of a vowel stimulus, complete with their harmonic structure, separated from the rest of the frequency components of the stimulus (i.e., F0, higher formant frequencies). These isolated formants had the same frequency as the tonal stimuli (i.e., 600 Hz and 2,100 Hz). Finally, a two-formant composite signal, which constituted a vowel, was also presented. Results indicated that the N100m source in response to the vowel stimulus was different in location from that predicted by both the puretone responses and by the superposition of responses to the component single-formant stimuli. These data indicate that formant structure is spatially represented in human cortex differently than the linear sum of responses to the component formant stimuli and suggest that formant structure is represented orthogonal to the tonotopic map. The authors of this work hypothesize that the different spatial representation of the vowel stimuli reflects the additional acoustic components of the vowel stimuli, including the harmonic and formant structures. The authors of this work refrain from stating a potentially more intriguing conclusion; that is, does the spatial representation of the vowel stimuli in some way reflect the behavioral experience of the subjects with these speech sounds? For example, it is possible that a larger, or different, population of cortical neurons is recruited for sounds that are familiar or have significant ecologic importance relative to the population recruited for puretones or single formant frequencies, and that the source location for the vowels reflects this phenomenon.

Additional studies have attempted to better describe the acoustic representation of vowels in the human brain. In one study, Obleser et al. (2003) addressed the neurophysiology underlying a classic study of speech acoustics in which it was shown that the distinction of vowels is largely carried by the frequency relationship of F1 and F2 (Peterson and Barney, 1952). To this end, cortical source locations were measured in response to German vowels that differ naturally in their F1-F2 relationships. Results indicated that the location of the N100m source reflects the frequency relationship of the F1-F2 formant components. This finding was replicated in a second study using 450 natural speech exemplars of three Russian vowels; again, the spectral distance between F1 and F2 was reflected in the dipole location of N100m responses (Shestakova et al., 2004). In both studies, the authors suggested that cortical sensitivity to F1-F2 differences can be explained by inhibitory response patterns in the auditory cortex; the closer the F1 frequency is to F2, the greater the

reciprocal neural inhibition, which, in turn, influences the location of the dipole source as measured by MEG (Obleser et al., 2003).

While these studies provide evidence that the cortex represents the formant structure of vowels in a manner that is (1) unrelated to the tonotopic map and (2) organized according to the perceptually essential formant frequencies, these findings require a number of caveats. First, the source locations described in these studies represent the center of gravity, as a single point in three-dimensional space in the cortex, of the neural contributors to a given N100m response (Naatanen and Picton, 1987). Because it is known that the N100 response has as many as six separate cortical generators, the N100m sources for even a simple cortical map (i.e., the tonotopic map), let alone a complex map such as the putative phonemotopic map, represent at least a partial abstraction of the underlying anatomy and should not be viewed as an exact representation of well-described auditory maps in animal models (Schreiner, 1998). This is particularly relevant given that the clear tonotopic gradient in the auditory cortex is no longer apparent when puretone stimuli are presented above 50 dB sound pressure level (SPL) (Schreiner, 1998), such as the levels used in the MEG experiments described in this section. In addition, it has not yet been definitively shown that the neural representations of phonemes described in these studies truly constitute a "phonemotopic" map. The presence of a phonemotopic map suggests behavioral relevance of phoneme stimuli beyond their acoustic attributes. None of the studies described here have tested whether cortical responses to the F1-F2 components for nonnative vowel sounds show similar sensitivity as native phonemes. Despite these limitations, these studies provide consistent evidence that a perceptually critical aspect of the formant structure of vowels, the F1-F2 relationship, is represented in a spatial map in the auditory cortex as early as approximately 100 ms after stimulus onset.

Another line of evidence has used functional imaging to show the particular regions of the temporal cortex that are sensitive to the formant structure of speech sounds relative to other natural and vocally generated (e.g., laughs, coughs) sounds (Belin et al., 2000). Cortical responses to natural vocal stimuli were compared to vocal stimuli in which the formant structure of speech was replaced by white noise and scrambled vocal sounds. All stimuli were matched for overall RMS energy. In both of these experimental conditions, the altered spectral information was modulated by the original amplitude envelope of the speech signal. Results from this experiment indicated that all stimuli activated regions along the superior temporal sulcus (STS), a cortical region consisting of unimodal auditory and multimodal areas that is hypothesized to be a critical speech processing center subsequent to more rudimentary acoustic processing in the superior temporal gyrus. However, responses to the natural vocal stimuli were significantly larger and more widespread throughout the STS, particularly in the right hemisphere, than for the spectrally manipulated vocal stimuli. These data indicate that the formant structure of speech deeply affects activity patterns in the STS, a speech-selective region of temporal cortex. Moreover, these data suggest a right hemisphere bias for processing the formant structure, which supports the more general hypothesis that the right hemisphere is dominant for resolving spectral components in acoustic signals (Zatorre and Belin, 2001; Zatorre et al., 2002).

An interesting consideration is how cortical asymmetries in response to the acoustic features of speech relate to well-established cerebral asymmetries for higher order language processing, such as phonemic and semantic processing (Geschwind and Galaburda, 1985; Binder et al., 1997; Hickok and Poeppel, 2004), which are strongly lateralized to the left hemisphere, although Hickok and Poeppel (2007) are less empathetic about assymetries, especially for phonemic processing. While a direct link between these forms of asymmetry has not been established, a plausible scenario is that the acoustic-level asymmetries precede and serve as the input to phonemic and semantic processing in left hemisphere language regions. If this is the case, it remains to be seen what physiologic advantage a right hemisphere preference for formant structure processing (Belin et al., 2000) might offer given that phonemic and semantic processing of speech stimuli takes place in the opposite hemisphere, thereby requiring transmission through the corpus callosum. Future studies investigating acoustic-level asymmetries and their interface with higher order language asymmetries would provide essential information regarding the functional neuroanatomy of speech perception.

In summary, the brainstem encodes lower formant frequencies, which are critical to vowel perception, with phase-locked responses. Converging evidence indicates that the cortex encodes a perceptually essential aspect of the formant structure of speech. Specifically, the F1-F2 relationship is spatially mapped in the cortex at approximately 100 ms after stimulus onset as measured by N100m source location. In addition, functional imaging data provide evidence that the STS, a nonprimary region of temporal cortex, is more responsive to speech stimuli that contain formant structure than speech in which the formant structure has been replaced with other sounds. Together, these results suggest that both primary and nonprimary regions of temporal cortex are sensitive to aspects of the formant structure that are essential for normal perception.

Frequency Transitions

ACOUSTIC DESCRIPTION AND ROLE IN THE PERCEPTION OF SPEECH

Frequency transitions of the fundamental and formant frequencies permeate ongoing speech. In English, modulation of the fundamental frequency does not provide segmental cues; rather, it provides suprasegmental cues such as the intent (e.g., question or statement) and emotional state of the

speaker. In other languages, such as Mandarin and Thai, modulations to the fundamental frequency provide phonetic cues. Formant transitions, on the other hand, are critical to speech perception of English, and most languages in the world, in that they serve as a cue for consonant identification and signal the presence of diphthongs and glides (Lehiste and Peterson, 1961). Moreover, formant transitions also have been shown to play a role in vowel identification (Nearey and Assmann, 1986). The movements of formant frequencies can be distilled to three basic forms that occur during an ongoing sequence of phonemes (taken from Lehiste and Peterson [1961]): (1) the movement of a formant from the initiation of the consonant until the beginning of the vowel in a consonant-vowel combination, (2) the movement of a formant from one vowel to another vowel (i.e., in a diphthong), and (3) formant movement from a vowel until vowel termination for a vowel-consonant combination. The frequency modulations that occur during formant transitions can occur at relatively fast rates (~40 ms) while spanning large frequency ranges (>2,000 Hz in F2 transitions).

PHYSIOLOGIC REPRESENTATION OF FREQUENCY TRANSITIONS IN THE HUMAN BRAIN

Auditory Brainstem

The short-latency FFR is able to "track," or follow, frequency changes in speech. This phenomenon was demonstrated in a study of FFR tracking of the fundamental frequency (F0) in Mandarin speech sounds (Krishnan et al., 2004). In this study, FFR to four different tonal permutations of the Mandarin word "yi" were measured in a group of native Mandarin speakers. Specifically, synthetic stimuli consisted of "yi" pronounced with (1) a flat F0 contour, (2) a rising F0 contour, (3) a falling F0 contour, and (4) a concave F0 contour that fell and then rose in frequency. In Mandarin, which is a "tonal" language, these four stimuli are different words; the F0 contour provides the only acoustic cue to differentiate them. Results indicated that the FFR represented the fundamental frequency modulations and harmonics for all of the stimulus conditions, irrespective of the form of the frequency contour. These data indicate that the FFR represents phase-locked activity in the brainstem for rapidly changing frequency components in speech. A recent study showed that it is also possible to distinguish different formant transitions present in stop consonants through brainstem timing (Johnson et al., in press).

A similar methodology was used in another study by Krishnan et al. (2005) to investigate the role of language experience on auditory brainstem encoding of pitch. FFRs to the "yi" stimuli described earlier were measured in native Mandarin speakers as well as native speakers of American English, to whom the stimuli bear no linguistic value. Results from this study indicate greater FFR pitch strength and pitch tracking in the Chinese subjects compared to the native English speakers across all four of the Mandarin tones. The FFR of the Chinese subjects also indicated increased harmonic representation of the fundamental frequency (i.e., larger neural representation of the harmonic content of the F0) compared to the English speakers. These data indicate that responses from the auditory brainstem reflect the behavioral experience of a listener by enhancing the neural representation of linguistically relevant acoustic features.

A hypothesis proposed by Ahissar and Hochstein (2004) may explain how experience engenders plasticity at low levels of sensory systems. Their "reverse hierarchy" theory proposes that when a naïve subject attempts to perform a perceptual task, the performance on that task is governed by the "top" of a sensory hierarchy. As this "top" level of the system masters performance on the task, over time, lower levels of the system are modified and refined to provide more precise encoding of sensory information. This can be thought of as an efferent pathway–mediated tuning of afferent sensory input. While the reverse hierarchy theory does not explicitly discuss plasticity of the brainstem, this theory could account for the findings of Krishnan, et al. Specifically, due to the importance of extracting lexical information present in pitch contours, native Mandarin speakers are "expert" at encoding this acoustic feature, which is accomplished, at least in part, by extreme precision and robustness of sensory encoding in low levels of the auditory system such as the brainstem. Native English speakers, who are not required to extract lexical meaning from pitch contours, are relative novices at this form of pitch tracking, and consequently, their brainstems have not acquired this level of modification.

An interesting question that was not addressed in this study but was proposed as a discussion item is whether native Mandarin speakers are better than English speakers at pitch tracking the F0 exclusively for familiar speech sounds or whether Mandarin speakers' superior performance would extend to all periodic acoustic signals, including nonnative speech sounds. This question would address whether a lifetime of experience using F0 to extract linguistic meaning generally improves the auditory system's ability to track all types of pitches or, alternatively, whether this phenomenon is exclusive to pitches present in familiar speech sounds. A recent study examined this particular question by measuring brainstem responses to speech-like stimuli characterized by linear F0 contours in native Mandarin and English speakers (Xu et al., 2006). Linear F0 contours are not characteristic of either English or Mandarin; however, they resemble the curvilinear contours in Mandarin. Results of this study showed that native English and Mandarin speakers had similar brainstem responses to the linear contours. This suggests that language experience specifically tunes the auditory brainstem to the pitch contours that are inherent to an individual's native language, and this tuning does not generalize to non-native pitch contours. Data from our lab suggest that another form of long-term auditory experience, musicianship, contributes to enhanced neural encoding of speech sounds in the auditory brainstem relative to nonmusicians

(Musacchia et al., 2007; Wong et al., 2004). This finding provides evidence that expertise associated with one type of acoustic signal (i.e., music) provides a general augmentation of the auditory system that is manifested in brain responses to another type of acoustic signal (i.e., speech) and indicates that auditory experience can modify basic sensory encoding.

Auditory Cortex

Similar to Krishnan's work involving the brainstem, multiple studies have investigated cortical processing of F0 pitch contours and its relationship to language experience (Chandrasekaran et al., 2007; 2008; Gandour et al., 1998; Klein et al., 2001; Wang et al., 2001). In one study, native Mandarin and native English speakers underwent PET scanning during passive listening and while performing a pitch discrimination task. Stimuli consisted of (1) Mandarin speech sounds that contained modulations of the fundamental frequency signaling lexical meaning and (2) English speech sounds that also contained modulations to the fundamental frequency; however, F0 modulations never provide lexical information in English. Imaging results indicated that native Mandarin speakers showed significant activation of the left anterior insular cortex, adjacent to Broca's area, only when discriminating Mandarin speech sounds (but not when engaged in passive listening); in contrast, the homologous right anterior insula was activated when this group discriminated English speech sounds, as well as when native English speakers discriminated both Mandarin and English speech sounds. These data suggest that the left anterior insula is involved in auditory processing of modulations to the fundamental frequency only when those modulations are associated with lexical processing. Moreover, these data suggest that the neural processing of acoustic signals is context dependent and is not solely based on the acoustic attributes of the stimuli.

In addition to studies of the neural representation of F0 modulations, a number of studies have also addressed the cortical representation of formant frequency modulation in humans. It is known that neurons in the auditory cortex do not phase-lock to frequencies greater than approximately 100 Hz (Creutzfeldt et al., 1980; Eggermont, 1991; Steinschneider et al., 1998; Lu et al., 2001), whereas the formant structure of speech consists of frequencies almost exclusively above 100 Hz. Consequently, the cortical representation of frequency modulation as measured by evoked potentials is abstract (i.e., not represented with time-locked responses) relative to that described for the auditory brainstem. One cortical mechanism that has received considerable attention for the processing of rapid formant modulations is that of asymmetric processing in the left hemisphere auditory cortex. A more general hypothesis proposes that the left hemisphere auditory cortex is specialized for all forms of rapid acoustic stimuli and serves as an early acoustic analysis stage at the level of the cortex. A significant piece of evidence in support of this hypothesis was provided in a study of cortical activation patterns for rapid and slow formant frequency modulations (Belin et al., 1998). In this study, nonspeech sounds containing temporal and spectral characteristics similar to speech sounds were presented to listeners as they were PET scanned. Nonspeech sounds were used so that any cortical asymmetry could not be associated with well-known asymmetries for language processing. Results indicated that the left superior temporal gyrus (STG), including primary auditory cortex, showed greater activation than the right STG for rapid (40 ms) formant frequency transitions but not for slow (200 ms) transitions. In addition, a left hemisphere region of prefrontal cortex was asymmetrically activated for the rapid formant transition, which was corroborated in a separate fMRI study that used nearly identical acoustic stimuli (Temple et al., 2000). Finally, it was shown that left-hemisphere preference for rapid acoustic signals is correlated to the timing of responses measured in the auditory brainstem (Abrams et al., 2006). These data suggest that left hemisphere auditory regions preferentially process rapid formant modulations present in ongoing speech.

In summary, results measured from the auditory brainstem indicate that modulations in the fundamental frequency of speech are faithfully encoded in the FFR. Moreover, these particular brainstem responses appear to be shaped by linguistic experience, a remarkable finding that indicates that cognitive processes (e.g., language) influence basic sensory processing. In the cortex, a mechanism for encoding frequency modulation is the specialization of left hemisphere auditory regions. Results indicate that rapid frequency changes in speech-like stimuli preferentially activate the left hemisphere relative to slower frequency changes. In addition, the anterior insular cortex is activated for the processing of F0 modulations; the left hemisphere insula is specifically activated when F0 modulations provide lexical information to a native speaker, while the right hemisphere insula is activated when F0 modulations do not provide lexical information. These cortical findings would appear to be contradictory; the former indicates that asymmetric activation by left hemisphere structures is based on physical parameters of the speech signal, irrespective of linguistic content, while the latter suggests that linguistic context is essential for left asymmetric insular processing of F0 modulations. However, Wong et al. (2004) stated that these results can be reconciled if the insular activity shown in their study occurs after the "acoustically specialized" cortical activity described by Belin et al. (1998) and Temple et al. (2000). If this were true, it would indicate two independent levels of cortical asymmetry: one based on the acoustic attributes of the signal and one based on the linguistic relevance to the listener. This hypothesis needs to be tested in future studies.

Acoustic Onsets

ACOUSTIC DESCRIPTION AND ROLE IN THE PERCEPTION OF SPEECH

Acoustic onsets are defined here as the spectral and temporal features present at the beginning (the initial ~40 ms) of

speech sounds. While the acoustics of phonemes are only slightly altered based on their location in a word (i.e., beginning, middle, or end of a word), an emphasis has been put on acoustic onsets in the neurophysiologic literature. Consequently, acoustic onsets are discussed here separately, despite some overlap with acoustic features (i.e., frequency transitions) discussed previously.

Onset acoustics of speech sounds vary considerably in both their spectral and temporal attributes. In some cases, the spectral features of the onset are essential for perception (e.g., the onset frequency of F3 for discriminating /da/ vs. /ga/), whereas in other cases, temporal attributes of onsets are the critical feature for perception. A frequently studied acoustic phenomenon associated with the temporal attributes of speech-sound onset is that of voice onset time (VOT), which is present in stop consonants. The VOT is defined as the duration of time between the release of a stop consonant by speech articulators and the beginning of vocal fold vibration. The duration of the VOT is the acoustic cue that enables differentiation between consonants that are otherwise extremely similar (e.g., /da/ vs. /ta/, /ba/ vs. /pa/, /ga/ vs. /ka/).

PHYSIOLOGIC REPRESENTATION OF ACOUSTIC ONSETS IN THE HUMAN BRAIN

Auditory Brainstem

The brainstem response to speech-sound onset has been studied extensively (Cunningham et al., 2001; King et al., 2002; Russo et al., 2004; 2005; Wible et al., 2004; 2005; Banai et al., 2005; Johnson et al., 2005; 2008; Kraus and Nicol, 2005). The first components of the speech-evoked ABR reflect the onset of the brainstem response to the stimulus (Fig. 26.2). Speech onset is represented in the brainstem response at approximately 7 ms in the form of two peaks, positive peak V and negative peak A.

Findings from a number of studies have demonstrated that the brainstem's response to acoustic transients is closely linked to auditory perception and to language-based cortical function such as literacy. These studies have investigated brainstem responses to speech in normal children and children with language-based learning disabilities (LD), a population that has consistently demonstrated perceptual deficits in auditory tasks using both simple (Tallal and Piercy, 1973; Reed, 1989; Hari and Kiesila, 1996; Wright et al., 1997; Hari et al., 1999; Nagarajan et al., 1999; Ahissar et al., 2001; Benasich and Tallal, 2002; Witton et al., 2002) and complex (Tallal and Piercy, 1975; Kraus et al., 1996; Bradlow et al., 1999; 2003; Ramus et al., 2003) acoustic stimuli. A general hypothesis proposes a causal link between basic auditory perceptual deficits in LDs and higher level language skills, such as reading and phonologic tasks (Tallal et al., 1993), although this relationship has been debated (Mody et al., 1997; Schulte-Korne et al., 1998; Bishop et al., 1999; Ramus et al., 2003). In support of a hypothesis linking basic auditory function and language skills, studies of the auditory brainstem indicate a fundamental deficiency in the synchrony of auditory neurons in the brainstem for a significant proportion of language-disabled subjects.

The brainstem's response to acoustic transients in speech features prominently in distinguishing LD from normal (control) subjects. A number of studies have provided compelling evidence that the representation of speech onset (Cunningham et al., 2000; King et al., 2002; Wible et al., 2004; 2005; Banai et al., 2005) is abnormal in a significant proportion of LD subjects. For example, brainstem responses to the speech syllable /da/ were measured for a group of 33 normal and 54 LD children; a "normal range" was established from the results of the normal subjects (King et al., 2002). Results indicated that 20 LD subjects (37%) showed abnormally late responses to onset peak A. Another study showed a significant difference between normal and LD subjects based on another measure of the brainstem's representation of acoustic transients (Wible et al., 2004). Specifically, it was shown that the slope between onset peaks V and A to the /da/ syllable was significantly smaller in LD subjects compared to normal subjects. The authors of this study indicate that the diminished V/A slope demonstrated by LDs is a measure of abnormal synchrony to the onset transients of the stimulus and could be the result of abnormal neural conduction by brainstem generators. The suggestion of abnormal neural conduction is consistent with anatomic findings of deficient axonal myelination in the temporal cortex of LD subjects (Klingberg et al., 2000). In another study (Banai et al., 2005), LD subjects with abnormal brainstem timing for acoustic transients were more likely to have a more severe form of LD, manifested in poorer scores on measures of literacy, compared to LD subjects with normal brainstem responses.

Taken together, these data suggest that the brainstem responses to acoustic transients can not only differentiate a subpopulation of LD persons from normal subjects, but can also differentiate the LD population in terms of the severity of the disability. Findings from the brainstem measures also indicate a link between sensory encoding and cognitive processes such as literacy. An important question is whether the link between sensory encoding and cognition is a causal one and, if so, whether brainstem deficits are responsible for cortical deficits (or vice versa). Alternatively, these two abnormalities may be merely coincident. Nevertheless, the consistent findings of brainstem abnormalities in a certain portion of the LD population have led to the incorporation of this experimental paradigm into the clinical evaluation of LD and central auditory processing disorders. The "BioMAP" (Biological Marker of Auditory Processing, Biologic Systems Corp., Mundelein, IL) measures and analyzes the brainstem response to speech and has been shown to be a reliable measure for the objective evaluation of children with learning and listening disorders.

Auditory Cortex

Cortical encoding of spectral features of speech-sound onset was recently reported by Obleser et al. (2006). In this paper, it was shown that a spectral contrast at speech onset, resulting from consonant place of articulation (e.g., front-produced consonant /d/ or /t/ vs. back-produced consonant /g/ or /k/), is mapped along the anterior-posterior axis in the auditory cortex as measured by N100m source location. This is significant because it indicates that phonemes differentially activate regions of auditory cortex according to their spectral characteristics at speech onset. It was also shown that the discrete mapping of consonants according to onset acoustics is effectively erased when the speech stimuli are manipulated to become unintelligible despite keeping the spectral complexity of the stimuli largely the same. This stimulus manipulation was accomplished by altering the spectral distribution of the stimuli. The authors argue that this latter finding indicates that the cortex is spatially mapping only those sounds that are intelligible to listeners. These data provide important evidence that cortical spatial representations may serve as an important mechanism for the encoding of spectral characteristics in speech-sound onsets. In addition to differences in spatial representations for place of articulation contrast, cortical responses also showed latency differences for these contrasts. Specifically, it was shown that front consonants, which have higher frequency onsets, elicited earlier N100m responses than back consonants. This finding is consistent with near-field recordings measured from animal models indicating earlier response latencies for speech onsets with higher frequency formants (McGee et al., 1996).

Cortical responses to temporal features of speech-sound onsets have also been reported in the literature, all of which have used VOT contrasts as stimuli. These studies were performed by measuring obligatory evoked potentials (N100 responses) to continua of consonant-vowel speech sounds that varied gradually according to VOT (Sharma and Dorman, 1999; 2000). Additionally, perception of these phonetic contrasts was also measured using the same continua as a means of addressing whether cortical responses reflected categorical perception of the phonemes. Neurophysiologic results indicated that for both /ba/-/pa/ and /ga/-/ka/ phonetic contrasts, one large negative peak was evident at approximately 100 ms in the response waveform for stimulus VOTs <40 ms. Importantly, a second negative peak in the response waveform emerged for stimulus VOTs of 40 ms, and this second peak occurred approximately 40 ms after the first peak and was thought to represent the onset of voicing in the stimulus. Moreover, as the VOT of the stimulus increased in duration, the lag between the second peak relative to the first increased proportionally, resulting in a strong correlation between VOT and the latency between the successive peaks ($r = {\sim}0.80$). The onset of double peaks in cortical responses with a VOT of 40 ms is consistent with neurophysiologic responses measured directly from the auditory cortex of humans (Steinschneider et al., 1999). An important consideration is that the onset of the double peak occurred at 40 ms for both the /ba/-/pa/ and /ga/-/ka/ phonetic contrasts. In contrast, behavioral results require different VOTs to distinguish the /ba/-/pa/ and /ga/-/ka/ phonetic contrasts.

Specifically, a VOT of ~40 ms was required for listeners to correctly identify /pa/ from /ba/, while a VOT of ~60 ms was required for correct identification of /ga/ from /ka/. Taken together, these data indicate that the cortical responses reflect the actual VOT at 40 ms irrespective of the categorical perception of the phonetic contrasts, which in the case of the /ga/-/ka/ contrast requires 60 ms.

Brainstem-Cortex Relationships

In addition to linking precise brainstem timing of acoustic transients to linguistic function, it has also been shown that abnormal encoding of acoustic transients in the brainstem is related to abnormal auditory responses measured at the level of cortex. In addition to their imprecise representation of sounds at the auditory brainstem, a significant proportion of LDs have also consistently demonstrated abnormal representations of simple (Menell et al., 1999; Ahissar et al., 2000) and complex (Kraus et al., 1996; Bradlow et al., 1999; Ahissar et al., 2001; Wible et al., 2002; 2005; Banai et al., 2005) acoustic stimuli at the level of the auditory cortex. Three recent studies linked abnormal neural synchrony for acoustic transients at the auditory brainstem to abnormal representations of sounds in the cortex. In one study (Wible et al., 2005), it was shown that a brainstem measure of the encoding of acoustic transients, the duration of time between onset peaks V and A, was positively correlated to the auditory cortex's susceptibility to background noise in both normal and LD subjects. Specifically, the longer the duration between onset peaks V and A, the more degraded cortical responses became in the presence of background noise. In another study, it was shown that individuals with abnormal brainstem timing to acoustic transients were more likely to indicate reduced cortical sensitivity to acoustic change, as measured by the mismatch negativity (MMN) response (Banai et al., 2005). Finally, a third study showed that brainstem timing for speech-sound onset and offset predicts the degree of cortical asymmetry for speech sounds measured across a group of children with a wide range of reading skills (Abrams et al., 2006). Thus, results from these studies indicate that abnormal encoding of acoustic onsets at the brainstem may be a critical marker for systemic auditory deficits manifested at multiple levels of the auditory system, including the cortex.

In summary, evidence from examining the ABR indicates that acoustic transients are encoded in a relatively simple fashion in the brainstem, yet they represent a complex phenomenon that is related to linguistic ability and cortical function. In the cortex, results indicate that spectral contrasts of speech onsets are mapped along the anterior-posterior axis in the auditory cortex, while temporal attributes of speech onsets, as manifested by the VOT, are precisely encoded with peaked N100 responses, the number of which (one or two) depends on whether VOT is less than 40 ms (one peak) or equal to or exceeds 40 ms (two peaks).

The Speech Envelope

DEFINITION AND ROLE IN THE PERCEPTION OF SPEECH

The speech envelope refers to the temporal fluctuations in the speech signal between 2 and 50 Hz. The dominant frequency of the speech envelope is at ~4 Hz, which reflects the average syllabic rate of speech (Steeneken and Houtgast, 1980). Envelope frequencies in normal speech are generally below 8 Hz (Houtgast and Steeneken, 1985), and the perceptually essential frequencies of the speech envelope are between 4 and 16 Hz (Drullman et al., 1994; van der Horst et al., 1999), although frequencies above 16 Hz contribute slightly to speech recognition (Shannon et al., 1995). The speech envelope provides phonetic and prosodic cues to the duration of speech segments, manner of articulation, the presence (or absence) of voicing, syllabication, and stress (van der Horst et al., 1999). The perceptual significance of the speech envelope has been investigated using a number of methodologies (Drullman et al., 1994; Shannon et al., 1995; Smith et al., 2002b), and taken together, these data indicate that the speech envelope is both necessary and sufficient for normal speech recognition.

PHYSIOLOGIC REPRESENTATION OF THE SPEECH ENVELOPE IN AUDITORY CORTEX

Only a few studies have investigated how the human brain represents the slow temporal information of the speech envelope. It should be noted that the representation of the speech envelope in humans has only been studied at the level of the cortex since measuring ABRs typically involves filtering out the neurophysiologic responses below ~100 Hz (Hall, 1992). Since speech envelope frequencies are between 2 and 50 Hz, the linear representation of the speech envelope in brainstem responses is removed with brainstem filtering.

In one MEG study, responses from the auditory cortex to natural and time-compressed (i.e., rapid) speech sentences were measured while subjects listened for semantic incongruities in experimental sentences (Ahissar et al., 2001). Results indicate that the human cortex synchronizes its response to the contours of the speech envelope, a phenomenon known as "phase-locking," and mimics the frequency content of the speech envelope, which the investigators called "frequency matching." Moreover, it was shown that these two neurophysiologic measures correlate with subjects' ability to perceive the speech sentences; as speech sentences become more difficult to perceive due to increased time compression, the ability of the cortex to phase-lock and frequency match is more impaired. A recent study has added to this literature by showing that right-hemisphere auditory cortex is dominant for processing speech envelope cues (Abrams et al., 2008). This study supports the hypothesis that human auditory cortex is asymmetric in processing acoustic rate information, with left-hemisphere regions showing preference for rapid acoustic features in speech (i.e., formant transitions) while the right-hemisphere is asymmetric for slow temporal features (i.e., the speech envelope; Poeppel, 2003).

A second line of inquiry into the cortical representation of speech envelope cues was described previously in this chapter in the discussion of cortical responses to VOT (Sharma and Dorman, 1999; 2000; Sharma et al., 2000). Acoustically, VOT is a slow temporal cue in speech (40 to 60 ms; 17 to 25 Hz) that falls within the range of speech envelope frequencies. As discussed earlier, neurophysiologic results indicate that for both /ba/-/pa/ and/ ga/-/ka/ phonetic contrasts, cortical N100 responses precisely represent the acoustic attributes of VOT. In addition, it was shown that neural responses are independent of the categorical perception of these phonetic contrasts (see the Acoustic Onsets section for a more detailed description of this study).

On the surface, it may appear that the findings from these experiments contradict one another since cortical phase-locking to the speech envelope correlates with perception in one study (Ahissar et al., 2001), while phase-locking fails to correlate with perception in other studies (Sharma and Dorman, 1999; 2000; Sharma et al., 2000). These data are not, however, in contradiction to one another. In both cases, an a priori requirement for perception is phase-locking to the speech envelope; there is no evidence for perception in the absence of accurate phase-locking to the temporal envelope in either study. The primary difference between the studies is that, despite phase-locking to the temporal envelope in the /ka/ stimulus condition at a VOT of ~40 ms, reliable perception of /ka/ occurs at approximately 60 ms. This suggests that accurate phase-locking is required for perception; however, perception cannot be predicted by phase-locking alone. Presumably, in the case of the /ka/ VOT stimulus, there is another processing stage that uses the phase-locked temporal information in conjunction with additional auditory-linguistic information (e.g., repeated exposure to /ka/ stimuli with 60-ms VOT) as a means of forming phonetic category boundaries. The questions of if and how category boundaries are established, irrespective of auditory phase-locking, require additional investigation.

CONCLUSION

Speech is a highly complex signal composed of a variety of acoustic features, all of which are important for normal speech perception. Normal perception of these acoustic features certainly relies on their neural encoding, which has been the subject of this review. An obvious conclusion from these studies is that the central auditory system is a remarkable machine, able to simultaneously process the multiple acoustic cues of ongoing speech in order to decode a linguistic message. Furthermore, how the human brain is innately and

dynamically programmed to use any number of these acoustic cues for the purpose of language, given the appropriate degree and type of stimulus exposure, further underscores the magnificence of this system.

A limitation of this chapter is that it has adopted a largely "bottom-up" approach to the acoustic encoding of speech sounds; neural encoding of acoustic signals is generally discussed as an afferent phenomenon with minimal consideration for the dynamic interactions provided by top-down connections in the auditory system (Xiao and Suga, 2002; Perrot et al., 2006). A notable exception to this includes work by Krishnan et al. (2004), which was described in the section on frequency modulation, in which the role of language experience was shown to affect sensory encoding in the auditory brainstem. Another limitation to this chapter is that it has also ignored the influence of other systems of the central nervous system, such as cognitive and emotional effects on auditory processing of speech, which most certainly have a role in shaping auditory activity.

To garner a greater understanding of how the central auditory system processes speech, it is important to consider both subcortical and cortical auditory regions. Across the acoustic features described in this review, the brainstem appears to represent acoustic events in a relatively linear fashion. The fundamental frequency and its modulation are represented with highly synchronized activity as reflected by the FFR; speech-sound onset is represented with highly predictable neural activation patterns that vary within fractions of milliseconds. Alternatively, the cortex appears to transform many of these acoustic cues, resulting in more complex representations of acoustic features of speech. For example, many of the cortical findings described here are based on the spatial representation of acoustic features (i.e., the relationship between F1-F2 required for vowel identification; the differentiation of speech transients; the encoding of periodicity). Because cortical neurons are not able to phase-lock to high-frequency events, it is tempting to propose that the cortex has found an alternative method for encoding these features based on the activity of spatially distributed neural populations. The extent to which these acoustic features are truly represented via a spatial organization in cortex is a future challenge that will likely be achieved using high-resolution imaging technologies in concert with EEG and MEG technologies.

ACKNOWLEDGEMENTS

We would like to thank Karen Banai, Patrick Wong, and Trent Nicol for their comments on a previous draft of this chapter. This work is supported by the National Institutes of Health grant R01 DC01510-10 and National Organization for Hearing Research grant 340-B208.

▨ REFERENCES

Abrams DA, Nicol T, Zecker S, Kraus N. (2006) Auditory brainstem timing predicts cerebral asymmetry for speech. *J Neurosci.* 26, 11131–11137.

Abrams D, Nicol T, Zecker S, Kraus N. (2008) Right-hemisphere auditory cortex is dominant for coding syllable patterns in speech. *J Neurosci.* 28, 3958–3965.

Ahissar M, Hochstein S. (2004) The reverse hierarchy theory of visual perceptual learning. *Trends Cogn Sci.* 8, 457–464.

Ahissar E, Nagarajan S, Ahissar M, Protopapas A, Mahncke H, Merzenich MM. (2001) Speech comprehension is correlated with temporal response patterns recorded from auditory cortex. *Proc Natl Acad Sci USA.* 98, 13367–13372.

Ahissar M, Protopapas A, Reid M, Merzenich MM. (2000) Auditory processing parallels reading abilities in adults. *Proc Natl Acad Sci USA.* 97, 6832–6837.

Banai K, Kraus N. (In press). The dynamic brainstem: implications for CAPD. In: D. McFarland D, Cacace A (eds). *Current Controversies in Central Auditory Processing Disorder.* Plural Publishing Inc: San Diego, CA.

Banai K, Nicol T, Zecker SG, Kraus N. (2005) Brainstem timing: implications for cortical processing and literacy. *J Neurosci.* 25, 9850–9857.

Belin P, Zatorre RJ, Lafaille P, Ahad P, Pike B. (2000) Voice-selective areas in human auditory cortex. *Nature.* 403, 309–312.

Belin P, Zilbovicius M, Crozier S, Thivard L, Fontaine A, Masure MC, Samson Y. (1998) Lateralization of speech and auditory temporal processing. *J Cogn Neurosci.* 10, 536–540.

Benasich AA, Tallal P. (2002) Infant discrimination of rapid auditory cues predicts later language impairment. *Behav Brain Res.* 136, 31–49.

Binder JR, Frost JA, Hammeke TA, Cox RW, Rao SM, Prieto T. (1997) Human brain language areas identified by functional magnetic resonance imaging. *J Neurosci.* 17, 353–362.

Bishop DV, Bishop SJ, Bright P, James C, Delaney T, Tallal P. (1999) Different origin of auditory and phonological processing problems in children with language impairment: evidence from a twin study. *J Speech Lang Hear Res.* 42, 155–168.

Bradlow AR, Kraus N, Hayes E. (2003) Speaking clearly for children with learning disabilities: sentence perception in noise. *J Speech Lang Hear Res.* 46, 80–97.

Bradlow AR, Kraus N, Nicol TG, McGee TJ, Cunningham J, Zecker SG, Carrell TD. (1999) Effects of lengthened formant transition duration on discrimination and neural representation of synthetic CV syllables by normal and learning-disabled children. *J Acoust Soc Am.* 106, 2086–2096.

Chandrasekaran B, Krishnan A, Gandour JT. (2007) Mismatch negativity to pitch contours is influenced by language experience. *Brain Res.* 1128,148–156.

Chandrasekaran B, Krishnan A, Gandour JT. (2008) Relative influence of musical and linguistic experience on early cortical processing of pitch contours. *Brain Lang,* [Epub ahead of print].

Creutzfeldt O, Hellweg FC, Schreiner C. (1980) Thalamocortical transformation of responses to complex auditory stimuli. *Exp Brain Res.* 39, 87–104.

Cunningham J, Nicol T, Zecker S, Bradlow A, Kraus N. (2001) Neurobiologic responses to speech in noise in children with learning problems: deficits and strategies for improvement. *Clin Neurophysiol.* 112, 758–767.

Cunningham J, Nicol T, Zecker S, Kraus N. (2000) Speech-evoked neurophysiologic responses in children with learning problems: development and behavioral correlates of perception. *Ear Hear.* 21, 554–568.

Diesch E, Luce T. (1997) Magnetic fields elicited by tones and vowel formants reveal tonotopy and nonlinear summation of cortical activation. *Psychophysiology.* 34, 501–510.

Drullman R, Festen JM, Plomp R. (1994) Effect of temporal envelope smearing on speech reception. *J Acoust Soc Am.* 95, 1053–1064.

Eggermont JJ. (1991) Rate and synchronization measures of periodicity coding in cat primary auditory cortex. *Hear Res.* 56, 153–167.

Galbraith GC, Amaya EM, de Rivera JM, Donan NM, Duong MT, Hsu JN, Tran K, Tsang LP. (2004) Brain stem evoked response to forward and reversed speech in humans. *Neuroreport.* 15, 2057–2060.

Galbraith GC, Threadgill MR, Hemsley J, Salour K, Songdej N, Ton J, Cheung L. (2000) Putative measure of peripheral and brainstem frequency-following in humans. *Neurosci Lett.* 292, 123–127.

Gandour J, Wong D, Hutchins G. (1998) Pitch processing in the human brain is influenced by language experience. *Neuroreport.* 9, 2115–2119.

Gardi J, Merzenich M, McKean C. (1979) Origins of the scalp recorded frequency-following response in the cat. *Audiology.* 18, 358–381.

Gehr DD, Komiya H, Eggermont JJ. (2000) Neuronal responses in cat primary auditory cortex to natural and altered species-specific calls. *Hear Res.* 150, 27–42.

Geschwind N, Galaburda AM. (1985) Cerebral lateralization. Biological mechanisms, associations, and pathology: I. A hypothesis and a program for research. *Arch Neurol.* 42, 428–459.

Hall JH. (1992) *Handbook of Auditory Evoked Responses.* Boston: Allyn and Bacon.

Hari R, Kiesila P. (1996) Deficit of temporal auditory processing in dyslexic adults. *Neurosci Lett.* 205, 138–140.

Hari R, Saaskilahti A, Helenius P, Uutela K. (1999) Non-impaired auditory phase locking in dyslexic adults. *Neuroreport.* 10, 2347–2348.

Hayes EA, Warrier CM, Nicol TG, Zecker SG, Kraus N. (2003) Neural plasticity following auditory training in children with learning problems. *Clin Neurophysiol.* 114, 673–684.

Hickok G, Poeppel D. (2004) Dorsal and ventral streams: a framework for understanding aspects of the functional anatomy of language. *Cognition.* 92, 67–99.

Hickok G, Poeppel D. (2007) The cortical organization of speech processing. *Nat Rev Neurosci.* 8, 393–402.

Houtgast T, Steeneken HJM. (1985) A review of the MTF concept in room acoustics and its use for estimating speech intelligibility in auditoria. *J Acoust Soc Am.* 77, 1069–1077.

Jezzard P, Matthews PM, Smith SM. (2001) *Functional MRI: An Introduction to Methods.* Oxford, United Kingdom: Oxford University Press.

Johnson K. (1997) *Acoustic and Auditory Phonetics.* Cambridge, MA: Blackwell Publishers Inc.

Johnson KL, Nicol TG, Kraus N. (2005) Brain stem response to speech: a biological marker of auditory processing. *Ear Hear.* 26, 424–434.

Johnson KL, Nicol TG, Kraus N. (2008) Developmental plasticity in the human auditory brainstem. *J Neurosci* 28, 4000–4007.

Johnson KL, Nicol TG, Zecker SG, Bradlow A, Skoe E, Kraus N. (In press). Brainstem encoding of voiced consonant-vowel stop syllables. *Clin Neurophysiol.*

King C, Warrier CM, Hayes E, Kraus N. (2002) Deficits in auditory brainstem pathway encoding of speech sounds in children with learning problems. *Neurosci Lett.* 319, 111–115.

Klein D, Zatorre RJ, Milner B, Zhao V. (2001) A cross-linguistic PET study of tone perception in Mandarin Chinese and English speakers. *Neuroimage.* 13, 646–653.

Klingberg T, Hedehus M, Temple E, Salz T, Gabrieli JD, Moseley ME, Poldrack RA. (2000) Microstructure of temporo-parietal white matter as a basis for reading ability: evidence from diffusion tensor magnetic resonance imaging. *Neuron.* 25, 493–500.

Kraus N, McGee TJ, Carrell TD, Zecker SG, Nicol TG, Koch DB. (1996) Auditory neurophysiologic responses and discrimination deficits in children with learning problems. *Science.* 273, 971–973.

Kraus N, Nicol T. (2005) Brainstem origins for cortical 'what' and 'where' pathways in the auditory system. *Trends Neurosci.* 28, 176–181.

Krishnan A. (2002) Human frequency-following responses: representation of steady-state synthetic vowels. *Hear Res.* 166, 192–201.

Krishnan A, Xu Y, Gandour JT, Cariani PA. (2004) Human frequency-following response: representation of pitch contours in Chinese tones. *Hear Res.* 189, 1–12.

Krishnan A, Xu Y, Gandour JT, Cariani P. (2005) Encoding of pitch in the human brainstem is sensitive to language experience. *Brain Res Cogn Brain Res.* 25, 161–168.

Lehiste I, Peterson GE. (1961) Transitions, glides, and diphthongs. *J Acoust Soc Am.* 33, 268–277.

Lu T, Liang L, Wang X. (2001) Temporal and rate representations of time-varying signals in the auditory cortex of awake primates. *Nat Neurosci.* 4, 1131–1138.

Makela AM, Alku P, Makinen V, Valtonen J, May P, Tiitinen H. (2002) Human cortical dynamics determined by speech fundamental frequency. *Neuroimage.* 17, 1300–1305.

McGee T, Kraus N, King C, Nicol T, Carrell TD. (1996) Acoustic elements of speechlike stimuli are reflected in surface recorded responses over the guinea pig temporal lobe. *J Acoust Soc Am.* 99, 3606–3614.

Menell P, McAnally KI, Stein JF. (1999) Psychophysical sensitivity and physiological response to amplitude modulation in adult dyslexic listeners. *J Speech Lang Hear Res.* 42, 797–803.

Mody M, Studdert-Kennedy M, Brady S. (1997) Speech perception deficits in poor readers: auditory processing or phonological coding? *J Exp Child Psychol.* 64, 199–231.

Musacchia G, Sams M, Skoe E, Kraus N. (2007) Musicians have enhanced subcortical auditory and audiovisual processing of speech and music. *Proc Nat Acad Sci* 104(40):15894–15898.

Musacchia G, Strait D, Kraus N. (2008) Relationships between behavior, brainstem and cortical encoding of seen and heard speech in musicians and nonmusicians. *Hear Res.* 241, 34–42.

Naatanen R, Picton T. (1987) The N1 wave of the human electric and magnetic response to sound: a review and an analysis of the component structure. *Psychophysiology.* 24, 375–425.

Nagarajan SS, Cheung SW, Bedenbaugh P, Beitel RE, Schreiner CE, Merzenich MM. (2002) Representation of spectral and temporal envelope of twitter vocalizations in common marmoset primary auditory cortex. *J Neurophysiol.* 87, 1723–1737.

Nagarajan SS, Mahncke H, Salz T, Tallal P, Roberts T, Merzenich MM. (1999) Cortical auditory signal processing in poor readers. *Proc Natl Acad Sci USA.* 96, 6483–6488.

Nearey TM, Assmann PF. (1986) Modeling the role of inherent spectral change in vowel identification. *J Acoust Soc Am.* 80, 1297–1308.

Nusbaum HC, Morin TM. (1992) Paying attention to differences among talkers. In: Tohkura Y, Sagisaka Y, Vatikiotis-Bateson E, eds. *Speech Perception, Production, and Linguistic Structure.* Tokyo: Ohmasha Publishing; pp 113–134.

Obleser J, Elbert T, Lahiri A, Eulitz C. (2003) Cortical representation of vowels reflects acoustic dissimilarity determined by formant frequencies. *Brain Res Cogn Brain Res.* 15, 207–213.

Obleser J, Scott SK, Eulitz C. (2006) Now you hear it, now you don't: transient traces of consonants and their nonspeech analogues in the human brain. *Cereb Cortex.* 16, 1069–1076.

Perrot X, Ryvlin P, Isnard J, Guenot M, Catenoix H, Fischer C, Mauguiere F, Collet L. (2006) Evidence for corticofugal modulation of peripheral auditory activity in humans. *Cereb Cortex.* 16, 941–948.

Peterson GE, Barney HL. (1952) Control methods used in a study of the vowels. *J Acoust Soc Am.* 24, 175–184.

Poeppel D. (2003) The analysis of speech in different temporal integration windows: cerebral lateralization as "asymmetric sampling in time." *Speech Commun.* 41, 245–255.

Ramus F, Rosen S, Dakin SC, Day BL, Castellote JM, White S, Frith U. (2003) Theories of developmental dyslexia: insights from a multiple case study of dyslexic adults. *Brain.* 126, 841–865.

Rauschecker JP. (1997) Processing of complex sounds in the auditory cortex of cat, monkey, and man. *Acta Otolaryngol Suppl.* 532, 34–38.

Reed MA. (1989) Speech perception and the discrimination of brief auditory cues in reading disabled children. *J Exp Child Psychol.* 48, 270–292.

Rosen S. (1992) Temporal information in speech: acoustic, auditory and linguistic aspects. *Philos Trans R Soc Lond B Biol Sci.* 336, 367–373.

Russo NM, Bradlow AR, Skoe E, Trommer BL, Nicol T, Zecker S, Kraus N. (2008) Deficient brainstem encoding of pitch in children with autism spectrum disorders. *Clin Neurophysiol.* 119, 1720–1731.

Russo NM, Nicol TG, Musacchia G, Kraus N. (2004) Brainstem responses to speech syllables. *Clin Neurophysiol.* 115, 2021–2030.

Russo NM, Nicol TG, Zecker SG, Hayes EA, Kraus N. (2005) Auditory training improves neural timing in the human brainstem. *Behav Brain Res.* 156, 95–103.

Sachs MB, Young ED. (1979) Encoding of steady-state vowels in the auditory nerve: representation in terms of discharge rate. *J Acoust Soc Am.* 66, 470–479.

Sachs MB, Voigt HF, Young ED. (1983) Auditory nerve representation of vowels in background noise. *J Neurophysiol.* 50, 27–45.

Sato S. (1990) *Magnetoencephalography* New York: Raven Press.

Schreiner CE. (1998) Spatial distribution of responses to simple and complex sounds in the primary auditory cortex. *Audiol Neurootol.* 3, 104–122.

Schulte-Korne G, Deimel W, Bartling J, Remschmidt H. (1998) Auditory processing and dyslexia: evidence for a specific speech processing deficit. *Neuroreport.* 9, 337–340.

Shannon RV, Zeng FG, Kamath V, Wygonski J, Ekelid M. (1995) Speech recognition with primarily temporal cues. *Science.* 270, 303–304.

Sharma A, Dorman MF. (1999) Cortical auditory evoked potential correlates of categorical perception of voice-onset time. *J Acoust Soc Am.* 106, 1078–1083.

Sharma A, Dorman MF. (2000) Neurophysiologic correlates of cross-language phonetic perception. *J Acoust Soc Am.* 107, 2697–2703.

Sharma A, Marsh C, Dorman M. (2000) Relationship between N1 evoked potential morphology and the perception of voicing. *J Acoust Soc Am.* 108, 3030–3035.

Shestakova A, Brattico E, Soloviev A, Klucharev V, Huotilainen M. (2004) Orderly cortical representation of vowel categories presented by multiple exemplars. *Brain Res Cogn Brain Res.* 21, 342–350.

Smith AJ, Blumenfeld H, Behar KL, Rothman DL, Shulman RG, Hyder F. (2002a) Cerebral energetics and spiking frequency: the neurophysiological basis of fMRI. *Proc Natl Acad Sci USA.* 99, 10765–10770.

Smith JC, Marsh JT, Brown WS. (1975) Far-field recorded frequency-following responses: evidence for the locus of brainstem sources. *Electroencephalogr Clin Neurophysiol.* 39, 465–472.

Smith ZM, Delgutte B, Oxenham AJ. (2002b) Chimaeric sounds reveal dichotomies in auditory perception. *Nature.* 416, 87–90.

Song JH, Banai K, Russo NM, Kraus N. (2006) On the relationship between speech- and nonspeech-evoked auditory brainstem responses. *Audiol Neurootol.* 11, 233–241.

Song JH, Skoe E, Wong PCM, Kraus N. (In press) Plasticity in the adult human auditory brainstem following short-term linguistic training. *J Cog Neurosci.* DOI:10, 1162/jocn.2008.20131.

Steeneken HJ, Houtgast T. (1980) A physical method for measuring speech-transmission quality. *J Acoust Soc Am.* 67, 318–326.

Steinschneider M, Reser DH, Fishman YI, Schroeder CE, Arezzo JC. (1998) Click train encoding in primary auditory cortex of the awake monkey: evidence for two mechanisms subserving pitch perception. *J Acoust Soc Am.* 104, 2935–2955.

Steinschneider M, Volkov IO, Noh MD, Garell PC, Howard MA 3rd. (1999) Temporal encoding of the voice onset time phonetic parameter by field potentials recorded directly from human auditory cortex. *J Neurophysiol.* 82, 2346–2357.

Stillman RD, Crow G, Moushegian G. (1978) Components of the frequency-following potential in man. *Electroencephalogr Clin Neurophysiol.* 44, 438–446.

Tallal P, Piercy M. (1973) Defects of non-verbal auditory perception in children with developmental aphasia. *Nature.* 241, 468–469.

Tallal P, Piercy M. (1975) Developmental aphasia: the perception of brief vowels and extended stop consonants. *Neuropsychologia.* 13, 69–74.

Tallal P, Miller S, Fitch RH. (1993) Neurobiological basis of speech: a case for the preeminence of temporal processing. *Ann N Y Acad Sci.* 682, 27–47.

Temple E, Poldrack RA, Protopapas A, Nagarajan S, Salz T, Tallal P, Merzenich MM, Gabrieli JD. (2000) Disruption of the neural response to rapid acoustic stimuli in dyslexia: evidence from functional MRI. *Proc Natl Acad Sci USA.* 97, 13907–13912.

van der Horst R, Leeuw AR, Dreschler WA. (1999) Importance of temporal-envelope cues in consonant recognition. *J Acoust Soc Am.* 105, 1801–1809.

Wang X, Merzenich MM, Beitel R, Schreiner CE. (1995) Representation of a species-specific vocalization in the primary auditory cortex of the common marmoset: temporal and spectral characteristics. *J Neurophysiol.* 74, 2685–2706.

Wible B, Nicol T, Kraus N. (2002) Abnormal neural encoding of repeated speech stimuli in noise in children with learning problems. *Clin Neurophysiol.* 113, 485–494.

Wible B, Nicol T, Kraus N. (2004) Atypical brainstem representation of onset and formant structure of speech sounds in children with language-based learning problems. *Biol Psychol.* 67, 299–317.

Wible B, Nicol T, Kraus N. (2005) Correlation between brainstem and cortical auditory processes in normal and language-impaired children. *Brain.* 128, 417–423.

Witton C, Stein JF, Stoodley CJ, Rosner BS, Talcott JB. (2002) Separate influences of acoustic AM and FM sensitivity on the phonological decoding skills of impaired and normal readers. *J Cogn Neurosci.* 14, 866–874.

Wong PC, Parsons LM, Martinez M, Diehl RL. (2004) The role of the insular cortex in pitch pattern perception: the effect of linguistic contexts. *J Neurosci.* 24, 9153–9160.

Wong PC, Skoe E, Russo NM, Dees T, Kraus N. (2007) Musical experience shapes human brainstem encoding of linguistic pitch patterns. *Nat Neurosci.* 10, 420–422.

Wright BA, Lombardino LJ, King WM, Puranik CS, Leonard CM, Merzenich MM. (1997) Deficits in auditory temporal and spectral resolution in language-impaired children. *Nature.* 387, 176–178.

Xiao Z, Suga N. (2002) Modulation of cochlear hair cells by the auditory cortex in the mustached bat. *Nat Neurosci.* 5, 57–63.

Xu Y, Krishnan A, Gandour JT. (2006) Specificity of experience-dependent pitch representation in the brainstem. *Neuroreport.* 17, 1601–1605.

Zatorre RJ, Belin P. (2001) Spectral and temporal processing in human auditory cortex. *Cereb Cortex.* 11, 946–953.

Zatorre RJ, Belin P, Penhune VB. (2002) Structure and function of auditory cortex: music and speech. *Trends Cogn Sci.* 6, 37–46.

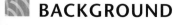

CHAPTER
27 Central Auditory Processing Evaluation: A Test Battery Approach

Kim L. Tillery

INTRODUCTION

The past 37 years has given us six editions of the *Handbook of Clinical Audiology*, including this edition. A review of chapters reveals 27 chapters related to assessment of central auditory processing disorders (CAPD) and two on remediation approaches. In the presence of this collection of information, there is inquiry as to why few in the field administer central auditory processing (CAP) testing. Audiologists routinely administer a peripheral hearing assessment; however, why so few in the field administer central auditory processing (CAP) tests is not a routine or comfortable task to all clinicians in our field. It seems logical that audiologists should assist individuals who exhibit difficulty in properly "hearing" the auditory message, whether it is due to a peripheral or central dysfunction. It is hopeful that with more educational training on this topic in clinical doctorate of audiology (AuD) programs and an increased awareness of the information that can be obtained through a test battery approach, many more audiologists will be performing CAP testing. After all, the hearing system is complex and we should be able to ascertain the integrity of the entire hearing system to better serve the population who struggle in communication, language, and learning functions.

BACKGROUND

CAPD was first officially described in 1992 by the American Speech-Language-Hearing Association (ASHA). The general definition described CAPD as having difficulty in retrieving, transforming, analyzing, organizing, and storing infor-

mation from audible acoustic signals (ASHA, 1992). This simple definition was later expanded when ASHA initiated a task force to discuss and derive the first professional consensus of several issues involving auditory processing disorders (APD) (ASHA, 1995; 1996). The issues included a definition, basic auditory science, assessment, clinical application, and developmental and acquired communication problems. CAPD was defined as involving deficits in localization, lateralization, auditory discrimination, pattern recognition skills, temporal processing, and performance decrements with competing or degraded auditory signals.

The consensus provided recommendations for determining the presence of CAPD and its functional deficits, emphasizing a team approach and the delineation of developmental or acquired CAPD deficits. Management approaches were focused on enhancing individuals' processing skills by increasing their language knowledge base and improving processing speed. Intervention goals were to bridge linguistic and cognitive perception (within the realm of the speech pathologist) and the acoustic properties of speech (within the realm of the audiologist), thus enabling the client with a CAPD to function better with a minimum of behavioral deficits. The consensus document encouraged collaborative efforts between clinicians and researchers to improve our understanding of CAPD.

ASHA provided an updated Technical Report on CAPD in 2005. This report recognized the previously accepted ASHA definition and detailed a number of additional topics, including a review of basic science advances, audiometric assessment, developmental and acquired communication problems associated with CAPD, and the use of diagnostic information to indicate specific interventions. While the

Bruton conference (Jerger and Musiek, 2000) suggested removing the word "central" from the title of this disorder, the ASHA (2005) report did not take a stand on the preferred title but rather indicated that both were acceptable. They recommended that the word "central" remain in the title, as (central) auditory processing disorder or (C)APD, because most of the tests administered for (C)APD diagnosis involve the central auditory nervous system (CANS).

A second clarification provided in the ASHA (2005) Technical Report addressed the "modality-specific" approach to diagnosing (C)APD (Cacace and McFarland, 2005; Jerger and Musiek, 2000). This approach, initiated by one group of researchers over the last decade (Cacace and McFarland, 2005; McFarland and Cacace, 1995; 1997), hinges on whether a (C)APD diagnosis is reliable without ascertaining the status of other sensory and supramodal systems, even if CAP tests indicate CANS dysfunction (Katz and Tillery, 2005; Musiek et al., 2005). The ASHA (2005) report provides substantial research and reasoning that a diagnostic criterion to rule out all other perceptual factors is not consistent with brain organization and central nervous system (CNS) processing and that assessment of multimodality function is not within the scope of one professional discipline. In addition, the report stated that influences of maturational delays, extent of neurobiologic disorders, social and environmental factors, and neurologic disorders or diseases most certainly can impact different individuals with the same auditory deficit in different ways. It was concluded that (C)APD involves a neural processing deficit of auditory stimuli that may "coexist with, but *is not the result of,* dysfunction in other modalities" (ASHA, 2005, p 3). Thus, (C)APD is described as a distinct clinical entity.

There is a range of functional behavioral limitations related to (C)APD and coexisting disorders (Chermak et al., 1999; Keller, 1992; 1998; Keller and Tillery, 2002). Questionnaires can be useful for indicating the types of functional limitations present and assisting in appropriate referrals (Tillery, 1998). Given the associated language, communication, and learning difficulties frequently associated with (C)APD, a multidisciplinary approach can lead to more accurate diagnoses, thereby enhancing effective treatment and management plans (Keller and Tillery, 2002). While a team approach is recommended to ascertain the functional behavioral limitations of the client's communication skills (Keller and Tillery, 2006), it is the audiologist who administers tests to ascertain the integrity of the CANS (ASHA, 1995; 2005).

■ CENTRAL AUDITORY PROCESSING TEST BATTERY APPROACH

As early as 1954, Mykelbust suggested that children with language disorders may have an auditory deficit beyond peripheral hearing and that the clinician should assess for such possibilities (Mykelbust, 1954). This early suggestion came

when there were no developed tests to ascertain functioning beyond the peripheral system. Today there are several central tests, and a test battery approach continues to be well recognized for CAP assessment (Bellis, 1996, Bellis and Ferre 1999, Chermak and Musiek, 1997; Domitz and Schow, 2000; Jerger and Jerger, 1975; Katz and Smith, 1991; Katz, 1992; Keith, 2000; Medwetsky, 2002b; Musiek and Lamb, 1994; Schow et al., 2000; Stecker, 1992; 1998; Willeford and Bilger, 1978).

The intent of CAP evaluations is to assess the CANS system at different levels. The efficacy of any test is determined by examining how it compares with different assessment tools (ASHA, 2005). Such comparisons may indicate that two or three auditory processing tests provide the same conclusions as six or seven other tests (Musiek and Lamb, 1994).

CAP tests have been in use for decades. The reader is referred to the following for a review of these tests: Bellis (2003), Katz (1994), Medwetsky (2002b) and Stecker (1992). Table 27.1 lists CAP tests with their targeted processes and CANS sensitivity.

Even with the knowledge that a test battery approach is necessary to efficiently tap into the CANS system, we are just now recognizing that such an approach should be determined by awareness of the underlying auditory mechanisms that are thought to be assessed. For example, Schow et al. (2000) analyzed various central tests in comparison to the ASHA (1996) processes listed and determined the following measurable auditory behaviors: (1) auditory pattern temporal ordering (APTO), (2) monaural separation/closure (MSC), (3) binaural separation (BS), and (4) binaural integration (BI). In addition, these authors suggested that (C)APD testing should also evaluate auditory discrimination, localization/lateralization, and temporal tasks (resolution, masking, and integration). Table 27.2 provides definitions of these measurable auditory behaviors with associated CAP tests.

The Schow et al. (2000) study is one example that illustrates the selection of tests, in this case based on auditory behaviors that should be assessed according to ASHA (1995; 2005). However, as detailed in following sections, different researchers have developed test batteries based on different conceptualizations of what they sought to examine.

■ CENTRAL AUDITORY PROCESSING TEST BATTERY MODELS

The application of CAP tests is seen in a variety of CAP models that have been in use for several years. These models vary in their construct. Some were developed to ascertain the underlying auditory deficit in relation to functional behavioral deficits (Bellis and Ferre, 1999; Katz and Smith, 1991), others tended to emphasize a medical framework (Jerger and Musiek, 2000), whereas others were based on the

TABLE 27.1 Summary of central auditory processing tests with targeted process and central auditory nervous system sensitivity to specific sites

	Monaural	Targeted processes	Sensitive to:
Low-Pass Filtered Speech Tests			
Band-Pass Filtered	X	Auditory closure	Brainstem/cortical lesions
Compressed Speech	X	Auditory closure	Primary auditory cortex
Speech Recognition in Noise	X	Auditory closure	Brainstem to cortex
Dichotic Speech Tests			
Dichotic Digits		Binaural integration	Brainstem/cortical/corpus callosum
Staggered Spondaic Word		Binaural integration	Brainstem/cortical/corpus callosum
Synthetic Sentence Identification w/Contra Competing Message		Binaural separation	Cortical vs. brainstem
Competing Sentences		Binaural separation	Language processing
Dichotic Sentence Identification		Binaural integration	Brainstem/cortical
Dichotic Rhyme		Binaural integration	Interhemispheric
Dichotic Consonant Vowels		Binaural integration	Cortical
Temporal Patterning Tests			
Pitch Pattern Sequence (PPS)	X	Temporal ordering Linguistic labeling	Cerebral hemisphere lesions Interhemispheric transfer
Duration Patterns	X	Temporal ordering Linguistic labeling Duration discrimination	Cerebral hemisphere lesions Interhemispheric transfer
Random Gap Detection Test		Temporal resolution	Left temporal/cortical
Frequency Pattern (FP)	X	Temporal ordering Linguistic labeling Frequency discrimination	Interhemispheric transfer Cerebral hemisphere lesions
Other Tests			
Binaural Fusion		Binaural interaction	Low brainstem
Masking Level Difference		Binaural interaction	Low brainstem
Rapid Alternating Speech		Binaural interaction	?Low or high brainstem

intertwining of cognitive, language, and auditory processes (Medwetsky, 2002a).

These models incorporate different tests depending on the desired outcome of the applied construct. Three of the four models deliver subtypes or profiles that describe the (C)APD, rather than a general CANS diagnosis, thus providing more information of an individual's functional limitations and, in turn, effective treatment opportunities. Regardless of the underlying construct, all of these models rely on CANS tests being administered in a manner that controls for fatigue and attention since these can affect test performance (Musiek, 1985; Tillery, 1998; Tillery et al., 2000).

Minimal Test Battery

Jerger and Musiek (2000) discussed a possible test battery that would include both behavioral and electrophysiologic testing. The authors suggested that clinicians should, at a minimum, consider the following tests:

- Immittance audiometry (tympanometry and acoustic reflex threshold testing) to ascertain the status of

the middle ear as well as auditory neuropathy differential diagnosis
- Otoacoustic emissions to diagnose inner ear problems
- Auditory brainstem and middle latency evoked responses to assess brainstem and cortical level integrity
- Puretone audiometry to evaluate the integrity of the peripheral hearing system
- Performance-intensity functions for word recognition ability
- A dichotic task consisting of dichotic words, dichotic digits, or dichotic sentences (assessing the communication between hemispheres)
- Duration pattern and a temporal gap detection test to assess (C)APD in the auditory temporal processing arena

The authors further elaborate that the above tests recommended in the minimal test battery (MTB) are a "reasonable compromise" (Jerger and Musiek, 2000, p 472) of tests until research can provide analogous measures in the

TABLE 27.2   Measurable auditory processing behavioral processes recommended by Schow et al. (2000) and adopted by the Bellis/Ferre model

Process	Measurable auditory processing performance	Types of tests	Bellis/Ferre profiles
Auditory pattern/temporal ordering (APTO)	Auditory discrimination of frequency or duration/order and sequencing/ temporal processes/ interhemispheric integration	1) Frequency pattern tests 2) Duration pattern tests 3) Pitch Pattern Sequence Test	Prosodic deficit
Monaural separation/ closure (MSC)	Performance with degraded signals	1) Filtered or time compressed speech 2) Ipsilateral competing signals	Auditory decoding deficit
Binaural integration (BI)	Ability to properly respond to all competing signals directed to both ears	Dichotic tests	Integration deficit
Binaural separation (BS)	Ability to attend to stimulus in one ear while ignoring the stimulus in the other ear	Competing sentences	Integration deficit
Sound localization/ lateralization	Ability to describe location of stimuli in relation to position of one's head	Brainstem-level binaural interaction tests (Masking Level Difference [MLD])	Integration deficit
Auditory discrimination	Ability to describe when two stimuli are different	1) Difference limens for frequency/duration/intensity or speech stimuli 2) Speech sound or word discrimination tests	Auditory decoding deficit
Temporal resolution Temporal masking Temporal integration	Discrimination of speech and nonspeech, prosodic elements of speech, localization/ lateralization	Need for research in developing more tests; possibly random gap detection/forward and backward masking	Auditory decoding deficit

visual modality and neuroimaging results can be applied to the clinical utility of (C)APD testing. Note that this model does not describe specific processing-related difficulties, but rather, the goal is to ascertain whether (C)APD is present.

Concerns were voiced about the MTB stating that a pure medical (diagnostic) model, as described in the Jerger and Musiek (2000) paper, would not delineate the CAP problems (Katz et al., 2002). Katz and colleagues pointed out that the tests lacked national CAP norms (at that time) and had limited clinical use (at that time) with the target population and that the MTB did not address the educational concerns of the children.

Bellis/Ferre Model

Initially, this model was called CATfiles (the CAT acronym stands for "categories" of CAPD) (Ferre, 1992). This was later developed into a broader expansion of profiles (Bellis, 1999; Bellis and Ferre, 1999) with even further published changes (Bellis, 2002; Ferre, 2002), based on the Schow et al. (2000) criteria (Bellis, 2002). The current Bellis/Ferre (C)APD subprofiles include three primary deficits—auditory decoding, prosodic, and integration—with secondary subprofiles that

include associative deficit and organization-output deficit. The profiles are based on a conceptualization of the underlying neurophysiology in the CANS for encoding the auditory signal with the goal of ascertaining dysfunction in the left hemisphere, right hemisphere, and interhemispheric pathways. Bellis (2003) suggests that by examining the pattern of results across auditory processing functions, cognition, language and learning, one can glean the underlying (C)APD difficulties/profile.

The Bellis/Ferre profiles may be seen in isolation or together, with Bellis (2002) cautioning that one profile is typically primary in nature; however, another profile can be present due to possible overlap in the adjacent cortical structures. Electrophysiologic tests are not used in the Bellis/Ferre Model. Table 27.2 outlines this model, while the reader is referred to Bellis (2003) for an in-depth review of these profiles. Following are descriptions of the various Bellis/Ferre (C)APD subprofiles.

Auditory Decoding Deficit

According to Bellis (2003, p 291), auditory decoding deficit is possibly "the only true (C)APD." This subprofile involves weak phonemic representations, poor discrimination and blending of sounds, and an inability to remember the learned phonemes. Determination of this profile is based on weaker right ear versus left ear test performance on low-redundancy speech and speech-in-noise tests (Bellis, 1996). Bellis (2002) describes the additional components of weak reading, vocabulary, and spelling skills, as well as concomitant behaviors such as auditory fatigue, and performance being improved with good visual perceptual skills. Site-of-lesion and electrophysiologic research has suggested the primary auditory cortex within the left hemisphere as the probable site of dysfunction (Bellis, 1996). A later report (Bellis, 2002) found this deficit to be associated with diminished right ear/both ear performance on the Dichotic Digits Test (Musiek, 1983) (labeled a BI weakness) and the Competing Sentence Test (Willeford and Burleigh, 1985) (labeled a BS weakness).

PROSODIC DEFICIT

Prosodic deficit is characterized by (1) difficulty in perceiving and recognizing nonverbal information, such as tonal patterns; (2) weak left ear test performance on dichotic tests showing weak BI and BS abilities; and (3) good speech-in-noise ability due to intact decoding ability (Bellis, 2002). Associated problems include weak singing ability (such as poor replication of melodies), poor social-communication skills, flat voicing patterns, and diminished ability on visual-spatial tasks. Academic concerns involve weakness in mathematics, reading, sequencing, and spelling and poor sight-word abilities.

INTEGRATION DEFICIT

Integration deficit is characterized as a struggle involving interhemispheric skills, such as drawing, understanding dictation, dancing, and multimodal tasking (Bellis, 1996). Integration Deficits may be the result of an immature corpus callosum or other structures related to the transfer of interhemispheric information. Auditory test results observed for this profile include weak left ear results on dichotic tasks and poor nonverbal test performance scores. Bellis (2002) further elaborates that BI and BS deficits are also often seen with this profile of (C)APD, with weak sound localization abilities.

SECONDARY PROFILES

Auditory Associative Deficit
The secondary profile known as an auditory associative deficit was observed in the original work of Bellis and Ferre (1999) as a (C)APD profile, but it more recently has been classified as a secondary profile of (C)APD (Ferre, 2002). This deficit consists of an inability to use rules of language with acoustic information, with the most severe cases replicating receptive childhood aphasia (Bellis, 1996). Performance on speech-sound discrimination tasks is normal; however, weak word recognition and dichotic test findings are observed bilaterally. Receptive language struggles are seen in vocabulary,

semantics, and syntax. Inefficient communication between primary and associative cortical regions may be the causal aspect of this category (Bellis, 1996) and realized as significant auditory–language-processing difficulties (Ferre, 2002).

Output-Organization Deficit
Another secondary profile is the output-organization deficit, which involves an inability to properly sequence, plan, and organize information (Bellis, 1996). Test performance requiring one simple response (e.g., monaural low-redundancy tests) will be good, whereas performance on tests with multiple components, such as those required on dichotic, frequency, or duration pattern tests, will be poor due to the use of complex stimuli (Bellis, 1996). Individuals with this type of deficit exhibit fine motor difficulties as well as sequencing and sound-blending errors. Reading comprehension is generally good for those who exhibit only this subprofile. At the time this subprofile was proposed, the site of dysfunction for this category was not known, although an efferent (motor planning) hypothesis was proposed due to the weak skills observed on motoric tasks seen with this type of (C)APD (Bellis, 1996).

Buffalo Model

This model, first reported in the early 1990s, consists of four (C)APD subtypes (Katz and Smith, 1991; Katz, 1992). The Buffalo Model is comprised of three tests, in which the Staggered Spondaic Word (SSW) test (Katz, 1962; 1968) is the center of the battery; the other two tests include the Phonemic Synthesis (Katz and Harmon, 1982) and Speech-in-Noise (Mueller et al., 1987) tests. This test battery provides 33 quantitative and qualitative indicators. Quantitative indicators are the number of errors seen in each of the three tests, while qualitative indicators refer to the behavioral struggles seen during testing. The combination of the test performance indicators and academic and social behaviors (particular clusterings of each being associated with cortical anatomic sites) results in four (C)APD subtypes: decoding, tolerance-fading memory (TFM), integration, and organization (Katz and Smith, 1991; Katz, 1992; Katz, 2001a; Medwetsky, 2002b). Clinicians may administer other tests (Medwetsky, 2002a; Stecker, 1998) in addition to the Buffalo Model tests. See Table 27.3 for the test indicators for the Buffalo Model types of CAPD.

DECODING

Decoding has been described as the most common type, but it may not be as prevalent as it was in the late 1980s and early 1990s because the whole language approach is no longer used in the school system (Stecker, 2004) and more emphasis is being placed on phonemic awareness now (Tillery, 2005). The decoding type involves a breakdown at the phonemic level, causing a weakness in identifying, manipulating, and remembering phonemes. Weak oral reading or word accuracy and spelling skills are usually found in this

TABLE 27.3 Qualitative and quantitative test indicators of Buffalo Model central auditory processing disorders (CAPD) types

CAPD Types	Primary indicators			Secondary indicators			Qualifying indicators		
	SSW	PS	SN	SSW	PS	SN	SSW	PS	SN
Decoding	RC errors LNC error Order L/H Ear H/L	Below normal	Mild		Nonfused, quiet rehearsals, delays		Delays Perseverations	Discrimination errors O/L	Mild/moderate in poorer ear
TFM	Order H/L Ear L/H		Moderate or severe in poorer ear	LC errors			Quick AYR/Y TTW Smush	Omission error on first sounds	Moderate in poorer ear
Integration type 1	Type A			Sharp LC peak of errors	See Decoding		Extreme delays	See Decoding	
Integration type 2	Type A		See TFM	Sharp LC Peak errors			Extreme delays and see TFM	See TFM	Moderate errors in poorer ear
Organization	Significant reversals	Significant reversals							

Abbreviations: SSW, Staggered Spondaic Word Test; PS, Phonemic Synthesis Test; SN, Speech-in-Noise Test (Katz, 2001a); RC, right competing; LNC, left noncompeting; H/L, high/low; L/H, low/high; O/L, whereby client produces an /o/ sound for the /l/ sound for the /l/ sound; TFM, tolerance-fading memory; AYR, "are you ready" response; Y, "yes" response; TTW, tongue twister.

subtype. Rapid incoming speech adds to the confusion of processing the message, and response delays are common due to the individual needing additional time to ascertain the verbal message. Weak discrimination and vocabulary are results of the misperceptions of the heard auditory stimuli. Reported site of dysfunction for this category is the phonemic zone (Luria, 1966) of the left posterior temporal lobe, also known as the auditory cortex. Test results associated with this subtype include weak SSW right competing (RC) and left noncompeting (LNC) scores and poor Phonemic Synthesis results (Katz, 1992). Qualitative signs include delayed responses, nonfused answers, and quiet rehearsals (described in Table 27.3).

TOLERANCE-FADING MEMORY

This (C)APD subtype has been considered the second most common in the general population (Katz, 1992). The theorized loci involve the frontal lobes and the anterior temporal region, which houses the hippocampus and amygdala, organs related to memory (Katz, 1992; Isaacson and Pribram, 1986). Functional behavioral limitations include a weak short-term memory and difficulty hearing auditory information in the presence of noise (the *tolerance* aspect of TFM); that is, individuals with TFM may exhibit significantly increased difficulty tolerating and understanding in noise as compared to individuals with other types. Other limitations associated with frontal lobe dysfunction include expressive language, motor programming (i.e., writing, articulation), and difficulty inhibiting impulsive responses. Qualitative signs include quick responses, smush responses (combining the competing words of an item into a single word, e.g., "sea *shore out*side" = "sea *shout*side"), an inability to refrain from repeating carrier phrases ("Are you ready?"), and omission or errors for the first set of stimuli presented. Individuals with attention deficit/hyperactivity disorder (ADHD) are commonly found to exhibit TFM (Keller and Tillery, 2002; 2006), probably because of the close association of the frontal and the anterior temporal lobes (Katz and Smith, 1991). The frontal lobe houses executive function that serves to regulate and coordinate behaviors to the environment, inhibit irrelevant responses, and oversee cognitive processes (Barkley, 1998), which are affected by ADHD.

INTEGRATION

One of the (C)APD subtypes (type 1) probably involves the posterior corpus callosum or the angular gyrus of the parietal-occipital region, which are regions thought to be associated with dyslexia (Geschwind and Galaburda, 1987), and another subtype (type 2) probably involves more anterior portions of the corpus callosum. Individuals with type 1 integration exhibit decoding signs on the test battery, whereas those with type 2 integration have TFM signs on the test battery. In 2001, Katz indicated that there may be two additional types of integration: type 3, which has both decoding and TFM signs, and type 4, which has neither

decoding nor TFM signs (Katz, 2001b). An integration sign is said to be present when one displays a type A pattern, that is, a severe peak of errors in one of two columns (out of eight total columns) on the SSW test performance form (the second or sixth columns labeled B and F). Type A indicates difficulty in transferring interhemispheric information. To ascertain the likely behavioral impact of the type A, one needs to look at the rest of the test battery findings. In addition, a qualitative sign in those with integration difficulties includes extremely long response times on the SSW items and that are generally seen in daily life activities as well. Functional behavioral limitations (decoding subtype) include significant reading problems and difficulty in integrating visual and auditory information. Integration is considered the most severe category and is often more resistant to therapy than the other three.

ORGANIZATION

This (C)APD subtype was first reported by Lucker (1981), who recognized that reversals on the SSW test are observed in individuals who are disorganized. A reversal is said to occur when stimuli (i.e., words, sounds) are repeated out of sequence. Both the SSW and Phonemic Synthesis tests have norms for determining the presence of a significant number of reversals (ages 5 or 6 years through adulthood). Reversals are considered an anterior sign (Katz, 1992). Note that those with attention disorders tend to exhibit weak organization, planning, and sequencing, all of which are associated with dysfunction in the prefrontal cortex (Barkley, 1998). Indeed, Tillery (1999) found SSW reversals to be very common in her studies of children with ADHD.

Spoken-Language Processing Model

This model expands on the Buffalo Model to include a broader perspective beyond auditory processing to better understand how one perceives and processes spoken language. Medwetsky (2002a; 2006) considers auditory processing to be a component of spoken-language processing (S-LP) and limited to those perceptual mechanisms involved in the initial acoustic analysis of the incoming signal. The reader is referred to Chapter 25 for a thorough explanation of this model and attention affects. Table 27.4 shows a summary of the S-LP Model. The (C)APD diagnosis may result in the following areas of concern: lexical decoding, fading memory, auditory-linguistic integration, sequencing, short-term memory span, prosodic perception, and attention and phonologic problems.

▨ ELECTROPHYSIOLOGIC MEASURES AND A CENTRAL AUDITORY PROCESSING TEST BATTERY?

The proposed MTB indicated a need for electrophysiologic testing to be included in all (C)APD test batteries (Jerger and

TABLE 27.4   Processes assessed through the spoken-language processing (S-LP) model (Medwetsky, 2002a)

Process	Definition	Test
Temporal resolution	Ability to detect rapid changes in the speech signal	Random Gap Detection Test; Gap-in-Noise Test
Lexical decoding speed	Ability to process words quickly and accurately	Staggered Spondaic Word (SSW) Test–Decoding Signs
Short-term memory (STM)/working memory	Severity/patterns of how information is maintained in conscious memory (i.e., initial vs. later presented information)	SSW Test–Fading Memory Signs
STM/working memory span	Amount of units/information retained in STM	Test of Auditory Perceptual Skills–Revised: (1) Auditory Number Memory–Forward; (2) Auditory Word Memory; (3) Auditory Sentence Memory
Sequencing	Ability to maintain speech sounds, words, and directions in order	SSW Test (organization), Phonemic Synthesis Test (reversals), Token Test, Pitch Pattern Sequences Test
Auditory-linguistic integration	Ability to integrate information (suprasegmental/visual/verbal) across processing regions	(1) Digit Span–Rhythm Task; (2) SSW Test–Integration Sign; (3) Competing Sentences Test–right ear dominance; (4) Pitch Pattern Sequences Test (nonverbal/verbal discrepancy)
Prosodic perception	Ability to perceive/replicate rhythmic patterns	Pitch Pattern Sequences Test (significant nonverbal sign) + flat voicing patterns
Selective auditory attention	Ability to focus and recall target stimuli in presence of competition	Figure-ground tests (i.e., speech embedded in noise) and binaural separation such as on Competing Sentences Test
Divided auditory attention	Ability to recall both competing stimuli presented	SSW Test, Competing Sentences Test, Competing Words from Screening Test for Auditory Processing Disorders (SCAN)/SCAN-Revised
Sustained auditory attention	Ability to maintain attention to verbally presented information over a period of time without a break	Auditory Continuous Performance Test
Higher order phonologic skills		
Phonemic synthesis	Ability to blend individually presented speech sounds and derive the target whole word	Phonemic Synthesis Test
Sound-symbol associations	Ability to discriminate/sequence/ represent speech sounds with symbols	Lindamood Auditory Conceptualization Test 3

Musiek, 2000). This recommendation was based on the fact that CANS neural synchrony in response to auditory stimuli is assessed through the application of a number of electrophysiologic procedures, including auditory brainstem response (ABR), middle latency response (MLR), mismatch negativity (MMN), and late evoked potentials (LEP), including P300. However, an abnormality of the CANS determined through electrophysiologic measures does not provide specific information as to the type of (C)APD or auditory behaviors that can be expected based on the results

obtained. That is, while electrophysiologic tests may show clinical utility in assessing the CANS (Jirsa, 2002), there is a paucity of research in understanding the abnormalities of these tests relative to the presence of learning disabilities (Cacace and McFarland, 2002). For example, clear relationships have not yet been found between the auditory behavioral limitations observed in individuals suspected of having (C)APD and neural dyssynchrony ascertained via electrophysiologic measures. In addition, research has revealed little evidence of an increased prevalence of abnormal ABRs or MLRs to click stimuli/tone bursts in (C)APD populations. Furthermore, it is questionable as to what information can be provided with application of traditional electrophysiologic testing when providing intervention recommendations (Bellis, 2003). Obviously, electrophysiologic tests control for attention, fatigue, and motivation influences when assessing the CANS, even though these areas can usually be identified and controlled for during behavior tests (Bellis, 2003; Katz and Tillery, 2005).

Some recent studies have investigated the application of electrophysiologic procedures to determine clinic utility in a (C)APD diagnosis. For example, MMN has been found to (1) verify neurophysiologic changes due to listening training that may accompany observable auditory behaviors (Tremblay et al., 1997); (2) assist in differentiating phonemic (low) levels and language (higher) levels during auditory processing (Dalebout and Stack, 1999); and (3) differentiate children with and without learning problems (Banai et al., 2005). It has also been suggested that LEP measures can: (1) differentiate attention disorders from other categorical problems (Kraus et al., 1995); (2) show increased latency and decreased amplitude on P300 for children with APD when compared to those without APD (Jirsa and Clontz, 1990); (3) be used to study developmental processes in children and adults with hyperactivity (Satterfield et al., 1984); and (4) examine children with language/speech disorders (Mason and Mellor, 1984). However, the most impressive research to date concerning the use of electrophysiologic procedures and speech processing comes from Krause and colleagues (Banai et al., 2005; Cunningham et al., 2002; Hayes et al., 2003; Johnson et al., 2005; King et al., 2002; Kraus and Nicol, 2005; Russo et al., 2005; Wible et al., 2004; 2005), who have evaluated speech-evoked brainstem response differences between children with and without learning problems. This has resulted in the development of a clinical tool called Biological Marker of Auditory Processing (BioMAP), which is discussed in the following section.

Biological Marker of Auditory Processing

The BioMAP, developed at the Auditory Neuroscience Laboratory at Northwestern University under the direction of Nina Kraus and distributed by Bio-logic Systems Corporation (Johnson et al., 2005), characterizes the neural response of the brainstem to a complex speech signal, /da/, in order to identify disordered auditory processing associated with learning problems. The auditory signal consists of both linguistic cues (vowel and consonant information) and paralinguistic (prosodic) information. These cues are derived through a source-filter model in which the source is related to the vocal cord vibrations, resulting in paralinguistic cues, and the filter is related to the shape of the vocal tract and articulator movements, resulting in linguistic information (Johnson et al., 2005). An abundance of research from Kraus's laboratory suggests that brainstem measures involving the encoding of filter information can serve as a marker for neural asynchrony in about one third of children with language-based learning disorders, such as dyslexia or (C)APD (Johnson et al., 2005). Furthermore, in the presence of noise or rapid stimulation, brainstem neural activity representing the filter information becomes degraded but significantly more so in the auditory processing–disordered population, whereas neural mechanisms that encode source information remain unchanged.

Specific brainstem markers include delayed peak latency or shallow slope measures of specific wave sets, indicating deficits in brainstem responses in the encoding of filter information. In addition to its utility for serving as an objective biologic auditory processing marker, BioMAP has also been used successfully in evaluating physiologic changes in the timing of specific peaks subsequent to auditory training with various commercial training programs (Hayes et al., 2003; Russo et al., 2005). (See Chapter 26 for specific stimulus and morphology responses of BioMAP.)

It is hopeful that the application of BioMAP will assist in determining those children who would benefit from auditory training programs specific to the initial decoding/encoding of speech sounds and assessing the benefits from such training. Other potential applications of BioMAP include (1) examining populations of individuals with known deficits in neural encoding to paralinguistic information, such as those with autism; (2) assessing auditory processing deficits in cochlear implant and hearing aid users; and (3) assessing preschool children to identify those who would benefit from early identification for subsequent auditory training (Johnson et al., 2005).

▧ CENTRAL AUDITORY PROCESSING SCREENING

CAP screening assesses the possibility of existence of a (C)APD and, in turn, can lead to possible referral for a comprehensive (C)APD evaluation. Psychologists and speech-language pathologists are two professional groups that would likely screen for CAP on a routine basis. As part of the screening process, teachers and parents may be asked to provide information on the child's behavioral functional limitations through the use of questionnaires.

Questionnaires

Questionnaires are a common tool for ascertaining the likelihood that an individual exhibits functional behavioral limitations in his or her communication, language, and learning. Because of possible bias, we must take into consideration who is rating the child's behaviors on the questionnaire. A teacher may give ratings that indicate weak attention or motivation of the student as being the possible culprit to "poor listening," whereas CANS tests may indicate that it is a (C)APD that is associated with that student's behavioral functional limitations of "listening difficulty." On the other hand, parents may insist that their child has a (C)APD and reflect this bias on the questionnaire ratings in order for their child to receive a referral for testing. Following is a list of a number of commercially available questionnaires, all available through the Educational Audiology Association:

1. Fisher Auditory Problems Checklist (Fisher, 1985). This was the first developed CAP screening questionnaire, with normative data available from kindergarten to grade 6. It has been designed to rate 25 items of concern. Many of the items listed on this questionnaire are commonly seen behaviors listed in the different types or profiles of (C)APD.

2. Children's Auditory Processing Performance Scale (CHAPPS) (Smoski et al., 1992). There are six listening situations (ideal, quiet, attention, memory, noise, and multiple inputs), and the rater (parent or teacher) compares the student to children of similar age and background. There are a total of 36 questions, and the choices vary from +1 (less difficulty than others) to –5 (cannot function in the situation). Scores can range from +36 to –180, and the more negative the score, the more difficulty that is noted. A child who receives a total score of –12 to –180 is at risk for (C)APD.

3. Screening Instrument for Targeting Educational Risk (S.I.F.T.E.R.) (Anderson, 1989). There are 15 questions over five category areas: communication, academics, attention, class participation, and social behavior. Scoring consists of 15 points per category, resulting in a failure if one is rated at or below 6 or 7 (depending on the category).

Screening Tests

Historically, screening test performance scores have sometimes been used to label a child with (C)APD, rather than to refer the child for further testing (Jerger and Musiek, 2000) by an audiologist to rule in or out the diagnosis of (C)APD. In general, screening tests have been designed to have high sensitivity (Jerger and Musiek, 2000) (i.e., those having CAPD are readily identified); however, this can also lead to a high false-positive rate (i.e., identify individuals as possibly having CAPD when, in fact, they do not).

Obviously, attention, fatigue, and status of an unchecked peripheral hearing system can influence screening test findings. It is recommended that screening tests be administered in a room without any noise distractions and during the morning in order to control for attention and fatigue. When possible, screening tympanometry and puretone thresholds should be obtained to improve the reliability of the screening results.

The Screening Test for Auditory Processing Disorders (SCAN) (Keith, 1986) and the Screening Test for Auditory Processing Disorders in Children–Revised (SCAN-C) (Keith, 2000) were considered the only audiologic screening tests for (C)APD until a conference on (C)APD (Jerger and Musiek, 2000) indicated promise for the Dichotic

Digits Test (DDT) (Musiek, 1983). Although psychologists and speech-language pathologists typically administer the SCAN or SCAN-C as a screening tool for (C)APD, audiologists sometimes use these instruments as a portion of their test battery. Currently, research is being conducted on the efficacy of SCAN-C as a diagnostic tool. The following is a description of some of the CAP screening tests available:

1. The SCAN, designed for children between ages 3 and 11 years, consists of three subtests: Auditory Figure Ground, Filtered Words, and Competing Words. The SCAN-C contains these three subtests, as well as a competing sentence test. A cassette player, headphones, and a quiet environment are necessary in order to administer these screening procedures. I have consulted and advised psychologists to administer the SCAN in the morning and that it be the first test in their test battery in order to control for fatigue and attention; otherwise, fatigue and lack of attention could influence the occurrence of false positives.

2. Recently, a new standardized screening tool, the Differential Screening Test for Processing (DSTP) (Richard and Ferre, 2006) was developed to differentiate skills associated with three neurologic levels of processing that are integrated depending on the communication task: (1) perception of primary acoustic characteristics of auditory signals; (2) identification of acoustic aspects related to the phonemic portion of language; and (3) the ability to attribute meaning within language.

   The authors indicate that the first level is evaluated by tests that target: (a) the ability to discriminate speech sounds (auditory discrimination); (b) binaural integration in which the client is asked to repeat numbers presented dichotically in order to assess communication between hemispheres, and (c) the ability to recognize acoustic patterns seen in verbal communication (temporal patterning) by verbally replicating the sequence of the two presented tones (high and/or low pitched).

   The second level is evaluated by using two subtests: "phonemic" manipulation and "phonic" manipulation. Phonemic manipulation provides two to four sounds in which the child must properly recognize (a) the number of discrete phonemes in a provided word, (b) blend the sounds in a word, and (c) change discrete sounds when asked. Phonic manipulation assess sound-symbol associations by providing three tasks that target (a) proper spelling with supplied tiles, (b) the ability to synthesize phonemes with the use of tiles, and (c) the ability to modify the tile representation when provided a new target word.

   The third level assesses meaning to the auditory signal by providing three subtests: antonyms, prosodic interpretation, and language organization. To assess antonym knowledge, the child must provide the opposite word to the provided target word. To assess prosodic interpretation, the child verbally responds with a "yes" or "no" to the sincerity of the message. For instance, the phrase "I am happy to be here" is provided in a sad tone of voice. The child would respond "no" because there is a discrepancy between the prosodic information and the provided statement. To assess language organization, the child must respond successfully to two different tasks. Task 1 provides eight different sentences, such as, "It's what you sit on at a table or a desk." The proper answer is chair, stool, or seat. For task 2, the child is provided pictures of objects and must describe the objects or what the objects do. For instance, a picture of a flower may be provided. The proper response can be any of the following: smells good, attracts bees, blooms, grows in a garden, has pollen, etc.

The DSTP was standardized by presenting the subtests to 509 students aged 6.0 to 12.11 years old, reflecting a balance across race, age, gender, grade, and all socioeconomic groups. Poor test performance in any area suggests the need for additional diagnostic evaluation(s) in order to establish the presence of a deficit.

3. Other possible screening tools. Speech-language pathologists routinely use the Test of Auditory Perceptual Skills–Revised (TAPS-R; Gardner, 1996), while psychologists typically use some form of digit span test (Wechsler, 1991) or the Visual-Aural Digit Span Test (Koppitz, 1975). Bellis (2003) indicates that the TAPS-R may be an instrument that can provide some indication of auditory perceptual ability, but it does not indicate the specific underlying auditory processing difficulties. Medwetsky (personal communication, November 2006) indicates that the Visual-Aural Digit Span test can identify individuals at risk for (C)APD because, in the absence of much contextual information, poor performance on this task is likely due to some form of processing-related difficulty (such as fading memory or poor decoding speed). Keller et al. (2006) found a correlation with test performance on digit span (Wechsler, 1991) and (C)APD, indicating that psychologists could refer individuals for a (C)APD evaluation when a client shows weakness on tests sensitive to short-term auditory memory span.

The DDT, administering two digits per ear, may also be a useful (C)APD screening tool because it is a very quick test to administer (4-minute task) and uses very familiar items (digits) that even young children will readily recognize (Musiek, 1983; Jerger and Musiek, 2000).

4. Combined screening measures may assist in minimizing overreferrals due to high false-positive findings (Jerger and Musiek, 2000). For example, this can be accomplished by using the combination of a questionnaire and CAP screening test measure. Another possibility posed by Jerger and Musiek (2000) is to administer both the DDT and a gap detection test; however, the authors stress the need for research to assess this possibility as a screening measure.

CENTRAL AUDITORY PROCESSING DISORDER TESTS

Auditory tasks administered to assess for auditory processing function consist of monotic (stimuli presented separately to each ear), diotic (same stimuli presented to both ears simultaneously), and dichotic (different stimuli presented to each ear simultaneously) tests. Audiologists generally choose their tests by the processes they wish to assess. Refer to the (C)APD Test Battery Model discussed in earlier sections of this chapter. Table 27.1 lists CAP tests with their associated targeted process and CANS sensitivity, whereas Table 27.2 defines the function assessed by the CAP tests. The reader is referred to numerous publications that provide a thorough description of the CAP tests seen in the various models (Bellis, 2003; Musiek and Chermak, 2006; Katz, 1994; Medwetsky, 2002b; Stecker, 1992).

REPORTING CENTRAL AUDITORY PROCESSING DISORDER TEST RESULTS

An evaluation report must be accurate, concise, and well written. These reports communicate to families and professionals (such as physicians, speech-language pathologists, teachers, tutors, occupational and physical therapists and psychologists) an explanation of the various test battery procedures, test performance results, and recommendations for remediation or compensations for the disorder. Professionals appreciate reports that are organized, consistent in format style, and provide details on the test performance data; in turn, this allows them to know exactly where to find a specific summary or fact, thus saving them time and effort. The reports should provide the raw scores, standard deviations (SD), and explanation of findings in terms that are understood by all those who read the report. When applicable, information should include both qualitative and quantitative results, severity of findings, overall implications (e.g., comorbidity associations, educational and medical aspects), and resources for the reader to consult. Reports should be sent within a reasonable time frame.

In summary, the report is likely the best opportunity to educate others about the diagnosis of (C)APD; facts regarding the administered test battery; social, medical, and educational ramifications; and recommendations for assisting with the client's auditory, learning, and communicative functional behavioral limitations.

THIRD-PARTY REIMBURSEMENT

The ASHA 2005 Technical Report of (C)APD is the first publication to provide information on how to submit for payment for (C)APD evaluations. Perhaps this is because

Current Procedural Terminology (CPT) codes implemented in January 2005 for the first time reflected the professional time and services provided in a (C)APD evaluation. The first hour of administering, interpreting, and/or providing test results falls under the CPT code 92620, with each additional 15-minute increments to be billed under code 92621. These codes preclude the peripheral hearing assessment, which is billed under each individual peripheral hearing measurement administered.

Previous history of reimbursement involved submitting for each central test administered, each with its own CPT code. Such billing was frustrating because some CAP tests would only allow a $3.00 reimbursement for a test that took 15 minutes to administer, while others provided a $25.00 reimbursement for a 10-minute test. Another billing problem in the past was that speech-language pathologists and audiologists had to bill for language and/or auditory processing evaluations under a single CPT code. Such procedures led to confusion and misrepresented (C)APD test assessment. In order to reconcile this billing dilemma, improved reimbursement procedures were developed for CAP assessment, which ultimately led to the new CPT codes.

Reimbursement Concerns

Insurance companies are not obligated to reimburse for testing, intervention sessions, and report writing that fall under an educational-related diagnosis or experimental applications. Some insurance companies indicate that (C)APD is related to educational factors (Excellus, 2002) and, therefore, is not covered, even under the diagnostic code 388.40 Abnormal Auditory Perception. When an educational-based reason is used as a reason for denial of payment of service or when an insurance company has outdated information and claims that (C)APD is experimental (Aetna, 2005), information should be provided to these insurance companies that includes the most current up-to-date facts, such as studies showing the clinical utility of (C)APD testing. During this interim period, the clinician would submit for payment to the insurance company for the peripheral hearing assessment procedures (considered medically based), while the client still would be responsible for payment of the (C)APD assessment.

Another concern is the need for evidenced-based research to address the types or subprofiles of (C)APD in terms of both medical and educational outcomes. Insurance companies rely on evidence-based research and technical reports to justify medical needs for services rendered. At the present time, all (C)APD models indicate some form of educational basis: poor reading and spelling, weak organization, poor or inconsistent academic performance, and weak expressive language written skill, etc. If this continues to be stressed in the models of (C)APD, without the medical counterpart, then insurance companies may prematurely conclude that there are only educational components of (C)APD and thus not realize the medical concerns. In turn, this will continue

to result in denials of reimbursement for services associated with 388.40 Abnormal Auditory Perception.

As professionals, we are obligated to provide evidence-based research regarding areas of concern related to differential diagnosis to indicate a medical need for testing and application of intervention. Differential diagnosis involves collaboration with the psychologist, speech-language pathologist, audiologist, and possibly the physician. The end result may be a child with only ADHD who may need medication to assist with the functional behavioral limitations associated with ADHD. However, the auditory problems of a child with (C)APD alone will not improve with medication (Tillery et al., 2000). The child with both (C)APD and ADHD will need a variety of therapeutic measures to assist ADHD (i.e., medication, tutoring, behavioral modification, counseling) and unique therapeutic measures for (C)APD. This example illustrates the concept of "win-win," with both the client and insurance company benefiting from the CAP evaluation and recommendations. The insurance company will not have to provide coverage for medication for someone with a diagnosis of (C)APD (which could cost the insurance company thousands of dollars over the course of many years), while the client hopefully will obtain the treatment that will best meet his or her needs.

▨ FUTURE CONCERNS IN AUDITORY PROCESSING TEST BATTERIES

The selection of CAP tests or a test battery approach relies on the comfort, experience, and education of the clinician, as well as the availability of a multidisciplinary team in the geographic area in which one resides. ASHA (2005) recommends that testing be done for children 7 years of age and older. However, the Buffalo and S-LP Models provide qualitative data congruent with quantitative data that can be administered to children as young as 5 years of age, resulting in the categorization of types of auditory processing problems that have educational and communication concerns. The identification of dysfunction among specific auditory processes is the basis of the Bellis/Ferre Model and provides specific categories of auditory problems that coincide with educational and communication concerns. Some clinicians broaden these models. For instance, Medwetsky's S-LP Model (2002a) uses the qualitative and quantitative data of the Buffalo Model as a foundation and further includes attention, memory span, and phonologic awareness/phonics test performance for further analysis (Medwetsky, 2006). Stecker (1998) discusses the application of additional tests to assess localization and/or low brainstem assessment beyond the Buffalo Model. Those who work with psychologists in a team approach may not need to administer attention tests such as the Auditory Continuous Performance Test (Keith, 1994) since it is routinely administered by the referring psychologist, as is the case in Western New York.

Perhaps in the future, there will be additional evidence-based research to validate the specific types of (C)APD (ASHA, 2005). In the meantime, clinicians will continue to administer (C)APD tests that are known to provide information regarding CANS dysfunction. As we work together to learn the "best of the best" in diagnosing (C)APD, here are some thoughts we should be aware of and try to answer:

- Can one test provide a diagnosis of (C)APD? ASHA (2005) indicates that one test failure at 3 standard deviations below the mean or a failure of two tests by a minimum of 2 standard deviations below the mean is sufficient for a diagnosis of CAPD in the presence of functional behavioral limitations. The use of one test failure used to be considered a lax approach, but most would agree that such a failure constitutes a dysfunction in only the specific auditory process being assessed. If the clinician controls for attention, motivation, and fatigue, then a failure of two tests at a minimum of 2 standard deviations below the mean or one test failure at 3 standard deviations below the mean would seem appropriate for the profession to consider as a criterion for the diagnosis of (C)APD.
- The various models for types or profiles of (C)APD have many commonalities and a few differences. Actually, it is interesting that there are more similarities versus differences. All of the models agree on an integration subtype of (C)APD. The TFM type of (C)APD is seen in the Buffalo Model, and FM is seen in the S-LP Model, whereas the prosodic category is only in the Bellis/Ferre and S-LP Models.
- There is agreement with respect to the organization category among the different models. However, only one CAP test (the SSW test) provides norms for reversals. What does it mean when one reverses on other tests, especially if those tests were developed to identify those with learning disabilities, such as the Pitch Pattern Sequence Test?
- Would the inclusion of electrophysiologic tests assist with profiling specific types of (C)APD? The inclusion of BioMAP may offer evidence of specific deficiencies in sound encoding in a certain percentage of individuals identified with learning disability. Thus, would BioMAP assist in the differentiation of types of (C)APD and the effectiveness of intervention?

SUMMARY

A test battery approach is recommended for assessment of the CANS when a client presents with functional behavioral limitations in auditory, learning, and communication skills. Currently, evaluating the CANS is not a routine application of assessment among audiologists; however, it is hopeful that this will change with the educational opportunities offered by AuD programs. Research should concentrate on the application and results of CAP tests that indicate specific types of (C)APD, as seen in the current models discussed, which would lead to appropriate intervention. Efforts should also be made to use electrophysiologic tests, as seen in the advent of BioMAP. These procedures would augment current behavioral test batteries by providing objective evidence of underlying processing deficits, help determine auditory training candidacy, and, in turn, evaluate the effectiveness of such therapy.

Questionnaires listed in this chapter are available at:
Education Audiology Association (EAA)
11166 Huron Street
Suite 27
Denver, CO 80234
800-460-7322
www.edaud.org

REFERENCES

Aetna. (2005) Clinical Policy Bulletins. Central auditory processing disorder (CAPD). Hartford, CT: Aetna; pp 1–4.

American Speech-Language-Hearing Association (ASHA). (1992) Issues in central auditory processing disorders: a report from ASHA Ad Hoc Committee on Central Auditory Processing. Rockville, MD: ASHA.

American Speech-Language-Hearing Association (ASHA). (1995) Central auditory processing: current status of research and implications for clinical practice. A report from the ASHA task force on central auditory processing. Rockville, MD: ASHA.

American Speech-Language-Hearing Association (ASHA) Task Force on Central Auditory Processing Consensus Development. (1996) Central auditory processing: current status of research and implications for clinical practice. *Am J Audiol.* 5, 41–54.

American Speech-Language and Hearing Association (ASHA). (2005) (Central) auditory processing disorders. A technical report. Rockville, MD: ASHA.

Anderson KL. (1989) *S.I.F.T.E.R.: Screening Instrument for Targeting Educational Risk.* Austin, TX: Pro Ed.

Banai K, Nicol T, Zecker S, Kraus N. (2005) Brainstem timing: implications for cortical processing and literacy. *J Neurosci.* 25, 9850–9857.

Barkley RA. (1998) *Attention-Deficit Hyperactivity Disorder: A Handbook for Diagnosis and Treatment.* 2nd ed. New York: Guilford and Press.

Bellis TJ. (1996) *Assessment and Management of Central Auditory Processing Disorders in the Educational Setting:* From Science to Practice. San Diego: Singular Publishing.

Bellis TJ. (1999) Subprofiles of central auditory processing disorders. *Educ Audiol Rev.* 2, 9–14.

Bellis TJ. (2002) Developing deficit-specific intervention plans for individuals with auditory processing disorders. *Semin Hear.* 23, 287–295.

Bellis TJ. (2003) *Assessment and Management of Central Auditory Processing Disorders in the Educational Setting: From*

Science to Practice. 2nd ed. Clifton Park, NY: Thompson Learning.

Bellis TJ, Ferre JM. (1999) Multidimensional approach to the differential diagnosis of central auditory processing disorders in children. *J Am Acad Audiol.* 10, 319–328.

Cacace AT, McFarland DJ. (2002) Middle-latency auditory evoked potentials: basic issues and potential implications. In: Katz J, ed. *Handbook of Clinical Audiology.* 5th ed. Philadelphia: Lippincott Williams & Wilkins; pp 349–377.

Cacace AT, McFarland DJ. (2005) The importance of modality specificity in diagnosing central auditory processing disorder (CAPD). *Am J Audiol.* 14, 112–123.

Chermak GD, Hall JW, Musiek FE. (1999) Differential diagnosis and management of central auditory processing disorder and attention deficit hyperactivity disorder. *J Am Acad Audiol.* 10, 289–303.

Chermak GD, Musiek FE. (1997) *Central Auditory Processing Disorders: New Perspectives.* San Diego: Singular.

Cunningham J, Nicol T, King C, Zecker SG, Kraus N. (2002) Effects of noise and cue enhancement on neural responses to speech in auditory midbrain, thalamus and cortex. *Hear Res.* 169, 97–111.

Dalebout SD, Stack JW. (1999) Mismatch negativity to acoustical differences not differentiated behaviorally. *J Am Acad Audiol.* 10, 388–399.

Domitz DM, Schow RL. (2000) A new CAPD battery-multiple auditory processing assessment (MAPA): factor analysis and comparisons with SCAN. *Am J Audiol.* 9, 101–111.

Excellus. (2002) Central auditory processing testing. New protocols recently approved by Corporate Protocol Committee. Universal medical policy. Rochester, NY: Excellus; p 4.

Ferre JM. (1992) CATfiles: improving the clinical utility of central auditory function tests. Paper presented at the American Speech-Language-Hearing Association Annual Convention. San Antonio, TX.

Ferre JM. (2002) Managing children's central auditory processing deficits in the real world: what teachers and parents want to know. *Semin Hear.* 23, 319–326.

Fisher L. (1985) Learning disabilities and auditory processing. In: Van Hattam RJ, ed. *Administration of Speech Language Services in Schools: A Manual.* San Diego: College-Hill Press; pp 231–290.

Gardner MF. (1996) *Test of Auditory-Perceptual Skills-Revised.* Hydesville, CA: Psychological and Educational Publications.

Geschwind ND, Galaburda AM. (1987) *Cerebral Lateralization: Biological Mechanisms, Associations, and Pathology.* Cambridge, MA: MIT Press; 1987.

Hayes EA, Warrier CM, Nicol TG, Zecker SG, Kraus N. (2003) Neural plasticity following auditory training in children with learning problems. *Clin Neurophysiol.* 114, 673–684.

Isaacson R, Pribram K. (1986) *The Hippocampus.* Volume 4. New York: Plenum Press.

Jerger J, Jerger S. (1975) Clinical validity of central auditory tests. *Scand Audiol.* 4, 147–163.

Jerger J, Musiek FE. (2000) Report of Consensus Conference on the diagnosis of auditory processing disorders in school-aged children. *J Acad Audiol.* 11, 467–474.

Jirsa RE. (2002) Clinical efficacy of electrophysiologic measures in APD management programs. *Semin Hear.* 23, 349–355.

Jirsa RE, Clontz K. (1990) Long latency auditory event-related potentials from children with auditory processing disorders. *Ear Hear.* 11, 222–232.

Johnson KL, Nicol TG, Kraus N. (2005) Brain stem response to speech: a biological marker of auditory processing. *Ear Hear.* 26, 424–434.

Katz J. (1962) The use of staggered spondaic words for assessing the integrity of the central auditory system. *J Aud Res;* 2: 327–337.

Katz J. (1968) The SSW test-an interim report. *J Speech Hear Disord.* 33, 132–146.

Katz J. (1992) Classification of auditory processing disorders. In: Katz J, Stecker N, Henderson D, eds. *Central Auditory Processing: A Transdisciplinary View.* Chicago: Mosby Yearbook; pp 81–92.

Katz J. (1994) *CAPD Test Battery.* Vancouver, WA: Precision Acoustics.

Katz J. (2001a) *Central Test Battery: Tester's Manual.* Vancouver, WA: Precision Acoustics.

Katz J. (2001b) INT-8 analysis: the ultimate. *SSW Rep.* 24, 2–6.

Katz J, Harmon C. (1982) *Phonemic Synthesis Program Training.* Vancouver, WA: Precision Acoustics.

Katz J, Johnson C, Brander S, Delagrange T, Ferre J, King J, Krossover-Wechter D, Lucker J, Medwetsky L, Saul R, Rosenburg G, Stecker N, Tillery K. (2002) Clinical and research concerns regarding the 2000 APD consensus report and recommendations. *Audiol Today.* April/May, 14–17.

Katz J, Smith P. (1991) The Staggered Spondaic Word Test: a ten-minute look at the central nervous system through the ears. *Ann N Y Acad Sci.* 620, 233–251.

Katz J, Tillery KL. (2005) Can central auditory processing tests resist supramodal influences? *Am J Audiol.* 14, 124–127.

Keith RW. (1986) *SCAN: A Screening Test for Auditory Processing Disorders.* San Diego: The Psychological Corp.

Keith RW. (2000) *SCAN-C: Test for Auditory Processing Disorders in Children–Revised.* San Antonio: The Psychological Corporation.

Keller W. (1992) Auditory processing disorder or attention deficit disorder? In: Katz J, Stecker N, Henderson D, eds. *Central Auditory Processing: A Transdisciplinary View.* St. Louis: Mosby; pp 107–114.

Keller W. (1998) The relationship between ADHD, CAPD and specific learning disorders. In: Masters G, Stecker N, Katz J, eds. *Central Auditory Processing Disorders: Mostly Management.* Needham Heights: Allyn and Bacon; pp 33–47.

Keller W, Tillery KL. (2002) Reliable differential diagnosis and effective management for auditory processing and attention deficit hyperactivity disorders. *Semin Hear.* 23, 337–347.

Keller W, Tillery KL. (2006) Intervention for individuals with (C)APD and ADHD: a psychological perspective. In: Chermak G, Musiek F, eds. *Handbook of Central Auditory Processing Disorders, Volume II: Comprehensive Intervention.* San Diego: Plural Publishing Inc.

Keller W, Tillery KL, McFadden S. (2006) Auditory processing disorder in children diagnosed with nonverbal learning disability. *Am J Audiol.* 15, 108–113.

King C, Warrier CM, Hayes E, Kraus N. (2002) Deficits in auditory brainstem pathway encoding of speech sounds in children with learning problems. *Neurosci Lett.* 319, 111–115.

Koppitz EM. (1975) Bender Gestalt Test, Visual Aural Digit Span Test and reading achievement. *J Learn Disord.* 6, 46–53.

Kraus N, McGee T, Carrell T, King C, Tremblay K. (1995) Central auditory system plasticity associated with speech discrimination training. *J Cogn Neurosci.* 7, 27–34.

Kraus N, Nicol T. (2005) Brainstem origins for cortical 'what' and 'where' pathways in the auditory system. *Trends Neurosci.* 28, 176–181.

Lucker JR. (1981) Interpreting SSW results of learning disabled children. *SSW Rep.* 3, 1–3.

Luria AR. (1966) *Higher Cortical Functions in Man.* New York: Basic Books; pp 103–108.

Mason BM, Mellor DH. (1984) Brainstem, middle latency and late cortical evoked potentials in children with speech and language disorders. *Electroencephalogr Clin Neurophysiol.* 59, 297–309.

McFarland DJ, Cacace AT. (1995) Modality specificity as a criterion for diagnosing central auditory processing disorders. *Am J Audiol.* 4, 32–44.

McFarland DJ, Cacace AT. (1997) Modality specificity of auditory and visual pattern recognition: implications for the assessment of central auditory processing disorders. *Audiology.* 36, 249–260.

Medwetsky L. (2002a) Central auditory processing. In: Katz J, ed. *Handbook of Clinical Audiology.* 5th ed. Baltimore: Lippincott Williams & Wilkins; pp 495–509.

Medwetsky L. (2002b) Central auditory processing testing: a battery approach. In: Katz J, ed. *Handbook of Clinical Audiology.* 5th ed. Baltimore: Lippincott Williams & Wilkins; pp 510–531.

Medwetsky L. (2006) Spoken language processing: a convergent approach to conceptualizing (central) auditory processing. *ASHA Leader.* 118, 6–7.

Mueller G, Beck G, Sedge R. (1987) Comparison of the efficiency of cortical level speech tests. *Semin Hear.* 8, 279–298.

Musiek FE. (1983) Assessment of central auditory dysfunction: the dichotic digits test revisited. *Ear Hear.* 4, 79–83.

Musiek FE. (1985) Application of central auditory tests: an overview. In: Katz J, ed. *Handbook of Clinical Audiology.* 3rd ed. Baltimore: Williams & Wilkins; pp 321–336.

Musiek FE, Bellis TJ, Chermak GD. (2005) Nonmodularity of the CANS: implications for (central) auditory processing disorder. *Am J Audiol.* 14, 128–138.

Musiek FE, Chermak GD. (2006) *Central Auditory Processing Disorders, Volume I: Auditory Neuroscience and Diagnosis.* San Diego: Plural Publishing Inc.

Musiek F, Lamb L. (1994) Central auditory assessment: an overview. In: Katz J, ed. *Handbook of Clinical Audiology.* 4th ed. Baltimore: Williams & Wilkins; pp 197–211.

Mykelbust HR. (1954) *Auditory Processing Disorders in Children: A Manual for Differential Diagnosis.* New York: Grune and Stratton.

Richard GJ, Ferre JM. (2006) *Differential Screening Test for Processing.* East Moline, IL: LinguiSystems, Inc.

Russo NM, Nicol GT, Zecker SG, Hayes EA, Kraus N. (2005) Auditory training improves neural timing in the human brainstem. *Behav Brain Res.* 156, 95–103.

Satterfield JH, Schell AM, Backs RW, Hidaka KC. (1984) A cross-sectional and longitudinal study of age effects of electrophysiological measures in hyperactive and normal children. *Biol Psychol.* 19, 973–990.

Schow R, Seikel J, Chermak G, Berent M. (2000) Central auditory processes and test measures: ASHA 1996 revisited. *Am J Audiol.* 9, 1–6.

Smoski W, Brunt M, Tannahill J. (1992) Listening characteristics of children with central auditory processing disorders. *Lang Speech Hear Serv Sch.* 23, 145–152.

Stecker N. (1992) Central auditory processing: implications in audiology. In: Katz J, Stecker N, Henderson D, eds. *Central Auditory Processing: A Transdisciplinary View.* St. Louis: Mosby; pp 117–127.

Stecker N. (1998) Overview and update of central auditory processing disorders. In: Masters G, Stecker N, Katz J, eds. *Central Auditory Processing Disorders: Mostly Management.* Boston: Allyn and Bacon; pp 1–14.

Stecker N. (2004) Challenging and changing times. *SSW Rep.* 26, 1–5.

Tillery KL. (1998) Central auditory processing assessment and therapeutic strategies for children with attention deficit hyperactivity disorder. In: Masters G, Stecker N, Katz J, eds. *Central Auditory Processing Disorders: Mostly Management.* Boston: Allyn and Bacon; pp 175–194.

Tillery KL. (1999) Reversals, reversals, reversals: differentiating information for CAPD, LD and ADHD. *SSW Rep.* 21, 1–6.

Tillery KL. (2005) CAPD characteristics in a large sample with and without CAPD. Paper presented at the American Speech-Language-Hearing Association (ASHA) Annual Convention. San Diego, CA.

Tillery KL, Katz J, Keller W. (2000) Effects of methylphenidate (Ritalin) on auditory performance in children with attention and auditory processing disorders. *J Speech Lang Hear Res.* 43, 893–901.

Tremblay K, Kraus N, Carrell TD, McGee T. (1997) Central auditory system plasticity: generalization to novel stimuli following listening training. *J Acoust Soc Am.* 102, 3762–3773.

Wechsler D. (1991) *Wechsler Intelligence Scale for Children.* 3rd ed. San Antonio, TX: Psychological Corporation.

Wible B, Nicol T, Kraus N. (2004) Atypical brainstem representation of onset and formant structure of speech sounds in children with language-based learning problems. *Biol Psychol.* 67, 299–317.

Wible B, Nicol T, Kraus N (2005) Correlation between brainstem and cortical auditory processes in normal and language-impaired children. *Brain.* 128, 417–423.

Willeford J, Bilger J. (1978) Auditory perception in children with learning disabilities. In: Katz J, ed. *Handbook of Clinical Audiology.* 2nd ed. Baltimore: Williams & Wilkins; pp 410–425.

Willeford J, Burleigh J. (1985) *Handbook of Central Auditory Processing Disorders in Children.* Orlando: Grune & Stratton.

28 Management of Central Auditory Processing Disorders

Larry Medwetsky, Laura Riddle, and Jack Katz

INTRODUCTION

As the lead author of this chapter, I will start off by recounting an event that took place in 1994 at the first American Speech-Language-Hearing Association (ASHA) consensus conference on central auditory processing disorders (CAPDs). At the end of the first day, a number of us went back to Jack Katz's hotel room to discuss what had been presented. One of the audiologists mentioned that although a number of tests were available to identify different underlying deficits, teachers and related school professionals often complained that management recommendations were always the same, irrespective of the underlying difficulties; at the time, this was often the case. However, there have been many developments in our conceptualization of central auditory processing and, in turn, how we can individualize a treatment regimen to address an individual's specific deficit areas.

In this chapter, the three authors discuss various approaches that can be used to address the specific needs of an individual with CAPD. As the lead author, I will present a background to the topic and then review various compensatory strategies and environmental modifications that can be easily implemented in a classroom setting (application of these can be generalized to the office setting as well as the home environment). Dr. Riddle will discuss the important collaborative role that speech-language pathologists can play in addressing the needs of children with CAPD through carefully chosen diagnostic instruments that can complement audiologic findings and application of various language processing intervention procedures to address the specific deficits that have been identified. Last, Jack Katz will describe three specific interventions that he has

developed to address phonemic decoding and speech-in-noise difficulties.

BACKGROUND

The key to any successful intervention of CAPD is (1) an understanding of how the brain typically processes spoken language and, in turn, how breakdown in any of these areas can be reflected in specific central auditory processing (CAP) deficits; and (2) a comprehensive test battery approach that can examine these various processes, thus enabling the clinician to derive a profile of the individual's processing strengths and weaknesses.

Susan Jerger (2007) has conceptualized the domains in which intervention can be applied:

- The first stage is known as "Form," which relates to the properties/clarity of incoming stimuli
- The second stage is referred to as "Transform," which relates to how successfully the incoming stimuli are processed
- The last stage is termed "Inform," which refers to the individual's ability to recognize and utilize the transformed input

In addressing the first stage, a number of approaches can be applied to enhance the quality of the signal delivered to the listener. These include environmental modifications as well as speaker delivery styles known to enhance signal quality/clarity. Deficits in the transform stage are addressed through perceptual/processing interventions, while the inform stage can be addressed by language processing interventions as well as compensatory strategies. The compensatory strategies, environmental modifications, and therapeutic interventions have been coined as the Tripod approach by Ferre (2002) and serve as a conceptual guide with which clinicians can address CAPD. I will start by providing an overview of various compensatory strategies and environmental modifications that can be implemented, followed by Dr. Riddle's and Dr. Katz's sections on therapeutic interventions.

Compensatory Strategies

This section will cover strategies that, if implemented, can greatly enhance the learning environment as well as reduce frustration and fatigue of the listener. What's great about compensatory strategies is that they have minimal or no costs and can easily be implemented as program accommodations in a 504 Plan or Individualized Education Plan (IEP). These are the two mechanisms whereby a child in the United States identified with a disability can receive services through a school in order to ensure that the child receives a free, appropriate public education (see Table 28.1 for definitions and general implementation). It should be noted that many of the strategies can be used by individuals with a processing disorder, individuals with hearing loss, second language learners, and even elderly individuals who are beginning to experience central presbycusis. That is, the same strategy may

be beneficial even though there may be different underlying causes.

CLEAR SPEECH AND LINGUISTIC ENHANCEMENTS

Perhaps the easiest way to assist individuals with CAPD is to use an effective speaking style that ensures maximum clarity of the speech signal as well as what I will term here as linguistic enhancements. It has been known for many years that talkers can effectively enhance the intelligibility of their speech by producing what has been referred to as "clear speech." In clear speech, a speaker consciously attempts to provide the clearest possible sample of the spoken utterance. The talker does this by (1) articulating all phonemes precisely and accurately, (2) slowing one's speech rate slightly (e.g., newscaster's style), (3) pausing slightly between phrases and thoughts (which provides the listener with additional processing time, while decreasing the amount that must be held in working memory at any one point), and (4) modestly increasing vocal volume. Research shows that clear speech results in longer vowel durations, greater frequency separations in vowel formants, and increased energy in the 1,000 to 3,000 Hz frequency region (Krause and Braida, 2004; Li and So, 2005; Ferguson and Kewley-Port, 2007). In analyzing the global acoustic properties of clear versus conversational speech, Liu et al. (2004) found that clear speech results in an overall slower rate of production, higher temporal amplitude modulations, and greater intelligibility than

---

TABLE 28.1   General descriptions of an individualized education plan (IEP) and 504 plan

IEP
- Under the Individuals with Disabilities Education Act (IDEA), a student is eligible for special education and related services if the student is properly evaluated as having one of 13 specified disabilities.
- IDEA is a federal funding statute, the purpose of which is to provide *financial aid* to states to ensure adequate and appropriate services for disabled children.
- To be eligible under IDEA, a student's disability must adversely affect the student's educational performance.
- There are specific guidelines regarding the testing administered, education, and placement; creation of a written IEP document with specific content; and procedural safeguards.

Thus, IEP provides funding toward the disabled child's education.

504 Plan
- A 504 Plan is another name for Section 504 of the Federal Rehabilitation Act of 1974, which is a broad civil rights law that protects the rights of individuals with disabilities in programs and activities that receive federal financial assistance from the US Department of Education.
- All school-aged children identified as disabled, who have a physical or mental impairment that substantially limits a major activity or who are regarded as disabled by others, can be covered under a 504 Plan.
- Under the 504 Plan, a free and appropriate education means an education comparable to the education provided to nonhandicapped students, requiring that reasonable accommodations be made; related services, independent of any special education services (as defined under IDEA), may be the reasonable accommodation.
- A student is eligible for a 504 Plan so long as s/he meets the definition of a qualified person with disability.
- Unlike the IEP, for an individual to qualify for a 504 Plan, the disability *does not have to adversely affect educational performance*, nor does the student need special education services in order to be protected.
- Similar to an IEP, there are testing/programmatic accommodation guidelines and procedural safeguards, including development of a written document (the 504 Plan).

Unlike IDEA, 504 Plans do not provide additional funds.

conversational speech. In both simulated and actual cochlear implant users, Liu et al. (2004) found a 3- to 4-dB enhancement in speech reception thresholds when clear speech was used. Bradlow and Alexander (2007) examined semantic and phonetic enhancements on speech-in-noise recognition by native and nonnative listeners. Phonetic enhancements were assessed by the production of clear speech versus typical conversational rate, while semantic enhancements were examined by the degree to which the final word was predicted by the preceding words. The authors determined that either condition resulted in improved intelligibility, with the greatest improvements occurring when both clear speech and high-predictability sentences were used (note that when only semantic enhancements were present, nonnative speakers did not reveal as much of an enhancement as native speakers, likely due to their not being able to access the semantic aspects in long-term memory as readily as native speakers because of less familiarity with the English language).

Extrapolating the findings from the aforementioned studies as well as from my own observations, it appears that one can greatly enhance the intelligibility of what is being presented, especially for novel material (i.e., improve intelligibility at lower speech-to-noise ratios), by doing the following:

- Articulate information carefully.
- Insert pauses between grammatical clauses.
- Stress key words and employ slightly more exaggerated prosodic variations.
- Employ the active tense (i.e., subject-verb-object; example, "The boy hit the ball") versus the passive tense (i.e., object-verb-subject; example, "The ball was hit by the boy").
- Use more familiar vocabulary/concepts.

An expression that I often include in my reports is, "The more novel/complex the material, the slower the rate one should use in presenting the material and the greater the number of repetitions and concrete examples that might be needed."

SPEECHREADING

Similar to individuals with hearing loss, most individuals with CAPD will benefit from attending to the talker's face for a visual complement to speech sounds and for facial expressions. However, for certain individuals with severe integration difficulties (such as those with autism or Asperger's syndrome), the combination of both speechreading and listening may result in sensory overload, and if so, we should not force them to speechread. For example, I heard an adult with Asperger's syndrome state, "Do you want me to look at your face, or do you want me to understand what you are saying?"

PREVIEWING

Sending information home prior to information being covered in class (e.g., any new vocabulary or topics) and highlighting/discussing key concepts prior to a lesson facilitate "top-down" processing. The ability to use linguistic context and world knowledge results in less reliance on "bottom-up" processing (i.e., auditory processing of the incoming acoustic stimuli). This "Funnel Approach" makes it easier to learn details by organizing and linking them to "general concepts." As mentioned earlier, semantic enhancements (i.e., more highly familiar material) result in an improved perceived signal-to-noise ratio. Consequently, individuals with CAPD may not be overwhelmed as often by the information being presented and may be better able to keep up with/comprehend the material being presented. Interestingly, this approach is often used in college. A course syllabus enables the students to read material on the topic prior to the class so that they will be in a better position to follow what is being presented. Unfortunately, this approach is rarely used in elementary, middle, or, high schools, where students usually are introduced to the topic for the first time within the classroom setting.

VERBAL DISSEMINATION OF INSTRUCTIONS

1. Presenting important events or information involving multiple steps:
   - For younger students, the talker can state one direction at a time and have the child repeat each direction and then have the child summarize these directions at the end; for somewhat older students, one can also ask them to internally visualize the directions as well. If any directions are missed, the talker can repeat that direction again. This approach ensures that the student has processed/retained all key information; in addition, this serves as a training technique.
   - For children in middle and high school, as well as for adults, one can present all of the directions but with sufficient pauses between each direction to allow for adequate processing time and then have the listener summarize the directions at the end.
2. On tasks where verbal instructions have been provided, the student will benefit from the teacher ensuring that instructions have been heard and understood. If there is any doubt, the teacher can have the student repeat what he or she thinks has been said, and if there were any errors, the teacher can reinstruct/clarify the information. Visual cues and handouts may also be helpful in supplementing the auditory information.
3. Instructions/directions should be given when it is quiet rather than when there may be commotion (such as children preparing to leave for recess or when changing classrooms). When presenting information to the class, for students in grade one or higher, the use of overheads with little fan noise (e.g., overhead projectors or PowerPoint presentations), rather than a blackboard (which is better than nothing at all), allows for

speechreading and an improved signal-to-noise ratio, while still providing a visual reference to the topic. If homework assignments are written on the board, students will benefit from being able to write these down before any clarifications are provided (thus avoiding any divided attention). The best method for those with significant attentional/organizational issues is to provide the homework assignments in a written format.

REDUCING PROCESSING DEMANDS AND FATIGUE

1. Listening Breaks
   Students with CAPD will benefit from occasional listening breaks if they appear to be becoming overloaded and their attention seems to be drifting. An example of this would be after the teacher has finished presenting material, the student is given a break of a few minutes prior to starting the next task.
2. Scheduling of Classes
   If possible, more difficult classes should be scheduled in the morning when the student is most likely to be alert (although this must be confirmed with the student and parents); an alternative is avoiding the back-to-back scheduling of difficult subjects. Note that flexibility in scheduling classes is more likely in middle and high school settings.
3. Extended Time
   Extended time for those with processing-related issues allows for more time to process written material, to analyze and integrate the content, and, if a written response is required, to retrieve, integrate, and organize concepts, with less resultant pressure in crafting the written response. The additional time also allows students to double check the accuracy of their work. Note that for older students, it is possible they will need encouragement/confidence and strategies to take their time since they may be feeling the need to rush through a task (either because they are afraid they will "lose their thoughts" or because they may not want to "stand out"). If this is the case, there are a number of options to address this issue, including the following: (1) parental or school counseling can help build up confidence and self-esteem; (2) have the student start the task earlier than his or her classmates so that the student finishes at approximately the same time as the others; or (3) the student can go to another room when tests are administered and thus will not be aware of how he or she is doing time-wise compared to the other students.

COMPENSATORY STRATEGIES AND THE OLDER STUDENT

In addition to the strategies delineated in the previous section, students in middle or higher academic settings may benefit from the following:

1. Reduced Workload/Homework Demands
   Students with more severe processing deficits may benefit from taking a reduced course load, thus decreasing the amount of homework and increasing ability to focus on core subjects. For those individuals with significant phonologic awareness/phonics-related issues impacting on reading, spelling, and writing, a foreign language waiver may reduce frustration and stress.
2. Spelling Variance
   For students with spelling-related difficulties, in subject matter/tests where content is the crucial element rather than spelling, a variance taking into account any spelling errors is a viable alternative (i.e., points should not be taken off for spelling errors). If spelling is deemed to be crucial, then the use of a notebook computer with a spell checker should be provided. Of course, this recommendation depends on the student's keyboarding skills, thus there may be an increased emphasis on keyboarding classes.
3. Note Taking
   Because note taking entails divided attention (i.e., writing down what someone has already presented, while still listening to the teacher), the listener must essentially process twice the amount of information per unit of time. Consequently, this task is one of the most difficult for students to handle. Therefore, many CAPD students will benefit from handouts, guided notes (such as printed PowerPoint slides with lines next to the slide for writing additional notes), and, if necessary, the use of a "designated" note taker.
4. Test-Taking Mode
   It should also be determined what the student's best mode of test taking is, and when possible, allowances should be made for that mode. For example, does the student do best on multiple choice quizzes, written essays, or when questions are read? Does the student have a chance to respond either verbally or via writing? Note that because of its multitask nature, written responses (especially essays) require significantly more mental load than multiple choice or even verbal responses.
5. Taping a Lecture
   Audio-taping of lectures is often recommended for CAPD students who attend college. This may not be a good approach for a variety of reasons. First, from talking with many students, many of them have often been too meticulous in getting the information down, so much so that a 1-hour lecture often becomes a 2- to 3-hour tortuous note-taking effort. Second and more importantly, if there is any noise in the background, it will become mixed in with the speech on the tape; unless the talker wears a microphone that is hardwired to the tape recorder, the speech-to-noise ratio subsequently suffers. In addition, unlike in real life where one can separate the designated talker from competing noise (via the ability to use binaural separation cues), this is usually not possible in most audio-taped formats. A preferred approach would be videotaped lectures; however, I believe that is a very rare occurrence. The approach

that will likely become the preferred method in the future will be real-time, computerized, voice-to-written text as computer software programs become more sophisticated in their ability to transcribe voice to text.

COMPENSATORY STRATEGIES FOR THE ADULT

Adults with CAPD often struggle in the workplace. Compensatory strategies can aid them in carrying out their work effectively. In addition to many of the aforementioned strategies, some of the following may also be beneficial:

Meetings

- Meeting rooms where minimal noise distractions are present
- Meetings held in the morning when the individual with CAPD is most likely to be alert
- If possible, provide copies of any handouts before the meeting (becoming familiar with the topics)
- Use of PowerPoint and/or overhead presentations
- If novel/complex material is to be presented, the speaker should be guided to: (1) use a slower talking rate, (2) use effective visuals, and (3) provide listening breaks every 30 to 45 minutes (even 1- to 2-minute breaks where attendees can just stand up and move around can be beneficial)
- Strategic seating, such as near the main talker (if the participant has a better processing ear, such as determined in speech-in-noise or binaural separation tasks, then seating should be with that ear closest to the main talker)
- Designation of an employee to be the note taker at each meeting, thus not only helping the individual with CAPD but also decreasing the processing demands of other individuals attending the meeting

Workplace Location

If the individual's work entails the use of an office or workstation, then he or she should be located in a quiet setting away from any major noise sources, such as a copy machine, waiting room, dining room, etc.

Communication Strategies

There are times when information will need to be conveyed in less than ideal listening conditions. In these instances, individuals with CAPD will often function as if they are "hard of hearing" and will benefit from strategies often used by those with hearing losses:

- Inform the speaker of the rate, talking level, and distance you feel would be best in that particular setting.
- Ask the talker to face you and have nothing obscure his/her lips so that you can speechread the talker.

- Move away from loud noise sources and strive to ensure good lighting on the talker's face, when possible.
- Position yourself on the side of your better ear.
- Use effective communication repair strategies to indicate what you heard and what part of the sentence was missed instead of saying "What?"

Section Summary

Effective compensatory strategies can go a long way in addressing many difficult listening situations or those that involve significant processing demands. For students, compensatory strategies often form the core of accommodations on the IEP or 504 Plan. In the next section, we look at environmental modifications. We have already discussed some aspects of environmental modifications (e.g., clear speech and positioning oneself relative to the talker).

ENVIRONMENTAL MODIFICATIONS

Most individuals with CAPD experience increased listening difficulty in background noise when compared to their normal-processing peers. The nature of this difficulty may be due to a poorer ability in filtering out speech stimuli embedded in nonlinguistic noise, decreased binaural separation abilities, or an overload in processing demands relative to the individual's capacity (see Chapter 25). Environmental modifications may range from something as simple as preferential seating arrangements to acoustic enhancements such as addressing room acoustics and providing assistive listening systems. The following are some of the ways we can implement environmental modifications to improve the listening environment for individuals with CAPD.

Preferential Seating

The goal of preferential seating is to minimize the distance between the teacher and the affected student. Sound intensity decreases significantly as a function of distance, decreasing approximately by 6 dB for every doubling of distance, although Medwetsky (1991) found that for speech, this estimate applies only to low-frequency vowels/consonants and varies as a function of the angle relative to the talker's mouth (e.g., /s/ drops only 3 dB/doubling of distance when measured at 0° relative to the talker's mouth, while dropping off significantly more than the 6 dB/doubling of distance when measured off-axis). Because of the possible effects of reverberation, one can approximate that the direct field (i.e., where the intensity of direct speech is greater or equal to the intensity of the reflected speech) is about 6 to 8 feet from the talker's mouth. Thus, preferential seating should be no more than this distance from the teacher. However, if the teacher moves around the room, in reality, preferential seating does not really exist. For example, if a student is seated in the first row of a traditional classroom and the teacher walks to the back of the classroom, it is as if the student is seated in the last row. Thus, if preferential seating is to provide any useful benefits, the teacher must remain in close proximity to that student.

Assessment of and Modification of Classroom Acoustics

In Chapter 34, Smaldino et al. indicate that most classrooms do not meet recommended criteria for classroom acoustics. The recommended criteria are +15 dB signal-to-noise ratio with a reverberation time of 0.4 seconds or less (ASHA, 2005). Smaldino et al. indicate that a major reason for noncompliance is that most of these classrooms do not have acoustic modifications in place. These authors state that the best way to ensure favorable listening conditions and low reverberant environments is in the planning stages of construction. However, it is often the case that many of the modifications occur after a student with CAPD has been identified and the audiologist is asked to assess the classroom acoustics.

Ferre (2007) highlighted a number of acoustic solutions that can be implemented, ranging from inexpensive/minor treatments to more extensive/expensive solutions. These are compiled in Table 28.2. In assessing classroom acoustics, an audiologist should:

- Assess the noise and reverberant levels in the various classrooms that the targeted student attends
- Determine the possible noise/reverberant sources
- Examine the teacher's speaking style and teacher movement within the classroom
- Devise a plan that can implement simpler/less expensive acoustic solutions

- Determine if more expensive solutions might be needed and, if so, how likely these can be implemented

After careful examination, the audiologist may determine that the acoustic modifications needed may not be economically practical or sufficient. If not, then consideration of an assistive listening system may be an alternative.

Assistive Listening Devices

Acoustic guidelines for classrooms are infrequently met, so methodologies such as assistive listening devices (ALDs) must be considered. ALDs increase the speech-to-noise ratio, thereby improving the audibility and quality of speech heard. Note that there is nothing magical about these systems. The improvement in the signal-to-noise ratio comes about by basically decreasing the effective talker-to-listener distance to as close as 1 to 2 inches away (i.e., the distance from the talker's mouth to microphone). There are a variety of systems available; the type chosen is based not only on the nature of the individual's listening difficulties, but also on the acoustics and room settings that the student encounters. For younger students, frequency modulated (FM) sound field systems generally are the systems of choice (i.e., where the student remains in one classroom for most of the day and the student does not manipulate the system). For those in middle school or higher, the use of a wearable personal system is generally recommended because it allows the student to take the system from class to class (i.e., the student can continue to wear the receiver but transports the transmitter to the various teachers). Descriptions and realized benefits from these systems are discussed in detail in Chapter 34. Please note that the degree of success can be mitigated somewhat by where the talker places the microphone. Medwetsky (1991) found that the best microphone placement is directly under the chin (thus, not directly in the air stream emitted from the mouth),

---

TABLE 28.2 Classroom acoustic abatement strategies

Relatively Inexpensive Classroom Abatement Strategies:
- Closing classroom windows
- Carpeting rooms
- Using curtains, drapes, and/or acoustic tiles
- Felt pads or rubber caps on the bottoms of chairs to minimize furniture-to-floor noise
- Placing bookcases perpendicular to each other or side to side but 6–8 inches apart to create baffles and minimize noise
- Cork bulletin boards and the use of fabric to cover hard surfaces to increase sound absorption and dampen reflective surfaces

Extensive and Often Expensive Solutions:
- Reduction or elimination of open classrooms
- Relocation of teaching classrooms away from playgrounds, gymnasiums, or cafeterias
- Infrastructural changes such as double-paned windows and noise control devices on heating, air conditioning, and ventilation systems
- Use of smaller and more irregularly shaped rooms
- Lowered ceiling levels

whereas microphone placements on the chest, ear level, and the shoulder result in reduced high-frequency components of speech. That is, because of head shadow and other body-related effects (including distance and angle relative to the talker's mouth), the high frequencies can be attenuated by as much as 15 dB depending on the placement of the microphone relative to the mouth position. Headset microphones are most beneficial because they position the microphone close to the mouth and when the person's head moves, the microphone is maintained in the same relative position to the mouth.

Miscellaneous Recommendations

Many CAPD students have difficulty focusing on the task at hand, such as when reading or writing when background noise is present. I know firsthand the impact of noise on processing, because when I do any task that involves significant processing demands, such as writing my section in this chapter, I need absolute quiet (the fan noise distracts me greatly when I need to concentrate). Because I am hard of hearing and wear hearing aids, this entails me turning them off. Because individuals with CAPD in many ways are similar to hard-of-hearing individuals, this has often led me to recommend the use of earplugs in test-taking situations and/or during study times to reduce competing auditory stimuli. Testing in a quiet room, separate from the rest of the class, is another alternative.

Section Summary

Implementation of environmental modifications can make a great difference in academic or vocational performance, and as audiologists, we need to be strong advocates of cost-effective, acoustic enhancements when appropriate. In the following sections, we turn our attention to direct interventions that can be implemented.

SPEECH-LANGUAGE PATHOLOGIST ROLE IN THE ASSESSMENT AND MANAGEMENT OF CENTRAL AUDITORY PROCESSING DISORDERS

Background

At a recent Committee on Special Education meeting at a New York State school district, the chair of the committee questioned the results of CAP testing. The chair believed that these results contradicted the speech-language pathologist's (SLP) testing results, which found that receptive and expressive language skills were developing typically. The audiologist was not willing to accept this conclusion and argued that the results were not a contradiction because the SLP did not assess the student's particular areas of weakness. If she had tested phonemic awareness or higher order language skills, she would have likely found areas of weakness that were consistent with the auditory processing findings. The lesson behind this brief story is that it is imperative that the SLP and the audiologist work together to discover the *consistencies* between the test results. In this section, I will attempt to elucidate the role of the SLP in the testing and management of CAPD.

SLPs play a critical role on an interdisciplinary team that provides assessment and intervention for children and adults with auditory processing disorders. According to ASHA's "Scope of Practice in Speech-Language Pathology" statement, the SLP's role involves "collaborating in the assessment of (central) auditory processing disorders and providing intervention where there is evidence of speech, language, and/or other cognitive-communication disorders" (ASHA, 2001, p 5). An effective collaboration will most certainly lead to an enhanced understanding of the problem and, in turn, a determination of the most effective management approach. The purpose of this section is to delineate the unique contribution that the SLP can offer to an interdisciplinary team, with the goal of fostering a better understanding of the SLP's assessment and treatment approaches.

The SLP's perspective on auditory processing often differs from the audiologist's, which can result in a breakdown in communication about test results and treatment recommendations. Therefore, I will begin by discussing some commonly held beliefs that an SLP can bring to the team. Second, the type of testing that the SLP can provide will be reviewed. A better understanding of the type of results that can be obtained should assist the audiologist in making a differential diagnosis. Finally, some treatment principles frequently implemented by SLPs will be highlighted. This should prove useful to the audiologist when making recommendations and talking with parents about management options. Ultimately, the audiologist and SLP should be able to construct effective IEPs after discussing the ways that the auditory processing and language assessment results complement each other. Please note that a Glossary (Appendix 28.1B) is included at the end of this chapter for terminology that may be unfamiliar to audiologists but that is typically referenced by SLPs. When the glossary terms are first encountered in the text, there will be an asterisk next to the term, thus letting the reader know that particular term is defined in the glossary section.

The Speech Language Pathologist Perspective on Auditory Processing

It is beyond the scope of this section to review the debate between individuals who believe that an auditory processing disorder is a viable construct versus those who believe auditory processing is a manifestation of a language processing disorder. However, many SLPs question whether the results of the auditory processing testing are useful to them in managing a child. I have had many debates with my colleagues in clinical practice who not only question the auditory processing findings, but also admit to not always understanding them.

There are many researchers in the field who take the view that the problem is a language processing issue rather than an auditory processing issue (see Newman-Ryan and Kamhi [2003] and Kamhi and Newman-Ryan [2004] for the most convincing arguments). In fact, many of the children referred for auditory processing testing have been diagnosed with a receptive and/or expressive language disorder. The question that begs to be answered is "Why are they referred for CAP testing?" In my experience, children are usually referred because:

- they have a gap between receptive and expressive language skills;
- they have a receptive language delay only;
- they are struggling with listening in the classroom; and/or
- they are not making progress in language therapy.

Additionally, parents, teachers, and SLPs want to determine whether there is an underlying cause for the child's language or learning difficulty.

Another view commonly held by SLPs is that auditory processing and language disorders are due to deficits in underlying general information processing mechanisms such as attention, memory, and executive functions (Johnston, 2006). There have been many research studies of children with language impairments over the past several years that support this idea. Studies of children with language disorders have found them to exhibit deficits in serial order memory, phonologic working memory, working memory capacity, attention, processing speed, and central executive functioning (Campbell and McNeil, 1985; Gillam et al., 1995; Hoffman and Gillam, 2004; Montgomery, 1995; 2000; Montgomery and Windsor, 2007; Tallal et al., 1985).

Medwetsky's model of spoken-language processing (see Chapter 25) takes a much broader information processing view of auditory processing. This model attempts to explain the testing results in terms of attention, memory, executive function, and even language, in addition to the auditory processing aspects. As such, it seems consistent with the view that auditory processing difficulties are due to deficits that involve general information processing mechanisms. It would seem that if audiologists and SLPs could view processing from this vantage point, we would indeed have a common reference point from which to examine and interpret our testing results. In the next section, I will discuss potential links between typical auditory processing test findings and language skills and suggest how language testing can complement these findings.

Speech-Language Pathologist's Role in the Evaluation of Children with Suspected Central Auditory Processing Disorders

One role of the SLP is to evaluate the language skills of children with suspected CAPDs. When CAP test findings are available, the SLP can use these results to make decisions about what type of testing to complete. See Appendix 28.1A for a summary of typical auditory processing test findings and related language assessment tools.

ASSESSMENT

Assessment of Phonologic and Morphologic Skills

One common test result of CAP testing is weak phonemic synthesis skills. With this result, SLPs would typically evaluate phonological and phonemic awareness, phonologic working memory, morphological awareness, reading, and spelling. Phonological awareness is defined as the awareness of the sound structure of a spoken word and often predicts reading and spelling ability (Gillon, 2004). Morphological awareness is defined as an individual's awareness of morphemes (meaningful word parts such as suffixes) in words and is frequently linked to spelling skills (Masterson and Apel, 2000; Gillon, 2004).

There are a number of standardized phonological awareness tests available. One frequently used instrument is the *Comprehensive Test of Phonological Processing* (CTOPP) (Wagner et al., 1999), which is used for individuals from 5 to 21 years of age. The CTOPP is useful because it evaluates phonemic awareness (e.g., elision* ["If I say the word /ball/ and I take away the /b/, what word do I now have left?"], sound blending, and sound segmentation ["What sounds make up the word /c-a-t/?"]), phonological working memory, and rapid naming skills. Phonological working memory is thought to be a short-term memory store where verbal information is processed (Gathercole and Baddeley, 1990; see page 650) and is assessed using nonword repetition tasks (see below). Rapid naming is the ability to rapidly and accurately name letters, numbers, colors, or objects and has been shown to predict reading ability. Children with both phonologic awareness and rapid naming difficulties are thought to exhibit a "double deficit" (Wolf and Bowers, 1999). Children with rapid naming speed deficits have difficulty quickly accessing and retrieving phonologically coded information from memory, which leads to poor sight word recognition (Roth, 2004). As a result, children with a "double deficit" will likely require intervention in word decoding, sight word reading, and reading fluency. Another commonly used test is the *Phonological Awareness Test* (Robertson and Salter, 1997), which is normed on children from 5 to 9 years of age. It covers a wide range of phonological awareness tasks including rhyming, syllable blending and segmentation, sound isolation* (e.g., "What is the first sound in the word 'cat'?"), sound blending, sound segmentation*, and sound substitution* (e.g., "Say 'bat' and change /b/ to /k/."). It also includes a letter knowledge task and a nonword decoding task (e.g., keb). Another well-known assessment tool of phonologic awareness is the *Lindamood Auditory Conceptualization Test-3* (LAC-3) (Lindamood and Lindamood, 2004). The LAC-3 has been used by both SLPs and audiologists and involves discriminating speech sounds, analyzing the number and order of speech sounds, and tracking speech sound changes at both the phoneme and syllable level. It is often used to predict spelling ability (Medwetsky L, personal communication, March 2006). At the preschool to early elementary level, the *Pre-Reading Inventory of Phonological Awareness* (Dodd et al., 2003) uses colorful pictures to evaluate rhyming, syllable segmentation, alliteration (production of two or more words beginning with the same sound), sound isolation, and speech sound segmentation. It also includes a letter-speech sound association task. SLPs also use other criterion referenced and informal tasks to evaluate phonological awareness (see Gillon [2004] for a more comprehensive review).

To evaluate phonological working memory, SLPs may use a nonword repetition task such as that found on the CTOPP (Wagner et al., 1999) or an informal version of the task (Dollaghan and Campbell, 1998). This task involves imitating an unfamiliar nonsense word such as "chasidoolid" or "bilidoge" (CTOPP) (Wagner et al., 1999). Research has shown that children with specific language impairments have difficulty repeating multisyllabic nonsense words, which, in turn, indicates deficits in phonologic working memory (Gathercole and Baddeley, 1990).

Morphological awareness skills involve "the ability to be conscious of and manipulate the morphological units of a language" (Masterson and Apel, 2000, p 56) and are typically evaluated by analyzing spelling skills. Masterson and Apel (2000) recommend the following ways to assess morphologic awareness:

- Spelling lists of words that are morphologically different (e.g., kicked, gladly)
- Cloze procedures in which children must produce a derived word (e.g., "define," the teacher gave the word's _____ "definition")
- Word judgment tasks (judge whether a pair of words represent a base word and a derived form; e.g., lead-leader)
- Suffix addition tasks (apply suffixes to nonsense words; e.g., teb/tebbed)

Children with language impairment will often omit morphologic endings such as past tense "–ed" or plural "–s," as well as more advanced derivational morphemes such as "–ly" or "–est."

It is recommended that reading and spelling skills also be evaluated for any children who have poor phonemic awareness skills. SLPs sometimes evaluate reading skills, although in school settings, this will generally be completed by educational diagnosticians, reading specialists, or special education specialists. Commonly used reading assessments used by SLPs include the *Woodcock Reading Mastery Tests–Revised* (Woodcock, 1987), the *Gray Oral Reading Test-4* (GORT-4) (Weiderholt and Bryant, 2001), the *Gray Silent Reading Test* (GSRT) (Weiderholt and Blalock, 2000), and the *Reading Miscue Inventory* (Goodman et al., 1987). Gillam and Gorman (2004) recommended the use of the Word Identification (assessed using real words) and Word Decoding (assessed using nonsense words) subtests on the *Woodcock Reading Mastery Tests–Revised* to assess word recognition skills. This test is useful in determining whether children are applying their phonemic awareness skills to reading. The GORT-4 and the GSRT use text-level reading tasks to assess accuracy, rate, fluency, and reading comprehension, while contrasting oral with silent reading ability. It is especially important to evaluate text-level reading and determine whether the child can read fluently and understand what he or she has read. The GORT-4 also includes an informal miscue analysis to determine what types of errors a child makes when reading. The *Reading Miscue Inventory* formally examines a child's reading errors to determine how discrepant they are from the targeted text (see Gillam and Gorman [2004] for a more detailed description of this assessment tool). A commonly used standardized spelling assessment is the *Test of Written Spelling-3* (Larsen et al., 1999), which evaluates the ability to accurately spell common words. A word of caution is that some children who score in age-appropriate limits on this test may still have a significant spelling disorder because the test does not sample a wide variety of spelling patterns. For a more thorough, criterion-referenced spelling assessment, SLPs may use the *Spelling Performance Evaluation for Language and Literacy* (SPELL) (Masterson et al., 2002), which is a computerized spelling assessment. SPELL is an in-depth assessment of spelling patterns that also identifies underlying linguistic deficits in the areas of phonological awareness, orthographic knowledge, vocabulary, morphological knowledge, and mental orthographic images (Masterson and Apel, 2000; Masterson et al., 2002). Writing samples are also frequently evaluated for more authentic evaluation of spelling skills. The audiologist should always refer the child with phonemic synthesis deficits to the SLP for an in-depth assessment of phonological awareness and reading and spelling skills because reading and spelling difficulties are one of the key presenting problems in children with processing delays.

Assessment of Lexical Decoding Speed
Another common auditory processing finding is lexical decoding speed difficulty. As defined by Medwetsky in Chapter 25, lexical decoding speed is the speed and accuracy with which one can decode the incoming speech stimuli into its corresponding words. The corollary of lexical decoding speed deficits is word retrieval difficulty. That is, the difficulties that slow down access to words in long-term memory when processing speech stimuli also make it more difficult to rapidly retrieve word labels from long-term memory. When this difficulty is present, SLPs should conduct a thorough evaluation

of (1) semantic skills of varying complexity, (2) morphologic and syntactical knowledge, and (3) word retrieval ability.

Semantic skills include the knowledge of word meanings and relationships between words. At the most basic level, an evaluation of semantic skills would include an assessment of single-word vocabulary skills using such tests as the *Peabody Picture Vocabulary Test-4* (Dunn and Dunn, 2007) or the *Receptive One-Word Picture Vocabulary Test* (Gardner, 2000). In addition to formal tests of vocabulary, an assessment of the child's understanding of the vocabulary of the school curriculum would provide information about how easily a child is acquiring word meanings related to school subject matter. This is typically completed through informal observation and tasks designed to test the vocabulary of particular academic units. Other aspects of semantics to explore include the ability to define words, knowledge of antonyms and synonyms, and the understanding and use of multiple meaning words. Higher level semantic skills such as figurative language* (e.g., similes*, metaphors*, proverbs*) should also be evaluated. One of the key aspects of evaluating semantics is to determine whether there is a lack of knowledge, a retrieval difficulty, or both. There are a variety of standardized tests available to assess semantic knowledge. The *Language Processing Test 3–Elementary* (Richard and Hanner, 2005) assesses different levels of semantic skills. There are two pretests (Labeling and Stating Functions) and six subtests (Associations, Categories, Similarities, Differences, Multiple Meanings, and Attributes). To assess slightly higher level semantic knowledge, the *Word Test 2–Elementary* (Bowers et al., 2004) can be used. It includes a variety of subtests that evaluate synonyms, antonyms, and semantic associations, as well as word definitions, semantic absurdities, and multiple meaning words that require oral explanation of word meanings and relationships. Other tests used to assess semantics include the *Clinical Evaluation of Language Fundamentals-4* (CELF-4) (Semel et al., 2003), the *Comprehensive Assessment of Spoken Language* (Carrow-Woolfolk, 1999a), and the *Test of Language Competence* (Wiig and Secord, 1989). Subtests to assess figurative language are included on the *Comprehensive Assessment of Spoken Language* and the *Test of Language Competence*. However, it should be noted that knowledge of figurative language is based in part on exposure to figurative expressions. It may be more accurate to assess this knowledge informally through the construction of tasks that require children to interpret figurative expressions commonly heard within their environment (Paul, 2007).

Once a child's level of semantic knowledge has been determined, the SLP should assess word retrieval skills. These skills are frequently deficient in children with lexical decoding speed deficits and language disorders. Children with word retrieval deficits have difficulty retrieving words that they are able to comprehend (Messer and Dockrell, 2006). Word retrieval difficulties can occur at the single word level and/or at the discourse level. At the discourse level, chil-dren exhibit such behaviors as interjections (such as /uh/, /you know/, or /like/), word repetitions and substitutions, and phrase repetitions and substitutions. Although these behaviors are not uncommon in individuals, it is significant when they are excessive. Messer and Dockrell (2006) suggested that word retrieval difficulty should be considered when "there are problems involving the production of words that are greater than would be expected given the children's ability to comprehend words" (p 310). An excessive amount of word retrieval difficulty can result in communication breakdown and frustration for that individual. The *Test of Word Finding-2* (German, 2000) is frequently used to assess word retrieval at the single-word level, whereas the *Test of Word Finding in Discourse* (German, 1991) is used to assess word retrieval skills in connected speech. Word finding at the single-word level is assessed by having children label pictures and provide category names, whereas word finding at the discourse level is evaluated during story retelling and conversational speech. An expressive language sample can also be used to observe word retrieval difficulties. When children exhibit lexical decoding speed difficulty, it is important to evaluate word retrieval ability because it is an area that is sometimes overlooked.

It is also important to evaluate morphologic and syntactical knowledge for children who exhibit lexical decoding speed deficits. As mentioned earlier, morphologic knowledge is defined as an individual's knowledge of grammatical morphemes* (i.e., meaningful word parts such as suffixes—grammatical markers attached to the ends of words). This knowledge is typically evaluated using a comprehensive test of receptive and expressive language such as the CELF-4 (Semel et al., 2003) or the *Test of Language Development–Primary: 3rd Edition* (TOLD-P3) (Newcomer and Hammill, 1997). A conversational or narrative expressive language sample can also be used to evaluate the functional use of grammatical morphemes and various sentence structures.

Assessment of Working Memory

Children with auditory processing weakness frequently exhibit deficits in working memory ability. The SLP can supplement the testing done by the audiologist by using a variety of memory span tasks such as digit and word repetition tasks and the nonsense word repetition task described earlier. One common test used by SLPs to assess memory is the *Test of Auditory Processing Skills-3* (Martin and Brownell, 2005), which includes a variety of memory span tasks. Montgomery (2002) provided several suggestions for assessing working memory ability. These measures include conventional memory span tasks, nonsense word repetition tasks, the *Competing Language Processing Task* (Gaulin and Campbell, 1994), and classroom observation and task analyses. Working memory deficits likely impact several aspects of language competency, including the ability to follow oral directions and the ability to comprehend sentences and text-level material. The ability to follow oral directions can be assessed using standardized tests such as the CELF-4 (Semel et al., 2003) or the *Token Test for Children-2* (McGhee et al., 2007). Since these tests are not always representative of oral directions within a functional setting, directions may be better assessed through informal tasks and observation in the classroom environment. There are a variety of tests available that assess sentence comprehension, including the *Test of Auditory Language Comprehension-3* (Carrow-Woolfolk, 1999b) as well as many of the comprehensive tests of language described earlier. It should be noted that children with auditory processing deficits will have most difficulty with long and elaborated syntax. Working memory deficits can also impact the ability to comprehend and tell narratives (see below for a discussion of narrative language).

Assessment of Organization/Sequencing and Integration Skills

Assessment of children with auditory processing deficits often reveals difficulty with organization and sequencing ability. This can impact the ability to comprehend and tell narratives. Narrative language is generally thought of as the ability to comprehend and tell personal events and stories. It requires the "coordination of phonologic, morphologic, syntactic, semantic and pragmatic (i.e., the appropriate use of language according to the situational context) knowledge" (Gillam and Pearson, 2004, p 1). It also involves sequencing and organizing a series of events into a coherent structure (see Naremore et al. [1995] for a review). Narrative language can be assessed using story retelling and story generation tasks, with analysis of story structure (see Paul [2007] for a review), or through standardized assessments such as *The Strong Narrative Assessment Procedure* (Strong, 1998) or the *Test of Narrative Language* (Gillam and Pearson, 2004). Another aspect of narratives to consider is the ability to go beyond the explicit information in the story and make inferences (which entails the ability to integrate, organize, and compare concepts). Inferential comprehension can be evaluated using the *Test of Narrative Language* (Gillam and Pearson, 2004) or by informally using stories with a series of implicit "why" and "how" questions (Westby, 2005). Westby (2005) also recommends the use of informal reading inventories such as the *Qualitative Reading Inventory-3* (Leslie and Caldwell, 2001) to assess both explicit and implicit knowledge about a story.

For children who demonstrate integration difficulties, it is hypothesized that they will also have difficulty with the prosodic (i.e., the use of suprasegmental aspects to convey the stress and intonation patterns of an utterance) elements of language. There is evidence that some children with language impairments have difficulty:

- producing various prosodic cues, such as intonation and stress patterns (Van der Meulen et al., 1997; Wells and Peppe, 2003);

- processing prosodic cues (Wells and Peppe, 2003; Fisher et al., 2007); and
- perceiving emotional prosody (Creusere et al., 2004).

The SLP makes judgments about the production of prosodic cues during conversational speech and language sampling, noting the child's ability to vary pitch and stress. SLPs can make observations about how a child comprehends sentences when stress and intonation are varied in various situations. In addition, some structured tasks of prosodic processing can be administered. For example, an SLP can produce two sentences varying the stress, such as "<u>fruit</u>, <u>cake</u>, and <u>pie</u>" versus "<u>fruit</u>-cake and pie," and determine whether the child can understand how many units are being produced (Wells and Peppe, 2003).

In addition to prosody, it is recommended that SLPs evaluate both conversational skills and figurative language knowledge. Many processing areas are activated when individuals engage in conversations with either one individual or a group of individuals. For example, conversations involve listening to a conversational partner, generating ideas that can contribute toward the topic of conversation, shifting attention to topic changes, shifting attention to speakers when in a group, and paying attention to facial cues and body language. Many children with language and processing impairments have difficulty managing conversations, as characterized by deficits in initiating and maintaining topics, asking for conversational repair when a message is not understood, repairing a misunderstood message, and generating cohesive ideas. Conversational skills are most effectively evaluated using conversational language samples in a variety of situations and with a variety of speakers. The samples can then be analyzed according to the elements discussed earlier. It may be difficult to judge whether individuals are having difficulty processing facial cues and body language; however, the SLP should keep this in mind if an individual is misunderstanding messages during conversation.

Another area to include in an assessment is knowledge of figurative language, which includes similes, idioms, metaphors, and proverbs. These forms commonly appear in textbooks, classroom discussion, lectures, and poems; informally in social situations; and when listening to jokes and other forms of humor (Nippold, 1998). Children as young as 7 years old have been shown to understand some figurative expressions, and this development continues into adulthood (Nippold, 1998). Figurative language expressions are interpreted using contextual cues, situational cues, and mental imagery (Nippold and Duthie, 2003). Figurative language is thought to involve integration because individuals must use situational cues as well as generate mental images of expressions they have heard. Assessment of figurative language was described earlier in the section on semantics.

Dynamic Assessment

In addition to the standardized testing noted earlier, Gillam et al. (2002) recommend dynamic assessment techniques to observe cognitive and language functions. Dynamic assessment procedures, consisting of a pretest, a teaching phase, and a posttest, can be used to investigate a variety of language forms and functions. Gillam et al. (2002) indicate that the SLP can obtain information about a child's attentional, perceptual, memory, and central executive abilities by observing his or her responses in the teaching phase of the assessment (see Gillam et al. [2002] and Miller et al. [2000] for descriptions of how to use dynamic assessment).

Summary of Speech-Language Pathologist's Role in Assessment

Because it is likely that individuals with CAP difficulties will exhibit deficits in many areas of processing, it is critical that SLPs complete a thorough language evaluation going beyond basic language skills. While many children can adequately comprehend and express ideas using age-appropriate vocabulary and syntax, they frequently have difficulty with more complex language such as narrative, conversation, complex semantic tasks, and figurative language. The SLP can use the results of the audiologic CAP assessment, along with behavioral information, to form hypotheses about what areas of language to investigate. The SLP can also refer children with language impairments and learning disabilities to the audiologist for assessment of auditory processing. The results of this testing can then be used to gain a better understanding of the child's processing abilities, which in turn will lead to more effective therapy. In the next section, I will discuss some general principles of intervention for children with auditory processing and language deficits.

Speech-Language Pathologist's Role in Management of Central Auditory Processing Disorders

The SLP will be responsible for direct management of children who have auditory processing and language difficulties. The SLP will use the CAP assessment data in conjunction with any language and/or educational assessment data to plan a treatment program. First, I will discuss some general treatment principles that can be incorporated, and second, I will discuss some specific treatment principles for the processing and language areas noted earlier. This review is intended to highlight key information and is not an in-depth review of the literature.

GENERAL TREATMENT PRINCIPLES

Gillam et al. (2002, p 43) report that "good language intervention is also good information processing intervention." Although SLPs will focus on semantic, syntactic, and pragmatic language goals, they should always be cognizant of the processing weaknesses these children bring to the table of language learning. Numerous studies have revealed that children with specific language impairment benefit from a slowed rate of speech (Ellis-Weismer and Hesketh, 1996) as well as the use of emphatic stress to highlight key words and language forms (Ellis-Weismer, 1997). Montgomery (2002) recommended that clinicians and teachers present language in smaller chunks with clear pauses between clauses. Gillam and Hoffman (2004) suggested that clinicians can facilitate attentional aspects of processing by explaining the purpose of the therapy session, using familiar concepts and scripts, making targets salient, and reducing distractions. Clinicians can also help children reach automatic levels of processing by providing frequent repetition and teaching language targets to high levels of accuracy (Montgomery, 2002; Snyder et al., 2002). While these general techniques can be highly beneficial, SLPs also use a variety of specific intervention approaches.

TREATMENT OF PHONOLOGICAL AWARENESS DISORDERS

One area of intervention used with children who exhibit auditory processing and language impairments is phonological awareness. Gillon (2004, p 134) indicates that "the goal of phonological awareness intervention is to enhance reading and writing performance." However, there are also studies that have shown that working on phonological awareness also improves phonological coding (Gillam and van Kleeck, 1996; van Kleeck et al., 1998). Phonological coding refers to the ability to form phonological representations of spoken or written words in short-term memory (Gillam and Hoffman, 2004). For example, when a child hears or reads a word, information about the speech sounds in the word is stored in working memory. Children then use those stored representations to perform phonological awareness tasks. There are many commercial programs available for children with phonological/phonemic awareness difficulty such as *The Phonological Awareness Kit–Primary* (Robertson and Salter, 1995) and *The Road to the Code* (Blachman et al., 2000). There are also a number of computer programs that are used to improve phonological awareness skills, including Fast ForWord (Scientific Learning, 1997) and Earobics (Cognitive Concepts, 2003). Medwetsky (2007) reviewed research regarding the treatment efficacy of these computer programs and found mixed results. While some children did show improvement in various language and processing skills, it is still unclear whether these programs are superior to traditional, curriculum-based approaches to phonemic awareness intervention (see Medwetsky [2007] for a thorough description of these programs and review of the relevant research).

SLPs can also design their own treatment programs. Gillon (2004) and the National Reading Panel (2000) offer a number of general treatment principles to guide clinicians. These include the following: (1) Children learn best when phonemic awareness is taught along with letter-sound knowledge and they are shown how to apply phonemic awareness skills to print. (2) Children learn best when they are taught one or two types of phonological awareness skills rather than several types at once. (3) For school-age children, training should focus on the phoneme level. (4) Segmentation and blending skills have a direct application to word decoding and spelling. (5) Phonological awareness training is most effective in individual or small group sessions. (6) Children benefit from the use of multisensory cues. Whether using a commercially developed program or a clinician-designed program, phonological awareness therapy has proved to be highly effective for children with language impairment and processing difficulty.

TREATMENT OF LEXICAL DECODING SPEED DEFICITS

Language intervention that will impact lexical decoding speed should focus on improving semantic knowledge, morphologic/syntactical knowledge, and word retrieval skills. A number of strategies can be used to improve knowledge of words and word associations. One of the most common techniques is the use of semantic mapping/graphic organizers to show the relationships among words and concepts (e.g., visual representation/organization of related ideas such as features of animals). A child's depth of word knowledge can be facilitated by focusing on antonyms/synonyms, word definitions, and multiple meaning words. In addition, older children should be taught strategies for learning unknown words they encounter when reading and listening. For example, in paragraphs in which the unknown word occurs, children can be taught to use both semantic and syntactic information to search for cues to meaning. They can also be encouraged to identify familiar word roots such, as "magic" in the word "magician." Morphologic/syntactical knowledge can be improved by strengthening the production of grammatical morphemes and derivational morphology*, expanding noun and verb phrases, and expanding clause structure. Direct syntax teaching techniques can be used, such as identifying parts of speech, paraphrasing concepts, formulating sentences with key words, or combining simpler sentences into more complex clause structure (Scott, 1995).

To address word retrieval deficits, SLPs may attempt to improve word associations through the semantic mapping techniques discussed earlier. German (2005) recommends that intervention address three areas: retrieval strategies, self-advocacy, and word finding accommodations. Retrieval strategies are memory strategies that can be used before and during speaking. They should be chosen based on the word finding profile of the individual and can include such strategies as mnemonic cueing*, syllable dividing*, alternate word strategy*, rehearsal, and pausing (German, 2005). As with all aspects of language processing, individuals must learn to understand their strengths and weaknesses and take responsibility for improving their skills. Accommodations that reduce the demands on retrieval in both oral and written work can also be helpful. German (2005) recommends a variety of accommodations such as extended time, multiple choice exams, and cue cards. Cue cards would consist of cards with prompts or key words used to aid recall. The SLP and audiologist together should advocate for these accommodations within the academic setting.

TREATMENT OF WORKING MEMORY DEFICITS

Working memory deficits comprise one of the more common difficulties exhibited by children with auditory processing disorders. Montgomery (2002) reviews a number of intervention techniques to facilitate working memory skills. He suggests that phonological awareness activities such as rhyming and phoneme blending can enhance phonological working memory skills. Children can also be encouraged to imitate nonsense words during interactive games. For older school-age children, he recommends taking a strategy-based approach. For example, there are many commercial programs designed to teach children various rehearsal strategies such as chunking information or using mnemonics to remember information. Other techniques include paraphrasing and organizing information using graphic organizers. These techniques involve taking a text, such as a story or factual passage, and breaking it down into smaller parts and identifying the main ideas. These can then be flowcharted onto paper so that one can see how the different story ideas relate to each other. This process facilitates integration of the material which, in turn, aids comprehension and ultimately the retention of the information.

The techniques noted earlier, as well as compensatory strategies such as clinicians and teachers slowing their rate of speech, stressing key words, and repeating information, all help to ease the memory load for children during online processing of language. Gillam and Hoffman (2004) recommend the use of cues to aid in recall such as key questions, summaries, or pictures. Visualization techniques can also be helpful for some children. One structured program frequently used by SLPs is *Visualizing and Verbalizing for Language Comprehension and Thinking* (Bell, 1991). Active listening techniques are also beneficial because children are taught to focus on key words regarding time, place, or person as well as transition words such as "because," "first," or "however." There are many techniques and programs available to work on memory skills. It is important that intervention for memory be based on easing the memory load while processing information (i.e., a compensatory strategy), while improving language knowledge and teaching strategy use in older children. It is the combination of these strategies that will make the greatest impact.

TREATMENT OF SEQUENCING AND ORGANIZATION DEFICITS

For children who have sequencing and organization difficulties, one of the most important areas of intervention is narrative language. Narrative language is thought to be important for reading comprehension and writing skills (Westby,

2005). Westby (2005) and Paul (2007) discussed a number of intervention strategies for children with narrative language difficulty. Children need to be taught how to sequence a series of events both temporally and in cause-effect relationships and to organize events into a coherent structure or story grammar*. Story maps* and flow charts are frequently used to show children the relationships among events and the key elements of a story. Various scaffolding* techniques such as key questions are used to assist the child in telling or writing a story. Narrative language development can be facilitated through comprehension tasks, the production of oral narratives, and the production of written narratives for the older child. Roth (2000) discussed various intervention techniques to facilitate narrative writing such as story maps, story frames*, story grammar cues, and story prompts*. Older school-age children should be taught to recognize text structure when reading to enhance their reading comprehension.

TREATMENT OF INTEGRATION DEFICITS

The last area and perhaps the area that is least understood by SLPs is integration. Although there are no commercially developed programs that work on integration, there are some techniques that SLPs use that address information flow across processing areas. I have suggested that SLPs address prosody, conversational skills, and figurative language as ways to facilitate the integration of multiple sources of information. There have been a few studies that have investigated intervention for prosodic difficulties in children with language impairment. Gerken and McGregor (1998) suggest that clinicians modify prosodic aspects of their own input to children. These modifications are typically used with preschool children and include speaking (1) at a higher pitch level with more exaggerated variability in pitch, (2) with increased loudness, and (3) at a slower rate. As previously discussed, these modifications can serve to direct a child's attention to the verbal input. Other potential treatment targets could include helping children to determine meanings of words based on syllabic stress and to become aware of pauses corresponding to clausal boundaries. Research is needed to determine whether interventions such as these improve an individual's linguistic processing.

RELATED AREAS OF INTERVENTION

SLPs frequently work on the conversational skills of children with language processing difficulty. Children with CAPD are particularly at risk in this area due to the fact that conversations require focusing on and processing multiple sources of information. Conversational intervention generally facilitates topic initiation and topic maintenance, including appropriate changes of topic, clarification requests, and the use of clear referents when speaking. It is recommended that one aspect of conversation be introduced at a time to avoid overloading a child's mental resources. School-age children with CAPD benefit from learning rules of conversation

because they frequently violate these rules. In addition, the use of conversational and social scripts* along with role playing can be beneficial. SLPs should also teach children to pay attention to prosodic features, facial expressions, and body language.

Another focus of intervention is improvement in the comprehension of figurative language such as similes, metaphors, idioms, and proverbs. Typically developing children infer the meaning of figurative expressions with repeated exposure to them in spoken and written language (Nippold, 1991). Figurative expressions develop gradually from elementary through adolescent years. Children with auditory and language processing difficulties have significant difficulty acquiring figurative language. Intervention research has investigated ways to facilitate the understanding of idioms* and proverbs and has frequently focused on teaching children strategies for determining the meaning of figurative expressions. Figurative expressions should be taught within a context such as a familiar story (Nippold, 1991). Techniques that have been found useful include contrasting literal to nonliteral meaning, explicit teaching of contextual cues, role-playing scenarios in which the expressions can be used, providing opportunities to use forms in a variety of spoken and written stories and activities, and teaching the communicative function of figurative expressions (Nippold, 1991; Abrahamsen and Smith, 2000; Power et al., 2001; Norbury, 2005; Paul, 2007). Nippold (1991) recommended that children be encouraged to keep a notebook or journal in which the child records figurative expressions that he or she hears or reads both at school and at home. Children should record the contextual information in which the expressions occur as well as the expressions themselves.

Summary of Assessment and Intervention Techniques Used by Speech-Language Pathologists

This brief review of assessment and intervention techniques commonly used by SLPs was intended to highlight the contributions that the SLPs can make to an interdisciplinary team serving children with CAPDs. It is imperative that SLPs and audiologists collaborate to understand how the audiologic and language test results can complement each other and clarify the complex processing deficits that many children exhibit. This understanding should lead to better recommendations regarding treatment. While there are many areas in both fields that we do not fully understand and that need well-developed research, we should strive to understand the research and clinical tools that are already available. The SLP should understand how the processing assessment findings can be used in intervention, whereas the audiologist should understand how the language findings can be used to further explain the processing deficit. Perhaps the first step is a realization that we are addressing a common disorder.

SOME DIRECT MANAGEMENT TECHNIQUES FOR CENTRAL AUDITORY PROCESSING DISORDERS

Decoding Therapies for Central Auditory Processing Disorders

This section will describe two phoneme-based procedures that effectively address decoding difficulty (i.e., slow and/or inaccurate phonemic processing) (Katz and Smith, 1991). Both methods teach individual speech sounds, incorporating words or nonsense syllables directly or in repair strategies. The Phonemic Training Program (PTP) is more basic than Phonemic Synthesis (PS), but in most cases, they can be carried out in the same session. The PTP has been effective as an initial entry point for individuals for whom the PS program was too difficult. These two programs are geared to help individuals who have difficulty processing speech quickly and accurately. In addition to those with CAPD, these programs can also be used with the mentally challenged, those with cochlear implants (Katz, 1998), and individuals with foreign dialects.

PHONEMIC TRAINING PROGRAM

The purpose of this program is to ensure accurate speech-sound perception. It assumes that those with phonemic decoding problems have vague, inaccurate, or overlapping concepts of various speech sounds. The therapeutic purpose is to clarify, correct, or disambiguate the phonemes. The materials needed are cards (e.g., $2^1/_2 \times 3$ inches) with a letter on each representing a sound. A fabric-covered cross-stitch hoop is used to conceal the clinician's lower face from view but leaving the acoustic signal unimpeded.

Generally, four speech sounds are introduced per session/week. They are spoken at a comfortably loud level while facing the client. The sounds are presented in isolation (e.g., /l/ or /b/) auditorily only. The following are the three basic PTP steps:

- *New Sounds* is the first step of the first lesson. The client is asked to listen to a sound (the listener does not know what sound is to be presented) that will be said a few times. The listener is not to say it back, just to listen. After two or three slow presentations that are given aperiodically, the card with the letter representing the sound is shown. The speaker says the sound a few more times with the speaker's face visible and may give a few words with the sound so that the person can also hear it embedded in words. Hearing a sound first without knowing what it will be is very useful because most people assume they know what the "L" sounds like, but they may come to realize that they need to revise their thinking if, in fact, they are surprised to find out that it actually differs from what they thought it would be. The per-

son is to point to the letter card on the table each time the sound is said. After one or two presentations, the card is withdrawn, and the second sound is introduced in the same way. With both cards on the table, the two sounds are then contrasted. Next, the third and fourth sounds are introduced as before and contrasted with the previous sounds. If more than a few repetitions of each sound are given, it is a good idea to change the position of the cards to keep the client's brain alert. It is also very helpful to introduce foils. These are sounds that are not represented on the table (e.g., /s/) and not easily confused with the available choices. The person is instructed to point to a certain place on the table when the sound is not one that is represented. The new sounds chosen for each lesson should be easily distinguishable from one another. For example, /t/, /ɛ/, /l/, or /n/ would be a good selection because each one is distinctly different, even if each is a difficult sound for the individual. Over time, clients hear the sounds in isolation many times, which, in turn, enables them to revise their built-in concepts. Gradually, new sounds are taught and reinforced until the individual is able to perceive them both quickly and accurately. During the first session, New Sounds is the only step in the PTP program.

- *Introduction & Review (IR)* is used to reinforce the sounds that were introduced in the previous session. Each sound is reintroduced more briefly than originally and contrasted with the others one at a time, as before. IR is given for the first time in the second session and subsequently in the following sessions, with the introduction of New Sounds always last.

- *Review.* For the third session and afterwards, the sounds that were already introduced and then reviewed (IR) are very briefly reviewed in this step. As the internally derived auditory concepts become clearer and clearer, more and more sounds are included in the review. For example, the /n/ might have been an early sound; although difficult at first, with practice, it becomes increasingly recognizable, especially from the other three sounds that were introduced at the same time (as there were no contrasting nasals). However, eventually /m/ is introduced, and two sessions later, both /m/ and /n/ may be among the sounds that are reviewed together. In time, /m/ and /n/ will be among the four or eight sounds that are presented together, which will test the success of the therapy to date. In each session, four more sounds reach review status. The sounds are generally placed on the table in groups of four in a random order all at once. Once they and the next group are reviewed separately, all eight sounds are contrasted. Usually eight sounds at a time is an efficient number, although some of the children will surely want to show their bravado by having more at a time. Having too many cards on the table, however, wastes time because of the visual challenge but can be done occasionally to maintain interest.

At the third session and afterwards, all three steps are given IR, then Review, and finally the New Sounds.

Phonemic Training Program Repair Procedure

PTP is a highly effective program. The most common error is that we try to achieve too much improvement too quickly. This can cause the person to become overloaded/confused, causing the individual to shut down and make errors on even the easiest material. If this should happen, change to a completely different task, and reduce the challenge when PTP is started again on the next visit. When ongoing confusions are observed, an effective method that can be used is Focus.

Focus reduces confusion in distinguishing two sounds (e.g., /ɛ/ vs. /æ/ or /f/ vs. /θ/). Generally, this suggests that the person's phoneme boundaries are highly overlapped. Show the two sound cards and tell the client you will say the /f/ sound three times and then the /θ/ once and point to the appropriate card each time. Next, try it again, always starting with the /f/, but indicate that you will not say how many /f/ sounds will be presented (vary the number of /f/ sounds presented from one to four times). After hearing the contrasted sounds several times, the client will be able to perceive the difference (perhaps vaguely at first). On the next visit, repeat the procedure; usually by the third visit, the person should have confidence in distinguishing the sounds. If not, try starting with the /θ/ three times followed by the /f/.

PHONEMIC SYNTHESIS

This time-honored approach has been used successfully for many years in many places and has been called by a variety of names (Monroe, 1932; Mulder and Curtin, 1955; Stovall et al., 1977; Katz, 1983). PS is a sound-by-sound presentation of words (or nonsense words). The listener is to say or point to pictures of the synthesized word. PS can be used in conjunction with the PTP to reinforce the speech sounds and to connect them to words. For those whose speech is not very clear, this training often results in spontaneous improvement (Katz and Medol, 1972). The PS CD/cassette therapy program is commercially available (Precision Acoustics 360-892-9367), but the same script can be used to present live voice when the recorded version is not desired. The PS program requires a good-quality cassette/CD player with stimuli delivered though loudspeakers or headphones and is presented at a comfortably loud level.

The program is made up of 15 lessons that are carefully designed to increase from easy to hard. It begins with simple words with easily recognizable phonemes in easy combinations and then gradually gets harder (Katz and Harmon, 1981). Instructions, repetition, and some humor are provided, and each lesson prepares the person for the next one.

PS was designed to provide relatively little feedback during the presentation to ensure that the individual is truly improving and understanding and not just remembering what to say, for example, when they hear *lem* or *bottle* (for the actual words *them* or *ball*, respectively). Most of the errors will be eliminated by repetition of the lesson itself or by branching (i.e., going off the program to address the specific challenge); branching is discussed in the following section. We have found it most helpful to graph the score for each lesson because it shows the person how he or she is doing.

■ The first three lessons have picture support, starting with easy words and only two picture choices. The second lesson uses the same words but has two or three picture choices, etc.
■ By the time children reach lesson four, they have heard the same five words broken up into their individual sounds many times and will likely be able to generate correct responses without picture support.
■ Gradually the words they have learned are lengthened to increase the challenge. For example, the word *cow* that was used in the previous four lessons is given again, followed by the *ch* sound to form the word *couch.*
■ Then harder sounds (e.g., /l/ and /w/) are introduced as well as consonant blends.
■ The program anticipates problems to ensure success and gradual improvement.
■ At the end of each lesson, the score is calculated and entered in the summary chart. This helps the clinician determine the next lesson and whether branching is in order.

Supportive Phonemic Synthesis Procedures

■ *Branching:* A process to speed up the therapy or when it seems that the client is stuck at a certain point. Branching means going off the program to address some specific challenge. For example, if a person says /f/ consistently for /s/ and there is no hearing loss or middle ear problem, and without additional training, it might take several repeats before this is learned. Therefore, it would be appropriate before the next administration of that lesson to teach the difference between /f/ and /s/. This could be done by Focus (see PTP) or Word Charts.
■ *Word Charts:* Six to eight words that are similar to the errors but not on the program may be written in large letters on a sheet of paper (usually in two columns) with the contrasting words opposite one another (e.g., fee/see, sore/for, calf/cass, flat/slat). Once the child can recognize the written words, these are presented one pair at a time in a random order, sound by sound, using a pointing response, and then all six or eight items are presented randomly. Then the PS lesson can be repeated to see if the learning

TABLE 28.3 Phonemic Synthesis (PS) normal limits for 8-year-old children and test results (number correct out of 25) before and after decoding therapies

	Normal limit	Test results: before training	Test results: after training
PS Quantitative Score	17	13.6	20.8
PS Qualitative Score	15	10.2	20.6

Qualitative score reduces correct scores for infractions (e.g., delays and quiet rehearsals).

was generalized; if not, one can go back to the actual error words and their substitutions on the Phonemic Synthesis Test and present them in the same way as discussed in this section.

DECODING THERAPY RESULTS

The two decoding therapies described in the previous sections have produced rewarding results. The data for 45 children with a mean age of 8.0 years (range, 6 to 16 years) are described below. The average length of therapy was 13 sessions, and only a total of about ≤6.5 hours was dedicated to the two decoding therapies.

Table 28.3 shows the results on the Phonemic Synthesis Test. When these scores are compared with 8-year norms, the mean improvement after therapy was 2.5 standard deviations for each measure, with the retest means falling well within normal limits. Table 28.4 shows parental/school ratings of change after therapy on the initial academic concerns. The results show that 86%, 94%, and 79% of the parents rated improvement as moderate or great in oral reading, phonics, and spelling, respectively, after this brief therapy program.

Speech-in-Noise Desensitization Training

Perhaps the most common complaint of those with CAPD or hearing loss is difficulty understanding speech in the presence of background noise. An analogy of what we try to achieve in speech-in-noise (SN) desensitization training is akin to what occurred many years ago when the author (J.K.) was getting desensitization shots for allergies. As in the case of allergies, we start with a low level of noise (instead of allergens) and work up gradually (Katz and Burge, 1971) to reduce the emotional impact and to increase the ability to pull the speech out of the background noise. Those who have difficulty understanding what is said in noise and have significant scores on SN (figure-ground) tests would be good candidates for this type of therapy. In the 50-minute auditory training sessions, we first administer the PTP, followed by SN desensitization training and then the PS program.

The current procedures expand and refine the original approaches used years ago. During the 13 therapy sessions, a total of approximately 3 hours of SN therapy is given. The procedure is administered from a CD player through a two-channel audiometer. This enables us to work in one or both ears through headphones or loudspeaker(s). Recorded speech is needed for this therapy. We use, for the most part, monosyllabic words instead of longer words, phrases, or sentences. However, follow-up with those other procedures is not precluded. We use 600 words divided into 10-word sublists. The noise should have a fairly consistent sound pressure level (SPL; e.g., ±5 dB) across the recording. The noise could be multitalker babble, cafeteria noise, or some other nonlinguistic competition. If free field training will be given, it is best not to work in a sound booth.

TABLE 28.4 Parent ratings of change in three academic areas that were noted as problems initially

	Improvement				Mean rating
	Great	Moderate	Slight	None	
Oral Reading	53%	33%	13%	0%	6.4 (0.7)
Phonetics	51%	43%	6%	0%	6.5 (0.6)
Spelling	42%	27%	23%	8%	5.9 (1.0)

A rating of 7 = great improvement, 6 = moderate improvement, 5 = slight improvement, and 4 = no improvement. There were no ratings below 4. The percentage of responses is shown in the center columns. On the right are the mean improvement ratings and standard deviations (in parentheses).

TABLE 28.5 Typical speech-in-noise series for an older child or adult as well as an alternating series

| Noise level (dB) | Typical series order | Alternating series order | |
		Right ear	Left ear
None	1	1	—
50	2	2	3
52	3	5	4
54	4	6	7
56	5	9	8
58	6	10	11
60	7	13	12

The second column from the left shows a typical speech-in-noise series for an older child or an adult with the specified noise levels on the left (assuming speech at 60 dB hearing level). The two columns on the right show an alternating series to compare the performance of the two ears for the same noise conditions. The numbers (1–13) show the sequence of the noise conditions with one sublist presented at each series. Note in this illustration of the alternating condition that the first presentation is to the right ear, and after two sublists, the ear is changed. If another alternate series is given at another time, it would be well to start in the left ear.

PROCEDURE

Choose a comfortable speech level for normal listeners; this can be changed for those who are hypersensitive or who are hard of hearing. During the session, the speech level is maintained at a constant level, but the noise levels are varied from no noise to a level equal to the speech level (0 dB signal-to-noise ratio). Ten words (one sublist) are presented at each noise condition. When working with young children or those who are fearful or stressed by noise, it is well to start with a milder signal-to-noise ratio early on. For example, for most normally hearing individuals, a +10 or +12 dB signal-to-noise ratio would be acceptable and not cause anxiety. Increase the noise level in 2-dB steps to the highest level (in which almost all of the words are audible if not fully intelligible). In children, if six or more errors occur at a noise level, generally we do not go to a higher level.

Some individuals have significantly poorer SN scores in one ear than the other. To remediate the interaural discrepancy, after a number of binaural sessions, we direct the therapy to the poorer ear for a few sessions and then check on the equality of the ears by using an "alternating" procedure under phones. That is, presentations are alternated from one ear to the other at the various noise levels (one sublist per ear-noise level) to determine if the discrepancy has been eliminated. For younger children, the right ear can be tested during one session, and the left ear can be tested the next. If one ear was poorer than the other, later on in the therapy, a few more series can be directed to the poorer ear. Table 28.5 shows a typical sequence for a series for an older child or adult as well as an alternating series.

RESULTS OF SPEECH-IN-NOISE DESENSITIZATION TRAINING

Therapeutic results have been impressive for SN. In one analysis of participants, overall improvement on the SN test in the two ears was 18%, bringing the mean score from below normal well into the normal range (Table 28.6). When the parents/schools were asked to rate improvement on three questions related to SN, the results were overwhelmingly positive (Table 28.7). Regarding specific questions, the results revealed the following:

- Change in "understanding SN": 94% indicated moderate or great improvement
- Children being "distracted by noise": 92% indicated moderate or great improvement
- Change in "hypersensitivity to noise": 77% indicated moderate or great improvement

The third way we studied the SN training progress was by examining the therapy materials themselves. The children typically started with an average of 19 errors at the first session. By the last noise series for the same noise levels, there were just six errors.

As in the case of decoding (PTP and PS) therapy, SN training was very effective in improving processing skills in children with CAPD.

TABLE 28.6 Speech-in-noise test results for 45 children who received auditory training

	Normal limit	Test	Retest
Speech-in-Noise Right	75%	64%	79%
Speech-in-Noise Left	73%	58%	77%

Eight-year-old speech-in-noise norms are shown for right and left ears as well as the test and retest scores.

TABLE 28.7   Parent/teacher ratings of change in three aspects associated with noise problems that were of initial concern

| | Improvement | | | | |
	Great	Moderate	Slight	None	Mean rating
Understands in Noise	56%	38%	6%	0%	6.5 (0.6)
Distracted by Noise	41%	51%	7%	0%	6.3 (0.7)
Hypersensitive to Noise	44%	33%	22%	0%	6.2 (0.8)

A rating of 7 = great improvement, 6 = moderate improvement, 5 = slight improvement, and 4 = no improvement. There were no ratings below 5. The percentage of responses is shown in the center columns. On the right is the mean improvement rating and standard deviation (in parentheses).

Summary of Direct Auditory Therapy for Children with Central Auditory Processing Disorders

For the past 50 years, the author (J.K.) has provided direct therapy for auditory processing deficits with impressive results. However, as the techniques have become more refined and modifications have been introduced, the results have gotten even better. It appears quite clear that these brief therapies that address decoding and SN skills are carried over into higher level activities by the children. This might suggest that, in the provision and ordering of therapies, it is most profitable to provide the basic therapies first to facilitate the learning and use of higher cognitive approaches.

REFERENCES

Abrahamsen EP, Smith R. (2000) Facilitating idiom acquisition in children with communication disorders: computer vs classroom. *Child Lang Teach Ther.* 16, 227–239.

American Speech-Language-Hearing Association. (2001) Scope of practice in speech-language pathology. Available at: http://www.asha.org/docs/html/SP2007-00283.html.

American Speech-Language-Hearing Association. (2005) Guidelines for addressing acoustics in educational settings. Available at: http://www.asha.org/docs/pdf/GL2005-00023.pdf.

Bell N. (1991) *Visualizing and Verbalizing for Language Comprehension and Thinking.* 2nd ed. San Luis Obispo, CA: Nancibell Inc.

Blachman BA, Ball EW, Black R, Tangel DM. (2000) *Road to the Code: A Phonological Awareness Program for Young Children.* Baltimore, MD: Brookes.

Bowers L, Huisingh R, LoGiudice C, Orman J. (2004) *The Word Test2: Elementary.* Moline, IL: Linguisystems.

Bradlow AR, Alexander JA. (2007) Semantic and phonetic enhancements for speech-in-noise recognition by native and nonnative listeners. *J Acoust Soc Am.* 121, 2339–2349.

Campbell TF, McNeil MR. (1985) Effects of presentation rate and divided attention on auditory comprehension in children with an acquired language disorder. *J Speech Hear Res.* 28, 513–520.

Carrow-Woolfolk E. (1999a) *Comprehensive Assessment of Spoken Language.* Bloomington, MN: Pearson.

Carrow-Woolfolk E. (1999b) *Test of Auditory Language Comprehension-3.* Bloomington, MN: Pearson.

Cognitive Concepts. (2004) *Earobics.* Evanston, IL: Cognitive Concepts.

Creusere M, Alt M, Plante E. (2004) Recognition of vocal and facial cues to affect in language-impaired and normally developing preschoolers. *J Commun Disord.* 37, 5–20.

Dodd B, Crosbie S, McIntosh B, Teitzel T, Ozanne A. (2003) *Pre-Reading Inventory of Phonological Awareness.* San Antonio, TX: Harcourt.

Dollaghan C, Campbell TF. (1998) Nonword repetition and child language impairment. *J Speech Lang Hear Res.* 41, 1136–1146.

Dunn LM, Dunn DM. (2007) *Peabody Picture Vocabulary Test.* 4th ed. Bloomington, MN: Pearson.

Ellis-Weismer S. (1997) The role of stress in language processing and intervention. *Topics Lang Disord.* 17, 41–52.

Ellis-Weismer S, Hesketh L. (1996) Lexical learning by children with specific language impairment: effects of linguistic input presented at varying speaking rates. *J Speech Lang Hear Res.* 39, 177–190.

Ferguson SH, Kewley-Port D. (2007) Talker differences in clear and conversational speech: acoustic characteristics of vowels. *J Speech Lang Hear Res.* 50, 1241–1255.

Ferre JM. (2002) Behavioral therapeutic approaches for central auditory problems. In: Katz J, ed. *Handbook of Clinical Audiology.* 5th ed. Philadelphia: Lippincott Williams & Wilkins.

Ferre JM. (2007) Classroom management: collaboration with families, teachers, and, other professionals. In: Chermak GD, Musiek FE, eds. *Handbook of (Central) Auditory Processing Disorder: Comprehensive Intervention, Volume II.* San Diego: Plural Publishing.

Fisher J, Plante E, Vance R, Gerken L, Glattke TJ. (2007) Do children and adults with language impairment recognize prosodic cues? *J Speech Lang Hear Res.* 50, 746–758.

Gardner MF. (2000) *Receptive One-Word Picture Vocabulary Test.* Novato, CA: Academic Therapy Publications.

Gathercole SE, Baddeley AD. (1990) Phonological memory deficits in language-impaired children: is there a causal connection? *J Mem Lang.* 29, 336–360.

Gaulin C, Campbell T. (1994) Procedure for assessing verbal working memory in normal school-age children: some preliminary data. *Percept Mot Skills*. 79, 55–64.

Gerken L, McGregor K. (1998) An overview of prosody and its role in normal and disordered child language. *Am J Speech Lang Pathol*. 7, 38–48.

German D. (1991) *Test of Word Finding in Discourse*. Austin, TX: PRO-ED.

German D. (2000) *Test of Word Finding-2*. 2nd ed. Austin, TX: PRO-ED.

German D. (2005) *Word Finding Intervention Program*. 2nd ed. Austin, TX: PRO-ED.

Gillam RB, Cowan N, Day LS. (1995) Sequential memory in children with and without language impairment. *J Speech Hear Res*. 38, 393–402.

Gillam RB, Gorman BK. (2004) Language and discourse contributions to word recognition and text interpretation: implications of a dynamic systems perspective. In: Silliman ER, Wilkinson LC, eds. *Language and Literacy Learning in Schools*. New York: Guilford Press; pp 63–97.

Gillam RB, Hoffman LM. (2004) Information processing in children with specific language impairment. In: Verhoeven L, van Balkom H, eds. *Classification of Developmental Language Disorders: Theoretical Issues and Clinical Implications*. Mahwah, NJ: Lawrence Erlbaum; pp 137–157.

Gillam RB, Hoffman LM, Marler JA, Wynn-Dancy ML. (2002) Sensitivity to increased task demands: contributions from data-driven and conceptually driven information processing deficits. *Topics Lang Disord*. 22, 30–48.

Gillam RB, Pearson NA. (2004) *Test of Narrative Language*. Austin, TX: PRO-ED.

Gillam RB, van Kleeck A (1996) Phonological awareness training and short-term working memory: clinical implications. *Topics Lang Disord*. 17, 72–81.

Gillon GT. (2004) *Phonological Awareness: From Research to Practice*. New York: Guilford Press.

Goodman YM, Watson DJ, Burke CL. (1987) *Reading Miscue Inventory: Alternative Procedures*. New York: Owen.

Hoffman LM, Gillam RB. (2004) Verbal and spatial information processing constraints in children with specific language impairment. *J Speech Lang Hear Res*. 47, 114–125.

Jerger S. (2007) Thoughts and issues on the management of auditory processing disorders. Presented at Contemporary Perspectives on Audiology: Celebrating Shlomo Silman's Clinical and Research Contributions. Graduate Center: City University New York, October 26, 2007.

Johnston J. (2006) *Thinking about Child Language: Research to Practice*. Eau Claire, WI: Thinking Publications.

Kamhi A, Newman-Ryan J. (2004). Auditory processing disorders as a misdiagnosed language disorder: implications for assessment and intervention. Paper presented at the Meeting of the American Speech-Language-Hearing Association, Philadelphia, PA.

Katz J. (1983) Phonemic synthesis and other auditory skills. In: Lasky E, Katz J, eds. *Central Auditory Processing Disorders: Problems of Speech, Language and Learning*. Baltimore: University Park Press.

Katz J. (1998) Central auditory processing and cochlear implant therapy. In: Masters MG, Stecker N, Katz J, eds. *Central Auditory Processing Disorders: Mostly Management*. Boston: Allyn & Bacon; pp 215–232.

Katz J, Burge C. (1971) Auditory perception training for children with learning disabilities. *Menorah Med J*. 2, 18–29.

Katz J, Harmon C. (1981) Phonemic synthesis: diagnostic and training program. In: Keith R, ed. *Central Auditory and Language Disorders in Children*. Baltimore: College Hill Park Press.

Katz J, Medol E. (1972) The use of phonemic synthesis in speech therapy. *Menorah Med J*. 3, 10–18.

Katz J, Smith PS. (1991) A ten minute look at the CNS through the ears: using the SSW test. In: Zappulla R, LeFever FF, Jaeger J, Bildern R, eds. *Windows on the Brain: Neuropsychology's Technical Frontiers. Ann NY Acad Sci*. 620, 233–252.

Krause JC, Braida, LD. (2004) Acoustic properties of naturally produced speech at normal speaking rates. *J Acoust Soc Am*. 115, 362–378.

Larsen SC, Hammill DD, Moats LC. (1999) *Test of Written Spelling*. 4th ed. Austin, TX: PRO-ED.

Leslie L, Caldwell J. (2001) *Qualitative Reading Inventory-3*. New York: Addison-Wesley Longman.

Li C, So CK. (2005) Acoustic properties of vowels in clear and conversational speech by female non-native English speakers. *J Acoust Soc Am*. 117, 2400–2401.

Lindamood PC, Lindamood P. (2004) *Lindamood Auditory Conceptualization Test, LAC-3*. 3rd ed. Austin, TX: PRO-ED.

Liu S, Del Rio E, Bradlow AR, Zeng FG. (2004) Clear speech perception in acoustic and electric hearing. *J Acoust Soc Am*. 116, 2374–2383.

Martin N, Brownell R. (2005) *Test of Auditory Processing Skills-3*. Novato, CA: Academic Therapy Publications.

Masterson JJ, Apel K. (2000) Spelling assessment: charting a path to optimal intervention. *Topics Lang Disord*. 20, 50–65.

Masterson JJ, Apel K, Wasowicz J. (2002) *Spelling Performance Evaluation for Language and Literacy*. Evanston, IL: Learning By Design.

McGhee RL, Ehrler DJ, DiSimoni F. (2007) *Token Test for Children-2*. Austin, TX: PRO-ED.

Medwetsky L. (1991) Effect of microphone placement on the spectral distribution of speech. Presented at the American Speech, Language, and Hearing Association Meeting, Atlanta, GA.

Medwetsky L. (2007) Utilization of computer software as a management tool for addressing CAPD. In: Geffner D, Ross-Swain D, eds. *Auditory Processing Disorders: Assessment, Management, and Treatment*. San Diego: Plural Publishing; pp 345–390.

Messer D, Dockrell JE. (2006) Children's naming and word finding difficulties: descriptions and explanations. *J Speech Lang Hear Res*. 49, 309–324.

Miller L, Gillam RB, Pena E. (2000) *Dynamic Assessment and Intervention of Children's Narratives*. Austin, TX: PRO-ED.

Monroe M. (1932) *Children Who Cannot Read*. Chicago: University of Chicago Press.

Montgomery JW. (1995) Sentence comprehension in children with specific language impairment: the role of phonological working memory. *J Speech Hear Res*. 38, 187–199.

Montgomery JW. (2000) Verbal working memory and sentence comprehension in children with specific language impairment. *J Speech Lang Hear Res*. 43, 293–308.

Montgomery JW. (2002) Information processing and language comprehension in children with specific language impairment. *Topics Lang Disord*. 22, 62–84.

Montgomery JW, Windsor J. (2007) Examining the language performance of children with and without specific language impairment: contributions of phonological short-term memory and speed of processing. *J Speech Lang Hear Res.* 50, 778–797.

Mulder ML, Curtin J. (1955) Vocal phonic ability and silent reading achievement. *Element Sch J.* 56, 121–123.

Naremore RC, Densmore AE, Harman DR. (1995) *Language Intervention with School-Aged Children: Conversation, Narrative and Text.* San Diego: Singular.

National Reading Panel. (2000) Teaching children to read: an evidence-based assessment of the scientific research literature on reading and its implications for reading instructions. Washington, DC: US Government Printing Office.

Newcomer DD, Hammill PL. (1997) *Test of Language Development-Primary.* 3rd ed. Bloomington, MN: Pearson.

Newman-Ryan J, Kamhi AG. (2003) Cases of auditory processing disorders: sudden epidemic, mis-diagnosis or good meme? Paper presented at the Meeting of the American Speech-Language-Hearing Association, Chicago, IL.

Nippold MA. (1991) Evaluating and enhancing idiom comprehension in language-disordered students. *Lang Speech Hear Serv Sch.* 22, 100–106.

Nippold MA. (1998) *Later Language Development: Ages Nine through Nineteen.* 2nd ed. Austin, TX: PRO-ED.

Nippold MA, Duthie JK. (2003) Mental imagery and idiom comprehension: a comparison of school-age children and adults. *J Speech Lang Hear Res.* 46, 788–799.

Norbury CF. (2005) Barking up the wrong tree? Lexical ambiguity resolution in children with language impairments and autistic spectrum disorders. *J Exp Child Psychol.* 90, 142–171.

Paul R. (2007) *Language Disorders from Infancy through Adolescence.* 3rd ed. St. Louis: Mosby.

Power R, Taylor CL, Nippold MA. (2001) Comprehending literally-true versus literally-false proverbs. *Child Lang Teach Ther.* 17, 1–18.

Richard GJ, Hanner MA. (2005) *Language Processing Test 3: Elementary.* Moline, IL: Linguisystems.

Robertson C, Salter W. (1995) *The Phonological Awareness Kit: Primary.* East Moline, IL: Linguisystems.

Robertson C, Salter W. (1997) *The Phonological Awareness Test.* East Moline, IL: Linguisystems.

Roth F. (2000) Narrative writing: development and teaching with children with writing difficulties. *Topics Lang Disord.* 20, 15–28.

Roth FP. (2004) Word recognition assessment frameworks. In: Stone CA, Silliman ER, Ehren BJ, Apel K, eds. *Handbook of Language and Literacy: Development and Disorders.* New York: Guildford Press; pp 461–480.

Scientific Learning. (1997) FastForward. Oakland, CA: Scientific Learning.

Scott CM. (1995) Syntax for school-age children: a discourse perspective. In: Fey ME, Windsor J, Warren SF, eds. *Language Intervention: Preschool through the Elementary Years.* Baltimore: Brookes; pp 107–145.

Semel E, Wiig EH, Secord WA. (2003) *Clinical Evaluation of Language Fundamentals-4.* San Antonio, TX: Harcourt.

Snyder LE, Dabasinskas C, O'Connor E. (2002) An information processing perspective on language impairment in children: looking at both sides of the coin. *Topics Lang Disord.* 22, 1–14.

Stovall JV, Manning WH, Shaw CK. (1977) Auditory assembly of children with mild and severe misarticulations. *Folia Phoniatrica.* 29, 162–172.

Strong C. (1998) *Strong Narrative Assessment Procedure.* Eau Claire, WI: Thinking Publications.

Tallal P, Stark RE, Mellits D. (1985) The relationship between auditory temporal analysis and receptive language development: evidence from studies of developmental language impairment. *Neuropsychologia.* 23, 527–534.

Van der Meulen S, Janssen P, den Os E. (1997) Prosodic abilities in children with specific language impairment. *J Commun Disord.* 30, 155–170.

van Kleeck A, Gillam RB, McFadden T. (1998) Teaching rhyming and phonological awareness to preschool-aged children with language disorders. *Am J Speech Lang Pathol.* 7, 66–77.

Wagner R, Torgeson J, Rashotte C. (1999) *Comprehensive Test of Phonological Processing, CTOPP.* Austin, TX: PRO-ED.

Weiderholdt JL, Bryant BR. (2000) *Gray Silent Reading Test.* Austin, TX: PRO-ED.

Weiderholdt JL, Bryant BR. (2001) *Gray Oral Reading Test.* 4th ed. Austin, TX: PRO-ED.

Wells B, Peppe S. (2003) Intonation abilities of children with speech and language impairments. *J Speech Lang Hear Res.* 46, 5–20.

Westby CE. (2005) Assessing and remediating text comprehension problems. In: Catts HW, Kamhi AG, eds. *Language and Reading Disabilities.* 2nd ed. New York: Pearson; pp 157–232.

Wiig EH, Secord W. (1989) *Test of Language Competence-Expanded Ed.* San Antonio, TX: Harcourt.

Wolf M, Bowers PG. (1999) The double-deficit hypothesis for the developmental dyslexias. *J Educ Psychol.* 91, 415–438.

Woodcock RW. (1987) *Woodcock Reading Mastery Tests-Revised.* Circle Pines, MN: American Guidance Service.

APPENDIX 28.1A
Auditory Processing Test Findings and Language Assessment Tools

Auditory processing deficit	Language domain	Assessment tools
Phonemic Synthesis	Phonologic Awareness	CTOPP, PAT, PIPA, LAC-3
	Phonologic Working Memory	CTOPP, Nonword Repetition Test
	Morphologic Awareness	Informal Tasks, Spelling Assessment
	Reading and Spelling	WRMT-R, GORT-3, Reading Miscue Inventory, TWS-3, SPELL
Lexical Decoding Speed	Semantic Skills	PPVT-4, ROWPVT, LPT3-E, WORD TEST2-E, CELF-4, CASL
	Word Finding	TWF-2, TWFD
	Morphologic/Syntactical Skills	CELF-4, TOLD-P3, Language Sample
Working Memory	Memory Span, Phonologic Working Memory	TAPS-3, CTOPP
	Oral Directions	Token Test, CELF-4
Sequencing	Narrative Language	TNL, Strong Narrative Assessment
Integration	Prosody	Informal
	Conversational Skills	Language Sample
	Figurative Language	TLC, CASL, Informal

See Appendix 28.1B for abbreviation definitions.

APPENDIX 28.2B
Glossary of Language Assessment Tools

Test abbreviation	Test name
CASL	Comprehensive Assessment of Spoken Language
CELF-4	Clinical Evaluation of Language Fundamentals-4
CTOPP	Comprehensive Test of Phonological Processing
GORT-3	Gray Oral Reading Test-3
LAC-3	Lindamood Auditory Conceptualization Test-3
LPT3-E	Language Processing Test 3–Elementary
PAT	Phonological Awareness Test
PIPA	Pre-Reading Inventory of Phonological Awareness
PPVT-4	Peabody Picture Vocabulary Test-4
ROWPVT	Receptive One-Word Picture Vocabulary Test
SPELL	Spelling Performance Evaluation for Language and Literacy
TAPS-3	Test of Auditory Processing Skills-3
TLC	Test of Language Competence
TNL	Test of Narrative Language
TOLD-P3	Test of Language Development–Primary: 3rd Edition
TWF-2	Test of Word Finding-2
TWFD	Test of Word Finding in Discourse
TWS-3	Test of Written Spelling-3
WORD TEST2-E	Word Test 2–Elementary
WRMT-R	Woodcock Reading Mastery–Revised

GLOSSARY

Alternate word strategy: substitution of a different word for a word that cannot easily be retrieved.

Derivational morphology: addition of a prefix or suffix that changes the grammatical category of a word (e.g., teach-teacher; love-lovely).

Elision: deletion of a sound from a word (e.g., say "soap" without the /s/ sound).

Figurative language: language that is not literal and uses figures of speech such as similes and metaphors defined below.

Idiom: an expression of a given language that cannot be understood from the individual meanings of its elements (e.g., skate on thin ice; let off some steam).

Grammatical morphemes: smallest unit of meaning that is formed by adding grammatical markers to words such as past tense "–ed" or present progressive "–ing."

Metaphor: figure of speech in which a characteristic is given to a person or thing by using the name of something else that has similar qualities (e.g., he is a bear when he is tired).

Mnemonic cueing: techniques used to aid in recall such as using an acronym or an associated word to retrieve the name of a word.

Proverb: a short popular saying, usually of unknown origin (e.g., the early bird catches the worm).

Scaffolding: a variety of supports that are designed to assist a child to learn optimally. Some examples include the use of questions and prompts and reducing the amount of material a child has to process at any one point in time.

Simile: figure of speech comparing two unlike things introduced by "like" or "as" (e.g., eats like a bird, smart as a whip).

Social scripts: a framework for a routine event (e.g., associated actions of dining in a restaurant or rules for participating in the classroom). It may include teaching a child the language to use in a particular situation.

Sound isolation: identifying the sound that occurs in the initial, medial, or final position of a word (e.g., What is the first sound in the word "cat"?).

Sound segmentation: division of a word into sound segments (e.g., tell me all the sounds in the word "soap," /s/ /o/ /p/).

Sound substitution: substituting one sound for another sound in a word (e.g., say "bat"; change /b/ to /k/).

Story frames: a set of cloze sentences (i.e., whereby a portion of a sentence is left out and the individual must use the sentence context to derive the missing portion) that serve as prompts for the parts of a story (e.g., The characters in the story were_____).

Story grammar: the organization of a story, which generally includes a setting, an initiating event or problem, actions to solve the problem, and a consequence.

Story maps: graphic organizer or flow chart in which the parts of a story are represented visually.

Story prompts: a series of questions that a child answers to identify the parts of the story (e.g., Where did the story take place?).

Syllable dividing: division of a word into syllables to aid in word retrieval.

CHAPTER 29
Individuals with Multiple Disabilities

Anne Marie Tharpe

 ## INTRODUCTION

Individuals with hearing loss and additional disabilities represent a widely diverse and complex population. They differ in the type and degree of their hearing loss, the type and degree of their accompanying disability, and their overall level of functioning. Approximately 30% to 40% of newborns who are deaf or hard of hearing have additional neurodevelopmental conditions, most often mental retardation (Fortnum and Davis, 1997; Mace et al., 1991; Van Naarden et al., 1999). Similarly, the Gallaudet Research Institute (GRI, 2005) indicated that approximately 42% of deaf or hard of hearing school-age children have additional disabilities. As seen in Table 29.1, the most prevalent conditions were intellectual disabilities, followed by learning disabilities and attention problems. It is also possible that some disabilities may not become apparent until well into childhood or adolescence, increasing these numbers even more.

There is also some evidence to suggest that the number of people with hearing loss who have additional disabilities is on the rise (Cano et al., 2001). Several reasons have been suggested to account for this increase including improved survival rates among very low birth weight infants (<1,500 g) who have a high risk of disability (Fortnum et al., 2001; Streppel et al., 1998). Heroic measures are now taken to save preterm infants who, even a decade ago, may not have survived. Most agree that those who do survive the traumas of birth are at higher risk of lifelong disorders than full-term infants (Hack et al., 1994; Wilson-Costello et al., 2005). However, some studies suggest that the technology and intervention that have improved survival rates have also resulted in improved overall outcomes for premature babies (O'Shea et al., 1997).

Genetic causes also contribute to the number of individuals with hearing loss and additional disabilities. Approximately one third of those with multiple handicapping conditions have a syndromic cause of hereditary deafness (Picard, 2004). The most common of these syndromes include Down, Usher, Pierre Robin, Treacher Collins, and CHARGE syndromes. Maternal infection remains a contributing causative factor of hearing loss. Although the prevalence of maternal rubella infection is down worldwide, cases of cytomegalovirus (CMV) are on the rise. CMV is associated with hearing loss and motor and cognitive deficits. Additional risk factors for developmental delays include environmental teratogens (i.e., factors that have adverse effects on embryos or fetuses), maternal substance abuse, and environmental deprivation.

Clearly, the high prevalence of infants and children with hearing loss and additional disabilities serves to emphasize the need for audiologists to acquire knowledge and competence to meet the challenges posed by their complex needs into adulthood. This chapter reviews some of the general characteristics of children and adults with hearing loss and additional handicapping conditions. Basic principles for assessment and suggestions for management of these special populations are offered. In considering these suggestions, a few points should be kept in mind. First, it is likely that patients with hearing loss and other disabilities will have some conditions that have not been identified at the time of the audiologic assessment. Therefore, audiologists should be mindful of the possibility that unknown conditions may influence the testing and management of some patients. This is especially true of more subtle conditions such as attention deficits and emotional problems. Second, the combined effects of some conditions may confuse or delay a diagnosis of hearing loss. For example, a child with autism and hearing loss may be nonresponsive to sound, in part, because of "tuning out" behavior and, in part, because he or she truly cannot hear some sounds. Third, a lack of training or experience may

TABLE 29.1   Percentage of disabilities that occur in children with hearing loss

Additional disabilities	% of children with hearing loss
No additional disabilities	57.6
Low vision/legal blindness	4.6
Intellectual disability	10.0
Autism	1.0
Orthopedic disability (including cerebral palsy)	3.7
Learning disability	9.2
Attention deficit disorder/ attention deficit hyperactivity disorder	6.3
Emotional disability	1.9
Other	6.9

Note: Values were taken from Gallaudet Research Institute. (2005). Regional and national summary report of data from the 2004–2005 Annual Survey of Deaf and Hard of Hearing Children and Youth. Washington, DC: Gallaudet Research Institute, Gallaudet University.

lead audiologists to think that some individuals with multiple disabilities are untestable by behavioral measures, which may result in a reliance on physiologic measures alone. Certainly, physiologic measures contribute valuable information about the integrity of the auditory system. However, we must bear in mind that behavioral tests provide an indication of how an individual uses his or her hearing, a very important factor when considering management needs. Collectively, physiologic and age-appropriate behavioral test methods can result in an accurate assessment of hearing in most individuals with multiple disabilities and will result in an improved ability for audiologists to develop management strategies.

CUSTOMIZING THE HEARING ASSESSMENT

When evaluating individuals who have multiple handicaps, consideration must be given to any physical or mental limitations that could affect the assessment procedures. A thorough case history, review of prior evaluations, and keen observation can often identify the potential obstacles to assessment and may highlight individual strengths or interests that can be used to enhance the evaluation process. Obtaining as much information about the patient before the evaluation can help the audiologist prepare appropriately for the test session. For example, prior developmental testing or the use of developmental checklists will help the audiologist determine the individual's ability to participate in behavioral tasks. Checklists are widely available and can be completed by parents or caregivers prior to their arrival at the clinic or while seated in the waiting room prior to the appointment.

Likewise, when physical limitations exist (e.g., cerebral palsy or other gross motor deficits), modifications to any behavioral task requiring a motor response must be considered.

At the clinic, an initial observation without the patient's awareness can be helpful in determining typical behavior of the individual. Discretely observing the interactions between the patient and the caregiver in a waiting area can provide insight into the type, amount, and quality of communication or accommodation that may be effective (Dean and Harris, 2003). These initial observations aid in predicting how much cooperation can be expected and thus determining how to proceed with the assessment. For example, pretest observations may demonstrate that an individual will not be able to participate in behavioral testing, and therefore, reliance on physiologic measures will be necessary. Whether testing adults or children, individuals with multiple disabilities are more likely than typically developing individuals to require a heavy reliance on physiologic measures over behavioral procedures. Observing the patient's behavior when his or her name is called in the waiting room can also provide some useful insight into the individual's level of functioning. Importance of the pretest interview cannot be overemphasized. Parents, care providers, therapists, and anyone who spends significant periods of time with the patient can provide valuable input about home and other environments, cognitive or physical limitations that might affect assessment or management, and potential compliance concerns.

Finally, based on the review of case history information, previous evaluations, and prior observations of the patient, audiologists should prioritize the tests in the battery so that those likely to yield the most useful information and that are most easily obtained for the patient are conducted first. The order of the tests in the protocol might be quite different than that used with typically developing individuals. The audiologist should be mindful of the distinction between hearing sensitivity and responses of young children or those with developmental disabilities when interpreting the results of a behavioral test. Noel Matkin (1977) coined the term *minimal response level* to describe the level at which a behavioral response to sound occurs but also recognizing that it may be elevated as a result of nonsensory factors such as attention, motivation, or behavior.

FUNCTIONAL AUDITORY ASSESSMENTS

It is not uncommon when assessing the hearing of some individuals with multiple disabilities to obtain little in the way of formal behavioral test results during an initial visit because of difficulty gaining a necessary level of cooperation. However, even without the patient's cooperation, useful information can be acquired through the use of functional auditory assessment tools. These assessments evaluate listening behaviors in real-world settings—outside the confines of the soundproof booth where most formal audiologic testing takes place. The goal of functional assessments is to tell us not only *what* an individual hears but, more importantly, how the individual *uses* what is heard in everyday situations. In addition, information can be obtained about how listening behavior might change in different settings, under different conditions, or with different speakers. This information can then be used to guide the evaluation and management plans for these patients. Typically, this information can be obtained from self-assessment, parent, teacher, or caregiver questionnaires. Although these tools have been designed for children, it is reasonable to adapt such questionnaires for information gathering purposes when assessing the needs of individuals of any age who have cognitive or behavioral disorders.

AUTISM SPECTRUM DISORDERS

Autism is a developmental disorder characterized by a triad of symptoms including qualitative impairments in social interaction, qualitative impairments in communication, and restricted, repetitive, and stereotyped patterns of behaviors, activities, and interests (American Psychiatric Association [APA], 1994). In addition to autism, autism spectrum disorder (ASD) includes pervasive developmental disorder (PDD), Asperger's syndrome, Rett's syndrome, and childhood disintegrative disorder. ASD is thought to have an early onset, with symptoms appearing before 30 months of age in most cases. However, a definitive diagnosis of autism is not generally made until the age of 4 to 4.5 years (Filipek et al., 2000; Siegel et al., 1988; Stone and Rosenbaum, 1988) as a result of overlapping conditions and scant information on behavioral characteristics at younger ages. More recently, diagnostic tools have become available that may contribute to a lower average age of identification (Lord et al., 2000; Wing et al., 2002). Prevalence estimates of autism have increased significantly over time from reports of one to five children per 10,000 in the 1970s (Brask, 1972; Treffert, 1970) to reports of five to 60 per 10,000 in the 1990s and 2000s (Bertrand et al., 2001; Kadesjö et al., 1999; Scott et al., 2002; Yeargin-Allsopp et al., 2003). Whether there has been a true increase in prevalence of autism over time or the reported changes in prevalence can be explained by changes in diagnostic criteria and increased awareness of the disorder by parents and professionals remains to be seen (Rutter, 2005; Wing and Potter, 2002). Boys are affected with autism more often than girls at a ratio of 3–4:1 (Van Bourgondien et al., 1987). Seventy to 80% of children with autism function intellectually within the range of mental retardation (Freeman et al., 1985; Ghaziuddin, 2000).

There is no strong evidence to suggest that individuals with autism have a greater risk of hearing loss than the general population. However, the presence of unusual sensory responses, including abnormal responses to sound, is considered an associated feature of autism. For example, individuals with autism often appear to be overly sensitive to

sound by covering their ears with their hands when loud or unexpected sounds occur. Other times, they may completely ignore sounds that would result in a reaction from typically developing individuals. Therefore, those with autism will likely be referred to audiologists for hearing assessments. Although little is known about the auditory abilities of adults with autism, young children with autism demonstrate essentially equivalent results on physiologic auditory tests compared to typically developing children. However, on average, behavioral responses of children with autism are elevated and less reliable relative to those of children in the general population (Tharpe et al., 2006).

Special Testing Considerations

Children with autism who have hearing loss are diagnosed, on average, almost 1 year later than those without hearing loss (Mandell et al., 2005). Therefore, it is reasonable for audiologists to be alert to the general behavioral characteristics of childhood autism in order to facilitate referral for evaluation when indicated. Several screening tools are available that can be used by audiologists. These include, among others, the Modified Checklist for Autism in Toddlers (M-CHAT) (Robins et al., 2001) and the Pervasive Developmental Disorder Screening Test II (PDDST-II) (Siegel, 1996).

Understanding the general behavioral characteristics of those with autism can also be helpful to audiologists as they consider modifications to the traditional test battery. For example, because the majority of those with autism exhibit cognitive deficits, behavioral abnormalities, and hypersensitivity to sensory stimulation, audiologists should be prepared to address those issues during the test session. Audiologists will want to minimize physical contact with autistic individuals who have tactile sensitivities. This may require initial testing in sound field because of the possibility of aversion to the tactile stimulation created by earphone placement. Regardless of the chronologic age of the individuals, audiologists will need to use behavioral test procedures that are appropriate for their cognitive level. This may mean that procedures typically used with infants and young children, such as visual reinforcement audiometry (VRA) or play audiometric techniques, will be used with older children or even adults. If VRA is used, one should consider minimizing the impact of the reinforcement by turning off the animation (if a lighted, animated toy is used) or using a video reinforcement. Other testing options for patients functioning at a developmental level of 2.5 years or greater are conditioned play audiometry (CPA) and tangible-reinforcement operant conditioning audiometry (TROCA) (Lloyd et al., 1968). TROCA requires the patient to press a bar or a button whenever a sound is heard, which is paired with the dispensing of a tangible reinforcement (e.g., small piece of food). TROCA is noted to be particularly effective with children having cognitive or behavioral (e.g., autism spectrum) disorders.

If a patient with autism will not allow the placement of earphones or probes for individual ear testing, audiologists may have to resort to sedated procedures. This is certainly true if one plans to fit hearing aids. Individuals with autism are known to be difficult to sedate with currently available pediatric sedating agents and are at risk for seizures while under sedation (Mehta et al., 2004). Therefore, consultation with the physician in charge of administering and monitoring the sedation process will need to include notification of the patient's diagnosis of autism.

Special Management Considerations

For individuals with autism, tactile sensitivities, and hearing loss, one can expect some resistance to wearing hearing aids. Therefore, maintaining consistent hearing aid use may take longer with this population than with typically developing individuals. One technique for introducing amplification is to start by having the parent or caregiver gently massage the patient's ears several times a day until little or no resistance is offered. This may take anywhere from a few days to weeks. From there, one can introduce, to one ear only, a soft earmold without the hearing aid connected and build up wear time starting with a few minutes until the patient is willing to wear it for longer periods of time. Once the earmold is tolerated with little resistance, the hearing aid can be coupled to the earmold, and eventually, both hearing aids can be introduced. Of course, this process will be slower or faster depending on the degree of tactile sensitivity and resistance offered. Hearing aids will need to be secured to the patient's clothing by use of retention devices designed specifically for hearing aids. Such devices will leave the hearing aids secured to the patient's clothing even if they are pulled from the ears.

Loudness discomfort or hypersensitivity to sound has frequently been documented in children with autism (Ohta et al., 1987; Monville and Nelson, 1994; Tharpe et al., 2006; Volkmar et al., 1986). As such, it is essential that audiologists carefully adhere to prescriptive formulae for the selection and verification of hearing aid gain and output characteristics. Because it may be difficult or impossible to measure the patient's comfortable loudness levels, audiologists will often need to use age-appropriate normative targets provided by the prescriptive formulae. It is reasonable for audiologists to consider initially lowering the gain and output levels below those prescribed and gradually raising them as the patient becomes accustomed to the amplified sound. However, gain levels should always make speech audible for the patient.

PHYSICAL DISABILITIES

Persons who are deaf or hard of hearing should have similar motor development and skills as those with normal hearing unless vestibular function is affected. That is, deafness alone does not affect motor abilities or balance function. In fact, 93% of deaf children have average to above average motor skills (Lieberman et al., 2004). Physical abilities are believed to be primarily influenced by environmental factors such as

TABLE 29.2 Gross motor milestones expected to be reached during the first 2 years of life

Skill	Expected age	Range
Holds head erect	4 months	3–6 months
Rolls front to back	4 months	3–6 months
Sits alone	6 months	5–8 months
Crawls	8 months	6–11 months
Stands alone	11 months	9–16 months
Walks alone	11 months	9–17 months
Runs	15 months	13–20 months
Walks up stairs (with railing)	16 months	12–23 months

emphasis of such skills in the school curriculum, opportunities for practice and play, and parenting styles. Table 29.2 provides a listing of gross motor milestones expected during the first 2 years of life. If a child with hearing loss is not walking by 15 months of age, a referral for further evaluation is warranted.

Vestibular abnormalities that can result in gross motor problems include cochlear malformations such as Mondini's deformity and cochlear hypoplasia. Other congenital causes of gross motor deficits in children with hearing loss include CHARGE syndrome, Usher syndrome type I, and cerebral palsy (CP). CP is a disorder of neuromotor function. Approximately 3% of children with hearing loss have also been diagnosed with CP, which is characterized by an inability to control motor function as a result of damage to or an anomaly of the developing brain (GRI, 2005; Roush et al., 2004). This damage interferes with messages from the brain to the body and from the body to the brain. The effects of CP vary widely from individual to individual. There are three primary types of CP:

- Spastic – characterized by high muscle tone (hypertonia) producing stiff and difficult movement
- Athetoid – producing involuntary and uncontrolled movement
- Ataxic – characterized by low muscle tone (hypotonia) producing a disturbed sense of balance, disturbed position in space, and general uncoordinated movement

These three types of CP can coexist in the same individual. CP can also be characterized by the number of limbs affected:

- Quadriplegia – all four limbs are involved
- Diplegia – all four limbs are involved and both legs are more severely affected than the arms
- Hemiplegia – one side of the body is affected and the arm is usually more involved than the leg
- Triplegia – three limbs are involved, usually both arms and a leg
- Monoplegia – only one limb is affected, usually an arm

CP is not a progressive condition. The damage to the brain is a one-time event. However, the effects may change over time. For example, with physical therapy a child's gross and fine motor skills may improve with time. However, the aging process can be harder on bodies with abnormal posture or that have had little exercise, so the effects may result in a gradual decline in motoric ability. It is important to remember that the degree of physical disability experienced by a person with CP is not an indication of his or her level of intelligence.

The brain damage that caused CP may also lead to other conditions such as learning disabilities or developmental delays. Approximately 20% of children with CP will also experience hearing or language problems (Robinson, 1973). The hearing loss is sensory-neural in nature. In addition, between 40% and 75% of individuals with CP will also have some degree of vision deficit.

Special Testing Considerations

Individuals with motor delays may not respond behaviorally to auditory stimuli because their physical disabilities limit their ability to orient to sound (Moore, 1995). When testing children, VRA can provide reliable information even for those with poor head and neck control. Modifications that may need to be made in the test arrangements for VRA include the use of an infant seat to provide additional head support. However, the audiologist must ensure that head supports do not block the ears and impede sound field stimuli. If children with motor difficulties cannot make a head-turn response to sound, response modifications can be made. Modifications include alternative responses such as localizing to the sound stimuli with their eyes as opposed to head turns. CPA (see Chapter 23) may also require modifications. Response modifications may need to include options that do not require the use of fine motor skills. Examples of such modifications could include asking a child to drop a ball into a large bucket rather than having the child insert a peg in a pegboard, partial hand raising, or even just a head nod. Additionally, a variety of gross motor responses (e.g., hand motion, etc.) can be used to trigger an electronic switch that will, in turn, activate a computer screen programmed for appropriate visual reinforcement.

If the physical disability has a neuromotor component, such as with cerebral palsy, physiologic measures might be affected. That is, abnormality in measures such as the auditory brainstem response (ABR) may be misinterpreted as indicating hearing loss when, in fact, the abnormality is in neurotransmission. Therefore, interpretation of the ABR must be made cautiously and in concert with the entire battery of auditory tests, behavioral and physiologic. Sedation may be required when conducting ABR with individuals who have CP in an attempt to relax their head and necks or to reduce extraneous muscle movements, thus reducing myogenic artifact.

Special Management Considerations

When selecting and fitting hearing aids on someone with physical impairments, there are a number of factors that must be considered, including the types of activities in which the individual participates (e.g., physical therapy) and his or her fine and gross motor ability (e.g., does the person sit in a wheelchair with head supports). If fitting children, it is important that the audiologist consider input from the parents and other professionals working with the child when determining amplification options. Children who require amplification for their hearing loss are typically fit with behind-the-ear (BTE) hearing aids. However, use of this type of aid may not be appropriate for children or adults with physical handicaps if they have poor head control (McCracken and Bamford, 1995; Tharpe et al., 2001). As seen in Figure 29.1A, the close proximity of head supports or the person's own shoulders if the head is leaning to one side may result in excessive feedback or discomfort from BTEs. The feedback problem may be reduced by selecting a hearing aid with a feedback cancellation feature. Another feature that may be beneficial for those with poor head control is a remote control. This can provide easier manipulation of the controls

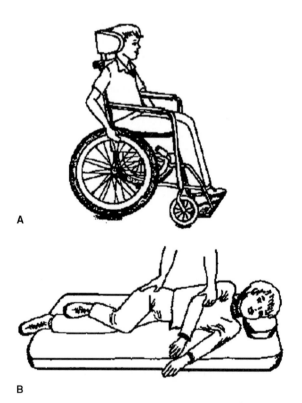

A

B

FIGURE 29.1 A and B. Head and neck braces can interfere with the placement of behind-the-ear hearing aids and may contribute to acoustic feedback (Reprinted with permission from Seewald RC, ed. [2000] *A Sound Foundation through Early Amplification*. Stäfa, Switzerland: Phonak AG).

(e.g., volume control wheel) of the hearing aid by caretakers (Roush et al., 2004).

Body-worn hearing aids provide another option and would eliminate many of the problems that BTEs pose for patients with poor head control. However, body-worn hearing aids also require special consideration when being used with patients who have physical disabilities. For example, for very young children and for those of any age with oral-motor difficulties, the microphone of the aid may be vulnerable to food and drink. Moreover, clothes may rub on the microphone port, resulting in extraneous noise, and wheelchair harnesses can rub or press against the aid, resulting in discomfort or damage. Although children are not typically fit with in-the-ear (ITE) hearing aids, they may be an appropriate solution for adults or children who spend part of their day in atypical positions such as during prone plinth work (Fig. 29.1B) or who use a wheelchair with headrests (McCracken and Bamford, 1995).

 MENTAL RETARDATION

Mental retardation, or intellectual disability, is a common co-occurrence with hearing loss and manifests prior to 18 years of age. Mental retardation is commonly defined as below average functioning both in objectively assessed cognitive ability (intelligence quotient [IQ] of ≤ 70) and in developmental or adaptive behaviors. Adaptive skill areas include:

- Communication
- Self-care
- Home living
- Social skills
- Community use
- Self-direction
- Health and safety
- Functional academics
- Leisure and work

As seen in Table 29.1, approximately 10% of children with hearing loss also have intellectual disabilities (GRI, 2005). Those with mental retardation are at an increased risk for visual or hearing impairment or both (Beange et al., 1995; Evenhuis, 1995; Kwok et al., 1996; MacFarland, 2003; van Schrojenstein Lantman-de Valk et al., 1997). Detection and treatment of hearing loss in adults and children with mental retardation are of utmost importance because hearing loss can exaggerate intellectual deficits by impeding the learning process (Roush et al., 2004).

Down syndrome, also referred to as trisomy 21, is the leading cause of hearing loss and intellectual disabilities. Therefore, audiologists are very likely to see a large number of children and adults with Down syndrome, a genetic disorder resulting from a chromosomal abnormality always associated with some degree of mental retardation. As individuals with Down syndrome age, there is a decline in intellectual ability. In fact, almost 100% of individuals with

Down syndrome over 40 years of age demonstrate degenerative neuropathologic changes consistent with Alzheimer-type dementia (Zigman et al., 1995). Furthermore, some have speculated that the precocious aging of individuals with Down syndrome results in early presbycusis in this population (Dille, 2003; Hassmann et al., 1998). Hearing loss progresses more rapidly in adults with Down syndrome than those with other forms of mental retardation or adults in the general population. Occurring in approximately one per 700 births, Down syndrome is also frequently associated with conductive hearing loss and, less often, sensory-neural hearing loss. Although the majority of the conductive hearing losses in those with Down syndrome are secondary to middle ear effusion, some are the result of middle ear anomalies such as ossicular malformations and damage to middle ear structures as a result of chronic infection. In contrast to the typically developing population, the prevalence of middle ear effusion tends to remain high in individuals with Down syndrome regardless of age. Marcell and Cohen (1992) found that adolescents with Down syndrome have poorer hearing and greater incidence of conductive hearing loss than their peers with mental retardation but without Down syndrome.

Special Testing Considerations

Little has been published on hearing assessment of adults with mental retardation. However, it is well documented that audiologists must use test techniques that will bridge the difference between the chronologic and developmental age of individuals with cognitive disabilities in order to obtain valid test results (Diefendorf, 2003; Roush, 2004). That is, the patient's mental or developmental age, not their chronologic age, should be considered when selecting appropriate test procedures and materials. Several investigators have evaluated the effectiveness of VRA with children having mental retardation, including those with Down syndrome (Greenberg et al., 1978; Thompson et al., 1979). With typically developing children and those with mental retardation, VRA is effective with infants as young as 6 months developmental age. However, children with Down syndrome require a developmental age of 10 to 12 months to participate in a VRA procedure. Furthermore, behavioral thresholds of infants with Down syndrome have been found to be 10 to 25 dB poorer than those of typically developing infants when all had normal hearing verified via ABR (Werner et al., 1996). This elevation of behavioral thresholds is presumed to be the result of more inattentive behavior on the part of the children with Down syndrome relative to their typically developing peers.

Although it is recommended that audiologists attempt to elicit a spontaneous head-turn response during the VRA conditioning process (Tharpe and Ashmead, 1993), some children with mental retardation may not have developed auditory localization ability. In such cases, several administrations of paired conditioning trials (pairing the stimulus and the reinforcer) may be required. If the patient does not respond to the auditory stimuli, the audiologist may be left with the question, "Does the patient not hear the stimuli, or can she or he not perform the task?" One method that can answer this question is for the audiologist to place a vibrator either in the patient's hand or on the head and, using a low-frequency stimulus at approximately 50 to 60 dB hearing level (HL), determine if the patient can perform the task using this vibrotactile cue. In this way, the patient is able to feel the stimulus and thus is not required to hear in order to participate. If the patient is able to cooperate for the task under these vibrotactile conditions, then the audiologist should return to the auditory stimuli and continue testing with the knowledge that the patient understands the task.

If using a play audiometric technique, it is often appropriate for the audiologist to demonstrate the play task to the patient with mental retardation rather than attempting to explain the instructions verbally. Because learning the desired response behaviors may take longer for children and adults with mental retardation, it may be useful to have them practice the listening task at home prior to coming to the clinic. It is important to keep the task as similar as possible to what will actually be expected in the clinical setting. Another approach is for the audiologist to demonstrate the task engaging the patient's parent or caregiver as the one being tested. The patient can then observe the procedure being conducted and see what is required. If the patient has some language, the audiologist should keep verbal instructions short, simple, and accompanied by gestures. Nonverbal expressions of reinforcement can be used generously (e.g., smiles, clapping, thumbs up) to indicate to the patient that he or she is complying with the task. Audiologists should keep in mind that the reinforcement is provided to support the response behavior of the patient, not to indicate if the patient is correct or incorrect (i.e., can hear or not hear the stimulus). Additional time will likely be needed to complete the play task, and the audiologist should expect response delays as a result of additional time needed for the patient to process the instructions and formulate a response. It is not unusual for patients with mental retardation to have to return for more than one visit in order to complete testing. It is important in these cases to keep the examiner and the test procedures the same so that a routine can be established with the patient.

Whether using VRA, CPA, or conventional test procedures, it is recommended that control trials (no sound trials) be included throughout the testing session. This is especially true if working with individuals who have Down syndrome because they have a remarkable desire to please others and this often results in a high number of false-positive responses. Control trials are inserted randomly into the testing procedure at times when the audiologist would otherwise present the auditory signal. If a response is noted during a control trial, it is evidence of a false-positive result and should not be reinforced. This lack of a reward for a false response should reduce their frequency.

Although important for complete evaluation of all patients, it is particularly important to monitor the middle ear status of those with intellectual disabilities because they are known to have a higher degree of abnormal tympanometry and conductive hearing loss than the general population. Those with Down syndrome have an even higher incidence of otitis media than others with mental retardation because of the anatomic anomalies of the head and neck including the cochlea, ossicles, Eustachian tube, and nasopharynx. In addition, those with Down syndrome are highly susceptible to impacted cerumen because of narrow or stenotic external ear canals. Therefore, all hearing test procedures (e.g., ABR, VRA, play or conventional audiometry) should include the use of bone conduction testing when possible. A conductive component can mask the presence of sensory hearing loss, thus delaying the fitting of amplification.

There will likely be a heavy reliance on physiologic measures during the hearing assessment of patients with mental retardation. One should be mindful of the impact of abnormal middle ear function on otoacoustic emissions (OAE) and ABR. That is, OAEs will be absent in the presence of impacted cerumen or middle ear effusion. Therefore, immittance audiometry will be an important component of the test battery. In a review of ABR studies in persons with Down syndrome, Dille (2003) concluded that ABR testing should be interpreted with caution because it is likely that those with Down syndrome demonstrate a neural developmental time course that is uniquely different than that of typically developing individuals. Thus, comparing latency-intensity functions to normative values might result in erroneous conclusions. Widen et al. (1987) suggested that the ABR interpretation be based on both threshold of the response and latency-intensity series.

Special Management Considerations

Because of the high incidence of middle ear disease in those with mental retardation, especially those who are institutionalized or have Down syndrome, it is most efficient to have otologic examinations prior to audiologic assessments. The otologic examinations can serve to ensure that the external canals are free of cerumen and that no active middle ear infection is present. Individuals with Down syndrome, regardless of age, should receive otologic and audiologic monitoring about every 3 months in order to manage cerumen and middle ear disease. By school age, between 30% and 50% of children with Down syndrome have had pressure-equalizing (PE) tubes. However, diligent audiologic and otologic monitoring is required because of the high failure rate of PE tubes in those with Down syndrome.

For those requiring amplification, several issues must be considered. First, the implementation of prescriptive amplification fitting is recommended for all children and adults. Individual or age-appropriate ear acoustics should be taken into account in the hearing aid selection and fitting process. This is accomplished by measurement and application of the real-ear-to-coupler difference (RECD) (see Chapter 38; Moodie et al., 1994). It is not uncommon for audiologists to use age-average RECD values as opposed to measuring them directly. However, one must consider the potential impact that any craniofacial anomaly (including Down syndrome) may have on this practice. Because of the typically smaller ear canals in individuals with Down syndrome, it is quite likely that an age-average RECD will result in an underestimation of ear canal sound pressure level, thus leading to over amplification.

Second, individuals with craniofacial anomalies or who have mental retardation may have difficulty keeping hearing aids in place for a number of reasons. The use of wig tape or other hearing aid retention devices can help them stay in place behind the patient's ears.

Third, bone-conduction hearing aids may need to be considered for patients with chronic or recurrent middle ear disease or stenotic canals. Bone-conduction hearing aids will be limited to those with mild to moderate levels of hearing loss because of power limitations of the hearing aid. In addition, for those with draining ears who use traditional air-conduction hearing aids, aids may need to be removed temporarily during times of active drainage.

Finally, the fitting of amplification may be delayed in individuals with mental retardation because of other health care needs and concerns of the family. However, the earlier amplification is introduced, the easier it may be to incorporate it into the patient's daily routine and the better the prognosis is for long-term acceptance. The parents or caretakers of patients with mental retardation should receive careful and frequent instruction on the use and care of the amplification devices. Of course, to the extent possible, patients should be included in this educational process and encouraged to participate in the care of the device.

VISUAL IMPAIRMENT

The combination of vision and hearing deficits may be congenital or acquired later in life. Although often referred to as "deaf-blindness," one should keep in mind that the term "deaf-blind" typically refers to persons with dual sensory impairments who have some residual hearing and usable vision (Miles, 2003; Moore, 1990). Possible etiologies include syndromes such as:

- CHARGE syndrome – A specific pattern of birth defects represented by the acronym CHARGE: "C" for coloboma, "H" for heart defects, "A" for atresia choanae, "R" for retardation of growth and development, "G" for genitourinary problems, and "E" for ear abnormalities.
- Usher syndrome – The most common condition that involves both hearing and vision problems; an autosomal recessive disorder with primary symptoms that include hearing loss and progressive

retinitis pigmentosa. The vision difficulties include the onset of night blindness, which may become apparent during a child's school years, followed by loss of peripheral vision typically leading to severe low vision or blindness.
- Bardet-Biedl syndrome – A complex disorder that affects many parts of the body including the retina. Individuals with this syndrome have a retinal degeneration similar to retinitis pigmentosa.
- Goldenhar syndrome – A congenital birth defect that involves deformities of the face. Characteristics include a partially formed or totally absent ear (acrotia or anotia) and one missing eye.

Other causative factors for vision and hearing deficits occurring together include congenital prenatal infections (e.g., rubella, toxoplasmosis, herpes, CMV). The rubella epidemic of 1963 to 1965 contributed to the birth of more than 2,500 children with deaf-blindness in the United States. By 2001, there were an estimated 10,000 children in the United States alone who were considered to be deaf-blind (Teaching Research Institute, 2001). There are also postnatal causes of vision and hearing deficits (e.g., meningitis, asphyxia, stroke). As seen in Table 29.3, a majority of individuals who are deaf-blind have additional disabilities such as physical impairments, cognitive impairments, and behavior disorders. In fact, more than 60% of individuals who are deaf-blind have IQs lower than 50 (Jensema, 1980).

Children with hearing loss are two to three times more likely to develop ophthalmic abnormalities than their normal-hearing peers (Guy et al., 2003; Regenbogen and Godel, 1985). The irony is that people with hearing loss have a greater reliance on their vision for communication and environmental monitoring than those with normal hearing. Therefore, audiologists should encourage families of patients with hearing loss to have their vision monitored on a regular basis.

TABLE 29.3	Additional disabilities in deaf-blind youth in 2000
Disability	**% of deaf-blind youth**
Physical impairments	54.4
Cognitive impairments	69.9
Behavior disorders	8.4
Complex health care needs	37.7
Other impairments	32.2

From Mascia J, Mascia N. (2003) Methods and strategies for audiological assessment of individuals who are deaf-blind with developmental disabilities. *Semin Hear.* 24, 211–221.

Special Testing Considerations

One of the first things that an audiologist should determine is the patient's preferred sense (typically, it is tactile), and then the audiologist should let the patient explore the test environment for a short period of time or until the patient appears to be comfortable. In addition to the environment, the patient must be given time to "find the audiologist," rather than the audiologist imposing on the patient's space. It is important to remember that individuals who are deaf-blind may explore their environments tactilely, but many are also tactile-defensive, so they must be approached slowly. As the patient becomes more comfortable in the environment and with the test situation, the rules about space and touching may change (Mascia and Mascia, 2003).

During activities that require the audiologist to touch the patient (e.g., otoscopic examination, insertion of earphones), it is recommended that the patient be given as much involvement as possible. That is, the patient should be allowed to examine the equipment (e.g., otoscope, earphones) tactilely. Then, with the patient's hand still in contact, the otoscope, probe, or earphone can be slowly guided to the patient's ear. This process will require patience by the audiologist and may require more than one visit (Mascia and Mascia, 2003).

Auditory responsiveness of individuals who are deaf-blind may be compromised by their lack of curiosity (Moore, 1990). Thus, they may not turn toward the source of sound for a VRA procedure. As discussed in the section on individuals with mental retardation, pairing the auditory stimuli with a vibrotactile stimulus may be necessary to condition the patient to the task (Mascia and Mascia, 2003; Moore, 1990). Once the patient has learned to respond consistently to the paired auditory and tactile stimulation, it can be assumed that the task is understood, and the tactile stimulation can be eliminated.

The selection of an appropriate reinforcement for behavioral tasks is critical. As previously mentioned, most individuals classified as deaf-blind have some residual vision. Therefore, even light perception can allow for successful implementation of visual reinforcement. This may require a slight dimming of the test suite lights to enhance the visual reinforcement for the patient. In some cases, a penlight positioned close to the patient and activated in response to a head turn or searching behavior can be implemented. If visual reinforcement is not possible, some patients may enjoy feeling specific textures, vibration, social praise, juice, food bits, or interesting toys (Moore, 1990). In any case, it will be important to consult with the patient's caregivers or teachers to assist in determining a desirable reinforcement.

It is also important when behaviorally assessing the hearing of a patient who is deaf-blind to determine an appropriate response to the stimulus. Parents, caregivers, and teachers may all be valuable resources in evaluating what kind of motor response can be expected from the patient in re- sponse to sound. Some possible responses include a head turn, reaching, arm raise, finger raise, or leg swing. Additionally, Moore (1990) suggested that it may often be necessary to physically "show" the patient when and how to perform the response by manipulating the patient's hand, leg, or foot into place when the auditory stimulus is presented. This assistance can gradually be decreased using successive approximations until the child is able to respond with no cuing or assistance from the clinician.

Special Management Considerations

It is likely that individuals with dual hearing and vision impairments will welcome the use of amplification when indicated. After all, the majority of this population has some degree of residual hearing ability (Michael and Paul, 1990), and enhancement of hearing could serve as an important supplement to less-than-optimal visual input. A recent survey of clinical audiologists confirmed the belief that those with vision and hearing difficulties could potentially benefit more from amplification than those with hearing loss alone (Tharpe et al., 2001). In addition, amplification for those with dual impairments has a role beyond that of only enhancing speech perception ability (Wiener and Lawson, 1997). That is, audiologists need to consider more than just enhancing speech perception and must also focus on the role hearing has in orientation and mobility, which is essential to the development of successful independent living skills (Tharpe et al., 2002).

Orientation and mobility refer to one's location relative to environmental features and moving safely through one's environment.

Much research has been conducted on hearing aid specifications designed to enhance speech perception ability, but considerably less research exists on enhancing the detection of environmental auditory cues. It is unknown whether there is a combination of hearing aid characteristics that can be used to enhance speech perception and also improve detection of environmental cues or that can possibly affect one or the other adversely. The need for an integrated approach is apparent for individuals with dual sensory impairments who need to coordinate the aspects of guiding, route instruction, and verbal communication. Even the limited research that has been done on sound localization with hearing aids has not considered the specific spatial hearing needs of persons with visual impairments. Because speech recognition is based mostly on frequencies above 500 Hz, it is common for hearing aids to attenuate frequencies below a cutoff level in the range of 500 to 1,000 Hz. This low-frequency cutoff is designed to reduce background sounds that may interfere with speech perception. However, that frequency range contains critical information for orientation and mobility with respect to traffic sounds (Wiener et al., 1997) and environmental surfaces such as walls (Ashmead et al., 1998). A third important property of hearing aids is the flexibility to switch between different configurations. That is, hearing aids that are programmable can be set to run in several different configurations. Assuming that different listening situations require different hearing aid settings for optimal perception, this flexibility will be important to consider in rehabilitation strategies for those with vision and hearing impairments.

Numerous investigators have found that directional microphones provide an advantage when listening to speech in noise under laboratory conditions. However, omnidirectional microphones appear to enhance localization ability under certain laboratory conditions and, perhaps, in real-world settings (Tharpe et al., 2002). A considerable amount of research is still needed in order to enhance our knowledge in this area. In the meantime, one should be cautious when selecting microphone options for use by individuals with significant vision and hearing deficits. It appears reasonable to offer a switchable directional/omnidirectional microphone option to those with significant visual impairments who must rely on their hearing for getting around their environments safely. Instruction regarding careful head positioning during communication, especially when using a directional microphone, appears warranted.

with some knowledge of the characteristics of a number of disabilities, early planning for and adjustments to diagnostic procedures, and careful consideration of individual and family needs, one can obtain valid and reliable test results that lead to meaningful audiologic management.

Part of facing this challenge requires recognizing and admitting that no one can be an expert on all disabilities. With these patients, probably more than most, we must acknowledge that our expertise may be limited and that we must work with a multidisciplinary team of professionals, the patient, and the patient's family in developing effective diagnostic and management strategies.

Finally, as with all patients, audiologists must consider the patient's and family's priorities as they relate to the hearing loss. For example, those with multiple disabilities may have other significant medical needs requiring substantial time and emotional energy. As such, the family may choose to defer the management of hearing loss until a time when they can more readily accept the challenge. Audiologists must be respectful of a family's decisions and be prepared to support and encourage families in their choices.

 ## SUMMARY

The assessment and management of individuals with multiple disabilities is a great challenge for audiologists. However,

 ## ACKNOWLEDGEMENT

The author would like to thank Jamie L. Watson for her assistance in the research and preparation of this chapter.

REFERENCES

American Psychiatric Association. (1994) *Diagnostic and Statistical Manual of Mental Disorders*. 4th ed. Revised. Washington, DC: American Psychiatric Association.

Ashmead DH, Wall RS, Eaton SB, Ebinger KA, Snook-Hill MM, Guth DA, Yang X. (1998) Echolocation reconsidered: using spatial variations in the ambient sound field to guide locomotion. *J Vis Impair Blind*. 92, 615–632.

Beange H, McElduff A, Baker W. (1995) Medical disorders of adults with mental retardation: a population study. *Am J Ment Retard*. 99, 595–604.

Bertrand J, Mars A, Boyle C, Bove F, Yeargin-Allsop M, Decoufle P. (2001) Prevalence of autism in a United States population: The Brick Township, New Jersey, investigation. *Pediatrics*. 108, 1155–1161.

Brask BH. (1972) A prevalence investigation of childhood psychoses. In: *Nordic Symposium on the Comprehensive Care of Psychotic Children*. Oslo: Barnepsykiatrist Forening; pp 145–153.

Cano A, Fons J, Brines J. (2001) The effects of offspring of premature parturition. *Hum Reprod Update*. 7, 487–494.

Dean J, Harris F. (2003) Adaptive hierarchical test procedures for developmentally delayed adults: taking the "difficult" out of "difficult to test." *Semin Hear*. 24, 247–262.

Diefendorf AO. (2003) Behavioral hearing assessment: considerations for the young child with developmental disabilities. *Semin Hear*. 24, 189–200.

Dille MF. (2003) Perspectives on the audiological evaluation of individuals with Down syndrome. *Semin Hear*. 24, 201–210.

Evenhuis HM. (1995) Medical aspects of ageing in a population with intellectual disability: II. Hearing impairment. *J Intellect Disabil Res*. 39, 27–33.

Filipek PA, Accardo PJ, Ashwal S, Baranek GT, Cook EH Jr, Dawson G, Gordon B, Gravel JS, Johnson CP, Kallen RJ, Levy SE, Minshew NJ, Ozonoff S, Prizant BM, Rapin I, Rogers SJ, Stone WL, Teplin SW, Tuchman RF, Volkmar FR. (2000) Practice parameter: screening and diagnosis of autism. *Neurology*. 55, 468–479.

Fortnum H, Davis A. (1997) Epidemiology of permanent childhood hearing impairment in Trent Region, 1985-1993. *Br J Audiol*. 31, 409–466.

Fortnum H, Summerfield Q, Marshall D, Davis A, Bamford J. (2001) Prevalence of permanent childhood hearing impairment in the United Kingdom and implications for universal neonatal hearing screening: questionnaire based ascertainment study. *Br Med J*. 323, 1–5.

Freeman BJ, Ritvo ER, Needleman R, Yokata A. (1985) The stability of cognitive and linguistic parameters in autism: a five-year prospective study. *J Am Acad Child Psychiatry*. 24, 459–464.

Gallaudet Research Institute. (2005). Regional and national summary report of data from the 2004-2005 Annual Survey of Deaf and Hard of Hearing Children and Youth. Washington, DC: Gallaudet Research Institute, Gallaudet University.

Ghaziuddin M. (2000) Autism in mental retardation. *Curr Opin Psychiatry*. 13, 481–484.

Greenberg DB, Wilson WR, Moore JM, Thompson G. (1978) Visual reinforcement audiometry (VRA) with young Down's syndrome children. *J Speech Hear Disord*. 43, 448–458.

Guy R, Nicholson J, Pannu SS, Holden R. (2003) A clinical evaluation of ophthalmic assessment in children with sensorineural deafness. *Child Care Health Dev.* 29, 377–384.

Hack M, Taylor HG, Klein N, Eiben R, Schatschneider C, Mercuri-Minich N. (1994) School-age outcomes in children with birthweights under 750 g. *N Engl J Med.* 331, 753–759.

Hassmann E, Skotnicka B, Midro AT, Musiatowicz M. (1998) Distortion products otoacoustic emissions in diagnosis of hearing loss in Down syndrome. *Int J Pediatr Otorhinolaryngol.* 45, 199–206.

Jensema C. (1980) A profile of deaf-blind children within various types of educational facilities. *Am Ann Deaf.* 125, 896–900.

Kadesjö B, Gillberg C, Hagsberg B. (1999) Brief report. Autism and Asperger syndrome in seven-year-old children. *J Autism Dev Disord.* 29, 327–332.

Kwok SK, Ho PC, Chan AK, Gandhi SR, Lam DS. (1996) Ocular defects in children and adolescents with severe mental deficiency. *J Intellect Disabil Res.* 40, 330–335.

Lieberman LJ, Volding L, Winnick JP. (2004) Comparing motor development of deaf children of deaf parents and deaf children. *Am Ann Deaf.* 149, 281–289.

Lloyd LL, Spradlin JE, Reid MJ. (1968) An operant audiometric procedure for difficult-to-test patients. *J Speech Hear Disord.* 33, 236–245.

Lord C, Risi S, Lambrecht L, Cook EH, Leventhal BL, DiLavor PC, Pickles A, Rutter M. (2000) The Autism Diagnostic Observation Schedule – Generic: a standard measure of social and communication deficits associated with the spectrum of autism. *J Autism Dev Disord.* 24, 659–686.

Mace AL, Wallace KL, Whan MQ, Stelmachowicz PG. (1991) Relevant factors in the identification of hearing loss. *Ear Hear.* 12, 287–293.

MacFarland SZC. (2003) Current trends and issues in understanding adults with developmental disabilities. *Semin Hear.* 24, 171–178.

Mandell DS, Novak MM, Zubritsky CD. (2005) Factors associated with age of diagnosis among children with autism spectrum disorders. *Pediatrics.* 116, 1480–1486.

Marcell MM, Cohen S. (1992) Hearing abilities of Down syndrome and other mentally handicapped adolescents. *Res Dev Disabil.* 13, 533–551.

Mascia J, Mascia N. (2003) Methods and strategies for audiological assessment of individuals who are deaf-blind with developmental disabilities. *Semin Hear.* 24, 211–221.

Matkin N. (1977) Assessment of hearing sensitivity during the preschool years. In: Bess FH, ed. *Childhood Deafness.* New York: Grune & Stratton.

McCracken WM, Bamford JM. (1995) Auditory prosthesis for children with multiple handicaps. *Scand Audiol.* 24 (suppl 41), 51–60.

Mehta UC, Patel I, Castello FV. (2004) EEG sedation for children with autism. *J Dev Behav Pediatr.* 25, 102–104.

Michael MG, Paul PV. (1990) Early intervention for infants with deaf-blindness. *Except Child.* 57, 200–210.

Miles B. (2003) Overview on deaf-blindness. DB-Link, The National Information Clearinghouse on Children Who Are Deaf-Blind. Sands Point, NY: Helen Keller National Center.

Monville DK, Nelson NW. (1994) Parental viewpoints on change following auditory integration training for autism. *Am J Speech Lang Pathol.* 3, 41–53.

Moodie KS, Seewald RC, Sinclair ST. (1994) Procedure for predict-ing real-ear hearing aid performance in young children. *Am Audiol.* 3, 23–31.

Moore JM. (1990) Hearing assessment of deaf-blind children using behavioral conditioning. *Semin Hear.* 11, 385–392.

Moore JM. (1995) Behavioral assessment procedures based on conditioned head-turn response for auditory detection and discrimination with low-functioning children. *Scand Audiol.* 24 (suppl 41), 36–42.

Ohta M, Nagai Y, Hara H, Sasaki M. (1987) Parental perception of behavioral symptoms in Japanese autistic children. *J Autism Dev Disord.* 17, 549–563.

O'Shea TM, Klinepeter KL, Goldstein DJ, Jackson BW, Dillard RG. (1997) Survival and developmental disability in infants with birth weights of 501 to 800 grams, born between 1979 and 1994. *Pediatrics.* 100, 982–986.

Picard M. (2004) Children with permanent hearing loss and associated disabilities: revisiting current epidemiological data and causes of deafness. *Volta Rev.* 104, 221–236.

Regenbogen L, Godel V. (1985) Ocular deficiencies in deaf children. *J Pediatr Ophthalmol Strabismus.* 22, 231–233.

Robins DL, Fein D, Barton ML, Green JA. (2001) The Modified Checklist for Autism in Toddlers: an initial study investigating the early detection of autism and pervasive developmental disorders. *J Autism Dev Disord.* 31, 131–144.

Robinson RO. (1973) The frequency of other handicaps in children with cerebral palsy. *Dev Med Child Neurol.* 15, 305–312.

Roush J, Holcomb MA, Roush PA, Escolar ML. (2004) When hearing loss occurs with multiple disabilities. *Semin Hear.* 25, 333–345.

Rutter M. (2005) Incidence of autism spectrum disorders: changes over time and their meaning. *Acta Paediatr.* 94, 2–15.

Scott FJ, Baron-Cohen S, Bolton PB, Brayne C. (2002) Brief report: prevalence of autism spectrum conditions in children aged 5-11 years in Cambridgeshire, U.K. *Autism.* 6, 231–237.

Siegel B. (1996) *World of the Autistic Child: Understanding and Treating Autistic Spectrum Disorders.* New York: Oxford University Press; p 107.

Siegel B, Pliner C, Eschler J, Elliott GR. (1988) How children with autism are diagnosed: difficulties in identification of children with multiple developmental delays. *J Dev Behav Pediatr.* 9, 199–204.

Stone WL, Rosenbaum JL. (1988) A comparison of teacher and parent views of autism. *J Autism Dev Disord.* 20, 513–522.

Streppel J, Richling F, Roth B, Walger M, von Wedel H, Eckel H. (1998) Epidemiology and etiology of acquired hearing disorders in childhood in the Cologne area. *Int J Pediatr Otorhinolaryngol.* 44, 235–243.

Teaching Research Institute. (2001) National deaf-blind child count summary. Available at: http://www.tr.wou.edu/.

Tharpe AM, Ashmead DH. (1993) A computer simulation technique for assessing pediatric auditory test protocols. *J Am Acad Audiol.* 4, 2.

Tharpe AM, Ashmead DH, Ricketts TA, Rothpletz AM, Wall R. (2002) Optimization of amplification for deaf-blind children. In: Seewald RC, Gravel JS, eds. *A Sound Foundation through Early Amplification. 2001: Proceedings of the Second International Conference.* St. Edmundsbury, United Kingdom: St. Edmundsbury Press.

Tharpe AM, Bess FH, Sladen D, Schissel H, Couch S, Schery T. (2006) Auditory characteristics of children with autism. *Ear Hear.* 27, 430–431.

Tharpe AM, Fino-Szumski MS, Bess FH. (2001) Survey of hearing aid fitting practices for children with multiple impairments. *Am J Audiol.* 10, 1–9.

Thompson G, Wilson WR, Moore JM. (1979) Application of visual reinforcement audiometry (VRA) to low functioning children. *J Speech Hear Disord.* 44, 80–90.

Treffert DA. (1970) Epidemiology of infantile autism. *Arch Gen Psychiatry.* 22, 431–438.

Van Bourgondien ME, Mesibov GB, Dawson G. (1987) Pervasive developmental disorders: autism. In: Wolraich ML, ed. *The Practical Assessment and Management of Children with Disorders of Development and Learning.* Chicago: Yearbook Medical Publishers; pp 326–351.

Van Naarden K, Decoufle P, Caldwell K. (1999) Prevalence and characteristics of children with serious hearing impairment in metropolitan Atlanta, 1991–1993. *Pediatrics.* 103, 570–575.

van Schrojenstein Lantman-de Valk HM, van den Akker M, Maaskant MA, Haveman MJ, Urlings HF, Kessels AG, Crebolder HF. (1997) Prevalence and incidence of health problems in people with intellectual disability. *J Intellect Disabil Res.* 41, 42–51.

Volkmar FR, Cohen DJ, Paul R. (1986) An evaluation of DSM-III criteria for infantile autism. *J Am Acad Child Psychiatry.* 25, 190–197.

Werner LA, Mancl LR, Folsom RC. (1996) Preliminary observations on the development of auditory sensitivity in infants with Down syndrome. *Ear Hear.* 17, 455–468.

Widen JE, Folsom RC, Thompson G, Wilson WR. (1987) Auditory brainstem responses in young adults with Down syndrome. *Am J Mental Defic.* 91, 472–479.

Wiener WR, Lawson GD. (1997) Audition for the traveler who is visually impaired. In: Blasch BB, Wiener WR, Welsh RL, eds. *Foundations of Orientation and Mobility.* 2nd ed. New York: AFB Press.

Wiener WR, Lawson GD, Naghshineh K, Brown J, Bischoff A, Toth A. (1997) The use of traffic sounds to make street crossings by persons who are visually impaired. *J Vis Impair Blind.* 91, 435–445.

Wilson-Costello D, Friedman H, Minich N, Fanaroff AA, Hack M. (2005) Improved survival rates with increased neurodevelopmental disability for extremely low birth weight infants in the 1990s. *Pediatrics.* 115, 997–1003.

Wing L, Leekam SR, Libby SJ, Gould J, Larcombe M. (2002) The Diagnostic Interview for Social and Communication Disorders: background, inter-rater reliability and clinical use. *J Child Psychol Psychiatry.* 43, 307–325.

Wing L, Potter D. (2002) The epidemiology of autistic spectrum disorders: is the prevalence rising? *Ment Retard Dev Disabil Res Rev.* 8, 151–161.

Yeargin-Allsopp M, Rice C, Karapurkan T, Doernberg N, Boyle C, Murphy C. (2003) Prevalence of autism in a US metropolitan area. *JAMA.* 289, 49–55.

Zigman W, Schupf N, Sersen E, Silverman W. (1995) Prevalence of dementia in adults with and without Down syndrome. *Am J Ment Retard.* 100, 401–412.

30 Noise Exposure and Issues in Hearing Conservation

James Feuerstein and Marshall Chasin

INTRODUCTION

Audiology tends to be a reactive profession. Generally, the audiologist identifies the presence of hearing loss and then develops a remedial plan either through referral for medical evaluation and treatment or by finding ways to offset the communicative difficulties imposed by those losses. On the other hand, the role of the industrial audiologist is one of being proactive and aimed at conserving hearing by protecting workers from the deleterious effects of noise exposure.

It is estimated that approximately 30 million people in the United States are exposed to hazardous levels of noise on a routine basis, with the majority of noise exposure occurring in the workplace (National Institute for Occupational Safety and Health [NIOSH], 2000). Sound levels capable of damaging hearing occur in manufacturing, farming, landscaping, construction, mining, music, transportation, and many other jobs. Figure 30.1 (Industrial Acoustics Company [IAC], 1970) shows the distribution of noise levels that may be expected in the manufacturing sector. Because workers in some industries are also exposed to ototoxic chemicals or chemicals that increase susceptibility to damage from noise exposure, the number of people at risk for work-related hearing loss may be as high as 30 million (Franks et al., 1996). Noise is considered to be a contributing factor to more than one in three people having an adult-acquired hearing loss (National Institutes of Health [NIH], 1990). With very few exceptions, hearing loss due to noise exposure is completely preventable.

Noise can affect hearing in a variety of ways. At low levels, noise can interfere with communication without causing either short-term or long-term damage to the auditory system (Kryter, 1985). At higher levels, noise can cause a temporary hearing loss that may last for a relatively short period after the cessation of noise. If the intensity of the sound increases beyond a critical level, the noise may cause damage to the internal structures of the cochlea, resulting in a permanent hearing loss, and may even damage structures of the peripheral mechanism such as the tympanic membrane and the ossicular chain (Melnick, 1978). Subsequent changes in more central areas of the auditory system may also occur (Miller et al., 1992). The amount of damage sustained is a function, primarily, of the intensity of the signal and the duration of the exposure. The nature of the noise (continuous vs. impulsive), the spectrum of the noise, and the presence of ototoxic chemicals also play a role (NIH, 1990; Franks et al., 1996). Industrial noise is measured using the dBA (Goldstein, 1978; Lipscomb, 1988; Gelfand, 1997).

This chapter will review the impact of noise exposure on hearing and the standards developed to protect workers from noise exposure, provide a detailed discussion of the Occupational Safety and Health Administration (OSHA) regulations on noise exposure, and briefly discuss nonoccupational noise exposure. It is important for audiologists to be cognizant of the effect of noise on hearing and to be familiar with hearing conservation issues. The audiologist can play a critical role in preventing noise-induced hearing loss.

CHANGES IN HEARING DUE TO NOISE

The three types of hearing changes that may occur following noise exposure are referred to as noise-induced temporary threshold shift, noise-induced permanent threshold

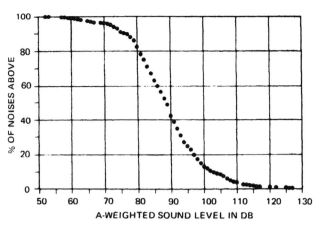

FIGURE 30.1 Distribution of sound levels in manufacturing industries. Each point on the vertical scale indicates the percentage of noises that exceeded the corresponding level on the horizontal scale. (Reprinted from Industrial Acoustics Company. [1970] *Hearing Conservation Notes.* **Bronx: Industrial Acoustics Company; Fig. 1.2, with permission.)**

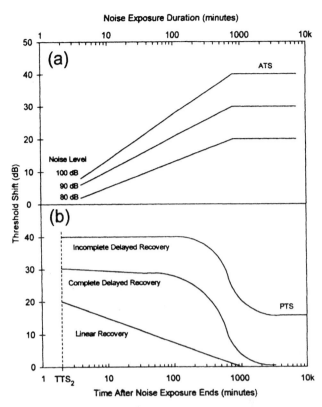

FIGURE 30.2 (A) Development of temporary threshold shift as a function of exposure duration (parameter is exposure level). **(B)** Patterns of recovery from temporary threshold shift following exposure. (Reprinted Gelfand SA. [1998] *Hearing: An Introduction to Physiological and Psychological Acoustics.* 3rd ed. New York: Marcel Dekker, Inc; p 330, Fig. 10.18, with permission.)

shift, and acoustic trauma (Melnick, 1978). Following is a brief overview of the nature of peripheral changes that take place in the auditory system in response to noise and some of the underlying factors that lead to those changes. More extensive coverage on this topic can be found in Lipscomb (1978), Kryter (1985), and Dancer et al. (1992). Physiologic changes in response to high-level noise have also been noted in the auditory nerve and central auditory system (Patuzzi, 1992).

Noise-Induced Temporary Threshold Shift

Noise-induced temporary threshold shift (NITTS) is a temporary reduction in hearing ability following exposure to loud sound. Typically, it is characterized by a reduction in sensitivity, a possible subjective fullness due to reduction in high-frequency sensitivity, and tinnitus. The symptoms of NITTS may be relatively brief, lasting less than 1 hour, or may extend up to several hours or days. The amount and duration of NITTS are related to the duration and intensity of the noise (Hirsh and Bilger, 1955; Mills et al., 1970; Melnick, 1978) and are summarized in Figure 30.2 (Gelfand, 1998). That is, lower levels of noise produce smaller amounts of NITTS than do higher noise levels. In addition, the shift grows as a function of the duration of the exposure during the first 8 hours, eventually reaching a plateau.

Stimulus frequency is also a factor in NITTS. For pure-tone stimuli, sounds in the 2,000- to 6,000-Hz range are the most effective at producing changes, with lower and higher frequency sounds producing lesser amounts of shift. For low-level NITTS, the shift in hearing occurs at the stimulus frequency. When greater amounts of NITTS are observed, the shift is typically observed at a frequency about one half to one full octave above the stimulus frequency (Ward, 1973; Schmiedt, 1984).

There are a variety of underlying physiologic changes associated with NITTS (Wenthold et al., 1992). Metabolic changes result from the hair cells being unable to maintain proper cell function (e.g., swelling of the hair cells). As swelling occurs, the hair cells may rotate, changing the orientation of the stereocilia to the tectorial membrane.

Although noise exposures causing permanent damage often have an overlaid NITTS component, susceptibility to NITTS is a poor predictor of risk for the development of permanent damage (NIH, 1990), especially in situations where noise exposure is intermittent or where impact/impulse noise is present (Gelfand, 1997).

Noise-Induced Permanent Threshold Shift

Noise-induced permanent threshold shift (NIPTS) occurs when there is less than a full recovery from NITTS. This may be a fairly common occurrence, with small amounts of permanent damage taking place following each of many NITTS experiences.

Swelling of the hair cells after noise exposure can lead to some cells rupturing and permanent loss. Hair cells may also become distorted, and the stereocilia may become fused (Durrant, 1978) or no longer transmit energy effectively to the hair cells (NIH, 1990). Progressive damage, in turn, may lead to degeneration of auditory nerve fibers and to changes within the central auditory system (NIH, 1990).

If the number of hair cells affected is small, there may be no perceptual change in hearing following early exposures. The effects of these very small changes appear to be cumulative, which is a key factor in the insidious nature of noise exposure. Although NITTS may be quite noticeable immediately after noise exposure, the small amount of NIPTS that remains after NITTS recovery may not be. That is, these small changes are often imperceptible relative to the subjective improvement from NITTS during the hours or days after exposure. As with other slowly progressive conditions, people with developing NIPTS may develop compensatory behaviors in the early stages (possibly unconsciously), or the hearing loss may not be acknowledged until a significant impact on lifestyle has occurred. It may take years of repeated exposures before the person perceives any change in hearing. Unfortunately, by then, it is too late.

The basic factors associated with NIPTS are intensity, duration, and spectrum. None of these factors is a stand-alone entity. They and other factors interact in significant and complex ways.

INTENSITY

The greater the intensity (above a minimum level of about 75 to 80 dBA), the greater is the risk of permanent damage (Passchier-Vermeer, 1974; Johnson, 1978). However, the impact of intensity is influenced greatly by the temporal pattern of exposure (i.e., moment-to-moment variation in intensity). Noise may be described as "steady-state," "fluctuating," "intermittent," or "impulsive." Steady-state noise is a continuous noise that does not vary by more than ± 5 dB and contains no impulse signals. Workers operating machinery that runs constantly or who work in areas with many machines running simultaneously will likely have this type of exposure. Fluctuating noise is continuous but varies by more than ± 5 dB over time, either gradually or rapidly. Workers who have mobility within their work settings frequently experience fluctuating noise levels. Intermittent noise is hazardous noise exposure mixed with periods of nonhazardous levels. This type of noise is very common for workers who use hand tools (e.g., welding, drilling) and for those who run equipment that is frequently turned on and off (such as machine processes with multiple set ups during the day); intermittent noise is also common in recreational activities. Impulse and/or impact noise may also be present in the industrial environment. Impulse noise is "a short duration sound that is characterized by a shock wave having nearly instantaneous rise time" (Hodge and Price, 1978). This type of noise is closely associated with explosions and does not last more

than one-half second. Impact noise has a longer rise time and duration. This is the type of noise associated with hammering or riveting (Hodge and Price, 1978).

Determining steady-state noise exposure levels is relatively easy. Levels of fluctuating or intermittent exposures are more difficult to quantify. One method is to equate the fluctuating sound to a steady-state noise of equal total acoustic energy. This method, the equalized sound level (Leq), is often used for measuring environmental noise and correlates fairly well with the physiologic effects of noise exposure (EPA, 1973; 1974). The Leq is based on an equal energy assumption. That is, a sound of 90 dB that lasts 2 minutes is assumed to have the same total energy as a sound of 93 dB that lasts for only 1 minute. In industrial settings, other methods tend to be used more (e.g., the principle of equal hazard). Examples of such measurement schemes are noise dose and the time-weighted average (TWA); these methods are described in more detail later on in this chapter. In all of these methods, the duration of the moment-to-moment sound levels must be known. They are best compiled by a noise dosimeter—sound measurement equipment designed to integrate the information into a single number.

DURATION

Longer exposure to noise above the minimum intensity level needed to induce NITTS (approximately 75 to 80 dBA) increases the risk of NIPTS. The risk of significant permanent damage from a single noise event is, actually, relatively rare. Slowly developing hearing losses associated with repeated daily exposure to noise are of more pressing concern and are more pervasive. Long-term exposure studies have shown a clear link between the number of years of daily exposure and the degree and configuration of hearing loss (Taylor et al., 1965; Baughn, 1973; Johnson, 1978). Therefore, it is necessary to evaluate the long-term exposure pattern of industrial workers. This need is one of the driving factors in the development of damage risk criteria (discussed below).

SPECTRUM

Most noise exposures are complex, variable, broadband signals. As with higher level NITTS, studies have shown that the damage from broadband signals typically occurs in the octave band above the noise (Ward, 1973; Kryter, 1985). Assuming industrial noise to be of relatively equal energy across the low to mid frequencies, the external ear's natural resonance in the 2,000- to 3,000-Hz range should result in maximal damage in the region between 4,000 and 6,000 Hz. This is consistent with the classic audiometric results for noise-induced hearing loss.

Acoustic Trauma

Acoustic trauma occurs following exposure to a single event involving extremely intense noise, such as an explosion. Even a brief exposure to a very intense sound can result in

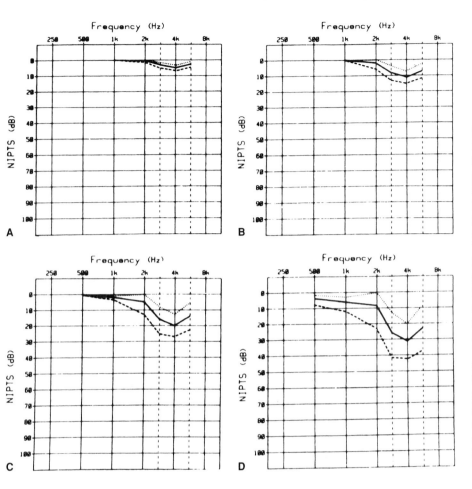

FIGURE 30.3
Noise-induced permanent threshold shift (NIPTS) graphed with audiogram format. NIPTS is shown for the 10th (*dotted line*), 50th (*solid line*), and 90th (*dashed line*) percentiles. The duration of exposure is 10 years. The individual graphs A to D represent the predicted results from exposure to 85, 90, 95, and 100 dBA, respectively, as derived by using ISO 1999. (Reprinted with permission from Melnick W. [1984] Auditory effects of noise exposure. In: Miller MH, Silverman CA, eds. *Occupational Hearing Conservation*. Englewood Cliffs, NJ: Prentice Hall; 100–131.)

permanent cochlear damage. In addition, the eardrum may be ruptured and/or the ossicular chain may be fractured. In these instances, the hearing loss is noticeable immediately (NIH, 1990).

Summary

The effects of workplace noise exposure are summarized in Figure 30.3, which represents the predicted hearing losses for workers exposed to different average sound levels over a 10-year period (Melnick, 1994). For low levels of noise exposure, there is minimal shift, and hearing remains within normal limits. For higher exposure levels, the degree of hearing loss increases, as does the variability in severity. Note also that the greatest amount of hearing loss occurs in the 2,000- to 6,000-Hz region, with the most hearing loss occurring at 4,000 Hz. This classic "noise-induced notch" is a function of the ear's response to broadband signals. As exposure levels increase and as factors such as age comingle with the noise exposure, hearing at frequencies outside the 2,000- to 6,000-Hz range will also be progressively affected. There appears to be at least some plateau effect with purely noise-induced hearing loss. Evidence suggests that the largest shifts in hearing occur during the first 10 to 15 years of noise exposure (Nixon and Glorig, 1961). While the characteristic hearing loss is one of a sloping configuration, the noise notch may disappear with progressively greater amounts of loss in the 8,000-Hz range, and the loss may flatten as the lower frequency regions of the cochlea become involved. The most common configuration of hearing loss due to long-term noise exposure is a bilaterally symmetric loss, but asymmetry is possible (NIH, 1990).

NONAUDITORY EFFECTS OF NOISE EXPOSURE

Nonauditory effects of noise exposure are those effects that do not cause hearing loss. Some of these are seen by changes in body functions, such as heart rate, and in learning/cognition in children. Nonauditory effects of noise exposure have been noted as far back as 1930 (Smith and Laird, 1930). In that specific study, nonauditory effects pertain to stomach contractions in healthy human beings when exposed to noise.

There are both laboratory and field studies of nonauditory effects. Laboratory studies set up well-controlled conditions and, therefore, are more suited to examine specific changes but are typically unsuited for examining long-term effects that may result in disease or cognitive/educational problems (Bronzaft, 1991). While laboratory studies can be more precise than field studies, they may or may not have any bearing on reality. In contrast, field studies are inherently less well designed in order to control for unwanted variables, but their conclusions may be more applicable to reality. Field studies are well suited to look at the long-term effects of disease and/or educational effects. For example, Stansfeld et al. (2000) demonstrate that, although transportation (truck) noise can disturb sleep patterns in a well-controlled laboratory setting, this is generally not the case in field studies because people tend to adapt over time to environmental noise. A major difficulty with all research into nonauditory factors is that subjective responses not based on intensity or duration may be quite significant. There are three classic studies from the early 1980s that provide an excellent overview for the interested reader: Thompson (1981), Cohen and Weinstein (1981), and DeJoy (1984). More recent studies have found similar results. High variability and questionable applicability continue to plague research in this very difficult area.

Cardiovascular Effects

In well-defined laboratory studies, the "noise/stress hypothesis is well understood: Noise activates the pituitary-adrenal-cortical axis and the sympathetic-adrenal-medullary axis. Changes in stress hormones including epinephrine, norepinephrine and cortisol are frequently found in acute and chronic noise experiments. The catecholamines and steroid hormones affect the organism's metabolism" (Babisch, 2002, p 1). However, few measurable biologic changes are directly or indirectly related to clinical changes in a population.

Most of the studies on cardiovascular effects have been performed in the laboratory on animals (mostly on rats). However, DeJoy (1984) commented that the rat may not be an appropriate model and that a primate species may be more appropriate. When primates were used in the laboratory, it was also found that blood pressure increased as the noise levels increased, but there was a large degree of variability in the studies.

In the few field studies on humans, blood pressure has been measured, but again, the level of variability is great. Sloan (1991, p 23), reviewing available data, notes that when taken as a whole "although there are inconsistencies in the findings . . . they generally support the assertion that exposure to noise is associated with higher levels of blood pressure." Data are still limited, however, and the results may depend on many uncontrolled factors, such as subjective response, the exact nature of physiologic assessment, and the animal model. In addition, it is still not known whether increased blood pressure in a noisy environment will lead to cardiovascular disease. Stansfeld et al. (2000) echo this concern and demonstrate that although laboratory studies show an association between noise and cardiovascular disease, field studies show only a weak relationship.

The physiologic rationales of the effects on body chemistry as a result of increased exposure to noise are beyond the scope of this chapter, but the interested reader is referred to Raymond (1991) and Babisch (2002).

Effects of Noise on Sleep

Pollak (1991, p 41) noted that "(1) noises are more annoying when they occur at times when people expect to rest or sleep, (2) noise can interrupt sleep, and (3) noise can also have subtle effects on sleep . . . that are detectable only with specialized instruments." Most laboratory studies use truck and aircraft noise as stimuli and measure the effect on a range of sleep study parameters. Noise can delay sleep and shift the sleep stages upward (i.e., more shallow sleeping). Upward sleep stage shifts have been observed even in relative quiet with 25 to 30 dB sound pressure level (SPL). Cardiovascular changes are usually not noted until the stimulus level is just below the arousal level for that individual. Thiessen (1978; 1983) found that as peak noise intensity increased, there was a linear increase in the probability of a change in sleep stage. Similar results have been found by Ouis (2002) and Matheson et al. (2003).

Effects of Noise on Fetal Development

There are some data suggesting an increased risk of noise-induced damage in fetuses, but this is still a very controversial issue. The interested reader is referred to Ryals (1990) and Stansfeld et al. (2000) for more information.

Nakamura (1977) noted low birth weights when the pregnant mother was exposed to high levels of occupational noise. Schell (1981) found that noise may in fact decrease birth weight. However, Edmonds et al. (1979) found that aircraft noise exposure had no significant effect on fetal development in pregnant women. Stansfeld et al. (2000), in laboratory studies, found no evidence that noise exposure contributes to congenital birth defects or low birth weight.

Effects of Noise on Learning

When speech is masked by background noise (e.g., at a noisy party), this is similar to having a hearing loss (with equivalent masked hearing thresholds). Children with even slight hearing losses have been shown to have decreased educational and cognitive performance. Davis (1985) found that children with a minimal (25 dB) hearing loss scored almost two full grade levels lower in reading comprehension by grade 4 (despite having minimal differences in grade 1).

Specifically with respect to normal-hearing children in a noisy school environment, Cohen et al. (1973) found that children whose classrooms were on the street level (nearer to truck and car noise) performed poorer in reading ability than children whose classrooms were in quieter locations. Bronzaft and McCarthy (1975) studied the reading ability of children in one school near elevated train tracks. Half the classrooms faced the train track, and the other half were on the quieter back part of the school. Students in the quieter classrooms did better on reading achievement tests, and by grade 6, those in the quieter classrooms were a full grade point ahead of those in the noisier classrooms. Green et al. (1982), in studying children near a New York airport, found that as noise level increased, the percentage of those children falling below grade reading level also increased. Wachs (1982) noted that children were slower to develop language skills in noisier homes. More recently, Matheson et al. (2003) noted similar results with low but significant correlations between neuroendocrine tests, blood pressure measurements, and educational success.

Again, it should be stressed that presence of biologic measures, such as heightened hormone or blood pressure levels, does not necessarily relate to long-term clinical changes in a population. While these changes may have long-term effects, there is no current evidence to support this extrapolation.

■ SOURCES OF NOISES IN THE MODERN WORLD

People recognize that the military and industry are high noise sources. In the military, there is equipment such as tanks, jet aircraft, and other heavy machinery, and personnel are exposed to rifle fire and explosions (in training and combat). Thus, noise exposure is an ongoing risk. In industrial settings, heavy equipment, machinery, printing presses, etc., also create an environment in which individuals may be exposed to hazardous noise levels. However, it is more difficult for the average person to recognize that everyday noise may be a contributing factor in the development of noise-induced hearing loss.

The largest potential source of noise exposure outside of occupational and military environments is from music exposure. This could be from listening to live music through amplifiers and speaker systems, listening through portable music players (such as CD or MP-3 players or Walkmans), and actual playing of music. By far, the largest contributor to a potential hearing loss is "portable music" because the CD, MP-3, or Walkman players can be used in noisy environments such as city streets where the volume needs to be turned up. In these situations, the most comfortable listening range is a higher SPL than in quieter or more controlled environments. Starting in the early 1970s, numerous studies have reported about the damaging effects of portable music (Wood and Lipscomb, 1972; Katz et al., 1982; Catalano and Levin, 1985; Lee et al., 1985; Rice et al., 1987; Turunen-Rise et al., 1991; Clark, 1991; Meyer-Bisch, 1996; LePage and Murray, 1998; Fligor and Cox, 2004). Of great interest is the Fligor and Cox (2004) study. In this well-controlled analysis of commercially available portable CD players, levels in excess of 121 dB SPL were measured depending on earphone. For example, with certain earphones, the outputs

were 7 to 9 dB greater than that same CD player with the manufacturer-supplied earphone. Peak SPLs were found in excess of 130 dB SPL. In general, Fligor and Cox (2004) found that greater outputs were produced when using physically smaller earphones. Fligor and Cox (2004, p 513) concluded that "based. . . on the noise dose model recommended by the National Institute for Occupational Safety and Health for protecting the occupational worker, a maximum permissible noise dose would typically be reached within 1 hr of listening with the volume control set to 70% of maximum gain using supra-aural headphones." In the interest of providing a straightforward recommendation, they state, "reasonable guidelines would [be] to limit headphone use to 1 hr or less per day if using supra-aural style headphones at a gain control setting of 60% maximum" (p 513). Based on their research, the maximum time that a CD player should be used if smaller insert earphones are used should be less than that recommendation.

Acoustic Trauma and the Musician

In addition to the overall long-term music exposure for musicians, exposure may include feedback squeals during sound checks, inappropriately set limiters, percussive blasts from cannons, and being stuck in front of a large stack of speakers for an extended performance. While there is scant research in the literature on the effects of single trauma impulses, clinical hearing loss has been confirmed where the source was a single or relatively short-duration blast. Reports of hearing loss due to long-term occupational noise exposure are numerous and, in some ways, better controlled because musical environments are much more poorly defined. In addition, unlike a worker in an occupational setting, musicians (and music lovers) may be subject to damaging levels of music exposure in their off-work hours.

Most models of noise-induced hearing loss are adequate for levels up to 115 dBA; however, they tend to break down for more intense impulse stimuli. Price and Kalb (1991) and Price (1994) investigated the effects of intense impulse sounds and found that the motion of the basilar membrane during the impulse sound was also important for the prediction of hearing loss (other than intensity and duration). Price (1994) noted "at lower SPLs losses are in all likelihood largely a function of the metabolic demand on the inner ear (it gets 'tired out') and that above some spectrally dependent critical level, the loss mechanism changes to one of mechanical disruption . . . (the ear gets 'torn up')." Price argues that if the basilar membrane is allowed to oscillate past the zero (atmospheric pressure) point, then more damage will be sustained by the hair cells in the organ of Corti. If impulses possess either completely positive or completely negative pressure waves, the displacement of the middle ear ossicles imparts sufficient energy to create a "tearing" action to the inner ear structures.

Although a cap pistol (at 30 cm) and two small wooden blocks (found in some Christmas carols) have almost identical peak SPLs (at 150 to 153 dB SPL), because of the shape of the pressure wave, the small wooden blocks would cause a 25-dB permanent hearing loss, but the cap pistol would only cause a 10-dB permanent hearing loss (Price, 1994).

The Audiometric Notch

Acoustic trauma typically shows up at, or near, the spectral peak frequency of the offending stimulus. A feedback squeal at 3,000 Hz will generate a sensory-neural hearing loss at about 3,000 Hz. In contrast to acoustic trauma, hearing loss from long-term noise or music exposure is typically in the 3,000- to 6,000-Hz region, and although there is a small dependence on spectral shape, this notched loss tends to be a hallmark of noise or music exposure. Coles et al. (2000) listed three primary criteria for the diagnosis of noise-induced hearing loss: (1) high-frequency sensory-neural hearing loss; (2) potentially hazardous amounts of noise exposure; and (3) high-frequency notch in the 3,000- to 6,000-Hz region. McBride and Williams (2001a) argued that although the 4,000-Hz notch is a well-established clinical sign of noise-induced hearing loss, the 6,000-Hz notch is variable and can be of limited value in correlating the loss to the noise exposure. McBride and Williams (2001b), in assessing the variability of this audiometric notch, noted that the "all rater index of agreement was 0.45" (p 106) and suggested that, because of this high clinician rating variability, other nonaudiometric factors such as case history be included in any diagnosis. Barrs et al. (1994), in a study of 246 workers, found that only 85% of those with noise exposure had a sloping high-frequency sensory-neural hearing loss. In addition, 20% of these workers had unexplained sensory-neural asymmetries that were subsequently investigated for retrocochlear pathology (with negative results).

Gates et al. (2000) found that, with older men (ages 58 to 80) who were exposed to noise earlier in their lives, 2,000 Hz decreased more than in a matched sample of men who were not exposed to noise. This implies that the effects of noise exposure may continue (at 2,000 Hz) long after noise exposure has ceased. The mechanism is reported to be unknown, but Gates et al. (2000) suspect that it is probably related to prior noise damage to the cochlea that did not show up on audiometric testing until much later, possibly due to a weakening of the support structures in the organ of Corti. However, Borg et al. (1995) found that, in reviewing a large number of studies with rabbits, an existing hearing loss does not make the ear more or less susceptible to future noise exposure.

What are the causes of the nonlinear monotonic nature of noise-induced hearing loss that creates an audiometric notch? Several explanations have been proposed for this notch. These include: (1) poor cochlear blood supply to the 3,000- to 6,000-Hz region (Crow et al., 1934); (2) greater susceptibility for damage of the supporting structures of hair cells in this region (Bohne, 1976); (3) orientation of the stapes

footplate aims its primary force toward those hair cells, causing eventual failure because of the constant hydromechanical action (Hilding, 1953; Schuknecht and Tonndorf, 1960); and (4) permanent noise exposure has its greatest effect approximately one-half octave above the peak frequency of the noise spectrum. Since all spectra are enhanced at 3,000 Hz by the outer ear canal resonance, the greatest loss will be in the 4,000- to 6,000-Hz region (Tonndorf, 1976; Pierson et al., 1994). Because of these phenomena, hearing losses due to noise or music exposure are relatively easy to spot.

However, many clinical cases of music or noise exposure do not have an audiometric notch. Indeed, Barrs et al. (1994) found that only 37% of workers suffering from noise exposure possessed an audiometric notch. It is quite possible that in advanced cases of exposure or advanced age where there is a significant age-related hearing loss ("presbycusis"), the hearing sensitivity at 8,000 Hz also may have deteriorated, leaving a flat audiometric configuration. In addition, depending on the noise spectrum, the damage may be above the audiometric test frequencies. For example, using data from violin players, the frequency of greatest damage can be at 8,000 Hz, and unless a higher frequency puretone is assessed (e.g., 10,000 Hz), a notch would not be apparent. Finally, the definition of a "noise notch" varies from study to study and has been defined as 15 dB worse than adjacent audiometric frequencies to over 30 dB worse.

Alberti (1982) argued that noise-induced hearing loss should be roughly symmetrical bilaterally. However, asymmetrical hearing losses are commonly found in those in the performing arts. Typical occupational environments for industrial workers are highly reverberant, with most of the sound pressure in the lower frequencies. Damaging sounds that emanate from one side may be almost as intense at the other side because of reverberations. In addition, because most of the sound is lower frequency, the head does not appreciably attenuate the sound from one side to the other. That is, there is no head shadow effect. Subsequently, even in asymmetrical noise situations, exposure tends to be symmetrical, with resulting symmetrical audiograms. In contrast, those in the performing arts work in relatively nonreverberant conditions where asymmetrical musical exposures (e.g., drummer near the right ear) may result in asymmetrical hearing loss. In addition, because of the significant mid- and high-frequency sound pressures (i.e., short wavelengths), the head acts to attenuate the off-side music exposure, producing acoustic shadow protection for the far ear. Nevertheless, audiometric asymmetries can be signs of serious medical problems and should be referred to the appropriate hearing health care professional for further assessment.

■ ASSESSING NOISE RISK

It is generally accepted that A-weighted SPLs less than 75 dB cause no measurable change in hearing, regardless of length of exposure (NIH, 1990). However, exposure to noise in excess of 80 dBA (of sufficient duration and exposure) on a routine basis over many years represents a general long-term exposure risk for developing significant hearing loss, for at least some individuals (Suter, 1988). Sound pressures exceeding 115 dB SPL are capable of causing at least some permanent damage following a single exposure of relatively short duration.

Because noise exposures do not affect all people to the same extent, estimates of the risk of developing hearing loss are necessary. These damage risk criteria (DRC) consider the intensity of the noise, the duration of the exposure (for either a single event or for repeated exposures over many years), and the percentage of people expected to develop significant hearing loss as a result of those exposures. They are designed as a predictive tool and serve as the basis for hearing conservation regulations.

It is possible to assess damage risk from at least two perspectives. The first is a prediction of the number of people at risk for developing hearing loss as a function of day-to-day noise exposure for various intensity levels. The second is the amount of time a given worker can spend in noise daily without incurring additional risk. It is beyond the scope of this chapter to examine fully these two options. The discussion that follows is designed to acquaint the reader with the basic issues involved in each type of risk assessment. More detailed information can be found in Hodge and Price (1978), Kryter (1985), and Henderson and Saunders (1998). Risk estimation as a function of noise exposure is a complex process. It is difficult to isolate the effects of noise over time at work from other factors affecting hearing, such as noise exposure during leisure activities. In addition, there is also the question of what constitutes a significant change in hearing. For instance, the Environmental Protection Agency (EPA, 1974) suggests that, as a general quality-of-life issue, a significant shift in hearing due to noise has occurred when there has been a change of greater than 5 dB at 4,000 Hz. Occupational regulations, on the other hand, are typically aimed at preventing the development of average hearing loss greater than 25 dB across the frequency range of 500 through 2,000 or 3,000 Hz and assess risk based on those criteria (United States Department of Labor [USDoL], 1981). Obviously, "safe" noise levels for these two end results are very different. Another complication arises when DRC are used in the regulatory process. It is an extension of the issue of how much protection is desired: How many people should be protected at what cost? Under the EPA guidelines, which call for daily exposure levels of less than 65 dBA, 4% to 10% of the population can be expected to develop a shift of greater than 5 dB at 4,000 Hz during their lives(EPA, 1974). Should these people be protected? Hearing loss sufficient to interfere with communication typically begins for some people who have daily exposure above 75 dBA, but only 5% of individuals with daily work exposure less than 85 dBA will develop such "material" hearing losses. Because the OSHA regulations (USDoL, 1983) regarding workplace noise apply to those individuals with daily exposure to levels at or above 85 dBA, it is likely that effective hearing con-

servation measures protect the vast majority of people with work-related noise exposures (Suter, 1988).

The process of determining how much time a worker can spend in noise of a given level without increased risk is also influenced by other factors associated with noise. The OSHA regulations are based on DRC that limit worker exposure to steady-state noise levels equal to or in excess of 90 dBA for a typical 8-hour workday. If exposure is less than 90 dBA, then the amount of time in the noise may be higher; if it is greater than 90 dBA, then the allowable exposure time is less than 8 hours. The International Organization for Standardization (ISO, 1990), on which many European noise regulations are based, and the National Institute for Safety and Health (NIOSH, 1974) in the United States have advocated for an equal energy approach to the regulation of worker exposure to noise. Because a doubling of sound energy equates to a change in SPL of 3 dB, these groups have suggested that the time spent in noise should be reduced by half for every three 3-dB increase in SPL in order to maintain similar hazard.

Steady-state noise exposure for a full 8-hour period is more the exception than the rule in most industries. Industrial noise tends to be fluctuating or intermittent, and most workers have noise-free, or at least noise-reduced, periods such as set up, clean up, coffee breaks, and lunch. Because breaks from noise have been shown to reduce the overall impact of the exposure, OSHA uses a 5-dB time-intensity trade-off (USDoL, 1983). That is, for every 5-dB increase in noise level, exposure time should be reduced by 50%. While the 5-dB trade-off is designed to accommodate the breaks from noise that may occur in the typical work day, the 3-dB rule is more appropriate in instances where the noise includes impulse/impact types of noise. This is because impulse/impact noises have been shown to have a greater than predicted effect on NIPTSs; therefore, a more stringent guideline is appropriate.

Finally, the DRC that are used to address long-term occupational noise exposure are not designed to address issues related to single-event exposures of the type typically encountered in nonoccupational settings. For persons relatively free from noise in most settings, the occupational DRC will tend to overestimate the effect of infrequent noise exposures. Persons with noise exposure at work, however, need to be especially careful with regard to avocational noise since that type of exposure will interact with their work exposure and, in turn, may increase the level of significant risk for noise-induced hearing loss.

The estimates of DRC for those who are exposed to nonoccupational noise sources (e.g., music) and/or are exposed to nonindustrial noise spectra can be difficult. Most of the research that forms the basis of DRC is based on steady-state, low-frequency emphasis noise spectra over a long period of time (see, for example, Burns and Robinson [1970] and ISO [1990]). However, little is known about DRC when the noise is non–steady-state or when the noise spectrum has significant mid- and high-frequency energy (e.g., music). Some insight can be gleaned by comparing two classic studies. Burns and Robinson (1970) used only subjects who were vigorously screened and who were only exposed to continuous steady-state industrial noise. In contrast, Passchier-Vermeer (1968) used subjects who were exposed to both steady-state and impulse (mid- and high-frequency) noise. Based on these models, the expected permanent hearing loss at 4,000 Hz for an exposure of 95 dBA would be 5 dB greater (23 dB vs. 18 dB) in the Passchier-Vermeer study than the Burns and Robinson study. Since the Passchier-Vermeer study allowed a more "music-like" exposure, one could argue that music exposure was slightly *more damaging* than the lower frequency steady-state noise exposure typical of many industries. However, in cases of intermittent noise (or music) exposure, the stapedial reflex does have the effect of reducing the overall noise level reaching the cochlea (Borg et al., 1995), so the potential damage for music-like stimuli would be *less damaging*. Clearly, more research needs to be performed on DRC with nonindustrial noise or music exposure, and caution should be exercised when making general statements about the potential of long-term hearing damage.

Musical instruments can generate low-frequency steady-state noises, high-frequency steady-state noises, low-frequency intermittent noises, and high-frequency intermittent noises. They can have low-frequency emphasis or high-frequency emphasis and can be quiet or intense. In short, no definitive statement can be made about the effects of musical instruments (Chasin, 2006). The same is true of portable recreational music such as iPods. Although this is more of a controlled spectrum, the choice of listening level and earphones makes prediction of potential damage a complicated task (Fligor and Cox, 2004). As far as intense impulse blasts are concerned, whether from cymbals or a rifle, models of hearing loss break down above 115 dBA for a number of reasons (e.g., lack of large-scale data, nature of damage to the cochlea, and specific characteristics of the impulse waveform), and very little can be said about the DRC (Price and Kalb, 1991).

■ REGULATION OF OCCUPATIONAL NOISE

In 1956, the United States Air Force established regulations on noise exposure for its personnel. Hearing protection was required if exposure in any of four frequency bands between 300 and 4,800 Hz exceeded 95 dBA or if personnel were exposed to overall noise levels above 85 dBA. Monitoring of hearing threshold levels was also required. In 1961, the ISO proposed limiting daily worker exposure to no more than 85 dB SPL for 4 hours in octave bands centered around 500, 1,000, and 2,000 Hz. In the early 1960s, the USDoL began to work toward regulation of noise levels as part of the Walsh-Healey Act. This goal was realized in 1969 with issuance of the Walsh-Healy Noise Standard (Suter, 1988).

In 1970, Congress passed the Occupational Safety and Health Act (OSHAct) (Williams and Steiger, 1970). This act established three groups with responsibility regarding work-related noise exposure. NIOSH was established to conduct health and safety research, develop criteria for assessing health and safety issues, and recommend regulations. An Occupational Safety and Health Administration (OSHA) was established with the responsibility of regulating health and safety and of enforcing those regulations. No longer limited to companies with federal contracts, OSHA regulations were to apply to all sectors of general industry, construction, and maritime workers. OSHA was also charged with assisting other federal agencies and state governments with development of their own regulations. Finally, the OSHAct established a separate review committee (Occupational Safety and Health Review Committee [OSHRC]) to act as an arbiter of regulatory disputes between OSHA and individual companies (Suter, 1988).

OSHA, as part of the Department of Labor, adopted the Walsh-Healey Noise Standard as the "new" OSHA General Industry Noise Standard (29 CFR 1910.95) and as the Construction Noise Standard (29 CFR 1926.52). Not covered under the OSHA mandates were mining and agriculture. The USDoL's Mine Safety and Health Administration (MSHA) also adopted the Walsh-Healey Noise Standard, while agricultural workers became exempt from noise regulation. The United States Department of Defense (DoD) developed their own noise standard, modeling the Walsh-Healey Noise Standard. In 1974, OSHA issued its proposed regulations on industrial noise (Melnick, 1992). After considerable comment, modification, legal challenges, and so forth, the OSHA regulations finally took effect in 1985 (Cherow, 1985).

NIOSH (1998) published revised criteria for occupational noise exposure. OSHA and other regulatory agencies are not bound to adopt the NIOSH recommendations but must consider these recommendations in future revisions of the existing regulations or during the promulgation of new regulations (Franks, 1999).

Individual states also have differing regulations regarding workplace safety, including noise exposure. All 50 states and the District of Columbia have Workers' Compensation statutes designed to recompense workers who have been injured while working, including those who have developed noise-induced hearing loss (American Speech-Language-Hearing Association [ASHA], 1992). Workers' Compensation claims are usually handled through insurance coverage. In addition to avoiding OSHA and state fines for compliance problems, companies can help keep their insurance premiums down by minimizing Workers' Compensation claims for hearing loss and other disabling conditions. Audiologists who are active in hearing conservation should be knowledgeable of their state's safety regulations as well as their state's Workers' Compensation statute. In turn, industrial audiologists can then help companies realize the benefits gained (hearing health of their employees and monetary savings) through implementation of a cost-effective hearing conservation program.

INTERNATIONAL STANDARDS

Most of the standards and regulations around the world are quite similar to those found in the United States. In many cases, the differences amount to varying action levels where hearing conservation measures should take place and the exchange rate (5 dB or 3 dB). Most parts of Europe use the ISO 4869 (parts 1 through 7), and DRC are based on the ISO R-1999 (ISO, 1990) model. In Canada, the federal standard is the Canadian Standards Association (CSA) Z94.2-94. However, noise control is both a provincial and a federal affair (rather than purely federal, as it is the United States), and the action level and exchange rates vary from province to province. Currently, they range from 80 to 90 dBA, and most provinces use a 3-dB exchange rate, although those regulations are continually being updated (Behar et al., 2000).

THE OCCUPATIONAL SAFETY AND HEALTH ADMINISTRATION REGULATIONS

OSHA has established an 8-hour TWA exposure level of 85 dB measured using the A-weighting filter (i.e., 85 dBA TWA$_8$) and the slow response mode of the sound level meter as the "action level" for hearing conservation activities. OSHA has also established 90 dBA TWA$_8$ as the maximum permissible exposure level (PEL), while impulse noise should not exceed 140 dBA. Once a worker's exposure equals or exceeds the action level, steps must be taken to ensure that the employee does not develop a work-related NIPTS. Additionally, workers must not be exposed to workplace noise levels equal to or in excess of the maximum PEL (USDoL, 1983).

There are five basic aspects to the OSHA regulations regarding noise exposure. They are:

1. Identification of exposure levels
2. Protection of workers from hazardous noise exposure
3. Annual hearing tests
4. Annual worker training
5. Record keeping

Identification of High Noise Levels (i.e., Monitoring)

All companies need to determine the sound levels to which their workers are exposed if there is any indication that the noise might equal or exceed the action level. Such determination is required to identify those workers who must be enrolled in a hearing conservation program. This determination is also needed to identify workers in need of

hearing protection and the amount of hearing protection required. Finally, monitoring provides both the company and the workers with information regarding the extent of the noise hazard (USDoL, 1983).

Factors posing a suspicion of risk include the type of noise source, worker complaints regarding noise levels (especially complaints of postexposure temporary hearing loss or tinnitus), and interference with communication (NIH, 1990). Probably, the single highest "predictor" index of likely noise exposure is the type of equipment being used in the manufacturing process. Machinery, especially tools involved in cutting, grinding, and shaping metal, typically produce noise in excess of the action level. Engine and motor noise within equipment, compressed air systems, conveyors, and other devices also produce high levels.

Sound levels must be measured in a manner appropriate to the setting, using equipment best suited for the task at hand. The three primary methods of measurement are area readings, short-term personal monitoring, and noise dosimetry. Each of these measurement strategies has advantages and disadvantages. Area readings involve the collection of sound level data at a number of locations within the workplace. This type of measurement is most effective when the noise is relatively homogeneous throughout the space, where there is little fluctuation in sound levels throughout the workday, where there is little or no impulse noise, and where worker mobility is relatively limited throughout each shift. Area readings are susceptible to inaccuracies if any of these conditions are not met. In areas where the noise is less homogeneous but where the levels are fairly constant throughout the day and worker mobility is limited, short-term personal monitoring is an option. These readings represent sound levels at specific workstations. They are made with the microphone of the sound level meter held at or near the worker's ear. Where the conditions of continuous noise are not met or where workers are highly mobile, these types of readings are subject to inaccuracies. In this case, personal dosimetry is the most accurate method of determining individual exposure levels. A dosimeter is a sound level meter capable of gathering sound level data over an extended period of time. The worker wears this instrument, usually with the microphone clipped to the clothing at the shoulder. Data are collected for part or all of a work shift and then retrieved from the instrument's memory. The final data may include (1) average sound level throughout the measurement period, (2) 1-second maximum level, (3) instantaneous peak level, (4) noise dose for the time of exposure (see below), and (5) projected dose for a full 8-hour shift. Some dosimeters are capable of providing minute-by-minute printouts of the data for detailed evaluation of the exposure period. In summary, dosimetry is the method of choice when the sound levels are variable during the day, when there is impulse noise, or when workers have a high degree of mobility within the job setting.

Lipscomb (1978) points out that dosimetry is not without its own special problems. Placement of the microphone in an appropriate position affects the data (the microphone should be in an unobstructed position on the shoulder several inches from the ear). Workers can contaminate the data (unintentionally or intentionally) by banging things against the microphone, shouting into the microphone, or covering the microphone. Such actions may lead to overestimation or underestimation of noise hazard. Dosimetry may underestimate the risk when impulse noise is present. For workers with a variety of work assignments or duties, dosimetry over several days may be necessary to obtain a true picture of the worker's exposure.

Two methods have been developed to assess noise exposure when fluctuating or intermittent noise occurs. The first of these is noise dose. Dose is based on the assumption that exposure to 90 dBA for an 8-hour period equals 100% of allowable exposure. Using the 5-dB trade-off rule, exposure to 85 dBA for 8 hours equals a dose of 50% and exposure to 95 dBA equals a dose of 200%. The formula for calculating dose is:

$$Dose = 100(C1/T1 + C2/T2 + \cdots + Cn/Tn)$$

Each C value equals the total time of exposure at a specific sound level, and T equals the allowable exposure time at that level. The T value is based on a 5-dB trade-off and is defined in Appendix A of the OSHA regulations. For instance, OSHA allows 16 hours of exposure at 85 dBA, 13.9 hours at 86 dBA, 12.1 hours at 87 dBA, etc. If a worker is exposed to 2 hours at 85 dBA, 2 hours at 87 dBA, 2 hours at 89 dBA, and 2 hours at 92 dBA during a given day, that employee's noise dose is calculated as follows:

$$
\begin{aligned}
Dose &= 100(2/16 + 2/12.1 + 2/9.2 + 2/6.1) \\
&= 100(0.125 + 0.165 + 0.217 + 0.328) \\
&= 100(0.835) \\
Dose &= 83.5\%
\end{aligned}
$$

This dose is above the 50% dose associated with the action level and below the 100% dose associated with the PEL. In this example, the worker needs to be included in the hearing conservation program but is not mandated to wear hearing protection unless a change in hearing takes place.

The second method of assessing noise exposure is to convert the dose value into a TWA equivalent for an 8-hour period (TWA_8). The TWA, expressed as a decibel value, is a basic figure that represents a steady-state noise exposure of equal hazard. It can help guide in the selection of appropriate hearing protection strategies. This conversion is completed using the following formula:

$$TWA_8 = 16.61 \log_{10}(D/100) + 90$$

D equals the noise dose. In the case of the worker described earlier, the TWA_8 would be 88.7 dB, which is above the action level of 85 dB and below the PEL of 90 dB.

Sound level measurements must include all sounds within the range from 80 to 130 dB. The industrial audi-

ologist needs to keep these parameters in mind when conducting noise dosimetry. Most modern dosimeters can be programmed to analyze the data using a variety of algorithms, and care must be taken to select the correct criteria. Another important factor in dosimetry is the trade-off value. Although a 3-dB increase represents a true doubling of sound power and, subsequently, exposure time should be halved to remain equally hazardous, OSHA uses a 5-dB doubling rule (USDoL, 1983). As mentioned earlier, the 5-dB trade-off is used because most workers have time away from noise in any 8-hour workday for activities such as coffee breaks and lunch. Therefore, there is downtime from the high-noise environment and a presumed reduction in the noise hazard.

OSHA requires that noise surveys be updated if there is any change in noise or if there is any suspicion that an increase in noise levels has occurred. Although sound level surveys need not be done if the noise has decreased, it is usually in the company's best interest to update the data in this situation. The OSHA-preferred method of protecting hearing is to engineer the noise out of the environment. If sound level reductions can be obtained, then fewer workers may need to wear hearing protection, and employees may no longer need to be enrolled in the hearing conservation program. Factors such as the addition or subtraction of machines, modification of machines (i.e., adding a noise-reduction hood), change in the manufacturing processes (i.e., using different stock material), or changes to the physical space all suggest that the noise survey should be updated. Because noise tends to increase as machinery ages, it is a good idea to obtain updated sound levels at least every few years. Updated sound levels are used to determine whether previously nonexposed employees are now at risk. In instances where workers were already at risk and using hearing protection, the updated sound level survey provides data that can be used in preliminary determination about what type of hearing protection should be used (see the discussion later in this chapter about noise reduction ratings of hearing protection) (USDoL, 1983).

OSHA requires that workers or a designated representative be allowed to observe the collection of data during the sound level survey. Once the sound level survey has been completed, the employer must notify all affected workers about their noise exposure status. There is no stipulation in the OSHA regulations about the nature of that notification. It may be in the form of individual or group meetings, included in the annual training program (see below), or through written notification (USDoL, 1983).

Protection of Workers from Noise Exposure

There are three methods of protecting workers from noise exposure. In the original proposed OSHA regulations (USDoL, 1974), in order of regulatory preference, these three methods were (1) engineered reduction of the noise, (2) limiting exposure time, and/or (3) use of personal hearing protection. In 1983, OSHA revised the hearing conservation regulations to what was referred to as a "performance approach." With this change, the priority of engineering controls was dropped, and employers were given the flexibility to develop their own approaches to meeting the requirements. The performance approach was established to allow employers to assess their own companies' unique environment and to develop cost-effective, efficient strategies for protecting their own workers.

The most effective way to limit noise risk is to prevent workers from being exposed to hazardous noise levels in the first place. By implementing engineered noise control, noise is reduced to "safe" levels. Engineered noise control is passive and relatively permanent. Subsequently, workers do not have to take active steps, such as using ear plugs, to be protected, and workers do not have to be scheduled in such a way that their exposures within a normal workday are time limited. Obviously, if the noise does not exceed safe levels, then all workers are protected from workplace-related NIPTSs, and there is no need for additional hearing conservation measures. Unfortunately, engineered control of noise can be very expensive, often requiring replacement or modification of existing equipment or structural changes to the workplace. Companies may be reluctant to expend the capital outlay necessary to reduce noise to nonhazardous levels. The *perceived* "low-cost" alternative of providing personal hearing protection and monitoring hearing levels through testing may be an attractive alternative.[1] In addition, in some situations, it may not be possible to engineer the noise down to safe levels.

Another method of preventing worker overexposure is to limit exposure time. If a worker must be exposed to 90 dBA or more of noise, the company may elect to limit that worker's exposure time so that the aggregate 8-hour dose is less than 100%. While time-limited exposures may be possible in highly automated processes, it is often difficult to achieve in other settings. Companies may also be reluctant to have skilled workers "off-line" during a substantial portion of the day. For example, to have an aggregate noise dose of less than 100%, a screw machine operator exposed to 100 dBA of noise from his machine would have to be in a quiet setting for 6 hours out of an 8-hour workday. Thus, four workers would be needed to run that machine in each 8-hour shift.

The third option, and the most widely used method of limiting noise exposure, is the use of personal hearing protection (i.e., personal hearing protective devices [PHPDs]). PHPDs may exist in the form of acoustic earmuffs, generic insert acoustic earplugs (e.g., foam plugs, flanged plastic plugs, etc.), or custom acoustic earmolds (Fig. 30.4)

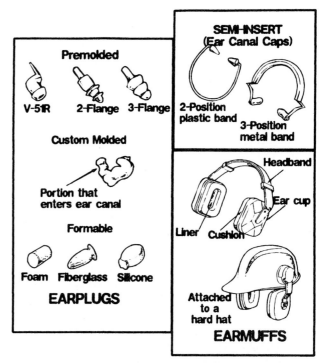

FIGURE 30.4 Sketches of hearing protectors, including premolded, custom-molded, and formable earplugs, and "semi insert" device (*upper right*). Earmuffs require less individualized sizing and fitting but are heavier than earplugs. Helmet-mounted earmuffs solve the compatibility problem between the headband and the hard hat but generally provide less protection. (Reprinted from Franks JR, Stephenson MR, Merry CJ, eds. [1996] *Preventing Occupational Hearing Loss: A Practical Guide.* Cincinnati: National Institute for Occupational Safety and Health; p 37, with permission.)

(Franks, 1999). The basic provisions of OSHA regulations are as follows: Hearing protection must be supplied at no cost to the worker, and it must be appropriate for the sound levels and the acoustic spectrum of the noise. Workers must also have a choice as to the type of hearing protection that they will use unless it can be demonstrated that one particular device is the only effective method of limiting noise to the required levels. When the PHPD option is used, all workers with *daily* exposure equal to or in excess of 90 dBA *must wear* PHPDs, and the protection must lower the exposure to below the 90-dBA TWA_8 level. Hearing protection must also be *available* to all workers with exposure equal to or in excess of 85 dBA TWA_8, and when in use, the PHPDs must lower exposure to below 85 dBA TWA_8.[2] In addition, hearing protection must be fit correctly, and each worker must be trained in the proper use and care of his or her hearing protection (USDoL, 1983).

---

[1] Hearing protection and hearing conservation testing costs are only a portion of the potential company costs associated with noise exposure. Increased lost work time, decreased efficiency, and higher Workers' Compensation insurance premiums are other factors to consider. Over the life of a machine or manufacturing process, the total costs associated with noise may be higher than they appear, and companies should be encouraged to perform a full projected cost analysis prior to opting away from engineering controls.

[2] Some workers with exposure between 85 dBA TWA_8 and 90 dBA TWA_8 must wear PHPD, as explained in the section on action following an STS.

Personal hearing protection has clear applicability in reducing noise exposure, but there are numerous, well-documented problems with the use of personal hearing protection (Berger, 1978). A distinct downside of personal hearing protection is that workers may unknowingly or knowingly fail to wear it properly. This reduces the effectiveness of the PHPD and potentially exposes the worker to noise damage. In 1979, the EPA adopted a single-number rating scheme for hearing protection—the Noise Reduction Rating (NRR) (Berger, 1978). The NRR is designed to provide users with an easy method of determining the applicability of a PHPD for a particular environment. Under normal use, however, the NRR overestimates the real-world effectiveness. Figure 30.5 (Berger, 2000) shows the difference between the protection provided under laboratory conditions versus real-world use for various styles of earplugs and earmuffs. These differences must be accounted for when selecting personal hearing protection designed to reduce exposures below specified target levels. It is likely best to err on the side of caution and select protection that has a "real-world" average attenuation sufficient to meet the situational objectives. The NIOSH (1998) recommendations are that hearing protection be "de-rated" to account for the differences between laboratory and real-world findings. NIOSH suggests that the NRR for acoustic muffs be de-rated by 25%, NRR for foam earplugs be de-rated by 50%, and NRR for all other earplugs be de-rated by 70%.

New methods for testing and labeling the effectiveness of PHPDs have been proposed, and the new regulations are anticipated sometime during 2007. It is hoped that the new

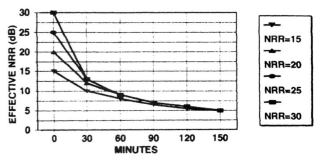

FIGURE 30.6   The protective function of hearing protectors is significantly reduced by failure to wear the protection for part of an exposure period. NNR, Noise Reduction Rating. (Reprinted from Franks JR, Stephenson MR, Merry CJ, eds. [1996] *Preventing Occupational Hearing Loss: A Practical Guide.* Cincinnati: National Institute for Occupational Safety and Health; p 39, with permission.)

regulations will more accurately reflect expected PHPD performance by redefining the NRR as the "noise reduction range," and thus eliminate the need for "de-rating" (ASHA, 2007). Annual instruction in the proper use and care of the protection, including actually observing the employee placing his or her protection in the ear, may help to raise the effectiveness of those devices on a day-to-day basis. A second important consideration in PHPD effectiveness is the consistency of use by each worker. As indicated in Figure 30.6 (Franks et al., 1996), failure to use hearing protection during a portion of an exposure period greatly affects the effective NRR. It should be noted that small periods of disuse have the greatest impact on effectiveness reduction; that is, threshold shift takes place rapidly during the early stages of any exposure period and then plateaus. Finally, some workers' attempts to use hearing protection may actually increase the risk of hearing loss. For example, the use of personal stereos or headset-mounted radios can actually increase noise exposure since the worker needs to turn the volume up to drown out the background noise that is present in the surrounding environment. The use of such systems cannot be condoned.[3]

It is important that each worker have a choice in determining the type of PHPDs that he or she will wear. Some employees like the convenience of acoustic earmuffs, while others may find that these get in the way of hard hats or that they tend to be uncomfortable during warm weather. Soft, formable plugs are preferred by other workers, while others

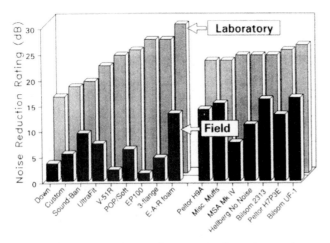

FIGURE 30.5   Noise Reduction Ratings for various kinds of hearing protectors in the laboratory (as labeled) versus in the field (in actual use in the field). The group on the left used earplugs; the group on the right used earmuffs. (Reprinted from Berger EH. [2000] Hearing protection devices. In: Berger EH, Royster LH, Royster JD, Driscoll DP, Layne M. eds. *The Noise Manual.* Fairfax, VA: American Industrial Hygiene Association, with permission.)

---

[3] The author has also seen instances where workers in noise below the action level (85 dBA TWA$_8$) have increased their exposure to above the action level and, in one case, to above the 90-dB TWA$_8$ permissible exposure level through use of a "boom-box" radio. While such a device may reduce boredom, it certainly cannot be endorsed from a noise exposure perspective.

may find that keeping them clean is a problem. Depending on the size and shape of the external ear, some employees have difficulty inserting some styles of plugs, or they find that the plugs work their way out of the ear over time. Workers who are forced to wear hearing protection they do not like will, almost inevitably, find ways to defeat the effort. When they do so, they only hurt themselves, while exposing the company to risks of OSHA fines and Workers' Compensation claims.

Audiometric Testing

If noise can be engineered to safe levels, there is no need to monitor workers for the development of hearing loss. In fact, if noise levels are below the 85-dBA TWA$_8$ level, there is no need for a hearing conservation program. Once noise levels equal or exceed the 85-dBA level, the alternative steps of either changing the worker's schedule so that the exposure time is reduced (administering out the noise) or using PHPDs must be instituted. However, these options are problematic and, if not carefully monitored, can be less than effective. How well the alternate methods are working must be assessed. The most efficient way to monitor the effectiveness of these measures is through periodic hearing testing. Additionally, as per the DRC on which the OSHA regulations are based, it is anticipated that at least some individuals with exposures between 85 and 90 dBA TWA$_8$ will also develop hearing loss. Early identification of susceptibility to NIPTSs is an effective way for instituting steps in avoiding the development of material hearing loss. Therefore, OSHA requires that all workers with noise exposure at or above the action level have routine hearing tests. The hearing testing program includes baseline testing, annual retests (with appropriate analysis to monitor for changes in hearing), worker training, and follow-up procedures (USDoL, 1983).

A professional must administer the audiometric testing program. The regulations stipulate that the professional must be an audiologist, otolaryngologist, or other physician. The administrator does not need to be the person who actually conducts the testing. OSHA allows for trained technicians to do the testing, with an administrator who oversees the program, supervises the technicians, reviews employee audiograms, and makes appropriate recommendations and referrals when needed (USDoL, 1983). It must be noted,

however, that while OSHA allows for the use of technicians, some states do not. Anyone responsible for a hearing conservation program that uses technicians should review the licensure laws and other applicable statutes of the states in which the hearing testing is being conducted. This is to ensure that they are adhering to state laws. OSHA does not require specific training for technicians but does recommend that the technician be certified by the Council for Accreditation of Occupational Hearing Conservationists (USDoL, 1983).

All hearing tests are puretone threshold procedures. They must include the following frequencies: 500, 1,000, 2,000, 3,000, 4,000, and 6,000 Hz, with each ear tested independently. The testing can be conducted manually or by using an automated audiometer calibrated to American National Standards Institute (ANSI) S3.6-1969 standards (ANSI, 1969). Steady-state or pulsed puretones may be used. Additionally, the testing must be conducted in a room meeting specified background levels as indicated in Table 30.1 (USDoL, 1983).

There are two basic types of audiograms that must be considered as part of a hearing conservation program. These are the baseline tests and the annual tests. The baseline test is the first test administered or the test results in which the most sensitive hearing thresholds have been obtained. Annual tests are conducted to monitor for changes in hearing. A standard requirement for all tests is that the preceding 14 hours be "noise-free." Usually this is the overnight period prior to the test. It is important that workers be cautioned to avoid noisy avocational activities (e.g., loud music, power tool use, gunfire, etc.) during that period. If noise cannot be avoided, either at home or at work, then the employee should attempt to keep the exposure time to a minimum and must use effective hearing protection while exposed to levels equal to or in excess of 85 dBA (USDoL, 1983).

The initial baseline test must be obtained within 6 months of the employee beginning work in noise that is at or above the action level. An allowance is made for companies that have their hearing testing conducted by a mobile testing service. In those cases, the initial baseline may be obtained up to 1 year following the first exposure at or above the action level, provided the worker uses effective PHPDs after the first 6 months in that setting (USDoL, 1983). Obviously, the closer the initial test is to the commencement of that

TABLE 30.1   Maximum allowable octave band sound pressure levels for audiometric test rooms used for testing in hearing conservation programs

Octave band center frequency (Hz)	500	1,000	2,000	4,000	8,000
Sound pressure level (dB)	40	40	47	57	62

Reprinted from United States Department of Labor. (1983) Occupational noise exposure: hearing conservation amendment: final rule. *Fed Reg.* 48, 9738–9785.

TABLE 30.2   When is a significant change in hearing not a standard threshold shift?[a]

		Frequency in hz			
		2,000	**3,000**	**4,000**	**Average**
Annual test	Hearing @ 58 years old	30	35	40	35
	Presbycusis adjustment	12	22	31	
	Adjusted threshold	18	13	9	13.3
Baseline test	Hearing @ 23 years old	5	10	10	8.3
	Presbycusis adjustment	3	4	6	
	Adjusted threshold	2	6	4	4

Actual change in hearing: 35 − 8.3 = 26.7 dB

Corrected change in hearing: 13.3 − 4 = 9.3 dB

[a] Using the Occupational Safety and Health Administration correction for presbycusis, this worker, who began work with normal hearing through 4,000 Hz and who is now developing a high-tone hearing loss, would not be identified as having had a significant change in hearing.

individual being employed in the high-noise setting, the less likely it is that the data will be contaminated.[4]

All workers with exposure at or above the action level must be retested at least annually. The results of the annual test are compared to the baseline test. The frequencies used for the comparison are 2,000, 3,000, and 4,000 Hz, with each ear evaluated independently. If the average hearing sensitivity at these frequencies is 10 dB or worse than the average obtained on the baseline audiogram, then a standard threshold shift (STS) has occurred (USDoL, 1983). This apparently straightforward process is complicated slightly by OSHA's allowance of an age adjustment to account for predicted presbycusis. Therefore, a frequency-by-frequency adjustment must be applied to each of the three comparison frequencies based on the workers age at the time of the baseline; adjustments are also made to the annual audiogram based on the current age. The averages are then calculated, and the comparison for STS is made (USDoL, 1983). As can be seen in Table 30.2, even though the raw data show a change of greater than 10 dB, the adjusted values may not constitute an STS.

The presence of an STS requires specific action be taken by the company, and it is in these actions that the process becomes rather complex. Under current regulations (29 CFR 1904.10, effective January 1, 2004), a shift needs to be recorded if the average age-corrected change in hearing at 2,000, 3,000, and 4,000 Hz is equal to or in excess of 10 dB

and the total average hearing loss at those frequencies in the same ear equals or exceed 25 dB hearing threshold level (HTL) (without age correction) (OSHA, 2006).

OSHA recognizes that some shifts in hearing may be temporary due to medical conditions, NITTS, lapses in attention during the test, or simple day-to-day fluctuations in hearing. For a basic STS, there is an allowance that the shift needs to be confirmed before specific action is taken. The confirmation retest must take place within 30 days of the company becoming aware of the shift. Often, the company is aware of the shift on the day the audiogram is conducted, and the retest deadline is based on that date. However, there may be times when the determination of shift is delayed, such as when an outside agency conducts the test. Under those circumstances, the retest deadline may, in fact, be more than 30 days after the test that first showed the shift.[5] If the retest confirms the shift, the employee's company must then notify the worker of the change in hearing. Notification must be in writing.[6] If the company decides not to use the retest option, then the company must notify the employee of the shift within 21 days of the date on which the company first became aware of the shift (USDoL, 1983).

All STSs are presumed to be due to work-related noise exposure unless a physician or other licensed health care worker determines that the shift is due to causes other than occupational noise exposure or that work-related noise did not have a significant role in the shift (OSHA, 2006). Additional steps must be taken unless this shift is determined medically to be non–work-related or not to have been

---

[4] Author's recommendation: The baseline should be obtained prior to the worker first being in noise, if possible. This allows for the identification of pre-existing hearing loss, which may be an important factor if a subsequent Workers' Compensation claim is filed. For instance, in New York State, companies can limit their exposure to that portion of the hearing loss that develops while the worker is employed by that company. If a loss is determined to be in existence at the time of hiring, the company may, through written notification, shift responsibility for the pre-existing portion of the loss to previous employers (Section 49-ee, NYS Workers' Compensation statute).

[5] Shifts equal to or in excess of 25 dB require retest within 30 days of the actual test on which the shift was noted. See text regarding 25-dB shifts for additional information.

[6] Author's recommendation: When a worker receives written notification of an STS, the company should keep a photocopy of the letter, signed and dated by the employee, as proof of notification.

exacerbated by workplace noise. If the worker has exposure of less than 90 dB TWA_8, and they are not currently wearing hearing protection, hearing protection must be fitted and the worker must be trained in the care and use of that protection. If the worker is currently using hearing protection, then he or she must be refit with equipment providing additional attenuation, if needed, and retrained in the appropriate use and care of hearing protection. In either case, PHPD use must reduce the exposure to less than 85 dB TWA_8. If there are signs that additional testing would be audiologically appropriate, then an audiologic referral is needed. If there are signs of a medical problem, either due to or made worse by PHPD use, then otologic referral is required. Otologic referral is also required for suspected medical problems unrelated to hearing protection use (USDoL, 1983).

For workers whose exposures are less than 90 dBA TWA_8, if a subsequent hearing test shows that an STS is not persistent, then the employee must be notified of the new results, and hearing protection use may be discontinued (USDoL, 1983).

STSs equal to or greater than 25 dB require additional action. These reportable shifts must be recorded by the employer on the OSHA Illness/Injury Log as soon as they are first identified (USDoL, 1986). These shifts are recorded in the category of occupational illness. Similar to the basic STS, discussed earlier, the company has a retest option to confirm the 25-dB shift, but the rules are different than for a basic (10-dB) STS. When the shift equals or exceeds 25 dB, the retest to confirm or refute a reportable shift must be done within 30 days of the *date of the annual audiogram* on which the shift was noted. This is different than the retest for a basic STS, which has to occur within 30 days of the company *becoming aware* of the shift.[7] If the retest fails to confirm the shift or if a subsequent medical evaluation indicates the shift to be due to non–work-related causes, then the Illness/Injury Log may be amended to reflect those findings. If the retest confirms the shift or if the retest option is not used, then the same follow-up procedures discussed earlier for a basic retest apply; that is, the worker must be notified in writing within 21 days, and the appropriate actions regarding hearing protection must be implemented.

Whenever an STS has occurred, the professional in charge of the hearing conservation program can revise the baseline audiogram to reflect current levels. This revised baseline audiogram serves as the basis for future comparisons to determine the occurrence of a new basic STS (USDoL, 1983). The rationale for this is as follows. If a worker shows a persistent STS, then each subsequent

annual test can be expected to show the same STS relative to the initial test. By continually referring back to the initial test, future basic STSs may not be identified easily. Revision of the baseline also avoids overreferral for additional attention. However, annual comparisons for reportable STS ($\geq$25-dB shift) should always be made relative to the *initial* test results. If comparison is not made to the initial results, a reportable shift could be missed. For example, Worker Smith develops a 15-dB shift after 10 years of work. This basic STS is confirmed by retest. Worker Smith is notified of the change, and the baseline is revised. Ten years later, Worker Smith develops another 15-dB basic STS (compared to the revised baseline). Unless comparison is made of the current test to the initial test, the 30-dB cumulative shift might be missed, and the company would be in violation of the OSHA regulations for failure to record the cumulative change.

Finally, if a worker shows a significant improvement in hearing, then revision of the baseline is also warranted (USDoL, 1983). For instance, some workers present with medical problems during their first test. Once those problems have been treated, hearing may improve significantly. Without a revision of the baseline following an improvement in hearing thresholds, any future noise-induced STS could go unnoticed, and initiation of (more) effective hearing protection could be delayed.[8]

Worker Training Program

Workers with noise exposure at or above the action level must have annual training with regard to hearing conservation measures. This training has three components. First, information on the effects of noise on hearing must be provided. Second, information must be discussed regarding hearing protection. The various forms of PHPDs must be reviewed, including the advantages and disadvantages of each and how much noise reduction is provided by the various styles of PHPDs. Third, each worker must also be instructed in how to use his or her hearing protection and how to care for that protection. Although not part of the direct training program, the OSHA noise regulations must be posted in the work place and available to workers (USDoL, 1983).

The line employee is the key to any successful hearing conservation program, and the training component can make or break the effectiveness of the conservation effort. If employees are not vested in the process, compliance with hearing protection strategies suffers. Workers are more likely to wear hearing protection and wear it appropriately when they understand the nature and long-term implications of hearing loss, the effects of noise on hearing, and why they are being required to wear hearing protection. The "pay-me-now or pay-me-later principle" is also helpful. That is, workers who understand that a bit of inconvenience now

---

[7] While it seems like splitting hairs, this is an important consideration for companies using mobile test vans. It is also important for larger companies, where testing may take place on several different dates. In both of these situations, there may be a delay between when the audiogram is obtained and when it is analyzed and reported back to the company by the audiologist. The reporting delay is less critical for a basic shift than it is when the shift equals or exceeds 25 dB.

[8] Author's recommendation: Revision of baseline should not be made until two consecutive annual tests show similar hearing levels.

(use of PHPDs) is far better than having to live with a hearing loss later on in life are more likely to take active steps to conserve hearing both at work and at home. Instead of having hearing protection "jammed down their ears," workers should have a justified feeling that management is concerned about their personal safety and welfare. This means that the entire company, from the executive suite on down, needs to support the hearing conservation effort. Having a voice in the PHPD selection process, seeing supervisors using hearing protection, and understanding that active participation in hearing conservation activities helps them preserve good hearing are all critical factors to workers buying into the process.

The hearing conservation effort should have as high a profile as any and all other safety efforts and should be ongoing throughout the year. A single, brief "pep talk" at the annual hearing test session is insufficient to ensure employee cooperation. In this regard, it is necessary for the industrial audiologist to interface with many individuals, including the industrial physician, occupational nurse, health and safety engineer, plant supervisory staff, and managers, to name a few. The audiologist should make a concerted effort to understand the roles these individuals play within the company and as part of the hearing conservation effort. Whenever possible, these individuals should be included in the planning and conduct of a training program. Line workers can also be helpful contributors to the process by persuading their fellow workers about the importance of hearing conservation.

Record Keeping

Companies are required to maintain records of noise exposure measurements and annual audiograms. All exposure records must be maintained for a period of at least 2 years.[9] Audiograms must be maintained for each worker's entire career with the company. Also, the audiograms must be provided to any worker (present or past) who requests his or her personal data.[10] Finally, in the event that the company is sold, the audiograms must be transferred to the new owners, and the data must be maintained as previously described (USDoL, 1983).

---

[9] Author's recommendation: Noise exposure records, including those that show no hazard, should be maintained as part of the company's permanent file. In the event of a subsequent Workers' Compensation claim for NIPTS, such records are helpful in documenting when a worker was or was not employed in a high-noise area.

[10] There is an inconsistency at this point in the regulations. If audiograms must only be maintained "for the duration of the employee's employment" (29 CFR 1910.20 Section m.3.ii), then those records will not be available when requested by former employees (29 CFR 1910.20 Section m.4). NIOSH recommends that audiograms be maintained for at least 30 years following termination (Frank et al., 1996). Author's recommendation: Audiograms should be on file permanently. Workers' Compensation claims are often filed many years after an employee leaves a company. It is important that the company have a record of hearing status as close as possible to the end date of employment. Although in some cases the audiograms will support a worker's claim, in other instances, the data will either refute the claim or limit exposure for hearing loss developed after the worker left the job.

▧ GOING BEYOND OCCUPATIONAL SAFETY AND HEALTH ADMINISTRATION REGULATIONS

The OSHA regulations on occupational noise exposure (USDoL, 1983) serve as the basis for the majority of hearing conservation programs in the United States. As indicated earlier, these regulations will protect most employees at risk from developing work-related noise-induced hearing loss, but by no means are they perfect. Some workers may develop significant amounts of NIPTS even if all aspects of the hearing conservation measures outlined earlier are instituted. One precautionary step is to include workers (e.g., through training) not currently considered at risk, which, in turn, may increase the protective function of the hearing conservation program. The OSHA regulations are the minimum guidelines that should be followed. There are no prohibitions regarding the development of more stringent protocols by individual companies or programs. It is wise for audiologists who are involved in industrial hearing conservation to consider the OSHA regulations as the starting point. From a standpoint of liability exposure, companies that adhere strictly to the OSHA regulations will continue to be at risk for compensation claims in at least some jurisdictions. They will also continue to have workers who develop significant amounts of hearing loss. That is, strict adherence to the OSHA guidelines will miss the development of materially significant hearing loss in 3% to 5% of the workers with noise exposure between 80 and 85 dB.

NIOSH (1998) has made a number of suggestions for increasing the effectiveness of hearing conservation efforts. A few examples include:

- The action level should be renamed the recommended exposure level (REL).
- All workers exposed at or above 85 dBA TWA should be required to use hearing protection,[11] and all hearing protection should reduce exposure to below 85 dBA TWA_8.
- A 3-dB trade-off should be used for all aspects of the program (i.e., where every increase by 3 dB requires half the exposure time).
- Workers should be tested within the first 30 days of noise exposure.
- Workers showing a shift of 15 dB or more at *any* frequency (500 to 6,000 Hz) should be considered to have an STS if the shift is present at the same frequency on an immediate retest of hearing.
- Program effectiveness should be judged based on no more than 5% of workers showing an STS.

---

[11] It is difficult to obtain consistent PHPD use by some workers who are in the 85 to 90 dB range and who have shown an STS. When that worker is the only one in an area required to wear protection, there is a peer pressure of sorts: "Why should I have to do this when no one else does?" In addition to protecting more people, this NIOSH recommendation would eliminate this problem.

Otoacoustic emission (OAE) testing has received widespread acceptance for screening in neonatal units of hospitals, and both distortion product and transient OAEs have been shown to be quite sensitive in the detection of hearing loss. Of late, several studies have demonstrated how OAEs can be used for assessing the effects of noise and music exposure. Davis et al. (2005) found that OAEs in chinchillas are more sensitive than audiometric threshold shifts for cochlear damage caused by noise exposure. LePage and Murray (1998) also demonstrated the same phenomenon in humans, with a change in OAEs showing up prior to a change in pure-tone audiometry. As such, one could argue that, if our role is in early prevention of noise- or music-induced hearing loss, then OAE testing should be a centerpiece of the test battery. However, OAE levels and OAE spectra in persons with normal hearing function (without excessive noise exposure) have been shown to demonstrate large intersubject variability. This would limit the clinical usefulness of the individual results obtained in cross-sectional studies. One reason for the large intersubject variability of OAEs is probably related to the intersubject variability of backward transmission function through the middle ear, as demonstrated by Trine et al. (1993). Whereas the afferent/efferent neurologic loop is probably of low variability, the mechanical transmission laterally to the outer ear canal is probably inherently variable.

However, the intrasubject variability of OAEs is quite small and, within an individual worker or musician, can be successfully used for longitudinal testing. This use has been valuable with musicians: Does a change occur over time within that musician or worker? This useful procedure has repeatedly been demonstrated in studies of both the temporary and permanent effects of noise exposure (Attias et al., 1998; Hamernik and Qiu, 2000; Fraenkel et al., 2003; Davis et al., 2004; 2005). The results of these studies do not support the hypothesis that OAEs may serve as an early warning of the onset of hearing loss induced by music noise if used over a large population. However, OAEs are quite useful for monitoring musicians and workers longitudinally.

Another useful tool is electrocochleography (ECoG). Kim et al. (2005) studied the relative sensitivity and specificity of ECoG and OAEs for detecting a music-induced temporary threshold shift. In this study, 20 normal-hearing young adults were assessed before and after 2 hours at a night club (90.3 dBA). The sensitivity and specificity of the ECoG test were 82% and 96%, respectively, whereas the values for OAEs were only 58% and 81%, respectively. Although both OAEs and ECoG demonstrated impressive specificities, the ECoG was found to be better at finding true-negative responses when compared with the sum of true negatives plus false positives. This was especially true for detecting temporary threshold shift when the baseline hearing was normal or near normal. However, the OAE test was more useful for those with mild permanent sensory-neural hearing losses up to 40 dB hearing level (HL). For very early detection, therefore, ECoG can be an effective early warning screener but loses its advantage over OAEs once there is a permanent, mild, sensory-neural hearing loss.

Evaluating Program Effectiveness

Lacking in the OSHA regulations are recommendations on determining the effectiveness of hearing conservation programs. Royster and Royster (1999) indicate that there are worker-related and workplace-related factors that affect STS rates and that these factors decrease the reliability of STS rates as a gauge of program effectiveness.

Because the OSHA STS is calculated as an average of three frequencies, considerable and significant shifts in hearing may occur before an STS is evidenced. Because of the plateau effect associated with NIPTS, workers with pre-existing high-frequency hearing losses may require a large shift at 2,000 Hz prior to being identified as having an STS. In these individuals, the change in hearing may have a significant impact prior to the STS being identified. In addition, factors such as the age of the workforce, the rate of retention among workers, how the testing is conducted, and so forth may also impact the STS rate (Royster and Royster, 1999).

Royster and Royster (1999) recommend using two measures other than STS to audit program effectiveness. Both procedures are based on standards suggested by the American National Standards Institute (ANSI). The first component is based on data contained in ANSI S3.44-1996 (ANSI, 1996) and involves matching the actual hearing levels of noise-exposed workers to those of nonexposed workers of the same age, sex, and race. When a group of workers has hearing worse than that of the control group, it suggests that the effectiveness of the hearing conservation program needs additional evaluation. This technique could be especially helpful when applied on an ongoing basis. For instance, if a group of workers is initially worse than the control group and there is no difference over time, then the hearing conservation program would appear to be accomplishing its goal. A decrease in the difference would suggest that the program is very effective, while a widening of the difference would suggest the need for improvements.

The second procedure recommended by Royster and Royster (1999) is to do an analysis of year-to-year audiometric variability as described in ANSI S12.13-1991 (ANSI, 1991). Using this procedure, each set of annual audiograms is compared to the previous year's data. The data are evaluated to determine the percentage of the population whose hearing is getting worse (W) over time (%W, based on a 15-dB decline at any frequency from 500 to 6,000 Hz) and the percentage of the population whose hearing is getting either better (B) or worse over time (%BW, based on either a decline or an improvement of 15 dB at any frequency from 500 to 6,000 Hz).

Changes in the %W group may be useful in tracking the effectiveness of changes in the program. For instance, introduction of a new style of hearing protection should result in either no change or an improvement (lower) in %W. If the %W increases, then the new hearing protection may not be adequate. Year-to-year changes up and down in the %W or differences between departments might signal variability in the enforcement of hearing conservation measures (Royster and Royster, 1999).

The %BW computation evaluates variability in hearing levels among the workers from year to year. Because group hearing levels should remain fairly stable, large %BW values are a cause for concern. Factors such as calibration problems, variability among testers, variability in the test environment, and so forth may need to be evaluated (Royster and Royster, 1999).

FINAL NOTES

Hearing conservation can be a rewarding area of professional practice. While considerable progress has been made in the past 25 years to prevent occupational hearing loss, much remains to be done. Additionally, work must be done to in-crease public awareness of the hazards of noise exposure. Tools such as chainsaws, gas-powered weed trimmers, and leaf blowers have become common additions in our per-sonal lives. Personal stereo systems, with their primary out-put through headphones, are often used at potentially haz-ardous levels. Car sound systems, with a few modifications, are capable of blowing out the windshield of the vehicle (as has happened during boom-car competitions). If shifting the occurrence of NIPTSs from the factory into the home is to be avoided, educational programs must continue to be expanded to include the general public.

And the next time you are working with employees on the graveyard shift and wondering how many other audiol-ogists are working at 4:00 AM, remember that there is a job to be done. Let's continue to be proactive and stop noise-induced hearing loss before it starts.

REFERENCES

Alberti PW, ed. (1982) *Personal Hearing Protection in Industry.* New York: Raven Press.

American National Standards Institute. (1969) ANSI specifications of audiometers. A report of the American National Standards Institute S3.6-1969 (R 1986). New York: Acoustical Society of America.

American National Standards Institute. (1991) Evaluating the ef-fectiveness of hearing conservation programs. Draft ANSI S12.13-1991. New York: Acoustical Society of America.

American National Standards Institute. (1996) Determination of occupational noise exposure and estimation of noise-induced hearing impairment. ANSI S3.44-1996. New York: Acoustical Society of America.

American Speech-Language-Hearing Association. (1992) A survey of state's workers' compensation practices for occupational hearing loss. *ASHA.* 34 (suppl 8), 2–8.

American Speech-Language-Hearing Association. (2007) EPA up-dates hearing protector regulations: new methods and labeling requirements included. *ASHA Leader.* 12, 5.

Attias J, Breshoff I, Reshef I, Horowitz G, Furman V. (1998) Evalu-ating noise induced hearing loss with distortion product otoa-coustic emissions. *Br J Audiol.* 32, 39–46

Babisch W. (2002) The noise/stress concept, risk assessment and research needs. *Noise Health.* 4, 1–11.

Barrs DM, Althoff LK, Krueger WW, Olsson JE. (1994) Work-related, noise-induced hearing loss: evaluation including evoked potential audiometry. *Otolaryngol Head Neck Surg.* 110, 177–184.

Baughn WL. (1973) Relation between daily noise exposure and hearing loss based on evaluation of 6,835 industrial noise ex-posure cases. Dayton, OH: Wright Patterson Air Force Base.

Behar A, Chasin M, Cheesman M. (2000) *Noise Control: A Primer.* San Diego: Singular Publishing Group.

Berger EH. (1978) Hearing protectors: specifications, fitting, use, and performance. In: Lipscomb DM, ed. *Noise and Audiology.* Baltimore: University Park Press; pp 145–191.

Berger EH. (2000) Hearing protection devices. In: Berger EH, Roys-ter LH, Royster JD, Driscoll DP, Layne M. eds. *The Noise Man-ual.* Fairfax, VA: American Industrial Hygiene Association.

Bohne BA. (1976) Safe level for noise exposure? *Ann Otol Rhinol Laryngol.* 85, 711–724.

Borg E, Canlon B, Engstrom B. (1995) Noise-induced hearing loss: literature review and experiments in rabbits. *Scand Audiol Suppl.* 40, 1–147.

Bronzaft AL. (1991) The effects of noise on learning, cognitive de-velopment, and social behavior. In: Fay TH, ed. *Noise and Hea-lth.* New York: The New York Academy of Medicine; pp 87–92.

Bronzaft AL, McCarthy DP. (1975) The effect of elevated train noise on reading ability. *Environ Behav.* 7, 517–528.

Burns W, Robinson DW. (1970) *Hearing and Noise in Industry.* London: Her Majesty's Stationary Office.

Catalano PJ, Levin SM. (1985) Noise-induced hearing loss and portable radios with headphones. *Int J Pediatr Otorhinolaryn-gol.* 9, 59–67.

Chasin M. (2006) Music and hearing aids. *Hear Rev.* March, 34–41.

Cherow E. (1985) Victory for OSHA: court upholds U.S. DOL's hearing conservation amendment. Audiology Update, Pro-fessional Practices Division, American Speech-Language-Hearing Association, p 1–2.

Clark WW. (1991) Noise exposure from leisure activities: a review. *J Acoust Soc Am.* 90, 175–181.

Cohen S, Glass D, Singer J. (1973) Apartment noise, auditory dis-crimination and reading ability in children. *J Exp Soc Psychol.* 9, 422–437.

Cohen S, Weinstein N. (1981). Non-auditory effects of noise on behavior and health. *J Soc Issues.* 37, 36–70.

Coles RR, Lutman ME, Buffin JT. (2000) Guidelines on the diag-nosis of noise-induced hearing loss for medicolegal purposes. *Clin Otolaryngol Allied Sci.* 25, 264–273.

Crow S, Guild S, Polvogot L. (1934) Observation on pathology of high-tone deafness. *Johns Hopkins Med J.* 54, 315–318.

Dancer AL, Henderson D, Salvi RJ, Hamernik RP. (1992) Noise-Induced Hearing Loss. St. Louis: Mosby Year Book, Inc.

Davis J. (1985) Hard of hearing children in the schools. Seminar presentation in St. Cloud, MN.

Davis R, Qiu W, Hamernik RP. (2004) The use of distortion product otoacoustic emissions in the estimation of hearing and sensory cell loss in noise-damaged cochleas. *Hear Res.* 187, 12–24.

Davis R, Qiu W, Hamernik RP. (2005) Sensitivity of distortion product otoacoustic emissions in noise-exposed chinchillas. *J Am Acad Audiol.* 16, 69–78.

DeJoy DM. (1984) The nonauditory effects of noise: review and perspectives for research. *J Aud Res.* 24, 123–150.

Durrant JD, (1978) Anatomic and physiologic correlates of the effects of noise on hearing. In: Lipscomb DM, ed. *Noise and Audiology.* Baltimore: University Park Press; pp 109–141.

Edmonds LD, Layde PM, Erikson JD. (1979) Airport noise and teratogenesis. *Arch Environ Health.* 34, 243–247.

Environmental Protection Agency. (1973) Public health and welfare criteria for noise: a report of the Environmental Protection Agency (EPA). Washington, DC: US Environmental Protection Agency.

Environmental Protection Agency. (1974) Information on the levels of environmental noise requisite to protect public health and welfare with adequate margin of safety: a report of the Environmental Protection Agency (EPA). Washington, DC: US Environmental Protection Agency.

Fligor BJ, Cox C. (2004) Output levels of commercially available portable compact disc players and the potential risk to hearing. *Ear Hear.* 25, 513–527.

Fraenkel R, Freeman S, Sohmer H. (2003) The use of ABR threshold and OAEs in detection of noise-induced hearing loss. *J Basic Clin Physiol Pharmacol.* 14, 95–118.

Franks JR. (1999) Historical highlights in the evolution of national standards for occupational safety and health. *Hear Rev.* 6, 18–27.

Franks JR, Stephenson MR, Merry CJ, eds. (1996) *Preventing Occupational Hearing Loss: A Practical Guide.* Cincinnati: National Institute for Occupational Safety and Health.

Gates GA, Schmid P, Kujawa SG, Nam B, D'Agostino R. (2000) Longitudinal threshold changes in older men with audiometric notches. *Hear Res.* 141, 220–228.

Gelfand SA. (1997) *Essentials of Audiology.* New York: Theme.

Gelfand SA. (1998) *Hearing: An Introduction to Physiological and Psychological Acoustics.* 3rd ed. New York: Marcel Dekker, Inc.

Goldstein J. (1978) Fundamental concepts in sound measurement. In: Lipscomb DM, ed. *Noise and Audiology.* Baltimore: University Park Press; pp 3–58.

Green KB, Pasternak BS, Shore RE. (1982) Effects of aircraft noise on reading ability of school-age children. *Arch Environ Health.* 37, 24–31.

Hamernik RP, Qiu W. (2000) Correlations among evoked potential thresholds, distortion product otoacoustic emissions and hair cell loss following various noise exposures in the chinchilla. *Hear Res.* 150, 245–257.

Henderson D, Saunders SS. (1998) Acquisition of noise-induced hearing loss by railway workers. *Ear Hear.* 19, 120–130.

Hilding AC. (1953) Studies on otic labyrinth: anatomic explanation for hearing dip at 4096 Hz characteristic of acoustic trauma and presbycusis. *Ann Otol Rhinol Laryngol.* 62, 950.

Hirsh IJ, Bilger RC. (1955) Auditory threshold recovery after exposure to pure tones. *J Acoust Soc Am.* 55, 117–121.

Hodge DC, Price GR. (1978) Hearing damage risk criteria. In: Lipscomb DM, ed. *Noise and Audiology.* Baltimore: University Park Press; pp 167–191.

Industrial Acoustics Company. (1970) *Hearing Conservation Notes.* Bronx: Industrial Acoustics Company.

International Organization for Standardization. (1990) *Acoustics— Determination of Occupational Noise Exposure and Estima-tion of Noise-Induced Hearing Impairment.* 2nded. Geneva, Switzerland: International Organization for Standardization.

Johnson DL. (1978) Derivation of presbycusis and noise-induced permanent threshold shift (NIPTS) to be used for the basis of a standard on the effects of noise on hearing. Dayton, OH: Wright Patterson Air Force Base.

Katz AE, Gertsman HL, Sanderson RG, Buchanan R. (1982) Stereo earphones and hearing loss. *N Eng J Med.* 307, 1460–1461.

Kim JS, Nam EC, Park S. (2005) Electrocochleography is more sensitive than distortion-product otoacoustic emission test for detecting noise-induced temporary threshold shift. *Otolaryngol Head Neck Surg.* 133, 619–624.

Kryter KD. (1985) *The Effects of Noise on Man.* 2nd ed. Orlando: Academic Press.

Lee PC, Senders CW, Gantz BJ, Otto SR. (1985) Transient sensorineural hearing loss after overuse of portable headphone cassette radios. *Otolaryngol Head Neck Surg.* 93, 633–625.

LePage EL, Murray NM. (1998) Latent cochlear damage in personal stereo users: a study based on click-evoked otoacoustic emissions. *Med J Aust.* 169, 588–592.

Lipscomb DM. (1978) *Noise and Audiology.* Baltimore: University Park Press.

Lipscomb DM. (1988) Basic principles of sound measurement. In: Lipscomb DM, ed. *Hearing Conservation in Industry, Schools and the Military.* Boston: College-Hill Press; pp 21–34.

Matheson MP, Stansfeld SA, Haines MM. (2003) The effects of chronic aircraft noise exposure on children's cognition and health: 3 field studies. *Noise Health.* 5, 31–40.

McBride DI, Williams S. (2001a) Audiometric notch as a sign of noise induced hearing loss. *Occup Environ Med.* 58, 46–51.

McBride DI, Williams S. (2001b) Characteristics of the audiometric notch as a clinical sign of noise exposure. *Scand Audiol.* 30, 106–111.

Melnick W. (1978) Temporary and permanent threshold shift. In: Lipscomb DM, ed. *Noise and Audiology.* Baltimore: University Park Press; pp 83–107.

Melnick W. (1992) Occupational noise standards: status and critical issues. In: Dancer AL, Henderson D, Salvi RJ, Hamernik RP, eds. *Noise Induced Hearing Loss.* St. Louis: Mosby Year Book; pp 521–530.

Melnick W. (1994) Industrial hearing conservation. In: Katz J, ed. *Handbook of Clinical Audiology.* 4th ed. Baltimore: Williams & Wilkins.

Meyer-Bisch C. (1996) Epidemiological evaluation of hearing damage related to strongly amplified music (personal cassette players, discotheques, rock concerts): high-definition audiometric survey on 1364 subjects. *Audiology.* 35, 121–142.

Miller JM, Altschuler RA, Niparko JK, Hartshorn DO, Helfert RH, Moore JK. (1992) Deafness-induced changes in the central nervous system: reversibility and prevention. In: Dancer AL, Henderson D, Salvi RJ, Hamernik RP, eds. *Noise Induced Hearing Loss.* St. Louis: Mosby Year Book; pp 130–145.

Mills JH, Gengle RW, Watson CS, Miller JD. (1970) Temporary changes in the auditory system due to noise exposure of one to two days. *J Acoust Soc Am.* 48, 524–530.

Nakamura R (1977). Gestation in noise (Abstract). In: Congress Handbook, Seventh Asian Congress of Obstetrics and Gynecology. S. Toongsuwan, T. Suvonnakoto (eds.). Bangkok.

National Institutes of Health. (1990) Noise and hearing loss. *Consens Statement.* 8, 1–24.

National Institute for Occupational Safety and Health. (1998) Criteria for a recommended standard—occupational noise exposure, revised criteria. NIOSH Publication No. 98-126. Cincinnati: National Institute for Occupational Safety and Health.

National Institute for Occupational Safety and Health. (1974) Occupational noise and hearing: 1968–1972: a report of the National Institute for Occupational Safety and Health (NIOSH). Cincinnati: National Institute for Occupational Safety and Health.

National Institute for Occupational Safety and Health (2000). Work Related Hearing Loss, DHHS (NIOSH) Publication No. 2001-103.

Nixon JE, Glorig A. (1961) A noise induced permanent threshold shift at 2000 cps and 4000 cps. *J Acoust Soc Am*. 56, 1585–1593.

Occupational Safety and Health Administration. (2006) Recording criteria for cases involving occupational hearing loss - 1904.10. Available at: http://www.osha.gov/pls/oshaweb/owadisp.show_document?p_table=STANDARDS&p_id=9641.

Ouis D. (2002) Annoyance caused by exposure to road traffic noise: an update. *Noise Health*. 4, 69–79.

Passchier-Vermeer W. (1968) Hearing loss due to exposure to steady-state broadband noise. Report No. 35. The Netherlands: Institute for Public Health Engineering.

Passchier-Vermeer W. (1974) Hearing loss due to continuous exposure to steady-state broad-band noise. *J Acoust Soc Am*. 56, 1575–1593.

Patuzzi R. (1992) Effect of noise on cranial nerve VIII responses. In: Dancer AL, Henderson D, Salvi RJ, Hamernik RP, eds. *Noise Induced Hearing Loss*. St. Louis: Mosby Year Book; pp 45–59.

Pierson LL, Gerhardt KJ, Rodriguez GP, Yanke RB. (1994) Relationship between outer ear resonance and permanent noise-induced hearing loss. *Am J Otolaryngol*. 15, 37–40.

Pollak C. (1991) The effects of noise on sleep. In: Fay TH, ed. *Noise and Health*. New York: The New York Academy of Medicine; pp 41–60.

Price GR. (1994) Occasional exposure to impulsive sounds: Significant noise exposure? Forum presented at the 19th Annual National Hearing Conservation Association Conference, Atlanta, GA.

Price GR, Kalb JT. (1991) Insights into hazard from intense impulses from a mathematical model of the ear. *J Acoust Soc Am*. 90, 219–227.

Raymond LW. (1991) Neuroendocrine, immunologic, and gastrointestinal effects of noise. In: Fay TH, ed. *Noise and Health*. New York: The New York Academy of Medicine; pp. 27–40.

Rice CG, Breslin M, Roper RG. (1987) Sound levels from personal cassette players. *Br J Audiol*. 21, 273–278.

Royster JD, Royster LH. (1999) How can we evaluate the effectiveness of occupational hearing conservation programs? *Hear Rev*. 6, 28–34.

Ryals BM. (1990) Critical periods and acoustic trauma. In: *National Institutes of Health (NIH) Consensus Development Conference on Noise and Hearing Loss, Program and Abstracts*. Washington, DC: National Institutes of Health.

Schell LM. (1981) Environmental noise and human prenatal growth. *Am J Phys Anthropol*. 56, 156–163.

Schmiedt RA. (1984) Acoustic injury and the physiology of hearing. *J Acoust Soc Am*. 76, 1293–1317.

Schuknecht H, Tonndorf J. (1960) Acoustic trauma of the cochlea from ear surgery. *Laryngoscope*. 70, 479.

Sloan RP. (1991) Cardiovascular effects of noise. In: Fay TH, ed. *Noise and Health*. New York: The New York Academy of Medicine; pp. 15–26.

Smith EL, Laird DA. (1930) The loudness of auditory stimuli which affect stomach contractions in healthy human beings. *J Acoust Soc Am*. 15, 94–98.

Stansfeld SA, Haines MM, Brown B. (2000) Noise and health in the urban environment. *Rev Environ Health*. 15, 43–82.

Suter AH. (1988) The development of federal standards and damage risk criteria. In: Lipscomb DM, ed. *Hearing Conservation in Industry, Schools and the Military*. Boston: College-Hill Press; pp 45–66.

Taylor W, Pearson J, Mair A, Burns W. (1965) Study of noise and hearing in jute weaving. *J Acoust Soc Am*. 38, 113–120.

Thiessen GJ. (1978) Disturbance of sleep by noise. *J Acoust Soc Am*. 64, 216–222.

Thiessen GJ. (1983) Effect of intermittent and continuous traffic noise on various sleep characteristics and their adaptation. In: Rossi G, ed. *Proceedings of the Fourth International Congress on Noise as a Public Health Problem (Turin), Vol. 2*. Milan, Italy: Edizioni Techniche a cura del Centro Ricerche e Studi Amplifon.

Thompson SJ. (1981) Epidemiology feasibility study: effects of noise on the cardiovascular system. Washington, DC: United States Environmental Protection Agency.

Tonndorf J. (1976) Relationship between the transmission characteristics of conductive system and noise-induced hearing loss. In: Henderson D, Hamernik RP, Dosanjh DS, Mills JH, eds. *Effects of Noise on Hearing*. New York: Raven Press; pp 159–178.

Trine MB, Hirsch JE, Margolis RH (1993). The effect of middle ear pressure on transient evoked otoacoustic emissions. *Ear Hear*. 14: 401–407.

Turunen-Rise I, Flottorp G, Tvete O. (1991) Personal cassette players ('Walkman'). Do they cause noise-induced hearing loss? *Scand Audiol*. 20, 239–244.

United States Department of Labor. (1974) Proposed requirements and procedures for occupational noise exposure. *Fed Reg*. 39, 37773–37778.

United States Department of Labor. (1981) Occupational noise exposure: hearing conservation amendment. *Fed Reg*. 46, 4078–4179.

United States Department of Labor. (1983) Occupational noise exposure: hearing conservation amendment: final rule. *Fed Reg*. 48, 9738–9785.

United States Department of Labor. (1986) Record keeping guidelines for occupational injuries and illnesses: a report of the US Department of Labor Statistics. Washington, DC: United States Department of Labor.

Wachs TD (1982). Relation of home noise-confusion to infant cognitive development. Paper presented at the Annual Meeting of the American Psychological Association, Washington, DC.

Ward WD. (1973) Adaptation and fatigue. In: Jerger, J ed. *Modern Developments in Audiology*. 2nd ed. New York: Academic Press; pp 241–286.

Wenthold RJ, Schneider ME, Kim HN, DeChesne CJ. (1992) Putative biochemical processes in noise-induced hearing loss. In: Dancer AL, Henderson D, Salvi RJ, Hamernik RP, eds. *Noise Induced Hearing Loss*. St. Louis: Mosby Year Book; pp 28–37.

Williams H, Steiger W. (1970) Williams-Steiger Occupational safety and health act. PL 91-596.

Wood WS, Lipscomb DM. (1972) Maximum available sound pressure levels from stereo components. *J Acoust Soc Am*. 52, 484–487.

31 Nonorganic Hearing Loss

Frederick N. Martin

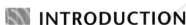

▨ INTRODUCTION

Not every patient seen in the audiology clinic is fully cooperative during the hearing evaluation. This lack of cooperation may be because the patient (1) does not understand the test procedure, (2) is poorly motivated, (3) is physically or emotionally incapable of appropriate responses, (4) wishes to conceal a handicap, (5) is deliberately feigning or exaggerating a hearing loss for personal gain or exemption, or (6) suffers from some degree of psychological disturbance. This chapter will describe some of the concepts underlying false or exaggerated hearing test results and the motivation for this behavior. It will also present some audiometric and nonaudiometric procedures that aid in the detection of inaccuracies and in the determination of a patient's true hearing thresholds.

Many terms have been used to describe a hearing loss that appears greater than can be explained on the basis of pathology in the auditory system. The most popularly used terms in the literature today are "nonorganic hearing loss," "pseudohypacusis," and "functional hearing loss." Such terms as "psychogenic hearing loss" and "malingering" suggest the motivation behind the behavior and may be oversimplifications. Williamson (1974) cautions that these terms may not be appropriate because clinicians typically do not know whether an exaggerated auditory threshold is the result of conscious or unconscious motivation. Therefore, it seems appropriate to use generic terms. In this chapter "nonorganic hearing loss" will be used to describe responses obtained on hearing examinations that are above the patient's true organic thresholds.

If one thinks of a hearing loss that is due to physical impairment in the auditory system as being "organic," then the term nonorganic is immediately clear. Many individuals with nonorganic hearing loss have nonorganic aspects superimposed on an organic hearing loss. Audiologists must remember that their function is to determine the extent of the organic component rather than to determine the precise reason for spurious test results.

▨ NONORGANIC HEARING LOSS IN ADULTS

A number of factors may encourage some persons either to feign a hearing loss that does not exist or to exaggerate a true hearing loss. One of these factors is financial gain. Altshuler (1982) reports that a significant amount of stress in the United States is directly attributable to economics. The very threat of the loss of income may drive some individuals to acts of "questionable honesty" that they might not otherwise consider. Disability compensation to veterans with service-connected hearing losses constitutes a significant portion of the many millions of dollars paid annually to beneficiaries of the Veterans Administration (VA) in an effort to compensate them for their disability.

Other factors that may contribute to nonorganic hearing loss are psychosocial and include the wish to avoid undesirable situations. There may be many other gains that the individual believes are afforded to hearing-disabled persons, including excuses for lack of success, advancement in position, poor marital situation, and so on (Altshuler, 1982).

The number of persons with nonorganic hearing loss may be increasing since the implementation of federal laws regarding hearing safety in the workplace. Some state laws regarding noise in industry are even more stringent than federal legislation. The promise of financial reward is bound to be a factor precipitating nonorganic hearing loss in workers who are in danger of incurring noise-induced hearing loss. Barelli and Ruder (1970) gathered data on 162 medicolegal patients and found that 24% of the 116 workers applying for compensation proved to have symptoms of nonorganic hearing loss.

Studying social and psychological characteristics of adult males with nonorganic hearing loss, Trier and Levy (1965) reported psychological and psychiatric evaluations of patients with and without hearing complaints. The group with nonorganic hearing loss achieved lower scores on all measures of socioeconomic status and scored significantly lower on measures of verbal intelligence. They showed a greater degree of clinically significant emotional disturbance. Trends of hypochondriasis were also noted, including many complaints of tinnitus. These findings are similar to other reports, which state that adults with nonorganic hearing loss also manifest a reliance on denial mechanisms. Such patients appear to have a diminished sense of confidence in their abilities to meet the needs of everyday life and may feel a sense of gain by appearing to have a hearing loss.

There is disagreement over whether nonorganic hearing loss may be psychogenic at all or whether all exaggerated hearing thresholds are deliberately and consciously manifested with an eye toward personal gain. Beagley and Knight (1968) stated that, although psychogenic deafness is rare, it does occur and can be diagnosed if careful attention is paid to the diagnostic criteria. They summarized 21 cases of nonorganic hearing loss and specified one case as fulfilling all of the criteria for a psychiatric motivation. Goldstein (1966) insists that psychogenic hearing loss does not exist as a clinical entity at all. He suggested that all nonorganic hearing loss is consciously simulated (malingered).

Two groups of servicemen were compared by Cohen et al. (1963). One group was consistent on auditory tests, and the other was not. The inconsistent group manifested deviant neurosensory signs and psychological abnormalities, gave reports of head injuries out of proportion to the actual extent of the injury, but showed no difference from the control subjects in predisposing factors. Cohen et al. (1963) concluded that individuals who present inconsistent results on hearing tests might be influenced by psychodynamic factors.

Gleason (1958), in a study of military personnel with nonorganic hearing loss, found that the patient who is inconsistent on audiologic tests is likely to be deviant psychologically but not necessarily psychiatrically ill. Fifty-five percent were judged to be emotionally immature, and 30% were judged to be neurotic. Of 278 consecutive cases, 30% showed inconsistencies and exaggerated hearing losses, and 86% of this subgroup had medically confirmed losses. The inconsistent group had many psychosomatic complaints, had deviant social behavior, and in general made poor adjustments to their hearing losses. Most of these men had done poorly in school. The conclusions of this study included: a nonorganic hearing loss may be on an unconscious level, motivation may be to obtain a favored goal, the patient may be attempting to mitigate blame for inadequate social behavior, hearing loss may be one symptom of a personality disorder. From this point of view, exaggerated hearing loss may be one symptom of a personality disturbance.

Katz (1980) cautions that certain neurologic problems can appear to be nonorganic in nature. For example, one patient who initially responded on puretone evaluation between 40 and 70 dB hearing level (HL) and eventually at levels of 20 dB HL responded immediately at 15 dB HL to spondees. This patient was neither a malingerer nor psychogenic. Rather, he was a volunteer for a study because he was terminally ill with a tumor of the corpus callosum. He did not claim to have difficulty with hearing, and he did not exhibit any difficulty in communication.

The question arises, "Why hearing loss?" Why does the patient with nonorganic hearing loss select this disorder rather than back pain, headache, whiplash, or some other more conventional malady? Altshuler's (1982) suggestions are logical, that some incident in the lives of these patients has focused their attention on hearing. The incident may have been an ear infection, physical trauma, noise exposure, or tinnitus or hearing loss in a relative or close friend. For whatever reason, this incident is the first step toward future nonorganic hearing loss.

■ NONORGANIC HEARING LOSS IN CHILDREN

A number of case reports of nonorganic hearing loss in children appear in the literature. Dixon and Newby (1959) reported on 40 children between the ages of 6 and 18 years with nonorganic hearing loss. Despite claimed hearing losses, 39 of these children were able to follow normal conversational speech with little difficulty. McCanna and DeLapa (1981) reported similar findings. Most experienced audiologists can report marked exaggeration of hearing thresholds for puretones in the presence of normal speech recognition thresholds.

There are also cases of apparent malingering with psychological undertones. For example, Bailey and Martin (1961) reported on a boy with normal hearing sensitivity who manifested a great many nonorganic symptoms. After the audiometric examination, he admitted a deliberate attempt to create the impression that he had a hearing loss. He claimed he did this so that he could be admitted to the state residential school for the deaf where his parents taught and his sister and girlfriend were students. Investigation into this boy's background revealed that he was a poor student in a high school for normal-hearing students. Hallewell et al. (1966) described a 13-year-old boy with a severe bilateral hearing loss who revealed essentially normal hearing sensitivity under hypnosis.

Cases of presumed psychogenic hearing loss in children have also been reported. Lumio et al. (1969) described three sisters whose hearing losses all appeared to develop over a period of a few months. Two of the three girls also had complaints of visual problems and were fitted with eyeglasses. All three apparently had their hearing return to normal in 1 day during a visit with their aunt. When the hearing returned, the visual disorders also disappeared. These authors reported that the nonorganic hearing loss was due to family conflicts. They believed that it was probable that the hearing loss of the youngest child was entirely unconscious, but the other two may have been deliberately simulated.

Thirty-two cases diagnosed as psychogenic hearing loss were reported by Barr (1963). Although puretone audiograms showed hearing levels in the 60- to 80-dB range, hearing for speech was considerably better than would be anticipated based on both formal and informal tests. Overall, these children were of normal intelligence but did not perform well in school. Because they were from homes where high scholastic performance was considered important, their parents willingly accepted the idea of hearing loss (based on failure of a school hearing test) as the explanation for poor academic achievement. It was believed that the attention paid to the children encouraged them, consciously or unconsciously, to feign a hearing loss on subsequent examinations. Barr (1963) stresses that nonorganic difficulty must be detected as early as possible before children realize that there are secondary gains to be enjoyed from a hearing disorder.

Austen and Lynch (2004) point out the obvious, that a dichotomy between acts of deliberate falsification (malingering) and those of unconscious motivation (psychogenesis) is an oversimplification of what may be a complex human dynamic. They propose another term, *factitious behavior*, and formulate a new nomenclature for the categorization of nonorganic hearing loss. Theirs is a detailed set of recommendations, and the reader is referred to this publication for greater specificity than can be addressed in this chapter.

Sometimes children who inadvertently fail school screening tests become the object of a great deal of attention. This may cause them to feign a hearing loss. Several such school children are discussed by Campanelli (1963). These children behaved on formal tests as if they had a hearing loss but behaved normally in other situations. This study further emphasized the need for caution against preferential seating, special classes, hearing therapy, and hearing aids until the extent of the hearing problem is defined by proper audiologic diagnosis. In a study evaluating one hearing conservation program (Leshin, 1960), quite a few cases of nonorganic hearing loss were discovered. A team including otologists, audiologists, medical social workers, and local health department staff worked to: (1) reconcile medical, audiologic, and psychosocial data to arrive at a diagnosis; (b) determine familial and environmental factors contributing to nonorganic loss; and (c) outline and implement courses of action to relieve a child's need to use nonorganic hearing loss as a personality mechanism.

Identification audiometry is a significant tool for discovering school children with hearing disorders. There is some reason to fear that a child may fail a school test despite normal hearing due to such factors as noisy acoustic environment, improper testing technique, insufficient motivation, or poorly calibrated equipment. If attention is attracted to this inadvertent failure, the child may get the notion that a hearing loss provides a variety of secondary gains, such as excuse for poor school performance. The end result may be referral to an otologic or audiologic clinic for further evaluation of hearing. Several authors (Ross, 1964; Miller et al., 1968) have stressed the need to uncover nonorganic hearing loss before referrals are made. Ross (1964) cited four cases that illustrate the problems of such referrals and the commitment this might give to the child to simulate a hearing loss.

Nonorganic hearing loss in children appears to occur with sufficient frequency to cause concern. Whether the notion of simulating a hearing loss comes out of a school screening failure or from some conscious or unconscious need, it must be recognized as early as possible by the audiologist to avoid a variety of unfortunate circumstances. Performance or supervision of hearing tests on young children by an audiologist, rather than a technician, may serve to avert what may later develop into serious psychological or educational difficulties. However, the audiologist should be alert to the possibility that the problem uncovered may be one of auditory perception and not true hearing loss (Wieczorek, 1979).

■ INDICATIONS OF NONORGANIC HEARING LOSS

The Nontest Situation

Frequently the source of referral will suggest the possibility of nonorganic hearing loss. For example, when an individual is referred by an attorney after an accident that has resulted in a client's sudden loss of hearing, it is only natural to suspect that nonorganicity may play a role in test results. This is also true of veterans referred for hearing tests, the results of which decide the amount of their monthly pensions. It must be emphasized that the majority of patients referred for such examinations are cooperative and well meaning; however, the VA population consists of a higher risk group for nonorganic hearing loss than self-referred or physician-referred patients. Nonorganic hearing loss must be on the minds of clinical audiologists, or they may miss some of the symptoms that indicate its presence.

A case history is always of value, but it is particularly useful in compensation cases. It is obviously beneficial for examining audiologists to take history statements themselves, so that they can observe not only the responses given to questions, but also the manner in which these responses are offered. The patient may claim an overreliance on lipreading, ask for inappropriate repetitions of words, or constantly readjust a hearing aid. It is usual for hard-of-hearing patients to be relatively taciturn about their hearing problems, whereas exaggerated or contradictory statements of difficulty or discomfort, vague descriptions of hearing difficulties, and the volunteering of unasked-for supplementary information may be symptomatic of nonorganic hearing loss.

We sometimes see, in patients with nonorganic hearing loss, exaggerated actions and maneuvers to watch every movement of the speaker's lips or the turning away with a hand cupped over the ear, ostensibly to amplify sound. As a rule, hard-of-hearing adults face the speaker with whom they are conversing, but their watching postures are not nearly so tortuous as those just described. Not all patients who intend to exaggerate their hearing thresholds create such caricatures, and even patients who do should not be condemned as having nonorganic hearing loss on the basis of such evidence alone.

The Test Situation

During the hearing examination, the patient with nonorganic hearing loss is frequently inconsistent in test responses. A certain amount of variability is to be expected of any individual; however, when the magnitude of this variability exceeds 10 dB for any threshold measurement, one must consider the possibility of nonorganicity. With the exception of some unusual conditions, it can be expected that the cooperative patient will give consistent audiometric readings.

Two types of patient error are frequently seen in the clinical testing of puretone thresholds. These are false-positive and false-negative responses. When the subject does not respond at levels at or slightly above true thresholds, this constitutes a false-negative response. False-negative responses are characteristic of nonorganic hearing loss. Frequently, the highly responsive patient will give false-positive responses, signaling that a tone was heard when none was presented at or above threshold. False-positive responses, although sometimes annoying, are characteristic of a conscientious responder.

Feldman (1962) pointed out that the patient with nonorganic hearing loss does not offer false-positive responses during silent periods on puretone tests. Chaiklin and Ventry (1965a) found that only 22% of their group of adult subjects with nonorganic hearing loss gave a "false alarm," whereas 86% of those with organic loss gave false-positive responses. Thus, one simple check for nonorganicity is simply to allow silent intervals of a minute or so from time to time. A false alarm is more likely to indicate that the patient is trying to cooperate and believes that a tone was introduced. Extremely slow and deliberate responses may be indicative of a nonorganic problem because most patients with organic hearing losses respond relatively quickly to the signal, particularly at levels above threshold.

The Audiometric Configuration

A number of authors have suggested that an audiometric pattern emerges that is consistent with nonorganic hearing loss. Some have described this pattern as a relatively flat audiogram showing an equal amount of hearing loss across frequencies (Fournier, 1958). Others have suggested that the "saucer-shaped audiogram" similar to a supraliminal equal loudness contour is the typical curve illustrating nonorganicity (e.g., Carhart, 1958). However, Chaiklin et al. (1959) observed that saucer-shaped audiograms can also occur in true organic hearing losses and that these curves are seen infrequently in nonorganic hearing loss. They concluded that there is no typical puretone configuration associated with nonorganic hearing loss. Because the patient with nonorganic hearing loss may attempt to give responses that are of equal loudness at all frequencies, ignorance of the manner in which loudness grows with respect to intensity at different frequencies does suggest that the result should be a saucer-shaped audiogram. The logic of this is apparently not borne out in fact.

In a study of 64 men with nonorganic hearing loss and 36 men with true organic loss, Ventry and Chaiklin (1965) asked a panel of three experienced audiologists to judge the configurations of the audiograms. Saucer-shaped curves appeared in only 8% of the nonorganic cases and were also seen in true organic losses. This research indicates, as many experienced audiologists have observed, that the saucer audiogram has limited use in identifying nonorganic hearing loss.

Test-Retest Reliability

One indication of nonorganicity is the lack of consistency on repeated measures. Counseling the patient about inaccuracies may encourage more accurate responses; however, if this counseling is done in a belligerent way, it can hardly be expected to increase cooperation. Sometimes a brief explanation of the test discrepancies encourages improved patient cooperation. By withholding any allegations of guilt on the part of the patient, the audiologist can assume personal responsibility for not having conveyed the instructions properly. This provides a graceful way out for many patients, even if they are highly committed to nonorganic loss. Berger (1965) found that some children can be coaxed into "listening harder," thereby improving results on puretone tests.

Although these suggestions are usually useful when working with civilian populations, exceptions exist when testing military personnel. When counseling and cajoling fail to eliminate symptoms of nonorganic hearing loss, direct confrontation has been made. Military patients have been told that exaggeration of thresholds is a violation of the Universal Code of Military Justice and therefore a court-martial offense. Personal communication with audiologists working in military installations reveals that such methods may be very effective in altering patient behavior. Veterans with service-connected hearing losses may have their pensions interrupted until examining audiologists are satisfied with test results. It is not known, however, whether this kind of open confrontation may have serious psychological effects on some patients. It can certainly be offensive if inappropriately used. A personal view is that the risk of psychological trauma in even a very small percentage of cases should be considered carefully before such aggressive tactics are used. A more prudent approach may be more time consuming but may also be safer.

The Shadow Curve

It may seem advantageous to a patient feigning a hearing loss to claim that loss in only one ear. Appearing to have one normal ear is convenient because individuals need not worry about being "tripped up" in conversation by responding to a sound that is below their admitted thresholds. In this way, all hearing can appear to occur in the "good ear," and the claim can be made that hearing is nonexistent in the "bad ear." Normal activities can be carried on for the unilaterally hearing-impaired individual without any special speechreading abilities.

It is generally agreed that a patient with a profound hearing loss in one ear will hear a test tone in the opposite ear by bone conduction if the signal is raised to a sufficient level during a threshold test. For an air-conduction signal, the levels required for contralateralization range from 40 to 70 dB when supra-aural earphones are used, depending on frequency (Zwislocki, 1953). The interaural attenuation, the loss of sound energy due to contralateralization, is much less for bone conduction than for air conduction. With the vibrator placed on the mastoid process, there is virtually no interaural attenuation. Therefore, if a person truly has no hearing for air conduction or bone conduction in one ear, then the audiogram taken from the bad ear would suggest a moderate unilateral conductive loss. Unless masking is applied to the better ear, a "shadow curve" should be expected. A more complete discussion of interaural attenuation, the shadow curve, and masking is presented in Chapter 6.

The naive patient with nonorganic hearing loss may give responses indicating no hearing in one ear and very good hearing in the other ear. The lack of contralateral response, especially by bone conduction, is a very clear symptom of unilateral nonorganic hearing loss and offers a good reason why all patients should be tested initially without masking,

even if it appears obvious at the outset of testing that masking will be required later in the examination.

Speech Recognition Threshold and Puretone Average Disagreement

The speech recognition threshold (SRT) is generally expected to compare favorably with the average of the lowest two of the three thresholds obtained at 500, 1,000, and 2,000 Hz. Lack of agreement between the puretone average (PTA) and the SRT, in the absence of explanations such as slope of the audiogram or poor word recognition/discrimination, is symptomatic of nonorganic hearing loss. Carhart (1952) was probably the first to report that, in confirmed cases of nonorganic hearing loss, the SRT is *lower* (better) than the PTA. Ventry and Chaiklin (1965) reported that the SRT-PTA discrepancy identified 70% of their patients with confirmed nonorganic hearing loss; in each case, the SRT proved to be at least 12 dB lower than the PTA. The lack of SRT-PTA agreement is often the first major sign of nonorganic hearing loss.

It is impossible to know the precise strategies patients use if they wish to deceive examiners on hearing tests. For one thing, simply asking them their methods would only result in rebuke, and since nonorganic hearing loss is, in many cases, an intrinsically deceitful behavior, an honest response would hardly be forthcoming. Martin et al. (2001) paid normal-hearing adults to feign hearing loss for puretones and motivated them by compensating them with more money as their actions became more convincing. Following a series of puretone tests, they were simply asked to describe the strategies they used. Most said that they initially responded randomly and then set a sort of loudness metric in their minds and tried to repeat it during retesting or at different frequencies. After they had taken the test for a short while and realized that a set procedure was being used (the American Speech-Language-Hearing Association method), they began to establish consistency by counting the number of tones, which were initially presented at 30 dB HL and then increased in 5-dB increments. Assuming that this methodology holds true for patients with actual nonorganic hearing loss, an obvious procedure would be to vary from an established technique and present tones at random intensities.

In attempting to remember the loudness of a suprathreshold signal previously responded to, one might easily become confused between puretone and spondaic word levels. Very little research has been carried out to explain why the discrepancy generally favors the SRT. It might be that the loudness of speech is primarily associated with its low-frequency components. According to the equal loudness contours, the low frequencies grow more rapidly in loudness than tones in the speech frequencies. This speculation is supported by the work of McLennan and Martin (1976), who concluded that when puretones of different frequencies are compared in loudness against a speech signal, the difference between them is a function of the flattening of the loudness contours. Hirsh (1952) likens the phon lines to loudness recruitment, in that the low-frequency sounds increase in loudness more quickly per decibel than the midfrequencies. Ventry (1976) explains the difference between the sensations of loudness for speech and puretones on the basis of their different sound pressure level references, but this theory has its limitations.

▩ SPECIAL TESTS FOR NONORGANIC HEARING LOSS

Qualitative Tests

One responsibility that audiologists bear is to determine the organic hearing thresholds for all of their patients, including those with nonorganic hearing loss. It is not simply a matter of gathering evidence against the patient to prove nonorganicity. This is sometimes necessary, but the unmasking of nonorganic cases should not be an end in itself. Although it is easier to make a diagnosis on cooperative patients in terms of their hearing thresholds, a lack of cooperation does not justify disinterest in the patient's true hearing status.

There are tests that prove the presence of nonorganic hearing loss, those that approximate the true threshold, and those that actually quantify the patient's threshold without voluntary cooperation. Discussion of tests for nonorganic hearing loss will follow.

Acoustic Immittance Measurements

Chapters 8 through 10 provide details on the subject of immittance measurements. Among the many valuable contributions that immittance testing brings to our field is the detection of nonorganic hearing loss. This section is devoted to measurements of use of tympanic membrane compliance and ways in which they may assist in the diagnosis of nonorganic hearing loss.

The acoustic reflex threshold is the immittance measurement that is of greatest value in the diagnosis of nonorganic hearing loss. The elicitation of this reflex at a low sensation level (SL) (60 dB or less above the voluntary threshold) has been construed to suggest the presence of a cochlear lesion. However, if the SL (the difference between the reflex threshold and the voluntary puretone threshold) is extremely low (5 dB or less), it is difficult to accept on the basis of organic pathology (Lamb and Peterson, 1967). Feldman (1962) cited a patient with unilateral nonorganic hearing loss who demonstrated acoustic reflexes in the "poor ear" below the patient's voluntary threshold. If the audiologist is certain that no artifact contaminates the readings, the suggestion that the acoustic reflex may be achieved by a tone that cannot be heard must be rejected, and a diagnosis of nonorganic hearing loss may be made.

More than merely identifying nonorganic hearing loss, acoustic reflex measurements may be useful in the actual estimation of thresholds. Jerger et al. (1974) describe a procedure based on the work of Niemeyer and Sesterhenn (1974) in which the middle ear muscle reflex thresholds for puretones are compared to those for wideband noise and low- and high-frequency filtered wideband noise. The procedure, which is referred to as SPAR (sensitivity prediction from the acoustic reflex), approximates the degree of hearing loss, if any, as well as the general audiometric configuration. Margolis (1993) has shown that this procedure can identify thresholds in a large number of cases with a high degree of specificity. Details of this procedure may be found elsewhere, but it certainly appears that this method may have use in estimating the thresholds of patients with nonorganic hearing loss.

There is no way to know how many patients with nonorganic hearing loss appear to have a conductive hearing loss, although I have never seen this. Of course, the middle ear muscle reflex measurement cannot be used in cases with nonorganic components overlying even mild conductive losses, since contralateral reflexes are absent in both ears when even one ear has a conductive disorder. Tympanometry is an objective method that may be used to suggest middle ear disorders in such cases.

The elaborateness of middle ear measurements, including the instructions for the patient to be quiet and immobile, may have the effect of discouraging nonorganic behavior if this test is performed early in the diagnostic battery. It is often good practice to perform middle ear measurements as the first test on adults and cooperative children. They are asked to sit quietly and are told that the measurements made will reveal a great deal about their hearing. I have no hesitancy in recommending this approach in general and believe it can be a useful deterrent to nonorganic hearing loss.

Stenger Test

Probably the best way to test for unilateral nonorganic hearing loss is by use of the Stenger test. The Stenger principle states that when two tones of the same frequency are introduced simultaneously into both ears, only the louder tone will be perceived.

Since its introduction as a tuning fork test over a century ago, the Stenger test has been modified many times. If unilateral nonorganic hearing loss is suspected, the Stenger test may be performed quickly as a screening procedure. This is most easily done by introducing a tone of a desired frequency into the better ear at a level 10 dB above the threshold and into the poorer ear at a level 10 dB below the admitted threshold. If the loss in the poor ear is genuine, the patient will be unaware of any signal in the poor ear and will respond to the tone in the good ear readily, because at 10 dB above threshold, it should be easily heard. Such a response is termed a negative Stenger, indicating that the poorer ear threshold is probably correct.

If patients do not admit hearing in the bad ear and are unaware of the tone in the good ear, they simply do not respond. This is a positive Stenger, which proves that the threshold for the "poorer" ear is better than the response given by the individual. A positive Stenger is the interpretation because the tone is actually above the true threshold in the "bad" ear and precludes hearing the tone in the good ear.

This screening procedure rapidly identifies the presence or absence of unilateral nonorganic hearing loss if there is a difference in admitted threshold between the ears of at least 20 dB. The test is most likely to be positive in nonorganic cases with large interaural differences (exceeding 40 dB) or large nonorganic components in the "poorer" ear.

A positive result on the Stenger test does not identify the true organic hearing threshold. To obtain threshold information, the Stenger test can also be performed by seeking the *minimum contralateral interference levels* (MCIL). The procedure is as follows. The tone is presented to the good ear at 10 dB SL. There should be a response from the patient. A tone is then presented to the bad ear at 0 dB HL, simultaneously with the tone at 10 dB SL in the good ear. If a response is obtained, the level is raised 5 dB in the *bad ear*, keeping the level the same in the good ear. The level is continuously raised in 5-dB steps until the subject fails to respond. Because the tone is still above threshold in the good ear, the lack of response must mean that the tone has been heard loudly enough in the bad ear so that the patient experiences the Stenger effect and is no longer aware of a tone in the good ear. Being unwilling to react to tones in the bad ear, patients simply stop responding. The lowest hearing level of the tone in the bad ear producing this effect is the MCIL and should be within 20 dB of the true threshold. An alert patient feigning a hearing loss may "catch on" to what the clinician is doing unless, from time to time, the tone in the good ear is presented without competition from the bad ear.

In one study (Peck and Ross, 1970), the Stenger test was performed on 35 normal-hearing subjects feigning a total hearing loss in one ear. Ascending and descending methods of tone presentation were used. No differences in the interference levels were observed between the two methods. The interference levels were found to be within 14 dB of the true thresholds, resulting in the general conclusion that the Stenger test can approximate the hearing thresholds of the poor ear in unilateral nonorganic hearing loss. This conclusion was supported by Kintsler et al. (1970), who found that the Stenger test correctly identified 25 of 31 cases of nonorganic hearing loss.

Because their results were better than suggested by the study of Chaiklin and Ventry (1965b), Kintsler et al. (1972) replicated the Chaiklin and Ventry study, which had found the Stenger test not to be a good identifier of nonorganic hearing loss. They noted a close correspondence between positive Stenger test results and nonorganic hearing loss. In conflict with this, Hattler and Schuchman (1971) found that,

of 225 patients with nonorganic hearing loss, the Stenger test was only applicable in 57% of the cases and had the poorest efficiency of all the tests tried even when applicable, correctly labeling only one half of the patients with nonorganic hearing loss.

Monro and Martin (1977) found that the Stenger test, using the screening method, was virtually unbeatable on normal-hearing subjects feigning unilateral hearing losses. Martin and Shipp (1982), using a similar research method, found that as sophistication and practice with the Stenger test are increased, patients are less likely to be confused by low contralateral interference levels.

The studies cited here illustrate that the accuracy and efficiency of the Stenger test continue to be contested. Although the Stenger test, like most tests, has certain shortcomings, most regard it as an efficient test for quick identification of unilateral nonorganic hearing loss. The only equipment required for the test is a two-channel, puretone audiometer with separate hearing level dials for the right and left ears. To be sure, if the test is performed by an inexperienced clinician, a series of patterns of tone introductions may betray the intentions of the test to an alert patient. The majority of respondents on a survey of audiometric practices (Martin et al., 1998a) named the Stenger test as their most popular test for nonorganic hearing loss, which is difficult to understand since unilateral cases are by far in the minority.

Modified Stenger Test

Taylor (1949) reported on the use of a modification of the puretone Stenger test with spondaic words. The Stenger principle holds for speech stimuli if words, like spondees, are presented via both channels of a speech audiometer simultaneously. All of the criteria for application of the puretone Stenger test apply to the modified version; that is, there should be at least a 20-dB difference between the SRTs of the right and left ears, and the greater the interaural difference and the closer to normal one ear hears, the better the test works. A two-channel audiometer with one volume unit (VU) meter is easiest to use with either monitored live voice or prerecorded presentation.

Subjects are instructed simply to repeat every spondee they hear. The words are presented 10 dB above the better ear SRT and 10 dB below the poorer ear SRT. If the patient continues to repeat the words, the modified Stenger is considered to be negative, providing no evidence of nonorganic hearing loss. If the patient does not repeat the spondees under these conditions, then the screening test has been failed and the MCIL should be sought.

To determine the MCIL, the SL of 10 dB should be maintained in the better ear. The hearing level dial controlling the intensity at the poorer ear should be set to the lowest limit of the audiometer. Each time a spondee is presented and repeated by the patient, the level in the poorer ear should be raised 5 dB. The lowest hearing level dial setting in the poorer ear at which the patient stops repeating two or more spondees correctly is considered to be the MCIL and is above the threshold for that ear. The precise threshold cannot be known, but MCILs have been noted as low as 15 dB above the SRT of the poorer ear. If the MCIL is as low as 30 dB HL, it may be assumed that hearing for speech is normal.

Experienced clinicians can manipulate the modified Stenger in a variety of ways. The speech itself can be less formal than spondaic words and may consist of a series of instructions or questions requiring verbal responses from the patient. The signal to the better ear may be randomly deleted on the chance that patients may be "on to" the test and may be repeating words they hear in their poorer ears but will not admit it because they believe that words are also above threshold in their better ears even though they do not hear them. To paraphrase an old saying, "experience is the mother of invention."

Martin and Shipp (1982) found that sophistication with the speech Stenger test resulted in higher MCILs, which can lead the unsuspecting clinician to accept an exaggerated SRT as correct. Because there is no way to control for any knowledge about the modified Stenger test that a patient brings to the examination, the alert clinician is wary of contamination of test results that such knowledge may cause.

Ascending-Descending Methods

The use of both an ascending and descending approach to puretone threshold measurements has been recommended as a rapid and simple procedure (Harris, 1958). A greater than 10-dB difference between these two measurements suggests a nonorganic problem because the two thresholds should be identical. Personal use of this procedure indicates that this difference is often as large as 30 dB for patients with nonorganic hearing loss. For these patients, the ascending method generally reveals lower (better) thresholds than the descending approach. The Harris test is quick and easy to perform with the simplest puretone audiometer and is the basis for the BADGE (Bekesy Ascending Descending Gap Evaluation) test using Bekesy audiometry (Hood, Campbell, and Hutton, 1964). Kerr et al. (1975) modified Harris' original procedure and suggested that the test is improved slightly by performing the descending portion in 10-dB rather than 5-dB steps. Cherry and Ventry (1976) have further altered this procedure using a modified method of limits. Most recently, Woodford et al. (1997) showed the ascending-descending gap to be an excellent screening tool for nonorganic hearing loss. In these studies, the stimuli included pulsing tones with standard off times.

Martin et al. (2000) used a combination of stimuli in the development of a screening procedure for nonorganic hearing loss. Using a standard diagnostic audiometer, they developed a procedure very much like the BADGE (Hood et al., 1964) but used standard instead of Békésy audiometry. They compared ascending and descending approaches using tones that were continuously on (CON), pulsing on and off with a standard off time (SOT), and pulsing with

a lengthened off-time (LOT). The CON-SOT-LOT test was described as being rapid and accurate in the detection of nonorganic hearing loss. Subsequent clinical use has borne this out.

Varying Intensity Story Test

The Varying Intensity Story Test (VIST) is based on the Swinging Story test used in the 1940s, which never became a popular approach to unmask unilateral nonorganic losses. The test required the use of a two-channel speech audiometer. A story was read to a patient with portions directed above the threshold of the normal ear (e.g., 10 dB above the SRT) through one channel, portions below the threshold of the "poorer ear" (e.g., 10 dB below the SRT), and portions through both channels simultaneously.

For the test to work, the story must be presented rapidly, including rapid switching from channel 1 to channel 2 to both channels. Although this can be done using monitored live voice, an easier method is to use a prerecording. Calibration tones for each channel allow for proper level setting before the test begins.

On completion of the recording, the patient is simply asked to repeat the story. Repetition of information directed to (and presumably heard in) the good ear or both ears is to be expected. Any remarks from the *bad ear* column must have been heard below the patient's admitted threshold for speech and show that the threshold for that ear has been exaggerated. All that can be determined from a positive result is that hearing is better in the poorer ear than what the patient has volunteered, providing evidence of nonorganic hearing loss.

The VIST (Martin et al., 1998b) is a major revision of the Swinging Story test. Two main advantages to the VIST are that it can be used in one or both ears (not limiting it to unilateral cases) and that it comes close, in many cases, to approximating the auditory threshold for speech.

Unlike the Swinging Story test (Martin, 1997), the theme in VIST changes when the *bad ear* column is included or excluded, adding to the complexity of the challenge for the patient with nonorganic hearing loss. Because the patient must concentrate on the story and commit it to memory, it is less likely that the individual will be able to remember which material was presented to the *bad* ear.

To perform the VIST, patients are advised that they will hear a story one time, after which they will be asked to respond to a series of 10 written questions. Part I of the story (see next page) is presented at 10 dB SL, and Part II is presented at 30 to 50 dB below the admitted SRT. The test is considered to be positive if questions resulting from information only supplied from Part II are answered correctly. Interpretation of a positive finding is that the SRT can be no poorer than the level for Part II. The VIST was shown to work well on subjects simulating nonorganic hearing loss, but it remains to be verified on true nonorganic cases.

PART I: Presented above threshold	PART II: Presented below threshold
China,	despite overpopulation,
is well known for its delicate beauty	and its rugged terrain.
Many popular styles of	cooking originating in
china exist today. Patterns	of beautiful gardens
of flowers and geometric	landscaping
designs are equally common	in many modern Chinese cities.
Hand-painted scenes	of the natural beauty of China
can be found	in many museums
if one knows where to look.	Books about
China owned by your grandmother probably	contain much misinformation because early 20th century China
	has arrived and
is quite different from modern China. The computer age	on all types of textiles. A new age has dawned
changed the way complex designs are printed	
on modern China.	

Low-Level Phonetically Balanced Word Tests

Phonetically balanced (PB) word tests are routinely performed at 30 to 40 dB above the SRT because most clinicians find that this usually approaches the PB max. Some clinicians routinely do performance-intensity functions for PB words (PI-PB), but this is usually reserved for special cases, such as for determination of site of lesion. Normally, low word recognition scores are expected at low SLs.

Hopkinson (1978), in interpreting the PI-PB functions reported by Harris (1965), suggests that normal-hearing individuals should reveal PB word scores approximately as shown in Table 31.1.

Snyder (1977) reported that unusually high PB word scores can be obtained on patients with nonorganic hearing loss at levels slightly above their admitted thresholds. Thus, if scores are substantially higher than those shown in Table 31.1 for these SLs above the admitted hearing level, then this would suggest exaggeration of threshold and essentially normal hearing for the speech range of frequencies.

Pulse-Count Methods

Some tests may be carried out by presenting a number of puretone pulses in rapid succession and asking the patient to count and recall the numbers of pulses that were heard. The intensity of the tones may be varied above and below the admitted threshold of the tone in one ear (Ross, 1964) or above the threshold in one ear and below the threshold in the other ear (Nagel, 1964). If the originally obtained thresholds are valid, the patient should have no difficulty in counting the pulses. Inconsistency should occur only if all the tone pulses are above threshold and the patient has to sort out the number of louder ones from the number of softer ones. This can be very difficult to do. A major advantage to this test is that it can be carried out quickly using any kind of puretone audiometer.

TABLE 31.1 Approximate word recognition scores at various sensation levels for normal listeners

Sensation level (dB)	Word recognition score (%)
5	25
10	50
20	75
28	88
32	92
40	100

When scores for those with apparent hearing loss exceed these values, this could suggest exaggerated hearing threshold levels (Hopkinson, 1978).

The Yes-No Test

Frank (1976) described a test for nonorganic hearing loss that would seem too simple to work; nevertheless, it often does. The test is intended for children but has occasionally been useful with naive adults. The patient is simply told to say "yes" when a tone is heard and "no" when a tone is not heard. The tone is presented at the lowest limit of the audiometer and increased in intensity in 5-dB steps. Some patients, in an attempt to convince the examiner of poor hearing, will say "no" to tones that are heard below the level selected to be "threshold." Of course, a "no" response that is time-locked with the introduction of a tone is clear evidence that the tone was heard, barring occasional false-positive responses. A similar procedure was described by Nolan and Tucker (1981). The audiologist must decide when such a procedure is best used with a given patient.

QUANTITATIVE TESTS

Despite the considerable interest that has been generated and the appeal of the previously mentioned tests, none so far has provided the most sought after information. They lack the ability to provide the true threshold of audibility in patients who will not or cannot cooperate fully. For measures of true threshold, our profession has tended to turn to electrophysiologic procedures.

Auditory Evoked Potentials

The enthusiasm for auditory evoked potentials (AEPs) (see Chapters 13 and 14) has resulted in the recommendation that they be used as objective tests for *all* patients complaining of noise-induced hearing loss (Heron, 1968), and AEP has been called the "crucial test" in the diagnosis of nonorganic hearing loss (Knight and Beagley, 1970). Alberti (1970) found that results obtained from this technique and from voluntary puretone testing agreed within 10 dB and recommended that AEP be used with all uncooperative patients.

The procedures that record the components of the evoked response that occur between 50 and 300 ms may, some day, become more popular because they provide threshold information at octave frequencies between 500 and 4,000 Hz. However, this test can easily take more than 1 hour. The earlier components, the auditory brainstem responses (ABR), thus far have proven to be more reliable than the later responses in detecting nonorganic hearing loss (Hall, 1992; Shulman-Galambos and Galambos 1975). A limitation of ABR is that it is less frequency specific because of the use of brief signals like clicks or tone bursts.

Berlin (1978) indicated that ABR, in combination with electrocochleography, tympanometry, and acoustic reflexes, forms a powerful test battery for noncooperative patients such as small children. It seems logical to extend this conclusion to patients with nonorganic hearing loss.

Even in the hands of experienced clinicians, high correlations between evoked response and voluntary thresholds are not always found (Rose et al., 1972). Although ABR is an important diagnostic tool for evaluating nonorganic hearing loss, it should be interpreted with caution.

Otoacoustic Emissions

Since their introduction into clinical audiologic practice, evoked otoacoustic emissions (EOAEs) have increased in popularity, and they serve as an important tool in the diagnosis of auditory lesion site, as well as in estimating hearing sensitivity in noncooperative patients (Musiek et al., 1995). See Chapter 21 for details on the otoacoustic emission (OAE) procedures. OAEs, especially transient-evoked otoacoustic emissions (TEOAEs), have been shown to be of value in cases of nonorganic hearing loss.

TEOAEs may reveal that hearing is normal or near normal in patients feigning a hearing loss but may be of little or no value for those with actual hearing levels greater than about 40 dB who wish the audiologist to believe that their hearing is poorer than that. The fact that the adult patient with nonorganic hearing loss is probably aware that some measures of hearing sensitivity are possible without patient cooperation may encourage individuals who arrive at the audiology clinic with plans to falsify test results to become more cooperative when they are prepared for TEOAE or AEP tests. This deterrent may be of greater value than the test itself.

Puretone Delayed Auditory Feedback

General dissatisfaction has been expressed with speech delayed auditory feedback (DAF) because it does not reveal the true threshold of the patient with nonorganic hearing loss. A procedure has been described that uses the delayed feedback notion with puretones and that can be administered to patients who appear unwilling or unable to give accurate readings on threshold audiometry (Ruhm and Cooper, 1964).

During puretone DAF, the patient is asked to tap out a continuous pattern, such as four taps, pause, two taps, pause, etc. The electromagnetic key on which the patient taps is shielded from the individual's visual field. After the patient has demonstrated the ability to maintain the tapping pattern and rhythm, an audiometer circuit is added so that, for each tap, a tone pulse is introduced into an earphone worn by the patient. The tone has a duration of 50 ms at maximum amplitude but is delayed by 200 ms from the time the key is tapped. If the tone is audible, its presence causes the subject to vary tapping behavior in several ways, such as a loss of rate or rhythm, the number of taps, or an increase of finger pressure on the key.

It has been demonstrated (Ruhm and Cooper, 1962) that changes occur in tapping performance at SLs as low as 5 dB and are independent of test tone frequency and manual fatigue (Ruhm and Cooper, 1963). Once a subject has demonstrated key-tapping ability, any alterations seen after introduction of a delayed puretone must be interpreted as meaning that the tone was heard.

Not all researchers have found the 5-dB SL change in tapping performance using puretone DAF. Alberti (1970) found that tapping rhythms were disturbed in general at 5 to 15 dB above threshold but has observed variations as great as 40 dB. He reported that some subjects are difficult to test with this procedure because they either cannot or will not establish a tapping rhythm, a problem that I have also observed. At times, patients appear to fail to understand the instructions, and at other times, they complain that their fingers are too stiff to tap the key.

Two studies (Monro and Martin, 1977; Martin and Shipp, 1982) show puretone DAF to be extremely resistant to effects of previous test knowledge and practice, with tones at low SLs. Experience apparently plays a role at suprathreshold levels with unpracticed subjects. The subjects without practice showed many more time and pattern errors than those with practice (Cooper and Stokinger, 1976). Practice notwithstanding, the puretone DAF procedure is considerably less time consuming than many of the electrophysiologic methods and has been found to be accurate, reliable, and simple (Robinson and Kasden, 1973). Despite these advantages, puretone DAF is not generally used, and commercial devices are not available for this procedure.

TEST SEQUENCE

During routine audiometrics, the precise order in which tests are done probably does not have a significant effect on results. However, patients with nonorganic hearing loss may attempt to set a level above threshold as a reference for consistent supra-threshold responses. For this reason, threshold tests should be performed before supra-threshold tests.

The following test order has proved useful in examining patients with suspected nonorganic hearing loss: (1) immittance measures; (2) SRT, including the modified Stenger test in unilateral cases; (3) air-conduction thresholds, including the Stenger test if indicated; (4) word recognition tests using PB word lists at low SLs; (5) bone-conduction thresholds; (6) puretone DAF; (7) OAE; and (8) ABR.

DISCUSSION

In the vast majority of cases, the detection of nonorganic hearing loss is not a difficult task for the alert clinician. The more challenging responsibility of the audiologist is to determine the patient's organic thresholds of hearing; however, the difficulty of this task increases as the cooperation of the patient decreases. Some patients with nonorganic hearing loss are overtly hostile and unwilling to modify their test behavior even after counseling.

It is not likely that a single approach to diagnosis and resolution of nonorganic hearing loss is forthcoming, although there are certain points on which we should all agree. For example, it is far better to discourage exaggeration of hearing thresholds at the outset of testing than to detect and try to correct these exaggerations later. Once nonorganicity is observed, the audiologist is faced with the responsibility of determining the true organic thresholds. Tests that may aid in deterring pseudothreshold responses include all the electrophysiologic and electroacoustic procedures. In my opinion, acoustic immittance measurements should be accomplished initially in all routine audiologic assessments, thereby discouraging some nonorganic hearing loss. Puretone DAF and the Stenger test are quick and easy to perform, where applicable, and allow the patient to realize that the examiner has methods of determining puretone thresholds, even without patient cooperation.

There are times when audiologists believe that their patients with nonorganic hearing loss should be referred for psychological or psychiatric guidance. Such decisions should not be made recklessly or arbitrarily, but rather after considerable thought. Suggestions of this nature must be made carefully because of the unfortunate stigma that may be associated with such referrals.

Great care must be taken in writing reports about patients with suspected nonorganic hearing loss. It must be borne in mind that once individuals have been diagnosed as "malingering," "uncooperative," or "functional," their reputations and prestige may be damaged. To label a patient in such ways is a grave matter because it implies deliberate falsification. Such labels are difficult to expunge and may be tragically unjust. The only way an audiologist can be absolutely certain that a patient with nonorganic hearing loss is truly a malingerer is for the patient to admit to the intent, and most experienced audiologists would probably agree with Hopkinson (1967) that such admissions are rare indeed. Value judgments are not within the purview of the audiologist and should be avoided.

Counseling sessions should be carried out after all audiologic evaluations. Counseling the individual with nonorganic hearing loss is naturally more difficult than counseling patients with an organic hearing disorder. Children may be told only that their hearing appears to be normal (if this is believed to be the case) despite audiometric findings to the contrary. Parents should be warned not to discuss their children's difficulties in their presence or to provide any secondary rewards that may accrue to a hearing loss. Adults with nonorganic hearing loss may simply have to be told that a diagnosis of the extent of the hearing disorder cannot be made because inconsistencies in response preclude accurate analysis. If a referral for psychological evaluation or guidance is indicated, clinicians must choose their words extremely carefully lest the patient be offended. It is at this juncture that audiology must be practiced as more of an art than a science.

REFERENCES

Alberti P. (1970) New tools for old tricks. *Ann Otol Rhinol Laryngol.* 79, 900–907.

Altshuler MW. (1982) Qualitative indicators of nonorganicity: informal observations and evaluation. In: Kramer MB, Armbruster JM, eds. *Forensic Audiology.* Baltimore: University Park Press; pp 59–68.

Austen S, Lynch C, (2004) Non-organic hearing loss redefined. Understanding, categorizing and managing non-organic behavior. *Int J Audiol.* 45, 283–284.

Bailey HAT Jr, Martin FN. (1961) Nonorganic hearing loss: case report. *Laryngoscope.* 71, 209–210.

Barelli PA, Ruder L. (1970) Medico-legal evaluation of hearing problems. *Eye Ear Nose Throat Mon.* 49, 398–405.

Barr B. (1963) Psychogenic deafness in school children. *Int Audiol.* 2, 125–128.

Beagley HA, Knight JJ. (1968) The evaluation of suspected non-organic hearing loss. *J Laryngol Otol.* 82, 693–705.

Berger K. (1965) Nonorganic hearing loss in children. *Laryngoscope.* 75, 447–457.

Berlin CI. (1978) Electrophysiological indices of auditory function. In: Martin FN, ed. *Pediatric Audiology.* Englewood Cliffs, NJ: Prentice Hall; pp 13–173.

Campanelli PA. (1963) Simulated hearing losses in school children following identification audiometry. *J Aud Res.* 3, 91–108.

Carhart R. (1952) Speech audiometry in clinical evaluation. *Acta Otolaryngol (Stockh).* 41, 18–42.

Carhart R. (1958) Audiometry in diagnosis. *Laryngoscope.* 68, 253–279.

Chaiklin JB, Ventry IM. (1965a) Patient errors during spondee and pure-tone threshold measurement. *J Aud Res.* 5, 219–230.

Chaiklin JB, Ventry IM. (1965b) The efficiency of audiometric measures used to identify functional hearing loss. *J Aud Res.* 5, 196–211.

Chaiklin JB, Ventry IM, Barrett LS, Skalbeck GS. (1959) Pure-tone threshold patterns observed in functional hearing loss. *Laryngoscope.* 69, 1165–1179.

Cherry R, Ventry IM. (1976) The ascending-descending gap: a tool for identifying a suprathreshold response. *J Aud Res.* 16, 281–287.

Cohen M, Cohen SM, Levine M, Maisel R, Ruhm H, Wolfe RM. (1963) Interdisciplinary pilot study of nonorganic hearing loss. *Ann Otol Rhinol Laryngol.* 72, 67–82.

Cooper WA, Stokinger TE. (1976) Pure-tone delayed auditory feedback: effect of prior experience. *J Am Audiol Soc.* 1, 164–168.

Dixon RF, Newby HA. (1959) Children with nonorganic hearing problems. *Arch Otolaryngol.* 70, 619–623.

Feldman AS. (1962) Functional hearing loss. *Marco Aud Lib Ser.* 1, 119–121.

Fournier JE. (1958) The detection of auditory malingering. *Trans Beltone Inst Hear Res.* 8.

Frank T. (1976) Yes-no test for nonorganic hearing loss. *Arch Otolaryngol.* 102, 162–165.

Gleason WJ. (1958) Psychological characteristics of the audiologically inconsistent patient. *Arch Otolaryngol.* 68, 42–46.

Goldstein R. (1966) Pseudohypoacusis. *J Speech Hear Disord.* 31, 341–352.

Hall JW. (1992) *Handbook of Auditory Evoked Responses.* Boston: Allyn and Bacon; pp 383–384.

Hallewell JD, Goetzinger CP, Allen ML, Proud GO. (1966) The use of hypnosis in audiologic assessment. *Acta Otolaryngol (Stockh).* 61, 205–208.

Harris DA. (1958) A rapid and simple technique for the detection of nonorganic hearing loss. *Arch Otolaryngol.* 68, 758–760.

Harris JD. (1965) Speech audiometry. In: Glorig A, ed. *Audiometry Principles and Practices.* Baltimore: Williams & Wilkins; pp 151–169.

Hattler KW, Schuchman GI. (1971) Efficiency of the Stenger, Doerfler-Stewart and lengthened off-time Békésy tests. *Acta Otolaryngol (Stockh).* 72, 262–267.

Heron TG. (1968) Industrial deafness and the summed evoked potential. *S Afr Med J.* 42, 1176–1177.

Hirsh I. (1952) *The Measurement of Hearing.* New York: McGraw-Hill; pp 212.

Hood WH, Campbell RA, Hutton CL. (1964) An evaluation of the Bekesy ascending descending gap. *J Speech Hear Res.* 7, 123–132.

Hopkinson NT. (1967) Comment on pseudohypacusis. *J Speech Hear Disord.* 32, 293–294.

Hopkinson NT. (1978) Speech tests for pseudohypacusis. In: Katz J, ed. *Handbook of Clinical Audiology.* 2nd ed. Baltimore: Williams & Wilkins; pp 291–303.

Jerger J, Burney L, Mauldin L, Crump B. (1974) Predicting hearing loss from the acoustic reflex. *J Speech Hear Disord.* 39, 11–22.

Katz J. (1980) Type A and functional loss. *SSW Newslett.* 2, 5.

Kerr AG, Gillespie WJ, Easton JM. (1975) Deafness: a simple test for malingering. *Br J Audiol.* 9, 24–26.

Kintsler DP, Phelan JG, Lavender RB. (1970) Efficiency of the Stenger tests in identification of functional hearing loss. *J Aud Res.* 10:118-123.

Kintsler DP, Phelan JG, Lavender RB. (1972) The Stenger and speech Stenger tests in functional hearing loss. *Audiology.* 11, 187–193.

Knight J, Beagley H. (1970) Nonorganic hearing loss in children. *Int Audiol.* 9, 142–143.

Lamb LE, Peterson JL. (1967) Middle ear reflex measurements in pseudohypacusis. *J Speech Hear Disord.* 32, 46–51.

Leshin GJ. (1960) Childhood nonorganic hearing loss. *J Speech Hear Disord.* 25, 290–292.

Lumio JS, Jauhiainen T, Gelhar K. (1969) Three cases of functional deafness in the same family. *J Laryngol.* 83, 299–304.

Margolis RH. (1993) Detection of hearing impairment with the acoustic stapedial reflex. *Ear Hear.* 14, 3–10.

Martin FN. (1997) *Introduction to Audiology.* 6th ed. Boston: Allyn & Bacon.

Martin FN, Champlin CA, Chambers JA. (1998) Seventh survey of audiometric practices in the United States. *J Am Acad Audiol.* 9, 95–104.

Martin FN, Champlin CA, Marchbanks T. (1998) A varying intensity story test for simulated hearing loss. *Am J Audiol.* 7, 39–44.

Martin FN, Champlin CA, McCreery TM. (2001) Strategies used in feigning hearing loss. *J Am Acad Audiol.* 12, 59–63.

Martin FN, Shipp DB. (1982) The effects of sophistication on three threshold tests for subjects with simulated hearing loss. *Ear Hear.* 3, 34–36.

Martin JS, Martin FN, Champlin CA. (2000) The CON-SOT-LOT test for nonorganic hearing loss. *J Am Acad Audiol.* 11, 46–51.

McCanna DL, DeLapa G. (1981) A clinical study of twenty-seven children exhibiting functional hearing loss. *Lang Speech Hear Serv Sch.* 12, 26–35.

McLennan RO, Martin FN. (1976) On the discrepancy between the speech reception threshold and the pure-tone average in nonorganic hearing loss. Houston: Poster Session at the American Speech and Hearing Association Convention.

Miller AL, Fox MS, Chan G. (1968) Puretone assessments as an aid in detecting suspected nonorganic hearing disorders in children. *Laryngoscope.* 78, 2170–2176.

Monro DA, Martin FN. (1977) Effects of sophistication on four tests for nonorganic hearing loss. *J Speech Hear Disord.* 42, 528–534.

Musiek FE, Bornstein SP, Rintelmann WF. (1995) Transient evoked otoacoustic emissions and pseudohypacusis. *J Am Acad Audiol.* 6, 293–301.

Nagel RF. (1964) RRLJ: a new technique for the noncooperative patient. *J Speech Hear Disord.* 29, 492–493.

Niemeyer W, Sesterhenn G. (1974) Calculating the hearing threshold from the stapedius reflex threshold for different sound stimuli. *Audiology.* l3, 421–427.

Nolan M, Tucker I. (1981) Functional hearing loss in children. *J Br Assoc Teachers Deaf.* 5, 2–10.

Peck JE, Ross M. (1970) A comparison of the ascending and the descending modes for administration of the pure-tone Stenger test. *J Aud Res.* l0, 218–220.

Robinson M, Kasden SD. (1973) Clinical application of pure tone delayed auditory feedback in pseudohypacusis. *Eye Ear Nose Throat Mon.* 52, 9l–93.

Rose DE, Keating LW, Hedgecock LD, Miller KE, Schneurs KK. (1972) A comparison of evoked response audiometry and routine clinical audiometry. *Audiology.* 11, 238–243.

Ross M. (1964) The variable intensity pulse count method (VIPCM) for the detection and measurement of the pure tone threshold of children with functional hearing losses. *J Speech Hear Disord.* 29, 477–482.

Ruhm HB, Cooper WA Jr. (1962) Low sensation level effects of pure tone delayed auditory feedback. *J Speech Hear Res.* 5, 185–193.

Ruhm HB, Cooper WA Jr. (1963) Some factors that influence pure tone delayed auditory feedback. *J Speech Hear Res.* 10, 223–237.

Ruhm HB, Cooper WA Jr. (1964) Delayed feedback audiometry. *J Speech Hear Disord.* 29, 448–455.

Schulman-Galambos C, Galambos R. (1975) Brain stem auditory evoked responses in premature infants. *J Speech Hear Res.* 18, 456–465.

Snyder JM. (1977) Characteristic patterns of etiologic significance from routine audiometric tests and case history. *Maico Aud Lib Ser.* 15, Report 5.

Taylor GJ. (1949) An experimental study of tests for the detection of auditory malingering. *J Speech Hear Disord.* 14, 119–130.

Trier T, Levy R. (1965) Social and psychological characteristics of veterans with functional hearing loss. *J Aud Res.* 5, 241–255.

Ventry IM. (1976) Pure tone-spondee threshold relationships in functional hearing loss: a hypothesis. *J Speech Hear Disord.* 41, 16–22.

Ventry IM, Chaiklin JB. (1965) Evaluation of pure tone audiogram configurations used in identifying adults with functional hearing loss. *J Aud Res.* 5, 212–218.

Wieczorek R. (1979) School-age malingerers. *SSW Newslett.*, 14.

Williamson D. (1974) Functional hearing loss: a review. *Maico Aud Lib Ser.* 12, 33–34.

Woodford CM, Harris G, Marquette ML, Perry L, Barhart A. (1997) A screening test for pseudohypacusis. *Hear J.* 4, 23–26.

Zwislocki J. (1953) Acoustic attenuation between the ears. *J Acoust Soc Am.* 25, 752–759.

Hearing Loss in the Elderly: A New Look at an Old Problem

Barbara E. Weinstein

▒ DEMOGRAPHIC CHANGES

One of the most significant demographic factors in America is the aging of the population. The number of persons age 65 and over was 36 million in 2003, with the number expected to more than double by 2030. Interestingly, approximately one in every eight Americans is over 65 years of age. The older population is getting older as well (Fig. 32.1), and the fastest growing segment is those over 85 years old. It is projected that, by 2030, 10 million persons will be 85 or over, which is nearly double the number reported in 2002 (Administration on Aging, 2008).

Of particular relevance to audiologists is that, in 2003, 52% of persons over 65 lived in one of the following nine states: California, Florida, New York, Texas, Pennsylvania, Ohio, Illinois, Michigan, and New Jersey. Because hearing is critical for individuals in the workforce, it is noteworthy that the Baby Boomers, the first set of whom turned 60 in 2006, are more often than not continuing in the workforce. The likelihood that employed individuals will continue to work as they get older is increasing. For example, in 2003, approximately 47% of employed men over 70 continued to work part time and nearly 67% of employed women over 70 continued to work part time (US Bureau of Census, 2005).

Hearing impairment is one physical disability that is increasing in prevalence in society in general and in older adults in particular. Approximately 31 million people have some degree of self-reported hearing difficulty, with the number projected to reach 44 million by 2030 (Kochkin, 2005a). This projected increase is due, in large part, to the growth in the older population. Within one generation, the hearing loss population will grow by one third (Kochkin, 2005a). Hearing impairment was the 13th most prevalent chronic condition affecting adults 65 years of age and older, with a 37% prevalence rate among persons 65 years and older and a 46% prevalence rate among those 75 years and older (Beers, 2005; Lethbridge-Cejku et al., 2002). It is noteworthy that dual sensory impairment (vision and hearing loss) affects about 20% of individuals 70 years of age and older. According to the recent 2005 US Census Bureau report, older adults with both vision and hearing loss were more likely than those without to have sustained a fall, to suffer from hypertension or heart disease, or to have suffered a stroke. They also reported fewer social engagements.

Older adults use health care services more frequently than do younger adults, and their health care costs are correspondingly higher. Health care utilization is highest among the oldest-old. Beers (2005) indicates that 30% of Americans 65 to 74 years of age reported that they had hearing impairment, whereas this percentage was 46% for those 75 and over. The average number of physician contacts in 2005 for those over 65 years had an average of almost 14 visits per 1000 Medicare enrollees (Administration on Aging, 2008). In light of the high number of physician visits among older adults, it is incumbent on audiologists to educate physicians about hearing loss, its consequences, and devices available to help overcome the handicap resulting from hearing impairment. Physicians should be encouraged to screen routinely for hearing handicap using valid, easy-to-administer tools.

Older adults with hearing impairment pose a real challenge to audiologists. Technological advances in the hearing

Population aged 65 and over: 2000 to 2050
(in millions)

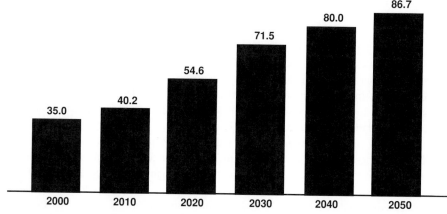

Note: The reference population for these data is the resident population.
Sources: 2000, U.S. Census Bureau, 2001, Table PCT 12; 2010 to 2050,
U.S. Census Bureau, 2004. For full citations, see references at end of chapter.

From: U.S. Bureau of Census, 2005.

FIGURE 32.1 Population aged 65 and over: 2000 to 2050 (in millions). (From United States Census Bureau [2005]) 65+ in the United States: 2005. Current Population Reports. Bethesda, MD: US Department of Health and Human Services, National Institutes of Health.)

aid industry are enormous, such that individuals with mild to profound sensory-neural hearing loss, unilateral hearing loss, and chronic middle ear disease can be well served by the variety of devices available. However, institutional barriers continue to interfere with the ability to serve this population: older adults wait more than 10 years before seeking audiologic assistance; there has been a decline in the proportion of physicians screening for hearing loss (<13%); the percentage of hearing instruments that remain in users' drawers has increased (16.7%); the average age of new hearing aid users has increased to nearly 70 years of age; and hearing instrument sales by audiologists have declined by 10% (Kochkin, 2005a; 2005b). It is within this framework that this chapter has been updated from the previous edition.

THE AGING AUDITORY MECHANISM

The entire auditory system undergoes changes with age. The field of "otogerontology" has made significant strides in documenting the anatomic, physiologic, and audiologic changes within the peripheral and central auditory mechanisms (Hnath-Chisolm et al., 2003). Age-related changes primarily take place in the sensory, neural, strial, and supportive structures within the inner ear and at each level along the central auditory pathways. Alterations in the outer and middle ear take place, as well, but on a lesser scale. There is a loss of elasticity and strength in the pinna and external auditory canal. The sebaceous and cerumen glands in the cartilaginous portion lose some of their secretory ability. The decrease in fat leads to significant changes in the skin lining the canal. Changes in the physical properties of the skin, including dryness and dehydration, make the canal prone to

trauma and breakdown. The cerumen becomes more concentrated, hard, and impacted due, in part, to inadequate epithelial migration (Ballachanda, 1995a; 1995b; Weinstein, 2000). The bony canal is especially susceptible to trauma from attempts at cerumen removal because the skin covering is very thin. This is also a concern when making ear impressions for hearing aids located completely in the canal (Ballachanda, 1995a) and may influence hearing aid fittings (Oliveira, 1995).

Cerumen impaction can occur in the outer ear because of increased activity of cerumen glands in the cartilaginous portion, physical obstruction due to a hearing aid, frequent use of cotton-tipped swabs, or the production of drier and less viscous cerumen. Combined with the presence of thicker and longer hair follicles oriented toward the tympanic membrane, the latter condition leads to a higher frequency of impaction (Gleitman et al., 1992). Mahoney (1987) reported that the prevalence of cerumen impaction may be as high as 34% in older adults.

The tympanic membrane, ossicular chain, and middle ear muscles and ligaments are susceptible to minor age-related changes. Rosenwasser (1964) and Etholm and Belal (1974) observed the following changes: (1) tympanic membranes appear to become stiffer, thinner, and less vascular with age; (2) thinning and calcification of the cartilaginous incudomalleal and incudostapedial joints; (3) atrophy and degeneration of the fibers of the middle ear muscles and of the ossicular ligaments; and (4) ossification and calcification of both the Eustachian tube cartilage and ossicles. Despite the variety of changes in the sound transmission mechanism, they do not appear to impact hearing sensitivity, immittance test results, or hearing aid outcomes.

The entire inner ear is vulnerable to the effects of aging. Most information about the pathology of human presbycusis stems from histopathologic studies of the temporal bone by Schuknecht (1955) and from supplementary studies in animal models (Gates and Mills, 2005; Hnath-Chisolm et al., 2003). The most critical risk factor for cochlear disorder is age (Moscicki et al., 1985). The structure most susceptible to age-related changes is the organ of Corti, with hair and supporting cell loss being the rule rather than the exception. Loss of hair cells is most severe in the basal region of the cochlea. The outer hair cells degenerate first, followed by the inner hair cells (Hnath-Chisolm et al., 2003; Weinstein, 2000). While the decrease in hair cell population is greatest in persons over 70 years of age and most pronounced for outer hair cells, inner hair cells do degenerate and do so independent of the outer hair cells. The loss of outer hair cells in the basal turn of the cochlea is responsible for the decline in hearing loss for high frequencies associated with age (Weinstein, 2000). Hypothesizing from their work with mice, Willott et al. (2001) speculated that the outer hair cells in the cochlea of older adults may be more susceptible to noise trauma and ototoxicity, accounting in part for the pattern of vulnerability in outer hair cell structures. Recent studies with mice suggest that atrophy of the outer hair cells may be mediated by genetic factors, suggesting the possibility for medical approaches to counteract the damage due to age (Hnath-Chisolm et al., 2003). Table 32.1 summarizes changes with age that occur throughout the auditory system.

TABLE 32.1   Summary of age-related changes in the auditory system

External Ear Canal
Walls are thin
Epithelium: dehydration,
Glands: loss of secretory ability
Cerumen: becomes drier, more tenacious

Middle Ear
Eardrum: thickens, appears duller, loses elasticity
Joints: arthritic changes
Ossicular chain: calcification and arthritic changes

Cochlea
Hair cells are lost, basilar membrane stiffens, auditory structures calcify, cochlear neurons are lost
Stria vascularis: capillaries thicken, endolymph production decreases, Na+ K+ ATPase activity decreases

Brain
Interhemispheric transfer of information through corpus callosum loses efficiency; degenerative changes throughout brainstem auditory pathways

From American Geriatrics Society. (2004) *Geriatrics Review Syllabus: A Core Curriculum in Geriatric Medicine.* 5th ed. New York: Blackwell Publishing.

Otte et al. (1978) and Suzuka and Schuknecht (1988) have reported a relationship between age and loss of ganglion cells, with spiral ganglion cell loss out of proportion to degeneration in the organ of Corti and occurring in all three turns of the cochlea. Neural histopathologic studies suggest that age-related loss in ganglion cells is greatest near the base of the cochlea. The aging process is also associated with a decrease in the average number of fibers in the cochlear nerve. The data of Crowe et al. (1934) demonstrated that nerve fiber loss is greatest within the basal 10 mm of the cochlea. Loss of nerve fibers in one turn of the cochlea or in all turns has been noted without severe hair cell loss (Hnath-Chisolm et al., 2003). Thus, loss of hair cells does not necessarily lead to age-related pathology of ganglion cells (Willott, 1991). There is a relationship between amount and location of ganglion cell loss and puretone thresholds, such that hearing loss first occurs once the neural unit population falls below that required for processing acoustic energy (Suzuka and Schuknecht, 1988; Schuknecht, 1989). In contrast, speech recognition ability is not predictive of spiral ganglion cell population (Pauler et al., 1988).

Schuknecht (1955) classified presbycusis into several types including sensory, neural, metabolic, cochlear conductive, mixed, central, and indeterminate, with the latter accounting for nearly 25% of all cases (Gates and Mills, 2005). Table 32.2 contrasts the varieties of presbycusis. Sensory presbycusis (outer hair cell loss) is difficult to distinguish histologically and clinically from acoustic trauma (Schuknecht, 1989). The hallmark of presbycusis, outer hair cell loss in the basal turn, probably has as much to do with noise toxicity as with age (Gates and Mills, 2005). The most consistent pathologic change associated with neural presbycusis is degeneration in the population of neural units (Schuknecht, 1989). Neuronal loss tends to be diffuse, involving all three turns of the cochlea and degeneration of the neurons (Schuknecht, 1989). Neuronal loss in the periphery is often accompanied by loss of neurons in the ventral and dorsal cochlear nuclei. According to Gates and Mills (2005), the most prominent feature of age-related hearing loss is atrophy of stria vascularis, which is characterized by loss of strial tissue and loss of strial cells primarily in the apical and middle turns of the cochlea. The hearing loss tends to be in the lower frequencies, flat in configuration, sensory-neural in nature, and mild to moderate in degree. Gates and Mills (2005) suggest that strial presbycusis has a high heritability factor and is associated with cardiovascular disease.

A classification of cochlear conductive presbycusis is made when the other varieties of presbycusis are histologically excluded and when decrements in hearing function appear in the high frequencies. Cochlear conductive presbycusis is associated with changes in the physical properties of the cochlea such as loss of elasticity of the basilar membrane, which affects its mechanical response. Mixed presbycusis is characterized by involvement of two or more of the four classic types of presbycusis. For example, the combination of sensory and strial presbycusis might present as an abrupt

TABLE 32.2   Classification of six types of presbycusis

Type of presbycusis	Criteria
Sensory	The presence of any total loss of hair cells beginning at the basal end of the cochlea that is at least 10 mm in length so as to involve the region of the speech frequencies on the cochlea
Neural	Loss of 50% or more of the cochlear neurons as compared to the mean number of cochlear neurons for neonates (i.e., 35, 500)
Strial	Loss of strial tissue cells in apical and middle turns of cochlea (e.g., atrophy of stria vascularis)
Cochlear conductive	Lack of gross histopathology; changes in physical properties of cochlea, loss of elasticity in basilar membrane
Mixed presbycusis	Presence of significant pathologic change in more than one structure
Intermediate presbycusis	Cochlear changes do not reach significant levels in any structure,and the audiometric profile of cochlear conductive presbycusis is not met

From Schuknecht H, Gacek J. (1993) Cochlear pathology in presbycusis. *Ann Otol Rhinol Laryngol.* 102, 1–16.

high-frequency hearing loss superimposed on a flat audiogram, whereas sensory and cochlear conductive presbycusis might emerge as an abrupt high-frequency loss superimposed on a descending puretone audiogram (Schuknecht and Gacek, 1993). Intermediate presbycusis, described by Schuknecht and Gacek (1993), is characterized by the presence of submicroscopic alterations in structures of the cochlea that control cell metabolism, a decrease in the number of synapses on hair cells, and chemical changes in endolymph (Hnath-Chisolm et al., 2003). Audiograms associated with presbycusis of this variety are primarily flat or mildly descending, without consistent or distinct pathologic correlates. Finally, central presbycusis, as described by Gates and Mills (2005), may be the result of degeneration secondary to loss of sensory cells in the cochlea.

The aging process impacts the central nervous system in general and the central auditory system in particular. Neuronal age-related atrophy is characterized by an overall loss of neurons; a change in neuron size; a decrease in size of the cell body, nucleus, or nucleolus; and a decrease in dendritic arborization along with a diminution or disappearance of dendrites (Powers, 1994; Willott, 1991). The magnitude of cell loss in the auditory cortex is greatest in the superior temporal gyrus. There is almost a one-to-one correlation between age and cell loss. There is a decrease in the thickness of the superior temporal gyrus with increasing age, which is not apparent in other cortical regions (Brody, 1955). In general, the age-related changes in the nervous system are not uniform across the nuclei within the central auditory nervous system and vary greatly among individuals.

MEDICAL CONDITIONS CONTRIBUTING TO HEARING LOSS IN OLDER ADULTS

In addition to age-related degeneration, a number of other factors can lead to hearing loss in older adults. These include excessive exposure to occupational or recreational noise, genetic factors, acoustic neuroma, trauma, metabolic disease such as diabetes, vascular disease, infections, autoimmune disease, and drug exposure, most notably aminoglycosides, antimalarial drugs including quinine and chloroquine, loop diuretics such as furosemide, antibiotics including vancomycin, salicylates such as aspirin or nonsteroidal anti-inflammatory agents, and antineoplastic agents such as cisplatin and methotrexate (Fausti et al., 2005). The pathogenesis of ototoxicity relates to the fact that medication is retained for a longer period and in a higher concentration in the inner ear fluids than in any other body tissue or fluid, especially in individuals with hepatic or renal dysfunction (Becker et al., 1989). Aminoglycosides appear to damage the outer hair cells first and then the inner hair cells if high enough concentrations of the drug are reached. Ototoxicity, which is related to sustained peak serum levels, varies considerably across the family of aminoglycosides. Prescription of medications that are ototoxic appears to be somewhat higher in the elderly, predisposing them to drug-induced sensory-neural hearing loss.

Cardiovascular disease (CVD) has recently been linked to hearing loss in older adults. Brant et al. (1996) found a relationship between CVD and hearing loss in their large sample of older adults who were free of noise-induced hearing loss and other hearing-related disorders. Specifically, their data demonstrated a significant relationship between systolic blood pressure and sensory-neural hearing impairment. Similarly, Gates et al. (1993) analyzed data from the Framingham cohort to determine the relationship between CVD and hearing loss. Low-frequency thresholds were more closely correlated to CVD than were high-frequency thresholds, suggesting a possible vascular or metabolic link. The association between CVD and hearing loss was impressive; however, the authors cautioned that a cause and effect relationship cannot be deduced from their findings.

Impacted cerumen, otitis media, glossopharyngeal tumors, and otosclerosis are not uncommon in older adults. The latter diseases, which are associated with conductive hearing loss, can occur in the presence or absence of cochlear involvement. Finally, affective disorders, such as depression, and cognitive disorders, such as senile dementia of the Alzheimer's type, are associated with hearing loss. It is noteworthy that inattention or confusion related to depression or dementia may give the impression of significant hearing loss. Complete audiometric studies can help identify the presence of hearing loss in older at-risk adults.

■ AUDIOLOGIC FINDINGS

Puretone Thresholds

Age-related changes throughout the auditory system are associated with decrements in hearing for puretone and speech stimuli. Age and frequency effects emerge in most cross-sectional and longitudinal studies of hearing loss, such that air-conduction thresholds became poorer with increasing frequency (e.g., >1,000 Hz). Recent studies on hearing loss in noninstitutionalized older adults confirm that age-related hearing has several distinct features. First, puretone hearing sensitivity tends to decline with increasing age, with the greatest loss in the frequencies above 1,000 Hz. Further, the hearing loss tends to be bilateral, symmetrical, and sensory-neural in origin and associated with deterioration of the sensory structures within the cochlea. The decline in high-frequency sensitivity appears to be greater in males, whereas the decline in low-frequency thresholds tends to be greater in females of comparable age. Hearing loss configuration in the higher frequency tends to be sharply sloping in males and gradually sloping in females (Gordon-Salant, 2005). The average hearing loss in older males can be described as mild to moderately severe, bilateral, and sensory-neural with a sharply sloping configuration. Older women tend to present with a mild to moderate,

gradually sloping, bilaterally symmetrical, sensory-neural hearing loss. Among residents of nursing facilities, the sensory-neural hearing loss tends to be moderately severely sloping to severely sloping (Weinstein, 2000).

Speech Understanding

Older adults have more difficulty understanding speech in noisy environments, when people speak quickly, in reverberant conditions, when there are multiple talkers, when the message is complex, or when there is reduced contextual information (Martin and Jerger, 2005; Wingfield et al., 1985). Loss of peripheral hearing sensitivity, declines in cognitive abilities, and age-related changes within the eighth nerve, auditory brainstem pathways, and auditory cortex account, in large part, for the nature of the speech understanding problems experienced by older adults (Martin and Jerger, 2005). Golding et al. (2006) reported the prevalence of central auditory processing disability to be approximately 50% in a clinical population and approximately 22% in a non–clinic-based population of older adults. The discussion below attempts to synthesize the factors and mechanisms that may underlie speech understanding difficulties experienced by some older adults.

The proportion of persons with problems in perceiving speech doubles per decade, from 16% at age 60 to 32% at age 70 to 64% at 80 (van Rooij et al., 1989). However, there are large individual differences in speech understanding among individuals over 60 years of age. Investigators have attempted to isolate the numerous factors that contribute to this variability. Several hypotheses have been posited to explain the mechanisms underlying the speech understanding problems experienced by older adults, including the peripheral hypothesis, the central auditory hypothesis, and the cognitive hypothesis (Humes, 1996; Humes et al., 1992). In the peripheral hypothesis, the auditory periphery is implicated; in the central auditory hypothesis, the brainstem pathways and auditory cortex are implicated; and in the cognitive hypothesis, the cortex that is responsible for information processing, labeling, and storage is implicated (Humes, 1996). The extent to which performance on measures of speech recognition can be accounted for by each of these mechanisms is discussed below.

Peripheral (i.e., cochlear changes) hypothesis. This hypothesis holds that speech recognition difficulties are attributable to individual differences in the encoding of sound by the outer ear through the inner ear and eighth nerve (Humes et al., 1992). The peripheral component is reflected in the frequency-specific sensitivity loss revealed by the audiogram, most notable in the high frequencies. The peripheral hypothesis has been further subdivided into two versions. One version suggests that simple changes in audibility, wherein sound energy falls below an individual's audible region, account for the speech understanding problems characterizing older adults. The other version suggests that re-duced physiologic processing associated with age-related changes in the cochlea creates distortions beyond loss of hearing sensitivity. Sources of distortion may arise from individual differences in other peripheral encoding mechanisms including loss of spectral and temporal resolution or loss of intensity discrimination.

Central auditory hypothesis. This hypothesis suggests that age-related changes in the central auditory system, including the auditory pathways of the brainstem or portions of the auditory cortex, degrade the speech signal, leading to central auditory processing disorders (CAPD) (Humes, 1996). The dysfunction within the brainstem or brain leads to impaired neural transmission, feature extraction, information processing, labeling, or storage, resulting in CAPD (Humes et al., 1992). According to this hypothesis, one is considered to have CAPD when scores on speech audiometric measures of central auditory processing ability are depressed relative to a given norm (Jerger et al., 1990).

Cognitive hypothesis. This hypothesis implicates higher centers in the auditory pathways as a source of individual variations in cognitive abilities and declines in cognitive performance. Cortical functions subsumed under these areas include information processing, storage, and retrieval. These cortical processes underlie performance on speech understanding tasks, and it follows that individual differences in speech understanding performance may be attributable to deficits in one or more of these areas. It is noteworthy that cognitive deficits are not confined to the auditory modality. Instead, short-term memory deficits may emerge on tasks involving both auditory and visual presentations of stimuli (Humes et al., 1992). The most notable changes in cognitive performance that influence speech understanding include age-related reductions in the speed of perceptual and mental processing (Martin and Jerger, 2005).

In sum, older adults tend to experience minimal difficulty understanding speech in ideal listening situations as long as the speech signal is audible enough to allow for reception of high-frequency speech cues (Gordon-Salant, 2005). Deficits in auditory temporal processing as revealed when the signal is degraded, such as in reverberant conditions or using time-compressed speech, appear to play a role in explaining the decrements that tend to emerge on selected tests of speech understanding. Age-related deficits in central auditory processing and global cognitive function, including reductions in working memory, may help to explain the speech processing problems of older adults. The role of speech-specific cognitive declines (e.g., absence of linguistic redundancy) in explaining the speech understanding difficulties experienced by older adults is noteworthy and has implications for design of technology (Wingfield, 1996). For example, the use of contextual information can reduce the difficulty older adults may have processing rapid speech. Interestingly, performance on objective tests of speech understanding and subjective self-report questionnaires of communicative, social, and emotional function demonstrate that older adults reveal a pattern of age-related differences. Specifically, older adults often perform more poorly than their younger counterparts on selected speech understanding tests designed to challenge the peripheral and central auditory systems. In contrast, older adults tend to underreport the extent of communicative problems and the social and emotional impact of hearing loss on self-report measures such as the Hearing Handicap Inventory for the Elderly (HHIE). These discrepancies or incomplete relationships between audiometric data and self-reported difficulties in communication underline the importance of assessing communicative function in a variety of ways.

Immittance Test Results

Structural changes in the middle ear mechanism due to aging have an effect on immittance tests. Wiley et al. (2005) conducted a longitudinal study of changes in tympanometric measures in older adults over a period of 5 years. Overall, changes in peak compensated static acoustic admittance, equivalent ear canal volume, tympanogram width, and tympanogram peak pressure over time were small and not considered clinically significant, indicating little change in middle ear function with age. Similarly, Wiley et al. (1996) reported little difference between younger and older adults in mean peak compensated static acoustic admittance measures. Holte (1996) noted a statistically significant correlation between age and tympanometric width; however, the correlation was slight, rendering the finding clinically insignificant. These findings do not appear clinically significant, and therefore, normative values used for adults can be applied to older adults during routine tympanometric testing.

Much of the evidence on the effect of age on acoustic reflex thresholds clearly shows that age has a negligible effect. For normal-hearing older adults, there is little change in acoustic reflex threshold for frequencies between 500 and 2,000 Hz (Osterhammel and Osterhammel, 1979; Thompson et al., 1979). Jerger et al. (1972) found that subjects with sensory-neural hearing loss had slightly higher acoustic reflex thresholds for high the frequencies.

PSYCHOSOCIAL CONSEQUENCES OF HEARING IMPAIRMENT

Literature that has emerged over the past 10 years has demonstrated conclusively that untreated hearing loss has detrimental effects on psychosocial well-being, communication, affect, cognitive status, and functional health status. In fact, the myth that hearing loss is harmless has been debunked, and it is becoming increasingly clear that, if untreated, hearing loss can be costly to the individual and family members. Results of the National Council on Aging (NCOA) survey (1999) revealed that untreated hearing loss is associated with sadness, depression, anxiety, paranoia, emotional turmoil, insecurity, and less social activity.

Dalton et al. (2003) conducted a population-based study of the relationship between hearing impairment and selected quality of life variables in a large sample of adults between the ages of 53 and 97 years old. More than half of the subjects had a hearing impairment, which was mild in 28% and moderate to severe in 24% of subjects. The quality of life indicators associated with hearing loss were social functioning, mental health, and physical functional status. Interestingly, significant hearing handicap and self-reported communication difficulties were significantly associated with reduced scores on each of the assessed domains of function.

These data confirmed the findings of Mulrow et al. (1990b) who demonstrated the adverse effect of hearing loss on functional health and psychosocial well-being. They conducted a study of 204 elderly male veterans selected from a primary care clinic designed to assess the association between hearing impairment and quality of life. Quality of life was defined according to responses to the (1) HHIE; (2) Quantified Denver Scale of Communication Function (QDS); (3) Short Portable Mental Status Questionnaire (SPMSQ), which yields information about cognitive function; (4) Geriatric Depression Scale (GDS), which assesses affect; and (5) Self-Evaluation of Life Function (SELF), which assesses function in several domains including physical disability, social satisfaction, aging, depression, self-esteem, and personal control. Hearing loss was associated with significant social, emotional, and communication handicaps on the HHIE and QDS. In contrast, scores for the hearing impaired and non–hearing impaired did not differ significantly on the depression scale (GDS) or the SELF. Because the extent of the perceived social and emotional dysfunction was considerable, the authors concluded that hearing loss has an adverse effect on quality of life. A follow-up randomized trial of hearing aid rehabilitation indicated that hearing aid intervention was effective at reducing the communication and psychosocial handicaps and the depressive and cognitive symptoms experienced by the majority of hearing-impaired subjects in their sample (Mulrow et al., 1990a).

According to Kochkin (2005b), untreated hearing loss is costly from an economic vantage point; it is associated with lost wages and lower income in retirement. Kochkin's data revealed a link between household income and hearing loss severity, with individuals reporting mild hearing loss reporting a household income of $36,400 and persons with severe loss reporting an income of $33,600 (Better Hearing Institute, 2005). Garstecki and Erler's (1996) observation that subjects in their economically advantaged sample of

300 older adults with mild to moderate hearing loss judged effective communication in the work setting to be more important than communication in social settings lends additional support to the importance of hearing in the workplace.

The adverse effects of untreated hearing impairment are global problems. Wu et al. (2004) evaluated the psychosocial consequences of self-perceived handicap in a sample of 63 older adults ranging in age from 62 to 90 years attending a geriatric medicine clinic in Singapore. In their study of subjects with self-reported hearing difficulty and a fail on the puretone screen, 70% of respondents indicated that they would be happier if their hearing were normal, 40% indicated that difficulty hearing made them feel frustrated, and 43% admitted to feeling sad because of their hearing handicap. Finally, the federal government in Australia is designing a comprehensive approach to managing age-related hearing loss because "as a cause of burden of disease, hearing impairment is the second highest disability for every Australian man" (Smith et al., 2005, p 2).

▨ A DIAGNOSTIC AND MANAGEMENT PROTOCOL

It is clear from research and clinical experience that older adults require a diagnostic and management protocol unique to their needs. The protocol proposed below is based on several premises coupled with the American Academy of Audiology Guideline for the Audiologic Management of Adult Hearing Impairment (2005).

Premise 1. The objectives of the initial audiologic assessment with an elderly client should be to: (1) understand the difficulties the individual is having from the perspective of the client and a significant other; (2) gain an objective feel for hearing status and speech understanding under a variety of conditions and at differing signal-to-noise ratios; (3) understand the client's stage of readiness to embrace some form of intervention; and finally, (4) determine candidacy for the most appropriate solution(s), be it hearing aid technology, hearing assistive technology (HAT), and/or some form of counseling.

Premise 2. Routine procedures are limited in their ability to enable audiologists to understand the complex speech understanding difficulties that are hallmarks of age-related hearing loss. Clinical measures of hearing are inadequate predictors of the difficulties older adults face in carrying out routine activities in their natural environments. The real-world impact of hearing impairment cannot be predicted from sensitivity loss alone. The correlation between puretone data, speech recognition scores, and self-assessed handicap is imperfect. In addition, the relationship between objective auditory tests and hearing aid satisfaction is weak. Presenting monosyllabic words in quiet is not going to enable us to quantify and understand our client's difficulties. Objective tests should be designed to uncover the listening difficulties the individual is experiencing, such as difficulty in the presence of noise, and to determine listening strategies being used (e.g., does the individual take advantage of visual cues when communicating). Self-report data as an adjunct to objective speech tests will help to shed light on specific listening difficulties and on readiness toward self-efficacy, especially in light of the incomplete relationship between audiometric data and handicap scale scores.

Premise 3. We should rethink our conceptualization of hearing technologies. Hearing technologies, such as a hearing aid or some type of HAT, are a way to lower some of the sensory and cognitive hurdles of aging; they are not merely devices that improve audibility and intelligibility. Their use should be encouraged early on. We must make the connection between hearing impairment, specific activity limitations, participation restrictions, and hearing technologies. We must help the patient realize that when it is easier to communicate, communication experiences become more stress free and natural. We can best serve the needs of our older clients by providing a customized solution for each client who walks in the door. We must accept that there is wide diversity among older adults, and we must focus on the individual, his or her spouse, any physical limitations, manual dexterity or visual problems, cognitive difficulties, and communication needs and desires. Important intervention outcomes should be independence, safety, and improved quality of life. Recommending hearing aids before considering HATs may be premature. Frequency modulated systems, infrared systems, and telecommunication devices are sometimes a good introduction to amplified sound, with later movement to hearing aids. Hearing aid recommendations must include features to enhance speech understanding in noise such as dual microphones and/or a telecoil for use with speakers, an induction loop system or silhouette, and possibly a frequency modulated boot.

Working from these premises, the audiologic evaluation for older adults should include the following: (1) the intake, (2) the evaluation, and (3) recommendations and counseling.

Step 1: The Intake

The purpose of the intake is to obtain a comprehensive history that encompasses medical and nonmedical aspects of the hearing loss. The traditional case history should focus on the evolution of the hearing loss, etiology of the hearing loss, and medical conditions that may be relevant. We should also get a feel for the impact of the hearing loss on the individual and the family. During the initial encounter with the patient, we must keep in mind what is important: What does it mean to this person to have this impairment at this time in his life, with his wife and children, in his environment, and with his peer group? To help gain some insight into the patient, the audiologist might administer the HHIE or a modified version of the International Outcome Inventory for Hearing Aids (IOI-HA). My modification of the IOI-HA is shown in Table 32.3. Responses to the self-report questionnaires completed during the intake will likely form the basis for counseling and decision making regarding the next step in the evaluative process.

Step 2: The Evaluation

The purpose of the evaluation is to determine type and severity of hearing loss and speech understanding ability in a variety of listening situations. Puretone air- and bone-conduction testing across octave and interoctave frequencies is the first part of the evaluation. Next, it is important

---

TABLE 32.3   Modified version of the international outcome inventory for hearing aids

1. How much hearing difficulty do you have?
   None   Moderate   Severe

2. Do you think other people are bothered by your hearing difficulties?
   Not at all   Somewhat   A good deal

3. How much have your hearing difficulties affected the things you can do?
   Not at all   Somewhat   A good deal

4. Considering everything, how much has your hearing difficulty changed your enjoyment of life?
   Not at all   Somewhat   A good deal

Note: Affirmative responses to these questions may lead to administration of a more in depth questionnaire such as the Hearing Handicap Inventory for the Elderly.

TABLE 32.4   The audiologic evaluation: income and outcome measures

Purpose of the audiologic assessment	Audiometric tools/ income measures	Sample outcome
Determination of puretone air and bone conduction thresholds	Use insert phones to obtain thresholds; check for collapsed canals, impacted cerumen; test interoctave frequencies	Mild to moderate sensory-neural hearing loss most pronounced in high frequencies
	Word recognition tests in quiet, in noise, with visual cues, at supra-threshold levels under earphones and in a sound field	Excellent supra-threshold word recognition scores; fair word recognition ability in sound field in quiet and extreme difficulty in sound field in noise; significantly greater difficulty in noise under earphones at right ear rather than left ear

to assess speech understanding ability using valid materials, presentation levels, and situations. For example, it is helpful to assess speech understanding (1) with and without visual cues; (2) with and without competing noise; and (3) at various presentation levels. Using this approach will shed light on situational difficulties and will be helpful during the counseling process. In my view, immittance tests are time consuming and costly and, therefore, should be administered in the event that there is suspicion of middle ear or retrocochlear involvement. The time previously spent on immittance testing can be better spent learning more about the patient's candidacy for intervention and to begin the counseling process. Table 32.4 summarizes the proposed steps in the evaluative process.

Step 3: Recommendations and Counseling

The rehabilitative process begins at the end of the evaluation when the audiologist shares results and makes recommendations for follow-up. The client has come for an evaluation and should walk away with concrete suggestions or an action plan because this will promote compliance with recommendations. At the conclusion of the evaluation, the audiologist should consider working with the patient and his/her family member to determine a rehabilitative roadmap. The audiologist should have a feel for the patient's readiness for some form of rehabilitation (stages of readiness questionnaire), and the patient should come away understanding the options available based on readiness and physical, sociologic, audiologic, and psychological variables. Table 32.5 provides a sample set of questions one might ask to determine readiness for intervention; the responses should guide the course of the counseling and future recommendations. Hence, an individual with a mild hearing loss with minimal handicap who experiences difficulty in very selected situations such as watching television might be a candidate for some form of HAT. Table 32.6 provides a matrix for discussing the different types of technology available for particular communicative difficulties. In contrast to the patient requiring some form of assistive technology, a patient who admits to a hearing loss and a significant self-reported handicap might be a candidate

for a hearing aid; the Hearing Aid Selection Profile (HASP) might help in determining the technology and style of the unit for the patient to consider when he or she returns for the evaluation. The audiologist might find it helpful to discuss the many benefits of hearing aids with the patient because this can help the patient to realize the value or cost benefit of current technology. Table 32.7 summarizes the areas in which hearing aids have proven beneficial.

■ HEARING SCREENING

Hearing screening has been a health promotion activity engaged in by audiologists to promote early identification of hearing loss and early intervention with HATs and hearing aids. Historically, compliance with traditional screening programs has been quite low, such that only a small proportion of individuals undergoing hearing screenings actually follow through with the recommendations. Hearing-impaired individuals have identified a number of significant barriers to following recommendations regarding a follow-up audiologic evaluation and possible use of an amplification device. These include the high cost of hearing aids, lack of insurance coverage for the evaluation and/or hearing aids, myths about hearing aids (e.g., amplify noise, not appropriate for persons with sensory-neural hearing loss), the stigma associated with hearing loss and use of hearing aids, ageism (e.g., belief that hearing loss is a normal concomitant of the aging process), and the false impression that hearing aids are not effective in remediating the psychosocial and communicative consequences of hearing loss.

Preventive hearing health care is an important initiative in which audiologists should become involved. Specifically, screening efforts targeting individuals with hearing impairments or dizziness that is associated with activity limitations and participation restrictions can assure that older adults receive the intervention services necessary to help promote quality of life. In recognition of the importance of preventive services for the elderly, including sensory declines, Medicare Part B Preventive Services began providing additional

TABLE 32.5   Recommendations and counseling

Purpose of the assessment	Audiometric tools/ income measures	Sample outcome
Determine patient's stage of readiness for intervention	Stage of Readiness Questionnaire	Identify the statement that best describes your perspective. *I do not think I have a hearing problem, and therefore nothing should be done about it.* Recommend: annual evaluation *I think I have a hearing problem. However, I am not yet ready to take any action to solve the problem, but I might do so in the future.* Recommend: HAT *I know I have a hearing problem, and I intend to take action to solve it soon.* OR *I know I have a hearing problem, and I am here to take action to solve it now.* Recommend: hearing aid
Determination of candidacy for hearing aids, HATs, and rehabilitative goals and baseline information against which to assess outcomes	COSI; HHIE	Five listening situations in which the patient has difficulty half of the time: friends; telephone; large groups; work; restaurants HHIE Score = 46%
Needs assessment to identify hearing aid technology most appropriate to the lifestyle, physical, status, cognitive status, affect, etc., of the patient	Hearing Aid Selection Profile[a]	Motivation – 15 Expectation –14 Appearance – 12 Cost – 15 Technology – 10 Physical Function – 16 Communication Needs – 13 Lifestyle – 10
Needs assessment to determine need for HAT	HATs Assessment Protocol (see Table 32.6)	Consider an infrared system for the television
Information sharing regarding results and recommendations	Synthesize information from above sources of data	Return for hearing aid

HAT, hearing assistive technology; COSI, Client Oriented Scale of Improvement; HHIE, Hearing Handicap Inventory for the Elderly.
[a] Subscales assess: motivation for and expectations of hearing aids, patient's perceptions of their personal appearance, cost of goods and services, patient's physical limitations, technology, communicative needs, and lifestyle.

coverage for new registrants (Solodar and Chappell, 2005). With the goal of promoting health and detecting diseases early, the following programmatic initiatives became available to new Medicare Part B beneficiaries as of January 1, 2005:

1. Physicians and nonphysicians are encouraged to use self-report screening questionnaires to review an individual's functional ability and level of safety in several areas, including hearing impairment and dizziness (Solodar and Chappell, 2005).
2. Service providers must offer education, counseling, and referral to individuals who do not pass the screening.

The new Medicare guidelines represent an opportunity for hearing health care providers to educate physicians about their role in hearing health care and to provide them with simple and acceptable screening tools for use with older adults (Hampton, 2005). According to Kochkin (2005a), the National Institutes of Health has endorsed the use of the HHIE and the Dizziness Handicap Inventory for screening purposes. Hopefully, the new Medicare guidelines will reverse the current trend toward a decline in the percentage of physicians screening for hearing difficulty. In 2004, 13% of physicians reported screening, which represents a decline of 5% since 1991 when 18% of physicians reported to be screening their patients. As is evident in Table 32.8, only 11.7% of physicians reported screening their patients who were 75 years of age and older (Kochkin, 2005a).

Recently, there have been a number of studies by physicians evaluating the efficacy of a variety of hearing screening protocols. Protocols usually include a physiologic measure of impairment, namely the audioscope; a measure of handicap

TABLE 32.6   Hearing assistive technologies (HATs) assessment

Goals of hearing assistive technology assessment	Environmental Influences (situations in which experience difficulties with and without hearing aids)	Technology	Outcomes in selected listening environments
Assess communication needs in face-to-face situations	Home Work Leisure Activities Restaurants Classrooms	Small/large group listening situations	Device recommended is easy to use; supplements hearing aids in situations in which patient continues to have difficulty
Assess difficulty understanding broadcast media	Television Radio Movies Theatre	Media technologies	Television voices are clear; can understand actors in movies and theatres
Assess telecommunication capabilities	Telephone Cell phone	Telephone assistive technologies	Can understand on the cell phone and land line
Assess ability to hear alerting signals and environmental stimuli	Smoke alarm Doorbell Telephone Child crying Alarm clock Appliances	Alerting devices	Alerting devices are audible

TABLE 32.7   Arenas in which the efficacy of hearing aids has been documented

Physical function	Social function	Psychological function	Communicative function	Financial
Physical health	Quality and nature of family relations	Self-esteem	Ease of communication	Earning power
Perceived mental function	Group interactions	Emotional stability	Reductions in compensatory communication behaviors (e.g., pretending to hear)	
	Independence	Reduce feelings of anxiety, depression, anger		

TABLE 32.8   Physician screening by year and age group

Age group	1991	1997	2004
20–44	14.8%	14.4%	14.3%
45–64	15.9%	14.6%	10.5%
65–74	20%	17.6%	10.7%
75+	24%	21.6%	11.7%
Total population	18%	16.6%	12.9%

From Kochkin S. (2005a) MarkeTrak VII: hearing loss population tops 31 million people. *Hear Rev.* 12, 16–29.

**Screening Protocol for Identifying Older Adults with Hearing Problems
Requiring Audiologic Intervention**

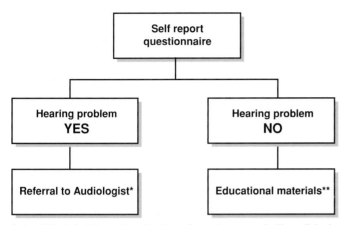

* Referral should include information about readiness to proceed with audiologic assessment and
management and educational materials appropriate to level of readiness

** Educational materials to promote readiness and awareness of effects of hearing loss

FIGURE 32.2 Screening protocol for identifying older adults with hearing problems requiring audiologic intervention.

such as the HHIE Screening version; a single question, such as "Do you have a hearing problem now?", or some combination of measures. There is ample evidence available to support use of these techniques alone or in combination. In my view, a preventive care protocol must be implemented in a context that will ensure that the patient is armed with information that will enable him or her to take an active role/interest in preventive care. When designing a hearing screening program, we should keep the following question in mind: How do we get people to seek and accept hearing care services, including hearing aids, assistive listening devices, and audiologic rehabilitation? Since most studies report that the yield from screening is higher using a self-report either in the form of a single question or a series of questions, I propose the protocol outlined in Figure 32.2, which includes an educational counseling component.

CASE PRESENTATION

Mr. R, an active 70-year-old man, recently returned to work part time after 1 year of full-time retirement. The case history reveals that he is in excellent health and enjoys being productive. He indicated that his work entails small group meetings with colleagues and that he has considerable difficulty when noise is present in the room and when he is sitting around large conference room tables. He also finds that he has more difficulty understanding female than male voices. Because of these problems, he scanned the internet for information on hearing loss and came to several websites that conducted hearing screenings. Mr. R completed an online screening version of the HHIE. His hearing profile revealed a score of 20, suggesting a mild self-perceived hearing handicap with a referral to a local audiologist. The site directed him to a list of audiologists in his geographic area. Mr. R scheduled an

appointment with the audiologist armed with considerable information about hearing loss and hearing aids and with questions regarding the virtues of hearing aid use.

The audiometric evaluation revealed that, indeed, Mr. R had mild bilateral sensory-neural hearing loss in both ears with excellent word recognition ability, which belied his experiences in the real world. The audiologist administered word recognition tests in the presence of noise bilaterally and word recognition testing at 50 dB hearing level (HL) in the sound field. Mr. R obtained scores of 72% on the speech tests in noise and 80% on the sound field test. Responses to the screening version of the HHIE revealed a score of 22, suggesting a mild handicap. In light of test results, the HASP was completed to help decide on the appropriate technology to recommend. His scores suggested that he was highly motivated to obtain hearing aids, had the manual dexterity to manipulate hearing aids, and had the financial resources to purchase digital hearing aids. The audiologist recommended bilateral digital hearing aids with a directional microphone. Mr. R returned to the audiologist after 3 and 6 weeks of hearing aid use for some fine tuning of his hearing aids, for assessment of his functioning with the units, and for judgments regarding satisfaction with the hearing aids and the services he received.

At the postfitting appointments, it was clear that Mr. R was quite satisfied with his hearing aids according to responses to the Knowles Satisfaction Survey. His score on the HHIE after 6 weeks of hearing aid use revealed a significant reduction in self-perceived handicap. His aided score was 8, suggesting with 95% confidence that this was a true change in the HHIE score from the unaided condition. Mr. R completed the HHIE 3 months after the fitting and continued to be deriving considerable benefit from the units (HHIE score increased to 10). This case was of interest because, despite a mild hearing impairment and excellent word recognition scores in quiet, the audiologist chose to do some additional speech testing to uncover some of the client's expressed communication difficulties. The more thorough examination confirmed the speech understanding difficulties in adverse listening situations and some psychosocial sequelae, which led to a decision to purchase hearing aids. The comprehensive client-centered examination enabled Mr. R to obtain the assistance he needed and, more importantly, to satisfy the communicative needs presented by his particular lifestyle. He is now a strong advocate for hearing aids and has been instrumental in helping some of his friends purchase hearing aids.

SUMMARY

The aging of the Baby Boomer generation brings with it challenges to which audiologists should be armed to respond,

namely a huge increase in the number of older adults in general and those with hearing impairments in particular. These individuals will need and want to hear and understand family, friends, and coworkers. They must be encouraged to seek out audiologic services early so that hearing loss does not interfere with the quality of their prolonged life. My goal in developing this chapter was to arm audiologists with information about hearing loss in older adults that will empower them to effectively identify, evaluate, and manage this growing and important population. Hearing health care services for older adults must be delivered with an understanding of the aging process and the biases older adults bring to their health care. A better understanding of aging in general and its impact on the hearing mechanism in particular will hopefully promote the delivery of more targeted audiologic services.

REFERENCES

American Academy of Aging. (2008) Older Americans: 2008—Key Indicators of Well Being. Washington, DC.

American Academy of Audiology. (2005) Guideline for the Audiologic Management of Adult Hearing Impairment. Available at: http://www.audiology.org/NR/rdonlyres/5DE475B4-58F3-40A7-934E-584AC11EABE9/0/haguidelines.pdf.

American Geriatrics Society. (2004) *Geriatrics Review Syllabus: A Core Curriculum in Geriatric Medicine.* 5th ed. New York: Blackwell Publishing.

Beers M. (2005) *Merck Manual of Geriatrics.* 3rd ed. Whitehouse Station, NJ: Merck.

Better Hearing Institute. (2005) Hearing solutions: the impact of treated hearing loss on quality of life. Available at: http://www.betterhearing.org/hearing_solutions/qualityOFLifeDetail.cfm.

Ballachanda B. (1995a) Ear canal acoustics. In: Ballachanda B, ed. *Introduction to the Human Ear Canal.* San Diego: Singular Publishing Group.

Ballachanda B. (1995b) Ear canal examination. In: Ballachanda B, ed. *Introduction to the Human Ear Canal.* San Diego: Singular Publishing Group.

Becker W, Naumann H, Pfaltz C. (1989) *Ear, Nose and Throat Diseases: A Pocket Reference.* Stuttgart, Germany: George Thieme Verlag.

Brant L, Gordon-Salant S, Pearon J, Klein L, Morell C, Metter E, Fozard J. (1996) Risk factors related to age-associated hearing loss in the speech frequencies. *J Am Acad Audiol.* 7, 152–160.

Brody H. (1955) Organization of the cerebral cortex: III. A study of aging in the human cerebral cortex. *J Compar Neurol.* 102, 511–556.

Crowe S, Guild S, Polvogt L. (1934) Observations on the pathology of high tone deafness. *Johns Hopkins Hospital Bulletin.* 54, 315–381.

Dalton D, Cruickshanks K, Klein B, Klein R, Wiley T, Nondahl D. (2003) The impact of hearing loss on quality of life in older adults. *Gerontologist.* 43, 661–668.

Etholm B, Belal A. (1974) Senile changes in the middle ear joints. *Ann Otol Rhinol Laryngol.* 83, 49–54.

Fausti S, Wilmington D, Helt P, Helt W, Konrad-Martin D. (2005) Hearing health and care: the need for improved hearing loss

prevention and hearing conservation practices. *J Rehabil Res Dev.* 42 (suppl 2), 45–62.

Garstecki D, Erler S. (1996) Use of the Communication Profile for the Hearing Impaired with mildly hearing impaired adults. *J Speech Hear Res.* 39, 28–42.

Gates G, Cobb J, D'Agostino R, Wolf P. (1993) The relation of hearing in the elderly to the presence of cardiovascular disease and cardiovascular risk factors. *Arch Otolaryngol Head Neck Surg.* 119, 156–161.

Gates G, Mills J. (2005) Presbycusis. *Lancet.* 366, 1111–1120.

Gleitman R, Ballachanda B, Goldstein D. (1992) Incidence of cerumen impaction in general adult population. *Hear J.* 45, 28–32.

Golding M, Taylor A, Cupples L, Mitchell P. (2006) Odds of demonstrating auditory processing abnormality in the average older adults: The Blue Mountains Hearing Study. *Ear Hear.* 27, 129–138.

Gordon-Salant S. (2005) Hearing loss and aging: new research findings and clinical implications. *J Rehabil Res Dev.* 42 (suppl 2), 9–24.

Hampton D. (2005) Hearing HealthCare News. Available at: http://www.hearinghealthnews.com/.

Hnath-Chisolm T, Willott J, Lister J. (2003) The aging auditory system: anatomic and physiologic changes and implications for rehabilitation. *Int J Audiol.* 42 (suppl), S3–S10.

Holte L. (1996) Aging effects in multifrequency tympanometry. *Ear Hear.* 17, 12–27.

Humes L. (1996) Speech understanding in the elderly. *J Am Acad Audiol.* 7, 161–168.

Humes L, Christopherson L, Cokely C. (1992) Central auditory processing disorders in the elderly: fact or fiction? In: Katz J, Stecker N, Henderson D, eds. *Central Auditory Processing: A Transdisciplinary View.* St. Louis: Mosby Year Book.

Jerger J, Jerger S, Maudlin L. (1971) Studies in impedance audiometry in normal and sensorineural ears. *Arch Otolaryngol.* 96, 512–523.

Jerger J, Oliver T, Pirozzolo F. (1990) Impact of central auditory processing disorder and cognitive deficit on the self-assessment of hearing handicap in the elderly. *J Am Acad Audiol.* 1, 75–80.

Kochkin S. (2005a) MarkeTrak VII: hearing loss population tops 31 million people. *Hear Rev.* 12, 16–29.

Kochkin S. (2005b) Hearing loss and its impact on household income. *Hear Rev.* 12, 16–24.

Lethbridge-Cejku M, Schiller J, Bernadel L. (2002) Summary health statistics for US adults: National Health Interview Survey, 2002. Vital and Health Statistics, series 10 (222). Hyattsville, MD: United States Department of Health and Human Services, Centers for Disease Control and Prevention, National Center for Health Statistics.

Mahoney D. (1987) One simple solution to hearing impairment. *Geriatr Nurs.* 8, 242–245.

Martin J, Jerger J. (2005) Some effects of aging on central auditory processing. *J Rehabil Res Dev.* 42 (4 suppl 2), 25–44.

Moscicki E, Elkins E, Baum H, McNamara P. (1985) Hearing loss in the elderly: an epidemiologic study of the Framingham Heart Study Cohort. *Ear Hear.* 6, 184–190.

Mulrow C, Aguilar C, Endicott J, Tuley M, et al. (1990a) Quality of life changes and hearing impairment: a randomized trial. *Ann Intern Med.* 113, 188–194.

Mulrow C, Aguilar C, Endicott J, Velez R, et al. (1990b) Association between hearing impairment and the quality of life of elderly individuals. *J Am Geriatr Soc.* 38, 45–50.

The National Council on the Aging. (1999) The consequences of untreated hearing loss in older persons. Washington, DC: National Council on the Aging.

Oliveira R. (1995) The dynamic ear canal. In: Ballachanda B, ed. *Introduction to the Human Ear Canal.* San Diego: Singular Publishing Group.

Osterhammel D, Osterhammel P. (1970) Age and sex variations for the normal stapedial reflex thresholds and tympanometric compliance values. *Scand Audiol.* 8, 153–158.

Otte J, Schuknecht H, Kerr A. (1978) Ganglion cell populations in normal and pathological human cochleae. Implications for cochlear implantation. *Laryngoscope.* 88, 1231–1246.

Pauler M, Schuknecht H, White J. (1988) Atrophy of the stria vascularis as a cause of sensorineural hearing loss. *Laryngoscope.* 98, 754–759.

Powers R. (1994) Neurobiology of aging. In: *Textbook of Geriatric Neuropsychiatry.* Washington, DC: American Psychiatric Press, Inc.

Rosenwasser H. (1964) Otitic problems in the aged. *Geriatrics.* 19, 11–17.

Schuknecht H. (1955) Presbycusis. *Laryngoscope.* 65, 402–419.

Schuknecht H. (1989) Pathology of presbycusis. In: Goldstein J, Kashima H, Koopman C, eds. *Geriatric Otorhinolaryngology.* Toronto: B.C. Decker.

Schuknecht H, Gacek J. (1993) Cochlear pathology in presbycusis. *Ann Otol Rhinol Laryngol.* 102, 1–16.

Smith J, Mitchell P, Wang J, Leeder S. (2005) A health policy for hearing impairment in older Australians: what should it include? *Aust New Zealand Health Policy.* 2, 31.

Solodar H, Chappell J. (2005) "Welcome to Medicare" preventative exam includes hearing and balance screening. *Audiol Today.* 17, 49.

Suzuka Y, Schuknecht H. (1988) Retrograde cochlear neuronal degeneration in human subjects. *Acta Otolaryngol Suppl.* 450, 1–20.

Thompson DJ, Sills J, Recke K, Bui D. (1979) Acoustic admittance and the aging ear. *J Speech Hear Res.* 23, 29–35.

United States Census Bureau. (2005) 65+ in the United States: 2005. Current Population Reports. Bethesda, MD: US Department of Health and Human Services, National Institutes of Health.

VanRooij J, Plomp R, Orlebeke J. (1989) Auditive and cognitive factors in speech perception in elderly listeners. I: Development of test battery. *J Acoust Soc Am.* 86, 1294–1309.

Weinstein B. (2000) *Geriatric Audiology.* New York: Thieme Medical Publishers, Inc.

Wiley T, Cruickshanks K, Nondahl D, Tweed T, Klein R, Klein B. (1996) Tympanometric measures in older adults. *J Am Acad Audiol.* 7, 260–268.

Wiley T, Nondahl D, Cruickshanks K, Tweed T. (2005) Five-year changes in middle ear function for older adults. *J Am Acad Audiol.* 16, 129–139.

Willott J. (1991) *Aging and the Auditory System.* San Diego: Singular Publishing, Co.

Willott J, Sundin V, Jeskey J. (2001) Effects of an augmented acoustic environment on the mouse auditory system. In: Willott JF, ed. *Handbook of Mouse Auditory Research: From Behavior to Molecular Biology.* Boca Raton, FL: CRC Press; pp 205–214.

Wingfield A. (1996) Cognitive factors in auditory performance: context, speed of processing and constraints of memory. *J Am Acad Audiol.* 7, 175–182.

Wingfield A, Poon L, Lombardi L, Lowe D. (1985) Speed of processing in normal aging: effects of speech rate, linguistic structure and processing time. *J Gerontol.* 40, 579–585.

Wu H, Chin J, Tong H. (2004) Screening for hearing impairment in a cohort of elderly patients attending a hospital geriatric medicine service. *Singapore Med J.* 45, 79–84.

33 Tinnitus and Hyperacusis

Richard S. Tyler, William Noble, Claudia Coelho, George Haskell, and Aditya Bardia

INTRODUCTION

Tinnitus and hyperacusis are two of the more challenging issues in audiology. Patients can be desperate, and there are no cures. Nonetheless, several forms of treatment are available, and audiologists possess a good educational foundation to provide the diagnosis and management of tinnitus and hyperacusis based on their knowledge of hearing loss, hearing measurement, and rehabilitation. We advocate a flexible approach, as appropriate, that includes collaboration with informed psychologists and physicians.

Tinnitus has been defined by McFadden (1982) as follows:

- A perception of sound (it must be heard)
- Involuntary (not produced intentionally)
- Originates in the head (not an externally produced sound)

Hyperacusis does not have a single widely accepted definition. Hyperacusis can involve perceptions and reactions of loudness, annoyance, and fear to acoustic stimuli. The link between the two conditions is not clear, but Tyler and Conrad-Armes (1983) noted that tinnitus is often accompanied by hyperacusis, and many current sound therapy protocols treat tinnitus and hyperacusis in parallel.

TINNITUS

Neurophysiologic Causes, Mechanisms, and Models

Virtually anything that produces hearing loss can also produce tinnitus. The most common causes are noise exposure, aging, head injury, and medications. Sometimes the causes are unknown. Estimates of prevalence vary, in part due to differences in the definitions used in surveys. In a prospective study in the United States, Nondahl et al. (2002) found that about 9% of adults reported "significant" tinnitus, and 2% reported "severe" tinnitus. This broadly agrees with earlier studies (Axelsson & Ringdahl, 1989; Coles, 1984; see Davis and Rafaie, 2000, for a review). The prevalence of tinnitus increases with age and hearing loss, but in particular it is influenced by noise exposure. As early as 1886, Barr noted that 42% of the boilermakers engaged in ship building reported occasional or continuous tinnitus. In a national survey in the United Kingdom (Davis, 1995), the prevalence of tinnitus approximately doubled with a history of noise exposure for all age groups. In our clinical experience, many workers in noisy situations report that the onset of tinnitus is gradual. Initially, tinnitus is heard only occasionally during the day or for brief periods after work. Subsequently, the duration of the tinnitus persists until it eventually becomes continuous. Typically (but not always), the onset of tinnitus occurs after the onset of hearing loss (sometimes years afterwards), but while the worker is still exposed to noise. Additionally, there are workers who report that tinnitus began after their exposure to noise had ended.

We classify tinnitus as either sensory-neural or middle ear (Tyler and Babin, 1986). Middle ear tinnitus is typically related to vascular or muscular dysfunction. Sensory-neural tinnitus originates in the cochlear and/or neural auditory pathway. It is important to remember that tinnitus is a symptom, not a diagnosis. There are likely several different subgroups of tinnitus arising from different mechanisms (Dauman and Tyler, 1992; Dobie, 1999). The mechanism responsible for coding tinnitus can originate in the cochlea, the brainstem, or the central nervous system (Fig. 33.1). Stevens

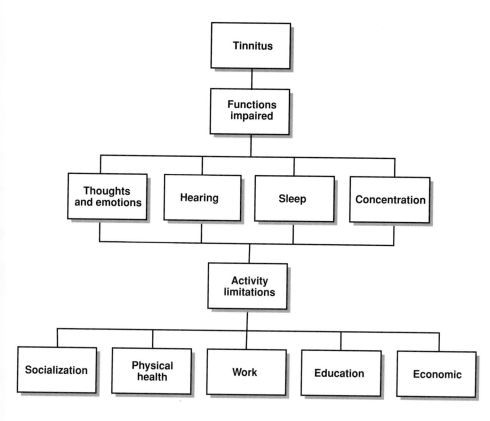

FIGURE 33.1 Domains where tinnitus can have an impact.

and Davis (1938, p 352) note that some forms of tinnitus are "...undoubtedly due to irritation of the higher auditory pathways and centers within the brain." We believe that the auditory cortex must be active in tinnitus, since that is where sound is "perceived." This cortical activity could be associated with:

- An increase in spontaneous activity (Kiang et al., 1970)
- Synchronous spontaneous activity across nerve fibers (Eggermont, 1984; Moller et al., 1984)
- More fibers tuned to the same best frequency (Salvi et al., 2000)

As noted by Hallam (1989), other parts of the brain must be involved in patients who are anxious or have emotional reactions to their tinnitus. This includes the autonomic nervous system and the amygdala (Cacace, 2003; 2004).

It is curious that other parts of the nervous system can also influence tinnitus. For example, some patients report a change in their tinnitus with eye movements, light touch, or voluntary muscle contraction (Cacace, 2003; Levine, 2001; Sanchez et al., 2002; Moller et al., 1992). In some patients, pressure around the head can change tinnitus, and jaw clenching can produce a high-pitch temporary tonal sound. How the stimulation of systems outside the auditory pathway changes tinnitus is not completely clear (see Kaltenbach et al., 2004). It is important to distinguish muscle contraction that changes tinnitus by contracting middle ear muscles rather than effects mediated by nonauditory neural pathways.

Some patients with "normal" hearing also report tinnitus (Nondahl et al., 2002). It should be remembered that "normal" hearing is somewhat arbitrary. Someone could have an audiometric "notch" of 20 dB hearing level (HL) at 4,000 Hz with 0 dB HL thresholds elsewhere. Although this might be considered "normal" by some, it likely represents an auditory pathology. Additionally, hearing thresholds are traditionally measured at octave frequencies from 250 Hz to 8 kHz, leaving large regions of the cochlea unexamined, including frequencies above 8 kHz.

Auditory Hallucinations

When someone reports hearing music or voices, it is important to determine if the person has a mental illness. Reports of imagined voices or music can occur as part of a psychosis-like schizophrenia (Davison et al., 2004). If there is no record of a psychiatric illness, but there is evidence of depression, anxiety, or unrealistic thoughts or actions, then these should be addressed with the client, and a referral should be made to an appropriately qualified psychologist or psychiatrist. In the absence of a mental illness, one could cautiously consider this tinnitus (Cole et al., 2002). Tinnitus can have a central origin. Some fibers or groups of fibers that are active produce the perception of crickets, whereas others might produce the perception of music or voices.

Patients without mental illness who hear music and voices should benefit from support, reassurance, and the counseling and sound therapy programs described on page

729–731. It is important not to overreact to their reports of hearing music and voices.

▧ EVALUATION

Medical

Referral to an otologist is appropriate for pulsatile, sudden onset, or worsening tinnitus, asymmetrical signs, and diseases of the auditory system (Perry and Gantz, 2000; Hegarty and Smith, 2000). When otologists see tinnitus patients, they will try to identify the etiology or etiologies. They begin with a clinical history and an examination of the head, neck, and neuro-otologic system. They might order laboratory examinations (e.g., cholesterol levels, glucose, zinc, screen for ototoxic drugs, etc.) and imaging tests (e.g., ultrasound, computed tomography scan, magnetic resonance imaging, magnetic resonance angiography). Generally, physicians are interested in identifying a possible treatable cause.

Middle ear tinnitus is associated with either abnormal blood flow or middle ear muscle contraction. Some call this "objective" tinnitus because it can be amplified and heard by the examiner. However, spontaneous otoacoustic emissions can also be heard but are produced in the cochlea, not the middle ear. Therefore, we prefer the term middle ear tinnitus. Otologists may determine whether the tinnitus sensation changes with manipulations of blood flow (by asking patients to perform a brief vigorous exercise or by partially constricting a blood vessel of the neck). These manipulations can change the pulsing sensation. Some vascular tumors also touch the eardrum and can be visually observed. Movements of the eardrum can sometimes be observed visually or with the help of measurements of air pressure in the external canal with tympanometry. Oral cavity examination may demonstrate myoclonic activity (palatal myoclonus). Signs of temporomandibular dysfunction might also be noteworthy.

Another focus is a search for treatable sensory-neural tinnitus. This includes some forms of sudden hearing loss, Ménière's disease, or a tumor of the auditory nerve. There is some evidence that tinnitus can be caused by metabolic diseases and deficiencies (e.g., anemia, diabetes, autoimmune disease, zinc and vitamin deficiency). Evaluations for these conditions would involve studies of the blood and urine.

Measuring the Tinnitus

The pitch, loudness, and amount of noise necessary to mask tinnitus can be measured to quantify the physical parameters of tinnitus, provide assistance for fitting maskers, and monitor changes in tinnitus perception (and often can be reimbursed using Current Procedural Terminology code 92625: Assessment of Tinnitus). Patients can usually compare the pitch produced by a puretone to the **most prominent pitch** of their tinnitus (Tyler, 2000; Henry et al., 1999). Pitch matching can be highly variable, and an indication of the variability

should be reported. For example, the results of three to six pitch matches can be reported. Patients can also adjust the intensity of a tone so that it has the same loudness as their tinnitus. Sensation level is not a measure of loudness. The results of a **tinnitus loudness match** can be reported in dB sensation level (SL), but this level can only be interpreted over time within a patient if the hearing threshold at that frequency does not change. An alternative approach is to convert the physical intensity of the sound into the subjective loudness scale based on sones using a formula (Tyler and Conrad-Armes, 1983). Sones represent an international standard; one sone represents the loudness of a 40-dB sound pressure level (SPL) 1,000-Hz tone in a normal listener. A sound that has a loudness of four sones is four times as loud. Another measure of the magnitude of tinnitus is the amount of noise required to mask the tinnitus, sometimes referred to as the **minimum masking level**. The noise level (specify the frequency characteristics of the noise, e.g., broadband 250 to 8,000 Hz) is increased until it just masks the tinnitus.

There are a few things that can contribute to the variability of tinnitus measurements. First, one should be aware that the test stimuli can change the tinnitus. This is probably more likely to happen for intense stimuli and when stimuli are presented ipsilaterally to the tinnitus. The ear receiving the stimuli should be reported. Second, in many patients, the perception of tinnitus is not constant but varies throughout the day or from day to day. A reasonable approach to this is to make multiple measurements and report each value. The variability of the measurements can be documented by replicating the measures and recording the results of each trial in the patient's chart. For example, we often use the average of three loudness matches, three minimum masking levels, and six pitch matches (because pitch tends to be more variable). In patients with highly variable tinnitus, additional measurements can be made, and the measurements can be repeated at subsequent visits (particularly for a patient whose tinnitus changes).

Measuring the Reaction to the Tinnitus

People's reaction to their tinnitus covers a broad range. Some appear to be not particularly bothered by it, whereas for others, the tinnitus can have a dramatic effect on their lifestyle. The impairment of tinnitus can result in difficulties with thoughts and emotions, hearing and communication, sleep, and concentration (Fig. 33.1) (Erlandsson, 2000; Tyler, 2006; Noble, 1998). Sleep disturbance is one of the most commonly reported problems (McKenna, 2000; McKenna and Daniel, 2006; Tyler and Baker, 1983). Some individuals have difficulty falling asleep, while others have difficulty falling back asleep once they wake up in the middle of the night.

When determining the impact tinnitus is having on an individual's life, an easy first step is to ask the person to "list all the problems you have that you associate with your tinnitus, starting with the problem that bothers you the most" (Tyler and Baker, 1983; Sanchez and Stephens, 1997). This can be done before the first appointment and can lead to an open discussion of the important problems as perceived by the patient.

Several questionnaires designed to quantify the problems caused by tinnitus are available (Tyler, 1993; Noble, 1998). Two of these, the *Tinnitus Effects Questionnaire* of Hallam et al. (1988) and the *Tinnitus Handicap Questionnaire* of Kuk et al. (1990), have been independently assessed (Henry and Wilson, 1998) and shown to be reliable. The *Tinnitus Reaction Questionnaire* of Wilson et al. (1991) focuses on general distress, interference with work and leisure, severe stress, and avoidance of activities. This is also a reliable scale and has been shown to relate to independent clinical ratings of coping ability and to be unrelated to measures of neuroticism. In other words, this scale assesses reactions that are specific to tinnitus. Tyler et al. (2006) have developed a new questionnaire, shown in Appendix 33.1, that specifically focuses on emotional, hearing, sleep, and concentration difficulties and assists in determining treatment needs.

TREATMENTS

There are two basic types of tinnitus treatment strategies: those designed to reduce or eliminate the physical perception and those designed to change the patient's reaction.

Counseling

There are a variety of counseling approaches that range from providing information to more engaged collaborative counseling (see Tyler [2006] for a review). Many of these are based on the early work of Hallam and colleagues (Hallam, 1989; Hallam and McKenna, 2006) known as Tinnitus Habituation Therapy. Others include strategies for improved coping, management, and behavioral change (Sweetow, 1986; Tyler et al., 1989; Davis, 1995). Among these are Tinnitus Activities Treatment (Tyler et al., 2004b; Tyler et al., 2006), Tinnitus Retraining Therapy (Jastreboff, 2000; Bartnik and Skarzynski, 2006), and Tinnitus Cognitive Behavior Therapy (Henry and Wilson, 2001; 2002). The aim of these procedures is to provide ways for the person suffering with tinnitus to adjust his or her reactions to the experience. It has been found that people who react with fear at the early signs of tinnitus are more likely to be distressed in the longer term (Langguth et al., 2003).

The goals of these psychologically based therapies can vary but often overlap (Tyler and Erlandsson, 2000; Tyler et al., 2006). For example, patients can be helped to habituate to their tinnitus by de-emphasizing the fear associated with it. Another approach is to decrease the attention given to the tinnitus, often with the help of background sound. The way a patient thinks about the tinnitus can influence his or her reactions to it. Therefore, some clinicians will help patients consider how they think about their tinnitus. These thoughts can be challenged and revised. Another approach

is to assist patients to change their focus away from their tinnitus. This can be facilitated by refocusing on other enjoyable and engaging activities. Having planned activities during which time it is known that the tinnitus is less intrusive can be very helpful. Andersson and Lyttkens (1999) have examined the outcomes from several independent studies and have shown that psychologically based therapy is a fruitful way to manage tinnitus reactions. It is our general view that many patients concerned about tinnitus can adapt to it after the explanation of its origin and its nonthreatening nature (where careful assessment has established that it is not a sign of anything more sinister). But there are a substantial number of patients for whom such reassurance is less effective, and a more elaborate intervention is needed. The descriptions in the following sections provide guidance on the sorts of counseling that may be considered as appropriate within the context of general audiologic practice. We do not assume that the average clinical audiologist has ambitions to pursue a parallel career as a clinical psychologist. Therefore, we advocate a flexible approach, such that in those cases that do not yield to reassurance or more elaborate counseling, reference to an appropriately qualified clinical psychology practice should be considered.

Basic tenets of good counseling that are helpful are:

- Ability to listen
- Patience
- Ability to be encouraging to the patient
- Emotional insightfulness
- Self-awareness
- Ability to laugh at the bittersweet aspects of life
- Positive self-esteem
- Emotional stability
- Ability to talk candidly about depression, anxiety, and other psychological issues

At the initial interview, it is helpful to determine if patients are curious, concerned, or distressed about their tinnitus (Fig. 33.2). Much of the anxiety associated with tinnitus stems from uncertainty regarding its source and consequences. Curious patients typically require only basic information regarding possible causes, mechanisms, prevalence, consequences, and likely outcomes. These patients find that once the mystery of tinnitus is explained to them, their reaction is largely resolved. Concerned patients require more detail and benefit from information regarding things they can do on their own or other treatment options. Depending on the level of concern, these patients can require a more formal evaluation that includes the questionnaires and psychoacoustical measurements discussed earlier. Distressed patients require specific tinnitus treatment. Patients with severe anxiety and depression should obtain help from psychologists or psychiatrists. Any patients who report suicidal thoughts or self-harm need to be questioned further regarding their intentions, and a referral to clinical psychology or psychiatric services should be made immediately if any concern exists.

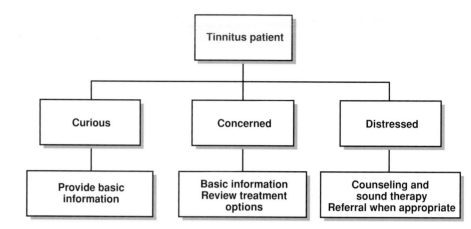

FIGURE 33.2 Broad categories of patients that reflect level of severity and therefore level of treatment needed.

While individual counseling approaches will vary, the common elements of successful counseling strategies include the items listed in the following sections.

PROVIDING INFORMATION

Most approaches provide information about hearing, hearing loss, and tinnitus. They usually include the causes, prevalence, and common consequences of tinnitus. For many people, the unknown aspects of tinnitus are the most alarming. They often find this basic information about tinnitus reassuring and may require no further assistance.

THOUGHTS AND EMOTIONS

It is helpful to distinguish the tinnitus itself from the person's reaction to the tinnitus. The way people think and feel about their tinnitus can have a major influence on their reactions. A major focus of cognitive behavior therapy, and other counseling strategies, is on challenging a person's thoughts about tinnitus and thereby facilitating changes to the reactions to the tinnitus (Hallam, 1989; Hallam and McKenna, 2006; Henry and Wilson, 2001; 2002; Sweetow, 1986).

CONSIDERING THE PERSON

Some counseling procedures go beyond providing information and attempt to understand and influence the overall emotional well-being of the patient. By necessity, these procedures are collaborative and require more time. Several approaches are available to help individuals understand and change the emotional consequences of their experience with their tinnitus. Mohr and Hedelund (2006) have developed a Person-Centered Tinnitus Therapy (trying to understand not just the tinnitus, but how the tinnitus fits into the larger scope of the individual's life).

COPING/MANAGEMENT STRATEGIES

Some counseling approaches include coping/management strategies to help patients understand and change their perceptions about tinnitus and to modify their reactions and behaviors. Activities are planned to determine situations in which tinnitus might be a problem and then to modify their specific situation to reduce these occurrences. For example, patients might report that their tinnitus is worse when they first get home from work. This might be a result of getting home and sitting in a quiet room reflecting on the day's activities. An alternative activity might be taking the dog for a walk while listening to music. Other activities are identified that can reduce the stress associated with an individual's tinnitus.

RELAXATION AND IMAGERY PROCEDURES

Some patients benefit from learning specific relaxation or imagery procedures. These can be used when people experience stress, and it can be helpful for them to learn relaxation strategies or to focus attention to other thoughts. Exercises to learn how to redirect attention away from the tinnitus are also employed. In a pair of excellent books (one for patients and one for clinicians), Henry and Wilson (2001; 2002) lay out programmatic exercises that patients can do on their own or that can be done in cooperation with the clinician.

Sound Therapies

Sound therapies include strategies that use background sounds to reduce the prominence of tinnitus or decrease its loudness or level of annoyance (Vernon and Meikle, 2000; Tyler and Bentler, 1987; Folmer et al., 2006).

THE USE OF HEARING AIDS

Most patients with tinnitus also have hearing loss. Properly fit hearing aids should help with communication and often also help with tinnitus by reducing the stress involved with intensive listening and by amplifying low-level background sounds. Hearing aids are often the first component of sound therapy for patients with tinnitus (Searchfield, 2006).

THE USE OF WEARABLE SOUND GENERATORS

Wearable ear level devices are available that produce low-level noise. Some patients prefer this to listening to their tinnitus, perhaps because it is more pleasant to listen to or because the devices may decrease the loudness or prominence of their tinnitus. Some patients wear devices while their tinnitus is particularly annoying, while others use these devices during all waking hours. These devices look like hearing aids and are worn either behind the ear or in the ear. The noise should be adjusted to a level so that it does not interfere with communication.

The level of the background noise that is suggested varies with different sound therapies. Two types of masking are available. Total masking covers tinnitus completely, so the person hears a "shhhhhh" instead of their tinnitus. With partial masking, the noise is set to a level so that both the tinnitus and the noise can be heard. This technique usually reduces the loudness, annoyance, or prominence of the tinnitus. Some protocols suggest that the ideal place for the noise should be at a level that is about equal to the tinnitus, where the tinnitus is just heard through the masking noise and mixes or blends with the tinnitus. Hazell (1987, p 40) recommended that "the masking sound does not completely cover the tinnitus." Jastreboff and Hazell (2004, p 210) recommended noise "below the level creating annoyance or discomfort." Other protocols focus on a lower level with the noise just in the background. For example, Coles and Hallam (1987, p 994) suggested that the masker be a "low-level background sound against which the loudness of the tinnitus is reduced." Tyler and Babin (1986, p 3213) suggested that patients should use the "lowest masker level that provides adequate relief."

Devices are available that combine a hearing aid and a noise generator in a single unit. They can provide the benefits of the hearing aids in combination with the noise generator.

THE USE OF NONWEARABLE SOUND GENERATORS

Many people also find it helpful to use sound in the background around the home or office or while they are going to sleep. Some use common devices, such as a fan, to produce the noise. There are also devices that are produced specifically for the purpose of producing background sounds, such as raindrops on leaves or waves on the shore. Pillows with tiny loudspeakers that connect into other sound devices are available to facilitate sleep. Radios and sound reproduction systems (e.g., CD players) have the advantage that they can be set according to preference. It is often helpful to have control of the level. Robb (2006) provides an excellent review of a variety of sound options.

THE USE OF MUSIC

Most people can enjoy some types of background music, and it is not surprising that many use a soft, light music in the background to help decrease the prominence of their tinnitus. Recently, Davis (2006) produced a counseling and sound therapy that combines background noise and modified music.

DURATION OF DEVICE USE

How long someone uses a device throughout the day and how many months someone should continue to use the device can vary across patients. Some patients will use a device only when their tinnitus interferes with an important task, such as reading for work. We never insist that patients have to "avoid silence" because their speech perception is often worse in noise and some will constantly monitor their environment and their tinnitus in this effort. Some will choose not to use the device when communicating with others. It is often advisable to set the device to a low partial masking level and leave it on all day. This can help the patient forget about it and avoids having the patient focus on the device and their tinnitus throughout the day. Some patients choose to use their noise generators for life, whereas others may choose to use them until they feel like they have attained some control and their reactions to the tinnitus are sufficiently reduced.

Tinnitus Activities Treatment

Our counseling approach has evolved over the years (Tyler and Babin, 1986; Tyler et al., 1989; Tyler and Erlandsson, 2000). We continue to prefer the partial masking strategy we recommended in the 1980s, although some patients benefit from total masking. We now call this approach Tinnitus Activities Treatment (Tyler et al., 2004b; 2006) which contains four separate modules.

THOUGHTS AND EMOTIONS

The way patients understand and think about their tinnitus influences their reactions to it. Providing information in a collaborative fashion to ensure understanding is essential. Key aspects of this area include:

- Listen to the patient and address issues that are important to them.
- Provide information about hearing, hearing loss, tinnitus, and attention.
- Understand reactions to unexpected, uncontrollable events.
- Suggest changes in behavior and lifestyle that can facilitate acceptance and habituation.

It is important to help patients recognize the difference between the tinnitus itself and their reaction to it. Cognitive therapy separates the tinnitus from the patients' reactions to it and may provide a sense of control over the impact tinnitus has on their lives.

HEARING AND COMMUNICATION

Tinnitus and hearing loss often occur together, but the patients cannot "hear" their hearing loss, so they project their communication problems on the tinnitus. Reviewing the patient's hearing loss and its impact on communication may redirect some of the anxiety to an area where treatment is more obvious. In addition to hearing aid information, a review of assertive communication versus passive and aggressive communication styles is useful.

SLEEP

Understanding normal sleep patterns is the first step in gaining control over the problem (McKenna, 2000; McKenna and Daniel, 2006). Other strategies include:

- Exploring factors that can affect sleep (e.g., stress, environmental noise, room temperature)
- Arranging the bedroom to promote sleep (e.g., comfortable bedding, remove distracting items from room)
- Avoid alcohol, smoking, and eating before bedtime
- Use of sound to mask tinnitus (e.g., noise generators or soft radio)
- Learning relaxation exercises (e.g., imagery, progressive relaxation)

CONCENTRATION

In our therapy, we discuss the importance of concentration and things that affect our concentration. We review factors in the environment (e.g., lighting, background noise, distractions, temperature) and personal factors (e.g., being tired, current health status, other stressors in our lives) that impact our ability to focus our attention for a sustained period of time.

Activities in "attention diversion" (Henry and Wilson, 2001) give patients practice switching attention from one engaging task or stimulus to another. This type of exercise shows people that they can control what sounds, images, or other stimuli they consciously focus their attention on. Repeated practice with this type of activity can help give patients a sense of control over their attention as well as their tinnitus.

Medical Approaches

PHARMACOLOGIC APPROACH

We believe that no medication has been shown to effectively eliminate tinnitus in repeated clinical trials, although there is continuing interest in this endeavor. Furthermore, it is likely that specific subgroups (as yet unidentified) of tinnitus patients benefit from some drugs. Potential medications include substances that have an action on blood circulation and viscosity, muscle relaxants, anticonvulsants, steroids, and diuretics (Murai et al., 1992; Dobie, 1999).

Pharmacologic approaches to treat tinnitus reactions include antidepressants, antianxiety drugs (anxiolytics), and drugs that facilitate sleep (benzodiazepine receptor agonists, herbal supplements, valerian, melatonin, and L-tryptophan) (Doghramji, 2006). They should be used in addition to counseling.

SURGICAL APPROACHES

Some forms of vascular abnormality can be treated by cutting away or restricting blood vessels. With myoclonus, surgical section of the tensor tympani and stapedial tendons can be successful.

In severe cases, cutting the eighth nerve (cochlear neurectomy) has been used, sacrificing hearing in that ear, but unfortunately, this has had only limited success in reducing tinnitus (House and Brachmann, 1981). Some physicians believe that tinnitus is a result of abnormal compression of the eighth nerve by a vessel (called vestibulocochlear compression syndrome) and have performed microvascular decompression operations of the vestibulocochlear nerve in the treatment of unilateral severe tinnitus (De Ridder et al., 2004).

Other Possible Treatments

Several other alternative approaches have been promoted to treat tinnitus. A guiding principal in judging these treatments should be that they have been shown to be effective in well-designed clinical studies that have been replicated. Chasing many different promised but ineffective cures can be detrimental to the patient's overall emotional state.

Herbal supplements, such as ginkgo and melatonin, and dietary supplements, such as zinc, magnesium, copper, niacin/vitamin B_3, and cobalamin/vitamin B_1, have been recommended (Seidman and Babu, 2003). Acupuncture has not been shown to be effective (Park et al., 2000).

Some patients also ask about the potential benefit of changing their eating and drinking habits. Maintaining healthy diets and exercising is good for all of us, but no data indicate that these changes necessarily will improve tinnitus.

Some have suggested that temporomandibular joint dysfunction can cause tinnitus and thus treatment with jaw manipulations can cure tinnitus. It is not obvious to us that this is possible. The value of this treatment is questionable.

Patients will ask about these treatments, and we recommend discussing the principle of documented effectiveness in well-designed replicated studies. We also note that individual differences might be important. Some options can be harmless (such as drinking less coffee), but some alternative treatments do have important risks or side effects, and these should be explained to the patient.

One of the most promising treatments for tinnitus is the use of electricity. Studies have included stimulation of the cochlea (Kuk et al., 1989; McKerrow et al., 1991; Rubinstein and Tyler, 2004) and brain (De Ridder et al., 2004). Electricity has also been successfully applied to the brain with transcranial magnetic stimulation (Langguth et al., 2003). Numerous studies have demonstrated the effectiveness of cochlear implants in reducing tinnitus in many patients. Thus, it seems that, in a few years, there will be devices available that reduce tinnitus via electricity. The proportion of patients for whom this will help is not known; the details of the appropriate stimulus parameters are also unknown.

 TINNITUS IN CHILDHOOD

Investigating tinnitus in childhood is challenging because of its subjectivity (Stouffer et al., 1991). It is rarely reported spontaneously by children (Fowler, 1955; Graham, 1965) and seldom routinely explored in pediatric otolaryngologic evaluation. Nonetheless, children do experience tinnitus. Most do not appear to be bothered (Baguley and McFerran, 2002), but remarkably, those who are bothered report similar suffering as adults (e.g., with emotional concerns, hearing, sleep, concentration) (Martin and Snashall, 1994), sometimes resulting in problems at school. Tyler and Smith (2002) cautioned about intervention with children when parents were more concerned than the child because this may increase the child's anxiety over the tinnitus. Kentish and Crocker (2006) have designed tinnitus counseling specifically for children.

 CONCLUSIONS REGARDING TINNITUS

There are likely many causes and mechanisms of tinnitus, and therefore, many treatments are likely to be necessary. It is important to distinguish differences between the tinnitus and the reactions to tinnitus. There are many counseling and sound therapies that likely help patients with their reactions. No medications or other treatments have been shown to be effective in well-designed and replicated trials.

 HYPERACUSIS

The concepts of **hyperacusis** include **loudness-hyperacusis, annoyance-hyperacusis,** and **fear-hyperacusis** (Table 33.1). One can imagine that sounds perceived as being very loud could easily become annoying. The anticipation of loud and/or annoying sounds could reasonably lead to the fear of these sounds. However, it is possible for sounds to be annoy-

ing or feared without being too loud. Patients also report that some sounds are physically painful, usually those perceived as loud. Occasionally, patients with tinnitus report that some sounds make their tinnitus worse (Tyler et al., 2003b). It is important to separate each of these symptoms, both for the patient and clinician, to understand the problems carefully and to offer treatment suggestions.

Neurophysiologic Causes, Mechanisms, and Models

Anything that causes a sensory-neural hearing loss likely can also cause hyperacusis. Hyperacusis can also occur without identifiable hearing loss.

As a stimulus is increased, the activity of individual nerve fibers increases, and the number of nerve fibers activated increases (and usually its perceived loudness also increases). Moderately intense sounds might result in loudness-hyperacusis if:

1. greater than normal activity was produced on individual nerve fibers
2. more nerve fibers were activated than normal, and/or
3. there was greater than normal synchrony across fibers

Salvi et al. (2000) suggested that **tinnitus** could result from brain plasticity following sensory-neural hearing loss. We suggest that hyperacusis might also be mediated by brain plasticity. Following a peripheral hearing loss, say at 4,000 Hz, nerve fibers in the brain that normally respond to 4,000 Hz begin to respond to other, nearby frequencies, for example 3,000 Hz. This results in more nerve fibers in the brain responding to 3,000 Hz than would be present normally. If hyperacusis is related to the number of fibers activated, this could account for hyperacusis.

Hazell (1987) suggested that hyperacusis might be the result of an "abnormal gain control." It is as if the brain receives a lack of information after hearing loss and therefore turns up some hypothetical gain control. While intriguing, there are several problems with this suggestion. First, such a gain control mechanism must not operate on acoustic signals because the hearing loss is not corrected. Second, our clinical experience is that some individuals without any apparent hearing loss also have hyperacusis. Third, most people with hearing loss do not get hyperacusis.

 EVALUATION

Medical

The medical evaluation for hyperacusis parallels that for tinnitus. Some conditions have been associated with hyperacusis, including facial paralysis, head trauma, and metabolic, infectious (Lyme disease), and genetic (Williams' syndrome) abnormalities (Katzenell and Segal, 2001).

TABLE 33.1	Definitions of different types of hyperacusis
Type	**Definition**
Loudness-hyperacusis	Moderately intense sounds are perceived as very loud
Annoyance-hyperacusis	Sounds are unusually annoying
Fear-hyperacusis	Unusual fear of sounds (phonophobia)

Measuring Hyperacusis

LOUDNESS-HYPERACUSIS

Loudness Discomfort Levels

Loudness discomfort levels (LDLs) can be performed with puretones at 500 and 4,000 Hz in each ear. We use the following instructions: "This is a test in which you will be hearing sounds in your right/left ear. We want you to decide when the sound first becomes uncomfortably loud."

Sherlock and Formby (2005) found that the variation in LDL among normal listeners without complaints of annoyance was very large, with many listeners having LDLs as low as 80 dB HL. This might have resulted from some subjects interpreting "uncomfortable" in a very different way than other subjects. Clearly, low LDLs do not always result in annoyance.

Magnitude Estimation of Loudness

It is possible to present tones and ask for a rating of loudness on a scale from 0 to 100, with 100 being the loudest sound a person can imagine.

We have developed the Hyperacusis Scales (Tyler et al., 2003a) to attempt to differentiate loudness and annoyance and to ascertain a general idea of the impact of hyperacusis on a patient's daily activities (see Appendix 33.2). The questionnaire asks individuals to consider several typical events they might encounter in their daily lives. They then separately rate the loudness and the annoyance for the same situations. For example, a patient may rate "Telephone ringing in the same room" as 40 out of 100 on the loudness scale (with 100 being unbearably loud), while rating it as 85 out of 100 on the annoyance scale (with 100 being unbearably annoying).

ANNOYANCE-HYPERACUSIS

As mentioned, a questionnaire is shown in Appendix 33.2 where we attempt to quantify annoyance of sounds. Appendix 33.3 shows a handicap scale that asks patients to respond to statements in terms of their hearing loss, tinnitus, and hyperacusis. The statements include items such as "You avoid shopping" or "You feel depressed" and allow clinicians to separate the impact on function that patients perceive from their hearing loss, tinnitus, and hyperacusis. Another approach we have tried is to have patients rate recorded sounds, but this is still in its pilot stage.

Dauman and Bouscau-Faure (2005) developed a multiple activity scale for annoyance-hyperacusis, providing 15 situations (e.g., concert, shopping center, work, church, children). Subjects rated from 1 to 10 each of the "relevant" activities, which were averaged for a total score. They also had patients rate annoyance-hyperacusis on a scale from 1 to 10.

FEAR-HYPERACUSIS

Patients can develop a fear of very specific sounds or categories of sounds (for example, those containing high frequencies) or of any intense sound. The simplest approach may be to ask the patients to make a list of sounds they fear to determine if a specific pattern exists.

▨ TREATMENT

Treatments for hyperacusis are less well developed than for tinnitus. First, a clear distinction needs to be made whether one is treating loudness, annoyance, or fear or a combination of these problems. The same basic tenants of good counseling mentioned earlier for tinnitus can be applied. Patients also have very different levels of distress associated with their hyperacusis. It is necessary to determine initially if they are just curious, somewhat concerned, or very distressed.

Counseling

We believe hyperacusis can influence a patient's emotional well-being, hearing and communication, sleep, and concentration. One approach would include a cognitive behavior modification model, thus focusing on response, emotions, and thoughts (Henry and Wilson, 2001; Hallam and McKenna, 2006). In Hyperacusis Activities Treatment, we include four sections.

EMOTIONAL WELL-BEING

Patients with hyperacusis are often anxious and distressed about being exposed to intense noise. We provide information about possible mechanisms. For example, we describe the coding of intensity by the number of nerve fibers and the activity on nerve fibers. We also review how our reactions are influenced by our expectations. For example, if we expect that a visit from a father-in-law will be trouble, we are more likely to react negatively even to reasonable events. Likewise, if we are expecting a situation to be unbearably loud, that raises our anxiety levels and influences how we react to sound. Some patients might have developed unreasonable expectations, so we provide some instruction on how we are able to change our reactions. It is important to help patients recognize the difference between the loudness of the sound and their reaction to it.

HEARING AND COMMUNICATION

Some patients avoid communication situations where they expect there to be intense sounds. Sound therapy to reduce loudness-hyperacusis should be able to provide some assistance with this. Others will avoid using hearing aids or use gain settings that are insufficient. Patients can set the maximum output of their hearing aids temporarily to a lower level (Searchfield, 2006) and gradually increase this over time.

SLEEP

Occasionally, hyperacusis patients will report that they are awakened from sleep by intense sounds or that they do not sleep as well because of the anticipation of an intense sound.

Partial masking sound therapy (for example, playing music throughout the night) can be helpful for some.

CONCENTRATION

Some patients report that they have difficulty concentrating in anticipation of an intense sound. Again, partial masking sound therapy can be helpful.

Sound Therapies

One fundamental issue is whether to protect the ears from moderately intense sounds, for example, with earplugs. Some patients with severe hyperacusis do this on their own. Of course, everyone (including hyperacusis patients) should protect their ears from potentially damaging high-intensity sounds. However, protecting a hyperacusis patient's ears from moderately intense sounds will not cure the patient's hyperacusis (Hazell, 1987). In fact, restricting one's exposure to moderately intense sounds might have a further negative impact. One can imagine that if it is uncommon to hear a sound at 85 dB SPL, then whenever a sound of this level is perceived, it might result in an overreaction.

There are currently five general sound therapy strategies that we are aware of for hyperacusis. Good evidence to suggest their effectiveness is lacking.

CONTINUOUS LOW-LEVEL BROADBAND NOISE

One approach is to expose the patient to continuous low-level broadband noise (Hazell and Sheldrake, 1992). The rationale is that the reduced input resulting from hearing loss is responsible for the hyperacusis. Correcting this reduced input by continuous noise exposure might reduce the hyperacusis. An advantage of this approach is that the noise can be provided during waking hours with wearable noise generators, and the patient does not have to focus on the device or treatments at times during the day. A possible disadvantage is that noise might interfere with speech perception. Formby and Gold (2002) have reported great success in some individual cases in loudness-hyperacusis (changes in the LDLs >50 dB). Dauman and Bouscau-Faure (2005) also used this procedure for annoyance-hyperacusis with some positive results; however, they concluded that "noise generators do not provide a rapid solution to the problem" (p 506) and that annoyance-hyperacusis "does not improve as rapidly as usually reported" (p 509).

SUCCESSIVE APPROXIMATIONS TO HIGH-LEVEL BROADBAND NOISE

A second approach is to allocate select times during the day for noise exposure and to gradually increase the duration and/or level of exposures over time. Vernon and Press (1998) suggested that patients should listen to pink noise daily for 2 hours under earphones. They indicated that patients reported relief, sometimes as briefly as after 3 months, and for as long as 2 years. This approach can be expanded. For example, a patient might listen to noise for 30 minutes at a soft loudness each night for 2 weeks. For the next 2 weeks, the noise might be increased by a few decibels. For the next 2 weeks, the duration of exposure might be increased by another 30 minutes. The level of the noise can be gradually increased over several weeks. An advantage is that the patient can participate in the strategy for increased exposure. The level should never be uncomfortable, but higher levels can be used because the patient can listen to these levels at times when speech perception is not required.

SUCCESSIVE APPROXIMATIONS TO TROUBLESOME SOUNDS

A third approach that we have used involves recording of specific sounds. These can be selected with the patient and obtained by direct recordings or by prerecorded sound samples. It can be particularly helpful for patients who experience hyperacusis for specific sounds. The patient can then replay the sounds at times when they are relaxed and at a much reduced (and not annoying) level. The patient can then successively increase the duration and level of listening periods over several weeks. The levels and categories of sounds can successively approximate the troublesome sounds.

PARTIAL MASKING

Partial masking (Tyler and Bentler, 1987) with a continuous background sound can be used to reduce the loudness and prominence of intermittent sounds that might otherwise be annoying. For example, low levels of music can partially mask background annoying traffic noise. Additionally, the low-level music can create a background whereby the patient is less likely to anticipate being disturbed while getting to sleep, sleeping, or concentrating.

GRADUAL INCREASE OF MAXIMUM OUTPUT OF HEARING AID

The maximum output of a hearing aid can be initially lowered to a level where sounds are not perceived as loud (Searchfield, 2006). Then, over several days or weeks, the maximum output can be gradually increased. This successively exposes the patient to sounds perceived as louder. If the patient experiences hyperacusis, the maximum output can be lowered again.

Medication

The use of medication to treat hyperacusis has not been investigated in clinical trials, but interest is high.

HYPERACUSIS IN CHILDHOOD

Hyperacusis also occurs in children and is frequently associated with tinnitus and noise exposure (Coelho, 2006).

Moderately intense sound from the television, games, and telephone rings can cause some children to cover their ears with their hands. The symptoms can be so severe that activities such as car rides, vacuum cleaning, and lawn mowing are avoided (Martin et al., 1984; Einfeld et al., 1997) (perhaps not a surprise among some teenagers!).

CONCLUSIONS REGARDING HYPERACUSIS

Hyperacusis can be related to disorders of loudness, annoyance, and fear, and it is critical to distinguish the particular problems involved with individual patients. Counseling to provide information and reassurance and to challenge beliefs about hyperacusis can be very useful. We have identified five different approaches to sound therapy, including the use of continuous low-level noise, the use of successive approximation of troublesome sounds, partial masking to reduce the loudness and/or prominence of sounds, and gradually increasing the maximum output of a hearing aid. These approaches all require controlled investigations. No medications have been shown to be effective.

SOME FINAL THOUGHTS ON TINNITUS AND HYPERACUSIS

Patients with tinnitus and hyperacusis often find themselves receiving little or no help from health care professionals. Dismissive responses to their concerns only exacerbate their frustration. This is unfortunate because many can be helped with brief, supportive counseling. Audiologists are in an excellent position with their training in hearing, hearing loss, and counseling to provide important assistance to these patients. The challenge is substantial, but so are the rewards.

Treatment methodologies for tinnitus and hyperacusis suffer from a lack of well-documented clinical research. Dobie (1999) provided a review of clinical trials on tinnitus treatments including medicinal, counseling, and sound therapies covering over 83 studies. His conclusions were well stated in his introduction: "The goal of this study is to review reports of randomized clinical trials in such [tinnitus] patients to determine whether there are well-established treatments (the answer is no), whether there are promising treatments that deserve further research (yes), and whether research procedures in this field can be improved (yes)."

Many cases of tinnitus and hyperacusis can be prevented by reducing noise exposure. This can be accomplished by reducing noise levels at the source, using hearing protection, reducing the duration of exposure to noise, and taking "rests" away from the noise. Never miss an opportunity to promote hearing loss, tinnitus, and hyperacusis prevention.

ACKNOWLEDGMENTS

We wish to acknowledge grant support provided by the American Tinnitus Association and the National Institutes of Health (Grant No. 5R01DC005972). Richard Tyler and William Noble are Obermann Scholars at the Obermann Center for Advanced Studies at The University of Iowa.

REFERENCES

Andersson G, Lyttkens L. (1999) A meta-analytic review of psychological treatments for tinnitus. *Br J Audiol*. 33, 201–210.

Axelsson A, Ringdahl A. (1989) Tinnitus—a study of its prevalence and characteristics. *Br J Audiol*. 23, 53–62.

Baguley DM, McFerran DJ. (2002) Current perspectives on tinnitus. *Arch Dis Child*. 86, 141–143.

Barr T. (1886) Enquiry into the effects of loud sounds upon the hearing of boilermakers and others who work amid noisy surroundings. *Proceedings of the Philosophical Society of Glasgow*. 17, 223–239.

Bartnik GM, Skarzynski H. (2006) Tinnitus retraining therapy. In: Tyler RS, ed. *Tinnitus Treatment: Clinical Protocols*. New York: Thieme Medical Publishers.

Cacace AT. (2003) Expanding the biological basis of tinnitus: Cross-modal origins and the role of neuroplasticity. *Hear Res*. 175, 112–132.

Cacace AT. (2004) The limbic system and tinnitus. In: Snow JB Jr, ed. *Tinnitus: Theory and Management*. Hamilton, Ontario, Canada: BC Decker.

Coelho CB. (2006) Tinnitus and hyperacusis in children: a prevalence study. PhD Thesis. Sao Paulo, Brazil: College of Medicine, University of Sao Paulo.

Cole MG, Dowson L, Dendukuri N, Belzile E. (2002). The prevalence and phenomenology of auditory hallucinations among elderly subjects attending an audiology clinic. *Int J Geriatr Psychiatry*. 17, 444–452.

Coles RRA. (1984) Epidemiology of tinnitus: prevalence. *J Laryngol Otol*. 9, 7–15.

Coles RRA, Hallam RS. (1987) Tinnitus and its management. *Br Med Bull*. 43, 983–998.

Dauman R, Bouscau-Faure F. (2005) Assessment and amelioration of hyperacusis in tinnitus patients. *Acta Otolaryngol*. 125, 503–509.

Dauman R, Tyler RS. (1992) Some considerations on the classification of tinnitus. In: Aran J-M, Dauman R, eds. *Proceedings of the Fourth International Tinnitus Seminar (Bordeaux, France)*. Amsterdam: Kugler & Ghedini Publications.

Davis A. (1995) *Hearing in Adults*. London: Whurr.

Davis A, Refaie A. (2000) Epidemiology of tinnitus. In: Tyler RS, ed. *Tinnitus Handbook*. San Diego: Singular Publishing Group.

Davis P. (1995) *Living with Tinnitus*. Woolahra, Australia: Gore & Osment Publications.

Davis PB. (2006) Music and the acoustic desensitization protocol for tinnitus. In: Tyler RS, ed. *Tinnitus Treatment: Clinical Protocols*. New York: Thieme Medical Publishers.

Davison GC, Neale JM, Kring AM. (2004). *Abnormal Psychology.* 9th ed. New York: Wiley.

De Ridder D, Ryu H, Moller AR, Nowe V, Van de Heyning P, Verlooy J. (2004) Functional anatomy of the human cochlear nerve and its role in microvascular decompression for tinnitus. *Neurosurgery.* 54, 381–388.

Dobie RA. (1999) A review of randomized clinical trials in tinnitus. *Laryngoscope.* 109, 1202–1211.

Doghramji PP. (2006) Trends in the pharmacologic management of insomnia. *J Clin Psychiatry.* 67 (suppl 13), 5–8.

Eggermont JJ. (1984) Tinnitus: some thoughts about its origin. *J Laryngol Otol.* 9, 31–37.

Einfeld SL, Tonge BJ, Florio T. (1997) Behavioral and emotional disturbance in individuals with Williams' syndrome. *Am J Ment Retard.* 102, 45–53.

Erlandsson S. (2000) Psychologic profiles. In: Tyler RS, ed. *Tinnitus Handbook.* San Diego: Singular Publishing Group.

Folmer RL, Martin WH, Shi Y, Edlefsen LL. (2006) Tinnitus sound therapies. In: Tyler RS, ed. *Tinnitus Treatment: Clinical Protocols.* New York: Thieme Medical Publishers.

Formby C, Gold SL. (2002). Modification of loudness discomfort levels: evidence for adaptive chronic auditory gain and its clinical relevance. *Semin Hear.* 23, 21–34.

Fowler EPJ. (1955) Somatopsychic and psychosomatic factors in tinnitus, deafness and vertigo. *Ann Otol Rhinol Laryngol.* 64, 29–37.

Graham J. (1965) Tinnitus aurium. *Acta Otolaryngol.* Suppl, 24–26.

Hallam RS. (1989) *Tinnitus: Living with the Ringing in Your Ears.* London: Harper Collins.

Hallam RS, Jakes SC, Hinchcliffe R. (1988) Cognitive variables in tinnitus annoyance. *Br J Clin Psychol.* 27, 213–222.

Hallam RS, McKenna L. (2006) Tinnitus habituation therapy. In: Tyler RS, ed. *Tinnitus Treatment: Clinical Protocols.* New York: Thieme Medical Publishers.

Hazell JWP. (1987) Tinnitus masking therapy. In: Hazell JWP, ed. *Tinnitus.* London: Churchill Livingston.

Hazell JWP, Sheldrake JB. (1992) Hyperacusis and tinnitus. In: Aran J-M, Dauman R, eds. *Tinnitus '91. Proceedings of the Fourth International Tinnitus Seminar.* Amsterdam: Kugler Publications.

Hegarty JL, Smith RJ. (2000) Tinnitus in children. In: Tyler RS, ed. *Tinnitus Handbook.* San Diego: Singular Publishing Group.

Henry JA, Meikle MB, Gilbert A. (1999) Audiometric correlates of tinnitus pitch: Insights from the Tinnitus Data Registry. In: Hazell J, ed. *Proceedings of the Sixth International Tinnitus Seminar.* London: The Tinnitus and Hyperacusis Centre.

Henry JL, Wilson PH. (1998) The psychometric properties of two measures of tinnitus complaint and handicap. *Int Tinnitus J.* 4, 114–121.

Henry JL, Wilson PH. (2001) *The Psychological Management of Chronic Tinnitus: A Cognitive Behavioral Approach.* Needham Heights, MA: Allyn & Bacon.

Henry JL, Wilson PH. (2002) *Tinnitus: A Self-Management Guide for the Ringing in Your Ears.* Boston: Allyn & Bacon.

House JW, Brackmann DE (1981). Tinnitus: surgical treatment. *Ciba Found Symp.* 85, 204–216.

Jastreboff PJ. (2000) Tinnitus habituation therapy (THT) and tinnitus retraining therapy (TRT). In: Tyler RS, ed. *Tinnitus Handbook.* San Diego: Singular Publishing Group.

Jastreboff PJ, Hazell JWP. (2004) *Tinnitus Retraining Therapy: Implementing the Neurophysiological Model.* New York: Cambridge University Press.

Kaltenbach JA, Zhang J, Zacharek MA. (2004) Neural correlates of tinnitus. In: Snow JB Jr, ed. *Tinnitus: Theory and Management.* Hamilton, Ontario, Canada: BC Decker.

Katzenell U, Segal S. (2001) Hyperacusis: review and clinical guidelines. *Otol Neurotol.* 22, 321–327.

Kentish RC, Crocker SR. (2006) Scary monsters and waterfalls: tinnitus narrative therapy for children. In: Tyler RS, ed. *Tinnitus Treatment: Clinical Protocols.* New York: Thieme Medical Publishers.

Kiang NYS, Moxon EC, Levine RA. (1970) Auditory-nerve activity in cats with normal and abnormal cochleas. In: Wolstenholme GEW, Knight J, eds. *Sensorineural Hearing Loss.* London: Churchill Livingston.

Kuk F, Tyler RS, Russell D, Jordan H. (1990) The psychometric properties of a tinnitus handicap questionnaire. *Ear Hear.* 11, 434–442.

Kuk F, Tyler RS, Rustad N, Harker LA, Tye-Murray N. (1989) Alternating current at the eardrum for tinnitus reduction. *J Speech Hear Res.* 32, 393–400.

Langguth B, Eichhammer P, Wiegand R, Maenner P, Jacob P, Hajak G. (2003) Neuronavigated rTMS in a patients with chronic tinnitus. Effects of 4 weeks of treatment. *Neuroreport.* 14, 977–980.

Levine RA. (2001) Diagnostic issues in tinnitus: a neuro-otological perspective. *Semin Hear.* 22, 23–36.

Martin K, Snashall S. (1994) Children presenting with tinnitus: a retrospective study. *Br J Audiol.* 28, 111–115.

Martin ND, Snodgrass GJ, Cohen RD. (1984) Idiopathic infantile hypercalcaemia—a continuing enigma. *Arch Dis Child.* 59, 605–613.

McFadden D. (1982) Tinnitus: facts, theories, and treatments. Report of Working Group 89, Committee on Hearing Bioacoustics and Biomechanics. Washington, DC: National Academy Press.

McKenna L. (2000) Tinnitus and insomnia. In: Tyler RS, ed. *Tinnitus Handbook.* San Diego: Singular Publishing Group.

McKenna L, Daniel HC. (2006) Tinnitus related insomnia treatment. In: Tyler RS, ed. *Tinnitus Treatment: Clinical Protocols.* New York: Thieme Medical Publishers.

McKerrow WS, Schreiner CE, Snyder RL, Merzenich MM, Toner JG. (1991) Tinnitus suppression by cochlear implants. *Ann Otol Rhinol Laryngol.* 100, 552–558.

Mohr AM, Hedelund U. (2006) Tinnitus person-centered therapy. In: Tyler RS, ed. *Tinnitus Treatment: Clinical Protocols.* New York: Thieme Medical Publishers.

Moller AR. (1984) Pathophysiology of tinnitus. *Ann Otol Rhinol Laryngol.* 93, 39–44.

Moller AR, Moller MB, Yokata M. (1992) Some forms of tinnitus may involve the extalemniscal auditory pathway. *Laryngoscope.* 102, 1165–1171.

Murai K, Tyler RS, Harker LA, Stouffer JL. (1992) Review of pharmacologic treatment of tinnitus. *Am J Otol.* 13, 454–464.

Noble W. (1998) *Self-Assessment of Hearing and Related Functions.* London: Whurr.

Nondahl DM, Cruickshanks KJ, Wiley TL, Klein R, Klein BE, Tweed TS. (2002) Prevalence and 5-year incidence of tinnitus among older adults: the epidemiology of hearing loss study. *J Am Acad Audiol.* 13, 323–331.

Park J, White AR, Ernst E. (2000) Efficacy of acupuncture as a treatment for tinnitus: a systematic review. *Arch Otolaryngol Head Neck Surg.* 126, 489–492.

Perry BP, Gantz BJ. (2000) Medical and surgical evaluation and management of tinnitus. In: Tyler RS, ed. *Tinnitus Handbook.* San Diego: Singular Publishing Group.

Robb MJA. (2006) Tinnitus device directory, part IV. *Tinnitus Today.* June, 9–11.

Rubinstein JT, Tyler RS. (2004) Electrical suppression of tinnitus. In (Ed.) Snow J, ed. *Tinnitus: Theory and Management.* Hamilton, Ontario, Canada: BC Decker; pp 326–335.

Salvi RJ, Lockwood AH, Burkard R. (2000) Neural plasticity and tinnitus. In: Tyler RS, ed. *Tinnitus Handbook.* San Diego: Singular Publishing Group.

Sanchez L, Stephens D. (1997) A tinnitus problem questionnaire in a clinic population. *Ear Hear.* 18, 210–217.

Sanchez TG, Guerra GCY, Lorenzi MC, Brandão AL, Bento RF. (2002) The influence of voluntary muscle contractions upon the onset and modulation of tinnitus. *Audiol Neurootol.* 7, 370–375.

Searchfield G. (2006) Hearing aids and tinnitus. In: Tyler RS, ed. *Tinnitus Treatment: Clinical Protocols.* New York: Thieme Medical Publishers.

Seidman MD, Babu S. (2003) Alternative medications and other treatments for tinnitus: facts from fiction. *Otolaryngol Clin North Am.* 36, 359–81.

Sherlock LP, Formby C. (2005) Estimates of loudness, loudness discomfort, and the auditory dynamic range: normative estimates, comparison of procedures, and test-retest reliability. *J Am Acad Audiol.* 16, 85–100.

Stevens SS, Davis H. (1938) *Hearing: It's Psychology and Physiology.* New York: John Wiley & Sons, Inc.

Stouffer JL, Tyler RS, Booth JC, Buckrell B. (1992) Tinnitus in normal-hearing and hearing-impaired children. In: Aran J-M, Dauman R, eds. *Proceedings of the Fourth International Tinnitus Seminar (Bordeaux, France).* Amsterdam: Kugler Publications.

Sweetow RW. (1986) Cognitive aspects of tinnitus patient management. *Ear Hear.* 7, 390–396.

Tyler RS. (1993) Tinnitus disability and handicap questionnaires. *Semin Hear.* 14, 377–384.

Tyler RS. (2000) Psychoacoustical measurement. In: Tyler RS, ed. *Tinnitus Handbook.* San Diego: Singular Publishing Group.

Tyler RS, ed. (2006) *Tinnitus Treatment: Clinical Protocols.* New York: Thieme Medical Publishers.

Tyler RS, Babin RW. (1986) Tinnitus. In: Cummings CW, Fredrickson JM, Harker L, Krause CJ, Schuller DE, eds. *Otolaryngology – Head and Neck Surgery.* St. Louis, MO: Mosby.

Tyler RS, Baker LJ. (1983) Difficulties experienced by tinnitus sufferers. *J Speech Hear Disord.* 48, 150–154.

Tyler RS, Bentler RA. (1987) Tinnitus maskers and hearing aids for tinnitus. In: Sweetow R, ed. *Seminars in Hearing, 8.* New York: Thieme Medical Publishers.

Tyler RS, Bergan C, Preece J, Nagase S. (2003a) Audiologische messmethoden de hyperakusis. In: Nelting M, ed. *Hyperakusis.* Stuttgart: Georg Thieme Verlag.

Tyler RS, Conrad-Armes D. (1983) The determination of tinnitus loudness considering the effects of recruitment. *J Speech Hear Res.* 26, 59–72.

Tyler RS, Erlandsson S. (2000) Management of the tinnitus patient. In: Luxon LM, Furman JM, Martini A, Stephens D, eds. *Textbook of Audiological Medicine.* Oxford, United Kingdom: Isis Publications.

Tyler RS, Gehringer AK, Gogel S. (2004a) *Loudness and Annoyance of Everyday Sounds.* Iowa City: The University of Iowa.

Tyler RS, Gehringer AK, Noble W, Dunn CC, Witt SA, Bardia A. (2006) Tinnitus activities treatment. In: Tyler RS, ed. *Tinnitus Treatment: Clinical Protocols.* New York: Thieme Medical Publishers.

Tyler RS, Noble W, Preece JP, Dunn CC, Witt SA. (2004b) Psychological treatments for tinnitus. In: Snow JB Jr, ed. *Tinnitus: Theory and Management.* Hamilton, Ontario, Canada: BC Decker.

Tyler RS, Preece JP, Noble W. (2003b) The management of tinnitus. *Geriatr Aging.* 6, 22–28.

Tyler RS, Smith RJ. (2002) Management of tinnitus in children. In: Newton VE, ed. *Paediatric Audiological Medicine.* Philadelphia: Whurr Publishers Ltd.

Tyler RS, Stouffer JL, Schum R. (1989) Audiological rehabilitation of the tinnitus patient. *J Acad Rehabil Audiol.* 22, 30–42.

Vernon J, Meikle M. (2000) Tinnitus masking: theory and practice. In: Tyler RS, ed. *Tinnitus Handbook.* San Diego: Singular Publications.

Vernon JA, Press L. (1998) Treatment for hyperacusis. In: Vernon, JA, ed. *Tinnitus: Treatment and Relief.* Boston, MA: Allyn and Bacon.

Wilson PH, Henry J, Bowen M, Haralambous G. (1991) Tinnitus reaction questionnaire: psychometric properties of a measure of stress associated with tinnitus. *J Speech Hear Res.* 34, 197–201.

APPENDIX 33.1
Iowa Tinnitus Activities Questionnaire (Tyler et al., 2006)

IOWA TINNITUS ACTIVITIES
QUESTIONNAIRE_{May 05}

Name: Date:

Please indicate your agreement with each statement on a
scale from 0 (completely disagree) to 100 (completely agree).

#	Statement	0–100
1	My tinnitus is annoying.	
2	My tinnitus masks some speech sounds.	
3	When there are lots of things happening at once, my tinnitus interferes with my ability to attend to the most important thing.	
4	My emotional peace is one of the worst effects of my tinnitus.	
5	I have difficulty getting to sleep at night because of my tinnitus.	
6	The effects of tinnitus on my hearing are worse than the effects of my hearing loss.	
7	I feel like my tinnitus makes it difficult for me to concentrate on some tasks.	
8	I am depressed because of my tinnitus.	
9	My tinnitus, not my hearing loss, interferes with my appreciation of music and songs.	
10	I am anxious because of my tinnitus.	
11	I have difficulty focusing my attention on some important tasks because of tinnitus.	
12	I just wish my tinnitus would go away. It is so frustrating.	
13	The difficulty I have sleeping is one of the worst effects of my tinnitus.	
14	In addition to my hearing loss, my tinnitus interferes with my understanding of speech.	
15	My inability to think about something undisturbed is one of the worst effects of my tinnitus.	
16	I am tired during the day because my tinnitus has disrupted my sleep.	
17	One of the worst things about my tinnitus is its effect on my speech understanding, over and above any effect of my hearing loss.	
18	I lie awake at night because of my tinnitus.	
19	I have trouble concentrating while I am reading in a quiet room because of tinnitus.	
20	When I wake up in the night, my tinnitus makes it difficult to get back to sleep.	

Scoring

Area	Questions	Score
Emotions and Thoughts	1, 4, 10, 12	%
Hearing and Communication	2, 6, 14, 17	%
Sleep	13, 16, 18, 20	%
Concentration	3, 7, 11, 15, 19	%
Total		%

APPENDIX 33.2

Loudness and Annoyance of Everyday Sounds (Tyler et al., 2003)

Some everyday sounds are loud and some are soft. Some everyday sounds are annoying and some are not. Please rate the **loudness** and the **annoyance** of the following sounds. Do not consider the annoyance when rating the loudness and do not consider the loudness when rating the annoyance.

For example, a sound may be very loud, but not annoy you. Likewise, a sound may be very soft, yet be very annoying. Rate the sounds using a scale from 0 (not loud/annoying) to 100 (unbearably loud/annoying).

	Sound	Loudness (0 to 100)	Annoyance (0 to 100)
1.	Standing next to a dog barking		
2.	Someone stacking dishes in the same room		
3.	Hearing music on the radio in a car when the volume is adjusted for normal-hearing listeners		
4.	Hearing music on the radio in a quiet room when the volume is adjusted for normal-hearing listeners		
5.	Telephone ringing in the same room		
6.	Television in the same room when the volume is adjusted for normal-hearing listeners		
7.	Standing next to a lawnmower		
8.	Standing next to a car door closing		
9.	Talking with someone in a noisy restaurant		
10.	Baby crying in the same room		

APPENDIX 33.3

The Relative Handicap of Hearing Loss, Tinnitus and Hyperacusis (Tyler et al., 2003a)

The following questions relate to hearing loss, tinnitus, and hyperacusis. Hyperacusis is either when sounds that are moderately loud for other people are *too* loud for you or when you find sounds annoying. Please rate your agreement/disagreement with the following statements, using a scale from 0 (completely disagree) to 100 (completely agree):

		Because of your hearing loss (0–100)	Because of your tinnitus (0–100)	Because some sounds are too loud or annoying (0–100)
1.	You avoid shopping			
2.	You do not go out with your friends			
3.	You have given up some hobbies			
4.	You do not go to restaurants			
5.	You avoid being in crowds			
6.	You feel depressed			
7.	You feel anxious			
8.	You are not able to concentrate			
9.	Your quality of life is poor			
10.	You are not able to perform tasks or jobs as well			

SECTION IV

MANAGEMENT OF HEARING DISORDERS

Room Acoustics and Auditory Rehabilitation Technology

*Joseph Smaldino, Carl Crandell, Brian Kreisman,
Andrew John, and Nicole Kreisman*

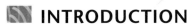 INTRODUCTION

Clearly sensory-neural hearing loss (SNHL) causes communicative difficulty, particularly in noisy or reverberant listening environments (Working Group on Speech Understanding and Aging, 1988; Crandell et al., 1991; Crandell, 1993; Needleman and Crandell, 1996). Due to the deleterious effects of SNHL on communication, individuals with hearing loss may exhibit reduced psychosocial function, including increased feelings of frustration, anger, fear, isolation, loneliness, and depression (Crandell, 1988; Bess et al., 1989; Christian et al., 1989; Vesterager and Salomon, 1991). In addition, perhaps as the result of reduced psychosocial functioning, persons with SNHL tend to exhibit a higher incidence of health-related difficulties, including hypertension, ischemic heart disease, arrhythmias, osteoarthritis, and reductions in activity level, quality of life, and physical mobility (Lichtenstein et al., 1988; Mulrow et al., 1990).

Due to the broad range of potential disruptions of communicative and psychosocial function as well as health-related quality-of-life (HRQOL) issues that can be caused by hearing loss, it is important that the audiologist not limit intervention to hearing aids alone. In many cases, particularly if there is excessive background noise, hearing aids alone may not be sufficient to restore effective communication. In these cases, other assistive listening technologies, communication strategies, and auditory rehabilitation training must also be considered and used in conjunction with the hearing aids. It is reasonable to speculate that, if communication function is improved, then the deleterious

psychosocial and/or HRQOL effects of reduced communication can be minimized. With these considerations in mind, the purpose of this chapter is to discuss rehabilitative technologies and communication strategies that have been shown to improve communicative efficiency in listeners with SNHL (and individuals with normal hearing who have difficulty processing auditory information) within the following environments: (1) room settings that are commonly used for communication, such as churches, restaurants, classrooms, meeting/conference rooms, and theaters; (2) face-to-face situations; (3) telecommunications; and (4) broadcast media (radio, television [TV], etc.). In addition, this chapter will address signal/alerting technologies that can assist individuals with hearing loss in the awareness of sounds within their listening environment. The term ***hearing assistance technology (HAT)*** will be used in this chapter, rather than the older term ***assistive listening device (ALD)***, to discuss technologies that improve communicative status through the transmission of an amplified auditory, tactile, or visual signal to the listener since many of these technologies are not limited to improvement of listening.

IMPROVING COMMUNICATION IN ROOM SETTINGS

Perhaps the most persistent complaint heard from listeners with SNHL is difficulty communicating in places used for verbal communication. Such environments include churches, restaurants, classrooms, therapy rooms, shopping establishments, meeting/conference rooms, and theaters. To understand why these difficulties occur, it is important that the audiologist have a basic understanding of acoustic variables that can interfere with the perception of speech. These acoustic variables include : (1) background noise; (2) speech signal level compared to background noise level; (3) reverberation time; (4) distance between the talker and the listener; and (5) interactions among these variables.

Background Room Noise

Background noise refers to any auditory disturbance within the room that interferes with what a listener wants to hear (Crandell et al., 1995). A common way of measuring noise in a room is with a sound level meter (SLM). An SLM can range from a compact, inexpensive, battery-operated unit designed to measure sound amplitude to a computer-based device that can measure and record numerous acoustic properties of a signal. SLMs are classified according to standards set forth in American National Standards Institute (ANSI) S1.14 (ANSI, 1983). Type I meters meet the most precise standards, type II are general purpose, and type III are for hobby use. Detailed measurement of room noise requires, at minimum, a type II (and preferably a type I) SLM. Many SLMs incorporate weighting filter networks. The A-weighting network is designed to simulate the sensitivity of the average human ear under conditions of low sound loudness (40 phons), the B-weighting simulates loud sounds (70 phons), and the C-weighting approximates how the ear would respond to very loud sounds. The convention for room measurements is the use of the A-weighting network. Unfortunately, the same single number obtained from a sound pressure measurement performed with the A-weighting scale can be obtained from a variety of very different sound spectra. Thus, a more accurate and complete way to measure room noise is to do a spectral analysis of the noise instead of attempting to use a single descriptor.

Noise criteria curves (NCC) are one way to measure the frequency content of background noise in a room. NCCs are a family of frequency and intensity curves based on the use of one-third octave-band sound pressure levels (SPLs). The NCC rating of a space is determined by plotting the SPLs within each frequency band relative to established NCC. Whenever possible, it is recommended that ambient noise levels in classrooms be measured using NCC measures since this procedure gives the examiner a more comprehensive assessment of the spectral characteristics of the noise.

Noise within an enclosure can come from several possible sources, including *external* sources (noise generated from outside the building), *internal* sources (noise originating from within the building, but outside the room), and *room* sources (noise that is generated within the room). Due to the many sources, relatively high background noise levels have been reported in many enclosures (Bess et al., 1986; Nober and Nober, 1975; Pearsons et al., 1977; Ross,

1978; Crandell and Smaldino, 1995; 2000). Pearsons et al. (1977), for example, reported that noise levels averaged 45 dBA for suburban residential settings and 55 dBA for urban dwellings; mean outdoor noise levels were 2 to 10 dB more intense than the indoor settings. Noise levels were measured at 54 dBA for department store environments and 77 dBA in transportation locations. Bess et al. (1986) measured background noise levels in 19 classrooms for children with hearing loss. Median occupied noise levels were 56 dBA, 60 dBB, and 63 dBC. In a similar investigation, Crandell and Smaldino (1995) reported that background noise levels in 32 unoccupied classroom settings were 51 dBA and 67 dBC. As will be discussed in a later section, such high levels of background noise can impair speech perception of not only listeners with SNHL, but also many with normal hearing sensitivity.

Background noise in a room can compromise speech perception by masking the acoustic and linguistic cues available in the message. Generally speaking, background noises in a room mask the weaker transient consonant phonemes more than the longer and more intense vowels (typically 10 to 15 dB more intense than consonants). A reduction of consonant information can have a significant impact on speech perception because approximately 80% to 90% of the acoustic information important for speech perception comes from the consonants (French and Steinberg, 1947; Licklider and Miller, 1951; Sher and Owens, 1974; Wang et al., 1978). The extent to which speech is masked by background noise is influenced by a number of factors, including: (1) the long-term acoustic spectrum of the noise; (2) the average intensity of the noise compared to the intensity of speech; and (3) fluctuations in the intensity of the noise over time. Often the most important factor for accurate speech perception is not the overall level of the background noise, but rather the relationship between the level of the signal as a function of frequency and the level of the background noise as a function of frequency. This relationship is often simplified and referenced as the signal-to-noise ratio (S/N), wherein the overall level of the signal and the overall level of the background noise are compared. Because the decibel is logarithmic, S/N can be stated simply as a difference between the overall level of the signal and the level of the noise. For example, if a speech signal is presented at 70 dB SPL and a noise is 60 dB SPL, the S/N is +10 dB. Due to high background noise levels, diminished S/Ns have been reported in many communication settings. Pearsons et al. (1977) reported that average S/Ns were +9 to +14 dB in urban and suburban residential settings, respectively. In outdoor settings, S/Ns decreased to approximately +5 to +8 dB. In department store settings, the average S/N was +7 dB, while transportation settings yielded an average S/N of −2 dB. Plomp (1978) reported that the average S/N found at cocktail parties ranged from +1 dB to −2 dB. In classroom environments, the range of S/Ns has been reported to be from +5 dB to −7 dB (Sanders, 1965; Blair, 1977; Markides, 1986; Finitzo-Hieber, 1988; Crandell et al., 1995).

Speech perception is generally greatest at favorable S/Ns and decreases as the S/N of the listening environment is reduced (Cooper and Cutts, 1971; Miller, 1974; Finitzo-Hieber and Tillman, 1978; Crandell et al., 1995). In general, speech perception ability in adults with normal hearing is not severely reduced until the S/N reaches 0 dB. However, this is not the case for listeners with SNHL. To obtain perception scores comparable to those of normal hearers, listeners with SNHL require the S/N to be improved by 4 to 12 dB (Crandell et al., 1995; Killion, 1997; Moore, 1997; Johnson, 2000); an additional 3 to 6 dB is required in rooms with moderate levels of reverberation (Hawkins and Yacullo, 1984).

Although a number of acoustic, linguistic, and articulatory factors influence the determination of appropriate S/Ns in a room, the literature suggests that, for young listeners with SNHL, the S/Ns in communication environments should exceed +15 dB (Finitzo-Hieber and Tillman, 1978; American Speech, Language, and Hearing Association, 1995; Crandell et al., 1995). To accomplish this S/N, unoccupied room noise should not exceed 30 to 35 dBA (Crandell et al., 1995; 2005). The recommendation of a +15 dB S/N is based on the finding that the speech perception of listeners with hearing loss tends to remain relatively constant at S/Ns in excess of +15 dB but deteriorates at poorer S/Ns. Moreover, when the S/N decreases to below +15 dB, those with hearing loss tend to expend so much attentional effort in listening to the message that they often prefer to communicate through other modalities. In addition to listeners with SNHL, some children with "normal" hearing sensitivity have greater than normal perceptual difficulties in noise and/or reverberation (Bess, 1985; Bess and Tharpe, 1986; Nabelek and Nabelek, 1994; Crandell et al., 1995). A list of populations that may or may not exhibit hearing loss but often find it difficult to listen and learn is presented in Table 34.1. A prominent feature of these populations is that they all have a developmentally delayed, incomplete, or distorted knowledge of language. Due to their language deficit, these individuals cannot always use the structure of language to fill in or predict speech information when the information is distorted or inaudible. Because of the important relationship between the quality of the acoustic signal and language development, a favorable S/N is widely recommended for children in the developmental stages of language acquisition as well as children with language knowledge deficits. The importance of a favorable S/N in the classroom was highlighted in the ANSI standard S12.6 entitled "Acoustical Performance Criteria, Design Requirements and Guidelines for Classrooms" (ANSI, 2002), which stipulated an unoccupied classroom background noise level of no more than 35 dBA. Applying the ANSI (2002) classroom acoustics standard, Knecht et al. (2002) found that most of the 32 elementary grade classrooms they studied did not meet the recommended background noise level of 35 dBA.

Reverberation

Another factor impacting on speech perception in enclosed settings is reverberation. Reverberation refers to the prolongation or persistence of sound within an enclosure when sound waves reflect off hard surfaces (e.g., bare walls, ceilings, windows, floors). Reverberation time (RT) is often stated as the amount of time it takes for a sound, at a specific frequency, to decay 60 dB after termination of the signal. For example, if a 120-dB SPL signal at 1,000 Hz takes 1 second to decrease to 60 dB SPL, the RT of that enclosure at 1,000 Hz is 1 second. Generally, RT increases as room volume increases and decreases as the amount of absorptive material in the room increases. Specifically, reverberation is decreased when surfaces in the room have a large sound absorption coefficient, or alpha (α), which is calculated as the amount of sound energy absorbed by surfaces in the room divided by the total sound energy from the signal source. The α of a room varies with the thickness, porosity, and mounting configuration of materials in a room and the frequency of the signal (Siebein et al., 1997). Materials with an α less than 0.2 are considered to be sound reflective, whereas materials with an α greater than 0.2 are considered to be sound absorbent. For instance, a brick wall has an α ranging from 0.03 at 125 Hz to 0.07 at 4,000 Hz, whereas a carpeted concrete floor ranges from 0.02 at 125 Hz to 0.65 at 4,000 Hz. Use of absorbent materials can decrease noise by 3 to 8 dB (Siebein et al., 1997). Note that rooms with irregular shapes (e.g., oblong) often exhibit longer RTs than rooms with more traditional quadrilateral dimensions.

All rooms exhibit some degree of reverberation. Audiometric test booths usually exhibit RTs of approximately 0.2 second (Crandell and Smaldino, 1994; 2000). Living rooms and offices often have RTs between 0.4 and 0.8 second (Nabelek and Nabelek, 1994). RTs for classrooms are usually reported to range from 0.4 to 1.2 seconds (Bradley, 1986; Crandell, 1992; Crandell et al., 1995; Crandell and Smaldino, 1995; 2000), whereas auditoriums, churches, and assembly halls may exhibit RTs in excess of 3.0 or 4.0 seconds (Crandell, 1992; Nabelek and Nabelek, 1994; Siebein et al., 1997).

TABLE 34.1	Populations that find it difficult to "listen and learn"

- Young children (<15 years old)
- History of recurrent otitis media
- Language disorder
- Articulation disorder
- Dyslexia or other reading disorders
- Learning disabilities
- Nonnative English
- Central auditory processing deficit
- Developmental delays
- Attentional deficits

Adapted from Crandell C, Smaldino J, Flexer C. (2005) *Sound Field Amplification: Applications to Speech Perception and Classroom Acoustics*. Clifton Park: Thompson Delmar Learning.

The presence of people in a room further affects RT. A room full of people will have an RT that is 0.05 to 0.1 second less than when it is empty (Boothroyd, 2005).

RT can be (1) measured using commercially available, handheld, special purpose reverberation meters that directly measure the decrease in intensity of a test signal as a function of time or (2) derived from the impulse response of the room. The impulse response methods require the introduction of controlled noise bursts to energize the acoustics of the room. The responses obtained from the bursts can be used to calculate nearly all standard acoustic performance measures, including reverberation. More recently, methods have been proposed that do not require a test signal to be employed and do not require any prior knowledge of room acoustic dimensions or absorptive characteristics of the room. These methods rely on passively received signals in the room and use of a sophisticated computer algorithm to estimate the most likely RT in the room (Ratnam et al., 2003).

Ideally, RT should be calculated at each octave interval from 63 to 8,000 Hz. More commonly, however, one low-, one middle-, and one high-frequency octave RT are calculated. For example, reports of RT often are obtained using the average of 500, 1,000, and 2,000 Hz (Siebein et al., 1997). Generally speaking, RT is longest at low frequencies (i.e., below 500 Hz), about equivalent in the range between 500 and 2,000 Hz, and shortest for higher frequencies (Nabelek, 1982). This is due to the fact that sound-absorptive materials have a greater α for higher frequency energy than for lower frequency energy.

Reverberation degrades speech perception through masking of the directly transmitted sounds (Bolt and Mac-Donald, 1949; Nabelek, 1982). To explain, reverberant speech energy reaches the listener some time after the corresponding direct sounds, overlapping subsequently presented speech sounds. This results in a "smearing" or masking of the directly transmitted speech signal. That is, reverberation causes a prolongation of the spectral energy of the vowel sounds, which tends to mask succeeding consonant phonemes, particularly consonants in word final positions. The masking effectiveness of reverberation involving vowels is greater than for consonants since vowels exhibit greater overall power and are of longer duration than consonants.

Speech perception tends to decrease as the RT of the environment increases (Lochner and Burger, 1964; Moncur and Dirks, 1967; Finitzo-Hieber and Tillman, 1978; Gelfand and Silman, 1979; Neuman and Hochberg, 1983; Crandell et al., 1995; Kreisman, 2003). Speech perception in adults with normal hearing is not compromised until the RT exceeds approximately 1.0 second (Nabelek and Pickett, 1974a; 1974b; Gelfand and Silman, 1979). Listeners with SNHL, however, need considerably shorter RTs (0.4 to 0.5 second) for maximum speech perception (Finitzo-Hieber and Tillman, 1978; Olsen, 1981; 1988; Crandell et al., 1995). In addition, studies have indicated that the populations of "normal-hearing" children discussed previously have greater speech perception difficulties in reverberation than were traditionally suspected (see Crandell et al. [2005] for a review of these studies).

Appropriate RTs (0.4 to 0.5 second) for persons with hearing loss are rarely achieved (Crandell, 1991; 1992; Crandell and Smaldino, 1995). Crandell and Smaldino (1995) reported that only nine of 32 classrooms (27%) examined in their study had RTs of 0.4 second or less. ANSI (2002) recommended an RT of 0.6 second for moderately sized learning environments. Knecht et al. (2002), applying the ANSI (2002) criteria for reverberation, found that most of the 32 elementary grade classrooms they studied did not meet the 0.6-second maximum RT recommended in the standard.

Effects of Noise and Reverberation

Noise and reverberation do not occur separately in a room. In most enclosures, both noise and reverberation combine in a synergistic manner (Nabelek and Pickett, 1974a; 1974b; Finitzo-Hieber and Tillman, 1978; Crandell et al., 1995). That is, the sum of the deleterious effects of noise and reverberation is greater than one would expect by simply adding these two variables together. It appears that this synergy occurs because reverberation fills in the temporal gaps in the noise. These gaps and modulations contribute significantly to speech perception for listeners with normal hearing (Festen and Plomp, 1990; Hygge et al., 1992; Gustafsson and Arlinger, 1994). However, reverberation eliminates these gaps, making the noise more steady-state in nature and, thus, a more effective masker. Similar to the findings obtained for noise and reverberation in isolation, research indicates that listeners with hearing loss and children with normal hearing (and even more so for children with processing-related deficits) experience greater speech perception difficulties in noise plus reverberation than do adults with normal hearing.

An example of the synergistic effects of noise and reverberation on the monosyllabic word perception of children with normal hearing and SNHL is shown in Table 34.2. Note that, even at the best S/N and RT conditions (S/N = +12 dB, RT = 0.4 second), 83% of children with normal hearing did not recognize speech perfectly, and children with hearing loss performed even more poorly (60%). As the S/N became poorer or as the RT lengthened, speech perception continued to decrease. In the listening condition of S/N = 0 dB and RT = 1.2 seconds, children with normal hearing achieved a score of 30% correct, while children with hearing loss achieved a score of only 11%. Each of the listening situations mentioned here have been reported in numerous classroom environments.

Distance

A final factor affecting speech perception in a room is the distance between the talker and the listener. Sound is distributed essentially in three different ways in a room (Fig. 34.1). The "direct" sound is the sound that travels from the speaker to a listener without striking other surfaces in the room. This is usually the first sound to arrive at the listener since it travels the shortest path between the speaker and the listener.

	Groups		
		Normal	Sensory-neural
Testing condition		hearing	hearing loss
RT = 0.0 second			
QUIET		94.5%	83.0%
+12 dB		89.2%	70.0%
+6 dB		79.7%	59.5%
0 dB		60.2%	39.0%
RT = 0.4 second			
QUIET		92.5%	74.0%
+12 dB		82.8%	60.2%
+6 dB		71.3%	52.2%
0 dB		47.7%	27.8%
RT = 1.2 seconds			
QUIET		76.5%	45.0%
+12 dB		68.8%	41.2%
+6 dB		54.2%	27.0%
0 dB		29.7%	11.2%

TABLE 34.2 Mean speech recognition scores (% correct) by children with normal hearing (n = 12) and children with sensory-neural hearing loss (n = 12) for monosyllabic words across various Signal-to-Noise ratios (S/Ns) and Reverberation Times (RTs)

Adapted from Finitzo-Hieber T, Tillman T. (1978) Room acoustics effects on monosyllabic word discrimination ability for normal and hearing-impaired children. *J Speech Hear Res.* 21, 440–458.

The power of the direct sound decreases with distance since acoustic energy spreads over a larger area as it travels from the source. Specifically, the direct sound decreases in accordance with the inverse square law, or approximately 6 dB SPL with every doubling of distance from the sound source. For example, if a speaker's voice is 80 dB SPL at 1 meter, then it will be 74 dB at 2 meters, 68 dB at 4 meters, and so on. Because the direct sound energy decreases so quickly, only those listeners who are seated close to the speaker will actually hear the direct sound energy.

The auditory system allows the listener to orient to the sound source using information from the first direct sound energy received. This ability is variously known as the "Haas effect" (after Helmut Haas, the first researcher to describe it in 1951), the "precedence effect," or the "law of the first wavefront" (Haas, 1972; Roberts, 2003). Using the precedence effect, the auditory system uses the physical characteristics of the head (two ears at different points in space with a barrier, the head, in between them) to determine the direction from which an incoming sound originates by analyzing the first sound energy to arrive at each ear. The precedence effect requires that the sound be discontinuous and be followed by reverberated sound energy no sooner than 1 ms and no later than about 40 ms after the first sound received (Moore, 1997). These conditions are usually met in reverberant rooms that are not very large, as sound reflecting off of solid surfaces in a room typically reaches the ear first at around 30 to 50 ms after the direct sound.

Slightly greater distances from the speaker result in early sound reflections reaching the listener. Early sound reflections are those sound waves that arrive at a listener within very short time periods (approximately 50 ms) after the arrival of the direct sound. In a typical room, most of the early reflections strike minimal room surfaces on their path from speaker to listener. Early sound reflections

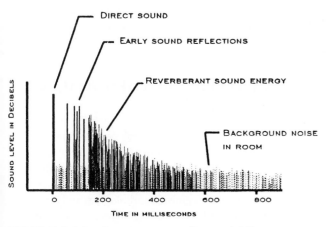

FIGURE 34.1 Components of sound (direct sound, early reflections, and late reflections or reverberation) within a room. (Siebein G, Crandell C, Gold M. [1997] Principles of classroom acoustics: reverberation. *Educ Audiol Monogr.* 5, 32–43, with permission.)

are usually combined with the direct sound and may actually increase the perceived loudness and intelligibility of the sound (Lochner and Burger, 1964; Bradley, 1986; Nabelek and Nabelek, 1994). This increase in loudness may actually improve speech perception in listeners with normal hearing.

Early reflections are dependent upon the intensity level of the original sound, the directionality of its source (tendency of the source to radiate energy in a forward direction rather than omnidirectionally), and the volume and RT of the room (Boothroyd, 2005). Early reflections are increased when the room is small and highly reverberant because these conditions allow the sound to reflect off of many surfaces before decaying. A source with low directionality also produces more reflected energy; that is, when sound is radiated omnidirectionally, less energy will be directed at the listener, and more energy will need to strike room surfaces to reach that listener.

As a listener moves farther away from the speaker, reverberation begins to dominate the listening environment. As discussed earlier, reverberation consists of sound waves that strike multiple room surfaces as they move from the speaker to the listener. As they strike multiple room surfaces, the sounds generally decrease in loudness due to the increased path length traveled and the partial absorption that occurs with each reflection from the room surfaces. Late reflected energy is more degraded than early reflections because this energy has traveled a greater total distance and undergone more partial absorption (especially high frequencies) subsequent to striking many surfaces (Nabelek, 1982). In addition to the change in spectrum, late reflections interfere with speech perception by masking meaningful parts of the signal.

Distance from the speaker can affect speech perception directly (Leavitt and Flexer, 1991; Crandell et al., 1995). Specifically, speech perception tends to decrease until the critical distance (i.e., the point at which the direct and reverberant sound energy is equal) of the room is reached. The critical distance in most rooms is approximately 2 to 6 meters from the speaker. Beyond the critical distance, perception ability tends to remain essentially constant unless the room is very large (e.g., an auditorium), where speech perception may continue to decrease as a function of increased distance. In general, direct sound is the major component of sound level within the critical distance, while reverberation is the dominant component beyond the critical distance (Bradley, 1986; Boothroyd, 2005).

These findings suggest that speech perception can be improved by decreasing the distance between a speaker and listener only if it is within the "critical distance" of the room. This explains why the simple recommendation of preferential seating in the classroom is often inadequate to ensure an appropriate listening environment. That is, teachers often move around the room, or turn their back to write on the blackboard, thus moving them out of the critical distance of the listener.

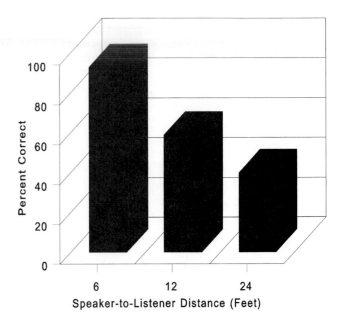

FIGURE 34.2   Mean speech recognition scores (% correct) of children with normal hearing in a typical classroom environment (signal-to-noise ratio = +6 dB; reverberation time = 0.6 second) as a function of speaker-to-listener distance. (Adapted from Crandell C, Smaldino J, Flexer C. [1995] *Sound Field FM Amplification: Theory and Practical Applications.* **San Diego: Singular Publishing Group, with permission.)**

Crandell and Bess (1986) examined the effects of distance, noise, and reverberation on the speech perception of 20 children (5- to 7 years old) with normal hearing in a classroom environment. The classroom had an S/N of +6 dB and an RT of 0.45 second. Multitalker babble served as the noise competition. Sentences were presented to the children at distances of 6, 12, and 24 feet. Results from this investigation are shown in Figure 34.2. As can be seen, a significant decrease in speech perception occurred as the speaker-listener distance increased (i.e., 89%, 55%, and 36% were obtained at 6, 12, and 24 feet, respectively).

ACOUSTIC MODIFICATIONS OF THE ROOM

The first strategy for improving speech perception within an enclosure is acoustic modification of that environment. The most effective procedure for achieving this goal is through appropriate planning with contractors, school officials, architects, architectural engineers, audiologists, and/or teachers of individuals with hearing loss *before* the design and construction of the building. Recall that acoustic guidelines for populations with hearing loss indicate that (1) S/Ns should be above +15 dB; (2) unoccupied noise levels should not exceed 30 to 35 dBA; and (3) RTs should not surpass 0.4 second. Unfortunately, as mentioned previously, such guidelines are rarely are achieved in most listening environments. One reason for the discrepancy between acoustic guidelines and actual room settings is that rooms often exhibit minimal degrees of acoustic modification. Bess et al. (1986) reported that, although 100% of the classrooms examined had acoustic ceiling tiles, only 68% had carpeting and only 13% had draperies. None of the classrooms contained any form of acoustic furniture treatment such as glides on the chair legs, projector tables of a height to keep the noise above ear level, or smaller desks to reduce the amount of sound reflective surface in the room. Findings of Crandell and Smaldino (1995) were even less favorable. For complete discussions on acoustic modifications and noise/reverberation reduction in rooms, the reader is directed to Barron (1993), Egan (1987), Harris (1991), and Siebein (1994).

PERSONAL AND GROUP AMPLIFICATION SYSTEMS

Due to a lack of appreciation of the impact of acoustics on communication and additional construction costs, compliance with favorable classroom acoustic guidelines is often not a priority during construction. Because of this, even with subsequent room modifications, noise and reverberation levels often remain excessively high. As noted earlier, appropriate planning prior to the design and construction of a building is the most effective procedure for meeting acoustic guidelines. Because of inappropriate room acoustics, other methodologies, such as the use of assistive technologies, should be implemented. One well-recognized strategy for improving speech perception in rooms is through the use of personal or group amplification systems. Investigations of room amplification systems have shown that they can improve significantly speech perception, listening, attention, academic performance, and on-task behaviors (see Crandell et al. [2005] for a review). The goals of room amplification systems are to: (1) maintain a high S/N with minimal reverberation at the listener's ears; (2) allow the signal to be modified to meet the acoustic needs of the individual(s); (3) provide wide frequency amplification with a minimal degree of distortion; (4) allow mobility for both the speaker and the listener; (5) allow listeners to hear not only the primary speaker, but also other speakers in the room as well as their own voices; and (6) accept inputs such as compact disc players, tape recorders, and TVs. Possible room amplification systems include personal hearing aids as well as personal frequency modulation (FM), sound field, induction loop, infrared, and hardwired systems.

Personal Hearing Aids

Numerous investigations have demonstrated that traditional hearing aids offer little speech perception benefit in noisy or reverberant environments (Duquesnoy and Plomp, 1983; Plomp, 1978; 1986; Van Tassell, 1993; Moore, 1997; Crandell

et al., 2005). This result should not be surprising because, although it is improving, traditional amplification technology does little to increase the S/N of the listening environment. Duquesnoy and Plomp (1983) indicated that minimal benefit occurred from personal amplification when background noise levels reached 60 dBA. Plomp (1986) reported that hearing aids offered limited speech perception benefit when background noise levels exceeded 50 dBA. A review of everyday background noise levels suggests that most environments exhibit background noise levels in excess of 50 to 60 dBA. These data strongly suggest that children wearing traditional amplification will require other technologies that enhance S/N and can augment the capabilities of the hearing aid. This situation has changed more recently, however, since several potential S/N-enhancing options for hearing aids have been introduced that may help the listener in noisy or reverberant environments. Some of these new technologies are described below (see also Chapter 35).

MODIFICATION OF FREQUENCY RESPONSE

One strategy for improving speech perception in noise with hearing aids is to shape the frequency response of the hearing aid by emphasizing the high frequencies and reducing the low frequencies. Such a shaping of the frequency response may reduce the upward spread of masking effects of low-frequency noise as well as offer improved S/Ns within the high-frequency regions. In a room with abundant steady-state low-frequency noise, such as air conditioning/ventilator noise, the ability to shift the frequency response of the amplification system in this way can effectively improve the S/N. However, as the interfering noise spectrum becomes more speech-like, the effectiveness of this strategy increasingly is diminished. Modification of the frequency response has been available for many years in hearing aids through the nonadaptive high-pass filter setting. Digital instruments are widely available that offer frequency response programs that are user selectable. Some modern hearing aid designs can amplify a wide band of frequencies, some as high as 6 to 8 kHz. By focusing amplification on frequencies associated with consonant identification and discrimination, these designs are likely to assist the listener in noisy environments.

DIRECTIONAL MICROPHONE TECHNOLOGY

Directional microphones, while often considered a new technology, were first used in hearing aids in 1972. The main design characteristic of a directional microphone is that it is differentially sensitive to acoustic spectra coming from specific azimuths around the head: specifically, more sensitive to spectra from in front of the head and less sensitive to spectra coming from other azimuths (the side or back). The differential sensitivity of a directional microphone can provide a 2 to 4 dB improvement in S/N if the desired signal is coming from a sensitive azimuth and the background noise is originating from a less sensitive azimuth. The advantages of a directional microphone, however, may be compromised in a reverberant room (Hawkins and Yacullo, 1984). Both the desired sound as well as reflections from the background noise can both arrive simultaneously at the microphone's most sensitive azimuth, thereby negating the beneficial effects of the directional microphone. Other microphone technologies have been developed to improve on typical directional microphone performance. **Dual microphones** use two closely matched omnidirectional microphones (microphones that essentially are equally sensitive to sounds coming from a wide range of azimuths) connected by an electronic delay. Improvements in S/N on the order of 6.6 to 7.8 dB, when compared to an omnidirectional microphone, have been reported for this technology (Valente et al., 1995). The **D-Mic** is also a dual microphone arrangement, with one of the microphones being directional and the other being omnidirectional. Improvements in S/N for the D-Mic over omnidirectional microphones on the order of 3.5 to 6.7 dB have been reported (Valente et al., 1999). Another new technology incorporates **multiple microphone arrays** of between two and 17 microphones that are electronically delayed and averaged according to specific design criteria. Improvements in S/N of 7.6 to 10 dB have been reported for these arrays (Valente et al., 1999). **Beamforming** refers to two microphones (one on each ear) whose outputs are digitally compared in the time and intensity domains (Valente et al., 1999). Beamformers can be adjusted to be sensitive to a wide variety of azimuths, and because they have memory capabilities, it is possible to optimize the microphone response for specific listening situations and environmental acoustic conditions. Because of the flexibility offered by beamformers, they hold the most promise for improving S/N in a variety of difficult listening environments (for more information on directional microphone technology, see Chapter 35).

ADAPTIVE SIGNAL PROCESSING STRATEGIES

Most hearing aids today use some form of adaptive signal processing in an attempt to enhance the listener's S/N. Recently, some hearing aids have been designed to reduce the effects of reverberation on the hearing-impaired listener. Adaptive signal processing strategies are often based on digital signal processing algorithms and can be simple or very complex. A review of the speech perception data concerning these strategies has been equivocal. That is, research has demonstrated that these strategies benefit some listeners in noise and in some reverberant environments, but not others. As these strategies are refined, more consistent and larger speech perceptual improvements are likely.

Hearing Aids May Not Be Enough

While there have been striking developments in hearing aid technology, this technology alone will not maximize speech perception for the most listening challenged in noise and reverberant environments. Fortunately, there are other tech-

nologies that can be used in these situations. Some of these are described in the following section.

Personal Frequency Modulation Amplification

FM systems have a long history of use and benefit with the hearing impaired and other special populations. FM systems have also been beneficial in improving communication in large room areas (conference rooms, theaters, churches) as well as in face-to-face settings (Montano, 1994).

An example of a personal FM system is shown in Figure 34.3. With a personal FM system, the voice is picked up by a FM wireless microphone located near the speaker's mouth where the detrimental effects of reverberation and noise are minimal (i.e., the microphone placement is well within the direct field). The acoustic signal is then converted to an electrical waveform and transmitted via FM signal to a receiver tuned to the same frequency. The electrical signal is separated from the FM signal and amplified, then converted back to an acoustic waveform and conveyed to the listener. The Federal Communications Commission (FCC) initially allocated the frequency region of 72.025 to 75.975 MHz for assistive listening devices used by individuals with hearing loss. This frequency region was subdivided into 40 narrowband or 10 wideband channels. More recently, the FCC also allocated the frequency range of 216 to 217 MHz for assistive device use, which has improved quality and reduced interference.

Figure 34.4 shows various FM coupling strategies for use with children who have hearing loss, while Figure 34.5 shows various FM microphone and transmitter options. As can be seen in Figure 34.4, the signal can be presented through headphones (or earbuds) or directly to the hearing aids via induction loop or direct auditory input (DAI) technology. The FM unit also can be coupled directly to the ear via a button or a behind-the-ear transducer. Furthermore, for children with

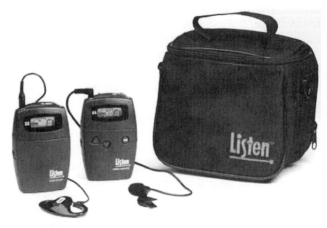

FIGURE 34.3   An example of a personal frequency modulation (FM) system. In this figure, the FM system is fitted to a hearing aid via direct audio input (DAI) technology. (Photo courtesy of Phonic Ear, Petaluma, CA.)

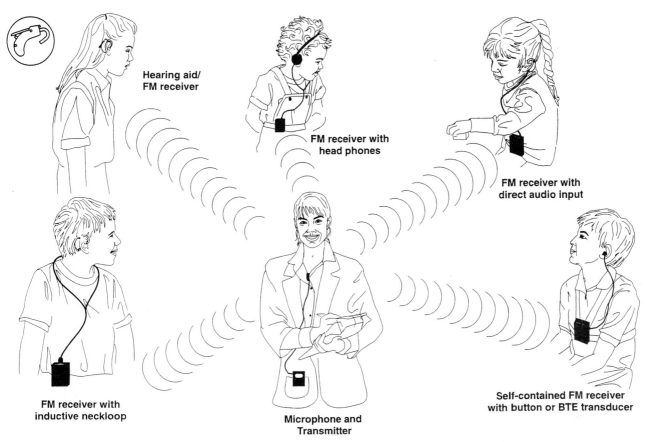

FIGURE 34.4 Various coupling options for use with frequency modulation (FM) systems for children with hearing loss. (Reprinted from Lewis D. [1998] Classroom amplification. In: Bess F, ed. *Children with Hearing Loss: Contemporary Trends*. Nashville: Bill Wilkerson Center Press; pp 277–298, with permission.)

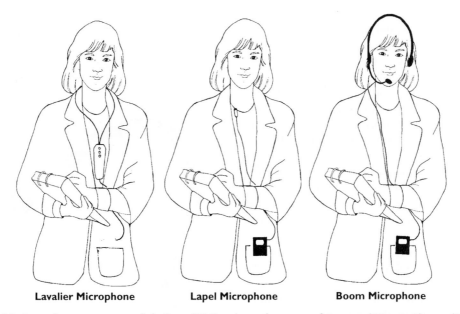

FIGURE 34.5 Various frequency modulation (FM) microphone and transmitter options. (Reprinted from Lewis D. [1998] Classroom amplification. In: Bess F, ed. *Children with Hearing Loss: Contemporary Trends*. Nashville: Bill Wilkerson Center Press; pp 277–298, with permission.)

conductive or mixed hearing losses, the FM system can be coupled to a bone-conduction transducer. However, it is recommended that, for children with hearing loss, the child's personal hearing aid or aids be incorporated with the FM system whenever possible. This allows the child's personal hearing aid, which is often more electroacoustically flexible than the FM system, to more accurately meet the child's pure-tone sensitivity requirements. By coupling the FM system to the child's hearing aid, a high S/N is provided for the child's listening environment. That is, it is best to allow the hearing aid to do what it does best (improve hearing sensitivity) and let the FM system accomplish what it does best (improve the S/N of the listening environment). Of course, one concern with this recommendation is that it assumes that the child has a completely functional hearing aid with the option of switching between the following various transmission modes: (1) FM only, for the purpose of focusing primarily on the talker; (2) environmental microphone (EM) only, for the purpose of listening to all individuals in the immediate listening environment as well as monitoring his or her own voice; and (3) FM + EM for listening to both the teacher as well as other individuals in that listening environment. For a more complete discussion on the advantages/disadvantages of various coupling systems, the reader is directed to Lewis (1998).

For children with "normal" hearing, the signal can be presented through earbuds or headphones (see Fig. 34.4). It is imperative to realize that there are personal FM systems manufactured for children with hearing loss as well as FM systems developed for children with normal hearing or slight degrees of hearing loss. Systems manufactured for children with hearing loss often offer the user a high degree of electroacoustic flexibility, including the potential for extended frequency response, high gain, and elevated SSPL90s. In addition, these latter systems usually have external controls that allow the child to switch between the various transmission modes (i.e., FM only, EM only, or FM + EM). In contrast, systems developed for children with "normal" hearing offer limited electroacoustic variability with limited gain and reduced OSPL90s. These systems are designed simply to provide the child an improved S/N with little to no amplification. Unfortunately, the authors have often seen children with "normal" hearing wearing FM devices designed for those with hearing loss. This form of FM use is alarming in that hearing loss could ensue if a child was wearing a device set for moderate gain and a high OSPL90. Thus, it is imperative that all children with "normal" hearing be fit with the appropriate FM system. In fact, since even these devices provide some gain, it is recommended that these children use an attenuated headphone when using FM technology in the classroom. An attenuated headphone will reduce the gain/output of the unit by approximately 10 to 20 dB, thus reducing the potential for overamplification. Moreover, Crandell and Ege (2000) found no significant decrease in speech perception between attenuated and nonattenuated headphones. Certainly no FM system (or any other HAT) should be fit prior to the veri-

fication of that fitting via real-ear measures. The reader is directed to Lewis (1998) for further information regarding selection and verification of FM systems.

Personal FM systems are also now available in ear-level models. The FM-only models are designed for children with auditory learning difficulties, auditory processing disorders (APDs), attention deficits, or mild conductive hearing loss. For children with hearing loss, integrated hearing aid/FM systems have been developed that provide the user with a combination of both a hearing aid and an FM system in the same ear-level device. For children with hearing within normal limits (WNL), the FM system is simply located in a behind-the-ear configuration, often in conjunction with an open earmold. In both cases, these systems allow the user the freedom of not having to use body worn receivers as required with the more traditional FM systems.

Recently, miniaturized personal FM devices even smaller than these ear-level behind-the-ear (BTE) units have been developed for classroom use. One of these, the Phonak EduLink (Fig. 34.6), is a lightweight FM device measuring 3.5 inches in length. A flexible receiver tube allows the device to be bent and hung over the ear with the end of the receiver tube in the concha (with an optional earmold) and the battery case behind the pinna. The EduLink was developed particularly for students with APD, attention deficit hyperactivity disorder (ADHD), and learning disabilities as a complement to auditory rehabilitation training. Unobtrusive devices like this one that are not only small but are also similar to popular mobile phone headsets may be more acceptable for classroom use by older, more image-conscious students. A clinical trial examining the speech-in-noise intelligibility effects of the EduLink device for elementary school–aged children began in March 2005.

With the continuing evolution of "boot technology," FM receivers can be added to virtually any BTE hearing aid or ear-level cochlear implant. The FM "boot" is a miniature FM receiver that permits a transmitting microphone to be

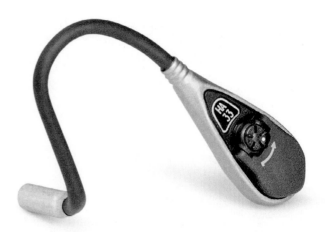

FIGURE 34.6 Example of an EduLink ear-level personal frequency modulation (FM) system. (Photo courtesy of Phonak, Warrenville, IL.)

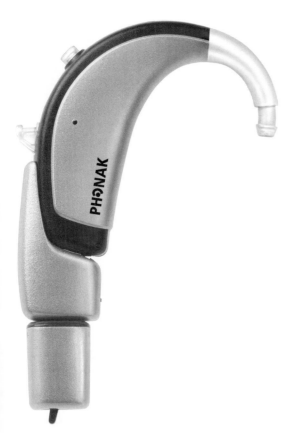

FIGURE 34.7   Frequency modulation (FM) system coupled to a hearing aid via a wireless "audio boot." (Photo courtesy of Phonak, Warrenville, IL.)

located close to a desired sound source. The FM "boot" usually attaches through a direct audio input connection to the hearing aid (Fig. 34.7). High-quality sound from an associated FM transmitter is received at the ear level by the FM boot, providing clear sound from a distance and in noisy environments.

Infrared Light Wave Systems

Infrared systems consist of a wireless microphone, infrared converter, and an infrared receiver. The microphone converts the acoustical signal to an electrical signal that is then transmitted to the converter. The converter transduces the electrical signal to an invisible infrared signal and transmits it to a receiver worn by the listener. The receiver (which also serves as an amplifier) contains photo detector diodes that pick up the infrared signal and transduce the infrared signal back into electrical energy. The electrical signal, in turn, is then changed into acoustic energy and routed to the listener via an induction loop/hearing aid telecoil setup or through headphones/insert earphones. Direct audio input can also be used by those listeners whose hearing aids have the required audio boot. Currently, the majority of infrared systems designed for individuals with SNHL use a narrowband carrier frequency of 95 kHz or a wideband carrier frequency of

250 kHz. Recently, other infrared carrier frequencies have been introduced, making system compatibility an issue. Infrared systems often are used in larger room settings, such as auditoriums, conference halls, theaters, and churches. For large rooms, such as theaters and auditoriums, arrays of transmitters must be used to ensure that all listeners are appropriately placed relative to the transmitted infrared light beams. In the home setting, infrared systems often are used for TV viewing. This application will be discussed in a later section.

For optimal sound quality with infrared systems, the listener must be in a direct line with the transmitter. Infrared light waves cannot pass through or bend around obstacles such as walls. Of course, this can be an advantage or a disadvantage. For example, in the classroom setting, it may not be practical to keep the child in direct line with the transmitter throughout the school day. That is, if other children move in front of the child using the infrared system, the signal may be blocked and not reach that child. Infrared systems also cannot be used outdoors or in highly sunlit rooms since they are susceptible to interference from sunlight. Because infrared light cannot penetrate solid barriers, this form of technology is excellent in large room settings (in which there is limited individual movement when the infrared is used) or adjacent room settings (e.g., multiplex cinemas) to avoid interference from the other room.

Sound Field Amplification

Another form of S/N-enhancing technology is sound field amplification. A sound field system is similar to a personal FM system; however, with this form of technology, the speaker's voice is conveyed to listeners in the room via one or more strategically placed loudspeakers (Fig. 34.8). The speaker's voice can be transmitted using an FM transmitting microphone or more recently via an infrared transmitting

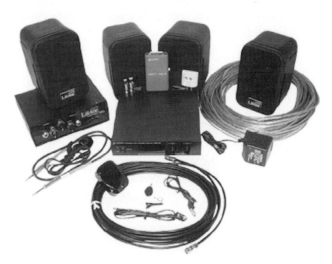

FIGURE 34.8   Components of a sound field amplification system. (Photo courtesy of Lifeline Amplification Systems, Platteville, WI.)

microphone. The radio or light signal is sent to an FM or infrared receiver connected to an amplifier. The amplified signal is distributed to loudspeakers in the room. Infrared has become the preferred technology in sound field amplification systems because of a major limitation of FM technology. There is a finite number of FM frequencies that can be used in proximity with one another without interference. If an entire school is outfitted with sound field technology, then there may not be enough available frequencies for all of the classrooms. Since infrared signals are confined by the walls of the classroom, interference with another classroom system is unlikely, and so the number of infrared systems that can operate in nearby rooms is virtually infinite. Additionally, if a second transmitting microphone (the pass-around microphone) is desired, another FM frequency is required, which further exacerbates the FM limitation. Infrared systems are typically stereo, and so there is another infrared channel available for the pass-around microphone. Sound field systems are generally used to assist children with "normal" hearing in the classroom who require a better S/N. The objectives when placing a sound field system in a classroom are twofold: (1) to amplify the speaker's voice by approximately 8 to 10 dB, thus improving the S/N of the listening environment; and (2) to provide amplification uniformly throughout the classroom. Sound field systems vary from compact, portable, battery-powered, single-speaker units to more permanently placed, alternating current (AC) powered speaker systems that use multiple (usually four) loudspeakers. Typically, loudspeakers are placed on stands and are strategically placed within the classroom. However, several companies now sell loudspeakers that can be placed in ceiling mounts (Fig. 34.9). In addition, portable sound field systems that can be placed on a student's desk and carried easily from classroom to classroom are also available (Fig. 34.10).

Numerous investigations have shown that when sound field amplification systems are positioned within the classroom, educational and psychosocial improvements occur for children with normal hearing sensitivity (Berg, 1993; Crandell and Smaldino, 1996; Crandell et al., 2005).

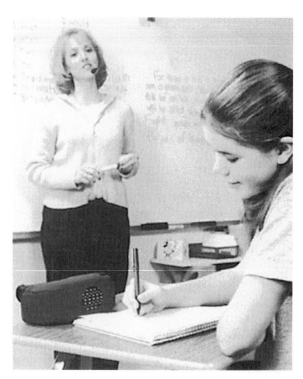

FIGURE 34.10   Portable sound field frequency modulation (FM) system on desk. (Photo courtesy of Lightspeed Technologies, Lake Oswego, OR.)

The original investigation concerning the effectiveness of sound field amplification was a 3-year longitudinal project called the Mainstream Amplification Resource Room Study (MARRS) (Sarff, 1981; Sarff et al., 1981). The project demonstrated that students with minimal hearing loss and children with learning disabilities (without any hearing loss) who received instruction using sound field amplification made significantly greater academic gains, at a faster rate, to a higher level, and at one-tenth the cost compared with students in unamplified classrooms receiving instruction with pull-out resource room intervention. Younger children tended to demonstrate greater academic improvements than older children. Furthermore, academic gains in the amplified group were obtained at a faster rate, to a higher level, and with reduced costs when compared with the unamplified group. A number of subsequent studies have reported similar findings (see Crandell et al. [2005] for a review of these studies).

It is reasonable to assume that these academic improvements were the result of the improved listening environment offered by the sound field FM amplification system. For example, Crandell and Bess (1987) examined the effects of sound field FM amplification on the speech perception of children without any history of learning difficulty or hearing loss in a classroom environment (S/N = +6 dB, RT = 0.45 second). Bamford-Kowal-Bench (BKB) sentences were recorded in both amplified and unamplified listening conditions at speaker-listener distances of 6, 12, and 24 feet. Multitalker babble was used as the noise competition. Subjects

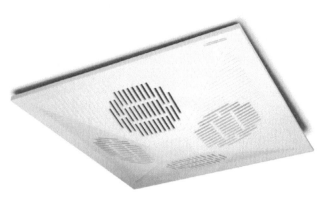

FIGURE 34.9   Sound field frequency modulation (FM) system placed in the ceiling. (Photo courtesy of Telex, Burnsville, MN.)

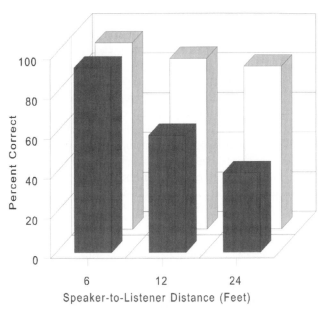

FIGURE 34.11 Mean speech recognition scores (% correct) of children with normal hearing in a "typical" classroom environment (signal-to-noise ratio = +6 dB; reverberation time = 0.6 second) without (*dark bars*) and with (*light bars*) sound field frequency modulation (FM) amplification. (Adapted from Crandell C, Smaldino J, Flexer C. [1995] *Sound Field FM Amplification: Theory and Practical Applications.* San Diego: Singular Publishing Group, with permission.)

consisted of 20 children, aged 5 to 7 years, who listened to the experimental tapes and repeated back the stimuli that they heard. Results from this investigation (Fig. 34.11) showed that sound field FM amplification improved speech perception at every speaker-listener distance, particularly at 12 and 24 feet.

Obviously, the same sound field unit and loudspeaker arrangement cannot be suitable for all classrooms. Consequently, Crandell et al. (1995; 2005) recommended a pragmatic approach to installing sound field equipment. The pragmatic approach takes into consideration the individual classroom, the individual teacher/teaching style(s), and the pupils in that particular classroom. For instance, if group learning is the primary mode of teaching, the goal is to have each student in the classroom perceive the teacher's voice maximally at all times during the school day. Typically, the larger the classroom, the more loudspeakers are need. If angled properly, three or four loudspeakers positioned about 5 feet up on the walls, or in a ceiling array, should provide "surround" sound for all students. If the classroom has specific learning centers/areas, a loudspeaker can be positioned close to each learning center for maximum effective amplification at each of the critical locations. If only one learning center is used at a time, then the other loudspeakers can be turned off. If a small resource classroom is used, two loudspeakers can provide an even and consistent S/N throughout

the area. In fact, if the room is quite small, with only a few students seated close to the teacher, even a single loudspeaker might be effective. If the classroom and class size are small, with only one teacher-instructed learning center in use at any given time, then a single battery-powered loudspeaker can be carried by the teacher to each teaching location to amplify that specific environment. In each of these cases, it is imperative that SPLs of the teacher's voice be measured via an SLM to ensure that a uniform, 8- to 10-dB improvement in S/N has been obtained in each of the specific learning areas.

Sound field FM amplification provides several benefits. First, sound field amplification provides benefit to virtually **all** children in the classroom. As previously noted, with a sound field amplification system, the teacher's voice is transmitted to **each** of the children in the classroom via one or more strategically placed loudspeakers. Consequently, while sound field FM amplification is usually recommended for "normal-hearing, at-risk" children, **all** of the children in that classroom receive, and subsequently can benefit from, an improved S/N. Second, a sound field system can provide benefit to children with mild degrees of SNHL while malfunctioning hearing aids or auditory trainers are being repaired (Blair et al., 1989). Logically, an increase in classroom S/N should augment, at least minimally, the perceptual cues available to these children until their own amplification systems are returned.

Third, sound field systems are often the most inexpensive procedure for improving speech perception in the classroom. Recall that guidelines for acoustic conditions in classrooms indicate that, for adequate communicative efficiency to occur in the classroom, RTs should not surpass 0.4 second, classroom S/Ns should not be less than +15 dB, and background noise levels should not exceed 30 to 35 dBA. Extensive acoustic modification of the classroom (acoustic ceiling tiles, acoustic wall panels, or acoustically modified furniture) can be cost prohibitive for schools (Crandell et al., 1995; 2005). Sound field amplification systems have been shown to be extremely cost effective in overcoming poor room acoustics. An illustration of the cost effectiveness of sound field amplification is shown in Table 34.3. If we estimate the average

TABLE 34.3	Example of the cost effectiveness of a sound field frequency modulation amplification system
Approximate initial cost of sound field unit	$1,000.00
Cost per child in classroom (25 children)	$40.00
Cost per child over 10-year time span	$4.00

Adapted from Crandell C, Smaldino J, Flexer C. (1995) *Sound Field FM Amplification: Theory and Practical Applications.* San Diego: Singular Press.

cost of a sound field system at approximately $1,000 and this cost is divided by all of the children in the classroom (since it will benefit the vast majority of children in the room), this equates to approximately $40.00 per child (considering a class size of 25 students). If this cost per student is prorated over a 10-year period (the estimated average life span of a sound field system), the annual unit cost per child is only $4.00. There are additional savings of sound field amplification that should be noted. Specifically, sound field systems have been shown to reduce the number of children requiring resource room assistance, which is often the most expensive assistance offered by schools. For instance, when the Putnam County school district in Ohio placed 60 sound field units in regular classrooms, the number of children with learning disabilities requiring resource room assistance decreased by 40% (Crandell et al., 1995).

Fourth, use of a sound field system does not stigmatize children, which can be the situation with auditory trainers or hearing aids (i.e., because the latter require the children to wear hardware). Children with "normal" hearing who demonstrate perceptual difficulties, particularly those in junior or senior high school, often experience negative reactions from their classmates when using personal FM systems that necessitate the use of headphones or earbuds. Due to this negative stigma, these students frequently choose to use FM devices sparingly. Thus, while personal FM systems offer an improved S/N compared to sound field FM systems, this technology is only useful if the student is motivated to wear it. Rosenberg and Blake-Rahter (1995) reported that 93% of students who used sound field technology in the classroom responded positively to the use of such systems. Moreover, by passing around the sound field microphone (for oral reports, oral reading, and asking/answering questions) students reported improved classroom interaction and participation.

Fifth, studies have found that teachers overwhelmingly accept sound field amplification systems once they have received in-service training on the instrumentation or have actually used the equipment (Allen, 1993; Berg, 1993; Crandell et al., 1995).

Sixth, teachers report lessened stress and vocal strain during teaching activities with sound field amplification. Vocal attrition has been reported to be one of the most frequent problems that teachers experience (Sapienza et al., 1999). With vocal rest, symptoms of vocal stress can be ameliorated and the teacher's voice can return to normal. However, most professionals cannot afford lengthy periods of time away from their job commitment. Therefore, an alternative mode of communication, such as sound field FM amplification, can assist in augmenting the teacher's voice projection and reducing vocal abuse. Sapienza et al. (1999) reported that sound field amplification can significantly reduce vocal strain in teachers, thus reducing the possibility of vocal attrition.

Seventh, sound field systems can be used to enhance other instructional equipment. Obviously, in the educational setting, all information presented to children should be au-

dible. Sound field systems can be connected to equipment such as TVs, cassette tape recorders, and compact disc players to make the output more audible in the classroom (Crandell et al., 1995).

Finally, parents willingly accept sound field amplification systems. Crandell et al. (1997) reported that more than 97% of parents willingly accept the concept of sound field technology, even if they have not seen the instrumentation used within the classroom. Presumably, parents overwhelmingly accept this technology not only because of the positive comments they hear from children and teachers, but also due to the significant improvements in academic performance noted by their children when sound field technology is implemented in the classroom.

It must be noted, however, that there are several potential disadvantages of sound field amplification. First, sound field amplification systems may not provide adequate benefits in excessively noisy or reverberant learning environments. While the exact levels of noise or reverberation that may negate the benefit of sound field systems is a topic of research, it is reasonable to assume that, if classroom noise levels are loud enough to mask the speech signal, a 10-dB improvement in the teacher's voice may not be enough to make all elements of speech audible. Moreover, sound field amplification systems are not appropriate in a highly reverberant classroom because these systems do not significantly reduce reverberation and, in fact, may increase the overall RT in some rooms. Therefore, it is imperative to know the acoustic characteristics of a room (noise levels and RT) and minimize these effects with acoustic modifications ***before*** the installation of sound field equipment is attempted.

Second, if the loudspeaker arrangement or number of loudspeakers(s) is not appropriate for the classroom, the level from the speakers may not be uniform throughout the classroom. In other words, the teacher's voice may be too loud for some children, while not loud enough for other children.

Third, sound field amplification may not be feasible in smaller classrooms. In smaller classrooms or learning environments, it may not be possible to amplify the teacher's voice by 10 dB because of feedback problems associated with the interactive effects of reflective surfaces and speaker closeness. While it is clear that a system that has frequent feedback will not be of benefit in a classroom setting, it is not clear whether an improvement in S/N of less than 10 dB still would warrant the installation of a system (Crandell et al., 1995; 2005).

Fourth, the teacher and students need appropriate in-service information and follow-up support if a sound field system is to provide maximum benefit in the classroom. As with any HAT, it is imperative that the teacher thoroughly understand why a sound field system is being recommended and placed in the classroom prior to installation. Specifically, it is critical to make the teacher comfortable with the instrumentation by explaining its theoretical and practical applications in nontechnological, easy-to-understand terminology. In instances when sound field amplification is not used effectively in the classroom, inadequate training of the teacher on its use is frequently at fault (Crandell et al., 1995; Crandell and Smaldino, 1996).

Fifth, sound field amplification systems may not benefit children with severe recruitment or hypersensitive hearing. By increasing the level of the sound in the classroom by even 10 dB, it is conceivable that a problem could be created for these children.

Finally, classroom-based sound field systems generally are not portable, which could prove to be a problem if the child uses several different classrooms during the day. However, as noted earlier, individual students may now use personal portable sound field systems that can be carried from class to class or benefit from the newer personal FM BTE units (such as the EduLink). Also with the growing acceptance of this technology, school districts often equip nearly every classroom in a school with this technology, so moving from classroom to classroom is less of a problem.

RECOMMENDING PERSONAL OR SOUND FIELD FREQUENCY MODULATION SYSTEMS

There is limited information comparing the effectiveness of sound field amplification to personal FM systems (Flexer, 1992; 1993). Clearly, the personal FM system should offer a more favorable S/N than the sound field system. Nabelek et al. (1986) examined speech perception through a public address system and through a personal FM unit in normal-hearing listeners and listeners with SNHL. While both systems provided improved speech recognition scores over unamplified conditions, results indicated that each of the groups obtained significantly higher speech recognition scores with the personal FM system.

Because sound field systems can be expected to provide only about 8 to 10 dB of amplification, such systems may not provide a sufficient communicative environment for students with moderate to severe degrees of SNHL. Thus, for children with greater than mild degrees of SNHL and/or severe perceptual difficulties in noise, a personal FM system may be the more appropriate amplification. In addition, these children are more likely to require an improved classroom S/N throughout their academic career (Flexer, 1992). It must be remembered, however, that many children, particularly those in junior or senior high school, may not use personal FM systems due to the potential stigma associated with such devices, necessitating the use of a sound field system. If a child with more than a mild degree of hearing loss uses sound field amplification, it is important that some measure of efficacy be obtained to evaluate the effectiveness of the system (see "Outcome Measures" section later in this chapter).

Electromagnetic Induction Loop Systems

An example of an induction loop amplification system (one of the oldest forms of room amplification) is shown in Figure 34.12. As can be noted from this figure, an induction loop system consists of a microphone connected via hard wire

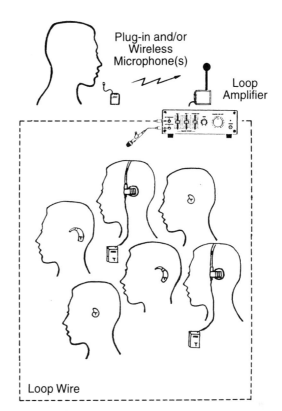

FIGURE 34.12 Components of a large-room electromagnetic induction loop system. Note that, in this figure, the electromagnetic signal is being received by listeners via telecoils located within an in-the-ear (ITE) hearing aid, behind-the-ear (BTE) hearing aid, and a portable induction receiver (for use without a hearing aid). (Photo courtesy of Oval Window, Nederland, CO.)

(or an FM transmitter) to an amplifier. A length of wire extends from the amplifier. This wire is placed either around the head of an individual (neckloop) or around a designated area, such as in a classroom or theater. When an electrical current flows through the wire loop, it creates an electromagnetic field that can be picked up by any device using telecoil technology. A telecoil is a special device often found in hearing aids that picks up and amplifies electromagnetic signals, and, in turn, converts these signals into acoustic energy that can be heard by the hearing aid user. Interestingly, for years, induction loop systems commonly have been used in international conferences to provide simultaneous translation service to conference attendees. In this case, the attendee uses an induction loop earbud or a handheld wand that contains a receiver/amplifier and speaker. The device can be turned on or simply held to the ear when language translation is required.

There are several advantages of induction loop systems over other forms of room amplification. First, induction loop systems tend to be the least costly of the room amplification systems. One reason for this cost reduction is that induction loop systems do not require additional receivers as do FM or infrared systems. Induction loop systems have relatively few components and are fairly easy to install. Troubleshooting and maintenance of such systems also tend to be relatively easy.

Unfortunately, there are several limitations of such systems in classroom settings. First, recall that induction loop systems require the student's hearing aid to have a functional telecoil that is sensitive enough to pick up the electromagnetic field throughout the classroom. It is incumbent upon the dispensing audiologist to be sure to include a strong telecoil in the student's hearing aid(s) if use of an induction system is expected. Failure to do so would make this technology unavailable or less effective to the student and perhaps force the use of more expensive technology to improve the S/N. Furthermore, even when the hearing aid has telecoil technology, past investigations have indicated that many children's hearing aids often malfunction (see Flexer [1992] for a review). Unfortunately, younger children may not be able to explain the resultant decreased acoustic signal when their telecoil is malfunctioning. Moreover, many telecoils do not provide enough gain to significantly improve perception with an induction loop system. Variables affecting telecoil gain include the absence/presence of a telecoil preamplifier and the position and/or orientation of the telecoil within the hearing aid. A second disadvantage of an induction loop system is that many hearing aids do not contain the microphone (M) + telecoil (T) option. Thus, the user without such switching capability would not be able to hear individuals other than the ones closest to the microphone. For example, a student may not hear other students' questions (or even be able to monitor his or her own voice) when receiving the signal from the induction loop system.

Third, the quality of the signal and, therefore, speech perception may decrease as the listener moves away from the induction loop. That is, depending on the orientation of the telecoil within their hearing aid and/or the placement of the induction loop itself, a child seated in the middle of a room may not be obtaining as high a signal quality as the child seated next to the induction loop. Moreover, in larger rooms, the induction loop may not be powerful enough to assist all of the listeners within that enclosure.

Fourth, although the induction loop system is relatively portable, it is not practical to move such systems to accommodate outdoor activities.

Fifth, since a hearing aid with an appropriate telecoil is required, the system often cannot be used for children with normal hearing.However, it should be noted that there are several devices on the market that use telecoil technology for individuals with normal hearing, such as handheld induction loop receivers with earbuds or a headset.

Sixth, the number of rooms in a building that can be equipped with induction loop technology is often limited because "spillover" (up to 50 to 100 feet) can occur across such systems. Spillover occurs when the electromagnetic signal generated in one room is picked up by a telecoil in an adjacent room.

Finally, the quality of the signal produced by induction loop systems and picked up via telecoils may be reduced by other electrical devices in the room that produce magnetic fields (and as a result generate a 60-Hz hum). Examples of such devices include fluorescent lighting and electric power lines.

To circumvent many of the difficulties associated with induction loop systems, Hendricks and Lederman (1991) developed a three-dimensional (3D) induction loop system. In a 3D induction loop system, a wireless microphone transmits the speaker's voice to an audio mixer, signal processor, and power amplifier. The amplified signal is then transmitted to specially designed induction loops that are placed within a floor mat that, in turn, may be placed under the room's carpet. Spillover has been shown to be significantly reduced with the use of the 3D induction loop system. Additionally, the strength of an inductance loop signal produced by the floor mats is more evenly distributed across the mats, thus eliminating the fluctuations in signal strength commonly encountered as a child moves closer and farther away from conventional loop systems.

Hardwired Systems

Hardwired systems are those assistive technologies that provide a direct physical connection between the sound source and the individual. Specifically, hardwired systems are so named because a wire connects the microphone to the amplifier, and the amplifier is connected directly to the receiver (headphones, earbuds). An example of such a system is shown in Figure 34.13.

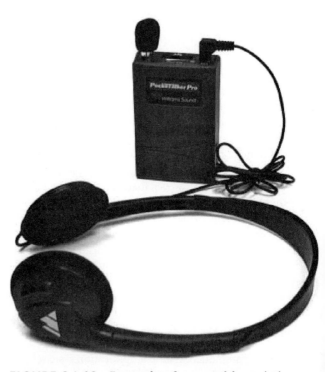

FIGURE 34.13   Example of a portable assistive listening device. (Photo cortesy of Harris Communications, Eden Prairie, MN.)

One advantage of such systems is that they provide an inexpensive approach for the amplification of sound. In addition, it often is easy for the consumer to purchase such equipment in electronics stores, through the mail, or over the internet. Such systems have been shown to be useful for some patients with hearing loss who may not be able to use conventional amplification (e.g., those with cognitive declines, physical disabilities, and/or severe manual dexterity difficulties). Weinstein and Amsel (1986), for example, reported that hardwired systems appeared to improve the communication status in nursing home–bound patients with dementia.

While inexpensive, there are a number of concerns with hardwired systems. First, such systems are not specified as medical devices by the Food and Drug Administration (FDA). Therefore, there are no standards for the electroacoustic characteristics (gain, frequency response, OSPL90, harmonic distortion) of such devices. The audiologist should perform comprehensive electroacoustic and real-ear measures prior to placing a hardwired system on an individual with hearing loss. A second concern with hardwired systems is the limitation of movement for the user. That is, since each part of the device is connected via a wire, the user can only be as far from the sound source as the wire length will allow. Hardwired systems generally are not used for larger rooms such as classrooms because they require the child to sit in predetermined locations and the microphone wire can restrict teacher movement.

COMMUNICATION STRATEGIES

While technology can improve significantly the acoustic environment in the classroom, it should not be entirely depended on to enhance listening and learning. Active participation of the teacher and students is necessary in order to optimize the effectiveness of the technology. Effort should be made to compliment the technology with physical positioning of teacher-student, the use of clear speech principles, optimization of visual speech cues, and learning to listen.

Reducing Speaker-Listener Distance

In the absence of any HAT, for optimal speech perception to occur, the listener needs to be in a face-to-face situation and in the direct sound field of the talker. Recall that speech perception can only be improved within the critical distance of the room. Beyond the critical distance, speech perception ability tends to remain constant. Therefore, in any listening environment, the speaker-listener distance should not exceed the critical distance of the room. Unfortunately, the critical distance in many rooms occurs only at close speaker-listener distances. To remain within the critical distance of a room, restructuring of the room dynamics may need to be considered. For example, small group instruction (where the speaker addresses one small group at a time) should be recommended over more "traditional" room settings (where the speaker is situated in front of numerous rows of students). Crandell et al. (1997) reported that speech perception scores of children were very good or excellent when such small group instruction was used in a classroom.

Clear Speech

Clear speech procedures may also facilitate speech perception in many enclosures. Clear speech refers to a process in which the speaker focuses attention on clearer pronunciation, while using a slightly slower rate of speech and a slightly higher intensity—a speech style used by most newscasters (Picheny et al., 1985a; 1985b). Several investigations have demonstrated that clear speech can improve significantly speech perception in noisy and reverberant environments (Crandell and Smaldino, 2000; Picheny et al., 1985a; 1985b; Schum, 1996). For example, Payton et al. (1994) demonstrated that, in poor listening environments, the average improvement in speech perception when clear speech was used was 20% for listeners with normal hearing and 26% for listeners with SNHL. It is reasonable to expect speakers, such as teachers, to learn clear speech procedures easily because talkers can be trained to produce clear speech continuously after a minimum amount of instruction and practice (Schum, 1996).

Optimizing Visual Communication

Face-to-face communication at relatively short speaker-listener distances also aids the listener with hearing loss by maximizing speechreading opportunities. Optimal speaker-listener distance is approximately 5 feet (Schow and Nerbonne, 1996). Speechreading ability tends to decrease significantly at 20 feet. Several investigators have also reported that speechreading benefit increases as a function of decreasing S/N (Erber, 1979; Middleweerd and Plomp, 1987; Rosenblum et al., 1996). That is, listeners rely more heavily on visually transmitted information as the acoustic environment becomes more adverse.

Improving Listening Strategies

Listening (as opposed to hearing) refers to the ability to detect, discriminate, identify, and comprehend various auditory signals. Listening is a major component of the communication process. Listening comprises 45% of daily communication for adults, while school children spend as much as 60% of the school day in the process of listening (Rosenberg and Blake-Rahter, 1995). Research has demonstrated that listeners who experience difficulty at any level of the listening process will find it more difficult to use auditory information in an efficient manner. Despite the importance of listening in communication, the process of listening is rarely taught to individuals with hearing loss (Rosenberg and Blake-Rahter, 1995). Erber (1979) emphasized the importance of a thorough audiologic and developmental speech assessment to determine the placement of a student on an auditory skill development continuum. This continuum, which includes sound awareness, sound discrimination, identification, and comprehension, forms the basis for the listening training activities that must be taught specifically to children with hearing loss but that develop normally without training in normal-hearing children. It is important to recognize, however, that listening training may also be necessary when new amplification devices are fit (because of the new signal characteristics) and if room acoustics reduce the intensity or distort the quality of the acoustic signal. It is also noteworthy that some normal-hearing children, such as those with APDs or nonnative speakers, may also benefit from listening training.

A recent and innovative approach to listening and cognitive training has been developed by Sweetow and Henderson-Sabes (2004). LACE (Listening and Auditory Communication Enhancement training) is a computer program composed of a series of interactive and adaptive exercises designed to strengthen listening and communication skills. Clinical trials have demonstrated improvements in listening in noise, self-perception of hearing handicap, and cognitive skills (such as auditory memory).

TECHNOLOGIES WITH APPLICATION TO INDIVIDUALS WITH HEARING LOSS/AUDITORY PROCESSING DEFICITS

Many new technologies recently have become available that can assist individuals with hearing loss; many of these same technologies are also useful for people with normal hearing who have processing-related difficulties and/or find themselves in adverse listening environments. It is beyond the scope of this chapter to overview all of these technologies. A web search will provide the interested reader with access to this ever-expanding list of assistive technologies. We have selected for review a cross section of prominent and promising technologies.

Reception of Broadcast Media

Individuals with SNHL often have a difficult time hearing and/or understanding the auditory broadcast over the TV or radio. As was outlined in the first section of this chapter, a number of factors, such as distance from the sound source, background noise, and poor room acoustics, can interfere with the signal to those with hearing losses. Add these factors to the often poor loudspeaker capabilities of the broadcast device and the distortion imposed by a damaged auditory system, and it becomes clear why simply turning up the volume of the TV or radio is not usually a satisfactory solution. Hearing aids alone often do little to reduce background noise or improve poor room acoustics and thus may not be a

viable solution. Assistive technologies, such as those discussed for large rooms (e.g., infrared systems), can also be used to link broadcast media to the individual with hearing loss and therefore effectively improve the quality of the audio signal. The use of assistive technologies to improve reception of the TV or radio can be accomplished with or without the use of a hearing aid. For example, one of the more popular TV listening devices (Fig. 34.14) sends the audio signal to a receiver worn by the user via infrared technology. The audio signal of the TV or radio may also be enhanced by coupling the individual's hearing aids to the receiving device through DAI or by an induction neckloop. In addition to the assistive technologies discussed previously, there are TV band radios that can be tuned to the channel being watched and placed close to the individual so that the volume can be increased and the effects of distance from the signal source reduced. Personal sound field FM systems also can be useful. In this case, the transmitting microphone is placed close to the TV or radio speaker and the receiving speaker amplifier is placed close to the listener. The increased volume and reduction of room acoustics improve sound reception. Additionally, TVs with audio output jacks can be connected to a stereo receiver. The listener can then plug earphones into the phone jack of the receiver and use the volume control and frequency adjustments to provide an amplified TV signal. If the listener's hearing loss is too great for the use of stereo headphones without feedback, then an inductance

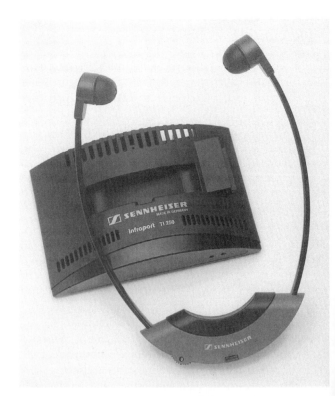

FIGURE 34.14 Personal infrared assistive device used to improve television listening. (Photo courtesy of Sennheiser, Old Lyme, CT.)

neckloop can be connected to the stereo receiver and the signal picked up by the telecoil in the listener's personal hearing aid.

Captioned Media

For the individual with a severe to profound SNHL (or an individual for whom English is a second language), TV viewing can be enhanced with various forms of captioned media (closed, real time, and open). With closed captioning, the text of the broadcast is encoded in the TV signal and must be re-coded in order to appear on the TV screen. Closed-captioned words appear in white uppercase format and are encased in a black box that usually appears in the lower portion of the TV screen, although recent innovations allow the captions to vary in location so as not to block any other text or the talker's face. A TV with a decoder chip or a separate decoder box is necessary to view the closed captioning. As a result of the Television Decoder Circuitry Act of 1990 (PL 101-431), all TV sets more than 13 inches must come equipped with a decoder chip so that individuals can have access to closed captioning when available. Most closed captioning is done "offline" and added to the recorded TV program before the broadcast.

Real-time captioning has become available for live broadcasts such as the news and sporting events. In real-time captioning, a trained stenographer-captioner follows the audio signal and, with a delay of 2 to 3 seconds, converts it to text that appears on the TV screen. Recently, voice-to-text technology has become refined enough to use as a real-time captioning device. Using sophisticated voice recognition technology, these devices hold promise of directly converting the speech signal into text that can be read by the individual with hearing loss.

Another form of captioned media is open captioning. With open captioning, the captions are permanently placed on to the videotape and always available to the viewer with no decoder needed. Open-captioned letters are usually white with a black shadow or border.

Two new captioning technologies promise to improve significantly access for people who are deaf or hard of hearing. Discrete personal captioning uses state-of-the-art electronic, optical, and voice recognition technologies to provide text in a "heads-up" display (similar to that found in fighter aircraft) built into a pair of glasses. A text readout seems to float in the air about 18 inches in front of the wearer. The second technology, called reflective captioning, is intended to help moviegoers follow the dialogue. This innovative technology uses an light-emitting diode (LED) display to project desired captions onto an acrylic panel positioned in front of hearing impaired viewers, thus projecting the captions into their lower visual field as they watch the movie. Both technologies are designed to provide equal access to public places by providing an inconspicuous and efficient transmission and text display of ongoing auditory signals.

Telephony

HEARING AID TELECOILS, REHABILITATIVE TECHNOLOGIES, AND TELEPHONE USE

A telephone induction pickup coil, or "telecoil," picks up the electromagnetic leakage from the telephone receiver. The signal is then amplified, transduced into acoustic information, and delivered to the individual's ear. Improved telephone communication is obtained because the hearing aid microphone is turned off, thus reducing the level of the background noise. In addition, the frequency response of most telecoils tends to be smoother than when the hearing aid is coupled acoustically to the telephone. Unfortunately, due to the miniaturization of hearing aids, many amplification systems are not equipped with telecoils at all or strong telecoils because of size restrictions. It is the view of the authors that hearing aids, whenever possible, should be equipped with telecoil technology because their use far exceeds telephone communication. It must be noted that there is great variability in telecoil power and frequency responses across hearing aids and even within hearing aid companies. Thus, the authors recommend that real-ear measures be conducted with telecoils to ensure their proper function. Certainly, whenever telecoil technology is implemented into a hearing aid, it is imperative that the patient be instructed concerning its proper use.

In addition to telecoil technology, a number of rehabilitative technologies can be used in conjunction with telephone use to improve communication in individuals with hearing loss. For example, one device consists of a disc-shaped microphone that attaches to the telephone handset. The signal is then routed into the listener's personal hearing aid via DAI (thus avoiding the use of the telecoil). Often, the use of individual personal rehabilitative technologies, particularly with DAI, can be beneficial in environments where electromagnetic interference (e.g., computers, fluorescent lights) is high.

TELEPHONE AMPLIFIERS AND ACCESSORIES

Telephone amplifiers and accessories designed specifically for individuals with hearing loss are readily available. Amplified phones offer an array of built-in features, such as hearing aid–compatible headsets, amplifiers with up to 50 dB of amplification, a volume control, and signal processing to maximize comfort and clarity; high-output adjustable ringers; a tone control to adjust the frequency response of the headset to improve intelligibility of words; background noise suppression circuitry to remove unwanted background noise; and visual ring indicators such as a strobe light. Many also have speakerphone capability. Stand-alone in-line amplifiers provide some of the features of the dedicated amplified phone but can be used with many modular unamplified phones.

Cell phone amplifiers are available that can be used with external headsets or earphones. The amplifier plugs into the 2.5-mm audio adapter of the cell phone, and the external headset then plugs into the amplifier. There are also Bluetooth devices that can interface with the cellular phone and be connected via DAI to the hearing aid (see section on Bluetooth). Also, portable telephone amplifiers can be strapped onto a nonamplified telephone to provide up to 30 dB of amplification.

TELECOMMUNICATION DEVICES FOR THE DEAF, TELETYPEWRITERS, TEXT TELEPHONE

Individuals with severe to profound hearing losses may not be able to use the telephone effectively, even with amplification devices. In addition, there are individuals with severe speech impairments or extremely poor speech perception who may not be able to use a conventional telephone. For these individuals, telecommunication devices for the deaf (TDDs), also called teletypewriters (TTYs) or text telephones (TTs), may be required (Fig. 34.15). Note that the preferred term at this time by the deaf community is TTY. Using typewriter technology, the TTY transmits a typed, visual message (in Baudot code) over standard telephone lines. The typed communication either appears on an LED display or can be printed on paper. Braille TTYs are also available to those with visual as well as hearing difficulties. The maximum rate of transmission is approximately 60 words per minute, depending on the sender's typing skills. In order for a TTY conversation to take place, both the sender and receiver must have TTY instrumentation that is compatible. Recent evidence indicates that users of TTYs that are connected directly to the telephone network experience more successful conversations with less message interference than with acoustic coupling (Spicer et al., 2005). The Americans with Disabilities Act (ADA; PL 101-336) mandates that all emergency access services have TTY accessibility. Unfortunately, it appears that many agencies and businesses do not use TTYs effectively.

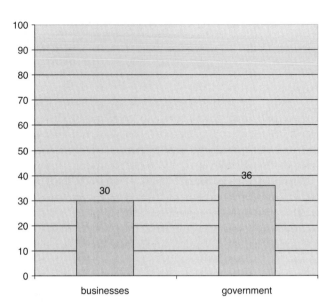

FIGURE 34.16   Percentage of correctly answered telecommunications device for the deaf (TDD) calls for businesses and government agencies. (Adapted from Davis W, Crandell C. [2000] TDDs: a survey of utilization and compliance. Paper presented at the Annual Meeting of the American Academy of Audiology, Chicago, IL.)

Davis and Crandell (2000) found that only 30% of businesses and 36% of governmental agencies correctly answered and/or responded to TTY calls (Fig. 34.16). A TTY system can be modified to communicate with a computer (i.e., one individual uses a TTY, while the other individual receives/sends transmissions on his or her computer). To allow this type of communication, an interface option is required to process the slower transmission rate of the Baudot code of the TTY to the faster transmission speed (American Standard Code for Information Interchange [ASCII]) of the computer. Several teletext computer programs have also become available over the past several years. These programs allow the user to communicate to TTY units, computers, or touchtone telephones via typewritten messages or synthesized voice. More recently, companies have developed portable units that can convert handheld devices to TTYs or to voice carryover (VCO) telephones. VCO allows individuals to use their own voice on the telephone, while allowing them to read the other person's response on a small LCD screen incorporated into the VCO telephone. People who are hard of hearing or deaf but have clear, understandable speech usually use VCO. A person wanting to make a VCO starts by calling a relay service. The relay service communication assistant acts as a go between by typing the called person's verbal responses so they appear on the caller's VCO telephone.

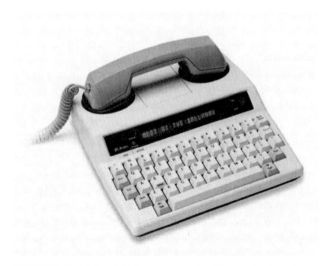

FIGURE 34.15   A telecommunications device for the deaf (TDD) that consists of a keyboard and a telephone cradle on top. (Photo courtesy of Silent Call, Clarkston, MI.)

MOBILE PHONE

The mobile phone quickly has become a pervasive multimedia platform for communication. Because these phones can connect to the internet, much of the assistive communication technology such as text messaging, e-mail, video conferencing, and Bluetooth interconnectivity is available in a highly compact and portable form. Downloads of text and video information to mobile phones from the internet are already possible, and the capabilities of these phones are sure to expand in the future.

Federal Communications Commission Rules Governing Telephony for the Deaf and Hard of Hearing

A common complaint of listeners with SNHL is difficulty understanding speech over the telephone. The Hearing Aid Compatibility Act of 1988 (HAC Act) requires that the FCC ensure that all "essential" telephones and all telephones manufactured or imported for use in the United States after August 1989 are hearing aid compatible. FCC rules require that phones subject to the HAC Act: (1) produce a magnetic field of sufficient strength and quality to permit coupling with hearing aids that contain telecoils; and (2) provide amplification with a volume control so the phone can be effectively used by individuals with hearing loss (with or without hearing aids). In 2003, the FCC adopted rules to make digital wireless telephones compatible with hearing aids and cochlear implants. The FCC's timetable for the development and sale of digital wireless phones that are compatible with hearing aids gradually increases the number of phones and types of services that will enable those who wear hearing aids to have effective access. The reader is referred to the FCC website (http://www.fcc.gov/cgb/consumerfacts/hac_wireless.html) for a complete description of these rules.

Communication through Facsimile Transmission

An older but still effective form of technology that can aid communication for individuals with hearing or speech difficulties is facsimile or fax machines. Facsimile transmission provides the ability to send a copy of a document almost instantly and inexpensively. With a standard fax machine, a hardcopy message is scanned, encoded, and compressed by the machine that is sending the fax. That information is then transmitted over telecommunication lines to the receiving fax machine. The receiving machine then decodes, decompresses, and prints the information. More recent technology enables faxing over the internet or via e-mail. With this method, a scanner and computer replace the standard fax machine. All-in-one printers with both traditional fax and scanners are also available for use with computers.

Communication through Video Conferencing

Video conferencing technology has become common for business situations, distance teaching and learning, and interpersonal communication. With such technology, a camera-based system is placed on the computer or TV. Both the caller and the person receiving the call must have the camera-based system and supporting software in order to use this technology and thus receive both the audio and video signals. Systems are also now available that provide for full motion video support for sign language. Keyboard-produced text and TDD capabilities are also available options. Video conferencing using more traditional telephone transmission has dramatically improved, but internet- and satellite-based telephony is growing in use and will probably eclipse the use of traditional phone transmission.

RECENT CROSSOVER TECHNOLOGIES WITH APPLICATION TO THE DEAF AND HARD OF HEARING

Multi-Use Handheld Devices

Over the past several years, handheld multi-use devices have become commonplace. For example, a single device may serve as a cell phone with video screen, text messenger, and digital camera. In addition, the device can access the internet, send and receive e-mail, receive internet broadcasts or webcasts, and contain technology that enables it to communicate with several other electronic devices at any given time. Although these features may be integrated within a single device, they are described individually in greater detail in the following sections.

BLUETOOTH

Bluetooth is a short-range wireless technology that can connect a wide variety of electronic devices. Bluetooth operates in the 2.4- to 2.5-GHz frequency range and has a range of approximately 10 meters. Due to the high frequency range and the method of transmission, Bluetooth requires only very small antennas and allows several devices to be connected simultaneously (Qian et al., 2003). Hundreds of products use this technology. For a current list of products, the reader is referred to www.bluetooth.com. One HAT product that has been made commercially available recently is an ear-level device that couples to BTE hearing aids through the DAI port. The device then can communicate with other Bluetooth-enabled devices, such as cell phones, TVs, and computers. For example, users can hear their cell phones ring through a hearing aid, push a button to activate the Bluetooth device, and receive the phone signal through the hearing aid via the Bluetooth device. Furthermore, the user's voice is picked up via a microphone built into the ear-level device, which is relayed to the cell phone. The device automatically ends the connection when the call is finished. Essentially, the cell phone itself is used only for dialing phone numbers. Individuals whose hearing aids do not have DAI can still couple their hearing aids to cell phones by plugging a compatible neckloop into the audio output jack of the cell phone.

TEXT MESSAGING/TEXT PAGER

These technologies enable individuals to send and receive text messages between handheld devices, such as cell phones, or from computers to cell phones. The allowable length of a text message depends on the type of messaging service, wireless network, and cell phone model; however, most text messages are limited to about 160 characters. Due to this limitation, text messages often include abbreviations. For example, "URGR8" is an abbreviation for "you are great." Research has demonstrated that text messaging is a popular form of communication between deaf individuals. As text-based communication continues to gain popularity, it may assist in breaking down barriers in communication between individuals with hearing loss and those with normal hearing. For further information regarding use of text messaging and text pagers, the reader is referred to Power and Power (2004), and Thurlow (2002).

RELAY SERVICES

Telephone relay services (TRS) are available to the TTY user who needs to communicate with a non-TTY user. With the TRS, the individual using the TTY types a message to a state-designated central telephone number that is picked up by a normal-hearing operator and, in turn, transmitted verbally to the non-TTY user. The non-TTY user can then respond to the TTY user by speaking to the relay operator, who, in turn, relays the message via written text to the TTY user. Thus, with TRSs, individuals with normal hearing ability can telephone individuals who use TTYs.

Video relay allows a person who is deaf or hard of hearing to make a call to a traditional voice phone number but allows them to use sign language transmitted via a camera or video phone instead of text. When using a computer, the person goes to the appropriate website, enters the number to be called, and can then begin the conversation. An interpreter watches the person signing and verbally translates to the person being called. Responses from the person being called are then translated into sign language by the interpreter. Several video relay services are available:

- Hands On Video Relay Services (http://www.hovrs.com)
- Communication Access Center (http://www.cacvrs.org/)
- Sprint VRS (https://www.sprintvrs.com/)
- Sorenson Video Relay Services (http://www.sorensonvrs.com)
- AT&T (http://www.attvrs.com/)
- Communication Services for the Deaf (http://www.csdvrs.org/)
- IP-Relay.com (http://www.ip-vrs.com/)

Relay calls can also be placed using certain instant messenger services or multi-use handheld devices. Federal Relay Conference Captioning (RCC) is also available. This government-mandated service allows individuals with hearing loss to participate in conference calls with users on voice lines by providing services including video relay and live captioning. The caption can then be read on any computer with an Internet connection. This service is free to all federal employees.

COMMUNICATION TECHNOLOGIES AND THE HOME COMPUTER

The home computer has enabled people with hearing loss (and people with normal hearing) to have better access to communications. Technologies that are available via a home computer that has network/Internet capabilities include electronic mail (e-mail), instant messaging (IM), video conferencing, and internet audio broadcasts or webcasts. E-mail allows a user to send and receive text messages that, in turn, can also have attachments of photos or electronic files. These messages can be sent and received almost instantly, and most can be of unlimited length. E-mail allows users to sort and store messages sent to them. Limitations of e-mail include total file size of the email (which may limit the size or number of attachments), available storage space on the home computer or remote server, spam (receiving unsolicited advertising via e-mail), and the spreading of computer viruses through e-mail.

Unlike e-mail, IM allows two computer users to communicate in real time via text messages sent through the IM software. Therefore, IM is more conversational in nature than e-mail. Many people with hearing loss are using IM more often because IM is faster than TTY. IM conversations can also be saved to an electronic file and can be printed via the computer printer.

Web telephone software use has increased in popularity recently. Generally, a broadband connection with access to voice-over internet protocol (VoIP) and a computer microphone and speakers are required for the use of web phones. Potential advantages of this technology include high-fidelity reproduction of sound compared to standard phone lines and the ability of each user to raise or lower the volume of the received message using the computer's speakers or internal volume control. One advantage of using computer speakers is that the volume can be adjusted more readily, and unlike standard telephones, the signal should not interfere with the use of hearing aids. The disadvantage of external speakers is that the other person may hear an echo of his or her own voice if the speaker volume is too high. This problem can be alleviated for the most part by using headphones or induction neckloops connected to the headphone slot.

Webcasts, or Internet broadcasts, enable the relatively low-cost distribution of prerecorded audio files for download to the computer, portable digital audio devices, and some mobile telephones. In an educational setting, netcasts may be used to reinforce classroom teaching and may enable individuals with hearing loss to access the material at their own speed. Debevc and Peljhan (2004) reported that adults and students who had access to web-based lectures performed better than adults using traditional lectures.

ELECTRONIC CHAT ROOMS AND DISCUSSION BOARDS

Internet chat rooms and discussion boards have become a very popular means of communication. Chat rooms can be formed based on a discussion topic and can be specially created for communication among individuals who are deaf or have hearing loss. The chat can be synchronous, meaning that everyone is online and communicating simultaneously. The discussion boards are asynchronous, meaning that messages and responses are posted by people online at different times. Both chat rooms and discussion boards can be used to reinforce classroom teaching or for distance education.

ALERTING SYSTEMS

For a person with hearing loss, common appliances that rely on sound to convey a signal to the user may not be useful. The term "alerting systems" is used to describe devices that can focus the user's attention and/or indicate the presence of sounds in the environment through one of three modalities: auditory (e.g., amplified or lowered pitch signal), visual (e.g., turning on/off lamp, strobe light, bright incandescent light), or vibrotactile (e.g., devices that vibrate, such as pocket pagers and bed shakers, or increases in airstream, such as a fan). These devices are widely available and are often thought to be appropriate for individuals with profound degrees of hearing loss; however, many such devices may also be beneficial for persons with milder degrees of hearing loss. For example, many persons with high-frequency hearing loss can exhibit difficulties hearing the microwave timer, doorbell, or telephone ringer, particularly if they are not in the same room as that device.

Direct Electrical Connect Systems

Direct electrical connect systems are interfaced permanently with, and activated directly by, the electrical system of the sound-activating device. For example, the alerting device may be connected directly to the telephone, alarm clock, microwave timer, or doorbell. When the device is activated, a visual, auditory, or tactile signal is transmitted to the individual. Generally speaking, such devices, while highly reliable for alerting purposes, are not portable.

Sound-Activated Systems

Sound-activated systems use a microphone to detect the presence of a particular environmental sound and relay the signal to an alerting system. For example, a microphone placed near the microwave or oven timer can inform the individual via an alerting system, such as a body-worn vibrotactile device or on/off activation of a lamp, when that timer has been activated. Another common example of this technology is the placement of a sound-activated microphone near a baby crib so that parents can be informed when the child cries or makes noises. Sound-activated systems generally have sensitivity settings to reduce the possibility of other environmental sounds activating the system. Sound-activated systems are portable and therefore may be advantageous to an individual with hearing loss who is traveling. Recent technologies have been developed that allow the user with hearing loss to monitor important traffic noises (such as emergency vehicles and car horns) when driving.

Induction-Based Systems

Induction-based systems use the electromagnetic field emitted from an activated electrical device to trigger a separate alerting device. An electromagnetic detector is typically placed via suction cup onto an electrical device such as a telephone. When the phone rings, the electromagnetic field that is generated triggers an alerting device such as a flashing table light. Although such systems are easy to use and portable, incorrect placement of the detector can cause the system to malfunction.

Hearing Dogs

In addition to traditional alerting systems, an individual with hearing loss may also choose to use a professionally trained hearing dog to indicate important environmental sounds. These dogs are trained to attract the attention of the person with hearing loss when particular sounds occur (such as a phone ringing) and to lead them to the source of the sound. In most states, restrictions on the use of hearing dogs in public places are similar to restrictions on guide dogs for individuals with loss of vision.

ASSESSING COMMUNICATION DEFICITS AND NEEDS

The aural rehabilitation process is designed to minimize the communication deficits caused by a hearing loss. The first step in this process is a thorough evaluation of the audiologic dimensions of the hearing loss. In addition to the usual comprehensive audiologic tests, which include pure-tone and speech audiometry and immittance measures, the individual's speech perception ability (using stimuli such as nonsense syllables, monosyllabic words, and sentences in quiet and noise) and central auditory processing capabilities should be evaluated. These procedures are discussed elsewhere in this handbook. Furthermore, a communication disability and needs assessment is a crucial component of the rehabilitative process. On the basis of the audiologic and communication assessments, audiologists can provide counseling regarding technologies and/or therapies that will minimize the impact of the individual's hearing loss in everyday activities. Evaluating communication needs or disability can be a daunting activity because it often is difficult to assess. Tye-Murray (2004) discussed four possible causes underlying this difficulty. First, communication handicap varies as a function of the communication setting and communication partner. For example, an individual may have a significant handicap in some situations when talking with unfamiliar people, yet have little handicap in quiet situations with a well-known family member. Second, handicap can vary as a function of the topic of conversation. A person may have no handicap when discussing the weather but may experience great obstacles during a discussion involving an unfamiliar topic. Third, handicap does not always manifest itself during conversations between the clinician and the individual with hearing loss. The office assessment is merely a snapshot in time that may not be representative of real communication ability or disability. Fourth, communication handicap is a construct made up of many dimensions; no single assessment measure is likely to capture all of these dimensions. As a result, several assessment measures should be taken in order to obtain a more comprehensive overview of an individual's communication handicap in various everyday life situations.

A number of procedures have been developed to quantify the extent of communication handicap imposed on the individual as a result of hearing loss. The same procedures can be used to monitor and document the effectiveness of interventions in reducing the communication handicap. Tye-Murray (2004) presents five general procedures. The first of these is the interview process, wherein specific information about a person's hearing problems is elicited through the use of informal or formalized questions. One of the problems with the interview process is that it is hard to quantify the responses of the individual with hearing loss. However, an interview approach called the Client Oriented Scale of Improvement (Dillon et al., 1997) requires the interviewees to rank order the five listening priorities they wish to address through the intervention process. The quantification of these problems can then be used as a measure for assessing whether the intervention has been effective. If the initial problem areas are no longer considered to be problematic or if the rank ordering changes to a lower ranking, the intervention might be considered to be successful.

A second procedure is the use of a questionnaire. Many hearing handicap questionnaires have been developed and can be quite useful if the questions match the everyday listening situations of individuals with hearing loss. A hearing handicap scale that is well matched to the individual can provide important information concerning the effectiveness of intervention. If after the intervention the individual reports a reduced hearing handicap, then the intervention can be considered effective.

A third procedure to evaluate communicative handicap is a daily log or diary, wherein the individual provides quantitative information about his or her communication difficulties. These logs provide an ongoing self-report of changes that occur as a result of the intervention and can be used to assess the intervention's effectiveness. In addition, in reporting use of communication strategies, the client may actually become more skilled at using the recommended strategies. For this reason, daily logs can be used as part of a training procedure.

A fourth procedure, group discussion, also can serve as an effective measure of communication handicap. The interactions that occur during a group discussion between persons with hearing loss often force individuals to reflect on their communication problems and possible solutions. Over time, group interactions can provide information and psychosocial support and thereby empower individuals to accept their hearing loss and encourage them to explore technologies that may maximize their potential.

The fifth procedure is called structured communication interactions, in which conversations between the individual with hearing loss and the evaluator are simulated to reflect communication situations typical for that person. The effectiveness of intervention can be assessed directly by simulating difficult communication situations with and without HAT.

Extended audiologic and communication handicap evaluations allow the audiologist to have a comprehensive picture of the auditory capabilities and communication needs of the client. This information is integrated into the counseling phase, and a rehabilitative plan is determined. Typically, such a plan would involve consideration of hearing aids, assistive devices, and a communication strategies training program (Compton, 1993; Tye-Murray, 2004). All three facets should be considered and integrated in order for communication handicap intervention to be most effective. Unfortunately, too often only one of the three options, the hearing aid evaluation, is suggested and implemented.

The technology requirements for effective communication for a particular individual will vary depending on setting and on the type of communication (e.g., face-to-face, over the telephone). The outcomes can be assessed through the assessment procedure as discussed earlier. Practical frameworks for this decision-making process have been presented elsewhere (Compton, 1993).

Communication Strategies Training

As a result of the audiologic and communication assessments, recommendations can be made regarding appropriate hearing aids and assistive devices. However, to have maximum impact on the communication handicap, the person must also be provided with the means to take ownership of his or her own communication environment and to have the psychosocial and behavioral tools to minimize miscommunication in everyday listening situations. The process by which the client is provided these tools is known as communication strategies training and is an important component of an overall audiologic rehabilitation plan. Tye-Murray (2004) conceptualizes communication strategies training as being composed of three stages. In the formal instruction stage, the client is provided with information about various types of communication strategies and appropriate listening and speaking behaviors. Included are presentations describing facilitative strategies (tactics a person can use to improve the reception of a message by varying the message, the speaker, the environment, and/or the listener), receptive and expressive repair strategies (tactics a person can use when a message is not understood), and instruction in using clear speech (a speaking technique for making speech highly intelligible).

The second stage is called guided learning. In this stage, the professional creates simulated real-life communication situations in which the strategies acquired in the formal instruction stage can be practiced. The audiologist provides feedback and tips to clients as they progress through the simulations.

The last stage requires the client to engage in prescribed real-world listening situations and to answer prepared questions regarding the effectiveness of the information learned in stage one and practiced in stage two. The reader is referred to Tye-Murray (2004) for a complete description of the communication strategies training component of the rehabilitative process.

OUTCOME MEASURES

Whenever HAT is recommended, it is important for the audiologist to identify and quantify the effects of the recommendation (Kane, 1997). Not only is this documentation often required by third-party payers, but also, as a profession, feedback for our recommendations is a means to establish best practices. In the realm of hearing aids, there are a number of approaches to measuring rehabilitative outcomes (see Weinstein [2000] for a review). Tools for measuring the efficacy of technology in the classroom are also available (Crandell et al., 2005). These and other measures can be used to document the changes that occur as the result of recommending or fitting an assistive device. For example, the Client Oriented Scale of Improvement (Dillon et al., 1997) could be used with assistive technologies as easily as hearing aids for which the assessment measure was designed. In either case, the client is required to list situations in which hearing help is needed and rate the difficulty experienced in each situation. After intervention (the fitting of a hearing aid or other HAT), the list is reviewed and re-rated to document changes as a result of the intervention.

REHABILITATION TECHNOLOGY IN THE AUDIOLOGY SETTING

Although this chapter has addressed the many advantages that assistive technologies can provide to listeners with hearing loss, research shows that these listeners are often unaware of assistive technology, and relatively few audiologists are actively dispensing such technologies. Mahon (1985)

suggested that individuals with hearing loss are generally unaware of HAT due to two factors. First, historically, audiologists (and hearing aid dispensers) have been somewhat indifferent to incorporating assistive technologies into their available product line. Second, audiologists often do not have an adequate knowledge base to inform their patients accurately about such technologies. Evidence supporting the first assumption is provided through Cranmer (1991) who reported that assistive technologies accounted for less than 2% of gross sales revenues for audiologists and hearing aid dealers. In an earlier study, Malinoff et al. (1990) surveyed 921 hearing aid dispensers and audiologists regarding the instruments and services those professionals felt were most beneficial in their practices. Discouragingly, assistive technologies and auditory rehabilitation were ranked last in order of importance. Support for the second assumption is found in a study by McCarthy et al. (1983). The authors showed that a majority of 50 individuals with hearing loss were unaware of the various assistive technologies available despite the fact they reported difficulties in most listening situations. When informed about assistive devices, many of the subjects were subsequently interested in purchasing the assistive technologies. More recently, Stika et al. (2002) reported that, in their survey, only 31% of hearing aid users recall being informed of HATs. Sadly, hearing assistive devices still represent only 2% of the gross revenues of hearing aid dispensers (Strom, 2004), which is unchanged from the gross revenues reported by Cramer in 1999. It is obvious that audiologists continue to underrate the importance and benefits of assistive technologies. This is unfortunate because there is ample evidence that integrating assistive technologies into our rehabilitative plans can be very effective when hearing aids are not enough (Chisolm et al., 2004; Wayner, 2004).

Consumer Acceptance of Assistive Technologies

Audiologists themselves must first be convinced of the value of assistive technologies in the overall rehabilitative plan for a client. Until now, great emphasis has been placed on the proper fitting of hearing aids, while little attention has been given to the benefits of HAT for addressing the rehabilitative needs of the individual with hearing loss. Therefore, the first step in creating consumer acceptance of these technologies is the development of a philosophy of rehabilitation that includes a multidimensional assessment of the individual's auditory and communication capabilities and needs. An outline of how this can be accomplished has been presented in this chapter. Within the context of the comprehensive rehabilitative plan, the value of assistive technologies is self-evident because these technologies are an integral part of the services provided in the rehabilitative plan for an individual, along with hearing aids and communication strategies training.

Outside of a carefully constructed rehabilitation program, there is a need to engage in activities for enhancing consumer acceptance of assistive technology. The same negative stigmas that are attached to hearing loss and hearing aids are likely to be attached to assistive devices and likely will occur to an even greater extent because assistive technologies are typically more noticeable and intimidating than a hearing aid. Sutherland (1995) details the following strategies for increasing consumer acceptance of assistive technologies: (1) educating consumers about technical devices, including their strengths and limitations; (2) training consumers to use technical devices; (3) helping consumers to make informed choices; (4) providing consumers with support; (5) encouraging experienced consumers to help others who are just learning about technical devices; (6) empowering consumers by working closely with them as part of a team or partnership; and (7) aligning with consumers to advocate for better laws and services and for universal accessibility for people with hearing loss. Wayner (2004) describes how assistive devices can be integrated into a hearing aid practice in order to increase awareness and acceptance. Wayner (2004) describes how an assistive device demonstration center was established in the classrooms where hearing aid orientations were performed. In this way, devices could be demonstrated in conjunction with hearing aids in difficult listening situations when hearing aids alone might not provide enough assistance. In a study of the effectiveness of the integrated center, Wayner (2004) reported that 86% of those surveyed found the center helpful and reported satisfaction with learning about assistive technologies and having the opportunity to try the technologies. In the same study, 75% of those purchasing HAT used the technology regularly and reported benefit in conjunction with their hearing aids or cochlear implants in daily activities. It is clear that integration of assistive technologies into our rehabilitative services is a best practice goal for our rehabilitative efforts. In order to accomplish this best practice goal, higher priority must be given to the evaluation, selection, and dispensing of assistive technologies.

■ LEGISLATION FOR HEARING ASSISTANCE TECHNOLOGY

During the 1980s and 1990s, the civil and education rights of individuals with disabilities were strengthened, and the important role that assistive technologies has in improving the quality of life of disabled individuals was recognized. Since 1988, federal laws specifically addressing the HAT needs of persons with disabilities have been passed.

Beginning in 1975 with the Education of All Handicapped Children Act and with the implementation of the Americans with Disabilities Act (1990) and, most recently, the 2004 reauthorization of the Individuals with Disabilities Education Act of 1997, there has been a sustained interest in removing barriers for persons with hearing loss and other disabilities. One of the ways that acoustic barriers to communication can be diminished is through the use of assistive listening technology. These technologies have been included as a reasonable accommodation under many federal laws

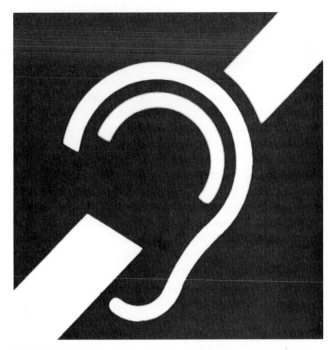

FIGURE 34.17   International symbol of access for individuals with hearing loss. (Photo courtesy of the National Association of the Deaf.)

(Access Board Website, 1998; Education of Handicapped Children, P.L., 94-142, 1977; Education of Handicapped Children, P.L., 99-457, 1986; Education of Handicapped Children, P.L., 101-476, 1990; Individuals with Disabilities Education Act, 1997; 2004). For example, in rooms that require permanently installed assistive technologies, the availability of such technologies must be posted using the international symbol of access for persons with hearing loss (Fig. 34.17).

■ HEARING ASSISTANCE TECHNOLOGY RESEARCH NEEDS

There is an ever-expanding need for research concerning assistive devices. This need is driven by the federally enforceable standards for accessibility and accommodations for hearing loss in the Americans with Disabilities Act, as well as an awareness on the part of many audiologists that, by including assistive technology in their rehabilitative plans, they can significantly improve the quality of care provided. Assistive technologies are constantly changing. As a result, one of the biggest research needs in the field of audiology is the development of protocols that can better evaluate the needs of individuals with hearing loss and a method for efficiently matching needs to technologies. Thibodeau (2004) describes a new assessment tool called the TELEGRAM to help meet a client's communication needs beyond the hearing aid. The acronym stands for communication areas assessed: Telephone, Employment, Legal issues, Entertainment, Group communication, Recreation, Alarms, and Members of the family. Information about a client's function in each of these areas is plotted on a multidimensional assessment form that rates the client's difficulty on a scale ranging from no difficulty to great difficulty. The multidimensional plot is analogous to an audiogram and can be used to identify areas in which additional technology or information is needed for clients to maximize their communication potential. Compton-Conley and Bernstein (2006) are in the process of developing a computerized needs assessment for assistive technologies. The online needs assessment tool, the Hearing Assistance Technology Needs Assessment Profile (HAT-NAP), will analyze an individual's receptive communication needs based on a needs questionnaire and generate a receptive communication "profile" for that individual. According to Compton-Conley and Bernstein (2006), the generated profile can be used to identify and select the most appropriate combination of technology/training that will provide the widest range of communication access to specifically address that individual's needs and lifestyle. An accompanying online tutorial designed to educate both consumers and audiologists regarding the various assistive technologies and communication strategies will also be available.

In addition to developing tools for the selection process, we must also have tools that allow us to measure the efficacy of the technology more accurately. Since any one technology might be used in a variety of situations, it is important to measure whether that technology is equally effective in all circumstances or if there are situations/populations for which that technology has a distinct advantage. Research is needed to explore ways that legislatures and rural school districts can make Internet resources and HAT more widely available in rural educational settings (for example, the use of electronic technology could be expanded to provide instructional services to individuals in rural areas who are deaf or have hearing loss). One final research area involves exploring ways to make assistive technologies more accessible and acceptable to those in need (e.g., telehealth). Telehealth is defined as the use of telecommunications and information technologies to share information and to provide clinical care, education, public health, and administrative services at a distance. Effective and efficient ways to use telehealth to inform individuals who are deaf or have hearing loss about available assistive technologies and perhaps make the technologies more acceptable to these consumers continues to be a research challenge.

SUMMARY

There is a growing awareness of the negative influence of room acoustics on the adequate perception of speech and on communication. The influences of distance, background noise, and reverberation are well documented. Various assistive technologies (such as induction loop, FM, and infrared assistive listening systems) and communication strategies can be used alone or together to reduce the influence

of poor room acoustics on communication. This chapter also covered other assistive devices that have been designed to improve receptive communication in situations such as those involving face-to-face communication, broadcast media, telecommunications, and alerting situations as well as methods to augment the capabilities of assistive devices. In order for HAT to be accepted and used by an individual with hearing loss, however, the communication needs and proper selection of assistive devices must be conducted within the context of an overall rehabilitative plan. Outside of the comprehensive rehabilitative plan, there is still a need to engage in activities to improve consumer acceptance of assistive devices and to help people understand the federal mandates that are already in place to remove acoustic barriers to communication. Research is needed to improve the type and quality of assistive devices available to individuals with hearing loss and to develop better methods of identifying the individuals who will benefit most from a particular technology. HAT offers the hearing health care professional a significant challenge but, at the same time, a wonderful opportunity to maximize the client's communication *and* human potential.

DEDICATION

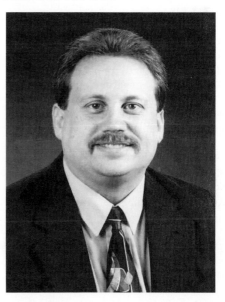

My dear friend and colleague, Carl Crandell passed away before he and I could finish revising this chapter. He was very excited about all of the new assistive technologies that have been developed since the chapter was first written in the previous edition of the Handbook. *It was Carl's wish to have some of his best students contribute to the revision. Brian and Nicole Kreisman and Andrew John ably filled in where Carl had left off. Still, much of Carl remains in the text, and I hope you will find inspiration and education in his words, for his words will not pass this way again.*

Joseph Smaldino

Sycamore, Illinois

REFERENCES

Access Board. (1998) Homepage. http:www.access-board.gov.

Allen L. (1993) Promoting the usefulness of classroom amplification. *Educ Audiol Monogr.* 3, 32–34.

American National Standards Institute. (1983) American National Standard Specification for Sound Level Meters. ANSI S1.14-1983 (R2006). New York: American National Standards Institute.

American National Standards Institute. (2002) Acoustic Performance Criteria, Design Requirements and Guidelines for Classrooms. ANSI S12.6-2002. New York: American National Standards Institute.

American Speech, Language, and Hearing Association. (1995) Guidelines for acoustics in educational environments. *ASHA.* 37 (suppl 14), 15–19.

Americans with Disabilities Act. Public Law 101-336-1990. Available at: http://www.usdoj.gov/crt/ada/adahom1.htm.

Barron M. (1993) *Auditorium Acoustics and Architectural Design.* London: E & FN Spon.

Berg F. (1993) *Acoustics and Sound Systems in Schools.* Boston: College-Hill Press.

Bess F. (1985) The minimally hearing-impaired child. *Ear Hear.* 6, 43–47.

Bess F, Lichtenstein M, Logan S, Burger C, Nelson E. (1989) Hearing loss as a determinant of function in the elderly. *J Am Geriatr Soc.* 37, 123–128.

Bess F, Sinclair J, Riggs D. (1986) Group amplification in schools for the hearing-impaired. *Ear Hear.* 5, 138–144.

Bess F, Tharpe A. (1986) An introduction to unilateral sensorineural hearing loss in children. *Ear Hear.* 7, 3–13.

Blair J. (1977) The effects of amplification, speechreading and classroom environments on reception of speech. *Volta Rev.* 77, 443–449.

Blair J, Myrup C, Viehweg S. (1989) Comparison of the effectiveness of hard-of-hearing children using three types of amplification. *Educ Audiol Monogr.* 1, 48–55.

Bolt R, MacDonald A. (1949) Theory of speech masking by reverberation. *J Acoust Soc Am.* 21, 577–580.

Boothroyd A. (2005) Modeling the effects of room acoustics on speech reception and perception. In: Crandell C, Smaldino J, Flexer C, eds. *Sound Field Amplification: Applications to Speech Perception and Classroom Acoustics.* 2nd ed. Clifton Park, NY: Thomson Delmar Learning.

Bradley J. (1986) Speech intelligibility studies in classrooms. *J Acoust Soc Am.* 80, 846–854.

Chisolm T, McArdle R, Abrams H, Noe C. (2004) Goals and outcomes of FM use by adults. *Hear J.* 57, 28–35.

Christian E, Dluhy N, O'Neill R. (1989) Sounds of silence: coping with hearing loss and loneliness. *J Gerontol Nurs.* 15, 4–10.

Compton C. (1993) Assistive technology. In: Alpiner J, McCarthy P, eds. *Rehabilitative Audiology: Children and Adults.* Baltimore: Williams & Wilkins.

Compton-Conley C, Bernstein C. (2006) RERC-HE Conference, September 2006, Washington, DC.

Cooper J, Cutts B. (1971) Speech discrimination in noise. *J Speech Hear Res.* 14, 332–337.

Crandell C (1988) Hearing aids: their effects on functional health status. *Hear J.* 51, 22–30.

Crandell C. (1991) Classroom acoustics for normal-hearing children: implications for rehabilitation. *Educ Audiol Monogr.* 2, 18–38.

Crandell C. (1992) Speech recognition in the elderly listener: the importance of the acoustical environment. *Texas J Audiol Speech Pathol.* 17, 25–30.

Crandell C. (1993) Noise effects on the speech recognition of children with minimal hearing loss. *Ear Hear.* 7, 210–217.

Crandell C, Bess F. (1986) Speech recognition of children in a "typical" classroom setting. *ASHA.* 28, 82.

Crandell C, Bess F. (1987) Sound-field amplification in the classroom setting. *ASHA.* 29, 87.

Crandell C, Ege L. (2000) Effects of attenuated and non-attenuated headphones on speech perception in personal FM systems. Unpublished Paper.

Crandell C, Henoch M, Dunkerson K. (1991) A review of speech perception and aging: some implications for aural rehabilitation. *J Acad Rehab Audiol.* 24, 121–132.

Crandell C, Smaldino J. (1994) The importance of room acoustics. In: Tyler R, Schum D, eds. *Assistive Listening Devices for the Hearing Impaired.* Baltimore: William & Wilkins; pp 142–164.

Crandell C, Smaldino J. (1995) An update of classroom acoustics for children with hearing loss. *Volta Rev.* 1, 4–12.

Crandell C, Smaldino J. (1996) Sound field amplification in the classroom: applied and theoretical issues. In: Bess F, Gravel J, Tharpe A, eds. *Amplification for Children with Auditory Deficits.* Nashville: Bill Wilkerson Center Press; pp 229–250.

Crandell C, Smaldino J. (2000) Room acoustics and amplification. In: Valente M, Roeser R, Hosford-Dunn H, eds. *Audiology: Treatment Strategies.* New York: Thieme Medical Publishers.

Crandell C, Smaldino J, Flexer C. (1995) *Sound Field FM Amplification: Theory and Practical Applications.* San Diego: Singular Press.

Crandell C, Smaldino J, Flexer C. (2005) *Sound Field Amplification: Applications to Speech Perception and Classroom Acoustics.* Clifton Park: Thompson Delmar Learning.

Crandell C, Smaldino J, Flexer C, Edwards C. (1997) An update on sound field FM amplification. Paper presented at the Annual Meeting of the American Academy of Audiology, Los Angeles, CA.

Cranmer KS. (1991) Hearing instrument dispensing – 1991. *Hear Instrum.* 42, 6–13.

Davis W, Crandell C. (2000) TDDs: a survey of utilization and compliance. Paper presented at the Annual Meeting of the American Academy of Audiology, Chicago, IL.

Debevc M, Peljhan Z. (2004) The role of video technology in on-line lectures for the deaf. *Disabil Rehabil.* 26, 1048–1059.

Dillon H, James A, Ginis J. (1997) Client oriented scale of improvement (COSI) and its relationship to several other measures of benefit and satisfaction provided by hearing aids. *J Am Acad Audiol.* 8, 27–43.

Duquesnoy A, Plomp R. (1983) The effect of a hearing aid on the speech-reception threshold of hearing-impaired listeners in quiet and in noise. *J Acoust Soc Am.* 73, 2166–2173.

Education of Handicapped Children. (1977) P.L. 94-142 Regulations. 1977, August 23. *Federal Register.* 42, 42474–42518.

Education of Handicapped Act Amendments of 1986. (1986) P.L. 99-457 Regulations. 1986, October 8. *United States Statutes at Large*. 100, 1145–1177.

Education of Handicapped Act Amendments of 1990. (1990) P.L. 101-476 Regulations. 1990, October 30. *United States Statutes at Large*. 104, 1103–1151.

Egan M. (1987) *Architectural Acoustics*. New York: McGraw-Hill Book Company.

Erber N. (1979) Auditory-visual perception of speech with reduced optical clarity. *J Speech Hear Res*. 22, 213–223.

Festen JM, Plomp R. (1990) Effects of fluctuating noise and interfering speech on the speech-reception threshold for impaired and normal hearing. *J Acoust Soc Am*. 88, 1725–1736.

Finitzo-Hieber T. (1988) Classroom acoustics. In: Roeser R, ed. *Auditory Disorders in School Children*. 2nd ed. New York: Thieme-Stratton; pp 221–233.

Finitzo-Hieber T, Tillman T. (1978) Room acoustics effects on monosyllabic word discrimination ability for normal and hearing-impaired children. *J Speech Hear Res*. 21, 440–458.

Flexer C. (1992) Classroom public address systems. In: Ross M, ed. *FM Auditory Training Systems: Characteristics, Selection and Use*. Timonium, MD: York Press; pp 189–209.

Flexer C. (1993) Management of hearing in an educational setting. In: Apliner J, McCarthy P, eds. *Rehabilitative Audiology: Children and Adults*. Baltimore: Williams & Wilkins; pp 176–210.

French N, Steinberg J. (1947) Factors governing the intelligibility of speech sounds. *J Acoust Soc Am*. 19, 90–19.

Gelfand S, Silman S. (1979) Effects of small room reverberation upon the recognition of some consonant features. *J Acoust Soc Am*. 66, 22–29.

Gustafsson HA, Arlinger SD. (1994) Masking of speech by amplitude-modulated noise. *J Acoust Soc Am*. 95, 518–529.

Haas H. (1972) The influence of a single echo on the audibility of speech. *J Audio Eng Soc*. 20, 146–159.

Harris C. (1991) *Handbook of Acoustical Measurements and Noise Control*. New York: McGraw-Hill.

Hawkins D, Yacullo W. (1984) Signal-to-noise ratio advantage of binaural hearing aids and directional microphones under different levels of reverberation. *J Speech Hear Dis*. 49, 278–286.

Hendricks P, Lederman N. (1991) Development of a three-dimensional induction assistive listening system. *Hear Instrum*. 42, 37–38.

Hygge S, Rönnberg J, Larsby B, Arlinger S. (1992) Normal-hearing and hearing-impaired subjects' ability to just follow conversation in competing speech, reversed speech, and noise backgrounds. *J Speech Hear Res*. 35, 208–215.

Individuals with Disabilities Education Act. (1997) Homepage. Available at: http://www.ed.gov/offices/OSERS/Policy/IDEA/index.html.

Individuals with Disabilities Education Act. (2004) IDEA 2004 News, Information and Resources. Available at: http://www.ed.gov/offices/OSERS/IDEA/.

Johnson C. (2000) Children's phoneme identification in reverberation and noise. *J Speech Lang Hear Res*. 43, 144–157.

Kane R. (1997) Improving outcomes in rehabilitation: a call to arms. *Med Car*. 35, JS4–JS7.

Killion M. (1997) SNR loss: I can hear what people say, but I can't understand them. *Hear Rev*. 4, 10, 12, 14.

Knecht HA, Nelson PB, Whitelaw GM, Feth LL. (2002) Background noise levels and reverberation times in unoccupied classrooms: predictions and measurements. *Am J Audiol*. 11, 65–71.

Kreisman B. (2003) The effects of simulated reverberation on the speech-perception abilities of listeners with normal hearing. Doctoral dissertation. Gainesville, FL: University of Florida.

Leavitt R, Flexer C. (1991) Speech degradation as measured by the Rapid Speech Transmission Index (RASTI). *Ear Hear*. 12, 115–118.

Lewis D. (1998) Classroom amplification. In: Bess F, ed. *Children with Hearing Loss: Contemporary Trends*. Nashville: Vanderbilt Bill Wilkerson Center Press; pp 277–298.

Lichtenstein MJ, Bess FH, Logan S. (1988) Validation of screening tools for identifying hearing-impaired elderly in primary care. *J Am Med Assoc*. 259, 2875–2878.

Licklider J, Miller G. (1951) The perception of speech. In: Stevens S, ed. *Handbook of Experimental Psychology*. New York: John Wiley.

Lochner J, Burger J. (1964) The influence of reflections in auditorium acoustics. *J Sound Vibrat*. 4, 426–54.

Mahon W. (1985) Assistive devices and systems. *Hear J*. 38, 7–14.

Malinoff R, Kisiel D, Kisiel S, Dygert P. (1990) The dispensing of hearing instruments: a study on industry structures and trends. *Hear Instrum*. 41, 12–14.

Markides A. (1986) Speech levels and speech-to-noise ratios. *Br J Audiol*. 20, 115–120.

McCarthy P, Culpepper N, Winstead T. (1983) Hearing impaired consumer's awareness and attitudes regarding auditory assistive devices. Paper presented at the Annual Meeting of the American Speech, Language, and Hearing Association, Cincinnati, OH.

Middleweerd M, Plomp R. (1987) The effect of speechreading on the speech reception threshold of sentences in noise. *J Acoust Soc Am*. 82, 2145–2146.

Miller G. (1974) Effects of noise on people. *J Acoust Soc Am*. 56, 724–764.

Moncur JP Dirks D. (1967) Binaural and monaural speech intelligibility in reverberation. *J Speech Lang Hear Res*. 10, 186–195.

Montano J. (1994) Rehabilitation technology for the hearing impaired. In: Katz J, ed. *Handbook of Clinical Audiology*. 4th ed. Baltimore: Williams & Wilkins; pp 638–649.

Moore B. (1997) *An Introduction to the Psychology of Hearing*. San Diego: Academic Press.

Mulrow C, Christine A, Endicott J, Tuley M, Velez R, Charlip M, Rhodes M, Hill J, DeNiro L. (1990) Quality-of-life changes and hearing loss. *Ann Intern Med*. 113, 188–194.

Nabelek A. (1982) Temporal distortions and noise considerations. In: Studebaker G, Bess F, eds. *The Vanderbilt Hearing-Aid Report: State of the Art Research Needs*. Upper Darby, PA: Monographs in Contemporary Audiology.

Nabelek A, Donahue A, Letowski T. (1986) Comparison of amplification systems in a classroom. *J Rehab Res Dev*. 23, 41–52.

Nabelek A, Nabelek I. (1994) Room acoustics and speech perception. In Katz J, ed. *Handbook of Clinical Audiology*. 4th ed. Baltimore: Williams & Wilkins.

Nabelek A, Pickett J. (1974a) Monaural and binaural speech perception through hearing aids under noise and reverberation with normal and hearing-impaired listeners. *J Speech Hear Res.* 17, 724–739.

Nabelek A, Pickett J. (1974b) Reception of consonants in a classroom as affected by monaura and binaural listening, noise, reverberation, and hearing aids. *J Acoust Soc Am.* 56, 628–639.

Needleman A, Crandell C. (1996) Speech perception in noise by hearing impaired and masked normal hearing listeners. *J Am Acad Audiol.* 2, 65–72.

Neuman A, Hochberg I. (1983) Children's perception of speech in reverberation. *J Acoust Soc Am.* 73, 2145–2149.

Nober L, Nober E. (1975) Auditory discrimination of learning disabled children in quiet and classroom noise. *J Learn Dis.* 8, 656–773.

Olsen W. (1981) The effects of noise and reverberation on speech intelligibility. In: Bess F, Freeman B, Sinclair J, eds. *Amplification in Education.* Washington, DC: Alexander Graham Bell Association for the Deaf.

Olsen W. (1988) Classroom acoustics for hearing-impaired children. In: Bess F, ed. *Hearing Loss in Children.* Parkton, MD: York Press.

Payton K, Uchanski R, Braida L. (1994) Intelligibility of conversational and clear speech in noise and reverberation for listeners with normal and impaired hearing. *J Acoust Soc Am.* 95, 1581–1592.

Pearsons K, Bennett R, Fidell S. (1977) *Speech levels in various noise environments.* EPA 600/1-77-025. Washington, DC: Office of Health & Ecological Effects.

Picheny M, Durlach N, Braida L. (1985a) Speaking clearly for the hard of hearing. I. Intelligibility differences between clear and conversational speech. *J Speech Hear Res.* 28, 96–103.

Picheny M, Durlach N, Braida L. (1985b) Speaking clearly for the hard of hearing. II. Acoustical characteristics of clear and conversational speech. *J Speech Hear Res.* 29, 434–446.

Plomp R. (1978) Auditory handicap of hearing loss and the limited benefit of hearing aids. *J Acoust Soc Am.* 75, 1253–1258.

Plomp R. (1986) A signal-to-noise ratio model for the speech reception threshold for the hearing impaired. *J Speech Hear Res.* 29, 146–154.

Power MR, Power D. (2004) Everyone here speaks TXT: deaf people using SMS in Australia and the rest of the world. *J Deaf Stud Deaf Educ.* 9, 333–343.

Qian H, Loizou PC, Dorman, MF. (2003) A phone-assistive device based on Bluetooth technology for cochlear implant users. *IEEE Trans Neural Sys Rehab Eng.* 11, 282–287.

Ratnam R, Jones DL, Wheeler BC, O'Brien WD, Feng AS. (2003) Blind estimation of reverberation time. *J Acoust Soc Am.* 114, 2877–2892.

Roberts RA. (2003) Effects of noise and reverberation on the precedence effect in listeners with normal hearing and impaired hearing. *Am J Audiol.* 12, 96–105.

Rosenberg G, Blake-Rahter P. (1995) In-service training for the classroom teacher. In: Crandell C, Smaldino J, Flexer C, eds. *Sound-Field FM Amplification: Theory and Practical Applications.* San Diego: Singular Publishing Group; pp 107–124.

Rosenblum L, Johnson J, Saldana H. (1996) Point-light facial displays enhance comprehension of speech. *J Speech Hear Res.* 39, 1159–1170.

Ross M. (1978) Classroom acoustics and speech intelligibility. In: Katz J, ed. *Handbook of Clinical Audiology.* Baltimore: Williams & Wilkins.

Sanders D. (1965) Noise conditions in normal school classrooms. *Except Child.* 31, 344–353.

Sapienza C, Crandell C, Curtis B. (1999) Effect of sound field FM amplification on vocal intensity in teachers. *J Voice.* 23, 101–110.

Sarff L. (1981) An innovative use of free field amplification in regular classrooms. In: Roeser R, Downs M, eds. *Auditory Disorders in School Children.* New York: Thieme-Stratton; pp 263–272.

Sarff L, Ray H, Bagwell C. (1981) Why not amplification in every classroom? *Hear Aid J.* 11, 44, 47–48, 50, 52.

Schow R, Nerbonne M. (1996) *Introduction to Audiologic Rehabilitation.* 3rd ed. Boston: Allyn and Bacon.

Schum D. (1996) Intelligibility of clear and conversational speech of young and elderly listeners. *J Am Acad Audiol.* 7, 212–218.

Sher A, Owens E. (1974) Consonants phonemic errors associated with hearing loss above 2000 Hz. *J Speech Hear Res.* 17, 656–668.

Siebein G. (1994) *Acoustics in Buildings: A Tutorial on Architectural Acoustics.* New York: Acoustical Society of America.

Siebein G, Crandell C, Gold M. (1997) Principles of classroom acoustics: reverberation. *Educ Audiol Monogr.* 5, 32–43.

Spicer J, Schmidt R, Ward CD, Pinnington LL. (2005) Evaluation of text telephones designed for people with impaired hearing or speech. *J Med Eng Technol.* 29, 137–144.

Stika C, Ross M, Cuevas C. (2002) Hearing aid services and satisfaction: the consumer viewpoint. *Hearing Loss.* May/June, 25–31.

Strom K. (2004) The HR dispenser survey. *Hear Rev.* Available at: http://www.hearingreview.com/issues/articles/2004-06_01.asp.

Sutherland G. (1995) Increasing consumer acceptance of assistive devices. In: Tyler RS, Schum DJ, eds. *Assistive Devices for Persons with Hearing Loss.* Needham Heights, MD: Allyn and Bacon; pp 251–256.

Sweetow RW, Henderson-Sabes J. (2004) The case for LACE: listening and auditory communication enhancement training. *Hear J.* 57, 32–40.

Television Decoder Circuitry Act. Public Law 101-431-1990. Available at: http://www.access-board.gov/sec508/guide/1194.24-decoderact.htm.

Thibodeau L. (2004) Plotting beyond the audiogram to the TELEGRAM, a new assessment tool. *Hear J.* 57, 46–51.

Thurlow C. (2002) Generation Txt? Exposing the sociolinguistics of young people's text-messaging. Discourse Analysis Online. Available at: http://www.shu.ac.uk/daol/articles/v1/n1/a3/thurlow2002003-paper.html.

Tye-Murray N. (2004) *Foundations of Aural Rehabilitation.* 2nd ed. Clifton Park, NY: Thomson/Delmar Learning.

Valente M, Fabry D, Potts L. (1995) Recognition of speech in noise with hearing aids using dual microphones. *J Am Acad Audiol.* 6, 440–449.

Valente M, Sweetow R, May A. (1999) Using microphone technology to improve speech recognition. *Hear Rev Suppl.* 3, 10–13.

Van Tassell D. (1993) Hearing loss, speech, and hearing aids. *J Speech Hear Res.* 36, 228–244.

Vesterager V, Salomon G. (1991) Psychosocial aspects of hearing loss in the elderly. *Acta Otolaryngol.* 476, 215–220.

Wang M, Reed C, Bilger R. (1978) A comparison of the effects of filtering and sensorineural hearing on patterns of consonant confusions. *J Speech Hear Res.* 24, 32–43.

Wayner D. (2004) Integrating assistive technology into a hearing aid practice. *Hear J.* 57, 43–45.

Weinstein B. (2000) Outcome measures in rehabilitative audiology. In: Alpiner J, McCarthy P, eds. *Rehabilitative Audiology.* Philadelphia: Lippincott Williams & Wilkins; pp 575–594.

Weinstein B, Amsel L. (1986) The relationship between dementia and hearing loss in the institutionalized elderly. *Clin Gerontol.* 4, 3–15.

Working Group on Speech Understanding and Aging. (1988) Speech understanding and aging. *J Acoust Soc Am.* 83, 859–894.

35 Hearing Aid Technology

Ruth A. Bentler and H. Gustav Mueller

INTRODUCTION

At one time, the practice of clinical audiology was heavily devoted to diagnostic testing. In the early years, using behavioral measures, the audiologist typically was given the task to determine whether the presumed hearing impairment was "conductive" or "sensory-neural." In the 1970s, immittance testing and electrophysiologic measures allowed the audiologist to not only differentiate middle ear versus sensory-neural pathologies, but also to further define the extent and locus of the auditory pathology medial to the cochlea. This era of audiology bred a wealth of discovery and excitement and to a great extent defined the profession. In the late 1970s, however, for political, ethical, professional, and economic reasons, more and more audiologists entered into a new area of audiology and began dispensing hearing aids. It's not that audiologists were not always *involved* with hearing aids and rehabilitative audiology, but in general, they had not been at the "front line" of fitting, dispensing, and dealing with postfitting problems.

As the scope of audiologic practice expanded into the hearing aid arena in the 1980s and 1990s, it also became apparent that training programs needed to stay abreast of the burst of electronic development within the hearing aid industry and related verification advances. It was not too many years ago when a Master's degree training program in audiology lumped the study of hearing aids together with speech audiometry in a single three-credit course. Today, with clinical audiology having moved to a 4-year clinical doctorate degree, two, three, or even four courses are offered solely for the selection and fitting of hearing aids. A large percentage of audiologists now consider hearing aids and hearing aid dispensing to be their primary professional activity. Modern hearing aids are become increasing complex, making hearing aid selection, fitting, and verification a challenging task

for the audiologist. Therefore, extensive training is necessary to provide critical groundwork in the technical aspects of hearing aids. This chapter provides an introduction to these technical aspects.

HEARING AID STYLE

This chapter focuses on the features of modern hearing aids; however, to some extent, the components and features vary depending on the specific style of hearing aid. In some cases, the style of the hearing aid that is selected is based on the signal processing used or the presence/absence of a telecoil, in other cases, the style chosen may depend on patient's cosmetic or functional requirements.

There are currently six primary styles of hearing aids available. These include: (1) body aid; (2) eyeglass aid; (3) behind-the-ear (BTE) aid; (4) in-the-ear (ITE) aid; (5) in-the-canal (ITC) aid; and (6) completely-in-the-canal (CIC) aid.

As reviewed by Mueller et al. (2006), the style of a hearing aid relates to its functional aspects and its cosmetic design and not the level of technology in the device. That is, when hearing aid manufacturers introduce new technology every other year or so, the technology usually can be implemented in any style of hearing aid. Still, some advanced features, such as directional microphones, or some user controls *cannot* be implemented on smaller ITE styles due to the limited space available on the faceplate (front) of the hearing aid.

Less Common Styles of Hearing Aids

BODY AID

Body aids are the largest hearing aid device. This style was more or less the only style available until the BTE models

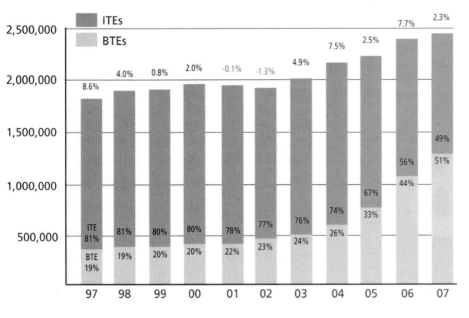

FIGURE 35.1 Percent of market share for behind-the-ear (BTE) and in-the-ear (ITE) styles of hearing aids from 1997 to 2007. (Courtesy of the *Hearing Review*, April , 2008.)

were introduced in the 1950s. While body aids do not represent much of the current hearing aid market in the United States or Europe (<1%), they have found a place in many developing countries. Because of their larger size and standard construction, they can often be manufactured less expensively. Because of their size and the size of the accompanying battery, body aids can provide a wide range of gain and output, as well as provide easier manipulation for individuals with motor or dexterity problems.

EYEGLASS HEARING AID

A second style of hearing aids is the eyeglass/hearing aid combination device. This has almost disappeared from the global hearing aid market but is still mentioned under available hearing aid styles because it was an innovative concept in its day during the 1960s. Once a year or so, a manufacturer will introduce a "new" eyeglass hearing aid concept; for example, enhancing directional effects through the use of several microphones placed in the temple of the eyeglass frame. While conceptually the combination eyeglasses and hearing aid unit sounds like a good idea, the combination of two prosthetic devices usually has proven to create more problems than benefit for the patient (see Sammeth and Levitt [2000] for review).

More Common Styles of Hearing Aids

In contrast to the two seldom used styles already mentioned, the following sections will review the four basic styles of hearing aids that generally are available from all the major hearing aid manufacturers. The market share for each of the current styles has fluctuated over the past 10 years (see Fig. 35.1) due to patient preference, feature availability, and new market penetration. The most common styles, as shown in Figure 35.2, are as follows.

BEHIND-THE-EAR STYLES

The BTE hearing aid is worn over the pinna and is typically coupled to tubing with an earmold that directs the amplified sound to the tympanic membrane. A schematic showing the major components of a modern BTE hearing aid is shown in Figure 35.3. The BTE may be less expensive than comparable custom-made hearing aids incorporating similar levels of technology. The BTE aid requires no special modifications to the shell case and, thus, can be completely manufactured in advance and maintained in stock by the hearing aid dispenser. In most instances, a custom earmold for channeling the sound into the ear canal is required (Mueller et al., 2006). However, in some cases, the BTE is connected to tubing only, which is inserted directly into the ear canal for a more open

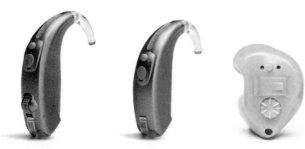

FIGURE 35.2 Sample of major styles of hearing aids. (Courtesy of Unitron Hearing)

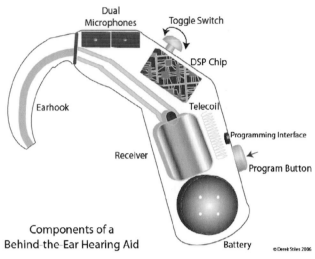

FIGURE 35.3 Schematic of a behind-the-ear (BTE) style hearing aid showing the major components of a modern hearing aid.

fitting. A recent variation of this style is referred to as an "open" fit or a mini BTE with micro-size tubing. Shown in Figure 35.4 with more standard-size BTEs, this model has become increasingly popular due to its small size and nonoccluding earpiece. Different manufacturers provide different earpiece/connectors, but most of these are referred to as a "mushroom" tip to hold the hearing aid in place. Several of the mini BTE models have the receiver placed within the ear canal as well.

IN-THE-EAR STYLES

The ITE hearing aid resides in the concha portion of the pinna with the receiver portion extending into the ear canal.

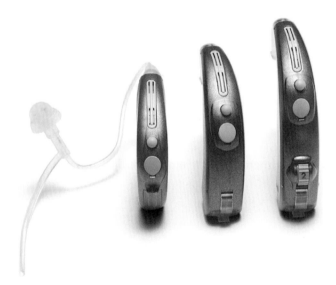

FIGURE 35.4 Sample of behind-the-ear (BTE) style hearing aids including the mini-BTE (open fitting) with narrow-diameter tubing. (Courtesy of Unitron Hearing)

The ITE style became commercially available in the 1960s and, in general, is considered more "modern" than the typical BTE hearing aid housing. There are three general variants of the ITE style: the full shell, low profile, and half shell (Fig. 35.2). The full-shell ITE fills the entire concha portion of the outer ear. The low-profile ITE fills the inner portion of the concha from top to bottom but does not protrude outwards as much as the full-shell ITE. The half-shell ITE style only fills the lower half of the concha near the ear canal. The full-concha ITE usually is used when more gain and output are required, although it does not produce as much gain as can be obtained with the BTE style.

The ITC hearing aid could be considered a subset of the ITE style. It only partially fills the lower approximate one quarter of the concha. Currently, it is the smallest style of hearing aid that can contain directional microphone technology because directional microphone ports need spacing of several millimeters on the faceplate to function effectively. The ITC hearing aid may be appropriate for patients who have cosmetic concerns and less severe hearing losses.

Another subset of ITE is the CIC hearing aid, which is completely contained within the ear canal and usually is considered the most cosmetically desirable of all styles. While it is the smallest hearing aid available, it does not offer as much gain and output or as many features as the larger hearing aids. Consequently, its popularity is not as great as might be believed, accounting for less than 20% of total hearing aid sales. Audiologists frequently counsel patients away from this hearing aid style in order to fit larger styles that have many advantages over the CIC.

OTHER STYLES

For the individual who has an unaidable hearing loss in one ear and normal hearing or an aidable hearing loss in the other ear, contralateral routing of signal (CROS) or bilateral contralateral routing of signal (BICROS) amplification, respectively, may be the most appropriate hearing aid arrangement. The CROS fitting places a microphone on the side of the poor ear, and its receiver is directed to the normal ear, so the good ear can receive sound from the opposite side of the head. The person, in effect, becomes a "two-sided" listener but, importantly, *not* a "two-eared" listener.

Somewhat different than the CROS fitting, BICROS hearing aids are used in cases where one ear is unaidable but there is some degree of aidable hearing loss in the other ear. This device has two microphones, one near the better ear and the other near the poorer ear. The acoustic signals from both sides are delivered to a single amplifier and receiver, with the output being directed into the better ear. For both CROS and BICROS fittings, the transmission of sound can be either via hardwire or FM. In the *hardwire* system, the signal is carried from one side of the head to the other by wires concealed within an eyeglass frame or by a tube or cord around the back of the neck when using ITE or BTE styles. The *frequency modulation (FM) system* is a wireless system

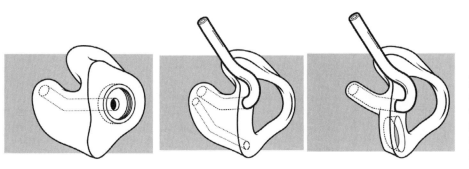

FIGURE 35.5   Various styles of earmolds used with behind-the-ear (BTE) styles of hearing aids. (Courtesy of Westone Laboratories)

that transmits the signals across the head to the better side by an FM transmitter and picked up by an FM receiver positioned near the better ear. The signal is then converted back to acoustic energy and presented to the better ear.

A final method of accomplishing the patient benefit desired from a CROS fitting is to use an implantable hearing aid on the poor ear side, with sounds subsequently transmitted to the cochlea of the good ear through skull vibrations. The earliest report (circa 1935) of a precursor to an implanted hearing device was the sprinkling of iron fillings onto the eardrum of a patient who was placed in a prone position on a couch (Goode, 1989). Applying a strong magnetic field resulted in the perception of sound due to the "flux of the magnetic field causing the iron fillings to vibrate in synchrony, which in turn vibrated the eardrum" (Chasin, 2001, p 34). Since that time, technology and surgical procedures have advanced significantly. Currently, bone-anchored hearing aids (BAHA) are surgically implanted for use with conductive, mixed, or sensory-neural hearing loss. Three components, (1) a titanium implant, (2) an external abutment, and (3) a sound processor, are used to bypass the external and middle ears. The titanium implant is placed into the skull behind the pinna during a short surgical procedure and, over time, integrates with the skull bone. The sound processor sits discreetly just behind the ear. Sound is picked up at the microphone of the processor and transmitted through the external abutment to the titanium implant. The external abutment serves as the connector from the processor to the implant. The vibrating implant sets up vibrations within the skull that stimulate the nerve fibers of the inner ear by bone conduction. This type of amplification has been used with unilateral deafness, chronic external and/or middle ear conditions, and congenital ear malformations. In the case of unilateral deafness, because the skull is set into vibration, the better ear (cochlea) can be stimulated by signals arriving on the side of the dead ear. And since no device or mold is inserted into the canal, ears with chronic ear disease or malformations get cochlear stimulation by way of bone, rather than air, conduction.

EARMOLDS

As the name suggests, *custom* hearing aids (those that fit within the ear itself) are fabricated from an impression of the ear. For hearing aids that are not custom, an earmold is used to direct the acoustic signal into the ear canal (and, in the case of the BTE instrument, also assist in maintaining the hearing aid on the ear).

As with custom hearing aids, custom earmolds come in various styles, ranging from large models that fill the entire concha of the outer ear to skeleton molds in which only a small piece of tubing extends into the ear canal. In fact, some aids simply have a small piece of tubing going into the ear canal and no earmold, *per se*. In general, the greater the hearing loss is, the larger the earmold needed. Figure 35.5 shows samples of many of the earmold styles that are available.

Once the earmold is coupled to the hearing aid, the properties of the sound reaching the user's ear are changed. The acoustic properties of the earmold itself and the length and diameter of the connecting tube play an important part in the final acoustical characteristics of the hearing aid system. To some extent, the signal can be modified by making changes to the earmold. The most common modification is called a *vent*, or a small hole drilled into the canal portion of the earmold. The vent is usually parallel to the sound bore, although in some instances, a diagonal (or "side branch") vent is used, usually when there isn't room for parallel. The acoustic effects provided are similar, although the diagonal vent can result in a reduction of amplification in the high frequencies as well as in the intended reduction in the low frequencies. Earmolds (and custom hearing aids) are vented for four primary reasons: (1) to allow unwanted amplified low frequencies to escape from the ear canal; (2) to release pressure to avoid a "plugged ear" sensation; (3) to reduce the occlusion effect (one's own voice sounds "hollow"); and (4) to allow the normal input of unamplified sound (Mueller et al., 2006). In recent years, there has been an increase in "open" fittings. In this case, a special nonoccluding earmold with a small tube is used. An example of this can be seen in Figure 35.4. Variable vents are also available that use small plastic plugs or different sizes of tubing that can totally occlude an existing vent or provide smaller openings of various diameters.

The effects of vent size can be observed in Figure 35.6. Observe that, as the size of the vent increases, the degree of "reduction" (leaking out of signal) increases, with the effect extending into higher frequencies. In general, it is believed that for frequencies where there is normal hearing, it is better to have the hearing aid user hear "natural" sound than

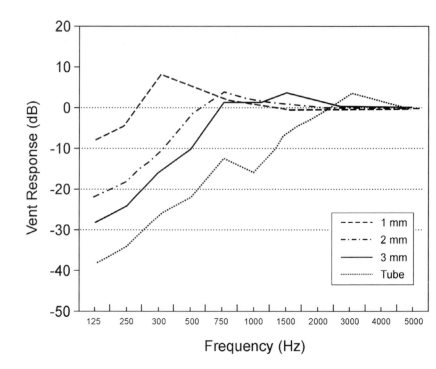

FIGURE 35.6 Example of venting effects. (Adapted from Lybarger S. [1985] Earmolds. In: Katz J, ed. *Handbook of Clinical Audiology.* 3rd ed. Baltimore: Williams & Wilkins; pp 885–910.)

amplified sound. Hence, the vent size is selected to correspond with the range of normal hearing in the low frequencies.

At one time, it also was common to use horn-shaped tubing to enhance the higher frequencies (termed "Libby horn" after the primary manufacturer). This horn tubing, in earmolds, usually provided a 3- to 5-dB boost in gain in the 3,000-Hz region. However, it is not possible to obtain the horn effect in custom instruments. Given the multiple channels and programming capabilities of today's hearing aids, horn tubing is not commonly used because it usually is possible to obtain desired gain without it.

Finally, as part of the overall plumbing of the BTE hearing aid, it is common for manufacturers to place a damper in the tone hook (that fits over the ear) to smooth the response in the 1,200 to 1,600 Hz range. Some manufacturers provide different hooks with different size dampers.

BASIC COMPONENTS AND FUNCTION

Hearing aids have basic components, common to all models and styles. The schematic in Figure 35.3 illustrates how these components fit together. A simplified description follows (from Mueller et al., 2006):

1. Sound waves enter the hearing aid through the *microphone or microphones*, which convert the sound waves into an electrical signal.
2. The *amplifier* increases the strength of the electrical signal.
3. The *receiver* converts the amplified signals back into an acoustic signal. The amplified sound is channeled from the *receiver* directly into the ear canal, via an earmold

or through tubing within the canal portion of a custom hearing aid.
4. The *battery* provides electrical energy to power the hearing aid.

There are other components that are common with certain styles of hearing aids or used for specific patient needs:

1. *On-Off Switch:* Allows the user to turn the hearing aid off when not in use. For many instruments, the on-off switch (if present) is part of the volume control wheel. The on-off switch can also be located on a remote control device.
2. *Volume Control:* The volume of the hearing aid can be controlled by a toggle switch, a button, or a rotating wheel, or through a remote control device.
3. *Telecoil:* A special circuit designed to enhance use of the hearing aid with the telephone. Electromagnetic signals are picked up by the telecoil from the receiver of the telephone (leakage), amplified, and transduced to acoustic energy before entering the ear. A telecoil switch may be incorporated into a toggle switch or exist as a separate control, or in some hearing aids, the switching is triggered by the input signal and occurs automatically. The telecoil can also be used to pick up electromagnetic fields generated by electric currents traveling through wires, such as induction loop systems (e.g., used in public facilities such as places of worship) or neck loops (e.g., connected to FM receivers). See Chapter 34 for more in-depth discussion of this topic.

HEARING AID FEATURES

The preceding section described the basic components of hearing aids. It would be unusual, however, to fit a hearing aid that only had these basic features. The following sections describe the numerous additional features and digital algorithms that are now available in modern technology.

Amplitude Compression

While amplitude compression typically is not considered a *basic function* of hearing aid circuitry, it is unusual to fit someone nowadays with hearing aids that do not have compression. Compression in hearing aids has been around since the 1930s. For a variety of reasons, however, for many years, compression was not considered a routine feature of hearing aid processing. Rather, it often was considered a "special feature" that was reserved for "special cases." For example, as recently as 1992, compression hearing aids had a market share below 20%. Today, however, the fitting decision usually does not involve *IF* we should fit compression, but rather, what type of compression is needed, how many *different* types of compression are needed, how many channels of compression are needed, and how should the various compression features be programmed. The understanding of compression and the correct programming of compression are vital to successful fittings and troubleshooting postfitting problems reported by the patient. We know that problems with loudness (both too loud and too soft) is a leading patient complaint and probably a leading reason for hearing aid rejection (Jenstad et al., 2003; Kochkin, 2004). With modern compression and judicious programming, loudness problems rarely are an issue.

There are many ways to classify compression, but it is first important to identify the two most basic types—input and output. As the name suggests, input compression means that the input signal to the hearing aid is analyzed and compressed *before* that signal reaches the final amplifier section (i.e., the amplifier consists of a number of amplifier circuits, with an initial amplifier and subsequent amplifier circuits). In contrast, output compression means that the signal is analyzed and compressed *after* it has been fully amplified (i.e., been processed through all of the amplifier sections). Both types of compression commonly are referred to as "automatic gain control" (AGC); basically, this is the patient's benefit of compression. Because compression can be either input or output, we use the terms AGCi and AGCo to differentiate the two different types. A block diagram illustrating these two different types is shown in Figure 35.7.

As mentioned earlier, compression has been available in hearing aids for 70 years, but only recently has there been a clear theoretical basis for its use. This theory has been strengthened by evidence-based research showing the positive patient benefits for compression.

AGCo

We know that loud sounds can be annoying for individuals and that less than 50% of hearing aid users are satisfied regarding how their hearing aids handle loud sounds. We also know that we cannot arbitrarily limit the output of all hearing aids to a single low level, as this would unneces-sarily limit the aided dynamic range for people with high loudness discomfort levels (LDLs) or thresholds of discomfort (TDs). Although we know that peak clipping (i.e., peaks of the signal or waveform are cut off at a level where the amplifying circuits are driven beyond their overload point) is an effective way to limit the output, research has shown that, for sound quality, patients prefer the limiting provided by AGCo (Mueller and Hornsby, 2002; Savage et al., 2006). There may be some exceptions to this for people with severe to profound hearing loss, especially if they are prior users of peak-clipping hearing aids (Marriage et al., 2005).

In theory, therefore, we need a patient-specific output setting that varies by frequency to match the patient's TDs. Moreover, we need to assure that the hearing aid settings correspond to real-world listening conditions. Research evidence has shown that the clinical procedure of adjusting the hearing aid output using AGCo to assure that loud sounds are not uncomfortable does indeed result in improved patient satisfaction (Mueller and Bentler, 2002; 2005). Therefore, from both a theoretical and practical standpoint, AGCo is the preferred method to limit hearing aid output.

AGCi

Unlike AGCo, the primary purpose of AGCi is *not* for output limiting. Rather, this form of compression is used to "reshape" or "repackage" the input signal, to allow a wide range of intensities to fit into the patient's restricted residual dynamic range.

To understand why this is necessary, we must first consider the typical loudness growth function of a person with a hearing loss. Individuals with cochlear hearing loss have a rapid loudness growth for supra-threshold signals (this is often referred to as "recruitment"). For example, someone with a hearing loss of 50 dB hearing level (HL) will probably have a TD of around 100 dB HL—the same level of someone with normal hearing (see Bentler and Cooley [2001] for review). This means that, within a 50-dB range (50 to 100 dB), this person has the same loudness growth that a normal-hearing person would experience from 0 to 100 dB HL. This loudness growth pattern is directly linked to outer hair cell damage in the cochlea—the type of hearing loss experienced by the vast majority of people fitted with hearing aids. One of the theoretical goals of using AGCi is to accomplish loudness restoration. To illustrate this, take a look at Figure 35.8 (see page 783). On the top panel, you can see the loudness growth for an individual with hearing loss compared to someone with normal hearing. Notice that, for soft sounds, there is a big difference in perceived loudness (as a result, this is where the maximum gain of instrument occurs); for loud sounds, the loudness ratings are fairly equal (in fact, the patient may not require any gain for loud sounds). If we measure the difference between these two curves, we then have the desired output as a function of input (Fig 35.8B) for a given input signal. If you want to think in terms of gain, subtract the input signal from the corresponding desired output. In the example given earlier, we would subtract the 40-dB input

Output controlled compression

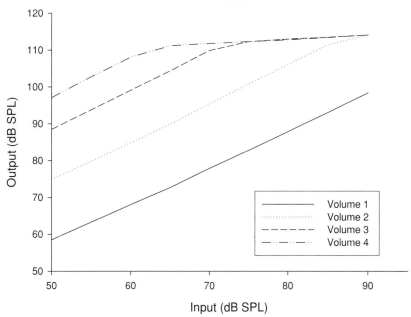

Input controlled compression

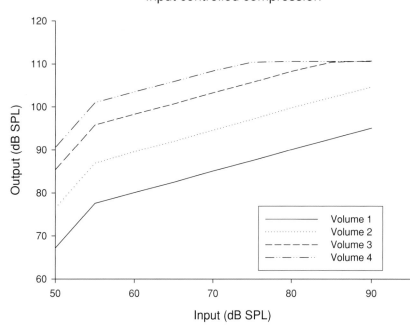

FIGURE 35.7
Input/output functions for automatic gain control–output (AGCo) and automatic gain control–input (AGCi). SPL, sound pressure level.

from the 65-dB output and conclude that this patient needs 25 dB of gain for soft sounds. We then can determine what compression settings best fit this entire function.

Kneepoints and Ratios

The way in which hearing aids alter gain is often displayed in an input/output function. The basic input/output amplifier function is linear, which in some ways can be thought of as the opposite of compression. With linear amplification, the output of the hearing aid increases in direct proportion to

the input (i.e., in a 1:1 manner). For example, for a hearing aid programmed with 30 dB of gain, the output will increase by 10 dB for every 10-dB change in input. Observe in the output-controlled compression in Figure 35.7 (at Volume 2) that, for a 50-dB input, the output is approximately 75 dB; for a 60-dB input, the output is approximately 85 dB; and so on. Notice that, when an output of 110 dB is reached, there is no further gain in output when input increases. That *could* occur because we have employed a circuit referred to as "peak clipping," which limits the output. As mentioned earlier, although peak clipping is effective in limiting the

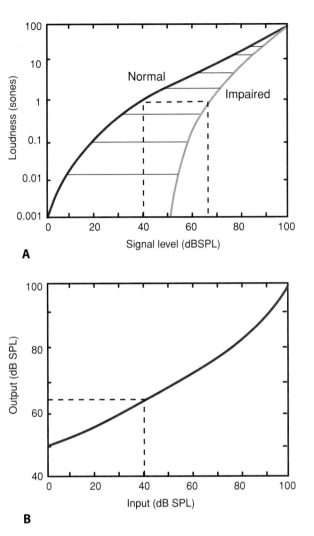

A

B

FIGURE 35.8 Example of loudness growth patterns for normal and impaired ears (top panel) and desired gain/output for the restoration of loudness for the limited dynamic range (bottom panel; refer to text). (Courtesy of Harvey Dillon, personal correspondence)

output, it introduces distortions that are annoying and can reduce the intelligibility and quality for loud speech. The desired alternative to peak clipping is AGCo.

The kneepoint of a compression function is the point where the output curve deviates from linear. The ratio of the function is the degree of deviation. For example, if the output of a hearing aid changes by only 5 dB for every 10-dB increase in input, this would be referred to as a compression ratio of 2:1. If the output changed by only 3.3 dB for every 10-dB increase in input, this would be a compression ratio of 3:1. As shown on Figure 35.7, we now have introduced AGCo with a kneepoint of 110 dB sound pressure level (SPL) and a ratio of 10:1. On an input/output chart, peak clipping and AGCo look similar; however, the quality of sound for high inputs is much different. Also notice that we have "linear processing" up to the point where the compression is acti-

vated. It is important to remember that, for some patients, we want linear processing, but yet we also employ compression for limiting the output. Hence, when we talk about hearing aid processing, compression and linear processing are not mutually exclusive.

Most individuals with cochlear hearing loss have a restricted residual dynamic range. Therefore, if we use linear processing of the signal, it is very difficult to fit both soft and loud sounds within the boundaries of this limited area. In order to make all sounds fit appropriately, we must employ different amounts of gain for different levels of input; this, in fact, is the purpose of AGCi. Also shown in Figure 35.7 is the input/output function for an AGCi hearing aid using a compression kneepoint of 55 dB SPL. Up to 55-dB input levels, the hearing aid provides linear gain. Observe that, when the input reaches 55 dB, the output of the hearing aid no longer changes in a linear manner. Also note that AGCo continues to be necessary when the output approaches 110 dB SPL, but the AGCo kneepoint is no longer reached for an 80-dB input as it was before.

When low kneepoints are used with AGCi, it is referred to as wide dynamic range compression (WDRC) because a wide range of the speech input signal is compressed. Usually when the kneepoint is 50 dB or lower, the term WDRC is used. It should also be obvious from Figure 35.7 that the volume control adjustment does *not* affect the kneepoint observed. That is, for AGCi, the kneepoint remains at approximately 55 dB *on the input* regardless of the volume setting; for AGCo, the kneepoint remains at approximately 110 dB *on the output* regardless of the volume setting.

To summarize the two most common types of compression: AGCo is a replacement for peak clipping and used to maintain high inputs below the patient's LDL or TD. AGCi is an alternative to linear processing and is used to reduce the dynamic range of the output signals so that these signals fit within the boundaries of the patient's residual dynamic range.

Compression Time Constants

Compression systems in hearing aids have time constants that can be defined as follows:

■ Attack time—Using a puretone input signal that changes abruptly from 55 to 90 dB SPL, attack time is the time required for the output to reach 3 dB of the steady-state value for the 90-dB input (American National Standards Institute [ANSI] S3.22-2003). Attack time is sometimes considered the time for the instrument to go "in" or "out" of compression; however, for AGCi with low kneepoints, the hearing aid may not go "out" of compression for most listening situations.

■ Release (recovery) time—The interval between the abrupt drop from 90 to 55 dB SPL and the point where the signal has stabilized to within 4 dB of the

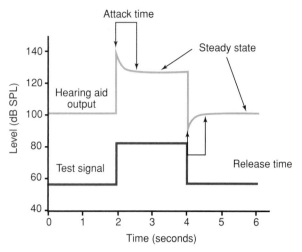

FIGURE 35.9   Schematic of the effect of attack and release of a compression circuit. (Courtesy of Harvey Dillon, personal correspondence)

steady-state value for the 55-dB input (ANSI S3.22-2003). In other words, release time is the time required for a circuit to respond to a decrease in the input and adjust to a lower compression characteristic (which, for some types of compression in some hearing aids, could be linear amplification).

Figure 35.9 illustrates the attack and release of a compression circuit. Although it is possible to have an attack time of a second or longer, this is not typically implemented in today's products. In fact, nearly all manufacturers have AGCi compression attack times that are very fast (e.g., <10 ms). The general thinking is that, if a loud input arrives, the hearing aid must react quickly so that the input is placed appropriately within the patient's dynamic range. This is especially important for annoying intense signals. The selection of compression release times is not as straightforward as for attack times. For this reason, there are products on the market with release times that are *very* short (<10 ms) and release times that are *very* long (>5 s). Proponents of short release times suggest that this is helpful to maintain audibility—that is, if a soft speech signal follows a loud speech sound, then the hearing aid recovers in time to apply the appropriate gain for the soft sound. On the other hand, long release times are better at maintaining the consonant-vowel relationship of speech, which some believe improves speech quality. For a review of the pros and cons of different release times, see Dillon (2001).

Expansion

Expansion is often described as the opposite of compression. Whereas compression is designed to decrease the gain as a function of increasing input, expansion is intended to increase the gain as a function of increasing input, when those inputs are below the kneepoint or threshold of the compressor.

Stated differently, expansion provides more "squash effect"—the softer the input, the more the gain is reduced. The intent has been to reduce the output of low-level environmental noises as well as internal noise generated by the hearing aid itself. Consider that many individuals need 30 to 40 dB of gain to make soft speech audible. However, amplifying low-level ambient noise and hearing aid microphone noise by 30 to 40 dB can be annoying. Therefore, the goal is to use WDRC to maximize audibility for soft speech and use expansion to minimize audibility of unwanted noises.

There has been little research published on the effect of this signal-processing scheme. Applied in a single-channel product, Plyler et al. (2005a; 2005b) reported improved listener preference using expansion in quiet listening situations but degraded speech perception in both quiet and noise when input levels were at or below the activation threshold (e.g., as expected, the expansion processing reduced the audibility of soft speech). The findings were not related to the configuration of the loss, as has been suggested by some manufacturers, but were related to the kneepoint and time constant of the expander. It remains unclear just what the ideal kneepoint and expansion ratio should actually be. In general, we can assume that, if the expansion kneepoint is below the level of soft speech throughout the speech range, then this processing should have little or no adverse effect on speech understanding and should continue to serve the purpose of reducing annoyance from soft background noise. Nearly all products today employ expansion. In some hearing aids, the effect can be adjusted by the audiologist by altering the kneepoint and/or the ratio, and if necessary, the expansion can be turned off. In other products, however, expansion is continually on and cannot be programmed by the audiologist.

Frequency Compression

It is generally accepted (with adults) that, when hearing thresholds exceed some critical level (e.g., 60 to 70 dB HL above 2,000 Hz), amplification may be ineffective due to "dead" regions in the cochlea (Ching et al., 1998; Hogan and Turner, 1998). This term refers to the loss of inner hair cell function, which, in turn, means that the corresponding auditory nerve fibers will not be stimulated. This tends to occur in frequency regions where the energy for many voiceless consonants critical for speech understanding lies (e.g., /s/, /th/, /f/, /sh/, /t/). Without transmission cells in these regions of the cochlea, any effort to provide gain cannot be successful. Although the actual diagnosis of "dead" regions is still clinically elusive, at least one tool has been forwarded to help clinicians determine when amplification is appropriate. Moore et al. (2000; 2004) have developed a Threshold Equalizing Noise (TEN) test that is designed to elicit masked thresholds over a relatively wide frequency range. By shaping the masker noise, thresholds for normal-hearing and hearing-impaired listeners *without* dead regions will be shifted by a known magnitude, whereas for those with dead regions, the shift in thresholds will be markedly higher. Although the test has limitations, it does provide the clinician with another tool to diagnose the severity of the hearing loss for a potential hearing aid candidate. In addition, because amplified sounds would remain inaudible to these individuals, even with amplification, several commercial attempts have been made to essentially move that high-frequency energy into a lower frequency range. Initially, frequency transposition or *shifting* was the scheme employed, wherein the higher frequencies' energy was lowered via a mixer. More recently, "frequency compression" hearing aids have become available, wherein both the frequency and the bandwidth are altered by a preset factor (or ratio). That is, incoming signals are analyzed and determined to be voiced or voiceless based on frequency and timing characteristics. If voiceless, which signifies a high-frequency consonant, the incoming sound is frequency compressed to the preset degree (anywhere from 1.5 to 5.0 in steps of 0.25). This action takes place extremely rapidly, in the order of 2 to 4 ms. When the next sound comes along, typically a vowel in the normal syllabic sequence, the aid reverts to its normal amplification pattern. The voiced (lower frequency) sounds are passed through and processed as determined during the initial programming. When the next voiceless sound is detected, the frequency compression circuit is again activated.

Multiple Channels

The frequency response of the processed input signal can be divided into bands or channels. While there is no standardized definition of these terms, it generally is accepted that bands represent regions where only gain can be adjusted, and channels are frequency regions where compression, expansion, digital noise reduction, directivity, and other signal processing can be independently programmed (via independent circuits) or be preprogrammed to have frequency-specific variances. That is, you could have many bands within a channel but could not have multiple channels within a band. The purpose of multiple channels is that, in many cases, the hearing aid user requires different degrees of signal processing in different frequency regions. For example, because soft speech is often more intense in the lower frequencies, it is usually desirable to use a higher expansion kneepoint (and concomitantly a higher compression kneepoint) in the low frequencies than in the high frequencies. Or, because people with increasing hearing loss in the higher frequencies have a narrower dynamic range in that region, it may be desirable to use a higher WDRC ratio for this frequency region. Each of these effects can be accomplished with separate channels of processing.

It is not known how many channels are enough or how many are too many. To some extent, this depends on the configuration of the audiogram and the signal-processing feature of interest. For the purposes of audibility and intelligibility, four to eight channels of gain and compression control probably are enough. Hearing aids today, however, commonly have 10, 15, 20, or more channels, although the channels are normally overlapping, which helps prevent artifacts and distortions because no single channel operates independently and, therefore, it is impossible to have a significant mismatch between adjacent channels. When more than four channels are used, it is common to employ "handles" in the fitting software. A handle can control several channels simultaneously, which, in turn, allows for easier programming and adjustment of the various parameters.

Multiple Memories

Many of today's products have multiple memories. Within a memory, certain hearing aid adjustments are stored, and various hearing aid features can be turned on or off. The patient can access a given memory through the use of a button on the hearing aid or using a remote control device. The presumed benefit of multiple memories is that very specific hearing aid settings may be desirable for one listening situation but not another. For example, many audiologists believe that the hearing aid settings for listening to music should be different from those for listening to speech in background noise. The patient, therefore, could simply switch the hearing aid to the "music program" whenever needed. As will be discussed later, hearing aids also have signal classification systems; that is, the hearing aid can detect the content of the input signal (e.g., music vs. speech vs. noise). Automatic adjustments to the signal processing can be made based on the content. As these algorithms become more advanced, there will be less need for multiple memories.

Telecoils

For people with hearing loss, using the telephone can be a frustrating experience. The signal emanating from the receiver of an ordinary telephone is band-limited from 300 to 3,000 Hz and slightly amplified to about 70 dB SPL. For those with mild hearing loss, this signal may be sufficient for effective telephone use. For a more severe hearing loss, some additional amplification is generally needed and is often achieved by the use of a telecoil.

How does a telecoil work?

In general, hearing aids and telephones do not work well together without some sort of interface. This is due to the feedback that results from placing the telephone receiver in close proximity to the hearing aid microphone (and receiver). There are several ways to effectively couple hearing aids and telephones. The most frequent is through a *telecoil*. A telecoil is a tiny coil of wire around a core that induces an electrical current when it is in the presence of a changing magnetic field. Originally, it was intended to "pick up" the magnetic signal generated by the older telephones, whose speakers were driven by powerful magnets. Newer phones often do not carry the strong magnetic signal but contain extra electronics to generate such a signal and are referred to as "hearing aid compatible" (HAC). In other words, the hearing aid can pick up the magnetic signal from the phone. The induction coil is formed by wrapping copper wire many times around a metal rod; the strength of the inductive pick up is determined by the number of turns of the copper wire around the metal axis rod. Larger rods permit more turns and more powerful telephone coils. By using an integrated amplifier to amplify the strength of the signal, the size can be reduced for hearing aid use. The strength of the electric current induced in the telecoil is directly proportional both to the energy in the magnetic field and to the relative positions of the induction coil in the hearing aid to the magnetic field generated from the telephone. This means that, in some positions, little or no electric current will be created in the induction coil. This is why hearing aid users must often experiment with the positioning of unfamiliar telephones to find the "hot spot" where the strongest signal is heard.

INTERFERING SIGNALS

When a hearing aid is in the telecoil mode, all nearby electromagnetic signals are detected and amplified. Some common sources of electromagnetic interference include powerful fluorescent lights, microwaves, televisions, computer monitors, power lines, and electrical transformers. Any of these electrical devices can produce strong electromagnetic "static" or noise. This electromagnetic static can interfere with the telecoil and with telephone reception in general. Because the strength of the electromagnetic field often varies considerably with small changes of position, it is sometimes possible to minimize the amount of the noise just by moving the telephone or hearing aid position slightly. However, often the length of the telephone cord limits the range of possible locations. When talking on the telephone in the vicinity of electromagnetic static, it is often necessary to change positions to determine where the interfering electromagnetic field is weakest. Sometimes, and in some places, effective

telephone communication with a telecoil is simply not possible given the strength of the interfering electromagnetic signals. As technology advances, many of the coupling and interference issues may be resolved with Bluetooth or similar wireless questions.

Directional Microphones

Directional microphones have been used in the broadcasting industry since the early 1940s (Bauer, 1942) and were first applied to prototype hearing aids during the same decade (Lybarger, 1947). Although commercial use of directional microphone hearing aids in the United States was realized in 1971, it was not until the 1990s that they became available in many different styles and models. A number of factors contributed to the surge in their use, including size miniaturization, market demand, digital signal processing for manipulation, and, generally, a clearer understanding of the physical and psychophysical advantages of the polar response patterns that could be derived.

In its basic design, a directional microphone operates on the principle that the microphone is more sensitive to forward-facing inputs (called *on-axis*) than to inputs from other azimuths (called *off-axis*). An omnidirectional microphone has a single opening to the diaphragm and, subsequently, has equal sensitivity to sounds arriving from all azimuths. Directional microphone schemes are achieved with one or more microphones and two or more ports. The inputs to the different ports are compared or subtracted, resulting in different sensitivity patterns dependent upon the physical spacing between the ports and the delay imposed between them. Figure 35.10 shows schematics of one- and

Directional microphone

· Single capsule
· Two ports

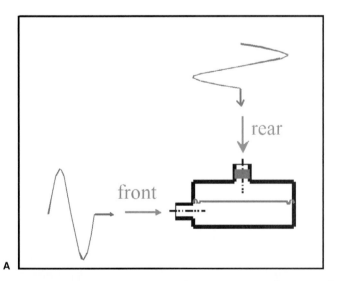
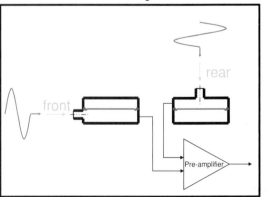

FIGURE 35.10   Schematics of (A) one-microphone and (B) two-microphone directional schemes.

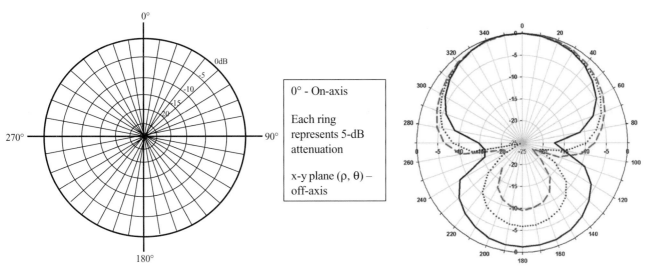

FIGURE 35.11   How to read a polar pattern. (Courtesy of Andrew Ditterner, personal communication)

two-microphone schemes. A polar response pattern, or *polar pattern*, is a graphical representation of the sensitivity of the microphone (or microphone system, since there may be more than one microphone in the design) for signals arriving at different angles, or azimuths. As shown in Figure 35.11, 0° represents signals arriving from directly in front of the listener (or microphone), 90° represents signals directly to the right, 180° represents signals directly behind, and so on. Although an infinite variety of responses can be achieved from directional microphones, three common first-order patterns (cardioid, hypercardioid, and, supercardioid) are shown in Figure 35.12 alongside the omnidirectional pattern. A fourth common shape is the dipole (or circle-eight) pattern. These patterns represent the theoretical limits of attenuation based on the physical design of two-input microphones (either two ports or two omnidirectional microphones). Second-order directional microphone hearing aids use more than two ports for comparison and typically exhibit narrower beams (towards the front) and wider nulls (i.e., regions of reduced sensitivity), thus theoretically providing increased attenuation to surrounding noise. From these patterns, a quantification of the directivity is obtained, referred to as the directivity index (DI) (ANSI, 2005). The DI quantifies the relationship between the microphone's (or hearing aid's) output response to frontal (on-axis) sound inputs and sound inputs from all other azimuths (off-axis). While theoretical DIs range from 5.4 to 6 dB for first-order microphone schemes and several dB higher for second-order schemes, the directivity is reduced when the microphone is installed in a hearing aid and placed on the head of the listener (Dittberner and Bentler, 2007a; 2007b). This is due to the disruption of the input levels and arrival times to the microphone ports imposed by the presence of a head and torso.

Recently, several manufacturers have introduced directional microphone hearing aids with frequency-specific polar patterns. For example, one manufacturer provides what it refers to as *split-directionality*: an omnidirectional

pattern in the low frequencies and a directional pattern in the high frequencies. Others allow for *multichannel* or *narrowband directionality*: a narrow-frequency range stimulus will result in a null for that frequency range only, while other frequencies maintain an omnidirectional polar pattern. Along with the trend toward increasing the number of processing channels, there is another trend toward channel-less directionality. In that design, there are no defined channels of processing; a polar pattern will show the null to occur in the frequency region of the single noise source, whatever that frequency may be. Some caution must be noted in these

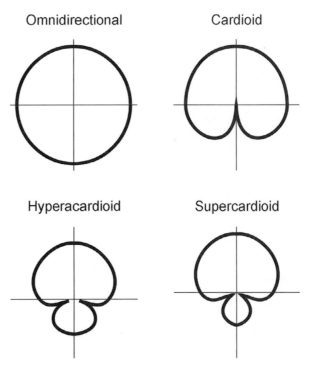

FIGURE 35.12   Sample of four common polar patterns.

measurement characteristics, however. Polar response patterns are typically obtained in anechoic chambers with precise characteristics and according to precise measurement standards (ANSI S3.35; ANSI, 2005). The directionality realized by any listener is altered by the location of the talker and noise (re: critical distance effects), the reverberation of the environment, and the presence of multiple noise sources.

Directional microphone hearing aids can be automatic and/or adaptive. *Automatic* refers to the automatic switching from an omnidirectional mode to a directional mode and vice versa. The goal of this design is to provide for a transition from omnidirectional to directional function, especially for those hearing aid users who either cannot make the adjustment themselves (e.g., children, persons with low cognitive function or physical disability) or cannot easily determine when the adjustment should be made. Although earlier versions of this design used environmental level as the trigger for switching, newer versions use algorithms that evaluate other characteristics of the environment such as the presence and level of amplitude modulations in the signal (signifying whether the signal is one of noise or speech) arriving at one or both microphone ports.

The term a*daptive* was used originally to refer to the *steering* or location switching of the null towards the primary noise source. The obvious intention of this design was to allow for alteration of the polar pattern—or null placement—to accommodate alterations in a listener's communication environment. An example of *null steering* can be seen in Figure 35.13, where the noise source (or *jammer*) is placed at three different azimuths and the polar patterns obtained indicate the null changes as a function of that placement.

Other versions of adaptive directional microphone technology are being developed and marketed. For example, in another design shown in Figure 35.14, the polar pattern that is dependent upon spacing and delay (the *fixed* pattern) is shown in the left panel. When the hearing aid is placed in its *adaptive* mode, shown in the right panel, the same patterns appear but at a reduced level. That is, in the adaptive mode in noise backgrounds, the nulls are not *steered* or altered, but the gain for sounds arriving from approximately 60° to 300° relative to the front (0°) is reduced. This interesting approach to directional microphone design represents an early era of combining polar nulls with active gain reduction in an effort to increase directional microphone effectiveness. Although standardized measurements exist for assessing the directional characteristics of *fixed* patterns (ANSI S3.35-2005), there is no current standardization of the terminology or measurement of these *adaptive* systems. It should be noted that issues of microphone drift, port alignment, and candidacy remain. In order to ensure that the intended polar pattern is realized in the directional hearing aid, the microphones must be carefully matched in both sensitivity and phase. That sensitivity can be misaligned by humidity, extreme temperature fluctuation, and debris in one or both ports. The challenge with microphone matching becomes even more critical with higher order systems. Small errors that can be tolerated in a first-order system create even larger errors when more than two microphones are used (Thompson, 2003). At least one hybrid system (second-order for high frequencies, first-order for low frequencies) is commercially available (Powers and Hamacher, 2002; 2004).

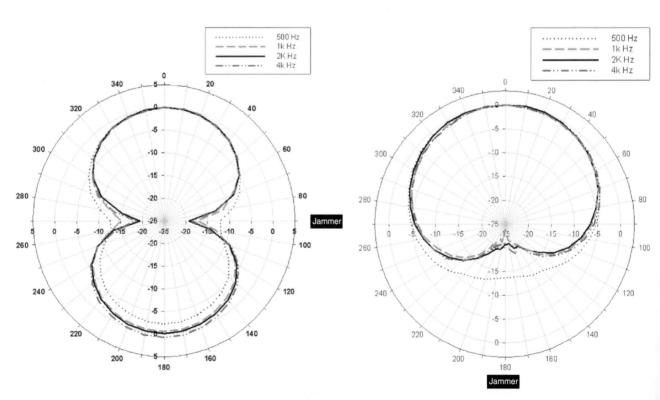

FIGURE 35.13 Example of null steering in an adaptive microphone scheme.

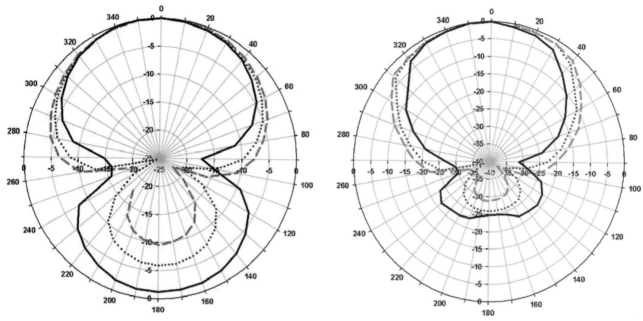

FIGURE 35.14 Example of side-band gain reduction in an adaptive microphone.

Port alignment refers to the alignment of the multiple ports in the horizontal plane. While ±20° variation is acceptable for maintaining the intended directivity pattern, more extreme variations have significant effect on the effectiveness of the design (Ricketts, 2000). Both clinician and manufacturer are responsible for ensuring this outcome, which is a challenge for pediatric and geriatric fittings, for sure, where the head may not always be aimed toward the primary talker. The reader is referred to Chapter 36 for assessing directional function via a hearing aid text box.

Candidacy should be determined on an individual basis. While the prospect of improving the signal-to-noise ratio (S/N) for all listeners seems appealing, the benefits of the technology must be balanced with the drawbacks. It is possible that the directional microphone system will reduce audibility for important off-axis inputs, result in more circuit noise, and be more costly than the alternative. It is also possible that the advantages of the directional microphone system will not be realized in real-world environments. In one series of studies, it was reported that the directional advantage obtained in the laboratory was not realized in field evaluations by the same subjects (Walden et al., 2003). Factors of training, visual cues, and reduced directivity (e.g., due to port misalignment or debris) were implicated.

Noise Reduction

Noise reduction as a feature has been available in hearing aids since the 1970s. Earlier analog versions included a tone switch (e.g., N-H) that was designed to switch on a low-frequency filter in order to reduce the low-frequency amplification of background interference. Other early processing schemes that were marketed as noise reduction included adaptive filtering (e.g., Manhattan Circuit™ [by Argosy]), Adaptive

Compression™ (by Telex), and low-frequency compression (ASP by Siemens). However, these systems did not provide the anticipated improvement in speech perception ability in background noise (Bentler et al., 1993).

With the availability of digital signal processing in ear-level hearing aids came a second era of noise reduction. Digital noise reduction (DNR) schemes are used by nearly every manufacturer of hearing aids. The algorithms developed by each differ in many ways; however, these algorithms share one common goal, which is to distinguish between speech and noise in the listener's immediate environment and reduce the "noise" component. In the first generation of DNR, most manufacturers use a modulation-based approach to accomplishing this goal. That is, the signal observed at the microphone is analyzed to determine whether modulations in the amplitude fluctuation (or waveform) are similar to those observed in speech. As early as 1930, H.W. Dudley at Bell Labs observed that the speech signal is formed by modulating (with the slowly changing vocal resonances) the spectral shape of the sound produced by the vocal mechanism. He observed that these modulations were both *periodic*, produced by vocal cord vibration, and *aperiodic*, produced by turbulent airflow at a constriction (AT&T, 2006). Researchers in the past 50 years have added to this understanding of the importance of amplitude modulations to speech perception. The modulated waveform, or temporal envelope of speech, contains information that is essential for the identification of the different parts of speech, such as phonemes, syllables, and words. However, reverberation in the listener's communication environment can reduce the clear delineation between speech and noise. As a result, the use of modulation-based algorithms to detect and eliminate noise has obvious limitations. Even if the noise *could be* identified and removed from the environment for specific spectral regions, the speech information in that same region would be removed as well. In fact, background "noise" for most listeners consists of multiple talkers talking! Recently, manufacturers have taken a multifaceted approach to identifying and reducing unwanted noise. By using algorithms with rules for the spectral make-up, fluctuations of level and frequency, and even the spatial separation of the incoming sounds (i.e., directional microphones), gain reduction rules are implemented. Several examples of the differences across manufacturers are shown in Figures 35.15A and 35.15B. Refer to Bentler and Chiou (2006) for further information on this feature.

Feedback Management

For decades, those who have fit hearing aids have had to contend with the difficult-to-resolve feedback issue. Generally,

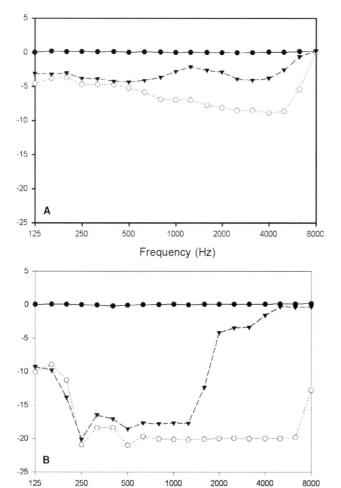

FIGURE 35.15 **Example of different outcomes for two different digital noise reduction schemes.**

feedback is the whistling sound that occurs when the gain of the hearing aid (at a particular frequency) is greater than the occlusion provided by the earmold (at that frequency) (Dillon, 2001). Kates (1988) modeled the feedback pathway in an effort to understand the limitations of gain provision. He noted that, in most traditional fittings, acoustic feedback limits the maximum possible gain to less than 40 dB. For more severe hearing losses, this limitation may not be acceptable. The management of that annoying outcome has been to (1) remake the earmold/shell to be fuller or deeper so that there is less leakage between the mold and the wall of the ear canal, (2) reduce the size of the venting, (3) roll off the high frequencies, and more recently, (4) reduce the gain in narrow frequency bands or through notch filtering centered in those bands. Each of these solutions may be counterproductive to the intent of the fitting. Solution #1 may result in an uncomfortable fit; solution #2 may impact on the acoustic characteristics desired; and solution #3 may decrease speech intelligibility. One possible negative outcome of solution #4 is the introduction of distortion for the listener. Even when the hearing aid gain is set to a level below the oscillation point, the signal feeding back may still cause alterations, or fluctuations, in the signal that are perceptible to listeners, especially when these alterations occur at formant transitions (Preves, 1988). It has been suggested that this gain be reduced 4 to 8 dB below the feedback onset to avoid these deleterious effects (Skinner, 1988). To do so, however, undermines the goal of providing optimal gain for audibility.

With the use of digital processing schemes, the management of this side effect of amplification has been reconsidered. Adaptive notch filters and/or phase (and frequency) shifting schemes have resolved many instances of the annoying squeal, without obvious signal distortion. Most recently, the use of adaptive feedback pathway cancellers has shown promise. This algorithm is currently employed in many hearing aids and includes three steps (that are either automatically activated or manually controlled by the clinician, depending on the manufacturer). A potential negative consequence of these algorithms is the occurrence of *entrainment* (Merks et al., 2006). Entrainment refers to the unintentional result of the filter attempting to cancel what appears to be feedback but, in reality, is some other tonal input to the microphone (e.g., from a musical production). The listener often reports hearing either an additional tone or a modulation-type distortion during entrainment.

The term *maximum stable gain* (MSG) has been used to quantify the gain that can be achieved following this adaptive filtering scheme. Any changes in the environment (e.g., head movement, hat or scarf placement, telephone use, and so on) may result in an inaccurate estimate of the feedback pathway with consequent (and inaccurate) alteration of the gain, producing unwanted distortion and/or perceptible noise to the listener (Joson et al., 1993). Even the introduction of reverberation has been shown to affect the accuracy with which these algorithms can model the feedback pathway. Since reverberation can persist for a much longer time than the short adaptive filter used to model the pathway, the reflections can cause changes in the pathway that are difficult to model (Kates, 2001; Dai and Hou, 2004). Since the number of computations required for updating the filter coefficients and applying the filter to the output signal is proportional to the filter length (or complexity), the limited computational power (low-voltage power source) requires that the filter be limited; that is, complex computations take additional time and power, neither of which are readily available in current hearing aids. As a result, the feedback pathway cancellation algorithm is limited in its ability to react to many fast changes in the feedback path, especially when the changes are related to reverberation. He and Bentler (2006) evaluated the effectiveness of two feedback algorithms in four conditions of reverberation using speech sounds as the input stimuli. They noted that the output of the hearing aid was most stable in the environment of least reverberation (sound booth), while reverberation had a significant impact on MSG headroom. Groth (2006) cautions that the provision of additional stable gain does not ensure that the fidelity of the amplified signal is maintained. For this reason, the clinician is cautioned to assess the outcome of the feature both acoustically (feedback canceller off vs. feedback canceller on) and perceptually. Acoustically, the hearing aid may provide more gain to the user, but perceptually, that amplified signal may be of reduced fidelity. Since each company/algorithm is somewhat different from the others, the clinician must experience the effectiveness across circuits by wearing/listening to the different models as often as possible.

Data Logging

Many of today's hearing aids have a feature referred to as data logging. This is more or less an electronic diary that can be used to collect data (1) on hearing aid use, (2) on program/memory use, and (3) to summarize the results of the input classification system (e.g., percentage of time the listener was in quiet, noise, speech-in-noise, etc.). Data logging is not a "processing" feature but can be helpful in patient counseling. For example, if the summary of the input classification system revealed that the patient was in high levels of background noise 40% of the time, but the data showed that the patient never used the program for the directional microphone, reinstruction concerning the benefits of directional technology would be appropriate. Data logging also plays a prominent role in trainable hearing aids that are becoming more prevalent in the marketplace; by logging the preferred settings in different environments, the data are subsequently used for automatic switching of parameters and features.

FREQUENCY MODULATION

The advantage of the FM system is that it improves the S/N at the listener's ear by transmitting the talker's voice from a microphone that is in close proximity to the talker's mouth.

The related, and positive, outcome is to reduce the apparent distance from talker to student/listener. FM systems are often beneficial for students in academic settings. The system consists of a microphone, transmitter, receiver, and some coupling scheme to get the signal from the receiver to the student's ear. This may take the form of (1) an induction neckloop connected to the FM receiver (creating an electromagnetic field that is picked up by the telecoil of the hearing aid); (2) an audio boot that connects directly to the hearing aid and interfaces with a wire connected with the FM system (thus, avoiding going into the T position of the hearing aid); and (3) an FM boot receiver connected directly to the hearing aid. For more information, the reader is referred to Chapter 34.

The teacher wears the microphone and transmitter. The transmitter changes the electrical signal from the microphone to the FM signal, which is then sent to the student's receiver. The teacher may use any one of several microphone options: a lavaliere microphone hung around the neck, a lapel microphone (wired or wireless) placed in a similar location, or a boom microphone positioned using a headband or ear-worn extender.

HYBRID (ACOUSTIC + ELECTRIC STIMULATION)

Cochlear implants have been under development since the early 1960s. The early work of Dr. William House helped refine the single-channel implant; current technology provides for 16 to 20 channels of electrical stimulation along the basilar membrane. With severe hearing loss, transmitting stimuli from the basilar membrane of the cochlea to the brain may be problematic due to damaged or missing inner hair cells. For those losses, a cochlear implant, which bypasses the basilar membrane vibrations and transductions of the inner hair cells, can be very effective (refer to Chapter 40 for a thorough discussion on this topic). With the common high-frequency hearing loss exhibited by many adults as a result of excessive noise exposure, the aging process, or even ototoxic drug ingestion, part of the frequency range (low frequency) may still exhibit relatively normal hair cell function, while the other part (high frequency) may be unaidable due to the resultant "dead regions" of the basilar membrane. One strategy that has evolved in the past few years to manage this type of hearing loss is referred to as a "hybrid" cochlear implant (Gantz and Turner, 2005). That is, the cochlear implant provides the high frequencies while the normal system is maintained for the low frequencies. An electrode array is implanted partially into the cochlea or a newly designed "short electrode" is inserted into the basal end of the cochlea to minimize damage to the apical (low-frequency) region of the cochlea (Keifer et al., 2005). Results have been promising in that many of the recipients of this *hybrid* amplification have better speech recognition ability compared with preimplant measures; in addition, the *hybrid* amplification provides better music perception (e.g., melody recognition) than most traditional cochlear implant schemes (Gfeller et al., 2006).

EVIDENCE-BASED PRACTICE CONSIDERATIONS

While it should be the goal of all disciplines to develop management schemes in alignment with the research evidence to support them, such is not always the case. In audiology alone, the number of papers published in the main audiology journals has grown from 200 a year to 1,700 a year since 1960 (Thorne, 2003). A clinician would need to read over five papers a day for 365 days a year in order to keep up! If hearing science literature is added, the total rises to 4,350 papers per year and requires reading 12 papers per day! Hearing health care is not unique in this dilemma. What may be unique in our field, however, is that the scientific basis for our clinical decision making has fallen far behind the technologic development of amplification devices (Cox, 2005; Medwetsky et al., 1999). Due in part to funding limitations, research relative to *efficacy* often falls into the hands of the manufacturer, and research relative to *effectiveness* occurs after the "new" technologic advancement has been replaced with something even newer. Thus the dilemma grows.

In current training programs, evidence-based practice is being incorporated into the curricula, either as a free-standing course, or embedded across clinical management courses. The concept embodies five steps: clearly defining the problem at hand, searching for evidence, critically appraising the evidence, formulating a recommendation, and assessing the outcome. Each step requires training and practice. Levels of evidence, grades of evidence, effect size, biases, and so on, all require study and practice. For further information on this topic, the interested reader is referred to American Speech-Language-Hearing Association (2004), Cox (2005), and Thorne (2003).

SUMMARY

The goal of this chapter was to summarize the state of the art relative to various types of hearing aid styles, technologies, capabilities, and advanced features. The intended audience includes students as well as practicing clinicians. No other realm of audiology changes more rapidly than amplification technology. As is the goal of any good teacher or program, we hope to encourage the interested reader to keep reading and learning, thus following new developments in technology over the years. This chapter should serve as a current starting point. There is much to be learned that has not yet been discovered.

REFERENCES

American National Standards Institute. (2005) American National Standard Method of Measurement of Performance Characteristics of Hearing Aids under Simulated Real-Ear Working Conditions. ANSI S3.35-2005. New York: American National Standards Institute.

American National Standards Institute. (2003) American National Standard Method Specification of Hearing Aid Characteristics. ANSI S3.22-1996. New York: American National Standards Institute.

American Speech-Language and Hearing Association. (2004) Evidence-based practice in communication disorders: an introduction. Available at: http://www.asha.org/members/deskref-journals/deskref/default.

AT&T (2006). 1936: synthetic speech. Available at: http://www.att.com/attlabs/reputation/timeline/36speech.html.

Bauer B. (1942) Super-cardioid directional microphone. *Electronics.* 1, 31–33.

Bentler RA, Anderson CV, Niebuhr D, Getta J. (1993) A longitudinal study of noise reduction circuits. Part I: objective measures. *J Speech Hear Res.* 36, 808–819.

Bentler RA, Chiou LK. (2006) Digital noise reduction: an overview. *Trends Amplif.* 10, 67–82.

Bentler RA, Cooley L. (2001) An examination of several characteristics that affect the prediction of OSPL90. *Ear Hear.* 22, 3–20.

Chasin M. (2001) The ins and outs of middle ear implants. *Hear J.* 54, 34–35.

Ching T, Dillon H, Byrne D. (1998) Speech recognition of hearing impaired listeners: predictions from audibility and the limited role of high-frequency amplification. *J Acoust Soc Am.* 103, 1128–1140.

Cox RM. (2005) Evidence-based practice in provision of amplification. *J Am Acad Audiol.* 16, 419–438.

Dai HP, Hou ZH. (2004) New feedback-cancellation algorithm reported to increase usable gain. *Hear J.* 57, 44–46.

Dillon H. (2001) *Hearing Aids.* Thieme: New York.

Dittberner AB, Bentler RA. (2007a) Predictive measures of directional benefit. Part 1: a three-dimensional, instrument-based approach to estimating the directivity index (DI). *Ear Hear.* 28, 26–45.

Dittberner AB, Bentler RA. (2007b) Predictive measures of directional benefit. Part 2: verification of different approaches to estimating directional benefit. *Ear Hear.* 28, 46–61.

Gantz BJ, Turner CW. (2005) Combining acoustic and electric hearing. *Laryngoscope.* 113, 1726–1730.

Gfeller K, Olszewski C, Turner C, Gantz B, Oleson J. (2006) Music perception with cochlear implants and residual hearing. *Audiol Neurootol.* 11 (suppl 1), 12–15.

Goode RL. (1989) Current status of electromagnetic implantable hearing aids. In: Maniglia AJ, ed. *Otology: Current Concepts and Technology. The Otolaryngological Clinics of North America.* Philadelphia: WB Saunders; pp 141–146.

Groth J. (2006) Improving sound quality with high-resolution hearing instruments. *Hear Rev.* 13, 44–48.

He S, Bentler R. (2006) Effects of reverberation on adaptive feedback pathway cancellation in hearing aids. *Unpublished technical paper.*

Hogan C, Turner CW. (1998) High frequency amplification: benefits for hearing impaired listeners. *J Acoust Soc Am.* 104, 432–441.

Jenstad LM, Van Tasell DJ, Ewert C. (2003) Hearing aid trouble shooting based on patient's descriptions. *J Am Acad Audiol.* 14, 347–360.

Joson HAL, Asano F, Suzuki Y, Sone T. (1993) Adaptive feedback cancellation with frequency compression for hearing aids. *J Acoust Soc Am.* 94, 3248–3254.

Kates JM. (1988) A computer simulation of hearing aid response and the effects of ear canal size. *J Acoust Soc Am.* 83, 1952–1963.

Kates JM. (2001) Room reverberation effects in hearing aid feedback cancellation. *J Acoust Soc Am.* 109, 367–378.

Keifer J, Pok M, Adunka O. (2005) Combined electrical and acoustical stimulation of the auditory system: results of a clinical study. *Audiol Neurootol.* 10, 134–144.

Kochkin S. (2004) MarkeTrak VII: customer satisfaction with hearing instruments in the digital age. *Hear J.* 58, 30–38.

Lybarger S. (1947) Development of a new hearing aid with magnetic microphone. *Electronic Manufacturer.* 11, 19–29.

Lybarger S. (1985) Earmolds. In: Katz J, ed. *Handbook of Clinical Audiology.* 3rd ed. Baltimore: Williams & Wilkins; pp 885–910.

Marriage JE, Moore BCJ, Stone MA, Baer T. (2005) Effects of three amplification strategies on speech perception by children with severe and profound hearing loss. *Ear Hear.* 26, 35–47.

Medwetsky L, Sanderson D, Young D. (1999) A national survey of audiology clinical practices: part 2. *Hear Rev.* 6, 14–22.

Merks I, Banerjee S, Trine T. (2006) Assessing the effectiveness of feedback cancellers in hearing aids. *Hear Rev.* 13, 53–57.

Moore BCJ, Glasberg BR, Stone MA. (2004) New version of the TEN test with calibration in dB HL. *Ear Hear.* 25, 478–487.

Moore BCJ, Huss M, Vickers DA, Glasberg BR, Alcantara JI. (2000) A test for threshold diagnosis of dead regions in the cochlea. *Br J Audiol.* 34, 205–224.

Mueller HG, Bentler RA. (2002) How loud is allowed revisited. *Hear J.* 55, 10–14.

Mueller HG, Bentler RA. (2005) Fitting hearing aids using clinical measures of loudness discomfort levels: a systematic review of effectiveness. *J Am Acad Audiol.* 16, 465–476.

Mueller HG, Hornsby B. (2002) Selection, verification and validation of maximum output. In: Valente M, ed. *Strategies for Selecting and Verifying Hearing Aid Fittings.* New York: Thieme; pp 23–66.

Mueller HG, Johnson E, Carter A. (2006) Hearing aids and assistive devices. In: Schow R, Nerbonne M, eds. *Audiologic Rehabilitation.* 4th ed. Needham Heights: Allyn and Bacon.

Plyler PN, Hill AB, Trine TD. (2005a) The effects of expansion on the objective and subjective performance of hearing instrument users. *J Am Acad Audiol.* 16, 101–113.

Plyler PN, Hill AB, Trine TD. (2005b) The effects of expansion time constants on the objective performance of hearing instrument users. *J Am Acad Audiol.* 16, 614–621.

Powers TA, Hamacher V. (2002) Three-microphone instrument is designed to extend benefits of directionality. *Hear Rev.* 55, 10–12.

Powers TA, Hamacher V. (2004) Providing adaptive directional technology works: a review of studies. *Hear Rev.* 11, 46–50.

Preves DA. (1988) Principles of signal processing. In: Sandlin RE, ed. *Handbook of Hearing Aid Amplification, Volume I: Theoretical and Technical Considerations.* Boston: College Hill Press; pp 91–120.

Ricketts TA. (2000) Directivity quantification in hearing aids: fitting and measurement effects. *Ear Hear.* 21, 45–58.

Sammeth CA, Levitt H. (2000) Hearing aid selection and fitting in adults: history and evolution. In: Valente M, Hosford-Dunn H, Roeser R, eds. *Audiology Treatment.* New York: Thieme; pp 213–259.

Savage I, Dillon H, Byrne D, Bachler H. (2006) Experimental evaluation of different methods of limiting the output of hearing aids. *Ear Hear.* 27, 550–562.

Skinner MW. (1988) Measuring for a successful fit. In: *Hearing Aid Evaluation.* Englewood Cliffs, NJ: Prentice Hall; p 285.

Strom K. (2006) Opinion: got BTEs? *Hear J.* 13, 6.

Thompson SC. (2003) Tutorial on microphone technologies for directional hearing aids. *Hear J.* 56, 14–24.

Thorne P. (2003) Evidence-based audiology and clinical evidence. *Aust N Z J Audiol.* 25, 10–15.

Walden BE, Surr RK, Cord MT. (2003) Real-world performance of directional microphone hearing aids. *Hear J.* 56, 40–47.

36 Troubleshooting Hearing Aids

Moneca Price, William Cole, and Marshall Chasin

░ INTRODUCTION

Many clients try hearing aids with great reluctance due to social stigma and the high cost associated with the devices. This reluctance is likely to be reinforced when common problems are not minimized or prevented during the prescription and fitting process. In a survey of hearing aid owners in the United States, one in six reported that they did not use their hearing aids at all (Kochkin, 2000). Common complaints included poor fit, occlusion, feedback, wax build-up, poor service, and sweaty ears. This chapter offers prevention and troubleshooting tips for hearing aid problems common among adult clients.

░ LOOKING FOR PATTERNS

A detailed and up-to-date case history and background are necessary for each client. This is especially important for new clients. Even changes in weight or occupation may affect hearing aid functioning. The clinician needs to determine the client's current level of knowledge and skill regarding the care and use of their hearing aids. A reported problem with a hearing aid may not be due to a technically related issue but, in fact, may be caused by a lack of knowledge on the client's part and may possibly be resolved with training and counseling.

The problem can result from many possible sources. The clinician needs to determine the nature of the problem: physical (pain in the ear); technical (hearing aid static, cutting out); acoustic (feedback); anatomic (occlusion, feedback); psychological (adaptation to hearing aid); or emotional (anxiety/fear about the hearing aid and stigma).

Remember that a client's complaint may have multiple underlying causes. Sometimes the problem is straightforward; other times, a client must be questioned closely over a series of visits. Table 36.1 lists a number of questions to guide the clinician in determining the underlying cause of a reported problem.

Patterns may point to the underlying cause of a problem. Problems may occur only in the evening, or when it is humid, or in certain locations. A client may complain that his or her hearing aid goes dead most afternoons or evenings, especially on a hot or rainy day, but usually works again the next morning. This pattern is typical for clients with persistent, dry flaky wax or skin. After several hours, the increasing levels of humidity can cause any dry wax or skin to expand enough to block the receiver tube. Overnight, the wax or skin dries out and shrinks, once again allowing sound to pass through. This pattern is also typical of drops of moisture condensing inside the hearing aid on a hot, humid day, which may cause a short circuit until the humidity level is low enough for the moisture to evaporate.

Another client may complain that whistling or feedback is heard only when he or she is visiting a particular person or location. It is possible that the hearing aid is fine and that what the client is hearing is the feedback of another person's hearing aid or simply some other high-pitched sound.

░ THE PROCESS OF HEARING AID TROUBLESHOOTING

Table 36.2 provides an overview of the various steps in effective troubleshooting of reported hearing aid problems.

TABLE 36.1   Patterns: determining the underlying cause of a problem

1. What is the problem?
2. How often does it happen?
3. How long does it last?
4. When did it start?
5. Is there a pattern?

It is meant to serve as a step-by-step guide to identifying and solving reported problems.

Performing a Visual Inspection

FIT IN THE EAR

Before proceeding with any other step, the clinician should observe the hearing aid while it is still in the client's ear. It is often possible to see common problems such as improper placement or loose fit. If the hearing aid is not properly placed, the client may experience pain or feedback. Clients require counseling and practice in the insertion of hearing aids. Clients should be counseled to recognize the signs of an improperly placed hearing aid, such as feedback, discomfort, or a decrease in sound quality or volume. If manual dexterity is an issue, a geriatric handle can be added to the aid or mold, or a caretaker can be trained to properly insert the hearing aid. For a full discussion on fit-related issues, see the section later in this chapter titled "Proper Fit."

Disinfection

Virtually every hearing aid has some kind of bacterial or fungal growth, and most have a combination of several microorganisms (Bankaitis, 2002). Handling multiple hearing aids risks passing bacteria, molds, and fungus such as *Staphylo-*

TABLE 36.2   The steps used in troubleshooting reported hearing aid problems

1. Look for patterns
2. Inspect the hearing aid in the client's ear
3. Disinfect the hearing aid before handling
4. Inspect hearing aid components:
   ■ Microphone
   ■ Receiver
   ■ Volume control
   ■ Program buttons and switches
   ■ Battery, battery door, and battery contacts
   ■ Ear hooks and tubing
   ■ Vents
5. Listen to the hearing aid
6. Perform American National Standards Institute tests on the hearing aid

coccus and *Candida* between clients. Associated diseases and infections include pneumonia, meningitis, and diphtheria.

The clinician must wash his or her hands using an established infection control protocol before handling any hearing aid. The hearing aid must be thoroughly disinfected with a germicidal wipe (such as Audiologist's Choice, Audio Wipes, or Assepto wipes). Ultraviolet light of a specific frequency (253.7 nm) is highly effective in infection control (Gates, 1929) and is used in devices such as the Dry & Store chambers. The following list indicates the most common microorganisms found on hearing aids and earmolds (Bankaitis and Kemp, 2003):

■ *Staphylococcus* (various)
■ Diphtheroids
■ *Pseudomonas* (various)
■ *Acinetobacter lwoffi*
■ *Enterobacter cloacae*
■ *Lactobacillus*
■ *Aspergillus flavus*
■ *Candida parapsilosis*

Inspecting the Hearing Aid and Component Parts

For a review of the basic anatomy of a hearing aid, consult Chapter 35, Hearing Aid Technology. The following sections list procedures for examining different parts of a hearing aid.

HEARING AID SHELL OR EARMOLD

Examine the hearing aid shell or the earmold for cracks or damage. Reshelling or a new mold may be indicated.

MICROPHONE

Check the microphone for debris. If there is a wind screen or wind hood, check to see if it is blocked. Look for signs of exposure to hair sprays or fine dust. Note that there may be moisture present even if water condensation is not visible (see section on moisture). Debris may be removed gently with a suction tool. Blocked or damaged wind screens and wind hoods should be replaced. Behind-the-ear microphone covers should be routinely replaced as specified by the manufacturer.

RECEIVER

Inspect the receiver. Remove any wax guard, and use an otoscope to look all the way down the receiver tube. To improve depth perception, back your eye off the otoscope view finder several inches and look down the otoscope view finder with both eyes. The receiver tube should be clear and the receiver clearly visible. Gently remove any debris, if possible. A vacuum chamber or suction tool can be used to remove small amounts of deeply seated wax, debris, or moisture (see following section on moisture).

For in-the-ear hearing aids, the receiver is particularly susceptible to damage by wax and moisture. Vigorous cleaning may also cause damage, dislodging the receiver tube and redirecting amplified output into the hearing aid cavity rather than into the ear canal. The presence of a basket-style wax guard can discourage mechanical damage from overzealous cleaning as well as prevent wax from reaching the receiver.

Effects of Moisture on a Hearing Aid

Much like a tropical jungle, the ear canal is hot, humid, and dirty. Humidity is increased due to the reduced ventilation caused by wearing hearing aids (Bailey and Valente, 1996); in addition, other sources can increase ear canal humidity, such as physical exertion, sweating, high humidity in the environment, and otitis externa (Gray et al., 2005). Behind-the-ear hearing aids are not directly exposed to the heat, humidity, and wax found inside the ear canal; however, they are exposed to sweat from the scalp and head.

The microphone and receiver must remain clear in order to pick up and transmit sounds accurately but can easily be clogged or damaged by dirt, wax, sprays, humidity, and sweat. The microphone diaphragm vibrates according to the frequency and volume of the incoming sound and can be significantly dampened by molecules of moisture. Because a wet diaphragm cannot vibrate fast enough to clearly transmit high frequencies, sound quality is compromised.

Moisture and sweat can also cause distortion, intermittent failure, faulty buttons and switches, corrosion of metal contacts and electronics, reduced battery life, and blocked vents, filters, and tubing. The regular use of a desiccant (such as a Dri-Aid kit or Dry & Store) and protective coverings for behind-the-ear hearing aids (such as sweatbands or Superseals) can significantly reduce the effect of sweat and humidity on hearing aids, both reducing the need for repair and lengthening service life.

VOLUME CONTROL

Examine the volume control if there is one. It should turn freely and not be too loose or too tight. A stiff volume control is often remedied by application of a contact cleaner. Remember that even if a volume control is present, it may be deactivated or may act as an on/off switch even when deactivated. A listening check will confirm the current functioning of a volume control.

PROGRAM BUTTONS AND SWITCHES

Examine program buttons, switches, or other controls on the hearing aid. Buttons and switches should move freely. Look for a build-up of debris or corrosion around the controls. A small brush will often remove most debris or dirt, and the careful use of a contact cleaner can loosen stiff buttons or switches. During the listening check (discussed later), listen to see if the buttons or switches are functioning correctly.

BATTERY, BATTERY DOOR, AND CONTACTS

The battery contacts should grip the battery snugly but not too tightly. Look for scratches on the battery caused by tight contacts. A battery door should open smoothly and not be too tight or loose. Check for cracks or breaks in the plastic of the battery door. The hinge of in-the-ear battery doors can break fairly easily, requiring replacement. With some practice, battery doors are easy to replace, although care must be taken that the correct replacement door is used. For some makes of hearing aids, there are right-hand and left-hand battery doors that cannot be interchanged. Also, battery doors may change from model to model within the same company. If in doubt, order the required battery door based on the serial number of the hearing aid.

When removing or replacing battery doors, always take great care not to damage the hinge pin. If the metal hinge pin is broken or dislodged, the hearing aid must be sent to the manufacturer for repair. For behind-the-ear and open-fit hearing aids, the hearing aid may need to be sent to the manufacturer if the battery door needs replacing.

Take a look at the battery and battery contacts for signs of corrosion. Use a cotton swab and contact cleaner to clean dirty contacts, if needed. Occasionally, the battery may be pushed into the internal cavity of the hearing aid rather than placed into the battery door. Typically, this happens with clients with poor vision or when caretakers or friends try to change the battery. Removing the battery can solve the problem; however, it is possible that the internal wiring or circuit may have been damaged. Unless an American National Standards Institute (ANSI) test of the hearing aid reveals that it is functioning within specifications, the hearing aid should be sent to the company for repair. For more information, see "Batteries" section later in this chapter.

EAR HOOKS (BEHIND-THE-EAR HEARING AIDS ONLY)

For behind-the-ear hearing aids, inspect the ear hook; loose ear hooks should be replaced. Check the tubing for any debris or moisture. If ANSI testing shows low gain, retest the hearing aid without the ear hook. Ear hooks with filters are particularly susceptible to partial or complete blockage by debris, wax, or moisture and should be replaced as needed. Care should be taken to avoid over-tightening when replacing an ear hook. Some ear hooks cannot be replaced in-house and must be sent to the manufacturer for replacement.

TUBING (BEHIND-THE-EAR HEARING AIDS ONLY)

If the tubing is hardened or cracked, it should be replaced because it can allow sound to cycle back to the microphone, causing feedback.

For open-fit hearing aids, inspect the tubing and dome for blockage or damage. Because the tubing for these hearing aids is so thin, wax blockage is the most common problem and should be cleared with the tool provided by the manufacturer for this purpose. Open fit tubing and tips should be changed regularly as recommended by the manufacturer. For those models with the receiver in the ear, there is generally a wax guard system that can be changed at the receiver.

VENTS

A vent is a passage through a hearing aid or mold that allows heat to escape from the ear canal, equalizes atmospheric pressure to the ear drum, and allows excess amplification at various frequencies to escape from the ear canal.

Check to see if the vent is occluded with wax or other debris. A plugged vent may cause sweaty ears, uncomfortable pressure, or occlusion. If a client complains that feedback started suddenly and an examination shows that the hearing aid has a large open vent, a vent plug may have been previously used but has since fallen out. A well-fitting vent plug should not fall out. When a vent plug is used, it should still provide a release of pressure if possible.

Performing a Listening Check

When listening directly to a hearing aid, use a custom listening ear piece for the best sound quality. Disinfect the flexible coupler of the listening piece (as described in the section earlier on infection control) before and after listening to a hearing aid.

With high-power hearing aids, always turn the volume to the lowest setting and do not insert the listening ear piece deep in the ear. Ensure a tight fit between the listening ear piece and the hearing aid to avoid painful feedback. Always remember that the sound pressure levels (SPLs) generated by power hearing aids are capable of causing damage to the clinician's inner ear.

Before doing a listening check or ANSI test, remove any wax guards, microphone protectors, ear hooks, or tubing. This will ensure that you are testing the hearing aid circuit. Always use a fresh battery to rule out battery-related issues. When performing a listening check of a hearing aid, listen for the following:

- Clear and consistent sound
- Smooth increase/decrease of sound when operating the volume control (if activated)
- Obvious distortion
- Cutting in and out
- Static or cutting out when operating the volume control
- Static or cutting out when operating the toggle switches or push buttons
- The hearing aid's frequency response, using the LING six sound test (Estabrooks and Birkenshaw-Fleming, 2003)

/m/   low frequencies
/oo/   low frequencies
/ah/   first and second formants, middle frequencies
/ee/   first formant low frequency, second formant higher frequency
/sh/   middle and high frequencies
/s/   high frequencies

A listening check may indicate that a hearing aid is functioning well, but it cannot replace an ANSI test, which determines whether the hearing aid is functioning according to manufacturer specifications.

Troubleshooting with Hearing Aid Analyzers

A typical hearing aid analyzer is shown schematically in Figure 36.1. A signal generator [6] provides test signals to a loudspeaker [1]. The level and spectrum of the signal is measured and controlled by a reference microphone [5] in conjunction with the signal generator. The output of the hearing aid [2] is coupled to a measuring microphone [3] and measuring system [7] by a coupler [4]. To reduce the impact of ambient noise on the intended stimuli or on the operation of the hearing aid, the sound source and hearing aid may be enclosed in a sound-isolating test chamber [8] that is lined with sound-absorbing material [9] to improve sound-field uniformity. In most cases, the stimulus is acoustic, but it may also be magnetic in cases where the performance of a telephone coil is to be tested.

TEST SIGNALS

A variety of test signals is available in the modern hearing aid analyzer. These include steady puretones, steady pseudo-random noise, modulated puretones, modulated noise, and real speech. It must always be remembered that, when testing

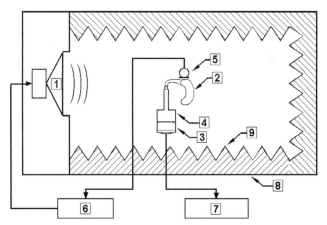

FIGURE 36.1 Schematic representation of a hearing aid analyzer. Acoustic test signals from loudspeaker [1] are generated and controlled by signal generator/control system [6] in conjunction with reference microphone [5]. Output of the hearing aid [2] is coupled to a measuring microphone [3] and measuring system [7] by a coupler [4]. Sound-isolating enclosure [8] is lined with sound-absorbing material [9] to reduce standing waves.

hearing aids with compression or any other adaptive processing features, the results obtained will be valid only for the test signal used. While it may be tempting and convenient to generalize performance for complex signals from measurements done with simpler signals, the error in doing so will be hearing aid dependent, and this error increases as the difference in signals increases (Henning and Bentler, 2005; Scollie and Seewald, 2002; Stelmachowicz et al., 1996).

In the configuration shown in Figure 36.1, the test signal is controlled by placing a small calibrated microphone very close to the hearing aid microphone port(s) and using the measured SPL to control the signal to the loudspeaker. This is known as the pressure method and is the preferred method in the American National Standard Specification of Hearing Aid Characteristics (ANSI S3.22-2003; ANSI, 2003). Alternately, a substitution method may be used to control the test signal. In this case, an equalization (leveling) step is performed prior to the test. In this step, the microphone is removed from the coupler and is used to measure the sound field near the hearing aid microphone port while a known electrical signal is applied to the loudspeaker. For greatest accuracy, all objects should be positioned in the test chamber just as they will be during the test, and a dummy microphone should be installed in the coupler. After the equalization step, the dummy microphone and the coupler microphone are interchanged for subsequent tests.

COUPLERS

The coupler that connects the hearing aid to the measuring microphone also serves as an acoustic load on the hearing aid. This acoustic load has a strong influence on the measured output of the hearing aid, and several have been standardized for hearing aid testing. The most common has a volume of 2 cm³ and is frequently referred to as a 2-cc coupler. The American National Standard Method for Coupler Calibration of Earphones (ANSI S3.7-1995; ANSI, 1995) defines this coupler and provides several variations to accommodate different hearing aid configurations. ANSI S3.22-2003 specifies which of these variations is to be used with different hearing aid types.

In-the-ear and in-the-canal devices, including deep insertion hearing aids, are to be tested in a type HA-1 coupler (Fig. 36.2), which has a direct entrance to the 2-cm³ cavity. The acoustic coupling between the sound outlet of the hearing aid and the coupler entrance must be made airtight by using an appropriate sealant. There is a rarely used provision in ANSI S3.22-2003 for modular in-the-ear hearing aids to be tested on an HA-3 coupler, a variation on the HA-2 coupler described in Figure 36.4.

Hearing aids that employ a button type receiver are to be tested using the type HA-2 coupler (ANSI S3.22-2003). This coupler (Fig. 36.3) has the entrance to the cavity through an earmold substitute having a 3-mm diameter sound bore that is 18 mm long. All hearing aids that couple to the ear by means of a length of tubing are to be tested using type HA-2

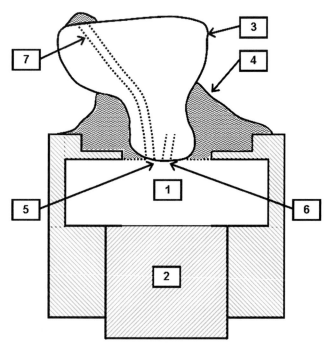

FIGURE 36.2   The HA-1 hearing aid coupler. The coupler microphone [2] is concentric with the cavity [1], which has a diameter between 18 and 21 mm and a volume of 2.0 cm³   ± 1%. Hearing aid [3] is sealed to the cavity with putty [4], such that the tip [5] is even with the cavity wall and the sound outlet [6] is approximately centered in the opening. Vent [7] is sealed at the faceplate.

with entrance through a tube. ANSI S3.22-2003 permits two variations on the tubing used in this coupler. The first is intended for most postauricular (behind-the-ear) hearing aids and consists of a rigid tube with a 2-mm inside diameter and a length of 25 mm between the earmold substitute and the tip of the ear hook (Fig. 36.4). The second variation (type HA-4) is like the first except that both the earmold substitute and the connecting tubing have a 1.93-mm diameter sound bore, creating a uniform sound path with a length of 43 mm. This was originally intended for use with eyeglass hearing aids, which used skeleton-type earmolds and a continuous length of #13 tubing (inside diameter of 1.93 mm).

A third variation of the HA-2 coupler is permitted by ANSI S3.22-2003 for testing modular in-the-ear hearing aids. In this variation, designated the HA-3 coupler, the tubing connects directly from the hearing aid receiver outlet to the entrance to the cavity. This tubing is required to have an inside diameter of 1.93 mm and a length from the receiver case to the cavity entrance of 10 mm.

The coupler to be used for postauricular hearing aids with the receiver in the ear canal is not explicitly indicated in ANSI S3.22-2003, but the HA-1 coupler is intended to be used with hearing aids having ear tips (ANSI S3.7-1995), and this is the logical choice for reporting test results for these devices. The tip and coupling system used should be of average size and should be stated.

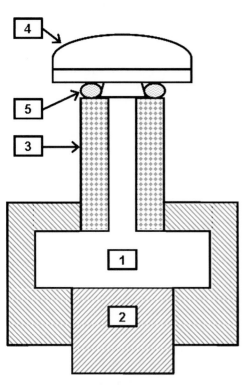

FIGURE 36.3   The HA-2 hearing aid coupler. The coupler microphone [2] is concentric with the cavity [1], which has a diameter between 18 and 21 mm and a volume of 2.0 cm^3 ± 1%. Entrance to the cavity is through an earmold substitute [3] having a 3-mm diameter sound bore with a length of 18 mm. The earphone [4] is sealed to the earmold substitute with a suitable sealing mechanism [5].

Vented or Open Fittings

There are no standardized couplers (see following "Ear Simulators" section) or test methods capable of characterizing hearing aids operating with large vents or in open ear canals. "Open-fit" hearing aids must be tested using one of the closed coupler configurations previously described. Postauricular hearing aids with thin coupling tubes are often provided with a standard ear hook; thus, they can be tested using the HA-2 coupler. If this is not the case, the open end of the thin tube must be sealed to the entrance of the HA-1 coupler using an adapter or an appropriate sealant. The exact configuration should be specified by the manufacturer, and any required adapters should be available from the manufacturer for test purposes.

EAR SIMULATORS

The 2-cc coupler does not accurately represent the acoustic impedance or resonances of a real ear, and its usefulness as a test load is confined to the 200- to 5,000-Hz range. Ear simulators are designed to more closely approximate the acoustic impedance and resonance characteristics of an average of ears over a wide frequency range. Their use is

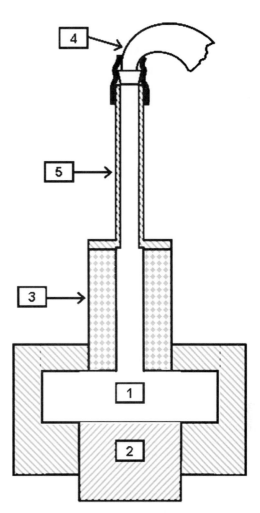

FIGURE 36.4   The HA-2 coupler with entrance through a rigid tube. The coupler microphone [2] is concentric with the cavity [1], which has a diameter between 18 and 21 mm and a volume of 2.0 cm^3 ± 1%. Entrance to the cavity is through an earmold substitute [3] having a 3-mm diameter sound bore with a length of 18 mm. Coupling from the tip of the hearing aid hook [4] to the earmold substitute is via a rigid tube [5] with a 2-mm inner diameter and a length of 25 mm.

required when realistic estimates of performance of deep insertion, vented and open fittings, and feedback suppression systems are desired. In some cases, a pinna may be part of the simulator, and the combination may be part of an acoustic manikin.

Simulators are more complex, more expensive, and more difficult to maintain than the 2-cc coupler, and this has confined their use to the laboratory. The Zwislocki coupler (Zwislocki, 1970; 1971), which is no longer commercially available, is one such ear simulator. The only simulator currently available commercially is the occluded ear simulator (OES), which is standardized in International Electrotechnical Commission (IEC) 60711-1981 (IEC, 1981) and often called the 711 coupler.

AMERICAN NATIONAL STANDARDS INSTITUTE HEARING AID TESTS

There are four standards published by the ANSI that relate to the testing of hearing aids. These are described here.

First is the ANSI S3.22-2003, Specification of Hearing Aid Characteristics (ANSI, 2003). This standard describes methods of measuring a number of hearing aid characteristics and provides allowable tolerances for those that are deemed important for the maintenance of product uniformity and compliance with published specifications. The use of portions of this standard is mandated by the Food and Drug Administration (FDA). This standard also contains procedures for many other tests that are not required by the FDA.

All hearing aid manufacturers are required to include in the product brochure or other labeling that accompanies the hearing aid the technical data listed in Table 36.3 with measurement conditions and tolerances as given in Table 36.4. When troubleshooting a hearing aid, these required

---

TABLE 36.3 Data obtained from ANSI S3.22-2003 that must be provided by the hearing aid manufacturer in a product brochure or in other labeling that accompanies a hearing aid

Requirement	Description of required data
Abbreviations	HFA: High-frequency average—the average of values at 1,000, 1,600, and 2,500 Hz SPA: Special purpose average—the average of values at three frequencies specified by the hearing aid manufacturer that are at one-third octave frequencies separated by two-thirds octave RTS: Reference test setting—setting of the gain control (i.e., volume control, master or overall gain control) required to produce an HFA gain within ±1.5 dB of the HFA-OSPL90 minus 77 dB for a 60-dB input sound pressure level (SPL) or, if the full-on HFA gain for a 60 dB input SPL is less than the HFA OSPL90 minus 77 dB, the full-on setting of the gain control AGC: Automatic gain control—means for controlling gain as a function of signal level; it includes various forms of compression
OSPL90 curve	Coupler SPL as a function of frequency for a 90 dB input SPL and gain control at full-on
HFA-OSPL90	The average of the OSPL90 values at the HFA or SPA frequencies
HFA full-on gain (HFA-FOG)	The average of the full-on gain at the HFA or SPA frequencies
Reference test gain (RTG)	The average of the gain at the HFA or SPA frequencies for a 60 dB input SPL, with gain control at RTS
Frequency response curve	The coupler SPL as a function of frequency for a 60 dB input SPL, with gain control at RTS
Frequency range	The range between the lowest and the highest frequency at which the frequency response curve is 20 dB below its HFA or SPA value
Total harmonic distortion (THD)	The ratio of sum of the powers of all the harmonics to the power of the fundamental
Equivalent input noise (EIN)	The SPL of an external noise source at the input that would result in the same coupler SPL as that caused by all the internal noise sources in the hearing aid
Battery current	The electrical current drawn from the battery when the input SPL is 65 dB at 1,000 Hz and the gain control is at RTS
Induction coil sensitivity (HFA-SPLITS)	For hearing aids with an inductive input coil (telecoil), the average of the coupler SPL at the HFA or SPA frequencies when the hearing aid, with gain control at RTS, is appropriately positioned on a telephone magnetic field simulator (TMFS)
Input-output curve	For hearing aids with AGC, the coupler SPL as a function of the input SPL at one or more of 250, 500, 1,000, 2,000, 4,000 Hz, with the gain control at RTS
Attack time	For hearing aids with AGC, the time between an abrupt change from 55 to 90 dB input SPL and the time when the coupler SPL has stabilized to within 3 dB of the steady value for a 90 dB input SPL, at one or more of 250, 500, 1,000, 2,000, or 4,000 Hz, with the gain control at RTS
Release time	For hearing aids with AGC, the time between an abrupt change from 90 to 55 dB input SPL and the time when the coupler SPL has stabilized to within 4 dB of the steady value for a 55 dB input SPL, at one or more of 250, 500, 1,000, 2,000, or 4,000 Hz, with the gain control at RTS

TABLE 36.4 **Food and Drug Administration–mandated ANSI S3.22-2003 tests and their parameters and tolerances**

Test	Gain Setting	AGC	Input	Frequency	Measure or Calculate	Tolerance
OSPL90 curve	Full on	Min	90 dB SPL	200–5,000 Hz	Coupler SPL	Unspecified
Maximum OSPL90	Full on	Min	90 dB SPL	Frequency of maximum	Maximum of OSPL90 curve	+3 dB
HFA- or SPA-OSPL90	Full on	Min	90 dB SPL	HFA or SPA	Average coupler SPL at HFA or SPA frequencies	±4dB
HFA or SPA full-on gain (HFA- or SPA-FOG)	Full on	Min	50 dB SPL	HFA or SPA	Average gain at HFA or SPA frequencies	±5dB
Reference test gain (RTG)	RTS	Min	60 dB SPL	HFA or SPA	Average gain at HFA or SPA frequencies	Unspecified
Frequency range	RTS	Min	60 dB SPL	From the lowest frequency (f1) to the highest frequency (f2) at which the frequency response curve is 20 dB below its HFA or SPA average		Unspecified
Frequency response curve	RTS	Min	60 dB SPL	From the higher of f1 or 200 Hz to the lower of f2 or 5,000 Hz; wider range may be shown	Coupler SPL or gain	±4dB from the lesser of 1.25 f1 or 200 Hz to 2 kHz. ±6dB from 2 kHz to the lesser of 4 kHz or 0.8 f2.
Total harmonic distortion (THD)	RTS	Min	70 dB SPL 65 dB SPL	500, 800, or ½ the lower two SPA frequencies 1,600 or ½ the highest SPA frequency		+3%
Equivalent input noise (EIN)	RTS	Min	OFF and 50 dB SPL	(Coupler SPL with no input) − (HFA or SPA gain with a 50 dB input SPL)		+3 dB
Battery current	RTS	Min	65 dB SPL	1,000 Hz	Battery current	+20%
SPL for an inductive telephone simulator (SPLITS)	RTS	Min	TMFS	200–5,000 Hz	Coupler SPL. Orient aid on TMFS for maximum output. Place BTE as flat as possible on test surface. ITE and ITC with faceplate as close as possible and parallel to test surface.	Unspecified
HFA or SPA SPLITS	RTS	Min	TMFS	HFA or SPA	Average SPLITS values at the HFA or SPA frequencies	±6dB

(Continued)

TABLE 36.4 *(Continued)*

Test	Gain Setting	AGC	Input	Frequency	Measure or Calculate	Tolerance
Input-output curves	RTS	Max	50 to 90 dB SPL in 5-dB steps	One or more of 250, 500, 1,000, 2,000, 4,000 Hz	Coupler SPL vs. input SPL	±5dB at 50 and 90 dB input SPL when matched at 70 dB input SPL
Attack time	RTS	Max	Step from 55 to 90 dB SPL	Same frequencies used for input-output curves	Time from input step until coupler SPL settles within 3 dB of its steady value for 90 dB input SPL	±5ms or 50%, whichever is greater
Release time	RTS	Max	Step from 90 to 55 dB SPL	Same frequencies used for input-output curves	Time from input step until coupler SPL settles within 4 dB of its steady value for 55 dB input SPL	±5ms or 50%, whichever is greater

AGC, automatic gain control; Min, minimum; Max, maximum; SPL, sound pressure level; RTS, reference test setting; HFA, high-frequency average; SPA, special purpose average; TMFS, telephone magnetic field simulator; BTE, behind-the-ear; ITE, in-the-ear; ITC, in-the-canal.

data are the benchmarks against which measured performance should be verified. It should be noted that, when verifying compliance with manufacturers' specifications, the indicated tolerance plus measuring equipment accuracy must be added to the value listed by the manufacturer. For example, if measurement equipment accuracy is ±1 dB and the tolerance given in the table for a particular test is ±4 dB, then a measured value within ±5 dB of the value listed by the manufacturer would be considered to be within specification.

When interpreting the results of the tests included in this ANSI standard, it is important to remember the following points:

1. ANSI S3.22-2003 is a quality control standard. The data apply only for the puretone signals and measurement conditions, hearing aid settings, and configuration employed when they were generated. They do not predict performance for other signals, conditions, settings, or configurations.
2. Measurements are defined only for the frequency range 200 to 5,000 Hz. A wider range may be shown for informational purposes.
3. Attack and release times include any processing delay through the hearing aid. For digital hearing aids, this will account for some fixed portion of the reported times,

typically between 3 and 10 ms. Given the allowed tolerances on these quantities, this is unlikely to be significant.
4. Attack and release times are very dependent on the hearing aid settings and the test protocol. Do not assume they represent times likely to be experienced in actual use.

The second standard is ANSI S3.35-2004, Method of Measurement of Performance Characteristics of Hearing Aids under Simulated Real-Ear Working Conditions (ANSI, 2004). This standard provides terminology and techniques for the precise determination of simulated insertion gain, three-dimensional directional response, and directivity index using a suitable manikin and ear simulator. It gives requirements for the test space (typically a large anechoic chamber) and the test equipment. Hearing aids must be placed in a linear, nonadaptive mode of operation. This is a voluntary standard, and its use is not mandated by any government regulation.

The third standard is ANSI S3.42-1992 (R2002), Testing Hearing Aids with a Broad-Band Noise Signal (ANSI, 2002a). This standard defines the spectrum of a broadband noise test signal and specifies analysis methods for obtaining the steady-state output and gain of hearing aids using this signal. It should be noted that the specified spectrum

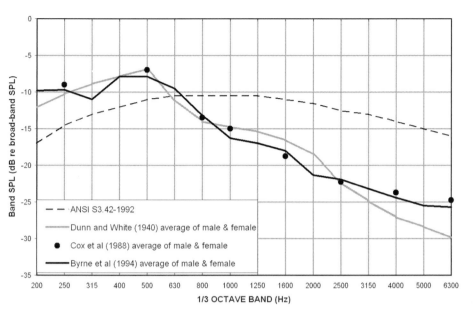

FIGURE 36.5 The ANSI S3.42-1992 noise spectrum and selected long-term average speech spectra.

of the test signal is that of the peaks of speech, not the long-term average speech spectrum (LTASS). As such, it has considerably more high-frequency content than is found in speech-weighted noise based on the LTASS (see Fig. 36.5 for a representation of the 1992 noise spectrum and LTASS). As noted in the standard, the steady-state gain and output obtained using this standard are not representative of the gain or output for real speech signals processed by compression hearing aids (Henning and Bentler, 2005; Scollie and Seewald, 2002; Stelmachowicz et al., 1996). This is a voluntary standard, and its use is not mandated by any government regulation.

Finally, the fourth standard is ANSI S3.46-1997 (R2002): Methods of Measurement of Real-Ear Performance Characteristics of Hearing Aids (ANSI, 2002b). This standard defines terms used in real-ear measurements and provides guidance on procedures for both closed and vented fittings, sources of error, and essential reporting and equipment requirements. This is a voluntary standard, and its use is not mandated by any government regulation.

Troubleshooting Using ANSI S3.22-2003 Tests

Most commercial hearing aid analyzers provide automated test sequences that make it easy to run the FDA-mandated hearing aid tests of ANSI S3.22-2003. Although these tests do not represent performance at "use" settings, it is good practice to run them for comparison with manufacturers' data when a hearing aid is first received, when it has been repaired, or when a malfunction is suspected.

The tests of ANSI S3.22-2003 are run with all adaptive features disabled and three different hearing aid setups (for more in-depth discussion of some of the hearing aid param-

eters discussed in the following list, the reader is referred to Chapter 35):

■ The Output Sound Pressure Level with a 90-dB Input (OSPL90) and full-on tests are run with any automatic gain control (AGC) function set for minimum effect (i.e., its most linear operation) and the maximum output and gain set to their highest values. Most programming software provides a setting that accomplishes this. If this is not the case, setting the AGC function for minimum effect may be accomplished by disabling the AGC (if possible), by setting the compression threshold to its highest setting, and/or by setting the compression ratio as close to 1.0 as possible, while still keeping maximum output and gain at their highest values.

■ All other tests are run with the gain control at the reference test setting. Most programming software provides a setting for this. If this is not the case, most commercial hearing aid test systems provide automated assistance in making this adjustment.

■ Attack and release times and input-output curve tests are performed with the AGC function set to have maximum effect. Some programming software may provide a setting that does this. If not, setting the AGC function for maximum effect may be accomplished by setting low-level gain as high as possible and setting high-level gain and maximum output as low as possible. This will typically result in a very low compression threshold, a very flat input-output curve above this threshold, and maximum attack and release times. These results should be interpreted as representing the extremes of what is attainable, not what is typical in use.

Manufacturers are required to indicate the control or software settings or provide test programs used for all tests. These settings must be used when verifying performance against test strips or specification sheets.

Before running the ANSI S3.22 tests, clinicians should do the following:

1. Install a fresh battery, or use the battery substitute in the analyzer.
2. For behind-the-ear aids, ensure that the plastic tubing on the HA-2 coupler is flexible, free from splits, and the correct length and diameter. The tubing between the tip of the ear hook and the entrance to the earmold simulator should be 2 mm in diameter and 25 mm in length. Some analyzers include all of this tubing within the HA-2 coupler, using a very short piece of earmold tubing only to seal the tip of the ear hook to the internal tubing. Others include varying amounts of the 2-mm section within the coupler, with the remainder (usually 15 to 25 mm) made up of flexible tubing added by the user. In these cases, both the internal diameter and the total length must be per the ANSI guidelines.
3. For behind-the-ear aids, ensure that the ear hook and dampers are as specified in the manufacturer's test data and that they are free of obstructions.
4. In-the-ear, in-the-canal, completely-in-the-canal, and other deep-insertion hearing aids should be well sealed to the HA-1 coupler with their tip flush with the entrance to the 2-cc cavity.
5. Any wax guards or microphone screens specified by the manufacturer must be in place and free of obstructions. Any not specified by the manufacturer should be removed.
6. Vents must be plugged at the faceplate (custom aids) or external (behind-the-ear) end.
7. The hearing aid should be set to the omnidirectional mode, its widest frequency response range, greatest high-frequency average (HFA) OSPL90 or special purpose average (SPA) OSPL90, and, if possible, greatest HFA or SPA full-on gain. The HFA frequencies are 1,000, 1,600, and 2,500 Hz; the SPA frequencies are specified by the manufacturer and are one-third octave frequencies separated by two-thirds octave. Any AGC function should be set to have minimum effect, and any adaptive features should be disabled. Settings or a program to achieve these conditions should be provided by the manufacturer.

Table 36.5 lists some potential deviations from manufacturers' specifications and their possible cause and remedy.

It is important to make sure that any given test has been run properly, with the hearing aid set exactly as specified, before attempting to draw any conclusions from the test results. Failing to close vents or improper sealing of the hearing aid or earpiece to the HA-1 coupler can result in curves like those in Figures 36.6 and 36.7. Please note that both curves are output SPL curves versus the typically displayed gain curves when illustrating the effects of venting on hearing aid performance.

Some "rules of thumb" for interpreting ANSI S3.22-2003 test results are as follows:

■ OSPL90 tests generally provide information about the output components of the hearing aid (i.e., receiver, hook, dampers, wax guards, etc.) or the power source.
■ Gain tests generally provide information about both the output and the input components of the hearing aid (i.e., microphones, wind filters etc.).
■ Distortion tests generally provide information about the receiver or power source.
■ Equivalent input noise tests will generally provide information about the microphone(s).
■ AGC tests may detect faulty components in analog circuits, but in digital hearing aids, these characteristics are controlled by software. Consequently, for digital circuits, it is extremely unlikely that these tests will be failed by themselves. Failures in digital circuits are more likely to impact many or all of the tests.

TROUBLESHOOTING WHEN ANSI S3.22 CANNOT BE USED

Sometimes data sheets or test strips are not available, programming software is not at hand, programming connectors are broken, cables cannot be readily obtained, or the hook is not the one used for the ANSI tests. In these cases, test results cannot be directly compared with ANSI specifications to determine if the hearing aid itself is functioning properly. The hearing aid analyzer then becomes a useful tool for probing the hearing aid to determine if it is performing in an acceptable fashion.

Perhaps the simplest deviation from the ANSI test conditions is the use of an ear hook different from the one used to generate the specifications. Running the ANSI tests with a different hook, especially one with different dampers, is likely to change the peaks in the OSPL90 and frequency response curves and the numerical data derived from them. However, the data should still indicate whether the hearing aid is performing reasonably close to expectations. If the ear hook is damaged or permanently blocked and a replacement is not readily available, it is still possible to determine if the hearing aid itself is functioning by replacing the hook with a length of earmold tubing that has the same length as the hook (this gets added to any tubing that would normally be attached to the coupler). Figure 36.8 shows frequency response curves for a behind-the-ear aid with the proper damped ear hook (lower curve) and with the hook replaced with earmold tubing having the same length as the ear hook but without dampers (upper curve). Although the peaks in the response curve are no longer damped, running an ANSI test battery in this case will still provide data that may be compared to the ANSI specifications to help decide if the hearing aid is functioning properly and simply needs a new

TABLE 36.5   Deviations from manufacturers' specifications and their possible cause and remedy

ANSI test	Result	Possible cause – *remediation*
OSPL90 curve	Large peaks or notches in the low to mid frequencies (see Figs. 36.6 and 36.7)	Open vent – *close at faceplate end* Poor seal of hearing aid tip to HA-1 coupler – *reseal* Cracked tubing on HA-2 coupler –*replace* Defective ear hook –*replace*
OSPL90 curve	Curve is very jagged	Aid is not set to test program – *correct settings*
OSPL90 curve, Maximum OSPL90, HFA-OSPL90	Curve is well below manufacturer's reported results Maximum and HFA-OSPL90 are below tolerance	Defective battery – *try new battery, different batch* Restricted airflow to zinc air battery – *clean air holes or grooves in battery compartment* Wrong or blocked ear hook – *replace/clean ear hook* Blocked wax guard – *clean or replace* Blocked receiver tube – *clean or repair* Defective receiver –*repair*
HFA-FOG	HFA-FOG is below tolerance, but OSPL90 tests are OK	Blocked microphone port(s) – *clean, replace filters* Defective microphone – *repair*
Frequency response curve	Curve is below tolerance at some frequencies, but OSPL90 tests are OK	Aid not in omnidirectional mode – *change settings* Blocked microphone port(s) – *clean, replace filters* Defective microphone – *repair*
Frequency response curve	Curve has sharp peaks at one or two frequencies	Feedback – *check seal to coupler and vent closure* Cracked tubing on HA-2 coupler – *replace* Defective hook – *replace* Internal feedback – *repair*
Total harmonic distortion	Levels are above allowed tolerance	Defective battery – *try new battery, different batch* Restricted airflow to zinc air battery – *clean air holes or grooves in battery compartment* Defective receiver – *repair* Defect in circuit –*repair*
Equivalent input noise	Levels are above allowed tolerance	Noise in the test environment – *repeat test in quiet* Blocked microphone port(s) – *clean, replace filters* Defective microphone – *repair* Specifications may be with expansion enabled – *check settings used by manufacturer for this test*
Attack and release times	Values are beyond tolerance limits	Noise in the test environment – *repeat test in quiet* Test settings do not match those specified by the manufacturer for these tests – *correct settings* Defect in circuit –*repair*

ANSI, American National Standards Institute; HFA, high-frequency average; FOG, full-on gain.

hook or if it has more serious problems and needs to be sent for repair.

If it is not possible to disable adaptive features as required for the ANSI tests or if it is simply desired to test the hearing aid at its "use" settings, consideration must be given to the response of the adaptive features to the test signal being used. Adaptive features are most likely to be activated by signals that are tonal or unchanging, and this activation may occur some time after the signal is applied. Running an ANSI test battery in this situation may produce erratic OSPL90 and frequency response curves. Tests of distortion or attack/release time are unlikely to be reliable because the relatively long duration of these tests will likely give the adaptive features time to react.

USE OF ACOUSTIC STIMULI TO ASSESS NONADAPTIVE HEARING AID CHARACTERISTICS

Tests Using Speech-Like Test Signals

There are a number of ways to extract useful information about the condition of the hearing aid without disabling adaptive features. The method with the least likelihood of inadvertently triggering noise reduction, feedback suppression, or adaptive directional features uses speech-like signals and determines gain or output. These may be real speech signals or signals such as modulated noise or International Collegium of Rehabilitative Audiology (ICRA) noise, a

FIGURE 36.6 Effect of an open vent on an OSPL90 curve for an in-the-ear hearing aid. The lower curve (1) is the correct curve, obtained with the vents sealed at the faceplate (outer) end; the upper curve (2) is obtained with the vent open; note that the low-frequency sound enters directly through the open vent unamplified, yielding more low-frequency energy in the output than if the vent was plugged. In addition, the open vent, in conjunction with the 2-cc cavity, forms a resonator for sounds entering directly through the vent, resulting in the boost observed at 500 Hz. This effect depends on vent dimensions, the hearing aid, and its settings.

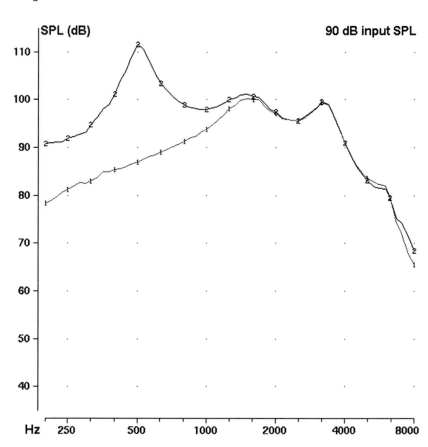

FIGURE 36.7 Effect of a poor seal to the coupler on the OSPL90 curve for an in-the-canal hearing aid. The smooth curve (2) is obtained with a good seal; the irregular curve (1) is obtained with a poor seal to the coupler. The magnitude of the effect depends on the hearing aid and its settings.

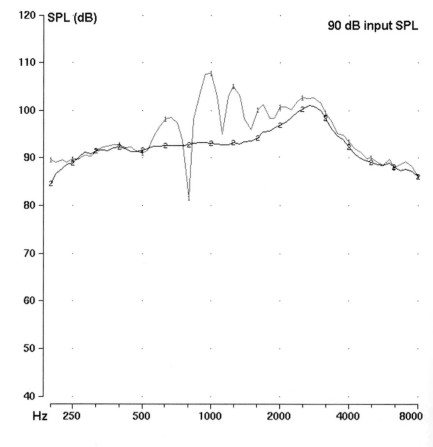

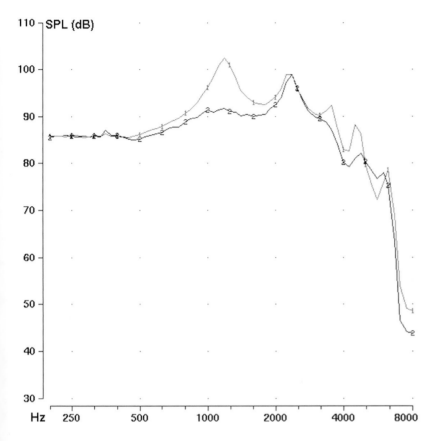

FIGURE 36.8 Effect of ear hook on frequency response curves. The lower curve (2) was obtained with the manufacturer-specified damped ear hook. The upper curve (1) was obtained with the hook replaced with earmold tubing having the same length as the ear hook and no dampers.

signal derived by digital manipulation of real speech (Dreschler et al., 2001). The amplified speech-like signal may be compared to the patient's hearing thresholds or to targets for amplified speech generated from the threshold data. Fitting methods such as Desired Sensation Level (DSL) and National Acoustics Laboratories – Non-Linear 1 (NAL-NL1) are based on amplifying speech to some desired level and yield targets for the amplified LTASS. Figure 36.9 shows the estimated ear canal SPL produced by a hearing aid amplifying real speech at 65 dB input SPL. The measured coupler SPL has been converted to ear canal SPL by adding the real-ear-to-coupler difference (see Chapter 37 for information on how this is measured) so that it may be compared with the SPL threshold and real-ear NAL-NL1 speech targets. Noise reduction is set for maximum effect and feedback suppression, and adaptive directional features are enabled. In Figure 36.9, the hatched area is the amplified speech region bounded by the peaks of speech at the top and the valleys at the bottom. The circles are the hearing thresholds converted to SPL and the elongated + marks are the NAL-NL1 targets for the amplified LTASS. Most of the speech region is above threshold, and the LTASS of the amplified speech is close to the NAL-NL1 targets, indicating that this hearing aid is providing adequate amplification for speech at this level. The test may be repeated at other levels to ensure that expansion does not reduce gain for low-level speech signals and that compression keeps loud speech well below levels that might cause discomfort.

It must be emphasized that, when testing hearing aids with compression or any other adaptive processing features, the results obtained will be valid only for the test signal used (Henning and Bentler, 2005; Scollie and Seewald, 2002; Stelmachowicz et al., 1996). Tests using speech-like test signals provide the most reliable indication that audibility goals are being met. If speech-like test signals are not available, the tests described in the following sections may provide estimates of electroacoustic parameters useful in deciding whether a hearing aid is performing as expected.

Tests Using Short-Duration Broadband Noise

If speech-like test signals are not available, tests that use short-duration broadband noise signals may be used to inspect the operation of the hearing aid. Since compression systems typically have millisecond attack times, while adaptive features usually have an onset time of several seconds, such signals will frequently show the operation of compression, free of the confounding effects of adaptive features. Figure 36.10 shows the gain obtained with a pink noise signal of 2 seconds in duration presented at (top to bottom) 45, 60, 75, and 90 dB SPL for the same hearing aid and same settings used in Figure 36.9.

■ Observe that the gain curves are free from sharp peaks or abrupt dips, and they resemble curves for similar hearing aids.

FIGURE 36.9   Using speech to check hearing aid operation with adaptive features enabled. The *hatched area* is the amplified speech region bounded by the peaks of speech at the top and the valleys at the bottom. The *heavy curve* is the long-term average speech spectrum (LTASS), the *circles* are the hearing threshold converted to sound pressure level (SPL), and the *elongated + marks* are the NAL-NL1 real-ear targets for the amplified LTASS. The input was real speech at 65 dB SPL. Ear canal SPL has been estimated by adding an average Real-Ear to Coupler Difference (RECD) to the coupler SPL. Noise reduction, feedback suppression, and adaptive directional features are enabled.

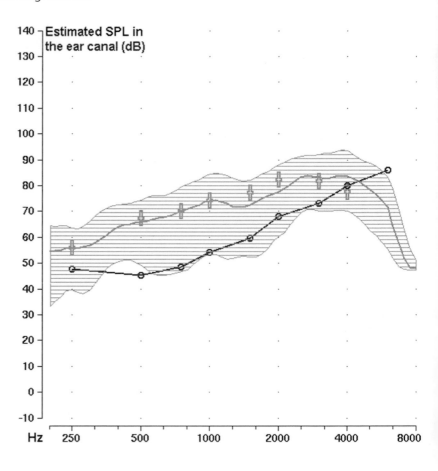

FIGURE 36.10   Using short-duration noise to check hearing aid operation. Curves are the coupler gain for pink noise presented for 2 seconds at (top to bottom) 45, 60, 75, and 90 dB sound pressure level (SPL) for the same hearing aid and same settings used in Figure 36.9. The *vertical lines* at 500, 1,000, 2,000, and 4,000 Hz indicate one-third to one-half the hearing loss for which this hearing aid was programmed.

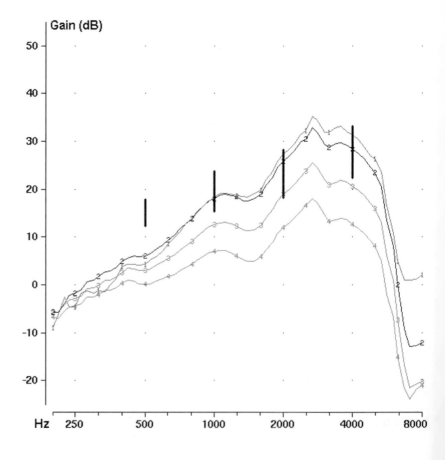

- The gain for 45 dB input SPL is 4, 18, 27, and 31 dB at 500, 1,000, 2,000, and 4,000 Hz, respectively. The half-gain rule would indicate that this hearing aid might be appropriate for a hearing loss of about 35 at 1 kHz, 55 at 2 kHz, and 60 at 4 kHz.
- The 45- and 60-dB curves are closely spaced, indicating a compression threshold below 60 dB SPL.
- The 60-, 70-, and 90-dB curves are separated by about 7 to 8 dB over much of the useful frequency range. This indicates wide dynamic-range compression with a compression ratio (input change/output change) of about 2.
- The 90-dB gain curve can be used to give a rough estimate of the OSPL90 of the hearing aid by adding 90 dB to the gain. This yields an estimated OSPL90 at 500 Hz, 1 kHz, 2 kHz, and 4 kHz of 90, 97, 102, and 103 dB, respectively, with a peak of about 108 dB at about 2.7 kHz.

These tests provide a good deal of information about this hearing aid and may be used to judge if it is functioning as intended. Refer back to Table 36.5 for a listing of possible causes and remediation of irregular response curves, low gain, and low maximum output.

Tests Using Short-Duration Tones

A test that can shed some light on hearing aid operation when it is not possible to change its programming is an input-output test. This test uses tones that are increased in 5-dB steps every few hundred milliseconds. The levels are maintained long enough to show the operation of compression but change frequently enough not be attacked by adaptive features. Figure 36.11 shows input-output curves at various frequencies for the same hearing aid and same settings used in Figures 36.9 and 36.10. In each panel, the horizontal axis is the input SPL, and the vertical axis is the output SPL.

1. For a 90 dB input SPL, the output at 500, 1,000, 2,000, and 4,000 Hz is 90, 94, 99, and 99 dB SPL, respectively.
2. The gain is the difference between the output SPL and the input SPL. For a 45 dB input SPL, the gain at 500, 1,000, 2,000, and 4,000 Hz is 5, 18, 28, and 25 dB, respectively.

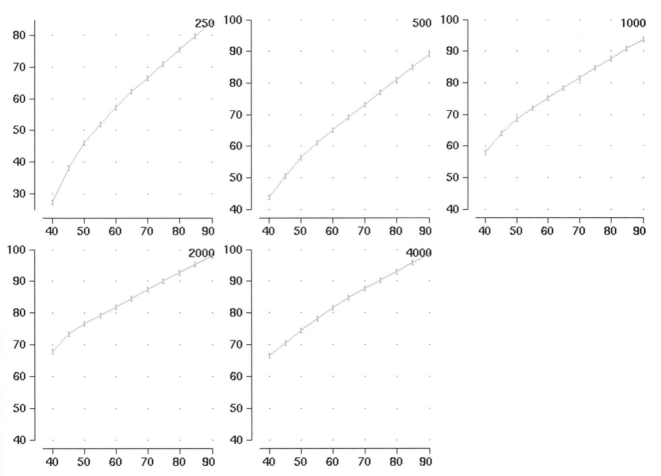

FIGURE 36.11 Using short-duration tones to generate input-output curves to check hearing aid operation. Curves are coupler sound pressure level (SPL; vertical) for varying input SPL (horizontal). The hearing aid and settings are the same as those for Figure 36.9.

3. The compression ratio is obtained by dividing a change in input SPL (e.g., 10 dB) by the corresponding change in output SPL. A compression ratio of 1 (a diagonal line) is linear amplification, less than 1 indicates expansion, and greater than 1 indicates compression. The 250-Hz panel shows a compression ratio of about 0.5 (expansion) below 50 dB SPL and about 1 (linear) above about 60 dB SPL input. The 2,000-Hz panel shows a compression ratio of about 2 above 50 dB SPL.

4. The lowest input SPL at which the compression ratio exceeds 1 is often referred to as the "compression threshold" or "kneepoint." The compression threshold at 500, 1,000, 2,000, and 4,000 Hz is about 55, 50, 45, and ≤40 dB SPL, respectively.

High-level short-duration tone bursts are sometimes used in real-ear measurement equipment to determine the maximum output capabilities of a hearing aid without causing discomfort to the patient or risking further hearing damage. These tone bursts are typically long enough to activate compression limiting but short enough to avoid triggering adaptive features. If such a signal is available in a hearing aid analyzer, it may be employed to estimate the OSPL90 of the hearing aid without the need to disable noise reduction, feedback suppression, or adaptive directional systems. Figure 36.12 shows the 2-cc coupler SPL in response to a series of 90-dB tone bursts at one-third octave intervals for the same

hearing aid and same settings used in Figures 36.9, 36.10, and 36.11. The estimated OSPL90 at 500, 1,000, 2,000, and 4,000 Hz is 86, 93, 98, and 100 dB, respectively.

Short-duration tone tests may be expected to produce somewhat different estimates of gain, maximum output, compression threshold, and compression ratio than those obtained using brief broadband noise signals because the two signals are likely to be treated differently by compression systems. However, either is sufficiently accurate when the goal is simply to determine whether a hearing aid is functioning as expected and it is not possible or desired to change settings.

▨ VERIFYING DIGITAL FEATURES USING HEARING AID ANALYZERS

The proliferation of digital technology in hearing aids has led to the introduction of features designed to address issues beyond amplification. These features may be significant factors in the selection and successful use of a hearing instrument, and their proper operation should not be taken for granted. These features are disabled for the standard tests of ANSI S3.22, but most hearing aid analyzers can be used to verify and document the functioning of noise reduction, adaptive directional microphones, and feedback

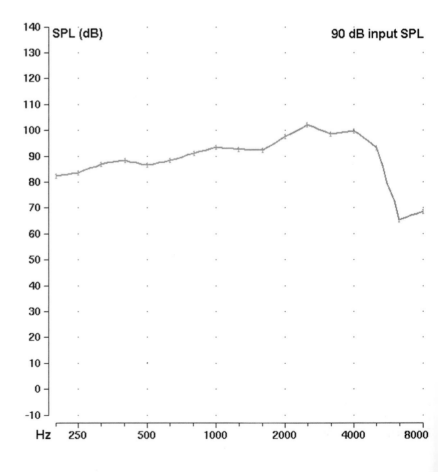

FIGURE 36.12 Using tone bursts to check maximum output with adaptive features enabled. Tone bursts were 128 ms in duration presented at 90 dB sound pressure level (SPL) at one-third octave frequencies. The hearing aid and settings are the same as those for Figure 36.9.

suppression features. The following tests have been found to work on many current hearing aids but may not be applicable to all hearing aids and may not work with future hearing aids.

Functional Check of Adaptive Noise Reduction

Most noise reduction algorithms operate by reducing gain in frequency bands in which the signals do not exhibit the modulation characteristics of speech (Chung, 2004a). A steady broadband noise signal may be used to verify the functioning of such systems. In Figure 36.13, the upper curve (1) shows the gain for a steady 60-dB SPL pink noise signal when it is first applied, while the lower curve (2) shows the gain when it has stabilized 10 seconds later. The noise reduction algorithm has reduced the gain by about 12 dB at 1 kHz. This test also provides some idea of the speed with which the hearing aid responds to the onset of noise. To avoid the confounding effects of adaptive directional response, it may be necessary to set the aid to omnidirectional mode before performing this test.

The noise reduction algorithm should not reduce the gain for a speech signal. This can be verified if the hearing aid analyzer provides speech-like test signals. That is, there should be no change in output for these signals when the noise reduction feature is toggled between minimum (or off) and maximum reduction.

Functional Check of Directional Hearing Aids

Accurately testing directional hearing aids requires a large test space and specialized equipment (ANSI S3.35-2004). However, it is possible to use a hearing aid analyzer to determine if the directional feature is functioning as expected. Note, however, that such tests performed in a small test chamber will not produce results that can be compared with published specifications. They will generally show less directionality, especially at lower frequencies.

It is usually recommended that the hearing aid be set for linear operation with a fixed directional pattern and to switch off any adaptive noise reduction and feedback suppression algorithms before attempting to measure directional performance. This is because gain or output for sounds from different directions is usually determined by making measurements from different directions at different times. Compression or adaptive features may change the gain or output of the hearing aid between successive measurements, resulting in erroneous measures of directional performance.

To test directional function, the hearing aid is set as indicated earlier, and a gain or output curve for a 50- to 65-dB broadband signal (e.g., pink noise) is obtained, with the hearing aid oriented so that its direction of maximum sensitivity is toward the loudspeaker (within 45°). Next, the hearing aid is oriented so that the direction of maximum sensitivity is away from the loudspeaker, and the test is repeated. The second

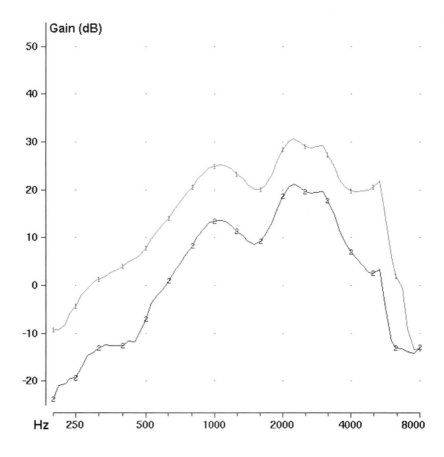

FIGURE 36.13 Functional check of adaptive noise reduction feature. The upper curve (1) shows the gain for a steady 60-dB sound pressure level (SPL) pink noise signal when it is first applied, whereas the lower curve (2) shows the gain when it has stabilized 10 seconds later.

curve should lie below the first, at least in the mid frequencies, with the separation between the curves being an indication that the directional feature is functioning. This is a functional test only, and the curve separation obtained in this way is not expected to correlate with standard measures of directional performance. As an additional check, the tests should be repeated with the hearing aid in omnidirectional mode. In this case, the two curves should be nearly coincident.

Some hearing aid analyzers provide special signals for testing directional function in a test chamber that has two speakers (Jonkman, 2006; Smriga, 2004). In this case, the test can be performed without setting the hearing aid for linear operation or switching off adaptive algorithms. This scheme delivers two separate signals, each containing over 500 different tones, from two directions simultaneously. Digital analysis separates the coupler signal into two frequency response curves, one for each direction, and the separation between these curves shows the functioning of the directional microphone(s). The operation of compression or noise reduction impacts both response curves, but their separation remains unaffected. Such a test may also reveal the signal level at which change is initiated and the time required for change to occur. The end result of such a test is shown in Figure 36.14. In each panel, the bold curve is the response from a source in the front hemisphere, while the lighter curve is the response from a source in the rear hemisphere obtained using two simultaneous pink noise signals. Panel A shows an omnidirectional response immediately after signal presentation, whereas panel B shows the directional response after the signals have been presented for 20 seconds. This test may be modified by adding speech to the sound source in the front hemisphere in order to test hearing aids that change their

directional response pattern as a function of signal-to-noise ratio rather than noise level.

A hearing aid may fail to show any appreciable directional function using these tests for the following reasons:

1. The hearing aid has been oriented so that gain is about the same for signals from both directions tested. Some directional patterns have rear or side lobes with gain comparable to the front lobe at some angles. This can be checked by changing the orientation used for the test.
2. The hearing aid is not set for directional operation. This may result from failure of a programming or directional switch, failure to enable the feature in the programming software, an automated decision within the programming software, or a failure of hardware or software.
3. Blockage of the microphone ports on the hearing aid.
4. Microphone drift in two-microphone directional systems. These systems rely on well-matched microphones for their directional performance. Microphone sensitivity changes with temperature, humidity, and time, all of which can degrade directional performance. Some hearing aids self-correct for these changes, but those that do not can cease to be directional hearing aids.
5. Miswired or improperly assembled microphones in the hearing aid.

Functional Check of Feedback Suppression Systems

Feedback occurs when the gain through the hearing aid (the forward path) plus the attenuation from the ear canal back to the hearing aid microphone (the feedback path) is greater

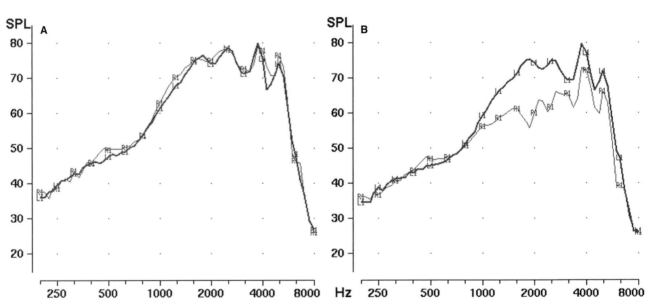

FIGURE 36.14 Functional check of adaptive directional feature. In each panel, the *bold curve* is the response from a source in the front hemisphere, while the *lighter curve* is the response from a source in the rear hemisphere obtained using two simultaneous pink noise signals. **(A)** An omnidirectional response immediately after signal presentation. **(B)** The directional response after the signals have been presented for 20 seconds.

than 0 dB, with a phase shift that is an integer multiple of 360°. The sum of the gain through the forward path and the attenuation (negative gain) through the feedback path is termed the open loop gain.

Feedback suppression systems operate by reducing the gain of the forward path at frequencies where the open loop gain would otherwise exceed 0 dB. This may be accomplished either through filters in the forward path or by subtracting from the microphone signal an estimate of the signal in the feedback path (called phase cancellation). In some systems, no action is taken to change the forward path gain until feedback, in the form of a persistent tonal signal, is detected. Freed and Soli (2005) have classed these as "detectors."

Other systems can measure the attenuation of the feedback path during the fitting process by internally applying a known electrical test signal to the hearing aid receiver and measuring the resulting signal at the hearing aid microphone. Freed and Soli (2005) have classed these as "initialized" systems. In the case of forward path filters, this information is used to reduce (or limit) the gain in frequency regions where the open loop gain would otherwise exceed 0 dB. In the case of phase cancellers, the same test signal being applied to the hearing aid receiver is also applied to a digital filter, which is automatically adjusted until its output approximates the signal being measured by the hearing aid microphone. The digital filter then effectively becomes a simulation of the feedback path. In operation, the output of this filter is subtracted from the microphone signal, canceling that portion of the microphone signal that is due to the feedback path. To avoid the initialization step and to accommodate changing feedback paths, some phase cancellers employ an adaptive digital filter that is continuously adjusted to minimize the difference between its output and the microphone signal, using ambient sound rather than an internally generated signal. Refer to Chapter 35 for a more detailed discussion of feedback suppression systems.

A number of laboratory measures have been proposed to characterize feedback suppression systems (Freed and Soli, 2005), but the test described here is intended only to determine whether the suppression system is working. It is based on a test described previously by Smriga (2004) and has been found to work on current hearing aids using different types of suppression systems. The difficulty in performing a test of a feedback suppression system in the test chamber of a hearing aid analyzer is getting feedback to occur on demand. Smriga (2004) described a way to do this in analyzers that provide a headphone for listening to the output of the hearing aid in the coupler. In the steps that follow, this method is used to induce feedback in the presence of a speech-like test signal. A speech-like signal is used to avoid engaging adaptive directional or noise reduction features and to ensure that changes in forward path gain caused by compression and/or expansion are representative of those achieved in actual use. Variations of this test are possible using a low-level noise signal or no input signal at all, but it may be necessary to

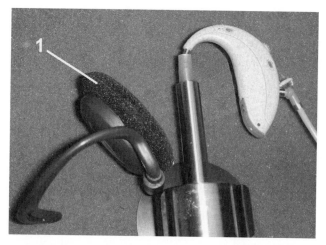

FIGURE 36.15 Setup for inducing controlled feedback in the test chamber. The monitor headphone (1), which is normally used to listen to the output of the hearing aid in the coupler, is placed near the hearing aid. The monitor gain is adjusted to induce feedback.

disable adaptive features and expansion, and the results may not represent real-use experience.

1. Program the hearing aid for normal use. Place the hearing aid in the test chamber as if for a standard hearing aid test.
2. Connect the monitor headphone, normally used for listening to the output of the hearing aid, and place it in the test chamber near the hearing aid (Fig. 36.15).
3. Present a speech-like signal at 60 dB SPL and display the coupler SPL.
4. Adjust the headphone volume control until one or more peaks appear in the response curve (Fig. 36.16).
5. Enable the feedback suppression and observe that the peaks are removed from the response curves. Observe also that there has been no significant loss of output at the frequencies of the peaks. This result may not be observed for some hearing aids that require an initialization step before enabling feedback suppression. In this case, perform initialization after Step 4 but with the sound source turned off. The sound source should be switched on before proceeding to Step 5.

▨ PROPER FIT

In a survey of hearing aid owners in the United States, the third most common reason for not using hearing aids was fit and comfort (Kochkin, 2000). Clients may complain that the hearing aids "are too big," "fall out of my ears," "hurt my ears," or "are uncomfortable." An accurate impression and proper fit in the ear are critical for effective hearing aid use.

Proper fit is often more critical and also more difficult to achieve in those with severe or profound hearing losses

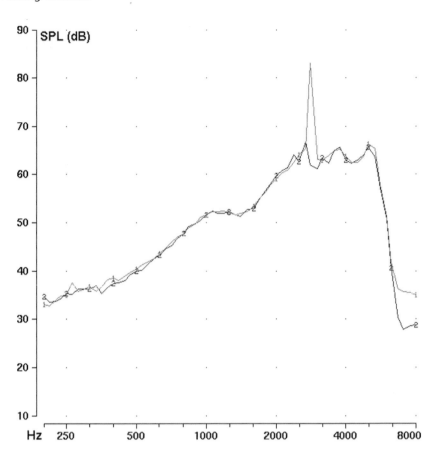

FIGURE 36.16 Functional check of adaptive feedback suppression. Shown is the long-term average speech spectrum for speech at 60 dB sound pressure level (SPL) obtained with the setup of Figure 36.15. Curve 1 was obtained by adjusting the gain of the monitor headphones, with feedback suppression disabled, until feedback occurred. Curve 2 was obtained after enabling feedback suppression without changing the gain.

and for those fit with completely-in-the-canal hearing aids. In some cases, two or three remakes of the hearing aid shell or mold may be required before a good fit is achieved. Depending on the material used and the degree of hearing loss, new molds may be required every 3 to 6 months, whereas others may not need to be remade for a year or more.

Pain

Hearing aids and earmolds should never cause pain or aching even after a full day of use. Clients should be cautioned to remove the hearing aid if there is pain and return as soon as possible to ensure a proper fit. While new users are more likely to give up when there is pain, some long-term users cannot manage without their hearing aids and will persist in wearing a painful hearing aid until there is a visible red, swollen sore that may take weeks to heal.

If proper placement in the ear is observed, it should be determined whether the pain experienced happens immediately or after a few hours of use. The ear needs to be inspected. Is a sore or red spot present in the helix, concha, or canal? Is the pain in one particular spot (indicating a possible pressure sore) or all over (indicating that the aid may be slightly too large and needs to be reduced in general by a small amount)? If the client experiences pain almost immediately or if the pain is felt in a widespread area, a complete remake of the shell or mold from a new impression is indicated. However,

if the pain occurs only after a few hours or only in one particular spot, then grinding and buffing the shell or mold is worth doing. Note that, with open-fit behind-the-ear hearing aids, pain may be caused by inappropriate tubing size or dome size.

If a sore is present, it is important to advise the client to leave the hearing aid out until all soreness, redness, or swelling is gone. Pressure sores can take days or weeks to heal completely and will not heal unless the hearing aid is not worn at all during the recovery period.

Excessive Hair in the Ear

Excessive hair growth in the concha or ear canal may cause chronic fit problems. The client may choose to keep the ear hair trimmed or switch to a behind-the-ear or open-fit model, if appropriate.

Change in Client's Weight

A change in the client's weight can affect the fit of a hearing aid. The shape and size of the ear can change with a weight increase or decrease of 10 pounds or more. In the case of weight loss, the hearing aid may become too loose and fall out of the ear or cause feedback. With significant weight gain, the hearing aid may become too tight and cause pain or sores. Reshelling for in-the-ear hearing aids or making a new mold in the case of behind-the-ear hearing aids usually alleviates the problem.

Effect of Climate

Hearing aids made from an impression in one season or climate may cause problems in another. To determine whether this may be a problem for a particular client, ask if rings and wrist watches are tighter in the summer and looser in the winter. This can be an issue for clients traveling to different climates. For behind-the-ear hearing aids, some clients may require a winter mold and a summer mold. For in-the-ear hearing aids, a shell made from an impression taken in the winter may feel tight in the summer but may avoid feedback or a loose fit in the winter. Table 36.6 lists various seasonal and climate problems.

Grinding and Buffing Shells and Molds

A hearing aid should be reshelled if the shell is quite thin or if there are cracks, holes, or signs of extensive grinding or previous application of coatings. However, sending a hearing aid or mold out for a remake means that the client will be without the hearing aid for several days or more. If a remake of the shell or mold is not required, grinding and buffing can be done in the office while the client waits. A Dremel-type tool with a flex-shaft is ideal for this kind of fine, delicate grinding and buffing. If one or two adjustments do not resolve the problem, it is advisable to take a new impression and have the shell or mold remade.

TABLE 36.6   Seasonal and climate problems

Summer issues
- High humidity can cause condensation in in-the-ear hearing aids, resulting in a short circuit
- High humidity can cause condensation in the tubing of behind-the-ear hearing aids, resulting in a blockage
- Client's ear tissues may swell (fluid retention), making fit snug or painful
- High temperatures (>122°F or 50°C) (common in cars on a hot day) may impair batteries (Energizer Application Manual, 2004)

Winter issues
- Dry air due to heating may shorten battery life
- Dry air due to heating may increase static electricity, which could damage the hearing aid circuit
- Cold or dry air may shrink client ear tissues, making the fit too loose and/or causing feedback
- Low temperatures (< −14°F or −10°C) may impair batteries (Energizer Application Manual, 2004)

There is a wide variety of materials available for earmolds such as acrylic, silicone, and polyvinyl chloride (PVC). The hardness (or Shore rating) of a material will determine the appropriate bit type and speed for grinding and buffing. Shore ratings and material descriptions are available from companies that make molds. For hard materials such as acrylic, a small bit and a medium speed are best. Hard materials are more difficult to smooth and need to be buffed well. For soft materials such as PVC, a medium bit and a higher speed work well and reduce the amount of shredding. Super-soft materials such as silicone require a larger bit and higher speed, and the mold must be braced to reduce vibration and increase the effectiveness of the grinding; softer materials, however, do not require buffing. If a large amount must be removed, soft materials such as PVC and silicone can be cut or trimmed before grinding, but care must be taken to ensure that there are no sharp edges.

OCCLUSION AND AMPCLUSION

"My own voice is too loud," "It sounds like I am shouting," and "Everything is hollow and echoing" are complaints often heard from clients trying new hearing aids. Sometimes the subjective discomfort is so pronounced that the client refuses to wear the hearing aids.

Shell-related occlusion is a common side effect of placing an object into the ear canal, particularly with binaural fittings. When talking, the voice projects primarily through the mouth, but some of the energy normally escapes through the ears. With the ears "plugged," however, a client's voice may resonate more within the head.

Ampclusion occurs when certain frequencies are over- or underamplified by the hearing aids, causing a hollowness or echoing effect. Some of the common causes of shell-related occlusion and ampclusion include:

- Too little venting in the hearing aid
- Inappropriate length of hearing aid in the canal
- Physical blockage of canals (e.g., wax, blocked vent)
- Inappropriate gain for hearing loss in low frequencies ("ampclusion")

Adapting to Initial Shell-Related Occlusion

Some shell-related occlusion effect should be expected when trying hearing aids for the first time. Clients should be counseled that their own voice and sounds, in general, will sound different at first. Mild cases of shell-related occlusion can disappear within a few minutes, although a few days of regular use are often needed as the client adapts to the new sound.

Persistent Occlusion: Shell-Related or Ampclusion?

When occlusion persists, the underlying cause must be determined. If the sense of occlusion is less when the hearing aids are turned off while still in the ear (by opening the battery door), then the problem is ampclusion (over- or underamplification provided by the hearing aids). If the occlusion effect is worse with the hearing aid off, then the problem is either underamplification (ampclusion) or shell-related occlusion. If the occlusion is unaffected by the hearing aids being on or off, then shell-related occlusion is the problem.

One needs to check whether the occlusion is present with just one hearing aid or with two. If the occlusion is primarily present in one ear, adjustments may be needed only in that ear. If the occlusion is observed only when both hearing aids are in place but not with either one alone, then the occlusion may be due to an increase in the resonance of sound within the head or underventing, both of which result in overamplification of low frequencies. Although the origin is shell-related, if shell-related solutions do not solve the problem, then it should be treated as ampclusion due to overamplification of the low frequencies.

Nonacoustic Occlusion due to Cranial Nerve Stimulation

The trigeminal nerve (cranial nerve [CN] V), vagus nerve (CN X), facial nerve (CN VII), glossopharyngeal nerve (CN IX), and many intermediary branches of nerves course through and around the external auditory canal, the tympanic plexus at the eardrum, and around the middle ear and Eustachian tube. Stimulation of any of these can trigger reflexes that may occasionally cause nonacoustic occlusion when fitting hearing aids. The vagus and trigeminal reflexes in particular may contribute to occlusion in some people; however, there is currently no easy way to determine whether this may be an underlying cause. Until a clinically feasible method for predicting and testing for cranial nerve stimulation is developed, this should be treated as a shell-related problem.

RESOLVING SHELL-RELATED OCCLUSION

During the assessment and prescribing process, the optimal venting for the hearing loss can be determined (Table 36.7)

TABLE 36.7   Optimal venting to minimize occlusion

Hearing loss at 500 Hz	Optimal vent size
<20 dB HL	Open fit (>3 mm)
20–30 dB HL	2–3 mm
30–40 dB HL	1.5–2 mm
>50 dB HL	<1 mm
With CICs	Reverse horn vent

HL, hearing level; CIC, completely-in-the-canal.
Adapted from Kuk F. (2005) Developing a hierarchy to manage the "own voice" problem. Session at American Academy of Audiology Conference, Washington, DC, April 2005.

to minimize shell-related occlusion. Shell-related occlusion may result from inappropriate venting in the hearing aid, too long a canal in the hearing aid, physical blockage of the hearing aid, or pressure on nerves in the ear canal, which, in turn, requires physical alteration of the hearing aid shell or earmold. An open-fit behind-the-ear hearing aid may solve occlusion for clients whose hearing loss is in the appropriate range.

Very deep insertion in the canal may also significantly reduce the occlusion effect, but the effective depth is 4 mm beyond the second bend, which is usually physically uncomfortable for the client (Pirzanski, 1998). The difficulty in inserting and removing these hearing aids, combined with physical discomfort, limits the clinical usefulness of very deep fits in the canal for reducing occlusion.

RESOLVING AMPCLUSION

Ampclusion may be resolved by adjusting low-frequency gain according to a client's perception of his or her own voice. If the problem is worse when the client speaks louder, overamplification is the issue, and low frequencies should be reduced. If the problem is worse when the client speaks softer, underamplification is the issue, and low frequencies should be increased.

▧ FEEDBACK

While many clients will persist in wearing a hearing aid that causes pain, most will refuse to wear one that squeals or buzzes. Feedback may occur with every head or jaw movement or may be occasional such as when putting on a hat or hugging family or friends.

Clients should be advised that there are times when feedback is expected and normal, such as when inserting or removing a hearing aid with both the power and volume on, or when the microphone is covered, such as by a hand, hat, or telephone. Some clients use feedback to confirm that the hearing aid is working and that the battery is good and to judge when the hearing aid has been correctly inserted based on when the feedback stops.

Understanding Feedback

A hearing aid is an amplifying system with a microphone, an amplifier, and a speaker (receiver). If the sound leaves the receiver and re-enters the microphone, it becomes reamplified and creates an oscillation. Low levels of acoustic feedback may not cause actual squealing but can disrupt frequency response and reduce speech clarity by creating an echo sensation. Feedback can progress into self-sustaining oscillation, which is the well-known, embarrassing whistle. When feedback drives the hearing aid into saturation, it generates multiple intense oscillations that are clearly audible and usually extremely uncomfortable for the wearer.

While both high- and low-frequency sounds can easily escape from the hearing aid through venting or poor fit, the shorter wavelengths of the high-frequency sounds allow them to more easily reflect off surfaces such as the pinna and concha, increasing the likelihood of re-entering the hearing aid at the microphone. High-frequency sounds exiting the receiver are also more likely to be in phase with the incoming sounds at the microphone.

In hearing aids with greater high-frequency gain, the escaping sound is more likely to be louder than the initiating sound when it finds its way back to the microphone. In addition, higher gain hearing aids may produce oscillations of multiple frequencies that result in a faster onset of acoustic feedback. Because peaks in the real-ear frequency response often occur at high frequencies and such peaks are often associated with rapid phase changes, it is clear how these factors interact to produce the oscillation of feedback.

Because high-frequency hearing loss is most common, clients may not hear the acoustic feedback even though it is audible to others around them.

IS IT REALLY FEEDBACK?

In some cases, it may be difficult to determine whether a problem experienced by a client is feedback. Clients will use a bewildering variety of terms and phrases to describe the problem, and it is not often clear what the actual issue is. Clients may describe a squealing and whistling that appear to indicate the presence of feedback or a buzz or other odd sound that could be an issue with the telephone coil in the hearing aid or the presence of a real sound in their environment. The various possibilities must be investigated to determine the underlying cause. One way to determine if feedback is the problem is to induce feedback by covering the hearing aid while it is in the client's ear. If the client reports that this is the sound he or she has heard, then feedback has been confirmed.

Patterns may help identify the source of feedback-related issues. If a client hears the disturbing sound in question only when he or she smiles or bends over, then feedback is likely the issue. However, if the sound in question is only heard at certain times or in certain locations, then the client may be hearing an unfamiliar sound in the environment. Main sources of feedback include:

- Improper fit in the ear
- Effect of impression materials
- Anatomy of the ear
- Improper placement in the ear
- Cracked or loose tubing in earmold
- Orientation of sound bore results in aiming sounds at the canal wall
- Presence of wax in the ear canal
- Reduced tympanic membrane compliance
- Large venting with high gain
- Low kneepoint (wide dynamic range compression [WDRC] circuit)

- Inappropriate style of hearing aid for the degree of hearing loss
- Distance between the microphone and receiver

Improper Fit

It is important to ensure the best physical fit possible in the ear before resorting to the application of software feedback managers. The more severe the hearing loss, the more amplification is usually prescribed and the more critical the fit will be in preventing feedback. With a new hearing aid or mold, it is worth the investment of time, energy, and resources in the first few months to achieve optimal fit and minimize future problems.

Feedback can be a major issue with older hearing aids, as well. Over time, the ear often changes slightly, and there may also be some shrinkage in the hearing aid shell or mold, depending on the properties of the material used and chemistry of the ear canal skin. Materials such as PVC can shrink significantly over 2 or 3 years. The fit of a hearing aid tends to become less precise after 2 or 3 years, usually getting looser in the ear over time. The resulting gaps between the hearing aid and the ear canal can allow sound to leak out of the ear and cause feedback. In some cases, the hearing aid becomes so loose that the shifting in the ear can easily be seen with normal jaw movement. One easy test is to apply a soft expanding material, such as Comply Soft Wraps, around the canal portion of the hearing aid. If the feedback is eliminated by the presence of the Comply Soft Wrap, then poor fit is likely the primary cause of the feedback, and a recoating or reshelling of the hearing aid often corrects the problem. If the hearing aid is 5 years old or older, it may be preferable to purchase a new hearing aid since repair and reshelling costs are higher for hearing aids over 5 years of age. With behind-the-ear hearing aids, a new earmold should be made if the fit is loose in the ear.

A significant change in the client's weight can also affect the fit and cause feedback. See earlier "Proper Fit" section.

Effect of Impression Materials

The type of impression material used for taking impressions can affect the ultimate fit in the ear. Standard viscosity silicone tends to give a more accurate impression of the ear, resulting in a better fit and less feedback (Pirzanski, 2000). When using injector guns for impression taking, keep in mind that many guns do not have enough power to push standard viscosity silicone; therefore, a standard syringe may be required. Low-viscosity materials reduce stretching of the ear tissue and can make a more comfortable though less accurate fit, increasing the chance of feedback in the hearing aid (Pirzanski, 2000). If feedback is a problem for a hearing aid made from a low-viscosity impression material, a reshelling from a medium- or high-viscosity material impression is worth trying.

Open-Jaw versus Closed-Jaw Impressions

Hearing aids and molds made from closed-jaw impressions or impressions taken while the client is chewing may lack a proper acoustic seal and result in retention and feedback problems (Pirzanski, 1996). Hearing aids and molds made from open-jaw impressions tend to have better anatomic definition of the ear, a more secure fit, less feedback, and better comfort (Chasin et al., 1997). Open-jaw impressions should be done one ear at a time, with a bite block as far back as possible on the same side and the longest axis kept vertical in order to maximize the openness of the jaw.

Anatomy of the Ear

Sometimes the cause of intermittent feedback can be traced to jaw movement. Look for patterns such as feedback that occurs after a meal or only later in the day. In some clients, the temporomandibular joint (TMJ) may significantly amplify the effect of jaw movement while talking and eating, resulting in the hearing aid shifting in the ear (Oliviera et al., 2005). Sometimes, the cumulative effect of chewing over several meals is needed before the jaw movement displaces the hearing aid enough to create feedback. In this case, the feedback tends to be experienced only later in the day. This effect is often greater in one ear than the other. A very straight ear canal tends to result in poor retention of the hearing aid as well, and jaw movement may shift the hearing aid out of the ear canal in some cases.

There is currently no way to predict whether the anatomy of a client's ear will have a negative effect on the fit of a hearing aid. For experienced users, ask if feedback has ever been a problem with previous hearing aids. If the problem is chronic ("I've always had problems with hearing aids in my right ear"), then the anatomy of the client's ear may be the root cause, and an open-jaw impression is recommended. For some clients, adding a canal or helix lock to in-the-canal or completely-in-the-canal hearing aids may solve the problem by improved retention.

Improper Placement in the Ear

Improper placement in the ear can cause feedback. See "Performing a Visual Inspection" section earlier in this chapter.

Cracked or Loose Tubing in Earmold

Cracked or loose tubing in earmolds allows sound to escape freely from the ear causing feedback. See "Inspecting the Hearing Aid and Component Parts" section earlier in this chapter.

Orientation of the Sound Bore

The orientation of the sound bore of the mold or hearing aid shell is also important. If the sound bore is pointed toward the wall of the ear canal rather than toward the eardrum, some of the sound may be reflected back toward the receiver, increasing the chance of feedback.

Presence of Wax in the Canal

The presence of a significant amount of wax in the ear can cause feedback. The sound from the receiver tube of the hearing aid can be deflected by the wax back towards the hearing aid. The sound can exit the ear via the vent and cause feedback. This can be exacerbated by an imperfect fit in the ear canal or improper placement of the hearing aid in the ear. In many cases, removal of the wax reduces or eliminates the feedback. If there is a significant amount of wax present, it should be removed before other causes of feedback are investigated and before other solutions (such as reshelling or running a software feedback manager) are attempted.

Open-fit behind-the-ear hearing aids are particularly susceptible to blockage by wax due to the small diameter of the tubing. Manufacturers provide a tool to keep the tubing clear.

Reduced Tympanic Membrane Compliance

A cold or middle ear infection may cause feedback due to the increased reflections of sound off a stiffened eardrum. In these cases, more sound would be reflected back out of the ear canal than would normally occur due to the increase in stiffness.

Venting with High Gain

If acoustic feedback is a problem, a vent may need to be reduced or closed completely; however, this may result in an increase in occlusion and humidity in the ear canals.

One way to retain some venting in a high-gain hearing aid is to choose a hearing aid with a smooth real-ear response or enough channels to achieve a smooth response. Feedback is less likely to occur if the peaks of the frequency response are minimized.

The large venting of open-fit behind-the-ear hearing aids allows high frequencies to escape easily, increasing the risk of feedback. More occlusive ear pieces are available from some companies for use with open-fit tubing that restrict the escape of high frequencies from the ear canal. Software feedback management can also be used to reduce feedback (see "Software Feedback Reduction Managers" section later in this chapter).

Feedback in Wide Dynamic Range Compression Circuits

Hearing aids using WDRC or other compression schemes that provide more gain for low-level input signals and less for higher level signals are more prone to feedback than linear hearing aids (Olsen et al., 2001). This is especially true when the input levels to the hearing aid are low. A hearing aid may be in feedback for quiet situations because of the relatively high gain, but the feedback may cease in noisier environments because of the lower amounts of gain (Chung, 2004b). Feedback in quieter locations can be partially reduced by increasing the threshold kneepoint, by increasing the amount of expansion, or by a binaural fitting (through loudness summation, thus reducing the amount of amplification required).

Inappropriate Hearing Aid Style for the Degree of Hearing Loss

Sometimes a person with a severe or profound hearing loss in the high frequencies is fit with an in-the-canal or completely-in-the-canal hearing aid. This can be an issue for persons with very straight ear canals or poor retention of the hearing aid. Feedback can be reduced or eliminated by increasing the distance between the microphone and receiver by increasing the canal length or switching from an in-the-ear model to a behind-the-ear model. Moving to a larger hearing instrument may increase the surface contact in the ear, thereby providing a more efficient seal. A behind-the-ear model also allows for use of softer materials, such as PVC or silicone, that can reduce feedback by providing a more snug fit in the ear.

Feedback can occur when open-fit behind-the-ear hearing aids are used with a severe hearing loss. A hybrid open fit with the slim tube attached to a custom-made earpiece may be effective in this case. The increasing effectiveness of software feedback managers may make the open-fit behind-the-ear hearing aid more useable for severe hearing losses (see earlier "Venting with High Gain" section; see also "Software Feedback Reduction Managers" section later in this chapter).

Distance between the Microphone and Receiver

If feedback persists with a behind-the-ear model, it is possible to route the signal contralaterally between two behind-the-ear hearing aids. In this configuration, the sound from the right hearing aid is routed to the left ear and vice versa. This can be accomplished either by a wire or a wireless (e.g., Wi-Fi) routing. The distance between the microphone and the receiver will be significantly increased and often eliminates feedback completely.

Body aids work on the same principle of maximizing the distance between the microphone and the receiver, with the microphone typically being worn at chest level. However, body aids are being phased out and are difficult to purchase.

The use of a frequency modulation (FM) system will also reduce or eliminate feedback, again due to the increase in distance between the microphone and the receiver.

Malfunctioning Battery

Batteries occasionally cause unusual problems with hearing aids, including feedback. Some hearing aid circuits will experience more feedback as the battery is about to expire. If no obvious cause for the feedback can be found, try a new battery from a different batch and/or brand.

Improper Mounting of Microphone and Receiver

In the course of normal operation, receivers generate a small amount of vibration. Any vibration transferred to the shell of the hearing aid may generate a small amount of sound that is sensed by the microphone, potentially causing feedback. If proper fit and venting have been ensured, persistent feedback may be due to the microphone or receiver not being mounted optimally to minimize vibration. In this case, the hearing aid would have to be returned to the manufacturer for verification.

Software Feedback Reduction Managers

Software feedback reduction managers should be the last resort for addressing persistent feedback problems. When running the feedback manager in a manufacturer's software, one needs to be aware of what the program is doing. There are many different methods employed within software feedback managers. Feedback management programs typically work by gain reduction, notch filtering, or phase shifting. It is well worth some investigation to determine the specifications of any software feedback manager before using it.

Gain reduction can eliminate feedback by reducing the gain in the high frequencies, but such a broad range of reduction can also decrease the ability to clearly understand speech, particularly for unfamiliar voices, for foreign accents, or in competing noise. For this reason, the gain reduction method of feedback reduction should be a last resort.

Notch filters work by gain reduction, but the frequencies reduced are limited to those known to cause feedback. This can be implemented at the hearing aid fitting, and there are some models of hearing aids that attempt to "seek out and destroy" the offending feedback signal. To date, this adaptive approach has met with limited success. A very narrow notch filter can reduce feedback without greatly altering the final output from the hearing aid. However, if the feedback occurs at multiple frequencies, several notch filters or a much wider notch filter may be required, and the resulting gain may be significantly lower than that required for the level of hearing loss.

Phase shifting or phase inversion, also known as "feedback cancellation," eliminates or reduces acoustic feedback without significantly reducing the prescribed gain of the hearing aid across the frequencies. This preserves the ability to hear speech and other sounds as clearly as possible. In phase shifting, the phase of any detected feedback is mirrored in a 180° phase shift, resulting in destructive interference. The goal is to achieve an exact 180° shift within an extremely short time in order to achieve near or complete cancellation of the feedback signal.

Feedback can build to saturation within 200 ms, so the ideal feedback-canceling system must be able to negate audible oscillations in real time. Some digital hearing aids incorporate high-speed real-time feedback cancellation systems that claim to completely stop feedback. As of yet, however, there are no independent, large-scale studies to substantiate these claims.

EAR WAX

An existing hearing loss can be exacerbated by the presence of ear wax. Ear wax can significantly reduce the transmission of sound by blocking the ear canal, blocking the sound from exiting the hearing aid, or causing damage to internal components of the hearing aid. Hearing aid manufacturers report that the majority of all hearing aid repairs are due to damage from ear wax (Price, 2005).

What Is Ear Wax?

Ear wax is a normal product of the ear. Ear wax is primarily composed of keratin (derived from dead skin) with a mixture of cerumen (secretions from the ceruminous and pilosebaceous glands), sweat, dust, and other debris (Hawke, 2002). The amount and consistency of ear wax vary from person to person. Ear wax can vary in color from yellow to orange or reddish-brown to dark brown or almost black. It may be nearly liquid or thick, sticky or dry, or soft or hard. Wax type is genetically inherited, although the appearance of wax may vary from time to time in the same person. Cerumen type has been used by anthropologists to track human migratory patterns, such as those of the Inuit (Bass and Jackson, 1977). There are two main types, wet and dry. Dry flaky wax is common in persons of Asian descent and Native Americans (Overfield, 1985). Dry wax contains by weight about 20% lipid. Wet wax is common in people of Western European descent (Caucasians) and people of African descent (Overfield, 1985) and consists of approximately 50% lipid (Burkhart et al., 2000). Wet wax can be either soft or hard, with hard wax being more likely to be impacted.

Why Do We Have Ear Wax?

Various hypotheses have been advanced as to the purpose of ear wax. It has been proposed that wax provides protection against foreign objects, assists in cleaning the ear canal, acts as a lubricant, acts as an antibacterial and antifungal agent, and promotes a healthy immune response.

Debris is removed from the ear canal by a "conveyor belt" process of epithelial migration that is aided by jaw movement (Alberti, 1964). Cells of the tympanic membrane migrate outwards from the umbo (at a rate equivalent to that of fingernail growth) to the walls of the ear canal. The speed of cell migration accelerates as the cells move outwards to the entrance of the ear canal. The cerumen in the canal is also carried outwards, taking with it any dirt, dust, and particulate matter that may have gathered in the canal. Jaw movement tends to dislodge any debris attached to the walls of the ear canal, although vigorous chewing may actually stimulate wax production in some people (Perry, 1957).

Wax can also act as a lubricant, preventing drying and itching of the skin in the ear canal (asteatosis). In wet-type cerumen, the lubricating effect is due to the presence of cholesterol, squalene, long-chain fatty acids, and alcohols produced by the sebaceous glands (Bortz et al., 1990; Harvey, 1989).

Studies have found that cerumen can provide protection against some strains of bacteria. Chai and Chai (1980), among others, have found cerumen to be effective in reducing the viability of a wide range of bacteria (sometimes by up to 99%), including *Haemophilus influenzae*, *Staphylococcus aureus*, and many variants of *Escherichia coli*. Megarry et al. (1988) discovered that cerumen significantly inhibited the growth of two types of fungi commonly present in otomycosis in humans. These antimicrobial properties are due to the presence of saturated fatty acids, lysozymes, and the relatively low pH of cerumen, which is typically around 6.1 in normal ear canals (Roland and Marple, 1997). Sirigu et al. (1997) also showed evidence of an antibody-mediated local immune response in the ear canal associated with the production and presence of cerumen, whereas Fairey et al. (1985) found that too little ear wax increases the risk of infection.

Removal of Ear Wax

If wax is hard and impacted in the ear canal, it may cause damage to the skin as it is removed and thus should be first softened. Wax removal is often more difficult for older people because their wax tends to be drier and harder (Roeser and Ballachanda, 1997). Ear wax can be softened by applying a few drops of mineral oil, baby oil, or glycerin in the ear for several days in a row. Oil should be administered at night time so that it can be absorbed into the wax and skin overnight. If oil is administered in the morning, the oil will likely get into the hearing aid when inserted and possibly disable the hearing aid.

Over-the-counter drops claiming to soften wax are available, most commonly with carbamide peroxide as the active ingredient. Other common active ingredients found in commercial wax removal preparations are triethanolamine oleate and docusate sodium. However, a recent study (Roland et al., 2004) found that triethanolamine oleate and carbamide peroxide were no more effective than a placebo (an isotonic salt solution) in aiding the removal of cerumen from occluded ear canals in an office setting. Docusate sodium and sodium bicarbonate have also been studied with conflicting results.

Once the ear wax has been softened, it can be removed with a minimum of discomfort. A standard protocol should be developed that includes obtaining informed consent and proper safety measures. The removal of wax may cause minor trauma to the ear canal, resulting in small amounts of blood. Since blood is a bodily fluid capable of transmitting various diseases, appropriate infection control measures should always be taken during cerumen removal.

SYRINGING WITH WATER

Syringing with water can be done by a client at home, by a trained audiologist, by a family doctor, or by another qualified person. Water pressure may, however, push the wax deeper into the canal (possibly touching the eardrum), while significant amounts of water may remain in the ear canal after syringing. When hydrogen peroxide (H_2O_2) is used, oxygen bubbles off, leaving water in the ear canal. A problem with wet, warm ear canals is that they make good incubators for growth of bacteria. In these instances, the ear canal may be flushed with isopropyl alcohol to displace the water and dry the skin but should be used sparingly to avoid excessive drying and itching.

PLASTIC SCOOPS

Small flexible, plastic scoops are commonly used by audiologists trained in wax removal. A good hands-free magnifier and light source are required. The basic technique is to gently scoop built-up wax from the canal. Care must be taken to minimize discomfort or trauma to the ear canal and to avoid contact with the tympanic membrane. This method is not recommended if wax is deeply impacted. Hairs in the ear canal may be embedded in the wax and can leave small amounts of blood in the canal when they are pulled out with the wax.

SUCTION

Suction is an effective way to remove wax and debris; however, there is a risk of damage to the ear canal and/or tympanic membrane. This method can be uncomfortable for the client, both physically because of the suction and acoustically due to the high SPLs. Suction should be used only by a qualified practitioner such as an otolaryngologist.

COTTON SWABS

Using cotton swabs to clean the ears is not recommended. Swabs tend to push wax deeper in the canal and may stimulate the production of more wax. Swabs irritate the skin of the ear canal and may damage the ear drum.

EAR CANDLING

Ear candling or coning is an ineffective and potentially dangerous method of cleaning the ears. A hollow candle is placed at the entrance of the ear canal and lit, supposedly sucking out ear wax. Despite many claims that ear candling is effective for wax removal, it has been proven that the substances appearing within the cone originate from the melted candle, not from the ears (Seely et al., 1996). The suction supposedly created by the candle's flame is insufficient to remove wax (Kaushall and Kaushall, 2000). There is a substantial risk of burns, infection, obstruction of the ear canal, and perforation of the eardrum (Seely et al., 1996). Ear candling is not recommended at any time, and federal health warnings have been issued in both the United States (FDA Important Alert #77-01; FDA, 1998) and Canada (Health Canada, 2002).

Cleaning Hearing Aids

Hearing aids should be cleaned regularly as a preventive measure. A thorough cleaning every 6 months is usually sufficient to reduce repairs due to wax damage. Some clients require deep cleaning of their hearing aids every month or even more frequently, whereas others may never have a problem with wax.

A vacuum chamber with a suction tip for cleaning hearing aids is essential for any hearing care practice. The vacuum chamber loosens and removes small particles of dust and wax, while the suction tip removes more recalcitrant debris. Care must be used when using a suction tip because the receiver can be easily damaged.

Prevention: The Use of Wax Guards

Wax guards are the first line of defense against wax damage in a hearing aid. Different kinds of wax guards have been developed, including covers, metal springs, vented plastic plugs, and vented plastic baskets. One of the most effective is the vented plastic basket type, which is also the simplest for clients to change on their own. When clients cannot change the wax guard themselves, encourage them to bring their hearing aids in for regular cleaning and to change the wax guards.

▨ HEARING AIDS AND TELEPHONES

The speech signal exiting from the receiver of an ordinary telephone is already slightly amplified to about 70 dB SPL, which may be sufficient for people with a mild hearing loss. For people with a severe hearing loss, using a telephone can be a frustrating experience due to a lack of amplification and visual cues and/or poor word recognition.

Feedback is also a common complaint for clients using a telephone. Feedback is generated when a hearing aid microphone is covered by the telephone receiver.

Foam Pads

For hearing aids without telecoils or acoustic telephone programs, feedback can be reduced or eliminated by adding a foam pad to a telephone receiver to increase its distance from the hearing aid microphone.

Telecoils

Hearing aids with telecoils can eliminate feedback caused when using a telephone by turning the hearing aid microphone off and allowing the telecoil to pick up the magnetic signal from the telephone receiver instead. The Hearing Aid Compatibility Act of 1988 required "essential" telephones made in the United States or imported into the United States from August 1989 onwards to be compatible with telecoils. The act defines "essential" phones as "coin-operated telephones, telephones provided for emergency use, and other telephones frequently needed for use by persons using . . . hearing aids"; this definition includes workplace telephones, telephones in hospitals and nursing homes, and telephones in hotel and motel rooms. For more information on telecoils, please refer to Chapter 35, Hearing Aid Technology.

Clients using telecoils may still run into problems using the telephone. Clients may have trouble operating the program button on their hearing aids, or the pressure of the telephone receiver can toggle the program button accidentally. With behind-the-ear hearing aids, a client must be shown how to hold the telephone to the hearing aid rather than to the ear in order for the telecoil to maximally pick up the magnetic signal. Also, there may be instances in which an older telephone model with insufficient electromagnetic leakage is used and, in turn, may result in a weak or nonexistent signal when used with the telecoil of a hearing aid.

Autocoils

Hearing aids with autocoils are switched into the telecoil mode automatically whenever a magnetic field is detected. The magnetic field must be very close to the hearing aid to trigger the autocoil. A typical problem with autocoils is that clients may not hold the phone close enough to trigger the autocoil. Counseling the client to hold the phone right up to the hearing aid should solve the problem. The initial feedback the client may hear should disappear quickly as the autocoil switches modes and the microphone is turned off.

A client may have a phone that does not have a strong enough magnetic field to trigger the autocoil. Adding a magnet to the telephone receiver may solve the problem, and a larger magnet or a second magnet may be added if required.

Magnetic Interference and Telecoils

When a hearing aid is in the telecoil mode, any strong or nearby electromagnetic signal may be detected and amplified, producing a buzzing sound. Common sources of electromagnetic interference include fluorescent lights, microwave ovens, televisions, tube-type computer monitors, power lines, and electrical transformers.

Because the strength of an electromagnetic field often varies considerably with small changes of position, it is sometimes possible to minimize interference by moving the head a few inches to one side. In some places, effective telephone communication with a telecoil is simply not possible given the strength of the interference.

Cell Phones

Historically, cell phones were not required under US law to be compatible with hearing aids; however, Section 255 of the U.S. Telecommunications Act of 1996 requires a phased improvement of compatibility according to ANSI-PC63.19 (ANSI, 2002c) in new cell phones sold after 2005.

For hearing aids with telecoils, a special neckloop may be plugged into the headset jack of the cell phone to transmit the signal to one or both of the hearing aids.

Bluetooth wireless technology can bridge the gap between hearing aids and cell phones. Hearing aids with Bluetooth can automatically receive wireless signals from Bluetooth-enabled cell phones. FM systems with Bluetooth can wirelessly forward signals from a Bluetooth-enabled cell phone to a hearing aid with an FM receiver. The future may see new technologies being used to communicate with cell phones, such as Falcon. Falcon is already being used in the hearing aid industry. Falcon may ultimately replace Bluetooth because Falcon uses a larger data rate and has lower power consumption (AudiologyOnline, 2007).

Modified Telephone Use

Modifications have been made to telephones to make them more accessible to the hearing aid user. There are many amplified telephones with built-in volume boost controls and high-quality speaker phones that allow for binaural listening. A direct connection from a telephone to a hearing aid via direct audio input (DAI) is also possible if the telephone has an output or headphone jack.

Frequency Modulated Systems

FM systems provide another way to access the telephone via a hearing aid as well as allow for binaural listening. Binaural listening on a telephone can significantly improve clarity and efficacy of communication for many people with hearing loss. With the correct connector cord, any telephone with an output or headphone jack can be routed to the auxiliary input of an FM transmitter. Many FM systems can be set to automatically switch into the telephone mode when the phone rings.

Acoustic Telephone Programs

Hearing aids without a telecoil may allow for an acoustic telephone program. Because telephones only transmit information at 3,000 Hz and below, amplification of the higher frequencies in the hearing aid can be reduced sufficiently to eliminate feedback. Significant reduction of higher frequencies may, however, impair effective speech discrimination. Therefore, hearing aids should have two or more programs with the primary program left unchanged.

Alternatives to the Telephone

Some people with severe hearing loss or poor word recognition cannot use the telephone at all. Many text-based alternatives are available including Voice Carry Over (VCO) telephones, e-mail, teletype devices, Blackberry communicators, pagers, and fax machines. The Blackberry and pagers usually have a vibration option to alert the owner to incoming messages.

BATTERIES

Clients may be shocked to learn that a battery will only last days or weeks—typically 150 hours of use. It might be useful to mention to a client that a battery would also only last 150 hours in a flashlight or radio as well. Chips for high-end hearing aids have become more and more sophisticated, incorporating more sound-processing features such as noise reduction, speech enhancement, adaptive directionality, and feedback cancellation, which, in turn, put a higher demand on the battery. However, even though the demands placed on batteries have increased, batteries have improved in strength and current drain, thus keeping overall battery life fairly constant.

The current standard is zinc air batteries. These are significantly more efficient than mercury or silver batteries and can be safely disposed of, unlike the mercury-based batteries.

How Do Batteries Work?

Zinc air batteries require oxygen to produce energy. Since they contain tiny air holes, environmental factors such as humidity can affect battery life. The batteries come with tabs to cover the air holes and may require several minutes to fully activate after the tab is removed.

Testing batteries

When using a battery tester, count to three slowly and look for any sign of decrease in power. A battery that initially appears to be at full power may begin to fade after a several seconds.

Most hearing aids have a low-battery warning; however, clients may not hear the warning beep if the hearing aid is blocked with wax or if the battery dies before emitting the warning signal. Clients should be advised to check for bad batteries and to recognize any low-battery warning given by their hearing aids. Most clients would benefit from purchasing their own battery tester.

Corrosion

Clients who sweat a lot or who live in a hot humid climate can experience chronic sweat-induced corrosion, a dark residue forming on the battery that has been described as "rust." This corrosion occurs when sweat enters the battery compartment and bridges the positive and negative terminals of the battery (Carpenter, 2003c). Salty sweat serves as an electrolyte that promotes ionic conduction, causing the battery to corrode. The corrosion is rapid, and severe "rusting" may be observed in a matter of minutes in some individuals. This problem is mostly associated with behind-the-ear hearing aids because the location of the aid allows for easy sweat access. A protective covering over the hearing aid, such as sweatbands or SuperSeals, or a waterproof or water-resistant hearing aid, such as the Rionet line, may solve the problem.

Clients who are regularly exposed to certain chemicals, such as high levels of chlorine in an indoor pool, may experience chronic chemical corrosion of their batteries. If the hearing aid must be worn in this environment, the use of a waterproof or water-resistant behind-the-ear model, such as the Rionet series, may be required.

Malfunctioning Battery

Batteries occasionally cause unusual problems with hearing aids. Some hearing aid circuits will experience increased distortion or feedback when the battery is about to expire. If no obvious cause for a problem can be found, a new battery from a different batch and brand may eliminate the problem.

Maximizing the Life of Batteries

Hearing aid batteries should be stored at room temperature and will operate best within the humidity range of 50% to 60% (Carpenter, 2003b). When humidity is above 60%, clients may use a dry-aid kit for both their hearing aid and batteries (Carpenter, 2003a). Batteries should also not be kept in locations where they may short out against metal objects.

Replacing the tab on the positive side of the battery may be beneficial if the typical battery life is longer than 10 days.

A tight-fitting battery compartment in a hearing aid that is made air-tight by debris build-up can result in shortened battery life. The Rionet water-resistant and waterproof hearing aids avoid this problem by using a ventilation window covered by a membrane on the battery compartment, which allows air to pass freely but repels liquids (Tateno, 2005).

PREVENTION

The importance of preventing common problems before they happen cannot be overstated. A positive, trouble-free experience for the client will reinforce the audiologist's message that hearing aids are supposed to make life easier and

---

TABLE 36.8 Prevention of common problems

Evaluation of listening needs and prescription:
Assess listening needs and physical abilities to ensure optimum prescription
Choose style and venting to minimize occlusion, sweat, and pressure
Include directional microphones whenever possible
Choose a circuit with fast real-time feedback cancellation whenever possible
Order appropriate wax guards
Take deep, accurate open-jaw ear impressions
Add canal or helix lock to overcome poor retention in the ear
Set adaptation levels as appropriate for each client

Expectations and training:
Discuss expectations with the client
Provide thorough training to the client during the initial fitting
Recommend regular cleaning for both the hearing aids and the client's ears
Provide Dri-Aid kit, battery tester, and appropriate accessories
Recommend the use of devices such as Dry & Store
Provide documentation and written instructions for new users
Provide aural rehabilitation (orientation classes, counseling, reading materials, etc.)

Follow-up:
Insist on timely and thorough follow-ups within the first months
Set up a call-back system to see how clients are doing during the first few days
Encourage clients to call if they are having any trouble

---

improve communication and the quality of life. Many of the common problems that discourage hearing aid use can be minimized or avoided during the prescription and fitting process. Refer to Chapter 37, Hearing Instrument Fitting and Verification for Children, and Chapter 38, Hearing Aid Fitting for Adults: Selection, Fitting, Verification, and Validation, for more detail on counseling new users and their families. Table 36.8 also lists a number of ways in which common problems with hearing aids can be prevented.

CONCLUSION

This chapter discussed many troubleshooting tips for hearing aids, as well as proper hearing aid assessment proto-cols. These included both formal and informal assessment of the hearing aids. Formal testing involves the use of hearing aid analyzers, different couplers, various test stimuli, different measures for testing digital hearing aids and advanced functions, and using the appropriate ANSI standard. Informal assessment focuses on visual assessment of the hearing aid and its components, the ear itself, and the fitting of the hearing aid to the ear.

As with a hearing assessment, a detailed up-to-date case history and background are necessary for each client. This is especially important for new clients. Even changes in weight or occupation may affect hearing aid functioning. The strategies, tips, and testing protocols in this chapter will assist you in helping your clients receive optimal benefit from their personal amplification.

REFERENCES

Alberti PWRM. (1964) Epithelial migration on the tympanic membrane. *J Laryngol Otol.* 78, 808–830.

American National Standards Institute. (1995) American National Standard Method for Coupler Calibration of Earphones. ANSI S3.7-1995. New York: American National Standards Institute.

American National Standards Institute. (2002a) American National Standard Method Testing Hearing Aids with a Broad-Band Noise Signal. ANSI S3.42-1992 (R2002). New York: American National Standards Institute.

American National Standards Institute. (2002b) American National Standard Method Methods of Measurement of Real-Ear Performance Characteristics of Hearing Aids. ANSI S3.46-1997 (R2002). New York: American National Standards Institute.

American National Standards Institute. (2002c) American National Standard for Methods of Measurement of Compatibility between Wireless Communications Devices and Hearing Aids. ANSI PC63.19-2002. New York: American National Standards Institute.

American National Standards Institute. (2003) American National Standard Specification of Hearing Aid Characteristics. ANSI S3.22-2003. New York: American National Standards Institute.

American National Standards Institute. (2004) American National Standard Method of Measurement of Performance Characteristics of Hearing Aids under Simulated Real-Ear Working Conditions. ANSI S3.35-2004. New York: American National Standards Institute.

AudiologyOnline. (2007). Interview with Dr. Franz J. Fink, President and CEO of Gennum Corporation. Available at: http://www.audiologyonline.com/interview/interview_detail.asp?wc=1&interview_id=408

Bailey JW, Valente M. (1996) Measurements of relative humidity and temperature in hearing aids. *Hear J.* 49, 59–63.

Bankaitis AU. (2002) What's growing on your patients' hearing aids? A study gives you an idea. *Hear J.* 55, 48–54.

Bankaitis AU, Kemp RJ. (2003) *Infection Control in the Hearing Aid Clinic.* St. Louis: Auban.

Bass EJ, Jackson JF. (1977) Cerumen types in Eskimos. *Am J Phys Anthropol.* 47, 209–210.

Bortz JT, Wertz PW, Downing DT. (1990) Composition of cerumen lipids. *J Am Acad Dermatol.* 23, 845–849.

Burkhart CN, Burkhart CG, Williams S, Andrews PC, Adappa V, Arbogast J. (2000) In pursuit of ceruminolytic agents: a study of ear wax composition. *Am J Otol.* 21, 157–160.

Byrne D, Dillon H, Tran K. (1994) An international comparison of long-term average speech spectra. *J Acoust Soc Am.* 96, 2108–2120.

Carpenter D. (2003a) Dry aid kits and hearing aid batteries. Available at: http://www.healthyhearing.com/library/ate_content.asp?question_id=155

Carpenter D. (2003b) Extending hearing aid battery life. Available at: http://www.healthyhearing.com/library/ate_content.asp?question_id=148

Carpenter D. (2003c) Battery rust. Available at: http://www.healthyhearing.com/library/ate_content.asp?question_id=133

Chai TJ, Chai TC. (1980) Bactericidal activity of cerumen. *Antimicrob Agents Chemother.* 18, 638–641.

Chasin M, Pirzanski C, Hayes D, Mueller G. (1997) The real ear occluded response (REOR) as a clinical predictor. *Hearing Rev.* 4, 22–26.

Chung K. (2004a) Challenges and recent developments in hearing aids. Part I. *Trends Amplif.* 8, 83–124.

Chung K. (2004b) Challenges and recent developments in hearing aids. Part II. Feedback and occlusion effect reduction strategies, laser shell manufacturing processes, and other signal processing technologies. *Trends Amplif.* 8, 125–164.

Cox RM, Metesich JS, Moore JN. (1988) Distribution of short-term RMS levels in conversational speech. *J Acoust Soc Am.* 84, 1100–1104.

Dreschler WA, Vershuure H, Ludvigsen C, Westermann S. (2001) ICRA noises: artificial noise signals with speech-like spectral and temporal properties for hearing instrument assessment. *Audiology.* 40, 148–157.

Dunn H, White S. (1940) Statistical measurements on conversational speech. *J Acoust Soc Am.* 11, 278–288.

Energizer Application Manual. (2004) Zinc Air batteries. Available at: http://data.energizer.com/PDFs/zincair_appman.pdf.

Estabrooks W, Birkenshaw-Fleming L. (2003) *Songs for Listening! Songs for Life!* Washington, DC: A.G. Bell Association for the Deaf and Hard of Hearing.

Fairey A, Freer CB, Machin D. (1985) Ear wax and otitis media in children. *Br Med J Clin Res Ed.* 291, 387–388.

Food and Drug Administration. (1998) FDA Important Alert IA #77-0: Detention without physical examination of ear candles. Issued September 1, 1998 with attachment May 23, 2005. Available at: http://www.fda.gov/ora/fiars/ora_import_ia7701.html.

Freed D, Soli S. (2005) An objective procedure for evaluation of adaptive antifeedback algorithms in hearing aids. *Ear Hear.* 27, 382–398.

Gates FL. (1929) A study of the bactericidal action of ultra violet light. *J Gen Physiol.* 13, 231–260.

Gray RF, Sharma A, Vowler SL. (2005) Relative humidity of the external auditory canal in normal and abnormal ears, and its pathogenic effect. *Clin Otolaryngol.* 30, 105.

Harvey DJ. (1989) Identification of long-chain fatty acids and alcohols from human cerumen by the use of picolinyl and nicotinate esters. *Biomed Environ Mass Spectrom.* 18, 719–723.

Hawke M. (2002) Update on cerumen and ceruminolytics. *ENT J.* Suppl 1, 23–24.

Health Canada. (2002) Medical bulletin on ear candling. Available at: http://www.hc-sc.gc.ca/iyh-vsv/med/ear-oreille_e.html.

Henning R, Bentler R. (2005) Compression-dependent differences in hearing aid gain between speech and nonspeech input signals. *Ear Hear.* 26, 409–422.

International Electrotechnical Commission. (1981) Occluded-ear simulator for the measurement of earphones coupled to the ear by ear inserts. IEC 60711-1981. Geneva: International Electrotechnical Commission.

Jonkman J. (2006) Directional hearing aid tester. U.S. Patent No. 7,062,056.

Kaushall PP, Kaushall JN. (2000) On ear cones and candles. *The Skeptical Inquirer.* 24, 12–13.

Kochkin S. (2000) MarkeTrak V: why my hearing aids are in the drawer: the consumer's perspective. *Hear J.* 53, 34–42.

Kuk F. (2005) Developing a hierarchy to manage the "own voice" problem. Session at American Academy of Audiology Conference, Washington, DC, April 2005.

Megarry S, Pett A, Scarlett A, Zeigler E, Canter RJ. (1988) The activity against yeasts of human cerumen. *J Laryngol Otol.* 102, 671–672.

Oliviera R, Babcock M, Venem M, Hoeker G, Parish B, Vasant K. (2005) The dynamic ear canal and its implications: the problem may be the ear, not the impression. *Hear Rev.* 12, 18–19, 82.

Olsen L, Musch H, Stuck C. (2001) Digital solutions for feedback control. *Hear Rev.* 8, 44–49.

Overfield T. (1985) Biologic Variation in Health and Illness: Race, Age, and Sex Differences. Menlo Park, CA: Addison-Wesley Publishing.

Perry ET. (1957) *The Human Ear Canal.* Springfield, IL: Charles C. Thomas.

Pirzanski C. (1996) An alternative impression-taking technique: the open-jaw impression. *Hear J.* 49, 30.

Pirzanski C. (1998) Diminishing the occlusion effect: clinician/manufacturer factors. *Hear J.* 51, 66–78.

Pirzanski C. (2000) Selecting material for impression taking: the case for standard viscosity silicones. *Hear J.* 53, 45.

Price M. (2005) Telephone poll of production floor managers of three major hearing aid manufacturers: Starkey, Siemens, and Oticon. November 2005. Unpublished phone survey.

Roeser RJ, Ballachanda BB. (1997) Physiology, pathophysiology, and anthropology/epidemiology of human ear canal secretions. *J Am Acad Audiol.* 8, 391–400.

Roland PS, Eaton, DA, Gross RD. (2004) Randomized, placebo-controlled evaluation of Cerumenex and Murine earwax removal products. *Arch Otolaryngol Head Neck Surg.* 130, 1175–1177.

Roland PS, Marple BF. (1997) Disorders of the external auditory canal. *J Am Acad Audiol.* 8, 367–378.

Scollie S, Seewald R. (2002) Evaluation of electroacoustic test signals. *Ear Hear.* 23, 477–487.

Seely DR, Quigley SM, Langman AW. (1996) Ear candles-efficacy and safety. *Laryngoscope.* 106, 1226–1229.

Sirigu P, Perra MT, Ferreli C, Maxia C, Turno F. (1997) Local immune response in the skin of the external auditory meatus: an immunohistochemical study. *Microsc Res Tech.* 38, 329–334.

Smriga D. (2004) How to measure and demonstrate four key digital hearing aid performance measures. *Hear Rev.* 11, 26–31.

Stelmachowicz P, Kopun J, Mace AL, Lewis DE. (1996) Measures of hearing aid gain for real speech. *Ear Hear.* 17, 520–527.

Tateno M. (2005) Membrane in Rion hearing aid battery compartment. Personal e-mail to William Cole, December 8, 2005.

Zwislocki J. (1970) *An acoustic coupler for earphone calibration.* Report LSC-S-7, Laboratory of Sensory Communication, Syracuse University, September, 1970. Syracuse, NY: Syracuse University.

Zwislocki J. (1971) *An ear-like coupler for earphone calibration.* Report LSC-S-9, Laboratory of Sensory Communication, Syracuse University, April 1971. Syracuse, NY: Syracuse University.

IN MEMORIAM

This chapter is dedicated to the memory of Moneca Price, whose sudden and unexpected death during its final revisions shocked and saddened all those who knew her. She was, without any doubt, the major contributor and the driving force behind what is printed here. It will endure as a tribute to her hard work, enthusiasm, and love of the field of audiology.

CHAPTER 37

Hearing Instrument Fitting and Verification for Children

Pat Stelmachowicz and Brenda Hoover

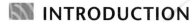

▨ INTRODUCTION

Studies have shown that infants with normal hearing are able to recognize and distinguish their mother's voice from others by 1 to 2 months of age (DeCasper and Fifer, 1980). After only 6 to 7 months of exposure to speech, they can discriminate the sounds and rhythmic patterns of their native language from other languages (Werker and Tees, 1984; Jusczyk and Luce, 2002). By 7 to 10 months, children are able to generalize across talkers, despite differences in gender, fundamental frequency, and formant frequencies (Kuhl, 1983; Houston and Jusczyk, 2000). And, by 12 months of age, first words begin to emerge. These remarkable accomplishments highlight the crucial need for early identification of hearing loss and, in turn, the fitting of appropriate amplification and implementation of effective habilitation programs as early as possible. Although newborn screening programs have enabled audiologists to identify hearing loss within the first few days of life, precise quantification of the degree and configuration of hearing loss may not be possible for many months. However, recent data have shown that children with hearing loss who undergo early intervention prior to 6 months of age outperform children who are identified later on (Yoshinaga-Itano et al., 1998). Thus, it is not considered reasonable to delay amplification until comprehensive behavioral audiologic data can be obtained (Bess et al., 1996; American Academy of Audiology [AAA], 2004). As such, it is important to use a systematic and theoretically based approach when fitting amplification to this population (Stelmachowicz, 2005).

▨ HEARING INSTRUMENT FITTING: ADULT-CHILD DIFFERENCES

The process of fitting hearing instruments to an infant or young child is qualitatively different from adults in a number of ways. Specifically, for infants and young children, the goal of amplification is to facilitate the *development* of speech and language. When hearing loss is acquired prelingually, language competency, cognitive abilities, and world knowledge cannot be used to supplement incoming acoustic information as is the case with adults. For example, it has been demonstrated that young children require higher sound pressure levels (SPLs) than adults to achieve equivalent speech recognition. Figure 37.1, adapted from Stelmachowicz et al. (2000), shows word recognition as a function of audibility index (AI) for adults and two groups of children with normal hearing. An AI of 0 indicates that no portion of the speech signal is above threshold, while a value of 1 indicates that the entire spectrum is above threshold. Note that, even at an AI of only 0.2, adults are able to identify 60% of words in meaningful sentences. In contrast, the 5- and 7-year-old children achieve scores of only 2% and 10%, respectively. Figure 37.2, adapted from Hall et al. (2002), illustrates the effect of masker type on spondee recognition threshold for adults and 5- to 10-year-old children. When the masker was speech-shaped noise, the average group differences were less than 3 dB, but when a two-talker masker was used, mean differences increased to 8 dB. This type of signal degradation, often referred to as "informational masking,"

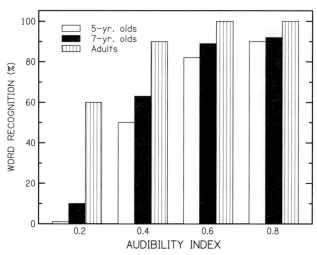

FIGURE 37.1 Word recognition in four-word high-predictability sentences as a function of audibility index for adults and two groups of children (5 and 7 year olds). (Adapted from Stelmachowicz PG, Hoover BM, Lewis DE, Kortekaas R, Pittman AL. [2000] The relationship between stimulus context, speech audibility, and perception for normal and hearing impaired children. *J Speech Hear Res.* 43, 902–914.)

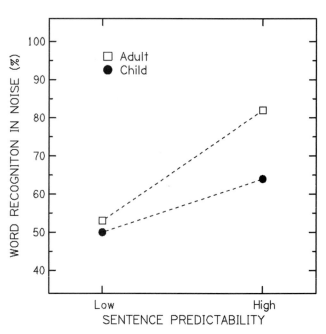

FIGURE 37.3 Word recognition in noise for low- and high-predictability four-word sentences. Data are shown for adults and 4- to 6-year-old children. (Adapted from Nittrouer S, Boothroyd A. [1990] Context effects in phoneme and word recognition by young children and older adults. *J Acoust Soc Am.* 87, 2705–2715.)

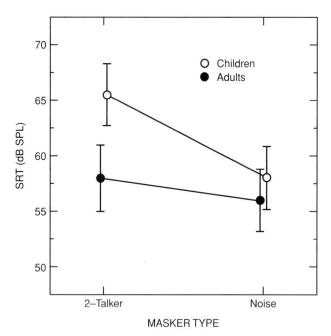

FIGURE 37.2 Spondee recognition threshold (SRT; in dB sound pressure level [SPL]) for two masker types (two-talker babble and speech-shaped noise). Data are shown for adults and 5- to 10-year-old children. (Adapted from Hall JW III, Grose JH, Buss E, Dev MB. [2002] Spondee recognition in a two-talker masker and a speech-shaped noise masker in adults and children. *Ear Hear.* 23, 159–165.)

is common in everyday listening situations. Figure 37.3 illustrates word recognition in noise for low- and high-predictability sentences (Nittrouer and Boothroyd, 1990). Performance for adults and 4- to 6-year-old children was similar for the low-context materials. When context was added, however, the increase in performance was significantly greater for the adults compared to the children, suggesting that young children cannot take full advantage of semantic knowledge. Similar adult-child differences have been reported for frequency and temporal resolution (Wightman et al., 1989; Hall and Grose, 1991), duration discrimination (Elfenbein et al., 1993), the manner in which acoustic cues are used (Morrongiello et al., 1984; Nittrouer and Studdert-Kennedy, 1987; Nittrouer, 1992; 1996), and selective attention (Oh et al., 2001; Wightman et al., 2003). As a result of these differences, several investigators have suggested that the prescriptive formulae used to fit hearing aids with adults (who generally acquire hearing loss later in life) may be inappropriate for infants and young children (Stelmachowicz, 1991; Scollie and Seewald, 2002b). In contrast, Dillon (2001) has argued that, because the available data are from normal-hearing (NH) children, they cannot necessarily be applied to children with hearing loss. Proponents of this viewpoint reason that NH children develop speech and language skills despite these early differences in performance relative to NH adults. However, it is important to recognize that, even with early amplification, the auditory input for young hearing-impaired (HI) children will be impoverished relative to their

NH peers due to reduced audibility, the likely greater negative effects of distance and reverberation, and the fact that, even with early identification, hearing aids may not be fitted until 4 to 6 months of age. Unfortunately, the necessary studies to examine the appropriateness of adult prescriptive formulae with children have not yet been conducted.

The basic audiologic information that is readily attainable from young children will be less complete and reliable than for adults. For infants less than 6 months of age, the initial hearing instrument fitting is generally based on information gleaned from evoked potential measures of auditory function. Supra-threshold measures of performance, such as speech recognition, loudness growth, and loudness discomfort levels cannot be obtained until much later (Kawell et al., 1988; Boothroyd et al., 1996). Factors such as middle ear disease, developmental delays, and additional handicapping conditions can further complicate the precision and interpretation of audiologic data. As a result, the type of information that is taken for granted in the adult hearing instrument fitting process is simply not attainable from young children.

The underlying etiologies, degree, configuration, and stability of hearing loss also have been shown to differ between children and adults. The most common causes of adult hearing loss are presbycusis and noise exposure. Pittman and Stelmachowicz (2003) categorized the audiologic configurations of 600 HI children and 600 adults with acquired hearing loss and found that 73% of the adult audiograms fell into the sloping (presbycusic) and U-shaped (noise-induced) categories, while the children's hearing losses were more evenly distributed across the six configuration categories defined in the study. The children also were more than three times as likely to exhibit asymmetrical hearing losses (defined as a difference in hearing thresholds of ≥ 15 dB at two or more frequencies).

In addition to the previously mentioned adult-child differences, numerous physical differences exist. The small size of the ear canal often limits options in terms of hearing instrument style, increases the likelihood of acoustic feedback, creates hearing instrument retention problems, and limits the scope of acoustic (earmold) modifications. Reduced ear canal volume also will result in an increase in the intensity of sound delivered to the cochlea (Feigin et al., 1989). Because young children are unable to provide subjective feedback regarding the comfort or clarity of amplified signals, it is important to account for these physical differences in order to avoid potential damage to hearing and/or hearing instrument rejection due to loudness discomfort.

Young children also have relatively little control over their acoustic environments. In difficult listening situations, adults can position themselves to maximize audibility or ask the talker to repeat what was said. Children are unable to optimize listening in the same way.

The noted differences between adults and children highlight the need for a well-designed and systematic approach to the fitting of amplification in this population. Our goals for this chapter are to discuss the theoretical and practical issues related to the fitting of amplification in the pediatric population, describe the process from the early stages of identification to the ultimate validation of hearing instrument benefit, and review relevant hearing instrument–related studies with children.

IDENTIFICATION AND QUANTIFICATION OF HEARING LOSS

The success of universal newborn hearing screening programs has had a dramatic effect on the age at which infants are referred for diagnostic audiologic tests, with children being referred at a much earlier age. As with older populations, diagnosing a hearing loss in the infant population involves a test battery approach. For the infant under 6 months of age, this includes frequency-specific auditory brainstem response (ABR) or steady-state evoked potentials, otoacoustic emissions, and immittance measures. Several studies have examined the relationship between behavioral puretone thresholds and evoked potential measures of threshold (Suzuki et al., 1982; Munnerly et al., 1991; Stapells et al., 1995; Gorga, 1999; Stapells, 2000; Purdy and Abbas, 2002; Rance and Briggs, 2002; Rance and Rickards, 2002; Gorga et al., 2005). In general, the relatively good agreement between evoked potential measures and behavioral thresholds suggests that these measures can be used to predict the magnitude and configuration of hearing loss. Recently, Bagatto et al. (2004) examined the validity of converting ABR thresholds into ear canal SPL thresholds by applying individually measured real-ear-to-coupler differences (RECD) across frequency. They concluded that evoked potential thresholds could be converted with a reasonable degree of accuracy, even for infants. These values can then be used to derive target values in hearing instrument prescriptive algorithms.

Beginning at approximately 6 months of age, visual reinforcement audiometry (VRA) can be used instead of or in addition to frequency-specific evoked potential measures. By 24 to 30 months, conditioned play audiometry (CPA) can be used. It is possible to achieve ear-specific thresholds for both of these procedures with the use of insert or supra-aural earphones. (See Chapter 23 for a review of behavioral test techniques.) At any age, subjective observations, such as parental or caregiver reports of auditory responsiveness, also should be used to corroborate and enhance the information obtained objectively. By using a battery of tests, the following questions should be answered for each ear, at least to a first approximation: (1) What is the degree of hearing loss in the low and high frequencies? (2) Is the hearing loss conductive, sensory-neural, or mixed? (3) Is there any evidence of neuropathy affecting the auditory brainstem pathways? Once these questions are answered, hearing instruments can be selected and fitted.

It is important to recognize that hearing loss in children can be associated with other medical or developmental problems. Referral to a pediatric otolaryngologist can help rule out concomitant medical problems and/or common syndromes. A child with a hearing loss also should be referred to a pediatric ophthalmologist to ensure that vision is normal. A genetic consultation can help to determine the etiology of hearing loss, identify associated medical problems, and give the family an estimate of recurrence risk. Once hearing loss is confirmed, the family should be referred to an early intervention program as soon as possible. Families also will benefit from parent-to-parent support groups and assistance in identifying sources of financial aid when necessary.

COUNSELING FAMILIES

Counseling the parents or caregivers of a child with newly identified hearing loss is fundamentally different than counseling adults. Surveys have shown that parents' major concerns at the time of diagnosis are: determining the cause of hearing loss, understanding the audiogram, understanding auditory function, gaining realistic timelines for speech and language development, and coping with the emotional aspects of hearing loss (Roush, 2000; Harrison and Roush, 2002). Several months later, priorities may shift to the development of audition and spoken language, the role of early intervention agencies, and the legal rights of children with hearing loss. It is important to recognize, however, that factors such as degree of hearing loss, cultural issues, parental education, family constellation, and financial resources are likely to influence parental priorities.

As universal newborn hearing screening programs and quality diagnostic services narrow the gap between the age at which hearing loss is first suspected and the age of amplification, parents will have less time to adjust to the diagnosis and its implications. As a result, some parents will be eager to proceed with amplification, while others may still be in a state of denial. Calmness, compassion, patience, and supportiveness are critical. It is important for the audiologist to respect the family's reactions and choices, including possible decisions to seek a second opinion. Parents want to learn about hearing loss and its implications for their child, but information must be given in a clearly formulated and unbiased manner. Information should be provided gradually and redundantly. Clearly and concisely written information about childhood hearing loss and amplification should also be available to supplement information given verbally. Meeting parents of other children with hearing loss may help families. Additional information on various aspects of counseling can be found in Chapter 43.

HEARING INSTRUMENT CANDIDACY

Studies have shown that even a relatively mild hearing loss can impact school behavior and performance in children

(Bess et al., 1998). Similarly, children with hearing loss restricted to the high frequencies (above 2 kHz) and those with unilateral hearing loss also are likely to demonstrate listening difficulties, particularly under adverse listening conditions. Several studies have also shown that approximately 30% to 35% of children with unilateral hearing loss failed at least one grade between kindergarten and sixth grade (Bess, 1982; Bess and Tharpe, 1988; Oyler et al., 1987; Lieu, 2004). Bess et al. (1998) reported that, in addition to academic delays, sixth-grade students with minimal hearing loss exhibited significantly greater dysfunction than NH peers in the areas of self-esteem and energy. As such, children with minimal sensory-neural hearing loss should be considered *potential* candidates for amplification. Even if amplification is not recommended at the initial diagnosis, these children should be monitored closely to identify any changes in hearing status and to quantify progress in terms of speech, language, and social development.

HEARING INSTRUMENT PRESELECTION

When recommending hearing instruments for infants and young children, there are several commonly accepted fitting premises. In general, binaural fittings of behind-the-ear (BTE) instruments with flexible electroacoustic characteristics are the standard. Instruments should be as small as possible, tamper resistant, easy to use, and durable. BTE hearing instruments are generally the style of choice with safety, durability of device, and rate of growth of the infant's ears as overriding concerns. Most young children have ears that are simply not large enough to accommodate in-the-ear (ITE), in-the-canal (ITC), or completely-in-the-canal (CIC) hearing instruments. In the rare case that a child's ear canals are large enough, the hard case of custom products poses a safety risk for active children. In addition, rapid growth of the ear canal in the first few years of life would necessitate frequent recasing of the device. In the interest of safety, a BTE device coupled to an earmold made of soft material is generally preferred. BTEs also require fewer repairs than custom devices and are more likely to be compatible with frequency modulated (FM) systems and other assistive devices. Body-style hearing instruments are rarely used unless all options to eliminate acoustic feedback have been exhausted.

It is generally accepted that a binaural fitting is preferable to a monaural fitting, even in cases of significant asymmetry between the ears. When there is no measurable hearing in one ear or an obvious contraindication, such as atresia, a monaural fitting will be necessary. Because "no response" on an ABR test does not conclusively prove the absence of residual hearing, two hearing instruments should be the starting point when fittings are based on ABR results alone. If subsequent behavioral testing demonstrates that one ear has no usable hearing (anacusis), that one ear has an extremely limited dynamic range, and/or that performance is degraded when wearing two hearing instruments, then a monaural fitting should be recommended.

At some point during the first 3 years of life, use of an FM system should be considered. Improvements of up to 18 dB in the signal-to-noise ratio (S/N) have been reported with FM use compared to personal hearing instruments (Hawkins, 1984). There is increasing evidence that the selective use of FM systems in nonacademic environments (e.g., car trips, shopping malls, parks, zoo) can improve auditory access and enhance language input to children with hearing loss (Gabbard, 2005). For this reason, FM system *compatibility* should be an essential feature of the first set of hearing instruments recommended.

While the features described previously are widely agreed upon, other factors such as type of signal processing, directional microphones, multiple memory devices, single microphone noise reduction, and frequency compression are more controversial. Although technologic advances in hearing instrument circuitry have been rapid and numerous, no research has been conducted involving the use of advanced technology with infants, and very few studies have involved children under the age of 5 years old. Fortunately, however, digital technology now allows great flexibility within a particular instrument, thus signal processing can be altered easily even after the initial hearing instrument fitting. Such flexibility allows the audiologist to adjust parameters as more information about hearing status is obtained or if the hearing loss progresses. A review of the literature related to the use of advanced technologies with young children will be provided in a later section.

PRESCRIPTIVE TARGETS

Because infants and young children cannot actively participate in the hearing instrument fitting process, an objective prescriptive strategy based on auditory thresholds is the method of choice for this population (Bess et al., 1996; AAA, 2004). It is important that the method account for factors known to differ between adults and children. These include age-related adjustments for ear canal size and the necessary transforms to compensate for the fact that various transducers are often used for threshold testing. Additionally, the approach should provide targets for maximum output, nonlinear hearing instruments, and, as will be discussed in detail in the next section, information regarding the degree of audibility of soft, average, and loud speech after amplification. It is important to recognize that the derivation of target values for any prescriptive approach will depend on the underlying theoretical assumptions. The two most commonly used prescriptive formulae are the Desired Sensation Level Multistate Input/Output (DSL [i/o]) method (Seewald et al., 1997; Seewald and Scollie, 2003) and the National Acoustic Laboratories (NAL-NL1) procedure (Dillon et al., 1998; Dillon, 1999; Byrne et al., 2001). The stated goal of DSL [i/o] is to fit the normal range of speech into the child's residual dynamic

range in order to optimize audibility of speech across both frequency and level. The stated goal of NAL-NL1 is to maximize speech intelligibility across typical input levels without exceeding the total loudness level experienced by listeners with normal hearing. In practice, there are many similarities between the two fitting algorithms.

Both procedures provide gain and maximum output targets for nonlinear hearing instruments, have similar prescribed Output SPL for 90 dB Input SPL (OSPL90) values, allow entry of individually measured RECDs, provide age-related mean RECD values, and display the amplified spectrum of speech. Recent descriptions of these fitting algorithms can be found in Ching et al. (2001; 2002), Seewald and Scollie (2003), Ching and Dillon (2003), Seewald et al. (2005), Bagatto et al. (2005), and Scollie et al. (2005).

Several investigators have attempted to compare the relative benefit of these hearing instrument fitting approaches in children. Unfortunately, the results of such studies are difficult to interpret. Specifically, findings generally have shown that children tend to prefer the prescriptive method used when their hearing instruments were originally fit (Snik et al., 1995; Ching et al., 1997; Scollie et al., 2000). Thus, the effects of acclimatization appear to influence preference judgments. To date, no studies comparing long-term speech and language outcomes for different fitting algorithms have been reported.

Regardless of the fitting strategy used to fit hearing instruments and the widespread use of digital technology, it is important to recognize that, in actual practice, it is extremely difficult to meet all target values across frequency over a range of input levels. Constraints include the degree and configuration of hearing loss, the number of bands that can be manipulated, and interactions among variables (e.g., compression threshold and/or compression ratio). As will be seen in the next section, the ability to view the amplified spectrum at multiple input levels can provide a common sense component to the hearing instrument fitting process when compromise is necessary.

ELECTROACOUSTIC VERIFICATION

The goal of verification is to confirm that the electroacoustic characteristics of the hearing instruments are optimal for a given child. Historically, the aided audiogram (sometimes referred to as functional gain) was used to quantify hearing instrument performance as a function of frequency. This procedure provides information regarding the lowest sound levels as a function of frequency that are audible with a particular hearing instrument configuration. As shown in Figure 37.4, the unaided and aided thresholds were often compared to the average level of speech sounds (converted to dB hearing level [HL]) to estimate their audibility. In this example, it appears that only a few speech sounds comprised of low-frequency energy would be audible to this child in the

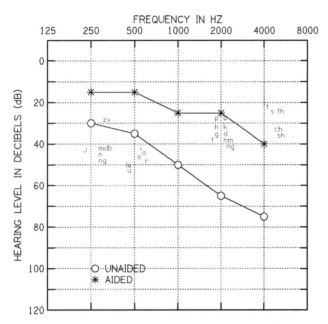

FIGURE 37.4 Aided (*asterisks*) and unaided (*open circles*) audiogram depicting the relationship between thresholds and various speech sounds at the level of average conversation.

unaided condition. With amplification, speech sounds with energy up to and including the 2,000-Hz region would be audible, but higher frequency fricatives and affricates would still be inaudible. In the early 1980s, the validity of the aided audiogram was questioned by several investigators (Macrae and Frazier, 1980; Macrae, 1982a; 1982b). Specifically, it was noted that the interpretation of aided thresholds can be complicated by noise floor problems in regions of normal or near-normal hearing. In such cases, amplified room noise will impose a lower limit on aided sound field thresholds. Stelmachowicz and Lewis (1988) also demonstrated that aided sound field thresholds cannot be used to estimate the degree of hearing instrument gain for supra-threshold signals such as speech. This is particularly true for nonlinear hearing instruments where gain varies as a function of input level. Additional criticisms of the functional gain method include poor test-retest reliability, limited frequency resolution (five to six test frequencies), and an inability to provide any information about real-ear maximum output levels (Balfour and Hawkins, 1993; Scollie and Seewald, 2001). The limitations of functional gain also apply in cases where evoked potential measures are used to estimate hearing instrument performance (Purdy et al, 2005). Aided sound field thresholds can be of value, however, to document performance for bone-conduction hearing instruments, frequency compression devices (instruments that shift high-frequency speech energy to lower frequency regions where hearing sensitivity is better), and cochlear implants and when thresholds are suspected to be vibrotactile (if unaided thresholds are vibrotactile, the improvements with amplification will be much less than expected).

It has been well established that 2-cm³ coupler measures of hearing instrument output do not adequately reflect

individual differences in factors that are known to affect hearing instrument performance (Larson et al., 1977; Mason and Popelka, 1986). These include acoustic impedance of the ear, earmold acoustics, ear canal size, leakage of sound from the ear canal, head diffraction effects, and hearing instrument microphone location effects. Discrepancies between real-ear and coupler measures may be particularly large for infants and young children (Nelson Barlow et al., 1988; Feigin et al., 1989; Westwood and Bamford, 1995; Martin et al., 1996). The results of these studies support the use of individualized real-ear measures in both children and adults in order to optimize the hearing instrument fit.

Fortunately, an approach for obtaining individual real-ear measures (probe-tube microphone technology) was introduced into clinical practice in the early 1980s. Placement of a small flexible probe-tube microphone into the ear canal allows individualized measures of aided real-ear gain and maximum output for test signals presented in the sound field. Studies have shown good test-retest reliability for probe microphone measures in 3- to 15-year-old children (Nelson-Barlow et al., 1988). Advantages of individualized probe-tube microphone measures over functional gain include a more detailed representation of gain across frequency, improved reliability, efficiency, direct measurement of real-ear maximum output, avoidance of noise floor effects, and a more valid representation of hearing instrument performance for nonlinear circuits (Hawkins et al., 1987; Stelmachowicz and Lewis, 1988; Hawkins and Northern, 1992; Scollie and Seewald, 2002a).

Because valid and reliable probe-tube microphone measures may not always be possible with infants and young children due to lack of cooperation, excessive movement, and vocalization, a clinically feasible technique to predict real-ear measures of hearing instrument gain and output was developed by Moodie et al. (1994). This procedure requires only a clinical probe-tube microphone system, an insert earphone (e.g., Etymotic ER3A), and the child's custom earmold. To obtain an RECD, the probe-tube microphone is placed into the ear canal adjacent to the earmold, and a broadband or swept-frequency stimulus is routed to the ear canal by connecting the output of the insert phone (or similar transducer) to the earmold tubing. Similar measures are then obtained with the transducer placed in a standard coupler. The mathematical difference between the two responses is the individual transfer function designated as the RECD. To estimate the real-ear amplified speech spectrum, these level-independent RECD values are added to coupler measures of hearing instrument output for different input levels. To predict the real-ear aided response (REAR), the following formula is used:

$$\text{REAR} = 2\text{-cm}^3 \text{ coupler response} + \text{RECD} + \text{HD} + \text{ML}$$

where HD and ML represent head diffraction and microphone location effects, respectively, as a function of frequency.

This procedure has many advantages over traditional probe-tube microphone measures with young children. The process requires only passive cooperation, and because the stimulus is presented via an insert earphone, head and body movements will have minimal effects on results. Stimulus presentation is brief (2 to 5 seconds), so multiple attempts to obtain the RECD can be made if necessary. An experienced clinician can obtain RECD measures for both ears in approximately 5 minutes. After the RECD is obtained, all subsequent measures of hearing instrument performance are obtained by adding the RECD to 2-cm³ coupler measures and do not require that the child be present. Studies have shown that the RECD procedure can provide a valid and reliable alternative to traditional probe-tube microphone measures (Westwood and Bamford, 1995; Sinclair et al., 1996; Seewald et al., 1999).

Adult hearing instrument verification protocols often define prescriptive targets in terms of real-ear insertion gain (REIG), which is calculated by subtracting the real-ear un-aided response (REUR) from the REAR. When testing children, however, it is preferable to evaluate hearing instrument performance in terms of the REAR for a several reasons. First,

this approach capitalizes on the accuracy of real-ear measures while minimizing test time and the amount of cooperation needed from the child since only one probe microphone measure is needed. Second, when test stimuli are speech-shaped noise or signals designed to mimic the spectral and temporal characteristics of speech, the REAR will provide a more valid representation of amplified speech for hearing instruments with complex digital signal processing than when swept puretones or steady-state noise is used (Stelmachowicz et al., 1990; Scollie and Seewald, 2002a; Scollie et al., 2002).

The REAR also can be used to visualize the audibility of speech for different input levels and/or listening situations. Figure 37.5 illustrates the amplified spectrum for four different speech input levels as depicted in the Situational Hearing Aid Response Profile (SHARP) (Stelmachowicz et al., 1996). In each panel, all variables are expressed in real-ear SPL based on probe microphone measures. The open circles represent thresholds for the right ear of a child with

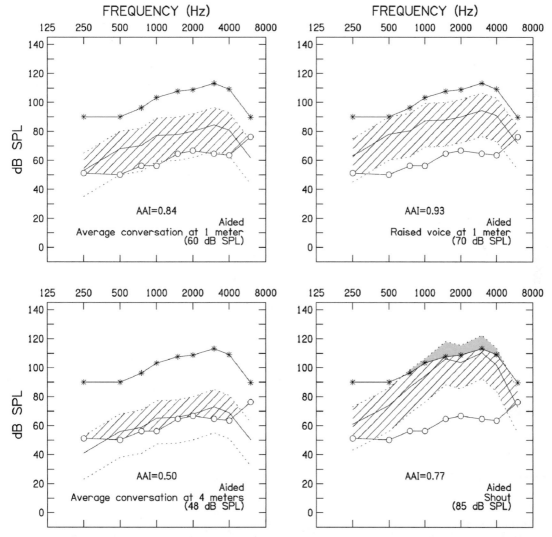

FIGURE 37.5 Amplified long-term average speech spectra (LTASS) in four listening conditions (average conversation at 1 meter, average conversation at 4 meters, shout, and own voice at hearing aid microphone). In each panel, *circles* indicate auditory thresholds; *solid line* indicates LTASS; *dotted lines* indicate +12/–18 dB range of speech; *cross-hatched region* indicates audible portion of signal; *asterisks* indicate real-ear saturation response. AAI, aided audibility index; SPL, sound pressure level.

a moderate to severe hearing loss. The solid line shows the long-term average spectrum at the designated overall level, and the dotted lines show the associated +12/−18 dB range of speech. The cross-hatched region shows the portion of the spectrum that is audible, whereas the asterisks show the real-ear maximum output measured with a swept puretone. Each panel also shows an aided audibility index (AAI) for each condition, where a value of 0 indicates that no portion of the speech signal is above threshold and a value of 1.00 indicates that the entire 30-dB range of speech is audible. Similar displays of audibility based on real-ear measures are provided in the DSL and NAL fitting software as well as in some real-ear measurement systems. Such displays provide a clear picture of the audibility of speech as a function of frequency for different input levels. These data can be used to guide clinical decisions regarding factors such as maximum output, compression threshold, and compression ratio. For example, if the audibility of high-level and average speech is adequate but soft speech produces low AAI values, compression threshold and/or compression ratio may be altered to improve overall audibility.

Although the relative differences in aided audibility provide the necessary information for comparisons across different listening conditions and/or hearing instrument settings, the AAI alone cannot provide an estimate of speech recognition. The relationship between AAI and speech recognition will depend on both the speech materials used and the characteristics of the listener. In Figure 37.6, average transfer functions for four-word meaningful sentences are shown for adults and 5-year-old children (Stelmachowicz et al., 2000). Because young children cannot take full advantage of semantic context, their function is shifted to the right. Figure 37.7 shows three displays of aided audibility for average conversational speech for a moderate to severe sensory-neural hearing

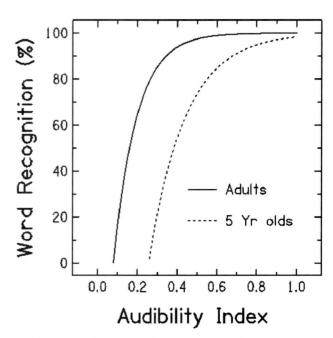

FIGURE 37.6 Recognition of words in high-predictability sentences as a function of the audibility index for adults and 5-year-old children. (Adapted from Stelmachowicz PG, Hoover BM, Lewis DE, Kortekaas R, Pittman AL. [2000] The relationship between stimulus context, speech audibility, and perception for normal and hearing impaired children. *J Speech Hear Res.* 43, 902–914.)

loss. The left panel shows the amplified spectrum using the manufacturer's algorithm for an adult who is a new user. Using the same hearing instrument, the middle and right panels show amplified spectra for a 5-year-old child using the manufacturer's algorithm and DSL [i/o], respectively. Note

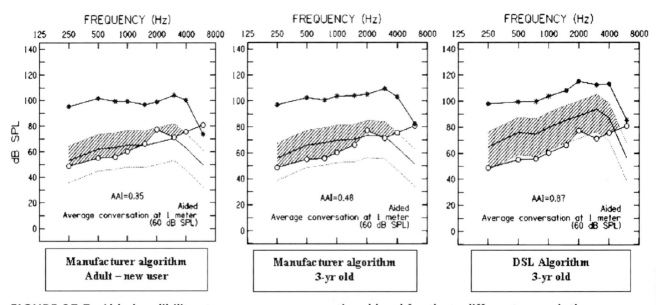

FIGURE 37.7 Aided audibility at an average conversational level for three different prescriptive algorithms. AAI, aided audibility index; SPL, sound pressure level. DSL, Desired Sensation Level.

that the AAI values for these three conditions range from 0.35 to 0.87. The transfer functions in Figure 37.6 can be used to estimate speech recognition scores from these AAI values. For adults, when the input is meaningful sentences, the relatively low AAI value of 0.35 corresponds to approximately 92% performance. This probably explains why many adults with hearing loss do not seem to require much gain. Using the transfer function for 5-year-old children, the manufacturer's fitting would result in 68% performance, and the DSL [i/o] fitting would correspond to 97% performance.

Many hearing instrument manufacturers now provide simulations of aided audibility in their fitting software. It is important to note that the validity of these displays is dependent upon the manner in which these calculations are made. In most instances, few, if any, details are provided regarding the conversion factors and the methods used to generate these graphs and associated audibility values (e.g., AAI, Speech Intelligibility Index). Highest validity is achieved when measures are based on real-ear (probe microphone) measures for an individual child. The use of average age-related RECDs is the next best choice.

ASSESSMENT OF SPEECH PERCEPTION

A variety of age-appropriate materials have been developed to assess speech perception abilities for children starting at approximately 3 years of age. A description of such tests can be found in Chapters 5 and 23. It is important to understand the limitations of speech perception measures as they relate to the hearing instrument fitting process. First, it has been well documented in studies with adults that word recognition tests are not sensitive enough to allow valid comparisons across various amplification schemes. There is no reason to assume that this would be different for young children. Second, it is important to match specific speech perception tests to the goals of the evaluation (Boothroyd, 2005). If one desires to assess the residual auditory capabilities of a child, it is important to use materials such as nonsense syllables because they are devoid of linguistic and semantic information. If, on the other hand, an estimate of how a child might function in a preschool environment is desired, age-appropriate meaningful sentence materials should be used.

A valuable tool for comparing aided and unaided speech perception has been developed and evaluated (Boothroyd, 2004; Mackersie et al., 2001). The Computer-Assisted Speech Perception Assessment (CASPA) was originally designed for sound field testing with and without sensory assistance, but it can also be used to compare performance in quiet and in noise. The software simplifies the process of presenting stimuli, scoring, data storage, and the construction of performance intensity functions. Stimuli can be routed from the computer directly to amplified loudspeakers or to loudspeakers via an audiometer. Test stimuli are consonant-vowel-consonant words. Results can be viewed and/or printed as either a graph or table. An example of the output from CASPA is shown in Figure 37.8, where phoneme recognition is

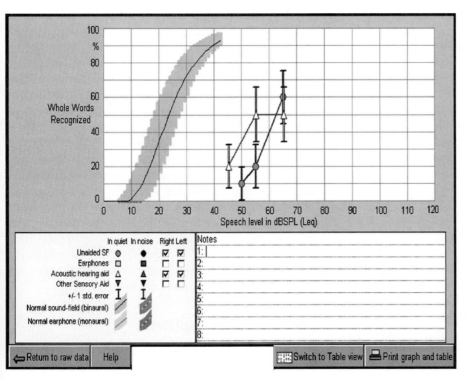

FIGURE 37.8 Graphic display from the Computer-Assisted Speech Perception Test developed by Arthur Boothroyd. (From Boothroyd A. [2004] Computer-Assisted Speech Perception Assessment. Available at: http://www.slhs.sdsu.edu/aboothro/.)

plotted as a function of stimulus level for both the unaided (circles) and aided (triangles) conditions. In this case, amplification results in 20% to 25% improvements in performance for low-level (<60 dB SPL) stimuli, but at higher levels, performance actually decreases slightly. Results can be scored by whole words, vowels, or consonants. A single 4- to 5-point performance intensity function can be obtained in approximately 10 minutes. The ability to compare aided and unaided performance across a range of input levels can provide valuable insights to guide the hearing instrument selection and fitting process.

Another useful option is the Bamford-Kowal-Bench Speech-in-Noise Test (BKB-SIN) (Bench et al., 1979). In this test, speech level is fixed while noise level is varied adaptively to obtain the level at which 50% performance is achieved for short meaningful sentences. A recent commercial implementation (www.etymotic.com) of this test procedure makes this easy to use in a clinical setting in order to demonstrate the benefit of amplification, assess the utility of directional microphones, and/or predict performance in noise over a range of speech levels.

■ SIGNAL PROCESSING AND ADVANCED TECHNOLOGY

Digital signal processing has quickly become the industry standard for hearing instruments. By definition, an analog signal is converted to a digital form, processed in some manner, and converted back to an analog signal. The introduction of digital processing has resulted in the ability to implement more complex and advanced types of signal processing than with analog technology. Although studies with adults have shown significant improvements in performance with specific processing schemes, no single type of processing has been shown to be beneficial for all individuals with hearing loss (Dillon, 2001). Precise information about these schemes is often deemed "proprietary" by manufacturers, and, for certain types of systems, standard clinical test signals (e.g., puretones, steady-state noise) will produce invalid results. Because objective measures are essentially the only option with infants, this limitation poses a significant problem unless test signals that simulate both the spectral and temporal characteristics of speech are available (Stelmachowicz et al., 1990).

Nonlinear Processing

Almost all hearing instruments use some form of nonlinear signal processing. Wide dynamic range compression (WDRC) circuits automatically adjust the gain of the instrument based on the level of incoming signals (see Chapter 35 for a detailed description of WDRC processing). To date, relatively few studies have addressed the efficacy of WDRC processing with children. Based on data from adolescents and young adults with hearing loss, Jenstad et al. (1999; 2000) found that, relative to linear circuitry, WDRC pro-

cessing improves the perception of low-level speech in quiet and results in aided growth of loudness functions that approximate NH individuals. Improved audibility of low-level speech, however, can only be achieved when low compression thresholds (≤40 dB SPL) are used. For some children with greater degrees of hearing loss, a low compression threshold may increase the likelihood of acoustic feedback. Christensen (1999) compared the performance of WDRC circuitry to linear peak clipping (LPC) and linear compression limiting (LCL) in 9- to 14-year-old children with mild to moderate hearing loss. In general, speech perception across a range of listening conditions was highest with the WDRC processor. LPC resulted in the poorest performance for most listening conditions. More recently, Marriage et al. (2005) compared speech scores for children (ages 7 to 15 years) with severe to profound hearing loss who were fitted with LPC, LCL, or WDRC hearing instruments. They also found significant benefit for the WDRC condition. To date, no direct studies have been conducted with infants or young children. There is, however, indirect evidence to support the use of WDRC processing in this population. As was seen in Figure 37.1, the relative differences in performance across the three age groups diminish as the AI increases. WDRC processing is ideally suited for addressing the problem of poor performance for low-level inputs (i.e., enhancing the AI function for low-level speech inputs) without influencing comfort for high-level signals. Thus, given the results obtained with older children and the improvement in audibility for low-level speech signals, it appears that there are no apparent reasons to not use WDRC processing with younger children.

Multiple Memories

Multi-memory hearing instruments have the capacity to store multiple processing schemes for use in different situations. Christensen (1999) investigated the ability of 9- to 14-year-old children to use multiple-memory devices. Results indicated that these children were willing and able to switch memories and that they reported subjective benefit from being able to do so. No studies of subjective or objective benefit in younger children have been published. It is not clear if the results of the Christensen study can be generalized to infants and young children. Obviously the parents or caregivers of these children would be responsible for switching from one memory to another. This requires that the responsible parties be well counseled regarding when and why to switch between programs. Other questions that are not easy to answer for this population include the following: (1) How many memories should be used? (2) What information is needed to determine the programs to be used? (3) How can the benefit of individual programs be measured?

Directional Microphones

The goal of directional microphones is to suppress signals arriving from the sides and rear, while retaining good sensitivity for sounds at 0° azimuth. Directional microphone technology has been shown to improve the ability for understanding speech in a background of noise in adults with mild to moderately severe hearing loss (see Chapter 38). Only two studies involving children have been published (Gravel et al., 1999; Kuk et al., 1999). In the Gravel et al. study, the performance of omnidirectional versus dual-microphone hearing instrument technology was evaluated in both preschool and school-age children. Objective benefit of directional microphone technology was demonstrated in children as young as 4 to 6 years of age, but the magnitude of benefit was smaller (3 to 5 dB) than that typically observed with adults (5 to 7 dB). In addition, the youngest children required a more advantageous S/N to achieve the same speech perception performance as older children. Kuk et al. (1999) assessed speech recognition in noise and subjective listener preferences in 20 school-aged children wearing digital directional hearing instruments versus their own analog omnidirectional hearing instruments. Results revealed improved speech recognition scores at multiple presentation levels with the directional hearing instruments as well as a subjective preference.

To date, no studies have been conducted with infants or early preschool children. Stelmachowicz (1996) has pointed out some possible contraindications to the use of directional microphones for these populations. They may pose a safety risk if environmental sounds cannot be detected and localized. They also limit the ability to "overhear" the conversations of others (a rich source of language input). Adults typically solve these problems by selecting a directional microphone configuration only when listening in noise; young children may not be able to make these decisions reliably. Recently, adaptive directional microphones have been developed. These systems are designed to determine the azimuth of the noise source and automatically modify the null point in the polar pattern to optimize S/N. Studies have demonstrated the benefit of adaptive directional microphones with adults (Ricketts and Henry, 2002; Maj et al., 2004). While this may seem like a good solution for infants and young children, the accuracy of such algorithms in typical environments currently is not known, so potential safety issues associated with the use of directional microphones would apply until further studies are conducted. At a minimum, the ability to switch from directional to omnidirectional should be available to the parent or caregiver.

Single-Microphone Noise Reduction

Although various forms of noise reduction (NR) have been available in hearing instruments for many years, the introduction of digital signal processing provided new possibilities in single-microphone systems. When characteristics of the interfering noise can be clearly defined (e.g., airplane cockpit noise), signal processing algorithms can easily be developed to improve the S/N (Levitt, 2001). In hearing instrument applications, however, this is rarely the case. Assuming

the target signal is speech, interfering signals may be random noise, another talker, or multiple talkers. The most common methods of NR use some variation of either spectral subtraction or an assessment of S/N in each band followed by gain reduction. Across NR systems, many different parameters (e.g., number of bands, time constants) are manipulated. In general, the ability of these systems to detect the presence of noise is good. The ability to separate speech from noise without altering the signal of interest, however, is much more challenging. Studies with adults have shown significant improvements in speech perception when the noise is restricted to a narrow frequency region (Van Dijkhuizen et al., 1991; Rankovic et al., 1992). When the long-term spectra of the target signal and noise are similar, however, most studies have failed to show improvements in speech perception, despite improvements in the physical S/N (Levitt et al., 1990; 1993; Boymans and Dreschler, 2000; Alcantara et al., 2003). One exception is a study by Hochberg et al. (1992) in which the influence of single-microphone NR on phoneme recognition was studied in NH listeners and cochlear implant users. NR had no effect on performance for either group at high S/Ns, but a significant improvement in performance occurred at poor S/Ns for the implanted group only.

Interestingly, Jamieson et al. (1995) reported that NR resulted in a reduction in test performance when stimuli were nonsense syllables. These results suggest that certain types of NR may actually degrade the speech signal. Because of the inherent redundancy of conversational speech, such alterations may have little influence on speech perception for adults with acquired hearing losses but may be detrimental to infants and young children who are developing speech and language skills.

It is important to recognize that, although most studies of single-microphone NR have failed to show objective improvements in speech perception, HI adults often report improved comfort and/or listening effort with this type of processing (Jamieson et al., 1995; Boymans and Dreschler, 2000; Walden et al., 2000). If similar effects were to occur for children, it is possible that reduced listening effort would improve attention to specific tasks. To date, however, no studies have investigated the effects of single-microphone NR circuitry for HI children.

Hearing Instrument Bandwidth

Recently, there has been some debate regarding the utility of providing high-frequency amplification to some HI listeners. Some studies with adults have shown that high-frequency amplification may fail to improve or actually decrease speech perception scores (Hogan and Turner, 1998; Ching et al., 1998), while other studies have shown improvement in performance for some listeners and/or conditions (Skinner, 1980; Sullivan et al., 1992; Turner and Cummings, 1999; Hornsby and Ricketts, 2003). These divergent results may be due to experimental differences such as test stimuli or subject inclusion criteria (degree and configuration of hearing losses). In the only study involving children, Stelmachowicz et al. (2001) investigated the effects of stimulus bandwidth on the perception of /s/ (in both consonant-vowel and vowel-consonant context with the vowel /i/) produced by three talkers (adult male, adult female, and child). This particular fricative was chosen because of its relative importance in the English language (denotes plurality, tense, and possession). Stimuli were low-pass filtered at seven frequencies from 2 to 9 kHz, and data were collected from normal and HI adults and children (5 to 8 years). Figure 37.9 shows the lowest cutoff frequency at which maximum performance was achieved as a function of talker for the four groups. For the male talker, a cutoff frequency of only 4 to 5 kHz was adequate for all groups. For the female and child talkers, however, a much wider bandwidth (6 to 9 kHz) was needed for maximum performance. These findings are consistent with the fact that the peak energy of /s/ is in the 5 to 6 kHz region for adult male talkers and 6 to 8 kHz region for adult female and child talkers (Stelmachowicz et al., 2001). Unfortunately, the majority of current BTE hearing instruments have an upper limit in the 5 to 6 kHz range. Because young children tend to spend most of their day with adult female caregivers and/or other children, the limited bandwidth of current hearing instruments may have a negative impact on early language development. Data from a longitudinal study of early speech production in NH and HI children conducted at Boys Town National Research Hospital provides evidence to this effect (Moeller et al., 2007). Data were obtained from 21 NH chil-

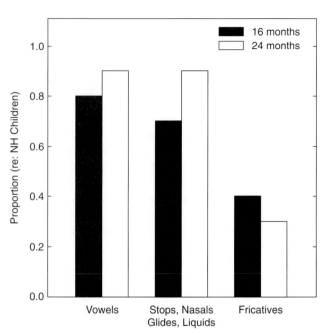

FIGURE 37.10 Production of vowels, nonfricatives, and fricative/affricates by hearing impaired (HI) children at 16 and 24 months. Values are expressed as the proportion of the normal hearing (NH) average score attained at each age.

dren and 12 children with moderate sensory-neural hearing loss who were identified and aided prior to 12 months of age (mean age: 4.2 months). Children were videotaped during play with their mothers at 4- to 6-week intervals beginning at 4 months of age. Figure 37.10 shows the production of vowels, nonfricatives, and fricative/affricates by HI children at 16 and 24 months. Values are expressed as the proportion of the NH average score attained at each age. Despite early intervention, preliminary data suggest that these HI children exhibited marked delays in the acquisition of all speech sounds relative to their NH peers. The delay was shortest for vowels and longest for the fricative class. This latter delay is consistent with the notion that these children may have had limited access to the high-frequency components of speech. In contrast to the earlier Stelmachowicz et al. (2001) study, which focused on /s/ (Fig. 37.9), these data show phonologic delays for the entire fricative class. Since approximately 50% of consonants in English are fricatives, these delays are likely to have marked influence on later speech and language development. As such, attempts to preserve the audibility of high-frequency speech sounds should be encouraged in children with usable residual hearing in this region.

Frequency Transposition and Frequency Compression

In cases of severe to profound high-frequency hearing loss where traditional amplification cannot provide adequate

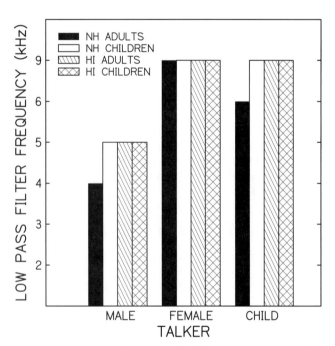

FIGURE 37.9 Low-pass cutoff frequency at which maximum performance was achieved for the phoneme /s/ spoken by an adult male, adult female, or child talker for four groups of listeners. NH, normal hearing; HI, hearing impaired.

gain, an alternative approach is needed. Over the years, several processing schemes have been devised in an attempt to improve the audibility of the high-frequency components of speech by "shifting" these components to lower frequencies (Ling, 1968; Beasley et al., 1976; Reed et al., 1985; Posen et al., 1993). Initially, frequency transposition was used only in cases of severe to profound high-frequency hearing loss. Early versions of "frequency transposition" shifted high-frequency components of speech to lower frequencies by a fixed value (in Hz). Many of the early attempts at frequency transposition met with limited success largely due to complications such as shifts in voice pitch, alterations in the time course of acoustic events, and unnatural sound quality.

The subsequent use of proportional frequency compression (using a fixed ratio) helped to preserve the normal frequency relations between the spectral components of speech, thus minimizing the problems described earlier. With proportional frequency compression, the entire bandwidth of speech is compressed to lower frequencies, and the spectrum is narrowed. The first commercially available device with this type of signal processing (AVR Transonic body aid) was introduced in 1991 and was designed primarily for individuals with minimal residual hearing sensitivity (left corner audiogram). With this device, the magnitude of frequency compression was adjustable, allowing voiced and voiceless speech sounds to be transposed with different fixed ratios (to help distinguish these sounds). In addition, added gain could be applied to voiceless sounds to improve audibility. In 1998, a BTE instrument (AVR Impact DSR 675) was introduced, followed by a smaller BTE and an ITE device in 2000. The most recent versions (DSP ImpaCt XP and Nano XP) were introduced in 2004 and include directional microphones, NR, and enhancements to the speech processing features. Additional details regarding this type of processing can be found in Davis (2001) and in Chapter 35. Recently, Widex Corporation has introduced a frequency compression hearing instrument. To date, no studies have been published using this device.

In general, studies of wearable frequency transposition/compression (FC) devices have shown mixed results that are often dependent on the study design, acclimatization/training time, speech materials, and subject characteristics (e.g., degree and slope of hearing loss). In a study with adults, Parent et al. (1998) reported improvement in speech perception over conventional hearing instruments for two of their four subjects. McDermott et al. (1999) reported small improvements in speech perception for two of their five adult participants. McDermott and Dean (2000) and McDermott and Knight (2001) found no significant differences between FC and conventional devices for the adults in their studies. In these two studies, however, the fitting strategy appeared to differ from that recommended by the manufacturer.

To date, only two studies have been reported with children. MacArdle et al. (2001) studied the effects of FC for 36 children (2 to 15 years old). After 4 years, only 11 of the 36 children continued to wear the devices. All of these children demonstrated significantly improved aided thresholds, but only three showed significant improvements on a 10-word list of monosyllabic words. Interestingly, the children in this subgroup were fitted at a younger age than the other subjects, and they were in oral communication programs. Recently, Miller-Hansen et al. (2003) reported results from a study conducted with 78 children (1.3 to 21.6 years old). In a subgroup of children (n = 16) who were able to perform a word recognition task (PBK words), the mean improvement over their conventional hearing aids was 12%. However, mean improvement varied by degree of hearing loss, with the greatest improvements in performance (relative to conventional hearing instruments) being achieved by those children with hearing loss in the severe range. Specifically, this group demonstrated an average improvement in speech recognition of 24%, compared to 8%, 5%, and 5% for children with mild, moderate, and profound hearing losses, respectively. It is important to note that these studies were conducted with earlier versions of this technology.

Frequency Modulated Systems

The goal of an FM system is to reduce the negative consequences of noise, distance, and reverberation on speech perception by placing a microphone close to the talker's mouth and transmitting the signal (via FM) to a receiver worn by an individual. When used properly, these devices can improve the S/N by as much as 18 to 20 dB in the FM-only condition. Despite numerous improvements in this technology over the past 20 years (e.g., miniaturization, reduced interference), these systems still are used primarily in educational settings. Although FM systems have been shown to improve auditory experiences in nonacademic settings, practical issues related to caregiver training, device misuse, and a lack of S/N improvements for nonprimary talkers have restricted widespread use (Moeller et al., 1996). Recent reports have suggested that part-time use of FM systems as an assistive device in selected environments (e.g., car, stroller, playground, museum) can provide a more consistent signal, improve listening in noise or at a distance, and potentially improve language skills (Gabbard, 2005). For more information on FM systems, please see Chapter 34.

■ SPECIAL POPULATIONS

Unilateral Hearing Loss

While the negative consequences of unilateral hearing loss support the use of amplification when residual hearing permits, in clinical practice, it is still relatively rare to provide amplification in the poorer ear of children with unilateral hearing loss. One reason for the lack of success is that the effects of unilateral hearing loss are not necessarily observable during the first several years of life. For many parents, potential long-term benefits are not sufficient to warrant the cost and effort required to maintain consistent hearing instrument use with a young child. Additional studies are needed with this population to determine if early provision of amplification improves long-term outcomes in children with unilateral hearing loss.

In cases where the poorer ear is unaidable due to anacusis, poor speech recognition, and/or loudness intolerance, amplification options are limited. While a contralateral routing of signals (CROS) fitting is usually considered under such circumstances for adults, the efficacy of this type of fitting has not been demonstrated for infants and young children. A better option might be a personal FM system fitted to the better ear with a nonoccluding earmold to improve listening in selected environments (Kopun et al., 1992). For school-age children, a classroom sound field FM system is another option.

Conductive and Mixed Hearing Loss

Children with recurrent otitis media, craniofacial anomalies, or other conditions that produce permanent conductive hearing loss may be candidates for some type of amplification. Unless contraindicated (e.g., atresia, drainage), a traditional (air-conducted) hearing instrument should be considered. Some hearing instrument fitting algorithms now provide gain and maximum output corrections for conductive and/or mixed hearing losses. In some cases, it may be necessary to deliver sound via bone conduction using either an externally worn bone-conduction transducer (either an ear-level or body-worn device) or a surgically implanted transducer known as a bone-anchored hearing aid (BAHA). However, the latter option is not approved by the Food and Drug Administration in the United States until 5 years of age. Age restrictions vary by country, so this surgical option is available at younger ages outside the United States. With the nonsurgical option, an external transducer is kept in place using a headband that has been designed or modified to accommodate the transducer and BTE hearing instrument. To minimize distortion of the skull, the placement of the transducer should be moved frequently during the first year of life. It has been suggested that the implantable device has a broader frequency response, a larger dynamic range, and a reduced potential for feedback (Gates and Valente, 1994; Snik et al., 1994). Several reports comparing the BAHA to conventional bone-conduction devices have shown improved subjective ratings in children (Granstrom and Tjellstrom, 1997) and improved speech recognition for adults (van der Pouw et al., 1998).

Progressive or Fluctuating Hearing Loss

Etiologies such as cytomegalovirus, hyperbilirubinemia, persistent pulmonary hypertension, extracorporeal membrane oxygenation (ECMO; a special procedure that involves the use of a heart-lung machine for patients whose hearts or lungs are failing), neurofibromatosis, Pendred syndrome, Usher syndrome, meningitis, and large vestibular aqueduct syndrome may be associated with progressive and/or fluctuating hearing loss (Joint Committee on Infant Hearing, 2000). In such cases, close monitoring of auditory thresholds is essential. Current hearing instruments typically are flexible enough from an electroacoustic perspective to accommodate substantial changes in threshold over time. When fluctuations are frequent, multi-memory devices may be useful.

Severe to Profound Hearing Loss

In recent years, both candidacy guidelines and the age at which cochlear implantation is considered have changed markedly. In general, children with hearing loss in the severe to profound range are considered to be *potential* candidates for cochlear implantation. Chapter 40 provides an overview of candidacy issues.

▨ DEVICE ORIENTATION

Optimal benefit from amplification can only be achieved with consistent and appropriate hearing instrument use. As such, parent education and device orientation are critical components of the fitting process. Ideally, this orientation process should include all individuals involved in the care of the child (e.g., parents, siblings, extended family members, daycare providers). All those involved should be fully familiarized with the parts of the hearing instruments, controls, functions, and safety issues (e.g., choke prevention, battery ingestion). Instruction and the required equipment to perform daily listening checks should be provided, along with simple troubleshooting steps. Because of the amount of new information that must be learned, it is critical to provide written materials (in lay terms) to supplement all verbal instruction.

▨ PRACTICAL ISSUES

Although the selected BTE device must be small enough to stay in place behind the child's ear, necessary electroacoustic features should not be compromised in favor of cosmetics. Larger devices can be kept in place with the help of retention clips, pediatric tone hooks, Huggie Aids, toupee tape, sweatbands, or caps. The size of a child's ear will increase dramatically between 3 months and 3 years of age, so strategies that may be necessary for retention in the early months of use can usually be eliminated at some point.

Although some parents may not be emotionally ready to accept device options that draw attention to their child's hearing loss, children often like the opportunity to select the color or pattern of earmolds and hearing instruments. Such involvement in the process can aid in the development of a child's self-esteem relative to having a hearing impairment and can help establish "ownership" of the situation.

VALIDATION/OUTCOME MEASURES

Numerous objective and subjective measures have been developed to document the efficacy of specific hearing instruments for adults and older children (see Chapter 38 for a review). For a variety of reasons, the tasks typically used with adults (e.g., subjective judgments, speech perception) are not applicable to infants and young children. Because improvements in speech production and/or language skills are not likely to occur immediately following the hearing instrument fitting, longitudinal monitoring may be necessary to identify changes in performance. Unfortunately, such an approach makes it difficult to separate the effects of normal development and/or the influence of other factors (e.g., therapy, family involvement) from those of amplification.

Despite the complexity of this issue, a variety of subjective outcome assessment tools have been developed for use with young children (see Dillon [2001] for a review). To date, relatively few metrics have been developed for children under 3 years of age (Zimmerman-Phillips et al., 1997; Palmer and Mormer, 1999). These tools can help to document auditory skill development over time for comparison to children with normal hearing. A lack of adequate progress over time can help to signal the need for changes in treatment (e.g., intervention program, amplification device) or the need to rule out additional developmental disabilities. Unfortunately, the necessary studies to determine the validity of various early outcome measures have not been conducted. There is a need to identify early markers that correlate highly with later outcomes. Such information could help determine the need to alter intervention strategies at an early age, thus optimizing the clinical decision-making process.

FOLLOW-UP AND MONITORING

Regardless of the degree and configuration of hearing loss, hearing status should be re-evaluated every 3 months for the first 2 years of life and every 6 months thereafter until school age, at which time an annual evaluation is generally adequate (Bess et al., 1996). If there are concerns about adequate progress or suspicion of progressing/fluctuating hearing loss, testing should be repeated more frequently. As the child matures, more details regarding auditory function will be possible. Measures of speech perception, loudness tolerance, and sound quality should be incrementally added to the test battery as appropriate.

SUMMARY

Over the past 20 years, tremendous gains have been achieved in the early identification and remediation of hearing loss. However, it has become apparent that the acoustic needs of young children with hearing loss are fundamentally different from those of their adult counterparts, and these needs are likely to change over time as children gradually learn to use linguistic knowledge to facilitate understanding in difficult listening situations. In addition, there is still much to learn about this population. For example, assessing device efficacy for infants and young children is considerably more complex than it is for adults. Continued studies are needed to address this issue as well as the many practical problems associated with hearing instrument use in this population.

ACKNOWLEDGEMENTS

The studies conducted at Boys Town National Research Hospital and cited in this chapter were supported by grants from the National Institute on Deafness and Other Communication Disorders, National Institutes of Health (R01 DC04300 and P30 DC04662).

REFERENCES

Alcantara JL, Moore BC, Kuhnel V, Launer S. (2003) Evaluation of the noise reduction system in a commercial digital hearing aid. *Int J Audiol.* 42, 32–42.

American Academy of Audiology. (2004) Pediatric amplification guidelines. *Audiol Today.* 16, 46–53.

Bagatto MP, Moodie S, Scollie S, Seewald R, Moodie S, Pumford J, Liu KP. (2005) Clinical protocols for hearing instrument fitting in the Desired Sensation Level Method. *Trends Amplif.* 9, 199–226.

Bagatto MP, Seewald RC, Scollie SD, Liu R, Hyde M. (2004) Integrating frequency-specific ABR thresholds into the hearing instrument fitting process. Presented at A Sound Foundation Through Early Amplification, Chicago, IL.

Balfour PB, Hawkins DB. (1993) Aided masked thresholds: case of deception. *J Am Acad Audiol.* 4, 272–274.

Beasley DS, Mosher NL, Orchik DJ. (1976) Use of frequency-shifted/time-compressed speech with hearing-impaired children. *Audiology.* 15, 395–406.

Bench J, Kowal A, Bamford J. (1979) The BKB (Bamford-Kowal-Bench) sentence lists for partially-hearing children. *Br J Audiol.* 13, 108–112.

Bess F. (1982) Children with unilateral hearing loss. *J Acad Rehab Audiol.* 20, 131–144.

Bess F, Chase P, Gravel J, Seewald R, Stelmachowicz P, Tharpe A, Hedley-Williams A. (1996) Amplification for infants and children with hearing loss (The Pediatric Working Group of the Conference on Amplification for Children with Auditory Deficits). *Am J Audiol.* 5, 53–68.

Bess F, Dodd-Murphy J, Parker R. (1998) Children with minimal sensorineural hearing loss: prevalence, educational performance, and functional status. *Ear Hear.* 19, 339–354.

Bess F, Tharpe AM. (1988) Performance and management of children with unilateral sensorineural hearing loss. *Scand Audiol Suppl.* 30, 75–79.

Boothroyd A. (2004) Computer-Assisted Speech Perception Assessment. Available at: http://www.slhs.sdsu.edu/aboothro/.

Boothroyd A. (2005) Measuring auditory speech-perception capacity in young children. In: Seewald RC, Bamford JM, eds. *A Sound Foundation through Early Amplification: Proceedings of the Third International Conference.* Stafa, Switzerland: Phonak AG; pp 129–140.

Boothroyd A, Eran E, Hanin L. (1996) Speech perception and production in children with hearing impairment. In: Bess FH, Gravel J, Tharpe AM, eds. *Amplification for Children with Auditory Deficits.* Nashville: Bill Wilkerson Press; pp 55–74.

Boymans M, Dreschler WA. (2000) Field trials using a digital hearing aid with active noise reduction and dual-microphone directionality. *Audiology.* 39, 260–268.

Byrne D, Dillon H, Ching T, Katsh R, Keidser G. (2001) NAL-NL1 procedure for fitting non-linear hearing aids: characteristics and comparisons with other procedures. *J Am Acad Audiol.* 12, 37–51.

Ching TY, Britton L, Dillon H, Agung K. (2002) RECD, REAG, NAL-NL1: accurate and practical methods for fitting non-linear hearing aids to infants and children. *Hear Rev.* 9, 12–20, 52.

Ching TY, Dillon H. (2003) Prescribing amplification for children: adult-equivalent hearing loss, real-ear gain, and NAL-NL1. *Trends Amplif.* 7, 1–9.

Ching TY, Dillon H, Byrne D. (1998) Speech recognition of hearing-impaired listeners: predictions from audibility and the limited role of high-frequency amplification. *J Acoust Soc Am.* 103, 1128–1140.

Ching TY, Dillon H, Katsch R, Byrne D. (2001) Maximizing effective audibility in hearing aid fitting. *Ear Hear.* 22, 212–224.

Ching TY, Newall P, Wigney D. (1997) Comparison of severely and profoundly hearing-impaired children's amplification preferences with the NAL-RP and the DSL 3.0 prescriptions. *Scand Audiol.* 26, 219–222.

Christensen LA. (1999) A comparison of three hearing-aid sound-processing strategies in a multiple-memory hearing aid for adolescents. *Semin Hear.* 20, 183–195.

Davis WE. (2001) Proportional frequency compression in hearing instruments. *Hear Rev.* 8, 34–42, 78.

DeCasper AJ, Fifer WP. (1980) Of human bonding: newborns prefer their mothers' voices. *Science.* 208, 1174–1176.

Dillon H. (1999) NAL-NL1: a new procedure for fitting non-linear hearing aids. *Hear J.* 52, 10–16, 32–38.

Dillon H. (2001) Special hearing aid issues for children. In: Dillon H, ed. *Hearing Aids.* Turramurra, Australia: Boomerang Press; pp 404–433.

Dillon H, Byrne D, Brewer S, Katsch R, Ching T, Keidser G. (1998) *NAL non-linear (NAL NL-1) User Manual, Version 1.01.* Chatswood, New South Wales, Australia: National Acoustic Laboratories.

Elfenbein JL, Small AM, Davis JM. (1993) Developmental patterns of duration discrimination. *J Speech Hear Res.* 36, 842–849.

Feigin J, Kopun J, Stelmachowicz P, Gorga M. (1989) Probe-tube microphone measures of ear-canal sound pressure levels in infants and children. *Ear Hear.* 10, 254–258.

Gabbard S. (2005) The use of FM technology for infants and young children. In: Seewald RC, Bamford JM, eds. *A Sound Foundation through Early Amplification: Proceedings of the Third International Conference.* Stafa, Switzerland: Phonak AG; pp 155–161.

Gates GA, Valente M. (1994) Fitting strategies for patients with conductive hearing loss. In: Valente M, ed. *Strategies for Selecting and Verifying Hearing Aid Fittings.* New York: Thieme Medical Publishers; pp 249–266.

Gorga MP. (1999) Predicting auditory sensitivity from auditory brainstem response measurements. *Semin Hear.* 20, 29–43.

Gorga MP, Johnson TA, Kaminski JK, Beauchaine KL, Garner CA, Neely ST. (2005) Using a combination of click- and toneburst-evoked auditory brainstem response measurements to estimate pure-tone thresholds. *Ear Hear.* 26, 593–607.

Granstrom G, Tjellstrom A. (1997) The bone-anchored hearing aid (BAHA) in children with auricular malformations. *Ear Nose Throat J.* 76, 238–237.

Gravel JS, Fausel N, Liskow C, Chobot J. (1999) Children's speech recognition in noise using omni-directional and dual-microphone hearing aid technology. *Ear Hear.* 20, 1–11.

Hall JW III, Grose JH. (1991) Notched-noise measures of frequency selectivity in adults and children using fixed-masker-level and fixed-signal-level presentation. *J Speech Hear Res.* 34, 651–660.

Hall JW III, Grose JH, Buss E, Dev MB. (2002) Spondee recognition in a two-talker masker and a speech-shaped noise masker in adults and children. *Ear Hear.* 23, 159–165.

Harrison M, Roush J. (2002) Information for families with young deaf and hard of hearing children: reports from parents and pediatric audiologists. In: Seewald RC, Gravel JS, eds. *A Sound Foundation through Early Amplification 2001: Proceedings of the Second International Conference.* St. Edmundsbury: St. Edmundsbury Press; pp 233–249.

Hawkins DB. (1984) Comparisons of speech recognition in noise by mildly-to-moderately hearing-impaired children using hearing aids and FM systems. *J Speech Hear Dis.* 49, 409–418.

Hawkins DB, Montgomery AA, Prosek RA, Walden BE. (1987) Examination of two issues concerning functional gain measurements. *J Speech Hear Dis.* 52, 56–63.

Hawkins DB, Northern JL. (1992) Probe-microphone measurements with children. In: Mueller HG, Hawkins DB, Northern JL, eds. *Probe Microphone Measurements: Hearing Aid Selection and Assessment.* San Diego: Singular Publishing Group Inc; pp 159–181.

Hochberg I, Boothroyd A, Weiss M, Hellman S. (1992) Effects of noise and noise suppression on speech perception by cochlear implant users. *Ear Hear.* 13, 263–271.

Hogan CA, Turner CW. (1998) High-frequency audibility: benefits for hearing-impaired listeners. *J Acoust Soc Am.* 104, 432–441.

Hornsby BW, Ricketts TA. (2003) The effects of hearing loss on the contribution of high- and low-frequency speech information to speech understanding. *J Acoust Soc Am.* 113, 1706–1717.

Houston DM, Jusczyk PW. (2000) The role of talker-specific information in word segmentation by infants. *J Exp Psychol Hum.* 26, 1570–1582.

Jamieson DG, Brennan RL, Cornelisse LE. (1995) Evaluation of a speech enhancement strategy with normal-hearing and hearing-impaired listeners. *Ear Hear.* 16, 274–286.

Jenstad LM, Pumford J, Seewald RC, Cornelisse LE. (2000) Comparison of linear gain and wide dynamic range compression hearing aid circuits II: aided loudness measures. *Ear Hear.* 21, 32–44.

Jenstad LM, Seewald RC, Cornelisse LE, Shantz J. (1999) Comparison of linear gain and wide dynamic range compression hearing aid circuits. I: Aided speech perception measures. *Ear Hear.* 20, 117–126.

Joint Committee on Infant Hearing. (2000) Year 2000 Position Statement. *Pediatrics.* 106, 798–817.

Jusczyk PW, Luce PA. (2002) Speech perception and spoken word recognition: past and present. *Ear Hear.* 23, 2–40.

Kawell M, Kopun J, Stelmachowicz P. (1988) Loudness discomfort levels in children. *Ear Hear.* 9, 133–136.

Kopun J, Stelmachowicz P, Carney E, Schulte L. (1992) Coupling of FM systems to individuals with unilateral hearing loss. *J Speech Hear Res.* 35, 201–207.

Kuhl PK. (1983) The perception of speech in early infancy: four phenomena. In: Gerber S, Mencher G, eds. *The Development of Auditory Behavior.* New York: Grune and Stratton; pp 187–218.

Kuk FK, Kollofski C, Brown S, Melum A, Rosenthal A. (1999) Use of a digital hearing aid with directional microphones in school-aged children. *J Am Acad Audiol.* 10, 535–548.

Larson VD, Studebaker GA, Cox RM. (1977) Sound levels in a 2-cc cavity, a Zwislocki coupler, and occluded ear canals. *J Am Audiol Soc.* 3, 63–70.

Levitt H. (2001) Noise reduction in hearing aids a review. *J Rehabil Res Dev.* 38, 111–121.

Levitt H, Bakke M, Kates J, Neuman A, Schwander T, Weiss M. (1993) Signal processing for hearing impairment. *Scand Audiol Suppl.* 38, 7–19.

Levitt H, Neuman A, Sullivan J. (1990) Studies with digital hearing aids. *Acta Otolaryngol Suppl.* 469, 57–69.

Lieu JE. (2004) Speech-language and educational consequences of unilateral hearing loss in children. *Arch Otolaryngol Head Neck Surg.* 130, 524–530.

Ling D. (1968) Three experiments on frequency transposition. *Am Ann Deaf.* 113, 283–294.

MacArdle BM, West C, Bradley J, Worth S, Mackenzie J Bellman SC. (2001) A study of the application of a frequency transposition hearing system in children. *Br J Audiol.* 35, 17–29.

Mackersie CL, Boothroyd A, Minniear D. (2001) Evaluation of the Computer-Assisted Speech Perception Assessment Test (CASPA). *J Am Acad Audiol.* 12, 390–396.

Macrae J. (1982a) Invalid aided thresholds. *Hear Instrum.* 33, 20, 22.

Macrae J. (1982b) The validity of aided thresholds. *Aust J Audiol.* 4, 48–54.

Macrae J, Frazier G. (1980) An investigation of variables affecting aided thresholds. *Aust J Audiol.* 2, 56–62.

Maj JB, Wouters J, Moonen M. (2004) Noise reduction results of an adaptive filtering technique for dual-microphone behind-the-ear hearing aids. *Ear Hear.* 25, 215–229.

Marriage JE, Moore BC, Stone MA, Baer T. (2005) Effects of three amplification strategies on speech perception by children with severe and profound hearing loss. *Ear Hear.* 26, 35–47.

Martin C, Westwood G, Bamford J. (1996) Real ear to coupler differences in children having otitis media with effusion. *Br J Audiol.* 30, 71–78.

Mason D, Popelka G. (1986). Comparison of hearing-aid gain using functional, coupler, and probe-tube measurements. *J Speech Hear Res.* 29, 218–226.

McDermott HJ, Dean MR. (2000) Speech perception with steeply sloping hearing loss: effects of frequency transposition. *Br J Audiol.* 34, 353–361.

McDermott HJ, Dorkos VP, Dean MR, Ching TY. (1999) Improvements in speech perception with use of the AVR TranSonic frequency-transposing hearing aid. *J Speech Lang Hear Res.* 42, 1323–1335.

McDermott H, Knight MR. (2001) Preliminary results with the AVR ImpaCt frequency-transposing hearing aid. *J Am Acad Audiol.* 12, 121–127.

Miller-Hansen DR, Nelson PB, Widen JE, Simon SD. (2003) Evaluating the benefit of speech recoding hearing aids in children. *Am J Audiol.* 12, 106–113.

Moeller M, Donaghy K, Beauchaine K, Lewis D, Stelmachowicz P. (1996) Longitudinal study of FM system use in non-academic settings: effects on language development. *Ear Hear.* 17, 28–41.

Moeller MP, Hoover B, Putman C, Arbataitis K, Bohnenkamp G, Peterson B, Wood S, Lewis D, Pittman A, Stelmachowicz P. (2007) Vocalizations of infants hearing loss compared with infants with normal hearing: part I – phonetic development. *Ear Hear.* 28, 605–627.

Moodie K, Seewald RC, Sinclair S. (1994) Procedure for predicting real-ear hearing aid performance in young children. *Am J Audiol.* 3, 23–31.

Morrongiello BA, Robson RC, Best CT, Clifton RK. (1984) Trading relations in the perception of speech by 5-year-old children. *J Exp Child Psychol.* 37, 231–250.

Munnerley G, Greville K, Purdy S, Keith W. (1991) Frequency-specific auditory brainstem responses relationship to behavioural thresholds in cochlear-impaired adults. *Audiology.* 30, 25–32.

Nelson Barlow N, Auslander M, Rines D, Stelmachowicz P. (1988) Probe-tube microphone measures in hearing-impaired children and adults. *Ear Hear.* 9, 243–247.

Nittrouer S. (1992) Age-related differences in perceptual effects of formant transitions with syllables and across syllable boundaries. *J Phonetics.* 20, 1–32.

Nittrouer S. (1996) Discriminability and perceptual weighting of some acoustic cues to speech perception by 3-year-olds. *J Speech Hear Res.* 39, 278–297.

Nittrouer S, Boothroyd A. (1990) Context effects in phoneme and word recognition by young children and older adults. *J Acoust Soc Am.* 87, 2705–2715.

Nittrouer S, Studdert-Kennedy M. (1987) The role of coarticulatory effects in the perception of fricatives by children and adults. *J Speech Hear Res.* 30, 319–329.

Oh EL, Wightman F, Lutfi RA. (2001) Children's detection of pure-tone signals with random multitone maskers. *J Acoust Soc Am.* 109, 2888–2895.

Oyler RF, Oyler AL, Matkin ND. (1987) Warning: a unilateral hearing loss may be detrimental to a child's academic career. *Hear J.* 18, 20–22.

Palmer CV, Mormer MA. (1999) Goals and expectations of the hearing aid fitting. *Trends Amplif.* 4, 61–71.

Parent TC, Chmiel R, Jerger J. (1998). Comparison of performance with frequency transposition hearing aids and conventional hearing aids. *J Am Acad Audiol.* 9, 67–77.

Pittman A, Stelmachowicz P. (2003) Hearing loss in children and adults: audiometric configuration, asymmetry, and progression. *Ear Hear.* 24, 198–205.

Posen MP, Reed CM, Braida LD. (1993) Intelligibility of frequency-lowered speech produced by a channel vocoder. *J Rehabil. Res Dev.* 30, 26–38.

Purdy S, Abbas P. (2002) ABR thresholds to tonebursts gated with Blackman and linear windows in adults with high-frequency sensorineural hearing loss. *Ear Hear.* 23, 358–368.

Purdy S, Katsch,R, Dillon H, Storey L, Sharma M, Agung K. (2005). Aided cortical auditory evoked potentials for hearing instrument evaluation in infants. In: Seewald RC, Bamford JM, eds. *A Sound Foundation through Early Amplification: Proceedings of the Third International Conference.* Stafa, Switzerland: Phonak AG; pp 115–127.

Rance G, Briggs RJ. (2002) Assessment of hearing in infants with moderate to profound impairment: the Melbourne experience with auditory steady-state evoked potential testing. *Ann Otol Rhinol Laryngol Suppl.* 189, 22–28.

Rance G, Rickards F. (2002) Prediction of hearing threshold in infants using auditory steady-state evoked potentials. *J Am Acad Audiol.* 13, 236–245.

Rankovic CM, Freyman RL, Zurek PM. (1992) Potential benefits of adaptive frequency-gain characteristics for speech reception in noise. *J Acoust Soc Am.* 91, 354–362.

Reed CM, Schultz KI, Braida LD, Durlach NI. (1985) Discrimination and identification of frequency-lowered speech in listeners with high-frequency hearing impairment. *J Acoust Soc Am.* 78, 2139–2141.

Ricketts T, Henry P. (2002) Evaluation of an adaptive, directional-microphone hearing aid. *Int J Audiol.* 41, 100–112.

Roush J. (2000) Implementing parent-infant services: advice from families. In: Seewald RS, ed. *A Sound Foundation through Early Amplification.* Chicago: Phonak AG; pp 159–165.

Scollie SD, Seewald RC. (2001) Electroacoustic verification measures with modern hearing instrument technology. In: Seewald RC, Gravel JS, eds. A *Sound Foundation through Early Amplification.* St. Edmundsbury: St. Edmundsbury Press; pp 121–137.

Scollie SD, Seewald RC. (2002a) Evaluation of electroacoustic test signals. I: Comparison with amplified speech. *Ear Hear.* 23, 477–487.

Scollie SD, Seewald RC. (2002b) Hearing aid fitting and verification procedures for children. In: Katz J, Burkhard RF, Medwetsky L, eds. *Handbook of Clinical Audiology.* Philadelphia: Lippincott Williams & Wilkins; pp 687–706.

Scollie SD, Seewald RC, Cornelisse L, Moodie S, Bagatto M, Laurnagaray D, Beaulac S, Pumford J. (2005) Desired Sensation Level Multistate Input/Output Algorithm. *Trends Amplif.* 9, 159–197.

Scollie SD, Seewald RC, Moodie KS, Dekok K. (2000) Preferred listening levels of children who use hearing aids: comparison to prescriptive targets. *J Am Acad Audiol.* 11, 230–238.

Scollie SD, Steinberg MJ, Seewald RC. (2002) Evaluation of electroacoustic test signals. II: Development and cross-validation of correction factors. *Ear Hear.* 23, 488–498.

Seewald RC, Cornelisse LE, Ramji KV, Sinclair ST, Moodie KS, Jamieson DG. (1997) DSL v4.1 for Windows: a software implementation of the Desired Sensation Level (DSL[i/o]). Method for fitting linear gain and wide-dynamic-range compres- sion hearing instruments. London, Ontario, Canada: Hearing Healthcare Research Unit, University of Western Ontario.

Seewald RC, Moodie K, Sinclair S, Scollie S. (1999) Predictive validity of a procedure for pediatric hearing instrument fitting. *Am J Audiol.* 8, 143–152.

Seewald RC, Moodie S, Scollie S. (2005) The DSL method for pediatric hearing instrument fitting: historical perspective and current issues. *Trends Amplif.* 9, 145–157.

Seewald RC, Scollie SD. (2003) An approach for ensuring accuracy in pediatric hearing instrument fitting. *Trends Amplif.* 7, 29–40.

Sinclair ST, Beauchaine KL, Moodie KS, Feigin J, Seewald RC, Stelmachowicz PG. (1996) Repeatability of a real-ear-to-coupler difference procedure as a function of age. *Am J Audiol.* 5, 52–56.

Skinner MW. (1980) Speech intelligibility in noise-induced hearing loss: effects of high-frequency compensation. *J Acoust Soc Am.* 67, 306–317.

Snik AF, Mylanus EAM, Cremers CWR. (1994) Aided free-field thresholds in children with conductive hearing loss fitted with air or bone conduction hearing aids. *Int J Pediatr Otolaryngol.* 30, 133–142.

Snik AF, van den Borne S, Brokx JP, Hoekstra C. (1995) Hearing-aid fitting in profoundly hearing-impaired children. Comparison of prescription rules. *Scand Audiol.* 24, 225–230.

Stapells DR. (2000) Threshold estimation by the tone-evoked auditory brainstem response: a literature meta-analysis. *J Speech Lang Pathol Audiol.* 24, 74–83.

Stapells DR, Gravel J, Martin B. (1995) Thresholds for auditory brain stem responses to tones in notched noise from infants and young children with normal hearing or sensorineural hearing loss. *Ear Hear.* 16, 361–371.

Stelmachowicz PG. (1991) Current issues in pediatric amplification. In: Feigin J, Stelmachowicz PG, eds. *Pediatric Amplification: Proceedings of the 1991 National Conference.* Omaha, NE: Boys Town National Research Hospital; pp 1–17.

Stelmachowicz PG. (1996) Current issues in pediatric amplification. *Hear J.* 49, 10–20.

Stelmachowicz PG. (2005) Pediatric amplification: past, present, and future. In: Seewald RC, Bamford JM, eds. *A Sound Foundation through Early Amplification: Proceedings of the Third International Conference.* Stafa, Switzerland: Phonak AG; pp 27–40.

Stelmachowicz PG, Hoover BM, Lewis DE, Kortekaas R, Pittman AL. (2000) The relationship between stimulus context, speech audibility, and perception for normal and hearing impaired children. *J Speech Hear Res.* 43, 902–914.

Stelmachowicz PG, Kalberer A, Lewis DE. (1996) Situational hearing aid response profile (SHARP). In: Bess F, Gravel J, Tharpe AM, eds. *Amplification for Children with Auditory Deficits.* Nashville: Bill Wilkerson Center Press; pp 193–213.

Stelmachowicz PG, Lewis DE. (1988) Some theoretical considerations concerning the relation between functional gain and insertion gain. *J Speech Hear Res.* 31, 491–496.

Stelmachowicz PG, Lewis DE, Seewald RC, Hawkins D. (1990) Complex and pure-tone signals in the evaluation of hearing aid characteristics. *J Speech Hear Res.* 33, 380–385.

Stelmachowicz PG, Pittman A, Hoover B, Lewis D. (2001) The effect of stimulus bandwidth on the perception of /s/ in normal and hearing-impaired children and adults. *J Acoust Soc Am.* 110, 2183–2190.

Sullivan JA, Allsman CS, Nielsen LB, Mobley JP. (1992) Amplification for listeners with steeply sloping, high-frequency hearing loss. *Ear Hear.* 13, 35–45.

Suzuki JI, Kodera K, Kaga K. (1982) Auditory evoked brainstem response assessment in otolaryngology. *Ann N Y Acad Sci.* 388, 487–500.

Turner CW, Cummings KJ. (1999) Speech audibility for listeners with high-frequency hearing loss. *Am J Audiol.* 8, 47–56.

van der Pouw KT, Snik AF, Cremers CW. (1998) Audiometric results of bilateral bone-anchored hearing aid application in patients with bilateral congenital aural atresia. *Laryngology.* 108, 548–553.

van Dijkhuizen JN, Festen JM, Plomp R. (1991) The effect of frequency-selective attenuation on the speech-reception threshold of sentences in conditions of low-frequency noise. *J Acoust Soc Am.* 90, 885–894.

Walden BE, Surr RK, Cord MT, Edwards B, Olson L. (2000) Comparison of benefits provided by different hearing aid technologies. *J Am Acad Audiol.* 11, 540–560.

Werker JF, Tees RC. (1984) Phonemic and phonetic factors in adult cross-language speech perception. *J Acoust Soc Am.* 75, 1866–1878.

Westwood G, Bamford J. (1995) Probe-tube microphone measures with very young infants: real ear to coupler differences and longitudinal changes in real ear unaided response. *Ear Hear.* 16, 263–273.

Wightman FL, Allen P, Dolan T, Kistler D, Jamieson D. (1989) Temporal resolution in children. *Child Dev.* 60, 611–624.

Wightman FL, Callahan MR, Lutfi RA, Kistler DJ, Oh E. (2003) Children's detection of pure-tone signals: informational masking with contralateral maskers. *J Acoust Soc Am.* 113, 3297–3305.

Yoshinaga-Itano C, Sedey AL, Coulter DK, Mehl AL. (1998) Language of early- and later-identified children with hearing loss. *Pediatrics.* 102, 1161–1171.

Zimmerman-Phillips S, Osberger MJ, Robbins AM. (1997) *Infant Toddler–Meaningful Auditory Integration Scale (IT-MAIS).* Sylmar, CA: Advanced Bionics Corporation.

Hearing Aid Fitting for Adults: Selection, Fitting, Verification, and Validation

Michael Valente and Maureen Valente

INTRODUCTION

Audiologists have a responsibility to achieve hearing aid fittings that provide the best possible "benefit" and "satisfaction." Surprisingly, these goals can often contradict each other. For example, patients commonly request hearing aids providing the best performance in noise (i.e., benefit), but this is quickly followed by the need for the hearing aids to be "invisible" (i.e., satisfaction). At this point, a conflict can immediately present itself because the technology capable of providing the greatest benefit in noise (directional microphone) may be in conflict with the desire for "invisibility" (i.e., completely-in-the-canal [CIC] hearing aids). The audiologist must either educate the patient on the technologies available providing the best benefit in noise and "convert" the patient to this technology or simply "give in" to the patient's demand for cosmetic appeal knowing the fitting will not provide the best benefit in noise. Ultimately, this patient might be fit with binaural hearing aids with directional microphones at one clinic, while the same patient could have been fit with binaural CIC hearing aids at another clinic. One fit will likely satisfy the goal of hearing better in noise, while the other fit will likely satisfy the cosmetic concerns of the patient.

To address the dilemma of "cosmetics" versus improved performance in noise, behind-the-ear (BTE) open-fit hearing aids with directional microphones have recently become available. Two recent studies examined the benefits of this technology. Kuk and Keenan (2005) evaluated eight subjects with one manufacturer's open-fit BTE using the Hearing in Noise Test (HINT) Reception Threshold for Sentences (RTS in dB). The sentences were presented at 0° azimuth, while HINT noise was delivered at 75 dB sound pressure level (SPL) with loudspeakers at 90°, 180°, and 270°. Valente and Mispagel (2008) evaluated 26 subjects with another manufacturer's open-fit BTE using HINT RTS in dB with sentences presented at 0° and uncorrelated restaurant noise presented at 65 dBA from eight loudspeakers set 45° apart. Results from both studies reported no significant differences between unaided and omnidirectional performance, but a directional benefit of slightly less than 2.0 dB was obtained compared to omnidirectional or unaided performance. The authors suggest that an anticipated 18% improvement in listening in a noisy listening situation is significant. For more information on recent advances in hearing aid technology, the reader is referred to Chapter 35.

These results seem to suggest that, when communicating in a noisy listening environment, patients require at least a directional microphone with an open-fit hearing aid to have aided performance better than unaided performance. These results also suggest that, despite the presence of an open fit, a directional microphone can provide significant benefit over omnidirectional and unaided performance in a noisy listening situation. Thus, assuming a 9% per dB improvement in sentence intelligibility of the HINT sentences (Soli and Nilsson, 1997), the directional microphone improved performance in noise, re: omnidirectional performance, by 18%. The authors suggest that an anticipated 18% improvement in listening in a noisy listening situation is significant.

This example illustrates one of the issues confronting audiologists when selecting hearing aids for their patients. To help readers achieve "the best fitting" for their adult

WASHINGTON UNIVERSITY QUESTIONNAIRE

Patient _____ Date _____ Aid _____ Ear(s) _____ Age _____

[X] Unaided   [O] Own Aid(s)   [+] New Aid(s)

Difficulty at Home	Always	Often	Sometimes	Rarely	Never	N/A
Communicate with spouse	[X]	[ ]	[O]	[ ]	[+]	[ ]
Family members/friends	[ ]	[X]	[O]	[ ]	[+]	[ ]
Children	[X]	[ ]	[ ]	[O]	[ ]	[ ]
TV, audio equipment	[X]	[O]	[ ]	[+]	[ ]	[ ]
Telephone	[X]	[ ]	[O]	[+]	[ ]	[ ]
Difficulty at work						
Telephone	[X]	[O]	[ ]	[+]	[ ]	[ ]
One-on-one in noisy situations	[X]	[O]	[ ]	[+]	[ ]	[ ]
Small meetings	[ ]	[X]	[ ]	[O]	[ ]	[ ]
Large meetings with speaker greater than 12 feet	[X]	[ ]	[O]	[ ]	[+]	[ ]
Difficulty in social situations						
Family gatherings	[ ]	[X]	[O]	[+]	[ ]	[ ]
Noisy restaurant	[X]	[O]	[ ]	[+]	[ ]	[ ]
House of worship	[ ]	[ ]	[ ]	[ ]	[ ]	[X]
Theater	[X]	[ ]	[O]	[+]	[ ]	[ ]
Party	[X]	[O]	[ ]	[ ]	[+]	[ ]

Comments/observations: _____
_____

FIGURE 38.1   Example of the Washington University Questionnaire.

patients, this chapter will provide a comprehensive overview of clinical procedures that audiologists can implement when selecting, fitting, verifying, and validating hearing aid fittings for adults. The procedures will be presented chronologically in the manner that hearing aids are typically selected, fitted, verified, and validated.

This process typically requires four visits. The *first* visit includes a comprehensive audiometric evaluation, counseling, and informally assessing patient motivation toward amplification. The *second* visit includes loudness judgments for puretones measured in dB SPL near the eardrum, counseling on fitting options, taking impressions, and obtaining unaided outcome measures, such as the Client Oriented Scale of Improvement (COSI) (Dillon et al., 1997) or the Washington University Questionnaire (Fig. 38.1). If time allows, the first and second visits can be collapsed into a single visit. The *third* visit includes assessing real-ear performance of the hearing aids and obtaining aided loudness judgments for speech. This visit also includes counseling on the use and care of the hearing aids. In addition, within 2 working days, the patient is contacted to determine initial reactions to the fitting. If problems are present, the patient is immediately scheduled to return to the clinic so the issue(s) can be resolved. The *final* visit, scheduled approximately 30 days after the initial fitting, includes obtaining the "aided" measure for the COSI or Washington University Questionnaire. This visit may also include fine tuning the hearing aids in response to the patient's assessment of performance during the 4-week trial period.

▨ PREFITTING DATA (FIRST VISIT)

Comprehensive Audiometry and Assessing Motivation

During the first visit, a case history is taken, and puretone (see Chapters 3 and 4) and speech audiometry (see Chapter 5) are measured in the conventional manner. Immittance measures (i.e., tympanometry, acoustic reflexes; see Chapters 9 and 10) are obtained if the audiometric results suggest conductive, mixed, or retrocochlear pathology. If the test data suggest that amplification would be appropriate, then candidacy for amplification is presented, and the patient is counseled to schedule an appointment with his/her physician for medical clearance for amplification. If the audiologist is questioned on the need for a medical examination, then the patient is informed that this examination is within his/her best interest, but the patient has the right to sign a medical waiver form.

In addition to candidacy, motivation toward amplification is observed. It is crucial during this initial visit that audiologists informally assess the motivation of the patient. The authors believe that dispensing hearing aids to unmotivated patients can do significantly more harm than good. If the experience with amplification is unsatisfactory, these feelings of dissatisfaction will probably be transferred to friends and/or family members who may also be considering amplification. Therefore, it would not be surprising if these other "potential" patients no longer pursue amplification because of the negative expression of their friend or family member. Thus, dispensing hearing aids to an unmotivated patient is strongly discouraged because this practice may lead to far more than simply a "return for credit." When counseling unmotivated patients, the authors suggest that this may not be the best time for them to consider amplification, but rather urge such patients to make an appointment when they feel more motivated.

HEARING AID EVALUATION (SECOND VISIT)

Real-Ear Measures of Loudness Discomfort

One of the most important facets of successful hearing aid fittings is to ensure that the amplified signal does not exceed a level where the patient reports it to be "loud, but okay." Munro and Patel (1998) reported that, if the measured real-ear saturation response with a 90-dB SPL puretone sweep ($RESR_{90}$) is below the individually measured loudness discomfort levels (LDLs), then subjects did not report "real-life" listening to be uncomfortably loud. This contrasted with subjects whose $RESR_{90}$ exceeded the individually measured LDL. Jenstad et al. (2003) reported that the primary complaint of patients newly fit with hearing aids who returned to the clinic for fine tuning was that the amplified sound was too loud.

As part of the hearing aid evaluation (HAE), measures are made to determine the intensity level where sound becomes "loud, but okay." To accomplish this, a probe tube, attached to a probe microphone, is placed in the ear canal approximately 4 to 6 mm from the eardrum to directly measure the SPL near the eardrum (Valente et al., 1990; 1991;

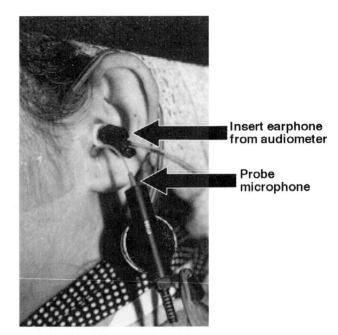

FIGURE 38.2 Placement of a probe tube, probe microphone, and insert earphone for measuring individual loudness discomfort levels (LDLs).

Mueller and Hornsby, 2002). To assure that the end of the probe tube is within 4 to 6 mm from the eardrum of an adult male patient, the probe tube is marked 30 mm from the tip (26 mm for an adult female). This mark is placed at the intratragal notch of the outer ear and taped into position.

Using this method, calibrated TDH series or ER-3A insert earphones are connected to the earphone output of a calibrated audiometer (American National Standards Institute [ANSI] S3.6-1996; ANSI, 1996) and placed in the ear canal along with the probe tube from the real ear analyzer (Fig. 38.2). At this point, a continuous puretone at 500 to 4,000 Hz in octave and mid-octave intervals is presented to the patient. The patient is asked to judge the loudness of the signal with choices of "very soft," "soft," "comfortable, but slightly soft," "comfortable," "comfortable, but slightly loud," "loud, but okay," and "uncomfortably loud" (Valente and Van Vliet, 1997).

Using an ascending procedure, the audiometer attenuator is increased in 5-dB steps to determine the intensity level where the patient consistently reports that the puretone signals are "loud, but okay." This level is read in dB SPL from a video monitor of the real-ear analyzer and is recorded as the patient's loudness discomfort level (LDL_{spl}) at each test frequency; these values are placed in the patient's chart (Fig. 38.3). In Figure 38.3, the LDL in dB hearing level (HL) is placed in the middle column (85 to 95 dB HL for this patient), and the measured LDL_{spl} is placed in the next column (96 to 106 dB SPL for this patient). The difference between these two measures is the real-ear-to-dial difference (REDD), and these values are placed in parentheses (10 to 15 dB for this patient). As part of the hearing aid fit at a

WASHINGTON UNIVERSITY SCHOOL OF MEDICINE
LOUDNESS MEASURES

Patient Name: _____

Date: _____

Right Ear:

	HL	SPL
500Hz	85	96 (11)
1 KHz	85	95 (10)
2 KHz	90	105 (15)
3 KHz	95	106 (11)
4 KHz	95	105 (10)

FIGURE 38.3 Example of a report form used to document a patient's measured loudness discomfort level (LDL) in dB HL and dB SPL and real-ear-to-dial difference (REDD; in parenthesis) at 500, 1,000, 2,000, 3,000, and 4,000 Hz. This form is placed in the patient's chart for future reference when measuring the real-ear saturation response with a 90-dB input (RESR$_{90}$).

subsequent visit, the audiologist, using the real-ear analyzer, measures the *output* (in dB SPL) from the hearing aid at the eardrum in response to a puretone sweep presented at 90 dB SPL (i.e., RESR$_{90}$; Fig. 38.4). Upon completing the RESR$_{90}$, the audiologist can determine the relationship between the measured RESR$_{90}$ and the previously measured LDL$_{spl}$. The audiologist needs to verify that the RESR$_{90}$ is *below* the measured LDL$_{spl}$; if so, this suggests the patient will not judge loud environmental sounds to be uncomfortably loud. As can be seen in Figure 38.4, this goal has been achieved for all test frequencies.

Patient Counseling on Realistic Goals

It is important that patients obtain information that will portray a realistic "picture" of the benefits they can expect from amplification; this may vary somewhat across patients. With these goals in mind, the patient is counseled on some or all of the following points:

a. Performance with hearing aids in "quiet" will be *significantly* better than performance without the hearing aids. At this point, the patient is reminded that the final judgment of *"significant benefit"* does not rely on the outcome of the numerous measures described in this chapter. Rather, the final decision concerning benefit lies exclusively with the patient.

b. Performance with the hearing aids in "noise" must be *significantly* better than the performance without the hearing aids (at least for patients with mild to moderate hearing loss). Achieving this goal is very important because most patients seek amplification because they experience difficulty recognizing speech in noise. Currently, it is our experience that fitting hearing aids incorporating directional microphones significantly increases the likelihood

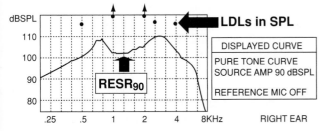

FIGURE 38.4 Example of the measured real-ear saturation response with a 90-dB input (RESR$_{90}$; *solid curve*) below the measured loudness discomfort levels (LDL) in dB SPL (*dots*). The ↑ symbol at 1,000 and 2,000 Hz means that the measured LDL in dB SPL, in this case, was greater than 120 dB SPL (*upper line on the ordinate*).

of achieving this goal (Valente et al., 1995; 2000; Gravel et al., 1999; Ricketts and Dhar, 1999; Kochkin, 2000; Pumford et al., 2000; Amlani, 2001; Compton-Conley et al., 2004; Lewis et al., 2004; 2005; Valente and Mispagel, 2004).

c. Patients should not expect performance in "noise" to be as satisfactory as performance in "quiet." The authors explain that listeners with normal hearing do not recognize speech as well in a noisy restaurant as they do in a quiet living room. Therefore, the patient is reminded that there is no reason for him/her to expect his/her hearing aids to perform as well in "noise" as they do in "quiet."

d. Input signals of "soft" intensity (i.e., 40 to 50 dB SPL) should be perceived as "soft, but audible."

e. Input signals of "average" intensity (i.e., 60 to 70 dB SPL) should be perceived as "comfortable."

f. Input signals of "loud" intensity (i.e., 80 dB SPL or greater) should be perceived as "loud, but not uncomfortable."

g. Earmolds or custom shells must be comfortable.

h. Patient's voice should not sound as if he/she is speaking at the bottom of a barrel (i.e., occlusion effect).

i. Patient should not experience acoustic or suboscillatory feedback.

j. It is common for patients purchasing "new" hearing aids to *expect* to hear as well as their normal-hearing friends in a noisy restaurant. To directly address this expectation, the first author asks the patient, when communicating in noisy situations, to mentally "score" the percentage of the conversation he/she has understood from his/her normal-hearing friend(s). Next, the patient then asks his/her normal-hearing friend(s) what percentage of *the patient's conversation* did the friend(s) understand? It has been the experience of the first author that, very often, the difference between these two "scores" is often not as great as the patient previously predicted they might be. That is, the patient now has a greater appreciation that even friends with normal hearing experience significant difficulty in noisy environments. After completing this simple exercise, the patient typically has a better "feel" for the benefit achieved with his/her aids, and his/her expectations are more realistic. Moreover, audiologists should counsel that even greater benefit in noise can be achieved with hearing assistive technology (HAT) (Lewis et al., 2004; 2005) and auditory rehabilitation.

k. If these expectations are not fulfilled, the patient *must* return to the office so that the hearing aids can be readjusted or replaced with another form of technology. If these problems cannot be addressed in a satisfactory manner, then the hearing aids should be returned for credit. The authors counsel patients that it is not our intent for these hearing aids to be another set of hearing aids lying in a dresser drawer!

To add to the accuracy of patient counseling and pairing patient needs with technology, one manufacturer recently introduced a device that is essentially a dosimeter that analyzes and stores the patient's listening environment (Flynn,

2005). The data from the body-worn device can be uploaded to a NOAH interface box, and the audiologist can determine what percentage of the time the patient was exposed to sound levels less than or greater than 80 dB SPL. Also, the audiologist can determine what percentage of time the patient was exposed to noise only, speech in noise, speech only, or quiet. This feature has recently been incorporated into many of the latest digital hearing aids offered by manufacturers.

Bilateral versus Monaural Amplification

Next, when appropriate, the authors counsel on the advantages of bilateral amplification. At our facilities, the authors strongly promote bilateral fittings to eliminate the *head shadow effect* and to yield a more "natural" amplified sound. During the 30-day trial period, patients are counseled to use the hearing aids equally as a monaural and bilateral fit. The authors want the *patient* to assess whether or not the addition of the second hearing aid proves beneficial. Using this approach, approximately 85% of patients in our practice have decided that the second hearing aid provides significant benefit and decide to keep the second hearing aid. The remaining 15% feel that performance was equal with one hearing aid in either ear in comparison to two. These relatively few patients decide to return one hearing aid for credit. Using a different strategy, the authors found that, if the initial monaural fitting was found to be successful, only 15% of our patients returned to convert their monaural fitting to bilateral. For these reasons, when the audiometric results and case history profile are appropriate, the authors fit bilaterally at the time of the initial fitting.

Hearing Aid Style, Technology, and Signal Processing

The authors counsel the patient on:

a. **Style:** BTE, in-the-ear (ITE), in-the-canal (ITC), and CIC.

b. **Microphone technology:** Omnidirectional, fixed directional, adaptive directional, and automatic adaptive directional. An adaptive directional microphone is designed to apply the most effective polar design automatically depending upon the azimuth of the noise. Thus, a cardioid design will automatically be in place when the noise is directly behind, and a bidirectional polar design will be in place if the noise moves from the back directly to the side. An automatic adaptive directional microphone is similar, with the exception that the microphones will automatically change from directional to omnidirectional when the environment switches from noisy to quiet. Also, when in the directional mode, as described earlier, the microphone is fully adaptive. Thus, an automatic adaptive microphone can provide the greatest convenience to the patient.

c. **Various benefits of digital signal processing (DSP):** *Feedback management, expansion* to reduce/eliminate circuit noise for those patients with normal low-frequency hearing, *noise reduction* for improved comfort in noisy listening situations, and *multiband processing* for greater precision in shaping the frequency gain/output response.

d. **Telephone communication:** Programmable telecoil; wireless Bluetooth communication (Yanz, 2005; Yanz et al., 2005).

e. **HAT:** Our facility has a fully stocked HAT display in two counseling rooms. In these rooms, patients can see and experience the benefits provided by such devices. The HATs displayed in the room include infrared television listening devices, amplified telephones, wireless Bluetooth communication systems, frequency modulated (FM) devices, alarm clocks, etc.

f. When applicable, the authors cover special applications:
   1. Open fittings.
   2. Wireless contralateral routing of signals (CROS)/bilateral CROS (BICROS).
   3. Bone-anchored hearing aid (BAHA) and TransEar for patients with one-sided deafness.

In addition, the authors discuss the various technologies available in the styles discussed in the previous list:

- Conventional analog (linear and nonlinear)
- Programmable analog/single memory (linear and nonlinear)
- Programmable analog/multiple memories (linear and nonlinear)
- Digital/single memory
- Digital/multiple memory
- Remote control and watches

Please note that it is the opinion of the authors that the only hearing aid technology currently available for significantly improving aided performance in noise is dual microphones (Valente et al., 1995; Kochkin, 1996; Lurguin and Rafhay, 1996; Agnew and Block, 1997; Voss, 1997).

For additional information on the various types of hearing aid technologies and signal processing, the reader is referred to Chapter 35.

Counseling Goals

The overall goals of this extensive counseling are three-fold. First, the audiologist must determine a hearing aid fitting that is the most appropriate for the patient in terms of addressing (1) the patient's *goals* (i.e., "hear better in noise," "improved communication on the telephone"), (2) *style* (i.e., BTE, ITE, ITC, CIC), and (3) *technology* (i.e., number of compression channels, feedback management, adaptive directional microphone, expansion, etc.). Second, the authors believe that a well-informed patient will more likely have greater user satisfaction than an uninformed or underinformed patient. Third, the patient needs to feel that he/she has as much a part in the decision in selecting the appropriate hearing aids as the audiologist. The final decision of which

hearing aids to pursue is based on the interaction of such issues as:

a. The magnitude, configuration, and symmetry of the hearing loss.

b. Listener lifestyle and its demands upon communication.

c. The patient's need or demand for the best and/or most convenient signal processing technology to reduce the deleterious effects of background noise. The authors cannot remember a single patient reporting that he/she hears better in "noise" than in "quiet." Therefore, the author's primary goal is to counsel the patient on the available technology that has been proven, via research (not manufacturer brochures and ads), to improve the recognition of speech in noise.

d. Importance of communication on the telephone and the sensitivity of the telecoil.

Unaided Outcome Measure

The authors believe that it is imperative that a comprehensive hearing aid fitting process include some outcome measure assessing the patient's impressions of hearing aid benefit (i.e., the degree of perceived improvement in the aided vs. unaided listening conditions). Numerous self-assessment questionnaires are available for audiologists to consider. These include the Profile of Hearing Aid Performance (Cox and Gilmore, 1990), Communication Profile of Hearing Impairment (Erdman and Demorest, 1990), Hearing Performance Inventory (Giolas et al., 1979), Hearing Handicap Inventory (Newman et al., 1990), Hearing Measure Scale (Noble and Atherley, 1970), Abbreviated Profile of Hearing Aid Benefit (APHAB) (Cox and Alexander, 1995), Hearing Handicap Inventory for the Elderly (Newman et al., 1990; 1991), Glasgow Hearing Aid Benefit Profile (Gatehouse, 1994; 1999), Satisfaction with Amplification in Daily Life (Cox and Alexander, 2001), and COSI (Dillon et al., 1997). Currently, the APHAB and COSI are available on the latest Hearing Instrument Manufacturers' Software Association module (Ingrao, 2005) as well as several manufacturer NOAH modules.

To satisfy the previously mentioned goal of having an outcome measure assess the patient's impressions of hearing aid benefit, initially the authors ask the patient to complete the "unaided" portion of either the COSI or the Washington University Questionnaire. With the COSI, the patient generates as many as five specific expectations (goals) he/she wants the hearing aids to achieve. For example, "hearing better in noise," "hearing better in church," "hearing better on the telephone," or "hearing better while communicating around the dinner table." By being "forced" to focus on *his/her* goals, the counseling can focus on the hearing aid technology that will most likely allow the patient to achieve his/her goals. In addition, the responses allow the clinician to gain further insight into the patient's expectations and, in turn, allow the clinician to determine if these expectations are realistic and attainable. After the patient has had the opportunity to wear the hearing aids for 4 weeks, he/she is asked to check the box on the COSI form that asks, "To what degree has the hearing aids changed your expectations?" The choices are "worse," "no difference," "slightly better," "better," or "much better." In addition, the patient is asked to check the box on the COSI form stating, "If, by using the hearing aids, you can hear satisfactorily: 'hardly ever (10%),' 'occasionally (25%),' 'half the time (50%),' 'most of the time (75%),' or 'almost always (95%).'" The COSI has proven to be a very useful clinical tool because it is easy to use and the goals are set by the patient rather than by the questionnaire.

With the Washington University Questionnaire (Fig. 38.1), the patient is asked to mark (placing a check in a column) the magnitude of difficulty ("always," "often," "sometimes," "rarely," "never," or "not applicable") both unaided ("X" in Fig. 38.1) and with his/her current aids (if experienced user; "O" in Fig. 38.1) for 14 listening situations divided into three areas (difficulty at home, difficulty at work, and difficulty in social situations). After patients have had the opportunity to wear the hearing aids for at least 4 weeks, they are asked to check the column corresponding to their perception of performance of the new aids compared to unaided and, if applicable, to their current hearing aids ("+" in Fig. 38.1). In this manner, the audiologist can quickly see whether these patients perceive the aided performance as being better than either their unaided or current hearing aid performance because the check marks would be placed in columns farther to the right compared with marks for the unaided and/or current aids. The Washington University Questionnaire has proven to be an efficient and useful clinical tool because of it is easy to use for both the patient and audiologist.

Earmold Impressions

Finally, at the end of this second dispensing visit, impressions are made for the purpose of ordering earmolds for BTE fittings or custom products. Figure 38.5 illustrates an important point concerning the benefits of ordering a Libby 3- or 4-mm horn for a BTE fitting. In this case, the first

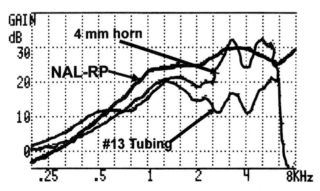

FIGURE 38.5 Difference in measured real-ear insertion gain (REIG) between #13 tubing and 4-mm Libby horn. The wider curve represents the NAL-RP prescriptive target for a 65-dB SPL input level.

author was fitting a patient who arrived at the clinic from another facility with a BTE coupled to the earmold with #13 tubing. Initial real-ear insertion gain (REIG) measures were performed to verify whether the measured REIG reasonably matched the prescribed National Acoustic Laboratories (NAL)-revised for profound hearing loss (RP) (solid curve) target. The initial REIG (lower curve) with the #13 tubing revealed that the measured REIG was significantly below the prescribed NAL-RP. Rather than attach the hearing aid to the programmer to increase the gain to match the target, it was decided to remove the #13 tubing and drill the bore to make it wider to accept the wider outside diameter of the 4-mm horn. A repeat REIG with the 4-mm horn (upper curve in Fig. 38.5) clearly indicates that the REIG with the 4-mm horn arrives much closer to the prescribed REIG than was possible with the #13 tubing! More importantly, the amplifier in the hearing aid was not programmed to achieve the greater required gain (i.e., maintained greater headroom). This leaves the amplifier available for future increases in gain should the patient's hearing loss decrease. In addition, by not programming the amplifier to provide greater amplification, there was probably less distortion at the output of the hearing aid, and the amplified sound was crisper. Thus, it is the strong belief of the authors that almost all patients should be fit with a 3- or 4-mm horn unless the hearing loss is of a rising configuration. In our clinics, virtually all of our patients are fit with a 3- or 4-mm horn! Also, the authors order earmolds and custom products with a select-a-vent (SAV) to provide greater flexibility for controlling the low-frequency response to reduce or eliminate the occlusion effect and maintain some control over feedback.

One of the most significant advances in earmold technology has been the manner in which impressions for earmolds *and* custom products are being processed after the impression has been made. In the past, the impression was placed in a box with the order form and forwarded to the hearing aid manufacturer or earmold laboratory (where a cast of the impression was made to create the end product). This process is still done but with one major change. Advances in computer and software technology allow the manufacturer to scan the impression and store it in its computer (Lesiecki, 2006). The scanned impression is then modeled, and decisions are made by the software for deriving the final product. Initially, scanning technology was only available by the leading hearing aid manufacturers (GNRe-Sound, Siemens, Phonak, Oticon, Widex, and Starkey) for the purpose of modeling custom products. In fact, one manufacturer (Siemens) recently introduced technology allowing the audiologist to scan an impression in the clinic and download the scanned image to the manufacturer via the Internet. Now, several earmold laboratories provide similar technology. One of the obvious advantages to this method is that it is no longer necessary to remake impressions when there is a problem with the initial impression. The remake can be manufactured from the scanned image. The day is not far off when this method of scanning will be replaced by the ability of audiologists to directly scan the ear and ear canal and send the scanned image over the Internet. In addition, the concerns and issues of placing oto-dams and impression material into the ear canal will become a thing of the past.

COUPLER MEASURES (BETWEEN THE SECOND AND THIRD VISIT)

ANSI-2003

When the hearing aids arrive from the manufacturer, they are placed on an HA-1 or HA-2 coupler, and their performance is compared to the ANSI S3.22-2003 (ANSI, 2003) (Fig. 38.6) measures supplied by the manufacturer. The performance of the hearing aids must adhere to the specifications provided by the manufacturer, and harmonic distortion must be less than 10% (Valente and Van Vliet, 1997). See Chapter 36 for a detailed discussion of ANSI S3.22-2003.

In addition to measuring the performance of the hearing aids with regards to ANSI S3.22-2003, the authors also evaluate the "smoothness" of the frequency-gain response to input levels of 50 or 60 dB up to 80 or 90 dB SPL in 10-dB steps (ANSI S3.42-1992; ANSI, 1992). Figure 38.7 illustrates the frequency-gain response of one hearing aid measured for input levels of 50 dB (upper curve) to 90 dB SPL

(lower curve) in 10-dB steps. Notice how the "smoothness" of the frequency-gain response for the 90-dB SPL input is the same as the "smoothness" of the frequency-gain response for the 50-dB SPL input. On the other hand, if the hearing aid yielded significant intermodulation distortion, then it would be expected that the frequency-gain response obtained with the 80- to 90-dB input (lower curves) would be "irregular" or quite "jagged" when compared to the frequency-gain responses at 50 to 70 dB SPL.

It is important for audiologists to be sure that the "morphology" or "smoothness" of the frequency-gain response remains the same for an input level of 80 to 90 dB SPL as it is for an input level of 50 to 60 dB SPL. Revit (1994) reports that the appearance of a "jagged" frequency-gain response at higher input levels is an indication of the presence of intermodulation distortion, which, in turn, can result in reduced recognition of speech. The authors feel that clinicians should return any hearing aids to the manufacturer for which a jagged frequency-gain response is obtained. It would also be wise to forward a copy of the coupler printout verifying the presence of the jagged frequency-gain response.

Special Tests

Since the last edition, there has been a significant increase in the number of hearing aids with multichannel DSP. As

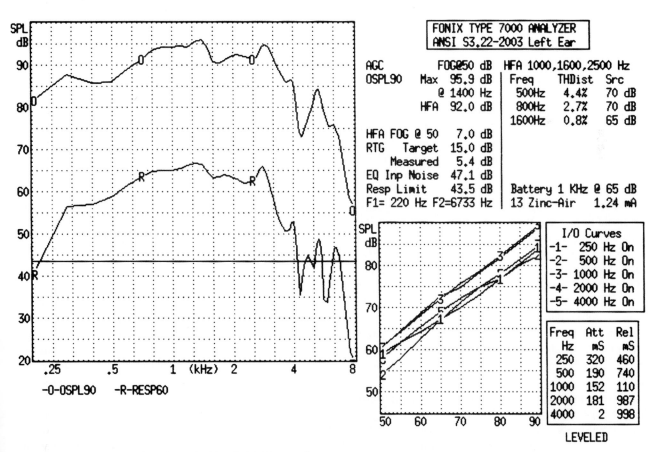

FIGURE 38.6   Example of ANSI S3.22-2003 coupler measure.

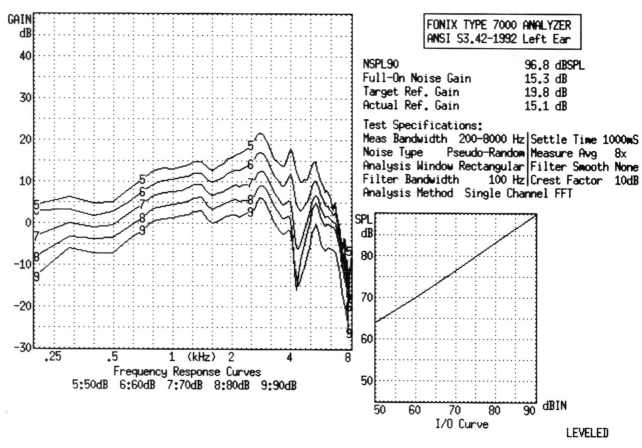

FIGURE 38.7 Example of ANSI S3.42-1992 coupler measure.

indicated earlier, there are many significant advantages provided by DSP when compared to analog signal processing. However, one potential disadvantage in increasing the number of signal processing channels is group delay. Processing time or group delay is defined as the finite time delay created as an input signal passes through a hearing aid from the microphone to the receiver (Agnew and Thornton, 2000). The group delay in digital hearing aids is considerably longer in comparison to analog hearing aids due to the complex conversion of the input sound signal into discrete quantities for signal processing. While the time required for a single-channel analog hearing aid to process input signals is a few tenths of a millisecond (ms), the time needed for DSP can vary widely depending on the DSP algorithm and number of processing channels. In general, the greater the degree of processing, the longer the processing time or "group" delay is (Frye, 2001). One major concern is the possibility of an unprocessed signal passing through a vent or leak around the earmold or shell and being heard earlier than the processed signal that is delayed due to the delay created by the hearing aid.

Previous research has demonstrated that long group delay can negatively affect speech recognition and perception for normal-hearing and hearing-impaired patients (Summerfield, 1992; Stone and Moore, 1999; 2000; 2005; Agnew and Thornton, 2000). Specifically, concerns of auditory confusion (Summerfield, 1992) and degradation of speech production and perception of subject's own voice (Stone and Moore, 1999; 2002; 2005; Agnew and Thornton, 2000) as a result of delay have been investigated.

Auditory confusion can occur when there is a delay between the hearing aid user observing the movement of the talker's lips and hearing the sound of the talker's voice. Summerfield (1992) reported that sound can lag the visual image by up to 80 ms before confusion will occur. Therefore, he recommended that processing for hearing aid users with severe to profound hearing loss be as short as possible, but group delays as long as 40 ms would be acceptable.

Stone and Moore (1999) reported on the effect of group delay on subjects' own speech productions and perceptions of their own voice for normal-hearing populations using a simulation of hearing loss. They reported that delays greater than 20 ms can lead to the perception of an "echo" in the subject's own voice, whereas delays less than 10 ms might lead to a perception of a subtle change in the timbre of the sound. In a follow-up study, Stone and Moore (2005) used hearing-impaired subjects to measure the effect of group delays (13 to 40 ms) on perception of the subjects' own voice and speech production. It was concluded that subjects' disturbance to their own voice increased with increasing group delay. Additionally, subjects with low-frequency (500, 1,000, and 2,000 Hz) hearing loss greater than 50 dB HL were significantly less disturbed than those subjects with less low-frequency hearing loss. They found that delays greater than 15 ms can be unacceptable to listeners with low-frequency hearing loss of approximately 35 dB HL, but listeners with more moderate to severe hearing loss in the low frequencies may be able to tolerate longer delays.

Stone and Moore (2002) also analyzed objective and subjective measures of the effects of hearing aid delay on speech production and perception in two different environments in order to define an upper limit to permissible processing delay. They concluded that normal-hearing subjects reported that the disturbing effects on perception became significant when delays exceeded 15 ms in an office environment and 20 ms in a test booth. Objective measures of speech production did not show any significant negative effects of delay until the delay reached 30 ms. As a result of these findings, Stone and Moore (2002) recommended that DSP hearing aids should be able to incorporate delays as long as 15 ms with few negative side effects. Additionally, the amount of tolerable processing delay decreased by about 5 ms in reverberant environments as compared to a near-anechoic environment.

Agnew and Thornton (2000) investigated the amounts of delay that were just noticeable and considered objectionable in 18 normal-hearing engineers to determine a worse-case limit for DSP hearing aid design. The listeners in this study reported that time delays greater than 10 ms were objectionable 90% of the time, which is a significantly shorter time delay than what was published by Stone and Moore (1999; 2005).

New Electroacoustic Procedures for Assessing Digital Signal Processing Features

Although not included as part of ANSI S3.22-2003, several tests are now available to verify several DSP features. Frye (2001) presents information on two tests that are included in the Frye equipment. These include measures of group delay and phase. Other measures (Frye, 2000) are modulated ANSI or International Collegium of Rehabilitative Audiology (ICRA) signals to assess the compression characteristics of the hearing aid and a bias signal to assess the effectiveness of the noise reduction (NR) algorithm.

Group Delay and Phase

In the Frye units, the group delay test uses a simple broadband impulse signal and a 20-ms time window. The measured group delay is calculated from the sampling rate (25.6 kHz), the internal analyzer delay (approximately 0.5 ms), and the characteristics from the hearing aid. Figure 38.8

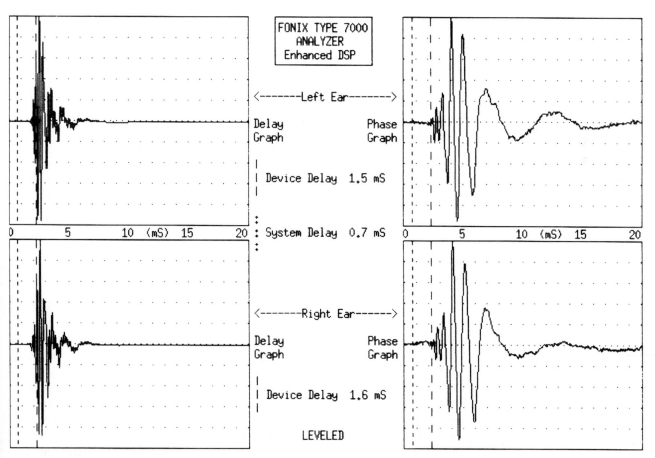

FIGURE 38.8 Example of measurement of group delay and phase for left and right hearing aids using the Frye 7000.

illustrates the group delay (curve to the left) for the left (1.5 ms) and right (1.6 ms) hearing aids as well as the phase (curves to the right) for each hearing aid. For reasons described earlier, ideally, the audiologist would hope to record a value of ≤15 ms. Also, this simple test can inform the audiologist if the hearing aid is analog or digital. If, when completing the test, the group delay is ≤1 ms, then the aid is probably analog. If, on the other hand, the group delay is ≥1 ms, then the hearing aid is probably digital.

As for phase, the Frye unit generates a 1,000-Hz cosine wave and turns it into a test signal by delivering this signal to the hearing aid. This wave is offset at the time of generation so that it starts at the baseline or "zero point." The signal then continues through a complete cycle and stops when the signal reaches baseline again. The data from this signal are displayed in graphical form 20 ms wide (Frye 7000 manual). The measure of phase is important only in bilateral fits, whether or not the signal processing is analog or digital. For the phase measures, the audiologist would like to see that the two curves on the right in Figure 38.8, in essence, superimpose each other if placed on top of each other. That is, when there is an upper deflection in the upper curve, then the same upward deflection should also be occurring in the

lower graph (other hearing aid). Also, when the upper curve is moving downward, the same should also be occurring in the lower graph. This indicates that the wiring of the receivers from the amplifiers for the two hearing aids is matched and the aids are "in-phase." Fitting hearing aids that are mismatched or "out-of-phase" can reduce the stereo effect and degrade sound quality.

Modulated Speech Signal

DSP hearing aids often react to a continuous speech signal as if it were noise and reduce gain/output. This can pose problems when trying to assess hearing aid gain characteristics. To resolve this problem, some manufacturers have developed *modulated* speech signals so the DSP processes the signal as speech and not reduce gain. With the Frye units, the usually continuous composite speech signal can be also be presented as a randomly amplitude-modulated speech signal in bursts 300 ms wide. To verify that the noise suppression (compression) feature of a DSP aid is operating correctly, a simple test is to examine the performance using the conventional continuous composite ANSI signal and then take a second measure with the modulated ANSI signal (Fig. 38.9). The

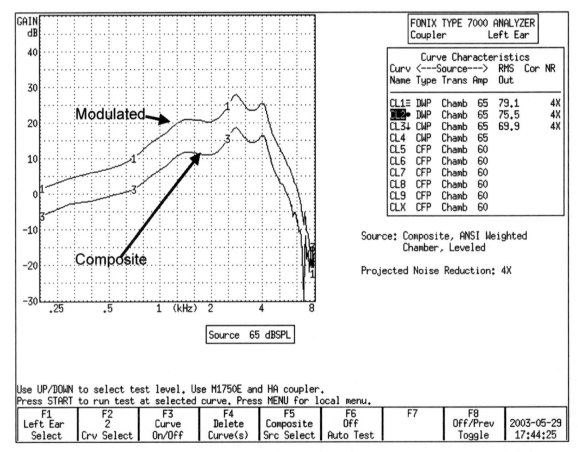

FIGURE 38.9 Example of the differences in measured coupler gain using a continuous American National Standards Institute (ANSI) composite signal (*lower curve*) and a modulated ANSI signal (*upper curve*) illustrating the compression of a digital signal processing (DSP) hearing aid.

difference between the two measures (typically the measure for the continuous signal will be lower than the measure for the modulated signal) reflects the amount of overall noise suppression provided by the hearing aid to a broadband noise. If the two curves are superimposed, it is a good indication that the noise suppression feature has been disabled or is not functioning properly or the hearing aid does not contain noise suppression. It is important to remember that significant differences may be present in the noise suppression feature between manufacturers. It is also possible that manipulation of the input level may be required to activate the noise suppression, or the audiologist may need to wait a few seconds before the noise suppression becomes active.

Several real-ear analyzers give audiologists the option of using various "speech-like" signals. With the Frye units, the audiologist has the option of using an ANSI (ANSI S3.42-1992) or ICRA speech signal. The spectrum of these two signals is quite different (Fig. 38.10). The ANSI signal decreases at a rate of 6 dB/octave above 900 Hz, while the ICRA signal is flat to about 500 Hz and then decreases more sharply at a rate of 10 dB/octave above 500 Hz. Below 900 Hz, ICRA is 3 dB more intense than ANSI, but above 900 Hz, ICRA rolls off more steeply than ANSI so that, at 2,000 Hz, ICRA is 8 dB less intense than ANSI and, by 8,000 Hz, ICRA is 16 dB less intense than ANSI. This means it is possible to measure significantly different gain and output values depending on the signal processing of the hearing aid. If the hearing aid has a low compression kneepoint in the high frequencies, it is likely that the measured gain/output using the ICRA signal will be considerably greater than if the ANSI spectrum was used (middle and upper curves in Fig. 38.11). The lower curve in Figure 38.11 is the response of the hearing aid to a continuous composite speech signal. This curve shows the least amount of gain because the hearing aid is processing this signal as noise.

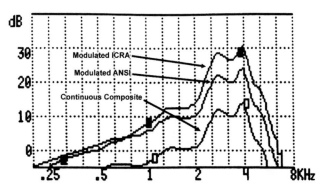

FIGURE 38.11 Difference in measured real-ear insertion gain (REIG) for a digital signal processing (DSP) hearing aid using continuous American National Standards Institute (ANSI) composite (*lower curve*), modulated ANSI (*middle curve*), and International Collegium of Rehabilitative Audiology (ICRA; *upper curve*) signals. (From Frye G. [2000] Testing digital hearing instruments: the basics. *Hear Rev.* 9, 20, 22, 24, 26–27.)

Bias Signal

To help audiologists verify the effectiveness of NR filters of a DSP hearing aid, Frye Electronics introduced a "bias signal" test. With this test, a randomly modulated speech spectrum signal (the audiologist can control the overall level of the speech signal) and a randomly modulated puretone signal are presented simultaneously (the audiologist can control the frequency and intensity of the bias signal). With this test, if the NR filter is functioning properly, the audiologist will see a reduction in gain/output in the frequency region surrounding the bias puretone signal, but the remaining portion of the frequency response above and below the bias signal will maintain full amplification. For example, in Figure 38.12, a

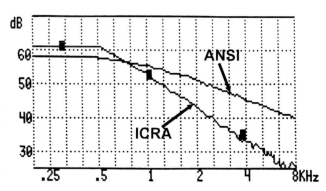

FIGURE 38.10 Difference in spectrum between the American National Standards Institute (ANSI) and International Collegium of Rehabilitative Audiology (ICRA) speech signals used in the Frye 6500 and 7000. (From Frye G. [2000] Testing digital hearing instruments: the basics. *Hear Rev.* 9, 20, 22, 24, 26–27.)

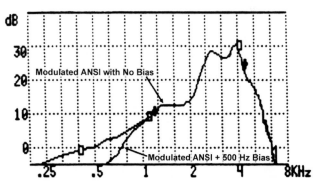

FIGURE 38.12 Illustration of the effectiveness of the noise reduction feature of a digital signal processing (DSP) hearing aid around 500 Hz using a 500-Hz bias signal plus modulated speech (*lower curve*) and modulated American National Standards Institute (ANSI) signal alone (*upper curve*). (From Frye G. [2000] Testing digital hearing instruments: the basics. *Hear Rev.* 9, 20, 22, 24, 26–27.)

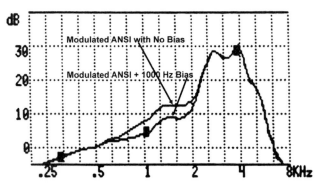

FIGURE 38.13   Illustration of the effectiveness of the noise reduction feature of a digital signal processing (DSP) hearing aid around 1,000 Hz using a 1,000-Hz bias signal plus modulated speech (*lower curve*) and modulated American National Standards Institute (ANSI) signal alone (*upper curve*). (From Frye G. [2000] Testing digital hearing instruments: the basics. *Hear Rev.* 9, 20, 22, 24, 26–27.)

500-Hz bias signal is presented with modulated ANSI speech. As can be seen, only the frequency region around 500 Hz reveals attenuation, whereas the frequency above approximately 500 Hz shows full amplification. Figures 38.13 and 38.14 illustrate the same point using a 1,000-Hz and 4,000-Hz bias signal, respectively. Note the mid-frequency attenuation in Figure 38.13, with full amplification above and below the mid-frequency region, and the high-frequency attenuation in Figure 38.14, with full amplification in the low- and mid-frequency regions. With this test, the more channels the DSP aid has, the narrower the frequency region is in which the reduction of gain/output occurs. On the other hand, in a hearing aid with fewer channels, the reduction

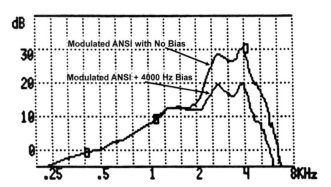

FIGURE 38.14   Illustration of the effectiveness of the noise reduction feature of a digital signal processing (DSP) hearing aid around 4,000 Hz using a 4,000-Hz bias signal plus modulated speech (*lower curve*) and modulated American National Standards Institute (ANSI) signal alone (*upper curve*). (From Frye G. [2000] Testing digital hearing instruments: the basics. *Hear Rev.* 9, 20, 22, 24, 26–27.)

in gain/output is broader. One must remember that, when there is a reduction of gain/output in response to a noise, there is also a reduction of gain/output in the same region of the speech signal. Thus, it can be assumed that a hearing aid with a greater number of channels may provide greater speech intelligibility/comfort in noise because a narrower slice of the speech signal is being reduced in response to the NR feature of the hearing aid.

▧ HEARING AID FITTING (THIRD VISIT)

Real-Ear Measures

The most reliable and efficient method for assessing the performance provided by amplification is real-ear measures. Research reports that the 95% confidence interval (CI) for repeatability of real-ear measures is approximately 3 dB (Valente et al., 1990; 1991). By comparison, the 95% CI for functional gain measures (i.e., unaided sound field puretone or spondee thresholds *minus* aided sound field puretone or spondee thresholds) is approximately 15 dB (Hawkins et al., 1987). If the audiologist were to incorporate a modification to a hearing aid (i.e., changes the vent size or tubing diameter; changes the damper in the ear hook; rotates a potentiometer or reprograms the aid), the difference between the gain measured *after* the change would have to be at least 3 dB different than the first real-ear measure in order for the difference to be considered statistically significant. Because of the greater variability inherent in functional gain measures, however, the difference between the second and first measure would have to be greater than 15 dB for the results to be statistically significant. One can readily see that real-ear measures are considerably more reliable than functional gain measures, and consequently, it is highly recommended that real-ear measures be used consistently instead of functional gain measures.

Typically, at least three real-ear measures are obtained clinically. The first involves the measurement of the response of the ear canal without the hearing aid in place. This is referred to as the real-ear unaided gain (REUG) and is an accurate and reliable measure of the resonance of the ear canal (lower curve in Fig. 38.15). To make this measure, the patient is seated in a chair directly facing a loudspeaker (i.e., 0° azimuth) that is placed at ear level (~45 inches from the ground) at a distance of 12 to 18 inches. The probe tube from the probe microphone is marked 30 mm from the tip for adult males and 26 mm for adult females. This mark is placed at the intratragal notch and taped in place. A short burst of a speech-weighted composite noise is presented at a level of 65 dB SPL and stored as the unaided response (lower line in Fig. 38.15). This measure represents the ear canal resonance. In the normal adult ear, the REUG has a peak amplitude of approximately 18 dB at 2,800 Hz (Valente et al., 1991).

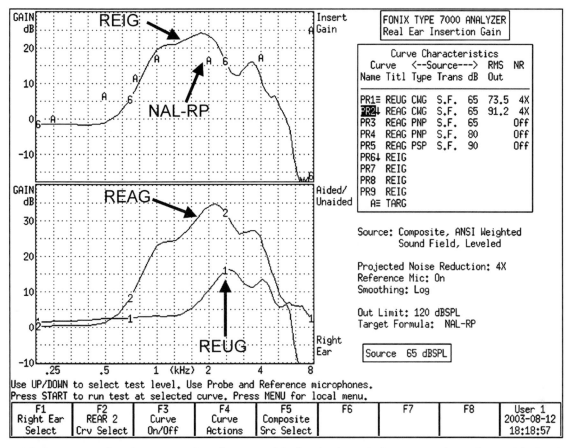

FIGURE 38.15   Example of measured real-ear unaided gain (REUG; *lower curve*), real-ear aided gain (REAG; *middle curve*), and real-ear insertion gain (REIG; *upper curve*) for a linear hearing aid to the NAL-RP ("A") prescriptive target using the Frye 7000.

Next, the hearing aid shell, or earmold coupled to a BTE, is placed in the ear canal, and the volume control is typically adjusted to the patient's most comfortable level. The resulting measure is the real-ear aided gain (REAG) provided by the hearing aid (middle curve in Fig. 38.15). The difference between the REAG and REUG is the REIG (upper curve in Fig. 38.15), or the gain provided by the hearing aid. The REIG is compared with the prescribed target ("A" in Fig. 38.15) to determine if the measured frequency-gain response is appropriate for the hearing loss.

To obtain the target REIG, the patient's audiometric data are entered into a real-ear analyzer to generate a "target" REIG ("A" in Fig. 38.15) to which the measured REIG is compared. For the hearing loss illustrated in Figure 38.15, most audiologists would agree that the measured REIG closely matches the prescribed NAL-Revised (R) (Byrne and Dillon, 1986) target.

Verification using a single input level, as illustrated in Figure 38.15, would be appropriate if the hearing aid has linear signal processing because gain remains constant and measuring gain and several input levels would provide little additional information. If, on the other hand, the hearing aid has nonlinear signal processing, then verifying gain should be done using several input levels. Figure 38.16 illustrates the

verification of a hearing aid with nonlinear signal processing where it is easy to see that the measured gain is greatest for the 50-dB input level and gain decreases as the input level increases from 50 to 90 dB SPL.

Measuring the Real-Ear Aided Response (dB SPL) to the Dynamic Range (dB SPL)

Since the previous edition was published, there has been a significant increase in the number of audiologists selecting to verify where the amplified output (real-ear aided response [REAR] in dB SPL measured near the eardrum) resides within the individual dynamic range (DR). Thus, using this method, the "prescriptive target" is the individual DR, and the purpose is to verify where the amplified output, in response to a wide range of input levels, falls within the DR.

Figure 38.17 illustrates how this is accomplished using the Frye 7000. In this figure, "T" represents threshold in dB SPL; "L" is the target for an input of 50 dB SPL; "M" is the target for an input of 65 dB SPL; "H" is the target for 80 dB SPL; and "U" represents the LDL. The space between "T" and "U" is the DR. Here the reader can see that the REAR for an input of 50 dB is very close to the "L" target for most of the frequency range. The REAR for the 65 dB input ("#3")

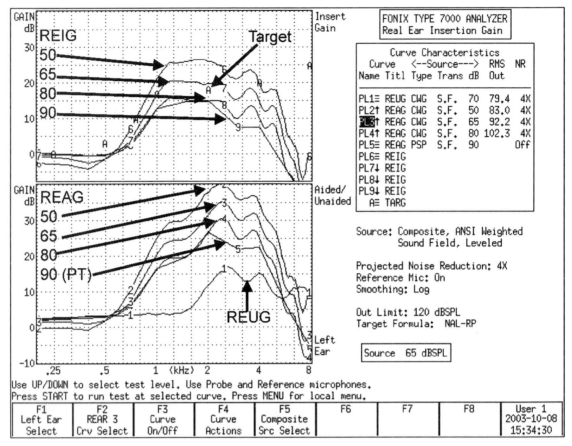

FIGURE 38.16   Example of real-ear unaided gain (REUG), real-ear aided gain
(REAG)50,65,80, and 90 (puretonesweep), **and real-ear insertion gain (REIG)**50,65,80, and 90 (puretonesweep) **for a nonlinear hearing aid to the NAL-RP ("A") prescriptive target using the Frye 7000. Shortly, Frye will introduce the NAL-NL1 prescriptive targets to the software. When this occurs, there will be separate targets for input levels of 50, 65, and 80 dB as well as the 90-dB puretone sweep.**

is at or near the "M" target. The REAR for the 80 dB input ("#4") is at or near the "H" target, and the REAR for the 90 dB SPL input is at or below the "U" target.

Figure 38.18 illustrates similar information using the MedRx Live-Speech Mapping unit. In this figure, the lower "O" line represents threshold, and the upper "U" line represents LDL. The lower curve is the REAR to an input of 56 dB SPL using live speech (e.g., spouse talking to the patient using a microphone in combination with the software), and the measured REAR is above the "O" target, indicating that soft speech is audible. The middle curve is the REAR in response to an input of 67 dB SPL using the same stimuli and method, whereas the upper curve is the REAR in response to an input of 89 dB SPL. Again, it can be verified that the REAR to the input range of 33 dB (56 to 89 dB) falls within the DR. Recently (Poe and Ross, 2005), MedRx released a unit that has been reduced in size to slightly larger than a cell phone.

Finally, Figure 38.19 illustrates similar information using the Audioscan Verifit system. In this example, the "X" and "O" in the left and right boxes represent threshold for the right and left ears, respectively; the "*" represents the

LDL; and the "+" represents the REAR target for an input of 65 dB SPL.

Although significant differences exist between these instruments, their commonality is in allowing the audiologist to measure how the output of the hearing aid lies within the DR range (measured in dB SPL near the eardrum) of the patient. These units allow audiologists to verify that the measured output to an input level of 50 dB SPL is above threshold; the measured output to an input level of 65 dB SPL falls approximately midway between threshold and LDL, and the measured output to a high input level (85 to 90 dB SPL) is below the LDL.

From the authors' perspective, one problem associated with these devices is the reliance upon predicted threshold (dB SPL) and LDL (dB SPL) based on the entered audiogram. For these units, after the audiologist enters the audiogram, the respective unit converts the entered thresholds (dB HL) into threshold in dB SPL by using *average* REDD transformations of dB HL to dB SPL. In addition, the software within these units will predict the LDL in dB HL based on the data published by Pascoe (1988) and then transform these into dB SPL using average REDDs. Unfortunately, research has

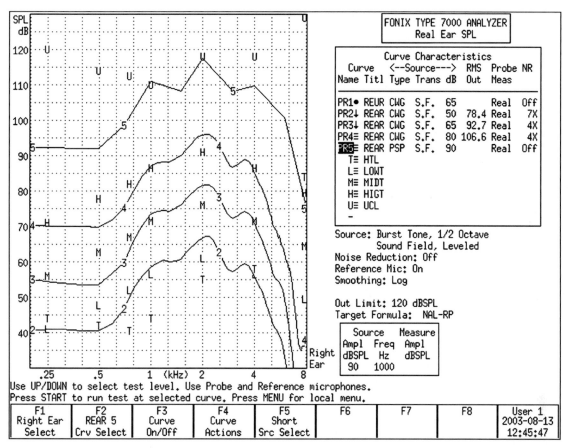

FIGURE 38.17 Example of real-ear aided response (REAR) measures for a nonlinear hearing aid using the Frye 7000. In this case, the "T" represents the predicted threshold in dB SPL, and "U" represents the predicted loudness discomfort level (LDL) in dB SPL. The area between the "T" and "U" is the residual dynamic range. The "L," "M," and "H" represent the targets for soft, average, and loud input levels, respectively. The 2, 3, and 4 curves represent the measured REAR for input levels of 50, 65, and 80 dB SPL, respectively.

shown that the intersubject variability of the combined factors of REDD and LDL can be up to 40 dB wide (Pascoe, 1988; Valente et al., 1994; 1997; Bentler and Cooley, 2001; Mueller and Hornsby, 2002). With such variability, it would be difficult to imagine, with any degree of confidence, that the *predicted* threshold and LDL in dB SPL would be the same as *individually measured* thresholds and/or LDLs. The major point being made here is that, if the advantage of these devices is that the "target" is the *patient's* DR and these units can report how the hearing aid output fits within that DR, then it would seem appropriate that the DR appearing on the monitor of these units should reflect the DR of the individual and not the DR of an average individual.

Figures 38.20 and 38.21 illustrate how this could be a potential problem. Figure 38.20 reports the *measured* hearing thresholds and LDLs in dB HL for the right ear of a patient. The LDLs are the same as those appearing in Figure 38.3 at 500 to 4,000 Hz. These audiometric thresholds were entered into the software of one commercially available real-ear system. From these entered thresholds, the software predicted thresholds in dB SPL by adding the average REDD. The

result is the "predicted threshold" illustrated in Figure 38.21. The "measured threshold" is the result of adding the patient's measured REDD (values in parentheses in Fig. 38.3). As can be seen, in this case, there was very little difference between "measured" and "predicted" threshold (dB SPL). The upper curve in Figure 38.21 is the "predicted LDL" that was calculated by the software of the real-ear system predicting the LDL in dB HL from the entered threshold of the patient based on the results of Pascoe (1988) and adding the average REDD. The lower-upper curve in Figure 38.21 is the "measured LDL" that was measured at the time of the HAE, as described earlier and reported in the table in Figure 38.3. As the reader might recall, the LDL measured by Pascoe (1988) was based on a loudness judgment of "too loud," whereas the loudness judgment for the measured LDL was "loud, but okay." In addition, the measured LDL uses measured REDD and not predicted REDD. As a result, even though the measured and predicted thresholds are quite similar, the differences between measured and predicted LDL are quite large. In turn, this results in a significant difference in DR between the measured and predicted curves; that is, the

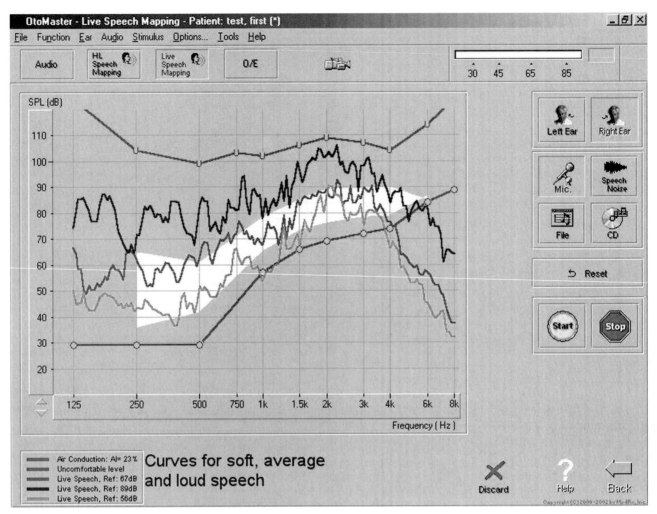

FIGURE 38.18 Example of real-ear aided response (REAR) measures for a nonlinear hearing aid using the MedRx. (Permission provided by MedRx.)

predicted DR is significantly wider than the measured DR. This can have a significant impact on the selection and programming of the compression and output limiting characteristics of the hearing aid. In addition, if the audiologist used the predicted LDL to determine where to place the RESR_90, then it can easily be seen how this patient would probably find the output of the hearing aid to be excessively loud and possibly lead to rejection of amplification.

SELECTION OF PRESCRIPTIVE FORMULAE

Prescriptive "Targets" for Linear Amplification

If the hearing aids provide linear amplification (i.e., constant gain for varying input levels), the authors determine whether the measured REIG "matches" the prescribed REIG by presenting an input signal level of 65 or 70 dB SPL (i.e., $REIG_{65-70}$). Figure 38.15 illustrates the measured $REIG_{65}$

(thin curve) in relation to the prescribed NAL-R REIG target ("A" in Fig. 38.15). Notice how well the measured $REIG_{65}$ compares to the prescribed target curve. If this goal is accomplished, the authors are reasonably assured that adequate amplification has been provided to allow average conversational speech, in a quiet environment, to be audible and comfortably loud. Please note that the authors are not overly concerned if the measured $REIG_{65-70}$ does not "hit" the prescribed REIG at each frequency but are more concerned about whether the "*shape*" of the measured $REIG_{65-70}$ "matches" the "*shape*" of the prescribed REIG. This is because the user has the ability to adjust the overall gain with the gain control.

In 1990, NAL-R (Byrne et al., 1990) was modified (NAL-RP) to provide greater gain for patients with severe to profound hearing loss (i.e., thresholds >60 dB HL). In the NAL-RP formula, when the hearing loss at 2,000 Hz is 95 dB or greater, greater gain is prescribed in the lower frequencies and less gain is prescribed in the high frequencies. Each of these formulae prescribe "use" gain (i.e., the amount of gain provided when the volume control is rotated to the point that

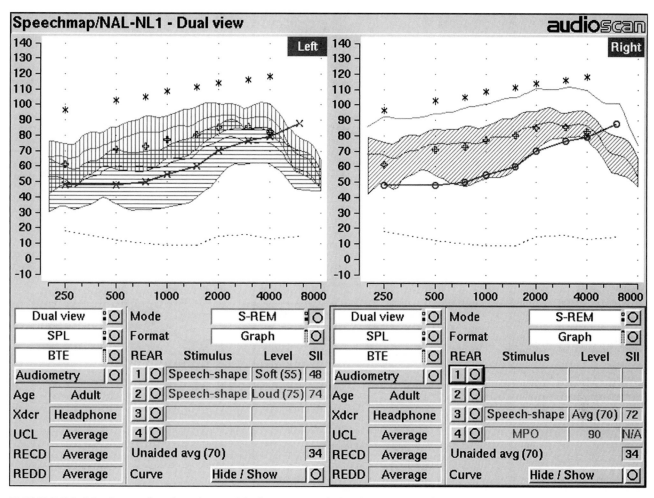

FIGURE 38.19   Example of real-ear aided response (REAR) measures for a nonlinear hearing aid using the AudioScan Verifit system. (Permission provided by Etymotic Research.)

amplification is comfortably loud). For example, to allow for variation in the volume control setting and for changes in hearing, prescription of gain/output (POGO) (McCandless and Lyregaard, 1983) assumes a reserve gain of 10 dB (i.e., rotation of the volume control from the use position to maximum rotation will provide 10 dB of additional gain), whereas NAL-RP assumes 15-dB reserve gain.

The most popular prescriptive "target" for linear aids appears to be the NAL-R (Byrne and Dillon, 1986), NAL-Nonlinear Version 1 (NL1) (Dillon, 1999), and Desired Sensation Level Multistate Input/Output (DSL [i/o]) (Cornelisse et al., 1995; Seewald et al., 1997). The NAL-R "target," however, is most appropriate for patients with mild to moderately severe hearing losses. If the magnitude of the hearing loss is greater than this, the audiologist is advised to select an alternative and more appropriate target (e.g., NAL-RP). Alternative prescriptive targets for linear aids include the POGO (McCandless and Lyregaard, 1983), POGO II (Schwartz et al., 1988), Libby 1/3-2/3 (Libby, 1986), Berger (Berger et al, 1989), or NAL-RP (Byrne et al., 1990). In addition, any selected target is often modified at our facilities for two reasons. First, if the patient has a conductive or mixed hearing

loss, the targeted gain is *increased* by 20% to 25% of the air-bone gap at the respective frequencies (Lybarger, 1944; Byrne and Dillon, 1986; Goebel et al., 2002). Second, when the hearing aid fitting is bilateral, we *decrease* the targeted gain for each ear by approximately 3 to 5 dB to compensate for binaural loudness summation. This is done because prescriptive formulas are based on a monaural fitting and patients often report binaural aided performance as too loud when the electroacoustic characteristics of the hearing aids are adjusted monaurally to match the prescribed REIG.

Prescriptive "Targets" for Nonlinear Amplification

INTRODUCTION

Typically, most hearing aids that have recently entered the commercial market use nonlinear signal processing (i.e., greater gain for low-input levels and less gain for high-input levels). Audiologists can also now program crossover frequencies, compression threshold(s), compression ratio(s), and time constants in one or more channels (bands) (see Chapter 35 for in-depth discussion of these parameters). As a

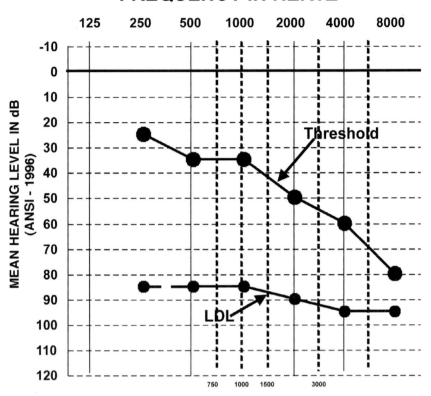

FIGURE 38.20 Measured threshold and loudness discomfort level (LDL; in dB HL) for a patient.

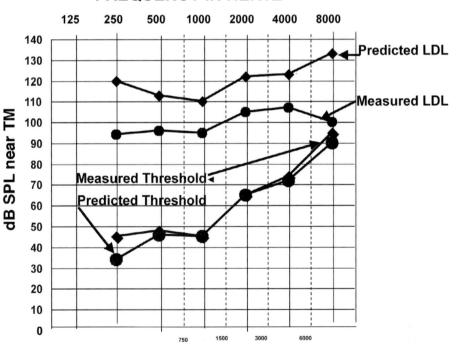

FIGURE 38.21 Measured and predicted threshold and loudness discomfort level (LDL; in dB SPL) for the same patient.

result, prescriptive procedures designed for linear signal processing (i.e., gain remains constant as input level changes) are no longer appropriate. To address this need, several prescriptive procedures for nonlinear signal processing have been recently introduced.

One approach incorporated into many of the new prescriptive procedures is to recreate the normal loudness patterns of speech and other complex sounds for the hearing-impaired listener (i.e., "normalization" approach) (Byrne, 1996). This approach is the major fitting goal of hearing aids using wide dynamic range compression (WDRC). Clearly, it may be difficult to normalize loudness patterns for complex sounds (i.e., speech) because abnormal loudness growth functions vary not only as a function of frequency, but also as a function of signal duration. An example of the new procedures using this approach includes DSL [i/o] (Seewald et al., 1997) for *variable* compression ratio circuit types.

Some argue that the normalization approach may not maximize speech intelligibility when compared to procedures whose fitting goal is to assure that all the frequency bands of speech are amplified to be equally loud at the most comfortable loudness level (i.e., "equalization" approach) (Byrne, 1996). Examples of the new procedures using this approach include NAL-NL1 (Dillon, 1999) and DSL [i/o] for *fixed* compression ratio circuit types.

In this section of the chapter, the authors provide a brief overview of the two procedures (DSL [i/o] and NAL-NL1) that are the most widely used to verify the performance of nonlinear hearing aids. The overview of the two procedures will be followed by recent research concerning the validity of these procedures.

DSL [i/o] Version 4.1

DSL [i/o] is a comprehensive software-based program (Cornelisse et al., 1995; Seewald et al., 1997) designed to help audiologists *select* (i.e., provide 2-cm^3 coupler targets for input levels of 20 to 100 dB SPL) and *verify* (i.e., provide REAR and REAG targets for input levels of 20 to 100 dB SPL) the performance of linear and nonlinear hearing aids. The primary goal of DSL [i/o] is to place conversational speech into the patient's most comfortable listening range. The comfortable listening range targets are approximately midway between the subject's threshold of audibility and the predicted (or measured) upper limit of comfort (one standard deviation below LDLs as reported by Pascoe [1988]).

In the DSL [i/o], the audiologist can enter data in dB HL (TDH earphones, insert earphones, or sound field) or real-ear dB SPL. When the audiologist enters data in dB HL, the software transforms the data into real-ear dB SPL by using average transformation data, corrected for age. If the audiologist is not comfortable with using "average" corrections, he/she can measure the individual's REUG, REDD, and the real-ear-to-coupler difference (RECD) and enter these data into the software. The RECD is the difference between the output of a hearing aid (or insert earphone) measured in the

ear canal versus what is measured in a 2-cm^3 coupler. The RECD is affected by individual differences in ear canal volume and eardrum impedance. In the authors' opinion, when fitting programmable devices for *adults*, it is not necessary to measure REUR, REDD, or RECD when using DSL [i/o] because the flexibility inherent within these DSP hearing aids allows the audiologist to "correct" for differences between the individual and "average" due to the ability to fine tune the hearing aids to match a prescriptive target.

Once these data are entered, the software illustrates *the auditory area* between threshold (lower limit) and LDL (upper limit) in dB SPL near the eardrum. Thus, in DSL [i/o], the "target" is the auditory area, in dB SPL, measured near the eardrum. The goal is to select hearing aids and then verify that the measured *output* is:

- Above threshold for a 50-dB SPL input signal,
- Below LDL for a 80- to 90-dB SPL input signal, and
- Between these two targets for a 60- to 70-dB SPL input signal.

The utilization of the DSL [i/o] prescription will become greater when the DSL [i/o] software is incorporated into the equipment used to measure the performance of hearing aids. Currently, DSL [i/o] is available in the AudioScan Verifit unit but is not currently available in the MedRx and some of the Frye units. When this occurs, threshold, LDL, REUR, REDD, and RECD can be entered into the real-ear analyzer and test box (for coupler measures). The software would generate and place on the monitor the targets as well as the other DSL [i/o] screens. All that the audiologist then has to do is simply place the hearing aid in the ear canal. The software would present input levels of 50, 65, 80, and 90 dB SPL to determine how closely the measured REAR matches the prescribed REAR for the nonlinear hearing aid.

NAL-NL1

NAL-NL1 is the most recent attempt to provide a tool to assist audiologists in fitting nonlinear hearing aids more accurately (National Acoustic Laboratories, 1998; Dillon, 1999). This procedure is reportedly based on the principle of providing a frequency-gain response that maximizes speech intelligibility, while keeping the overall loudness of the input signals at a level that is no greater than that perceived by a listener with normal hearing.

To use this program, the audiologist enters the patient's audiometric thresholds. In addition, as with DSL [i/o], the audiologist can enable the software to predict the REUG and RECD, or the audiologist can enter the individual REUG and RECD. After the audiologic data have been entered, the software calculates and displays up to two curves to illustrate various *gain* and/or *output* prescriptive targets from a menu of nine possible choices. For example, the software displays the prescribed REIG and coupler gain for input levels of 50, 65, and 80 dB SPL (the user can select other input levels). Other *gain* curves are the REAG, 2-cm^3 coupler gain, input/output curves, and SPL-O-Gram. Similar curves can be presented in terms of *output.* In addition, the software will calculate and display calculated crossover frequency(s), compression threshold(s), compression ratio(s), and low-level (50 dB input) and high-level (80 dB) gains for single- or multiple-channel hearing aids. In addition, the user can have the software calculate these parameters based on either a speech-weighted or puretone signal. The calculated compression threshold and 50- to 80-dB gains will change depending upon the selected signal (speech-weighted or pure-tone) and display (REIG, REAG, and coupler). All of these are provided so the audiologist can determine whether the measured performance (coupler or real-ear) agrees with the prescribed performance. The audiologist can also observe the prescribed NAL-NL1 targets in comparison to what would have been prescribed using either the NAL-RP or POGO II (Schwartz et al., 1988).

SMOOTHNESS OF REAL-EAR AIDED RESPONSE MEASURES FOR MULTIPLE INPUT LEVELS

Earlier, the authors emphasized the need for hearing aid coupler measures to be as smooth for input levels of 80 to 90 dB SPL as for input levels of 50 to 60 dB SPL. The same goals also need to be achieved for hearing aid performance when actually worn by the patient. At this point, our emphasis shifts to observing the "smoothness" of the REAR at 50 to 90 dB SPL (Fig. 38.16) for the goal of ensuring that the morphology of the REAR$_{90}$ curve is as smooth as the REAR$_{50}$ curve (Valente and Van Vliet, 1997). If the REAR$_{90}$ curve is "jagged," then it has been suggested that the hearing aid is generating an excessive amount of intermodulation distortion (Revit, 1994).

Real-Ear Saturation Response with a 90-dB Input

With the hearing aid still in place and the volume control at the same position, the authors measure the RESR$_{90}$ using a 90-dB puretone sweep (200 to 8,000 Hz) to measure the SPL near the eardrum. At the completion of the sweep, the authors observe whether the measured RESR$_{90}$ is below the LDL measured at the initial evaluation. If it is, then this assures the audiologist that intense environmental sounds should not be perceived as uncomfortably loud (Mueller and Hornsby, 2002; Munro and Patel, 1998). As mentioned earlier, Figure 38.4 illustrates the RESR$_{90}$ in relation to the measured LDL ("dots") at 500 to 4,000 Hz for a patient. Note that, at each test frequency, the measured RESR$_{90}$ (thin line) is below the measured LDL. The dots with an arrow pointing up indicate that the measured LDL$_{spl}$ was greater than 120 dB SPL at that frequency. According to Mueller and Hornsby (2002) and Munro and Patel (1998), if the results reported in Figure 38.4 are achieved, then the audiologist can be reasonably

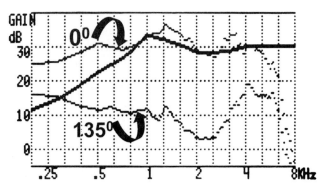

FIGURE 38.22   Using real-ear measures to verify the performance of a hearing aid with a directional microphone.

assured that environmental sounds at high input levels will not be judged as uncomfortable by the patient.

Verification of Performance of Directional Microphones

Figure 38.22 illustrates the use of real-ear measures to verify that the directional microphone is performing correctly. In the author's experience, it is not uncommon to receive new hearing aids where either (1) the functions of the microphones are reversed so that the rear microphone is amplifying and the front microphone is attenuating, or (2) the rear microphone is not working at all, resulting in the hearing aid having only omnidirectional capability. In Figure 38.22, the top curve was measured with the patient facing the real-ear loudspeaker (0°) and the signal (modulated ANSI composite) presented at 65 dB SPL. With the signal remaining on, the patient is slowly rotated so the rear microphone is facing the loudspeaker. As the patient is rotated (making sure the distance between the loudspeaker and the microphone is the same for this measure as it was for the 0° measure), the audiologist views the monitor of the real-ear system to determine the azimuth where there is the least amount of amplification. In Figure 38.22, this occurred at 135° (hypercardioid polar design), showing about a 20- to 25-dB decrease in gain when the rear microphone is facing the loudspeaker in comparison to when the front microphone is facing the loudspeaker. This verifies that the rear microphone is working properly. When the rear microphone is not working, the front and rear measures will superimpose, suggesting no reduction in gain caused by the activation of the rear microphone (omnidirectional performance). When the microphone function is reversed, the 0° curve would be an example of a measure for the rear microphone, and the 135° curve would be an example of a measure for the front microphone.

Verification of the Effectiveness of Feedback Management

Figure 38.23 illustrates how real-ear measures can be used to verify the efficacy of the feedback manager of a commercially

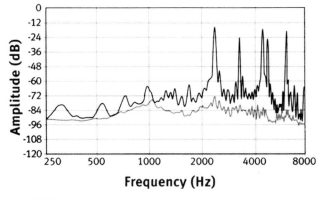

FIGURE 38.23 Using real-ear measures to verify the feedback management feature of a digital signal processing (DSP) hearing aid. (Permission provided by MedRx.)

available DSP hearing aid. The upper curve clearly illustrates the presence of feedback in the output signal as illustrated by the five major peaks in the 2,500- to 6,000-Hz region. After this measure was made, a feedback test was implemented, and the real-ear measure was repeated. The lower curve illustrates the output of the hearing aid after the feedback test was completed. Clearly, the feedback manager of this hearing aid effectively eliminated the feedback because the lower curve does not include the peaks seen in the upper curve.

Loudness Judgments for Speech

In the previous section, the authors described a method to validate that a frequency-specific signal (puretone sweep), presented at a high input level (90 dB SPL), was not uncomfortable to the patient. However, in the "real world," the listener is often exposed to varying levels of speech that have much broader bandwidths than frequency-specific stimuli. Therefore, it is important to include in the protocol a method to assess loudness judgments for a "speech-like" signal (Valente and Van Vliet, 1997).

To accomplish this goal in a clinically efficient manner, the authors present speech composite noise from a real-ear analyzer at 50, 65, and 85 dB SPL. While wearing both aids for a bilateral fit (or one aid for a monaural fit), the authors ask the patient to judge the loudness of the speech-weighted noise using the same loudness scaling categories described earlier. If the hearing aids are adjusted properly, the patient should rate the 50-dB SPL input as "very soft," "soft," or "comfortable, but slightly soft." For an input level of 65 dB SPL, the patient should rate the loudness as "comfortable, but slightly soft," "comfortable," or "comfortable, but slightly loud." For the input level of 85 dB SPL, the patient should never report a rating of "uncomfortably loud." If the patient reports the high input level to be "uncomfortably loud," then the audiologist must consider reducing the output and/or compression threshold. Another alternative would be to provide a more aggressive compression ratio.

Aided Sound Field Thresholds

One quick and reliable measure is to obtain aided sound field thresholds using warble-tones at 250 to 8,000 Hz presented in a calibrated (ANSI, 1996) sound field. With the patient facing the loudspeaker, he/she is asked to press a button when he/she hears a sound no matter how loud or soft. Research has suggested that, if it can be demonstrated that the aided sound field threshold is 20 dB HL or better, then this is indicative that the patient can hear the softest components of speech (Skinner et al., 2002; Mueller and Killion, 1990).

Hearing Aid Counseling: Use and Care of the Hearing Aids

Assuming that the fitting goals have been achieved, the authors then counsel the patient on the use and care of the hearing aids. Items typically covered include the following:

1. Inform the patient about the length (1 to 3 years) and terms of the warranty (damage or loss and damage). Also, the patient is informed that he/she will receive a card in 1 year to remind him/her of the need to check his/her hearing and the function of the hearing aids.
2. Remind the patient that the hearing aids are purchased on a 30-day trial period (varying across different states). If the patient should decide to return the hearing aids, then the patient will receive a full refund minus a small "professional fee."
3. Operation of the volume control for those hearing aids that have volume controls.
4. Operation of the remote control (volume, switching between programs, etc.) if the hearing aids use a remote control.
5. Operation of any buttons or switches that may be necessary to operate the hearing aids.
6. Insertion and removal of the batteries.
7. The type of battery and expected battery life. The authors also counsel the patient if the hearing aids have a feature informing him/her when the battery drainage is low.
8. Insertion and removal of the shells or earmolds.
9. Problems related to moisture. Each patient is provided a Dry and Store at the time of the fitting. If the patient has been dispensed BTE aids, then he/she is also provided with an air blower to quickly remove moisture from the tubing.
10. Problems related to cerumen plugging the vent and/or sound channel. Counseling is also extended to other options for combating cerumen. These may include extended receiver tubing, spring guards, and tools to remove cerumen from the vent. The patient is also counseled on the correct use of the brush and wax removal device accompanying most custom products.
11. Use of the telecoil. Whenever possible, the patient is counseled on using the microphone of the hearing aid as

an "acoustic" telecoil. Typically, we dial the local weather line and observe as the patient typically moves the telephone receiver around the entrance to the ear canal and pinna. We counsel the patient on the need to place the receiver of the telephone *adjacent to the microphone of the hearing aid*. In many cases, this is the position typically preferred by patients for using the telephone with hearing aids. When this is not successful, we then counsel the patient on the operation of the telecoil switch on the hearing aids. Several programmable hearing aids allow the audiologist to program a stronger telecoil response. Recently, several manufacturers have incorporated the EasyPhone feature into their hearing aids. With this technology, the hearing aid automatically switches to telecoil when the circuit detects an electromagnetic signal and then switches back to microphone when it detects that the electromagnetic signal is no longer present.

12. Discuss HAT and aural rehabilitation (our facilities have full-time audiologists providing aural rehabilitation).

13. Finally, inform the patient that he/she will be called in 2 days to determine how he/she is doing. The patient is also scheduled to return within 4 weeks for a hearing aid assessment.

OUTCOME MEASURES (FOURTH VISIT)

Hearing Aid Assessment

At this visit, the authors are interested in the patient's overall satisfaction with the hearing aids. For example, the authors want to know how well the patient performed during the intervening 3 to 4 weeks as he/she listened to speech in a variety of listening situations. Other questions relate to judgment of sound quality; presence/absence of feedback; ease of communication on the telephone; ability to remove and insert the earmolds, hearing aids, or batteries; the duration of battery life; issues related to the comfort of the hearing aids; and finally, issues related to the presence or absence of the occlusion effect. It is during this interview process that decisions

are made relative to the need for readjusting the electroacoustic characteristics or transmission line characteristics of the hearing aids.

At this visit, the patient is also asked to complete the "aided" portion of the COSI or Washington University Questionnaire (Fig. 38.1).

CONCLUSIONS

The American Speech-Language-Hearing Association (ASHA, 1998) has published their "Guidelines for Hearing Aid Fitting for Adults." This chapter's first author had the honor of chairing that committee. Recently, the first author had the pleasure of chairing a national task force for the American Academy of Audiology (AAA) to develop a national guideline for selecting, sitting, verifying, and validating the hearing aid performance in adults using evidence-based principles. In both of these guidelines, several important points were made. These include the following:

1. Real-ear measures are the preferred method for verifying the performance of hearing aids.
2. Patients need to be counseled on the realistic benefits to be derived from hearing aids.
3. Thresholds of discomfort, or LDLs, should be directly measured using frequency-specific stimuli when possible to accurately assess/adjust the output and/or compression characteristics of the hearing aids.
4. Outcome measures need to be included in the hearing aid fitting process.
5. HAT needs to be integrated into the fitting and counseling.

This chapter has provided a comprehensive overview of procedures to select and fit hearing aids for adults. Many of the requirements of the guidelines suggested by ASHA and AAA are included in the procedures outlined in this chapter. The authors feel that incorporating some or all of these suggestions provides a high probability of a successful hearing aid fitting.

REFERENCES

Agnew J, Block M. (1997) HINT thresholds for a dual-microphone BTE. *Hear Rev.* 4, 26, 29–30.

Agnew J, Thornton J. (2000) Just noticeable and objectionable group delays in digital hearing aids. *J Am Acad Audiol.* 11, 330–336.

American National Standards Institute. (1992) American National Standard for Testing Hearing Aids with a Broad-Band Noise Signal. ANSI S3.42-1992. New York: American National Standards Institute.

American National Standards Institute. (1996) American National Standard: Specification for Audiometers. ANSI S3.6-1996. New York: American National Standards Institute.

American National Standards Institute. (2003) American National Standard: Specification of Hearing Aid Characteristics. ANSI S3.22-2003. New York: American National Standards Institute.

American Speech-Language-Hearing Association. (1998) Guidelines for hearing aid fitting for adults. *Am J Audiol.* 7, 5–13.

Amlani A. (2001) Efficacy of directional microphone hearing aids: a meta-analytic perspective. *J Am Acad Audiol.* 12, 202–214.

Bentler R, Cooley L. (2001) An examination of several characteristics that affect the prediction of OSPL90 in hearing aids. *Ear Hear.* 22, 58–64.

Berger K, Hagberg N, Rane R. (1989) *Prescription of Hearing Aids.* 5th ed. Kent, OH: Herald Publishing.

Byrne D. (1996) Hearing aid selection for the 1990s: where to? *J Am Acad Audiol.* 7, 178–186.

Byrne D, Dillon H. (1986) The National Acoustic Laboratories (NAL) new procedure for selecting gain and frequency response of a hearing aid. *Ear Hear.* 7, 257–265.

Byrne D, Parkinson A, Newall P. (1990) Hearing aid gain and frequency response requirements for the severely/profoundly hearing impaired. *Ear Hear.* 11, 40–49.

Compton-Conley C, Neuman A, Killion M, Levitt H. (2004) Performance of directional microphones for hearing aids: real-world versus simulation. *J Am Acad Audiol.* 15, 440–455.

Cornelisse LE, Seewald RC, Jamieson DG. (1995) Wide-dynamic-range compression hearing aids: the DSL (i/o) approach. *Hear J.* 47, 23–24, 26, 28–29.

Cox RM, Alexander GC. (1995) The abbreviated profile of hearing aid benefit. *Ear Hear.* 16, 176–186.

Cox RM, Alexander GC. (2001) Validation of the SADL questionnaire. *Ear Hear.* 22, 151–160.

Cox RM, Gilmore C. (1990) Development of the Profile of Hearing Aid Performance (PHAP). *J Speech Hear Res.* 33, 343–357.

Dillon H. (1999) NAL-NL1: a new procedure for fitting non-linear hearing aids. *Hear J.* 52, 10, 12, 14, 16.

Dillon H, James A, Ginis J. (1997) Client oriented scale of improvement (COSI) and its relationship to several other measures of benefit and satisfaction provided by hearing aids. *J Am Acad Audiol.* 8, 27–43.

Erdman SA, Demorest ME. (1990) *CPHI Manual: A Guide to Clinical Use.* Simpsonville, MD: CPHI Services.

Flynn M. (2005) Envirograms: bringing greater utility to data logging. *Hear Rev.* 12, 32, 34, 36, 38.

Frye G. (2000) Testing digital hearing instruments: the basics. *Hear Rev.* 9, 20, 22, 24, 26–27.

Frye G. (2001) Testing digital and analog hearing instruments: processing time delays and phase measurements.*Hear Rev.* 10, 36–42.

Gatehouse S. (1994) Components and determinants of hearing aid benefit. *Ear Hear.* 15, 30–50.

Gatehouse S. (1999) Glasgow hearing aid benefit profile: derivation and validation of a client-centered outcome measure for hearing services. *J Am Acad Audiol.* 10, 80–103.

Giolas TG, Owens E, Lamb S, Schubert E. (1979) Hearing performance inventory. *J Speech Hear Dis.* 44, 169–195.

Goebel J, Valente M, Valente M, Enrietto J, Layton K, Wallace M. (2002) Fitting strategies for patients with conductive or mixed hearing loss. In: Valente M, ed. *Strategies for Selecting and Verifying Hearing Aid Fittings.* 2nd ed. New York: Thieme Medical Publishers; pp 272–286.

Gravel J, Fausel N, Liskow C, Chobot J. (1999). Children's speech recognition in noise using omnidirectional and dual-microphone hearing aid technology. *Ear Hear.* 20, 1–11.

Hawkins D, Montgomery A, Prosek R, Walden B. (1987) Examination of two issues concerning functional gain measurements. *J Speech Hear Dis.* 52, 56–63.

Ingrao B. (2005) HIMSA module puts evidence-based care only a mouse click away. *Hear J.* 58, 5052–5053.

Jenstad L, Van Tasell D, Ewert C. (2003) Hearing aid troubleshooting based on patients' descriptions. *J Am Acad Audiol.* 14, 347–360.

Kochkin S. (1996) Customer satisfaction and subjective benefit with high performance hearing aids. *Hear Rev.* 3, 16–26.

Kochkin S. (2000) Customer satisfaction with single and multiple microphone hearing aids. *Hear Rev.* 7, 24, 26, 28–29, 32–34.

Kuk F, Keenan D. (2005) Efficacy of an open-fitting hearing aid. *Hear Rev.* 12, 26–30, 32.

Lesiecki W. (2006) Does the in-office electronic scanning of the impression really change everything? *Hear Rev.* 13, 32, 34–35, 94.

Lewis M, Crandell C, Valente M, Horn J. (2004) Speech perception in noise: directional microphone versus frequency modulation (FM) systems. *J Am Acad Audiol.* 15, 426–439.

Lewis M, Valente M, Horn J, Crandell C. (2005) The effect of hearing aids and frequency modulation technology on results from the communication profile for the hearing impaired. *J Am Acad Audiol.* 16, 250–261.

Libby ER. (1986) The 1/3–2/3 insertion gain hearing aid selection guide. *Hear Instrum.* 37, 27–28.

Lurguin P, Rafhay S. (1996) Intelligibility in noise using multi-microphone hearing aids. *Acta Otol Rhinol Laryngol.* 50, 103–109.

Lybarger S. (1944) Method for fitting hearing aids. U.S. Patent Application SN 543,278.

McClandless G, Lyregaard P. (1983) Prescription of gain/output (POGO) for hearing aids. *Hear Instrum.* 34, 16–21.

Mueller HG, Killion M. (1990) An easy method for calculating the articulation index. *Hear J.* 49, 1–4.

Mueller HG, Hornsby B. (2002) Selection, verification and validation maximum output. In: Valente M, ed. *Strategies for Selecting and Verifying Hearing Aid Fittings.* 2nd ed. New York: Thieme Medical Publishers; pp 23–65.

Munro K, Patel R. (1998) Are clinical measurements of uncomfortable loudness levels a valid indicator of real-world auditory discomfort? *Br J Audiol.* 32, 287–293.

National Acoustic Laboratories. (1998) *NAL Non-Linear. NAL-NL1 v1.01 User Manual.* Chatswood, New South Wales, Australia: National Acoustic Laboratories.

Newman CW, Weinstein BE, Jacobson GP, Hug GA. (1990) The hearing handicap inventory for adults: psychometric adequacy and audiometric correlates. *Ear Hear.* 11, 430–433.

Newman CW, Weinstein BE, Jacobson GP, Hug GA. (1991) Test retest reliability of the hearing handicap inventory for adults. *Ear Hear.* 12, 355–357.

Noble WG, Atherley GR. (1970) The hearing measure scale: a questionnaire for the assessment of auditory disability. *J Aud Res.* 10, 229–250.

Pascoe D. (1988) Clinical measurement of the auditory dynamic range and their relation to formulas for hearing aid gain. In: Jensen J, ed: *Hearing Aid Fitting, Theoretical and Practical Views.* Copenhagen: Danavox Jubilee Foundation; pp 129–152.

Poe G, Ross T. (2005) A "small" change in verification: a compact live speech REM system. *Hear Rev.* 12, 38–40.

Pumford J, Seewald R, Scollie S, Jenstad L. (2000). Speech recognition with in-the-ear and behind-the-ear dual-microphone hearing instruments. *J Am Acad Audiol.* 11, 23–35.

Revit LJ. (1994) Using coupler tests in the fitting of hearing aids. In: Valente M, ed. *Strategies for Selecting and Verifying Hearing Aid Fittings.* New York: Thieme Medical Publisher; pp 64–87.

Ricketts T, Dhar S. (1999) Comparison of performance across three directional hearing aids. *J Am Acad Audiol.* 10, 180–189.

Schwartz D, Lyregaard P, Lundh P. (1988) Hearing aid selection for severe-to-profound hearing loss. *Hear J.* 41, 13–17.

Seewald R, Cornelisse L, Ramji K, Sinclair S, Moodie K, Jamieson D. (1997) DSL v4.1 for windows. A software implementation of the Desired Sensation Level (DSL [i/o]) Method for fitting linear gain and wide-dynamic-range compression hearing instruments. London, Ontario, Canada: University of Western Ontario.

Skinner M, Binzer S, Potts L, Holden L, Aaron R. (2002) Hearing rehabilitation for individuals with severe and profound hearing impairment: hearing aids, cochlear implants, and counseling. In: Valente M, ed. *Strategies for Selecting and Verifying Hearing Aid Fittings*. 2nd ed. New York: Thieme Medical Publishers; pp 311–344.

Soli S, Nilsson M. (1997) Predicting speech intelligibility in noise: the role of factors other than pure-tone sensitivity. *J Acoust Soc Am*. 101, 3201.

Stone MA, Moore BCJ. (1999) Tolerable hearing aid delays. I. Estimation of limits imposed by the auditory path alone using simulated hearing losses. *Ear Hear*. 20, 182–192.

Stone MA, Moore BCJ. (2002) Tolerable hearing aid delays. II. Estimation of limits imposed during speech production. *Ear Hear*. 23, 325–238.

Stone MA, Moore BCJ. (2005). Tolerable hearing aid delays. IV. Effects on subjective disturbance during speech production by hearing-impaired subjects. *Ear Hear*. 26, 225–234.

Summerfield Q. (1992) Lipreading and audiovisual speech perception. *Philos Trans R Soc Lond Biol*. 335, 71–78.

Valente M, Fabry D, Potts L. (1995) Recognition of speech in noise with hearing aids using dual-microphones. *J Am Acad Audiol*. 6, 440–449.

Valente M, Meister M, Smith P, Goebel J. (1990) Intratester test-retest reliability of insertion gain measures. *Ear Hear*. 11, 181–184.

Valente M, Mispagel K. (2004) Performance of an automatic adaptive dual-microphone ITC digital hearing aid. *Hear Rev*. 11, 42–46, 71.

Valente M, Mispagel K. (2008) Unaided and aided performance with a directional open-fit hearing aid. *Int J Audiol*. 47, 329–336.

Valente M, Potts L, Valente M. (1997) Differences and intersubject variability of loudness discomfort levels (LDL) measured in sound pressure level and hearing level for TDH-50P and ER-3A earphones. *J Am Acad Audiol*. 8, 59–67.

Valente M, Potts L, Valente M, Vass W, Goebel J. (1994) Intersubject variability of the real-ear SSPL90: conventional versus insert earphones. *J Am Acad Audiol*. 5, 390–398.

Valente M, Schuchman G, Potts L, Beck L. (2000). Performance of dual-microphone in-the-ear hearing aids. *J Am Acad Audiol*. 11, 181–189.

Valente M, Valente M, Goebel J. (1991) Reliability and intersubject variability of the real ear unaided response REUR. *Ear Hear*. 12, 216–220.

Valente M, Van Vliet D. (1997) The independent hearing aid fitting forum (IHAFF). *Trends Amplif*. 2, 6–35.

Voss T. (1997) Clinical evaluation of multi-microphone instruments. *Hear Rev*. 4, 36, 45–46, 74.

Yanz J. (2005) Phones and hearing aids: issues, resolutions, and a new approach. *Hear J*. 58, 41–42, 44, 48.

Yanz J, Roberts R, Sanguino J. (2005) A wearable Bluetooth device for hard-of-hearing people. *Hear Rev*. 12, 38–41.

Building and Growing a Successful Audiology Practice

David Cunningham and James Baer

▧ INTRODUCTION

This chapter will focus on establishing and growing an audiology practice. Many audiologists receive little or no business management training, but this should not dissuade the clinician from an entrepreneurial undertaking. Generally speaking, those individuals who are drawn to audiology have an ability to organize, plan, and lead. Our intent is to take the perspective of a relatively junior clinician who is considering opening his or her own practice and help the reader develop the skills to be a successful practitioner, manager, and entrepreneur. Any skills that are not inherent to the novice clinician can be developed.

This chapter, while discussing some basic business principles and theories, will be written from a practical rather than a theoretical perspective. It is important to note that, although the intent of this chapter is to provide a comprehensive overview of practice management, our advice will need to be supplemented by consultants such as an attorney, financial advisor, and accountant.

Caveat Emptor

This chapter will be as beneficial to an individual who has absolutely no interest in developing a practice as to the person who intends to build a multilocation chain of audiology practices. The truth of the matter is that, wherever you go or whatever you do, the principles outlined in this chapter are applicable. Whether you are an owner of a practice, an employee in a small single-site clinic, or a pediatric audiologist in a children's hospital, someone somewhere is "counting the beans." Inevitably, you will be held

accountable for controlling costs, understanding the "bottom line" of a Profit and Loss (P&L) statement, maximizing profits, or justifying the cost associated with expanding the practice.

At this point, it may be prudent to issue a caveat to the reader. This chapter could very well dampen your entrepreneurial spirit. Writing a business plan, making educated guesses about the projected profit and loss of your business, creating a marketing plan, and securing capital can seem overwhelming. As an entrepreneur, one is required to constantly monitor the financial solvency of the practice, assess and reassess competition, maintain a thorough understanding of the changing scope of practice and regulations, learn reimbursement procedures, create adaptive marketing plans, track marketing results, manage collections, and much more. While doing all of these things, it is also necessary for the clinician-manager-owner to stay abreast of emerging technologies and standards of practice. Without a doubt, being a clinician in the employ of someone else is far less risky and more stable and predictable than opening one's own practice. For some, however, the rewards of owning and successfully managing their own practice far outweigh the associated risks and additional work.

Recommended Readings

In addition to reading this chapter, the authors highly recommend the following supplemental readings: *The E-Myth Revisited* by Michael Gerber (1995) and *Selling the Invisible* by Harry Beckwith (1997). These books, while not written as audiology-specific texts, are invaluable resources for any entrepreneur.

Selling the Invisible focuses on the importance of "fixing your service" and stresses the fact that, at all times, the service you provide must be critically examined not only for flaws, but also for opportunities to set your offerings apart from competitors. Providing outstanding service is critical to the success of your business and also to your patients' satisfaction.

The E-Myth Revisited discusses the "entrepreneurial seizure," the exact moment when the individual in the employ of another comes to the realization, "I can do this better, so why am I working for someone else?" The book further discusses the multiple roles that must be played but are seldom considered by the would-be entrepreneur. One of these roles is the "Technician." This is the part of our personality that knows how to perform a given job with absolute technical proficiency and is completely content doing so. The "Entrepreneur" is the portion of our persona who has a "dream." The Entrepreneur sees into the future and plans for that future. The "Manager" is initially the most often ignored aspect of our persona when undertaking a new business. The unfortunate Manager is the "middle man" who runs interference between the Entrepreneur and the Technician trying to persuade each to pay some attention to the business. The Technician is content to perform diagnostic testing, prescribe and fit hearing aids, and counsel patients. The Entrepreneur is dreaming of a bigger and better future. Both are content with their respective endeavors and have little interest in spending time working on the business. This is not to suggest that either of these roles is less important than the Manager's; however, it is critical to realize that each of these roles must be maintained in balance. This is a key point. If you open your own practice, you must plan to not only work **IN** your business, but also to devote time to working **ON** your business. Working on your business involves taking care of daily managerial responsibilities such as billing; accounts payable and receivable; marketing; detailing job responsibilities; following up on assigned responsibilities with your staff; creating, maintaining, and updating clinical protocols; planning short- and long-term goals to help achieve the entrepreneurial dream; and organizing, organizing, organizing.

No Margin, No Mission

Organization is the key to a successful business. Most of us have heard the accurate, if clichéd, phrase "Location! Location! Location!" However, before location, comes organization. At its core, management is organization and leadership. Again, anyone who has completed a higher education degree and is a successful audiologist must have some organizational and leadership skills. Think of all of the times you have had to prioritize, organize, and juggle your schedule in order to meet deadlines, either academic or vocational. The point is that all of the skills to be an entrepreneur and manager can be learned.

Individuals who are drawn to audiology are generally caring and giving. Many seem to feel that there is a disparity between helping people and being a successful business person. It is imperative to realize that if you are not "minding the store" by paying attention to profits, you will quickly find yourself in the position of being unable to help anyone, including yourself. The more successful you can make your practice, the more you can help those in need of audiology services. We like the old expression, "No margin, no mission!" If you don't have an adequate profit margin, it is impossible to fulfill your mission: helping others hear.

▨ PERSONAL ISSUES, ROLES, AND RESPONSIBILITIES

Sure He's Smart but His Personality...

You've spent years and countless dollars acquiring a degree in audiology and are a skilled technician. Now you want to open your own practice, and you may mistakenly believe that technical proficiency is your most valuable professional asset. You couldn't be more wrong. Managers must be intelligent, but more important than IQ is your emotional quotient (EQ). You can test your EQ at http://quiz.ivillage.co.uk/uk_work/tests/eqtest.htm.

As an owner/manager, you will be required to assume multiple, sometimes conflicting, roles, most of which you will *not* have been prepared for by formal education. Managers manage people, not products. In the course of your career as a clinician-manager-owner, you will encounter countless personality types and will need to learn to work with all of them. One tool, the Myers-Briggs Type Indicator (MBTI), based on the work of Karl Jung (famous psychologist and one-time student of Sigmund Freud), has often been employed as a team-building tool. Jung theorized that there are 16 archetypical personality traits that exist in all of us in varying degrees. Jung's theory applies to the clinician-manager-owner triad and to practical business management. Log onto www.teamtechnology.co.uk/mbti.html to discover your personality type for a nominal fee. There are also a multitude of websites that are designed to help you understand your personality type and how it applies to management and leadership skills.

The Small Business Administration's (SBA) website (http://www.sba.gov/) lists many of the qualities of a good manager; it is worth your time to visit this informative site. The first quality is emotional stability. A good manager is able to maintain his or her composure under stress, during conflicts, and while embroiled in frustrating situations. Essentially, the good manager is able to put on a "poker face" that may belie his or her internal emotional state.

The second personal quality of the effective manager as cited by the SBA is dominance. Managers are faced with dozens if not hundreds of decisions on a daily basis. Being decisive and assertive is critical to effective management. Dominance is a skill that must be developed carefully. The SBA recommends that the effective manager learn to be assertive, but it is important to recognize the difference between assertiveness and aggressiveness. Dominance should always be tempered by active listening. The manager must also seek the advice and counsel of others including employees, consultants, and patients. While dominance is a critical skill in decision making, it is also important to recognize that managers do not push people toward a goal, *they lead.* Leadership entails helping others to share the vision of the manager and to become active and enthusiastic participants in attaining clearly articulated goals. If you make your expectations known to associates and colleagues at the outset, you eliminate the need for guesswork and a large potential source of confusion.

The third quality of management is enthusiasm! The manager is the cornerstone of the team's morale. If a manager is listless, unenthusiastic, bored, and uninvolved, the team will quickly assume the same characteristics. However, if the manager is an active participant in daily business, is excited about team achievements, recognizes and rewards individual contributions, and is the quintessential "cheerleader," then the team will be more motivated to produce and achieve. Enthusiasm is contagious!

The fourth quality is conscientiousness. The effective leader is conscientious to a fault, often working late or working harder than anyone would expect in striving to perfect his or her service. The conscientious individual has high expectations and the drive to continually strive toward excellence in all endeavors.

The fifth quality is social boldness. Entrepreneurs and managers alike are calculated risk takers. Often, taking calculated risks requires the development of a "thick skin" and the ability to assess, critically analyze, and move on when risk-taking leads to failure. One of our favorite quotes is as follows: to paraphrase Samuel Beckett (1983), "Try. Fail. Try again. Fail better!"

The final quality is being tough-minded. This skill relates to the ability to be doggedly pragmatic and logical, to critically analyze every interaction and situation, and to sort the wheat from the chaff when making decisions. This ability ties in with the compulsive aspect of personality that requires highly developed organizational skills. Nothing is left to random chance, and precision is fundamental. Planning is an integral part of this aspect of the manager's personality. The compulsive portion of the manager's personality lives by the credo, "If you fail to plan, you plan to fail."

In order to apply all of these skills in real-world interactions, it is important to have a degree of self-assurance and confidence. Even bad decisions executed properly lead to a good outcome if you are able to accept failure, critically analyze the situation, and move on. Once again the maxim "Try. Fail. Try again. Fail better" is apropos.

As the clinician-manager-owner, you will wear many hats. Your roles will be varied, and at times, you will find that these roles come into conflict. Part of your responsibility is to balance these roles, prioritize, and make decisions taking all factors into account. Some of the roles you need to play are: human resource manager/personnel director, marketing strategist/media manager, public relations director, risk manager, buyer, salesman, merchandiser, planner, billing specialist, collections agent, accountant, insurance broker/negotiator, and clinician. This is where your management skills come to bear. You must prioritize not only the work that you do on a daily basis, but also the needs and demands of each of these roles. For example, the marketing strategist may demand that you spend $5,000.00 on a promotion, while the collections agent, accountant, and billing specialist insist that there are insufficient funds to do so. You as the manager must find a reasonable compromise that will allow you to continue to market your service while working within the confines of your budget. It is no mean feat to balance all of these roles, but with the application of common sense, most conflicts between roles can be resolved through compromise.

Who's the Boss?

So who is responsible to whom? In an organizational chart, you might see each individual in the practice as having an immediate supervisor with the clinician-manager-owner at the top of the food chain. The reality of the situation is that, despite the fact that you have opened your own practice in order to avoid having a boss, your new bosses (note plural) are your patients. Every patient who walks through your door forms an opinion about you, your clinic, and your service. Those patients are also your customers, and customer satisfaction is of paramount importance. To this end, you, the clinician-manager-owner, must strive toward continuous quality improvement (CQI). CQI examines the current protocols and standards and continuously questions methods while looking for any means to improve the current standard. CQI is proactive and is related to foresight. It correlates with Beckwith's (1997) observation of continually fixing your service. If you think there is nothing wrong with your service, look again; there is always some way to improve, to differentiate yourself from your competitors, and to excel beyond your patients' expectations.

To examine the effectiveness of patient care, the Doctor of Audiology program at the University of Louisville uses a health care matrix adopted by the American Council of Graduate Medical Education (ACGME) and the Institute of Medicine (IOM). The health care matrix was developed by Quinn and Bingham (Bingham et al., 2005) at Vanderbilt University (Fig. 39.1). The core rationale behind the matrix is CQI. As you can see in Figure 39.1, there are six IOM quality-related categories across the top of the form. They are designed to assess the clinician–patient interaction for safety,

ACGME \ IOM	SAFE[1]	TIMELY[2]	EFFECTIVE[3]	EFFICIENT[4]	EQUITABLE[5]	PATIENT-CENTERED[6]
Assessment of Care						
I. PATIENT CARE[7] (Overall Assessment) Yes/No	Yes	Yes	No. Patient returned to learn how to put batteries in her hearing aid. Instruction may need to be reviewed or supplemental written materials added.	No. Pt. was seen in an hour but instruction was insufficient to meet her needs.	Yes. Pt treated fairly	No. Patient's learning needs were not met. Tx was not adapted to meet the patient's specific needs.
II. a MEDICAL KNOWLEDGE[8] (What must I know)			We need to critically assess our fitting protocol. May need to add a cognitive processing screening test or learn to better adapt to pt. needs.	Yes. Inefficient at communicating that knowledge	Yes.	Yes.
II. b INTERPERSONAL AND COMMUNICATION SKILLS[9] (What must I say)	Yes	No. Time ineffectively used. Taking 10 more minutes at initial fitting would have saved the patient an extra trip to the clinic and an extra available clinic hour from the clinician.	No. Did not teach pt. effectively. Review other means and modalities of presentation.	No. Ineffective communication interfered with efficacy.	Yes.	No. Need to adjust personal communication skills to each patient's level of ability. Supplemental tools?
II. c PROFESSIONALISM[10] (How must I act)	Yes	Yes.	No. Professional behavior would include more sensitivity to pt. needs and ability to adjust accordingly.	Yes.	Yes.	Yes.
II. d SYSTEM-BASED PRACTICE[11] (On whom do I depend and who depends on me)	Yes	No. Implement fitting protocol with instructions for pt.'s. Written handout may reduce or eliminate unnecessary visits.	No. Waste of practice resources with visits that could be avoided.	No. Pt. requires additional visits due to lack of effective protocol / handouts.	Yes.	Yes.
Improvement						
III. PRACTICE-BASED LEARNING AND IMPROVEMENT[12] (How must I improve)		Time management is not a matter of simply being faster. It also includes being thorough.	Improve effectiveness through implementation of additional resources for pt.'s.	Increase efficiency via implementation of new procedures to decrease unnecessary follow-ups.		
Information Technology						

[1] Safe: Avoiding injuries to patients from the care that is intended to help them.
[2] Timely: reducing waits and sometimes harmful delays for both those who receive and those who give care.
[3] Effective: providing services based on scientific knowledge to all who could benefit and refraining from providing services to those not likely to benefit (avoiding underuse and overuse, respectively).
[4] Efficient: avoiding waste, including waste of equipment, supplies, ideas, and energy.
[5] Equitable: providing care that does not vary in quality because of personal characteristics such as gender, ethnicity, geographic location, and socio-economic status.
[6] Patient-Centered: providing care that is respectful of and responsive to individual patient preferences, needs and values and ensuring that patient values guide all clinical decisions.
[7] Patient care that is compassionate, appropriate, and effective for the treatment of health problems and the promotion of health.
[8] Medical Knowledge about established and evolving biomedical, clinical, and cognate sciences (i.g. epidemiological and social-behavioral) and the application of this knowledge to patient care.
[8] Interpersonal and communication skills that result in effective information exchange and teaming with patients, their families and other health professionals.
[10] Professionalism, as manifested through a commitment to carrying out professional responsibilities, adherence to ethical principles, and sensitivity to a diverse patient population.
[11] System-based practice, as manifested by actions that demonstrate an awareness of and responsiveness to the larger context and system of health care and the ability to effectively call on system resources to provide care that is of optimal value.
[12] Practice-based learning and improvement that involves investigation and evaluation of their own patient care, appraisal and assimilation of scientific evidence, and improvement in patient care.

FIGURE 39.1   Health care matrix. (Reprinted with permission from Bingham JW, Quinn DC, Richardson MG, Miles PV, Gabbe SG. [2005] Using a healthcare matrix to assess patient care in terms of aims for improvement and core competencies.*Journal on Quality and Patient Safety*. 31, 98–105.)

timeliness, effectiveness, efficiency, equitability, and patient centeredness. Along the y-axis are the ACGME core competencies. These assess overall patient care, medical knowledge, interpersonal and communication skills, professionalism, system-based practice, and practice-based learning and improvement. Each of the categories is filled in as in the example. The function of the health care matrix is not to assign blame, but to constantly gauge our level of quality.

W. Edwards Deming is famous for his understanding of CQI. Table 39.1 lists Deming's 14 points (Hosford-Dunn et al., 1995). These are essential to all aspects of effective management.

TABLE 39.1	Deming's 14 points of continuous quality improvement
1	Create constancy of purpose for improvement of product and services. The marketing goal of the practice is not to make money; the goal is to stay in business and provide jobs through innovation, research, constant improvement, and maintenance.
2	Adopt the new philosophy. Mistakes and negativism are unacceptable.
3	Cease dependence on inspection to improve quality. Quality comes from improving the process, not from inspection of what is already done. Properly instructed workers can contribute to this improvement.
4	End the practice of awarding business on price tag alone. Price has no meaning without consideration of quality (as perceived by the practitioner as well as the consumer).
5	Improve constantly and forever the system of production and service. Again, quality is not a one-time event. Always strive to improve quality and productivity, thereby reducing costs.
6	Institute training on the job.
7	Institute leadership. Help employees do a better job, and identify those who need individual help.
8	Drive out fear. Everyone in the practice needs to feel secure in order to do their best and ask enough questions to be sure they "know where they are going."
9	Break down barriers between staff areas. Make sure everyone in the practice works together as a team.
10	Eliminate slogans, exhortations, and targets for the work force (e.g., "THINK" doesn't help!!).
11	Eliminate numerical quotas. Selling on commission or doing "X" number of audiograms per day is antithetical to the marketing of quality.
12	Remove barriers to pride of workmanship. Be sure the practice is properly equipped and that everyone is encouraged for doing their best.
13	Institute a vigorous program of education and retraining.
14	Put everyone in the practice to work to accomplish these steps.

Adapted from Hosford-Dunn H, Dunn DR, Harford ER. (1995) *Audiology Business and Practice Management*. San Diego: Singular.

Outcome Measures

In order to assess progress toward established goals, it is important to have a list of "best practices" and policies in place. As an effective manager, you leave nothing to chance and do not put your staff in the position of having to guess about your goals and expected outcomes. Every process should have a written procedure. Every patient should be seen in accordance with established protocols and be evaluated from a CQI perspective.

Business-oriented outcome measures allow you to determine the degree to which you have been able to meet desired business objectives and include: projected versus earned income; marketing efficacy tracking, also known as return on promotion; cost control; percentage of growth; and return on investment. Most audiologists have experience applying outcome measures to patient interactions but enter a business endeavor with little or no knowledge of how to read a P&L statement, how to measure the value of a promotion, or how to perform other managerial functions. The key point is that it is every bit as important to track these items as it is to perform treatment outcome measures. If you invest the time and resources in a marketing push, for example, it is critical to have some means of tracking the result of that venture so that you can analyze the outcome and make educated decisions about using a similar campaign at a later date. Needless to say, tracking your income on a monthly, quarterly, and annual basis is essential. You cannot take a "hope for the best" approach. If you wait to see the outcome at the end of the year, you may find yourself in the unenviable position of closing your doors forever.

■ THE NEW BUSINESS MINDSET

Thus far, we've stressed the importance of organization in general terms. Gerber (1995) discusses business organization on a different level. Gerber stresses the importance of having an organization chart. The clear delineation of duties for each manager, associate, and employee is critical to the successful operation of your practice. In Gerber's words, "if everybody's doing everything, then no one's accountable for anything?" The lack of delineated responsibilities leads to chaos, resentment, and poor quality of service.

All businesses, big or small, would be well advised to think of themselves as a corporation when creating an organization chart. Despite the fact that you may begin your practice with only yourself and one full- or part-time receptionist, it is critical to create an organization chart from the outset *and to realize that each of the positions in the chart will be and **must** be filled by you!* As new employees are hired, the owner can delegate these roles to others. A sample organization chart is shown in Figure 39.2.

According to Gerber, the first step in creating your organizational chart is to establish a "strategic objective" that defines how the company will be doing business. For

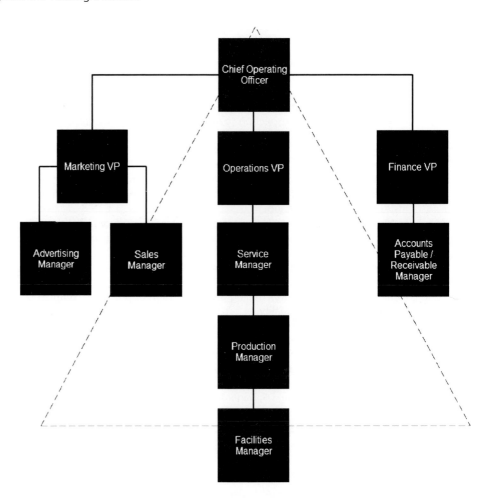

FIGURE 39.2 Sample organizational chart. VP, vice president.

example, when you plan your first practice, you will most likely have one location providing a set list of services to a given target population within a specified geographic marketing area. It will then be necessary to decide on the number and type of departments and positions that will be required in order to meet demand and to provide the highest quality of service. Examples of positions that may be included in your organization chart include: President/Chief Operating Officer (COO), Vice President of Marketing, Vice President of Operations, and Vice President of Finance. Each of these positions will have individuals or departments that report to them. These are included in Figure 39.2. Despite the fact that, at the outset, there may be only two or three people or contracted (out-sourced) service providers listed on the organization chart, it is still important to begin to conceptualize your practice as a larger corporation.

For each position listed on the organization chart, a "position contract" must be completed (Gerber, 1995). A position contract is not a job description, but rather outlines the company's rules and expectations. The position contract describes the nature of the position and delineates the responsibilities for which the individual will be held accountable.

As you become accustomed to performing the duties associated with each position, it will become necessary to

begin to replace yourself with a **system**. If you begin to try to create a system for the COO, you will quickly find yourself at an impasse. A large portion of your responsibilities as COO lies in the supervision of the various positions that report to you. How can you supervise positions that have yet to be created? In order to effectively describe each job and to create a system that will stand the test of time, you must begin at the *bottom* of the chart. The foundation of any business is in the technical work. Notice in Figure 39.2 that the organization chart takes on the general shape of a pyramid. Any engineer can tell you that, in order for a pyramid to be structurally sound, it must have a firm, broad-based foundation. Proficient technical work is the basis of your business organization. If you fail to do good technical work in your practice, you will not need to worry about a system for the position of COO. You must look at each position within your organizational structure as a "franchise" from which you are contracting services (Gerber, 1995) and organize it in a way that would entice you to use the services offered by that franchise.

Before you begin writing your business plan, you need to critically analyze your motives for creating your own practice. If your intent is to create a job for yourself, then you would be well advised to save the time, expense, and effort of writing a business plan and starting a practice. A legitimate goal is to create a business that can accommodate the given *lifestyle* that you've chosen or that you wish to achieve. *Ultimately, you create a practice to duplicate and eventually sell.* Based on *The E-Myth Revisited* by Gerber (1995), there are multiple strategies that will help you to succeed in this endeavor.

When we addressed the issue of an effective organizational chart, we discussed the issue of replacing yourself with a system. The technical aspect of your work is where you need to begin creating your system. Customers crave constancy and consistently high-quality service. You have prepared yourself by education and experience to provide that level of service. But what happens when you begin to expand and you have other associates providing the "technical" services that you gave personally at the outset? Does this new associate approach customer service with the same intensity of care that you have put so much time into perfecting? Will your new associate care as deeply as you do? Are you willing to gamble all of your hard work and time on the hope that your new associate will strive to provide the same level of service that you have?

Gerber (1995) discusses the phenomenon of the "turn-key revolution." Perhaps the most effective means of elucidating this concept is with an example. McDonald's is the largest restaurant chain in the world. McDonald's is run by teenaged employees. How can the largest restaurant chain be run by people with little or no real work experience? The answer is that McDonald's is a turn-key operation. Turn-key operations are ones in which every aspect of the business is organized to such an extent that all functions of each position can be written out precisely and concisely in manuals. Nothing is left to chance or guesswork. French fries are always prepared in the exact same manner and cooked for the exact same amount of time and salted to the same degree each time, no matter who the fry-cook is. Hamburgers always have X number of pickles on them, X quantity of mustard, and X amount of catsup. Customers in Iowa receive the same hamburgers as those in New York. Giving associates clearly defined protocols is highly beneficial to the associate, to the patient, and ultimately to you as the clinician-owner-manager. The best manager-owners are those who can walk away from the practice and know with absolute certainty that the daily function of the clinic will not suffer from their absence. If your practice requires your constant presence, you have not organized it sufficiently or have not written your manuals appropriately.

The same organization that will allow your business to run smoothly in your absence will afford you the ability to duplicate the practice with ease when you are ready to expand to other sites. Duplicating a highly organized and efficient practice is a simple matter of printing additional sets of manuals and training the new staff to follow the procedures.

As a counterpoint to this idea, audiologic service is not quite the same as hamburgers and french fries. While you will undoubtedly want to write clinical protocols and procedures for your practice, you may also wish to provide your associates with some professional leeway. Part of being a good

clinician is the ability to adapt. Diagnostic audiology is frequently based upon clinical judgement and will require some flexibility. It may behoove the owner to create a protocol that allows the clinician to perform additional testing to assure the highest quality care.

If decision making and procedures are reduced to a systematic process, it will lighten your load as manager. In essence, you will be required to "manage the exceptions" that cannot be foreseen or addressed with a simple procedure or protocol. Essentially, this is an effective means of time management so that you can fulfill your major roles of entrepreneur, manager, and technician. Protocol and procedure manuals must be written for all business functions as well.

Another means of effective time management is to know your own limitations. There will certainly be tasks that you can perform on site with relative ease, while other tasks might be out-sourced by necessity. Examples of services that may be contracted include: billing and collections, human resources, management, and accounting and legal services. It is important to remember that, although these services may not be performed within your clinic, it is your responsibility to understand the processes involved and to keep your finger on the pulse of what these consultants are doing for you and how much they are costing you.

Tracking data provides valuable information. Tracking revenue, expenses, and profit margin by Current Procedural Terminology (CPT) code, by clinician, and by site of service provides information about productivity. This can help you make important business decisions about incentive programs for associates, client mix, and the type of services provided. Of course, this is not to suggest that critical services be dropped based solely on the fact that they yield a smaller margin, but it can help you choose between two clinical procedures that yield essentially the same information, but with different reimbursement rates.

Another beneficial business tool is tracking referrals. This can be achieved in numerous ways and can help you to understand why a patient chose your site over another. Once you know what patients like about your service, you can do more of it to attract a larger patient base. Conversely, if you find out why referral sources are not sending patients to your site, you can fix the problem in an attempt to build a stronger image and draw more referrals. Tracking referrals can be as simple as having your receptionist ask why a patient chose your clinic, or it can be incorporated into intake paperwork.

Give 'Em More Than They Expect!

Each time a patient steps through your door, you have a "marketing moment" (Beckwith, 1997). Marketing is all about the impression you make on the patient. You have a single chance to make a good impression. Marketing begins before the patient steps through the front door. Your first line of marketing "offense" is your reception staff. The receptionist gives patients their first chance to form an opinion about you and your service. . . *and they will form an opinion!* Scripted phone protocols can help to promote a positive image to potential patients and to reduce or eliminate negative impressions. Reception staff can make or break you. When choosing to hire receptionists, *choose wisely*!

Your service is your marketing. The patient who leaves with a bad impression of you or of your clinic *will* spread the word. The patient who is satisfied may or may not spread the word but will most likely return for future service. Patients have an acutely tuned sense of good service. While "service" is intangible, it is clearly perceptible. The first question you should ask yourself is *not* how the rest of the profession is offering the service, but how you can offer it in a unique, higher quality manner. If you copy the service of the audiologist down the street, you have failed to distinguish yourself. Good service plans should follow the example of Walt Disney by giving the consumer more than they expect. If your marketing is not working, you need to work on your service (Beckwith, 1997).

LEGAL ISSUES

Where Structure, Form, and Function Meet

One of the first things you'll need to do is choose a business structure for your practice. There are several types of business structures, each with inherent advantages and disadvantages. Before continuing, it is important that we remind you that seeking legal and accounting expertise is important. It is also important to realize that you may find it beneficial to change your structure as your business matures. All forms of business require licenses and other legal formalities to be completed prior to commencing business. Visit the Internal Revenue Service's (IRS) website at www.irs.gov to find a complete listing of all tax-related documents that must be filed. These are listed by type of business structure. You will also need to check with state and local government for information on obtaining licenses, business permits, tax identification numbers, etc. The SBA is an excellent resource for information of this nature. We recommend that you visit the SBA's website at www.sba.gov to take advantage of this excellent resource.

According to Thomas Stemmy (2004), there are two main questions that the aspiring entrepreneur needs to consider when choosing a business structure. The questions center around legal liability and tax benefits. Legal liability, according to Stemmy, is best addressed by the business owner(s) and their legal counsel. Tax considerations should be discussed with a Certified Public Accountant (CPA) before choosing your structure. For ease of comparison, Table 39.2 is a compilation and adaptation of Stemmy (2004) and Hosford-Dunn et al. (1995).

The simplest form of business structure is the *sole proprietorship*. A sole proprietorship is one in which there is one person (or a married couple) operating as the owner. Sole proprietorship is easy to establish. If you are operating the business under a name other than your own legal name, you would be required to file a DBA, or "doing business as," document (Hupalo, 1999). Some of the potential drawbacks of operating as a sole proprietorship are the fact that your personal assets are linked to the business and are subject to foreclosure should your business fail. Although no one plans to fail, it can happen. Additionally, as a practitioner providing health care services, your personal assets are subject to liability in a malpractice claim due to the fact that the business is not considered an "entity" in and of itself (Hosford-Dunn et al., 1995). As mentioned earlier, the second factor is tax considerations. The revenue generated or lost in a sole proprietorship is reported on the owner's income taxes. For the first year or two, a new small business should not expect to make money, which will provide a tax benefit to you as the sole proprietor when you file your personal taxes. When the business does begin to show a profit, this too will be reported on your personal income tax as personal gain (Hupalo, 1999).

The next basic structure is a *general partnership*. A partnership is similar to a sole proprietorship in that it is a relatively simple to establish (Stemmy, 2004). There are no significant costs or cumbersome processes involved, but "wise counsel...will give you about a dozen reasons why you should have a detailed partnership agreement drafted whenever you put yourself on the line with any other individual" (Stemmy, 2004). The following items must be considered:

- An investment agreement that specifies the initial capital investment of each partner
- The rights, duties, and responsibilities of each partner
- The method in which dividends will be paid to each partner
- Salary agreements
- Dispute resolution procedures
- A dissolution agreement in the event that the business is closed, the partnership is dissolved, or a partner dies or becomes disabled

According to Hosford-Dunn et al. (1995), these items would be included in a legal agreement known as "articles of partnership." Advantages of partnerships include collaboration between colleagues and less financial risk for each partner. One of the disadvantages of a partnership is the inability to make quick decisions and the fact that one partner's poor judgment may impact the finances of all partners (Hosford-Dunn et al., 1995).

Two other forms of partnerships are the *limited partnership* and the *limited liability partnership* (QuickMBA, 2005). Limited liability partnerships are very similar to a partnership, except that one partner is "limited" both in liability and in his/her personal activity in the business. The "limited" partner *is* still liable to the extent of his or her investment provided that partner never takes an active role in the practice (Stemmy, 2004). Similarly, limited partnerships have silent partners who act in the capacity of investors but take no active role in the operation of the business. The investors have no liability and risk only their investment (QuickMBA,

TABLE 39.2 Comparison of the most common business structures

	Formation	Duration	Liability	Simplicity of operation	Taxation	Pass-through income	Cost of creation
Sole Proprietorship	Simple to form by obtaining licenses and applying for a tax ID number	Life of the owner or until transferred	Proprietor is 100% liable	Few legal requirements; owner and business are considered one entity	Owner is taxed at individual rates; dividends are fully taxable to the owner	Yes; no double-taxation	Nominal
General Partnership	Agreement of parties involved only	Dissolved by death of a partner or bankruptcy	Partners are 100% liable	Minimal legal requirements	Partners pay taxes on their own share of dividends	Yes; no double-taxation	Nominal
Limited Liability Company (LLC)	Similar to a partnership; registration with the state in which you do business is mandatory	Typically limited to a fixed amount of time	Members are not liable for debts of the LLC	Some formal requirements; less involved than a corporation	If properly structured, no tax at the individual level	Yes; no double taxation	Filing fee with the state
Corporations							
Close Corporations (C-Corp)	File with state for permission	Perpetual	Shareholders are not typically liable for debts of the corporation	Formal; board of directors, officers, directors, etc.	Corporation is a taxable entity	No; double taxation (income taxed at the corporate level and each shareholder pays taxes on dividends)	Filing fees with the state
Subchapter Corporations (S-Corp)	File with state for permission	Perpetual	Shareholders are not typically liable for debts of the corporation	Formal; board of directors, officers, directors, etc.	Not taxed as a separate entity	Yes; no double-taxation	Filing fee with the state

Adapted from Stemmy TJ. (2004) Business structure basics. Available at: http://www.entrepreneur.com/startingabusiness/startupbasics/businessstructure/article75118.html; and Hosford-Dunn H, Dunn DR, Harford ER. (1995) *Audiology Business and Practice Management*. San Diego: Singular.

2005). The limited partnership also has partners who are active and who expose themselves to liability. This type of partnership is "especially useful for raising capital since [it] permits investors to participate financially in the business without incurring personal liability" (QuickMBA, 2005).

Corporations are legal entities recognized under the law. They are considered to be corporeal, that is, having a body that protects the owners from personal liability. Corporations provide the additional benefit of easily transferable shares and perpetual existence (QuickMBA, 2005). Taxation may be problematic because the corporation will pay taxes on profits and, if those profits are then disbursed to shareholders, they will also pay personal income tax on the revenue (Elgin, 2002). This will depend on the type of corporation (for further information on types of corporations and advantages/disadvantages of each type, see Hupalo [1999]).

CYA: Cover Your "Assets"

For audiologists, there are two types of liability insurance that are prerequisites to opening your practice. The first of these is general liability insurance. General liability insurance covers your practice in the event of a lawsuit regarding an accident that occurs on your property. This coverage is limited to bodily injury or property damage. It covers you, your clients, and your employees (see www.techinsurance.com). It is important to understand that general liability insurance does not cover professional errors or error of omission claims related to the delivery of professional services. This is where professional liability insurance comes into play. As the practice grows, your insurance needs will change. Involve your attorney and accountant in decisions regarding the type and amount of insurance you and your business require. While it is important to shop for the best possible insurance rates, this is not the time to be penny wise and pound foolish.

The Health Insurance Portability and Accountability Act

You need to consider how the Health Insurance Portability and Accountability Act (HIPAA) affects your practice. Not only do all patients need to read and sign an HIPAA-compliant privacy agreement, but the HIPAA law needs to be visibly posted in your office. Most clinicians choose to post these rules on the wall of the waiting room. You need to consider HIPAA regulations when constructing office space. An enclosed area for your receptionist is a wise investment. Files must be stored in such a way as to provide a reasonable assurance of patient privacy.

In addition to protecting your patients' files, it may be necessary to encrypt or encode your patient database. Additionally, you will be contracting certain services from business partners. According to HIPAA law, the "covered entity" (i.e., health care provider, health plans, or clearinghouse) is responsible to ensure that business associates who have access to Protected Health Information (PHI) are capable of complying with the law (Swartz, 2003). Examples of business associates include: vendors, consultants, lawyers, auditors, accountants, clearinghouses, billing firms, and records storage organizations.

FINANCIAL MANAGEMENT

The first thing to know about managing your finances is that you are not qualified to do it yourself. You might not even be qualified to hire a competent CPA to advise you. According to Edwards (1992), "frequently, owners of very small businesses lack even a rudimentary understanding of accounting and financial management subjects, which leaves them unable to judge the differences in accountants' skill levels." This brings to light the importance of educating yourself on at least the elementary aspects of accounting and financial management. It is critical that you at least know how to check into the background, references, and skill level of your CPA prospects. Do not allow your own inability to understand accounting procedures force you to "farm out accounting functions to anyone willing to perform those functions for a reasonable fee" (Edwards, 1992). Choosing your accountant wisely can, in a very real sense, make or break your practice. Remember, you are not simply hiring a "bookkeeper" but are partnering with a financial advisor. Viewing the agreement in this light will help you to avoid the pitfall of ineffectively defining the services contracted (Edwards, 1992). All contracts should have clearly defined terms and conditions and unambiguously define the services that will and will not be provided by your accountant.

Many small business owners make the mistake of waiting to contract accounting services until the end of the fiscal year when income tax time rolls around. This is an egregious error in judgment that may well end up costing you money or your business itself. Keeping your financial records in an organized manner will help you avoid the "shoe box syndrome" (Bacon, 1991). The shoe box syndrome occurs when financial records and receipts are mounded into an old shoebox until tax season arrives. This exposes your business to potential fiscal liability and short-circuits decision making throughout the year. For example, you cannot successfully track or control expenses if you do not know where your money is being spent.

Accountants can also help you to file the paperwork to obtain the licenses and permits that are necessary to begin your practice and, as discussed earlier, to advise you in matters of business structure including the potential tax benefits of each (Wolitzer and Wolitzer, 1991).

Ask potential accountants if they have represented other medical professionals. Accounting consultants who represent medical professionals face some unique challenges and have a degree of expertise that may not be required for other businesses. Financial consultants of medical professionals must, for example, be familiar with International

Classification of Diseases, Ninth Revision, Clinical Modification (ICD-9-CM) coding, billing third-party payers, malpractice insurance procedures, and referral patterns (Teitelman, 2005).

Tracking Expenses and Revenue

You must know where your money is coming from and where it is going. Expenses must be broken down into various categories. This facilitates an understanding of which expenses are variable and which expenses are fixed, that is, what expenses can be controlled with effective management and what expenses are costs of doing business.

Variable costs are those that fluctuate with sales and the volume of service provided. Examples of variable costs for your practice include hearing aids purchased for resale (cost of goods sold), employee bonuses, disposable supplies, etc. Estimating variable costs will be covered in depth later in the chapter. Fixed costs are costs that do not fluctuate as a function of volume. Examples of fixed costs include mortgage or rent payment, loan repayments, and utilities.

Expenses and revenue must be tracked by CPT code so that you can accurately assess reimbursement rates/revenues and expenses associated with each clinical service. Expenses and revenues should also be tracked by clinician, site, and referral source and over time (in monthly, quarterly, semi-annual, or annual epochs).

Tracking, along with cost accounting analysis, assesses the viability of clinical offerings and supports proposals for expansion (Sides, 2000). Sides recommends two steps that should be followed in order to institute cost accounting analysis.

1. Determine revenue and cost centers.
2. Calculate costs per procedure to evaluate operational cost efficiency.

Creating cost and revenue centers will help you to understand how cash is flowing into and out of your practice. This can also help you to determine which services should be developed and which are less cost effective. It will also help you to determine which services help to counterbalance the costs of services on which little revenue is generated or that are performed at a loss (Sides, 2000). Note that some services performed at a loss (i.e., loss leader) still serve a valuable function in that they may lead to more profitable services; for example, the revenue engendered by a hearing assessment may not cover all of its costs (direct and indirect) but may result in the dispensing of a hearing aid with an ensuing large profit margin.

Accounts Receivable and Aging Reports

Accounts receivable are monies that are owed to your practice by consumers and third-party payers. Collecting on receivables can be a difficult and time-consuming process but is critical to the success of your practice. The people to whom you owe money will not wait patiently for payment, and your bank account may become somewhat lean if you are not managing your accounts receivable.

One of the tools necessary when generating billing is an "aging report." Aging reports are typically generated on a monthly basis and show how long a patient's charges have been "on the books." It is a well-established fact that the longer an account is left unpaid, the less likely that you will actually collect on the debt. Many corporations have a cutoff date, such as 90 days past due, at which point they turn the account over to a collection agency. Some ways suggested by Graves (2004) to improve collection rates and reduce collection time include:

1. Offering small discounts as incentives to customers who pay in a timely manner
2. Assessing late fees for accounts that are delinquent
3. Generating an invoice and sending it to the customer earlier rather than later
4. Calling or making some other form of contact with the customer *before* the account is past due
5. Keeping detailed notes on each contact with the customer in case of litigation. This may also help to make appropriate credit decisions.

We also suggest decreasing the age of accounts receivable by focusing on "payment at the window." Be certain to accept all major credit cards as forms of payment. Although you will be assessed a fee for each transaction, the fee is negligible compared to the cost of trying to collect on past due accounts.

In addition to credit card payments, most states offer low interest rate loans for patients to purchase amplification. These loans are established to be easily affordable and may greatly reduce the financial stress associated with buying amplification. Many states also have vocational rehabilitation programs that will purchase amplification as a form of assistance to those with little or no income. Appropriate referral to these types of programs may not yield the return that would typically be generated by full private-pay transactions, but a certain amount of community service work is warranted.

Accounts Payable Report

Accounts payable is what you owe to other vendors or contracted services. Paying the bills in a timely fashion is obviously very important. Accounts payable must also be tracked. Should you fail to pay your debts in a timely manner, late fees can be assessed, and you risk damaging your credit. Paying your account in full at the end of each month might help you negotiate lower wholesale prices on products and services. The value of a strong reputation and good payment history should not be underestimated.

Statement of Assets and Liabilities

A statement of assets and liabilities, also known as a "balance sheet," is an assessment of the practice's financial health at a fixed point in time (Hosford-Dunn et al., 1995). According to Hosford-Dunn et al. (1995), assets are categorized into three subsets:

1. Current assets: Cash, accounts receivable, and inventory
2. Fixed assets: Land, buildings, equipment, furniture and fixtures, and vehicles

3. Intangible assets: Trademarks, copyrights, and goodwill

Figure 39.3 is an example of a balance sheet from CCH Business Owners Toolkit (http://www.toolkit.com/tools/bt.aspx?tid=balshe_m). CCH allows consumers to download the template, modify it as needed, and use it free of charge.

[Your Business Name] Balance Sheet [Mmmmm Dd, 2000x]			
Assets			
Current Assets:			
Cash		$0	
Accounts Receivable	$0		
Less: Reserve for Bad Debts	0	0	
Merchandise Inventory		0	
Prepaid Expenses		0	
Notes Receivable		0	
Total Current Assets			$0
Fixed Assets:			
Vehicles	0		
Less: Accumulated Depreciation	0	0	
Furniture and Fixtures	0		
Less: Accumulated Depreciation	0	0	
Equipment	0		
Less: Accumulated Depreciation	0	0	
Buildings	0		
Less: Accumulated Depreciation	0	0	
Land		0	
Total Fixed Assets			0
Other Assets:			
Goodwill		0	
Total Other Assets			0
Total Assets			$0
Liabilities and Capital			
Current Liabilities:			
Accounts Payable		$0	
Sales Taxes Payable		0	
Payroll Taxes Payable		0	
Accrued Wages Payable		0	
Unearned Revenues		0	
Short-Term Notes Payable		0	
Short-Term Bank Loan Payable		0	
Total Current Liabilities			$0
Long-Term Liabilities:			
Long-Term Notes Payable		0	
Mortgage Payable		0	
Total Long-Term Liabilities			0
Total Liabilities			0
Capital:			
Owner's Equity		0	
Net Profit		0	
Total Capital			0
Total Liabilities and Capital			$0

FIGURE 39.3 Sample balance sheet. (Reprinted with permission from Business Owner's Toolkit. [2005] Balance sheet template. Available at: www.toolkit.cch.com/tools/balshe_m.asp.)

Profit and Loss Statement

P&L statements are perhaps best known from the term "bottom line." The P&L shows positive or negative cash flow by month over the course of a year. The P&L statement is similar to the balance sheet except that it provides the benefit of allowing you to see business trends over an extended period of time. The longer your practice is in existence, the better you will be able to see the development of trends. One of the positive aspects of this is financial planning based on performance history. As a clinician-manager-owner, you can adjust your marketing activities in an attempt to boost sales in months that have traditionally been slow. We further suggest that, as soon as possible, the practice should focus on making more lasting changes through marketing to eliminate sharp increases and decreases in income. This will be addressed in more detail later.

SETTING FEES AND PRICES

Arguably, the most important decision that you will face as a new practice owner will be the determination of your fees and prices. Not only will this determine the public's perceived value of the products and services you provide, but it will also determine whether or not you remain in business. Several factors contribute to the prices and fees you set. Among them are the exclusivity of your service, the geographic location, the socioeconomic climate in which your practice is set, your level of expertise and experience, and the costs that you incur by providing the goods and services.

Some price determinants are intangible and must be assessed by reasoned judgment after getting to know the marketplace. It is critical to understand your market before you establish a practice. There are also tangible price determinants that must be taken into account. One factor that will help to determine your pricing is the competition in your area. Vendors are a good source of information about the prices being charged by competitors, but the wise practice owner will remember that those same vendors will most certainly share your pricing with your competitors as well.

A more tangible price determinant is the actual cost of providing your service. This is something that is frequently underestimated or not accounted for at all by novice clinicians. There are a multitude of expenses associated with providing services. Among these are the costs of your personnel including your own professional services, operating expenses including rent, utilities, cost of insurance, depreciation of the equipment, the cost of your money (i.e., loan repayments), the wholesale cost of goods sold, and your desired profit margin.

Figure 39.4 is a "Worksheet for Calculating Fees" provided by Whitmyer et al. (1989), as cited in Hosford-Dunn et al. (1995). Performing this exercise is illuminating. The result may surprise the novice clinician. It would not be unusual to discover that a small practice must collect, not just bill, *between $175.00 and $200.00 per hour when all costs and a reasonable profit margin are considered.* This will help determine your fee structure for all services that you render. For example, if you must collect $175.00 per hour and you estimate that the average adult hearing aid patient will require 3.5 hours of your time for assessment, fitting, follow-up visits, and counseling, you must factor $612.50 (3.5 hours × $175.00 hourly) of collections into the product price. This cost must be added to the cost of goods sold (wholesale price of the product) to arrive at the retail price. You'll notice that we have included some specific costs of doing business in our adaptation of the Whitmeyer et al. (1989) version of the worksheet. Although the original worksheet is highly detailed, we recommend setting up your own version in a computer spreadsheet so that it can be custom tailored to your practice.

Another component of pricing is a break-even analysis. Figure 39.5 from Hosford-Dunn et al. (1995) shows an example of a completed break-even analysis. The break-even analysis is a graphic demonstration of how many units of goods or services must be sold/completed in order to cover your operational costs. The break-even point occurs when you have neither made nor lost revenue. Any units sold or services provided above the break-even point yield profit that can be reinvested in the business, paid out as bonuses, or paid on the principle of loans.

To calculate the break-even point, you must first know the associated cost of each service provided. This is best accomplished by performing an evaluation of service by CPT code. Figure 39.6 is a list of common CPT codes. In Figure 39.7, you will notice that we first calculated the anticipated percentage of patients who were private pay versus Medicare or private insurance. After establishing the total percentage of the patient load assigned to each of those categories (i.e., "patient mix"), we then anticipated the expected reimbursement percentage from each of those sources. The Milliman USA report requisitioned by the American Speech-Language-Hearing Association (ASHA) in 2005 provides cost data for Medicare averages (McCarty, 2005). The Milliman USA report can be acquired for a nominal fee from ASHA. All test batteries were then broken down by CPT codes, which were grouped into procedures along with anticipated reimbursement levels. Figure 39.8 shows the total calculated reimbursement rate per service and reimbursement type. After total revenues were calculated, they were multiplied by a factor of 0.75 to account for *actual* collections. Remember, no matter how efficient your collections process is, you will *never* collect 100% of what is owed to you.

Another question that must be considered when setting up fee schedules is whether or not you will "bundle" your services. Bundling has traditionally been the choice of

WORKSHEET FOR CALCULATING FEES

1 Yearly Salary	$37,000	(Supply the salary you wish to earn)	
2a Days worked per month	22	(Supply the number of days you wish to work)	
2b Days worked per year	264	(Multiply 12 months by the number of days you work per month)	
3 Desired percent profit	12	(Supply the percent of profit you want)	

4 EXPENSES (Fill in the lines below for your expenses)
Operating Overhead Office Expenses

Rent	$2,300.00	x 12 =	$27,600.00
Office Help	$2,100.00	x 12 =	$25,200.00
Postage	$100.00	x 12 =	$1,200.00
Telephone	$80.00	x 12 =	$960.00
Utilities	$190.00	x 12 =	$2,280.00
Office Supplies	$75.00	x 12 =	$900.00
Repairs/Maint.	$350.00	x 12 =	$4,200.00
Subtotal	$5,195.00	x 12 =	$58,140.00

Support Services

Insurance	$30.00	x 12 =	$360.00
Marketing	$500.00	x 12 =	$6,000.00
Legal/Accounting	$300.00	x 12 =	$3,600.00
Other	$40.00	x 12 =	$480.00
Subtotal	$870.00	x 12 =	$10,440.00

Additional Expenses

Equip. Loan Pmt	$1,200.00	x 12 =	$14,400.00
DLOC Payment	$1,500.00	x 12 =	$18,000.00
Tuition Reimbur.	$1,200.00	x 12 =	$14,400.00
Business Travel	$100.00	x 12 =	$1,200.00
Licenses / Dues	$60.00	x 12 =	$720.00
Miscellaneous	$40.00	x 12 =	$480.00
Subtotal	$4,100.00	x 12 =	$49,200.00

5 Total expenses (Add the expense figures and put total here)

Monthly	$15,135.00	Annual	$177,420.00

6 Daily Overhead	$672.05	(Divide total yearly expenses by number of days worked per year)
7 Daily Salary	$140.15	(Divide total yearly salary by number of days worked per year)
8 Revenue Requirement	$812.20	(Sum of Daily Overhead (6) and Daily Salary (7).)
9 Daily Profit	$97.46	(multiply Desired Percent Profit (3) by Revenue Requirement(8) and divide by 100.)
10 Required Billing Rate	$909.66	(Add Daily Overhead (6), Daily Salary (7), and Daily Profit (9).)
11 Equivalent Hourly Rate	$101.07	(Divide Required Billing Rate by the number of billable hours worked per day).

FIGURE 39.4 Worksheet for calculating fees. (Reprinted with permission from Whitmyer C, Rasberry S, Phillips M. [1989] *Running a One Person Business.* **Berkeley, CA: Ten Speed Press.)**

dispensing audiologists. The benefit of bundling diagnostic and follow-up care costs into the hearing aid price is simplicity. Another consideration, however, is that bundling diminishes the patient's perception of the "value" of your professional services. The hearing aid becomes the focal point of the transaction.

Some audiologists are now unbundling pricing. Unbundling not only takes the focus off of the piece of plastic in the patient's ear, but also allows the audiologist to recover expenses associated with patients who require more than the "average" follow-up care. Unbundling may help the patient appreciate your professional services as distinct from the product.

Some audiologists use a hybrid of bundling and unbundling in which a given number of follow-up visits are included in the original price of the hearing aid. For patients who do not choose to purchase amplification, billing for audiologic evaluation is priced separately. There are many ways in which hybridization of bundling and unbundling can be achieved. It is up to you as the owner-manager-clinician to

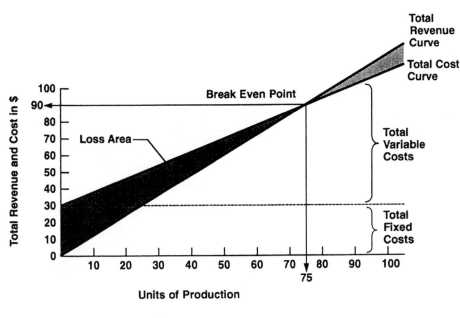

FIGURE 39.5 Break-even analysis. (Reprinted with permission from Hosford-Dunn H, Dunn DR, Harford ER. [1995] *Audiology Business and Practice Management.* **San Diego: Singular.)**

choose a pricing structure that is best suited to the needs of your practice and your patients.

Choosing a price and fee structure also requires you to have at least a rudimentary understanding of the supply and demand curve for your market. If your pricing is too high, you will obviously achieve a higher profit margin but most likely have fewer patients. If your pricing is too low, you will draw many patients but will make very little margin on each hearing aid dispensed or service provided. In this scenario, you and your staff will work very hard for minimum return on investment. That is, what you give up in price, you must make up in volume.

Other considerations related to the demand curve are that of marginal cost and marginal profit (Hosford-Dunn et al., 1995). Marginal cost can best be explained with the example of hearing aids. Imagine that the cost of goods sold (COGS) for a single hearing aid is $400.00 and your other fixed costs are $700.00. Your total cost then is $1,100.00 to dispense that hearing aid. When you dispense two hearing aids to a patient, the fixed costs remain the same, but the COGS doubles (Hosford-Dunn et al., 1995). Other fixed costs can change as the practice expands and more staff is required to meet the demand. This is a good example of why costs and pricing must be reviewed on a regular basis.

There are several general pricing strategies that can be used. Among them are: Economy, Skimming, Penetration, and Premium (marketingteacher.com, 2005). These are graphically represented in Figure 39.9, which depicts "Price" with the qualitative descriptors of "high" and "low" on the x-axis and "Quality" with the same qualitative descriptors on the y-axis (marketingteacher.com, 2005). If the product quality and the price point are low, it is an economy pricing strategy that is designed to drive business in the door. As discussed previously, this will result in high-volume, low-profit sales. When the quality is low and the price is high, it

is referred to as "market skimming." We do not recommend either of these two strategies as a general rule because either of them can, and probably will, quickly destroy your practice. When quality is high and the price is low, one is attempting to achieve market penetration. While this strategy will drive patients to your practice, the cost to the practice can be overwhelming if not carefully controlled. This type of strategy is frequently employed during a marketing push and will result in a sharp short-lived spike in sales. As stated previously, it may well prove to be a myopic strategy that adds no real long-term growth to the practice. Used carefully, however, it can be an effective marketing tool. The final general pricing strategy is premium pricing. Premium pricing offers high-quality products at high prices. This general strategy can be effective depending upon your market. In some geographic regions, paying top dollar for a product is a status symbol and helps the patient to feel that he or she is getting the most for his or her money. Figure 39.10 was adapted from Hosford-Dunn et al. (1995) and summarizes additional pricing strategies.

In regards to pricing, most people are probably not "purists." Most business owners employ some combination of these strategies or maintain a carefully calculated equilibrium between two or three of them.

One thing that the novice practitioner must bear in mind is that antitrust laws prohibit price fixing. Price fixing is a form of collusion in which pricing is fixed by a large number of service providers. This stems the competitive nature of the market (McCarty, 2005). The Milliman USA actuarial analysis requested by ASHA provides a summary of average costs of audiologic service and product fees. It cannot be used to determine pricing but might be referred to in order to ascertain how your pricing structure compares to the national average (McCarty, 2005). Again, the reader is ***strongly cautioned*** to avoid any behavior that could be construed as price fixing.

CPT Codes and Reimbursement Rates

Type	CPT Code	Test	Charge	M-Care	Private Ins.	60% Un-Ins.
ENG	92541	Spontaneous Nystagmus Test	$115.00	$32.77	$46.00	$69.00
	92542	Positional Nystagmus Test	$142.00	$29.19	$56.80	$85.20
	92543	Caloric Irrigation (per unit)	$70.00	$10.35	$28.00	$42.00
	92544	Optokinetic Nystagmus Test	$64.00	$16.83	$25.60	$38.40
	92545	Oscillating Tracking Test	$70.00	$23.34	$28.00	$42.00
	92547	Vertical Electrodes w/ above	$63.00	$22.05	$25.20	$37.80
	92584	Electrocochleography	$280.00	$98.00	$112.00	$168.00
	97110	Epley Maneuver	$51.00	$17.85	$20.40	$30.60
	97550	Physical Performance Test	$58.00	$20.30	$23.20	$34.80
ABR	92585	Brainstem Evoked Responses	$343.00	$117.45	$137.20	$171.50
Peripheral	92587	OAE - limited	$166.00	$61.98	$66.40	$99.60
Diagnostic	92567	Tympanograms	$59.00	$22.19	$23.60	$35.40
	92568	Acoustic Reflexes	$43.00	$15.69	$17.20	$25.80
	92579	Visual Reinforced Audiometry	$80.00	$29.84	$32.00	$48.00
	92582	Conditioned Play Audiometry	$72.00	$29.84	$28.80	$43.20
	92552	Basic Audio (air)	$51.00	$18.36	$20.40	$30.60
	92553	Basic Audio (air & bone)	$74.00	$27.16	$29.60	$44.40
	92555	Speech Audiometry Threshold	$43.00	$15.69	$17.20	$25.80
	92556	SAT with Speech Recognition	$64.00	$24.10	$25.60	$38.40
	92557	Comprehensive Audiometry	$135.00	$49.35	$54.00	$81.00
	92583	Picture SRT	$60.25	$36.73	$44.07	$36.15
	92599	Tinnitus Evaluation	$100.00	$35.00	$40.00	$60.00
Hearing	92590	HAE and selection (monaural)	$285.00	$0.00	$114.00	$171.00
Aids	92591	HAE and selection (binaural)	$570.00	$0.00	$228.00	$342.00
	92592	HA Check (monaural)	$40.00	$0.00	$16.00	$24.00
	92593	HA Check (binaural)	$55.00	$0.00	$22.00	$33.00
	29594	Electroacoustic Eval of HA (mon)	$38.00	$0.00	$15.20	$22.80
	19595	Electroacoustic Eval of HA (bin)	$56.00	$0.00	$22.40	$33.60
	69210	Cerumen Removal	$30.00	$0.00	$12.00	$18.00
	v5010	Assessment of HA	$285.00	$0.00	$114.00	$171.00
	v5011	HA Fitting/Orientation	$200.00	$0.00	$80.00	$120.00
	v5014	HA repair/Modification	$29.00	$0.00	$11.60	$17.40
	v5020	Conformity Evaluation	$75.00	$0.00	$30.00	$45.00
	v5090	Dispensing fee, unspecified HA	$250.00	$75.00	$100.00	$150.00
	v5160	Dispensing fee, binaural	$250.00	$115.00	$100.00	$150.00
	v5299	Earmold, single	$55.00	$16.00	$22.00	$33.00
	v5299	Earmold, binaural	$110.00	$32.00	$44.00	$66.00
	v5299	Swim molds	$75.00	$0.00	$30.00	$45.00
		HA Cost/per unit	$2,000.00	$400.00	$800.00	$1,200.00
APD	92589	APD Test (per test)	$60.00	$22.57	$24.00	$36.00
Testing	92576	Synthetic Sentence Identification	$30.00	$10.00	$12.00	$18.00

FIGURE 39.6   Sample Current Procedural Terminology (CPT) codes.

PURCHASING PRODUCTS FOR RESALE

It has been said that success in business is dependent *not on how well you sell, but on how well you buy.* There are many purchasing options, each with associated benefits and detriments. It is important that you understand the perquisites and pitfalls associated with each so that you are well informed when negotiating wholesale prices.

One of the options available to you is to join a buying group in order to take advantage of the buying power associated with mass quantity purchasing. Buying groups offer discount pricing due to cooperative purchasing. Most offer various other "membership benefits."

Expected Pay Rates Per Patient Type & Annual Billings

	% Patients:	M-Care 40%	Private 58%	Un-Ins*** 2%

AE OM Pt.*	Protocol	M-Care	Private	Un-Ins
OAE	92587	$61.98	$66.40	$99.60
Tymp.	92567	$22.19	$23.60	$35.40
Reflexes	92568	$15.69	$17.20	$25.80
CPA Audio	92582	$29.84	$28.80	$43.20
SAT	92555	$15.69	$17.20	$25.80
CPA Total:		$145.39	$153.20	$229.80

Predicted total Patients / Yr			43
M-Caid	17 x	$145.39 =	$2,471.63
Private	25 x	$153.20 =	$3,830.00
Un-Insured	1 x	$229.80 =	$229.80
Expected Gross from CPA AE:			**$6,531.43**

*AE OM Pt. = Auditory Assessment for patient with Otitis Media

	% Patients:	M-Caid 35%	Private 35%	Un-Ins 30%

AE HA Pt.*	Protocol	M-Care	Private	Un-Ins
OAE	92587	$61.98	$66.40	$99.60
Tymp	92567	$22.19	$23.60	$35.40
Reflexes	92568	$15.69	$17.20	$25.80
Comp. Audio	92557	$49.35	$54.00	$81.00
AE Total:		$149.21	$161.20	$241.80

Predicted total Patients / Yr			435
M-Care	152 x	$149.21 =	$22,679.92
Private	152 x	$161.20 =	$24,502.40
Un-Insured	131 x	$241.80 =	$31,675.80
Expected Gross from AE:			**$78,858.12**

*AE HA Pt. = Auditory Assessment for patient requiring Hearing Aids

HA Sales Pt	M-Care	Private	Un-Ins.
HA Sale	$800.00	$1,600.00	$2,400.00
v5299	$32.00	$44.00	$66.00
v5160	$115.00	$100.00	$150.00
19595	$0.00	$22.40	$33.60
Total:	$947.00	$1,766.40	$2,649.60

Predicted total Patients / Yr			121
M-Care	23 x	$947.00 =	$21,781.00
Private	30 x	$1,766.00 =	$52,980.00
Un-Insured	1 x	$2,649.60 =	$2,649.60
Expected Gross from HA:			**$77,410.60**

HA Pt	M-Care	Private	Un-Ins.
92593	$0.00	$22.00	$33.00
19595	$0.00	$22.40	$33.60
Total:	$0.00	$44.40	$66.60

Predicted total Patients / Yr			121
M-Care	46 x	$0.00 =	$0.00
Private	60 x	$44.40 =	$2,664.00
Un-Insured	2 x	$66.60 =	$133.20
Expected Gross from HA F/U:			**$2,797.20**

*** These titles refer to the following:

M-Care	Medicare or Medicaid patient
Private	Patient who has private insurance
Un-Ins	Patient with no insurance who will pay out-of-pocket

FIGURE 39.7 Sample of estimated reimbursements.

Benefits include assistance with marketing, practice management, business training, patient referral, practice valuation, and human resources management. These services can be an asset to the novice entrepreneur. Other benefits associated with buying groups are "greenhouse seminars," which are designed to increase the business acumen of the professional.

There are, however, other considerations to take into account before choosing to participate in any of the buying groups. Each of the buying groups purports to allot a certain amount of profit and membership dues to marketing in order to increase sales and raise public awareness of hearing loss. The critical reader will note that we did not say that these buying groups intend to promote audiology, per se.

Gross Billings Per Year

OM AE CPA	$6,531.43
OM AE	$1,450.80
HAE	$31,675.80
HA Sales	$77,410.60
HA F/U	$2,797.20
APD	$22,730.79
ABR	$47,822.96
ENG	$160,640.36

Total Gross Billings: **$351,059.94**

Expect to collect about .75 of total Billings   75%

Total Collected Billings/ Profit: **$263,294.96**

Figure Legend

OM AE CPA		Conditioned Play Auditory Assessment for patient with otitis media
HAE		Hearing Aid Evaluation Testing
HA Sales		Revenue from sale of hearing aids
HA F/U		Ancillary Accessory Sales from Hearing Aid follow up
APD		Auditory Processing Disorder Evaluation
ABR		Neurodiagnostic / Tone Burst Threshold Search ABR
ENG		Electronystagmography / Vestibular assessment

FIGURE 39.8 Sample of gross billings sheet.

Only one of the buying groups currently sells exclusively to audiologists. Groups like this are more likely to promote the profession of audiology. Some buying groups also maintain company-owned stores that could become direct competitors in your region. By buying from them, you are helping the competition to thrive.

A second purchasing option is to buy through a wholesaler. Wholesalers offer discount pricing based on quantity purchasing in much the same manner as the buying groups. One of the negative aspects of buying through wholesalers is that they will sell directly to anyone, including selling directly to patients over the internet. This is only problematic in that patients can "price shop" and will fail to consider the fact that part of the price of hearing aids is the cost of your expertise.

Finally, one may choose to buy directly from manufacturers. As mentioned previously, it is in your best interest to negotiate a pricing structure that will allow you to maximize profits while delivering quality service that your customers will perceive as a good value. One method of reducing prices is to create volume discounts for yourself. For this reason, it is wise to choose two to three vendors only. This will allow you the flexibility of finding products to fit any patient, while developing greater expertise with each product line.

In the grand scheme of things, there is relatively little difference between vendors or product lines from a technical standpoint. Most of the major vendors provide similar product lines with similar features despite claims to the contrary. With a few possible exceptions, the product quality at a given price point is essentially equivalent. The major deciding factors that will determine the vendors you choose are: the manufacturer's research and development initiatives, the reputation of the manufacturer for quality product lines, and most importantly, the company's customer service to you. We often think of the quality of service that we provide our patients, and we are no less entitled to excellent customer service from manufacturers. Once you have

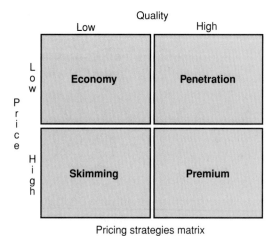

Pricing strategies matrix

FIGURE 39.9 Pricing matrix. (Reprinted with permission from Marketingteacher.com. [2005] Pricing strategies. Available at: http://marketingteacher.com/Lessons/lesson_pricing.htm.)

Pricing Approach	Bundling	Unbundling	Time-period Pricing	Image Pricing	Value-added price packages	Pay-one Price	Constant promotional pricing	Captive Pricing	Product Line
Example	Combining services into a grouped package at discounted rates	Charging for each service or product individually	Purchases which include a trial period	Pricing based upon high quality image.	Free services included in purchase. "Gift-with" purchases.	Unlimited access to services at a flat rate	No one ever pays the "regular" price which is set as a point to increase perceived discount	Sell the product nearly at cost and make margin on "add-on" value services	Use a non-linear multiplier to increase margin of entry level products while offering the quality of higher end products. Encourages customers to purchase entry level where margin is greatest.
As Applied to Audiology	Not charging for audiometric testing if the patient purchases hearing aids	Charging for each component of testing / amplification at individual rates	Free hearing screen during "May is Better Speech / Hearing Month"	High end digital hearing aids at high prices	Free office visits for a year with purchase of hearing aids	Free follow-up visits for the life of the hearing aid	Discount on all hearing aid sales	Free hearing test to promote hearing aid sales	Higher margin on entry level digital hearing aids while still offering highest end digital hearing aids.

FIGURE 39.10   Pricing strategies comparison. (Adapted from Hosford-Dunn H, Dunn DR, Harford ER. [1995] *Audiology Business and Practice Management.* **San Diego: Singular; Fig. 14-5.)**

chosen your manufacturers, it is important to keep records of the frequency of repair requests, the speed with which repaired hearing aids are returned to you, and the overall quality of repair work. Tracking your repairs is as important as any other tracking, and a simple computer spreadsheet can be established in order to facilitate record retrieval for analysis.

MARKETING YOUR PRACTICE

Marketing can simply be defined as anything you do to grow your practice. As we have discussed earlier in this chapter, it is important that *audiologists understand that they are not marketing a product but a service.* In the words of Beckwith (1997), audiologists are "selling the invisible."

Beckwith (1997) states, "the core of service marketing is the service itself." Beckwith stresses the importance of a continuous focus on service in a service-dominated business such as audiology. This is not to suggest that using multiple media and marketing strategies is unimportant, but simply that these marketing activities are secondary to "marketing management." Marketing management is the process of creating and following a specific marketing plan to *maximize your opportunities to provide excellent service.* Remember that service is of paramount importance. "First, before you write an ad, rent a [mailing] list, dash off a press release – fix your service" (Beckwith, 1997). Providing excellent customer service will ensure positive "word of mouth" advertising that is worth far more than all other forms of marketing com-

bined. Remember, each time you see a patient, you have a "marketing moment."

Media Marketing

Once you are satisfied that your service is at a good initial level (again, we stress that service is dynamic and should be under constant evaluation), you are ready to begin marketing in the more traditional sense. There are several media that can be chosen as marketing tools. These include: newspaper, radio, television, direct mail, website advertising, open house events, e-mail to existing patients, and free public seminars.

When choosing a form of media, there are several considerations to be taken into account. First, you must consider your market. In some areas, television may be the most cost-effective means of reaching the largest portion of your target market, whereas in other markets, newspaper may be the media of choice. This brings us back to the idea of being familiar with your target market and knowing the habits of your potential customers. Next, you must be familiar with the concept of "shelf-life." Shelf-life refers to how long the media will remain in circulation. Obviously a newspaper advertisement's shelf-life is 1 day. An ad in the yellow pages of the telephone directory has a shelf-life of approximately 1 year. Typically, advertising space is purchased in blocks with price breaks depending on the number and placement of promotions; the more you buy, the lower the cost.

A third consideration for your marketing plan will be the media mix for a given advertising campaign. Iacobucci et al. (2002) studied marketing strategies to help ameliorate the negative image associated with hearing aids. The study used three types of messages in a marketing campaign. The three types of messages were categorized as "warm and emotional," "educational," and "wedge of doubt" (Iacobucci et al., 2002). Emotional appeal messages are those intended to direct the market subject's attention to the difficulty and frustration caused to those closest to the individual with hearing loss. Educational messages are intended to provide information regarding the necessity of annual hearing checkups, and "wedge of doubt" messages bring to the fore the fact that those with hearing loss may choose to deny it or suggest that others might feel that "you've lost your mental edge." The messages were delivered in multiple combinations through mixed mass media, such as television and print ads, and through direct telemarketing and direct mailings, also known as "private media" (Iacobucci et al., 2002). The best combination of messages and media style was the "wedge of doubt" message through private media. The authors hypothesize that private media may produce the best results due to the public's opinion that hearing aids are an "embarrassing product." The second best combination was the "warm and emotional" message delivered through private media. This is not to suggest that these are the best messages and media choices in all markets and circumstances. It simply demonstrates the need to know your market and to give due diligence to these considerations.

The same authors completed another study in 2003 that investigated hearing aids as an "embarrassing product" in relation to other medical services. A strong negative stigma was clearly associated with hearing aids. The authors demonstrated several reasons why hearing aid candidates do not purchase hearing aids. In rank order from most to least common, these reasons include: denial of need, cost of consultation, lack of interest in hearing aids, and a negative previous experience with hearing aids (Iacobucci et al., 2003). This study also showed that the same patients were more willing to use other assistive interventions such as eyeglasses, pain relievers, and canes than to use hearing aids. These results exemplify other research and anecdotal data that have been known to audiologists for many years. The authors then examined the impact of advertisement and advice from physicians on the individual's buying intention. It was shown that, although advertising did enhance the consumer's opinions about hearing aids, it did not change purchasing behaviors. Advice from physicians and increased physical need were the two factors that demonstrated a statistically significant impact on purchasing intentions (Iacobucci et al., 2003).

Sergei Kochkin has been conducting a longitudinal study of the hearing aid market and consumer opinions toward amplification for many years. The data collected and the wealth of conclusions and inferences that can be drawn from this large pool of data are not to be overlooked when considering your marketing strategy. We refer you to a list of Kochkin's published works at http://www.picosearch.com/cgi-bin/ts.pl?index=211668&query=Market+Trak. The key points of Kochkin's work are too numerous to cover in this chapter. It is important to note that Kochkin's surveys are mailed to 20,000 homes that are known to be representative of the United States (Kochkin, 1990). Furthermore, Kochkin uses the PRIZM system to segment the market into 40 distinct neighborhood subtypes. The data in Kochkin's extensive publications are invaluable in determining your market subtype and in assisting you in understanding which marketing media is most appropriate for your particular market. In the article entitled "Introducing MarkeTrak: A Consumer Tracking Survey of the Hearing Instrument Market," Kochkin (1990) presents a series of tables that outline activities, census/demographic information, media habits, and magazine preferences of hearing instrument users versus nonusers. This is just one of the many valuable pieces of information to be obtained from the MarkeTrak series.

Physician Referral Marketing

This brings us to another method of marketing your practice. Successful practitioners often market their practice directly to primary care physicians. Kochkin's (2005) data demonstrate the fact that the number of physicians performing hearing screenings for their patients has decreased over the past 20 years. Currently, only 12.9% of physicians are performing any form of hearing screening. Kochkin (2005) makes multiple recommendations for increasing the number of physicians performing hearing screenings. Chief among them is the suggestion to provide a satisfactory screening tool to physicians. Kochkin further notes that the Better Hearing Institute's "Physician Referral Program," which did not include an actual screening tool, did create a modest increase in physician referrals in the early 1990s. This should provide sufficient inducement to the audiologist to foster positive relationships with primary care physicians and otolaryngologists as potential referral sources.

One might be tempted to believe that marketing to physicians is "free." After completing the worksheet for calculating fees discussed earlier in this chapter, you will realize that your time is most decidedly not free. Still, physicians are an excellent source of referrals and should be included in the comprehensive marketing plan.

Public Education Seminars

An additional marketing strategy is to provide public education seminars. These advertised events can draw many potential patients to your practice. We have employed this method of marketing and achieved very positive results. Not only are you drawing more patients to your practice, but you are also providing valuable education to the public about the services that audiologists provide. These seminars should be educational in nature with ample time for individual

Retail sales from Promotion		$30,000.00
20 units at $1500.00 each		
Cost of Promotion		
20 units @ $600.00 each		$12,000.00
Advertisement		$1,200.00
Total Cost of Promotion		**$13,200.00**
ROP Calculation		$30,000.00
		($13,200.00)
		$16,800.00
Product		$16,800.00
Divided by cost of promotion		÷ $13,200.00
		1.27
		x 100
		127%

FIGURE 39.11   Sample return on promotion (ROP) calculation.

questions from the attendees. Typically, these sessions are not focused on specific products, and no "selling" occurs. Those attendees interested in acquiring additional information can make an appointment to visit the clinic for an audiologic assessment. It is reasonable to perform this type of marketing activity three or four times per year. Choosing a venue is an important component of these seminars. Hotels often have conference rooms that can be rented at reasonable rates. Choose an attractive venue that is within a reasonable driving distance of your practice site(s). Offering simple refreshments is a good idea.

Bearing in mind the fact that these seminars are a marketing tool, it is wise to track the return on promotion for future reference. In order to do this, you will need to calculate all costs, including rental of the conference room, clinician time, refreshments, and advertising costs. An appointment book should be taken to the seminar in order to schedule appointments for those who express an interest without inconveniencing the patients by forcing them to call the office to schedule a visit. Offering a door prize allows you to capture potential patient names for your database. It is also a good practice to send a follow-up letter to all attendees to thank them and to invite them to contact you with any questions they may have.

No matter which promotional strategies you choose to employ, it is important to estimate the cost of the activity. Knowing the cost is important not only for planning, but also for calculating the "return on promotion" (Staab, 2000). Return on promotion (ROP) is a means of calculating the efficacy of a given promotion. ROP can be estimated before a given marketing campaign and then recalculated based upon actual data after the promotion. To calculate ROP, simply estimate the retail sales less all costs involved in generating the sales and then divide the result by the cost of the

sale. An example is provided in Figure 39.11. ROP can be based on daily, weekly, monthly, or cyclic sales (Staab, 2000). Of course, in order to gather the required data, it will be necessary to track referrals generated from each promotion.

When writing copy for promotions, it is vital to consider your image. You need to be mindful of "branding" when promoting your practice. Branding is making your name synonymous with better hearing health care. Frequently, novice practitioners encounter the pitfall of marketing a product rather than service. We do not recommend tying the name of your practice to any one brand of product. If, for example, you make a strong public association between your practice and a given manufacturer and that manufacturer is the recipient of some negative publicity, it may well impact your practice. Focus your marketing efforts on excellent service and professional hearing health care.

In-House Marketing

The receptionist is the first impression of your practice that most patients will encounter. The old adage that states "you never get a second chance to make a first impression" is particularly important in business. This means that choosing the correct person to work as your receptionist is critical. Training your receptionist is of paramount importance. Until the receptionist is fully trained, prepared "scripts" may be in order. Scripts help the receptionist to know exactly what to say and how to reply to patient comments and questions.

Using reception staff to the fullest extent possible can be very rewarding. The cost of reception staff is considerably less than the cost of an audiologist. Therefore, it behooves you to train your receptionist to perform basic skills such as cleaning or performing minor repairs to hearing aids. The ability to affect basic repairs in-house is a huge benefit to the patient and will help to shape the patient's perception of your practice. Reception staff should also be trained in the sale of basic supplies, warranties, and assistive listening devices. Providing incentives for selling supplies, batteries, accessories, assistive listening devices, warranties, appointment bookings, and repairs can help to encourage better service for your patients and to motivate the receptionist to continue to learn about the practice.

Coordination of Marketing Activities

Timing is important when planning marketing activities. An example of poor timing would include doing a massive advertising campaign every month of the year. This may confound tracking and calculation of ROP. Saturation marketing can become stale and lose its impact. At the other end of the spectrum, planning two large-scale marketing pushes a year may not provide sufficient market penetration and will interfere with your ability to brand your service. It is important to understand seasonal fluctuations in the market and to advertise accordingly. A well-timed advertisement can take advantage of natural fluctuations in sales. Again, we emphasize the importance of creating a marketing plan for the entire year. Remember, marketing is not limited to ad copy. You may decide to make telephone contact with every patient within 24 hours of being fit with amplification. Activities such as this are as much a part of your marketing plan as is a block of television or radio time.

As your practice grows and your marketing plan becomes more involved, it will be advantageous to employ a marketing manager on a part-time basis. Marketing managers should be well versed in marketing and should be eager and willing to learn about marketing for audiology practices. Finding a marketing manager who has experience in marketing medical practices may be useful, but you should plan to allow time for the individual to learn about audiology. It is important that your marketing manager understand audiology well enough to be able to explain your services to a physician or to a layperson. Paying a marketing manager may seem to be a significant investment, but it is important that you remember the value of your time. Bringing in a marketing manager is essentially no different than hiring an attorney or accountant. You are contracting with a specialist for expert advice and direction. The marketing manager employed by our audiology clinics devised and implemented a marketing strategy to eliminate sharp transient dips in sales and to create long-term linear growth. The new marketing plan incorporated public education seminars and direct marketing to primary care physicians.

Providing incentives for patient referrals is another means of encouraging word of mouth referrals. For example, you can offer a year's supply of batteries to the referring patient. Alternately, you may provide a free year of extended warranty if the patient refers at least three patients to your clinic. These incentives are relatively inexpensive to you but are a great value to the patient. Remember, the greatest incentive for a patient is excellent service. Another reminder: If your marketing isn't working, work on your service (Beckwith, 1997).

■ THE RIGHT PLACE AT THE RIGHT TIME

Choosing a location and site for your practice is one of the first steps in preparing your business plan. An important consideration in choosing a location is to determine where you would like to live and practice. Being content with the city or town in which you live and practice is not inconsequential (Hosford-Dunn et al., 1995). Remember, the whole purpose of owning a practice is to create a comfortable lifestyle for yourself and your family.

Several factors will need to be considered. These include the competition in the area, demographics, potential referral sources, population growth, the cost of doing business, and many others. All of these are outlined in the accompanying figures.

When considering potential locations, it is wise to create a comparison chart to help you sort out the pros and cons for the geographic regions under consideration (Windmill et al., 2000). Understand that location should be broken down into three main categories: "macro-location," "micro-location," and "site" (Windmill et al., 2000).

Macro-location refers to the larger geographic region. Windmill et al. (2000) have provided a comparison chart, an adapted version of which is shown in Figure 39.12. Some of the items in the chart focus on the personal amenities in the region, and some focus on business factors such as competition, population changes, cost of doing business, cost of living, etc. Once you have chosen a geographic region, you will want to focus on the micro-location. Figure 39.13 is adapted from Windmill et al. (2000). Use it to compare three or more potential communities.

Choosing a specific site is the next step. Consider the convenience of the location to your patient base. How accessible is the site? Is the site close to anchor points and referral sources? Anchor points are major landmarks that make finding your practice easier.

Cost of the site is a major consideration. This is not to suggest that the least expensive site is always the best choice. Rather, it is a matter of value. In much the same way that our patients assign value to our services, you will need to decide whether the cost of the site will be justified by growth potential, patient convenience, and even your "image." You will need to discuss the costs of finishing the commercial site if the option exists; this is known as "build-out" or "leasehold improvements." Commercial realtors may give an allowance for build-outs or amortize these costs in your monthly lease. Other costs that will need to be considered are Common Area Maintenance (CAM) fees. Snow removal, security, building maintenance, and lawn care are examples of CAM services.

Choosing a macro-location

Competition			
Regional Economic Outlook			
Main Industries			
Unemployment Rate			
Overall Population			
Target Population as a Percent of Overall Population			
Population Growth			
Health Insurance Trends			
Healthcare Trends			
Population Diversity			
Access to Higher Education			
Public Transportation			
Shopping and Entertainment			
Estimated Economic Potential			
Per Capita Income			
Disposable Income			
Proximity to Family and Friends			
Housing Costs			
Taxes			
School Systems			
Climate			
Proximity to Places of Worship			
Amenities			
Cost of Living			
Recreational Opportunities			
Licensure Laws			
Other			

*Rate each area on a scale of 1 to 10 with one being least favorable and 10 being most favorable. Total the points for each region.

FIGURE 39.12 Macro-location comparison chart. (Reprinted with permission from Windmill IM, Cunningham DR, Johnson KC. [2000] Designing an audiology practice. In: Hosford-Dunn H, Roeser R, Valente M, eds. *Audiology Practice Management.* **New York: Thieme; pp 291–311.)**

This should be clearly outlined in the lease. Before signing any lease, you need to know the term (length) of the lease, the cost per square foot, estimated utility bills, sublease options, etc. (Hosford-Dunn et al., 1995). Consult your attorney before signing a lease agreement.

This brings us to space requirements. We believe that investing in space and site is more important than investing in equipment. After all, you can upgrade equipment a lot easier than you can change your site/space. If you are planning for the eventual expansion of your practice but do not need the space immediately, consider subleasing to other professionals such as a speech-language pathologist or a physical therapist. A fuller treatment of space needs will be given later in this chapter.

As your practice grows, you may find that there are opportunities to expand to another site. You will need to complete a new demographic analysis in order to determine the appropriateness of opening a satellite facility. We caution you to complete a new business plan that includes the proposed site. Pay particular attention to the cost of expansion as well as return on investment. The satellite site should be far enough away from your current site so that you are not merely relocating your current patients from one office to the next. Study the demographics of the proposed satellite site carefully. Literally draw a 5-mile radius around the current and proposed sites, look for overlap, and try to avoid it as much as possible. Experience has shown that typical consumers prefer to travel in a 5-mile radius around a "home base" in order to receive services in an urban location. Patients in rural settings are accustomed to travel much farther to receive services.

■ DESIGNING AN OFFICE

Whether you are having a practice built or redesigning leased space, the first things you must consider are patient and practitioner comfort, safety, patient flow, and HIPAA privacy issues. Safety issues can be addressed by reducing the distance patients must walk. Long distances and/or stairs could be problematic for elderly patients or patients with vestibular disorders. Floor coverings can also pose a safety risk. Carpets that are not secure can create a fall risk. Keeping patient files confidential is paramount. Deciding where patient charts will be stored is not only an HIPAA consideration, but also a matter of ease of accessibility for your office personnel. An investment that will help you to lay out your office space is a Computer-Aided Design (CAD) software package. If you are leasing a space that is already defined, you might need to reconfigure the space in order to accommodate patient flow, HIPAA considerations, and patient safety. If you are building a new facility, this becomes even more important so that you can estimate the number of square feet needed and have a rough draft blueprint before you begin searching

Evaluating Community Potential

FAMILY LIVING	Community 1	Community 2	Community 3
Nice Residential Area			
Housing Availablity			
Property Taxes			
Schools			
Parks and Recreation Areas			
Proximity to Amenities			
Cultural Activities are Available			
Shopping			
Progressive Community			
General Appeal of the Community			
Climate / Weather			
Proximity to Family and Friends			
Availability of Work for Significant Other			
Place of Worship is Available			
Subtotal of Points for Family Living			

Professional Considerations	Community 1	Community 2	Community 3
Eligibility for Licensure			
Commercial Property is Available and Desirable			
Availability of Potential Personnel			
Hospitals and Healthcare Providers Opinions			
Continuing Education is Available and Costly			
Collaboration with other Audiologists is Viable			
Referral Sources can be Obtained			
A niche is open			
SWOT analysis is reasonably positive			
Subtotal for Professional Consierations			

Economic Potential	Community 1	Community 2	Community 3
Population Increases are Likely			
Audiologist to Target Market Population is Favorable			
Income Level / Disposable Income is High			
Retail Sales Show Steady Growth			
Industry is Stable and Growing			
Local Residents Look Favorably on Addition of Audiologist			
Potential for Business and Referral Contacts			
Accessibility to HMO, PPO Contracts Exists			
Favorable Patient Mix Exists			
Unemployment Rate is Low			
Subtotal for Economic Potential			
Grand Total			

FIGURE 39.13 Micro-location comparison. (Reprinted with permission from Windmill IM, Cunningham DR, Johnson KC. [2000] Designing an audiology practice. In: Hosford-Dunn H, Roeser R, Valente M, eds. *Audiology Practice Management.* New York: Thieme; pp 291–311.)

for an architect or contractor. You can visualize the interior of your space before beginning construction by drawing it on your computer. We recommend that, after you have designed your space in the computer, you go to the location with a roll of masking tape to mark the areas where walls and major units will be located. This can give a perspective on the office space that a two-dimensional model will not reveal. Once the space is taped off, walk through the office from the perspective of a clinician trying to provide services. Recreate a typical patient interaction for the services you will provide. Verify the ease of accessibility to the equipment you will need and the flow from room to room. Repeat this procedure for each type of patient assessment you intend to perform. Also keep in mind the approximate amount of time that each room will be in use. As you add clinicians to your staff, you will need to keep room availability in mind when scheduling appointments. Try to take on the roll of every working individual in the practice so that you can assess the adequacy of room size and layout.

There have been many psychological studies on the impact of color on individual mood. It is important to take color scheme into account when planning your office space. Work areas, for example, should be painted in bold colors that make workers feel comfortable but energized. Waiting rooms should be painted in warmer color tones that are soothing and comforting (Tom, 2005). It is also important to consider the overall palette of the entire space. Rapid changes in color scheme from room to room can be disorienting and disquieting and should be avoided.

You will want to give careful consideration to lighting when designing your office. Natural lighting is still the gold standard due to its energy-efficient nature and its natural enhancement of productivity (Tom, 2005). If natural lighting is not easily attained, uplights and light emitting diode (LED) lighting are growing in popularity due to increased energy efficiency and color tone when compared to traditional fluorescent lighting (Tom, 2005).

Windmill et al. (2000) discuss four major interior design images that might be employed. These are defined in Figure 39.14. It is important that you know your patient demographic when choosing a style. If, for example, your patient base is generally comprised of lower income unskilled laborers, a "gracious living" style is incongruent and will convey the message that your services are overpriced and inaccessible. If you intend to cater to a primarily pediatric patient population, you would be well advised to consider the comfort of both the caregiver and the child. A play area that is within view of parents would be apropos.

The interior of the site is not the only factor to be considered. You must also consider parking availability and the proximity of handicapped parking spaces to your front door. Wide doorways and sidewalks and ample handicap-accessible parking spaces will be critical to ease of patient access. Patients prefer "at-the-door" surface parking to parking garages. If you must use a garage structure, consider offering to pay for valet parking with patient drop-off and pick-up at your building's entrance.

Style	Gracious Living	Modern and Efficient	Spare and Basic	Cold and Untouchable
Essential Ambiance	Quiet and subdued.	Contemporary Healthcare office.	Relaxed.	Distant and clinical.
General Characteristics	Elegant furnishings. Professional cards, brochures, pamphlets and newsletters. Staff activity is apparent, but discreet. Amenities such as coffee and light refreshments are offered.	Contemporary furnishings with designer fabrics, colors and lighting. Current popular magazines are present as is a display of professional information. Amenities such as food and beverage are not offered. Staff activity takes place out of sight of the waiting room.	Furnishings are nondescript and adequate. Popular magazines are available. Staff activity is audible but not discernible from the examination rooms. Food and beverages are not offered.	Furnishings are angular and metallic. A lack of color predominates. Glossy magazines are present but no professional information is displayed. Seating is adequate.
Demographic	This style works well in affluent neighborhoods.	This style works well in a variety of markets including those that cater to white collar professionals.	This style is appropriate for predominantly middle class marketplaces.	None. Though some practices convey this image, it is not one that should be actively pursued and should be avoided at all costs.
Script	The patient is warmly greeted by a well-informed associate. Staff are busy but always courteous. Pre-registration information is confirmed and the patient is informed of how soon they will be seen.	The patient signs in at the front desk upon arrival in the clinic. A receptionist confirms pre-registration information and the patient is seated until called to the examination room.	The patient is greeted when someone is available. The patient seats herself and waits until he or she is called.	The patient is greeted with a request for information of pre-registration information confirmation, method of payment, and insurance information. The patient seats herself and waits to be called.

FIGURE 39.14 Interior design styles. (Compiled from Windmill et al. [2000] and Hosford-Dunn et al. [1995].)

A practical approach is the wisest course when preparing to purchase equipment for your practice. You must consider the equipment cost as a function of the revenue that will be generated as a result of the purchase. For example, a tympanometer is an indispensable piece of equipment. You know that tympanometry will be performed on nearly every patient. Consider the collections that will be generated. A posturography unit, on the other hand, is a piece of equipment that many practices may want to own but that may not be required immediately. When the time comes to add a posturography unit, you will complete a cost/revenue analysis as a part of your annual business plan. In the new plan, you will estimate the number of patients who will require posturography and estimate the benefit of adding this piece of equipment to the practice. We would like to point out that "benefit" is not simply a matter of collections; you must also take into account the potential to expand into a new part of the market. Although it may be tempting to the novice clinician to purchase every piece of equipment as brand new and to buy the newest technology on the market, this is not advisable. Spending excessive amounts of capital on "state of the art" equipment initially can jeopardize the financial well-being of your practice. Beginning with only the equipment that is absolutely necessary and that has been previously owned or factory refurbished can save the practice tens of thousands of dollars. This will allow you to expand in a logical manner as the capital to do so becomes available.

If the base price of your used tympanometer is $4,000.00 and you know that you will collect (remember, collections and billings are not synonymous) $20.00 per procedure, you can easily calculate the number of procedures that will be required in order to amortize the equipment. Simply divide the price of the equipment by the collections per procedure to arrive at the answer. In our example, $4,000.00/$20.00 results in 200 procedures to amortize the equipment. If you believe that you will provide 120 tympanometry procedures per month, you can arrive at the number of months required to amortize the equipment. Therefore, 200/120 brings us to the conclusion that 1.6 months will be required to amortize the equipment. At this point, the tympanometer is generating margin. The following is a list adapted from Hosford-Dunn et al. (1995). It is a recommended list of questions that the novice owner-manager-clinician must ask before purchasing equipment.

- Do I NEED this or just WANT it?
- Will it generate revenue?
- Is there a less expensive alternative?
- Will it continue to generate revenue in 5 years' time?
- Is it reasonably priced?
- How long until the equipment has paid for itself and begins to generate profit?
- How much could I sell it for?
- Can I buy it secondhand?
- Will this piece of equipment disrupt clinical flow?

■ DRAFTING THE BUSINESS PLAN

Before you begin to think about writing a business plan, we advise you to do a self-assessment. Figure 39.15 includes a set of criteria that all new entrepreneurs should meet before opening a practice. It is important that you answer these questions as honestly as possible. In addition to your professional education in audiology, you would be well advised to take continuing business education courses offered by the American Academy of Audiology (AAA), ASHA, and the Academy of Dispensing Audiologists (ADA). Additionally, the SBA and the Service Corps of Retired Executives (SCORE) have tremendous amounts of educational information at their websites (www.score.org; www.sba.gov). Although some universities offer practice management courses as a part of the Au.D. curriculum, many do not, and even those that do cannot possibly teach you all that you need to know in a single graduate-level course. We also advise enrolling in general business courses and seminars offered through your local community college. Whether you are still in the earliest stages of entrepreneurship or a seasoned veteran, there is much to be learned. Continuing business education can also be obtained through "greenhouse" seminars offered by manufacturers and buying groups.

When traveling, make a point of visiting other private practices. It has been our experience that successful

NECESSARY SKILL	UNDERDEVELOPED	EMERGING	ACQUIRED
Can you appreciate the exigencies of working in a cost-sensitive environment?			
Have you acquired at least two years of experience beyond the Au.D externship in all areas in which you intend to practice?			
Have you learned what to do from observation of those with experience, how to be an effective manager?			
Have you learned through direct observation what not to do from managers with whom you have worked?			
Have you learned about the market in the area in which you intend to practice through direct patient contact?			
Have you made contacts with other professionals and referral sources in the area in which you intend to practice?			

FIGURE 39.15 Criteria to be met before opening a practice.

audiologists are eager to share their knowledge and to help you avoid pitfalls. Although much can be learned from visiting other practices, you must be mindful of the fact that there are regional differences that affect how practices are run. Examples of regional differences include the penetration of managed care into the market, the influence of labor union contracts, and regional differences in insurance coverage for products and services. The savvy practitioner will be aware of these issues and create a proactive management style. You should bear in mind that, although a given strategy may have failed in one practice, it may succeed at a later date in the same practice or may prove highly beneficial in your market. Although it is wise to listen attentively to the advice offered by well-meaning and successful practitioners, it is also advisable to consider advice as opinion and to critically assess its application to your particular situation.

To expand on the advice offered in Figure 39.15, we recommend that you have *at least* 2 years of experience beyond the Au.D. externship before you consider starting a private practice. The experience gained in university clinics, while invaluable, is not completed in a cost-sensitive environment. Typically, university training clinics are "sheltered workshops," especially when it comes to real-world billing and collection issues. There is no substitute for learning through direct experience in a cost-sensitive clinical environment. Much can be learned about purchasing at the best possible prices, managing overhead costs, and staff supervision in "real-life" settings. Although most directors/managers of private practices that have been in existence for several years are probably doing more things correctly than incorrectly, there is as much to be gained in terms of learning what **not to do** as there is in learning what **to do**.

S.W.O.T Analysis

S.W.O.T. analysis is a good first step in completing a business plan. S.W.O.T. stands for "strengths," "weaknesses," "opportunities," and "threats." The first step in completing a S.W.O.T. analysis is to compile a complete and thorough list of the strengths, or areas that might give your practice an edge over others. Strengths associated with the new enterprise might include your skills as a clinician and any business education you have acquired. It should also include the strengths associated with the area in which you intend to practice and any anticipated economic boons. Although you may not know the "micro-location" while completing the S.W.O.T. analysis, you most certainly will have a "macro-location" chosen. Strengths may include the fact that you intend to offer vestibular services in your practice and there are currently no audiologists offering those services in the general vicinity. Weaknesses are any areas that could potentially prove hazardous to the enterprise. Weaknesses associated with the endeavor might include areas in which your skills are limited, successful competitors, potential economic declines, and/or lack of confirmed referral sources.

Opportunities are areas that can be developed in the future to ensure the success of the practice. Opportunities might include potential for expansion of the practice, the possibility of purchasing another practice, or the potential to expand into services that are currently underrepresented in the area. Threats are obstacles to be overcome in order to achieve your objectives. Threats can include new competitors, access limitations to your practice, rumors that the major industry in the region is relocating, or declining income for a segment of your target population. Figure 39.16 is a sample S.W.O.T. analysis.

Mission Statement

The mission statement is the most succinct declaration of your goals. It is the rudder with which you steer your practice. It should be a concise statement that lays out your business purpose and enduring principles. Figure 39.17 is a sample of a mission statement that can be used as a guide to writing your own. It is important to note that the mission statement remains essentially unchanged throughout the life of your business.

Rationale for the Proposal

The rationale for the project should cover the necessity of adding your services to the market. It should also include information on incidence of hearing loss in your target population, the demographics of the area, a list of current providers, and a statement that indicates what additional services you will offer to the community. It should also discuss in some detail the consequences of not adding your practice to the market and the impact that neglecting to add your services would have on the patients in your demographic. Figure 39.18 is an example of a rationale.

Demographic Analysis

When conducting a demographic analysis, you must first identify your target population(s). Demographic information can be downloaded from the internet and is available in several formats. A simple internet search will provide demographic information from the latest US Census. Completing the demographic analysis requires a working knowledge of the geographic region and the attitudes and opinions of the population you intend to serve. As you begin to find a potential micro-location and site, you should plot the site on a map and then draw a series of concentric circles with your site at the epicenter. If you are practicing in a rural area where people are accustomed to driving an hour or more to receive services, you may quantify the target area represented inside the concentric circles as 15-, 30-, and 50-mile radii. In a larger urban area, your circles may need to encompass a much smaller geographic region of 3, 5, and 10 miles for example. There are consultants that perform these types of analyses as a part of a comprehensive demographic analysis.

SWOT Analysis
SWOT Subject: Initial Analysis for Sound Solutions

Strengths – All patients at Sound Solutions receive the highest possible level of audiologic care from a doctoral level professional. Patients are made to feel that they are a part of the practice and are encouraged to be active participants in their auditory rehabilitation and treatment planning. The personal interest and investment of the staff provides patients with a sense of belonging. Follow up care, audiologic rehabilitation and personal counseling are all areas of frequent neglect in other audiology practices but are of paramount importance at Sound Solutions. Sound Solutions is located in a professional medical building on a busy thoroughfare. This increases the number of referrals from otolaryngologists and primary care physicians due to proximity and the outstanding level of care provided.

Weaknesses – More attention needs to be paid to following up with patients who do not return to Sound Solutions following an initial evaluation. A database will be created that will prompt Sound Solutions staff to call patients from whom we have not heard in 6 to 12 months. Furthermore, when a suggestion is made to a patient that (s)he return to Sound Solutions to have his or her hearing monitored at a future date, a note will be made in a directory that will prompt the staff to call the patient 2 months prior to the suggested follow-up appointment for monitoring. This is not only better business practice, but provides the patient follow-through that is necessary for any successful business.

Opportunities – Within 5 years, Sound Solutions will continue to expand into the marketplace by seeking potential sites that are affordable and located in prime sites. This will not only help the business to grow, but will expand the excellent level of care to a larger portion of the population. Once the second site is well-established, Sound Solutions will again begin to look at potential sites for further expansion into the market. Sound Solutions will volunteer to serve as an educational site for doctoral level students from the local university. This will not only help to serve the field of audiology by contributing to the education of future doctors of audiology, but will help to keep the staff at Sound Solutions abreast of the most current research. Students will not only learn the clinical application of audiologic techniques, but will learn all aspects of the business including customer care, provision of follow-up care, and the challenges of staffing and audiology practice. A full time audiology extern student will be employed by Sound Solutions by month 5 after opening. The practice has been designed to support this type of expansion.

Threats – A large audiology practice in the vicinity provides similar services to those provided at Sound Solutions and has retrained a doctoral level audiologist on staff. This competitor is well-established and has referral sources firmly in place. Due to the fact that this area is rapidly developing, the potential for other competitors to move into this growing marketplace exists. The students who have been trained as interns and externs through Sound Solutions will have access to tremendous amounts of information regarding the practice. This provides potential future competitors with a wealth of private information about Sound Solutions' business practices.

FIGURE 39.16 Sample strengths, weaknesses, opportunities, and threats (S.W.O.T.) analysis.

There are nominal costs for these services. A demographic analysis can easily be completed without employing outside services. Figure 39.19 is a sample of a demographic analysis of Durham, North Carolina.

You should know the number of individuals who are within your target population by age, income level, estimated prevalence of auditory-vestibular pathology, and type of insurance coverage, if any. This can provide valuable information for you and powerful information for potential investors or financiers.

Taken together with the number of service providers in the identified geographic area, this information will help to establish a case supporting the need for your practice. If the demographics do not support the addition of your practice and services, you would be wise to consider alternate locations. If you "massage" your numbers or are not completely honest about the necessity of adding a practice to your chosen location, you are putting your reputation and financial

well-being at risk. The business plan should be an ***accurate*** representation of the market and not simply a necessary evil in order to attain financing.

Referral Sources

Figure 39.20 is a sample of a referral source chart that has been adapted from Windmill et al. (2000). In our adapted version, the referrals are listed as estimates as a function of probability. In Figure 39.20, you will note that Dr. Jones is listed as the first referral source. There is a low probability that Dr. Jones will refer five patients, a moderate probability that she will refer three patients, and a high probability that she will refer at least one patient to our practice in any given month. Tally the number of estimated referrals to create a "best," "average," and "worst" case scenario for inclusion in your pro forma P&L statement. The P&L statement will be explained later in this chapter.

Mission Statement

Sound Solutions is an audiology clinic dedicated to providing full-range audiologic, vestibular diagnostic assessment, and, hearing aid dispensing services to the residents of the community in which it is located. These services will be provided in a consistently professional and ethical manner that adheres to the "Gold-book Policy" outlined below.

Gold Book Policy

Sound Solutions and its representatives will operate within the following parameters and guidelines:

    1) Continuously strive for excellence in customer service and patient care.

    2) Always provide professional level hearing care to our consumers and adhere to the established "gold standard" protocols.

    3) Maximize company profit while minimizing the cost of hearing healthcare to the patient through the conscious and active control of expenses.

    4) Recognize that patients and consumers have the privilege of choosing the source of their hearing healthcare and incessantly strive to show that we appreciate their confidence and trust in our staff and practice.

    5) Adhere to professional ethics and standards and never place the "sale" before the customer.

    6) Subscribe to the belief that our patients are, first and foremost, people with individual and varied needs. Sound Solutions associates will always think of the person from a gestalt perspective and not simply as a person with a disability.

FIGURE 39.17   Sample of a mission statement.

Rationale for Project

It is a well known fact that the baby boomer generation is beginning to reach the age at which they will begin to require more services for the aging and aged. Among these services are hearing testing, hearing aid fitting, vestibular diagnostics, and full prevention assessments. By the year 2025 there will be twice as many people over the age of 65 as there will be teens.

According to recent employment growth projections in the U.S. Bureau of Labor Statistics' (BLS.) 2002-2003 Occupational Outlook Handbook, audiology ranked among the top 30 (out of 700) fastest growing occupations over the next decade, with the number of audiology positions expected to climb by 45% between 2000 and 2010. This is a prime time to enter the field of audiology and to open a practice. The following statistics support this statement:

- Baby boomers are now approaching middle age, a time when the possibility of neurological disorders and associated speech, language and hearing disorders, increases.

- Medical advances have improved the survival rate of premature infants, trauma, and stroke victims, increasing the need for speech, language and hearing assessment and treatment.

- About 28 million people in the U.S. have some degree of reduced hearing sensitivity. Of this number, 80% have irreversible hearing loss (Better Hearing Institute, 1999). Facts about hearing disorders.

- 4.6% of individuals between the ages of 18 and 44 years have hearing loss.

- 14% of individuals between the ages of 45 and 64 years have hearing loss.

- 54% of the population over age 65 has hearing loss

FIGURE 39.18   Sample project rationale.

Cohort	Pop. in Durham	% Hearing Impaired	Hearing Impaired in Durham	Percent Seeking Amplification	Total Patients	Anticipated Market Share	Total Potential Patients
18 – 44	86,115	4.6%	3,961	20%	792	20%	158
45 – 64	33,763	14%	4,727	20%	945	20%	189
65 – 74	8,548	23%	1,966	20%	393	20%	79
75+	8,807	31%	2,730	20%	546	20%	109
Total:	**137,233**	**Total:**	**13,384**	**Total**	**2,676**	**Total:**	**535**

FIGURE 39.19 Sample demographic analysis for Durham, North Carolina.

Analysis of the Competition

It is very important to identify the competition. The analysis should delineate competitors' hours of operation, including days of the week they are open; the types of services/products they provide; their qualifications; etc. The analysis of competition must include a detailed statement of any unmet needs in the area, statements about underserved populations, and issues related to convenience, location, and extended hours of operation. In essence, you are trying to identify your "market niche" with this analysis.

The Business Organization

The business organization section should include a list of all of the principle owners as well as an organizational chart. The business organization section will also detail the business type (e.g., corporation, sole proprietorship, etc.) with which you choose to begin. It is important to remember that you can change your business type at any time by filing the correct paperwork.

Measurable Goals and Objectives of the Business

Establishing and explaining the goals and objectives of your business is vital. Creating short-, intermediate-, and long-term goals and *measurable* objectives for the practice keeps you on track and helps convince your banker that you have been very thorough in planning to be successful. Short-term goals should cover a 1-year period. We recommend that, as you create your business plan, you complete a short-term goal sheet listing all of the marketing activities and other duties that must be completed before opening. Essentially, your initial short-term goal statement may extend from 6 months prior to opening throughout the first year of business. Short-term goals can include marketing activities, financial goals, hiring schedules, referral source meetings, and any of the other steps you will take to build your practice. Remember, you will be rewriting all of your goals on an annual basis. Figure 39.21 is one example of how short-term goals can be written. Intermediate goals should cover a 1- to 3-year period and may include anticipated expansion of

Referral Source Chart

SOURCE	LOW	LIKELY	HIGH	AVG. / MONTH
OTOLARYNGOLOGISTS				
Edward Jones, D.O.	5	3	1	3
John Timms, M.D.	3	5	7	5
Elton Lee, M.D.	1	3	5	3
George Smythe, M.D.	0	2	4	2
Physicians ENT Group	3	6	9	6
SKILLED NURSING FACILITIES				
Respite Center	5	3	1	3
Sunnyside Nursing Home	0	1	2	1
Best Care Inc.	3	2	1	2
PRIMARY CARE PHYSICIANS				
Jeff Johnson, M.D.	5	3	2	3
Adam Groves, M.D.	1	2	3	2
Tim Robinette, M.D.	0	0	1	0
Phyllis Sisk, M.D.	6	3	1	3
Grand Totals	32	33	37	33

FIGURE 39.20 Sample referral source chart. (Reprinted with permission from Windmill IM, Cunningham DR, Johnson KC. [2000] Designing an audiology practice. In: Hosford-Dunn H, Roeser R, Valente M, eds. *Audiology Practice Management*. New York: Thieme; pp 291–311.)

Short Terms Goals and Objectives Planner

Task	Priority	Person Responsible	Implemtation Date	Current Status	Next Evaluation Date	Next Action
Place advertisement for office manager/receptionist	High		Nov. 2010	Planning	Oct. 2010	Write ad and obtain classified ad pricing from local paper
Contact various universities with Au.D programs to find potential students for May 2011	Mod.		Dec. 2010	Planning	Jan. 2011	Mail out advertisement to Universities with Au.D. programs
Increase heaing aid sales to 15 units per month	High		Jan. 2011	Planning	Feb. 2011	Increase sales through excellent customer service, active marketing to potential customers and referral sources
Contact hearing aid manufacturers and discuss pricing and contracts to evaluate the most cost effective product	High		Nov. 2010	Planning	Dec. 2010	Evaluate information provided from all manufacturers and choose at least 2 with which to begin contracting

FIGURE 39.21   Sample of short-term goals.

staff and clinical services, financial projections, equipment purchasing schedules, returns on investments, and increasing market penetration. Intermediate goals are built upon the short-term goals and should show the progression from the initial status of the practice to a higher level of success. Figure 39.22 shows some examples of intermediate goals. Long-term goals should be written in keeping with your entrepreneurial vision. If your vision is to own five offices, then your long-term goals should reflect that. Figure 39.23 is a sample of some reasonable long-term objectives.

Start-Up Costs

Calculating start-up costs requires some research and a detail-oriented mindset. You must think of all of the equipment needs, supplies, and incidentals. Start-up costs also include leasehold improvements (build-outs), equipment,

furnishings and decorations, supplies, inventory, signage, and other essentials.

Capital equipment is loosely defined as that equipment that you use to deliver products and services. Capital equipment, for our purpose, refers to the "big ticket" items such as an audiometer, tympanometer, sound booth, real-ear measurement equipment, etc. Again, the wisest course of action is to seek out used or refurbished equipment that will adequately meet your needs. There will be some pieces of capital equipment that you are unwilling to compromise on, but essentially, a serviceable audiometer is an audiometer whether it is this year's model or 5 years old. All capital equipment should be very briefly explained/justified to the lender.

Supplies and inventory have been discussed earlier in terms of general supplies and audiology-specific supplies. Carefully thinking through a typical patient visit while writing down each item that will be needed in order to

Intermediate Goals and Objectives Planner

Task	Priority	Person Responsible	Implementation Date	Current Status	Next Evaluation Date	Next Action
Meet 6 physicians from the referral source list each week	High		Aug. 2010	Planning	Sept. 2010	Implement Plan ad pricing from local paper.
Meet at least 2 SNF directors each week for 10 weeks prior to opening the practice	High		October prior to opening	Planning	Nov. 2010	Implement Plan
Purchase "Coming Soon" banner at least 10 weeks prior to opening	High		October prior to opening	Incomplete	Oct. 2010	Visit Office supply store to order an outdoor, durable banner at a cost of approximately $160.00
Send announcement letters to area secondary schools to make them aware of our presence	Mod.		December prior to opening	Incomplete	Jan. 2011	Follow-up calls to secondary school

FIGURE 39.22   Sample of intermediate goals.

Long Term Goals and Objectives Planner

Task	Priority	Person Responsible	Implementation Date	Current Status	Next Evaluation Date	Next Action
Increase market share to 25%	High	All associates	Immediate	Ongoing	Dec. 2011	Evaluate current market share
Increase awareness of the Au.D and the benefits of doctoral level hearing care	High	All associates	Immediate	Ongoing	Jun. 2012	Exemplify excellent care level given by doctors of audiology
Open a second site within 25 miles of the initial site within 5 years of opening	High		Ongoing	Ongoing	Dec.2017	Continually monitor practice progress by reviewing P&L and business plan
Open a third site within 10 years of opening the initial site	High		Ongoing	Ongoing	2017	Evaluate progress of initial 2 sites and monitor feasibility and profitability of opening a third site

FIGURE 39.23   Sample of long-term goals.

successfully complete the interaction will help you to avoid miscalculating your start-up costs. Fortunately, our practices do not require an inventory of hearing aids. Keeping inventory levels low keeps your capital free so that it can work for you. General office supplies and equipment will include computers, paper products, photocopying machine, pens, patient forms, file folders, etc. All of these things must be included in the calculation of start-up costs so that you are not forced to borrow from your reserve funds. While visiting your local office supply store, inquire about the cost of having professional signage printed. You will also need to contact a graphic artist in order to have your practice's sign and logo made. The SBA has some excellent tools available to small business that can help to calculate start-up costs and other aspects of the business plan. We *strongly* recommend that you visit their website at http://www.bplans.com/contentkit/index.cfm?s=tools&affiliate=sba.

Third-Party Reimbursement Estimates

Again, we cannot emphasize enough the importance of knowing your market before opening a practice. Regional differences in insurance coverage and third-party reimbursement rates will affect your revenue projections. Some regions of the country have high levels of industry and trade union contracts for amplification, for example. When calculating third-party reimbursements, it is essential to estimate the approximate percentage of your patient population that has the various types of coverage (i.e., private insurance or Medicare/Medicaid). Often these numbers are only attainable through experience and are not published data that can be readily extracted from an outside source. In Figure 39.7, we estimated the percentage of the total patient base that would be covered by private pay, Medicare/Medicaid, or private insurance. These statistics were then applied to the total reimbursement per service type as listed by the CPT codes. You will notice that CPT codes have been compiled by type of patient (pediatric vs. adult) and by test battery. In our

example, hearing aids and assistive listening devices were presumed not to be covered by Medicare or most private insurance policies. After establishing the anticipated number of patients in each category, we then applied the estimated reimbursement rates from each source. As a final parameter, we estimated a 75% collection rate on all billed transactions. This may be somewhat disheartening to the budding entrepreneur, but it is far better to underestimate the amount of collections than to overestimate. This type of analysis shows the lender that you have thoroughly investigated your sources of payment and your revenue estimates are realistic.

Fees for Service

Use the information from the "Worksheet for Calculating Fees" (see Fig. 39.4) to give the lender an idea of what your time is worth. Prepare a list of services by CPT code, and assign a dollar value to each. Create two or three typical patient encounters (e.g., a complete audiologic evaluation, an adult hearing aid evaluation and fitting, and a diagnostic workup for a dizzy patient), and show the lender your billing rate for each situation. Include an "average" collection for a typical patient in the business plan. (Reminder: Billings and collections are *not* the same thing; you will be fortunate to collect 70% to 80% of the amount you bill). Multiply the "average" collection by the number of anticipated patients per month and include that figure on the "revenue from services" line in your pro forma P&L.

Cost of Goods Sold

To complete the COGS section, you must estimate your product mix. Product mix refers to the number of products you will dispense by price category. If you have arranged a differential pricing scale based on style (i.e., completely-in-the-canal, in-the-canal, in-the-ear, or behind-the-ear), then you will need to first calculate how many of each style you might

Entry Level Digital

	Cost	Markup	Retail		COGS
Hearing Aid	$400.00	50%	$800.00		$807.50
Dry Aid	$7.50	50%	$15.00		
Fitting / Follow-up	**3.5	$101.70	$355.95		Price / pair
	$1,163.45		$1,170.95		$1,970.95

Mid-Line Digital

	Cost	Markup	Retail		COGS
Hearing Aid	$700.00	50%	$1,400.00		$1,480.00
Dri and Store	$80.00	50%	$160.00		
Fitting / Follow-up	**3.5	$101.70	$355.95		Price / pair
	$1,835.95		$1,915.95		$3,315.95

High-End Digital

	Cost	Markup	Retail		COGS
Hearing Aid	$1,300.00	50%	$2,600.00		$2,680.00
Dri and Store	$80.00	50%	$160.00		
Fitting / Follow-up	**3.5	$101.70	$355.95		Price / pair
	$3,035.95		$3,115.95		$5,715.95

* The $101.70 that is used in the Fitting / Follow-up row was obtained from the completed Worksheet for Calculating Fees

** For the purposes of this figure, it was estimated that the average patient would require 3.5 hours of follow-up care. Therefore, 3.5 hours is multiplied by the required billing rate of $101.70

FIGURE 39.24 Sample pricing calculation.

dispense. We do not recommend a price differential based on style, but rather on the technologic features of the product. In the interest of simplicity, Figure 39.24 shows three levels of technology with estimated prices applied to each. It is reasonable to assume that given a choice of "good, better, or best" technology, most people will choose the middle product because it will be perceived as the most sensible. When faced with such a choice, most people will choose the mid-level technology (Decker, 2005). Use the COGS of your "better" technology product to calculate the average revenue line of the P&L statement. As you collect real data and experience, you will have better estimates of the average COGS and revenue for your practice.

Pro Forma Profit and Loss Statement

The first step in creating a pro forma P&L statement is to begin to estimate the number of people who will seek out your services. Demographic data will provide the number of residents in your region broken down into broad age ranges. If, for example, you intend to provide services to adult and geriatric patients, you must find research that estimates the number of people who have hearing loss in each age range. Data from the National Health Interview Survey (Centers for Disease Control and Prevention, 1995) indicate that approximately:

- 4.6% of individuals aged 18 to 44 have hearing loss
- 14% of individuals aged 45 to 64 have hearing loss
- 23% of the population aged 65 to 74 have hearing loss
- 31% of the population aged 75 and older have hearing loss

A simple application of these percentages to the real numbers obtained through your demographic research can be used to estimate the number of people who might require services. It is important to note that only approximately 20% of those who require services ever seek them. Multiplying the products of your previous calculations by 20% will provide the total potential pool of patients. Next, you must consider the competition in order to estimate your "market share." The most simplistic application is to divide the market share equally between your practice and those of your competitors. Although there will undoubtedly be a "ramp up" time until you achieve an equal market share, this calculation can provide excellent information about the potential pool of patients. These data can be taken into consideration with your short-term, intermediate, and long-term goals. For example, if there are currently three other practices in the area in which you intend to practice, you may estimate that, for the first year, you will only achieve 15% of the total market share rather than an equal 25% (100% ÷ 4 practices). Your short-term goals can include marketing strategies that will help you achieve 18% of the market share in your second year of practice and a full 25% of the market share by the end of your third year. The long-term goal could be to market your practice in such a way that you achieve 32% of the market share by the middle of your fifth year of practice. Figure 39.19 is an example of applying the National Health Survey statistics to your demographic data.

Now that you have some data to work with, you can begin to write a P&L. It is advisable to involve your accountant in this process. The P&L is set up with line items listed along the ordinate and months listed along the abscissa. All activities that generate income are listed in the upper rows of the P&L statement, with a subtotal of all estimated income as the final row of that section. Within that section, you will list all income-generating activities by type. For example, if you anticipate dispensing 12 hearing aid units in the month of February, you will multiply the number of units by the average collections per aid. Use the averaged data that you have compiled for various services provided in order to estimate the number of units of service you will provide in a given month and the average collection per service type. At the bottom of the "Income" portion of the P&L statement, you will total your cash sales and anticipated collections.

The lower portion of the P&L statement considers your expenses. All costs, both fixed and variable, are tallied. Subtotaled expenses will include COGS, all overhead costs, salaries and benefits, loan repayments, rent or mortgage payments, insurance costs, CAM charges, office supplies, etc. Figure 39.25 shows a standard layout for a P&L statement. Costs are subtracted from collections in order to find the "bottom line," that is, a statement of the net profit (or loss) of the business for a given period. Your accountant will be able to help you create a pro forma P&L statement that is easily accessible, functional, and informative.

Marketing Plan

The most practical approach to writing a marketing plan is to create a monthly planner similar to Figures 39.26 and 39.27, which show a yearly marketing calendar and an expanded monthly view for the month of May, respectively. The marketing plan should always be consistent with the mission statement and should include all activities of marketing including cultivating referral sources, presenting public education seminars, direct mailings, and other traditional marketing activities. It should outline your plan to evaluate, re-evaluate, and improve your daily service since this is one of the most critical aspects of marketing. While direct mailings and advertising campaigns through mass media can be effective marketing tools, we reiterate the necessity of creating steady growth by marketing to primary care physicians and directly to the public through educational seminars.

In order to successfully market your practice, you must know your target market and choose a marketing method that is well suited to both the target population and to the products and services you provide. Second, you must identify what you are selling. In the audiology culture, "selling" is sometimes viewed with distaste. In this case, we remind you that what you are "selling" is not hearing aids, aural therapies, or diagnostic test procedures. You are selling better hearing, better balance, and a better quality of life through your professional service.

Next, you must calculate the cost of each marketing activity. You will need this information to ensure adequate funding and to later calculate the ROP. Calculating the ROP will enable you to hone your marketing activities to your specific practice and marketplace.

Request for Funding/Annual Budget

The request for funding is the summary of all of the costs you have calculated by category. It should include an organized spreadsheet that shows one-time start-up costs for capital equipment, supplies and furnishings, personnel costs including salary and benefits, and operating expenses for the early phase of your business. You will include a "grand total" request and calculate a loan repayment schedule. It should be clarified at this juncture that many banks will only extend a small business loan for amounts linked to tangible items such as capital equipment and furnishings; some will extend credit to cover intangibles such as salaries and benefits, several months of operating expenses, and marketing. The "grand total" request should be phrased succinctly but should be comprised of a sentence or two reaffirming the benefits of granting the loan request and the projections that support the fact the investment is sound. If you have followed our recommendations and performed a "good," "better," and "best" P&L analysis, demonstrate to the lender that, even in the worst case scenario, the practice will remain solvent and will not default on the loans. Figure 39.28 provides a sample of a request for funding.

Appendices and Supporting Materials

Appendices should include references to all data and information sources, a copy of your demographic data, a copy of the site lease, a copy of the national trends and incidence of hearing disorders, your resume, a copy of the CAD design for the site, a photograph of the site (if available), and personal and professional references and letters of recommendation from former employers, faculty, or coworkers. Letters of recommendation from successful small business/practice owners with whom you have worked can be very powerful tools. Letters from vendors with whom you have already

INCOME	JAN	FEB	MAR	APR	MAY	JUN	JUL	AUG	SEPT	OCT	NOV	DEC
AE Diagnostic Eval	8	6	9	5	8	9	11	7	13	15	8	10
Fee for Service	156.30	156.30	156.30	156.30	156.30	156.30	156.30	156.30	156.30	156.30	156.30	156.30
Diagnostic Cash Intake	1250.40	937.80	1406.70	781.50	1250.40	1406.70	1719.30	1094.10	2031.90	2344.50	1250.40	1563.00
Vestibular Diagnostic Eval	2	2	3	4	2	3	2	5	2	3	5	4
Fee for Service	293.30	293.30	293.30	293.30	293.30	293.30	293.30	293.30	293.30	293.30	293.30	293.30
Diagnostic Cash Intake	586.60	586.60	879.90	1173.20	586.60	879.90	586.60	1466.50	586.60	879.90	1466.50	1173.20
ABR Diagnostic Evaluation	2	3	5	2	2	4	2	2	2	1	3	4
Fee for Service	218.00	218.00	218.00	218.00	218.00	218.00	218.00	218.00	218.00	218.00	218.00	218.00
Diagnostic Cash Intake	436.00	654.00	1090.00	436.00	436.00	872.00	436.00	436.00	436.00	218.00	654.00	872.00
Hearing Aid Evaluation	6	4	7	6	9	9	8	6	6	1	12	10
Fee for Service	293.00	293.00	293.00	293.00	293.00	293.00	293.00	293.00	293.00	293.00	293.00	293.00
Diagnostic Cash Intake	1758.00	1172.00	2051.00	1758.00	2637.00	2637.00	2344.00	1758.00	1758.00	3223.00	3516.00	2930.00
Hearing Aid Units Sold	6	4	10	8	9	10	8	9	7	14	12	10
Avg. Price Per Unit	2588.50	2588.50	2588.50	2588.50	2588.50	2588.50	2588.50	2588.50	2588.50	2588.50	2588.50	2588.50
Hearing Aid Sales Intake	15531.00	10354.00	25885.00	20708.00	23296.50	25885.00	20708.00	23296.50	18119.50	36239.00	31062.00	25885.00

COLLECTIONS												
Cash Sales	15531.00	10354.00	25885.00	20708.00	23296.50	25885.00	20708.00	23296.50	18119.50	36239.00	31062.00	25885.00
Diagnostic Billings	4031.00	3350.40	5427.60	4148.70	4910.00	5795.60	5085.90	4754.60	4812.50	6665.40	6886.90	6538.20
Collections (.75 of billings one month delayed)	0	3023.25	2512.8	4070.7	3111.525	3682.5	4346.7	3814.425	3565.95	3609.375	4999.05	5165.175
Batteries, supplies, ALD's etc	776.55	517.7	1294.25	1035.4	1164.825	1294.25	1035.4	1164.825	905.975	1811.95	1553.1	1294.25
Total Sales	16307.55	13894.95	29692.05	25814.10	27572.85	30861.75	26090.10	28275.75	22591.43	41660.33	37614.15	32344.43
PURCHASES (C.O.G.S)	4680.00	3120.00	7800.00	6240.00	7020.00	7800.00	6240.00	7020.00	5460.00	10920.00	9360.00	7800.00
PAYMENTS FOR PURCHASES												
Paid First Month	0	4680.00	3120.00	7800.00	6240.00	7020.00	7800.00	6240.00	7020.00	5460.00	10920.00	9360.00
TOTAL PAYMENTS	0	4680.00	3120.00	7800.00	6240.00	7020.00	7800.00	6240.00	7020.00	5460.00	10920.00	9360.00
Gross Profit / Loss	16307.55	9214.95	26572.05	18014.10	21332.85	23841.75	18290.10	22035.75	15571.43	36200.33	26694.15	22984.43

CASH EXPENSES												
Accounting / Legal	300.00	300.00	300.00	300.00	300.00	300.00	300.00	300.00	300.00	300.00	300.00	300.00
Advertising / Promotion (10% of Gross Profit)	1630.755	921.495	2657.205	1801.41	2133.285	2384.175	1829.01	2203.575	1557.1425	3620.0325	2669.415	2298.4425
Capital Expenditures	0	0	0	0	0	0	0	0	0	0	0	0
Charitable Contributions	40.00	40.00	40.00	40.00	40.00	40.00	40.00	40.00	40.00	40.00	40.00	40.00
Dues and Subscriptions	30.00	30.00	30.00	30.00	30.00	30.00	30.00	30.00	30.00	30.00	30.00	30.00
Insurance - Malpractice	10.75	10.75	10.75	10.75	10.75	10.75	10.75	10.75	10.75	10.75	10.75	10.75
Insurance - Office	300.00	300.00	300.00	300.00	300.00	300.00	300.00	300.00	300.00	300.00	300.00	300.00
License	30.00	30.00	30.00	30.00	30.00	30.00	30.00	30.00	30.00	30.00	30.00	30.00
Office Expenses	100.00	100.00	100.00	100.00	100.00	100.00	100.00	100.00	100.00	100.00	100.00	100.00
Rent / Utilities	2,470.00	2,470.00	2,470.00	2,470.00	2,470.00	2,470.00	2,470.00	2,470.00	2,470.00	2,470.00	2,470.00	2,470.00
Repairs / Maintenance	350.00	350.00	350.00	350.00	350.00	350.00	350.00	350.00	350.00	350.00	350.00	350.00
Salary - Audiologist	3,083.34	3,083.34	3,083.34	3,083.34	3,083.34	3,083.34	3,083.34	3,083.34	3,083.34	3,083.34	3,083.34	3,083.34
Salary - Receptionist	2,100.00	2,100.00	2,100.00	2,100.00	2,100.00	2,100.00	2,100.00	2,100.00	2,100.00	2,100.00	2,100.00	2,100.00
Salary - Second Audiologist	0	0	0	0	0	0	0	0	0	0	0	0
Phone	80.00	80.00	80.00	80.00	80.00	80.00	80.00	80.00	80.00	80.00	80.00	80.00
Equipment Loan Payment	1,500.00	1,500.00	1,500.00	1,500.00	1,500.00	1,500.00	1,500.00	1,500.00	1,500.00	1,500.00	1,500.00	1,500.00
Line of Credit Payment	1,500.00	1,500.00	1,500.00	1,500.00	1,500.00	1,500.00	1,500.00	1,500.00	1,500.00	1,500.00	1,500.00	1,500.00
Misc. Expenditures	80.00	80.00	80.00	80.00	80.00	80.00	80.00	80.00	80.00	80.00	80.00	80.00
TOTAL EXPENSE OUTFLOW	13604.85	12895.59	14631.30	13775.50	14107.38	14358.27	13803.10	14177.67	13531.23	15594.12	14643.51	14272.53
NET CASH FLOW	2702.71	-3680.64	11940.76	4238.60	7225.48	9483.49	4487.00	7858.09	2040.19	20606.20	12050.65	8711.89
Plus Beginning Balance	50,000.00	52702.71	49022.07	60962.83	65201.43	72426.90	81910.39	86397.39	94255.47	96295.66	116901.87	128952.51
ENDING CASH BALANCE	52702.71	49022.07	60962.83	65201.43	72426.90	81910.39	86397.39	94255.47	96295.66	116901.87	128952.51	137664.40
REQUIRED FINANCING												
NET PROFIT	2702.71	-977.93	10962.83	15201.43	22426.90	31910.39	36397.39	44255.47	46295.66	66901.87	78952.51	87664.40

FIGURE 39.25   Sample profit and loss (P&L) statement.

JANUARY	FEBRUARY	MARCH	APRIL
Mass Direct Mailing	Contact ENT's on referral source chart	Open House Event	*Calculate ROP on Jan. Direct Mailing
Follow-up calls to all patients	Follow-up calls to all patients	Follow-up calls to all patients	Follow-up calls to all patients
Birthday cards to all patients	Birthday cards to all patients	Birthday cards to all patients	Birthday cards to all patients

MAY	JUNE	JULY	AUGUST
Public info Seminar on hearing loss @ Ramada Inn Physician Marketing events Radio spots begin w/ free battery incentive	Purchase additional mailing list	Set up booth at Senior Expo for Sr. Health Fair!!!	Contact PS112 re: hearing screen to be conducted at the school
	Follow-up calls to all patients	Follow-up calls to all patients	Follow-up calls to all patients
	Birthday cards to all patients	Birthday cards to all patients	Birthday cards to all patients

SEPTEMBER	OCTOBER	NOVEMBER	DECEMBER
Calculate ROP on radio spots		TV Commercial spots -- emotional appeal messages begin	Advertisement spot in the Yellow Pages final ad copy due
Follow-up calls to all patients	Follow-up calls to all patients	Follow-up calls to all patients	Follow-up calls to all patients
Birthday cards to all patients	Birthday cards to all patients	Birthday cards to all patients	Birthday cards to all patients

FIGURE 39.26   Sample of an annual marketing planner.

established credit along with a personal credit score may also be useful.

Executive Summary

The executive summary should be a well-written, succinct, one-page summary of the business plan. Loan managers receive many business proposals and will often read the executive summary first in order to determine the worthiness of the project. The executive summary needs to capture the reader's interest and be convincing. We have included a sample executive summary in Figure 39.29 for your perusal. Although the executive summary is written last, *it should appear at the beginning of the business plan.*

■ BUYING OR SELLING A PRACTICE

Whether you are considering buying a practice or preparing to sell your practice, the single most salient and confounding question is, "How much is the practice worth?" Determining the value of the practice is a process known as "valuation." There are several means of establishing a practice's value, the first of which is essentially heuristic and emotional in nature (Fisher, 2000). This method employs "guesstimates" and is largely determined by the seller's personal investment and attachment to the business. This method is tempting due to the appeal of setting a price based on the hours of due diligence invested in the practice by the owner. Some owners may choose a reasonable market value using this approach. Many times the practice will be overpriced, discouraging

serious bids, or underpriced, providing limited benefit to the seller.

Several other options are more practical both from the perspective of the seller's investment and buyer's confidence in the accuracy of the valuation. Most of these options involve the seller and his or her financial advisor determining the practice value through applied study of the practice's finances. The application of formulae reduces the potential for overestimating or underestimating the true fair market value of a practice. According to Tarantino (2002), there are several pieces of information that will be required before performing a valuation. These include detailed information about the legal structure of the practice including articles of incorporation or partnership agreements, if such exist. Of course, it will be necessary to have tax records, financial statements, and evidence of the debt structure, equity, income, and cash flow. You will also need to provide a list of all tangible assets that details the anticipated useful life expectancy of the equipment and a list of equipment acquisitions anticipated prior to the transfer of ownership. Copies of lease agreements, existing contracts including their expiration dates, and a thorough accounts receivable report are also required. Table 39.3 is a summary of the homework that must be undertaken by the seller.

Although a number of approaches have been developed to determine the value of an existing practice, we will focus on only a few here. The first of these is the "new versus established practice approach." It takes into account the financial standing of the practice being valuated and what would be required of a new practice to grow to a similar level of success. A theoretical growth pattern is then established for the "new practice" for as many years as are required until the "new"

May		
Monday	1st	Book room at Hampton Inn for Public Education Seminar
Tuesday	2nd	
Wednesday	3rd	Radio Spots begin!!!
Thursday	4th	
Friday	5th	Meet with Drs Newmann, Collins, Smythe and Lee for lunch to discuss referrals
Saturday	6th	
Sunday	7th	Meet with Principal Reeves of PS119 re: school screenings this fall
Monday	8th	
Tuesday	9th	Call Jim Edwards at Newbury Nursing Home re: auditory screenings
Wednesday	10th	
Thursday	11th	Review ROP results from Jan. marketing push
Friday	12th	
Saturday	13th	
Sunday	14th	
Monday	15th	Confirm refreshments with Hampton Inn staff (coffee, light refreshments)
Tuesday	16th	
Wednesday	17th	
Thursday	18th	
Friday	19th	
Saturday	20th	Interview with Mary Epstein for marketing strategist position (Part Time)
Sunday	21st	
Monday	22nd	Review ad for Sunday newspaper
Tuesday	23rd	
Wednesday	24th	
Thursday	25th	
Friday	26th	
Saturday	27th	Reminder calls to all registrants for the seminar
Sunday	28th	
Monday	29th	SEMINAR 10AM - 12PM Remember to take appointment book to schedule
Tuesday	30th	
Wednesday	31st	

Notes: Remember: Every patient encounter is a "MARKETING EVENT!"

FIGURE 39.27 Sample of expanded month of May marketing planner.

practice achieves the same level of success as the established practice. For each year of business during this "catch up" period, the theoretical income is subtracted from the income of the established practice. The differences for each year of "growth" are summed to arrive at the sale price of the new practice (Kamara, 1988).

Some practices use a valuation method based on the number of active files (Hosford-Dunn et al., 1995). This method assigns a monetary value to each active patient file and simply generates a sum. For example, if each active file is worth $200.00 during the course of the next 5-year period and there are 1,500 active files, then the practice would sell for $300,000.00. This method is highly subjective, and arriving at a price per active chart may be very difficult. Undoubtedly, estimating the real value of active patient charts may be incorporated into other valuation methods.

Yet another approach to valuation is known as the Discounted Cash Flow Approach (DCFA). This approach is based on the presumed income of your practice for a set period of time. This assumed income is estimated to be available to the new owner as profit. The figure is then reduced by a given amount of money on the premise that the value of the money will be reduced with the passage of time (Fisher, 2000). In other words, a dollar today is worth less than 10 years ago, so the profit that would be earned by the practice at the current rate will be worth less than it is today.

The work of valuating a practice to sell does not all fall exclusively on the shoulders of the seller. An interested buyer must also do a lot of preparatory work and research before committing to a purchase. The buyer must ascertain the real value of the practice for sale and approximate the profitability and potential return on investment associated with the purchase. Much of the work the buyer completes is similar to completing a business plan. All of the components of a good business plan outlined previously in this chapter must

As can be clearly seen from the data presented in this proposal, {*insert name of your practice here*}is a sound financial investment which will yield a high return on investment. Furthermore, the services offered by {*insert name of your practice here*} are in high demand in {*insert name of town where practice will be located*} and will serve to enrich the community and help to promote economic growth as the practice continues to grow and expand. Dr. {*insert your name here*}'s vision is to expand to a multi-site practice as the market will bear, thereby creating employment and contributing to the economic growth of the region.

Start-up Costs Summary:

Description	Total Cost
TANGIBLES:	
Equipment	$100,500.00
INTANGIBLES:	
Lease (first year of payments)	$33,720.00
Cleaning and Maintenance fees (first year)	$5,820.00
Salaries with benefits	$65,200.00

The total cost of tangibles is $100,500.00 of which the lending institution will finance approximately 70%. This amounts to $70,350.00. The interest on this loan currently amounts to 6.25%.

In order to cover the balance of the tangible expenses, as well as the intangible expenses for the first year of operation, a Direct Line of Credit loan of $150,000.00 is required. The interest on this type of financing is 5.75%. The term of the loan is to be 60 months and loan repayment has been accounted for in the Pro Forma Profit & Loss Statement. Even in the worst case scenario, loan repayment does not cause an undue burden on the practice.

FIGURE 39.28   Sample request for funding.

EXECUTIVE SUMMARY

{*Insert name of practice*} is a Subchapter Corporation founded by {*insert your name here*} which will offer a full range of audiologic and vestibular diagnostic services including: adult and pediatric audiologic assessment, hearing aid evaluations, workers' compensation evaluations, neurodiagnostic services, vestibular assessment and fall prevention to a wide segment of the {*insert name of city*} population. {Your name here} has extensive experience in hearing aid dispensing as well as a broad array of diagnostic skills.

{Name of practice} will begin offering services on January 5, 2011. It will be located at {insert address of practice} which is central to the majority of the population of {city }. At the outset, {your name} will provide all audiologic services assisted by a receptionist. {Your name} holds a Certificate of Clinical Competence (CCC) and is fully qualified to supervise students including fourth-year doctoral students in Au.D. programs. {Practice name} will offer an externship to a student who will become a second staff member as of May 2011. Externs from Au.D. programs require half-time supervision and provide a means whereby multiple patients can be seen. Although {practice name} will offer services to all individuals from school-aged children through late adulthood, the primary focus of the practice will be on the aged and aging.

{Practice name} is in the unique position of having the opportunity to offer a range of services that are currently underrepresented in {city. Though there are currently {#} main competitors in the {city} area, only one other offers vestibular assessment and none offer full assessments/ prevention, which is a growing field of interest and necessity. The market continues to grow and develop in {city}, further providing opportunities for {practice name} to expand and to position itself in the public perception as equivalent to "hearing healthcare".

{Practice name} will request an initial loan of ${insert loan request amt}for tangible equipment and supplies. Additionally, a Direct Line of Credit of ${insert DLOC request amt} will be required in order to meet start-up costs and additional expenses.

FIGURE 39.29   Sample executive summary.

TABLE 39.3   Homework for the seller

1. Establish a clear statement for the purpose of the sale. Buyers will want to know why you are selling the practice. Your job is to give a clear, concise, and honest statement explaining why the practice is being sold.
2. Establish a timeline to announce the sale of the practice. A timely announcement will avoid confusion and prevent demoralization of the staff and patients. The announcement must provide ample opportunity for staff and patients to adjust to the idea of a transition.
3. Once the announcement to sell is made, the seller must have a clear timeline for transition of the practice. A prolonged state of "limbo" will reduce the value of the practice. A natural consequence of being "mentally finished" is to allow the practice to languish and stagnate.
4. Decide how to advertise the sale of the practice. Relying solely on "word of mouth" may be insufficient and extend the time between the decision to sell and the actual sale.
5. Assemble a portfolio of the following information:
   - Demographics
   - Local/regional growth trends
   - Analysis of the competition
   - Special circumstances/situations that are unique to the practice/area
   - Copy of the Mission Statement
   - Copy of short-term, intermediate and long-term goals with updates
   - Blueprint of the office
   - Copy of the deed or lease
   - List of services by Current Procedural Terminology (CPT) code
   - Inventory of tangible products with estimated values
   - Pricing structure
   - Aging report of active patient files seen within the past 12, 18, and 24 months
   - Computer printout of "inactive patient files"
   - Statistics on the average number of patients seen per day, annual percentage of increase in total patients etc.
   - List of referral sources with average number of referrals per month filled in
   - Promotional materials complete with return on promotion calculations
   - Samples of all practice forms, policy manuals, and other documentation

Adapted from Hosford-Dunn H, Dunn DR, Harford ER. (1995) *Audiology Business and Practice Management*. San Diego: Singular.

be completed in order to understand the practice's current financial status as well as its future prospects.

In some cases, the seller will finance all or part of the sale of the practice. This allows the buyer more flexibility in financing the purchase, while affording the seller a "reliable stream of income without placing too heavy a financial burden on the younger professional" (Northey and Fisher, 2000). Naturally, this type of arrangement must conform to the law and to a strictly defined agreement between the buyer and the seller (Hosford-Dunn et al., 1995). An agreement would include such items as the amount of the down payment, monthly payments, and scheduled balloon payments (a large lump-sum payment scheduled at the end of a series of smaller, periodic payments); the length of the payoff period; and assessed penalties for late payments or default on the loan. The down payment must be substantial in order to guarantee that the seller will have enough capital to cover the tax assessed with the sale (Hosford-Dunn et al., 1995). Hosford-Dunn et al. (1995) further recommend the use of a title company to both record the sale and to collect the monthly payments for the seller. Using a title company encourages a professional relationship between the buyer and seller. This is particularly important if part of the negotiation includes the employment of the selling audiologist in the practice during a transition period to promote continuity.

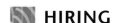 HIRING

The initial selection of employees is a critical aspect of building a practice. Many new interviewers will go with "gut" instinct as the primary determinant of employability. However, there are services available that will provide "vetting" services for a fee. Vetting is simply a term that means "screening." If you do not wish to employ the services of an outside contractor, you can perform your own vetting. In order to engage in effective interviewing and hiring, you must first identify work roles and key competencies that are critical to the successful performance of the job. Furthermore, use telephone screening techniques before ever scheduling a face-to-face interview. This will save time not only for the potential employer, but also for the applicants. We suggest you provide adequate time for the interviewee to pose questions. The entrepreneur who takes hiring and training lightly is foolish indeed. It has been estimated that turnover (the necessity of replacing a lost or terminated employee) can be an expense in excess of 1.5 times the annual salary and benefits of the position in question. This is a result of clinic "down time," the costs of advertising, the time spent interviewing applicants, the time invested in training the new applicant, and the cost of mistakes made by the replacement individual while learning the position. Human capital is the most valuable asset in any business. The cost of replacing employees is so exorbitant that it behooves the entrepreneur to not only be cautious in hiring employees, but also to ensure that employees are relatively happy in their work and invested in the practice.

Succession planning is as important to your practice as creating a well-defined organization chart. In fact, the two are closely related. As the organization grows, there will be a shift in duties and responsibilities. You may find that there will be additional duties due to higher patient volume and that some of the subordinate boxes in the organizational chart will need to be split into two or more positions. You must bear this in mind when interviewing potential employees. Assess not only the applicant's ability to perform his or her current job, but also his or her potential for growth and change. The receptionist you hire today may be the office manager in 2 years. For each candidate you consider, you should contemplate the candidate's potential career path. There are multiple ways to make a bad hiring decision. These can be looked upon as a set of commandments. As such, they may be read as, "**Thou shalt not...**"

- ■ ...use an unstructured interviewing approach
- ■ ...allow physical attractiveness to unduly influence your decision
- ■ ...allow personal similarity between yourself and the applicant to unduly influence your decision
- ■ ...allow the necessity of filling the position to influence your decision
- ■ ...allow verbal ability to unduly influence your decision
- ■ ...hire extremely overqualified individuals
- ■ ...use intuition as your primary guide
- ■ ...make a decision based on the applicant pool rather than on the requirements of the position
- ■ ...rely too heavily on network or political influence
- ■ ...rely on personal stereotypes
- ■ ...attempt to attract a top candidate by overselling the job and altering the reality of the position

Incentives

Employee motivation also involves incentives. Most frequently, we think of incentives as monetary in nature, but this is not always the case. Many employees crave advancement and recognition, and some desire time off or more flexible work schedules. It is appropriate to negotiate incentive packages for each employee and to assess which incentive(s) will provide the most motivation. We recommend using a variety of motivational tools and incentives to demonstrate your appreciation for the work that your staff does.

Termination

We conclude the chapter with a few words about termination of employment. Terminating an employee is never easy, no matter how necessary. We cannot emphasize enough the importance of consulting with a human resources specialist who is familiar with local state and federal laws on the topic. There are several things that must be done in order to terminate an employee correctly. It all starts with documentation. Although we advocate a counseling approach when reprimanding employees, it is important to document the discussion and to place a signed copy of the discussion in well-maintained and confidential personnel files. Copies of documentation must be signed both by the supervisor and by the employee. Different businesses use different sets of criteria for termination, and a well-written and clearly defined policy on the topic is imperative. For example, you may choose to define just cause for termination as a series of two documented verbal counseling sessions and two written counseling sessions for the same offense.

At times, it may be necessary to terminate employment in the absence of employee negligence or inappropriate behavior. For example, you may experience an unanticipated decline in patient flow and a consequent reduction in the need for staffing. In these cases, you may offer the employee incentives to help ease the transition. For example, some employees may desire a letter of recommendation. For others, you may offer a severance package. These are a means of easing the transition and expressing gratitude for services rendered. At all costs, embarrassing the employee must be avoided. Depending on the circumstance, escorting the employee from the premises may be a wise course of action after all company property has been returned. It is unwise to allow much lag time between informing the employee of your decision to terminate and the actual moment of their leaving. This gap in time is an opportunity for the employee to sow ill will among other staff and patients. It also gives a disgruntled person a chance to damage the practice in more malicious ways such as corrupting computer files/programs, expunging their personnel records, and the like. Once you have made the decision to terminate, move forward quickly with as much grace as possible.

▨ CONCLUSION

No single source exists that covers all aspects of practice development and management. This chapter merely provides a framework for considering the tasks involved in starting and sustaining a successful audiology practice. The reader is encouraged to adopt the philosophy that management is a learned process and that learning never stops. Ask any long-time practice owner how they have survived the rough and tumble world of business, and they will surely tell you that their dedication to learning, flexibility, and continuous quality improvement are at the top of their list of survival skills. Go forth and do likewise.

REFERENCES

Bacon V. (1991) Show your small business clients how to get and stay organized: curing the shoe box syndrome. *The CPA Journal.* 61, 67.

Beckett S. (1983) Westward Ho: the complete short prose of Samuel Beckett. 1995. New York: Grove Press.

Beckwith H. (1997) *Selling the Invisible. A Field Guide to Modern Marketing.* New York: Warner Books.

Bingham JW, Quinn DC, Richardson MG, Miles PV, Gabbe SG. (2005) Using a healthcare matrix to assess patient care in terms of aims for improvement and core competencies. *Journal on Quality and Patient Safety.* 31, 98–105.

Centers for Disease Control and Prevention. (1995). The national health interview survey. Available at: http://www.cdc.gov/nchs/nhis.htm.

Decker S. (2005) Marketing lesson from a cop: offering a lesser alternative. Available at: http://decker.typepad.com/welcome/2005/03/marketing_lesso.html.

Edwards ED Jr. (1992) What financial problems? *Management Accounting.* 74, 54–58.

Elgin J. (2002) Choosing a legal form for your franchise. Available at: http://www.entrepreneur.com/franchises/buyingafranchise/franchisecolumnistjeffelgin/article55206.html.

Fisher M. (2000) The value of valuations. Available at: http://www.audiologyonline.com/articles/article_detail.asp?article_id=220.

Gerber ME. (1995) *The E-Myth Revisited. Why Most Small Businesses Don't Work and What to Do about It.* New York: Harper Business.

Graves EG. (2004) Capital ideas. *Black Enterprise.* 35, 65.

Hosford-Dunn H, Dunn DR, Harford ER. (1995) *Audiology Business and Practice Management.* San Diego: Singular.

Hupalo PI. (1999) *Thinking Like an Entrepreneur: How to Make Intelligent Business Decisions That Will Lead to Success in Building and Growing Your Own Company.* Minneapolis: HCM Publishing.

Iacobucci D, Calder BJ, Malthouse EC, Duhachek A. (2002) Consumers tune in to multimedia marketing. *MHS.* Summer, 16–20.

Iacobucci D, Calder BJ, Malthouse EC, Duhachek A. (2003) Psychological, marketing, physical, and sociological factors affecting attitudes and behavioral intentions for consumers resisting the purchase of an embarrassing product. *Advances in Consumer Research.* 30, 236–240.

Kamara CA. (1988) Buying and selling a private practice. *ASHA.* 30, 35–36.

Kochkin S. (1990) Introducing Marketrak: a consumer tracking survey of the hearing instrument market. *Hear J.* 43, 1–8.

Kochkin S. (2005) Marketrak VII: hearing loss population tops 31 million people. *Hear Rev.* 12, 16–29.

Marketingteacher.com. (2005) Pricing strategies. Available at: http://marketingteacher.com/Lessons/lesson_pricing.htm.

McCarty J. (2005) How do I evaluate my fees? Available at: http://www.asha.org.

Northey TJ, Fisher M. (2000) Don't roll-over for roll-ups. Available at: http://www.audiologyonline.com

QuickMBA. (2005) Business legal structures. Available at: http://www.quickmba.com/law/org/.

Sides RW. (2000) A cost-accounting analysis can help group practices assess their costs of doing business and determine the profitability of managed care contracts. *Healthcare Financial Management.* 54, 63–66.

Staab WJ. (2000) Marketing Principles. In: Hosford-Dunn H, Roeser R, Valente M, eds. *Audiology Practice Management.* New York: Thieme; pp 137–172.

Stemmy TJ. (2004) Business structure basics. Available at: http://www.entrepreneur.com/startingabusiness/startupbasics/businessstructure/article75118.html.

Swartz N. (2003) What every business needs to know about H.I.P.A.A. *Information Management Journal.* March/April, 26–36.

Tarantino DP. (2002) How much is your practice worth? Part I: nuts and bolts of business. *Physician Executive.* Available at: http://www.encyclopedia.com/doc/1G1-90317139.html?Q=valuators.

Teitelman GE. (2005) Prescription for working with health care providers. *Pennsylvania CPA Journal.* 75, 18.

Tom K. (2005) Trends in office design: flexibility, technology and security continue to drive corporate spaces. *Interiors and Sources.* Available at: http://www.isdesignet.com/articles/detail.aspx?contentID=3992.

Whitmyer C, Rasberry S, Phillips M. (1989) *Running a One Person Business.* Berkeley, CA: Ten Speed Press.

Windmill IM, Cunningham DR, Johnson KC. (2000) Designing an audiology practice. In: Hosford-Dunn H, Roeser R, Valente M, eds. *Audiology Practice Management.* New York: Thieme; pp 291–311.

Wolitzer P, Wolitzer R. (1991) New small business formation and the CPA. *The CPA Journal.* 61, 42–48.

Webliography

http://www.irs.gov/businesses/small/article/0,,id=98359,00.html
http://www.windustry.com/basics/06-business.htm
http://www.tded.state.tx.us/guide/STEP1.html
http://www.hg.org/busstructure.html
http://medc.michigan.org/services/startups/structure/
http://www.picosearch.com/cgi-bin/ts.pl?index=211668&query=Market+Trak
http://www.score.org/leg_6
http://www.thinkinglike.com/Small-Business-Book/Business-Structure.html
http://www.quickmba.com/law/org/
http://www.companiesinc.com/structures.asp
http://www.paopen4business.state.pa.us/paofb/cwp/view.asp?a=3&Q=440562

http://money.howstuffworks.com/biz-structure2.htm
http://www.activefilings.com/en/information/faq_structures.htm
http://www.techinsurance.com/
http://www.allbusiness.com/articles/Insurance/389-30-1801.html
http://www.tannedfeet.com/business_insurance.htm
http://sbinformation.about.com/od/insurance/a/liability.htm
http://www.insurepro.net/
http://www.toolkit.cch.com/text/P12_9625.asp
http://www.mostchoice.com/business_insurance_overview.html
http://www.aaiaudiology.com/whyAAI.html
http://www.hpso.com/about/endorsers.php
http://www.audiologyonline.com/articles/arc_disp.asp?id=384

INTRODUCTION

Cochlear implants are considered to be one of the most significant technologic achievements to have occurred in the 20th century for the treatment of deafness. Prior to the introduction of cochlear implants, the only treatment options available for profoundly deaf individuals included visual communication (lipreading and/or sign language), tactile devices, or reliance on amplification systems that provided limited auditory information. Presently, cochlear implants are widely accepted as a safe and effective treatment for children and adults with hearing losses ranging from moderate to profound. They consist of surgically implanted electronic components coupled to external components and provide most users with the ability to detect speech sounds covering the frequency range of 100 to 6,000 Hz at levels of approximately 20 to 40 dB with present day devices. Thus, cochlear implants provide profoundly deaf individuals with access to high-frequency information that usually is not available with hearing aids. This enhanced ability to detect sound has fostered great improvements in the postoperative outcomes experienced by cochlear implant recipients, including improvements in expressive and receptive spoken language skills (Geers, 2006), academic and vocational achievement (Geers, 2006; Stacey et al., 2006), and quality of life and cost-effectiveness findings (Cheng et al., 2004; Stacey et al., 2006). In fact, many children who receive cochlear implants today demonstrate speech and language outcomes similar to their peers with normal hearing (Geers, 2006).

Many changes have taken place in the field of cochlear implants since they were first introduced in the early 1980s, including improvements in internal and external device technology, expansion of candidacy, and improvements in outcomes. This chapter will provide a brief historical overview of cochlear implants, describe the internal and external components of currently available cochlear implant systems, describe pre- and postoperative procedures used in the evaluation process, and provide information regarding outcomes achieved by children and adults. The chapter will conclude with discussions regarding future directions in this field.

HISTORICAL OVERVIEW OF COCHLEAR IMPLANTS

The first published report of electrical stimulation of the auditory system in a deaf individual was provided by Djourno and Eyries in 1957. This early implant consisted of an active lead placed on a segment of the auditory nerve and an induction coil and indifferent electrode surgically implanted in the patient's temporalis muscle. Although this pioneer patient was not able to develop speech discrimination skills with this device, he reported an improvement in his awareness of background sounds and improved speechreading skills (Luxford and Brackman, 1985). In 1961, William House performed the first single-channel operation in the United States in an adult. This device consisted of a hardwire gold electrode placed in the scala tympani via the ear canal and round window (Doyle et al., 1964). William House also performed the first single-channel operation on a child in the United States, which took place in the early 1980s (Luxford et al., 1987). Graham Clark developed and implanted the first multiple-channel cochlear implant in an adult in 1978 and in a child in 1985 in Melbourne, Australia (Clark et al., 1987).

There are three different cochlear implant manufacturers who currently offer products in the United States. These include Cochlear Americas (Cochlear Pty. Limited, Sydney, Australia), Advanced Bionics Corporation (a subsidiary of Boston Scientific, Boston, MA), and MED-EL GmBH (Innsbruck, Austria).

HOW COCHLEAR IMPLANTS WORK

Currently available cochlear implant systems have several common components that work together to provide the hearing-impaired individual with sound. These include surgically implanted internal components and an externally worn speech processor and headset components.

Internal Device Components

The internal device consists of a receiving coil/internal processor and tiny contacts (electrodes) that deliver the electric signal to the inner ear. The receiving coil is the largest portion of the internal device and is surgically placed in the mastoid bone. It is composed of a magnet (for attachment of the external headset) and an antenna that receives the transmitted signal. Currently available devices use either silastic or ceramic casing to house the receiving coil/internal processor.

All of the currently available systems are multichannel, meaning that they deliver information to more than one channel (electrode) in the cochlea. Early devices, such as the 3M-House single-channel cochlear implant, processed sound along a single channel and stimulated nerve fibers using a single electrode that was located within the cochlea. The speech perception abilities of patients implanted with single-channel devices were limited. Although some single-channel users were able to obtain some open-set speech recognition skills when using hearing alone (Hochmair-Desoyer et al., 1980; Tyler et al., 1989), most patients were not able to recognize words or sentences in a sound-only condition. Single-channel devices were important because they demonstrated the safety, feasibility, and efficacy of cochlear implants.

In present day devices, the electrodes are attached to the receiver and can be either extracochlear or intracochlear. Extracochlear electrodes are located in areas outside the cochlea, such as on the plate of the receiving coil, or surgically placed under the temporalis muscle. Extracochlear electrodes are mainly used as a ground source for monopolar stimulation. Intracochlear electrodes are housed along a carrier referred to as the electrode array and can be programmed to serve as either an active (stimulating) or indifferent (ground) component of the electrical charge. Intracochlear electrodes are surgically placed inside the cochlea and may vary in number, material, shape, size, and spacing along the electrode array.

Multichannel devices take advantage of the tonotopic organization of the cochlea and provide differently processed information to electrodes positioned at different locations within the cochlea. When stimulated, these electrodes provide localized excitation of cochlear nerve fibers, resulting in place pitch information used to understand speech. The number of stimulating electrodes used in current systems varies from 12 to 22. Several options are available regarding the length and structure of the desired electrode array. A standard array is most often used when the recipient presents with a normal cochlea. Shortened or medium-length arrays may be used for cases where deep insertion is not desired or is not possible due to anatomic restrictions. Compressed arrays, which contain electrodes spaced over a shorter distance, are used when the patient presents with anomalies such as cochlear ossification or a cochlear malformation that may make complete insertion of a longer array impossible. This enables the implant user to utilize most or all of the electrodes. Split arrays, which are constructed of two separate electrode branches designed for insertion into different areas of the cochlea, also maximize the number of channels available to recipients.

There are two primary methods of stimulation used to drive the electrodes. Bipolar stimulation occurs when the active and indifferent electrodes are close together. In currently available devices, bipolar stimulation occurs when current flows between two neighboring electrodes, both of which are located within the cochlea. Monopolar stimulation occurs when the current flows between an active electrode that is distant from the indifferent electrode. In most cases, the indifferent electrode is placed in a remote location outside the cochlea, while the active electrodes are located within the cochlea. Due to the greater spread of current throughout the cochlea, monopolar stimulation requires lower current levels to operate than bipolar stimulation. This results in lower (better) thresholds and increased battery life for the speech processor and has facilitated greater miniaturization of external components. The specific mode of stimulation used with a patient will depend on several factors, such as the preferred mode of stimulation for a particular strategy and the patient's response to electric stimulation. All of the recently introduced speech-encoding strategies use monopolar stimulation.

External Components

Currently available cochlear implant systems have several common external components. These components work together to collect, analyze, process, and transmit auditory information to the internal components. External components include a microphone, speech processor, connecting cables, and a transmitter coil (Fig. 40.1). The microphone captures sound from the environment and sends it to the speech processor, where it is converted into digital information that is coded for transmission to the internal device. The signal is then sent via a wire to the transmitter located on the outside of the implant user's head. The transmitter is aligned with the internal receiving coil and is held in place by external and internal magnets. The integrated circuit within the cochlear implant internal processor receives the information, decodes the signal, and delivers electrical stimulation to the implanted

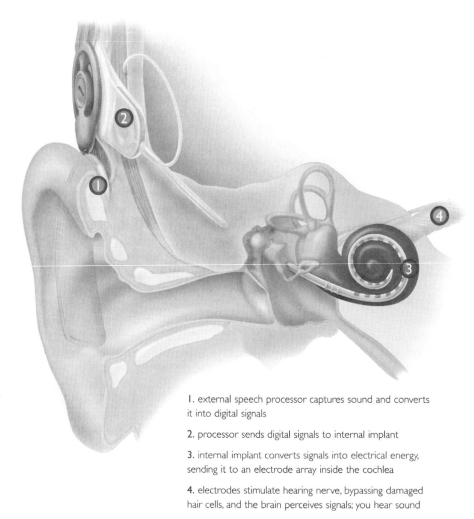

1. external speech processor captures sound and converts it into digital signals

2. processor sends digital signals to internal implant

3. internal implant converts signals into electrical energy, sending it to an electrode array inside the cochlea

4. electrodes stimulate hearing nerve, bypassing damaged hair cells, and the brain perceives signals; you hear sound

FIGURE 40.1   Schematic diagram of how a cochlear implant works. Courtesy of Cochlear Americas.

electrodes. All of the currently available devices use transcutaneous transmission, which means the signal is delivered across intact skin using a radiofrequency link. Some of the early devices, such as the Symbion/Richards Ineraid device, used percutaneous transmission, which involved a direct, hardwired connection through the skin via an external plug mounted on the implant user's skull.

Currently available devices offer several options that enable the clinician to provide optimum efficiency and fit of the external equipment for individual patients. Cords come in a variety of lengths, and magnets come in a variety of strengths to accommodate the needs of both adults and children. Additionally, speech processors, cords, and headset components are offered in a variety of colors to maximize cosmetic appearance.

Processor Features

All of the currently available systems offer both body-worn and ear-level speech processors. Ear-level processors are modular and include a battery pack that can be worn in one of two ways; it can be attached to the processor and worn behind the ear, or it can be attached to the processor with a cable and worn on the recipient's clothing. Such detachment decreases the size of the unit worn behind the ear and helps prevent loss or damage to the speech processor. All processors are able to store multiple programs and have special features that decrease their susceptibility to electrostatic discharge (ESD). The number of memories or programs that the processor is able to contain varies from two to nine. Having more than one memory is advantageous because it provides the user with the ability to experiment with different programs and/or different processing strategies outside the clinic setting. Such flexibility helps decrease the number of follow-up appointments needed to adjust the patient's program.

All of the currently available devices have separate dials to control on/off and volume and sensitivity, as well as provide private and public alarms. The role of the volume control is to increase or decrease how loud the sound can become for the implant user. The sensitivity control, on the other hand, determines the softest sounds that will be picked up and detected by the microphone. A private alarm can only be heard by the implant user and indicates when something is wrong with the processor, such as a low battery. A public alarm provides an audible signal that parents or teachers can hear and can be set to indicate if there is a low battery or if the child has changed the processor settings. Some manufacturers offer a "lock" feature that prevents the child from changing the settings on the speech processor.

All processors have an external input port that enables the implant recipient to use various assistive listening devices. Such accessories are useful for connecting to handheld external microphones, telephone adapters, television (TV)/high fidelity (HI-FI) connectors, and/or personal audio connectors.

The speech processors are powered by various sizes of batteries, depending on the processor used. The specific amount of battery life obtained by a patient will vary depending on the battery size, speech processing strategy, characteristics of the incoming signal, and patient's psychophysical requirements. Most processors use either standard alkaline or rechargeable batteries.

Specific information regarding the internal and external components of currently available cochlear implant systems will be briefly described below. Additional information can be obtained from each manufacturer's website, which is provided at the conclusion of discussion of each device.

1. Advanced Bionics

The **HiResolution Bionic Ear System** is manufactured by Advanced Bionics Corporation of Sylmar, California. The first commercial device (Clarion) was introduced in 1987 by MiniMed Technologies, which later became Advanced Bionics Corporation (Valencia, CA). Advanced Bionics became a subsidiary of Boston Scientific in 2004, but recently left Boston Scientific to again become The Advanced Bionics Corporation.

Several different versions of the Clarion internal device have been introduced over the past several years. A description of these devices is provided here because many recipients continue to use these devices today. In 1991, the Clarion 1.0 device was introduced. The internal device was downsized and introduced as the Clarion 1.2 in 1995 and received Food and Drug Administration (FDA) approval for use in adults in 1996 and for children in 1997. In 2000, the HiFocus 1 array was introduced as part of the 1.2 device and received FDA approval for use in adults in 2000. The Clarion CII with the HiFocus 1 array was released in 2001. The HiResolution 90K (HR90K) device, Clarion's currently available device, was introduced in 2003. The HR90K device differs from previous Clarion devices because it has a thinner case, is housed in silastic, and has a removable magnet. The HR90K received FDA approval for use in adults and children in 2003. As of May 1, 2008,

over 26,000 children and adults have been implanted with Clarion devices worldwide (Patricia Trautwein, Advanced Bionics, personal communication, 2008).

Components of the HiResolution Bionic Ear system are displayed in Figure 40.2. This system includes the HR90K implant, the HiRes Harmony processor, and the Platinum Sound body-worn processor. The HR90K implant consists of a hermetically sealed silastic case that contains an integrated circuit, antenna coil, external ground electrodes for monopolar stimulation, electrode array, and a removable internal magnet. The electrode array consists of 16 electrodes each independently controlled by digital signal processor (DSP) driven output circuits. The electrodes are square shaped rather than round for added current control and are oriented towards the modiolus. The HR90K contains an integrated chip and ICCE (independent computer controlled electrodes) technology to permit software upgrades as future HiResolution sound processing modes become available.

Speech processors manufactured for previously available Clarion systems include the 1.0, 1.2, and S-Series body-worn processors and the Platinum BTE and CII BTE ear-level processors. The 1.0 speech processor was made obsolete in 1996, while the 1.2, S-Series, Platinum BTE, and CII BTE processors are still used by many recipients.

Presently, patients who receive a **HiResolution Bionic Ear System** receive a Harmony ear-level or a Platinum body-worn speech processor. The Harmony processor contains two primary components: the processor and the battery compartment. The ear-level version of the Harmony processor is attached to the battery compartment and worn completely behind the ear. With the modular version, the processor is worn behind the ear but is attached to the battery compartment via a cable. The battery compartment is attached to the recipient's clothing, decreasing the size of the processor worn on the ear and decreasing the risk of loss or damage that may occur if the processor falls off the recipient's ear. The speech processor is constructed of sturdy plastic and comes with a variety of different-colored attachments that change the overall appearance of the device. It has a three-way switch for setting of program number, an adjustable volume dial, programmable sensitivity setting, built in telecoil, and several pediatric-friendly features such as built in light-emitting diode (LED) to monitor system status during device use that provides parents and educators with information to assist with troubleshooting. Three different types of ear hooks are available for use with the Harmony processor: an ear hook with an adjustable microphone that is placed near the opening of the external ear (t-mic), an ear hook with a port for built-in connection to wireless frequency modulation system (FMs; iConnect), and an ear hook with a port for connection to personal audio

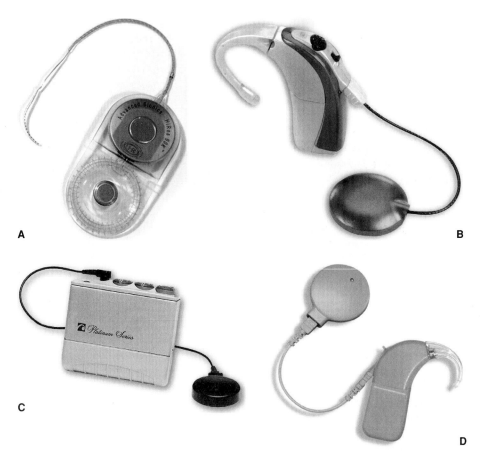

FIGURE 40.2 The HiResolution Bionic Ear System. (A) HiResolution 90K (HR90K) cochlear implant. **(B)** HiRes, Harmony behind-the-ear speech processor. **(C)** Platinum speech processor (PSP). **(D)** CII behind-the-ear speech processor. Courtesy of Advanced Bionics, LLC.

devices such as MP3 players (Direct Connect). The transmitter coil is held in place by varying strengths of magnets and attaches to the processor via a short cable.

The Platinum processor is a body-worn unit that has separate rotary controls for selection of program number, volume, and sensitivity and has a programmable audible alarm that indicates a low battery charge or indicates when the data/power transmission link has been interrupted. The processor casing is made of metal. The Platinum speech processor (PSP) headset, which is connected to the processor via a cable, consists of a single unit that houses a microphone, magnet, and transmitting coil.

There are three speech processing strategies currently available with the HiResolution Bionic Ear System:

- HiResolution (HiRes-S, HiRes-P, HiRes-S with Fidelity 120, HiRes-P with Fidelity 120)
- Continuous Interleaved Sampling (CIS)
- Multiple Pulsatile Sampler (MPS)

A description of the various Advanced Bionics speech processing strategies (as well as those provided with Nucleus and MED-EL devices) are discussed in the

next section. Additional information regarding the Advanced Bionics HiResolution Bionic Ear System can be found at www.bionicear.com.

2. **The Nucleus Freedom Device**
The Nucleus Freedom cochlear implant device is distributed in the United States by Cochlear Americas and is manufactured by Cochlear Pty. Ltd. of Australia. Several earlier versions of this device have been available. The Nucleus CI22 received FDA approval for use in adults in 1985 and for use in children in 1990. The CI22M was released in 1986 and was also known as the Mini 22. This device was a smaller version of the CI22 that incorporated use of a magnet to hold the external transmitter in place. In 1997, Nucleus released the CI24M receiver-stimulator coupled to a 22-electrode straight array that used both bipolar and monopolar stimulation. The CI24M received FDA approval for use in adults and children in 1998. In 2000, the FDA granted approval for use of the Nucleus 24 Contour, a device that consisted of the CI24R receiver-stimulator and the Contour precurved, perimodiolar electrode array. This was followed by introduction of the Contour Advance (CA) electrode, consisting of 22 half-banded electrodes,

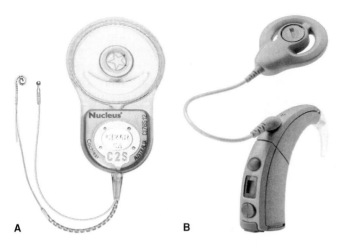
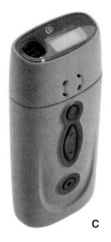

A   **B**   **C**

FIGURE 40.3 The Nucleus Freedom cochlear implant system. **(A)** Nucleus Freedom (CI24RE) receiver-stimulator and electrode array. **(B)** Nucleus Freedom behind-the-ear speech processor. **(C)** Nucleus Freedom body-worn controller.

and the Advance Off-Stylet (AOS) insertion technique in 2003. The Contour Advance is similar to the Contour but has a softer tip to guide insertion and minimize insertion trauma. The CI24RE receiver-stimulator was released in 2005. This receiver-stimulator has the same external shape and size characteristics as the CI24R but has improvements in internal mechanical design, package strength, and electronic capabilities and improved strength against external impact (Patrick et al., 2006). The current device offered by Cochlear Americas, the Nucleus Freedom, uses the CI24RE receiver stimulator. The Freedom was first introduced in the United States in a clinical trial involving adults in August 2004, and received FDA approval for use in adults and children in March 2005. As of June 1, 2007, more than 44,000 children and more than 40,000 adults have been implanted with various versions of the Nucleus device worldwide.

Internal and external components of the Nucleus Freedom device are displayed in Figure 40.3. The pre-curved, perimodiolar electrode array is made up of 22 banded intracochlear electrodes and 10 nonstimulating support rings housed along a flexible silicone rubber carrier. The electrode array is connected to the body of the implant, which is referred to as the receiver-stimulator. The receiver-stimulator is a hermetically sealed titanium case that is covered with a biocompatible silicone material. It contains an integrated circuit, antenna coil, and removable magnet. The implant additionally has two extracochlear ground electrodes that enable use of monopolar or bipolar stimulation. The first ground electrode is a small ball electrode that is placed under the temporalis muscle during surgery. The second ground is a plate electrode housed on the receiver-stimulator package. Although the Freedom uses the same electrode array as the Nucleus Contour Advance, the receiver-stimulator package has been upgraded to contain the SmartSound digital microchip, which is designed to handle future speech processing upgrades.

Presently, the Nucleus Freedom system offers the Freedom speech processor, which is a modular device that can be worn on either the body or behind the ear. The Freedom processor attaches to a controller that can be worn behind the ear or as a body-worn processor. Both the ear-level and body-worn controllers are constructed of sturdy plastic, come in a variety of colors, and have a liquid crystal display (LCD) that provides the patient with information regarding the program number that is in use. With manipulation, the display will also provide information regarding the volume and sensitivity setting in use, settings for the personal or public alarms and lock feature, and various informational icons to assist with troubleshooting. The processor contains dual microphones, a built-in telecoil, and a built-in connector port for use with a FM device. The transmitter coil attaches to the processor via a short cable and contains a magnet that helps keep the transmitter coil in place.

Previous models of Cochlear body speech processors include the Wearable Speech Processor (WSP), Mini Speech Processor (MSP), Spectra, and Sprint. The WSP and MSP are obsolete. Previous models of Nucleus ear-level processors include the Esprit 24, the Esprit 22, and the Esprit 3G. The Esprit 22 is used by recipients of the Nucleus 22 or Mini 22, whereas the Esprit 24 can only be used by patients with Nucleus 24 devices. The Esprit 3G can be used by recipients of the 22 or 24 devices as well as by recipients of the Freedom device. The speech processing strategies currently available with the Nucleus Freedom include Spectral Peak (SPEAK), Advanced Combined Encoder (ACE), and CIS. Additional information about devices manufactured by Cochlear Americas can be found on their website at www.cochlear.com.

3. **MED-EL Combi PULSAR$_{CI}^{100}$ Cochlear Implant**
The MED-EL device is manufactured by MED-EL GmBH of Innsbruck, Austria. Previous generations of the MED-EL device include the MED-EL COMBI 40 and the MED-EL COMBI 40+. Both devices were

straight electrode arrays with eight and 12 intracochlear electrode pairs, respectively. The MED-EL COMBI 40+ device was first introduced in Europe in 1996, was introduced in the United States in 1997, and received approval from the US FDA for use in adults and children in 2001. MED-EL's present device, the PULSAR$_{CI}^{100}$, was introduced in the United States as an FDA-approved device in 2005. To date, thousands of children and adults have received MED-EL devices worldwide.

Internal and external components of the MED-EL PULSAR$_{CI}^{100}$ device are displayed in Figure 40.4. The PULSAR$_{CI}^{100}$ consists of a flexible electrode array that is made up of 24 stimulating contacts arranged as 12 connected electrode pairs. The standard electrode array is 31 mm in length and is connected to the body of the implant, which is housed in a ceramic receiver. The receiver contains an integrated circuit, antenna coil, and magnet. An extracochlear ground electrode is attached to the receiver that enables the device to use monopolar stimulation. This ground electrode is a small cloverleaf electrode that is placed under the temporalis muscle during surgery. MED-EL offers several different configurations of the electrode array, including arrays designed to fit various anatomic variations of the cochlea.

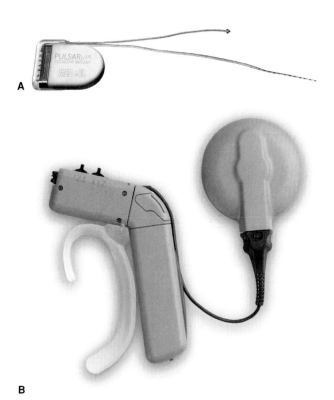

FIGURE 40.4 The MED-EL PULSAR$_{CI}^{100}$ multichannel cochlear implant system. (A) MED-EL PULSAR$_{CI}^{100}$ COMBI 40+ electrode array. (B) Tempo+ speech processor. Courtesy of MED-EL Corporation.

Like the Nucleus and Advanced Bionics ear-level units, the MED-EL TEMPO+ speech processor is a modular unit that can be worn completely behind the ear or can be detached from the battery pack for attachment to the recipient's clothing. Four different battery packs are available for use with the MED-EL TEMPO+ speech processor. The TEMPO+ speech processor stores up to nine different programs and is constructed of sturdy plastic. It comes in a variety of colors and includes a sensitivity control, an indicator light with four different patterns for troubleshooting, an optional locking battery compartment for child safety, and capability for connection to assistive listening devices (from two of the four battery packs). A speech processor previously available with the MED-EL device includes the CIS Pro+, a body-worn unit. Speech processing strategies currently available with the MED-EL device include CIS+ and N-of-M.

Additional information regarding products offered by MED-EL can be found on their website at www.medel.com.

HYBRID DEVICES

Hybrid devices are new devices that use both electric and acoustic stimulation in the same ear. Candidates for these electric-acoustic stimulation (EAS) devices include individuals with a mild to moderate hearing loss in the low-frequency range (<1 kHz) and a severe to profound hearing loss in the higher frequencies (Hochmair et al., 2006). Hybrid devices present high-frequency information via the implant and low-frequency acoustic information via an ipsilateral hearing aid. EAS devices are based on the premise that it is possible to preserve low-frequency hearing after cochlear implant surgery when one uses careful surgical techniques and certain electrode designs that minimize trauma to inner ear structures (Hochmair et al., 2006). Gstoettner et al. (2006a; 2006b) report long-term hearing preservation rates of 70% and 83.2%, respectively, with EAS devices, indicating that hearing preservation is possible following cochlear implant surgery. Previously, it was assumed that patients would experience a total and complete loss of residual hearing following insertion of the electrode array.

At the time of this writing, Cochlear Americas and MED-EL are conducting clinical trials to investigate the use of hybrid cochlear implants. Cochlear Americas has collaborated with the University of Iowa to develop a 10-mm Hybrid electrode array containing six contacts designed to preserve the hearing of recipients who present with low-frequency hearing (Gantz et al., 2005). MED-EL's FLEX^{eas} electrode is a 20.9-mm electrode array with a flexible tip designed to reduce the force placed on the cochlea during electrode insertion, increasing the chances for preservation of residual hearing (Hochmair et al., 2006). In 2005, MED-EL introduced the DUET EAS hearing system, which combines the features of the MED-EL TEMPO+ speech processor with digital hearing aid circuitry (Hochmair et al., 2006).

SPEECH PROCESSING STRATEGIES

The specific type of information delivered to the internal array will vary depending on the speech processing strategy used as well as on the capabilities of the internal components, such as the integrated circuit within the implant and the characteristics of the electrode array. All of the strategies offered in systems in current production are pulsatile and include: (1) CIS, HiRes, and MPS from Advanced Bionics; (2) ACE, CIS, and SPEAK from Nucleus; and (3) CIS and N-of-M from MED-EL. The only analog strategy currently in use is the Simultaneous Analog Stimulation (SAS) strategy that is used by some recipients of early versions of the Clarion device. Each strategy will be briefly described in this section.

Wilson et al. (1991) developed the CIS strategy. Although versions of this strategy are used with all three of the commercially available cochlear implant systems, details of its implementation vary considerably. CIS is a sequential, interleaved pulsatile strategy that presents high fixed rates of stimulation to a relatively small number of fixed channels. This strategy differs from spectrally based strategies where channels are selectively based on their spectral content. With CIS, a bank of band-pass filters spectrally separates the incoming signal into a number of frequency bands. The energy of each band is independently determined and is used to modulate the amplitude of a fixed high-rate pulse train that is delivered to a designated electrode on a place-coding basis. Stimuli derived from channels with low center frequencies are directed to apical electrodes, while stimuli from channels with high center frequencies are directed to basal electrodes (Wilson, 2000). As with many other strategies, stimuli are delivered nonsimultaneously to the electrodes (Wilson et al., 1995). Although the order of stimulation can be varied, it frequently occurs in a basal to apical direction (Wilson, 2000). In the MED-EL device, this strategy is referred to as CIS+. The MED-EL implementation includes a dual-loop automatic gain control (AGC) that provides an input dynamic range of 75 dB and implements the Hilbert Transform, a mathematical algorithm that estimates the envelope of the incoming signal.

The SPEAK strategy is currently available with the Nucleus 24 and Nucleus Freedom devices. This strategy uses a DSP that performs spectral analysis using fast Fourier transform (FFT). The incoming signal is analyzed, and the electrodes corresponding to the bands with the greatest amount of spectral energy (spectral maxima) are stimulated. Although the average number of maxima per scan is six, this number can range from one to 10. SPEAK is a spectrally based strategy that is contingent upon a relatively large number of stimulation sites. With this strategy, the site of stimulation varies and is dependent on the spectral content of the incoming signal (Parkinson et al., 2002). Cycles of stimulation are presented at rates between 180 and 300 per second. The time needed to complete each cycle is dependent on several factors, including the number of electrodes in use, number of channels included in the cycle, and the pulse amplitude and duration for each of the electrodes (Wilson, 2000). Thus, inclusion of only a few electrodes will increase the rate of stimulation, whereas inclusion of many electrodes will reduce the rate (Wilson, 2000).

The ACE strategy is currently available with the Nucleus 24 and Nucleus Freedom devices. ACE uses both spectral representation (like SPEAK) and high-rate temporal representation (like CIS). Like the SPEAK strategy, ACE uses a DSP that performs spectral analysis using FFT. The electrodes corresponding to the bands with the greatest amount of spectral energy (spectral maxima) are stimulated. The number of electrodes stimulated in a particular sequence is larger than with the SPEAK strategy due to its ability to stimulate at faster rates and can vary from two to 20. Each sequence is repeated at a fixed rate that can vary from 250 to 2,400 Hz (Staller, 1998). Thus, the primary advantage that ACE offers over SPEAK is its ability to stimulate a greater number of maxima in a sequence and its ability to stimulate at rates beyond 250 Hz.

The N-of-M strategy is currently available with the MED-EL PULSAR$_{CI}^{100}$ device. Blake Wilson and colleagues at the Research Triangle institute developed this strategy (Wilson et al., 1991). With N-of-M, a total of "m" frequency bands are analyzed, and only the "n" electrodes corresponding to the "n" highest energy bands are stimulated on a given processing cycle (Wilson, 2000). The N-of-M strategy uses wider frequency bands and fewer stimulation sites than the SPEAK strategy. Additionally, the number of "n" (highest energy bands) bands stimulated in a given cycle is constant for N-of-M, whereas this number varies from cycle to cycle for SPEAK. The fixed number of "n" bands can be changed but is usually dependent on the number of electrodes available for stimulation.

The MPS strategy is currently available with the Advanced Bionics device. This is a partially simultaneous strategy that presents pulsatile stimulation to a minimum of two channels at the same time. It differs from SAS because it uses pulsatile rather than analog stimulation and only stimulates nonadjacent electrodes (Zimmerman-Phillips and Murad, 1999).

The SAS strategy is the only analog strategy currently being used in a commercially available device. This strategy continues to be used by recipients with Clarion 1.2 and HiFocus arrays but is not presently available with the Advanced Bionics HiResolution Bionic Ear System. SAS uses stimulation signals composed of continuous, analog waveforms that are simultaneously transmitted to the electrodes along the array. With SAS, a full spectrum of the input signal is spectrally separated into a set number of frequency bands that correspond to the number of active electrode pairs in use. The energy of each band is independently determined and is used to modulate the amplitude of a pulse train that is delivered to a designated bipolar electrode pair.

The HiRes strategy is presently available with the Advanced Bionics HR90K device. This strategy uses dynamic bin averaging for each channel (rather than envelope or spectral peak extraction). Additionally, narrow pulse widths are used, so information can be transmitted at very fast rates to all 16 of the available channels during each stimulation cycle. This strategy can be programmed to deliver information using either paired simultaneous stimulation (HiRes-P) or sequential stimulation (HiRes-S) (Koch et al., 2004). In HiRes-P, two electrodes are stimulated at the same time. In HiRes-S, all available electrodes are stimulated sequentially.

One of the most recently introduced speech processing strategies is HiRes 120. This is the first commercially available speech processing strategy to use current "steering." This strategy is based on the finding that varying the proportion and amplitude of current delivered to adjacent pairs of simultaneously stimulated electrodes results in unique sound percepts that are not available with earlier strategies (Firszt et al., 2007; Koch et al., 2007). Manipulation of the simultaneous stimulation delivered to the two adjacent electrode pairs results in an average of seven new percepts (i.e., virtual channel) for each electrode pair (Spahr and Emadi, 2005). With HiRes 120, depending on the spectrum of the incoming signal, the processor "steers" the current to any one of the 15 electrode pairs or to one of the seven "virtual channel" locations. This results in up to 120 different percepts. HiRes 120 received FDA approval for use with adults in 2007.

▨ DETERMINING CANDIDACY FOR A COCHLEAR IMPLANT

Candidacy requirements for a cochlear implant have changed greatly since cochlear implants were first introduced. This is primarily due to the results of clinical trials that have been performed to evaluate device efficacy and safety. In the United States, the FDA oversees the selling, distribution, labeling, and marketing of drugs, medical devices, and other products. It also determines if the specific wording used in device labeling, including information regarding indications for its use, is appropriate. All of the presently available cochlear implant systems provide information regarding FDA-approved indications for their use on labels that are used in packaging the internal array.

One of the greatest influences on selection criteria has been the increasing amount of open-set speech recognition obtained by recipients with their cochlear implants. In early clinical trials, only patients who demonstrated no benefit from amplification (i.e., scored 0% correct on open-set tests of sentence recognition) were considered to be candidates for a cochlear implant. Today, most clinics define limited benefit from amplification as a score ≤50% correct in the ear to be implanted on taped sentence recognition tests and ≤60% in the best-aided listening condition. Because the current criteria include patients with open-set speech recognition, it is important for clinicians to ensure that all measures have been taken to determine if an individual can benefit from appropriate amplification prior to providing him or her with a cochlear implant. The recommendation to proceed with a cochlear implant should only be made if the clinician believes the patient will demonstrate improved communication skills with implant use. Additionally, it is important for clinicians to remain informed about the changing guidelines that continue to evolve as advances are made in device technology, surgical technique, and speech processing strategies. General selection guidelines for children and adults are provided in Tables 40.1 and 40.2.

TABLE 40.1   Candidacy criteria guidelines for children to receive a cochlear implant

1. Severe to profound bilateral sensory-neural hearing loss (unaided thresholds should be ≥90 dB hearing level [HL] beyond 1,000 Hz). In younger children, the hearing loss should be confirmed using electrophysiologic measures such as the auditory brainstem response (ABR) test.
2. 12 months of age or older.
3. Little or no benefit from hearing aids. In young children, this is demonstrated by lack of progress in the development of simple auditory skills in conjunction with appropriate amplification and participation in an intensive auditory habilitation program. This is also demonstrated by parental response to client-administered questionnaires such as the Meaningful Auditory Integration Scale (MAIS) (Robbins et al., 1991) or the Infant-Toddler MAIS (Zimmerman-Phillips et al., 1998). In older children, minimal benefit from amplification is demonstrated by scores ≤30% correct on open-set speech recognition measures such as the Lexical Neighborhood Test (LNT) (Kirk et al., 1995) or the Multisyllabic Lexical Neighborhood Test (MLNT) (Kirk et al. 1995). A 3- to 6-month hearing aid trial is recommended for children with no previous hearing aid experience.
4. No medical or radiologic contraindications to surgery.
5. Placement in an educational setting that is able and willing to provide a concentrated auditory skill development program.
6. Motivated family and consent of the child if appropriate.

TABLE 40.2 **Candidacy criteria guidelines for adults to receive a cochlear implant**

1. At least a moderate hearing loss in the low frequencies and a profound hearing loss (unaided thresholds ≥90 dB hearing level [HL]) in the mid to high speech frequencies bilaterally.
2. Little or no benefit from hearing aids. This is currently defined as a score of ≤60% correct in the best-aided listening condition on tape-recorded tests of open-set sentence recognition when using hearing alone and a score of ≤50% correct on tape-recorded tests of open-set speech recognition in the ear to be implanted.
3. No medical or radiologic contraindications to surgery.
4. Motivated patient and possession of appropriate expectations.

Preoperative Testing to Determine Candidacy for a Cochlear Implant

The primary purpose of the preoperative evaluation is to determine if the patient is medically and audiologically suitable for a cochlear implant. Additionally, such information should be compared to postoperative results to evaluate recipient progress and device efficacy. The determination of candidacy for a cochlear implant is most often made by a group of qualified professionals, including a surgeon, audiologist, speech-language pathologist, deaf educator, and psychologist. The opinions of other professionals, such as school personnel, are also taken into account.

Test procedures commonly included in the preoperative process for determining implant candidacy are described here:

A. **Medical Evaluation**

During the preoperative medical evaluation, the physician obtains a complete medical history and performs a physical examination. The surgeon attempts to identify the cause of the hearing loss if it is not already known and determines if treatment options other than a cochlear implant are more suitable, such as performing a stapedectomy in cases of far-advanced otosclerosis. The cochlear implant candidate's general health is also evaluated to determine if he or she is healthy enough to participate in the surgery required for cochlear implantation.

B. **Cochlear Imaging**

Computed tomography (CT) or magnetic resonance imaging (MRI) of the temporal bone is routinely performed as part of the preoperative evaluation process to visualize development of the mastoid and inner ear structures. These procedures identify any inner ear anomalies, determine if cochlear ossification is present, and help determine the most suitable ear for implant. Knowledge regarding the presence of cochlear anomalies is important prior to surgery because it may affect the type of electrode array selected for surgery (i.e., compressed, straight, or split array), the surgical approach used to access the cochlea, the insertion depth of the electrode array, selection of the ear for implantation, and final placement of the electrode array. Cochlear malformations rarely preclude placement of a cochlear implant (Balkany et al., 1996; Tucci et al., 1995), although severe anomalies may limit the insertion depth of the electrode array to a degree that would compromise the anticipated benefit from the device. Furthermore, associated anomalies of the temporal bone, particularly absence of the eighth nerve, may render cochlear implantation unwise. To avoid unnecessary risks to the patient, disappointment for the family, and delay in the initiation of alternative communication modes, the preoperative assessment of patients with anomalous temporal bones should include MRI and electric auditory brainstem response (EABR) testing. These results will allow the clinician to assess both the structural and functional integrity of the auditory neural pathways and to counsel the family accordingly.

C. **Audiologic Evaluation**

The primary purpose of the preoperative audiologic evaluation is to determine the type and severity of hearing loss. This evaluation typically includes unaided testing of air- and bone-conduction thresholds, speech reception threshold (SRT), if possible, or speech detection threshold (SDT), word recognition, otoacoustic emissions (OAEs), and tympanometry and acoustic reflexes. Current FDA guidelines regarding audiometric candidacy vary slightly for the available FDA-approved devices. The most lenient recommendations regarding audiometric status indicate that adults with a moderate hearing loss in the low frequencies and a profound hearing loss (≥90 dB hearing level [HL]) in the mid to high speech frequencies may be a candidate for a cochlear implant (Cochlear Americas, 2006). For children, audiometric criteria may be dependent on the child's age and may be more stringent for very young children due to the inability to evaluate their speech perception skills. For example, indications for the Nucleus Freedom state that this device "... is intended for use in children 12 to 24 months of age who have bilateral profound sensory-neural deafness," whereas "children two years of age or older may demonstrate severe to profound hearing loss bilaterally" (Cochlear Americas, 2006).

D. **Electrophysiologic Testing**

Several implant centers include electrophysiologic tests in their preoperative test battery. Auditory brainstem response (ABR) testing is used to verify behavioral audiometric test results, help identify patients with auditory dyssynchrony, and rule out the possibility of functional deafness. Such testing is particularly important when testing young children. Additionally, some centers perform Electrically Evoked Auditory Brainstem Responses (EABR) (Kileny et al., 1994; Kileny and Zwolan, 2004) testing prior to implantation to verify electric stimulability of an ear. Such testing is usually performed in the operating room immediately prior to cochlear implant surgery and involves the presentation of current pulses via a transtympanically placed promontory needle electrode (Kileny et al., 1994; Stypulkowski et al., 1986). The EABR is particularly useful when questions arise regarding presence or stimulability of the eighth nerve in the ear to be implanted.

E. **Hearing Aid Evaluation and Speech Perception Testing**
The preoperative hearing aid evaluation (HAE) is used to evaluate the patient's performance with appropriate amplification and typically includes evaluation of aided detection and aided speech perception skills. It should begin with an examination of the patient's personal amplification to determine if the aids meet the manufacturer's specifications and to determine if it is suitable and appropriate for the patient's hearing loss.

Typically, the HAE includes determination of aided warble tone sound field detection thresholds at 250, 500, 1,000, 2,000, 3,000, and 4,000 Hz; determination of the aided most comfortable loudness level, uncomfortable loudness level, aided SDT, aided SRT, and speech perception testing. These procedures should be performed with each ear aided separately as well as in a binaural aided condition. On average, cochlear implant recipients demonstrate postoperative sound field warble tone detection thresholds of 25 to 40 dB HL for the test frequencies ranging from 250 to 4,000 Hz when their speech processor is set to an average use setting. The aided detection thresholds obtained preoperatively by possible candidates with hearing aids can be compared to the earlier mentioned levels to determine if detection skills will improve with a cochlear implant. When making such a comparison, it is important to keep in mind that such measurements represent simple detection; they provide no information regarding the discriminability of the sounds presented.

When evaluating candidacy for a cochlear implant, it is important to consider the amount of time the candidate has used appropriate amplification. This is particularly true with children, prelingually deafened adults, and adults and children who demonstrate some open-set speech recognition because experience with amplification can greatly influence auditory detection and speech recognition skills. In most cases, a 3-month trial with appropriate amplification and rehabilitation is recommended to ascertain the potential for aided benefit. A shorter trial with amplification is justified, however, if there is radiologic evidence of cochlear ossification or if the patient clearly receives no benefit from amplification. A longer trial may be needed if the clinician observes good improvement in auditory skills during the trial period.

The primary purpose of preoperative speech perception testing is to determine if the patient qualifies for a cochlear implant based on hearing-alone speech perception skills. In addition, documentation of preoperative speech perception skills is important, since such data will influence future expansion of cochlear implant candidacy.

Speech perception testing should be performed in a sound field using recorded test materials whenever possible (this is often not feasible, however, when testing small children). Most clinics and most clinical trials presently use a presentation level of 60 dB sound pressure level (SPL) for test stimuli (Firszt et al., 2004).

When administering speech perception tests, patients should be seated in a sound-treated room that contains minimal visual and auditory distractions. The presentation level should be calculated using a calibration microphone placed at the center of the listener's head. Test materials should be presented a single time only, and feedback should not be provided.

Speech perception materials can be broken down into various categories based on the type and number of choices provided to the listener. Closed-set materials provide the listener with a set of choices from which to select a response. The difficulty of the closed-set task and its chance level are determined by the number of choices available to the listener. For example, a test item containing two possible responses will have a 50% chance of being correct and is easier than tests containing four possible choices. Open-set materials, on the other hand, provide the listener with an infinite set of choices because none are provided. Therefore, chance scores for open-set tests are considered 0%.

With adult patients, the speech perception evaluation should include assessment of the ability to understand phonemes and words when presented in isolated monosyllables and an assessment of ability to perceive words when presented in the context of a sentence. Additionally, one may want to consider a measure of lipreading ability. Monosyllabic word tests commonly used by implant centers include the NU6 Monosyllabic Words Test (Tillman and Carhart, 1966) and the Consonant-Nucleus-Consonant (CNC) Monosyllabic Words Test (Peterson and Lehiste, 1962). Frequently used sentence materials include the Hearing in Noise Test (HINT) (Nilsson et al., 1994), City University of New York (CUNY) Sentences (Boothroyd et al., 1985), and Bamford-Kowal-Bench (BKB) Sentences (Bench et al., 1979). Closed-set consonant and vowel recognition tests may also be used and provide information regarding specific features of the speech signal that are or are not being perceived by the listener.

In terms of speech recognition skills, candidates are no longer required to demonstrate scores of 0% correct on open-set speech recognition measures. Current candidacy criteria for all of the commercially available devices indicate that patients should demonstrate minimal benefit from amplification. In the recently approved indications for use of the Nucleus Freedom device, limited benefit from amplification for an adult is defined as a test score less than or equal to 60% correct in the best aided listening condition on tape-recorded tests of open-set sentence recognition (Cochlear Americas, 2006). Indications for the HiResolution Bionic Ear System define limited benefit as a sentence score ≤50% (Advanced Bionics Corporation, 2007), while the MED-EL Pulsar device recommends a sentence score ≤40% correct on such measures (MED-EL, 2007).

It is important to keep in mind that the previously mentioned scores are guidelines approved by the FDA for particular products and that specific wording of each product is influenced by several factors, including the timeframe of FDA approval and design of the clinical trial. Thus, some patients who have received cochlear implants have demonstrated preoperative speech recognition scores that are better than the previously mentioned recommendations. Additional factors that go into a decision regarding implant candidacy include the patient's willingness and/or ability to use hearing aids and the effect that reduced speech recognition has on the patient's ability to function in occupational and social settings. In some instances, insurers will only preauthorize payment for the device if the patient meets FDA indications, limiting any flexibility the clinic may have regarding candidacy.

It is important to note that Medicare, the national health insurance program that provides health insurance to US citizens age 65 and over, has specific criteria that clinics need to follow if a patient is enrolled in Medicare. Presently, these criteria differ from those of the FDA. The Centers for Medicare and Medicaid Services (CMS), which administers the Medicare program, presently states that, "Cochlear implantation is reasonable and necessary for treatment of bilateral pre-or-postlinguistic, sensory-neural, moderate-to-profound hearing loss in individuals who demonstrate limited benefit from amplification. Limited benefit from amplification is defined by test scores of ≤40% correct in the best-aided listening condition on tape recorded tests of open-set sentence recognition." CMS also states, "a cochlear implant is reasonable and necessary for individuals with hearing test scores of >40% and ≤60% only when the provider is participating in and patients are enrolled in either an FDA-approved category B IDE clinical trial, a trial under the CMS Clinical Trial Policy, or a prospective, controlled comparative trial approved by CMS as consistent with the evidentiary requirements for National Coverage Analyses and meeting specific quality standards." Additional information regarding this matter can be obtained from the CMS website (http://www.cms.hhs.gov/).

Selection criteria for children have also been expanded to include candidates with minimal open-set speech perception skills. Like adults, the specific wording used in FDA-approved guidelines is different for currently approved devices. FDA-approved indications for use of all devices state that, in younger children, limited benefit is defined as lack of progress in the development of simple auditory skills in conjunction with appropriate amplification and participation in intensive aural rehabilitation over a 3- to 6-month period, and all recommend that hearing aid benefit be quantified in young children using measures such as the Meaningful Auditory Integration Scale (MAIS) (Robbins et al., 1991) or the Early Speech Perception (ESP) test (Moog and Geers, 1990). With older children, all three manufacturers recommend use of the open-set Multisyllabic Lexical Neighborhood Test (MLNT) (Kirk et al., 1995) or Lexical Neighborhood Test (LNT) (Kirk et al., 1995), depending on the child's cognitive and linguistic skills. Like adults, the particular score used to define lack of benefit varies. For the Nucleus Freedom, lack of aided benefit is presently defined as a score ≤30% correct, while the Advanced Bionics HiResolution and the MED-EL Pulsar systems define this as a score ≤20% correct on such measures.

With both children and adults, preoperative speech perception testing should include different tests that measure a variety of speech perception skills. The specific tests used with children are often dependent on the child's age and linguistic ability. However, there needs to be some flexibility with children because they vary in their ability to participate in certain tests.

Pediatric speech perception tests can be broken down into three general areas: (1) closed-set tests that measure prosodic cue, speech feature, or word perception; (2) open-set word and sentence tests that provide an estimate of the child's ability to communicate in the "real world," and (3) objective report scales, such as the MAIS (Robbins et al., 1991), that use parental report to evaluate the child's listening skills in his or her daily environment. Speech perception tests commonly used with children in pre- and postoperative cochlear implant evaluations are listed in Table 40.3. For a comprehensive review of these test procedures, the reader is referred to Iler Kirk et al. (1997).

F. **Speech and Language Evaluation**

Speech-language evaluations are performed at most centers as part of the pediatric pre- and postoperative evaluations. This evaluation is essential because it provides information regarding the child's development of speech and language skills—a critical factor when considering pediatric candidacy for a cochlear implant. During this evaluation, the speech-language pathologist may evaluate the child's developmental expressive and receptive language skills, articulation skills, and speech intelligibility. Importantly, the child's communicative status is evaluated with respect to normative models of language

TABLE 40.3   Tests commonly used to evaluate speech perception skills of pediatric cochlear implant users

Early Speech Perception Test (ESP) (Moog and Geers, 1990):
The *standard version* was designed to obtain accurate information about the progression of speech discrimination skills in children with profound hearing loss. Test stimuli include 36 words presented in an auditory-only condition (three subsets of 12). The format involves a closed-set picture identification task. Each item is randomly presented twice. The first subtest includes a total of 12 words that fall into one of three categories: one-, two-, or three-syllable words. In the first subtest, the child receives pattern credit if he or she chooses any word within the correct syllable pattern category and word credit if it is the correct word. The second subtest contains 12 spondees, and the third subtest contains 12 monosyllabic words (i.e., assessing the word percent correct score for these two subtests). For each subtest, the child is presented with a card containing pictures of all 12 possible words and is asked to point to the correct picture. The material can be presented live voice or via a recording.

The *low verbal version* was designed to estimate speech perception abilities in very young children (2 years and up) with limited verbal abilities. The number of choices in the closed set is smaller (4 vs. 12) than in the standard version, and all three levels of the low verbal version use objects (toys) instead of pictures. Like the standard version, stimuli for the first level include words that vary in number of syllables or stress pattern. The second level contains only spondaic words, and the third level contains only monosyllabic words. The material can be presented via live voice or a recording. Minimum age for this test is 2 years or when vocabulary has been acquired.

Meaningful Auditory Integration Scale (MAIS) (Robbins et al., 1991):
This questionnaire assesses a child's meaningful listening skills in everyday situations. There are 10 questions scored on a scale of 0 to 4 (0 = never, 4 = always). Parental response to client-administered questions is sought to determine the child's history with their hearing device. Minimum age for this test is 2 years. For children younger then 2 years, the Infant-Toddler Meaningful Auditory Integration Scale (IT-MAIS) has been developed.

Word Intelligibility by Picture Identification (WIPI) Test (Ross and Lerman, 1979):
This test was designed to evaluate the child's ability to perceive words. Stimuli consist of four lists of 25 single-syllable words with similar vowels but different consonants. Carrier phrase "Show me. . ." is used to present stimuli. Format is a closed set containing six possible picture stimuli. Minimum age for administration is 5 to 6 years for children with moderate hearing loss and 7 to 8 years for children with severe to profound hearing losses.

Northwestern University-Children's Perception of Speech (NU-CHIPS) Test (Elliott and Katz, 1980):
This test assesses word recognition abilities in children. Stimuli consist of monosyllabic words. Stimuli are presented in a closed set containing four different pictures. Presentation can be a live voice or a recording. Minimum age requirement is an age equivalency of 2.5 years on the Peabody Picture Vocabulary Test.

Phonetically Balanced Kindergarten (PBK)-50 Word List (Haskins, 1949):
Stimuli consist of three lists of 50 monosyllabic words. Each response is scored for word and phoneme accuracy. Format is open set. Presentation can be a live voice or a recording. Minimum age is 6 years. This test was not specifically designed for children with hearing loss.

Bamford-Kowal-Bench (BKB) Sentences (Bench et al., 1979):
This test assesses speech recognition at a sentence level. Stimuli consist of key words in sentences, which are used to derive a percent correct score. Format is open set. Presentation is either a recording or a monitored live voice. Minimum age is 6 years.

Glendonald Auditory Screening Procedure (GASP) (Erber, 1982):
This test was designed to assess a child's open-set speech recognition abilities using both words and sentences that are familiar. Stimuli consist of three lists of 12 words and two lists of 10 sentences. Sentences are in the form of questions. Presentation is via monitored live voice.

Lexical Neighborhood Test (LNT) (Kirk et al., 1995):
This test was designed to assess a child's open-set speech recognition abilities using monosyllabic words. Stimuli consist of 25 words presented via either a monitored live voice or a recording. The test contains lexically "easy" words (those high in frequency of occurrence but phonemically dissimilar to other words) and lexically "hard" words (those low in frequency of occurrence but phonemically similar to other words).

Multisyllabic Lexical Neighborhood Test (MLNT) (Kirk et al., 1995):
This test was designed to assess a child's open-set speech recognition abilities using multisyllabic words. Stimuli consist of either 12 or 24 words presented via either a monitored live voice or a recording. The test contains lexically "easy" words (those high in frequency of occurrence but phonemically dissimilar to other words) and lexically "hard" words (those low in frequency of occurrence but phonemically similar to other words).

development, and this provides information regarding expectations for speech and language improvements that may or may not be seen following intervention with a cochlear implant. Occasionally, the speech-language pathologist may recommend participation in structured therapy before making a recommendation regarding the patient's candidacy for a cochlear implant. Such therapy may be particularly helpful in borderline cases, in cases where the child has received little therapeutic intervention or has been inappropriately fit with amplification, and also in cases of auditory dyssynchrony. Some centers require prelingually deafened adults, and some postlingually deafened adults, to participate in such testing or preoperative therapy.

Similar to speech perception materials, the specific tests used in the speech and language evaluation are dependent on the child's age and language level. Postoperatively, children with cochlear implants should continue to participate in regularly scheduled speech and language evaluations. Postoperative speech and language evaluations help determine which speech cues are or are not being perceived by the child, help identify lack of progress that may be due to internal device failure, provide information that may aid in programming the child's device, and help determine auditory training goals.

G. Psychological Evaluation

The psychological evaluation is primarily performed with pediatric patients but also may be necessary with adults who present with concerns regarding cognitive status or mental function. With children, a preoperative evaluation should include nonverbal assessment of cognitive, social, emotional, and adaptive abilities in order to determine if factors other than hearing impairment are hindering the child's auditory development. Depending on the patient's age and the presenting concerns, the ability of the child to attend to and remember information also may be assessed, and recommendations may be made regarding educational services. The presence of a cognitive impairment may impact the child's ability to develop spoken language skills and will influence the counseling provided to parents regarding the expected outcomes for their child. Parents of very young children should be informed that some psychological deficits (e.g., autism) are not typically identified until the child is 2 years of age or older and that performance with the device may be hindered later on if there is cognitive impairment.

In recent years, greater numbers of children presenting with a disability in addition to their hearing loss have been evaluated for a cochlear implant (Donaldson et al., 2004; Waltzman et al., 2000; Wiley et al., 2005). This has increased the need for preoperative psychological evaluations. This evaluation helps determine how effectively the child will be able to utilize the auditory signal, which will influence the decision of whether or not to provide the child with a cochlear implant. Importantly, the input

of the psychologist is essential when determining if referrals to other professionals are necessary prior to and after the child receives an implant.

H. Counseling

Counseling is an ongoing part of the pre- and postoperative evaluation process. When the patient is first seen, information should be provided regarding device options, cochlear implant technology, candidacy requirements, expectations of performance, appointments involved in the evaluation process, and financial obligations. Many centers make arrangements for patients to meet with a cochlear implant recipient or meet with the parents of a pediatric cochlear implant recipient to discuss the implant evaluation process.

I. Coordination of Services within the Child's Educational Setting

Ideally, a visit to the child's school should occur prior to implantation. During such visits, the audiologist and/or speech-language pathologist meets with the child's teacher(s) to provide instruction regarding care, use, and troubleshooting of the device and to discuss the child's language and auditory curriculum. The child may be observed in his/her classroom setting, and recommendations may be made regarding management of the child's auditory needs in the classroom.

J. Determination of Implant Ear

The determination of which ear to implant can be influenced by several factors. Many clinics routinely implant the ear with the least amount of residual hearing, while other clinics routinely implant the patient's "best" hearing ear. Some clinics determine the ear of implant on a case-by-case basis, while others leave this decision up to the patient and/or the parents. Research indicates that there are no known factors that help professionals predict which ear will respond best to the implant.

Recently, many clinics have begun to offer bilateral implants, eliminating the need to make a decision about which ear to implant. A cochlear implant can be placed in each ear during a single surgery (simultaneous bilateral implantation) or during separate surgeries (sequential bilateral implantation) that take place weeks, months, or even years apart. Recent studies indicate numerous benefits of bilateral implantation, including benefits for speech perception resulting from overcoming the head shadow effect, improved speech understanding in noise, and improved sound localization (Patrick et al., 2006). One of the benefits of bilateral simultaneous implantation is that such a strategy ensures that the better ear is always implanted. Unfortunately, many factors make it difficult or impossible for clinics to provide bilateral implants to their patients. These factors include poor reimbursement by insurers for unilateral and/or bilateral implants, poor insurance reimbursement for rehabilitative services, and an increase in the number of audiologists needed to program two devices. It is likely that bilateral cochlear implants will become the standard of care once these issues are resolved.

Summary of Preoperative Testing

In summary, preoperative testing is used to determine if a patient is a suitable candidate for a cochlear implant. Three primary questions that should be addressed in the preoperative evaluation include: (1) Can we increase the patient's auditory detection skills? (2) Can we improve the patient's speech understanding when compared to that obtained with a hearing aid? (3) In the pediatric population, is there a good chance that implant use will facilitate or improve spoken language more than would be expected with continued hearing aid use?

The specific criteria used to determine candidacy have changed greatly over the past several years and will continue to evolve and be influenced by patient results. Thus, it is important for clinicians to remain current regarding candidacy guidelines. Updates can be obtained by contacting local cochlear implant programs or by accessing cochlear implant manufacturer websites.

▨ SURGICAL PROCEDURE

Surgery begins with administration of general anesthesia. Hair is shaved above and behind the ear, the skin is prepared with an antiseptic solution, and sterile drapes are placed around the ear. A postauricular incision is made, and a well is created in the skull behind the mastoid bone in order to accommodate the receiver-stimulator portion of the internal device. The surgeon drills through the mastoid air cells and removes bone between the tympanic membrane and the facial nerve until the round window and the cochlear promontory are visualized. An opening (called a cochleostomy) is made into the basal turn of the scala tympani just anterior to the round window, and the electrode array is inserted into the scala tympani. If a ground electrode is attached to the receiver, it is then placed under the temporalis muscle. The receiver-stimulator is placed and secured into the well behind the mastoid, the incision is closed, and a pressure dressing is placed over the ear for 24 hours.

Some special considerations are needed when implanting young children because surgical intervention with this age group requires specific knowledge of temporal bone anatomy and the impact of skull growth on the implanted device. Although temporal bone growth has been shown to continue through adolescence, anatomy of the facial recess is fully developed at birth (Eby, 1996). The most significant developmental changes are in the size and configuration of the mastoid cavity. Eby and Nadol (1986) recommend that the surgeon leave approximately 2.5 cm of additional electrode lead in the mastoid area to accommodate for head growth. Additionally, modifications to the surgical technique may be necessary when the patient presents with anatomic anomalies, such as cochlear ossification or malformation.

Cochlear implant surgery lasts between 2 and 5 hours depending on the surgeon's experience, the device selected, and the complexity of the anatomy encountered in each patient. Most clinics perform this as an out-patient procedure, enabling patients to return home in less than 24 hours. Children and adults return to their normal routines when they feel well enough to do so, often within 1 week of surgery.

Cochlear implantation has the same risks as other procedures conducted under general anesthesia and those of other surgeries of the middle or inner ear. In centers with considerable experience performing cochlear implant surgery, such risks are quite limited and are greatly outweighed by the advantages that the properly selected patient will obtain from the implant. Risks include a remote possibility of infection, temporary or permanent facial paralysis on the operated side, mild temporary taste disturbances, tinnitus, and vertigo. In traditional cochlear implant surgery, one may expect loss of any residual hearing in the implanted ear, as well as mild pain and numbness at the site of the incision following the surgery. Removal of the cochlear implant may become necessary if the internal device suffers electrical or mechanical damage, if an infection at the site cannot be successfully treated with medication, or if the device or the electrode array becomes displaced. Such surgical intervention is similar in scope to initial placement of the device, although generally less risky due to the drilling having been completed at the original operation.

Cochlear implant recipients must avoid various medical/surgical procedures that could damage the implanted device or the functioning auditory nerve fibers that transmit the electrical signal to the brain. The use of monopolar electrosurgical instruments in the region of the head or neck, diathermy, neurostimulation, ionizing radiation therapy involving the area of the implant, electroconvulsive therapy, and MRI must all be avoided because they can cause excessive magnetic and electromagnetic interference, which may result in demagnetization of the internal magnet, displacement of the device, and/or disruption of the device electronics. Two commercial cochlear implant devices, the Nucleus Freedom and Advanced Bionics HR90K, are manufactured with a removable internal magnet and may be preferable for patients who are expected to need MRI in the future, such as those who suffer from multiple intracranial tumors related to neurofibromatosis type II. The MED-EL Cochlear Implant System, which does not have a removable magnet, is FDA approved for use with MRI at a maximum strength of 0.2 Tesla.

▨ POSTOPERATIVE MANAGEMENT: PROGRAMMING THE DEVICE

After surgery, patients return to their implant center for initial programming of their device. The recommended amount of time between surgery and device programming varies; some centers activate the device within days, while others may wait several weeks. Waiting for device activation allows for healing and reduction of swelling around the incision, which will enable the headset magnet to adhere properly. The particular procedures followed for the activation will vary depending on the patient's age as well as on the device that was implanted.

For all devices, initial programming begins with connection of the patient's speech processor to the audiologist's computer. This interface of hardware to the internally implanted device enables the clinician to perform objective and subjective measurements needed to appropriately set the device. First, telemetry is performed and provides valuable information regarding the status of the internal device. Telemetry systems work by sampling, digitizing, and reporting back to the clinician information about the voltage generated on the internal electrodes during stimulation. Telemetry measurements provide information about electrode impedances, short-circuited electrodes, and voltage compliance for each of the electrodes in the array (Abbas et al., 2006). Such measurements guide clinicians in their determination of which electrodes to include or exclude from the recipient's program.

Next, the clinician works with the patient to determine the softest level of sound that results in hearing for each of the electrodes. This level is referred to as "threshold" and is recorded on a computer using programming software. Additionally, the upper level of stimulation is determined for each active electrode. Depending on the type of device used, the level of stimulation is increased until the patient reports the sound is "most comfortable" (M level) or is loud but comfortable (C level). This results in creation of a speech processor program tailored to the hearing of the individual being tested.

Programming of the electrodes and creation of the speech processor program can be particularly challenging with young children and with patients who are unable to provide feedback regarding the perceptibility and loudness of the electrical signal. With young children, traditional behavioral test techniques, such as behavioral observation audiometry (BOA), visual reinforcement audiometry (VRA), and conditioned play audiometry (CPA) (see Chapter 23), are used to determine threshold and comfort level measurements. Additionally, objective measures, such as neural response telemetry (NRT), neural response imaging (NRI), EABR, and measurement of electrically evoked stapedial reflexes (ESRT), may aid in determination of programming levels.

Various programming techniques are used to refine the patient's psychophysical measures, such as loudness balancing, pitch scaling, and sweeping of the active electrodes. The finalized psychophysical data are applied to a particular speech processing strategy using programming software. Once it is determined that the program is appropriate, it is transferred to the patient's speech processor, and the patient takes it home to use following completion of the initial programming session.

The total number of electrodes used by a patient may be less than the number of electrodes available on the array.

Determination of which electrodes to use may be influenced by factors such as telemetry test results, mode of stimulation, the patient's response to electrical stimulation, encoding strategy, and surgical placement of the electrode array. For example, the patient may experience discomfort, dizziness, or facial nerve stimulation when one or more of the electrodes are stimulated. When this occurs, the electrode is simply deactivated, which means it will not be used in the patient's map and will not cause discomfort. Additionally, the optimal number of electrodes differs for the various speech processing strategies. Thus, several of the electrodes along the array may be deactivated in order to use only the optimal number needed for a particular speech processing strategy. Lastly, an incomplete insertion of the electrode array may limit the number of electrodes that can be stimulated. Such incomplete insertions may occur with cochlear malformations or cochlear ossification.

Both the Nucleus Freedom and the Advanced Bionics HiResolution devices offer objective assessment of the response of the auditory nerve to electrical stimulation in the form of the auditory nerve compound action potential. NRT or NRI testing is a measure of the synchronous primary afferent neural response to electrical stimulation. In order to obtain these measures, one electrode within the cochlea stimulates the nerve, while a different intracochlear electrode records the response of the nerve (Abbas et al., 2006). Various aspects of this measurement provide information that can be used to guide the clinician when setting threshold and comfort levels.

The number of times patients return to their implant center for continued programming varies greatly and can be affected by factors such as the patient's psychophysical/programming needs, distance traveled to reach the implant facility, and occupational demands. In most cases, children are seen twice a month for the first 3 months, monthly for the next 3 months, and then every 6 to 12 months to program their speech processor. During such visits, warble tone thresholds should be obtained in a sound field to verify the appropriateness of the patient's program. At many centers, speech perception testing is performed every 6 to 12 months with children. Adult patients are usually seen twice a month the first month, and then at 3, 6, and 12 months postactivation. Patients are subsequently seen annually for programming and speech perception testing. Such testing is valuable because it can be compared to previous speech perception test results to determine if performance has improved or declined. Decreases in scores are unusual and may indicate that the current program is not optimal for the patient.

Often, the same measures that were used to evaluate speech perception preoperatively are used in the follow-up evaluations. If the patient uses a hearing aid in the contralateral ear, this evaluation should include testing while the patient uses the implant alone, the hearing aid alone, and implant and hearing aid together. This testing enables the clinician to perform a pre- versus postoperative comparison and identify cues that are misperceived by the recipient and provides information regarding further rehabilitative needs. Importantly, postoperative test results enable the clinician to monitor the function of the internal device. For example, comparisons may show the internal device declining in function, which could go unnoticed by the implant recipient. This may result in reduced speech perception or speech-language skills over time. Documentation of such reduced performance is valuable when determining the recommended intervention, such as a decision to explant the malfunctioning device and replace it with a working device. Lastly, postoperative results provide information that can be used in future selection criteria.

(RE)HABILITATION

The goal of postoperative rehabilitation and training is to teach patients how to use their devices to maximize their oral communication ability. The amount of rehabilitation provided to recipients varies greatly and will depend on several factors, including performance with the device, length of deafness prior to implantation, and primary communication mode.

Postlingually Deafened Adults

Most postlingually deafened adults have only mild rehabilitative needs following adequate adjustment of their device. Such rehabilitation primarily focuses on training in the proper care and use of the device, utilization of assistive listening devices with the cochlear implant, and training to maximize communication ability in difficult listening situations, such as listening in the presence of background noise and using the device on the telephone. Some adults enroll in classes to improve their speechreading skills. Many recipients demonstrate profound improvements in their communication skills immediately following device activation, reducing their need for formalized rehabilitation and training.

Prelingually Deafened Adults

Prelingually deafened adults demonstrate greater rehabilitative needs than postlingually deafened adults. Because they tend to demonstrate a higher nonuse rate than postlingually deafened adults, it is recommended that they be seen more often than postlingually deafened adults for the first year following activation. Such visits provide an opportunity to provide ongoing counseling regarding issues related to dissatisfaction with the device. Additionally, adjustments can be made to patients' programs in order to maximize the clarity of the electrical signal they are receiving. This is often needed because prelingually deafened adults may demonstrate more frequent changes in their hearing ability than postlingually deafened adults. These changes often include increased consistency in their ability to detect sound, gradual increase

in the upper level of the dynamic range (increased C or M levels), and an improved ability to do loudness balance scaling. Many prelingually deafened adults report that initial stimulation of their device results in a sensation of feeling, rather than hearing. This feeling may occur in the forehead, sternum, throat, or the area around the ear. Increased experience with sound, however, often facilitates a transformation from feeling to hearing.

There are several rehabilitative programs designed for use by both pre- and postlingually deafened adults. All three implant manufacturers offer computer programs for purchase that are aimed at improving the speech perception skills of adults and children. Thomas and Zwolan (2006) found that use of the Rosetta Stone language learning software (Fairfield Language Technologies, Harrisonburg, VA) fostered statistically significant improvements for speech intelligibility, auditory comprehension, and reading level for prelingually deafened adults when the program was used consistently at home for a period of 3 months. Home-based computer programs appear to be particularly beneficial for prelingually deafened adults because they are self-paced and provide the implant recipient with a nonthreatening learning partner.

Children

The (re)habilitative needs of children with cochlear implants are great. This is an important part of the implant process that must be provided if the child is to receive maximum benefit from the device. Such (re)habilitation should include parent training and parental involvement; speech perception training and assessment; speech and language assessment and training, including speech production and receptive and expressive language; and involvement of the child's teachers. In many instances, the child's school is the primary provider of (re)habilitative services. The audiologist and/or speech-language pathologist on the cochlear implant team may work additionally with the child on rehabilitative tasks and make recommendations to the child's school regarding (re)habilitative needs. In some cases, children attend private therapy in addition to that provided by their school system. For specific information regarding rehabilitation therapy techniques commonly used with children with cochlear implants, the reader is referred to Allum (1996) and Estabrooks and Birkenshaw-Fleming (2006). Additionally, each cochlear implant manufacturer provides excellent resources for parents, educators, and hearing professionals regarding pediatric aural (re)habilitation and device troubleshooting.

Use of a Hearing Aid in the Contralateral Ear

Cochlear implant recipients receive a variety of recommendations regarding use of a contralateral hearing aid with a cochlear implant. Such recommendations should be made on a case-by-case basis and take into consideration the amount of hearing in the nonimplanted ear, appropriateness of the hearing aid for the patient's loss, the willingness of the recipient to give up use of the aid, and the patient's early level of performance with the cochlear implant. Some professionals recommend continued use of the aid, while others believe that use of a contralateral hearing aid may actually increase the amount of time it takes for some patients to adjust to the sound quality of the implant. Such professionals may recommend cessation of hearing aid use for brief or prolonged periods of time following device activation, followed by reintroduction of the aid once the recipient has accepted the sound quality of the cochlear implant.

AN OVERVIEW OF CURRENT SPEECH PERCEPTION AND SPEECH AND LANGUAGE RESULTS

Adults

Performance of adults with cochlear implants is greatly affected by several factors, including age at onset of deafness, length of deafness, and primary communication method. Patients who lost their hearing prior to the development of speech and language skills (prelingually deafened adults) typically demonstrate poorer speech perception skills with an implant than postlingually deafened adults (Skinner et al., 1992; Waltzman, and Cohen, 1999; Zwolan et al., 1996). Postimplant changes in speech recognition scores vary greatly for prelingually deafened adults. Some demonstrate progress, while others demonstrate little or no change in scores over time, even when combined with intensive rehabilitation. Because of these factors, prelingually deafened adults demonstrate a higher device nonuse rate than postlingually deafened adults. However, many prelingually deafened adults use their device regularly, report that they are satisfied with their device, and report that using the cochlear implant improves both their expressive and receptive communication skills (Zwolan et al., 1996).

The speech recognition performance currently obtained by postlingually deafened adults far exceeds that envisioned when cochlear implants were first introduced and far exceed the results obtained by prelingually deafened adults. At minimum, most postlingually deafened adults demonstrate greatly enhanced lipreading skills when using their implant, and most hear so well that they are able to converse interactively over the telephone. Results of the most recent multichannel clinical trial for the Nucleus Freedom device in adults indicate a mean group score of 57% correct for CNC words, a mean score of 78% correct for HINT sentences in quiet, and a mean score of 64% correct for HINT sentences in noise (Balkany et al., 2007).

Children

Several factors are known to impact children's performance with a cochlear implant, including age at onset of profound deafness, age at which the child receives the implant, status of the cochlea, amount of residual hearing prior to implantation, presence of additional disabilities, and the child's educational environment. Recent publications indicate that many children who receive cochlear implants at a young age approach levels of speech perception and speech-language performance similar to those attained by children with normal hearing (Eisenberg et al., 2006; Geers et al., 2003; Taitelbaum-Swead et al., 2005). Such outcomes far exceed those anticipated when cochlear implants were first introduced.

AGE AT ONSET OF DEAFNESS

Several investigators have demonstrated that the age at onset of profound deafness has a strong impact on performance with a cochlear implant. In general, postlingually deafened children tend to demonstrate quicker postoperative gains in speech recognition than prelingually deafened children, although such differences are not as great as those observed between pre- and postlingually deafened adults. Most prelingually deafened children demonstrate profound gains in speech perception and speech production skills within 18 to 24 months of receiving a cochlear implant, while most postlingually deafened children tend to demonstrate immediate improvements (Fryauf-Bertschy et al., 1992; Osberger et al., 1991). These differences are likely due to the fact that postlingually deafened children have had greater experience with sound.

AGE AT WHICH THE COCHLEAR IMPLANT IS RECEIVED

Current FDA guidelines for the three commercially available devices indicate that it is appropriate to implant children as young as 12 months of age. There appear to be several arguments that support such an early age for implantation. First, providing an implant at an early age maximizes the amount of auditory information available to the child during the critical period for learning language (Cairns, 1986; Dale, 1976). Additionally, providing the child with sound decreases the length of auditory deprivation, which has a positive effect on the outcome (Young, 1994). Numerous investigators report that patients implanted at younger ages attain better speech perception scores and oral language capabilities than children implanted at older ages (Geers et al., 2003; Kileny et al., 1999; Miyamoto et al., 2003; Waltzman et al., 2002) and that children seem to perform optimally if provided with a cochlear implant prior to the age of 2.5 years (Connor et al., 2006).

STATUS OF THE COCHLEA

Recipients who present with abnormal cochleae, such as those with congenital malformations or cochlear ossification, may experience reduced performance because of incomplete insertion of the electrode array or insufficient loudness growth. However, patients who present with such anomalies are still considered to be candidates for a cochlear implant (Balkany et al., 1996; Tucci et al., 1995). El-Kashlan et al. (2003) found that, although prelingually deafened children with postmeningitic hearing loss and ossified cochleae received significant benefit from cochlear implants, their mean overall performance was poorer than that of children with cochlear implants and nonossified cochleae. Eisenman et al. (2001) found that some children with radiographic cochlear malformations performed as well as their matched counterparts with normal cochleae, although their improvements occurred more slowly over time. Children with more severe malformations demonstrated poorer performance than children with mild abnormalities or normal cochleae. It is important to provide preoperative counseling regarding anticipated outcome when such anomalies are identified with the preoperative CT or MRI.

AMOUNT OF RESIDUAL HEARING

Some studies indicate that children with greater amounts of residual hearing at the time of implant tend to demonstrate greater overall gains in speech perception with an implant than children who demonstrate little or no residual hearing (Geers, 2006; Zwolan et al., 1997). This is probably due to the increased auditory experience that such children have when compared to other children who have had little or no experience with sound.

ADDITIONAL DISABILITIES/DIAGNOSES

Some children may demonstrate disabilities secondary to their deafness that may affect performance with a cochlear implant. Noncognitive disabilities, such as blindness and cerebral palsy, are not likely to impact the decision to implant or to impact the child's eventual performance with a cochlear implant. Cognitive disabilities, on the other hand, are likely to impact performance (Waltzman et al., 2000) and may affect the decision regarding candidacy. These conditions include children diagnosed with learning disabilities secondary to meningitis and children diagnosed with mental impairments such as autism (Donaldson et al., 2004). If a child with cognitive disabilities receives a cochlear implant, appropriate expectations must be set at home and at school regarding expected performance with the device.

Additionally, there has been a large increase recently in the number of children with auditory dyssynchrony (AD) who receive cochlear implants. AD is a term used to describe an auditory disorder characterized by recordable otoacoustic emissions and/or cochlear microphonics, absent or atypical ABRs, and speech recognition skills that are poorer than would be expected based on the audiogram (Rapin and Gravel, 2003). Determination of candidacy for a cochlear implant in patients with AD can be difficult because such patients may meet candidacy criteria based on their poor speech recognition skills but may fail to meet criteria based

on their audiometric thresholds being better than current criteria indicate. Determination of cochlear implant candidacy for patients with AD is additionally complicated by the finding that some patients demonstrate improvement of detection and speech recognition skills over time (Neault, 2003) and that many children who present with AD also present with additional medical diagnoses that may affect expected performance outcomes (Rance et al., 1999).

Several investigators have reported that cochlear implant recipients with AD demonstrate postoperative outcomes that are similar to those obtained by more traditional cochlear implant recipients (Mason et al., 2003; Peterson et al., 2003; Sininger and Trautwein, 2002). Some investigators hypothesize that cochlear implantation is successful in such recipients because it provides a supraphysiologic electrical stimulation to the auditory nerve, with the hope of reintroducing synchronous neural activity that cannot be achieved with acoustic stimulation (Mason et al., 2003). Because of the potential loss of residual hearing, determination of implant candidacy for a child with AD should be made carefully and be determined on a case-by-case basis. One factor that should receive strong consideration is the child's spoken language skills. The presence of a severe language delay demonstrates a need for intervention.

COMMUNICATION METHODOLOGY

When a child is identified with a hearing loss, parents must select a treatment plan that determines the child's primary method for communicating with others. These communication options include American Sign Language (ASL), Simultaneous (Total) Communication (TC), Oral Communication (OC), and the Auditory-Verbal (AV) approach. Such options vary greatly in the amount of emphasis they place on the child's use of spoken language, and therefore, can affect outcomes with a cochlear implant.

Several investigators have compared the speech perception and speech and language skills of children with cochlear implants who use these various methods of communication. Studies that include a TC approach is particularly difficult to control because educational settings vary greatly in regard to the emphasis placed on oral versus manual communication. Many recent studies report that children trained to use either AV or OC demonstrate more rapid gains in spoken communication abilities than children who use TC (Geers et al., 2003; Tobey et al., 2004). Geers et al. (2003) compared speech and language and speech perception measures of children who received a cochlear implant prior to the age of 2 and found that most children with average learning ability who used OC produced and understood the English language at a level comparable to that of their peers with normal hearing.

With regard to educational placement, it is well agreed that children will perform optimally with a cochlear implant if their school supports the child in his or her use of the device, offers aggressive auditory management and treatment, and provides an optimal auditory environment that promotes and encourages auditory development.

SURGICAL COMPLICATIONS AND DEVICE FAILURES

Occasionally, patients will experience failure of the internal device or surgical complications that will necessitate surgical revision or replacement of the internal device. Possible reasons for such intervention include mechanical device failure, less than optimal electrode placement, skin flap complications, need for technological upgrade, or intratemporal pathologic conditions (Donatelli et al., 2005). Mechanical failures of the internal device are often referred to as either "hard failures," which are unequivocal device failures identified or verified by integrity testing performed by the device manufacturer, or "soft failures," which are failures that occur when the implant recipient experiences discomfort or an unexplained decrease in clinical benefit, even though manufacturer-conducted integrity testing indicates that the device is functioning within normal limits. The "hard" failure rates reported by clinics vary and range from a low of 2.9% (Donatelli et al., 2005) to a high of 11% of all patients (Parisier et al., 1991) and 14.9% of pediatric patients

(Parisier et al., 1991). Fortunately, many studies have found that reimplantation following device failure is a viable option and that many cochlear implant recipients show improved or stable benefit following reimplantation (Buchman et al., 2004; Donatelli et al., 2005; Ray et al., 2004).

FUTURE DIRECTIONS

Future advances in the field of cochlear implants are highly anticipated and expected. Some implant manufacturers are evaluating techniques for drug delivery to the cochlea via the electrode array. Such drugs could prevent further degeneration of the auditory system or may help keep electrode impedances and power requirements low by preventing tissue growth within the cochlea following implantation (Hochmair et al., 2006). Internal and external components of cochlear implant systems will continue to decrease in size while their design, flexibility, and function will continue to improve. Additionally, it is likely that completely implantable cochlear implant systems will be available in the future and that recipients will continue to demonstrate even greater speech recognition skills and enhanced hearing enjoyment in quiet and in noise as new and improved speech processing strategies are developed.

REFERENCES

Abbas PJ, Brown CJ, Etler CP. (2006) Electrophysiology and device telemetry. In: Waltzman SB, Roland JT, eds. *Cochlear Implants*. 2nd ed. New York: Thieme Medical Publishers.

Advanced Bionics Corporation. (2007) HR90K package insert. Boston: Advanced Bionics Corporation.

Allum DJ, ed. (1996) *Cochlear Implant Rehabilitation in Children and Adults*. San Diego: Singular Publishing Group.

Balkany T, Gantz BJ, Steenerson RL, Cohen NL. (1996) Systematic approach to electrode insertion in the ossified cochlea. *Otolaryngol Head Neck Surg*. 114, 4–11.

Balkany T, Hodges A, Menapace C, Hazard L, Driscoll C, Gantz B, Kelsall D, Luxford W, McMenomy S, Neely JG, Peters B, Pillsbury H, Roberson J, Schramm D, Telian S, Waltzman S, Westerberg B, Payne S. (2007) Nucleus Freedom North American clinical trial. *Otolaryngol Head Neck Surg*. 136, 757–762.

Bench J, Kowal A, Bamford J. (1979) The BKB (Bamford-Kowal-Bench) sentence lists for partially-hearing children. *Br J Audiol*. 13, 108–112.

Boothroyd A, Hanin L, Hnath T. (1985) A sentence test of speech perception: reliability, set equivalence, and short term learning (Internal Report RCI 10). New York: City University of New York.

Buchman CA, Higgins CA, Cullen R, Pillsbury HC. (2004) Revision cochlear implant surgery in adult patients with suspected device malfunction. *Otol Neurotol*. 25, 504–510.

Cairns H. (1986) *The Acquisition of Language*. Austin, TX: Pro-Ed.

Cheng AD, Grant GD, Niparko JK. (2004) Meta-analysis of pediatric cochlear implant literature. *Ann Otol Rhinol Laryngol Suppl*. 177, 124–128.

Clark GM, Blamey PJ, Busby PA. (1987) A multiple-electrode intracochlear implant for children. *Arch Otolaryngol*. 113, 825–828.

Cochlear Americas. (2006) Nucleus Freedom [CI24RE(CA)] package insert. Sydney, Australia: Cochlear Americas.

Connor C, Craig C, Raudenbush S, Heavner K, Zwolan T. (2006) The age at which young deaf children receiver cochlear implants and their vocabulary and speech production growth: is there an added value for early implantation? *Ear Hear*. 27, 628–644.

Dale P. (1976) *Language Development: Structure and Function*. 2nd ed. New York: Holt, Rinehart, & Winston.

Djourno A, Eyries C. (1957) Prothese auditive par excitation electrique a distance du nerf sensoriel a l'aide d'un bobinage inclus a demeure. *Presse Medicale*. 35, 14–17.

Donaldson AI, Heavner KS, Zwolan TA. (2004) Measuring progress in children with autism spectrum disorder who have cochlear implants. *Arch Otolaryngol Head Neck Surg*. 130, 666–671.

Donatelli A, Zwolan TA, Telian S. (2005) Cochlear implant failures and revision. *Otol Neurotol*. 26, 624–634.

Doyle JH, Doyle JB, Turnbull FM. (1964) Electrical stimulation of eighth cranial nerve. *Arch Otolaryngol*. 80, 388–391.

Eby TL. (1996) Development of the facial recess: implications for cochlear implantation. *Laryngoscope*. 106 (suppl 80), 1–7.

Eby TL, Nadol JB. (1986) Postnatal growth of the human temporal bone: Implications for cochlear implants in children. *Ann Otol Rhinol Laryngol*. 95, 356–382.

Eisenberg LS, Johnson KC, Martinez AS, Cokely CG, Tobey EA, Quittner AL, Fink NE, Wang NY, Niparko JK; CDaCI

Investigative Team. (2006) Speech recognition at 1-year follow-up in the childhood development after cochlear implantation study: methods and preliminary findings. *Audiol Neurootol.* 11, 259–268.

Eisenman DJ, Ashbaugh C, Zwolan TA, Arts HA, Telian SA. (2001) Implantation of the malformed cochlea. *Otol Neurotol.* 22, 834–841.

El-Kashlan HK, Ashbaugh C, Zwolan T, Telian SA. (2003) Cochlear implantation in prelingually deaf children with ossified cochleae. *Otol Neurotol.* 24, 596600.

Elliott L, Katz D. (1980) *Development of a New Children's Test of Speech Discrimination.* St. Louis: Auditec.

Erber NP. (1982) *Auditory Training.* Washington, DC: Alexander Graham Bell Association for the Deaf.

Estabrooks W, Birkenshaw-Fleming L. (2006) *Hear & Listen! Talk & Sing!* Washington, DC: Alexander Graham Bell Association for the Deaf.

Firszt JB, Holden LK, Skinner MW, Tobey EA, Peterson A, Gaggl W, Runge-Samuelson CL, Wackym PA. (2004) Recognition of speech presented at soft to loud levels by adult cochlear implant recipients of three cochlear implant systems. *Ear Hear.* 25, 375–387.

Firszt JB, Koch DB, Downing M, Litvak L. (2007) Current steering creates additional pitch percepts in adults cochlear implant recipients. *Otol Neurotol.* 28, 629–636.

Fryauf-Bertschy H, Tyler RS, Kelsay DM, Gantz B. (1992) Performance over time of congenitally deaf and postlingually deafened children using a multichannel cochlear implant. *J Speech Hear Res.* 35, 913–920.

Gantz BJ, Turner C, Gfeller KE, Lowder ME. (2005) Preservation of hearing in cochlear implant surgery: advantages of combined electrical and acoustical speech processing. *Laryngoscope.* 115, 796–802.

Geers AE. (2006) Factors influencing spoken language outcomes in children following early cochlear implantation. *Adv Otorhinolaryngol.* 64, 50–65.

Geers AE, Nicholas JG, Sedey AL. (2003) Language skills of children with early cochlear implantation. *Ear Hear.* 24, 46S–58S.

Gstoettner W, Helbig S, Maier N, Kiefer J, Radeloff A, Adukna O. (2006a) Ipsilateral electric acoustic stimulation of the auditory system: long term preservation of acoustic hearing. *Audiol Neurootol.* 11 (suppl 1), 49–56.

Gstoettner W, Van de Heyning P, O'Connor AF, Morera C, Sainz M. (2006b) Results from a multi-centre EAS clinical investigation. *Wien Med Wochenschr.* 156 (suppl 119), 121.

Haskins HA. (1949) A phonetically balanced test of speech discrimination for children. Unpublished master's thesis. Evanston, IL: Northwestern University.

Hochmair I, Nopp P, Jolly C, Schmidt M, Schober H, Garnham C, Anderson I. (2006) MED-EL cochlear implants: state of the art and a glimpse into the future. *Trends Amplif.* 10, 201.

Hochmair-Desoyer IJ, Hochmair ES, Fischer R, Burian K. (1980) Cochlear prostheses in use: recent psychophysical data and speech comprehension results. *Arch Otorhinolaryngol.* 229, 81–98.

Iler Kirk K, Diefendorf AO, Pisoni DB, Robbins AM. (1997) Assessing Speech Perception In Children. In: Mendel LL, Danhauer JL, eds. *Audiologic Evaluation and Management and Speech Perception Assessment.* San Diego: Singular Publishing Group; pp 101–131.

Kileny PR, Zwolan TA. (2004) Perioperative, transtympanic electric ABR in pediatric cochlear implant candidates. *Cochlear Implants Int.* 5 (suppl 1), 23–25.

Kileny PR, Zwolan TA, Ashbaugh CJ. (1999) The influence of age at implantation on performance with a cochlear implant in children. Presented at the annual meeting of the American Otological Society, Desert Springs, CA.

Kileny PR, Zwolan TA, Zimmerman-Phillips S, Telian SA. (1994) Electrically evoked auditory brain-stem response in pediatric patients with cochlear implants. *Arch Otolaryngol Head Neck Surg.* 120, 1083–1090.

Kirk KI, Pisoni DB, Osberger MJ. (1995) Lexical effects on spoken word recognition by pediatric cochlear implant users. *Ear Hear.* 16, 470–481.

Koch DB, Downing M, Osberger MJ, Litvak L. (2007) Using current steering to increase spectral resolution in CII and HiRes 90K users. *Ear Hear.* 28 (suppl 2), 38S–41S.

Koch DB, Osberger MJ, Segel P, Kessler DK. (2004) HiResolution and conventional sound processing in the HiResolution Bionic Ear: using appropriate outcome measures to assess speech recognition ability. *Audiol Neurotol.* 9, 214–223.

Luxford WM, Berliner KI, Eisenberg MA, House WF. (1987) Cochlear implants in children. *Ann Otol.* 96, 136–138.

Luxford WM, Brackman DE. (1985) The history of cochlear implants. In: Gray R, ed. *Cochlear Implants.* San Diego: College Hill Press; pp 1–26.

Mason JC, De Michele A, Stevens C, Ruth RA, Hashisaki GT. (2003) Cochlear implantation in patients with auditory neuropathy of varied etiologies. *Laryngoscope.* 113, 45–49.

MED-EL. (2007) MedEl PULSAR$_{CI}^{100}$ package insert. Innsbruck, Austria: MED-EL.

Miyamoto RT, Houston DM, Kirk KI, Perdew AE, Svirsky ME. (2003) Language development in deaf infants following cochlear implantation. *Acta Otolaryngol.* 123, 241–244.

Moog JS, Geers AE. (1990) *Early Speech Perception Test for Profoundly Hearing-Impaired Children.* St. Louis: Central Institute for the Deaf.

Neault M. (2003) Auditory dys-synchrony of infancy: implications for implantation. Presented at the Ninth Symposium on Cochlear Implants in Children, Washington, DC.

Nilsson MJ, Soli SD, Sullivan JA. (1994) Development of the Hearing in Noise Test for the measurement of speech reception thresholds in quiet and in noise. *J Acoust Soc Am.* 95, 1085–1099.

Osberger MJ, Todd SL, Berry SW, Robbins AM, Miyamoto RT. (1991) Effect of age at onset of deafness on children's speech perception abilities with a cochlear implant. *Ann Otol Rhinol Laryngol.* 100, 883–888.

Parisier SC, Chute PM, Weiss MH, Hellman SA, Wang RC. (1991) Results of cochlear implant reinsertion. *Laryngoscope.* 101, 1013–1015.

Parkinson A, Arcaroli J, Staller SJ, Arndt PL, Cosgriff A, Ebinger K. (2002) The Nucleus 24 contour cochlear implant system: adult clinical trial results. *Ear Hear.* 23 (suppl 1), 41S–48S.

Patrick JF, Busby PA, Gibson PJ. (2006) The development of the Nucleus Freedom cochlear implant system. *Trends Amplif.* 10, 175.

Peterson A, Shallop J, Driscoll C, Breneman A, Babb J, Stoeckel R, Fabry L. (2003) Outcomes of cochlear implantation in children with auditory neuropathy. *J Am Acad Audiol.* 14, 188–201.

Peterson GE, Lehiste I. (1962) Revised CNC lists for auditory tests. *J Speech Hear Disord.* 27, 62–70.

Rance G, Beer DE, Cone-Wesson B, Shepard RK, Dowell RC, King AM, Rickards FW, Clark GM. (1999) Clinical findings for a group of infants and young children with auditory neuropathy. *Ear Hear.* 20, 3.

Rapin I, Gravel J. (2003) "Auditory neuropathy": physiologic and pathologic evidence calls for more diagnostic specificity. *Int J Pediatr Otorhinolaryngol.* 67, 707–728.

Ray J, Proops D, Donaldson I. (2004) Explanation and reimplantation of cochlear implants. *Cochlear Implants Int.* 5, 160–167.

Robbins AM, Renshaw JJ, Berry SW. (1991) Evaluating meaningful auditory integration in profoundly hearing-impaired children. *Am J Otol.* 12 (suppl), 144–150.

Ross M, Lerman J. (1979) *Word Intelligibility by Picture Identification.* Pittsburgh, PA: Stanwix House, Inc.

Sininger YS, Trautwein P. (2002) Electrical stimulation of the auditory nerve via cochlear implants in patients with auditory neuropathy. *Ann Otol Rhinol Laryngol.* 189 (suppl), 23–31.

Skinner MW, Binzer SM, Fears BT, Holden TA, Jenison VW, Nettles EJ. (1992) Study of the performance of four prelinguistically or perilinguistically deaf patients with a multi-electrode intracochlear implant. *Laryngoscope.* 102, 797–806.

Spahr AJ, Emadi G. (2005) Preliminary results of pitch strength with HiRes 120 Spectral Resolution. *Advanced Bionics Auditory Research Bulletin*, Biennial Edition. Boston: Advanced Bionics.

Stacey PC, Fortnum HC, Barton GR, Summerfield AQ. (2006) Hearing-impaired children in the United Kingdom. I: Auditory performance, communication skills, educational achievements, quality of life, and cochlear implantation. *Ear Hear.* 27, 161–186.

Staller S. (1998) Clinical trials of the Nucleus 24 in adults and children. Presented at the 10th Annual Convention of the American Academy of Audiology, Los Angeles, CA.

Stypulkowski PH, van den Honert C, Kvistad SD. (1986) Electrophysiologic evaluation of the cochlear implant patient. *Otolaryngol Clin North Am.* 19, 249–257.

Taitelbaum-Swead R, Kishon-Rabin L, Kaplan-Neeman R, Muchnik C, Kronenberg J, Hildesheimer M. (2005) Speech perception of children using Nucleus, Clarion or Med-El cochlear implants. *Int J Pediatr Otorhinolaryngol.* 69, 1675–1683.

Thomas E, Zwolan T. (2006) Benefit of language software for prelingual/teen adult CI users. Presentation at the Ninth International Conference on Cochlear Implants and Related Sciences, Vienna, Austria.

Tillman TW, Carhart R. (1966) An expanded test for speech discrimination utilizing CNC monosyllabic words. Northwestern University Auditory Test No. 6. (USAF School of Aerospace Medicine Technical Report). Brooks Air Force Base, TX: US Air Force.

Tobey EA, Rekart D, Buckley K. (2004) Mode of communication and classroom placement impact on speech intelligibility. *Arch Otolaryngol Head Neck Surg.* 130, 639–643.

Tucci DD, Telian SA, Zimmerman-Phillips S, Zwolan TA, Kileny PR. (1995) Cochlear implantation in patients with cochlear malformations. *Arch Otolaryngol Head Neck Surg.* 121, 833–838.

Tyler RS, Moore BCJ, Kuk FK. (1989) Performance of some of the better cochlear implant patients. *J Speech Hear Res.* 32, 887–911.

Waltzman SB, Cohen NL. (1999) Implantation of patients with prelingual long-term deafness. *Ann Otol Rhinol Laryngol Suppl.* 177, 84–87.

Waltzman SB, Cohen NL, Green J, Roland JT. (2002) Long-term effects of cochlear implants in children. *Otolaryngol Head Neck Surg.* 126, 505–511.

Waltzman SB, Scalchunes V, Cohen NL. (2000) Performance of multiply handicapped children using cochlear implants. *Am J Otol.* 21, 329–335.

Wiley S, Jahnke M, Meinzen-Derr J, Choo D. (2005) Perceived qualitative benefits of cochlear implants in children with multihandicaps. *Int J Pediatr Otorhinolaryngol.* 69, 791–798.

Wilson BS. (2000) Strategies for representing speech information with cochlear implants. In: Niparko J, ed. *Cochlear Implants: Principles and Practices.* Philadelphia: Lippincott Williams & Wilkins.

Wilson BS, Finley CC, Lawson DT, Wolford RD, Eddington DK, Rabinowitz WM. (1991) Better speech recognition with cochlear implants. *Nature.* 35, 236–238.

Wilson BS, Lawson DT, Zerbi M, Finley CC, Wolford RD. (1995) New processing strategies in cochlear implantation. *Am J Otol.* 16, 669–675.

Young NM. (1994) Cochlear implants in children. *Curr Prob Pediatr.* 24, 131–138.

Zimmerman-Phillips S, McConkey-Robbins A, Osberger MJ. (1998) Assessing device benefit in infants and toddlers. Poster presentation at the Seventh Symposium on Cochlear Implants in Children, Iowa City, Iowa.

Zimmerman-Phillips S, Murad C. (1999) Programming features of the Clarion Multi-Strategy cochlear implant. *Ann Otol Rhinol Laryngol.* 108, 17–21.

Zwolan TA, Ashbaugh CJ, Zimmerman-Phillips S, Hieber SJ, Kileny PR, Telian SA. (1997) Cochlear implantation of children with minimal open-set speech recognition skills. *Ear Hear.* 18, 240–251.

Zwolan TA, Kileny PR, Telian SA. (1996) Self report of cochlear implant use and satisfaction by prelingually deafened adults. *Ear Hear.* 17, 198–210.

Intervention, Education, and Therapy for Children Who Are Deaf or Hard of Hearing

Arlene Stredler Brown

▨ INTRODUCTION

Intervention and education for children with hearing loss has changed dramatically in recent years. There are many reasons for this change. Newborn hearing screening is now common practice (Green et al., 2007), while advanced hearing aid technology and cochlear implants provide better access to auditory information. In addition, age-old arguments about the best communication approach are starting to fade.

Starting in 1975, public laws have supported the provision of individualized intervention and education. These laws give students with hearing loss more opportunities to receive an appropriate education in their neighborhood schools. The Individuals with Disabilities Education Act (IDEA) (1997) was reauthorized by Congress in 2000 and again in 2004. As a result, the education of students with hearing loss today occurs more frequently in public schools than special schools for the deaf (Lang, 2003).

Until recently, educators were not very successful in improving the reading skills of deaf students. The Babbidge Report (Babbidge, 1965) indicated that the average reading level of a child who was deaf or hard of hearing at high school graduation was at the third-grade level. As of 2000, despite new methods for remediation and education, the average child with a profound hearing loss still graduated from high school with a fourth-grade reading level (Traxler, 2000). Educators look forward to the impact of early identification and early intervention to reverse this trend. Johnson (2006a) reported on the reading scores from 2001 to 2005 of a cohort of children with hearing loss. Results were reported for children tested from third grade to tenth grade. The percentage of children scoring unsatisfactorily had dropped from 40% to 32%. Children with partial reading proficiency had

increased from 28% to 30%, whereas those with proficient reading scores had increased from 22% to 31%. There was even a small percentage of children (approximately 2%) who exhibited reading scores in the advanced category. Even more encouraging was the amount of growth in reading these students had made over time. Of 751 students in the study, in 1 year, 40% attained 1 year of growth, 41% achieved more than 1 year of growth, and 18% showed less than 1 year of growth. In analyzing the findings, variables correlating with better reading scores included early intervention, student participation in extracurricular activities, and higher socioeconomic level.

The trends reported here support the impact of technological advances, early identification, an early start of intervention, and advances in educational programming. All of these factors contribute to the recent success of many children with hearing loss. It is now reasonable to expect children with hearing loss to have developmental and academic skills that are commensurate with their hearing peers.

Audiologists play a key role in the early intervention and education of children with hearing loss and thus can contribute greatly to the success of these children. This chapter reviews the important role of the clinical audiologist in early intervention and education.

▨ AFTER DIAGNOSIS

Diagnosing hearing loss shortly after birth is now a standard. The Early Hearing Detection and Intervention (EHDI) initiative supports the 1-3-6 rule (White, 2003). That is, children should receive a newborn hearing screening by 1 month of age, diagnosis should be confirmed by 3 months of age, and any necessary early intervention should start by 6 months of age. When these guidelines are met, children are more likely to have communication and language skills that are within normal limits for their age (Yoshinaga-Itano et al., 1998; Moeller, 2000). This reverses a trend that persisted for many years, one in which children with hearing loss lagged behind their peers in both communication and language development. The benefit of early identification and associated early intervention has given these children an opportunity to enter school with achievement levels never seen before (Allen, 1986; Holt, 1994).

The Walsh Bill that was first approved in 1999 is seeking reauthorization. This bill supports the establishment of programs for early detection, diagnosis, and intervention for newborns and infants with hearing loss. The fact that there are currently 40 states with legislation (Diggs, 2006) and eight others that are screening voluntarily (Green et al., 2007) is testimony to the success of this federal initiative. One additional benefit from this initiative has been the attempt to collect increasingly accurate information on the incidence of hearing loss in the newborn population (Eichwald and Gaffney, 2007). The website for the National Center for Hearing Assessment and Management (2007) reports an overall incidence of one to three per thousand babies with bilateral hearing loss of all degrees in the neonatal population. In addition, approximately one in 1,000 newborns has been shown to have a unilateral hearing loss (Clinical Health Information Record for Patients, 2005).

State EHDI programs depend on the participation of many agencies to create their state systems. There is also growing agreement that early intervention requires interagency or multiagency support to adequately fund services. The Part C agency in a state is of paramount importance (Part C will be discussed in depth later in this chapter).

At 36 months of age, children with hearing loss transition out of early intervention programs and enter their local school districts. There are approximately 2 million school-age children with hearing loss (Schow and Nerbonne, 2002). An analysis of the degree of hearing loss in the school-age population indicates the following prevalence figures (Gallaudet Research Institute, 2005):

- Minimal hearing loss   17.1%
- Mild hearing loss   12.4%
- Moderate hearing loss   13.4%
- Moderate-severe hearing loss 12.2%
- Severe hearing loss   15.0%
- Profound hearing loss   29.9%

The etiology of hearing loss falls into these categories (Gallaudet Research Institute, 2005):

- Genetic   22.7%
- Pregnancy related   12.0%
- Postbirth disease or injury   15.2%
- Cause cannot be determined   53.7%

Note that the total exceeds 100%, with some overlap across categories.

Special education services are provided in a variety of school settings. The setting can be a public school, a private school, or a state school for the deaf. In order to qualify for special education services, the hearing loss must have an adverse affect on learning. This is defined in the law as "a hearing loss that impairs the ability of a child to process linguistic information through hearing, with or without amplification, as to significantly affect a child's educational performance" (IDEA 34CFR300.8[b][3]).

Children with hearing loss can also receive related support services so that they can benefit more fully from their special education (IDEA Sec. 300.34[a]). The support includes speech-language pathology and audiology services, interpreting services, and parent counseling and training. Of special interest are the specific audiologic provisions that are listed as support services (IDEA Sec. 300.34 [b][1]):

- Identifying children with hearing loss
- Determining the range, nature, and degree of hearing loss
- Providing (re)habilitative activities such as language habilitation, auditory training, and speechreading
- Counseling and guidance of children, their parents, and teachers regarding hearing loss
- Determining a child's needs for group and individual amplification

A TEAM APPROACH

The treatment and education of a child with hearing loss often require a team of professionals who, with the child's parents, convene at regular intervals to create a plan. For children under 3 years of age, the team develops an Individual Family Service Plan (IFSP). An Individual Education Plan (IEP) is generated for children older than 3. (The IFSP and IEP will be discussed in depth in following sections.) The team works together to determine placement, provide services, and monitor developmental and educational outcomes. Communication between the audiologist and related personnel is critical. An audiologist can be the service coordinator for an infant or toddler, an instructional team member, and/or a consultant (Johnson et al., 1997). The audiologist shares diagnostic information, makes recommendations for amplification, may provide direct (re)habilitation services, and provides family support.

IDEA: THE LAW SUPPORTS SERVICES

The Individual Family Service Plan

For children from birth to 36 months of age, Part C of IDEA assures that each child has access to services. A description of these services is identified in the IFSP. The IFSP is a written plan. It documents the desired outcomes for the infant or toddler's development and services to be provided to the child and the child's family. The IFSP includes statements of the child's present level of development, the family's resources and their priorities and concerns, the major outcomes expected, and a statement of necessary early intervention services.

The service coordinator is an integral participant in this process. As defined by statute, the service coordinator serves as the single point of contact to help parents obtain the services and assistance they need. The law identifies the service coordinator as a professional who meets the family soon after the hearing loss is diagnosed. The role of the service coordinator, as defined in IDEA Sec. 303.22, includes the following responsibilities:

- Coordinating services across agency lines
- Serving as the single point of contact to help parents obtain the services and assistance they need
- Assisting parents to access early intervention services and other services identified in the IFSP
- Coordinating the provision of early intervention services and related services
- Facilitating the timely delivery of available services
- Continuously seeking the appropriate services

The law further states that it is appropriate for the service coordinator to be from the profession most immediately relevant to the infant's, toddler's, or family's needs. With this in mind, some states have created a role for a specialty service coordination (i.e., trained relative to the presenting disability). The specialty service coordinator serves as a conduit between the diagnosing clinical audiologist and the early intervention system. This specialty system of service coordinator has, in some states, effectively reduced the age at which children with hearing loss start early intervention. For example, in one state, the average age for starting early intervention is 3.5 months (Clinical Health Information Record for Patients, 2005). This age is well below the national average.

A survey of one state's specialty service coordinators (Sedey and Stredler-Brown, 2004) identified the type of information parents of children with hearing loss requested most frequently. Of the 13 topics listed, the ones families asked for most often were: (1) communication approaches; (2) language development; (3) speech development; (4) sign language; (5) hearing aids; and (6) the development of functional auditory skills. Only when using a model of specialty service coordination, can one assure that this information will be delivered.

The Individual Education Plan

When children turn 3 years of age, they leave the Part C early intervention system and enter the school system. Under special education law, Part B of IDEA, there is no require-

ment that a service coordinator be designated for a child and his or her family. Rather, Child Find coordination includes many components that are part of service coordination. One professional is identified as the liaison among educators, therapists, and the parents. The individual with this responsibility is often assigned by the local education unit.

Parents continue to have an active role in the development of their child's education program. They participate in the development of the IEP. The IEP must include a statement of the child's present levels of educational performance, a statement of measurable annual goals, short-term objectives to meet these goals, and a statement of the special education, related services, and supplementary aids that will be provided to the child.

Part B of IDEA provides guidelines for delivering a "free and appropriate public education" (FAPE) (IDEA 1997 612[a][1]) for children with disabilities. FAPE applies to preschool, elementary school, and secondary school education. This part of the law requires the local education agency to provide special education services and related services at no expense to the parents.

The audiologist's information is of much interest to the educators and to the specialty providers. Of primary importance are the findings related to the child's use of hearing aids, cochlear implant(s), and/or assistive listening technology. Ideally, the audiologist presents the audiologic assessment findings and information on amplification in person at the IEP. This authenticates the role of the audiologist.

Many states have initiatives to reform deaf education. In Colorado, the deaf education reform initiative advocates for the following services for school-age children with hearing loss (Johnson and Jaitly, personal communication, February 25, 2002):

1. **Services must be communication accessible.** Students who are deaf and hard of hearing have diverse communication needs and abilities. Whether auditory/oral, manual, or a combination, full communication access must be the foundation for placement decisions.

2. **Regional and center-based programs for students who are deaf and hard of hearing are necessary as part of the continuum of services.** In order to accommodate the diverse communication needs of students and to create sufficient numbers of students to effectively provide a full continuum of service options, a statewide system of programs and services should be implemented. Center-based and regional programs expand the geographic boundaries for enrollment. Children do not necessarily attend their home school. Rather, center-based and regional options bring together more students with hearing loss. This, in turn, creates a critical mass of language peers. These programs also bring the professionals together in one teaching environment.

TABLE 41.1   Delivery of education, instruction, and therapy

Developmental/curricular area	Definition	Professional responsible
Audiologic Rehabilitation	Instruction or therapy teaching specific speech skills, functional auditory skills, and/or speechreading skills	■ Rehabilitation audiologist ■ Speech-language pathologist ■ Teacher of the deaf/hard of hearing ■ Speech-language pathology assistant (SLP-A)
Developmental and Academic Instruction	Instruction; monitoring progress; administration of developmental or academic tests	■ Teacher of the deaf/hard of hearing ■ Sign language interpreter ■ Para-professional
Environmental/Classroom Acoustics	Identifying the acoustic characteristics of the environment and proposing appropriate accommodations	■ Audiologist

Adapted from Pichora-Fuller K, Schow RL. (2007) Audiologic rehabilitation for adults and elderly adults. In: Schow RL, Nerbonne MA, eds. *Introduction to Audiologic Rehabilitation.* Boston: Pearson Education Inc.

3. **Support personnel are needed who are trained to work with students who are deaf and hard of hearing.** Communication specialists, a hybrid of professionals trained as speech-language pathologists, audiologists, and deaf educators, are needed to guide the communication development for these students.

Curricular areas such as audiologic rehabilitation, developmental and academic instruction, and environmental and classroom acoustics are defined in Table 41.1.

Section 504 of the Rehabilitation Act of 1973

There are occasions when a child with a hearing loss does not need to be enrolled in special education but still needs specific accommodations to facilitate learning. These children may be eligible for a 504 Plan. The Rehabilitation Act of 1973 is a civil rights law that prohibits discrimination on the basis of a disability when programs, public and private, receive federal funds. A student who qualifies for a 504 Plan can receive accommodations in the way of supplemental aids and services. The 504 Plan assures an educational experience that is comparable to that provided to students without disabilities. The services identified in the plan must be provided at no cost to the child or to the family.

■ DEGREE OF HEARING LOSS AND IMPLICATIONS FOR TREATMENT

One must not be misled by thinking that the degree of hearing loss equates, in a linear way, with the impact on a child's

development. Rather, the degree of hearing loss is just one factor of many that contribute to the developmental profile of each student.

Minimal Hearing Loss

Historically, the term "minimal" has implied that the developmental impact of hearing loss is "inconsequential" (Bess, 2004). Carol Flexer (personal communication, September 7, 1995) stated that "implicit in the term 'minimal' is permission to provide the least possible intervention and the fewest management strategies." However, as discussed later in this section, the effects of even a mild or unilateral hearing loss may have a significant impact on a child's language or education.

As a result of newborn hearing screening, many more children with minimal hearing loss are being identified in the newborn period. The Centers for Disease Control and Prevention (CDC) conducted a review of the literature (Ross, 2006) to identify the prevalence of minimal hearing loss in both the newborn and school-age populations. The CDC adopted the working definitions of minimal hearing loss that were published by Bess et al. (1998). Hearing levels are based on the standards developed by the American National Standards Institute in 1996.

- Unilateral Sensory-Neural Hearing Loss (USHL): Average air-conduction thresholds (500, 1,000, and 2,000 Hz) ≥ 20 dB hearing level (HL) in the impaired ear, with an average air-bone gap no greater than 10 dB at 1,000, 2,000, and 4,000 Hz. Average air-conduction thresholds in the good ear ≤ 15dB.

- <u>Mild Bilateral Sensory-Neural Hearing Loss (BSHL)</u>: Average puretone thresholds between 20 and 40 dB HL bilaterally with average air-bone gaps no greater than 10 dB at frequencies of 1,000, 2,000, and 4,000 Hz.
- <u>High-Frequency Sensory-Neural Hearing Loss (HFSHL)</u>: Air-conduction thresholds >25 dB HL at two or more frequencies above 2,000 Hz (i.e., 3,000, 4,000, 6,000, or 8,000 Hz) in one or both ears with air-bone gaps at 3,000 and 4,000 Hz no greater than 10 dB.

The incidence of minimal hearing loss in newborns ranges from 0.36 to 1.3 (per 1,000) births for mild bilateral hearing loss and 0.8 to 2.7 (per 1,000) births for unilateral hearing loss (White et al., 1994; Watkin and Baldwin, 1999; Dalzell et al., 2000; Johnson et al., 2005). For school-age students, the prevalence figures for minimal hearing loss vary greatly and are likely higher than those for younger children who have not yet enrolled in school. Bess et al. (1998) report that three in every 100 school-age students in their sample had a unilateral hearing loss and a total of 5.4% of students had a minimal hearing loss, including unilateral hearing loss. "In a sample of 1218 children, prevalence of Minimal Sensorineural Hearing Loss (MSHL) was 5.4%. Stated otherwise, 1 in 20 school-age children exhibited MSHL. USHL was the most prevalent form of MSHL in children followed by HFSHL and BSHL, respectively. When all forms of hearing loss were considered, the prevalence was 11.3% — approximately 2 times the 5 to 6% prevalence rate typically reported in the schools using as the criterion an average of 25dB or more through the speech frequency range" (Bess et al., 1998, p 346).

The research on the impact of minimal hearing loss on language and academic skills in school-age children is compelling. Many studies have identified a subset of students with minimal hearing loss, including unilateral hearing loss, and determined the presence of academic, social, and behavioral difficulties (Blair et al., 1985; Bess and Tharpe, 1986; 1988; Culbertson and Gilbert, 1986; Davis et al., 1986; Klee and Davis-Dansky, 1986; Oyler et al., 1987; Bovo et al., 1988; Brookhouser et al., 1991; Bess et al., 1998; Davis et al., 2001; Lieu, 2004). The common challenge for children with minimal hearing loss is their inability to hear speech and language adequately in typical listening situations. For instance, classrooms typically have high levels of noise that can interfere with speech perception (Bess, 2000; Crandell and Smaldino, 2000). Wake and Poulakis (2004) indicated that mild hearing loss has a significant impact upon children, especially during the primary school years. For example, young children with minimal hearing loss report increased difficulties listening under adverse conditions and have less energy. For children with unilateral hearing loss, the ability to localize and focus on "target" sounds can be challenging when listening at distances and in noisy or reverberant environments. One study determined the impact of unilateral hearing loss in the birth

to 3 years period (Sedey et al., 2002). In this study, one out of three toddlers with unilateral hearing loss demonstrated a delay in communication, speech, or language. However, with ongoing, direct early intervention services, the language outcomes for these children were shown to be comparable to their hearing peers (Sedey, 2006).

Based on these findings, more aggressive management and monitoring of children with minimal hearing loss is recommended for very young children before academic difficulties arise. For example, some states have recognized the potential impact of bilateral hearing loss of mild degrees on infants and toddlers by making these children eligible for early intervention services.

There are many functional assessments that can be used to identify students who are experiencing problems in school as a result of a minimal hearing loss. The Screening Inventory for Targeting Educational Risk (SIFTER) (Anderson, 1989), the Pre-School SIFTER (Anderson and Matkin, 1996), the Listening Inventories For Education (LIFE) (Anderson and Smaldino, 1998), and the Auditory Behavior in Everyday Life (Purdy et al., 2002) all assess, in an informal way, the communication competence of a student with minimal hearing loss. An evaluation of the developmental skills of individual children with minimal hearing loss can assure that these children are not overlooked and receive appropriate interventions in a timely manner.

Some clinicians recommend personal amplification for children with minimal hearing loss. This practice is more common for students with bilateral hearing loss and is being investigated for children with unilateral hearing loss (McKay and Iyer, 2005). Personal or sound field frequency modulation (FM) systems also offer potential benefit.

Moderate, Severe, and Profound Hearing Loss

Statistics indicate that more than two-thirds of children with a hearing loss have moderate, severe, or profound degrees of loss bilaterally (Gallaudet Research Institute, 2005). Because access to sound is compromised, the development of functional auditory skills is compromised. In turn, both receptive and expressive language learning and spoken language are affected. Table 41.2 lists and describes various components of language.

Delays in vocabulary development are pervasive and persistent. Yoshinaga-Itano and Downey (1986) report that children with hearing loss tend to have a reduced vocabulary. As a group, they demonstrate limited understanding of metaphors, idioms, figurative language, and jokes. In addition, they are generally challenged by multiple meanings of words (e.g., "*run* the stats," "go for a *run*," "*running* water").

The development of syntax, or grammar, is also affected. Children with hearing loss, to varying degrees, exhibit a shorter mean length of utterance (MLU), tend to use simpler sentence structure, overuse the subject-verb-object sentence pattern, and demonstrate infrequent use of specific word

TABLE 41.2   Components of language

Components of language learning	Description
Semantics	The study of word meanings and word relations
Syntax	The aspect of language that governs the rules for how words are arranged in sentences
Morphology	The study of the minimal units of language that are meaningful, such as /-s/ for plural nouns or third-person verb tenses, /-ing/ for present progressive, and /–ed/ for past tense
Pragmatics	The functional use of language

Adapted from Schow RL, Nerbonne MA. (2002) Overview of audiologic rehabilitation. In: Schow RL, Nerbonne MA, eds. *Introduction to Audiologic Rehabilitation.* Boston: Allyn and Bacon.

forms (e.g., adverbs, auxiliaries, conjunctions). A curious observation about the language of children with more severe degrees of hearing loss is their use of inappropriate syntactic patterns. For example, a child may say, "I want you go get eat things." In this example, the message is understood, but the syntactic patterns do not follow the rules for English.

Pragmatic characteristics of language are also usually affected. Most pragmatic skills are accomplished by hearing children by the time they reach preschool. However, a sample of children with all degrees of hearing loss demonstrates challenges on the use of pragmatics during these preschool years (Yoshinaga-Itano, 1999). This study showed that children with hearing loss have the most success using language when they make requests and express their feelings. As a group, they demonstrated moderate success initiating and maintaining topics in conversation, giving directions, making polite commands, expressing their state of mind, and asking questions to gather information. The children demonstrated the most difficulty apologizing for or explaining their behavior, revising an unclear message or asking for clarification of a message that was not understood, offering and supporting their own opinion, giving biographical information, and explaining cause and effect.

The effect on speech production and speech intelligibility is a direct result of a child's auditory access to sound. Normal hearing infants are able to discriminate their mother's voice shortly following birth. Their ability to discriminate other speech sounds is fine tuned during the first year of life (Marean et al., 1992; Kuhl, 2000).

By 12 months, a normal hearing baby starts to discriminate speech sounds. A child with a moderate hearing loss has access to vowels and some consonants. However, depending on the specific audiogram and performance in the aided condition, the child may not have full access to these sounds. A child with a profound hearing loss may only be able to access duration patterns.

In turn, challenges in these language domains lead to difficulties in reading and writing. When a child has a low literacy level, graduation from high school and later vocational opportunities are adversely affected. In order to offset these problems and thereby succeed, appropriate intervention and educational accommodations are needed. Diagnosis, intervention, and education programs are covered in depth later in this chapter.

Auditory Neuropathy/Auditory Dyssynchrony

This relatively new diagnosis presents particular challenges to professionals. Some of the classic behaviors observed in a student with auditory neuropathy (AN)/auditory dyssynchrony (AD) are as follows: speech perception is poorer than would be expected based on the student's audiologic results, inconsistent responses to sound, and fluctuating hearing loss. Some of these children have the ability to understand what they hear better than would be expected based on the abnormal auditory brainstem response (Cone-Wesson et al., 2001).

The goal, as for all children with hearing loss, is to define an appropriate treatment protocol. However, consensus has not yet been reached on what exactly constitutes "appropriate" treatment for children with AN. There is a wealth of research that supports, to varying degrees, the fitting of amplification. Rance et al. (1999) found that approximately 50% of affected children benefited from amplification. In the sample of Berlin et al. (2002), 50% of the sample tried amplification. However, of this group, only 17% reported benefit. Rance (2005) studied 18 subjects with AN/AD who were fit with amplification by 18 months of age. Anecdotal and formal speech perception data suggested that at least some children with AN/AD benefited from conventional amplification.

The benefit of cochlear implants has been quite remarkable for some children with AN/AD (Berlin, 2001; Neault, 2001; Shallop et al., 2001), with improvements in sound detection, speech perception, and oral communication skills reported. Before advancing to a cochlear implant, it is important to allow sufficient time to determine if the child will develop neural synchrony or receive sufficient benefit from auditory stimulation to develop speech and language without the implant.

Children with AN/AD present with unique profiles of auditory, speech, and language development, which heightens the importance of having an individualized intervention/education plan. First, a baseline of the child's developmental skills, in all developmental domains, needs to be obtained. A comprehensive evaluation includes an assessment of cognition, functional auditory skills, communication and language, speech, and the mode of communication that is benefiting the child. The success of visual forms of communication such as sign language, cued speech, and/or speechreading is often related to the child's ability to positively benefit from auditory input as well. In order to evaluate the child's most effective communication mode, testing can be conducted in the auditory mode, in the visual mode, and using a combination of auditory and visual stimuli (Stredler-Brown, 2002a).

Children with Multiple Disabilities

Children with hearing loss are at an increased risk for additional disabilities (Moores and Martin, 2006). These conditions can include visual impairments, motor disabilities, cognitive delay, attention deficit disorder, learning disabilities, and others. To address these conditions, children with hearing loss may be treated by a physician and/or may receive additional therapies such as occupational therapy, physical therapy, vision therapy, or mental health services. One study has shown that up to 38% of children, birth to 3 years of age, have an additional developmental disability (Schildroth and Hotto, 1993). Data from the Gallaudet Research Institute (2005) surveying school-age children with hearing loss show that 42.4% of the student population has an additional disability.

It is important to recognize that a child with multiple disabilities does not require multiple treatment programs. Rather, the various therapies can be integrated into one treatment program to address the developmental needs of the child. A transdisciplinary model is one example of a coordinated program that integrates the expertise of different professionals to serve children with complicated needs (Linder, 1993; Orelove and Sobsey, 1996). This service delivery model gives the audiologist the opportunity to educate other professionals about the impact of hearing loss on development in other domains.

▧ EDUCATIONAL STAGES

Early Intervention

As discussed earlier in the chapter, the 1-3-6 rule, which is promoted by the CDC, sets standards for screening, audiologic evaluation, and the start of early intervention. A hearing screening should be done by 1 month of age, an audiologic

diagnosis confirmed by 3 months of age, and the start of any necessary early intervention (EI) by 6 months of age. When children are enrolled in EI by 6 months of age, they are more likely to learn language at a rate that is commensurate with their hearing peers (Yoshinaga-Itano et al., 1998; Moeller, 2000). It should be noted that, although Yoshinaga-Itano et al. (1998) reported that children starting EI by 6 months of age exhibited language skills within normal limits, a detailed analysis of the performance of these children indicates that many still had persistent language delays specific to concept vocabulary, early world knowledge, and syntax (Sedey, 2004). Thus, although children with hearing loss are coming to school with better language than ever before, specific language skills still may not match those of their hearing peers.

For those entering EI, a parent-centered approach to intervention is supported by statute (IDEA, 2004) and is currently the most common. This approach focuses on the parents and other caregivers by:

- providing parents with information about hearing loss,
- supporting the parents' emotions associated with the diagnosis of hearing loss, and
- teaching specific strategies to parents and caregivers that can be used to facilitate a child's development.

The parents and the early interventionist form a collaborative partnership. Haley (1987) describes a guideline for "joining" a family. Even the first contact with the family is critical because it sets the tone for subsequent contacts and can influence families' attitudes about professionals in general. The professional is encouraged to focus discussions on the issues most pertinent to the family, such as (1) how much they know about hearing loss and how much they *want* to know, (2) listening to family members as they discuss the feelings they have and responding to the feelings of each family member, (3) helping the family identify their supports, and (4) partnering with family members as they conduct intervention.

Child-centered therapy is an alternative approach to family-centered intervention. In child-centered therapy, the professional works directly with the child to investigate, identify, and implement specific interventions. The content areas remain the same: use of amplification and development of functional auditory skills, speech, prelinguistic communication, language, and cognition. While parents may observe these therapy sessions, the professional provides direct one-on-one instruction to the child. Although Part C of IDEA supports a parent-centered paradigm, child-centered therapy remains a viable option.

Part C of IDEA states that early intervention services "to the maximum extent appropriate, are provided in natural environments, including the home, and community settings in which children without disabilities participate" [34 CFR 303.12(b)]. Following these guidelines, the interventionist commonly provides services to the family in locations that are typical for that family. This could be the home, a community park, or a neighborhood store. The intent of the law is to teach the skills families will use in familiar settings. This increases the likelihood that follow-through will occur.

The Western States Early Intervention Administrators Coalition for Young Children with Sensory Disabilities issued a statement in 1999 on this subject of natural environments. This statement, outlined in Table 41.3, provides an interpretation of natural environments specifically for young children who are deaf or hard of hearing. It is based on the premise that children with hearing loss benefit from a "language-rich environment" in order to learn to communicate (DesGeorges et al., 2006; Colorado Department of Education, 2002). A language-rich environment supports language learning, provides free and natural access to communication, and promotes communication with the adults and peers in the child's environment. Typical peers may not be included in these treatment environments, and typical family routines may not provide an optimal environment. Fortunately, federal law does allow the intervention team to justify when intervention should be conducted in settings other than natural environments [34 CFR 303.12(2)].

Professionals providing (re)habilitation services to children with hearing loss receive their preservice training from a variety of disciplines, including educators of the deaf/hard of hearing, speech/language pathology, educational audiology, and early childhood special education. The curriculums in

---

TABLE 41.4   Competencies for an early interventionist providing parent-centered intervention

- Communicating with family members
- Forming collaborative partnerships
- Working with families
- Assessing, interpreting assessments, and progress monitoring
- Developing and implementing a therapy plan
- Managing sensory devices
- Maximizing auditory potential
- Facilitating communication development
- Facilitating cognitive development

Adapted from Colorado Infant Hearing Advisory Committee. (2003) *Guidelines for Infant Hearing Screening, Audiologic Assessment, and Early Intervention.* Denver, CO: Colorado Department of Public Health and Environment.

---

each preservice training program fulfill, to varying degrees, the competencies needed by an early interventionist. Table 41.4 identifies a list of skills and knowledge for early interventionists working with infants and toddlers who are deaf or hard of hearing.

As mentioned earlier, as a result of newborn hearing screening programs, many more infants are identified with hearing loss. In some states (Colorado Department of Education, 2006), the number of children enrolled in early intervention has more than tripled since the start of its universal newborn hearing screening program. There is an emergency need to train more early interventionists to serve this growing population. In addition, there is a critical need for in-service training opportunities.

Preschool Education for Children 3 to 5 Years of Age

The transition from early intervention to preschool services starts when a child is 2.5 years old. The early interventionist is encouraged to support parents as they learn about different preschool placements. When a child enters preschool, instruction focuses on preacademic skills with most services being child centered. However, there is still an opportunity for parents to receive parent counseling and training. Parent counseling and training is an important related service in special education; this is discussed in more detail later in this chapter.

There are many venues for preschool. One option, the one considered the least restrictive, is to mainstream the child with hearing loss into a preschool program with hearing children. This could be a publicly funded preschool program or a private preschool. A second option is to enroll the child with hearing loss in a noncategorical preschool program. This type of program operates within a public school and enrolls children with different types of disabilities in the same

---

TABLE 41.3   Natural environments: considerations for infants and toddlers (Birth–3 Years) who are deaf/hard of hearing

- Minimizing a family's isolation by increasing the family's sense of involvement; this is done by providing a network of other parents of children who are deaf or hard of hearing
- Assuring equal access to communication through a visual or auditory communication system specific to that child/family
- Encouraging and assisting families in identifying their child's and family's strengths and resources
- Supporting families as they build relationships that enhance their child's communication
- Supporting families to develop meaningful communication, using a visual or auditory communication system, so the child may become a fully participating member of the family
- Providing typically developing children with positive interactions with children who are deaf or hard of hearing

Adapted from Western States Early Intervention Coalition for Sensory Impairments. (1999) Natural environments for infants and toddlers who are deaf and hard of hearing. Available at: http://www.asha.org/about/legislation-advocacy/federal/idea/nat-env-child-facts.htm.

TABLE 41.5   Considerations for selecting a preschool program

- Total number of students in the classroom
- Number of students with hearing loss in the classroom
- Adult-to-child ratio
- Communication approach used by each child in the classroom
- Accommodations for amplification
- Related services (e.g., speech-language pathologist, educational audiologist, occupational therapist, physical therapist, psychologist)
- Parent support
- Physical environment
- Acoustic accommodations
- Curriculums
- Communication between school and home
- Family involvement in day-to-day preschool activities
- Role models who are deaf or hard of hearing
- Assessment

Adapted from Johnson CD, Beams D, Stredler-Brown A. (2005) Preschool/Kindergarten Checklist. Colorado Department of Education, Special Services Unit. Available at: http://www.cde.state.co.us/cdesped/download/pdf/dhh-PS-KPlcmntCklst.pdf.

classroom. A third option, often found in larger metropolitan areas, is a center-based program. A center-based program attempts to enroll a critical mass of children with hearing loss in one classroom. In order to assemble a critical mass, children from different schools are transported to one school. All of these options, to varying degrees, may enroll typically developing children. These peers do not have disabilities and serve as models for typical language development.

Parents are encouraged to visit preschools as they make their selection. A checklist can guide parents' decisions. Considerations for selecting a preschool program are listed in Table 41.5.

An increasing number of states have created legislation to support education placements and education programs. At the time of this publication, six states have legislation, and an additional 10 have documentation that is often referred to as a "Deaf Child's Bill of Rights." Information about these legislative initiatives is posted on the website of the National Association of the Deaf (www.nad.org). This legislation includes a communication plan. This plan is a legal document and provides a mechanism to discuss critical issues that will likely impact the development and communication of the child. A sample communication plan used in one western state is shown in Figure 41.1.

Early Elementary Education

There are a variety of program options for school-age children. It is important to note that the goal of any placement is to meet specific learning criteria for each child. What works well for one child may not be productive for all children. Marschark et al. (2002) report that there is no evidence to indicate that one educational setting is uniformly better than another.

Residential schools have a long history in the United States of providing educational as well as social opportunities for children. However, Lang (2003) reported that, in 1986, only three out of 10 deaf children in the United States still attended state-run residential schools; the majority attended public schools, either in special classes for deaf students or in regular classes with an interpreter or an itinerant teacher of the deaf. This trend continues, with even more students attending regular classes with their hearing peers (Karchmer and Mitchell, 2003). Recently, there have been increasing opportunities for children to be educated in public schools close to their homes. This trend first started with federal legislation that was passed in the 1970s and has continued to gain momentum since that time. At first, placement in the mainstream was encouraged. In the mainstream, a student attends some classes with their hearing peers and receives some of their education in a special classroom, or Resource Room, specifically for children with hearing loss. After several years, the term "inclusion" replaced "mainstreaming." An inclusive environment encourages delivery of *all* services within a regular classroom. Table 41.6 provides a brief explanation of these educational settings.

The factors that need to be considered when making a placement decision are the communication needs of the child, opportunities for direct communication with peers, contact with professionals, the student's academic skills, and the supports required to deliver instruction to maintain or achieve age-appropriate skills.

PARENT COUNSELING AND TRAINING

Because receptive and expressive communication start at birth, the family continuously experiences the impact that hearing loss has on communication. In family-centered intervention, for children birth to 36 months of age, the focus on family members is of primary importance (Jones, 1993). Parents receive information from their audiologist, service coordinator, and/or early interventionist. This information might include topics such as child development, the value of intervention, specific intervention programs, the various communication approaches that help develop language, and parent-to-parent support. This information may be delivered in writing, through video or DVD, or, most importantly, through discussion. However, information alone cannot correct a situation. Personal adjustment counseling can be effective in helping the parents acknowledge their feelings and engage in problem solving. The early interventionist can be an advocate for the parents and their child, assist the parents as they learn to observe their child's behavior, and lend

Communication Plan
For Child/Student who is Deaf/Hard of Hearing

The IEP team has considered each area listed below, and has not denied instructional opportunity based on the amount of the child's/student's residual hearing, the ability of the parent(s) to communicate, nor the child's/student's experience with other communication modes.

1. The child's/student's primary communication mode is one or more of the following:
   (check all that apply)
   - ❏ aural, oral, speech-based
   - ❏ American Sign Language
   - ❏ English-based manual or sign system

   Issues considered:

   Action plan, if any:

2. The IEP team has considered the availability of deaf/hard of hearing adult role models and peer group of the child's/student's communication mode or language.

   Issues considered:

   Action plan, if any:

3. An explanation of all educational options provided by the administrative unit and available for the child/student has been provided.

   Issues considered:

   Action plan, if any:

4. Teachers, interpreters, and other specialists delivering the communication plan to the child/student must have demonstrated proficiency in, and be able to accommodate for the child's/student's primary communication mode or language.

   Issues considered:

   Action plan, if any:

5. The communication-accessible academic instruction, school services, and extracurricular activities the child/student will receive have been identified.

   Issues considered:

   Action plan, if any:

FIGURE 41.1
Communication Plan. IEP, Individual Education Plan. (From the Colorado Department of Education, 2006.)

support to the parents as they make their decisions. Some professionals are also comfortable providing psychosocial counseling to help parents through the emotional grief often associated with the diagnosis of their child's hearing loss.

When the family members resolve their grief, they are ready to learn specific techniques and strategies to support their child's development. This training teaches parents specific auditory, speech, and language activities that they can incorporate into their routines. For the very young child, parents are taught using a three-step process (Stredler-Brown et al., 2004; Stredler-Brown, 2005). First, the parents identify, with the early interventionist, the strategies that are priorities for them and their child. Next, the early interventionist

demonstrates each strategy. The parents join the interventionist, practicing the strategy that has been demonstrated. After that, the parents and professional assess and evaluate, in an informal way, the effectiveness of the strategy. Each strategy is to become a natural and ongoing part of the family's routines.

For children over 36 months of age, the parents are entitled, by law, to parent counseling and training when it is identified as a related service on the child's IEP (IDEA 1997 300.24 [b][7]. This part of the law engages parents as collaborators with their educational partners. Parent counseling and training are considered a related service only when the IEP team, which includes the parents, determines that these

TABLE 41.6 Educational placements	
Educational placements	**Definition**
Residential school	This is usually a state-sponsored program with a large number of children with hearing loss and many teachers of the deaf. Some children live on campus; some attend as day students.
Center-based program	A school dedicates space, staff, and related services to a program that is located within a public school for children who are deaf or hard of hearing. Children receive services within this program for a designated number of hours per week.
Self-contained classroom	This program includes only children who are deaf or hard of hearing.
Resource room	Instruction is provided in specific curricular areas in a room designated for children who are deaf or hard of hearing. Children spend part of their day in regular (mainstreamed) classrooms.
Mainstream education	Children who are deaf or hard of hearing attend classes with their typically hearing peers.
Itinerant support	Itinerant teachers work in several schools, providing support services to children who are deaf or hard of hearing and consultative services to the general education teachers.

services are required to assist the child in benefitting from special education. The purpose of parent counseling and training is to assist parents in acquiring skills to support the implementation of their child's IEP. While most often the prescribed services are provided face-to-face, they can also be provided through other methods such as phone calls or written lessons.

Generally, parent counseling is defined as the provision of information and support. Counseling services may help parents receive information about their child's disability or to identify community resources that offer support.

Parent training focuses on developing skills. This includes instruction and demonstration of effective techniques that are used in school. It is often beneficial for the student if these techniques are also provided in the home. This training can include the use of amplification, sign language training, implementation of auditory training techniques, and/or literacy techniques.

■ CURRICULAR AREAS

1. Functional Auditory Skill Development

Auditory skill development, also commonly known as auditory training, is not new. For example, auditory-oral therapy has been the hallmark of therapy provided at the Clark School for the Deaf and Central Institute for the Deaf, among others, since their establishment in the beginning of the 20th century. Acoupedic therapy (Pollack, 1970) was started in the 1960s, with the approach now being referred to as auditory-verbal therapy. The common feature of these approaches is to teach children to use their residual hearing. In so doing, the child learns to listen. The goal is to provide better access to all sounds, the most important of which is speech. The success of auditory skill development lies in appropri-

ate amplification and rigorous and systematic training of a hierarchy of listening skills.

Professionals can access a countless number of auditory skill checklists and curriculums (Erber, 1982; Stout and Windle, 1992; Tye-Murray, 1992; Watkins, 1993; Razack, 1994; Johnson, Benson, and Seaton, 1997; Estabrooks, 1998; Stredler-Brown and Johnson, 2004). While these checklists may ascribe different names to the stages of auditory skill development, they are essentially the same when it comes to the discrete tasks that are included. Hierarchal auditory skills typically included in various checklists are described in Table 41.7 as part of the Functional Auditory Performance Indicators (FAPI) (Stredler-Brown and Johnson, 2004).

There are two unique features of the FAPI. First, each skill listed is assessed in multiple listening conditions. For instance, although a child may be able to respond at an awareness level to a speech stimulus in a *quiet* environment, the child may not be able to respond to the same stimulus in a *noisy* situation. The FAPI is designed to identify the degree to which each skill is accomplished in a variety of listening conditions. Some of these conditions are as follows:

- Responses to auditory stimuli that are paired with *visual cues*, contrasted with responses to an *auditory stimulus alone*
- Responses to auditory stimuli that are presented in *close proximity* to the child versus responses to stimuli that are presented *far away*
- Responses to auditory stimuli in a *noisy situation* versus responses to stimuli in a *quiet environment*
- Responses to auditory stimuli that are observed when the child is *prompted* to listen versus *spontaneous* responses to auditory stimuli

The second unique characteristic of the FAPI is the scoring paradigm. A skill can be scored as "not present," "emerging," "in process," or "acquired." Having a quantifiable

TABLE 41.7   Hierarchy of auditory skills in the Functional Auditory Performance Indicators (FAPI)

Stages of auditory development	Definition
Awareness and meaning of sounds	The child is aware that an auditory stimulus is present. The child may demonstrate awareness of loud environmental sounds, noisemakers, music, and/or speech. The child further demonstrates that sound is meaningful by associating a variety of auditory stimuli with their sound source. The stimuli include loud environmental sounds or noisemakers, music, vocalizations (nontrue words), and speech stimuli.
Auditory feedback and integration	The child changes, notices, and monitors his/her own vocal productions. A child may demonstrate this skill by responding to sound when amplification is turned on, by vocalizing to monitor when amplification is working, and/or by noticing his/her own vocalizations. Furthermore, the child uses auditory information to produce a spoken utterance that approximates or matches a spoken stimulus.
Localizing sound source	The child searches for and/or finds the auditory stimulus. Searching is a prerequisite skill for localizing. Children with hearing in only one ear may not be able to localize to the sound source.
Auditory discrimination	The child distinguishes the characteristics of different sounds as being the same/different, including environmental sounds, suprasegmental characteristics of speech (e.g., intensity, duration, pitch), nontrue words, and true words.
Auditory comprehension	The child demonstrates understanding of linguistic information that is heard by identifying what is said, identifying critical elements in the message, and following directions.
Short-term auditory memory	The child can hear, remember, repeat, and recall a sequence of units (e.g., digits, unrelated words, sentences, etc.). This skill is developmentally appropriate for children who are 2 years of age and older.
Linguistic auditory processing	The child uses auditory information to process language. This category measures the ways in which audition is used to sequence language, to learn and use morphemes, to learn and use syntactic information, and to understand spoken language.

Adapted from Stredler-Brown A, Johnson CD. (2004) Functional auditory performance indicators: an integrated approach to auditory development. Colorado Department of Education, Special Education Services Unit. Available at: http://www.cde.state.co.us/cdesped/download/pdf/FAPI_3-1-04g.pdf.

score allows the interventionist, teacher, and/or parents to measure progress. The objective measures of functional listening can also be used by the audiologist to adjust amplification settings.

2. Preverbal or Nonverbal Communication

How and why does a baby communicate? Babies coo, babble, and make a variety of pleasant vocalizations. They make repetitive movements such as kicking or rhythmically extending and flexing the arms or hands. Babies look intently at the adult who is looking at them, which is referred to as mutual gaze. As the baby grows, symbolic gestures emerge. Gestural communication is an important stage in the acquisition of language (Schirmer, 1994) because babies communicate their intentions using these nonverbal methods. They may repeat, answer, request an action or an object, protest, or comment using their vocalizations, gestures, or intentional body movements (Coggins, 1988).

It is crucial for parents to interact with their baby during these early months, long before real words are ever spoken by the child. Papousek and Papousek (1987) describe the communication strategies used by parents as they interact with their hearing babies. They report that many of these behaviors are not conscious but are ideally suited to support the baby's inclination to adapt to its social world. For instance, parents need to respond to the communicative attempts of their baby in order to reinforce the baby's communicative bids. Jamieson (1994) reports that some parents of children with hearing loss find this to be a challenge. It is the role of the early interventionist to teach the parents adaptive strategies to use with their baby who is deaf or hard of hearing. Parents can be taught to repeat, answer, request, or comment on their child's initiations. The parents can use their own gestures and vocalizations to create an interactive "conversation." Early intervention teaches family members to recognize the early communicative attempts of their child and to learn specific ways to encourage preverbal and verbal communication. While the interventionist looks carefully at the characteristics of communication, the audiologist has the crucial role of fitting amplification to provide access to spoken language. The audiologist can validate the fitting based on information the audiologist receives about the child's communication.

3. Speech

Irrespective of the communication approach a child uses, because a child is exposed to speech, the child is likely to attempt some oral communication. However, the child's ability to develop intelligible speech is highly correlated with several factors. One factor is the degree of hearing loss (Levitt et al., 1987). Another is the range, in decibels and frequencies, of the residual, aided hearing (Tye-Murray et al., 1995). Yet another factor is the extent of the child's functional listening ability. To identify specific sounds that are likely to be audible to the student at a typical talker-listener distance (approximately 6 feet), the child's audiogram can be superimposed on the Familiar Sounds Audiogram (Northern and Downs, 2002), which is shown in Figure 41.2.

Speech development is enhanced by (1) maximizing the audibility of sounds, (2) training the child to use speechreading cues, and (3) teaching precise auditory and speech skills. Speech training programs can use an analytic or a synthetic approach. Using an analytic or tutorial format teaches specific speech phonemes, syllables, or words. In a synthetic approach, the use of dialogue incorporates specific speech skills into longer phrases and natural language in real-world communication settings. It is often a combination of the two approaches that provides the best results (McConkey-Robbins, 1998).

There are several components of a comprehensive speech production program. Each of these components contributes to speech intelligibility. These include evaluating and working on the following:

- The impact of voice quality on speech intelligibility
- The use of suprasegmental features such as intensity, duration, and pitch
- A phonetic inventory of vowels, consonants, and consonant blends
- An analysis of the accuracy of the segmental features (vowels and consonants) that are used in actual words
- The total number of utterances spoken by the child

The professional responsible for implementing the speech program can be a speech-language pathologist who has expertise and experience working with students who are

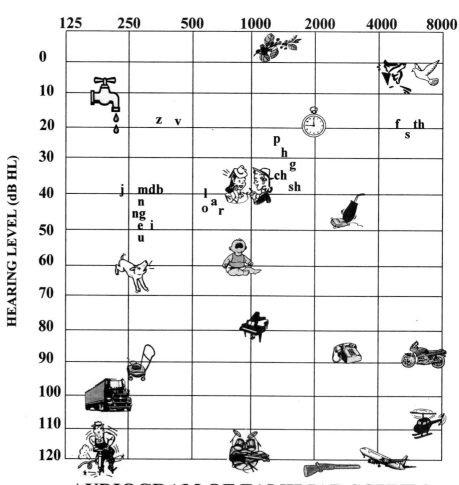

FIGURE 41.2 Familiar sounds audiogram. (Used with author's permission from Northern J, Downs MP. [2002] *Hearing in Children.* **5th ed. Baltimore, MD: Lippincott Williams & Wilkins; p 18.)**

AUDIOGRAM OF FAMILIAR SOUNDS
FREQUENCY IN CYCLES PER SECOND (HZ)

deaf or hard of hearing. Sometimes, it is the teacher of the deaf/hard of hearing who has this knowledge. It is essential to consider the competencies and experience of the professional who is working on the development and/or remediation of voice, articulation, and speech intelligibility.

4. Language

A primary goal for children with hearing loss is to develop language that is commensurate with their hearing peers. All communication approaches include a focus on semantics, syntax, morphology, and pragmatics. Each of these is described in Table 41.2.

One goal for students who are deaf or hard of hearing is to develop language according to the "one-to-one rule" (Johnson, 2006b). This benchmark expects a young child or student to develop skills at the same rate as his or her hearing peers. In 1 month, 1 month of growth is expected. In 6 months, 6 months of language growth will be attained. This is a relatively new way of thinking and has become more popular since the inception of newborn hearing screening programs and early intervention. School programs are often challenged by this expectation, with many teachers needing to change their practices because they are now often working with students who have language quotients that are well within normal limits.

5. Visual Support for Communication

The combination of auditory and visual information is known to result in more than a simple additive effect (Hipskind, 2002). Two types of oral cues can be provided. These are cued speech (Cornett, 1967; Cornett and Daisey, 1992) and speechreading. Cued speech is the use of specific hand shapes at locations around the mouth that are paired with lip movements of spoken language to visually represent speech. Speechreading, while less systematic, provides visual support for speech reception. It has been estimated that as many as 60% of the English phonemes are not readily visible on the lips (Woodward and Barber, 1960). However, for some students who are deaf or hard of hearing, the combination of speechreading cues and functional listening improves speech reception dramatically.

Manual support for communication, represented by a variety of signed systems and American Sign Language, provides another type of visual representation of language. A complete discussion about communication approaches, including sign language, is discussed later in this chapter.

▨ QUANTITATIVE AND QUALITATIVE ASSESSMENT

To prepare an individualized intervention or education program, one must collect information, analyze it, share it with team members at the IFSP or IEP, and establish goals to meet the child's needs. This entire process depends on collecting data.

In parallel to the audiologist collecting clinical information about the hearing loss, the intervention/education team can be collecting information about the developmental skills of the child. The information in the curricular areas, as identified earlier, can be collected in a variety of ways. These include using checklists, surveys, criterion-referenced tests, and norm-referenced tests. The data are collected using observation, interview, and/or clinician-administered tests. The people providing the developmental information can be parents, educators, special educators, or specialty providers such as speech-language pathologists, physical therapists, psychologists, or social workers. The goal is to collect objective information and to interpret this information according to existing benchmarks for hearing children.

There has been reluctance to compare the skills of a child with hearing loss to their typically developing, hearing peers. In the 1970s, it was common to compare a child's development at one point in time to the child's own development at a previous point in time. Using this strategy, it is easy to observe developmental gains from one testing session to the next. However, this type of testing does not compare the child's development to that of his or her hearing peers. As a result, one might have false confidence that the child's accomplishments are age appropriate.

As a result of newborn hearing screening, early intervention provides a *habilitative* approach, rather than a *rehabilitative* approach. A habilitative approach is competency based, with the intervention team creating an intervention program to reduce the potential of developmental delays. With this goal in mind, it is appropriate to use diagnostic tests that are normed on hearing children. These testing procedures measure progress quantitatively as well as qualitatively.

Once in school, current federal initiatives continue to require ongoing quantitative assessment. The No Child Left Behind Act (2004) is one example. All children, including those with hearing loss, are tested annually. Although accommodations for test administration are offered, the students receive the same tests as hearing children. Under this law, children with hearing loss will continue to be evaluated on standardized tests that measure reading, writing, math skills, and language.

▨ COMMUNICATION APPROACHES

There has been a long-standing debate that attempts to identify the best approach to language learning in children who are deaf or hard of hearing, but no consensus has been reached. Perhaps the debate has been misdirected. This long-debated argument about communication approach will not be discussed here because it is basically an academic exercise that cannot be resolved in this chapter. However, a relatively new methodology for selecting a communication approach, using an objective and prescriptive procedure, will be presented. This procedure includes a number of steps. The professionals must partner with the parents to make this decision. First, family members are provided access to information describing the various communication approaches. Next, the professionals engage family members in discussions to identify the family's unique circumstances and answer their questions. Probably the most important stage involves the gathering of information about the child. In this stage, parents can be taught to observe their child; in addition, professionals can take the opportunity to collect objective information about the child's developmental profile. By collecting this objective information about the child's development and combining it with the parents' observations, parents can make an informed choice.

There is consensus on the specific characteristics that make an approach successful (Stredler-Brown, 2002b). Common to all approaches is providing early access and, subsequently, full access to the approach. It is important for the child to have multiple role models using the approach, both within the family and in the community. For infants and toddlers, dedicated time needs to be given to teach parents the strategies they can use to implement the approach successfully. For infants, toddlers, and school-age children alike, the professionals working with the family and the child must have expertise in using the selected approach. Parental commitment to the approach goes a long way towards its success.

Building on early identification and the early start of intervention, a proposed model for selecting a communication approach for a very young child follows these five steps:

1. Parents select an approach after engaging in an informed decision-making process.
2. Professionals and parents conduct informal and formal observations of the child's developmental profile.
3. The modalities used by the child during spontaneous communication are observed.
4. Professionals document, analyze, and share their observations.
5. Parents actively review the approach they are using, revising it if they see that progress has not been satisfactory.

Many families change the communication approach during the first few years of their child's life (Sedey, 2003). These changes may reflect new information the parent has obtained. Or, the objective information describing the child's communication and language skills may provide justification to adapt the approach being used. The premise held here is that all approaches provide opportunities for learning. As stated by a parent organization, Families for Hands and Voices, "what works for your child is what makes the choice right" (Families for Hands and Voices, 2006).

Lane et al. (1997) developed the Family Communication Self-Evaluation Checklist. Parents can use this checklist periodically to reflect on the success of the approach they

---

TABLE 41.8   Family communication self-evaluation checklist

Does my child feel successful communicating with others in his/her life?

Does my child understand most of what I say?

Can we communicate easily enough so that I am able to talk with my child about what is happening?

Does my child have access to the same information as his/her hearing siblings?

Am I continuing to use an approach because of what I have been promised will happen or because of what I have observed?

Adapted from Lane S, Bell L, Parson-Tylka T. (1997) *My Turn to Learn: A Communication Guide for Parents of D/HH Children.* Burnaby, British Columbia, Canada: Elks Family Resource Centre.

---

have selected. The goal is for a child with hearing loss to be able to communicate freely and effectively in all settings. The questions listed in Table 41.8 provide parents with some quality indicators to monitor the success of their choice.

In summary, the selection of a communication approach considers the parents' preferences, the child's developmental profile, the child's communication skills, and objective input from the intervention/education team (Stredler-Brown, 1998).

■ DEFINITIONS OF APPROACHES, METHODS, SYSTEMS, AND PHILOSOPHIES

There are a variety of communication approaches, methods, and modes. Each one has been proven effective for some children. The traditional communication approaches and communication philosophies are defined in Table 41.9. Each approach or philosophy is further defined by delineating the specific characteristics of communication employed by each approach. Table 41.10 identifies the language, system, and/or communication strategies that are part and parcel of each approach.

There have been many attempts to provide a structure for parents and professionals to use to select the communication features that are best suited to a particular child. A current representation of the range of choices is being developed at Gallaudet University (Nussbaum et al., 2006). This novel depiction looks at both expressive and receptive communication. Receptively, the degree to which the child listens or watches is represented along a continuum from fully visual to fully auditory. There are five stages along the continuum:

■ Fully visual (e.g., depends on visual information via American Sign Language or other signs)
■ Mostly visual with some benefit from auditory information

TABLE 41.9 Communication approaches and philosophies

Communication approaches and philosophies	Definition
Bilingual model	A person who achieves fluency in American Sign Language (ASL) and English (or another language) is bilingual. ASL is often the first language, with English being taught as a second language to develop literacy skills. English can be taught using a sign system or through print. Spoken English is not included in the bilingual model that is currently promoted by the deaf community.
Simultaneous communication	This is the use of signs and speech at the same time. In order to provide language simultaneously, a sign system, rather than a signed language, is used to depict the oral language while using manual symbols or signs.
Sign-supported speech and language	The use of signs to support spoken language development can be used as a "bridge" to completely oral communication or as a "back-up" in certain situations, such as noisy environments or when a hearing device is not in use. (Lane et al., 2006)
Auditory/oral approach	This approach combines oral spoken language to express oneself and speechreading, accompanied by active listening, to receive information. The use of natural gestures is acceptable.
Auditory-verbal approach	An educational approach in which technology is paired with specific techniques and strategies that teach children to listen and understand spoken language. A primary emphasis is placed on access to learning through the auditory modality. This refinement of the oral-aural approach makes a concerted effort to remove visual cues during therapy sessions so the child can develop the auditory system through directed listening practice. Speechreading is not a primary teaching strategy, and this visual information is reduced or eliminated during therapy by covering most of the face while presenting speech stimuli (Estabrooks, 1994).
Total communication	Introduced in the 1960s by Roy Holcomb, this philosophy was adopted by the Maryland School for the Deaf as the official name for their educational philosophy. This "philosophy" aims to make use of a number of strategies or modes of communication including sign, oral, auditory, written, and other visual aids. The choice of modalities depends on the particular needs and abilities of the child and professes to provide whatever is needed to foster communicative success.
Multisensory approach	Uses both vision and hearing to recognize speech and uses speech and/or sign language to express oneself.
Unisensory approach	Students using this approach traditionally rely only on residual hearing to receive spoken messages. The child is expected to recognize the signal auditorily.

- Equally dependent on and able to use visual information via sign and auditory information via spoken English
- A primary reliance on auditory information via spoken English with some visual information delivered through sign or speechreading to clarify spoken English (the responsibility for understanding the content relies on the use of techniques, such as speechreading, that the child has learned)
- Fully auditory (e.g., primarily depends on auditory information delivered through spoken English with limited assistance from visual cues)

A companion continuum describes expressive communication. The degree to which the person signs or uses oral communication is represented on another five-point continuum. A child may be a fully signing communicator or a fully oral communicator. The five steps along this expressive language scale are as follows:

- Fully signing communicator
- Using mostly sign with some oral communication
- Using sign and oral communication equally
- Primarily using oral communication along with some signs for clarification
- Fully oral communicator

It is notable that this model does not identify the methods themselves. Rather, the focus is on the child and the characteristics of the child's communication.

TABLE 41.10   Languages, systems, and strategies

Communication approach	Characteristics of communication
American Sign Language (ASL)	ASL is a visual-gestural language that is used by many deaf people in the United States and Canada. It has its own set of rules that are separate from spoken or written English. It is not possible to speak English and sign ASL at the same time.
Conceptually Accurate Signed English (CASE) or Pidgin Signed English (PSE)	Signs from ASL are used in English word order. The focus is on conceptual accuracy to aid understanding, and no attempt is made to provide a one-to-one relationship with spoken English. Specific features of ASL, such as facial expression and use of space, may be used. These sign systems rely on context and mechanisms such as initialization to support meaning.
Manually Coded English (MCE): Signed English (Bornstein et al., 1983); Signing Exact English (Gustason et al., 1993)	These systems were constructed by educators to teach English. The sign systems attempt to represent English by combining ASL signs, English word order, and some invented signs to represent grammatical markers (e.g., plurals, possessives, tenses, etc.) in English. Each word, including each morpheme, is signed. An example would be to sign the word "working" by signing the word "work" and then signing the ending "ing." All structure words, such as "the" and "to," are signed in this system.
Cued Speech	A supplement to spoken English, cued speech is intended to make important features of spoken language fully visible, since approximately 60% of the phonemes are not visible through speechreading. This system enhances speechreading by employing phonemically based gestures to distinguish between similar visual speech patterns.

THE ROLE OF THE AUDIOLOGIST

Audiologists are in a vital position because they screen newborns for hearing loss. They continue to be the professional who takes the reins when diagnosing hearing loss and fitting amplification. However, at this time, the role of the audiologist in the intervention and education of a child who is deaf or hard of hearing is relatively ambiguous.

Audiologists can have a key role in the intervention and educational programming, a role that will enhance the quality of services to children. Professionals and parents often look to the audiologist to provide counseling and guidance. Some audiologists provide auditory training. The information provided by the audiologist is of great importance to educators, speech-language pathologists, and other professionals working with young children. Whether a clinical audiologist or an educational audiologist, the audiologist validates his or her role by being actively involved in the intervention and education of young children with hearing loss.

SUMMARY

As a result of newborn hearing screening programs and burgeoning advancements in technology, children with hearing loss can achieve academic levels never seen before.

Children with all types and all degrees of hearing loss are eligible, to varying degrees in each state, to specialized services. Federal and state initiatives support the provision of these services.

For infants, early intervention should start within weeks of the diagnosis of hearing loss. Preschool services are a standard for children 3, 4, and 5 years of age. In addition, special programs in elementary schools are growing in number.

It is now the responsibility of educators, speech-language pathologists, and audiologists to set a high standard for achievement for children with hearing loss. No longer should we hear, "This child is doing well for a deaf child." Rather, services and accommodations can provide opportunities for children with hearing loss to achieve academic levels comparable to their hearing peers.

In order to meet this goal, commitments must be made to secure appropriate services. Professionals must work with parents as they select a communication approach. All approaches are considered to be viable options.

Curricula address many facets of communication development including the acquisition of functional auditory skills, preverbal communication, language skills, speech, and, for some, the use of sign language. There is a growing trend to monitor progress using outcome data. By collecting the evidence, one can be certain each child is attaining the skills he or she needs to learn, to communicate, to learn, and to succeed.

REFERENCES

Allen T. (1986) Patterns of academic achievement among hearing impaired students: 1974 and 1983. In: Schildroth A, Karchmer M, eds. *Deaf Children in America.* Boston: College Hill Press; pp 161–206.

Anderson K. (1989) Screening Instrument for Targeting Educational Risk (SIFTER). Tampa, FL: Educational Audiology Association. Available at: www.hear2learn.com.

Anderson K, Matkin N. (1996) The Preschool Screening Instrument for Targeting Educational Risk. Tampa, FL: Educational Audiology Association. Available at: www.hear2learn.com.

Anderson K, Smaldino J. (1998) The Listening Inventories for Education (LIFE). Tampa, FL: Educational Audiology Association. Available at: www.hear2learn.com.

Babbidge J. (1965) The Babbidge Committee Report. ERIC Document Reproduction Service No. ED 014 188. Washington, DC: Department of Health, Education and Welfare.

Berlin C. (2001) Auditory neuropathy: etiology and management. Presented at RIHAP 7th Annual Seminar, Providence, RI.

Berlin C, Taylor-Jeanfreau J, Hood L, Morlet T, Keats BJB. (2002) Managing and re-naming auditory neuropathy (AN) as part of a continuum of auditory dys-synchrony (AuDys). Powerpoint Presentation.

Bess F. (2000) Classroom acoustics: an overview. *Volta Rev.* 101, 1–14.

Bess F. (2004) Children with minimal sensorineural hearing loss. Presented at the Wyoming EHDI Conference, Laramie, WY.

Bess F, Dodd-Murphy J, Parker R. (1998) Children with minimal sensorineural hearing loss: prevalence, educational performance, and functional status. *Ear Hear.* 19, 339–354.

Bess F, Tharpe A. (1986) Case history data on unilaterally hearing-impaired children. *Ear Hear.* 197, 14–19.

Bess F, Tharpe A. (1988) Performance and management of children with unilateral sensorineural hearing loss. *Scand Audiol Suppl.* 30, 75–79.

Blair J, Peterson M, Viehwed S. (1985) The effects of mild sensorineural hearing loss on academic performance of young school-age children. *Volta Rev.* 87, 87–93.

Bornstein H, Saulnier KL, Hamilton LB. (1983) *The Comprehensive Signed English Dictionary.* Washington, DC: Gallaudet University Press.

Bovo R, Martini A, Agnoletto M, Beghi D, Carmignoto D, Milani M, Zangaglia AM. (1988) Auditory and academic performance of children with unilateral hearing loss. *Scand Audiol Suppl.* 30, 71–74.

Brookhouser PE, Worthington DW, Kelly WJ. (1991) Unilateral hearing loss in children. *Laryngoscope.* 101, 1264–1272.

Clinical Health Information Record for Patients [Electronic data]. (2005) Denver, CO: Colorado Department of Public Health and Environment.

Coggins TE. (1988) Communicative intention scale. In: Olswang L, Stoel-Gammon C, Coggins T, Carpenter R, eds. *Assessing Prelinguistic and Early Linguistic Behaviors in Developmentally Young Children.* Seattle, WA: University of Washington Press; pp 78–97.

Colorado Department of Education. (2002) A blueprint for closing the gap: developing a statewide system of service improvements for students who are deaf and hard of hearing. Available at: http://www.cde.state.co.us/cdesped/download/pdf/dhh-blueprint.pdf.

Colorado Department of Education. (2006) Communication plan. Avialable at: http://www.cde.state.co.us/cdesped/download/pdf/dhh-DeafChildBillRts.pdf.

Colorado Infant Hearing Advisory Committee. (2003) *Guidelines for Infant Hearing Screening, Audiologic Assessment, and Early Intervention.* Denver, CO: Colorado Department of Public Health and Environment.

Cone-Wesson B, Rance G, Sininger Y. (2001) Amplification and rehabilitation strategies for patients with auditory neuropathy. In: Sininger Y, Starr A, eds. *Auditory Neuropathy: A New Perspective on Hearing Disorders.* San Diego: Singular; pp 233–249.

Cornett RO. (1967) Cued speech. *Am Ann Deaf.* 112, 3–13.

Cornett RO, Daisey ME. (1992) *The Cued Speech Resource Book.* Raleigh, NC: National Cued Speech Association.

Crandell CC, Smaldino JJ. (2000) Classroom acoustics for children with normal hearing and with hearing impairment. *Language, Speech, and Hearing Services in the Schools.* 31, 362–370.

Culbertson JL, Gilbert LE. (1986) Children with unilateral sensorineural hearing loss: cognitive, academic, and social development. *Ear Hear.* 7, 38–42.

Dalzell L, Orlando M, MacDonald M, Berg A, Bradley M, Cacace A, Campbell D, DeCristofaro J, Gravel J, Greenberg E, Gross S, Pinheiro J, Regan J, Spivak L, Stevens F, Prieve B. (2000) The New York State universal newborn hearing screening demonstration project: ages of hearing loss identification, hearing aid fitting, and enrollment in early intervention. *Ear Hear.* 21, 118–130.

Davis A, Reeve K, Hind SBJ. (2001) Children with mild and unilateral hearing loss. In: Seewald RC, Gravel JS, eds. *A Sound Foundation through Early Amplification: Proceedings of the Second International Conference.* St. Edmundsbury, United Kingdom: St. Edmundsbury Press; pp 179–186.

Davis JM, Elfenbein J, Schum R, Bentler RA. (1986) Effects of mild and moderate hearing impairments on language, educational, and psychosocial behavior of children. *J Speech Hear Dis.* 51, 53–62.

DesGeorges J, Johnson CD, Stredler-Brown A. (2006) Natural environments: a call for policy guidance for infants and toddlers (0-3) who are deaf/hard and hearing. Unpublished manuscript.

Diggs C. (2006) State of the states 2006: legislatures address qualified providers, early hearing detection, and more. *The ASHA Leader.* 11, 1, 39–41.

Eichwald J, Gaffney M. (2007) The new EHDI screening and follow-up survey. Presented at the Annual Early Hearing Detection and Intervention Conference, Salt Lake City, UT.

Erber NP. (1982) *Auditory Training.* Washington, DC: Alexander Graham Bell Association for the Deaf.

Estabrooks W. (1994) *Auditory-Verbal Therapy.* Washington, DC: Alexander Graham Bell Association for the Deaf.

Estabrooks W. (1998) Auditory-verbal ages and stages of development. In: Estabrooks W, ed. *Cochlear Implants for Kids.* Washington, DC: Alexander Graham Bell Association for the Deaf.

Families for Hands and Voices. (2006) Homepage. Available at: www.handsandvoices.org.

Gallaudet Research Institute. (2005) Regional and national summary report of data from the 2004-2005 annual survey of deaf and hard of hearing children and youth. Washington, DC: Gallaudet Research Institute, Gallaudet University.

Green DR, Gaffney M, Devine O, Grosse SD. (2007) Determining the effect of newborn hearing screening: an analysis of state hearing screening rates. *Public Health Rep.* 122, 198–205.

Gustason G, Zawolkow E, Lopez L. (1993) *Signing Exact English.* Los Alamitos, CA: Modern Signs Press.

Haley J. (1987) *Problem Solving Therapy.* 2nd ed. San Francisco: Jossey-Bass.

Hipskind NM. (2002) Visual stimuli in communication. In: Schow RL, Nerbonne MA, eds. *Introduction to Audiologic Rehabilitation.* Boston, MA: Allyn and Bacon.

Holt JA. (1994) Classroom attributes and achievement test scores for deaf and hard of hearing students. *Am Ann Deaf.* 139, 430–437.

Individuals with Disabilities Education Act Amendments of 1997. (1997) Public law #105-17, 111 Stat. 38. (Codified as amended at 20 U.S.C. Sections 1400-1485.)

Individuals with Disabilities Education Improvement Act of 2004. (2004) 20 U.S.C. §1400 et seq.

Jamieson JR. (1994) Teaching as transaction: Vygotskian perspectives on deafness and mother-child interaction. *Exceptional Children.* 60, 434–449.

Johnson CD. (2006a) CSAP analysis: students who are deaf or hard of hearing. Paper presented at the American Academy of Audiology Annual Meeting, Minneapolis, MN.

Johnson CD. (2006b) One year's growth in one year, expect no less. *Hands and Voices Communicator.* 9, 3.

Johnson CD, Beams D, Stredler-Brown A. (2005) Preschool/Kindergarten Checklist. Colorado Department of Education, Special Services Unit. Available at: http://www.cde.state.co.us/cdesped/download/pdf/dhh-PS-KPlcmntCklst.pdf.

Johnson CD, Benson PV, Seaton JB. (1997) *Educational Audiology Handbook.* San Diego: Singular Publishing Group.

Jones EA. (1993) Partnering with families: a clinical training manual. Unpublished manuscript, University of Colorado at Boulder.

Karchmer M, Mitchell R. (2003) Demographics and achievement characteristics of deaf and hard-of-hearing students. In: Marschark M, Spencer P, eds. *Oxford Handbook of Deaf Studies, Language, and Education.* New York: Oxford University Press; pp 21–37.

Klee TM, Davis-Dansky E. (1986) A comparison of unilaterally hearing-impaired children and normal-hearing children on a battery of standardized language tests. *Ear Hear.* 7, 27–37.

Kuhl PK. (2000). A new view of language acquisition. *Proc Natl Acad Sci.* 97, 11850–11857.

Lane S, Bell L, Parson-Tylka T. (1997) *My Turn to Learn: A Communication Guide for Parents of D/HH Children.* Burnaby, British Columbia, Canada: Elks Family Resource Centre.

Lane S, Bell L, Parson-Tylka T. (2006) *My Turn to Learn: A Communication Guide for Parents of Deaf or Hard of Hearing Children.* Burnaby, British Columbia, Canada: Bauhinea Press.

Lang HG. (2003) Perspectives on the history of deaf education. In: Marschark M, Spencer P, eds. *Oxford Handbook of Deaf Studies, Language, and Education.* New York: Oxford University Press.

Levitt H, McGarr N, Geffner D. (1987) *Development of Language and Communication Skills in Hearing-Impaired Children. Monograph of the American Speech-Language-Hearing Association.* Rockville, MD: American Speech-Language-Hearing Association.

Lieu JE. (2004) Speech-language and educational consequences of unilateral hearing loss in children. *Arch Otolaryngol Head Neck Surg.* 130, 524–530.

Linder TW. (1993) *Transdisciplinary Play-Based Intervention: Guidelines for Developing a Meaningful Curriculum for Young Children.* Baltimore, MD: Paul H. Brookes Publishing Company.

Marean GC, Werner LA, Kuhl PK. (1992). Vowel categorization by very young infants. *Dev Psychol.* 28, 396–405.

Marschark M, Lang HG, Albertini JA. (2002) *Educating Deaf Students: From Research to Practice.* New York: Oxford University Press.

McConkey-Robbins A. (1998) Two paths of auditory development for children with cochlear implants. *Loud and Clear Newsletter.* 1, 1.

McKay S, Iyer A. (2005) Management guidelines for children with unilateral hearing loss. *The ASHA Leader.* May 24, 4, 10.

Moeller MP. (2000) Early intervention and language development in children who are deaf and hard of hearing. *Pediatrics.* 106, 1–9.

Moores DF, Martin DS. (2006) Overview: curriculum and instruction in general education and in education of deaf learners. In: Moores DF, Martin DS, eds. *Deaf Learners: Developments in Curriculum and Instruction.* Washington, DC: Gallaudet University Press.

National Center for Hearing Assessment and Management. (2007) Prevalence of congenital hearing loss. Available at: http://www.infanthearing.org/summary/summary.html#prevalence.

Neault M. (2001) Cochlear implants for children with auditory neuropathy: who, why, and when. Presented at RIHAP 7th Annual Seminar, Providence, RI.

No Child Left Behind Act of 2001, Pub. L. No. 107–110, 115 Stat. 1425 (2002). Available at: http://www.ed.gov/nclb/landing.jhtml.

Northern J, Downs MP. (2002) *Hearing in Children.* 5th ed. Baltimore: Lippincott Williams & Wilkins.

Nussbaum D, Scott S, Waddy-Smith B, Koch M. (2006). Spoken language and sign: optimizing learning for children with cochlear implants. Presented at Laurent Clerc National Deaf Education Center, Washington, DC.

Orelove FP, Sobsey D. (1996) *Educating Children with Multiple Disabilities: A Transdisciplinary Approach.* Baltimore: Paul H. Brookes.

Oyler RF, Oyler A, Matkin N. (1987) Warning: a unilateral hearing loss may be detrimental to a child's academic career. *Hear J.* 9, 18–22.

Papousek H, Papousek M. (1987) Intuitive parenting: a dialectic counterpart to the infant's precocity in integrative capacities. In: Osofsky JD, ed. *Handbook of Infant Development.* 2nd ed. New York: Wiley; pp 669–720.

Pichora-Fuller K, Schow RL. (2007) Audiologic rehabilitation for adults and elderly adults. In: Schow RL, Nerbonne MA, eds. *Introduction to Audiologic Rehabilitation.* Boston: Pearson Education Inc.

Pollack D. (1970) *Educational Audiology for the Limited Hearing Infant.* Springfield, IL: Charles C. Thomas.

Purdy SC, Farrington DR, Moran CA, Chard LL, Hodgson SA. (2002) A parental questionnaire to evaluate children's auditory behavior in everyday life (ABEL). *Am J Audiol.* 11, 2, 72.

Rance G. (2005) Auditory neuropathy/dys-synchrony: clinical presentation, perceptual consequences and management options. Presented at Frontiers in Hearing: Emerging Practices, Breckenridge, CO.

Rance G, Beer D, Cone-Wesson B. (1999) Clinical findings for a group of infants and young children with auditory neuropathy. *Ear Hear.* 20, 238–252.

Razack Z. (1994) *The Development of Listening Function.* Kitchener, Ontario, Canada: The Waterloo County Board of Education; pp 26–30.

Ross DS. (2006) Mild and unilateral hearing loss: summaries of research articles. Available at: http://www.cdc.gov/ncbddd/ehdi/unilateralhi.htm#summaries.

Schildroth A, Hotto S. (1993) Annual survey of hearing impaired children and youth: 1991-1992 school year. *Am Ann Deaf.* 138, 163–168.

Schirmer BR. (1994) *Language and Literacy Development in Children Who Are Deaf.* New York: Macmillan.

Schow RL, Nerbonne MA. (2002) Overview of audiologic rehabilitation. In: Schow RL, Nerbonne MA, eds. *Introduction to Audiologic Rehabilitation.* Boston: Allyn and Bacon.

Sedey A. (2003) Communication approach used by children in Colorado. Unpublished raw data.

Sedey A. (2004) Language of young deaf and hard-of-hearing children: what's missing? Presented at the Colorado Symposium on Deafness, Language and Learning, Colorado Springs, CO.

Sedey A. (2006) What early interventionists can learn from research. Presented at the Colorado Symposium on Deafness, Language and Learning, Colorado Springs, CO.

Sedey A, Carpenter K, Stredler-Brown A. (2002) Unilateral hearing loss: what do we know, what should we do? Presented at the National Symposium on Hearing in Infants, Breckenridge, CO.

Sedey A, Stredler-Brown A. (2004) Summary of facilitator survey. Unpublished raw data.

Shallop J, Peterson A, Facer G, Fabry L, Discoll C. (2001) Cochlear implants in five cases of auditory neuropathy: postoperative findings and progress. *Laryngoscope.* 111, 555–562.

Stout GG, Windle JVE. (1992) *The Developmental Approach to Successful Listening.* 2nd ed. Englewood, CO: Resource Point, Inc.

Stredler-Brown A. (1998) Early intervention for infants and toddlers who are deaf and hard of hearing: new perspectives. *J Educ Audiol.* 6, 46–49.

Stredler-Brown A. (2002a) Developing a treatment program for children with auditory neuropathy. *Semin Hear.* 23, 239–249.

Stredler-Brown A. (2002b) Identifying early: a state model for early intervention. Panel facilitated at Oklahoma Speech and Hearing Association Convention, Oklahoma City, OK.

Stredler-Brown A. (2005) The art and science of home visits. *ASHA Leader.* 6-7, 15.

Stredler-Brown A, Johnson DeConde C. (2004) Functional auditory performance indicators: an integrated approach to auditory development. Colorado Department of Education, Special Education Services Unit. Available at: http://www.cde.state.co.us/cdesped/download/pdf/FAPI_3-1-04g.pdf.

Stredler-Brown A, Moeller MP, Gallegos R, Corwin J, Pittman P. (2004) *The Art and Science of Home Visits* (DVD). Omaha, NE: Boys Town Press.

Traxler CB. (2000) The Stanford Achievement Test (9th edition): national norming and performance standards for deaf and hard-of hearing students. *J Deaf Stud Deaf Educ.* 5, 337–348.

Tye-Murray N. (1992) *Cochlear Implants and Children: A Handbook for Parents, Teachers and Speech and Hearing Professionals.* Washington, DC: Alexander Graham Bell Association for the Deaf.

Tye-Murray N, Spencer L, Woodworth G. (1995) Acquisition of speech by children who have prolonged cochlear implant experience. *J Speech Hear Res.* 38, 327–337.

Wake M, Poulakis Z. (2004) Slight and mild hearing loss in primary school children. *J Pediatr Child Health.* 40, 11–13.

Watkin PM, Baldwin M. (1999) Confirmation of deafness in infancy. *Arch Dis Child.* 81, 380–389.

Watkins S. (1993) *The SKI*HI Resource Manual.* Logan, UT: Hope, Inc.

Western States Early Intervention Coalition for Sensory Impairments. (1999) Natural environments for infants and toddlers who are deaf and hard of hearing. Available at: http://www.asha.org/about/legislation-advocacy/federal/idea/nat-env-child-facts.htm.

White KR. (2003) The current status of EHDI programs in the United States. *Ment Retard Dev Disabil Res Rev.* 9, 79–88.

White KR, Vohr BR, Maxon AB, Behreus TR, McPherson MG, Mauk GW. (1994) Screening all newborns for hearing loss using transient evoked otoacoustic emissions. *Int J Pediatr Otorhinolaryngol.* 29, 203–217.

Woodward MF, Barber CG. (1960) Phoneme perception in lipreading. *J Speech Hear Res.* 3, 212–222.

Yoshinaga-Itano C. (1999) Assessment and intervention of preschool-aged deaf and hard-of-hearing children. In: Alpiner J, McCarthy P, eds. *Rehabilitative Audiology: Children and Adults.* Baltimore: Williams & Wilkins.

Yoshinaga-Itano C, Downey DM. (1986) A hearing-impaired child's acquisition of schemata: something's missing. *Topics Lang Disord.* 7, 45–57.

Yoshinaga-Itano C, Sedey A, Coulter DK, Mehl AL. (1998) The language of early- and later-identified children with hearing loss. *Pediatrics.* 102, 1161–1171.

APPENDIX 41.1

National Resources

These agencies provide information and support to parents and professionals. Each organization is dedicated specifically to children with hearing loss.

- Alexander Graham Bell Association for the Deaf and Hard of Hearing (AG Bell) – http://www.agbell.org
- American Society for Deaf Children – http://www.deafchildren.org
- Auditory-Verbal International – http://www.auditory-verbal.org
- Boys Town National Research Hospital – http://www.babyhearing.org
- Beginnings for Parents of Children Who Are Deaf or Hard of Hearing – http://www.beginningssvcs.com
- Centers for Disease Control and Prevention - Early Hearing Detection and Intervention – http://www.cdc.gov/ncbddd/ehdi
- Hands & Voices – http://www.handsandvoices.org
- John Tracy Clinic – http://www.jtc.org
- National Association for Hearing Assessment and Management (NCHAM) – http://www.infanthearing.org
- National Association of the Deaf – http://www.nad.org
- National Cued Speech Organization – http://www.cuedspeech.org
- National Deaf Education Center at Gallaudet University – http://clerccenter.gallaudet.edu/infotogo

CHAPTER 42 Management of Adults with Hearing Loss

Dean Garstecki and Susan Erler

INTRODUCTION

The number of adults who experience hearing loss is large and growing. Kochkin (2005a) estimates that there are currently 31.5 million individuals in the United States with impaired hearing, and that number is expected to increase to 41 million by 2025. It is well documented that the prevalence of hearing loss increases with age, with hearing loss prevalence estimates falling in the 35% and higher range for older adults. In a recent study, Cruickshanks et al. (2003) reported hearing loss prevalence among adults averaging 65.8 years of age to be 45%. Recent popular press reports (e.g., http://www.earfoundation.org/downloads/baby_boomer_survey.pdf) suggest that more than half of Baby Boomers (i.e., adults born between 1945 and 1964) report hearing problems compared with 20% of similarly aged adults in 1990; this suggests that Baby Boomers are losing their hearing at a more rapid pace than past generations. The estimated annual cost in terms of lost earnings due to untreated hearing loss is currently at $122 billion; the cost to society in unrealized federal taxes is $18 billion (Kochkin, 2005b). Clearly, the number of adults who may require assistance with managing their hearing loss is significant and growing, while the cost of untreated hearing loss is staggering and must be contained.

Audiologists assume responsibility for the prevention, identification, evaluation, and treatment of hearing loss and its associated problems. Audiologists are required to practice within the scope of their competence, education, and experience (American Speech-Language-Hearing Association [ASHA], 2004) and abide by the ethical standards of their professional organization, ASHA (ASHA, 2003) and/or the American Academy of Audiology (Hamill, 2006). It is essential that audiologists hold paramount the welfare of the individuals they serve.

HEARING LOSS IN OLDER ADULTS

Changes in the auditory system due to aging include increased cerumen production and degradation of external canal skin. These rarely result in permanent hearing loss but possibly affect testing and treatment. Changes within the middle ear occur infrequently but may include stiffening of the tympanic membrane, deterioration of the middle ear muscles, and arthritic stiffening of ossicular joints. More commonly, over time, adults experience changes in inner ear function that are likely to affect hearing sensitivity and speech processing ability, resulting in a need for rehabilitative intervention (see Chisholm et al. [2003] for a review).

Age-related hearing loss, or presbycusis, has multiple causes and manifestations. For most adults, the onset of hearing loss is insidious, advancing over a 15- to 20-year period before corrective action is taken. Hearing loss due to the normal process of aging is typically permanent, bilateral, and sensory-neural in nature. Among men, the high frequencies are typically affected first, whereas women initially experience greater low-frequency loss (Jerger et al., 1993). Conditions resulting in hearing loss in adults are first manifested by a filtering effect on incoming auditory signals, a particular concern in everyday speech perception. Aging adults with characteristic high-frequency sloping hearing loss tend to encounter more difficulty recognizing differences among consonants, which contributes to generalized word confusions. Over time, this difficulty may be increased by natural physiologic deterioration of the entire auditory system. As this occurs, a common complaint is that one is able to hear but not understand spoken messages.

A number of interacting factors have been suggested as contributing to age-related hearing loss (Willot, 1991). These include biologic and genetic factors, exposure to noise, exposure to ototoxic agents, and some medical conditions. Atrophy of the organ of Corti and/or stria vascularis, loss of cochlear neurons, diminution of blood vessels, and deterioration of other structures can occur, resulting in hearing loss of various degrees and configurations. Poor speech discrimination, particularly in the presence of background noise, is common. Some individuals are genetically destined to experience impaired hearing in their lifetime, while others may suffer the consequences of long-term exposure to environmental, occupational, and recreational noise. Additionally, some may be exposed to ototoxic drugs, contract ear diseases or disorders, or experience ear trauma that negatively impacts their hearing. Regardless of the cause, inner ear changes are likely to result in permanent hearing loss that is not medically or surgically reversible.

Added to these biologic or genetic factors are so-called nonauditory factors (e.g., age, gender, socioeconomic status, personality) that are known to influence the personal impact of hearing loss. When hearing loss results in communication difficulty, it potentially diminishes quality of life. It may have a broad and devastating impact on physical health, emotional and mental well-being, mental acuity, social communication, family relationships, self-esteem, and work performance/employment, particularly among those with severe to profound loss (Mulrow et al., 1990). These negative consequences to quality of life may be mitigated through the successful use of hearing prostheses (e.g., hearing aids, implantable aids, and assistive listening devices) and participation in an aural rehabilitation (AR) program.

Successful hearing loss management is highly related to self-sufficiency in daily living (Carabellese et al., 1993). Adult AR programs provide direction and training in ways to facilitate effective and efficient communication. These programs typically include identification and evaluation of hearing problems, vision screening, counseling, and referral. They help participants to understand hearing loss and options for medical, surgical, and prosthetic solutions to hearing problems. Through comprehensive interviews and assessment, AR programs also help consumers optimize the use of sensory aids, maximize communication skills, and establish independent self-management of hearing loss.

Components of an AR program may include: (1) information on the acquisition and use of assistive listening devices beyond hearing aids; (2) speechreading instruction and auditory training to maximize use of residual hearing; (3) information on implantable prostheses; (4) information on the legal rights to communication access guaranteed under the Americans with Disabilities Act (Public Law 101-336;

1990); and (5) information on how to access community support groups. AR programs may be located in universities, hospitals, community centers, and private practices and may provide opportunities whereby adults and their families can: (1) socialize with others with hearing loss and their family members; (2) share strategies for dealing with difficult communication circumstances; and (3) receive peer support. In addition to AR programs, adults can glean information on available products and services from the Internet as well as from library holdings. Equipped with such information, individuals with hearing loss are in a good position to take control of their hearing loss management concerns.

Other problems common among adults with hearing loss, such as tinnitus and balance disorders, may be addressed, at least in part, through audiologic management. It is estimated that 8% to 20% of the adult population in the United States experiences tinnitus (Noell and Meyerhoff, 2003), with adults 40 to 70 years of age being the most likely to report this problem. Although most report that the ringing, buzzing, and tones they perceive cause little or no disruption to their daily activities, 1% to 2% of the population indicate that they are debilitated by severe tinnitus. As a result, millions of adults seek treatment to relieve symptoms of tinnitus and reduce its impact on daily activities, reduce feelings of anxiety and depression, and minimize its disruption of sleep.

Like tinnitus, dizziness and balance disorders are common among adults with hearing loss. Nearly one-third of adults age 60 and older experience dizziness (Sloane et al., 2001). The prevalence of dizziness (including vertigo) increases with age and is more commonly diagnosed among women. Chronic and acute bouts of dizziness have been associated with labyrinthitis, Ménière's disease, trauma, neurologic disorders, exposure to ototoxic agents, and psychological disorders. Dizziness and balance disorders contribute to falls, fear of falling, and limitation of daily activities. Further discussion of treatment of tinnitus and dizziness is provided later in this chapter.

■ IMPORTANCE OF HEARING LOSS MANAGEMENT

Despite the pervasive impact of hearing problems, relatively few adults actively attempt to manage them. For example, less than 20% of adults who could benefit from the use of amplification, which is the most common approach to hearing loss management, choose to purchase hearing aids. Adults often wait years between the time they first notice a hearing problem and when they finally consult an audiologist. Adults are most likely to purchase hearing aids for the first time because the severity of their hearing loss has progressed or they are responding to the urging of family members to take action (Kochkin, 2005a). Unfortunately, nearly one-fifth of purchased hearing aids are rarely, if ever, worn. Other rehabilitative interventions, such as communication training, counseling, or participation in self-help groups, are used even less than amplification.

Treatment of hearing-related problems is complex due to the heterogeneity of the affected population. Not surprisingly, numerous investigators report a mismatch between objectively measured hearing loss and self-assessed hearing handicap (Cox and Alexander, 2000). Degree of hearing loss, age, gender, socioeconomic status, personality traits, and employment status individually or in combination influence how a person is affected by hearing loss (Gatehouse, 1990; Garstecki and Erler, 2001). For example, social impact has been shown to vary with gender. Women typically place higher value on social competence than men, which may increase the perceived negative impact of a hearing loss (Garstecki and Erler, 1999).

Hearing loss can result in significant disruption of day-to-day activities. A recent survey (http://www.earfoundation.org/downloads/baby_boomer_survey.pdf) revealed that, for adults age 40 to 59 (the so-called Baby Boomers) who experience hearing problems:

- 46% said they were most affected at home
- 44% said that the hearing loss caused them problems in social situations
- 35% said they had difficulty hearing and understanding telephone conversations
- 24% said their hearing loss made them feel misunderstood
- 9% felt socially isolated by their hearing problem

One can easily understand these consequences by examining the impact of hearing loss in everyday communication. Hearing loss may result in frustrating misunderstandings and requests for repetitions. It may disrupt communication and, in turn, social interaction. Subsequently, interpersonal relations may be challenged (Kochkin and Rogin, 2000). Arlinger (2003) asserts that persons with hearing loss may become isolated because the need to articulate clearly, repeat, rephrase, or provide visual cues creates too great a communication burden for family and friends. In the extreme, because of the hearing loss, individuals may withdraw from usual and valued activities, which ultimately may reduce intellectual stimulation.

Hallberg (1999), in a study of the consequences of hearing loss on family life, found that some significant others may perceive a need to "overprotect" (i.e., tolerate denial of the severity of the hearing problem) in an attempt to maintain normalcy as a couple. Individuals with hearing loss may come to find themselves dependent on others and feel diminished in social stature (Hetu et al., 1996). Perceived threats to social identity, in turn, may lead to denial of hearing loss and rejection of recommendations to use amplification. Communication partners may also tire of the effort required to interact with someone with impaired hearing. Morgan-Jones (2001) reported that some adults attributed the failure of their marriage to hearing loss.

The emotional impact of untreated hearing loss must be considered. Compared to adults who use hearing aids, those without amplification are more likely to report feelings of sadness, worry, depression, anger, and paranoia (Kochkin and Rogin, 2000). Although most of these symptoms do not reach a level of clinical significance, clearly negative reactions may affect daily function, productivity, and interpersonal relationships. Garstecki and Erler (1998) found that women with untreated hearing loss reported poorer personal adjustment to hearing loss than men and women who used amplification, as well as to men who chose not to use hearing aids. Significant others note improvement in emotional state (i.e., reduction in frustration, anger, annoyance) when partners use amplification (Kochkin and Rogin, 2000).

Finally, there are financial implications. As mentioned earlier, Kochkin (2005b) placed a price tag of $122 billion in lost income annually that could be attributable to untreated hearing loss. Estimated lost income varies with degree of hearing loss, increasing from $1,000 per year for adults with mild hearing loss to $12,000 annually for those with profound hearing loss.

Benefits from amplification/cochlear implantation and participation in audiologic rehabilitation as demonstrated by (1) improved communication, (2) decreased negative emotional response, (3) increased earning potential, (4) improved interpersonal relationships, (5) reduction in hearing aid returns, and (6) overall enhanced quality of life support the need to provide hearing loss management services to adults of all ages. These benefits underscore the importance of educating the public regarding available services and devices, as well as promoting the need for continuing development of appropriate assessment and treatment methods and provision of individualized services.

PROSTHETIC DEVICES

Hearing Aids

Among hearing loss management options when prosthetic solutions are sought, first consideration typically is given to the use of hearing aids. However, hearing aid adoption rates are astoundingly low. Of adults with impaired hearing, less than one-fourth own a hearing aid, and far fewer use their hearing aid(s) on a regular basis. In addition, more than 80% of all hearing instruments are owned by adults age 65 and older, and the average age of new hearing aid users is 70 years (Kochkin, 2005a).

Although the majority of hearing aid users report that they are satisfied with their device, most adults with hearing loss continue to resist their use. A combination of factors influences the utilization of amplification (Garstecki and Erler, 1998). Adults indicate that decline in self-perceived hearing sensitivity is the most common reason for purchasing hearing aids (Kochkin, 2005a); those who reject recommendations to use amplification typically do not believe their hearing loss is severe enough to warrant hearing aid use

(Garstecki and Erler, 1998; Gussekloo et al., 2003). Another factor influencing hearing aid use is social support; encouragement from spouses, family, physicians, and audiologists strongly influences acceptance of amplification. In contrast, financial burdens and stigma associated with hearing aid use are frequently cited as barriers to their use. Recent reports, however, suggest that cost may be of less importance than issues related to personality, health, and demographic factors. In a recent study of Swedish older adults in which hearing aids were available free of charge to those who were appropriate candidates, only 6% took advantage of this offer (Rosenhall and Karlsson Espmark, 2003). Studies of stigma and hearing aid use indicate that negative reactions to hearing aid use are more common among younger adults (Erler and Garstecki, 2002). Personality variables such as self-esteem, extroversion, and anxiety can influence perceptions of stigma (Saunders and Cienkowski, 1996), whereas coping styles and locus of control (LOC) also influence acceptance of amplification. LOC refers to how individuals perceive their ability to ensure a desired outcome. Those who are internal in LOC believe life events are contingent upon their own behavior. In contrast, an external LOC is demonstrated by individuals who believe outcomes are determined by chance, fate, or powerful others. Adults who seek help for their hearing problems and those who use amplification tend to be more analytical and insightful problem solvers and more internal in their LOC (Cox et al., 2005; Garstecki and Erler, 1998). Finally, familiarity with hearing loss and use of amplification may also influence decisions to use or reject hearing aids.

With so many barriers to hearing aid use, what can be done to increase their adoption and maximize user satisfaction? Clearly, audiologists must consider the influence of individual physiologic, social, and personality factors on decisions to accept and acquire amplification. Hearing aid candidates must have realistic expectations regarding the benefits and limitations of hearing aid use (Cox and Alexander, 2000; Garstecki and Erler, 1996). Counseling tools, such as the Expected Consequences of Hearing Aid Ownership Scale (Cox and Alexander, 2000), can be useful in assessing expectations and stimulating discussion with patients. Selection of an appropriate hearing aid that ensures comfort and ease of manipulation is essential. Multiple memories, directional microphones, and compression options offer exciting options that were not available until recently but should be chosen carefully to meet individual needs. Although many adults report a preference for new technologies (Kochkin, 1996), physical and/or cognitive limitations may reduce the benefit of such devices. See Chapter 35 for more information concerning hearing aids and the latest in technological features.

Implantable Devices

An increasing number of adults with severe to profound hearing loss are opting for cochlear implantation, particularly those who are postlingually deafened. As many as 10% of adults with hearing loss may be candidates for a cochlear

implant (CI) (Havlik, 1986). Criteria for implantation do not stipulate a maximum age for implantation, with adults in their 80s and 90s having been implanted successfully. A number of factors may impact an older adult's ability to benefit from a CI. It has been suggested that older adults might have poorer outcomes due to deterioration of the spiral ganglion, central presbycusis, and surgical risks. Surgical complications to be considered include issues of wound healing and presence of diabetes, hypertension, or other circulatory problems. Some medical conditions, such as pulmonary and renal disorders, may confound the use of anesthesia. As with all individuals considered for implantation, care must be taken to caution the patient regarding such risks.

The good news is that recent reports refute many of these concerns. Chatelin et al. (2004) compared adult CI users older than 70 years of age with a younger group and found significant improvement in auditory function regardless of age and no surgical complications in either group. Francis et al. (2002) found significant improvements in speech perception, level of social activity, and confidence among adult CI users 50 years and older. Studying three groups of adults ($\leq$55 years, 56 to 69 years, and $\geq$70 years), Vermeire et al. (2005) found improvement in speech recognition and measures of quality of life for all groups; however, the amount of improvement among the oldest group of participants was less than that of the other groups, including postoperative aided puretone averages. Advancements in implant technology as well as better understanding of the effect of implantation on the central auditory mechanism should further increase the benefits to adults with CIs. For an in-depth discussion of CIs, the reader is encouraged to read Chapter 40.

An additional benefit to implantation among adults is relief from tinnitus. In a review of the CI literature (Quaranta et al., 2004), results of 17 studies revealed that the majority of adult CI patients reported a reduction in the intensity of the tinnitus they experienced and that only a small number (<9%) reported an increase in tinnitus. Interestingly, although CIs typically are used unilaterally, some wearers report contralateral suppression of tinnitus (McKerrow et al., 1991; Souliere et al., 1992).

A second category of implantable device is the bone-anchored hearing aid (BAHA). These may be appropriate for adults with conductive and mixed hearing loss, as well as those with unilateral sensory-neural hearing loss who cannot benefit from traditional hearing loss management techniques. Like CIs, BAHA is a Food and Drug Administration (FDA)–approved treatment. Compared to conventional bone-conduction hearing aids, BAHA systems provide improved sound quality and greater comfort (Hakansson et al., 1990). Benefit has been demonstrated for adults with a variety of etiologies, including malformations of the outer or middle ear, chronic middle ear disease, otosclerosis, acoustic neuromas, and trauma. Enhanced sensitivity to sound and speech discrimination have been reported (Lustig et al., 2001). Significantly improved localization by individuals with unilateral sensory-neural hearing loss, unfortunately, has not been demonstrated (Wazen et al., 2005). Despite such limitations, patients with unilateral hearing loss report satisfaction with the BAHA device, no doubt due to their reports of improved communication in a variety of settings. As with other implantable devices, candidates for BAHA must be advised regarding potential surgical risks. For more information on BAHA, the reader is referred to Chapter 35.

Hearing Assistive Technology

Assistive technology is available to mitigate problems created by hearing loss (Weinstein, 2000) and includes devices such as personal amplifiers, telecommunication systems, large-area amplification systems, television listening aids, and alerting appliances. Some assistive listening devices can be used in conjunction with hearing aids to "close the gap" when communicating across large areas and in noisy settings (Compton, 2000), whereas many devices are "stand alone" units that do not require a companion device. Assistive device development has been motivated by consumer interest and needs, as well as by the Americans with Disabilities Act (ADA) of 1990, which ensures communication access for all people with disabilities (Williams and Carey, 1995).

Under Title III Public Accommodation of the ADA, access is guaranteed to information in public buildings and outdoor space, including places of lodging, establishments serving food and drink, places of exhibition or entertainment and recreation, places of public gathering, stores, service establishments, and public transportation stations. Text telephones, television program decoders, large-print texts, sign language interpreters, and assistive listening devices may be useful in these settings. Title IV Telecommunications ensures telephone communication access for all individuals with impaired hearing, including use of relay systems, that combine use of conventional telephone hardware with a text telephone and operator assistance, i.e., acting as an intermediary, the operator voices typed text received from a TTY to the normal hearing listener and, in turn, types text of the spoken information to the hearing impaired TTY user. There are a variety of device options available, including:

- **Personal amplifiers** that are compact, portable, and battery powered and can be used in face-to-face communication and as television listening aids. They function essentially as generic amplification systems and may provide up to 50-dB gain. Some are available with high-frequency emphasis. When equipped with a remote microphone (wired or wireless), they are effective in reducing the effects of background noise on message reception (Compton, 2000).
- **Telecommunication technology**, such as amplified and text telephones. Telephone amplification may be provided in the form of (1) hardwired (self-contained) telephones, (2) receiver cord (in-line) amplifiers, and (3) amplifiers coupled to the telephone receiver. Amplified corded and cordless telephones may provide as much as 55-dB gain (Slager, 1995). Some amplified telephones are equipped with

such features as high- or low-frequency emphasis, volume controls, ring flashers, loud ringers, large buttons, telecoil-compatible handsets, and multiple memory functions. In-line amplifiers may provide up to 40-dB gain, and some are equipped with tone controls to shape the amplified signal characteristics to the listener's preference. Finally, portable amplifiers attached to the telephone handset by means of a durable rubber strap may provide up to 30-dB gain (Compton, 2000). For those whose level of hearing ability precludes benefit from amplification, text telephones (TTYs and TDDs) are available. Moreover, personal computers and text messaging devices are popular ways of transmitting typed messages (Compton, 2000).

- **Large-area individual and group communication systems**, such as frequency modulation (FM), infrared, and induction loop systems (see Compton [2000] for comparison of benefits and limitations of large-area amplification systems).
- **Television aids**, using both amplifying and decoding technology. One type of amplifying device uses radio frequency (RF) technology, transmitting signals wirelessly over distances of up to 300 feet. Closed captioning is available on all televisions manufactured for sale in the United States after 1993 when the picture tube is 13 inches or larger (Schum and Crum, 1995).
- **Alerting devices**, include a range of electromechanical hardware such as alarm clock signalers, telephone signalers, visual alert smoke alarms, and door bell signalers. Acoustic, electronic, or inductive sensing systems are used to activate these signaling aids (Garstecki, 1995).

Assistive devices may be purchased from manufacturer or distributor catalogs, from online sources (see Appendix 42.2), and from retail outlets specializing in the needs of individuals with communication disorders and disabilities. Device purchase and replacement typically are not covered by public or private health insurance plans. Community hearing societies and hearing clinics often maintain a modest inventory of popular devices for sale. Telephone amplifiers may be acquired from telephone and radio supply outlets.

Assistive device selection should take into consideration user preferences and needs in addition to device advantages and limitations (Compton, 1995). Consideration should be given to the potential user's hearing capabilities and ability to purchase and afford upkeep and operation of the device. It must be determined whether or not the intended user has sufficient visual acuity and manual dexterity to independently operate the device, turn it on and off, change batteries, and adjust settings, as well as to couple it to a companion device when necessary. Consideration should be given to the need to maintain privacy when using personal amplifiers and telephone amplifying systems. Overall compatibility of current telephone, television, doorbell, and other systems with the assistive device also needs to be considered. Keeping these factors in mind when selecting a device helps to ensure its acceptance and optimal use. It is good practice to conduct a formal needs assessment to guide device selection (Palmer, 1992). Communication needs at home, in the workplace, in educational settings, and while traveling need to be considered. (See Appendix 42.1 for a sample needs assessment.) For in-depth discussion of assistive listening devices, the reader is referred to Chapter 34 of this text.

▨ COMMUNICATION TRAINING

The first adult AR programs, developed in hospitals serving World War II veterans, provided the context for developing formal instruction in management of hearing loss and related communication problems. The approach was to provide instruction in communication training, specifically lipreading/speechreading and auditory training (Ross, 1997). Today, communication training continues to be a central component of adult hearing loss management (Wayner and Abrahamson, 1996).

Lipreading/Speechreading

Lipreading is the act of identifying a spoken message by observing the message sender's lip, tongue, mouth, and jaw movements. Lipreading is a fundamental component of speechreading, the process of synthesizing visible speech and nonspeech elements deemed relevant to spoken message identification. In addition to lipreading, speechreading may include consideration of a message sender's facial expression, body movement, and hand gestures. Speechreading takes into account selected contextual, environmental, and situational cues (Alpiner and Schow, 2000). While individuals with impaired hearing benefit from using all available message identification cues, with increasing hearing loss, there tends to be growing dependence on lipreading cues. Lipreading and speechreading form the basis of the visual communication system relied on by most individuals with impaired hearing. The visual communication process is influenced by the sender (speaker), receiver (listener), message, and environmental or situational variables.

Sender variables include facial characteristics (e.g., presence of facial hair, unique mouth shape and tongue movements), facial expression, familiarity with the receiver, speaking rate, and other mannerisms and features (e.g., dialect, language). Senders who fail to maintain eye contact with the receiver, speak while chewing food, or cover their mouth with objects or their hands are likely to jeopardize successful visual communication.

Receiver variables include visual acuity, visual perception skills, aided or unaided residual hearing, visual communication skills, attention to the communication task, and familiarity with the idiosyncrasies of the sender, such as their language skills and manner of speaking. Receiver assertive-

ness in "stage managing" the communication situation to optimize the opportunity for successful communication (e.g., minimizing interfering noise, avoiding glare) also may vary.

Message variables include linguistic complexity and redundancy. Simple messages are easier to lipread/speechread. Shorter messages are easier to understand than longer messages, which tend to become diminished through coarticulation effects. Homopheneity, or confusion among visually similar words (e.g., man, pan, ban), may create a problem in isolated word recognition. Messages with predictable content (e.g., instructions on how to drive a car, grow vegetables, paint a room) are easier to identify than messages with few or no cues from context (e.g., names of people and places, telephone numbers, addresses).

Environmental or situational variables include visible obstructions between senders and receivers (e.g., conversation partners speaking from different rooms and/or at a distance) that would preclude use of lipreading cues, distractions (e.g., conversing in a situation where attention is focused on an unusual event), poor lighting (e.g., bars or night clubs), and competing noise (e.g., automobile traffic, background music, construction noise).

Difficulty in identifying and defining the influence of these variables on communication and in reducing them to a representative sample (i.e., average sender, average receiver, everyday message, and common environmental condition) has negatively impacted development of standardized clinical assessment tools to the point where essentially no new universally accepted measures have been developed since around the time of World War II! As a result, there is little recourse for clinicians but to assess lipreading/speechreading skills using (1) dated test material (e.g., Utley, 1946) administered live with little or no control over sender variables; (2) material developed and standardized for assessment of auditory word or sentence recognition, such as the Northwestern University Auditory Test No. 6 (NU-6) monosyllabic word lists (Tillman and Carhart, 1966), administered live or by recording; (3) clinician-created material developed for pre-post treatment purposes to satisfy clinical program, funding agency, or client interests in demonstrating the need for and benefit from clinical intervention; and (4) material developed by hearing product developers to demonstrate the practical benefit of emerging technology.

Regardless, to plan a comprehensive lipreading/speechreading training program, every effort should be made to directly assess the analytic skills (i.e., the ability to identify phonemes, syllables, and monosyllabic words) required for lipreading and the synthetic skills (i.e., the ability to comprehend phrases, sentences, and connected discourse) necessary for speechreading. This should be preceded by screening of binocular visual acuity to establish the basic physical ability to visually perceive speech and/or to justify referral for further examination by an ophthalmologist or vision specialist. Self-perceived visual communication difficulty should be surveyed using an appropriate hearing handicap questionnaire such as the Hearing Performance Inventory

(Lamb et al., 1983). Handicap scales, such as the Communication Profile for the Hearing Impaired (Demorest and Erdman, 1987), can also be used to identify challenging communication environments and to screen knowledge and use of appropriate communication strategies.

A variety of methods to teach lipreading/speechreading have been proposed over the years (French-St. George and Stoker, 1988). Early techniques included both analytic approaches emphasizing syllable drills (e.g., Meuller-Walle Method) and synthetic approaches using sentence-length stimuli and contextual cues (e.g., Nitchie Method). Jeffers and Barley (1971) identified key psychological constructs important for successful lipreading/speechreading. These included emphasis on peripheral perception (the physical process of identifying visual speech information), perceptual proficiency (the ability to draw and revise perceptual and conceptual closures), and speed of perception. Perceptual closure referred to identification of message elements such as parts of words, while conceptual closure referred to recognition of message meaning. Together, they formed the basis of message synthesis, a vital process in everyday message understanding.

The synthetic approach to speechreading often begins with viseme analysis, a form of lipreading calisthenics involving identification of different consonants paired with common vowels. A viseme is defined as the visual equivalent of a phoneme, the smallest recognizable element of a visual speech signal. Viseme identification exercises employed use of consonant-vowel (CV), vowel-consonant (VC), and consonant-vowel-consonant (CVC) syllables (Binnie et al., 1974). On this base, a hierarchy of stimuli was developed, increasing in redundancy of information at each step from words that inherently contained a semantic component that syllables lacked (e.g., NU-6 word list) to sentences that provided syntactic cues to message perception (e.g., Utley Lipreading Test) to paragraph and story material. An alternative to this approach was introduced by De Filippo and Scott (1978) who developed speechtracking as a method for developing skill in identifying and following dialogue. Contrary to popular interest in message synthesis, speechtracking was a highly analytic task in that verbatim repetition of visually presented message units was expected.

Graduated skill-building exercises help those with impaired hearing to develop an understanding of the lipreading/speechreading process. Techniques also can be taught for controlling and/or overcoming negative influences and thus increase the likelihood of success. For example, in recent years, additional emphasis has been directed toward developing anticipatory and repair strategies to facilitate successful communication.

Auditory Training

Auditory training refers to the process of refining use of one's residual hearing, often with a sensory aid (e.g., hearing aid, CI), to improve awareness of acoustic cues to speech perception (Blamey and Alcantara, 1994). The need for and potential benefit from auditory training depends on the integrity of one's auditory system, which may change over time due to the cumulative effects of, for example, age, noise exposure, and ototoxic drug use that may impact auditory skills beyond the hearing loss per se. In general, anyone who has difficulty hearing an average voice of 65 dB sound pressure level (SPL) in intensity in quiet at 1 meter can be considered to be a possible candidate for auditory training, as can anyone using a hearing aid, CI, or other sensory aid for the first time.

Erber (1982) suggested a hierarchy of auditory skill development that guides the organization of auditory training programs. The most elementary skill in this hierarchy is signal detection; that is, one must be able to detect the presence or absence of sound in order to engage in higher order auditory signal processing. Relevant training tasks might include identification of the number of sound units presented in a listening task, demonstrating awareness of sounds of varying intensity, or recognition of when sounds stop. The next critical skill in the hierarchy involves differentiation among auditory signals, a skill labeled "auditory discrimination." This could include exercises to recognize environmental sounds, speech sounds (including suprasegmental features such as number of syllables, number of words, word length, sentence emphasis, sentence forms, and segmental features such as the target word in a pair and familiar word in a list), and voices. The third level in Erber's hierarchy is identification of or the ability to understand object names or labels. Finally, the highest skill is auditory comprehension, or the ability to comprehend numbers in open-set presentation, understand words-sentences-stories, and understand everyday conversation.

Auditory training programs can be organized to highlight development and refinement of these skills as well as related skills such as distance hearing, sound localization, understanding in noise, auditory closure (filling in the missing elements of a misheard or poorly transmitted message), and auditory memory (recalling spoken messages, names, phone numbers, etc.).

Auditory training materials are commercially available as "listening programs." Materials used in speech audiometry and for speechreading training are commonly used in clinical training. They may be presented in "bottom up" paradigms, beginning with analytic tasks involving perception of environmental sounds and isolated speech elements (e.g., syllables) and progressing to larger speech units (i.e., monosyllabic words, sentences, paragraphs, short stories). Alternately, auditory training may proceed following a "top down" strategy, progressing from perception of lengthier to shorter message units. Again, syllable materials may be used to develop analytic skills, whereas word, sentence, paragraph, story, and conversational dialogue materials may be used to develop auditory synthesis skills. An underlying premise is that the tasks are ordered from easier to more difficult (e.g., from closed-set to open-set tasks, supra-threshold to competing background noise), capitalizing on the momentum of success to progress through the more difficult tasks.

Finally, in an effort to place responsibility for communication skill development directly on the person with impaired hearing, the Listening and Communication Enhancement (LACE) program (Sweetow and Henderson-Sabes, 2004) was developed. LACE is a computer-based interactive training program that is useful for improving comprehension of degraded speech signals (speech presented with competing noise or time-compressed speech), development of cognitive skills including auditory memory and maximum processing speed, and development of communication strategies (tips to stage manage communication experiences). Although some adults may be uncomfortable with the computer format or lack the self-motivation required to complete the program, preliminary results are promising (Sabes and Sweetow, 2007).

Auditory-Visual Training

When audible speech information is combined with lipreading, the term auditory-visual speech perception commonly applies. Studies comparing analytic and synthetic methods support a combined approach to communication training (Alcantara et al., 1990). Materials for developing auditory communication skills may be identical to those used in speechreading training. Speechreading and auditory training alone emphasize unisensory perception. In reality, effective communication requires integration of auditory and visual information, particularly when speech signal presentation is degraded. Although speechreading facilitates communication in situations where the message is inaudible and auditory communication facilitates message understanding when the message sender is not visible, it is the case that simultaneously occurring visual and auditory cues facilitate message understanding (Binnie et al., 1974). Auditory-visual speech perception skills may be assessed using such clinical measures as the Iowa Consonant Confusion Test (Tyler et al., 1986a), the Iowa Sentence Test (Tyler et al., 1986b), the Computer-Aided Speechreading Training (CAST) system (Pichora-Fuller and Benguerel, 1991), and Auditrain (Plant, 2001). Again, as with visual and auditory communication assessment, training in combined auditory-visual perception should include consideration of a self-report of perceived communication difficulty such as the Hearing Performance Inventory (Lamb et al., 1983) and the Communication Profile for the Hearing Impaired (Demorest and Erdman, 1987).

Communication Strategy Training

It is not enough to have auditory, visual, and combined auditory-visual communication skills to communicate effectively. It is necessary to be appropriately assertive in applying communication strategies to help ensure effective and efficient communication. One technique includes "stage managing," or positioning oneself in optimal viewing and listening proximity to a speaker. Environmental management strategies are used to enhance room lighting and reduce noise or other distractions. Note taking and other recording strategies may be used to guarantee message understanding. Other types of strategies may be used to capture missed information, including requests for message clarification, repetition, and rephrasing. Asking for key words to be written or, in some cases, fingerspelled or signed, also may be useful.

Home Study

Finally, a variety of home communication training exercises are available. These include the following:

1. **LACE** (Sweetow and Henderson-Sabes, 2004) is an interactive, computerized program that helps develop improved listening skills, increased speed of thought processing, improved auditory memory, better use of language skills, and greater facility in use of interactive strategies.
2. **Sound and Beyond**, which was developed by the House Ear Institute and marketed by the Cochlear Corporation, is an interactive, computerized program consisting of eight modules: puretones, environmental sounds, male/female identification, vowel recognition, consonant recognition, everyday sentences, and music appreciation.
3. **Seeing and Hearing Speech** computerized lipreading and listening lessons were developed by Sensimetrics and are intended to provide practice in auditory-visual speech perception.
4. **Conversation Made Easy**, which was developed by Tye-Murray (2002), is intended for use by children and adults with hearing loss. Sound and sentence items and everyday situation scenarios are presented in closed-set format.

▨ MANUAL COMMUNICATION

Most adults with hearing loss are able to use residual and/or amplified hearing to communicate orally. The proportion of adults in the United States who cannot hear well enough to understand any speech is quite small. Because adult hearing loss typically is acquired, adults are most likely to continue to rely on spoken communication. Although introducing a formal method of manual communication would be unnecessary for most adults with impaired hearing, use of visual cues, namely gestures, will facilitate communication. Gesturing is natural and pervasive. Gestures can be used to facilitate language comprehension and production, convey emotion, or regulate behavior. Most investigations have relied on behavioral measures to determine the effect of gestures on the processing of speech. Recently, Kelly et al. (2004) used event-related potentials to measure how gesture influences speech processing. Their findings provide important objective evidence that gesture plays an important role in the way speech is encoded. Adults with hearing loss easily recognize gestures that are described as "emblems" (Goldin-Meadow, 1999). Gestural emblems are those that are understood without speech (e.g., index finger to the lips indicating quiet). Other recognizable gestures may be iconic, demonstrating what is said. Such gestures match what is uttered and contribute to comprehension. Deictic, or pointing, gestures provide spatial information and direct attention. Children with impaired hearing often use gestures and home signs to communicate. Similarly, adults with impaired hearing may rely on certain gestures to interpret what is being said. Significant others often report that they have developed a system of gestures to alert and inform their partner. Adults with impaired hearing and their communication partners may benefit from training that formalizes the use of gestures. Such training might include development of a set of gestures that can alert the individual with hearing loss to acoustic information as well as direct their attention.

▓ COUNSELING

Counseling facilitates the acceptance of, adjustment to, and management of problems created by hearing loss (Erdman, 2000). It provides an opportunity for audiologists to support, guide, and provide information to individuals with hearing loss and their families. As mentioned earlier in this chapter, there is no reliable correlation between hearing loss and self-perceived hearing handicap (Hawes and Niswander, 1985). For example, severely impaired individuals may find hearing loss frustrating, whereas moderately hearing-impaired individuals may be devastated. Reaction to hearing loss is based on a combination of the degree and type of hearing loss, speech recognition skills, presence of associated problems (e.g., tinnitus or vestibular dysfunction), personal variables (e.g., age, gender, intelligence, education, occupation, socioeconomic status, psychoemotional attributes, general health), communication skills, and compensatory ability (e.g., benefit from use of sensory aids, visual communication skills, risk taking behavior, ability to manage environmental obstacles).

Assessment

Clinical management of counseling should begin with an assessment of hearing disability and handicap. Ideally, individuals engage in problem identification and resolution along with the audiologist. In doing so, there is likely to be greater adherence to professional recommendations and strategies for change, and in turn, overall treatment effectiveness is likely to be enhanced (Erdman, 1994).

Since it is the perception of disability and handicap that prompts individuals to seek intervention, the counseling evaluation should include subjective measurements. Self-assessment scales are designed to measure the disability (i.e., impairment on functional performance and activity) and handicap (i.e., how the individual interacts with and adapts to the surroundings) domains of auditory dysfunction. The responses help in identifying and evaluating rehabilitation goals, charting clinical progress, and assessing effectiveness of treatment procedures. There are a number of different scales, including:

1. **Communication Profiles**
   - Revised Hearing Performance Inventory (Lamb et al., 1983)
   - Communication Profile for the Hearing Impaired (Demorest and Erdman, 1987)
   - Performance Inventory for Profound and Severe Loss (Owens and Raggio, 1988)
   - Self-Assessment of Communication/Significant Other Assessment of Communication (Schow and Nerbonne, 1982)
2. **Psychosocial Effect Scales**
   - Hearing Handicap Inventory for Adults (Newman et al., 1990)
   - Hearing Handicap Inventory for the Elderly (Ventry and Weinstein, 1982)
3. **Hearing Aid Benefit Scales**
   - Abbreviated Profile of Hearing Aid Benefit (Cox and Alexander, 1995)
4. **Informal Measures**
   - Client Oriented Scale of Improvement (Dillon et al., 1997).

Self-assessment scales should be selected on the basis of need, anticipated usefulness, and cost versus benefit.

Treatment

Counseling intervention may focus on information giving, adjustment to hearing loss, and emotional acceptance of hearing loss. Information giving covers topics such as general information on hearing loss, the hearing evaluation results, and hearing loss management options; information concerning availability of community self-help and support groups should also be provided. Personal adjustment counseling may focus on reducing the negative psychological impact of hearing loss, such as helping individuals develop a positive self-image and attitude in dealing with hearing loss (Schum, 1994). Emotional adjustment counseling focuses on how to help individuals respond to the grief experienced in hearing loss adjustment, with the goal of helping to improve overall quality of life (Van Hecke, 1994).

A person-centered, Rogerian approach to counseling is typically favored over psychoanalytic or behavioral models (Clark and English, 2004), enabling the participants to determine program direction and topics to be addressed. The format may allow for individual or group sessions and may incorporate bibliotherapy and online resources. Wylde (1987) describes eight steps involved in adult counseling:

1. Entry (i.e., opening an avenue for assistance, establishing the groundwork for a trusting relationship, and encouraging discussion of the hearing loss management problem)
2. Clarification (i.e., review of the effect of hearing loss on one's overall life situation)
3. Structure (i.e., determination of requisite counselor skills to handle the need)
4. Relationship (i.e., the decision by both parties to proceed with committing to a counseling relationship),

5. Exploration (i.e., identification of intervention strategies and review of alternative approaches to problem solving)

6. Consolidation (i.e., agreement on a course of action and practice of newly learned skills)

7. Planning (i.e., development of ongoing treatment, eventual program termination, and possible referral)

8. Termination (i.e., summary of accomplishments, initiation of referrals, follow-up plans, and offer to stand by if needed)

Another approach is to encourage individuals to participate in support groups for adults with impaired hearing and their families. Support groups offer a peer-driven approach to management of hearing loss, providing an opportunity to share experiences and collaborative problem solving. Some groups are nationally based (with local chapters), including the Association of Late-Deafened Adults (ALDA) and the Hearing Loss Association of America (HLAA), formerly called Self-Help for the Hard of Hearing. Other support vehicles may be established by community groups and senior centers. No data exist to validate the efficacy of hearing loss support groups. However, anecdotal evidence strongly supports the contention that adult participants find them highly beneficial. They serve to instill feelings of empowerment and confidence. They are cost effective and help enhance self-efficacy.

Online health care and telehealth/telemedicine programs provide additional sources for hearing loss management information. Online support groups, chat rooms, and listserves place individuals with hearing loss in contact with one another and with information resources across the world. Opportunities for interaction with others via the Internet are limitless. For more information on counseling, the reader is referred to Chapter 43 of this text.

CLINICAL MANAGEMENT OF RELATED CONDITIONS

Tinnitus

Adult audiology patients frequently complain about tinnitus. In fact, millions of adults report the perception of ringing, roaring, and/or buzzing in their ears or head without the presence of an external sound. Although most report only mild irritation caused by tinnitus, a significant number consider their tinnitus to be debilitating (Sindhusake et al., 2003). The findings from the Epidemiology of Hearing Loss Study (Nondahl et al., 2002) suggest that the prevalence of tinnitus declines with age. Age changes in prevalence may reflect the impact of other health conditions or improvement in coping strategies or may possibly be related to the specific populations tested.

The causes of tinnitus are varied. Exposure to noise, cardiovascular disease, high cholesterol, and other preventable or controllable conditions are some risk factors for developing tinnitus. The relationship between gender and tinnitus is less clear, with some investigators reporting greater risk for women (Nondahl et al., 2002) and others reporting greater risk for men (National Center for Health Statistics, 1998). Some patients experience vibratory (objective) tinnitus, which may result from real sounds such as muscle spasms, the person's pulse, or vascular disorders (Noell and Meyerhoff, 2003). In contrast, the more common nonvibratory tinnitus is subjective in nature and not associated with a mechanical source. Nonvibratory tinnitus may be associated with presbycusis, exposure to noise, and inner ear and cardiovascular diseases.

Severity of tinnitus is typically assessed through interviews and questionnaires (e.g., Iowa Tinnitus Handicap Inventory [Kuk et al., 1990], Tinnitus Handicap Inventory [Newman et al., 1996]). The goal should be to determine how often and to what degree the individual is bothered by tinnitus, the activities that are impacted, and negative feelings associated with the tinnitus (Folmer and Carroll, 2006). Affected individuals should be queried about difficulty concentrating, hearing, sleeping, and completing tasks, as well as the psychosocial impact of tinnitus. Descriptions of the loudness, severity, quality, and fluctuations of tinnitus are useful. History of use of ototoxic medication, exposure to noise, vestibular complaints, head trauma, otologic disorders and treatment, and associated medical conditions (e.g., hypertension, obesity, diabetes) should be obtained. Those with severe complaints should be referred for medical evaluation to identify medically treatable conditions. A complete audiometric evaluation should be conducted for adults with complaints of tinnitus to determine its loudness and frequency, when possible, using matching techniques.

It is not considered a good idea to simply advise a person to learn to live with the condition. That approach may actually exacerbate the impact of tinnitus (Jastreboff and Jastreboff, 2000). For example, some may feel guilty that they complained or feel angry that nothing can be done.

A variety of interventions, including medical and surgical treatments, may relieve tinnitus symptoms. Pharmacologic treatments have been suggested as possible tinnitus treatments, but little or no efficacy information for such approaches has been found (Dobie, 1999). However, when feasible, reduction or elimination of some medications such as aspirin or anti-inflammatory drugs may offer tinnitus relief. Also, the use of tranquilizers to alleviate anxiety and stress and antidepressants to relieve depression and sleep disturbance has been beneficial. However, alternative treatments, such as the use of ginkgo biloba and acupuncture, have not been effective (Davies, 2001). Surgical treatment of otosclerosis and severe cases of Ménière's disease can be beneficial. In addition, dietary restrictions of caffeine and salt may also be useful.

Other options for tinnitus management rely on prosthetic approaches, counseling, or a combination of the two. Folmer and Carroll (2006) suggest that the purpose of treatment is not to eliminate tinnitus, but rather to allow individuals to "pay less attention to their tinnitus" (p 134).

Hearing aids, noise generators, and other maskers have been used for many years to treat tinnitus. The concept is to use an external sound to reduce awareness of tinnitus. Some patients find relief by listening to background music or environmental sounds, such as running water. For adults with sensory-neural hearing loss, hearing aids may provide sufficient masking to relieve the impact of tinnitus. For others, an ear-level masking device or a device that combines masking and amplification may be beneficial. Use of CIs also results in reduction in tinnitus severity for the majority of users (Mo et al., 2002; Souliere, et al, 1992). Moreover, many tinnitus sufferers report temporary reduction in or absence of tinnitus (i.e., residual inhibition) after cessation of the use of a masker or CI. A secondary benefit reported by patients is a feeling of increased control over their tinnitus with the use of hearing aids and maskers.

In a study of neuro-otology patients seeking treatment for tinnitus, McKenna et al. (1991) reported that 45% experienced significant psychological distress. Counseling may be effective in reducing distress. Methods ranging from relaxation techniques to biofeedback and cognitive behavioral therapy have been recommended (Reynolds et al., 2004). One of the more widely discussed approaches to tinnitus treatment is Tinnitus Retraining Therapy (TRT) (Jastreboff and Jastreboff, 2000). Based on a neurophysiologic model in which consideration is given to both auditory perception and emotional associations, TRT combines directive counseling that addresses the causes of and reactions to tinnitus along with sound therapy that optimally results in reduction in awareness of tinnitus. Clearly, a variety of treatments offer hope of tinnitus relief. See Chapter 33 for an in-depth discussion of tinnitus.

Dizziness

Comprehensive hearing loss management for adults should include consideration of balance and dizziness. As many as half of all adults age 65 and older fall each year. Conservatively, it is estimated that 30% of falls are attributable to balance and dizziness disorders (Rubenstein and Josephson, 2002). In fact, Lesser (2006) reports that, of 428 older adults who had fallen, 80% had experienced symptoms of vestibular impairment during the year before their fall. Although audiologists typically play a greater role in diagnosis than treatment of vestibular problems, it is important to be aware of their causes and treatment options.

Dizziness and balance problems may be caused by a variety of factors. Balance relies on central integration of cues from the vestibular, visual, and proprioceptive systems. Unlike children and younger adults who rely more on vestibular and proprioceptive cues, older adults rely more on visual and proprioceptive cues to maintain balance. Unfortunately, older adults may experience decreases in sensory receptors in all three systems. Sensory discrepancies, poor central integration, limited muscle strength, reduced processing speed, abnormal motor function, and cognitive decline, individually or in combination, can contribute to dizziness and balance problems. Adults with labyrinthitis, Ménière's disease, vascular disease, neurologic disorders (e.g., Parkinson), peripheral neuropathy, tumors of the central nervous system, and exposure to ototoxic drugs may report symptoms of dizziness and disequilibrium. Dizziness may also be related to psychological factors, such as anxiety and phobic disorders.

Treatment varies by etiology and symptom and is usually provided by physicians and physical therapists, although some audiologists also provide treatment. Some conditions may resolve spontaneously, while others will respond to manipulation (e.g., Epley or Brant-Daroff exercises), gaze adaptation exercises, medication (e.g., steroids, antivertigo drugs, diuretics), or surgery (Eaton and Roland, 2003). Balance training, strength and flexibility exercises, and improvement of posture have been demonstrated to reduce risk of falls, decrease dizziness, and increase confidence (Whitney and Wrisley, 2004). Patients reporting symptoms of dizziness and balance disorders, including history of falls, should be referred to a physician and counseled regarding benefits of appropriate treatment.

Summary

Adults experiencing hearing-related problems constitute a heterogeneous population. Onset, etiology, and impact vary widely. The number of adults who may benefit from professional and self-directed hearing loss management is large and growing. Audiologists must be prepared to provide comprehensive services that address these complex needs. This chapter has provided an overview of various approaches and technology that can be used to help adults overcome the emotional/physical barriers imposed by hearing loss and improve their quality of life. Audiologists can make an important difference in the lives of these individuals.

▧ REFERENCES

Alcantara JI, Cowan RSC, Blamey PJ, Clark GM. (1990) A comparison of two training strategies for speech recognition with an electrotactile speech processor. *J Speech Hear Res*. 33, 195–204.

Alpiner JG, Schow RL. (2000) Rehabilitative evaluation of hearing-impaired adults. In: Alpiner JG, McCarthy PA, eds. *Rehabilitative Audiology: Children and Adults*. Philadelphia: Lippincott Williams & Wilkins.

American Speech-Language-Hearing Association. (2003) Code of ethics (revised). *ASHA Suppl*. 23, 13–15.

American Speech-Language-Hearing Association. (2004) Scope of practice in audiology. *ASHA Suppl*. 24, 1–9.

Arlinger S. (2003) Negative consequences of uncorrected hearing loss—a review. *Int J Audiol*. 42, 2S17–2S20.

Binnie CA, Montgomery A, Jackson P. (1974) Auditory and visual contributions to the perception of consonants. *J Speech Hear Res.* 17, 619–630.

Blamey PJ, Alcantara JI. (1994) Research in auditory training. In: Gagne JP, Tye-Murray N, eds. *Research in Audiological Rehabilitation. J Acad Rehabil Audiol Monogr Suppl.* 27, 161–191.

Carabellese C, Appollonio I, Rozzini R, Bianchetti A, Frisoni GB, Frattola L, Trabucchi M. (1993) Sensory impairment and quality of life in a community elderly population. *J Am Geriatr Soc.* 41, 401–407.

Chatelin V, Kim EJ, Driscoll C, Larky J, Polite C, Price L, Lalwani, AK. (2004) Cochlear implant outcomes in the elderly. *Otol Neurotol.* 25, 298–301.

Chisholm TH, Willott JF, Lister JJ. (2003) The aging auditory system: anatomic and physiologic changes and implications for rehabilitation. *Int J Audiol.* 42, S3–S10.

Clark JG, English KM. (2004) Audiologic counseling defined. In: Clark JG, English KM, eds. *Counseling in Audiologic Practice.* Boston: Pearson Education, Inc.; pp 11–13.

Compton C. (1995) Selecting what's best for the individual. In: Tyler RS, Schum DJ, eds. *Assistive Devices for Persons with Hearing Impairment.* Needham Heights, MA: Allyn & Bacon.

Compton CL. (2000) Assistive technology for the enhancement of receptive communication. In: Alpiner JG, McCarthy PA, eds. *Rehabilitative Audiology: Children and Adults.* 3rd ed. Philadelphia: Lippincott Williams & Wilkins.

Cox R, Alexander G. (1995) The abbreviated profile of hearing aid benefit. *Ear Hear.* 16, 176–186.

Cox R, Alexander G. (2000) Expectations about hearing aids and their relationship to fitting outcome. *J Acad Rehabil Audiol.* 11, 368–382.

Cox R, Alexander G, Gray GA. (2005) Who wants a hearing aid? Personality profiles of hearing aid seekers. *Ear Hear.* 26, 12–26.

Cruickshanks KJ, Tweed TS, Wiley TL, Klein BE, Klein R, Chappell R, Nondahl DM, Dalton DS. (2003) The 5-year incidence and progression of hearing loss: the epidemiology of hearing loss study. *Arch Otolaryngol Head Neck Surg.* 129, 1041–1046.

Davies WE. (2001) Future prospects for the pharmacological treatment of tinnitus. *Semin Hear.* 22, 89–99.

De Filippo CL, Scott BL. (1978) A method for training and evaluating the reception of ongoing speech. *J Acoust Soc Am.* 63, 1186–1192.

Demorest ME, Erdman SA. (1987) The Communication Profile for the Hearing Impaired. *J Speech Hear Disord.* 52, 129–143.

Dillon H, James A, Ginis J. (1997) Client Oriented Scale of Improvement (COSI) and its relationship to several other measures of benefit and satisfaction provided by hearing aids. *J Am Acad Audiol.* 8, 27–43.

Dobie RA. (1999) A review of randomized clinical trials in tinnitus. *Laryngoscope.* 109, 1202–1211.

Eaton DA, Roland PS. (2003) Dizziness in the older adult. Part 2: treatments for causes of the four most common symptoms. *Geriatrics.* 58, 46–52.

Erber N. (1982) *Auditory Training.* Washington, DC: Alexander Graham Bell Association for the Deaf.

Erdman SA. (1994) Self-assessment: from research focus to research tool. In: Gagne JP, Tye-Murray N, eds. *Research in Audiological Rehabilitation: Current Trends and Future Directions* (monograph supplement). *J Acad Rehabil Audiol.* 27, 67–90.

Erdman SA. (2000) Counseling adults with hearing impairment. In: Alpiner JG, McCarthy PA, eds. *Rehabilitative Audiology: Children and Adults.* 3rd ed. Philadelphia: Lippincott Williams & Wilkins.

Erler SF, Garstecki DC. (2002) Hearing loss- and hearing aid-related stigma: perceptions of women with age-normal hearing. *Am J Audiol.* 11, 83–91.

Folmer RL, Carroll JR. (2006) Long-term effectiveness of ear-level devices for tinnitus. *Otolaryngol Head Neck Surg.* 134, 132–137.

Francis HW, Chee N, Yeagle J, Cheng A, Niparko JK. (2002) Impact of cochlear implants on the functional health status of older adults. *Laryngoscope.* 112, 1482–1488.

French-St. George M, Stoker R. (1988) Speechreading: an historical perspective. In: De Fillippo CL, Sims DG, eds. *New Reflections in Speechreading* (monograph). *Volta Rev.* 90, 17–31.

Garstecki DC. (1995) Alerting devices for the hearing impaired. In: Tyler RS, Schum DJ, eds. *Assistive Devices for Persons with Hearing Impairment.* Boston: Allyn and Bacon.

Garstecki DC, Erler SF (1996) Older adult performance on the Communication Profile for the Hearing Impaired. *J Speech Lang Hear Res.* 39, 28–42.

Garstecki DC, Erler SF. (1998) Hearing loss, control, and demographic factors influencing hearing aid use among older adults. *J Speech Hear Res.* 41, 527–537.

Garstecki DC, Erler SF. (1999) Older adult performance on the Communication Profile for the Hearing Impaired: gender difference. *J Speech Lang Hear Res.* 42, 785–796.

Garstecki DC, Erler SF. (2001) Personal and social conditions potentially influencing women's hearing loss management. *Am J Audiol.* 10, 78–90.

Gatehouse S. (1990) Determinants of self-reported disability in older subjects. *Ear Hear.* 11 (suppl), 57–65.

Goldin-Meadow S. (1999) The role of gesture in communication and thinking. *Trends Cogn Sci.* 3, 419–429.

Gussekloo J, de Bont LE, von Faber M, Eekhof JA, de Laat JA, Hulshof HI, van Dongen E, Westendorp RG. (2003) Auditory rehabilitation of older people from the general population: the Leiden 85 Plus study. *Br J Gen Pract.* 53, 536–540.

Hakansson B, Liden G, Tjellstrom A, Ringdahl A, Jacobsson M, Carlsson P, Erlandson BE. (1990) Ten years of experience with the Swedish bone-anchored hearing system. *Ann Otol Rhinol Laryngol.* 151 (suppl), 1–16.

Hallberg LRM. (1999) Hearing impairment, coping, and consequences on family life. *J Acad Rehabil Audiol.* 32, 45–59.

Hamill T. (2006) *Code of Ethics of the American Academy of Audiology. Ethics in Audiology.* Reston, VA: American Academy of Audiology.

Havlik R. (1986) Aging in the eighties: impaired sense for sound and light in persons age 65 years and over. Preliminary data from the supplement on aging to the National Health Interview Survey, United States, January–June 1984. Washington, DC: National Center for Health Statistics, Department of Health and Human Services.

Hawes NA, Niswander PS. (1985) Comparison of the revised Hearing Performance Inventory with audiometric measures. *Ear Hear.* 6, 93–97.

Hetu R, Jones L, Getty L. (1993) The impact of acquired hearing impairment on intimate relationships: implications for rehabilitation. *Audiology.* 32, 363–381.

Jastreboff PJ, Jastreboff MM. (2000) Tinnitus Retraining Therapy (TRT) as a method for treatment of tinnitus and hyperacusis patients. *J Am Acad Audiol.* 11, 162–177.

Jeffers J, Barley M. (1971) *Speechreading (Lipreading)*. Springfield, IL: Charles C. Thomas.

Jerger J, Chmiel R, Stach B, Spretnjak M. (1993) Gender affects audiometric shape in presbyacusis. *J Am Acad Audiol*. 4, 42–49.

Kelly SD, Kravitz C, Hopkins M. (2004) Neural correlates of bimodal speech and gesture comprehension. *Brain Lang*. 89, 253–260.

Kochkin S. (1996) MarkeTrak IV: 10-year trends in the hearing aid market—has anything changed? *Hear J*. 49, 23–34.

Kochkin S. (2005a) MarkeTrak VII: hearing loss population tops 31 million people. *Hear Rev*. 12, 16–29.

Kochkin S. (2005b) *The Impact of Untreated Hearing Loss on Household Income*. Alexandria, VA: Better Hearing Institute.

Kochkin S, Rogin CM. (2000) Quantifying the obvious: the impact of hearing instruments on quality of life. *Hear Rev*. 7, 6–34.

Kuk F, Tyler R, Russell D, Jordan H. (1990) The psychometric properties of a tinnitus handicap questionnaire. *Ear Hear*. 11, 434–445.

Lamb SH, Owens E, Schubert ED. (1983) The revised form of the Hearing Performance Inventory. *Ear Hear*. 4, 152–157.

Lesser T. (2006) Elderly fallers and the ENT surgeon. *ENT News*. 15, 59–60.

Lustig LR, Arts HA, Brackmann DE, Francis HF, Molony T, Megerian CA, Moore GF, Moore, KM, Morrow T, Potsic W, Rubenstein JT, Srireddy S, Syms CA, Takahashi G, Vernick D, Wackym PA, Niparko JK. (2001) Hearing rehabilitation using the BAHA bone-anchored hearing aid: results in 40 patients. *Otol Neurotol*. 22, 328–334.

McKenna L, Hallam RS, Hinchcliffe R. (1991) The prevalence of psychological disturbance in neuron-otology outpatients. *Clin Otolaryngol*. 16, 452–456.

McKerrow WS, Schreiner CE, Snyder RL, Merzenich MM, Toner JG. (1991) Tinnitus suppression by cochlear implants. *Ann Otol Rhinol Laryngol*. 100, 552–558.

Mo B, Harris S, Lindback M. (2002) Tinnitus in cochlear implant patients: a comparison with other hearing-impaired patients. *Int J Audiol*. 41, 527–534.

Morgan-Jones R. (2001) *Hearing Differently: The Impact of Hearing Impairment on Family Life*. London: Whurr.

Mulrow CD, Aguilar C, Endicott JE, Velez R, Tuley MR, Charlip WS, Hill JA. (1990) Association between hearing impairment and the quality of life of elderly individuals. *J Am Geriatr Soc*. 38, 45–50.

National Center for Health Statistics. (1998) Vital and health statistics: current estimates from the National Health Interview Survey, 1995. DHHS Publication No. (PHS) 98-1527, Series 10; No. 199 (10/98). Hyattsville, MD: National Center for Health Statistics; pp 77–92.

Newman CW, Jacobson GP, Spitzer JB. (1996) Development of the Tinnitus Handicap Inventory. *Arch Otolaryngol Head Neck Surg*. 122, 143–148.

Newman CW, Weinstein B, Jacobson G, Hug G. (1990) The Hearing Handicap Inventory for Adults: psychometric adequacy and audiometric correlates. *Ear Hear*. 11, 430–433.

Noell CA, Meyerhoff WL. (2003) Tinnitus: diagnosis and treatment of this elusive symptom. *Geriatrics*. 58, 28–34.

Nondahl DM, Cruickshanks KJ, Wiley TL, Klein R, Klein BE, Tweed TS. (2002) Prevalence and 5-year incidence of tinnitus among older adults: the epidemiology of hearing loss study. *J Am Acad Audiol*. 13, 323–331.

Owens E, Raggio MW. (1988) Performance Inventory for Profound and Severe Loss. *J Speech Hear Disord*. 53, 42–56.

Palmer CV. (1992) Assistive devices in the audiology practice. *Am J Audiol*. March, 37–57.

Pichora-Fuller MK, Benguerel AP. (1991) The design of CAST (Computer-Aided Speechreading Training). *J Speech Hear Res*. 34, 202–212.

Plant G. (2001) *Auditrain: An Auditory and Auditory-Visual Training Program*. Innsbruck, Austria: MED-EL GmbH.

Quaranta N, Wagstaff S, Baguley DM. (2004) Tinnitus and cochlear implantation. *Int J Audiol*. 43, 245–251.

Reynolds P, Gardner D, Lee R. (2004) Tinnitus and psychological morbidity: a cross-sectional study to investigate psychological morbidity in tinnitus patients and its relationship with severity of symptoms and illness perceptions. *Clin Otolaryngol*. 29, 628–634.

Rosenhall U, Karlsson Espmark AK. (2003). Hearing aid rehabilitation: what do older people want, and what does the audiogram tell? *Int J Audiol*. 42 (suppl 2), S53–S57.

Ross M. (1997) A retrospective look at the future of aural rehabilitation. *J Acad Rehabil Audiol*. 30, 11–20.

Rubenstein LZ, Josephson KR. (2002) The epidemiology of fall and syncope. *Clin Geriatr Med*. 18, 146.

Sabes J, Sweetow R. (2007) Variables predicting outcomes on listening and communication enhancement (LACE) training. *Int J Audiol*. 46, 374–383.

Saunders GH, Cienkowski KM. (1996) Refinement and psychometric evaluation of the Attitudes Toward Hearing Loss questionnaire. *Ear Hear*. 17, 505–519.

Schow RL, Nerbonne MA. (1982) Communication screening profile: use with elderly clients. *Ear Hear*. 3, 135–147.

Schum DJ, Crum L. (1995) Television viewing for persons with hearing impairment. In: Tyler RS, Schum DJ, eds. *Assistive Devices for Persons with Hearing Impairment*. Needham Heights, MA: Allyn & Bacon.

Schum RL. (1994) Personal adjustment counseling. In: Gagne JP, Tye-Murray N, eds. *Research in Audiological Rehabilitation: Current Trends and Future Directions* (monograph supplement). *J Acad Rehabil Audiol*. 27, 223–236.

Sindhusake D, Mitchell P, Newall P, Golding M, Rochtchina E, Rubin G. (2003) Prevalence and characteristics of tinnitus in older adults: The Blue Mountains Hearing Study. *Int J Audiol*. 42, 289–294.

Slager RD. (1995) Interfacing with the telephone system. In: Tyler RS, Schum DJ, eds. *Assistive Devices for Persons with Hearing Impairment*. Boston: Allyn and Bacon.

Sloane PD, Coeytaux RR, Beck RS, Dallara J. (2001) Dizziness: state of the science. *Ann Intern Med*. 134, 823–832.

Souliere CR, Kileny PR, Zwolan TA, Kemink JL. (1992) Tinnitus suppression following cochlear implantation: a multifactorial investigation. *Arch Otol Head Neck Surg*. 118, 1291–1297.

Sweetow RW, Henderson-Sabes J. (2004) The case for LACE: listening and auditory communication enhancement training. *Hear J*. 57, 32–40.

Tillman T, Carhart R. (1966) An expanded test for speech discrimination utilizing CNC monosyllabic words. Northwestern University Auditory Test No. 6 (Technical Report No. SAM-TR55). Brooks Air Force Base, TX: USAF School of Aerospace Medicine.

Tye-Murray N. (2002) *Conversation Made Easy: Speechreading and Conversation Strategies Training for People with Hearing Loss*. St. Louis, MO: Central Institute for the Deaf.

Tyler RS, Preece J, Tye-Murray N. (1986a) *The Iowa Phoneme and Sentence Tests.* Iowa City, IA: The University of Iowa Hospitals and Clinics.

Tyler RS, Preece J, Tye-Murray N. (1986b) *The Laser Videodisc Sentence Test.* Iowa City, IA: University of Iowa, Department of Otolaryngology-Head and Neck Surgery.

Utley J. (1946) A test of lipreading ability. *J Speech Hear Dis.* 11, 109–116.

Van Hecke ML. (1994) Emotional responses to hearing loss. In: Clark JG, Martin FN, eds. *Effective Counseling in Audiology: Perspectives and Practice.* Englewood Cliffs, NJ: Prentice-Hall; pp 92–115.

Ventry I, Weinstein BE. (1982) The Hearing Handicap Inventory for the Elderly: A new tool. *Ear Hear.* 3, 128–134.

Vermeire K, Brokx JP, Wuyts FL, Cochet E, Hofkens A, Van de Heyning PH. (2005) Quality-of-life benefit from cochlear implantation in the elderly. *Otol Neurotol.* 26, 188–195.

Wayner DS, Abrahamson JE. (1996) *Learning to Hear Again: An Audiological Rehabilitation Curriculum Guide.* Austin, TX: Hear Again.

Wazen JJ, Ghossaini SN, Spitzer JB, Kuller M. (2005) Localization by unilateral BAHA users. *Otol Head Neck Surg.* 132, 928–932.

Weinstein B. (2000) Hearing aids and assistive listening devices. In: Weinstein BE, ed. *Geriatric Audiology.* New York: Thieme Medical Publishers, Inc.

Whitney SL, Wrisley DM. (2004) Vestibular rehabilitation. In: Kent RD, ed. *The MIT Encyclopedia of Communication Disorders.* Cambridge, MA: The MIT Press; pp 564–567.

Williams J, Carey AL. (1995) Impact of the Americans with Disabilities Act on audiologists. In: Tyler RS, Schum DJ, eds. *Assistive Devices for Persons with Hearing Impairment.* Boston: Allyn and Bacon.

Willott JF. (1991) *Aging and the Auditory System: Anatomy, Physiology, and Psychophysics.* San Diego, CA: Singular Group Publishing.

Wylde MA. (1987) Psychological and counseling aspects of the adult remediation process. In: Alpiner JG, McCarthy PA, eds. *Rehabilitative Audiology: Children and Adults.* Baltimore: Williams & Wilkins.

APPENDIX 42.1
Northwestern University Needs assessment questions

a. How important is it for you to improve your success in hearing in face-to-face communication situations?

      Not at all _ _ _ _ _ Very Important

b. How important is it for you to improve your success in hearing in small group settings?

      Not at all _ _ _ _ _ Very Important

c. How important is it for you to improve your success in hearing in an automobile?

      Not at all _ _ _ _ _ Very Important

d. How important is it for you to improve your success in hearing in noisy settings?

      Not at all _ _ _ _ _ Very Important

e. How important is it for you to improve your success in hearing on the telephone?

      Not at all _ _ _ _ _ Very Important

f. How important is it for you to improve your success in hearing your television?

      Not at all _ _ _ _ _ Very Important

g. How important is it for you to improve your success in hearing your doorbell?

      Not at all _ _ _ _ _ Very Important

h. How important is it for you to improve your success in hearing your alarm clock?

      Not at all _ _ _ _ _ Very Important

i. How important is it for you to improve your success in hearing your telephone ring?

      Not at all _ _ _ _ _ Very Important

j. How important is it for you to improve your success in hearing your smoke alarm?

      Not at all _ _ _ _ _ Very Important

k. How important is it for you to improve your success in hearing in large meeting rooms?

      Not at all _ _ _ _ _ Very Important

APPENDIX 42.2
Sample Internet Sources for Hearing Loss Management Resources

www.advanceforaud.com
www.asha.org
www.harcmercantile.com
www.harrsiscomm.com
www.hitec.com
www.radioschack.com
www.sonicalert.com
www.soundbytes.com
www.ultratec.com
www.wheelockinc.com

43 Counseling: How Audiologists Can Help Patients Adjust to Hearing Loss

Kris English

INTRODUCTION

Like other health care professions, audiology is a combination of "hard" and "soft" sciences. Audiology's hard sciences include the anatomy and physiology of the auditory system, the physics of sounds, etc. We must master these hard sciences to understand a patient's auditory functions and structures, as described by The World Health Organization's *International Classification of Functioning, Disability, and Health (ICF)* (2002) (Fig. 43.1).

However, the ICF model does not "stop at the ear," nor should the audiologist. The ICF model also requires the audiologist to consider how a hearing loss impacts a patient's activities, the level of participation in those activities, and the range of environmental and personal factors that both influence, and are influenced by, living with a hearing loss.

Significantly, only one component of the ICF model uses the knowledge base taught by the hard sciences. The remaining components require mastery of the soft sciences: psychology, sociology, cultural studies, etc. That said, it is important to note that "soft" science does not mean "easy to learn" or "less important" science. If these were easy to learn, we would fully understand human nature by now! While much is known in general, each patient will present a unique blend of resources, fears, motivations, and reactions to life's stressors. To serve patients well, audiologists should not only understand these responses, but also develop interpersonal skills to help patients address them. This kind of active patient support is called *audiologic counseling* (Clark and English, 2004). This chapter will describe a range of patient responses to hearing loss, as well as provide strategies that audiologists can use to help patients' adjustment process.

COUNSELING IN AUDIOLOGY

Most audiologists who entered the field with a master's degree did not receive specific training in counseling (Culpepper et al., 1994). Many audiologists assumed that *counseling* simply meant *explaining*: test results, hearing aid function, hearing aid limitations, use of assistive devices, and so on. Graduate students were advised to "avoid jargon," but otherwise were given little guidance on how to communicate effectively with every patient.

Kennedy and Charles (2001) proposed a broader definition of counseling, first by making the distinction between *professional* and *nonprofessional* counseling. Readers are familiar with counseling professionals (e.g., psychologists, psychiatrists, social workers) who are trained to provide long-term therapy to patients by examining and challenging personal history and by analyzing the meanings of one's responses (Cormier and Hackney, 1999; Crowe, 1997). Psychotherapy searches for the cause of a person's problems, which might be rooted in family relationships or childhood trauma. Nonprofessional counselors, however, are those in other "helping professions" who assist patients confront a range of psychological and emotional reactions *as they relate to their own specialty area*. In other words, audiologists as nonprofessional counselors can help patients who are angry, hostile, depressed, or anxious about how their hearing loss is affecting their lives. If concerns unrelated to hearing loss present themselves (e.g., domestic abuse, familial

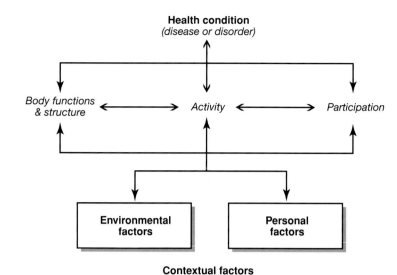

FIGURE 43.1   The International Classification of Function, Disability, and Health (ICF). (From World Health Organization. (2002) *International Classification of Function, Disability, and Health.* **Geneva: World Health Organization.)**

unemployment, other health problems, medications), then audiologists must recognize their "professional boundaries" and refer these patients to appropriate agencies or colleagues (Stone and Olswang, 1989). When an audiologist begins to feel uncomfortable with either the content or the intensity of the interaction, he or she can assume that a boundary is being approached, and it is probably an appropriate time to refer the patient or parent to a professional counselor.

Within the domain of nonprofessional counseling, two distinctions can be made: nonprofessional counseling can take the form of either *informational* counseling or *personal adjustment* counseling. Examples of informational counseling were provided earlier (i.e., the act of explaining or conveying content to patients and families). Informational counseling is vital but is often done poorly; evidence indicates that, in general, patients understand only about 50% of what a health provider tells them and remember only 50% of that information (Margolis, 2004). In other words, if we are not alert to this risk, only 25% of our informational counseling may be effective, and the other 75% will be wasted. When conveying information, audiologists must be very sensitive to the "learning readiness" of a patient as information is conveyed. We must remember that people do not learn or understand much when they are upset or in shock, and we need to provide back-up information with handouts, videos, etc., for later reference, when the patient attempts to recall and understand the information conveyed.

Personal adjustment counseling will be the focus of this chapter. What steps do patients need to work through as they seek hearing help, and how can we help in that process? What are patients' psychological and emotional reactions to hearing loss, and how might we help patients adjust to and transcend these reactions? (Hint: We will explore the counseling model of "helping patients help themselves.") Because patients do not live in a vacuum, throughout this chapter, we will also consider how patients' hearing loss affects their relationships with loved ones and community members.

Update: With the introduction of the Audiology Doctorate, almost all graduate training programs now include a counseling course or actively integrate counseling into other courses (English and Weist, 2005). Students are being prepared to support patients through the help-seeking process, as described in the next section.

THE HELP-SEEKING PROCESS

Two psychological conditions must be met before patients will adhere to an audiologist's recommendations for hearing help: acceptance of one's problem and willingness to make a change. Audiologists will usually be mistaken if they assume that these conditions are in place when patients make initial appointments.

The help-seeking process (adapted from Hill and O'Brien [1999]) has four steps. Each of the first three stages represents a psychological struggle for the patient. If we forge ahead with recommendations for hearing help before the patient is at the last stage, the recommendations may very well be perceived as adversarial interference—the last impression we want to give.

We will take a look at each stage and give an example of how that stage presents itself in audiologic practice. We will also discuss different approaches to help the patient advance through these stages. These approaches are based on a premise developed by Rogers (1961): when patients are in a supportive environment and feel free to consider options, patients will "choose growth"; in other words, when people do not feel compelled to defend themselves and their previous, less effective decisions, they will be more likely to make choices that are in their best interests.

Stage 1: I Don't Have a Problem

This stage is often described by clinicians as denial. This kind of shorthand thinking does not serve the clinician well, however. We need to understand that when a patient says, "I don't have a hearing problem," she does not actually mean what she says. The patient lives with the problem and knows full well that her hearing has changed and she is starting to struggle. This comment only means that, at this moment, the patient is not ready to talk to us about it, or does not trust us yet to share this personal problem. Facing the hearing loss is unacceptable right now. There is a truism about human nature: "If you push me, I will push back." The most ineffective approach to take at this point is to "push" the patient into acceptance.

In this stage, a patient will usually inform us that, "I'm only here because my spouse (or other loved one) asked me to get my hearing checked." The audiologist will find out some important information by asking two questions: "What does your spouse say about your hearing?" (allow that story to be told, without taking sides), and then, "How would *you* describe your hearing today?" Notice that we do not ask the patient to describe any hearing *problems*; we are neutral.

We are now at a fork in the road, and the patient's answer will advise us which direction to take. If the patient says, "I disagree with my spouse, I think my hearing is fine," then we proceed by respecting the patient's perceptions. "Okay, then, let's get the hearing test done and see what we find." When the testing is done, we present the results carefully: "I did find that you have a moderate hearing loss in both ears; you missed about 40% of those words, for instance. Whether that's perceived as a *problem*, only you can say."

Our intent is to respect the patient's dilemma: The audiometric results are inconsistent with the patient's earlier position, so he might feel defensive about it. He will either retreat with a comment such as, "Just send me the report; I did what I promised I would do," or he may be willing to consider the next step (described in the next subsection). If he retreats and makes no decision at that time, he will at least depart feeling that the audiologist appreciated his point of view and did not pressure him to change when he was not ready. If and when he chooses to pursue hearing help, he will feel he can trust this audiologist.

Having this patient walk out the door without hearing help is not a failure on the audiologist's part. We are not responsible for patients' decisions; we are only responsible for supporting their decisions (e.g., providing optimal hearing help when they want it). In fact, it would be unethical to move ahead with amplification when the patient is telling us in no uncertain terms that he is not interested. The real failure in audiology is the percentage of hearing aids resting in drawers instead of being used (17%, per Kochkin [2005]). These data tell us that some aspect of the help-seeking process was overlooked for a large number of patients.

Earlier, we mentioned being at a fork in the road when asking a patient, "How would *you* describe your hearing today?" The patient might just as likely have said, "I hate to admit it, but my wife may be right. She's not the only one who has mentioned problems, and I've noticed some things. It's not easy to admit one is getting older."

If this response occurred after the hearing assessment and a hearing loss was confirmed, the reader may be wondering: Why didn't the patient just say so in the first place? The answer is probably this: We often need to ease our way into what Stone et al. (1999) call a "difficult conversation." Appreciating the fact that these conversations are personal and uncomfortable for the patient helps the audiologist remember to listen deeply, *to attend to the messages behind the words*. Reik (1948) calls this attention "listening with the third ear."

Stage 2: I Do Have a Problem but I Don't Need Help

A patient in this stage is willing to acknowledge the situation; granted, she is not hearing as well as she used to. In her mind, however, she has conducted a "cost-benefit" analysis: the hearing loss causes minor inconveniences, she misses a few words, but she is not feeling a great deal of stress because of it; in other words, the benefits of maintaining the status quo outweigh those small costs.

As always, we would want to learn, "How can I help you today?", and the answer will likely be the same as in Stage 1, "I told my loved one I'd find out what is going on," or perhaps, "I would like to find out just how bad it is for myself—you know, establish a baseline."

Stage 3: I Have a Problem, I Need Help, but I Don't Want Help

Stages 2 and 3 are very similar, but the difference is in terms of recognizing and vocalizing the need for help. We are not comfortable asking for help in our culture; we pride ourselves on self-reliance and self-sufficiency. In this case, asking for help also means acknowledging not just a problem, but a disability, a health failing. And the help audiologists provide most often will be hearing aids—a recommendation tied with stigma, cosmetic concerns, and aging. These patients may be quite aware that they need help, but accepting our type of help is another matter altogether. How can we help patients in Stages 2 and 3 "choose growth"?

One way is to provide an opportunity to "talk out" one's concerns. We can use existing audiologic self-assessments as counseling tools in providing these opportunities. Self-assessments not only give patients a vehicle to describe their reactions and perceptions of living with impaired hearing, but they can also be used as a springboard into counseling conversations. For instance, the Self-Assessment of Communication (Schow and Nerbonne, 1982) is short (10 items) and includes not only questions about listening conditions, but also one's reactions to them, as well as perceptions from significant others. Question 8 is intentionally open-ended: "Is there anything about your hearing that upsets you?" If a patient indicates Agree or Strongly Agree, the audiologist now has an opening: "Can you tell me more about this answer?" We will not know what is on the patient's mind until we give them an opportunity to tell us; self-assessments are a nonthreatening, neutral way of providing that opportunity.

Another way to help patients in Stages 2 and 3 is to bring up the concept of readiness. Patients may agree to "go through the motions" of seeking help in order to keep peace in the family or for other reasons, but genuine commitment to change only occurs when one is ready for it. The simple concept of a 1-10 Readiness Scale can tell us clearly where a patient stands: "Mrs. Quigley, we've reviewed your test results and related them to the problems you described in the beginning. My recommendation to help you hear better would be to amplify your world with hearing aids. Before we go further, though, I need to know from you, on a scale from 1 to 10, 1 being No Way and 10 being Completely Ready, how ready are you for hearing aid help?"

The answers are always interesting and sometimes not at all what we would predict. If the answers fall in the range from 1 to 7, we know the patient still has reservations, doubts, and unexpressed worries. These need to be explored! Investing time in these conversations will pay off because patients are far more likely to be satisfied with their care. As Stone et al. (1999) put it, "People almost never change without feeling understood" (p 29).

To help with this process, we can ask patients to consider directly those costs and benefits mentioned before. By taking a blank piece of paper and drawing a line to divide it in half, we might place a plus sign in one column and a minus side in the other and say, "You say you are a 3 in readiness, but other things you've said suggest ongoing concerns about not hearing well. Could you tell me the pluses and minuses about hearing help. I will jot them down, and this will help me understand better." This process actually helps the *patient* understand the following questions better: What are my barriers? Why am I stalling? What can I face, and what do I find intolerable? The discussion can lead to the following type of "self-cure" recently witnessed by the author.

"Well, in the minus column, I would put how I would look. I would look so old! That makes me very uncomfortable, yet even saying that out loud makes me sound silly and vain. People do get old, and I am usually okay about it, actually, but not this time. I've been my own worst enemy when it comes to change; I refused to get my vision checked and then almost hit a pedestrian [while driving] because I didn't see him! That scared the daylights out of me. It's possible not hearing well could also put me or someone in danger; now that is NOT acceptable, is it? I'm just going to have to get over this mental block of mine. What do we do next?"

The audiologist later reported mixed reactions; in one respect, "All I did was just listen." Yet the audiologist also realized that by "just listening," nonverbally conveying respect and care, the patient felt safe in confiding these personal reactions. When the patient heard her own thoughts, she was able to perceive the barriers she had created and was then more able to address them.

Stage 4: I Have a Problem, I Need and Want Help, and I Am Ready to Accept Help

A patient in this stage has let us clearly know that the costs of the hearing loss are too high, and the benefits of nonaction are not acceptable. The patient has reached full "ownership" of her hearing problem. Ownership of any life problem is a prerequisite before one will commit to the solution to the problem (Brammer, 1993) and will be discussed in more depth in a subsequent section.

Throughout this help-seeking process, patients are experiencing a host of psychological reactions to living with impaired hearing. The following section will consider a few typical reactions.

PSYCHOLOGICAL REACTIONS TO HEARING LOSS

Most individuals acquire some degree of hearing loss as part of the aging process, although this fact is small consolation to patients. Patients often wait up to 7 years or more before they seek help for their hearing problems, and even then, as mentioned earlier, their initial appointments are often made at the behest of family members, not because they are personally ready to seek help.

Understanding this delay is the first step in understanding our patients. Why do patients wait? What are their fears? What are the barriers?

Reactions to Stressors

When we are faced with a situation that creates stress, we either *approach* the situation (by solving it, or finding help to solve it), or we *avoid* it. Avoidance can take the form of *cognitive avoidance* ("I will think about this later"), *emotional redirection* (e.g., expressing anger about an unrelated situation), or *cognitive distortion* (making assumptions on false premises: "I can't have a hearing problem because I am in perfect health").

When patients start to experience hearing problems, psychological avoidance is a natural reaction. Patients can defer "thinking about it" because they still hear quite a bit, and no pain is involved. They can "explain it away" by blaming others for poor speaking habits. As the hearing loss increases, however, so does the stress, and those initial coping strategies become less effective. Patients' first audiology appointments are the beginning steps to approaching the hearing problem.

"Owning" the Hearing Loss

So far, we have considered steps that patients work through before consulting with an audiologist (i.e., moving from avoidance to approach). However, anecdotal evidence suggests that perhaps *only half of initial audiology appointments are made by patients because they perceive a hearing problem.* More often, spouses and family members, frustrated with communication problems, insist that the patient be tested. Patients understandably express resentment about the situation and will likely be suspicious of the audiologist's motivation to help. Although the patient has kept this appointment, the audiologist cannot genuinely help until the patient "owns" the hearing problem, that is, not only accepts the reality of a permanent, untreatable health problem but also decides to improve the situation. This "ownership" requires a patient's active engagement.

When we have a toothache, or our car has broken down, or the plumbing is clogged, we do not hesitate to get help; we pick up the telephone and call an expert immediately. Why is it different when the problem is a hearing loss? The author once asked this question of a group of successful hearing aid users, and the audience took a few moments to think about it. Finally, a gentleman said, "With the hearing problem, you have to take responsibility." He went on to explain that, in the first examples, once we make the phone call, our role is passive; the expert fixes the problem and we are not actively engaged in the process, except to pay for the service at the end. In these examples, the problem is not perceived as personal. Rather, we are a consumer of goods or services, and we expect the expert to "own" (stand by) the solution.

When patients have a hearing loss, they may assume this passive role will suffice and expect that taking the initiative and paying for devices/services are all that they need to do. If this consumer orientation is not addressed, patients will be chronically dissatisfied. As mentioned earlier, patients have to "own" the hearing loss as a personal problem before they will commit to managing it.

Threat to Self-Concept

Only 20% of the population who would benefit from the use of hearing aids actually obtain and use them. When asked, people in the remaining 80% indicate cosmetic concerns as second only to the cost of hearing aids (Kochkin, 1996). What do cosmetic concerns mean to patients? Worrying about how one looks may seem superficial; after all, hearing aids are "just" plastics and electronics, in one sense. However, an involuntary change in how one looks (body image) represents a very real threat to the core of our psychological existence: our *self-concept.*

Self-concept is defined as the perception of one's traits, attitudes, abilities, and social natures; that is, the way we describe ourselves (James, 1892; Nichols, 1995). Individuals initially are dependent on the messages given by caretakers to define themselves (I am loved/not loved; I am capable/not capable; I am/am not a worthy person). Over time, individuals decide for themselves how to define their self-concept by threading in their cumulative life experiences into a developing tapestry. This tapestry represents a lot of hard work, with insights obtained through trials, mistakes, and successes. Self-concept has been described as a vital personal possession, the heart of one's personality (Breslin, 1974).

Once we appreciate the importance of one's self-concept, it is easy to see that the prospect of needing to *change* one's self-concept is not going to be welcomed; in fact, it will be resisted if the change is perceived as a negative one. When we first inform patients that in fact they do have a hearing loss, their self-concept ("I am a person with normal hearing") is under attack; when we add that, to help the problem, we recommend using hearing aids (change one's body image), the attack intensifies. The redefinition in one's self-concept from "I am a person with normal hearing" to "I am a person who needs hearing aids" can take some patients a great deal of time and support.

Part of the resistance to this particular change comes from the phenomenon called the "hearing aid effect." Our society has yet to accept hearing aids as a neutral technical device; instead, there tends to be a negative association with hearing aid use, with biased assumptions of reduced abilities, attractiveness, and intelligence. Many studies have examined this phenomenon, first identified by Blood et al. (1977). In their study, they showed subjects a set of pictures of individuals, some wearing visible hearing aids and some not. When the instruments were visible, individuals were given lower scores in almost every category of intelligence, personality, attractiveness, and capability. They concluded that the very presence of a hearing aid can stimulate negative reactions.

Patients are well aware of these reactions and struggle with the prospect of putting themselves in this kind of situation, to present to the public a persona that might not be respected or considered attractive. This is not an insurmountable barrier, but it is a real one that audiologists must respect.

Loss and Grief

Most audiologists are already familiar with the "grief cycle" as developed by Kubler-Ross (1969). Her model considered our general reactions to death and dying: denial, anger, bargaining, depression, and acceptance. Tanner (1980) later applied these reactions to a broader consideration of communication disorders. He pointed out that death is not the only kind of loss; any change in the status quo is a loss, and our reactions will likely work through the same stages. When we inform patients that their hearing abilities have changed, we will likely trigger the same reactions.

Other Reactions

In addition to avoidance, attempts to protect one's self-concept, and subtle expressions of grief, adults have reported a full range of other emotional and psychological reactions to hearing loss, including anxiety, insecurity ("What will this mean about my future?"), stress (especially before the effects of the hearing loss are well understood, e.g., in understanding speech in restaurants), resentment, and depression.

A Downward Spiral

Family members take the brunt of the stress when a member has to deal with the fact that his or her hearing is changing. They are blamed for not speaking clearly or for purposefully leaving the person with hearing loss out of the conversation. Because communication is difficult, families do tend to "talk around" the patient or, if asked to repeat something, to minimize the effort by responding, "Never mind, it wasn't really important." Significant others (particularly spouses) often assume the responsibility of "hearing" for the family member, by explaining what was missed, covering up for miscommunications, taking responsibility for all telephone contacts, or worrying about possible social embarrassment when a response is unrelated to the comment made.

The person with hearing loss may not realize the burden the spouse carries. When the patient and spouse take identical surveys to describe the effects of the hearing loss on their lives, the spouse usually reports greater problems before a hearing aid fitting and greater benefit after the hearing aid fitting, compared to the patient's perceptions. These reports tell us a great deal about the stress of the hearing loss on the nonimpaired spouse or significant other.

Other family members may also experience frustration and disappointment when communication by phone or in person is ineffective, and the person with the hearing loss may internalize these problems as a rejection of themselves rather than as a consequence of the communication problems. A downward spiral can occur: "It's too hard to talk to Dad, so I'll keep the details to a minimum." Dad resents the limitation and contributes even less to the communication efforts. These reactions obviously will extend to the patient's social and work world as well.

The previous paragraphs remind us that patients are social beings and their hearing loss will impact their personal relationships. Therefore, audiologists need to include significant others in the treatment process to the fullest extent possible. Persons identified by the patient as significant others—spouses, partners, family, friends—should be encouraged to attend appointments, provide input, offer insights, and participate in the development of the treatment plan. Audiologists are only one part of the patient's support system; the more support the patient receives from loved ones, the more likely he or she will commit to the treatment plan.

Summary

Acquiring hearing loss in adulthood is usually a gradual, insidious process and is usually recognized by family and friends before being recognized by the person whose hearing is becoming impaired. Before, during, and after confirmation of hearing loss, adults may experience any of the reactions described earlier, all of which should be perceived as a "legitimate response to being shut out of social contexts" (Duchan, 2004, p 352).

Up to this point, we have considered the patient familiar to most audiologists: the adult who acquires hearing loss over time. The next section will consider the unique needs of parents of children with impaired hearing and then the children themselves.

■ CHILDREN, PARENTS, AND HEARING LOSS

Informing Parents of Their Child's Hearing Loss

More than 90% of children with hearing loss are born into families with normal-hearing parents (Gallaudet Research Institute, 2005). The vast majority of these parents have little or no experience with hearing loss, so the diagnosis of hearing loss is unexpected and upsetting news, a moment frozen in time that they never forget. Even if parents have suspected hearing loss for some time before the diagnosis, they still report experiencing sadness as well as relief for having their suspicions confirmed.

From their personal reports, it appears that most parents experience emotional reactions consistent with the stages or phases of the grief cycle discussed earlier (Kubler-Ross, 1969). The traditional grief cycle includes an additional first stage when the hearing loss is identified via newborn screening: shock. Because infants are now being tested in the first couple days of life, their parents have had no opportunity to observe and wonder about their children's hearing abilities (Luterman, 2001). One of audiology's greatest challenges is informing parents that their child has a hearing loss when they had no reason to suspect it.

To help audiologists "break the news" to parents about their child's hearing loss, the following guidelines have been developed (English et al., 2004):

1. Ensure privacy and adequate time.
2. Assess parents' understanding of the situation.
3. Encourage parents to express feelings.
4. Respond with empathy and warmth.
5. Give a broad timeframe for action.
6. Arrange for a follow-up appointment.
7. Briefly discuss treatment options.
8. During follow-up appointments, review treatment options, answer questions, and provide information about support systems.
9. Document thoroughly.

Steps 1 to 6 should be done even when time is limited. Sites should keep "fast-track" appointments open so parents can return within a week for more information and decision making. Although this suggestion seems like common sense and common courtesy, it is not a universal practice. A parent of a newly identified baby recently reported being told the next available appointment was 2 months later; only when he expressed anger did the clerk make an appointment within the week (Shigio, 2006).

Adjusting to a New Reality

When the reality of the situation begins to sink in, parents may find themselves feeling depressed or helpless for a time, while they attempt to cope with the implications of the diagnosis. Other reactions include depression, sorrow, confusion, and vulnerability and are known to resurface at unexpected times in the family's development. Luterman (2001) reminds us that it is inappropriate for a professional to expect families to be "over their grief by now"; families have the right to feel the way they feel, and professionals must refrain from passing judgment. Over time, most parents can work their way past their own anticipated self-concept of being parents of a "perfect" child to the "new reality" of being parents of a child who has a hearing loss, although this process can be harder for some parents than for others.

Professionals may unintentionally contribute to parental stress by emphasizing issues that are not the parents' primary concerns. For instance, upon first fitting hearing aids on a child, audiologists have been observed to insist, "Mrs. R, you will want to make sure that your son wears these hearing aids every waking hour. That way, he will have the best conditions to develop speech and language." While an accurate statement, this clinical approach may miss the mark; "developing speech and language" may mean nothing to parents, or it may suggest to them that they are to surrender their role as loving parent and become their child's therapist. If we attempt to "speak parents' language," we might instead say something like this: "Mrs. R, the more your son wears his hearing aids, the more he will learn from your voice how much you love and cherish him; the more he will learn when you are teasing and when you are serious about obeying you; the more he will be part of your family's life ...." At the same time all this is happening, the child will also have optimal conditions to develop speech and language, but within a context that families can understand and use. In addition, the undue pressure of "pleasing the professional" has been removed; instead, the parent has been acknowledged as a competent adult who has a lot to manage and who will do her best for her child as her energy level allows.

Growing Up with Hearing Loss

Even a mild degree of hearing loss can adversely affect vocabulary development and the subtle intricacies of language use. When language development is delayed, there is a cascading effect on many aspects of a child's psychosocial development, including self-concept, emotional development, and social competence.

SELF-CONCEPT

Self-concept was mentioned earlier relative to adults whose self-concept is threatened with change. Interestingly, individuals are not born with their self-concepts intact; rather, *self-concept is learned* by absorbing the input and feedback and reactions from those around us. Children typically internalize such reactions without question and allow others'

attitudes to "define themselves to themselves." Children are likely to think: "I see myself the way you tell me you see me."

Children with hearing loss are at risk for developing a relatively poor self-concept, most likely from negative reactions regarding their communication difficulties and also from being perceived differently as hearing aid users. One study (Cappelli et al., 1995) collected information from 23 hard of hearing children, ages 6 to 12, as well as from 23 children with no hearing loss, matched by sex and classroom. From a "Self Perception Profile for Children," it was found that children with hearing loss perceived themselves as less socially accepted than their non–hearing-impaired peers. Another study (Bess et al., 1998) asked more than 1,200 children with mild hearing loss to answer questions such as, "During the past month, how often have you felt badly about yourself?" Overall, children with mild hearing loss exhibited significantly higher dysfunction in self-esteem than children without hearing loss (self-esteem or self-regard being an evaluative component of self-concept). The researchers concluded that "even mild losses can be associated with increased social and emotional dysfunction among school aged children" (Bess et al., 1998, p 350).

Children who grow up with hearing loss often receive negative feedback and reactions not only because of their communication difficulties, but also because of the cosmetic issue of "looking different." It is encouraging to note that preschool children seem less likely to hold these negative and preconceived notions (Riensche et al., 1990) and that teens may be becoming more accustomed to and accepting of hearing aids among their peers (Stein et al., 2000). But, in general, if the appearance of a device on or in the ears creates a negative reaction among people who see it, their reaction is likely to be perceived by the hearing aid user, which can adversely impact the user's self-concept. We would do a disservice to children growing up with hearing loss to dismiss society's reactions to hearing aids as a "nonissue" or to downplay it as "only the other person's problem." Edwards (1991) reminds us that "it is the wearing of the device which 'amplifies' the difference between the child with hearing loss and his or her peers" (p 7), and children deserve our honesty in acknowledging that this difference does exist. (To experience the hearing aid effect firsthand, readers with normal hearing are encouraged to wear a highly visible pair of hearing aids for a full day around their community and record their subjective impressions of those around them as well as their own reactions.)

Since "the acquisition of language is essential for the development of self" (Garrison and Tesch, 1978, p 463), it follows that a delay in language acquisition would adversely affect the development of self. This correlation in fact has been demonstrated in several studies, as described in the next section.

EMOTIONAL DEVELOPMENT

An individual uses language to describe, interpret, and ultimately understand the abstract nature of his or her emotions. Because of concomitant language deficits, children growing up with hearing loss may have limited experience in self-expression and a subsequent delay in awareness and understanding of their own emotions, as well as the emotions of others. By virtue of having a hearing loss, they frequently miss overhearing adults and older children talking about and verbally managing their feelings about situations.

Researchers have shown that, when language development is delayed due to hearing loss, children are often less accurate in identifying others' emotional states and have a poorer understanding of affective words than children without hearing loss. Affective vocabulary describes how one feels, including adjectives such as frustrated, confused, overwhelmed, insecure, confident, satisfied, or reluctant.

The author Amy Tan (2003) provides insight as to how words provide meaning. Growing up in a bilingual home, she was aware that she often learned some words later than usual. In her early adult years, she learned the word for the color "mauve." Once she learned the word, she saw mauve everywhere! The color was always there, of course, but without a word for it, she hadn't noticed it before. The same principal holds true for understanding how one feels: one cannot really understand it until a word is assigned to name it (Greenberg and Kusche, 1993). (For further information about the importance of general emotional development, readers are referred to Goleman [1995].)

As children grow up, their social world expands to include same-age peers. Here, too, difficulties have been observed among children with hearing loss; because of their delay in developing communication skills, children with hearing loss have fewer opportunities for peer interactions, making it difficult to learn "the social rules governing communication" (Antia and Kreimeyer, 1992, p 135). Poor and limited communication results in poor social competence, which includes the following skills (Greenberg and Kusche, 1993):

- The capacity to think independently
- The capacity for self-direction and self-control
- Understanding the feelings, motivations, and needs of self and others
- Flexibility
- The ability to tolerate frustration
- The ability to rely on and be relied upon by others
- Maintaining healthy relationships with others

It would appear that children with hearing loss are at risk in developing these social competencies. For instance, a group of 40 parents completed a questionnaire and, overall, indicated that their children with hearing loss typically had more problems when interacting with others and establishing friendships than their normal-hearing siblings (Davis et al., 1986). The children themselves were interviewed, and 50% expressed their own concerns about peers and social relationships. Most children stated that they would not mention wearing hearing aids because of "a fear of being teased

and embarrassed, and many others reported spending most of their time alone" (Davis et al., 1986, p 60). The researchers wondered if these social problems were typical among most preadolescents, so they conducted the same interview among 58 children without hearing loss. After factoring out the responses from two children who had just moved to a new school, only 12% of these children reported having difficulty making friends or getting teased.

SPECIAL ISSUES IN ADOLESCENCE

Most of the information reviewed so far has focused on elementary school children. The teen years present new challenges, as well as heighten the intensity of existing ones. Adolescence is a stage of life with important developmental factors, including peer group affiliation, identity formation, occupational preparation, and adjustment to physiologic changes (Altman, 1996). During these turbulent times, self-consciousness increases, as well as uncertainty and mood swings. All teens, with or without hearing loss, may feel besieged with emotions that they find hard to articulate, and the presence of a hearing loss can exacerbate teens' struggles for self-awareness and self-expression.

As indicated earlier, peer relationships take paramount importance for teens, yet these relationships may be strained when hearing loss is involved (Oliva, 2004). Mothers have reported that their teenage children seemed less emotionally bonded to their friends when hearing loss was a variable and also rated these friendships as more fragile (Henggeler et al., 1990). Being with other teens with hearing loss may be more important than expected, when we consider how peer relationships help teens define themselves. Most of the 220 mainstreamed students in one study indicated that they preferred to spend most of their time with other students with hearing loss, finding these relationships deeper and more satisfying (Stinson et al., 1996).

The desire to conform to group expectations seems to peak in ninth grade (Kimmel and Weiner, 1995). For teens with hearing loss, this desire will probably include the desire to reject amplification for the sake of conformity. This desire may also represent a struggle to accept oneself as a person with a disability. The "hearing aid effect" is probably still in play in society, although there is some evidence that the magnitude of this negative effect has been lessening in the last 10 years (Stein et al., 2000). Overall, however, it is agreed that "during adolescence, being different is generally not valued" (Coyner, 1993, p 19).

During these years, students also need to develop appropriate social or interpersonal skills to advocate for their needs as they transition to college or work settings. This developmental task frequently is not supported by educational programs, resulting in high school graduates who move on to higher education or work placements without learning how to describe and request the services they need to succeed (English, 1997; Flexer et al., 1990). That is, professionals who serve adolescents face both the challenge of helping with the here-and-now issues of self-identity as well as concerns of the imminent future, and often, the former may seem so paramount that the latter is overlooked.

SUMMARY

This section described a range of possible psychosocial and emotional difficulties that might occur as a result of growing up with a hearing loss. Self-concept as well as parental attachment, emotional development, and social competency can all be impacted because of communication limitations. Interventions are available to help reduce these effects and should be used when concerns arise (English, 2001). The following section will describe the role of the audiologist in providing some of these interventions.

Counseling Children and Teens: What to Talk About

Who will talk to children and teens about their "hearing" challenges? It is well within audiology's scope of practice to provide personal adjustment support to children as well as adult patients. One way to do so is to provide opportunities to talk through the indirect approach; rather than putting someone on the spot about their reactions and fears, the audiologist can present a "third thing" to react to: a survey, a quote, a book, an idea.

The following "talking points" are taken from Clark and English (2004) and English (2002). A small group format is recommended to give children an opportunity to learn from and identify with peers. However, if that format is not feasible, one-on-one conversations are also helpful and appropriate.

TALKING POINT #1: "HOW WOULD *you* ANSWER THESE QUESTIONS?"

One activity could involve discussion of some results obtained by a fairly recent survey (see Appendix 43.1). It was developed by a hard of hearing 11th-grade student, and its distribution was supported by his educational audiologist (Lambert and Goforth, 2001). When they surveyed 64 middle school students with hearing loss, they obtained some interesting answers. The majority of respondents indicated feeling different from peers, and almost half felt that they were "less than" people without hearing loss.

These survey items can be posed one at a time to a child (or a team of children) and with the challenge to predict the survey results. They can then choose to discuss why their predictions agreed or did not agree with the survey. Using reflective listening and nonjudgmental responses, an audiologist may be able to help children and teens articulate their worries, doubts, and other burdens and serve as a sounding board as they talk through some realizations that they are "not alone" in their experiences and reactions. Self-disclosure does not come easily to many children and teens, so starting off by discussing others' responses can reduce that natural reluctance.

TALKING POINT #2: "WHAT WOULD YOUR BEST FRIEND SAY?"

Another way to facilitate a conversation with a child is to include a good friend and to use a questionnaire as a springboard for discussion. Elkayam and English (2003) describe this concept in a study with 20 hard of hearing (HoH) adolescents, using their best friends as significant others. The first author modified an adult instrument mentioned earlier (the Self-Assessment of Communication [SAC] and the Significant Other Assessment of Communication [SOAC]) (Schow and Nerbonne, 1982) to reflect adolescent situations. When comparing their responses to those of their friends, the HoH teens were not very surprised that even their best friends did not fully understand what their lives were like with hearing loss. These differences then served as a conversation starter, a point from which to talk about what life was like for them. Subsequent interviews revealed themes of inherent isolation and struggles with identity, cosmetics, self-acceptance, and problem solving.

A follow-up questionnaire indicated that the HoH teens found these conversations to be very helpful. However, they indicated little change in their problem-solving strategies, suggesting that HoH teens need more than a one-time interaction with a receptive audiologist to develop the self-confidence and the skills needed to solve one's problems.

The SAC-A(dolescents) and SOAC-A are currently undergoing the validation/reliability process, but they can serve as a model for audiologists looking for a starting point for conversations with teens with hearing loss. The outcomes of the conversation are impossible to predict, but the potential for insight and growth is vast.

TALKING POINT #3: PRACTICING "COST-BENEFIT" ANALYSES

A third approach is to set up a discussion on the costs and benefits of one's decisions. Teens could begin by discussing this quote, "Hiding a disability is one of the most serious threats to selfhood" (Morris, 1991, p 36). Teens could then create two tables—one that shows the costs and benefits associated with the decision NOT to disclose having a hearing loss and one to show the costs and benefits of disclosing having a hearing loss (Smart, 2001). The role of the audiologist in this setting would be simply to organize and summarize teens' opinions. No judgment is necessary as to the wisdom or folly of these opinions. By openly communicating their rationales and by considering the implications, teens will be challenged to consider their own best interests. Over time, they are more likely to make decisions that will meet these interests compared to never having the opportunity to express and evaluate them.

ADDITIONAL TALKING POINTS

Audiologists can facilitate productive discussions by simply presenting a case or a statement, such as:

- What does it mean to "own" a problem? What does it mean to own a hearing problem?

- A young woman has stopped using her hearing aids and is really struggling at her job, but she is willing to accept this. Now she is engaged but has not yet told her fiancé about her hearing problems. She thinks that if she tells him, he will not love her any more. What is going on?
- A high school student tells his teachers that he has left his hearing aids at home, and at home, he tells his parents he accidentally left them at school. What is going on?

TWO POTENTIAL PITFALLS

When counseling patients, audiologists should be aware of two communication behaviors that could inhibit our ability to provide personal adjustment support. The first is called communication mismatch; the second is the "Don't Worry– Be Happy" response.

Communication Mismatch

Early in the chapter, we made the distinction between *informational* counseling and *personal adjustment* counseling. When a person expresses a personal adjustment concern ("I feel very self-conscious when I wear these hearing aids"), that person is asking for help with that concern. But what if we miss the point? If we focus only on information, do we only hear requests for information?

If we reply with content or facts ("The important thing is these hearing aids are helping you hear better"), we have caused a *communication mismatch*. This patient was

saying, "I feel self-conscious"; she did not say, "Do they improve my hearing?" A more appropriate response would be a direct acknowledgement of her expressed concern. An encouraging head nod and repetition of the key words ("Self-conscious?") lets the patient know we are listening, following her train of thought, and waiting for her to expand upon it if she so chooses (and she probably does have more to say). This type of response "matches" her communicative intent.

One study tested the hypothesis that, without training, audiologists will not perceive requests for personal support and instead provide information although it was not requested (English et al., 2000). To find out, five statements were created and judged by professional counselors to be highly affective in nature (e.g., "My family says Ashley was born deaf because I worked until the last week of pregnancy"). These statements were presented to 11 of the students enrolled in a distance education counseling course before the semester began, with the request that they submit responses to each statement. All 23 students in the course completed the same exercise at the end of the term. Ten students from another course comprised a control group; all 10 gave responses before and after the term.

All responses were randomly organized and then rated by two reviewers on a 1 to 5 scale, with 1 representing a highly technical/information-based response and 5 representing a response that perceived the affective component to the statement. The average ratings for all groups are shown in Figure 43.2.

This graph shows that all 10 students in the control group provided technical or informational responses

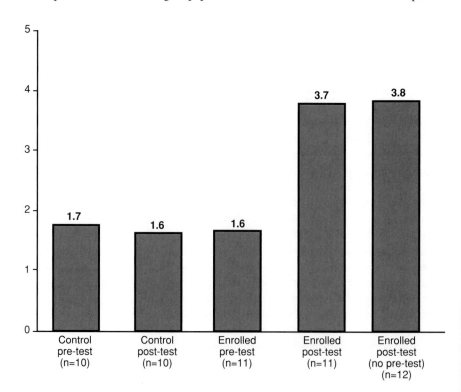

FIGURE 43.2 Responses to affective statements.

(e.g., "There are several studies indicating that working during pregnancy is not related to children's hearing loss") before the term (first bar) and after the term (second bar). The 11 students enrolled in the counseling course also gave technical responses before the course (third bar). However, after the course, their responses indicated an improved ability to perceive and respond to the affect in these comments (fourth bar).

There is always the possibility that the experience of completing this exercise before the term could influence the responses at the end of the term (called a "pre-test effect"). However, the students in the counseling course who did not participate in the exercise before the term (last bar) were rated virtually the same as those who did; in addition, a pre-test effect would have impacted the post-test responses from the control group. So it would appear there was no pre-test effect. It also appears that, although there was a strong tendency toward communication mismatch before the course, students were able to identify the tendency and reduce that mismatch significantly after the course.

How does the listener know what the speaker is asking for? How does the listener become aware that the question or comment is more than about information? The mindful listener will want to develop a skill called *differentiation* (Cormier and Hackney, 1999), which requires a few seconds of consideration and observation. Is this parent literally asking about when the school bus will arrive to take her child to a special education program, or is there something more? Is this older patient casually mentioning that his only son is moving his family to another state to make conversation, or is there something more? The skill of differentiation can be learned, as the study mentioned earlier indicates, but one never fully masters it.

"Don't Worry–Be Happy"

Imagine a patient saying with a certain amount of stress, "This sudden change in my hearing is really bothering me." Now imagine an audiologist saying, "It's only 10 dB different from last time; it's not actually a big change."

The audiologist, with all good intentions, was hoping to make the patient feel better. However, this response actually presents a problem. Not only is the response a communication mismatch (providing facts when facts were not requested and missing the affect altogether), but the audiologist also is dismissing what the patient reports as being important to her. The audiologist is giving the patient no credence about how she is feeling and, in fact, is *telling the patient how she should feel*. This kind of response is called "inappropriate reassurance"; the intention was to reassure the patient, but the outcome was subtly harmful. An appropriate response might attempt to understand how the patient feels. For instance, if the audiologist acknowledged, "Even a small change is worrisome," the patient will likely expand upon her fears of losing even more hearing, her concerns about her current hearing aids, or about needing new hearing aids.

But when the audiologist responds, "It's only 10 dB from last time; it's not actually a big change," the patient is likely to reply (but only to herself), "It's big to me! But apparently you don't care about that."

Clark (1990) was the first to point out to audiologists that they may be inclined to give inappropriate reassurance, or a "don't worry–be happy" response. A typical exercise in counseling is to imagine being in this patient's shoes: how would *you* react if a health care professional tells you, "It's not as bad as you indicate," or "Other people have it worse than you do"? You will likely feel even less understood than before and now also belittled.

Reassurance has its place, of course, specifically when one is asking about facts that we can confirm. "I think I forgot to pack my medicine." "Don't worry, I checked the suitcases before we closed them, I saw your medicine." Compare that situation (confirmable) to this one: A high school senior says, "I will be so depressed if I don't get into my first-choice college," and an adult says, "You will certainly get in! You are the smartest kid in the family." This situation is not confirmable, and the reassurance overlooks the student's anxiety. Surprisingly, it only makes the adult feel better; the teen now has additional pressure, not less.

It is likely that we confuse the concepts of hope and reassurance. Hope implies having a reason to be positive about the future, whereas reassurance conveys the message, "Someone else has told me I can be positive about the future." Hope is discovered by the patient; reassurance is provided by professionals. If we say to patients, "The road ahead will be a challenge, but I will be with you every step of the way and will provide as many supports as I can for you," the patient can depart knowing the audiologist is confident in how to help, is committed to the process, and is not unfamiliar with the road mentioned (I have a reason to be hopeful). If the audiologist says, "Keep every appointment and follow all recommendations and everything will turn out fine," patients are now put in a passive role that requires them only to trust the audiologist, not themselves. They will depart feeling uneasy or worried—certainly not hopeful.

When the concern expressed is about how a patient feels, we do well to follow Lundberg and Lundberg's (1995) advice and "let patients feel the way they are feeling," rather than try to "make it better." The "don't worry–be happy" response is a hard habit to break; even conscientious audiologists will occasionally find "don't worry" responses coming out of their mouths.

■ DOES COUNSELING MAKE A DIFFERENCE?

Audiology uses evidence to support its practices. Evidence is collected from many sources, ideally from the most rigorously controlled experimental studies. When those studies are lacking, we rely on descriptive studies, case studies, and other sources for evidence to confirm that our practices achieve the intended results on a systematic basis.

Because audiology is a relatively small field, and counseling is a relatively new interest in audiology, we must look to other health care data to determine if nonprofessional counseling makes a difference. The answer seems to be *yes*; for instance, the medical literature is replete with outcome data indicating that, when practitioners attentively listen to their patients' stories, actively acknowledge their emotional state, and respect their abilities to handle their problems (fundamental counseling strategies), patients are more likely to adhere to their recommendations (Squier, 1990; Stewart, 1995; Wilson, 1995; Stewart et al., 1999; Smith, 2002). If patients will follow strict diets or difficult medical regimes, lose weight, or stop smoking as a result of the counseling support they receive from their physicians, then it stands to reason that our patients, with counseling support, will adjust to a new self-concept, put less value on society's reactions to hearing aids, and make choices that are in their best interests.

We have anecdotal evidence from private practitioners who contend that the key to their success is their ability to develop supportive relationships with their patients (Tresolini, 1994). Other anecdotal evidence suggests that, when appropriate counseling is provided at the initiation of patient care, fewer problems emerge later (English, 2001). More compelling evidence, however, is needed to confirm our hypothesis that audiologic counseling has a positive effect on a patient's decision to follow our recommendations regarding amplification and hearing conservation.

COUNSELING PATIENTS OF DIFFERENT CULTURES

The counseling strategies described earlier are based on the assumption that the audiologist and patient share the same Western cultural background. This is not the safest of assumptions. As Roberts (2004) indicates, the demographics in the United States are rapidly changing, and patients from across the globe may be seeking the audiologist's help. When cultures differ, there is an even greater risk of miscommunication and not just because of language differences. A patient's value system and worldview will influence his or her reason to seek or not seek help and to accept or not accept help. For instance, cultures have different views on how a disability affects the patient's role in the family and community. There is also a wide range of views about the role of the clinician. Fadiman (1998) described how a Hmong tribe family's perception of disease was diametrically opposed to that of the health care professionals working in the neighborhood hospital. Those professionals' lack of interest in understanding the family resulted in tragedy. Our patients' cultural values and worldviews need to be understood before we can hope to be effective.

Stone (2005) advises us that there are two kinds of understanding that we need in order to provide effective services

to patients from other cultures. One is *knowledge about the specific culture*. Several chapters in his book are written by individuals who attempt to provide introductory information about different cultures, with the caveat that the information is necessarily cursory. Readers are also encouraged to read Lynch and Hanson (2004) for additional background information.

Berrera and Corso (2003), however, suggest that we really can only start with one family and try to understand their perspective to the best of our abilities—but to take care not to draw too general an assumption about all families from that culture. We should expect to build our cultural competence one family at a time.

Stone's (2005) "second type of understanding" relates to the "general *process* of working with persons with disabilities from different cultures, whatever those cultures may be" (p xiv). The process is often called "cultural brokering" and is defined as the act of "bridging, linking, or mediating between groups or persons of differing cultural backgrounds for the purpose of reducing conflict or producing change" (p 37). Berrara and Corso (2003) call this process "creating a third space." The act of understanding across cultures creates a new (third) entity, from which insight and solutions can develop.

These few paragraphs obviously cannot do justice to such a complex topic as the development of cultural competence and associated counseling skills. The reader will realize that this field will be part of one's lifelong learning process.

FINALLY: WHEN TO REFER?

It is not uncommon for patients and parents to present with difficulties that cannot be attributed to the hearing loss alone. Marital problems, family dissension, parenting dilemmas, financial or legal stress, and fragile emotional and mental health can be exacerbated by the presence of hearing loss, but treating the hearing loss alone will not resolve the fundamental problems. There is no simple answer to the question, "When should I refer to a professional counselor?" However, the answer is apparent when the audiologist sees a situation beyond one's expertise and scope of practice. It is strongly recommended that a referral system be established in advance so that, when the need to refer arises, a phone contact is immediately provided to the patient. This preparation will suggest to the patient that an outside referral is not rare and that the professional is aware of and is adhering to his or her professional boundaries. The audiologist will want to ask for the clinical site's procedures for referring patients and, additionally over time, to review those procedures and to ensure that the contact information is up to date.

CONCLUSION

As mentioned in the first paragraph, audiology includes the "soft science" of counseling. We have seen that the word *counseling* is a somewhat "shorthand" way of referring to a wide range of interpersonal communication skills. It includes careful teaching of information (knowing when and how much to teach), as well as perceiving the emotional and psychological reactions that our patients experience (mindful listening) and responding to those reactions to facilitate in their adjustment process. This one chapter will not make the reader a skilled counselor, nor will one book or even a counseling course; learning to become an effective audiologic counselor is a lifelong commitment. Readers are encouraged to read, observe, reflect, and discuss these concepts during the course of their careers and to seek guidance from other audiologists about one of the most challenging aspects of audiology—helping patients accept and transcend the effects of hearing loss on their lives.

▧ REFERENCES

Altman E. (1996) Meeting the needs of adolescents with impaired hearing. In: Martin F, Clark JG, eds. *Hearing Care for Children.* Needham Heights, MA: Allyn & Bacon; pp 19–210.

Antia S, Kreimeyer K. (1992) Social competence intervention for young children with hearing impairments. In: Odom S, McConnell S, McEvoy M, eds. *Social Competence of Young Children with Disabilities: Issues and Strategies for Intervention.* Baltimore: Paul H. Brookes Publishing Co; pp 135–164.

Berrara I, Corso R. (2003) *Skilled Dialogue: Strategies for Responding to Cultural Diversity in Early Childhood.* Baltimore: Paul H. Brooks Publishing.

Bess FH, Dodd-Murphy J, Parker R. (1998) Children with minimal sensorineural hearing loss: prevalence, educational performance, and functional status. *Ear Hear.* 19, 339–355.

Blood GW, Blood M, Danhauer JL. (1977) The hearing aid "effect." *Hear Instrum.* 20, 12.

Brammer LM. (1993) *The Helping Relationship: Process and Skills.* 5th ed. Boston: Allyn & Bacon.

Breslin F. (1974) *The Adolescent and Learning.* 2nd ed. New York: Collegium Book Publishers, Inc.

Cappelli M, Daniels T, Durleux-Smith A, McGrath PJ, Neuss D. (1995) Social development of children with hearing impairments who are integrated into general education classrooms. *Volta Rev.* 97, 197–208.

Clark JG. (1990) The "don't worry–be happy" professional response. *Hear J.* 4, 21–23.

Clark JG, English K. (2004) *Counseling in Audiological Practice: Helping Patients and Families Adjust to Hearing Loss.* Boston: Allyn & Bacon.

Cormier S, Hackney H. (1999) *Counseling Strategies and Interventions.* 5th ed. Boston: Allyn & Bacon.

Coyner L. (1993) Academic success, self-concept, social acceptance, and perceived social acceptance for hearing, hard of hearing, and deaf students in a mainstream setting. *J Am Deaf Rehabil Assoc.* 27. 13–20.

Crowe T. (1997) Approaches to counseling. In: Crowe T, ed. *Applications in Counseling in Speech-Language Pathology and Audiology.* Baltimore, MD: Williams & Wilkins; pp 80–117.

Culpepper B, Mendel LL, McCarthy P. (1994) Counseling experience and training offered by ESB-accredited programs. *ASHA.* 36, 55–58.

Davis J, Elfenbein J, Schum R, Bentler R. (1986) Effects of mild and moderate hearing impairments on language, educational, and psychosocial behavior of children. *J Speech Hear Disord.* 51, 53–62.

Duchan JF. (2004) Maybe audiologists are too attached to the medical model. *Semin Hear.* 25, 347–354.

Edwards C. (1991) The transition from auditory training to holistic auditory management. *Educ Audiol Monogr.* 2, 1–17.

Elkayam J, English K. (2003) Counseling adolescents with hearing loss with the use of self-assessment/significant other questionnaires. *J Am Acad Audiol.* 9, 485–499.

English K. (1997) *Self-Advocacy for Students Who Are Deaf and Hard of Hearing.* Austin, TX: Pro-Ed.

English K. (2001). Integrating counseling skills into existing audiology practices. Available at: http://www.audiologyonline.com/articles.

English K. (2002) *Counseling Children with Hearing Impairments and Their Families.* Boston, MA: Allyn & Bacon.

English K, Kooper R, Bratt G. (2004) Informing parents of their child's hearing loss: "breaking bad news" guidelines for audiologists. *Audiol Today.* 16, 10–12.

English K, Rojeski, T, Branham K. (2000) Acquiring counseling skills in mid-career: outcomes of a distance education course for practicing audiologists. *J Am Acad Audiol.* 11, 84–90.

English K, Weist D. (2005). Growth of AuD programs found to increase training in counseling. *Hear J.* 58, 54–58.

Fadiman A. (1998) *The Spirit Catches You and You Fall Down.* New York: Noonday Press.

Flexer C, Wray D, Leavitt R. (1990) *How the Student with Hearing Loss Can Succeed in College: A Handbook for Students, Families, and Professionals.* Washington, DC: Alexander Graham Bell Association.

Gallaudet Research Institute. (2005) Regional and national summary of data from the 2003-2004 annual survey of deaf and hard of hearing children and youth. Washington, DC: Gallaudet Research Institute, Gallaudet University.

Garrison WM, Tesch S. (1978) Self-concept and deafness: a review of research literature. *Volta Rev.* 80, 457–466.

Goleman D. (1995) *Emotional Intelligence: Why It Can Matter More Than IQ.* New York: Bantam Books.

Greenberg MT, Kusche CA. (1993) *Promoting Social and Emotional Development in Deaf Children: The PATHS Project.* Seattle: University of Washington Press.

Henggeler SW, Watson SM, Thelan JP. (1990) Peer relations of hearing-impaired adolescents. *J Pediatr Psychol.* 15, 721–731.

Hill C, O'Brien K. (1999) *Helping Skills: Facilitating Exploration, Insight, and Action.* Washington, DC: American Psychological Association.

James W. (1892) *The Principles of Psychology.* New York: Holt.

Kennedy E, Charles S. (2001) *On Becoming a Counselor: A Basic Guide for Nonprofessional Counselors.* New York: Consortium.

Kimmel DC, Weiner IB. (1995) *Adolescence: A Developmental Transition.* New York: Wiley and Sons.

Kochkin S. (1996) MarkeTrak IV: 10-year trends in the hearing aid industry: has anything changed? *Hear J.* 48, 23–34.

Kochkin S. (2005) MarkeTrak VII: hearing loss population tops 31 million. *Hear Rev.* 12, 16–29.

Kubler-Ross E. (1969) *On Death and Dying.* New York: McMillan Publishing Co.

Lambert D, Goforth D. (2001) Middle school hard of hearing survey. *Educ Audiol Rev.* 18, 13–19.

Lundberg G, Lundberg J. (1995) *"I Don't Have to Make Everything All Better:" Six Principles That Empower Others to Solve Their Own Problems while Enriching Your Relationships.* New York: Penguin Books.

Luterman DL. (2001) *Counseling Persons with Communication Disorders and Their Families.* 4th ed. Austin, TX: Pro-Ed.

Lynch E, Hanson M, eds. (2004) *Developing Cross-Cultural Competence: A Guide for Working with Children and Their Families.* Baltimore: Paul H. Brooks Publishing.

Margolis R. (2004) What do your patients remember? *Hear J.* 57, 10–17.

Morris J. (1991) *Pride against Prejudice: Transforming Attitudes to Disability.* Philadelphia: New Society.

Nichols M. (1995) *The Lost Art of Listening.* New York: Guilford Press.

Oliva G. (2004) *Alone in the Mainstream: A Deaf Woman Remembers Public School.* Washington, DC: Gallaudet University Press.

Reik T. (1948) *Listening with the Third Ear.* New York: Farrer, Strauss.

Riensche L, Peterson K, Linden S. (1990) Young children's attitudes toward peer hearing aid wearers. *Hear J.* 43, 19–20.

Roberts S. (2004) *Who We Are Now: The Changing Face of America in the 21st Century.* New York: Times Books.

Rogers C. (1961) *On Becoming a Person.* Boston: Houghton Mifflin.

Schow R, Nerbonne M. (1982) Communication screening profile: use with elderly clients. *Ear Hear.* 3, 135–147.

Shigio L. (2006) Audiologists working with parents. Unpublished doctoral project, Central Michigan University.

Smart J. (2001) *Disability, Society, and the Individual.* Gaithersburg, MD: Aspen Publications.

Smith R, (2002) *Patient-Centered Interviewing.* 2nd ed. Philadelphia: Lippincott Williams & Wilkins.

Squier R. (1990) A model of empathic understanding and adherence to treatment regimens in practitioner-patient relationships. *Soc Sci Med.* 30, 325–339.

Stein R, Gill K, Gans D. (2000) Adolescents' attitudes toward their peers with hearing impairment. *J Educ Audiol.* 8, 1–6.

Stewart M. (1995) Effective physician-patient communication and health outcomes: a review. *Can Med Assoc J.* 152, 1324–1433.

Stewart M, Brown J, Boon H, Galajda J, Meredith L, Sangster, M. (1999) Evidence in patient-doctor communication. *Cancer Prev Control.* 3, 25–30.

Stinson MS, Whitmore K, Kluwin TN. (1996) Self perceptions of social relationships in hearing-impaired adolescents. *J Educ Psychol.* 88, 132–143.

Stone D, Patton B, Heen S. (1999) *Difficult Conversations: How to Discuss What Matters Most.* New York: Viking Press.

Stone J, ed. (2005) *Culture and Disability: Providing Culturally Competent Services.* Thousand Oaks, CA: Sage Publications.

Stone JR, Olswang LB. (1989) The hidden challenge in counseling. *ASHA.* 31, 27–31.

Tan A. (2003) *The Opposite of Fate: A Book of Musings.* New York: Putnam.

Tanner D. (1980) Loss and grief: implications for the speech-language pathologist and audiologist. *ASHA.* 22, 916–928.

Tresolini CP. (1994) *Health Professions Education and Relationship-Centered Care.* San Francisco: Pew-Fetzer Professions Commission.

Wilson B. (1995) Promoting compliance: the patient-provider partnership. *Adv Renal Replace Ther.* 2, 199–206.

World Health Organization. (2002) *International Classification of Function, Disability, and Health.* Geneva: World Health Organization.

APPENDIX 43.1

Responses from 64 Middle School Students with Hearing Impairment (Lambert and Goforth, 2001)

Do you feel that you are different from other kids?

Yes	27%
Sometimes	51%
No	22%

Does anyone ever tease you because you talk different?

Yes	34%
No	27%
N/A	48%

Do you ever get teased because you are hard of hearing?

Yes	25%
Sometimes	27%
No	48%

Do you ever think you are less than people who can hear

Yes	14%
Sometimes	31%
No	55%

How often do you wish you didn't have a hearing disability?

All the time	30%
Sometimes	48%
Almost Never	13%
Never	9%

Do you ever get angry because of your hearing disability?

Yes	30%
Sometimes	37%
No	33%

Do you feel that your hearing disability makes it harder for you to make friends?

Yes	38%
No	62%

Do you wear your hearing aids?

All the time	44%
Most of the time	27%
Sometimes	19%
Never	10%

Do people ask you what your hearing aid(s) are?

Yes	54%
Sometimes	28%
No	18%

Do you think your hearing aid(s) is an important part of your life?

Yes	45%
Semi-important	19%
Somewhat	18%
Not so important	5%
Don't think about them	13%

Which of the following do you feel about your hearing aid(s)?

They're OK	29%
Fine with me	25%
Love them, help me learn	22%
Don't care	24%

When you don't have your hearing aid(s), do you feel like you are missing a part of you?

Yes	52%
No	48%

Do you feel stupid when you ask a question because you are afraid it was already asked?

Yes	50%
No	50%

How often do you think your peers give up talking to you if you say "What?"

All the time	8%
Most of the time	10%
Sometimes	42%
Hardly ever	32%
Never	8%

Do you ever NOT say "What?" so that the other person does not get mad?

Yes	50%
No	50%

AUTHOR INDEX

SUBJECT INDEX

Page numbers in italics denote figures; those followed by a t denote tables